Pediatric Predicted Weight, BSA, and Equipment Needs

	Age												
	Birth	6 mo	1 yr	2 yr	3 yr	4 yr	5 yr	6 yr	8 yr	10 yr	12 yr	14 yr	Adult
Weight (kg)	3.5	7	10	12	14	16	18	20	25	30	40	50	70
Body surface area (m²)	0.25	0.38	0.49	0.55	0.64	0.74	0.76	0.82	0.95	1.18	1.34	1.5	1.73
Endotracheal tube size (mm)	3-3.5	3-5.4	4	4.5	4.5	5	5	5.5	6	6.5	7	7	7.5-8
Teeth to mid-trachea (cm)	9	11	12	13	14	14	15	15	16	17	18	20	20
Nares to mid-trachea (cm)	10	12	14	15	16	17	18	19	20	21	22	23	24
Suction catheter size (Fr)	6-8	8	8	8-10	8-10	10	10	10	10-12	12	12	12	12-14
Nasogastric tube size (Fr)	5-6	8	8-10	10	10-12	12	12	14	14-18	18	18	18	18
Urinary catheter size (Fr)	5-6	8	8-10	10	10	10-12	10-12	10-12	12	12	12	12-16	16

Normal Heart, Respiratory Rates, and Blood Pressures in Children

	Normal Heart Rates in Children		Normal Respiratory Rates in Children (breaths/min)	Normal Blood Pressures in Children	
Age	Awake Heart Rate (beats/min)	Sleeping Heart Rate (beats/min)		Systolic Pressure (mmHg)	Diastolic Pressure (mmHg)
Neonate	100-180	80-160	30-60	60-90	20-60
Infant	100-160	75-160	30-60	87-105	53-66
Toddler	80-110	60-90	24-40	95-105	53-66
Preschooler	70-110	60-90	22-34	95-110	56-70
School-age child	65-110	60-90	18-30	97-112	57-71
Adolescent	60-90	50-90	12-16	112-128	66-80

Estimated systolic blood pressure norms (for infants and children beyond 1 year of age): 50th percentile systolic blood pressure = 90 mmHg + (2 × age in years); 5th percentile systolic blood pressure = 70 mmHg + (2 × age in years).

Maintenance Fluid and Caloric Requirements

Body Weight Maintenance Formula

Weight	Formula
Neonate (<72 hr)	60-100 ml/kg
0-10 kg	100 ml/kg
11-20 kg	1000 ml for first 10 kg + 50 ml/kg for kg 11-20
21-20 kg	1500 ml for first 20 kg + 25 ml/kg for kg 21-30

Body Surface Area Formula

1500 ml/m² body surface area/day

Insensible Water Losses

300 ml/m² body surface area

Daily Caloric Requirements by Age

Infant	100-150 Calories/kg
1-2 yr (Toddler/Preschooler)	90-100 Calories/kg
School-age	70-80 Calories/kg
10-12 yr	50-60 Calories/kg

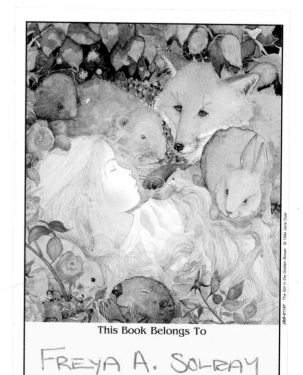

This Book Belongs To

FREYA A. SOLRAY

CRITICAL CARE NURSING

of Infants and Children

SECOND EDITION

Freya Angelica Solray,

Congratulations on finishing Nursing School 12/2005!
Best wishes on your career, I know
you will do well. Your patients will
be lucky!

Sincerely,

Bachireu

CRITICAL CARE NURSING

of Infants *and* Children

Second Edition

MARTHA A.Q. CURLEY, RN, PhD, CCNS, FAAN

Critical Care Clinical Nurse Specialist
Multidisciplinary Intensive Care Unit
Children's Hospital Boston
Boston, Massachusetts

PATRICIA A. MOLONEY-HARMON, RN, MS, CCNS, CCRN

Advanced Practice Nurse/Clinical Nurse Specialist
The Children's Hospital at Sinai
Baltimore, Maryland

SAUNDERS

An Imprint of Elsevier

Vice President, Nursing Editorial Director: *Sally Schrefer*
Executive Editor: *Barbara Nelson Cullen*
Senior Developmental Editor: *Cindi Anderson*
Project Manager: *John Rogers*
Designer: *Kathi Gosche*

SAUNDERS
An Imprint of Elsevier
The Curtis Center
Independence Square West
Philadelphia, PA 19106

Printed in the United States of America

Library of Congress Cataloging in Publication Data

Critical care nursing of infants and children / [edited by] Martha A.Q. Curley, Patricia Moloney-Harmon.—2nd ed.
     p. ; cm.
  Includes bibliographical references and index.
  ISBN 0-7216-9031-9
    1. Pediatric intensive care. 2. Pediatric nursing. 3. Intensive care nursing. I. Curley, Martha A.Q., 1952- II. Moloney-Harmon, Pat.
  [DNLM: 1. Critical Care—Child. 2. Critical Care—Infant. 3. Pediatric Nursing—methods. 4. Critical Illness—nursing. 5. Intensive Care Units, Pediatric—standards. WY 159 C934 2001]
  RJ370 .C87 2001
  610.73'62—dc21   00-067021

        05 GW/MV 9 8 7 6 5 4 3

To the patients and families
we've had the privilege to come to know.

To my nursing colleagues:

It's NOT Invisible

Today, I saw you . . .

*Make room for more than 20 family members at the bedside all at once,
so that everyone could be together with Billy one last time.*

*Ask Billy's grandfather to plug the extension cord in; you knew he
needed to do something*—anything.

*Give options to Billy's parents about "being there" during resuscitation attempts and help
them choose words to talk with him, considering he was only 8 years old.*

*Speak very softly to Stephen while removing the tape from his eyelids
only to find his pupils blown and unequal . . . , you didn't even change
your facial expression—you didn't want to upset mom . . . , not any more
. . . not just then.*

*Ask Stephen's mom what she was thinking as she stood near his bed
looking out the window just before support was withdrawn. . . . "He was
always very quiet, but I knew something was wrong; I should have taken him to the hospital—
but, he didn't want to go". . . , wipe your tears as you listened and convincingly say that she
did the best that she could.*

*Take a deep breath before you spoke up at team conference . . . "We ought to be more vigilant
about the conversations we hold at the bedside—we don't know what Stephen's level of
consciousness is under the sedation and chemical paralyzing agents". . . , whisper in Stephen's
ear that the new ventilator might be scary because of the noise it made, then dry his tears.*

*Take the time to sit with Rachel's mom while others resuscitated her
daughter, your patient, because you knew she was alone—her husband was on his way in.*

*Resuscitate Rachel because you knew that Rachel's mom needed your
colleague right then.*

*Care enough to take the time to "orchestrate" death . . . , to make the
worst-thing-in-the-world-anyone-could-ever-experience . . . , a little more tolerable.*

*It may be very hard for others to hear what we do . . . it can just be so sad. We eventually stop
telling them. Eventually, we might think that our caring becomes invisible. But, it is not invisible—
not to Billy, not to Stephen, not to Rachel, or their parents, or to one another.*

MARTHA A.Q. CURLEY, RN, PhD, CCNS, FAAN

CONTRIBUTORS

PATRICIA ADAMS, RN, BSN, MS
Staff Nurse
Pediatric Critical Care
CCN Incorporated
Laurel, Maryland
Chapter 28: Trauma

CHRISTINE ANGELETTI, RN, BSN
Pediatric ICU Nurse Coordinator
Pediatric Intensive Care Unit
Children's Hospital of Pittsburgh
Pittsburgh, Pennsylvania
Chapter 26: Organ Transplantation

ANNETTE L. BAKER, MSN, RN, PNP
Pediatric Nurse Practitioner
Cardiovascular Program
Children's Hospital Boston
Boston, Massachusetts
Chapter 18: Cardiovascular Critical Care Problems

DEBBIE BRINKER, RN, MS, CCNS, CCRN
PICU Clinical Nurse Specialist
Pediatric Intensive Care Unit
Deaconess Medical Center
Spokane, Washington
Chapter 24: Hematologic Critical Care Problems

JANET CRAIG, RN, MS, CS, CCRN
Pediatric Nurse Practitioner
Pediatric Cardiology
Primary Children's Medical Center
Salt Lake City, Utah
Chapter 7: Tissue Perfusion
Chapter 18: Cardiovascular Critical Care Problems

MARTHA A.Q. CURLEY, RN, PhD, CCNS, FAAN
Clinical Nurse Specialist
Multidisciplinary ICU
Children's Hospital Boston
Boston, Massachusetts
*Chapter 1: The Essence of Pediatric Critical
    Care Nursing*
*Chapter 3: Caring Practices: The Impact of
    the Critical Care Experience on the Family*
Chapter 8: Oxygenation and Ventilation
Chapter 19: Pulmonary Critical Care Problems
Chapter 27: Shock

SANDRA J. CZERWINSKI, RN, MS
Administrative Director
Department of Nursing
All Children's Hospital
St. Petersburg, Florida
Chapter 5: Facilitation of Learning

CATHY H. DICHTER, RN, PhD, FCCM
Clinical Nurse Specialist
Pediatric Critical Care Center
Clarian Health Partners, Inc.
Riley Hospital for Children
Indianapolis, Indiana
Chapter 27: Shock

MARY J. FAGAN, MSN, RN
Acting Vice President, Inpatient Services/Designated
    Nurse Executive
Children's Hospital, San Diego
San Diego, California
Chapter 4: Leadership in Pediatric Critical Care

LORI D. FINEMAN, RN, MS
Clinical Nurse Specialist
Pediatric Critical Care
University of California—San Francisco
San Francisco, California

MARY JO C. GRANT, PNP, PhD
Pediatric Critical Care Nurse Practitioner/
    Nurse Researcher
Pediatric Intensive Care Unit
Primary Children's Medical Center
Salt Lake City, Utah
Chapter 15: Host Defenses
Chapter 19: Pulmonary Critical Care Problems

LAUREN SORCE GREHN, RN, MSN, CCRN, CPNP
Pediatric Nurse Practitioner
Pediatric Critical Care
Children's Memorial Hospital
Chicago, Illinois
Chapter 21: Renal Critical Care Problems

TAMMARA L. JENKINS, MSN, RN, CCRN
Clinical Nurse Specialist, Pediatric Critical Care
Warren G. Magnuson Clinical Center
National Institutes of Health
Bethesda, Maryland
Chapter 25: Oncologic Critical Care Problems

PATRICK KADILAK, RN, MSN, CNS
Clinical Nurse Specialist
Patient Care Services
Shriners Hospital for Children—Boston
Boston, Massachusetts
Chapter 29: Thermal Injury

ANDREA M. KLINE, RN, MS, PCCNP, CCRN
Pediatric Critical Care Nurse Practitioner
Pediatric Intensive Care Unit
Children's Memorial Medical Center
Chicago, Illinois
Chapter 21: Renal Critical Care Problems

DONNA M. KRAUS, PHARMD
Associate Professor of Pharmacy Practice
Pediatric Clinical Pharmacist
Departments of Pharmacy Practice and Pediatrics
University of Illinois at Chicago
Chicago, Illinois
  Chapter 13: Clinical Pharmacology

PATRICIA M. LYBARGER, MSN, RNC
Clinical Information Specialist
Patient Care Services
Shriners Hospitals for Children—Burns Hospital
Boston, Massachusetts
  Chapter 29: Thermal Injury

AIMEE C. LYONS, RN, MSN, CCRN
Clinical Coordinator Multidisciplinary Intensive Care Unit
  and Pediatric/Neonatal Transport Team
Department of Nursing
Children's Hospital, Boston
Boston, Massachusetts
  *Chapter 31: Resuscitation and Transport of Infants
    and Children*

MAUREEN A. MADDEN, MSN
Pediatric Critical Care Nurse Practitioner
Division of Pediatric Critical Care
Infants and Childrens Hospital of Brooklyn
Maimonides Medical Center
Brooklyn, New York
  Chapter 30: Toxic Ingestions

EUGENE D. MARTIN, RN, MS
Advanced Education Specialist
Nursing Education, Research and Program Development
All Children's Hospital
St. Petersburg, Florida
  Chapter 5: Facilitation of Learning

SARA A. MARTIN, RN, MS, CPNP, PCCNP, CCRN
Pediatric Critical Care Nurse Practitioner
Pediatric Intensive Care Unit
Rush–Presbyterian–St. Luke's Medical Center
Chicago, Illinois
  *Chapter 2: Caring Practices: Providing
    Developmentally Supportive Care*

ELAINE C. MEYER, PHD, RN
Staff Psychologist
Children's Hospital of Boston
Assistant Professor of Psychology
Department of Psychiatry
Harvard Medical School
Boston, Massachusetts
  *Chapter 3: Caring Practices: The Impact of
    the Critical Care Experience on the Family*

PATRICIA A. MOLONEY-HARMON, RN, MS, CCNS, CCRN
Advanced Practical Nurse/Clinical Nurse Specialist
The Children's Hospital at Sinai
Baltimore, Maryland
  Chapter 24: Hematologic Critical Care Problems
  Chapter 28: Trauma

PAULA MOYNIHAN, RN, BSN, CCRN
Clinical Coordinator
Cardiovascular Intensive Care Unit
Children's Hospital
Boston, Massachusetts
  Chapter 18: Cardiovascular Critical Care Problems

LINDA OAKES, RN, MSN, CCRN, CCNS
ICU/Pain Clinical Nurse Specialist
Department of Nursing
St. Jude Children's Research Hospital
Memphis, Tennessee
  Chapter 17: Caring Practices: Providing Comfort

PATRICIA O'BRIEN, RN, MSN, PNP
Nurse Practitioner
Cardiovascular Program
Children's Hospital, Boston
Boston, Massachusetts
  Chapter 26: Organ Transplantation

MARY FRANCES D. PATE, DSN, RN
Clinical Nurse Specialist
Pediatric Intensive Care Unit
The Children's Hospital of Alabama
Birmingham, Alabama
  Chapter 14: Thermal Regulation

ANN POWERS, MS, RN, CPNP
Pediatric Nurse Practitioner
Long Pond Pediatrics and Osteopathy, P.C.
Plymouth, Massachusetts
  Chapter 9: Acid-Base Balance

SANDY QUIGLEY, MSN, CPNP, CETN
Clinical Nurse Specialist in Enterostomal Therapy
Patient Services
The Children's Hospital
Boston, Massachusetts
  Chapter 16: Skin Integrity

KATHRYN E. ROBERTS, RN, MSN, CCRN
Clinical Nurse Specialist
Pediatric Intensive Care Unit
The Children's Hospital of Philadelphia
Philadelphia, Pennsylvania
  Chapter 11: Fluid and Electrolyte Regulation

CYNDA HYLTON RUSHTON, DNSc, RN, FAAN
Assistant Professor of Nursing; Clinical Nurse Specialist
in Ethics; Coordinator, Pediatric Palliative Care
Program; Faculty, Phoebe Berman Bioethics Institute
The Johns Hopkins University and Children's Center
Baltimore, Maryland
*Chapter 6: Advocacy/Moral Agency: A Road Map for
Navigating Ethical Issues in Pediatric Critical Care*

GREGORY J. SCHEARS, MD
Assistant Professor of Anesthesia and Pediatrics
Department of Anesthesia and Critical Care Medicine
Children's Hospital of Philadelphia, University
of Philadelphia
Philadelphia, Pennsylvania
Chapter 12: Nutrition Support

LYNN M. SEWARD, DIPLOMA
RN Coordinator
7 South—Transplants
Children's Hospital of Pittsburgh
Pittsburgh, Pennsylvania
Chapter 26: Organ Transplantation

SHARI L. SIMONE, RN, MS, CRNP, CCRN
Pediatric Critical Care Nurse Practitioner
Pediatric Intensive Care Unit
University of Maryland Medical System
Baltimore, Maryland
Chapter 22: Gastrointestinal Critical Care Problems

PEGGY SLOTA, RN, MN
Director, Critical Care Services
Administration
Children's Hospital of Pittsburgh
Pittsburgh, Pennsylvania
Chapter 26: Organ Transplantation

MARY FALLON SMITH, RN, MSN
Clinical Nurse Specialist
Emergency Department
Children's Hospital Boston
Boston, Massachusetts
*Chapter 31: Resuscitation and Transport of Infants
and Children*

JANIS BLOEDEL SMITH, RN, MSN
Case Manager
Systems Support Services
Vanderbilt University Medical Center
Nashville, Tennessee
*Chapter 2: Caring Practices: Providing
Developmentally Supportive Care*
Chapter 7: Tissue Perfusion

KATHY L. SWARTZ, RN, MS, CCRN
Care Manager
Pediatric Intensive Care Unit
Children's Hospital
Columbus, Ohio
Appendix

JOHN E. THOMPSON, RRT
Director of Clinical Technology
Children's Hospital
Associate in Anesthesia
Department of Respiratory Care
Harvard Medical School
Boston, Massachusetts
Chapter 8: Oxygenation and Ventilation

TARA TRIMARCHI, MSN, RN, CRNP
Nurse Practitioner
Pediatric Intensive Care Unit
The Children's Hospital of Philadelphia
Lecturer
University of Pennsylvania, School of Nursing
Pediatric Critical Care Nurse Practitioner Program
Philadelphia, Pennsylvania
Chapter 23: Endocrine Critical Care Problems

JUDY VERGER, RN, MSN, CCRN
Pediatric Nurse Practitioner
Pediatric Critical Care
School of Nursing, University of Pennsylvania
The Children's Hospital of Philadelphia
Philadelphia, Pennsylvania
Chapter 12: Nutrition Support

PAULA VERNON-LEVETT, MS, RN, CCRN
Staff Nurse II
Pediatric Intensive Care Unit
University of Iowa Hospitals & Clinics
Iowa City, Iowa
Chapter 10: Intracranial Dynamics
Chapter 20: Neurologic Critical Care Problems

JOYCE WEISHAAR, RN, MSN
Clinical Nurse Specialist
Pediatric Intensive Care Unit
Children's Memorial Hospital
Chicago, Illinois
Chapter 21: Renal Critical Care Problems

DARLENE E. WHITNEY, RN, BSN, CCRN
Staff Nurse Level Two
Patient Services
The Children's Hospital
Boston, Massachusetts
Chapter 16: Skin Integrity

FOREWORD

This publication of the second edition of *Critical Care Nursing of Infants and Children* is another important milestone in the evolving development of pediatric critical care nursing. It often surprises students and colleagues when I discuss my experiences in the days "before pediatric intensive care units." They cannot conceive of a time when these specialized units, along with their highly technologic treatments, were not available to facilitate the care of critically ill children. During this "before" period, seriously ill children were cared for on regular hospital units with minimal technology. Staff nurses were often assigned to "special" the child, unless the family provided a private duty nurse. Sometimes a separate room was set aside for care of several seriously ill children so that one nurse could care for several children. The level of expertise of these staff and private duty nurses, however, was not adequate for the intensive care needs of critically ill children. Obviously children with serious health problems or children recovering from major surgery were at high risk of dying because adequate treatments and monitoring measures were not available.

The development of pediatric critical care units alongside the development of more-sophisticated treatments and related technology was highly effective in reducing the mortality of acutely ill children. As these units developed, it soon became obvious that the nurses working in these units needed advanced training to adequately monitor and care for these seriously ill children. It was essential that nurses have access to the developing knowledge about critical care and develop the skills to apply that knowledge. Staff education, advanced critical care modules, and graduate education were some of the approaches used to prepare nurses for roles in pediatric critical care. In addition, nurses themselves began to become involved in the development of knowledge about critical care nursing through the conduct of nursing research and the synthesis and application of knowledge through the publication of clinical articles and textbooks.

The publication of *Critical Care Nursing of Infants and Children* was another important step in the evolution of nursing knowledge related to pediatric critical care. This state-of-the-art textbook was unique in its strong nursing perspective, and the organization of the textbook was highly innovative. The first two sections provide a comprehensive background for the book, including a focus on historical, developmental, and family issues, as well as issues related to the practice environment. This section has been improved with a greater depth of information about development. Given the current complexities of treatment options in the PICU, the ethics section also has been expanded. The next section, on phenomena of concern, thoroughly covers the major phenomena that pediatric critical care nurses must deal with on a daily basis. This content is then pulled together by focusing in depth on problems involving the major body systems as well as multisystem problems. All of these sections have been updated to reflect current knowledge and practice.

The end result is a reference and teaching textbook that provides comprehensive and holistic content related to pediatric critical care nursing. Furthermore, the book has very high standards for scholarship. Content is well validated through reference to research and the latest clinical and theoretical knowledge in the field. Putting this material together in an organized, cohesive, reader-friendly manner was truly a challenging and exciting endeavor.

Having watched and participated in the evolution of pediatric critical care nursing over the past 35 years, I am astounded at the knowledge explosion in the field and at the comprehensive and complex scope of this specialty area of nursing. To be a pediatric critical care nurse takes knowledge and skills in both the art and the science of nursing. All nurses who take the step toward becoming pediatric critical care nurses should have a copy of this book to guide their development as professionals in this exciting and ever-challenging field. Nurses who are already experienced pediatric critical care nurses can gain new ways of conceptualizing their practice and will find the book extremely valuable as a resource in caring for challenging patients on their units. The text will also be invaluable for students enrolled in advanced practice pediatric graduate programs. One would hope that every pediatric intensive care unit in the country will have copies available for staff reference.

Critical Care Nursing of Infants and Children continues to be a milestone in nursing textbooks because of its excellence and creativity. It serves as a model for future approaches in knowledge synthesis for practice. It certainly can serve to strengthen the specialty of pediatric critical care nursing by providing a strong framework and background for practice.

MARGARET SHANDOR MILES, PhD, RN, FAAN
Professor, School of Nursing
The University of North Carolina at Chapel Hill

PREFACE

Critical Care Nursing of Infants and Children is a state-of-the-art textbook, written to provide a comprehensive reference for experienced nurses caring for critically ill pediatric patients and their families. It is based on the broad clinical experiences of its contributors in the care of seriously ill or injured children and in nursing research aimed at improving and perfecting care. The strong nursing focus of this book is apparent in its structural approach—*phenomena of concern* and *final common pathways*. Phenomena of concern address nursing care issues common to all critically ill pediatric patients regardless of their primary problem. Final common pathways cluster patient problems in such a way that allows them to be reframed from a perspective that guides nursing care.

Pediatric critical care nursing has experienced extraordinary development since the advent of intensive care units designed specifically for the care of critically ill children. Nurses who care for critically ill infants and children are continuously challenged by diversity in patient age and diagnosis. Skilled clinical practice requires knowledge about a wide variety of illnesses and injuries integrated with an awareness of the continuums of growth and development. Pediatric critical care nurses also require comprehensive information about maturational anatomy and physiology, physical and psychosocial development, pathophysiology and disease, critical instrumentation and patient management, and the most current pediatric critical care research findings.

The foundation for the text is provided in the chapters that detail children's and families' responses to the experiences of critical illness and intensive care, because this aspect of pediatric critical care nursing is inherent to the practice. Practical information supporting the evolving role of the nurse as tender of the care milieu is unique. Chapters on nutrition, clinical pharmacology, thermal regulation, host defenses, skin integrity, and comfort management provide hard-to-find, clinically relevant information specific for the critically ill pediatric patient. A comprehensive review of physiology, with emphasis on the impact of maturation on system structure and function, is provided for each body system. The pathophysiologic mechanisms, clinical manifestations, and diagnosis of disease in infants and children are presented in detail. Multisystem problems, including oncology, organ transplantation, shock, trauma, thermal injury, toxic ingestions, and resuscitation and transport, are presented separately. Instrumentation appropriate to caring for critically ill children and critical care management of infants and children is discussed from a collaborative framework. Appendixes are provided as a clinically useful reference. A complete reference list is found at the end of each chapter, and tables and figures provide support to the entire text.

Critical Care Nursing of Infants and Children is divided into six sections that encompass all aspects of pediatric critical care nursing.

Section I: Holistic Pediatric Critical Care Nursing

presents essential concepts that provide a foundation for the practice of pediatric critical care nursing. The evolution of pediatric critical care nursing as a specialty is presented. Discussion of the impact of critical illness on children and families provides nurses with an appreciation of the magnitude of this experience and guides interventions aimed at mitigating stress and promoting individual and family growth.

Section II: The Practice Environment focuses on the milieu affecting nursing care delivery. The broadening professional responsibilities of the nurse as leader, teacher, and mentor are acknowledged and supported. Ethical issues are illuminated from a pediatric critical care nursing perspective.

Section III: Phenomena of Concern focuses on the unique care needs of all pediatric patients regardless of their primary problem. Nurses play a major role in optimizing the patient's potential outcome through a deliberative proactive process that integrates skilled clinical knowledge about tissue perfusion, oxygenation and ventilation, acid-base balance, intracranial dynamics, fluid and electrolyte regulation, nutrition, clinical pharmacology, thermal regulation, host defenses, skin integrity, and comfort. Within each phenomenon of concern, essential embryology, maturational anatomy and physiology, and instrumentation are discussed.

Section IV: Final Common Pathways presents state-of-the-art nursing care for patient problems within each body system. A focus on the final common pathways of many disease states is presented so that system dysfunction is viewed broadly and addressed within a nursing framework. For example, the numerous pathophysiologic states that result in increased intracranial pressure become similar to the nurse who is responsible for managing moment-to-moment changes in cerebral compliance in an effort to prevent secondary brain injury. The etiology, incidence, and pathogenesis of specific disorders that lead to development of a final common pathway are also presented when appropriate. Critical care management is focused on the final common pathways of system dysfunction and specifically on patient care unique to a particular disorder.

Section V: Multisystem Problems addresses the needs of patients experiencing multiple system dysfunction and their complicated demands and unique needs. Because these patients' illnesses involve more than a single body system, they present a distinctive challenge to the care team.

Critical care nursing of infants and children is a dynamic specialty necessitating nurses to ensure their practice is evidenced-based. Our goal in writing this text will be realized if readers are provided the knowledge they need to ensure excellent care to critically ill children and their families. The goal of excellence in the critical care nursing of infants and children is based on commitment to children as our most precious resource and to families as the agents of developing human potential. Also necessary is genuine respect for the unique contributions of each member of the multidisciplinary team and for our nursing colleagues as sources of immeasurable humanity and healing.

MARTHA A.Q. CURLEY
PATRICIA A. MOLONEY-HARMON

ACKNOWLEDGMENTS

We express our gratitude to the clinical experts who are our contributors. The excellence of their work is evident in the pages that follow, in which they share the wealth of their knowledge and expertise. We are grateful to our reviewers, who took the time and made the effort to comment constructively and thoughtfully on the manuscript. We are also grateful to the diligence of the research librarians and graphic artists who either found or created the impossible. Finally, inspiration has always come from the children, families, and professionals with whom we have worked. Some of them may work with us still, perhaps others have a memory of some time or some experience we shared, others may be unaware that we carry their echoes with us. Thank you all.

We would also like to acknowledge the following contributors to the first edition of *Critical Care Nursing of Infants and Children*. This second edition builds upon the solid foundation their work provided.

Mary Allen Craig Alter
June Levine Ariff
M. Claire Beers
Anne Milligan Browne
Cheryl Cahill-Alsip
Elaine Caron
Sylvia Chin-Caplan
Christine M. Dickenson
Patricia Dillman
Kathryn M. Dodds
Neil Ead
E. Marsha Elixon
Arthur J. Engler
Barbara J. Few
Barbara Gill
Peggy C. Gordin
Donna H. Groh
Nancy Hagelgans
Twila W. Harmon
Carol J. Howe
Diane S. Jakobowski
Kimmith M. Jones

Patricia Lawrence Kane
Lori J. Kozlowski
Mary Berry LeBoeuf
S. Jill Ley
Patricia Lincoln
Cathleen B. Longo
Wendy Ludwig
Susan Morgan Madder
Kimberly Mason
Beth McDermott
Pamela M. Milberger
Joyce Molengraft
Regina Muir
Kathryn M. Murphy
Kathleen M. Ouzts
Susan N. Peck
Wendy Roberts
Linda F. Samson
Claire E. Sommargren
Judith J. Stellar
Michele Topor
Karen Zamberlan

MARTHA A.Q. CURLEY
PATRICIA A. MOLONEY-HARMON

CONTENTS

Holistic Pediatric Critical Care Nursing

This section presents essential concepts that provide a foundation for the practice of pediatric critical care nursing. The evolution of pediatric critical care nursing as a specialty is presented. Discussion of the impact of critical illness on children and families provides nurses with an appreciation of the magnitude of this experience and guides interventions aimed at mitigating stress and promoting individual growth.

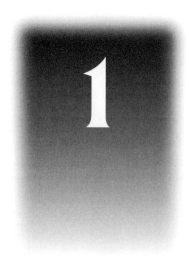

The Essence of Pediatric Critical Care Nursing

Martha A.Q. Curley

EVOLUTION OF THE DISCIPLINE
  First Units
  Patient Population
  Levels of PICU Care
  Literature
  Professional Organizations
  Certification in Pediatric Critical Care Nursing

DESCRIBING WHAT NURSES DO: THE SYNERGY MODEL
  Patient Characteristics of Concern to Nurses
  Nurse Competencies Important to the Patient
  Optimal Patient Outcomes

CURRENT ENVIRONMENT

Nurses are privy, like almost no one else, to the body's secret bruises and disfigurements, the mind's unuttered worries, the heart's sweetest emotions, and the spirit's last glimmer.

Angela McBride[1]

Pediatric critical care nurses create an environment in which critically unstable, highly vulnerable infants and children benefit from the vigilant care and the coordinated efforts of a team of highly skilled pediatric healthcare professionals. Indeed, the art and science of pediatric critical care have matured tremendously over the past three decades. Still vivid are memories of small rooms, minimum technology, changing boundaries of professional practice, and little clinical expertise. As noted by Diers,[2] nursing is what is intense about intensive care unit (ICU) care; the constant within the pediatric critical care environment is the pediatric critical care nurse. This chapter introduces the reader to both the genesis and essence of the practice of pediatric critical care nursing.

EVOLUTION OF THE DISCIPLINE

Nursing's historical practice of watchful vigilance and triage provided the model for the care of critically ill patients in ICUs.[3] In the late nineteenth century, Louisa May Alcott wrote:

> My ward was divided into three rooms. . . . I had managed to sort out the patients in such a way that I had what I called "my duty room, my pleasure room, and my pathetic room," and worked for each in a different way. One, I visited, armed with a dressing tray, full of rollers, plasters, and pins; another, with books, flowers, games, and gossip; a third, with teapots, lullabies, consolation, and, sometimes, a shroud. . . . wherever the sickest or most helpless man chanced to be, there I held my watch.[4]

First Units

North Carolina Memorial Hospital opened the first "special care unit" for acutely ill patients in 1953.[5] This unit was created to meet the challenge of improving patient care while simultaneously saving time for nursing personnel. Before creating the special care unit, patients were assigned beds by virtue of their financial status. Nurses would care for patients with varying levels of acuity on the same unit; the almost constant attention required of acutely ill patients prevented nurses from adequately caring for less acute patients.[5] Of interest to pediatrics, the idea of putting all critically ill patients in one room with everything available in case of an emergency was generated by an assistant director of nursing, chief of anesthesia, medical director of the hospital, and otolaryngologist after a near-miss life-threatening respiratory event involving a 4-year-old patient.[6] This young patient survived only by chance; a nurse passed her door (a private room at the end of a hallway), noted her distress, and gave her emergency treatment.

The first pediatric-specific ICUs opened after improved patient outcomes were realized when specialized care was provided to critically ill neonates and adults. From the 1920s to early 1950s, epidemics of acute poliomyelitis necessitated the use of assisted ventilation for polio victims (Fig. 1-2). First described was negative pressure ventilation by Drinker and Shaw[7] in Boston, followed by tracheal intubation and positive pressure ventilation by Lassen[8] in Copenhagen.

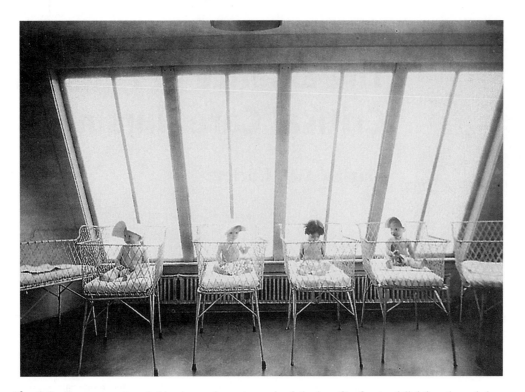

Fig. 1-1 Sun room where babies in sun bonnets received the benefit of natural lighting through large windows, 1930. (Courtesy Children's Hospital, Boston.)

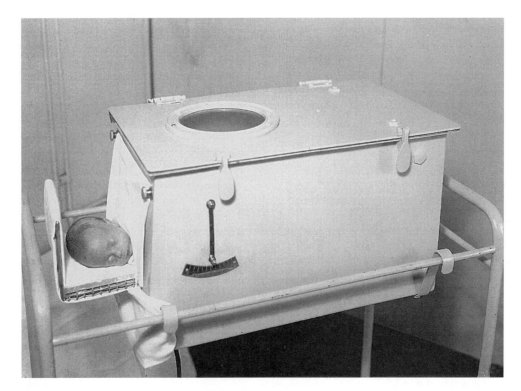

Fig. 1-2 Infant in respirator, 1934, Infant's Hospital, Boston. (Courtesy Children's Hospital, Boston.)

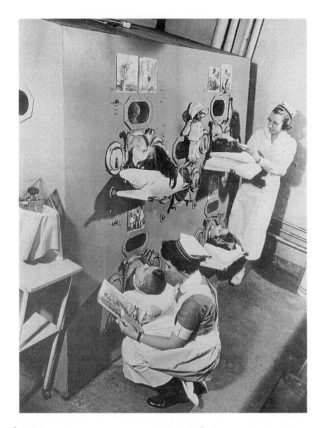

Fig. 1-3 Nurses reading to children in a four-unit respirator, c. 1955. (Courtesy Children's Hospital, Boston.)

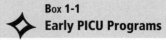

Box 1-1

Early PICU Programs

Abroad

1955 Children's Hospital of Goteburg, Sweden
1961 Stockholm, Sweden
1963 Hospital St. Vincent de Paul, Paris
1963 Royal Children's Hospital, Melbourne
1964 Alder Hey Children's Hospital, Liverpool

United States

1967 Children's Hospital of Philadelphia
1969 Children's Hospital of Pittsburgh
1969 Yale-New Haven Medical Center
1971 Massachusetts General Hospital, Boston

From Downes JJ: The historical evolution, current status, and prospective development of pediatric critical care, *Crit Care Clin North Am* 8:1-22, 1992.

James Wilson, a pediatrician at the Children's Hospital of Boston, designed the four-bed negative pressure ventilator in 1952 (Fig. 1-3).[9] As noted by Downes,[10] this was "probably the first unit in the world to cohort and support pediatric patients with vital organ failure." Later in Scandinavia, it was recognized that children had higher mortality rates than adults in these special poliomyelitis respiratory units. Responding to this, separate pediatric respiratory units were developed to specifically care for children in Uppsala and Stockholm.[11]

In January 1967, John J. Downes[10] and his colleagues from Children's Hospital of Philadelphia opened the first multidisciplinary pediatric intensive care unit (PICU) in the United States (Box 1-1). This unit consisted of six fully monitored beds with an adjacent procedure room and intensive care chemistry laboratory (Fig. 1-4). As recalled by Downes, Erna Goulding, then director of nursing, became convinced that opening the ICU would be the right decision. Willing to err on the side of what was best for patients, Ms. Goulding recruited a number of high-caliber nursing staff for the unit. The unit's first nurse manager was Janet Johnson, followed by Joan Alessio. According to Downes, Johnson's tenure was short. Alessio contributed creativity, drive, and spark to build a self-directed cohesive team that adapted well to the new PICU environment.[12]

By the end of the 1970s, medical training programs for pediatric intensivists developed. In 1985, the American Board of Pediatrics recognized the subspecialty of Pediatric Critical Care Medicine and set criteria for subspecialty

certification. The American Boards of Medicine, Surgery, and Anesthesiology gave similar recognition to the subspecialty. By the mid-1980s, advanced practice nursing programs in acute care pediatrics were established at Yale University, the University of Pennsylvania, and the University of California at San Francisco. Currently, PICUs are found in every major center that provides care to seriously ill pediatric patients. In 1992 the American Hospital Association listed 328 PICUs,[13] and in 1998, this number increased to 411 PICUs.[14]

Patient Population

Although many PICUs care for critically ill surgical neonates and maturing young adults with a congenital or childhood disease, the pediatric critical care population traditionally consists of patients who range in age from full-term neonates to adolescents and their families. Unlike system-specific adult critical care units, a wide spectrum of illnesses are found in most PICUs. Extremes in age and illness require pediatric critical care nurses to function as generalists within a subspeciality area.

Levels of PICU Care

Although patients with a wide variety of illness can be found in most PICUs, Guidelines and Levels of Care for Pediatric Intensive Care Units have been promulgated by the Pediatric Section of the Society of Critical Care Medicine, the American Academy of Pediatrics Section on Critical Care Medicine, and the Committee on Hospital Care.[15,16] The guidelines recommend that level I PICUs provide multidisciplinary definitive care for a wide range of complex, progressive, rapidly changing, medical, surgical, and traumatic disorders, occurring in pediatric patients of all ages, excluding premature newborns. The guidelines also recommend that level II PICUs provide stabilization of critically ill children before transfer to another center or, to avoid long-distance transfers, provide

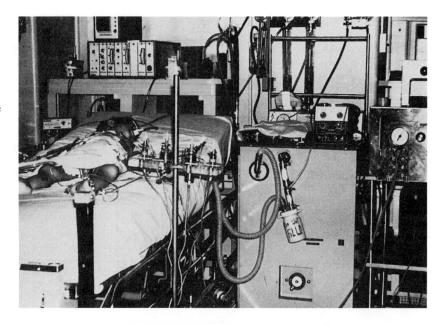

Fig. 1-4   Patient in the first pediatric intensive care unit in the United States (Children's Hospital of Philadelphia, 1970.) Note Emerson PV-1 ventilator, Gorman-Rupp water mattress, Stratham monitoring system, and strain-gauge transducers. (From Downes JJ: The historical evolution, current status, and prospective development of pediatric critical care, *Crit Care Clin North Am* 8:1-22, 1992.)

care for disorders of less complexity or lower acuity. Although the same standards of quality are applied to patients managed in both level I and level II PICUs, requirements for level II PICUs differ from those for level I PICUs in respect to the type and immediacy of physician presence and hospital resources. Cooperation between hospitals and professionals within a given region is essential to ensure that an appropriate number of level I and II units are designated. Duplication of services leads to underuse of resources and inadequate development of skills by clinical personnel and are costly.[17]

Literature

The rapid evolution of pediatric critical care required nurses to be self-motivated learners accountable for their own education. Before the early 1980s, educational materials specific to pediatric critical care nursing were nonexistent. Pediatric critical care nurses would occasionally find an additional chapter on pediatrics or an appendix on normal pediatric vital signs placed at the end of a critical care nursing text. In 1981, the first pediatric critical care nursing texts were published: *Pediatric Critical Care Nursing,* edited by Katherine W. Vestal, and *Critical Care Nursing of Children and Adolescents,* edited by Annalee R. Oakes and sponsored by the American Association of Critical-Care Nurses (AACN).[18,19] These were followed by Janis Bloedel Smith's *Pediatric Critical Care* and then Mary Fran Hazinski's AACN-endorsed first edition of *Nursing Care of the Critically Ill Child.*[20,21] Journal articles about pediatric critical care nursing are sporadically found in both pediatric and critical care journals.

As we enter a new millennium, pediatric critical care nurses have many options. In addition to a selection of nursing and medical pediatric critical care textbooks, the Society of Critical Care Medicine and the World Federation of Pediatric Intensive and Critical Care Societies released its inaugural journal *Pediatric Critical Care Medicine* at the Third World Congress in Pediatric Critical Care. In addition to print media, pediatric clinicians now have the World Wide Web. *PCCMeds* (http://PedsCCM.wustl.edu/) provides a multidisciplinary educational and practical resource for the subspecialty. The web site contains original peer-reviewed content and is linked to numerous associated sites on the Internet.

Professional Organizations

The AACN, first organized in 1969 as the American Association of Cardiovascular Nurses, has a long history of supporting critical care nursing across the lifespan.[22] The mission of AACN is to provide and inspire leadership to establish work and care environments that are respectful, healing, and humane. AACN is committed to providing the highest quality resources to maximize nurses' contribution to caring and improving the healthcare of critically ill patients and their families. AACN's vision is to create a healthcare system driven by the needs of patients and families whereby critical care nurses make their optimal contribution (see http://www.aacn.org for more information).

In 1982 the AACN introduced Special Interest Groups (SIGs) to respond to members' expressed needs for specialized information, networking, and education.[23] The pediatric SIG, later known as the Neonatal and Pediatric Special Interest Group (NAP SIG), provided the first opportunities for pediatric critical care nurses to collectively gather and share their expertise. The first members of this group included Mary Fran Hazinski (coordinator), Nan Smith-Blair, Margaret Slota, Karen Killian, Holly Weeks-Webster, Janet Wintle, Linda Miers (AACN board liaison), and James Niebuhr (AACN staff liaison).

Priorities for the NAP SIG included the provision of high-level programming to meet the specific educational needs of its members. Before this initiative, pediatric critical care nurses attended adult or neonatal programs and extrapolated perceived relevant information when caring for the pediatric patient population. Other priorities of the NAP SIG included developing a resource file of consultants, audiovisual programs, policies and procedures, care plans, and teaching programs and support of separate critical care certification examinations for neonatal and pediatric critical care nurses.[24,25]

In 1989 AACN restructured all SIGs into a national network of Special Interest Consultants (SICs). Acknowledging the unique and separate needs of neonatal and pediatric nurses, distinct neonatal and pediatric SIC positions were established. Pediatric SICs specifically focused on issues related to pediatric critical care nursing and were readily available to AACN as regional experts on issues related to pediatric critical care nursing practice. The pediatric SICs have now been phased out and replaced the pediatric Board Advisory Team (BAT), who communicate electronically using e-mail.

Other organizations of interest to pediatric critical care nurses include the Society of Pediatric Nurses (SPN) and the Society of Critical Care Medicine (SCCM). Established in 1990, the mission of the SPN is to promote the optimal health of children and excellence in nursing care of children and their families (see http://www.pednurse.org for more information). Established in 1970, the SCCM is a multidisciplinary multispecialty, international organization whose mission is to secure the highest quality care for all critically ill patients by promoting the superiority of a multidisciplinary, ICU-based, intensivist-directed team for delivery of the highest quality, cost-efficient critical care (see http://www.sccm.org for more information).

Certification in Pediatric Critical Care Nursing

In 1975 the AACN Certification Corporation was established to formally recognize the professional competence of critical care nurses. The mission of the AACN Certification Corporation is to certify and promote critical care nursing practice that optimally contributes to desired patient outcomes. The program establishes the body of knowledge necessary for CCRN certification, tests the common body of knowledge needed to function effectively within the critical care setting, recognizes professional competence by granting CCRN status to successful certification candidates, and assists and promotes the continual professional development of critical care nurses.

Certification is attractive to both the critical care nurse and the consumer of critical care nursing services. State licensure signifies that an individual has the basic knowledge needed for the general practice of nursing, whereas certification provides a means of recognizing professionals who have specialized knowledge and experience and assures the public that they are receiving care from practitioners who meet a defined level of competence.[26]

Because critical care nursing practice is constantly changing, a Role Delineation Study (RDS) is conducted every 3 to 5 years to define the dimensions of current critical care nursing practice and to identify the actual tasks required

TABLE 1-1   Percentage of Time Caring for Patients With Alterations in Body Systems

System Dysfunction	Pediatric Practice	Neonatal Practice	Adult Practice
Pulmonary	28%	39%	22%
Cardiovascular	24%	15%	39%
Neurologic	15%	6%	8%
Multisystem	12%	22%	10%
Hematology/ Immunology	75%	5%	4%
Renal	5%	3%	5%
Gastrointestinal	5%	7%	8%
Endocrine	4%	3%	4%

Data from Certification Corporation, American Association of Critical-Care Nurses: *Role delineation study,* Laguna Niguel, Calif, 1990.

of a competent critical care nurse. The tasks serve as a framework for the CCRN examination blueprint. Examination questions are linked to the study data and evaluate the knowledge and skills required of a nurse to perform the tasks at a competent level of critical care nursing practice.

Before 1992 content and construct validity of the CCRN examination was established for critical care nurses who primarily cared for adult patients. Pediatric critical care nurses who sat for the CCRN examination were tested on content that did not reflect their practice. For example, the cardiovascular system, which reflected 19% of the CCRN examination, contained questions on myocardial infarctions and angina/atherosclerosis, a rare phenomenon in pediatric critical care. For years, pediatric critical care nurses recognized both the similarities *and* differences between their practice and that of neonatal and adult critical care but found them difficult to articulate.

In 1989 AACN Certification Corporation began a new RDS. The purpose of the 1989-1990 study was to refine the existing adult CCRN examination and define the tasks, knowledge, and skills fundamental to neonatal and pediatric critical care nursing. Major differences among neonatal, pediatric, and adult critical care nursing practice were identified in the types of patient care problems for which direct bedside care is provided and in the amount of time spent caring for the patients with specific problems (Table 1-1). The results, for the first time, described the practice of pediatric critical care nursing and justified the need for separate pediatric, neonatal, and adult CCRN examinations. The 1989-1990 RDS described the diverse practice of pediatric critical care nursing and communicated it in terms that could be equated with neonatal and adult critical care nursing practice. The first CCRN examination, specific for pediatric critical care nursing, was administered in July 1992. Almost 75% of the first 848 pediatric critical care nurses who sat for the examination passed it.[27]

In 1997 the unique competencies of pediatric, neonatal, and adult critical care nurses were rearticulated using the Synergy Model as a conceptual framework.[28] Again, differences across the lifespan were described, and the separate CCRN programs still exist (Table 1-2). To date, over 1200 pediatric critical care nurses hold CCRN-Pediatric certification.

In 1999 AACN also initiated a certification program for clinical nurse specialists in pediatric critical care (CCNS-Pediatric). The CCNS program validates an advanced practice nurse's qualifications and knowledge for practice as a clinical nurse specialist. The examination also uses the Synergy Model as a conceptual framework and consists of questions designed to reflect general knowledge needed in the CNS role and questions covering age-specific content (Table 1-3). To date, 14 pediatric clinical nurse specialists hold CCNS-Pediatric certification. It is anticipated that a

TABLE 1-2   CCRN Blueprints Using the Synergy Model as a Conceptual Framework

	Pediatric Practice*	Neonatal Practice*	Adult Practice*
Clinical Judgment	**80%**	**80%**	**80%**
Pulmonary	24%	31%	17%
Cardiovascular	19%	13%	29%
Neurologic	10%	4%	7%
Multisystem	11%	17%	10%
Hematology/immunology	4%	3%	3%
Renal	3%	3%	5%
Gastrointestinal	5%	6%	6%
Endocrine	4%	3%	3%
Caring Practices	**20%**	**20%**	**20%**
Advocacy/Moral agency	4%	4%	4%
Caring practices	4%	4%	4%
Collaboration	4%	4%	4%
Systems thinking	2%	2%	2%
Response to diversity	2%	2%	2%
Clinical inquiry	2%	2%	2%
Facilitation of learning	2%	2%	2%

Data from Certification Corporation, American Association of Critical-Care Nurses: *Role delineation study 1997,* Aliso Viejo, Calif, 2000.
*Percent of examination questions.

TABLE 1-3   Pediatric CCNS Exam Blueprint

Dimension	Percent of Examination Questions
Clinical judgment	25%
Facilitation of learning	18%
Collaboration	14%
Clinical inquiry	13%
Caring practices	10%
Systems thinking	8%
Advocacy/agency	7%
Response to diversity	5%

Data from Certification Corporation, American Association of Critical-Care Nurses: *CCNS Exam Blueprint,* Aliso Viejo, Calif, 2000.

Pediatric Acute Care Nurse Practitioner certification program will soon be initiated.

DESCRIBING WHAT NURSES DO: THE SYNERGY MODEL

Given the current demands of the healthcare environment, a clear sense of the unique contributions of nursing to patient outcomes is critical. The synergy model describes nursing practice based on the needs and characteristics of patients.[28] The fundamental premise of this model is that patient characteristics drive nurse competencies. When patient characteristics and nurse competencies match and synergize, optimal patient outcomes result.

Synergy is an evolving phenomenon that occurs when individuals work together in mutually enhancing ways toward a common goal. The Synergy Model recognizes the combined actions of both patient and nurse. Within this model the patient and family are active participants in the patient-nurse interaction. Patient-nurse synergy results in a better outcome than what could be achieved independently.

The following presents the major tenets of the Synergy Model: patient characteristics of concern to nurses, nurse competencies important to the patient, and patient outcomes that result when patient characteristics and nurse competencies are mutually enhancing.

Patient Characteristics of Concern to Nurses

Contextually, each patient and family is unique with varying capacities for health and vulnerability to illness. Each individual possesses a singular genetic and biologic makeup that establishes a capacity for health. Each individual practices various degrees of healthy behaviors, for example, diet, exercise, and stress reduction. Each lives within a community with different institutions, economic structures, government, social organization, and community perceptions. All exist within a macrosocial structure consisting of societal infrastructure, the physical environment, cultural characteristics, and population perceptions. All of these factors place the patient within the context of an individual, unique environment and impact the nursing care required for a particular patient and family.

Each person brings a unique cluster of personal characteristics to a healthcare situation. These characteristics—stability, complexity, predictability, resiliency, vulnerability, participation in decision making, participation in care, and resource availability—span the continuum of health and illness. *Stability* refers to the person's ability to maintain a steady-state equilibrium. *Complexity* is the intricate entanglement of two or more systems (e.g., body, family therapies). *Predictability* is a summative patient characteristic that allows the nurse to expect a certain trajectory of illness. *Resiliency* is the patient's capacity to return to a restorative level of functioning using compensatory and coping mechanisms. *Vulnerability* refers to an individual's susceptibility to actual or potential stressors that may adversely affect outcomes. *Participation in decision making and in care* is the extent to which the patient and family engage in decision making and in aspects of care. *Resource availability* refers to resources the patient, family, or community bring to a care situation; resources include personal, psychologic, social, technical, and fiscal.

These eight continua are applicable to patients in all practice settings, which is important for nurse-to-nurse communication of patient characteristics across traditional unit and system boundaries. For example, a healthy uninsured 4-year-old girl undergoing a preschool physical examination could be described as an individual who is (a) stable, (b) not complex, (c) very predictable, (d) resilient, (e) not vulnerable, (f) parent able to participate in decision making and care, but (g) has inadequate resource availability; whereas a critically ill infant in multisystem organ failure can be described on the other end of the continuum in some areas but very similar in others, for example, as an individual who is (a) unstable, (b) highly complex, (c) unpredictable, (d) highly resilient, (e) vulnerable, (f) unable to become involved in decision making and care, but (g) has adequate resource availability.

Individuals vacillate at different points along these eight continua. For example, in the case of the critically ill infant in multisystem organ failure, stability can range from a high to low risk of death; complexity, from atypical to typical; predictability, from uncertain to certain; resiliency, from minimal to strong reserves; vulnerability, from susceptible to safe; family participation in decision making and care, from no capacity to full capacity; and resource availability, from minimal to extensive. At any point in time, various combinations of these eight continua paint a different picture of the patient. From a clinical perspective, this makes sense. Patient characteristics evolve over time; what might seem very important one day may be less important the next. Compared with traditional patient classification systems that count nursing tasks, for example, partial or complete bath, frequency of vital signs, and so on, these eight dimensions better describe the needs of patients.

Nurse Competencies Important to the Patient

Nursing competencies, derived from the needs of patients, are also described in terms of essential continua: clinical judgment, advocacy/moral agency, caring practices, facilitation of learning, collaboration, systems thinking, response to diversity, and clinical inquiry. *Clinical judgment* is clinical reasoning that includes clinical decision making, critical thinking, and a global grasp of the situation, coupled with nursing skills acquired through a process of integrating formal and experiential knowledge. *Advocacy/moral agency* is defined as working on another's behalf and representing the concerns of the patient, family, or community. The nurse serves as a moral agent when assuming a leadership role in identifying and helping to resolve ethical and clinical concerns within the clinical setting. *Caring practices* are a constellation of nursing activities that are responsive to the uniqueness of the patient and family and create a compassionate and therapeutic environment with the aim of promoting comfort and preventing suffering. Caring behav-

iors include but are not limited to vigilance, engagement, and responsiveness. *Facilitator of learning* is the ability to use one's self to facilitate patient learning. *Collaboration* is working with others (patients, families, healthcare providers) in a way that promotes and encourages each person's contributions toward achieving optimal, realistic patient goals. Collaboration involves intradisciplinary and interdisciplinary work with colleagues. *Systems thinking* is appreciating the care environment from a perspective that recognizes the holistic interrelationships that exist within and across healthcare systems. *Response to diversity* is the sensitivity to recognize, appreciate, and incorporate differences into the provision of care. Differences may include but are not limited to individuality, cultural practices, spiritual beliefs, gender, race, ethnicity, disability, family configuration, lifestyle, socioeconomic status, age, values, and alternative care practices involving patients and families and members of the healthcare team. *Clinical inquiry* is the ongoing process of questioning and evaluating practice, providing informed practice based on available data, and innovating through research and experiential learning. The nurse engages in clinical knowledge development to promote the best patient outcomes.

These competencies reflect a dynamic integration of knowledge, skills, experience, and attitudes necessary to meet patients' needs and optimize patient outcomes. Nurses become competent within each continuum at a level that best meets the fluctuating needs of their patient population. Logically, more compromised patients have more severe or complex needs; this in turn requires the nurse to possess a higher level of knowledge and skill in an associated continuum. For example, if the gestalt of a patient were stable but unpredictable, minimally resilient, and vulnerable, primary competencies of the nurse would be centered on clinical judgment and caring practices (which includes vigilance). If the gestalt of a patient were vulnerable, unable to participate in decision making and care, and inadequate resource availability, the primary competencies of the nurse would focus on advocacy/moral agency, collaboration, and systems thinking. Although all eight competencies are essential for contemporary nursing practice, each assumes more or less importance depending on a patient's characteristics. Synergy results when there is a match between patient's needs/characteristics and nurse competencies.

Clinical Judgment. Pediatric critical care nursing practice is based on a unique body of knowledge that integrates the individual effects of system maturation on physiology, pathophysiology, sociology, psychology, and human development. Clinical expertise—that is, skilled clinical knowledge, use of discretionary judgment, the ability to integrate complex multisystem effects and understand the expected trajectory of illness and human response to critical illness—embellishes competent practice. In critical care, Funk notes that the clinician first masters then transcends the technology and uses it as a means to an end in providing holistic care. With experience, personal mastery develops, enabling the competent nurse to balance the art and science of care. The expert nurse anticipates the needs of patients, predicts the patient's trajectory of illness, and envisions the patient's level of recovery.

Aiken, Smith, and Lake[29] note that the current expectations for professional nursing practice are high: "Care has become increasingly complex; the exercise of professional judgment by nurses is ever more important in preventing adverse and sometimes catastrophic events." Clinical expertise creates *safe passage* for patients. In fact, excellent nursing care is often invisible, and from a perspective of preventing untoward effects and complications, it should be. Nursing's unique contribution to patients within the healthcare environment, the one that encompasses all nursing's competencies, is that nurses create safe passage for patients and families. Safe passage may include helping the patient and family move toward greater self-awareness, self-understanding, competence, and health and through transitions and stressful events or a peaceful death.

Safe passage requires that the nurse "know the patient." Tanner and colleagues[30] described "knowing the patient" as a primary caring practice that includes knowing the patient as a person and having in-depth knowledge of that individual's typical responses. Knowing the patient refers to how a nurse understands a patient, grasps the meaning of a situation for a patient, or recognizes the need for a particular intervention. Knowing the patient requires clinical judgment and creates the possibility for advocacy, which limits patient vulnerability.

Advocacy/Moral Agency. "Agency"—an expression of responsibility for a patient's outcome—includes reading the situation based on expected changing relevance, including action based on the significance inherent in the situation, and a practical grasp of other clinicians' perception of the situation.[31] Moral agency is a competency that acknowledges the unique trust inherent within nurse-patient relationships, a trust gained from nursing's long history of speaking on the patient's behalf in an effort to preserve a patient's "lifeworld."[32]

Each discipline offers a *unique* and *necessary* perspective in advocating for patients. Visintainer[33] applied an analogy of maps to contrast each discipline's unique approach to clinical problem solving. Various maps exist to describe a geographic location, for example, road maps, air traffic maps, weather maps, and mineral distribution maps. Although all of these maps represent the same geographic area, they differ in what they represent as relevant. A traveler would find a mineral distribution map completely irrelevant, as would an air traffic controller when using a road map. Similar to geographic maps, maps of a discipline provide a framework for selecting and organizing information. In determining what is relevant and what is not relevant for that specific discipline, the nursing map reflects an illness perspective—to care, helping patients and families. The medical map reflects a disease perspective—to cure.

In the PICU, it is especially challenging to balance technology with values that emphasize the quality of life, consumer choice, risk-benefit decisions, access, and integrity of human life.[34] Nursing's moral sensitivity reflects a holistic view of the patient. Nursing practice values and empowers the patient's and families' right to make informed choices consistent with autonomy, personal values, life-styles, plans, or self-determination.

When cure becomes futile, nurses assume a leadership role in focusing care to ensure death with dignity and comfort. When parents must make difficult decisions about their child's life, what they require from nursing is a real presence that will support them, empower them, and give them the courage to decide.[35] Through experience, we know which activities might be helpful to families, and we provide options when death is imminent. Nurses "orchestrate" death, supporting parents and family members through the worst thing in the world anyone could ever experience, the death of a loved one.

It is extremely difficult to "orchestrate death" and then continue on with the day as if nothing happened. Often nurses are not able to share their day (like the rest of the world) with nonnurse friends because of the difficulty in talking about and listening to the topic. As one continues to experience the death of patients, one personally recovers much more quickly—death may become too routine, although it shouldn't be. It is emotionally exhausting to orchestrate death, and traditionally, nurses learn how to do so by watching their colleagues. This almost never-talked-about intimate aspect of care, which is learned through role modeling—colleague to colleague—is nursing's most profound contribution to humankind.

Caring Practices. Caring practices optimize and make clinical competence and expertise more visible. As a basic value, caring embodies a spiritual and metaphysical dimension concerned with preserving, protecting, and enhancing human dignity.[36,37] Caring practices include not only *what* nurses do but also *how* they do it. From the patient's perspective, caring practices are expressive activities that help the patients and families *feel cared for*.[38] Essential to the process of caring is nurse recognition and appreciation of the patient's and parent's worth and competency to know and attend to self and congruence of the nursing action with the patient's or parent's perception of need.[39-41]

Demonstration of professional knowledge and skill, surveillance, and reassuring presence have been identified as important caring practices when there is perceived threat to an individual's physical well-being.[38] Extremely vulnerable patients require a high level of nursing vigilance. From a patient's perspective, vigilance is a highly valued caring practice unique to critical care. In critical care, caring is vigilant behavior that embodies nurturance and highly skilled and technical practices.[42] Vigilance preserves, protects, and enhances human dignity. Alert and constant watchfulness, attentiveness, and reassuring presence are necessary to limit potential problems and complications.

The unique significance of nursing is in making a difference for patients; understanding the impact of critical illness on the infant's or child's person, development, and entire family; and helping so that patients and their families can tolerate the experience. This aspect of practice, our presence with patients, is unique to nursing.

Nurses coordinate the patient's and family's experiences by continuously focusing on the person beneath all the high technology. Nursing's concept of vigilance includes the "illness perspective," or the patient's experience of being ill. It takes courage to acknowledge the person of someone critically ill—those patients, surrounded by technology, therapists, physicians, and nurses, chemically paralyzed, narcotized, and apparently lifeless except for the rhythm of monitors, ventilators, and occasional alarms. We acknowledge their person by surrounding them with their possessions—for example, family pictures, cards from friends, their music. We make them human by talking with them, orientating them, and telling them what's going on. Occasionally the communication is not only one way. The person responds by increasing heart rate or blood pressure or dropping intracranial pressure or sometimes by just shedding a tear. Not only are nurses sensitive to this level of communication, but also they take it one step further by teaching this level of communication to family members so that they too can interact with their critically ill loved one.

Through our vigilance, we coordinate the individual experience of illness and create the environment, making it bearable. Not only do we make it bearable, but also in some cases, we make it growth provoking. Numerous nursing research studies now exist to help guide nursing practice in the neonatal ICU to support the development of preterm infants. Nursing research has changed the environment from one that was provider suited to one that is patient driven. The bright, noisy, and sterile neonatal ICUs of long ago now facilitate "kangaroo care"—the practice of giving preterm infants skin-to-skin contact with their parents, enabling them to share warmth and natural closeness. In addition to easing the pain associated with parent-infant separation, kangaroo care helps premature infants grow; leave their isolettes sooner; and achieve a deeper, more peaceful sleep.[43] Lights are dimmed, isolettes are covered with blankets to decrease both light and noise, and blankets provide appropriate boundaries. Patient survival mandates that neonatal critical care nurses be responsive to the behavioral clues of newborns and assist parents in interpreting and responding to their baby's behavior. Care is focused at supporting the entire family unit, not just a piece of it that can be biologically but never emotionally separated from the rest.

Critical care nurses have always prided themselves on having empathetic practices that value the family and provide close, attentive care to the patient.[44] More than any other subspeciality, pediatric critical care nurses have made significant progress in role modeling family-centered care in critical care. An abundance of nursing research describes family stress associated with critical illness. Regardless of the population, the themes are similar: the need for hope, information, proximity; to believe that their loved one is receiving the best care possible; to be helpful; to be recognized as important; and to talk with others with similar issues.

Pediatric critical care nurses have moved beyond just describing what is upsetting to families to describing interventions that the recipients of our care, themselves, find helpful.[28,40,45] We have improved our dialogue with families so that we provide families what they need to make

responsible care decisions—to be educated consumers of critical care. Parents note that the most significant contribution pediatric critical care nurses make in their care is to serve as "interpreter" of their critically ill child's responses and of the PICU environment.[45]

When nurses develop mutually respectful trusting relationships with parents, families become empowered to choose and to take responsibility for their choices. Creating a humanistic, empowered environment that recognizes parents as unique autonomous individuals who, when supported, are capable of providing vital elements of care to their children forms the foundation for family-centered care. Different for each individual, humane care incorporates the hopes, dreams, values, cultural preferences, and concerns of patients and their families into the daily practice of critical care.[46] The only time parents should ever have to be placed in a situation in which they must ask permission to see their children is when the privacy of other patients must be protected. However, ICUs should be designed to provide all patients with privacy. Parents are not visitors to their children.[40] Family-centered care implies more than just that open visiting hours exist.[39]

Facilitator of Learning.   Providing patients and families the opportunity, accountability, and responsibility to make their needs explicit requires consumer education. Nurses facilitate patient learning so that patients can understand the healthcare system and make informed choices. Pediatric critical care nurses infuse teaching into each and every patient encounter. Learning helps alley patient and family fear and helps individuals accommodate to and transition from the PICU environment.

Collaboration.   Jacques,[47] an organization theorist who studied the structural dimensions of nurses' work, noted: "The nurse is the one person on the unit whose job is to care about anything that might happen in the universe of the patient and to connect any parties who need to be connected in order to assure a successful outcome for the patient." Although it is critically important for the novice nurse to learn, come to know, then articulate nursing's independent contributions, only through the work of the entire team will patient outcomes be optimized.

Optimal collaboration requires multidisciplinary socialization. Interpersonal team skills include conflict resolution and consensus building. Senge[48] notes that team learning begins with dialogue, in which members suspend assumptions and think together to solve problems or chart the future.

Knaus and associates[49] found an inverse relationship between actual and predicted patient mortality and the degree of interaction and coordination of multidisciplinary intensive care teams. Hospitals with good collaboration and communication and a lower mortality had a comprehensive nursing educational support program that included a clinical nurse specialist and specific educational programming to support the use of clinical protocols in which staff nurses were independently responsible. AACN's demonstration project also documented a low mortality ratio, low complication rate, and high patient satisfaction in a unit that had a high perceived level of nurse-physician collaboration, highly rated objective nursing performance, positive organizational climate, and job satisfaction and morale.[50]

Systems Thinking. Nurses are leaders in creating and managing systems. Back in the 1960s, only nurses who gave direct patient care were considered "real" nurses. Today, as Angela McBride notes, real nurses also design, implement, and evaluate whole programs of caregiving; manage units in which care is provided; monitor whether the healthcare system as a whole is sensitive to patient needs; and play a role in ethical decision making around caregiving.[1]

Current expectations for professional nursing practice are high. Although professional skill and technologic capability are vital, these essential traits must exist in a patient-centered culture that emphasizes strong leadership, coordination of activities, continuous multidisciplinary communication, open collaborative problem solving, and conflict management.[51] Nurses have learned to manipulate the system to work for the patients, systems thinking,[48] whereas the ability to understand the interrelationships and patterns involved in complex problem solving is a new but required skill in assuming overall responsibility for the environment in which care is provided.

Managing multidisciplinary high-performance teams focused on outcomes requires systems savvy. Nurses are comfortable as team leaders, team members, and colleagues while providing supervision of unlicensed employees. Delegation is a new activity for those with singular experience within a primary nursing model.

The role of case/care manager "ups the ante" on professional practice by ensuring a level of professional accountability not always apparent within the actual, not intended, primary nursing model.[52] The case management model outlines and activates strategic management of quality patient outcomes and costs. Transforming primary nurses into case managers moves the focus of practice from the nursing process to multidisciplinary outcomes.

Creating a safe environment includes managing complex systems. Schumacher and Meleis[53] gave evidence to support "transitions" as a central concept in nursing. Nurses-patient relationships generally occur around transitional periods of instability brought on by the demands of developmental, situational, or health-illness changes. Facilitating transitions across traditional healthcare system boundaries, for example, into and out of the community, requires systems savvy and intradisciplinary collaboration.

Response to Diversity. Response to diversity celebrates the individual differences that exists in everyday life. At a minimum, care is delivered in a nonjudgmental, nondiscriminatory manner. This approach requires effective communication with patients and families at their level of understanding and, perhaps, tailoring the healthcare culture to meet the diverse needs and strengths of families. At a higher level, the expert clinician anticipates differences and beliefs within the team and negotiates consensus in the best interest of the patient and family.

Clinical Inquiry. Clinical inquiry helps push the limits of current practice so that patients receive evidence-based care. Studying the clinical effectiveness of care and how it impacts patients will provide information that helps determine where to draw the line between cost and quality.

Quality improvement methods continue to progress from single-department joint commission mandates to multidisciplinary teams working together to integrate systems in the best interests of patient care. Parallel processes working with outdated management tools (e.g., nursing care plans) continue to give way to collaborative practice groups working with clinical practice guidelines.

Clinical practice guidelines (CPGs)—patient-centered, multidisciplinary, multidimensional plans of care—help the team move toward evidence-based practice and improve the process of how care is delivered. CPGs encourage practitioner accountability, encourage highly coordinated care, decrease unnecessary variation in practice patterns, increase high-quality cost-effective services, and provide a mechanism to systematically evaluate the quality and effectiveness of practice in moving patients toward desired outcomes. Effective CPGs are driven by the patient's needs and the evidence that the intervention truly does make a difference in patient outcomes. CPGs guide the appropriate use of resources in that, if any intervention does not directly benefit the patient, it's probably not worth doing.

Nursing's primary model for knowledge generation has been the empirical/analytic model of the traditional sciences.[54] When instituting new therapies, the nursing focus is on the illness aspect of care—the human response to disease and therapy. For example, although our medical colleagues may design a randomized study to investigate the effects of high-frequency oscillatory ventilation in pediatric patients with diffuse alveolar disease and air-leak syndrome, nursing may focus on what bed to nurse the patient on (the chest shakes differently on an air than on a conventional mattress); the noise level, which is still quite high with this mode of ventilation; how to maintain skin integrity, which is challenging with the rigid arm of the ventilator; and how to suction the patient without compromising lung volume.

Numerous caring behaviors that create safe passage for patients, especially those behaviors mentored by peers, for example, clinical leadership, creating trust, comforting behaviors, and orchestrating death, are best investigated using qualitative methodologies. Yet, although qualitative methods more accurately describe the essence of nursing, they lack a causal, predictive requirement. This limits their use as a sole strategy of inquiry for nursing.

Optimal Patient Outcomes

According to the Synergy Model, when patient characteristics and nurse competencies match and synergize, optimal patient outcomes result. Many outcome measures have been proposed including: physiologic status, psychologic outcomes, functional measures, behavior, knowledge, symptom control, quality of life, home functioning, family strain, goal attainment, utilization of services, safety, problem resolution, and patient satisfaction.[55]

Making pediatric critical acute care nursing *visible* by delineating "nurse-sensitive" outcomes is challenging.

Nurse-sensitive outcomes, a term first coined by Johnson and McCloskey,[56] define a dynamic patient or family caregiver state, condition, or perception that is responsive to nursing interventions. Quite recently, Mitchell, Ferketich, and Jennings[57] described a quality health outcomes model that aligns more closely the dynamic processes of patient care and outcomes. To best capture the unique contribution of nursing and care delivery models to patient and family well-being, Mitchell and co-workers[58] proposed that outcome measures should *integrate* the functional, social, psychologic, physical, and the physiologic aspects of patients' experiences in health and illness. Outcome measures were further proposed to be operationized in five categories: (1) achievement of appropriate self-care, (2) demonstration of health-promoting behaviors, (3) health-related quality of life, (4) patient perception of being cared for well, and (5) symptom management.

Numerous mediating factors impact nurse-sensitive outcomes. First, optimal patient outcomes require both the unique and collective contributions of the patient and family, the nurse, the entire multidisciplinary team, the healthcare system, and the community. According to Mitchell,[59] outcomes should be "relevant to the individual's goals in seeking care, the institution's social contract in providing care, and the society's value and understanding of elements relevant to public as well as private health." The Synergy Model views patients in the context of their environments and as active participants in the care process. Thus the responsibility and accountability for optimal patient outcomes are shared.

Isolating nursing from the unique contributions of the patient and family and other practitioners is problematic. Brooten and Naylor[60] note: "The current search for 'nurse-sensitive patient outcomes' should be tempered in the reality that nurses do not care for patients in isolation and patients do not exist in isolation." What might be influenced by nursing care in one context may be influenced by another discipline or family in another.

Fearing that changes in both the structure and composition of the nursing workforce would jeopardize patient safety, the American Nurses Association published *Nursing Report Card for Acute Care Settings.*[61] The purpose of this report was to begin to explore the nature and strength of linkages between nursing care and patient outcomes. From an initial pool of 21, six major nursing quality indicators were identified; they include patient and family satisfaction, adverse incident rate, complication rate, patient adherence to discharge plan, mortality rate, and patient length of stay. Adverse incident rates include medication errors and patient injuries not directly related to their primary healthcare problem. Total complication rates include additional healthcare problems, for example, pressure ulcers and nosocomial infections that are unrelated to the patient's primary healthcare problem. Both these factors alter safe passage and increase patient suffering, risk of mortality, length of stay, and healthcare spending.

The Synergy Model is congruent with the *Nursing Report Card for Acute Care Settings* and provides a framework for outcome analysis. Three levels of outcomes are delineated: patient level outcomes, patient-nurse level outcomes, and patient-system level outcomes. Keeping the patient in a primary position, "optimal patient outcomes" are what patients (or the people of significance to the patient), themselves, define as important. Safe passage is reflected in a number of these outcome variables.

Patient Level Outcomes. From the patient's or family's perspective, illness is associated with perceived vulnerability and powerlessness, which stimulates the need for both competence and caring that could inspire immediate and unqualified trust.[62] In part, trust results from the nurse knowing the patient and patient knowing the nurse. Trust is a product of the nurse's clinical competency and moral agency. Patients and families will be vigilant if concerned about caregiver competence or agency. Fidelity to patient concerns, family empowerment, and coaching honors the outcomes of moral agency.

Caregiver trust is a prerequisite for the dispensing and the receiving of information. Knowledge in and of itself is not an outcome, whereas the associated change in patient health behavior related to the knowledge is. Patients and families have grown in their knowledge about health and its promotion and have gradually assumed a greater responsibility for their own health.[63]

From the patient's perspective, care that comforts them, especially when they are acutely ill, is one of the most basic services that caregivers can provide.[62] Caring practices create a compassionate and therapeutic environment with the aim of promoting comfort and preventing unnecessary suffering. The patient's experience of comfort is a quality-of-care outcome.[64] Patient and family satisfaction and ratings are subjective measures of individual health or quality of health services. Although patient and family satisfaction measures query individuals about their expectations and the extent to which they were attained, ratings include individual assessment of fact, for example, level of overall health or time one waited for services. Patient satisfaction measures involving nursing typically include technical-professional factors, trusting relationships, and education experiences.[65]

Patient-perceived functional change and quality of life are multidisciplinary outcome measures. Nurses uniquely help patients manage through transitions of functional health and quality of life. Both of these generic outcome measures can be used across all patient populations, but when analyzed separately, they provide information specific to a patient population. Precise longitudinal measures, for example, use of the *Child Health Questionnaire,*[66] is important so that real change in status can be detected over time. Measuring functional status at intermediate steps will map the trajectory of a patient's recovery. Linking patient satisfaction, functional status, and quality of life is important because the three are often related.

Patient-Nurse Level Outcomes. Patient-nurse level outcomes include physiologic changes, the presence or absence of complications, and the extent to which care or treatment objectives are attained. Monitoring and managing instantaneous therapies by trending physiologic changes are a specific phenomenon of critical care nursing. For example, when weaning a patient from mechanical ventilation, the nurse expects to find a gradual transference of the work of breathing from the ventilator to the patient. A certain trajectory of physiologic changes, for example, arterial blood gases and the percent of minute ventilation assumed by the patient can be predicted, monitored, and then evaluated.

Outcomes related to limiting iatrogenic injury and complications to therapy acknowledge the potential hazards inherent in illness and the healthcare environment. Again, nurses through their vigilance and clinical judgment create healing environments that provide safe passage for vulnerable individuals. Safe passage mandates preventive care, for example, the prevention of iatrogenic injury, infection, and hazards of immobility (e.g., pressure ulcers).

The extent to which care or treatment objectives are attained within the predicted period also serve as outcome variables. Nurses coordinate the day-to-day efforts of the entire multidisciplinary team. The nurse's role as the integrator of numerous services is critical for optimal patient outcomes and abbreviated lengths of stay. As discussed, nurse-physician collaboration and positive interaction are associated with lower mortality rates, high patient satisfaction with care, and low nosocomial complications.[48,49]

Patient-System Level Outcomes. To economically survive, healthcare systems must tighten resources *and* maintain quality that is collaboratively defined by both users and providers in the system. The goal is high-quality care at moderate cost for the greatest number of people. Important patient-system outcome data include recidivism and costs/resource use.

Recidivism, that is, *re*hospitalization and *re*admission, is rework that adds to the personal and financial burden of providing care. In addition to patient and system factors, nurses can decrease the patient's length of stay through coordination of care, prevention of complications, timely discharge planning, and appropriate referral to community resources. Reducing length of stay and tracking rehospitalization and acute care visits ensure that cost shifting is not occurring.

Payers are not interested in spending more for similar clinical outcomes. They are also not interested is assessing the unique contributions of a specific discipline but, rather, the entire outcome from an episode of care. Clinical effectiveness questions are answered by linking patient outcomes to cost data. Strong data serve as the safety net to protect against too little care. Benner[31] notes, that cost-effective care will only exist in situations in which the patient is known and continuity of care is provided by *expert* caregivers. Continuity in care and clinical judgment stabilize care within chaotic environments.

CURRENT ENVIRONMENT

Acuity within intensive and acute care units continues to rise. Care, traditionally provided in inpatient settings, is being transferred to the outpatient setting. Much of the technology used in the ICU has been adapted for use in the home. All this challenges our traditional understanding of intensive care; describing critical care nursing practice by location or by its technology seems passé. In a patient-driven system, nursing practice is described from a patient-needs perspective. Critically ill patients are characterized by the presence of, or being at high risk for developing, life-threatening problems.[67] Benner[31] notes that critically ill patients need astute clinical judgment applied to problems that have very little margin for error. Redefining critical care of nursing from a concept of vigilance allows us to maintain our focus on the patient's needs and not on geography and technology.

Critical illness is just one point on the health-illness continuum. Caring for patients in isolation from where they came or where they are going will interrupt the fluidity of care. Desperately needed is a balanced healthcare system that equally values prevention; health maintenance and education; and primary, chronic, and acute care. Pediatric critical care practitioners have long supported the value of primary prevention (e.g., pool and bicycle safety and helmet legislation). Caring for chronically ill infants and children during acute episodes of their illness, pediatric critical care practitioners appreciate the continuum of care.

Ensuring continued competence of healthcare professionals is critical to consumer protection.[68] Across the country, hospitals are experiencing a shortage of nurses. Many units, in dire distress, are offering new incentives, such as sign-on bonuses for experienced nurses and new graduates or critical care internship programs for new or inexperienced nurses. What started out as a scattered regional issue is rapidly becoming a widespread phenomenon.

The AACN's Registered Nurse Statistics Fact Sheet demonstrates that this trend has been building since the mid-1990s.[69] For example, almost 2 million registered nurses (RNs) were employed in 1996; the prediction is that there will be 2.3 million RN jobs in 2006 (21% increase). In 1996, 1.2 million RNs were employed in hospitals; the prediction is that there will be 1.3 million RN hospital jobs in 2006 (7.4% increase). The most critical shortages and thus the highest needs are for those critical care nurses in the most specialized areas; for example, requests to fill open pediatric ICU positions increased 50% from 1997 to 1998.[70]

The bottom line is that our patient population is sicker and we have fewer nurses entering and staying within nursing. Creative strategies to recruit and retain experienced critical care nurses are a priority for the profession.

Workplace redesign requires innovation, an imagination to see what is possible, and a willingness to try something new. When creating new realities, everyone is accountable for innovation and change. This is begun by challenging the givens, which are fundamentally unsupportive to a patient-driven system and unsupported by clinical research. The "givens" are similar to what Senge[51] describes as mental models—notions or assumptions that have the power to move us forward or hold us back. Stellar changes have occurred when the status quo or basic "givens" were challenged.

Innovation requires both risk taking and collegial support. Nursing and risk taking appear to be dichotomous terms.[71] The American Nurses Association Code for Nurses states that the nurse acts to "safeguard the client," which may be perceived as limiting opportunities in taking risks.[72] However, the code also challenges us to participate in the development of new knowledge and in improving our standards of care. This aspect of practice definitely involves risk taking in identifying innovations or changes in the care we deliver to groups of patients.

Change—any change—can be risky. Advocating for change, especially when it may appear to buck the system or be unpopular with colleagues, is risky. However, in taking risks, having the courage to move out of a "comfort zone" to value diversity in thought is the essential element for both personal growth and innovations in care. Defeo[73] notes that personal and professional growth requires courage to move ahead despite doubts or opposition. Three types of courage have been described: (1) social courage, to invest in open relationships; (2) creative courage, the willingness to instigate change and allow innovation; and (3) moral courage, the courage to care enough to become involved, that is, the courage to take a risk for a matter of principle.[74]

Many nurses have never learned how or when to take risks. Critically important is timing—being strategic in taking risks for what is really important to the profession. Again, what is right for patients and their families is right for the profession. Ask, then really listen to the consumers of care—they know their needs. Be a leader. True nursing leaders support a learning environment because, as Burns[75] points out, successful leaders are comfortable enough with their own fallibility in that they allow themselves to be vulnerable and are willing to take risks. Giving oneself permission to make mistakes empowers one to take risks.

By continuing the historic tradition of creating safe passage for patients, nurses make a significant contribution to the quality of patient care services, containment of costs, and patient outcomes. By reducing mortality rates, length of stay, costs, and complications and by increasing family satisfaction and readiness and ability to function upon discharge, nurses make significant contributions to both the quality of hospital services and the containment of hospital costs.[76]

In conclusion, as Donna Diers[77] pointed out in 1984:

> Believe in nursing, in the wildest possible expanse of role and function, and believe so strongly that your beliefs can sustain you through the battles with the unknowing, unthinking, deluded, and barefoot pragmatists who wish to restrain the ideas and talents of nurses.

REFERENCES

1. McBride AB: How nursing looks today, *Indiana University Alumni Magazine,* Jan-Feb:64, 1994.
2. Diers D: Nursing: implementing the agenda for social change. Paper presented at the Fiftieth Anniversary Symposium: Nursing as a force in social change, University of Pennsylvania School of Nursing, Philadelphia, Pa, Sept 20, 1985.
3. Fairman J: Watchful vigilance: nursing care, technology, and the development of intensive care units, *Nurs Res* 4:56-60, 1992.
4. Alcott LM: *Hospital sketches,* Boston, 1863, James Redpath.
5. Cadmus RR: Special care for the critical case, *Hospitals* 28:65-66, 1954.
6. Cadmus RR: Intensive care reaches silver anniversary, *Hospitals* 54:98-102, 1980.
7. Drinker P, Shaw LA: An apparatus for the prolonged administration of artificial respiration, *J Clin Invest* 7:229, 1929.
8. Lassen HCA: A preliminary report on the 1952 epidemic of poliomyelitis in Copenhagen with special reference to the treatment of acute respiratory insufficiency, *Lancet* January 3, 37-41, 1953.
9. Smith CA: *The Children's Hospital of Boston: "Built better than they knew,"* Boston, 1983, Little, Brown.
10. Downes JJ: The historical evolution, current status, and prospective development of pediatric critical care, *Crit Care Clin North Am* 8:1-22, 1992.
11. DeNicola LK, Todres ID: History of pediatric intensive care in the United States. In Fuhrman BP, Zimmerman JJ, eds: *Pediatric critical care,* St Louis, 1992, Mosby.

12. Downes, personal communication, June 17, 1994.
13. American Hospital Association: Hospital statistics 1993-1994 edition, p 231, Table 13A, Chicago, 1993.
14. American Hospital Association: Hospital statistics 1998 edition (p 151, Table 7; Facilities and Services in the US Census Divisions and States), Chicago, 2000, Health Forum LLC.
15. Committee on Hospital Care and Pediatric Section of the Society of Critical Care Medicine: Guidelines and level of care for pediatric intensive care units, *Pediatrics* 92:166-175, 1993.
16. Committee on Hospital Care and Pediatric Section of the Society of Critical Care Medicine (In Press).
17. Yeh TS: Regionalization of pediatric critical care, *Crit Care Clin North Am* 8:23-35, 1992.
18. Vestal KW: Pediatric critical care nursing, New York, 1981, Wiley Medical.
19. Oakes AR: *Critical care nursing of children and adolescents,* Philadelphia, 1981, WB Saunders.
20. Smith JB: *Pediatric critical care,* New York, 1983, Wiley Medical.
21. Hazinski MF: *Nursing care of the critically ill child,* St Louis, 1984, Mosby.
22. Lynaugh J: Four hundred postcards, *Nurs Res* 39:254-255, 1990.
23. Disch J: Special Interest Groups—providing opportunities for AACN members, *Focus on AACN* 41-43, April 1982.
24. Christopherson D: Priorities established for special interest groups, *Focus on AACN* 35, August 1982.

25. Griffin J, Hitchens M, Smith-Blair N: Certification for pediatric intensive care nurses, *AACN: Neonatal and Pediatric SIG Newsletter* 1:6, 1984.
26. Niebuhr BS: Credentialing of critical care nurses, *AACN Clin Issues Crit Care Nurs* 4:611-616, 1993.
27. Ramseyer K, Jones P: Passing point determined for neonatal and pediatric exam, *CCRN News* 6, Fall 1992.
28. Curley MAQ: Patient-nurse synergy: optimizing patients' outcomes, *Am J Crit Care* 7:64-72, 1998.
29. Aiken LH, Smith HL, Lake ET: Lower Medicare mortality among a set of hospitals know for good nursing care, *Med Care* 32:771-787, 1994.
30. Tanner CA, Benner P, Chesla C et al: The phenomenology of knowing the patient, *Image J Nurs Sch* 25:273-280, 1993.
31. Benner P, Tanner C, Chesla C: From beginner to expert: gaining a differentiated clinical world in critical care nursing, *Adv Nurs Sci* 14:13-28, 1992.
32. Patricia Hooper-Kyriakidis, personal communication, 1996.
33. Visintainer MA: The nature of knowledge and theory in nursing, *Image J Nurs Sch* 18:32-38, 1986.
34. Pew Health Professions Commission: *Healthy America: practitioners for 2005,* October 1991. (Available from Pew Charitable Trusts, 1388 Sutter Street, Suite 805, San Francisco, CA 94109.)
35. Marsden C: Real presence, *Heart Lung* 19:540-541, 1990.

36. Watson J: New dimensions of human caring theory, *Nurs Sci Q* 1:175-181, 1988.

37. Caine RM: Incorporating CARE into caring for families in crisis, *AACN Clin Issues Crit Care Nurs* 2:236-241, 1991.

38. Brown L: The experience of care: patient perspectives, *Top Clin Nurs* 8:56-62, 1986.

39. Curley MAQ: Effects of the nursing mutual participation model of care and parental stress in the pediatric intensive care unit, *Heart Lung* 17:682-688, 1988.

40. Curley MAQ, Wallace J: Effects of the nursing mutual participation model of care on parental stress in the pediatric intensive care unit—a replication, *J Pediatr Nurs* 7:377-385, 1992.

41. Wolf ZR, Giardino ER, Osborne PA et al: Dimensions of nurse caring, *Image J Nurs Sch* 26:107-111, 1994.

42. Burfitt SN, Greiner DS, Miers LJ et al: Professional nurse caring as perceived by critically ill patients: a phenomenologic study, *Am J Crit Care* 2:489-499, 1993.

43. Ludington SM: Energy conservation during skin-to-skin contact between premature infants and their mothers, *Heart Lung* 19:445-451, 1990.

44. Alspach G: Giving voice to the vision—achieving the patient-driven system, *Crit Care Nurse Suppl* June 2, 1994.

45. Curley MAQ: Effects of the nursing mutual participation model of care and parental stress in the pediatric intensive care unit. Unpublished master's thesis, New Haven, Conn, 1987, Yale University School of Nursing.

46. Harvey MA, Ninos NP, Adler DC et al: Results of the consensus conference on fostering more humane critical care: creating a healing environment, *AACN Clin Issues Crit Care Nurs* 4:484-507, 1993.

47. Jacques RW: Untheorized dimensions of caring work: caring as a structural practice and caring as a way of seeing, *Nurs Admin Q* 17:1-10, 1993.

48. Senge PM: *The fifth discipline: the art and practice of the learning organization,* New York, 1990, Doubleday.

49. Knaus WA, Draper EA, Wagner DP et al: An evaluation of the outcome from intensive care in major medical centers, *Ann Intern Med* 104:410-418, 1986.

50. Mitchell PH, Armstrong S, Simpson TF et al: American Association of Critical-Care Nurses Demonstration Project: Profile of excellence in critical care nursing, *Heart Lung* 18:219-237, 1989.

51. Zimmerman JE, Shortell SM, Rousseau DM et al: Improving intensive care: observations based on organizational case studies in nine intensive care units: a prospective, multicenter study, *Crit Care Med* 21:1443-1451, 1993.

52. Zander K: Nursing case management: strategic management of cost and quality outcomes, *J Nurs Admin* 18:23-30, 1988.

53. Schumacher KL, Meleis AI: Transitions: a central concept in nursing, *Image J Nurs Sch* 26:119-127, 1994.

54. Norbeck JS: In defense of empiricism, *Image J Nurs Sch* 19:28-30, 1987.

55. Lang NM, Marek KD: Outcomes that reflect clinical practice. National Institutes of Health. Patient outcomes research: examining the effectiveness of nursing practice, Department of Health and Human Services, NIH publication No 93-3411, 27-38, 1992.

56. Johnson M, McCloskey JC: *Quality in the nineties.* In *Series on nursing administration.* Vol III. *Delivery of quality health care,* St Louis, 1992, Mosby.

57. Mitchell PH, Ferketich S, Jennings BM: American Academy of Nursing Expert Panel on Quality Health Care, *Image J Nurs Sch* 30:43-46, 1998.

58. Mitchell PH, Heinrich J, Moritz P et al: Outcome measures and care delivery systems conference, *Med Care* 35(suppl 11)NS124-127, 1997.

59. Mitchell P: Perspectives on outcome-oriented care systems, *Nurs Admin Q* 17:1-7, 1993.

60. Brooten D, Naylor MD: Nurses' effect on changing patient outcomes, *Image J Nurs Sch* 7:95-99, 1995.

61. American Nurses Association. Lewin-VHI: *Nursing care report card for acute care settings,* Washington, DC, 1995, American Nurses Publishing.

62. Gerteis M, Edgman-Levitan S, Daley J et al: Medicine and health from the patient's perspective. In *Through the patient's eyes: understanding and promoting patient-centered care,* San Francisco, 1993, Jossey-Bass.

63. American Nurses Association: Nursing's Social Policy Statement, Washington, DC, 1995, American Nurses Foundation.

64. Ferrell BR, Wisdom C, Rhiner M et al: Pain management as a quality of care outcome, *J Nurs Qual Assur* 5:50-58, 1991.

65. Hinshaw AS, Atwood JR: A patient satisfaction instrument: precision by replication, *Nurs Res* 31:170-175, 1982.

66. Langraf JM, Abetz L, Ware JE: *Child Health Questionnaire (CHQ): a user's manual,* Child Health Questionnaire Project, 1996, The Health Institute, New England Medical Center, Box 345, 750 Washington St, Boston, MA.

67. Gordon S: Inside the patient-driven system, *Crit Care Nurse Suppl* June, 3-28, 1994.

68. AACN: *Outcome standards for nursing care of the critically ill,* American Association of Critical-Care Nurses, 1990, PO Box 30008, Laguna Niguel, CA 92607.

69. Pew Health Professions Commission: The nursing profession. In *Health professions education for the future: schools in service to the nation,* February 1993. (Available from Pew Charitable Trusts, 1388 Sutter St, Suite 805, San Francisco, CA 94109.)

70. AACN FAQ: FAQ: can you provide information about the current critical care nursing shortage? FAQ 99-4. Nursing Shortage, April 6, 2000, AACN Website, at http://www.aacn.org/AACN/practice.nsf/.

71. Gillam T: Legal notes: risk-taking: a nurse's duty, *Nurs Standard* 5:52-53, 1991.

72. American Nurses Association: *Code for nurses with interpretive statements,* Washington, DC, 1985, The Association.

73. Defeo DJ: Change: a central concern for nursing, *Nurs Sci Q* 3:88-94, 1990.

74. Nyberg J: Roles and rewards in nursing administration, *Nurs Admin Q* 13:36-69, 1989.

75. Burns SP: Determining the qualities of a leader, *Aspens Advis Nurse Exec* 4:4-5, 8, 1989.

76. Prescott PA: Nursing: an important component of hospital survival under a reformed health care system, *Nurs Econ* 11:192-199, 1993.

77. Diers D: Commencement address, *Yale Nurse,* 3, Fall 1984.

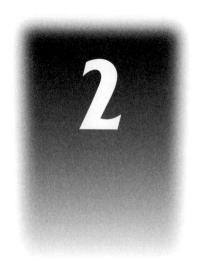

2 Caring Practice: Providing Developmentally Supportive Care

Janis Bloedel Smith
Sarah A. Martin

CONCEPTUAL FOUNDATION FOR CARING PRACTICE

Hospitalization during childhood is a situational crisis for children and their families. Illness, disability, disfiguring treatment, disrupted family relationships, and unsupportive environments threaten development. Behavioral disturbances after brief, scheduled hospital admissions are not uncommon and include regression in achievement of developmental milestones, feeding difficulties, and altered sleep and rest cycles. Nurses have been actively involved in identifying aspects of hospitalization that are difficult for children and their families and in implementing developmental practices aimed at mitigating stress during the experience. In fact, managing the emotional aspects of critical illness and intensive care is a unique aspect of the nurse's role. A foundation for effective intervention to meet the developmental needs of children in the pediatric intensive care unit (PICU) is an appreciation of the impact of critical illness on the individual child's experience. This chapter discusses the concepts of stress, coping, and adaptation related to critical care hospitalization. Stresses of a PICU hospitalization are reviewed, and the developmental significance for children from infancy through adolescence is discussed. Interventions to assist children in the PICU to manage stress, cope with illness, and achieve mastery are presented.

Stress

Stress is the result of a problem or an especially demanding situation that cannot be easily solved, that taxes or exceeds an individual's resources, and endangers personal well-being. Selye[1] and Lazarus[2] have provided the foundation for understanding the human stress response from both physiologic and psychologic perspectives.

Stress results in a complex physiologic response. Selye[1] described the physiologic response as mediated by the action of a stressor on the anterior pituitary, which stimulates production of somatotropin and adrenocorticotropic hormone (ACTH). Somatotropin augments the inflammatory response and combats the pathogen; ACTH stimulates the adrenal cortex to produce both mineralocorticoids and glucocorticoids. Catecholamine production by the adrenal medulla is also increased. Epinephrine and norepinephrine production increases in stressful experiences, increasing metabolic rate and influencing a wide range of physiologic functions. The autonomic nervous system also influences production of the catecholamines by the adrenal medulla in the stress response. Designed to regulate physiologic defense mechanisms, the stress response is a multifactorial hormonal and nervous system protective reaction.

Psychologic stresses activate this same pituitary-adrenal response. Increased stress hormone production occurs in response to failing ego defenses, punishment, sleep deprivation, noxious stimulation, and general anxiety. However, psychologic sources of stress and the individual's psychologic responses are not as uniform and predictable as physiologic stresses and responses. Consequently, psychologic stress cannot be defined in completely objective terms. A unique relationship exists between the individual and the stressful experience, mediated by cognitive appraisal. Cognitive appraisal determines the meaning of an event for individuals and shapes their emotional and behavioral response to it. Through cognitive appraisal, individuals evaluate the significance of what is happening in terms of their own well-being. Cognitive appraisal is not always a conscious, obvious mental operation. Defense mechanisms or routine problem-solving processes may operate unperceived on a conscious level.

Stress appraisal is influenced by factors related to the individual experiencing the stressful event and by characteristics of the event. The most important personal factors are commitments and beliefs. The more meaningful and important a commitment, the greater the threat and challenge in a stressful situation that menaces that commitment. Greater threat also can motivate the person to action and help sustain hope. Beliefs, particularly those about self-control and control over the stressful event, affect emotion and coping. Existential beliefs enable individuals to find meaning and maintain hope in difficult situations.

Interdependently influencing the cognitive appraisal are characteristics of the stressful situation. Situations that are uncertain or ambiguous are threatening. Individual tolerance of ambiguity or uncertainty varies between persons. Ambiguity can intensify threat because it limits the individual's sense of control over the situation and increases feelings of helplessness. On the other hand, ambiguity can reduce threat because it permits individuals to consider alternative interpretations of a situation and maintain hope.

The timing of a stressful event influences its appraisal. Generally, imminent events are more urgent. Delay before a stressful event can heighten anxiety, but delay also provides opportunity to marshal coping efforts and reduce stress. A lengthy event may lead to exhaustion but also permits emotional habituation through coping.

The timing of events over the life cycle can affect cognitive appraisal. Normal life events may be stressful crises if they occur "off time" or out of sequence. When events occur off time, they are often unexpected, and individuals do not have the opportunity to prepare. In addition, they may not have the support of compatible peers. The timing of a stressful event in relation to other events may magnify the cumulative stress experienced. Accumulated stressful events can increase distress because of the added weight of additional events or because of links between events.

An individual's perception of stress is influenced by past experience in coping, both with a particular stress and by general coping ability. Stress-resistant people have a certain "hardiness"—a set of attitudes that leaves them open to change, feeling involved, and in control of events. These characteristics, even under very stressful circumstances, are linked to positive coping ability.

The perceived magnitude of a stress also influences coping ability. Perception of stress as minimal, requiring only a simple response, is likely to result in effective coping behaviors. When stress is perceived as complex and large, the coping response must be similarly complex. The individual's coping abilities may be overwhelmed, unless the stress can be divided into manageable pieces.

For children, the ability to appraise a stressful situation is linked to cognitive development. In addition, each developmental phase is characterized by concerns unique to that stage. Appraisal of a situation is determined by both cognitive maturity and developmental age. Each child's view of a stressful situation or event is most meaningful from the vantage point of individual development.

Coping

Coping involves cognitive and behavioral efforts to minimize, tolerate, or manage external or internal stresses that tax or exceed the individual's resources. Automatic thoughts and behaviors that do not require effort are useful in situations that do not burden an individual's resources. Coping is process oriented, and effort is required to manage stressful demands regardless of the outcome. Consequently, no coping strategy can be considered inherently better or worse than another. Some situations cannot be mastered and require that the individual minimize, avoid, deny, tolerate, and accept the stressful conditions.

Coping during childhood is influenced by a variety of factors. Most significant is the individual child's developmental stage, which largely determines the range of responses available to the child. As young children come to understand the world, they learn complex ways of coping. However, despite changes in the details of coping that are related to maturation and development, evidence shows that patterns in coping responses are apparent early in life and remain constant across life. Likewise, sources of stress change with age, but it is doubtful that coping changes in basic ways across the lifespan.

Resources. Resources determine, in part, individual coping. Resources include health, energy, problem-solving skills, social skills, social support, commitments, beliefs, and material resources. Effective use of resources may be constrained by a variety of factors. Personal constraints are internalized cultural values that define acceptable ways of behaving. Environmental constraints include institutions that thwart coping efforts. In addition, when a high level of threat is present, as in the PICU, individuals may be unable to use coping resources effectively. This is of particular concern because the critically ill patient obviously lacks fundamental coping resources: health and energy. Box 2-1 illustrates resources found to contribute to positive coping in children.

Parental Coping. The level of parental coping during the stress of a child's illness and hospitalization affects how children cope. Because of the close relationship between parents and their children and the dependence normally experienced during childhood, children tend to accept what their parents accept. Parental anxiety, despite attempts to conceal it, is often transmitted to children. Termed "emotional contagion," the transmission of parental anxiety to children has been identified and effectively treated by providing parents information about what will occur and how they can assist their child.[3,4] These interventions not only are effective in reducing the child's distress but also increase parents' feelings of comfort and competence.

Because parents are the most important individuals in a child's support system, characteristics of the parent-child relationship are correlated with the child's coping abilities. When the relationship is characterized by a high degree of compatibility, parents are able to provide their children with a great deal of emotional support. Conversely, parent-child relationships that are unreliable and tenuous may result in children receiving limited support from their parents. There is no substitute for parental love, encouragement, and support.

Coping Experiences. Cognitive maturation permits children to recall previous experiences with stressful or challenging situations. A child who has coped successfully with a demanding situation in the past is able to recall the experience with pride and self-confidence. However, the child who has had little opportunity or has been unsuccessful in attempts to master new experiences may lack the confidence necessary to succeed when challenged. Doubtful about their personal abilities, these children are likely to react negatively to new or challenging situations.

Temperament. Innate qualities that determine individual temperament can be identified during infancy and are characteristics remarkably stable across the lifespan. Regularity of body functions and daily schedule, confident responses to new stimuli, pleasant mood, and persistence in challenging activities characterize children who cope well with new situations. A positive, outgoing attitude toward life is evident in children likely to have a broad range of positive

Box 2-1
Factors That Contribute to Positive Coping in Children

Individual Child Factors

Positive temperament
Above-average intelligence
Good academic achievement
Ability to relate well to others
Participation in activities

Family Factors

Supportive parents
Family closeness
Adequate rule setting

Community Factors

Availability of friends
Availability of extended family
Good schools

From Byrne C, Hunsberger M: Stress, crises, and coping. In Betz CL, Hunsberger M, Wright S, eds: *Family-centered nursing care of children,* ed 2, Philadelphia, 1994, WB Saunders, p 635.

coping resources and the pride, courage, and resilience to mobilize resources despite disappointment and frustration. Children who feel secure about themselves and confident about the adults around them are tolerant of retreat and regression, which may be necessary in very stressful situations.

Defense Mechanisms. Defense mechanisms are intrapsychic ways of thinking or behaving unconsciously employed in coping with stress. Because the range of defense mechanisms increases with cognitive development (Table 2-1), young children have a limited repertoire of mechanisms available for coping. Some are considered undesirable or even pathologic in older children, adolescents, and adults; however, the stress of critical illness justifies, at least for limited periods, the use of any mechanism that assists with coping.

For example, *regression* is a defense mechanism often identified in children that may be difficult for others to accept. Regression is a temporary retreat or reversion to an earlier stage of behavior to retain or regain mastery of a stressful, anxiety-producing, or frustrating situation, thus achieving self-gratification and protection. Regression allows the child to conserve energy and strength for recuperation and accept caring provided by others. The child who regresses during a period of stress usually gives up the most recently acquired skill. For example, toilet training may be "forgotten" or the child may revert to thumb sucking or drinking from a bottle. The regressed child may also cry a great deal, especially when parents are present. Rather than constituting a negative behavior, crying with parents permits the child to release tension and demonstrates a feeling of safety in relating strong emotions. Lost skills are generally rapidly relearned as recuperation and recovery restore available energy. Regression is an unhealthy response to a

TABLE 2-1	**Defense Mechanisms Available by Developmental Age**
Stage	**Defense Mechanism**
Infants	Discrete defense mechanisms not identifiable
Toddlers and preschoolers	Regression: Return to an earlier stage of development in thought, feeling, or behavior
	Denial: Mental refusal to acknowledge a stressful reality
	Repression: Unpleasant experiences or thoughts are barred from conscious awareness
	Displacement: Transfer of emotionally charged thoughts or feelings to a more acceptable substitute object
School-age children	Preceding mechanisms, plus the following:
	Projection: Attribution of unacceptable thoughts or impulses to another person or out into the environment
	Reaction formation: Expression of an unacceptable impulse or feeling by transforming it into the polar opposite
	Sublimation: Transformation of unpleasant, blocked, or unacceptable thoughts or wishes into socially acceptable pursuits
Adolescents	Preceding mechanisms, plus the following:
	Rationalization: Application of logical, socially acceptable reasons for behavior or events that do not reflect the real reasons behind the action
	Intellectualization: Excessive reasoning is applied to allay disturbing feelings or thoughts and to permit isolation

stressful situation only if the child is unable to remaster previously learned skills.

Denial is another defense mechanism often regarded as pathologic. However, when stress is acute, denial is necessary for at least short periods. Denial allows the child to ward off threatening aspects of the environment and to maintain hope. For example, the child who closes or covers the eyes during a stressful procedure, such as suctioning the endotracheal tube, or one who indicates dismissal, turning the head away when a parent must leave, uses denial in a protective way. Like regression, denial is an unhealthy defense only if it persists unreasonably and interferes with a child accepting a permanent aspect of reality.

Adaptation and Mastery

Adaptation implies that an individual experiencing stress undergoes change that facilitates interaction with the envi-

ronment. Assimilating aspects of the environment that are new, different, or challenging into previously learned behaviors and accommodating or modifying behavior in response to new or different demands are essential aspects of adaptation. In fact, Piaget[5] viewed the ability to adapt as key to the survival and subsequent development of the human infant. Adaptation is based on *accommodation* (modification to conform to environmental demands) and *assimilation* (incorporation of previously learned activities in current behavior). The two processes together comprise the key techniques that children and adults use to interact successfully with the world. Adaptation is a key process in maintaining health. The concepts of development, stress, and adaptation emphasize change as the constant feature of life.

Mastery is possession or development of the skills needed to overcome and defeat a specific challenge. For critically ill children, the challenge is the experience of the illness or injury and the subsequent intensive care hospitalization, with all its inherent stresses. Adaptation may well be required in this circumstance. Mastery is the outcome when caring interventions identify and supply the tools necessary for each child to experience a level of success that surpasses adaptation; that is, the child has the feelings of pride, self-esteem, and self-reliance associated with sure success in a challenging encounter.

Stressors During Hospitalization

Despite the individual nature of stress, events characteristic of critical illness and intensive care are predictable stresses. The PICU environment itself, separation from family and significant others, pain, intrusive procedures, and developmental disruption necessitate caring intervention to mitigate stress and promote coping.

The PICU Environment. Little in the intensive care environment bears resemblance to the everyday world of infants and children. The environment is one of high activity around the clock and is crowded with equipment and people. The noise level is often excessive, as equipment alarms sound, telephones ring, and voices of caregivers— sometimes raised in anxiety—contribute to a technologic symphony. The mean noise level recorded in a busy PICU was measured at 55.1 decibels, with sudden, sharp increases to 90 decibels[6]; these levels are significantly in excess of the 35 decibels considered necessary for adequate rest.[7] Noise was the most significant cause of sleep deprivation in one study on sleep disturbance in intensive care units.[8] Unlike the critical care nurse, who knows the significance of each beep and buzz, children in a PICU can make no sense of these sounds.

Visual stimulation is also excessive because of continuous overhead lighting. Lights can create sensory confusion, cause patients to lose day-night orientation, and interrupt sleep. Sleep-wake cycles are disturbed by environmental stimulation, by pain and discomfort, and also by caregiving interventions. Sleep deprivation is a common problem for children in the PICU. Children in the PICU sleep far less than is normal and have seriously disturbed sleep patterns.[6,7,9-10] In the recent Cureton-Lane and Fontaine study,[6] children slept a mean total of 4.7 hours, in intervals that averaged only 28 minutes. Their sleep was interrupted nearly 10 times during a 10-hour night by noise, light, and contact with caregivers.

Unfamiliar sights and people characterize the PICU. Children as young as those beginning their school years are aware of other patients and are concerned for their welfare.[11] Unable to understand the meaning of what they observe, children may become anxious for another child and concerned that they too may undergo a painful or distressing procedure.

The "Intensive Care Unit syndrome" (also called ICU psychoses) has been described in adult patients. Contributing factors include sensory overload or monotony, sleep deprivation, and use of medications. Manifestations include fear, anxiety, depression, hallucinations, and delirium. In the PICU environment, children have been subjectively described as withdrawn, passive, anxious, egocentric, negative, and demanding.[12,13] Objectively measurable behavioral expression of anxiety, depression, agitation, and withdrawal occurs in children in the PICU.[14] PICU patients in the study exhibited apprehension about routine nonpainful procedures, anxiety and worry, detachment with staff, sadness and weeping, and tremulousness and shakiness. Positively correlated with the presence of these behaviors were the duration of the intensive care hospitalization, the number of previous hospitalizations, increasing severity of illness, and preexisting psychiatric disorders. Critically ill children are at high risk for the development of stress-related behavioral disturbances.

Separation. Nurses are instrumental in ensuring liberal visiting policies for parents of children who are hospitalized. However, children in the PICU often experience periods of separation from those who are their most important source of emotional support. As recently as 1994, a survey of 125 hospitals in ten southeastern states found that 57% restricted visits to pediatric patients in intensive care units.[15] Parents may be asked to leave the unit when procedures are performed on their child or others and are often excluded during resuscitative efforts.

Separation is a painful experience at any age. The normal passages of life include leaving familiar and comforting people and surroundings as individuals move through school, career, intimate relationships, and the eventual death of parents and other older relatives and friends.

The significance of parents for children has been demonstrated in both animal and human studies. Although hospitalization at the start of the twenty-first century will not likely include extremes of separation of children from their parents, historical studies illustrate the importance of that close and continuing relationship.

Harlow and Zimmerman[16] showed that newborn monkeys provided adequate nutrition from a cloth and wire-mesh "mother" became antisocially aggressive and unable to interact within a clan. Spitz[17] observed children separated from their mothers for both short and long periods in penal nurseries and orphanages. After 6 months of separation, the children had fixed changes: they were silent, their measured intelligence fell, previously acquired motor skills were lost,

TABLE 2-2 Phases of Separation Anxiety in Infants and Young Children

Phase of Anxiety	Behavioral Responses
Protest	Loud, vigorous protest at the absence of parents Restlessness; expectant watching for the parents' return Refuses care or attention from others
Despair	Loud crying ceases Less activity, withdrawn, disinterested in play or food Apathetic and isolated appearance Hopeless and grieving
Resignation/ detachment	Resigned to loss and appears to have adjusted Shows some interest in surroundings, begins new relationships but is detached

and their faces were rigid and expressionless. Although these children were fed and kept clean, by age 4 years, of the 21 children still in the institutions, only 1 could talk in sentences, 6 could not talk at all, 5 could not walk, and 16 walked only by holding onto furniture.

In his study of hospitalized children, Robertson[18] provided the labels for the stages of separation that Spitz[17] had observed. Young children in the hospital demonstrated three stages of "separation anxiety," characterized by protest, despair, and resignation (Table 2-2). Bowlby[19] studied children who had been separated from their London families during World War II and placed in physically safe English countryside homes when nightly bombing raids threatened. These children, although physically safe, suffered deprivation and were characterized as emotionally flat and expressionless. Children deprived of parental contact demonstrate persistent long-term manifestations of their deprivation: impaired trust, diminished intellectual and motor functioning, and disturbed behavior. Children are dependent on the close and reliable presence of their parents under normal circumstances; their need for parental closeness when they are ill is still greater. Maintaining the parent-child relationship and preventing stress related to separation is the standard of care in the PICU.

Fagin[20] noted that the quality of the parent-child relationship influenced children's responses to separation. Assured of the fact that parents return after they have "disappeared," through the development of object permanence (the knowledge that the object or person has an independent, individual, and permanent existence), older infants and toddlers learn to tolerate periods of separation when well as their parents reliably return after a period of absence. When parents have an inconsistent relationship with their child and are unable to provide consistent substitute caregivers, the child may have difficulty learning to tolerate periods of separation. Consequently, separation may affect the child who has an insecure relationship with parents to a greater extent than those children with a secure and confident relationship with their parents.

Pain and Intrusive Procedures. Pain and painful or invasive procedures are potentially destabilizing and demoralizing experiences for critically ill patients (see Chapter 17). Pain induces fear because it evokes unpleasant physical sensations and because of the emotional responses common to the experience of pain. Critically ill children may not be able to articulate their experiences or their fears of pain but are afraid of both physical sensations and threats to self-integrity and self-esteem.

Fear of body intrusion and mutilation is a stress related to pain and common to the experience of critical illness and intensive care. Like pain, intrusive procedures threaten self-esteem and self-integrity. Consequently, children respond similarly to both. They fear that body injury and mutilation may result from invasive procedures and equipment.

Developmental Disruption. Social and emotional development provides children with increasing ability for self-control—an essential part of ego integrity. Emotional self-control is a marker of self-confidence and self-esteem. Children who feel confident and proud of themselves and their abilities are more likely to be self-controlled. New situations challenge an individual's ability to maintain self-control, particularly when the situation is threatening. The experiences of critical illness and intensive care disrupt familiar routines and the opportunities for physical activity, independence, and productivity that children need to maintain developmental progress toward self-control.

All individuals establish routines that provide a sense of order in their daily lives. The need to maintain an orderly, predictable environment safe from threat is ageless and universal. The need for a safe, stable environment is ranked just above the need for food, water, shelter, and other physiologic needs. Young children are dependent on routines and rituals to view the world as safe, predictable, and subject to their control. Serious illness and intensive care dramatically alter daily routines. The ability of children to maintain self-control despite the loss of trusted people, objects, and routines relied on for stability is tenuous.

Children who are hospitalized experience fear and anxiety about the unknown. Children actively engage their world by learning about it and mastering its sometimes complex, challenging parts. When understanding is achieved, control follows. Young children in the hospital often have vague, generalized fears related to their stage of development, whereas older children tend to have more specific fears related to events or procedures for which they are unprepared. An event or procedure does not need to be potentially or actually painful to induce stress; unfamiliar settings, equipment, and machines may be threatening and challenge children's ability to maintain self-control.

Coping during childhood is aided by the discharge of anxious energy in physical activity. Illness necessitates some restriction of activity to conserve energy for recuperation, whereas a variety of procedures required by a critically ill child may necessitate actual physical restraint and immobility. Physical restrictions limit sensory stimula-

tion and threaten self-control. Physical restraints to prevent the child from dislodging needed critical care paraphernalia and immobilization techniques used by healthcare providers during a procedure have the potential to produce high anxiety and near panic.

Infants and young children are accustomed to depending on others for care. Consequently, the enforced dependency of hospitalization, particularly if familiar caregivers play a substantial role in providing aspects of care, may not threaten the self-esteem and self-control of these youngsters. On the other hand, even toddlers assert their independence when they are well, as their sense of autonomy develops. Older children and adolescents, accustomed to independence in self-care activities, have increased stress by the necessary dependence of the sick role. By the school-age years, these characteristics are often an internal source of self-control and may lead to feelings of inadequacy, powerlessness, and anxiety when illness requires dependency on others. Illness must not only require that sick children be dependent. The environment must permit and provide recovery opportunities to regain independence.[21]

Children also experience feelings of loss of self-control and powerlessness because they are unable to enact the social roles that provided them status in their families, their school settings, and peer groups. Sick children fear that their status and position within the family may be preempted by a sibling if they are not present to perform certain tasks. Loss of status with schoolmates and peers is feared by children absent from these social groups.

Critical illness and intensive care are stressful for infants and children. Mitigating the effects of the stress imposed by the PICU environment, separation from family and significant others, pain and intrusive procedures, and developmental disruption define caring critical care nursing practice. Pain and illness are not simply physiologic phenomena, leaving the mind and the spirit unaffected. The total patient—physiologic, psychologic, sociocultural, and developmental—is the concern of nursing.

THE INFANT (0 TO 12 MONTHS)

Developmental Characteristics of the First Year of Life

The rapid development and magnitude of change across the first year of life warrant considering this stage in two phases: the neonatal period (the first month of life) and infancy. The following section and Table 2-3 describe the most significant aspects of development for the infant.

Parent-Infant Attachment. During the neonatal period, the foundation for parent-infant attachment established during the prenatal period is solidified and strengthened. Parent-infant attachment is a reciprocal process in which the parents and their infant become acquainted and bond with one another. Attachment is a process, not a spontaneous occurrence, in that it does not occur instinctively but is the result of the unique relationship that develops between parents and infants. From the infant's perspective, the process of attachment permits a view of the world as reliable

◆ TABLE 2-3 Infant Development				
Developmental Characteristic	**0-3 Months**	**3-6 Months**	**6-9 Months**	**9-12 Months**
Cognitive Piaget's stages[5]	Sensorimotor Stage 1 (birth-1 month) • Continued practice with reflex activities leads to a sense of order • Understands through direct sensations and motor actions	Sensorimotor Stage 2 (1-4 months) • Primary circular reactions stimulate effort to repeat a behavior • Able to fixate, conjugate, differentiate size and shape, can see clearly at a distance	Sensorimotor Stage 3 (4-8 months) • Secondary circular reactions stimulate effort to re-create an interesting effect in the environment • The basis for play is established	Sensorimotor Stage 4 (8-12 months) • Coordination of secondary circular reactions to intentionally form new, more complex behaviors
Social-emotional • Erikson[22]—developmental progression through mastery of tasks and subtasks and negative component	Sense of trust (vs. mistrust) is gained with consistent, quality care		Has definite likes and dislikes	Shows emotions: anger, fear, and affection
• Fears/death According to Johnson,[23] the concept of death (not returning) can develop without mastering the cognitive tasks of object/person permanence and separation anxiety. Separation anxiety and person permanence provide the foundation for the concepts of fear and death.		Fears: Stranger anxiety develops at 6-7 months and peaks at 18 months	Fears: Separation anxiety develops at 8-9 months Greatest fear is separation from parents	Fears: pain
Language	Responds to sound (birth)	Smiles and coos Babbles (5-6 months)	"Dada" and "mama" (8-9 months) Responds to own name	Two words other than "dada" and "mama" Understands simple commands
Gross motor	Good head control (2-3 months)	Rolls front to back (4-5 months) Rolls back to front (5-6 months)	Sits alone (6 months) Crawls Pulls self to stand	Stands alone Toddling
Fine motor	Grasp and shake rattle (2-3 months)	Reaches for objects or persons (3-4 months) Hand-to-hand transfer of objects (5-6 months)	Raking grasp (6-7 months) Pincer grasp (7-9 months)	Holds a spoon Makes marks on paper with pencil or crayon (10-12 months)

Data from the American Academy of Pediatrics. In Shelov SP, Hannemann RE, eds: *Caring for your baby and young child: birth to age 5*, New York, 1998, Bantam Books; Green M, ed: *Bright futures: guidelines for health supervision of infants, children, and adolescents pocket guide*, rev ed, Arlington, Va, 1998, National Center for Education in Maternal and Child Health; Millonig VL, Baroni MA, eds: *Pediatric nurse practitioner certification review guide*, ed 3, Potomac, Md, 1999, Health Leadership Associates.

Continued

TABLE 2-3 Infant Development—cont'd

Developmental Characteristic	0-3 Months	3-6 Months	6-9 Months	9-12 Months
Growth	Average U.S. newborn weighs 3.1 kg (7 pounds), is 51 cm (20-21 inches) in length, and head circumference is 33-35.6 cm (14 inches) Growth spurts at 6 weeks and 3 months	Newborn loses 10% of birth weight during the first 3 days of life; weight regained by 14 days Gains 180-240 grams (6-8 ounces) per week Head circumference increases 1.27 cm (½ inch) per month for the first 6 months	Gains 180-240 grams (6-8 ounces) per week Birth weight doubles by 4 months	Gains 90-120 grams (3-4 ounces) per week Head circumference increases 0.64 cm (¼ inch) per month through 12 months	Triples birth weight by 1 year Length increases 50% from birth by 1 year
Dentition	Eruption timing can vary, but sequence is generally consistent To estimate expected number of teeth during the first 2 years (age of child in months − 6 = expected number of teeth)		Mandibular central incisors (5-7 months)	Maxillary central incisors (6-8 months), mandibular lateral incisors (7-10 months) Initiate brushing teeth	Maxillary lateral incisors (8-11 months) Mandibular and maxillary first molars (10-16 months)
Diet	Require 100-120 calories/kg/day Breast-feed or formula for the first 4 to 6 months All prepared formulas should contain iron No milk before 1 year, as contributes to allergies and iron deficiency No honey before 2 years because of the risk of botulism	Breast-feeding intake, feeding times vary; breast milk is preferred and should be used if available (encourage pumping during periods of critical illness and administer by gavage); breast-feeding is contraindicated only in HIV-positive mothers Parents instructed to hold the infant for feeding; avoid bottles in bed or propping the bottle Intake variable: 0-1 month: 60-120 ml every 3-4 hours; 2-4 months: 150-210 ml every 4-5 hours	Introduce rice cereal at 4-6 months (mix cereal with breast milk or formula and feed with a spoon) Introduce pureed fruits or vegetables next (one new food every 3-5 days) Avoid common allergenic foods (cow's milk, egg whites, wheat, and citrus)	Initiate drinking from a cup at 6 months with water or juice (<120 ml/day)	Finger foods, mashed table foods begun at 9 months Avoid "choke foods": peanuts, popcorn, carrot sticks, whole grapes, hot dogs, raisins, and hard candy

Sleep				
Supine or side-lying sleep position recommended by the American Academy of Pediatrics (AAP) to decrease the incidence of sudden infant death syndrome Critically ill infants may appear to sleep for long periods; sleep is of poor quality as compared with healthy infants[24]	Neonates sleep an average of 18 hours/day 2-4 months: 8-12 hours at night; 2 or 3 daytime naps	At 4 months, start bed routine, put infant to sleep awake	11-12 hours at night; 2-3 naps (6-12 months)	At 1 year, sleep approximately 12-14 hours/day
Health Maintenance **Anticipatory Guidance**	First month: Breast-feeding, bottle feeding Crib and bath safety Position on back to sleep Car seat use Smoke-free environment 2-4 Months: Introduction of solids Anticipation of rolling	4-6 Months: Discourage walkers Reaching for objects begins Keep hot liquids, cigarettes away	Introduction of table foods Use of cup Teething Crawling, reaching Childproofing Syrup of Ipecac available for emergency use	Progression of table foods Use of cup Self-feeding Increased mobility-hazards
Immunizations	Birth: hepatitis B (#1) 1 month: hepatitis B (#2) 2 months: DTaP (#1), HiB (#1), IPV (#1)	4 months: DTaP (#2), HiB (#2), IPV (#2)	6 months: DTaP (#3), HiB (#3)	9 months: hepatitis B (#3) 12 months: IPV (#3), varicella
Approach to Physical Examination[25] and Interventions Strive to provide continuity with caregivers to support a consistent care routine	Conduct from noninvasive to invasive (auscultate first) Approach slowly Use distraction and engaging facial expression Ask parents to provide a transitional object	Restraints are stressful because the infant cannot explore and play Liberal visitation	Keep parents within visual field	

Data from the American Academy of Pediatrics. In Shelov SP, Hannemann RE, eds: *Caring for your baby and young child: birth to age 5*, New York, 1998, Bantam Books; Green M, ed: *Bright futures: guidelines for health supervision of infants, children, and adolescents pocket guide*, rev ed, Arlington, Va, 1998, National Center for Education in Maternal and Child Health; Millonig VL, Baroni MA, eds: *Pediatric nurse practitioner certification review guide*, ed 3, Potomac, Md, 1999, Health Leadership Associates.
DTaP, Diphtheria, tetanus, pertussis; *HiB*, *Haemophilus influenzae* type B; *IPV*, polio vaccine.

and trustworthy. When parents reliably respond to their infant's needs, the baby learns trust. Mistrust is the negative counterpart of the task of infancy.

The innate, awakening senses of infants equip them for interaction with their parents and their environment. Tactile sensation is obvious at birth, as demonstrated by the rooting reflex and sensitivity to pain and temperature extremes. Affectionate and comforting touch from parents confirms feelings of reassurance and builds trust. At birth, infants demonstrate a preference for staring into a human face rather than at an inanimate object. In addition, the senses of taste, smell, and hearing are present within hours of birth. The infant sucks when a pleasant taste is introduced. Babies can differentiate between the smell of their mothers and others and prefer the familiar maternal scent. Hearing is present even before birth. The healthy infant is equipped from the moment of birth to engage in the processes that promote attachment and the development of trust.

The Neonatal Period. In the first month, infants spend as much as 80% of the time sleeping. Their waking hours are spent exercising the activities with which they are born: sucking, looking, grasping, and crying. Through repeating and perfecting these activities, the infant gains control over small aspects of the environment and becomes expert at a limited repertoire of activities by the end of the first month. Coordination between activities is undeveloped; neonates can look at a visually appealing object but are unable to reach out for it.

Infancy. Infants are engaged in establishing the differences between themselves and the rest of their world. By the middle of the first year, infants recognize themselves as separate from their parents. Simultaneously, parents become the strongly preferred caregivers. By 4 to 6 months of age, the attachment of infants for their parents has grown beyond the assurance that needs for food and comfort will be met. Infants begin to prefer their parents for the sake of their company alone, apart from the satisfaction of physical needs. The responsive smile that greets familiar caregivers signals infants' preference for these individuals.

Their developing physical abilities permit infants to have greater interaction with the world that surrounds them. Infants learn new behaviors as the result of accidental responses. For example, the baby accidentally gets a hand, finger, or thumb into the mouth, triggering the sucking response and the sensation of the thumb in the mouth. The response and the sensation lead to repetition of the behavior until it is intentional, rather than accidental. Similarly, infants learn that kicking makes a mobile sway and move.

Tremendous learning takes place in the second half of the first year of life. Infants learn to use signs to anticipate events. For example, putting on an infant's jacket signals that the family is going out. Rituals at bedtime—a bath, putting on pajamas, stories in the rocking chair—become increasingly important as the infant learns to view the world as reliable and predictable.

Infants in the second 6 months of life are able to coordinate their activities to bring about a desired end. They can now look at an object, reach for it, grasp it, and bring it to the mouth. An important consequence is the development of the realization that objects exist separately and apart from the actions of the baby. Piaget[5] referred to this development as the acquisition of the object concept.

The beginnings of the cognitive knowledge of object permanence follow. Object permanence refers to the ability of infants to separate objects from their perception of them and realize that an object continues to exist even when it is out of sight. The delight that infants in the first year demonstrate at peek-a-boo games provides evidence of their progress at mastering this concept. However, infants have not sufficiently mastered the concept of object permanence to face separation from their parents with relaxed ease. Stranger anxiety is often evident in infants between 6 and 9 months of age. The anxiety displayed by infants toward strangers is related to anxiety regarding separation from parents who are not established as having a permanent existence when out of sight. Under usual circumstances, infants in the last part of the first year of life awaken at night and cry for the comfort and reassurance of their parents.

The primary mode of activity during infancy is sensorimotor. Motor control is developed through nearly constant muscle activity during an infant's waking hours. Motor activity is also the primary mechanism by which the infant learns to distinguish between self, others, and the environment.

Impact of Hospitalization

Research with neonates has demonstrated the impact of the stressful, hectic PICU environment on newborns.[26-29] Stress during intensive care hospitalization affects neurobehavioral organization, physiologic stability, and both short-term and long-term outcomes. Bright lighting, noise, and caregiving activities have been linked to stress in the newborn intensive care patient. Strategies to mitigate stressful aspects of the PICU environment by structuring caregiving and modifying the environment have been associated with improved outcomes for neonates.[26,27,30]

Signs of distress in the infant resulting from environmental overstimulation are nonspecific, requiring that the critical care nurse be alert to their presence because early intervention can prevent physiologic and behavioral decompensation. Distressed newborns may be jittery, frequently agitated, and unable to quiet themselves. Vital signs are altered; heart rate, blood pressure, and respiratory rate are elevated. Breathing may be irregular, and oxygenation and skin color may be altered. Digestion is affected, and hiccuping, gagging, and feeding intolerance may develop. Level of consciousness may change, with some infants demonstrating "shut down," that is, becoming unreactive to the environment. Consistency in the assignment of caregivers to critically ill infants assists each to know individual patients on a more sophisticated level and enables the accurate identification of subtle, nonspecific behavioral and physical signs of distress.

As the infant proceeds from the newborn period across the first year of life, recognition of signs that the baby is distressed becomes steadily clearer. Often parents recognize distinguishable differences in how the baby cries when hungry, tired, fearful, in pain, or when needing comfort and support for some other reason. Critical care nurses receive valuable input from parents to assist them in recognizing these signs. In addition, infants experience tremendous refinement of fine and gross motor skills throughout the first year, enabling them to express distress and displeasure far more articulately than earlier.

Turning away from an unpleasant stimulus is a simple coping tool. Older infants even attempt to remove a noxious stimulus. Autonomic nervous system stability develops steadily in the first months of life. Characteristic changes in vital signs persist in the face of overstimulation and distress, but changes in oxygenation and skin color are not antici- pated beyond the newborn period, unless the infant is premature or gravely ill.

Illness and hospitalization disrupt the infant's usual existence. Regularity and reliability in the environment and freedom to explore the environment are important require- ments for the development of trust in themselves and others that engages infants across the first year. Predictable daily routines provide infants the stability necessary for them to view their environment as safe and reliable. Immobilization and restraint limit motor activity and alter the amount and the variety of environmental stimuli the infant receives.

Developmental Care

Modifying the PICU environment is a necessary first step to prevent neurobehavioral disorganization. Overhead lighting is dimmed and augmented with individually controlled bedside lighting. When procedures necessitate bright light- ing, a light blanket shielding the infant's eyes mitigates distress. Staff awareness of the auditory impact of loud conversation, telephones, stereo equipment, overhead inter- com announcements, and mechanical equipment and alarms is crucial. Monitor and equipment alarms are kept at a safe minimum volume, which ensures that they are heard but do not startle infants when they sound. Reduction of the overall noise level effectively minimizes stress for infants. An environmental assessment by each nurse at the start of each shift ensures that the environment is appropriately modified for infants in the PICU.

The isolette or infant bed requires modification to avoid overstimulation and promote neurobehavioral organization. Isolettes shield infants from the environment, especially if partially covered to decrease both light and noise stimula- tion. Parents can assist the critical care staff to create a bed space that is personalized and soothing for their infant. The goal is to enhance the infant's ability to rest and sleep be- tween caregiving episodes. A calm, relaxing environment is the ideal. Selected toys, music, and pictures are to comfort, not overstimulate. Any combination of containment, swad- dling, and supportive positioning promotes neurobehavioral organization (Figure 2-1). Containment can be provided during routine handling, as well as during stressful proce- dures. "Containing" the infant's extremities close to the trunk with the caregiver's or parent's hands or with swad- dling diminishes extraneous, disorganized motor activity. Light swaddling of the infant with hands free to reach the face enables hand-to-mouth maneuvers. Successfully bring- ing the hands to the mouth assists in the development of motor organization and the ability to self-comfort. Support-

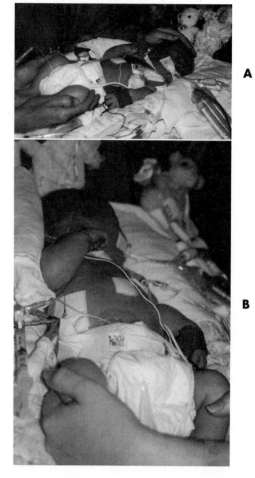

Fig. 2-1   Containment. **A,** Infant's mother is providing physical and emotional support by placement of her hand on the infant's head. The mother applies gentle firm pressure while the infant's grandmother uses both hands to gather the lower extremities and hold them in a supported position close to the body. **B,** Infant's lower extremities are being contained by the mother, while bedding and blanket rolls around the infant provide containing support to the infant's upper extremities and trunk. Containment can be offered during stressful procedures or as a method of comforting and calming the infant.

ive positioning promotes comfort and rest in a firm nest, maintains a balance of muscular flexion and extension, and prevents abnormal posturing or malformation. The infant is positioned with neck, trunk, and extremities flexed and in the midline position. Positioning is maintained with rolls, swaddling, foam supports, or commercially available posi- tioning devices. Inappropriate arousal and exaggerated mo- tor responses to stimuli are minimized.[30]

Direct caregiving activities are best begun slowly and very gently, maintaining containment and flexion and allowing the infant to grasp or suck during care. Startling the infant is avoided by close attention to the infant's state as care is initiated and by gentle arousal. Swaddling during stressful procedures helps to prevent disorganization and maintains physiologic stability. A period of rest and recovery is provided after stressful procedures, such as blood sampling or endotracheal tube retaping, before another intervention is carried out. Rest and sleep facilitate organization. Sleep is promoted by providing supportive positioning, ending interaction with the infant, and modifying the environment to ensure quiet and dim lighting.

Involving parents in their baby's care is the foundation to alleviating environmental stress for the older infant in the PICU. Infants require the close and reliable presence of their primary caregivers to relax, rest, and recuperate. Ensuring that the environment is warm, quiet, and dimly lit also minimizes environmental stress for infants beyond the newborn period. Comforting and familiar objects from home may support an infant's coping abilities during distressing procedures, as does distraction with a rattle or small toy and use of a pacifier or the fingers or thumb for sucking, rocking, and swaddling.

Very young, very ill infants cannot demonstrate distinct behavioral responses to separation from their parents. Nonspecific changes in behavior, such as increased gross motor activity, frequent crying, poor feeding, insomnia, emotional withdrawal, and self-stimulating behaviors may indicate distress. Older infants, if well enough, are likely to demonstrate the phases of separation anxiety (see Table 2-2).

Parents can provide data regarding how their infant has responded in the past to strangers and new situations. With that information in mind, the critical care nurse develops an approach to the individual baby and assesses responses to separation from parents and to substitute caregivers. Subtle cues indicating distress are evaluated, as the baby may well be too young or too ill to protest at separation or stranger. Critical care nurses demonstrate that they recognize parental presence is crucial by welcoming parents in the PICU and including them in both the planning and implementation of the care required by their infant.

Infants are assisted to cope with temporary separation from their parents, when unavoidable, by assignment of consistent substitute caregivers. In addition, a quiet, gentle approach to the sick infant helps to establish trust, as does the prompt and consistent response of caregivers to signs that the infant is distressed. Trust develops with a combination of consistency, continuity, and sameness.[31] Transitional or security objects can ease periods of separation for the infant, as can familiar musical or story tape recordings.

Very ill or very young infants respond to immobilization and restraint with little physical resistance. However, infants recovering from critical illness and those who are older may protest vigorously when restrained. Nurses assess the amount of physical restriction required by an individual infant to maintain safety and perform procedures effectively. Not only is motor activity limited by physical restraint, but the infant is unable to move away from sources of environmental sensory overload or appreciate fully a range of sensory experiences. Assessing the PICU environment for factors that contribute to sensory overstimulation or deprivation is a first step in the process of evaluating the infant for distress related to physical restriction. When restraints are necessary for safety, they are regularly removed to permit the infant to move freely while supervised. Restraints are applied in a manner that permits the infant to self-comfort (e.g., to get the thumb to mouth) whenever feasible. Infants who are ill require frequent position changes within their bed.

Ensuring appropriate infant stimulation is an important corollary to the physical care of the baby in the PICU. While the infant is ill, stimulation must be gently planned to protect the baby from environmental overstimulation. As the infant recovers, social stimulation is of particular importance because it encourages relationship formation and trust in others. All stimulation is designed to mitigate sensory deprivation with sights, sounds, or activities that appeal to infants.

THE TODDLER (1 TO 3 YEARS)

Developmental Characteristics of Toddlers

Toddlers are among the most challenging children cared for in the critical care setting. The toddler period represents only about 3% of the average human lifespan but encompasses more physical, intellectual, and emotional change than any other period. Table 2-4 summarizes development during the toddler period.

The beginning of toddlerhood is marked by the development of object permanence, an elementary concept of cause and effect, and actions that demonstrate deliberate intention. Through assimilation, tactile stimulation, manipulation, and interaction with the environment, toddlers are intent on figuring out how things work. Toddlers are driven by a nearly insatiable curiosity. Nonetheless, verbal ability is limited, and toddlers tend to act out much of what they feel. Their thinking is egocentric, and their world view is absolute and animistic.

The social and emotional task of individuating and separating from parents, with the ultimate goal of autonomy, evolves over the 2 years of the toddler period. The struggles for independence characteristic of toddlers are evidenced in battles over holding their own spoon and squirming against a restraining parent's hand. The inevitable passage through a "no" stage also marks the quest for autonomy. The successful establishment of toddlers' sense of autonomy opposes feelings of shame and doubt that are the negative counterpart of development at this stage.

These social developmental tasks require tremendous emotional growth and change, which often produce ambivalence and aggression in toddlers. Change is managed by dependence on aspects of daily life that are stable and consistent. The sense of security derived from the sameness of certain routine aspects of living is so important to toddlers that routines become rituals. Repetition and mimicking are commonplace in both language and action.

Impact of Hospitalization

Hospitalization is likely to be particularly threatening in the evolution of autonomous toddlers. Their limited intellectual ability renders preparatory explanations of upcoming events ineffective. Logical explanations likewise prove ineffective because toddlers are not logical. Because newly acquired independence is founded on the security of a trusting relationship with their parents, this relationship is

TABLE 2-4   Toddler Development

Developmental Characteristic	Attributes
Cognitive/Language	
• Piaget's stages[5]	Sensorimotor: 0-2 years
	Stage 5 (12-18 months):
	Tertiary circular reactions to attain a goal
	Rudimentary trial-and-error behavior with active experimentation
	Object permanence achieved
	Stage 6 (18-24 months):
	Can remember, plan, imitate, and imagine
	Use mental symbols
	See themselves as separate from others
	Onset of magical thinking
	Preoperational: 2-7 years
	Stage 1 (2-4 years):
	Preconceptual stage; reason dominated by perception and linkage to events
	Play is symbolic and imitative
	Egocentrism influences perception of objects, events, and language
	Use two-word phrases, 10 or more words in vocabulary (18 months)
	900-word vocabulary (3 years)
Social-Emotional	
• Erikson[22]	Autonomy vs. shame and doubt
	A sense of autonomy and realization of will develop, giving opportunities to gain some self-control
	Acceptance of reality develops
	Striving for independence
	Negativism and temper tantrums are common
• Fears/death	Awareness of ownership/"mine" (18 months)
	Fears: separation from parents/abandonment, intrusion of body orifices, bodily injury, loss of control, and pain; stranger anxiety
	Death: Unable to comprehend the concept of death; may show fear or sadness as displayed by parents
Motor	
	Uses a cup well (15 months)
Years of Exploration	
	Kneels without support (15 months)
	Runs (3 years)
	Most children are psychologically and physically ready to begin toilet training between 18-30 months
Growth	
	Reduced rate of growth
	Gains approximately 1.8-2.7 kg (4-6 pounds)/year
	Grows approximately 7.5 cm (3 inches)/year
	Head circumference 2.5 cm (1 inch)/year up to 3 years (measure head circumference until 2 years)
	First molars 10-16 months, second molars 20-30 months; has approximately 20 teeth by 3 years
Diet	
Nutritional requirements 100 cal/kg/day	"Anorexia" and food jags are common
	Provide foods from the five major food groups: one fourth to one third of adult portions or 1 tablespoon for each year
	Whole milk until 2 years of age (potential for iron deficiency anemia if drinks more than 24 ounces of milk/day)
	Self-feed, bottle to cup transition at about 1 year
	Start using utensils (18 months)
	Eat meals as a family

Data from the American Academy of Pediatrics. In Shelov SP, Hannemann RE, eds: *Caring for your baby and young child: birth to age 5,* New York, 1998, Bantam Books; Green M, ed: *Bright futures: guidelines for health supervision of infants, children, and adolescents pocket guide,* rev ed, Arlington, Va, 1998, National Center for Education in Maternal and Child Health; Millonig VL, Baroni MA, eds: *Pediatric nurse practitioner certification review guide,* ed 3, Potomac, Md, 1999, Health Leadership Associates. *Continued*

TABLE 2-4 Toddler Development—cont'd

Developmental Characteristic	Attributes
Health Maintenance Anticipatory Guidance	Immunizations: HiB (#4), MMR (#1) (15 months); DTaP (#4) (18 months)
	Sleep 10 to 12 hours at night; take 1-2 naps
	Safety: check for hazards at toddler walking level, keep medications and poisons out of reach (highest poisoning incidence at 2 years), parents should have syrup of Ipecac, emphasize street safety
	Develop strategies to deal with nightmares (2-3 years)
	First dental examination by 3 years
Approach to Physical Examination[25] and Interventions	Noninvasive to invasive sequence
	Use a slow gradual approach
	Talk quietly and calmly about what will occur just before the event
	Allow child to touch and hold equipment
	Give choices when possible; reinforce limits
	Praise the toddler often; need to be told they are "good"
	Distraction is helpful
	Limit number of caregivers, if possible
	Allow to sit up when possible (allows them to gain familiarity with caregivers and environment)
	Familiar toys and family photos can serve as transitional or security objects

Data from the American Academy of Pediatrics. In Shelov SP, Hannemann RE, eds: *Caring for your baby and young child: birth to age 5,* New York, 1998, Bantam Books; Green M, ed: *Bright futures: guidelines for health supervision of infants, children, and adolescents pocket guide,* rev ed, Arlington, Va, 1998, National Center for Education in Maternal and Child Health; Millonig VL, Baroni MA, eds: *Pediatric nurse practitioner certification review guide,* ed 3, Potomac, Md, 1999, Health Leadership Associates.
DTaP, Diphtheria, tetanus, pertussis; *HiB, H. influenzae* type B; *MMR,* measles, mumps, rubella.

key to managing the stress inherent in a critical care hospitalization.

In the PICU, a cold chrome crib replaces the familiar warmth of a wooden crib filled with comforting toys. The environment is intimidating with bright lighting, strange noise (often loud and offensive), and unknown equipment and people around the bed. Toddlers, who adventure out into the unknown on short excursions from the safely known, are thrust into a completely foreign environment.

If able, toddlers may cry fearfully. Some may react to the unfamiliarity of the environment with increased vigilance, rarely closing their eyes even when exhausted. Sicker toddlers are likely to withdraw from the environment. Their withdrawal is essential to coping because it allows them to take in the environment a little at a time.

Toddlers require the close and consistent presence of their parents to manage distress. The security of their relationship with trusted parents permits them to rest and recuperate. Separation from parents is a major source of stress for toddlers who are hospitalized. When separation is unexpected and enforced, toddlers fear abandonment. Egocentric thinking may lead toddlers to conclude that some misdeed of theirs is the cause of their parents' absence.

Toddlers react to impending separation from their parents with vigorous verbal protest and clinging. The seriously ill toddler lacks the ability to protest but may cry inconsolably when left alone. When a behavioral response is impossible for the toddler, separation is no less frightening. Toddlers who are denied the dependable and consistent presence of their parents for an extended period may demonstrate the behaviors associated with separation anxiety: protest, de-

spair, and resignation. Even when parents are reliably present, toddlers are not relieved of all distress. Parents may be subjected to avoidance behaviors, aggression, and ambivalence.

Denial and regression are the primary defense mechanisms available to toddlers. Denial is evidenced in avoidance of the parents when they are present. Behaviors including gaze aversion and refusal to seek physical comfort or initiate contact with their parents may be observed, particularly as critically ill toddlers recover. Regression is necessitated by the stress of critical illness and high anxiety.

Developmental Care

The ability of the hospitalized toddler to maintain self-control is threatened by altered routines and physical restriction. The development of an autonomous toddler who is able to separate from parents is dependent on the toddler's ability to move away from them physically. As the growing toddler's world widens, self-control is maintained chiefly through routine and ritual, which permit these youngsters to view their expanding world as reliable and subject to control. The usual routines toddlers rely on to maintain self-control separate from their parents are likely disrupted by hospitalization. The world is no longer reliable. Fear of the unknown and enforced dependency may affect the older toddler.

Nurses learn of the individual child's routines and habits, particularly those related to eating, sleeping, bathing, and toileting, from the toddler's parents. Disruption in all of these areas is likely during a PICU admission. Bedtime is an especially vulnerable time for the toddler, with difficulty settling for sleep and sleep disturbances common among these young children. Regression is a common response to altered routines. Negativism may also be evidenced as toddlers protest disruption. Incorporating as many of the toddler's routines and habits into the hospital schedule as possible provides the foundation for individualized care. Parents play a key role in maintaining routine and are the greatest source of stability for their child. When parents cannot be present, transitional objects and tape recordings, particularly of bedtime stories or songs, assist toddlers to relax and maintain self-control.

Toddlers lack the cognitive development necessary for specific fears of the unknown aspects of hospitalization. However, the unfamiliarity of the entire environment is likely to intimidate even the bravest toddler. Toddlers can recall past experiences that were painful or frightening, and fearful anticipation often precedes a procedure or event. In fact, fearfulness may prevent the toddler's maintaining much, if any, self-control.

Transitional or security objects also provide a measure of reassurance in the unfamiliar PICU environment or when new and unknown procedures or events occur. Preparation of toddlers for events is best provided only shortly before the experience and, because of the egocentric nature of toddlers' thought processes, is depersonalized. Parents are thoroughly prepared for the events their child will experience to facilitate their support and comfort of the child.

Illness slows the typical active pace of the toddler's life, but immobilization and restraint result in protest if physical energy is available. Sensory deprivation and immobilization are likely to result in regression and aggression in toddlers. Aggression may be evidenced by general restlessness, physical resistance, or struggling. Aggression, which permits the release of tension and energy, may be impossible until the toddler is less ill. Limiting immobilization and restraint whenever possible diminishes their impact on the recuperating toddler in the PICU. Parents can provide watchful eyes and ensure that their child is safe. Recuperation can also provide outlets for aggression if the toddler is permitted activities such as throwing soft balls, exploring, manipulating toys, and the like. Enforced dependency can be mitigated by providing toddlers with choices when there is an option they can safely choose. Choices are not offered when none exist. Recuperation also permits the toddler to accomplish some aspects of care independently, such as self-feeding. Liberal praise is in order when toddlers complete tasks.

THE PRESCHOOLER (3 TO 5 YEARS)
Developmental Characteristics of Preschoolers

Preschool children, through the development of initiative, become active members of their world. Successful transition through the toddler years produces a self-confident and separate person who has overcome fears of abandonment. Rapid progress in cognitive function, language develop-

ment, and motor abilities leads to the acquisition of a distinctive, individual personality. Each preschooler develops a "self." Table 2-5 provides a summary of preschool development.

Cognitive development is reflected in increasing awareness of themselves and others. Preschoolers are aware of their own sex and that of others, understand kinship, and become aware of cultural differences at 5 years. However, preschool logic is preoperational. Preschoolers are unable to apply the principle of conservation and cannot classify objects. They focus attention on the most obvious, immediate single aspect or characteristic of a situation. For example, healthcare providers may be classified together as individuals who wear white coats and give shots. Egocentrism, animism, magical thinking, and fantasy characterize the preschooler's view of the world. They are unable to separate fantasy from reality and may fear ghosts, monsters, supernatural forces, robbers, kidnappers, and people in white coats. Consequently, preschoolers are most often not as mature as might be thought from their verbal ability.

Conscience begins developing during the preschool years and is tied to identification of what behaviors are acceptable to parents. Behavior is refined in taking turns, sharing, and following the rules to games. Rules are absolute during the preschool years, determined by parents who are always right. Preschoolers strive to be similar to their parents, particularly the parent of the same sex. Sexual curiosity is characteristic of the preschool years. The development of longing for the opposite-sex parent and its resolution in identification with the same-sex parent occurs.

Emotional and social development is characterized by egocentrism and is related to the preschooler's developing sense of self. Preschoolers are unable to see the viewpoint of others and unable to understand another's inability to see their own point of view. Their sense of self provides security and competence, which motivates them to accomplish the tasks and activities that lead to the development of initiative. Initiative is the boldness or courage to take on great projects. If initiative does not develop and the preschooler lacks the self-confidence to tackle new opportunities, guilty feelings are the negative counterpart of preschool developmental tasks.

Impact of Hospitalization

Hospitalization interrupts the preschooler's efforts to master control of the environment and develop initiative through mastery of physical and social skills. The restrictive hospital environment causes considerable distress for preschoolers who experience guilt when their accomplishments are obstructed. Guilty feelings may also be related to egocentric thinking, which leads to the conclusion that "wrong" or "bad" thoughts or actions have caused their illness. Treatment and hospitalization are seen as punishment. Preconceptual and magical thinking create exaggerated fears. Despite resolution of fears of abandonment, preschool children fear being left alone. Separation anxiety is expressed more subtly, and protest when parents must leave is less aggressive. Distress may be evidenced in sleep distur-

TABLE 2-5 **Preschooler Development**

Developmental Characteristic	Attributes

Cognitive/Language
• Piaget's stages[5]
	Preoperational stage
	    Stage 2 (4-7 years):
	      • Intuitive stage, reason is not governed by logic
	      • Reasoning is transductive, from one particular to the next
	      • Able to focus on one aspect of an object or event only
	      • "Magical thinking" places at risk for accidental injury and increase in fears
	      • May see illness as retribution for "bad" thoughts
	      • Continually questions "why?" (4 years)
	      • Can count, identify colors and geometric shapes, and memorize nursery rhymes
	      • Speech is intelligible (4 years)
	      • 2100-word vocabulary used in meaningful sentences (5 years)

Social-emotional
• Erikson[22]
	Initiative vs. guilt
	    • A sense of initiative and the realization of purpose develop given opportunity to do for self
	    • A period of questioning and exploring the environment and own body
	    • Sexual differences noted
	    • Feels guilty for negative events
	    • Mood swings and verbal tantrums (4 years)
	    • Conscience develops and is tied to the identification of what behaviors are acceptable to parents
	    • Follows "the rules" (5 years)
	    • Multiple fears as have active imaginations (bodily injury, the dark, monsters, robbers, kidnappers, and being left alone)

• Fears/Death	Fears: the unknown related to inability to maintain self-control when distressed Death[23]: Between the ages of 3-6 years, reality and magic are mixed when thinking about the causes of death; believe that death is reversible
Motor	Skips, hops on one foot (4 years) Skips, hops on alternate feet (5 years) Usually daytime toilet trained (3 years) Usually nighttime toilet trained (3-5 years)
Growth	Gains approximately 2.3 kg (5 pounds)/year Grows approximately 7.5 cm (2 to 3½ inches)/year May begin to lose primary teeth
Diet Requirements: 90 cal/kg/day	Strong food preferences Provide food from the five food groups in realistic amounts and nutritious snacks Low-fat milk recommended; may use whole milk
Anticipatory Guidance **Health Maintenance**	Immunizations: DTaP (#5), IPV (#4), MMR (#2) at 4-6 years Sleeps 8-12 hours/night, gradually eliminates nap Sleep disturbances persist as these children are sensitive to sensory input and dependent on bedtime routines May have dreams and nightmares Safety: stranger danger, use bike helmet, reinforce pedestrian safety, and use seat belt Annual dental appointment Brush teeth after each meal and at bedtime
Approach to Physical Examination[25] and Interventions	Needs feedback during assessments Provide concrete, truthful information; emphasize events to be expected, regardless of the child's clinical condition (unclear neurologic status, chemical sedation, neuromuscular blockade, etc.) Provide consistent caregivers Play therapy may be therapeutic

Data from the American Academy of Pediatrics. In Shelov SP, Hannemann RE, eds: *Caring for your baby and young child: birth to age 5,* New York, 1998, Bantam Books; Green M, ed: *Bright futures: guidelines for health supervision of infants, children, and adolescents pocket guide,* rev ed, Arlington, Va, 1998, National Center for Education in Maternal and Child Health; Millonig VL, Baroni MA, eds: *Pediatric nurse practitioner certification review guide,* ed 3, Potomac, Md, 1999, Health Leadership Associates.
DTaP, Diphtheria, tetanus, pertussis; *IPV,* polio vaccine; *MMR,* measles, mumps, rubella.

bances, eating difficulties, quiet crying, and withdrawal from others. Without parental presence, preschoolers may be unable to cooperate with healthcare personnel during procedures. They may not cooperate with their parents, either, if they leave for a period. Aggression is usually not experienced with this age group, although younger preschoolers may still have temper tantrums.

Regression is the most common coping response for preschoolers dealing with separation. Thumb sucking may be resumed, or baby talk may replace the typical language of the preschooler. Self-care skills and control of body functions, often recently acquired, may be threatened.

The critical care environment remains a source of distress for hospitalized preschoolers. Egocentricity, magical thinking, and preconceptual logic may lead to exaggerated fears of equipment, procedures, and personnel. Older preschoolers are often aware of others and may, as a consequence, have fears from information they overhear and do not understand or for other patients around them. Sleep disturbances persist among these young children who are exquisitely sensitive to sensory input (sights, sounds, odors) and still reasonably dependent on bedtime routines.

Fearful behaviors may not be detected in those preschoolers who are very ill. During recuperation, some exhibit fearfulness related to the PICU environment, procedures, or personnel by tense behaviors such as nail biting or whining. Others exhibit distress in regressed behavior, such as clinging to their parents or a security object, dependency, and withdrawal. Concrete evidence of the fears that some preschool children experience is sometimes obtained from their drawings or by requesting that they tell a "story" about hospital procedures or experiences. Nightmares occurring after recovery and hospital discharge are sometimes related to lingering fears and are reported by many parents after young children are hospitalized. Sleep or night terrors in preschoolers following hospitalization occur when usual sleep patterns have been disorganized.[7,32]

Developmental Care

Preschoolers can be protected from at least some of the fears associated with the critical care unit. All procedures are explained in concrete, understandable terms, with emphasis on events to be expected. This practice is ensured even when a child's condition is critical, neurologic status unclear, and responses prohibited by chemical sedation or paralysis. When preschoolers are less ill, they benefit from therapeutic play and education.

Shielding preschoolers from disturbing sights and sounds offers protection from the PICU environment and from other patients around them. Conversations about the child between caregivers or with parents are not held within earshot of the preschooler unless the child is included. Not only may unintentionally overheard conversations be frightening to preschoolers who are unable to completely understand the content, but they may also inadvertently induce guilty feelings. The preschooler may feel guilty and responsible based on comments such as "she failed to wean," in reference to a patient's inability to tolerate a decrease in

mechanical ventilation, or "he's certainly not doing any better," to describe a patient's condition. It is crucial to remember that the preschooler understands concretely and literally.

Preschoolers require the close and consistent presence of their parents when ill. Because they have learned to extend trust to other adults, providing consistent caregivers is especially advantageous for this age group, particularly when parents must leave. Transitional or security objects are valuable to ease distress when separation from parents occurs. Parental participation in caretaking is comforting for these young children. Parents can also assist their preschooler to maintain contact with siblings and peers through audiotape or videotape recordings. Even the sickest child can benefit from the comforting voices or images of family members and friends.

Because of the tremendous cognitive development that occurs during the preschool years, children of this age group who are successfully gaining initiative feel extremely powerful. These feelings are instrumental in the preschooler's ability to maintain self-control despite serious illness and hospitalization in an unfamiliar and threatening environment. Loss of self-control may result when preschoolers' omnipotent feelings are confronted by fears of the unknown and enforced dependency. Physical restriction and altered routines continue to contribute to distress for preschoolers in the PICU.

Dependency on routines diminishes across the preschool years, but bedtime remains a vulnerable time. All preschoolers relate their sense of time to routine daily activities and may feel disruption of their sense of time and need routine and ritual more when ill. Regression also increases dependence on rituals. Fears are vague and generalized and may be exaggerated by the thought processes characteristic of the age group (magical thinking, animism, etc.).

Preschoolers require explanation of the equipment around them and of all procedures just before they are done. Information about what they are experiencing and who the people are around them orients them to reality and helps to avoid or correct fantasy and misperception. Preschoolers who are well enough to interact verbally are encouraged to ask questions. They can be questioned to elicit fears or misconceptions about illness and its treatment. Restraint during procedures may be minimized if the preschooler is adequately prepared. Preschoolers can cooperate if they are calm, have had adequate explanation, and are permitted to participate.

Restraint may be perceived as punishment. Both limited mobility and restraint in the critical care environment result in altered sensory stimulation. The impact of physical restriction and restraint may not be significant if only briefly necessary. Longer periods of immobilization may result in quiet, passive submission or active protest and aggressive behavior. Enforced dependency also often results in extremes of behavior if illness and critical care are lengthy. Preschoolers may become overly dependent as a consequence of regression or may actively protest and aggressively act out their frustration with lost independence. Limiting physical restriction and restraint, while maintaining a safe environment, encourages cooperation and self-control. When restraint is necessary, its need is simply stated and the child reassured that immobilization is not a punishment. Child participation in self-care or hygiene and participation in treatments encourages maintenance of self-control and mastery of the environment while it limits dependency. With the exception of the most seriously ill children, all children most likely can participate in some aspect of their care.

THE SCHOOL-AGE CHILD

Developmental Characteristics of School-Age Children

Although physical growth and neuromuscular development are fairly slow and steady during the school years, cognitive and social skills explode (Table 2-6). The school-age period is a time of mastering an ever-expanding world as the foundation for adult roles is established. Cognitive development is characterized by dramatic shifts. The young school-age child uses intuitive thought based on immediate, unanalyzed relationships between particular elements of the environment and the child. Reasoning is not logical. Thought processes become concrete at 7 or 8 years of age, and by the end of the school-age years, cognitive operations have moved toward formal operations.

Concrete operations strongly influence knowledge acquisition. School-age children work hard to discover how the world around them functions. Conservation of matter, weight, and volume are achieved. The various parts of a whole can be considered while the concept of the whole is maintained. Classification, seriation, and numerical concepts are mastered. Concrete and personal observation are the foundation for learning. Abstract or hypothetical thinking is not yet possible.

Concrete operations also profoundly influence emotional and social development as children's experiences broaden and their intellectual capacity increases. During this stage, children emerge from their egocentric view of the world and realize that their way of thinking is not the only way. They can mentally retrace the steps they took to reach a conclusion and realize that there may be more than one way of reaching the same end point. They also recognize the role of chance in the occurrence of events as egocentricity diminishes. They are no longer the cause of every action and reaction around them. Cooperation with others in a group effort leads to an appreciation of the democratic principles of mutual consent and consensus, as well as respect for others and for self. Rules are more flexible; reasoning and discussion can lead to their being reconsidered and reworked.

The major challenge of Erikson's fourth stage of development is the establishment of a sense of industry—a sense of being useful and able to make and do things well. The negative counterpart of this stage is a sense of inadequacy or inferiority, rather than competence, which may develop if children view their physical and intellectual skills as deficient. School-age children learn to recognize

their limitations and accept them, as they also recognize and capitalize on their abilities to develop a sense of competence and self-esteem.

The peer group, especially same-sex peers, increases in importance across the school-age years. Interest in the opposite sex begins at the end of the school-age period, but a best friend is more important at this stage. Clubs, teams, camp, and group projects are enjoyed. Team loyalty is intense at the end of the school years. The competent and industrious school-age child becomes productive within a social group of peers in preparation for being a productive member of society as an adult. Cooperation and collaboration based on mutual respect are evidenced in the pride school-age children feel for each other's accomplishments, as well as those of the group. Group activities teach children that individual strengths and weaknesses are balanced in a group.

The absolute rules that guide action for the preschooler become tempered by the realization that the same act can be viewed differently by different individuals. Intentions prompting an act are taken into consideration. Through cooperative and competitive interaction with peers, school-age children develop rules by consensus and mutual consent. Rules are no longer unbendable but can be changed in a democratic process or by extenuating circumstances. Moral judgment becomes increasingly independent of adults as peer groups grow in solidarity. Morality is based on cooperation, developed in discussion with peers.

Increasing independence from adults peaks at age 11 or 12, with the child wanting unreasonable independence and demanding privacy. Relationships with parents and family are ambivalent; children are often self-conscious about their parents. Unruliness, sloppiness, and secretive behavior may impede reasonable increases in the independence permitted children in the transitional period that concludes the school-age years.

Impact of Hospitalization

School-age children are better equipped, from a developmental perspective, to cope with hospitalization. Short-term hospital admissions are associated with less distress for children older than 5 years of age. Although intellectually more mature and capable of sophisticated language and communication, school-age children focus on reality and are unlikely to have had specific experiences that will mitigate all the stress of hospitalization. Their abilities to solve problems and learn are likely to be thwarted when they are seriously ill. Illness restricts opportunities for individual achievement, as well as group accomplishments.

School-age children have low rates of mortality and serious morbidity when compared with other age groups. Chronic illness, which may be a factor in a school-age child's admission to the PICU, places concomitant demands on the child and family and may influence the coping responses of both when critical care is necessitated.

Generally, for school-age children, the unfamiliar PICU environment is less intimidating than it is for those who are younger. During the school years, unreasonable fears and

TABLE 2-6   School-Age Development

Developmental Characteristic	Attributes
Cognitive	
• Piaget's stage[5]	Concrete operations (7-11 years)
	Reasons with inductive logic; comprehends conservation and reversibility
	Able to classify and order; comprehends multiple aspects of object, event, or situation
	Problem-solving requires that the problem involve identifiable (concrete) objects
	The future and the abstract are still beyond comprehension
	• Can consider various parts of the whole, while retaining the concept of the whole
	• Achieves understanding of conservation of matter, weight, and volume
	• Defines common objects in terms of their use (6 years)
	• Tells time (7 years)
	• School performance great indicator of development (9-10 years)
	• May view illness as a form of punishment
	• Vocabulary of 2500 words, learns to read, learns correct grammar, and uses language as a tool in riddles, jokes, chants, and word games
	• Steady increase in vocabulary, with words used in complex sentences
Social/Emotional	
• Erikson[22]	Industry vs. inferiority
	A sense of industry is gained given opportunities to achieve success and recognition, which fosters self-esteem
	Competence, responsibility, social and work skills, cooperation, and fair play is learned
	Relates closely with same-sex peers
	Can share and cooperate (6 years)
	6-7 years: egocentric thinking, nervous mannerisms, restless activity
	8-10 years: takes on idols and heroes; friends serve as allies against adults
	10-12 years: increased self awareness and self-consciousness, body image concerns, mood swings, need for independence
	Lying and cheating common
• Fears/death	Fears: bodily injury, loss of control, failure to attain expectations, and death
	May have specific fears related to unfamiliar aspects of hospitalization
	Death (7-11 years)
	Aware that death is irreversible, permanent, and universal; able to state examples of causes of death, express logical thoughts about death
	Linked to external forces (e.g., illness, violence, and old age)
	Recognized as a source of sadness; characterized as dangerous, scary, and mean
Growth	
	Gain approximately 1.4-2.2 kg (3-5 pounds)/year; at 10 years, may gain 10 pounds/year
	Grow approximately 4-6 cm (1½-2½ inches)/year
	Deciduous teeth are lost, and most permanent teeth erupt during these years
Diet	
Requirements are 80 cal/kg/day	Teach how to choose healthy foods, including fruits and vegetables
	Eat some meals as a family
Motor	Refinement of dexterity (6 years)
	Good eye-hand coordination (9 years)
Health Maintenance Anticipatory Guidance	Growth rate has slowed, and sleep needs decrease to 8-11 hours
	Reinforce seat belt use
	Encourage discussions about drugs, smoking, and alcohol
	Sex education: anatomy and physiology, sexual activity, contraception, prevention of sexually transmitted diseases and acquired immunodeficiency syndrome
	Annual dental appointment
	Brush teeth after every meal and before bedtime
Approach to Physical Examination and Interventions	Likes to help and have choices
	Respects the need for privacy
	Provides clear and factual information
	Provides positive feedback as builds evolving self-esteem and encourages self-esteem
	About one half of school-age children have a special attachment object
	During recovery, play therapy may be therapeutic

Data from the American Academy of Pediatrics. In Shelov SP, Hannemann RE, eds: *Caring for your baby and young child: birth to age 5,* New York, 1998, Bantam Books; Green M, ed: *Bright futures: guidelines for health supervision of infants, children, and adolescents pocket guide,* rev ed, Arlington, Va, 1998, National Center for Education in Maternal and Child Health; Millong VL, Baroni MA, eds: *Pediatric nurse practitioner certification review guide,* ed 3, Potomac, Md, 1999, Health Leadership Associates.

fantasies lessen, and these children actively master that which is unknown or unfamiliar through concrete cognition. However, school-age children do fear bodily injury, loss of self-control, and death, and they may be intimidated by the critical care environment. In addition, school-age children in the PICU have demonstrated worry for other patients. Anxiety, depression, agitation, and withdrawal have been reported among school-age children requiring intensive care. These occur with greater frequency in the PICU environment than in other hospital settings.[14]

Little overt fearfulness is demonstrated by children past the earliest school-age years (6 or 7 years of age). Maintenance of self-control is of vital importance, but anxiety may lead to nail biting or hair twirling in children who are well enough. Behavioral expression of anxiety may be exhibited in apprehension with routine nonpainful procedures, worried detachment with staff, sadness, and weeping. Some patients demonstrate tremulousness, shakiness, and motor agitation. The length of hospital stay correlates positively with these findings. Increasing severity of illness is positively correlated with the presence of confusion and disorientation and apprehension or fearfulness about staff and routine procedures.[14] Serious illness may necessitate regression, with behaviors and fears similar to those of preschoolers. Crying, excessive fearfulness, or difficulty separating are examples of regressive behaviors.

A concrete concept of time develops across the school years, permitting more accurate appraisal of time spent alone. Despite this developmental progress toward independence, school-age children continue to need close, reliable contact with parents. Familiar articles from home remain important, particularly during the early school years. About one half of school-age children continue to have a special object to which an attachment was formed during early childhood.

Young school-age children may have lingering fears of being left alone and demonstrate fearfulness when their parents leave them, clinging to a transitional object, if available, or crying. By the middle school years, such fearfulness is less common, but when alone, older school-age children may feel threatened, rejected, isolated, depressed, lonely, and bored. Their tolerance of the PICU environment and necessary procedures diminishes without the supportive presence of their parents. Anxiety or hostility may be evidenced in irritability or verbal aggression. Some children withdraw from contact with others, longing to ask their parents to stay but afraid of appearing to be "a baby."

Separation from siblings, friends, and schoolmates, which includes the concomitant loss of their productive roles in the family, neighborhood, and classroom, affects hospitalized school-age children. These children value the roles they play within their families, peer groups, and schools. Actual or perceived changes in the roles they play threaten self-esteem and self-control. Fear of being displaced from their usual position within their families and among friends provokes stress and anxiety. Fear of falling behind at school is the consequence of the student role being disrupted during hospitalization. Being displaced from productive roles at home and school results in feelings of

sadness and fearfulness about school failure. Withdrawal and depression are common responses.

School-age children are actively engaged in their world. Self-control is normal for them. New experiences carry a high sense of adventure for school-age children when they are well. Industrious school-age children thrive on their steadily increasing ability to be independent. However, independence is limited by hospitalization. Feelings of loss are experienced when they are placed in the dependent role of a hospitalized patient for a period beyond a day or two. Self-control is diminished by limited opportunities for independence in self-care and the pursuit of industry and its associated feelings of worthiness and importance.

Immobility or physical restraint limits the discharge of energy and anxiety in physical activity. The sensory burden of the PICU may be overwhelming to immobilized children who are unable to turn away from it. Immobilization or physical restraint may result in depression, frustration, or hostility among school-age children. If physical restraint is viewed as a significant threat, anger, hostility, and aggression are common responses. Regression is likely if physical restriction is prolonged or permanent. When dependency is prolonged, regression and overdependency are common responses. Serious illness may limit displays of hostility and aggression but not the angry, hostile feelings. Their release in agitated behavior or their sublimation in regressed behavior may be detected.

School-age children usually have very specific fears related to the unfamiliar aspects of hospitalization and are anxious about matters that they do not know or understand. Enhancing their sense of personal control through cognitive mastery of the unknown is an essential component of caring for them.

Developmental Care

The nursing history provides data regarding routines to which a school-age child is accustomed. Their incorporation into the hospital routine, whenever possible, assists the youngest school-age children in maintaining self-control and normalizes the PICU environment to an extent. Bedtime routines are often most important for young school-age children and warrant special effort. Recuperation provides increased opportunity to incorporate the child in developing comfortable daily patterns like those followed at home. The provision of consistent caregivers helps school-age children to maintain self-control. Support of their close bonds to parents is key to managing distress during hospitalization. The family also serves as a conduit for information about friends and classmates, easing school-age children's sense of absence from important social groups. Letters and cards from classmates or videotapes of family and school activities assure school-age children that they have not been forgotten if hospitalization is lengthy.

School-age children are information seekers. The ability of children to understand their illness, treatment, and procedures increases steadily across the school years. The youngest children may still relate illness to bad behavior, a misunderstanding that requires correction. The information that school-age children have received in preparation for hospitalization is assessed to develop an effective teaching plan. The child's perception of events to come is elicited, if possible, and verbalization of fears and questions is encouraged. Fears of unknown aspects of illness and critical care are addressed by providing accurate, concrete, and scientific descriptions of the illness and its treatment. Because school-age children may be disturbed by unfamiliar body responses, these too are explained in scientific terms. An explanation and a rationale for procedures assist school-age children to maintain self-control and are important even when verbal or physical interaction is prevented by illness or its treatment. School-age patients in the PICU are likely to hear and appreciate explanation of what they are experiencing, even if unable to participate in discussion. As recovery occurs, children are encouraged to verbalize concerns and ask questions. Misinformation or misunderstanding is corrected with complete, truthful information provided in a caring and supportive manner.

School-age children are accustomed to external appraisal of their accomplishments and are supported in coping with the PICU environment when they receive praise. Positive feedback is a primary intervention with school-age children in the PICU; it builds self-esteem and encourages self-control. Praise is offered for efforts at cooperation, self-care, and participation in procedures or treatments. Providing opportunities for success several times daily gives the child a sense of accomplishment. Regression is tolerated without negative comment or criticism, and the child is reassured that crying or fearfulness is not unusual when someone is very ill.

Physical restrictions are limited to those imposed by illness, as well as those necessary for safety, because school-age children usually cooperate. Thorough preparation for procedures and treatments may limit the amount of restraint necessary. When actively held down for a procedure, the school-age child may abandon all attempts at self-control and cooperation. During recovery, quiet activities are enjoyed, but creative outlets for frustration normally discharged in physical activity are also needed.

School-aged children can direct procedures, participate in self-care, and make decisions regarding their care to mitigate the negative aspects of enforced dependence as soon as they are physically able. Children age 7 years or older, in the stage of concrete operations, are able to assent (agree or concur with a decision made by others). Maturation through the school years increases knowledge, understanding, and competence, preparing children by about age 10 to dissent (disagree and withhold assent). Dissent should be taken seriously when the child displays sufficient knowledge and understanding of the illness and its treatment. Additional discussion, at a minimum, is necessary when school-age children indicate disagreement with their treatment plan. Involving children in healthcare decisions is not without practical problems, including determining competence and cognitive development, legal ramifications, and potential conflict with parental rights.[33,34]

If hospitalization is lengthy, peer relationships within the hospital setting are fostered. Provision for continuing schoolwork is also important during lengthy hospitalization.

THE ADOLESCENT (12 TO 21 YEARS)

Developmental Characteristics of Adolescents

Adolescence begins at approximately 12 years of age and ends when the child is independent of the family. Physical growth, which once marked the end of adolescence, is complete at about 18 years of age. Cognitive, emotional, and social development are considered to extend the period of adolescent life until the emancipation of an independent young adult. Table 2-7 provides a summary of adolescent development.

Physical growth increases significantly during adolescence. Around puberty, both boys and girls attain the final 20% of their mature height. At 18 years, nearly all growth is complete. Growth is typically uneven, with the legs lengthening first, followed by broadening of the thighs and then the shoulders, and trunk growth occurring last. Lack of coordination is often evident, resulting from uneven growth. Sexual maturation is generally not completed until 20 or 21 years of age. The hormones produced by the ovary and testes are the consequence of hypothalamic and pituitary secretion and are responsible for the development of the secondary sexual characteristics. Tanner[36] described and labeled these stages as guidelines to the progression of normal development.

Piaget[5] describes the cognitive development of the adolescent years as a progression and reconstruction of concrete operations to a new level called formal operations. With formal operations, adolescents can imagine possibilities, form and test a hypothesis, and interpret the results. Unexpected results are not as confusing as they are to school-age children because the adolescent has considered several possibilities. Adolescents are able to mentally reverse a sequence of events to understand why something has happened. Piaget[37] notes that in addition to the ability to form hypotheses and the capacity for deductive reasoning, adolescents' thought processes become more flexible, and new problems stimulate the use of previous learning.

As adolescents contemplate the future, they construct ideals, sometimes leading to a critical view of the adults around them. Their ability to think about thinking leads to introspection, accompanied by a resurgence of egocentricity and preoccupation with self. Adolescents believe that everyone is observing their appearance and behavior, noting their flaws, and taking measure of their assets. Teenage egocentricity also leads adolescents to consider their experience as unique. They accuse adults of lack of understanding, believing that no one has ever been through what they are experiencing. Egocentricity diminishes by late adolescence as young adults discover that although they are individuals, their experiences and emotions are not unique. The audience teens once believed was watching fades, enabling them to act and react genuinely.

Erikson[22] described the central task of adolescence as the development of identity, with role confusion the possible negative outcome of unsuccessful teen social and emotional development. Formal operations permit the internalization

◆ TABLE 2-7 Adolescent Development			
Developmental Characteristic	**Early Adolescence (11-14 Years)**	**Middle Adolescence (15-17 Years)**	**Late Adolescence (18-21 Years)**
Cognitive • Piaget's stage[5]	Early adolescence: a period of transition from concrete to formal operations	• Formal operations (11 years on) • Logical reasoning based on deductive logic • Able to consider the hypothetical and abstract; understand symbolism • Problem analysis is systematic • Can think about past, present, and future • Pure thought independent of action • Develops strong idealism	• Consolidation of formal operations, which allow planning for the future
Social/Emotional • Erikson[22]	Identity vs. role diffusion Sense of identity is established through experiences that build self-esteem and foster independence Fidelity is realized Moves toward heterosexuality, selects vocation, begins separation from family Emergence of independence from family; peer group provides important social support Interest in sexuality	• Major task is achievement of sexual identity Preoccupation with self Increased interest in member of the opposite sex Engages in some sort of sexual experimentation	• Intimacy vs. isolation Intimacy and solidarity are established in close, shared relationships Love is realized with individuals of the same and the opposite sex Creativity and productivity are achieved Major task is identification of an occupational identity
• Fears/death	Fears: Adopt an "it can't happen to me" attitude Death[23]: Differences between the adolescent and adult reaction to death Death viewed only as a remote possibility	• Fears/death: potential for loss of control is predominant Fears death	• Fears/death: understands death as a final and universal experience that is intensely personal Capacity to think about the future allows consideration of impending death
Growth	Period of rapid change; varies regarding timing and between sexes Girls gain 7-25 kg (15-55 pounds) Girls grow 5-20 cm (2-8 inches) Boys gain 7-30 kg (15-65 pounds) Boys grow 10-30 cm (4-12 inches) Puberty onset for girls between 8-10 years and for boys usually 10-12 years Menarche at 10.5-15 years, with ovulation occurring 6-12 months later		

Anticipatory Guidance		
Health Maintenance	Immunizations: dT booster (12-14 years, at least 5 years after last DTaP); dT booster recommended every 10 years Review immunization status: hepatitis B required after 1992; many adolescents are not immunized Adolescents are the highest-risk group for nearly all sexually transmitted diseases (STDs)[35] Sex education: anatomy and physiology, sexual activity, contraception, prevention of STDs and acquired immunodeficiency syndrome Encourage discussions about drugs, smoking, and alcohol	Sex education should include discussion about sexual intercourse and contraception Discuss substance abuse because often increased exposure with dating Discuss use of seat belt because many are driving
Approach to Physical Examination and Interventions	Provide feedback and reassurance about assessment findings; emphasize normalcy Ensure privacy during examinations and procedures	Provide specific, detailed, accurate, and scientific information about events and procedures

Data from the American Academy of Pediatrics. In Shelov SP, Hannemann RE, eds: *Caring for your baby and young child: birth to age 5*, New York, 1998, Bantam Books; Green M, ed: *Bright futures: guidelines for health supervision of infants, children, and adolescents pocket guide*, rev ed, Arlington, Va, 1998, National Center for Education in Maternal and Child Health; Millonig VL, Baroni MA, eds: *Pediatric nurse practitioner certification review guide*, ed 3, Potomac, Md, 1999, Health Leadership Associates; Felice ME: Eleven to thirteen years: early adolescence—the age of rapid changes. In Dixon SD, Stein MT, eds: *Encounters with children: pediatric behavior and development*, St. Louis, 1992, Mosby, pp 347-357; Rice LI, Felice ME: Fourteen to sixteen years: mid-adolescence—the dating game. In Dixon SD, Stein MT, eds: *Encounters with children: pediatric behavior and development*, St. Louis, 1992, Mosby, pp 359-369; Rice LI, Felice ME: Seventeen to twenty-one years: late adolescence. In Dixon SD, Stein MT, eds: *Encounters with children: pediatric behavior and development*, St. Louis, 1992, Mosby, pp 371-382.
dT, Diphtheria, tetanus; *DTaP*, diphtheria, tetanus, pertussis.

of self-image, self-concept, or identity. Potential sources of confusion are the rapid body changes that the adolescent undergoes and the reality of the future and adulthood, with the accompanying loss of the comfortable familiarity of childhood.

Peer alliances formed in early adolescence ease the way toward comfort with their own bodies for young teens. Joking and teasing about voice changes or discussing menstrual cramps assure most adolescents that their experiences are normal. However, the invariable comparisons with those around them may produce anxiety in those who develop slightly earlier or later than the majority of the peer group.

Peer relationships help the adolescent avoid role confusion. Peer alliances are firmly established in middle adolescence, but early in the adolescent years, changes in groups of friends, as well as the accepted style of dress and manner of speech, are common. Once established, the peer group provides a sort of safety net for teens trying out social roles and behaviors. In fact, isolated or disconnected teens may appear self-reliant but are likely feeling that they have no one to depend on or trust and must insulate themselves because their emotional pain is too much to bear.[38] The sometimes violent and traumatic world may be a personal reality for some teens, whereas it is an existential truth for others. Strategies to deal with its reality in either circumstance are a necessity for effective intervention with adolescents. By late adolescence, the peer group naturally diminishes in importance, and roles and behavior are individually determined.

Independence from parents and family assists adolescents to develop their individuality and identity. Early adolescents have incorporated the values and standards of their parents, usually viewing them as role models and accepting their authority. However, adolescence is a progressive test of parental limit setting as more and more independence is demanded. Some adolescents engage in rebellious behavior. Middle adolescents also often confide in an adult other than one of their parents, limiting the influence parents exert as their adolescent progresses. Consistent and trustworthy adults who value adolescents and what they have to say may help them to establish connections and trust.[38] Older adolescents may return to parents for consultation, once they are secure outside the home when parents are no longer seen as a threat to independence or autonomy. Parents and their children ideally develop an adult relationship across the years of adolescence.

Impact of Hospitalization

Critical illness during adolescence is a potentially serious threat to the successful transition from childhood to adulthood. Young adolescents are less troubled by enforced dependency and better able to permit their parents and others to care for them. Middle adolescents (15 to 17 years of age) tolerate illness the least well because their drive for independence is at its peak. Young and middle adolescents experience anxiety related to physical appearance, function, and mobility when ill. Older adolescents have often achieved sufficient maturity to tolerate some temporary dependence and are individually secure enough to use their families for support. Older adolescents fear that illness will disrupt their career and other future goals. All are distressed by disruption of their usual lifestyle. Fear of death is pervasive across the adolescent years.

Like adult patients, an adolescent ill enough to require admission to a PICU will manifest an emotional response. Anxiety and fear are usual emotional responses to critical illness and intensive care. Adolescents realize there is a danger of death. Anxiety may be evidenced by agitation, excessive verbosity, or complete withdrawal. High anxiety is not tolerable, usually resulting in some degree of denial, which is indicated by withdrawal or regression. When illness and intensive care are prolonged, anxiety is often followed by despondency and depression. Some adolescent patients deal with stress and depression by constant talk, whereas others withdraw. Serious illness requiring lengthy critical care is also associated with disorientation.

Withdrawing from contact with others may also indicate feelings of depersonalization. Adolescents in the PICU are isolated from their important peer associations and activities and are at high risk for such feelings. Staff communication about personal topics within earshot of the adolescent is particularly distressing because it also depersonalizes the individual. Individual identity is threatened, particularly if the adolescent needs to communicate with staff. Adolescents may be embarrassed by overhearing details of the personal lives of staff who are caring for them.

Separation from home and family is usually tolerated without distress by adolescents who require hospitalization. Separation from the peer group, however, causes significant anxiety. Illness and hospitalization are clear deviations from the accepted group norm. Adolescents feel deprived when separated from their peers and are threatened by potential loss of status within their social groups, particularly if they have achieved leadership status and must relinquish that position. The absence of peer acceptance and approval may threaten emerging individual identity. Separation anxiety may be evidenced by withdrawal, uncooperativeness, and ambivalence about visitors, especially family members. Defense mechanisms may mask the verbal acknowledgment of the importance of peers or family because the adolescent is adept at intellectualization and rationalization.

Chronic illness ties adolescents to their families—physically, emotionally, and financially. Some respond with active rebellion, whereas others are passive and overdependent. The chronically ill adolescent in the PICU may react to separation from the family more intensely than others. The stress of critical illness may delay progress at learning to manage a chronic illness independently, a vital transition for the chronically ill teenager. Regressed behavior is not uncommon among chronically ill adolescents who may, for example, want their parents to stay with them until they fall asleep. Critical illness may exacerbate overdependency, but when survival itself is questioned, independence is a lower priority.

Adolescents generally adapt to brief interruption of their typical routines without difficulty but are threatened by the possibility that their lifestyle may be permanently altered. Anxiety results from the fact that seriously ill adolescents can do little to exert control over the events happening around and to them. Routines for every aspect of life are altered and controlled. Loss of control of daily routines forces dependency on an age group struggling for independence. Fear of unknown events and procedures in the critical care environment is stressful. For some, the uncertainty of treatment efficacy and eventual recovery is even more significant, heightening anxiety. Serious illness forces adolescents to reexamine their present and future lifestyle, as well as their potential for adult fulfillment.

Adolescents are unlikely to be unduly anxious about brief periods of immobility or limited physical restrictions. Most procedures do not require restraint if the adolescent is aware of events that will occur and is sufficiently cognizant to cooperate. Immobility that persists beyond a brief period or repetitive procedures may cause distress for even the most resilient adolescent. Adolescents facing lengthy immobilization often are angry and aggressive during the early stages of dealing with their illness or injury. Withdrawal and depression often follow, particularly when dependence on others is necessary. Enforced dependence, and the concomitant depersonalization experienced by adolescents, may result in episodes of resentment, anger, and acting out from an otherwise withdrawn teenager. Loss of productive roles contributes to feelings of depersonalization and may exacerbate depression or anxiety.

Critical illness or injury permits adolescents to temporarily release self-control to others. However, if recovery does not provide opportunity for reexerting control, most adolescents demonstrate distress. For example, overly rigid hospital routines or regulations are likely to result in resentment, anger, and hostility as adolescent patients protest the alterations in their usual lifestyle.

Developmental Care

Like adult patients, adolescents require orientation to their environment, as well as to date and time. Some relief of anxiety and distress is provided by verbal explanation of what is happening, how it is anticipated to feel, what it will accomplish, and how long it will last. Even when patients cannot communicate, explanation is reliably provided. When adolescent patients are able to communicate, they are encouraged to verbalize questions and concerns. Some may need their caregivers to broach the topics of anxiety, fear, or feelings of sadness to begin to express their own concerns. Positive reassurance can be therapeutic. Pharmacologic management of anxiety and psychiatric consultation may be indicated for adolescents who have marked emotional reactions in the PICU.

Assignment of consistent caregivers for adolescent patients in the PICU can mitigate some of the depersonalization and dependence experienced by teenage patients. Trust is established, and a personal, but respectful, relationship develops, providing an atmosphere for optimal recognition of individual identity. Most adolescents strive to regain self-control and independence after serious illness.

Mitigating the stress associated with separation from peers and family members is accomplished by ensuring contact with parents and liberal visits from siblings and friends, particularly if an adolescent has a prolonged PICU stay. Peer visitation is a significant event for these patients.

As progress occurs throughout adolescence, teenagers develop the cognitive skills necessary for informed consent for treatment and procedures. The stage of formal operations encourages a sense of internal control and recognition that decision-making authority about events in an individual's life should lie with the individual. Informed consent requires that adolescents receive sufficient information, comprehend it, and voluntarily consent. Adolescents are assured opportunities to exert control over decisions regarding their treatment regimen.

Adolescents need to express frustration via physical activity. Innovation is necessary to develop ways for adolescents to move out of bed and around the unit as they recover from serious illness. Physical and occupational therapy are encouraged to build independence, strength, and mobility during recuperation. When serious or chronic illness prolongs limited mobility and dependency, some adolescents regress because the need to be cared for outweighs the need to be independent. When immobilization is the permanent consequence of illness or injury, significant adaptation is required. Long-term rehabilitation deals with the emotional aspects of this life change, as well as its physical consequences.

Setting flexible limits and encouraging participation in self-care as adolescents recover restore a measure of control over daily routines. Adolescents are also provided opportunities to participate in setting goals, planning their care, and choosing options to promote self-control and independence. Feelings of depersonalization are avoided when the staff attends to the emotional needs of patients with the same energy and commitment demonstrated in the intense care of physical needs. Willingness to talk and listen to patients and know them as individuals is essential.

THE CHRONICALLY CRITICALLY ILL CHILD

Advances in pediatric critical care continue to result in decreased mortality and increased survival of infants and children who require repeated, sometimes prolonged, PICU admission and depend on technology for survival. Children who are ventilator dependent, have significant neurologic impairment or neuromuscular disease with respiratory complications, and are seriously, but chronically, ill are often transitioned from hospital to home or long-term care setting after a prolonged PICU hospitalization. Improved management of resuscitation, acute injury, and rehabilitation technology and the development of improved technologies have resulted in a rise in the number of chronically ill children at home and in school requiring technology. The Presidential Task Force on Technology Dependent Children[39] reported in 1988 that some 2300 to 17,000 children in the United States were dependent on ventilators, parenteral nutrition, intravenous medications, or other respiratory or nutritional support.

Children who require lengthy PICU admission are often the sickest and youngest patients. Feldman and co-workers[40] examined the incidence and cause of hospital stays longer than 30 days among children less than 3 years of age. They reported that although only 2% of the inpatient population required such lengthy hospitalization, their hospital stays represented 23% of the patient days for children from newborn to 3 years and 11% of the total patient days for children of all ages. Chronically ill children and their families present special issues for the PICU care team. The social and emotional needs of these children and their families are complex, as their life experiences are distorted by prolonged hospitalizations.

Impact of Chronic Illness on the Child

Chronic illness influences the cognitive, social, emotional, and physical development of children. The diagnosis, symptoms, treatment, and prognosis are factors influencing the impact of a specific illness on an individual child. All face separation from their families, home, school, and other familiar environments when hospitalized. The critical care experience is unlikely to provide a developmentally nurturing environment. Although all critically ill children adopt the "sick role" and display illness behaviors; children with chronic illness are unable to fully recover and discard the sick role.

Chronic illness shapes a child's foundation and limits developmental opportunities at every age. During infancy, repeated hospitalizations may interfere with the parent-infant attachment and acquisition of trust. For chronically ill toddlers and preschoolers, acquiring autonomy and initiative is difficult as illness erects barriers to independence. Preschoolers who are chronically ill are aware that they are different from their peers. By school age, parents describe chronically ill children as lacking skills for social interaction, self-care, and compliance, often exhibiting aggressive and self-destructive behaviors.[41] School is often a source of stress for these children rather than an environment in which they thrive because academic and social progress is interrupted by their illness. Peers are often unsupportive, if not unkind. Chronically ill adolescents may react to separation from the family more intensely and experience an increased dependency on their families as their peers are achieving independence. The stress of critical illness may delay progress at learning to manage their illness, which is a vital transition for the chronically ill teenager. Adolescents may be blocked from establishing independence and forced to consider limitations on social, educational, and vocational plans.

Impact of Chronic Illness on the Family

Chronic illness affects many aspects of family life: cognitive, social, emotional, behavioral, and financial. Chronic illness increases obligations, tasks, commitments, and expenses for the family. Chronically ill children may cause anxiety and confusion in social situations when others are uncertain how to interact with the child or family. Families with a chronically ill child strive to lead a "normal" family life. They must actively reconstruct family life following the diagnosis of a child's chronic illness, engage in parenting activities and family routines, and interact with others from a perspective that permits normalization.[42] Normalization is complex as it changes and evolves with family situations, processes, and developmental transitions. Parents may have feelings of guilt, blame, and personal grief because of their child's illness. The grieving process may be exacerbated or reactivated by new medical issues or developmental transitions, such as starting school. Hospitalization often brings renewed or additional sadness. Mastering guilt and grief is necessary for each parent's emotional well-being, influences the self-esteem and emotional development of the chronically ill child and siblings, and affects the normalization of the family.

Impact of Critical Care

The potential for distress is high when an acute illness necessitates intensive care for the chronically ill child. Critical illness may negate family efforts at normalization. Managing uncertainty and stress is the new priority. Chronically ill children in the PICU require a supportive environment that will protect the family and child's growth and development. For the technologically dependent child, prolonged hospitalization requires multidisciplinary team intervention. An identified primary physician and nurse coordinate the efforts of the multidisciplinary care team and facilitate communication. These individuals are primarily responsible for identifying specific family and patient needs and formulating comprehensive plans to facilitate achieving desired outcomes.

Developmental Care

Environmental factors in the PICU affect care of long-term or chronically ill patients. Ongoing evaluation of the need for critical care for the chronically ill child is crucial because the care of these children should be deescalated as soon as possible. Jansen and associates[43] contend that a change in the philosophy of care for chronically ill patients who are medically stable is necessary to optimize psychosocial and cognitive development of both the patient and the family. Many PICU staffs face caring for alert, active children with normal intelligence in the midst of the hectic critical care setting because the PICU may be the only unit equipped to care for ventilator-dependent children. To minimize the exposure to the harshness of the environment, the child may be located in a corner, by a window, and away from heavily traveled areas. Plugging electrical outlets, removing sharp objects and possible hazardous equipment, and devising play areas in the child's bed space or room provide safety and may enhance cognitive development as these children have greater freedom to interact with their environment.[43]

Regression to an earlier and safer period of development or lack of developmental progress are common responses to the demands of a chronic illness. Critical illness further necessitates some degree of regression, but motivation for developmental progress may be nearly nonexistent for chronically ill children even during recovery. Exclusion from activity, learned inferiority, and nonacceptance take a toll on the emotional well-being of children who are chronically ill.[44] Table 2-8 lists responses commonly identified among chronically ill children and the needs that typically underlie each response. Critical care staffs who consistently meet those needs offer an opportunity for chronically ill children to adapt and progress.

As the number of advanced practice nurses (APNs) practicing in the PICU continues to increase, assignment of chronically ill children to their caseload ensures continuity of care. Developmentally supportive care is enhanced through multidisciplinary involvement coordinated by the APN. Patient care conferences with involved disciplines permit planning a daily schedule and supporting routines. Needed changes in the schedule are accommodated, as occurs in the outpatient or home setting.

Federal law (PL 99-457) and state regulations provide infants and children requiring prolonged hospitalization with eligibility for early intervention programs that may commence during hospitalization and for schooling. Consultation with child life specialists, social workers, and psychologists may lead to services that benefit chronically ill or disabled children and their families as they transition to home and the community.

Family Care

Families are an asset and source of support for chronically ill children in the PICU. However, parents of chronically ill children often experience conflict with staff members during their child's hospitalization. According to Anderson,[45] 70% to 90% of illness episodes in chronically ill children are managed at home, outside the formal healthcare system. Parents are knowledgeable and skilled in providing their child's care, sometimes providing care more often within the scope of professional healthcare practice. Clearly, these parents are capable of assessing and making some management decisions for their children. PICU staff may feel threatened by such parental knowledge and parents' expectations for complete and accurate information about their child. Parents of chronically ill children are often viewed as excessively demanding by the staff in a busy PICU. Their insistence on care performed in a manner they designate may be viewed as inappropriate or even uncooperative. Their emphasis on normal routines for their child may be seen as unrealistic.

Modification of usual PICU routines, such as decreasing the frequency of vital sign measurement and suctioning, can

 TABLE 2-8 Responses to Chronic Illness From Children

Child's Behavior	Child's Needs
Fear	
Frightened of everything	Self-confidence
Exaggerated normal fears	Independence
Few friends	
Gives up easily	
Fantasy	
Creates imaginary world	Reality
Escapes undesired thoughts	Problem-solving skills
Neglects real needs	
Helpless, dependent	
Alone	
Invisibility	
Unobtrusive	Security
Indifferent, passive	Structure
Withdrawn	Encouragement
Humor	
Appears happy	Express anger, sadness
Keeps everyone laughing	Closeness
Insecure, immature	Independence
Fears others do not like him or her	
Keeps a distance from others	
Overinvolvement in Medical Care	
Aloof, rigidly independent	Express anger, depression
Adept at medical jargon	Normal peer relationships
Verbally assertive	
Pleases others	
Friendships with health-care personnel	
Explosive Anger	
Temper tantrums and rages	Understand anger
Clings to others	Reasonable expectations
Blames others; jealous of others	
Believes life is unfair	
Irresponsible	
Giving Up	
Unmotivated, helpless	See personal potential
Ostracized by peers	Realistic goals
Blames others	Gain attention in achievement
Expects to be waited on	
Overdependence	
Extreme awareness of limitations	Encouragement, praise
Afraid to try	Independence
Fear of failing	

Data from Siemon M: Patterns of impairment: cognitive/emotional. In Rose MH, Thomas RB, eds: *Children with chronic conditions: nursing in a family and community context,* Orlando, Fla, 1987, Grune & Stratton; Stevens M: Adolescents' perceptions of stressful events during hospitalization, *J Pediatr Nurs* 1:303-313, 1986.

TABLE 2-9 **Family Power Resources Model**	
Power Resource/Definition	**Interventions**
Positive Self-Concepts Family emphasis on the normality of the sick child	Recognize coping skills Support maintenance of "normalcy"
Physical Strength and Reserve Family physical functioning, strength of the marriage, strength of sibling support, health of the family system	Promote family involvement in child's care Promote parent/child control
Psychologic Stamina Psychologic strength and resiliency of individual family members and the family system	Encourage family sharing of the child's illness Divide and share family tasks
Support Networks Significant others in the community, parent groups, social services	Identify sources of strength Maximize support systems
Energy Capacity to do work	Ensure adequate nutrition, rest, equitable distribution of labor
Knowledge Information; realistic view of the child's situation	Provide detailed, up-to-date information Provide question-and-answer sessions
Motivation Spiritual or philosophical orientation that overcomes inevitable losses, maximizes potential, and develops positive self-esteem	Provide support Recognize achievements Focus on the present Support family decisions

Adapted from Ferraro AR, Longo DC: Nursing care of the family with a chronically ill, hospitalized child: an alternative approach, *Image J Nurs Sch* 17:77-81, 1985.

be negotiated with families and home routines incorporated in the plan of care for chronically ill children. Daily communication with the families by a hospital staff member is essential. Ferraro and Longo[46] described a model of family power that increased coping and adaptation with chronic, disabling illness in a child. Table 2-9 summarizes components of the model and suggests interventions with families while their chronically ill child is hospitalized. Nurses who must balance the demands of physiologically unstable patients and the expectations of parents of chronically ill children may need an opportunity to participate in patient rounds and care conferences to optimize the plan of care for long-term patients.

DEATH IN THE PEDIATRIC INTENSIVE CARE UNIT

The death of a child is not an uncommon experience in pediatric critical care. Knowledge of the experiences of terminally ill children, the responses of parents and siblings to the death of a child, and the process of bereavement guide practices in the PICU.

Development of Concepts About Death

Children learn about death through the course of regular life events. Children younger than 2 years of age have little awareness of death. Between the ages of 3 and 5 years, death is usually thought of as temporary and reversible, like sleep. Although death is seen as departure, those who have died are thought of existing in some other place, most often in heaven, and are attributed with life processes, actions, and thoughts. There is lack of realization of its finality. Often these young children associate death with old age.

School-age children gradually move toward the concept of death as permanent and irreversible when they gain firsthand experience and exposure to death. Death is most often identified with the dead object; the process of dying remains elusive. Death is linked to external forces and violence or associated with illness and old age. Because death is recognized as a source of sadness, it is also considered dangerous, scary, or mean. Near the end of the school years, children who are 10 to 12 years old recognize that death is universal and final and that death happens to all living things. The process of dying is identified and associated with pain and suffering. Death is fearful and brings feelings of sadness and loneliness.

Adolescents develop an understanding of death similar to adults. Death is the final and universal experience of all living things but is also an intensely personal experience. The capacity of adolescents to think about the future allows them to consider impending death, thereby increasing its impact. Periods of rapid physical and emotional change during adolescence are often periods of vulnerability to fears about loss. Adolescents are especially fearful about death.

Talking to Children About Death

Terminally ill children come to know that they are dying, although no one may directly inform them. Often they conceal this information from their families and from healthcare personnel. Because children do not often tell what they know or ask questions about what will happen to them, some adults believe that children do not know that they are gravely ill. If they do, adults believe that children do not want to talk about it or that they are silent because they sense the reluctance of the adults around them to discuss the situation. Children interpret the behavior of others, especially those they trust, in their view of themselves. They are adept at identifying inconsistencies between verbal and nonverbal messages. Tearful, anxious parents and staff members who speak in hushed voices come to have meaning across time and with experiences in healthcare settings.

Evidence that children are knowledgeable about death does not ease the task of talking with them about their own impending death. Few guidelines are available. Children who are dying need to share their knowledge, and they need to have their parents with them. Terminally ill children conceal their knowledge of their prognosis from their parents, leading to the conclusion that their need for parental closeness is greater than their need to talk about dying. However, their preoccupation with death is evidenced in their play and art, in avoidance of conversation about the future and concern that things be done immediately, in anxiety, and in acting out or withdrawing from others to establish emotional distance. Children do share their knowledge if given the opportunity. They talk with those adults who listen to them carefully, taking cues from the child and answering only what is asked on the child's terms. Parents and healthcare professionals are guided by this principle.

Application in the PICU

Some patients in the PICU may be physically and neurologically able to talk with parents and caregivers. Discussion with them is particularly important if, for example, an aggressive treatment plan is considered. However, many children in the critical care unit are too ill to participate in discussion. Death most often occurs only after aggressive, lifesaving interventions have been attempted and ultimately are deemed futile. Death is unavoidable and imminent, expected within moments or days, and aggressive interventions no longer appropriate.

Families and caregivers may not know what to say to these children. They have no way of knowing with certainty whether terminally ill children can hear or understand. Some parents continue to talk with their unconscious children, often acknowledging that the child is dying and that they are saying good-bye. Caregivers can follow the parents' lead in talking with children who are dying in the PICU. Caregivers may also show an example of such behavior to parents who may need unspoken permission to continue to interact with their dying child.

When aggressive intensive care is discontinued, care is directed toward maintaining the child's comfort and dignity. Many tools among the personal and caring resources of professional caregivers can ensure humane care to dying children and to their families. Ensuring cleanliness and comfort, providing privacy, and speaking with the child are only a few examples. Dying children, if they are able, maintain some sense of control by choosing care or therapies that enable them to make each day as comfortable as possible. Pain control is a priority because fear of pain with death is common among children and is a worry for parents of dying children. Parents are logically the individuals who also benefit from participating with or for their child in care that ensures comfort. Parents may perform caregiving tasks if they wish for this sort of physical closeness to their child.

Helping After a Child's Death

Parents may need practical assistance with making funeral arrangements and contacting their extended families. They also face the sizable task of talking with their other children. Siblings are best told about the death as soon as possible in clear and truthful terms. A parent or another trusted adult share information, as well as their feelings of sadness, in a controlled manner. Some parents find books that describe talking to children about death helpful or are assisted by books written for children. Others may find community support groups, such as Compassionate Friends or the Candlelighters, beneficial in the bereavement process. Programs established in the PICU for families who lost a child in death, institutional memorial services, and the like are beneficial for families and caregivers.

REFERENCES

1. Selye H: *Stress without distress,* Philadelphia, 1974, JB Lippincott.
2. Lazarus RS: *Psychological stress and the coping process,* New York, 1966, McGraw-Hill.
3. Skipper JK, Leonard RC: Children, stress and hospitalization, *J Health Soc Behav* 9:275-287, 1968.
4. Youngblut JM, Shang-Yun PS: Characteristics of a child's critical illness and parents' reactions: preliminary report of a pilot study, *Am J Crit Care* 1:80-84, 1993.
5. Piaget J: *The origins of intelligence in children,* New York, 1952, International Universities Press.
6. Cureton-Lane RA, Fontaine DK: Sleep in the pediatric ICU: an empirical investigation, *Am J Crit Care* 6:56-63, 1997.
7. Slota MC: Implications of sleep deprivation in the pediatric critical care unit, *Focus Crit Care* 15:35-43, 1988.

8. Schwab RJ: Disturbances of sleep in the intensive care unit, *Crit Care Clin* 10:681-694, 1994.

9. Richards KC, Bairnsfather L: A description of night sleep patterns in the critical care unit, *Heart Lung* 17:35-42, 1988.

10. Fontaine DK: Measurement of nocturnal sleep patterns in trauma patients, *Heart Lung* 18:402-409, 1989.

11. Barnes C: *School-age children's recall of the intensive care unit: ANA Clinical Sessions,* Norwalk, Conn, 1975, Appleton-Century-Crofts.

12. Carty RM: Observed behaviors of preschoolers to intensive care, *Pediatr Nurs* 6:21-25, 1980.

13. Thompson RH: *Psychological research on pediatric hospitalization and health care.* Springfield, IL, 1985, Charles C Thomas.

14. Jones SM, Fiser DH, Livingston RL: Behavioral changes in pediatric intensive care units, *Am J Dis Child* 146:375-379, 1992.

15. Whitis G: Visiting hospitalized patients, *J Adv Nurs* 24:261-265, 1994.

16. Harlow HF, Zimmerman R: Affectional responses of the infant monkey. In Mussen P, Conger J, Kagan J, eds: *Readings in child development and personality,* New York, 1965, Harper & Row.

17. Spitz RA: Hospitalism: An inquiry into the genesis of psychiatric conditions in early childhood. *Psychoanalytic Study of the Child,* pp. 153-166, 1945.

18. Robertson J: *Young children in hospitals,* London, 1958, Tavistock.

19. Bowlby J: *Maternal care and mental health,* New York, 1966, Schocken Books.

20. Fagin C: Pediatric rooming-in: its meaning for the nurse, *Nurs Clin North Am* 1:83-93, 1966.

21. Vessey JA, Farley JA, Risom LR: Iatrogenic developmental effects of pediatric intensive care, *Pediatr Nurs* 17:229-232, 1991.

22. Erikson EH: *Childhood and society,* New York, 1964, WW Norton.

23. Johnson SE: The development of a child's concept of death. In Johnson SE, ed: *After a child dies: counseling bereaved families,* New York, 1987, Springer.

24. Whitley SL, Cowan M: Developmental intervention in the newborn intensive care unit, *NAACOGS Clin Issu Perinat Womens Health Nurs* 2:23-26, 1991.

25. Yoos L: A developmental approach to physical assessment, *MCN Am J Matern Child Nurs* 6:168-170, 1981.

26. Als H, Lawhon G, Duffy FH et al: Individualized developmental care for the very low birth weight preterm infant: medical and neurobehavioral effects, *JAMA* 272:853-858, 1994.

27. Als H, Lawhon G, Brown E et al: Individualized behavioral and environmental care for the very low birth weight preterm infant at high risk for bronchopulmonary dysplasia:neonatal intensive care and developmental outcome, *Pediatrics* 78:1123-1132, 1986.

28. Gorski PA: Premature infant behavioural and physiological responses to caregiving intervention in the intensive care nursery. In Call JD, Galenson E, Tyson RL, eds: *Frontiers in infant psychiatry,* New York, 1983, Basic Books.

29. Gorski PA: Promoting infant development during neonatal hospitalization: critiquing the state of the science, *Child Health Care* 20:250-257, 1991.

30. Taquino LT, Lockridge T: Caring for critically ill infants: strategies to promote physiological stability and improve developmental outcomes, *Crit Care Nurse* 19:64-79, 1999.

31. Washington GT: Trust: a critical element in critical care nursing, *Focus* 17:418-421, 1990.

32. Ferber R: *Solve your child's sleep problems,* New York, 1985, Simon & Schuster.

33. Erlen JA: The child's choice: an essential component in treatment decisions, *Child Health Care* 15:156-160, 1987.

34. Leiken SL: Minor's assent or dissent to medical treatment, *J Pediatr* 102:169-176, 1983.

35. Biro FM, Rosenthal SL: Adolescents and sexually transmitted diseases: diagnosis, developmental issues, and prevention, *J Pediatr Health Care* 9:256-262, 1995.

36. Tanner JM: *Growth at adolescence,* Oxford, 1962, Blackwell Scientific.

37. Piaget J: *The psychology of intelligence,* Totowa, NJ, 1976, Littlefield, Adams.

38. Hunter AJ, Chandler GE: Adolescent resilience, *Image J Nurs Sch* 31:243-247, 1999.

39. Report of the Task Force on Technology Dependent Children, Washington, DC, 1988, US Government Printing Office, 1988-210-048/80264.

40. Feldman HM, Ploof DL, Hofkosh D et al: Developmental needs of infants and toddlers who require lengthy hospitalization, *Am J Dis Child* 147:211-215, 1993.

41. Beavers J, Hampson RB, Hulgus YF et al: Coping in families with a retarded child, *Fam Process* 25:365-378, 1986.

42. Deatrick JA, Knafl KA, Murphy-Moore C: Clarifying the concept of normalization, *Image J Nurs Sch* 31:209-214, 1999.

43. Jansen MT, DeWitt PK, Meshul RJ et al: Meeting the psychosocial and developmental needs of children during prolonged intensive care hospitalization, *Child Health Care* 18:91-95, 1989.

44. Siemon M: Patterns of impairment: cognitive/emotional. In Rose MH, Thomas RB, eds: *Children with chronic conditions: nursing in a family and community context,* Orlando, Fla, 1987, Grune & Stratton.

45. Anderson JM: The social construction of illness behavior: families with a chronically ill child, *J Adv Nurs* 6:427-434 1981.

46. Ferraro AR, Longo DC: Nursing care of the family with a chronically ill, hospitalized child: an alternative approach, *Image J Nurs Sch* 17:77-81, 1985.

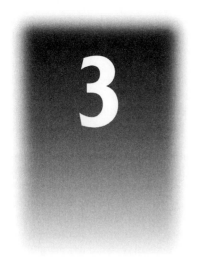

3 Caring Practices: The Impact of the Critical Care Experience on the Family

Martha A.Q. Curley
Elaine C. Meyer

It is a good professional rule to let a mother work at her own level, supporting her in her skills and understanding and bolstering her confidence in herself, quietly supplementing her effort instead of giving detailed directions and cautions which may undermine her confidence.

James Robertson[1]

Inherent in the practice of pediatric critical care nursing is helping families to endure the stressful and unspeakable experience of an infant's or child's critical illness. This humanistic aspect of practice is essential so that families can continue to function in vitally important roles that are ther-apeutic to them and their critically ill children. Factors compromising the care of families include gaps in nurses' knowledge and skill in working with families, unclear lines of responsibility for various aspects of family care, and insufficient support or mentoring for the difficult emotional work inherent in caring for families.[2,3] This chapter reviews the evolution of family interactions in pediatric settings and the rationale for psychosocial intervention in the intensive care setting. We then review the research on pediatric intensive care unit (PICU)–related parental stress, the trajectory of parental stress, and parental needs during the pediatric critical care hospitalization. The unique role of nursing in helping families to cope and alleviate stress is emphasized. The nursing mutual participation model of care is presented, which provides a framework for supportive psychosocial interventions for parents of critically ill children. This is followed by a review of issues of particular concern to nursing staff, including the support of other family members, transition from the PICU, bereavement in the context of the intensive care setting, and referral and collaboration with ancillary psychosocial support personnel.

EVOLUTION OF FAMILY-CENTERED CARE PRACTICES

The parental role in the care of hospitalized infants and children has evolved over time. Not too long ago, parents were neither welcomed nor allowed in pediatric inpatient units primarily because of concerns about infection control. Bowlby's and Robertson's classic work[1,4,5] describing the stages of separation trauma experienced by young children in hospitals—protest, despair, then detachment—supported the hypothesis that parent-child separation is detrimental to the child and to the parent-child relationship. We now acknowledge that parents are crucial to a child's healthy psychosocial and physical well-being and that parental support during a stressful event, such as critical care hospitalization, is essential for the child's continued socio-emotional growth and development.

Family-centered care is currently considered "best practice" in pediatric healthcare settings. The central tenet of family-centered care is that the family is the constant in the child's life and, ultimately, holds the responsibility for ensuring that the child's physical, social, and emotional needs are met.[6] Thus parents are now encouraged to continue parenting during the entire period of their infant or child's hospitalization.

The basic tenets of family-centered care are outlined in Box 3-1. Family-centered care is a philosophy of care that recognizes, respects, and supports the essential role of the family in the lives of children. It is a philosophy that acknowledges and supports diversity among families—diversity that encompasses varied family structures and sociocultural backgrounds; family goals and priorities; strategies and actions; as well as diversity in family support, service, and informational needs.[7] Family-centered care

strives to support families in their natural caregiving roles by building on their unique strengths as individuals and families. It is a philosophy that views parents and professionals as equals in a partnership committed to excellence at all levels of healthcare.[6] Shelton[8] notes that the key to family-centered care is a fundamental commitment to a helping style that truly embodies partnerships. Box 3-2 reviews the values and beliefs identified as critical for developing positive parent-professional partnerships.

Although pediatric nurses have long recognized the fundamental importance of caring for infants and children within a family context, the operationalization or "how to" of family-centered care in the clinical setting is less clear and is often based on intuition and untested assumptions with few empirical guidelines.[9,10] At times, particularly in intensive care settings, parents may be only marginally involved in the decision-making process and care of their children. Parents may be considered as "visitors," thus forcing a temporary or perhaps permanent disruption in the parent-child relationship. Rushton[10] has identified several barriers to family-centered care in pediatric critical care settings, including the highly technologic environment, ethical dilemmas, range in patient population, staff shortages, professional attitudes, the intensive care organizational culture, and economic trends.

Despite the greater expectations that parents participate as partners in their child's care to the extent that they wish, paternalistic attitudes and behaviors can be prevalent within the PICU as a result of underlying assumptions that parents are incapable of complex decision making under the circumstances. There may be the tendency to "protect" parents and to present a "consistent picture," which, although well-intended, limits parents from fully participating as equal-status partners in the decision-making process and care of their child.[9,11] Information that is incomplete, biased, or otherwise not understandable can diminish the parents' status relative to professionals and cripples full participation in healthcare decision making. Bogdan, Brown, and Foster[12] address the complexities of parent-professional communication within the intensive care setting and advise that professionals be "honest but not cruel."

Box 3-1
Key Elements of Family-Centered Care

- Incorporating into policy and practice the recognition that the family is the constant in a child's life, while the service systems and support personnel within those systems fluctuate
- Facilitating family-professional collaboration at all levels of hospital, home, and community care:
  –Care of an individual child
  –Program development, implementation, evaluation, and evolution
  –Policy formation
- Exchanging complete and unbiased information between families and professionals in a supportive manner at all times
- Incorporating into policy and practice the recognition and honoring of cultural diversity, strengths, and individuality within and across all families, including ethnic, racial, spiritual, social, economic, educational, and geographic diversity
- Recognizing and respecting different methods of coping and implementing comprehensive policies and programs that provide developmental, educational, emotional, environmental, and financial supports to meet the diverse needs of families
- Encouraging and facilitating family-to-family support and networking
- Ensuring that hospital, home, and community service and support systems for children needing specialized health and developmental care and their families are flexible, accessible, and comprehensive in responding to diverse family-identified needs
- Appreciating families as families and children as children, recognizing that they possess a wide range of strengths, concerns, emotions, and aspirations beyond their need for specialized health and developmental services and support

From Shelton TL, Stepanek JS: *Family-centered care for children needing specialized health and developmental services,* 1994, Association for the Care of Children's Health, 7910 Woodmont Avenue, Suite 300, Bethesda, MD 20814, 301/654-6549.

Box 3-2
Beliefs and Behaviors Critical for Parent-Professional Partnerships

- A presumption of and respect for the inherent capabilities and strengths of families
- A commitment to and valuing of diversity
- An ability to communicate and share information in ways that are affirming and useful
- An ability to treat others with dignity and respect
- An ability to build on family strengths to enhance feelings of control and independence
- An ability to provide assistance in ways that match family priorities

From Shelton TL: Family-centered care in pediatric practice: when and how? *J Dev Behav Pediatr* 20:117-118, 1999.

Parental needs, parental roles within the PICU, and the establishment of therapeutic nurse-parent relationships are aspects of family-centered care that continue to present challenges to pediatric critical care nurses. Fundamentally, family members are not visitors but part of nursing's sphere of concern—the people nurses take care of. Specifically, pediatric nurses participate in therapeutic relationships with individual patients and their families. The concept of "mutuality" articulates the nurse-parent relationship that embodies the philosophy of family-centered-care.[13]

Mutuality is defined as a synchronous, co-constituting parent-nurse relationship that stimulates the process of personal growth. Two attributes characterize mutuality: (1) a synchronous co-constituted relationship and (2) evolution of both individuals toward personal growth. The synchronous co-constituted relationship speaks to the responsive interdependence, intersubjectivity, shared commonality, and equity within the relationship. The feelings engendered by mutual respect belong to each respectively. Movement toward personal growth speaks to the goal of the interaction—to benefit each participant in the relationship. Through the relationship, participants develop greater self-awareness and self-understanding, which contribute to their personal growth.

Nurse-family mutuality may help contribute to optimal family outcomes. Outcomes of concern include the perception of being well cared for, achievement of appropriate self-care, demonstration of health-promoting behaviors, improved symptom management, and quality of life.[14]

CHANGING AMERICAN FAMILY DEMOGRAPHICS

Any discussion of family-centered care would be incomplete without recognizing the great variability among families with respect to family structure, function, and role responsibilities. The "traditional" two-parent family is no longer the norm, in which mother serves as child caregiver, nurturer, and homemaker and father serves as economic breadwinner, protector, and disciplinarian. Indeed, many of our assumptions about family membership and organization are no longer applicable and must be adjusted to effectively serve and support children and their families. It is recommended that in psychosocial assessments, nurses inquire directly about family member composition, parental role assignments, employment, and child-care arrangements rather than inaccurately assuming traditional family structure and function.

Family members include anyone who is important in the life of the child. Consider the following facts as evidence of changing American family demographic characteristics.[15] It is estimated that only 22% of American families are structured in which the father is employed outside of the home and the mother stays at home full time. As further evidence of the changing parental role responsibilities within families, approximately 73% of all mothers with children between the ages of 6 and 13 years are employed outside of the home. One in five families currently has a female head of household. Twenty-five percent of all infants

are born to unwed mothers. Approximately 500,000 infants each year are born to teenage mothers. Twenty-one percent of our nation's children are being reared amid poverty conditions. Chronic, persistent poverty is overrepresented among minority children and families in the United States.[16] From conception, minority children are directly or indirectly exposed to a host of problems associated with socioeconomic disadvantage, including differential access to healthcare, residential segregation, unsafe neighborhoods and violence, substandard housing, and parental unemployment or underemployment.[17]

The projections of population growth for the twenty-first century emphasize the need for healthcare providers to understand the parenting processes and family characteristics among ethnic and minority families. Demographers project that the proportion of minority children and families will continue to increase over the next 20 years, as the result of immigration and higher fertility rates in those groups, among other factors.[18,19] African Americans currently make up approximately 12% of the population and constitute the largest ethnic minority group in the country. Hispanic Americans now constitute approximately 8% of the population but are projected to become the largest minority group in the country.

The values, attitudes, and parenting behaviors of ethnic and minority parents vary widely and influence their experience and coping with childhood critical illness and intensive care hospitalization. Factors that are important to consider include the family's cultural heritage and ancestral world views, language preference, degree of acculturation, access to societal institutions, socioeconomic status, exposure to poverty, and other life stressors in the context of racism, prejudice, and discrimination.[17]

BASIS FOR INTERVENTION

It is simply impossible to care for infants and children without caring for them in the context of their families. From a family systems perspective, family members are interconnected, and consequently, events that befall a single member affect all family members.[20-24] Although infants and children can be physically separated from their parents, they cannot be separated emotionally or legally. Mahler, Pine, and Bergman[25] proposed that mothers and infants are psychologically inseparable until completion of the separation-individuation process, which occurs at about 3 years of age. They note that "the biological birth of the human infant and the psychological birth of the individual are not coincident in time. The former is a dramatic, observable, and well-circumscribed event; the latter a slowly unfolding intrapsychic process." Mahler and colleagues[25] note that developmental readiness for independent functioning is the driving force behind this normal process.

Historically, parents have served as the primary decision makers for their infants and children.[11] From a legal perspective, parents who have custody must provide consent for their child's procedures. For parents to provide informed consent, they must understand their child's condition and the proposed treatment plan and procedures, and they must have the opportunity to ask questions. Consent forms should be available in the parent's primary language.

In general, critical illness is extremely stress provoking for infants, children, and their families. Parents are confronted with the possible or actual mortality of their offspring, which represents a great violation of the natural order, whereby children are expected to outlive their parents. Intensive care hospitalization violates the parents' usual role in caring for and protecting their child, which may be experienced by parents as displacement, enforced passivity, and profound helplessness. Circumstances surrounding the child's admission (e.g., accident, planned surgery, new diagnosis) and the family's previous experience with illness and hospitalization influence the parental experience of stress and coping responses.[26] The most prominent sources of parental stress include the fear of death, brain damage, and physical handicap.[27,28] Specific fears depend on the characteristics of the child's illness, including acuity, condition, and prognosis. Uncertainty, that is, ambiguity, lack of clarity, conflicting information, and unpredictability over various aspects of the illness or outcome, can also be extremely stress provoking for parents.[29,30,31]

Anxiety and stress may be transferred from the parent to the infant or child through what Skipper and Leonard[32] first described as the "emotional contagion" hypothesis. Infants and children can be exquisitely sensitive to the emotions and moods of their parents. Children's moods often reflect their own internal states, as well as the feelings of their parents. Nursing care that facilitates adaptive functioning in the parents will, theoretically, decrease both parent and child emotional disequilibrium and stress.

The crisis inherent in hospitalization can severely impair parental sense of confidence and control, thereby compromising parental coping and performance. Hebb[33] described the relationship between stress and behavioral functioning as an inverted U-shaped curve; that is, moderate degrees of stress are related to optimal behavioral functioning and performance, and very low and very high degrees of stress are related to poor functioning and performance. Thus helping parents to reduce their own levels of stress into the moderate range enables parents to better fulfill their natural parenting roles, which can be therapeutically useful at the bedside.[34]

Effective parental functioning can be both supportive and

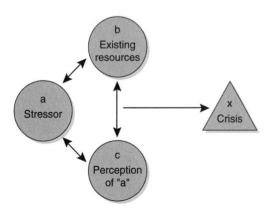

Fig. 3-1 ABCX model of crisis.

stabilizing to critically ill children. Some preliminary evidence now supports the therapeutic value of parental involvement in the PICU environment. For example, Mitchell and colleagues[35] noted that parental stroking reduced children's intracranial pressure (ICP). Compared with an investigator's touch, the researchers noted an occasional, rather profound decrease in the ICP with apparent stabilization following parental touch. Similarly, increased parental caregiving and visitation with preterm infants in the neonatal intensive care unit have been found to improve weight gain and reduce the length of hospitalization.[36] Nursing research has also documented the positive effects on neonatal growth and development of "kangaroo" care, in which mothers have early and regular skin-to-skin contact with their preterm infants.[37]

SOURCES OF PARENTAL STRESS

The critical illness of an infant or child is clearly recognized as stressful to parents. Understanding the basis and progression of that stress is necessary so that care can be focused to help parents modulate PICU-related stress. The nature of the nurse-family relationship can be instrumental in reducing the stress experienced by parents of critically ill children, enabling parents to function effectively in their supportive and therapeutic roles with their children.

Crisis Theory

Hill's ABCX model of crisis[38] provides a basis for understanding the individual responses and needs of parents of critically ill infants and children (Fig. 3-1). Hill described family crises as those situations that create a sense of sharpened insecurity or that block the usual patterns of action or call for new ones. Three interacting variables determine whether and to what degree an event becomes a crisis (X) for a family. The variables include the hardship of the situation or the event itself (A); the family's crisis-meeting resources, such as role structure, flexibility, and previous history with crises (B); and the meaning the family ascribes to the event according to their goals, sociocultural background, and religious affiliation (C).

Thus the ABCX model of crisis can help to explain individual differences among family members and why family members have different perceptions, needs, and coping styles when confronting similar illnesses in their children. It is important to note that parental responses to the PICU admission of their child are not well predicted by objective measures of the child's severity of illness.[39] Rather, parental perceptions of the child's illness and hospitalization appear to have greater use in understanding and predicting parental responses and coping. Hospitalization often precipitates changes in a family's social support network and view of themselves as protectors and nurturers and can disrupt the balance between available resources and presenting demands.[40]

Expanding on Hill's work, the double ABCX model proposed by McCubbin and Patterson[41] incorporates post-crises events that may affect family stress and coping over time (Fig. 3-2). The double ABCX model provides a useful conceptual model for families of chronically critically ill children who require ongoing treatment and periodic hospitalization. This model includes the cumulative nature, or pileup, of demands for change within a family as the crisis extends over time (aA); family system resources that may include family members, the family unit, and the community (bB); and the family's perception of the illness-related experience, which includes the family's definition of the major stressor event, the meaning of the resulting hardships, and the family's effort to redefine the event (cC). The resultant crisis (X) may be perceived differently by family members as an opportunity, challenge, or an overwhelming burden. Coping strategies, which are defined as the cognitive, behavioral, or emotional processes that individuals use to adapt to the demands of stressful and associated events, result from interactions between aA, bB, and cC.

Through cognitive appraisal of the perceived meaning of the event, a crisis sets forth basic adaptive tasks to which varied coping skills can be applied.[42] Five major adaptive tasks to be confronted in managing crises have been identified (Box 3-3). Coping skills focus on the meaning of the crisis, the reality of the crisis, or the emotions associated with the crisis. Parents of critically ill children typically use both problem-focused and emotion-focused forms of coping almost equally.[43-45] Problem-focused coping behaviors include attempting to modify or eliminate the source of stress, to deal with the tangible changes, to actively change oneself, and to develop a more satisfying situation. Emotion-focused coping behaviors include managing the emotions aroused by the stressors. The constellation of coping strategies used by parents varies according to parental age, perception of the illness, locus of control, anxiety level, and parental involve-ment in caregiving activities.[46] Philichi[47] noted that an important role for nurses is the identification and facilitation of the various coping strategies used by families.

Stress Unique to the PICU

Rothstein[26] noted that the family's stress level is increased when the child's illness is severe, when little or no preparation for hospitalization has occurred, when the cause is unclear, and when the outcome is uncertain. Miles and Carter[48] were the first to empirically describe parental stress in the PICU setting. They identified three major sources of stress specifically experienced by parents of children in the PICU, including situational variables, personal characteristics, and the PICU environment. The first two sources of stress identified by Miles and Carter are congruent with Hill's ABCX model of crises. Situational variables corre-

---

> **Box 3-3**
> **Adaptive Tasks in Managing Crises**
>
> 1. Establish the meaning of and understand the personal significance of the crises
> 2. Confront reality and respond to the requirements of the crises
> 3. Sustain relationships with family and friends and others who may be helpful in resolving the crises
> 4. Maintain a reasonable emotional balance by managing upsetting feelings
> 5. Preserve a positive self-image and maintain a sense of competence and mastery

Data from Moos RH: *Coping with life crises: an integrated approach,* New York, 1986, Plenum Medical Books, pp 3-28.

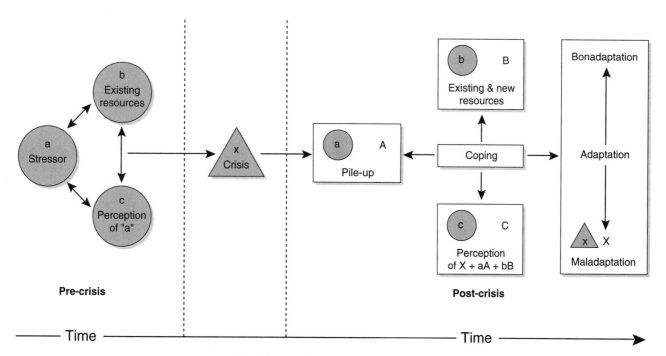

Fig. 3-2 Double ABCX model of crisis.

spond to Hill's "A" component of the model, for example, the child's critical illness and hospitalization. Personal characteristics correspond with Hill's "B" and "C" components of the model, for example, the family's existing resources and individual perceptions of what is occurring. The third factor, environmental sources of stress, is unique to the PICU setting and potentially within nursing's role to manipulate.

Miles and Carter[48] delineated seven dimensions of the PICU experience that parents find stressful (Table 3-1). These dimensions, derived from observational data, parent and staff nurse interviews, and the literature, form the basis of the Parental Stressor Scale: Pediatric Intensive Care Unit (PSS:PICU). These dimensions may be conceptually divided into two major categories of stress including (1) the physical aspects of the intensive care environment and (2) the psychosocial aspects, which include parent-staff relationships and the parent-child relationship. Alterations in parental role, and the subsequent disruption in the parent-child relationship, have consistently been identified as the most stressful aspect of the PICU environment.[49-54,60] Changes in the child's behavioral and emotional reactions, which can challenge the parents' ability to know and care for their child, are ranked second in degree of stressfulness following parental role alteration. Rennick[55] noted that when the parental role is threatened, the parent as a whole person is at risk.

Under usual circumstances, parents provide a safe and constructive environment for their child, which fosters their growth and development. Traditionally, parents nurture, protect, educate, and advocate for their children. Parents are usually considered to be the "expert" on their child, in that they know their child better than anyone else. Although parents take for granted their usual control over their children's lives, critical illness and hospitalization often threaten that sense of control, competence, and stability.[56] Parents can find themselves displaced from their familiar roles and, in many cases, dependent on healthcare providers for the very survival of their child. It is not uncommon, over the course of a PICU hospitalization, for parents to lose confidence in their ability to know or to comfort their child in meaningful ways.

Parent-child interactions are often compromised as a result of barriers created by life support equipment, sedating medications, precaution policies designed to reduce the risk of infection (e.g., surgical masks), prolonged hospitalization, and visitation restrictions (e.g., during change of shift).[57,58] The critically ill child does not look or act the same to the parent when, for example, paralyzing agents distort the child's facial features. A child might respond to the parent with an increased heart rate, causing monitoring alarms to sound—this can be not only unnerving but also serve to squelch future attempts to interact with the child. It can be discouraging and frustrating to parents that the familiar methods of comforting their child are not feasible or effective. Parents may become unsure of themselves during caregiving activities and tasks that they had previously completed hundreds of times. Not only must parents face the uncertainty of their child's critical illness, but also they may feel helpless and ineffectual because they believe that they can do little or nothing to improve the situation.

Susan Jay[59] first identified role revision, the process of giving up the familiar role of "parent-to-a-well-child" and taking on a new role as "parent-to-an-acutely-ill-child," as a stressor to parents of critically ill children. Jay noted that during the crisis of a sudden acute illness, parents first grieve for their previous role and "need time to resolve the fact that others have their child's life in their hands, that they are no longer in control, and that they may no longer know what is best for their own child." Transition to their new role occurs by first imitating the caretaking responses of others available to them. They watch parents of other children in the PICU and also watch nurses caring for their own infant or child. Parents slowly assume their revised identity as parent-to-an-acutely-ill-child. Variability in parental role attainment will normally occur. The spectrum is wide and ranges from abandonment, keeping a distance, passive involvement, and active involvement to hypervigilance. Rennick[55] has questioned whether role revision would occur in parents who spent only brief periods in the PICU before transfer of the infant or child to another unit.

Mothers generally report higher levels of stress than fathers in the PICU. Miles and colleagues[53] concluded that stress is associated with alterations in parental role and is the

---

◆ **TABLE 3-1   Environmental Sources of PICU-Related Stress**

Dimension	Items
Sights and sounds	Monitors, alarms, other sick children
Child's appearance	Puffiness, color changes, appearing cold
Child's behaviors and emotional responses	Confusion, uncooperative, crying, demanding, pain, restless, inability to talk, frightened, angry, sad
Child's procedures	Injections, tubes, suctioning, IV, pulmonary care, ventilator, incisions
Staff communication	Explaining too fast, using words that are not understood, inconsistent information, not saying what is wrong, not talking enough
Staff behavior	Not introducing themselves, laughing, joking, too many people
Parental role revision	Not seeing, not holding, not taking care of the child themselves, not visiting, not with crying child, not knowing how to help child

Data from Carter MC, Miles MS: *Parental stressor scale: pediatric intensive care unit,* Kansas City, KS, 1983, School of Nursing, University of Kansas.

result of changes in the child's behavior and emotional reactions. Parents who experience an unexpected admission of their child are usually more stressed than parents who are prepared for their child's admission.[50,51,60] Similarly, parents who are unprepared for the admission are more stressed than parents who had formal preparation before the experience.[49]

Advanced preparation for parents whose children will be hospitalized typically includes providing parents with information about (1) a child's anticipated response to the illness or procedure based on their developmental stage; (2) a preadmission tour, informal interview, or information session; (3) preadmission parent-child interaction guidelines; and (4) printed resources for the child and parent.[61] Miles and Mathes[62] noted that parents of critically ill children were seldom prepared for the perceived alterations in the parent-child relationship, which is the most stressful aspect of the PICU hospitalization.

Trajectory of Parental Stress

Research to date has delineated phases and characteristics of the trajectory of parental stress in the PICU. Awareness of the normal trajectory of PICU-related parental stress enables nurses to focus intervention strategies and to identify extreme parental behavior. Parents who experience stress responses that are outside the expected range or extreme may benefit from early consultation or referral for more intensive intervention with psychosocial support staff.

Rothstein[26] studied parents of children admitted to the PICU after catastrophic illnesses and described a pattern of parental reactions. Within the first 12 hours of admission, parents often exhibit overwhelming shock associated with feelings of helplessness. Within 24 hours, this period is followed by a phase in which parents grapple for explanations. This behavior supports the parent's search for explanations to ascribe meaning to the illness.[29,31] Rothstein[26] noted that parents are "responsible" for their children and thus may experience real or imagined guilt or blame themselves for their child's critical illness.

Rothstein[26] next described an anticipatory waiting phase, lasting hours to days, which coincides with the child's medical stabilization. During this phase, parents frequently express concerns about the long-term effects of the illness; focus on seemingly insignificant changes, hoping to see improvement; and become more demanding of and perhaps angry at the staff. Specific uncertainties during this time include the child's likelihood of survival, future appearance, anticipated level of functioning, and duration of illness and hospitalization. Parental helplessness continues during this period of waiting. Anticipatory waiting is then followed by either the elation of discharge or the bereavement process if the outcome is death.

Lewandowski[63] was the first to describe the initial responses and coping strategies of parents of children undergoing open-heart surgery. Lewandowski reported that despite preoperative teaching and a preadmission tour of the PICU, parents often express shock and feel unprepared for their first postoperative visit at the bedside. Parents may experience helplessness and powerlessness because they are unable to function in their familiar role of protector. Lewandowski described several parental coping strategies, which are presented in Table 3-2. Restructuring, sometimes referred to as a time to focus on little things, allows the parent to focus on one thing at a time, which prevents parents from becoming overwhelmed by the overall condition of the child.

Curley[51,60] found that changes in a child's appearance and PICU-related procedures were more stressful to parents during the first few days of hospitalization than later in the course of hospitalization. As the hospitalization progresses, issues related to staff communication and behavior become greater contributors to the parental experience of stress. Supporting Rothstein's notion of the anticipatory waiting phase, Curley documented an overall increase in parental stress after the first few days of PICU hospitalization.[26,51,60] Most importantly, parental stress related to role alterations was significant throughout the entire PICU hospitalization. Parents, accustomed to their protector role, report helplessness in protecting their child from pain and in knowing how best to help their child. Curley and Wallace[52] noted that the trajectory of child illness and concomitant trajectory of parental stress vary across different patient populations. The "typical" trajectory of parental stress differs significantly between parents of surgical patients and medical patients. The trajectory for surgical patients often begins with a hyperacute phase that predictably improves over time, whereas the trajectory for medical patients is often more variable and can be just the opposite of the surgical patients.

As the child's condition stabilizes and the parents gradually adjust to the role of parent-to-a-critically-ill-child, parents frequently express the need to become personally involved in their child's care. Although parents may initially have been relieved that they were not solely responsible for the care of the child, they wish to play a more active role as their child improves[27] or as they gain self-confidence within the PICU setting.[51,60] Curley[51,60] has postulated that increases in perceived parental stress relate specifically to nursing communication and nursing behavior and, in general, may reflect parents' unmet needs to participate in

◆ TABLE 3-2 Initial Coping Strategies

Immobilization	Delay in parental approach to the bedside
Visual survey	Visually scanning the environment and orienting self before attending to verbal explanations
Withdrawal	Nonresponsive passive behaviors or actual physical withdrawal from the bed space
Restructuring	Focusing on one physical detail or on the care provided
Intellectualization	Dealing with the child's illness on an intellectual level

Data from Lewandowski LA: Stressors and coping styles of parents of children undergoing open heart surgery, *Crit Care Q* 3:75-84, 1980.

caregiving and to fulfill meaningful roles. Parents may experience displacement by staff and usurpation of their traditional parental caregiving role. Similarly, Rothstein[26] noted that the helplessness experienced by parents is heightened when parents are discouraged or excluded from taking an active role in the care of their child. Despite the high levels of technology in the PICU environment and the seriousness of the child's illness, most parents wish to be informed, to have input into the plan of care, to help with their child's physical care, and to be recognized as important in their child's recovery.[64,65]

IDENTIFIED PARENTAL NEEDS AND COPING STRATEGIES

Numerous researchers have described the perceived needs of parents during the course of PICU hospitalization. Perceived needs support parents' individual coping efforts and, ultimately, the ways in which they are able to manage the threat of their infant's or child's illness. Psychosocial intervention that addresses the parents' identified needs serves to support their individual coping. Commonly cited parental needs are summarized in Box 3-4.

Even when parents are stressed within the PICU setting, Kirschbaum[64,65] found that they are still readily able to identify their own needs when asked. Needs that are most important to parents included believing that there is hope, knowing that the child is receiving the best care possible, and believing that they are getting as much information as possible. One half of the 10 most important needs identified by parents are informational in nature. Thus excellence in clinical care and provision of information are major factors that support families. Accurate information is necessary for parents to cognitively appraise the situation, to construct meaning of the illness, to make informed decisions, and to help their children understand events. Rothstein[26] noted that parental trust develops when information is honest, consistent, and anticipatory in nature.

Melnyk and colleagues[66,67] designed Creating Opportunities for Parent Empowerment (COPE), a two-part intervention that provides parents with (1) information about their child's behavior during recovery from critical illness and how parents could help facilitate their child's adjustment and (2) a parent-child workbook containing three parent-child activities designed to assist parents in enhancing their children's coping during and after the hospital experience. They found that mothers who received the COPE program provided more support to their children during intrusive procedures; provided more emotional support to their children; reported less negative mood states and less parental stress related to their children's emotions and behaviors; and reported fewer posttraumatic stress symptoms and less parental role changes for weeks following hospitalization.

Compared to relatives of acutely ill adult patients, parents of acutely ill children report a greater need to be recognized as vital to their ill child's recovery, to visit anytime, and to help with the child's physical care.[64,65,68] These findings make intuitive sense because parents nor-

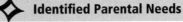

> **Box 3-4**
> **Identified Parental Needs**
>
> - Getting as much information as possible
> - Assurance that their child is receiving the best possible care
> - Feeling that there is hope
> - Vigilance
> - Being near their child as much as possible
> - Help with physical care
> - Being recognized as important to child's recovery
> - Talking with other parents
> - Prayer
> - Instrumental resources (e.g., transportation, meals)

mally "take care of" their children. Parents need to feel important to their children regardless of how sick they are. For example, parents generally tend to put their child's needs above their own needs. Parents consistently rate their own personal needs (e.g., "having someone concerned about my health") as less important than any child or parent-child need.[65] Some parents, however, do acknowledge a physiologic and psychologic need to curtail the amount of time they spend with their child in the PICU.[69]

Miles and Carter[44] identified five coping strategies perceived as most helpful to parents of critically ill children. Coping strategies included (1) seeking help or comfort from others, (2) believing that the child is getting the best possible care, (3) seeking as much information as possible, (4) having hope, and (5) being near the child as much as possible. The use of prayer, asking questions of the staff, and talking with other parents were also cited as important. Similarly, Kasper and Nyamathi[69] identified the most common parental needs as proximity to the child; frequent, accurate, and truthful information about the child's condition; participation in the child's caregiving; sleeping accommodations near the PICU; and reassurance that the child is receiving needed care and treatment.

In addition, parents need to know that their child is being treated as a person.[70] Parents assessed this parameter by noting whether staff called their child by name or talked to their child at an appropriate developmental level, even if their child was comatose or heavily medicated. Verbally preparing even an unresponsive child for procedures conveyed the message to parents that the nurse cared about, not just for, their child. Parents perceived staff efforts to treat their children with such dignity as the "best possible care."

Although parents have consistently identified proximity to their infants and children as a very important need, some PICUs limit parental access to children several times during the day. Notwithstanding 24-hours-a-day visitation policies, nurses and other staff often excuse parents from the bed space during activities such as nursing reports, medical rounds, and procedures.[71] This exclusion is inconsistent with family-centered, humane care in the PICU. Furthermore, mothers who have the benefit of individualized visitation have significantly lower anxiety scores and perceive their child's illness as less severe than mothers who experience structured visitation.[72] Carnevale[73] notes that even the word *visitation* marginalizes the significance of family presence. The most salient component of family visiting guidelines is flexibility. An individual approach that enables the family's informal social support system to be involved during the hospitalization is also recommended.[74] This not only includes parents, but also siblings, grandparents, and child-care workers, among others, whom the family identifies as important.

The coping strategy of vigilance serves to reduce the parental sense of helplessness and to maintain the parental role of protector.[75] The vigilant parent of a critically ill infant or child is one who stays with the child as much as possible but who is also able to leave to meet the needs of self and family. The vigilant parent asks questions to keep informed, checks to ensure that the child is receiving proper care, and may request to remain with the child during procedures for the purpose of supporting the child. Vigilant parental behavior increases when the child and parents are exposed to many different caregivers.[51] One could hypothesize that parents will remain vigilant until they feel confident that their assigned nurse "knows" them and their child.

In some cases, parents may manifest hypervigilance, in which the positive aspects of vigilance are outweighed by the negative or even the well-being of the child is jeopardized.[75] Several factors have been associated with hypervigilance (Table 3-3). The hypervigilant parent overuses or exaggerates the use of vigilance. Parents never or rarely leave the bedside. They may demand detailed information before agreeing to even minor changes in the child's treatment plan, sometimes delaying or denying medications or treatments. Hypervigilant parents may continually monitor staff, attempt to control how care is provided, or assume total care of the child. These parents may trust only a few staff and wish to select the nurses assigned to care for their child. They might examine the medical record to identify problems or discrepancies and then record them in a logbook.

Our society generally values and rewards the vigilant parent but not necessarily in the PICU setting. Hypervigilant parents can be unnerving or even threatening to nursing staff. Nursing interventions should be focused to decrease the parent's sense of helplessness and provide the parent with some degree of control. Positive nursing interventions include welcoming parents and their assistance at the bedside, reinforcing parental questioning, providing information on a consistent basis, reinforcing the parental role, and being receptive to their telephone calls. Nurses need to support each other when providing care for hypervigilant parents and to remember that, although it may be difficult, the parents are doing the best that they can under the circumstances. Negative staff behavior that can further fuel parental hypervigilance includes acting defensively, withholding information, maintaining power and control, failing to include parents in the decision-making process, avoiding the parents, and resenting their questions.

Parents have also identified the importance of parent-to-parent support as a means of coping in the PICU. Parents can offer perspectives and support to each other that

TABLE 3-3 Factors That Influence Parental Vigilance

Parent-family issues	Parent's personality
	Family relationships
	Cultural/parental role
Parent-child issues	Child's meaning to parent
Illness-related issues	Parent's perception of the infant's or child's vulnerability
	Parent's usual level of responsibility for the child's care at home
	Parent's understanding about the illness
	Acuity of the illness
	Illness trajectory
	Pain; painful or invasive procedures
Environmental issues	Parent-staff communications
	Level of trust
	Quality of communication
	Quality of care
	History of misdiagnosis, improper care or treatment
	Continuity of nurses and physicians
	Response of the staff to vigilant behaviors

Data from Miles MS: Vigilance as a parental coping strategy when a child is seriously ill. Abstract for poster presentation. Biennial meeting of the Society for Research in Child Development, Baltimore, Md, 1987.

professionals are not able to provide.[15] Although parents spontaneously interact in waiting rooms, Halm[76] studied the effect of formal support groups on the anxiety levels of family members during critical illness. Family members perceived many benefits of the group milieu, such as sharing with other people in similar situations, instilling hope, reducing anxiety, and learning new coping strategies. Nursing staff can be instrumental in facilitating parent-to-parent support.[10]

Parent-professional trust is the necessary foundation from which all supportive care can build. Trust develops in the context of the parents' perception that their child is receiving excellent care, from the nurses' reassuring presence, and through recognition of parents as unique autonomous individuals who have important contributions to make toward the child's care. Continuity of nursing and medical care allows strong alliances to form with parents, which further contribute to the development of trust.[55]

Although competence is the most highly valued quality of nursing care, parents also prefer nurses who are sensitive and caring.[77] For example, nurses are considered caring when they talk with parents, provide information without asking, do not make parents feel intrusive, help parents feel that they are part of the team, enable parents to feel comfortable in leaving, and reassure them that everything will be taken care of and communicated.[51] In general, parents can more willingly relinquish their child's care to someone they trust.

INTERVENTION STRATEGIES

Most of the nursing research generated on parental stress has been descriptive in nature. Many consistent recommendations for interventions intended to minimize parental stress in the PICU setting have been offered. Interventions may be divided into three major categories: (1) those that nurture a trusting environment, in parents themselves, their children, and PICU staff; (2) those that establish effective communication patterns and provide information and anticipatory guidance; and (3) those that limit parental powerlessness by reestablishing a parental relationship through visitation and participation in caregiving activities. Such interventions are consonant with the Parents' Bill of Rights (Box 3-5).

Nurses tend to intervene in a similar manner with all families whose needs are perceived to be essentially the same.[78] This approach is problematic because there is significant variability in parental perceptions and experiences, stress levels, and needs among individuals that require individualized nursing interventions. Interventions that may be helpful to one parent may not be helpful or even useful to another parent, even within the same family.

Nursing perceptions and interventions may be well intended but may not be accurate. Researchers have noted differences between what nurses perceive parental needs to be and what parents perceive as their own needs within the PICU setting.[79] Indeed, additional parental stress may result from mismatches between nurses' understanding of parental needs and parents' own understanding.[80] Generalized or generic family supportive intervention strategies intended to meet nonexistent needs or needs already met by others often lead to much wasted time and energy.[81]

NURSING MUTUAL PARTICIPATION MODEL OF CARE

Models that emphasize an individual approach to nursing interventions are preferred, given the individualized nature of PICU-related parental stress and findings that generic

family support models are not adequate and may even exacerbate parental stress. The nursing mutual participation model of care (NMPMC) represents such an example (Box 3-6). Szasz and Hollender[82] first described a "mutual participation" model for use with chronically ill adults. The model, fundamentally different from others practiced at the time, was based on the premise that the healthcare provider could not profess to know what is best for an individual. The search for that which may be considered individually helpful was the essence of the therapeutic interaction. The individual was assisted to help himself or herself as his or her own experiences and beliefs provided reliable and important clues to therapy. In 1980, Brody[83] further elaborated the model as a four-step process for use with adults in outpatient settings. The foundation of the intervention process was conceptualized as agenda seeking; the patient was enlisted and invited into the healthcare decision-making process by asking, "How can I help you today?"

Curley[51,60] adapted the model for nursing care of critically ill children and their parents because it provided the philosophical foundation to incorporate many of the therapeutic interventions recommended from descriptive research. The model supports the view that the nature of PICU-related stress requires individualized nursing interventions. The model is based on the premise that nurses have something of value to offer parents and acknowledges

---

Box 3-6
Nursing Mutual Participation Model of Care

Admission

Extend our care to include parents
Acknowledge their importance

Daily Bedside Contact

Enabling strategies that provide parents with system savvy
• Information—teach and clarify
• Anticipatory guidance—illness trajectory
• Provide instrumental resources
Facilitate transition to "parent-to-a-critically-ill-child"
• Enhance parent—child unique connectedness
• Role model interactions
• Invite participation in nurturant activity
• Provide options during procedures
Communication pattern
• Establish a caring relationship with the parent
  How are you doing today?
• Assess parental perception of the child's illness
  How does s/he look to you today?
• Determine parental goals, objectives, and expectations
  What troubles you most?
• Seek informed suggestions and preferences, and invite participation in care
  How can I help you today?

Data from Curley MAQ: Effects of the nursing mutual participation model of care and parental stress in the pediatric intensive care unit, *Heart Lung* 17: 682-688, 1988; Curley MAQ, Wallace J: Effects of the nursing mutual participation model of care on parental stress in the pediatric intensive care unit-A replication, *J Pediatr Nurs* 7:377-385, 1992.

Box 3-5
A Pediatric Bill of Rights

In this hospital you and your child have the right to:
• Respect and personal dignity
• Care that supports you as a family
• Information you can understand
• Quality healthcare
• Emotional support
• Care that respects your child's growth and development
• Make decisions about your child's care

Data from Association for the Care of Children's Health: *Bill of rights for parents: a pediatric bill of rights,* Bethesda, Md, 1991, Association for the Care of Children's Health.

that parents also have something of value to contribute to the caregiving process of their children. Nurses have some expertise in knowing what might generally be helpful to parents who are experiencing the critical illness of a child, but nurses do not specifically know what might be best for an individual parent. Parents, on the other hand, know what may be helpful to them and their infant or child, but they do not know what is unique about the PICU or what strategies have helped other parents in similar situations.

The NMPMC provides a framework for individualized nursing interactions in the PICU. It clarifies the parental role, supports active parental involvement with their critically ill child, and fosters parental confidence in performing their role in a foreign setting. The process is individually determined and evolves to meet the expressed needs of each parent. Nurse-parent relationships are characterized by a high degree of empathy and partnership, and expert knowledge is imparted to limit perceived helplessness and passivity. Critical features of the model include the equal status of parent and professional in the relationship, mutual interdependency, and mutual satisfaction between nurses and parents.

The effects of the NMPMC on helping parents to alleviate their stress have been supported in two separate nursing research studies. In the first study, the principal investigator, functioning in the role of a clinical nurse specialist, implemented the model.[51,60] Parents reported significantly less overall stress in the areas of child's behavior and emotions, parental role revision, child's procedures, and nursing communication and behavior. In the second study,[52] primary nurses implemented the model. Parents who had the benefit of NMPMC intervention reported significantly less stress associated with the hospitalization, particularly in the area of parental role alteration.

The NMPMC is consistent with Greeneich and Long's nursing taxonomy of family satisfaction (NTFS).[84] Within the NTFS, family satisfaction results from an interaction between the family, nurse, and healthcare system. Nurses can influence family satisfaction by (1) optimizing critical juncture incidents, (2) accommodating parental personality styles, (3) determining family expectations, and (4) adapting the environment to the family's needs. Critical juncture incidents are episodes in which a nurse's behavior and intervention significantly affect the patient at a time when the family perceives the patient to be most vulnerable. Nurse personality attributes include social courtesy, acceptance, kindness, helpfulness, empathy, and advocacy. The ability of the nurse to develop a trusting relationship with the family is also considered to be an element of personality fit. Trust is inherently linked to effective communication (matched to the family's style) and nursing proficiency. Nurses create a milieu to adapt to the family's expectations and needs. Family satisfaction results when the parent's expectations of care match with the reality of care.

Initial Contact

For parents, admission is a very stressful period, during which they experience a significant loss of control.[32,34] Acknowledging the parent's valuable and irreplaceable role

in actions and words during this critical period helps to set the tone for the entire PICU hospitalization. Also important is an acknowledgment of the individuality of a family's experience as its relates to their present and past experiences of illness. The nurse should state the obvious, for example, "Here at Children's Hospital we believe parents to be very important to their children, especially when they're sick. We would like to work with you to help you find ways that you can continue to be important to your child while she or he is in the ICU." These words broaden the perspective of care to include parents. Right from the start, parents are invited as partners into the caregiving process, thus establishing an atmosphere in which parents feel that their contributions are valued, expected, and essential. Parents feel less anxious when they sense that their role is valued, that their child still belongs to them, and that someone will help them to get through the experience with their child as a welcomed participant.

As soon as information is available, the nurse and the physician should provide it. This demonstrates multidisciplinary collaboration and communication to the family. After any period of separation or change in their infant's or child's appearance or behavior, parents require preparation for what they will see or hear before reuniting them. Information may need to be repeated several times because high levels of parental stress can interfere with the parent's ability to process, understand, and remember information.

If parent-child separation is necessary, parents are provided with privacy and a telephone so that they may contact extended family members. During this period of separation, it is imperative that nursing staff maintain contact with the parents. Right from the beginning, staff should seek the parent's preference about the level of information and frequency of contact. Parents usually request information about stabilizing methods, and they wish to be reunited with their infant or child as soon as possible. If prolonged periods of separation are unavoidable, opportunities are sought to provide parents with brief updates or visits between procedures.

Daily Bedside Contact

After openly acknowledging the importance of the parental role, the model provides a framework for daily interventions that are supportive to and guided by the unique perceived needs of each parent. The model (1) incorporates enabling and empowering strategies to equip the parent with healthcare system savvy, (2) facilitates the parent's transition to parent-to-a-critically-ill-child, and (3) delineates a consistent nurse-parent communication pattern. An accurate family assessment, such as that suggested by Miles,[27] helps to guide effective intervention strategies (Box 3-7). Family characteristics such as the degree of adaptability (rigid, structured, flexible, chaotic) and cohesion (disengaged, separated, connected, enmeshed) are important considerations in psychosocial intervention planning.[47]

Enabling Strategies That Provide Parents With System Savvy. It has been said that parents do not need to be empowered within the clinical setting; they just

Box 3-7

Parameters of a Family Assessment

1. History of child's illness: when and how diagnoses were made; previous hospitalizations and treatments
2. Parental perception and understanding of illness
3. Feelings engendered by the child's illness: fear, guilt, remorse, helplessness, hopelessness, anger
4. Family history and significant events: past experiences with illness, divorce, death
5. Current family functioning: family membership, structure, and roles, current marital relationship, communication patterns within family, patterns of expressing feelings, siblings and their relationship within the family, religious background, cultural values, financial problems
6. Parental roles and relationships with child: identification of the child as "special" as a result of having been the only child, only daughter, only son, youngest, eldest, most vulnerable
7. Unmet parental needs: lack of sleep, lack of privacy, poor nutrition, untreated health problems, poor hygiene, lack of opportunity for sexual expression

Data from Miles MS: Impact of the intensive care unit on parents, *Issues Compr Pediatr Nurs* 3:72-90, 1979.

need their inherent power recognized. Socializing parents to the PICU and hospital system serves to empower them, especially those skills that improve their access to information and resources.

Provide Information That Instructs and Clarifies. In addition to information about the infant's or child's illness and the standard PICU equipment (monitors, catheters, endotracheal tubes, etc.), specific information is vital about the changes in the child's appearance, behavior, and emotional reactions and in the parental role. When discussing the technologic devices surrounding the patient, including a discussion about alarm systems is important. Although nurses know that there is a hierarchy of alarm systems about which to be concerned and how quickly to respond, parents do not necessarily understand these distinctions. Unfamiliar alarms are feared equally by parents, such as those that signal hypotension to those that signal the end of an antibiotic infusion or artifact on a cardiac monitor.

After addressing these immediate needs, parents require an understanding of the PICU and hospital environment. Written materials, such as orientation booklets, are effective in assisting families to remember discrete pieces of information.[85] The process of how parents gain access to their infants and children is critically important. It should be stressed that the only reason parents are asked to request permission to see their child in the PICU is for the protection and privacy of other patients.

Information including the routines of the unit, who is in charge of their child's medical and nursing care, and when and where parents get information enables them to effectively function within the system's hierarchy. Parents of children who require multiple services and parents of

chronically critically ill children are at high risk for communication problems related to insufficient, incorrect, or contradictory information about their child's care and management. It is essential that the nurse coordinate the informational needs of parents by delineating, together with the attending physician and parents, a daily communication plan. Routinely scheduled weekly multidisciplinary team meetings can be very helpful to the entire team and to parents of chronically critically ill children.

Only after (1) sharing information about their infant or child, (2) providing information about the hospital environment, and (3) answering questions that the parents have should dialogue progress to the perceived alterations in parental role and responsibility.

Provide Anticipatory Guidance About the Illness Trajectory. Information about what parents will see or experience should be shared before it happens, if at all possible. If feasible, nurses should meet with parents and patients before a planned admission to the PICU. Describing the illness trajectory, as far as it can be reasonably predicted, is extremely helpful in allowing parents to understand and distinguish what is "normal and expected" from what is "life threatening." Although videotapes may be helpful, tours (except to empty bed spaces) should be avoided because they violate the privacy of existing patients and may frighten the future patient.

Provide Instrumental Resources. Provision of adequate instrumental resources is also necessary so that families are able to maintain both physical and emotional accessibility to their critically ill child 24 hours a day. Necessary resources include sleep facilities, showers, telephones, data ports, nutritious food, transportation, and parking.[86,87,88] Providing beepers to parents can help to ease their separation anxiety and conveys a message about the importance of communication and access to staff. Physical barriers to the welcoming process, including activities that make parents feel like visitors to their own infants and children, should be eliminated.

Facilitate Transition to Parent-to-a-Critically-Ill-Child. Alterations in parental role and the subsequent disruption in the parent-child relationship are the most stressful aspects of the PICU environment. Assisting parents to formulate a role with which they are personally comfortable and supporting them in their decision-making capacity help parents in a successful transition to parent-to-a-critically-ill-child.

Enhance Parent-Child Unique Connectedness. Because of changes in their child's appearance and behavior, parents may need help reconnecting to a child who appears to be so much different. Strategies include finding some characteristic of the child that has not changed (that is, some enduring feature) and emphasizing it to the parents. Examples may include hair or eye color or evidence of the child's increased heart rate in response to the parent's voice. Creativity is sometimes needed to help reestablish the unique parent-child connection when significant disfigurement is present. Parents may need "permission" and demonstrations of how to touch and interact with their critically ill infant or child. Rubin's maternal touch progression,[89] for example, can be demonstrated in the PICU regardless of the age of the infant or child.

Parents can also be encouraged to bring in the child's favorite blanket, toy, doll, or family pictures to comfort the child and to individualize the bed space. All of these reminders of life at home provide nonverbal cues of the valued nature of the family, and they are as important as direct verbal communication. Macnab and colleagues[90] noted that displaying pictures might open an avenue for communication, allow parents to express unspoken concerns, and give parents comfort or a goal to strive for, thus alleviating some stress associated with having a child in the ICU.

Role Model Interactions. Parents have reported that their initial fears are lessened by observing and imitating nursing care activities. Parents notice and sort observed nursing activities into two categories: those that are familiar activity (bathing, diaper changing, holding, etc.) and those that are different activity (dressing changes, endotracheal suctioning, etc.).[59] Parents watch what nurses do to learn, not to make judgments on the correctness of how care is done, because the majority of parents are not healthcare professionals. Acknowledging that one's nursing care activity is being observed provides an opportunity for the nurse to role model care through nonverbal communication. For example, knowing that their actions are being observed, nurses can role model where parents can safely touch their instrumented child during a bedside conversation with parents. Typically, parents can be observed following the nurses lead in safe touch after the conversation is over.

Invite Participation. After the initial period of shock and disbelief, parents are usually able to identify those activities in which they wish to participate. When offered caregiving options and opportunity, parents typically wish to participate. Such participation can renew their sense of self-esteem and help them to feel instrumental in their child's recovery. Suggesting ways in which parents can assist their child in coping helps to reduce parental anxiety.[91] Ideally, special aspects of parental care and comforting can be distinguished from things that others can do for the child (e.g., provide breast milk, voice, touch). Nursing staff should help parents to identify the range of options by suggesting appropriate diversional, nurturing, comforting, caregiving, and monitoring activities.

The social and emotional needs of infants, in particular, are met in close association with their bodily needs. With a new caregiver, the infant loses much of what is familiar. Physical care constitutes an essential element of the very intimate relationship between parents and infants. Usurping this role from parents is generally not welcomed by the infant, nor is it helpful, especially when the infant is stressed. Nursing practice that directly involves the primary caregiver is more therapeutic than care that replaces the primary caregiver. Efforts should be extended to welcome parents; they should never be made to feel out of place or in competition for their infant or child.[92]

Parents generally enjoy helping with activities that they find personally rewarding and participating in new activities with nursing guidance. A developmental approach

is a starting point, for example, consideration of what parents normally do for their baby, toddler, child, or adolescent.[52] Reading, massages, bathing, and hairbrushing are familiar and comforting activities for both parents and child. Sociocultural influences will likely affect the parent's selection of activities. Communication, teaching, anticipatory guidance, and mutual trust and support are essential during this process. Parents frequently feel uncomfortable performing tasks that they had previously mastered as a parent of a well child. Clearly, bathing an infant at home is different than bathing an infant who is attached to numerous pieces of equipment. Once the child's condition is stabilized, it is important to incorporate parent-child "private time" in the management plan to sustain the parent-child relationship.

With time, some parents may ask to participate in daily bedside rounds. In practice, most parents can be observed listening in (at a distance) whenever any team rounds on their child. If the system can support the parent's request, nursing can support the parent's success by reviewing the structure of rounds (who presents what information) and, in teaching institutions, the educational mission of the hospital as healthy debate often permeates rounds. As with any new experience, the nurse should mentor the parent and provide feedback and debriefing as necessary.

Provide Options During Procedures. Traditionally, parents have been asked to step out of the PICU during their or another child's procedures or treatments. Enforced separations, sometimes lasting hours, and related conflicts in values about the approaches used to obtain the child's cooperation are significant sources of stress for parents.[45] Currently, great variability is seen among institutions regarding parental presence during special procedures. Inconsistency among staff and unclear policies about visitation and parental presence during procedures can provoke further anxiety for parents, as well as the staff.[10]

Parents may be dismissed from treatments because of staff fear and apprehension that they may interfere with the procedure or make their child more upset. Sevedra[93] studied 60 children, ages 2 weeks to 6 years, who had blood drawn in the presence of their parents. The study suggested that even when the procedure was difficult and stressful, parents were not disruptive but instead were supportive of their child as directed by personnel. A variety of verbal and nonverbal strategies were used by parents to help the child to better cope. Similarly, Shaw and Routh[94] compared 18-month-old and 5-year-old children's reactions to immunizations in the presence and absence of mothers. They found more upset behavior when mothers were present, but the researchers hypothesized that the children's increase in negative responses reflected a disinhibitory response. That is, the mother's presence allowed the child greater expression of his or her feelings in an unfamiliar and threatening environment. Behavioral difficulties including crying, terror, uncooperation, or violent protest can be expected when the infant or toddler is stressed by the parent's absence, let alone by a painful procedure. Lack of expected distress responses may reflect deterioration in the child's level of functioning, detachment, or severe emotional withdrawal.

Expecting cooperative behavior or a diminished negative response when parents are present is probably unrealistic.

Parental presence can potentially support the child's coping efforts and provide the child with a familiar source of comfort. The recommendation is that parents be offered a choice regarding their presence or participation, as well as support for their decision. In fact, Robinson and colleagues[95] found little evidence to support the exclusion of relatives who wish to be present during resuscitation. Meyers and co-workers[96] supported these findings in their study of family presence during invasive procedures and resuscitation. Families described their presence as helpful and noted that they would do it again. Instead of functioning as passive observers, families perceived themselves as active participants, caring for the patient with staff. Flexible policies based on the needs and preferences of individual patients and their parents are ideal.

Developmentally appropriate, honest preparation should precede all procedures. It is important to remember that young children's receptive language generally exceeds their expressive language abilities. Simple explanations that can be easily understood are always offered. For parents to be supportive during a procedure, they need to know the importance of the procedure, what to expect during the procedure, normal age-related reactions that may occur, and how they can best help. Parents should not be placed in a position of restraining their child during any procedure.

Parent support is also important when parents choose to excuse themselves during a procedure. It is likely that parents can anticipate the ways that they and their child can best be helped through a given procedure. Parents may need help to articulate the fears that may block their ability to believe that they are the best possible parent under the circumstances. Parents may find it especially difficult to be present during painful procedures because this seems in conflict with their protective and nurturant roles. Parents may benefit from information about their child's developmental level, efforts to prepare the child, and means of pain control, should that be necessary.

Parents also serve as their child's teachers. Using parents as the primary source of information for their children may enhance communication and may also limit misconceptions and misinterpretation. Gutstein and Tarnow[97] found that children's active involvement in preparatory play was significantly related to lower levels of distress after elective surgery. They also found that the child's active involvement in preparatory play with stress-related objects was significantly related to parent helping behaviors. For example, a child may try on several types of oxygen masks if their parent participates in the activity.

When parents must wait during procedures, they often make assumptions that the longer the wait, the more difficult the procedure or that something is wrong. Parents of sick children spend much time waiting together. This can be a source of either comfort or additional stress. Comfort can be had when another parent is one step ahead and can share in the experience "with someone who really understands." Stress can be exacerbated when another family's child is not doing well. Upset and grieving parents require privacy for themselves and for other parents.

Communication. The NMPMC delineates a four-step communication process that is helpful and demonstrates caring toward the parent, assesses parental perceptions, determines the parental agenda, and invites participation in care. This communication process is congruent with the ABCX model of crisis in that nursing interventions should depend on the family's perception of the stressful event. This communication strategy is helpful in the PICU because interventions can be specifically focused when time is limited. In addition, Scott[98] found significant differences in what parents identify as important and what nurses identify as important. When help is rationally directed to what parents identify as important and purposefully focused at the right time, it is perceived as more effective than more help given at a period of less emotional accessibility.

Establish a Caring Relationship. This first aspect adds a humanistic touch by extending the focus of our care to include parents. Asking the parents, for example, "How are you doing? Were you able to sleep?" helps to convey the message that parents, too, are important. An interesting note is that parents often answer queries based on their child's state, for example, "I feel better today. Paul was able to get off his blood pressure medication." Unless assessed and validated, parental affect or behaviors may be misinterpreted in the intensive care setting. For example, a father's body language may be misinterpreted as anger, but when queried, he may remark how scared and upset he feels. Interventions for angry parents versus scared parents are quite different.

Assess Family's Perceptions of the Child's Illness. To assess the parental perception of illness severity, ask, "How does your child look to you today? How serious do you think his illness is? How are other family members dealing with everything?" Here, the nurse builds trust by providing accurate, concise, and complete information and by clarifying any misconceptions. In addition, nurses often make assessments and judgments about a child's pain, activity, and behavior based on PICU experience but without familiarity with an individual child. Parents are often well aware of their child's subtle behavioral and communicative cues that can be helpful in individualizing care. Nurses and parents working together can better understand and address an individual child's needs.

Help Families Participate. The third step helps parents to rank their concerns. It also sanctions the expression of feelings that parents may otherwise consider inappropriate to express. Here, the nurse may ask, "What troubles you most? Do you have any questions? Is this what you expected? Do you have any suggestions or preferences concerning the care your child is receiving? Is there anything that you personally want to do for your child?"

Seek Informed Suggestions and Preferences and Invite Participation in Care. The last step invites parental participation in determining how nursing interventions can be provided. Here, the nurse may ask, "How can I help you? How can we do this together?" Interventions are then focused on parent-specific issues rather than nurse-speculated problems. Note that failure to address a parent's agenda, especially after it has been elicited, may often lead to an increase in stress and parental dissatisfaction.

Providing a humanistic PICU environment that recognizes parents as unique autonomous individuals who, when supported, are capable of providing vital elements of care to their critically ill child helps to alleviate parental stress. The NMPMC is effective in helping to decrease parental stress by assisting parents to formulate a role that is individually comfortable and supportive of them in their decision-making capacity. Not all parents have the desire or capability to actively participate in the care of their child; however, the NMPMC provides a means to assess and individualize psychosocial interventions.

FAMILY CONTEXT OF CHILDHOOD CRITICAL ILLNESS

Traditionally, hospitals have had an approach that emphasizes the treatment of individuals in isolation from their broader family and sociocultural context.[99] By contrast, family-centered care embraces a systems approach in which the child's illness is viewed in context. Family-centered care advocates for the child and family as the appropriate focus of healthcare intervention, thus necessarily broadening the care perspective and traditional interventions.

Entire families are affected when an infant or child is critically ill. Parents find themselves thrust into unfamiliar roles, including negotiating an often overwhelming healthcare setting, integrating information about the child's illness, and participating in emotionally laden decision making.[48,56] Family routines are suddenly disrupted, and traditional roles are altered. In addition, parents must balance multiple demands, including traveling to the hospital or temporarily residing at the hospital, maintaining a home, caring for other children, meeting financial obligations, and negotiating employment circumstances, among others. Parents may feel torn between the needs of children at home and their critically ill child's immediate needs. As described earlier, parents often experience diminished competence and helplessness relative to their critically ill child, and their inability to adequately meet the needs of their healthy children may compound these self-deprecating feelings. This sense of conflict may be long-standing and particularly difficult for parents when their child is chronically critically ill.

To a great extent, families adjust their priorities and family life when a child requires hospitalization. Hospital staff members tend to view parents primarily as parents of a hospitalized child, however, with less than adequate recognition of the parents' broader family, employment, and community responsibilities (see Box 3-7).[9,99] Problems arise, for example, when staff members assume that parents can be available at any time for meetings and care conferences. Similarly, convenient visiting times for parents may conflict with unit rounds or nursing report. Thus flexibility and mutual respect are necessary on the part of both staff and family members to facilitate a collaborative parent-professional partnership.

For the majority of parents, the most important potentially supportive relationship during this time is with their spouse.[56,100] The crisis of critical illness and hospitalization is emotionally charged and represents fertile ground for conflict that may strain even strong spousal relationships. For example, parents may need to come to consensus on issues such as how far to pursue treatment or whether the child's organs may be donated. Aspects of successful adaptation include how parents develop and negotiate their new roles amid the challenges of the PICU and how they manage to support each other. Parents need to communicate with many healthcare providers and with each other, to grapple with potentially difficult ethical decisions, to negotiate being parents with little privacy, and to keep family and friends informed of the child's condition.[101] The unanticipated and fearsome financial burdens inherent in PICU hospitalization may represent an additional, although often unspoken, stressor for parents. Preexisting vulnerabilities in the couple's relationship may be seriously challenged by the child's illness. Spousal conflicts that were present but compensated for before the child's critical illness may now resurface and threaten to disrupt the couple's equilibrium.

Supporting the Siblings of a Critically Ill Child

Siblings of hospitalized infants and children often have concerns and questions regarding the well-being of their brother or sister and their parents.[102,103] Multiple factors influence a sibling's responses and adjustment to critical illness, including the sibling's developmental stage, nature of illness, the sibling's perception of the illness, number and type of other operative stressors, and available situational supports.[104] Children may experience disruption in usual family routines, separation from parents, and changes in caregiving arrangements, all of which may contribute to their degree of stress. Siblings may experience feelings of helplessness, fear, guilt, and anger that they may or may not be able to communicate to parents.[105]

It is not uncommon for parents to request help for siblings who are perceived to be having difficulty coping with the illness. Parents may also wish guidance about how and how much to explain to their children about the illness, visitation in the PICU, ways to meaningfully involve their other children in the hospitalization, and, in some cases, preparation for the child's death. It may be that enlisting supportive services for their other children is more acceptable to parents than the alternative of direct psychologic service for themselves. At the same time, it may also serve to bolster parents in their familiar roles of protector and provider for their children.

In a study investigating the impact of critical care hospitalization on the perceptions of adult patients, spouses, children, and nurses, Titler, Craft, and Cohen[106] noted that parents frequently shielded their children from anxiety-provoking information. Parents perceived that their children, ranging in age from 5 to 18 years of age, did not comprehend much about the parental illness or hospitalization. However, children provided accurate descriptions of the hospitalized parent and of both parents' feelings. These findings suggest that children are keenly aware of illness-related experiences and, to the extent possible, construct their own meanings despite limited access to information and healthcare providers.

Formal sibling programs can be facilitated through collaborative efforts between nurses, child life specialists, and volunteers. Developmentally appropriate interventions are recommended that prepare siblings for what they might see and hear.[107] Educational, supportive visitation programs may include preparation of siblings for visitation, follow-up contact, individual or group activities in the waiting area, and a sibling library.[74,102,108] Children who had the benefit of Facilitated Child Visitation Intervention (FCVI), which includes educational and supportive components, experienced fewer parent-reported behavioral and emotional problems after visitation.[109] Before visitation, children need to be carefully screened for signs of illness and exposure to communicable diseases. Sibling visitation enables children to experience the reality of the situation firsthand and to participate in family problem solving and support of their ill brother or sister.[74,105,107] Overall, sibling visitation can contribute to greater family cohesion, adaptation, and satisfaction.

Professional Relationships

Intervening with families while maintaining appropriate professional nursing boundaries has been addressed by Barnsteiner and Gillis-Donovan.[110] The goal of a professional relationship is to have caring, well-defined boundaries between a nurse and the patient and family, that is, boundaries that are positive and therapeutic and that promote the family's control over the child's healthcare.[111] Professional nursing is emotionally complicated, requiring the ability to stay meaningfully concerned about a patient and family but, at the same time, separate enough to distinguish one's own feelings and needs. Extremes in inappropriate professional relationships include overinvolvement or underinvolvement with individual patients and their families.[112]

Relatively inexperienced nurses and those who are new to the intensive care unit necessarily tend to concentrate on technical skill attainment and mastery rather than psychosocial aspects of care. Within the highly technical and demanding PICU setting, nurses may have little time to devote to psychosocial aspects of care. Moreover, nurses may feel ill-prepared to address the often highly charged emotional aspects of PICU hospitalization. In general, as professionals gain clinical experience, they become increasingly willing and comfortable to formulate collaborative relationships with parents that are consistent with the model of family-centered care.[113]

In a study investigating critical care nurses' perceptions of their role with families, in which 20% were pediatric critical care nurses, Hickey and Lewandowski[114] found that most critical care nurses believed it was emotionally exhausting to repeatedly become involved with families in need of support. Despite this, nurses report becoming involved with families regardless of their ambivalence and the possible emotional costs to themselves. More than one third of the nurses believed that they did not have the requisite knowledge to meet the emotional and psychosocial

needs of families. This underscores the need for ongoing nursing education and collaboration with psychosocial support staff, including advanced practice nurses, social work, pediatric psychology, psychiatry, and child life specialists. Among the factors that most influenced nurses' involvement with families were situations relating to the child's death and subjective feelings and responses toward the patient and family.

Collaborative Relationships With Psychosocial Support Staff

Nursing staff who care directly for the child and family generally have the greatest degree of familiarity and regular contact with families. The role of staff nurses in acknowledging and systematically integrating psychosocial aspects of care, as in the NMPMC, usefully broadens the focus of intervention from the child alone to the child-in-family. Thus nurses play a pivotal role in expanding the traditional medical-technologic orientation and language of the intensive care unit to include psychosocial aspects of care.[115] Through inquiry and attention to parental perceptions and experiences, the nurse emphasizes that these are legitimate aspects of clinical concern and conveys the message that family members, too, are important.

In addition to the nurse's role in psychosocial assessment and intervention, several psychosocial support staff members are available within the intensive care setting who may play a role in psychosocial service delivery to the family (Box 3-8). Social workers are assigned to each family in the ICU and fulfill a varied role, including psychosocial assessment, family support and advocacy, instrumental support, and accessing legal and protective services, if required. Although considerable variability exists among PICUs, other professionals who are available to meet the family's psychosocial needs may include pediatric psychologists, psychiatrists, child life specialists, discharge planners, ethicists, chaplains, child-abuse specialists, and parent volunteers. Appleyard and colleagues[116] described using a nurse-coached volunteer program to help support families of critically ill patients. After implementation of the program, families believed that nurses were more willing to accept families as members of the care team.

In many cases, the nursing staff and unit-based social worker can adequately address the family's psychosocial needs. However, when the child's or family's needs demand additional services or consultation, support staff should be readily incorporated in the psychosocial planning and intervention efforts. Introducing support staff to parents and letting them know that support staff have something valuable to offer for many hospitalized children help to facilitate the consultation process.

The nurse plays a pivotal role in contacting and mobilizing these additional services or consultations when needed on behalf of families. It is important that the nurse have a good working knowledge about the various roles of these disciplines, including what they have to offer families and how they may be consulted.[117] To facilitate psychosocial service delivery and referral, the unit can establish

Box 3-8
Psychosocial Support Staff

Advanced practice nurse/clinical nurse specialist
• Assesses family coping capacities
• Provides short-term family support
• Consults with staff regarding expected trajectory of parental stress and coping and interventions with families in crisis related to the critical illness of their child

Social worker
• Performs psychosocial family assessments
• Provides family support and advocacy
• Promotes client access to financial and community services
• Serves as liaison with child protection team

Child life specialist
• Provides developmental and therapeutic play activities
• Supports patient and sibling coping
• Consults with parents regarding normal child development and adjustment
• Initiates tutoring referrals

Patient care coordinator
• Facilitates comprehensive discharge plan
• Serves as liaison for family with third-party payers
• Performs utilization review
• Accesses community support services for family

Psychologist, psychiatrist
• Performs diagnostic assessments of children and families
• Facilitates management and discharge planning of suicidal patients
• Provides short-term family counseling
• Provides crisis intervention
• Facilitates psychopharmacology referrals

Parent volunteer
• Welcomes family to the PICU
• Orients parents to the family area
• Assures family comfort in the waiting area
• Provides information about hospital resources (meals, telephone, sleep facilities, etc.)

Chaplain
• Provides spiritual support
• Performs sacraments as requested by family (e.g., baptism)

Ethics committee
• Consults with families and staff on ethical issues
• Educates staff about ethical and legal issues

regular psychosocial rounds in which representatives from these disciplines are present. Note that ancillary personnel may provide direct service to children and families or may merely consult with nursing and social work staff in the context of psychosocial rounds. An organizational chart that delineates the various roles and collaborative relationships of psychosocial support staff and details regarding contact and referral information can be helpful.

PREPARING FOR PATIENT TRANSFER

Transition from the intensive care setting to a general hospital unit or to home can be fraught with apprehension. On one hand, parents may derive comfort from the fact that their child has achieved another step toward recovery.[51,52,60]

On the other hand, the transfer requires adjustment to new staff members who do not yet know their child and to a new environment. Parents may be concerned about their child's readiness for transfer or the lower staff-to-patient ratio on the prospective unit. Parents who have come to trust the PICU staff members may be reluctant to reinitiate the process with yet another set of healthcare providers. Anticipatory guidance to assist parents in the transition from the PICU to the general inpatient unit may help to alleviate parental stress related to PICU discharge. Bouve, Rozmus, and Giordano[118] demonstrated that a straightforward preparatory letter explaining the impending transfer from the PICU to a general pediatric floor significantly lowered parental anxiety. Parents need to know that the staff of the receiving unit will be fully informed about the child's history and progress, preferably by the primary nurse or another staff member who knows the child well. This not only ensures optimal clinical care but also reduces parental anxiety about the transfer.

Formal care conferences that involve the PICU primary nurse, family members, and a nurse from the receiving unit have also been demonstrated to significantly reduce the transfer-related anxiety of families.[119] In this particular study, the care conference lasted 15 to 30 minutes and consisted of three phases. First, there were introductions and a discussion about the purpose of the meeting. Second, the group discussed the physical environment of the new unit and the child's degree of recovery and progress and addressed mutual goals and expectations. The third phase provided an opportunity for the group to establish child-centered goals. Conferences such as these serve to mark the transfer from the PICU as a significant event and have the advantage of focused communication, mutual goal setting, and parent participation.

BEREAVEMENT

The death of a child is one of the most stressful and traumatic events that a family may ever experience and endure.[120-122] The death of a young child is generally perceived in our society as unnatural, untimely, and particularly tragic. Compared with other deaths, the grief of parents can be particularly severe, complicated, and long lasting as a result of the nature of the parent-child relationship, the circumstances of the death, and societal expectations.[122,123] Parents typically remember the events surrounding the child's death, including the responses of healthcare providers, with great clarity, detail, and emotion.[120,124-126] The immediate responses and subsequent adjustment of bereaved parents are significantly influenced by the attitudes, psychosocial interventions, and bereavement support offered by healthcare professionals.[121,127,128] Thus positive experiences in the intensive care setting have the potential to facilitate parental bereavement and adjustment, whereas negative experiences may compromise or even derail the parental bereavement and coping process.

Stage models of grief and bereavement have been proposed,[129,130] including an adaptation specifically for parents who have suffered the loss of a child.[121,131-133] Expanding on Parkes' original model, Miles[131,132] has usefully described three broad phases of parental grief, including numbness and shock, intense grief, and reorganization. Although stage models offer a "blueprint" with which to understand the bereavement process, it is important to recognize the inherent limitations of linear models to fully explain such complex processes.[100] How intense and enduring the pain of bereavement is for any given parent is more a function of idiopathic factors rather than the mere passage of time.

In the intensive care setting, parents may experience emotional turmoil and anticipatory grief before the child's death and a combination of disbelief, shock, and intense grief responses upon the death of the child. In retrospective semistructured interviews conducted 1 to 3 years after their children's deaths, parents frequently reported "numbness," accompanied by difficulty integrating information, listening to healthcare providers, and making decisions during the time at the hospital.[125] Initial emotional and behavioral responses vary greatly among parents, depending on personality style, sociocultural background, social support, and circumstances of the death.[122,131,132] Emotionally, parents may experience sadness, despair, anger, rage, regret, frustration, guilt, resentment, or relief, among others. Behavioral responses may include crying, withdrawal, hysteria, or physical acting out, such as clinging to the child's dead body or aggression toward objects or people.[133] During the subsequent phase of intense grief, parents may experience intense loneliness and yearning for the child, helplessness, guilt, anger, fearfulness for the safety and well-being of other children, depressive symptoms such as sleep and appetite changes, and disorganization.[121] During the reorganization phase, bereaved parents gradually begin to remember the child with less emotional pain, commemorate the child and focus on happier memories, reinvest in new relationships, and return to their usual life activities and responsibilities. Some bereaved parents report that they never truly recover from the death of their child, but rather that they learn to go on and, as a result of the loss, they can never truly be the same persons again.[120]

When the decision has been made to discontinue intensive treatment efforts and the child's death has been declared imminent, the burden of comfort care rests with the nursing staff.[134] During this time, the priorities for nursing intervention include comfort and dignity for the dying infant or child and his or her family.[135] The most important aspects of care for families during this time is to demonstrate a caring and genuine attitude, to extend kindness and understanding, and to be present with the family.[121,122,125,136] Although nurses sometimes worry about what to say and specifically how to say it to families, a caring and genuine approach is most important and more likely to be remembered by families than any particular thing that might be said. Johnson and Mattson[137] have addressed the issue of communication with families before and after the child's death, including suggestions for open-ended questions and responses that may be helpful to families and anxiety containing for nurses.[137] Key elements of parent-professional communication at the end of life include validation of feelings, empathy, and support.

Nurses do indeed help to "orchestrate" the death and early bereavement process for families in the context of the hospital setting. When curative interventions become futile, care shifts to ensure death with dignity and comfort. Suggestions for intervention include providing accurate and ongoing information to parents, preparing parents for what to expect relative to the child's bodily functions and the dying process, and listening to and honoring parental stories about the child and parental expressions of grief.[121,125] Parents often need and seek reassurance from nursing staff that everything possible has been done for the child and that the child will not experience pain. Parents remember and acknowledge the importance of caring for the child with respect, addressing the child by name, attending to the "little kindnesses" (e.g., combing the child's hair), welcoming family members and friends, and individualizing aspects of care according to the family's wishes (e.g., child wearing own pajamas, favorite sleeping positions). Nurses may facilitate referrals for hospital chaplains; however, parents emphasize that it is important to be given a choice about this beforehand.[125]

Choices about whether and how to hold and view the body during discontinuation of life support equipment and following death are highly individual decisions for parents that are remembered long after the death. Parents should be offered an explanation of how life support is discontinued (e.g., child will be extubated), including what they can expect and who, if anyone, may be in attendance, according to their wishes. Parents report that viewing the child's dead body serves as a means of closure.[125] Parents may also like the infant's footprints, lock of hair, or hospital identification band as keepsakes. The parents' final good-bye to staff and exit from the unit, with its symbolic finality, may be eased with the escort of a familiar nurse.

Some units have developed standardized care plans for terminally ill patients that may be modified according to the child's circumstances and family wishes.[136] Care plans such as these serve to assist nursing staff in delivering comprehensive care, facilitate the psychosocial aspects of care, coordinate communication and referrals, and ensure individualized aspects of care. Guidelines such as these help the staff to orchestrate the many aspects of providing care to a dying child and also ease the burden on individual nurses. In addition, in an effort to provide the best practice and to support families during the early bereavement process, many hospitals have implemented bereavement support and follow-up programs.[138-140] In general, families and staff alike note the benefits of bereavement support programs as a means to cope with childhood death. Educational and support programs, designed specifically to address the needs of staff nurses, have also been developed with the goals of better preparing nurses for caring for dying children and their families and preventing "bereavement overload."[141-143]

SUMMARY

Continued nursing research is needed to describe the possible differences in perceived parental stress in relation to the age of the parent and in relation to a constant primary nurse provider and the trajectory of parental involvement in relation to the child's clinical status. Studies investigating the relationship between nursing staff attitudes toward parental involvement on parental stress and participation in care are also needed. Studies that illuminate how specific parental involvement can be therapeutic in the PICU setting can guide clinical practice. Few studies describe the long-term effects of PICU hospitalization on parents and children.

Pediatric critical care nurses must continue to challenge and improve traditional practice. Nurses traditionally serve as the gatekeepers, that is, the people who directly control parental access and involvement with their children. Parents are the ultimate consumers of pediatric healthcare. It is imperative that parental- and consumer-driven satisfaction be accomplished to economically survive in a highly competitive healthcare delivery system. Care must be inherently supportive to parents. Parental involvement must be encouraged and welcomed because family-centered care implies an ongoing parent–professional partnership, not merely that 24-hour visitation is allowed.[51,60] Nurses must continue to accept the challenge of developing strategies that assess parental needs, establish therapeutic nurse-parent relationships, provide care that is flexible and individualized, and support the parents' role in the care of their critically ill child. Nurses can make a significant positive difference for parents of critically ill children. By providing care that is inherently supportive to parents, we help to make the experience of parent-to-a-critically-ill-child as positive as possible.

REFERENCES

1. Robertson J: *Young children in hospitals,* Great Britain, 1958, Tavistock Publications.
2. Bruce B, Ritchie J: Nurses' practices and perceptions of family-centered care, *J Pediatr Nurs* 12:214-222, 1997.
3. Chesla CA, Stannard D: Breakdown in the nursing care of families in the ICU, *Am J Crit Care* 6:64-71, 1997.
4. Bowlby J: *Maternal care and mental health,* Geneva, 1952, World Health Organization.
5. Bowlby J: *Attachment and loss,* vol 2, *separation,* New York, 1973, Basic Books.
6. Shelton TL, Stepanek JS: *Family-centered care for children needing specialized health and developmental services,* ed 3, Bethesda, Md, 1994, Association for the Care of Children's Health.
7. Ahmann E: Family-centered care: the time has come, *Pediatr Nurs* 20:52-53, 1994.
8. Shelton TL: Family-centered care in pediatric practice: when and how? *J Dev Behav Pediatr* 20:117-118, 1999.
9. Meyer EC, Bailey DB: Family-centered care in early intervention: community and hospital settings. In Paul JL, Simeonsson RJ, eds: *Children with special needs: family, culture, and society,* New York, 1993, Harcourt Brace Jovanovich College Publishers.
10. Rushton CH: Family-centered care in the critical care setting: myth or reality? *Child Health Care* 19:68-78, 1990.
11. Zaner RM, Bliton MJ: Decisions in the NICU: the moral authority of parents, *Child Health Care* 20:19-25, 1991.
12. Bogdan R, Brown MA, Foster SB: Be honest but not cruel: staff/parent communication on a neonatal unit, *Human Organ* 41:6-16, 1982.
13. Curley MAQ: Mutuality: an expression of nursing presence, *J Pediatr Nurs* 12:1-6, 1997.
14. Mitchell PH, Ferketich S, Jennings BM: American Academy of Nursing Expert Panel on Quality Health Care, *Image J Nurs Sch* 30:43-46, 1997.
15. Shelton TL, Jeppson ES, Johnson BH: *Family centered care for children with special health care needs,* ed 2, Washington, DC, 1987, Association for the Care of Children's Health.
16. *Current population reports,* Washington, DC, 1991, Department of Commerce, Economics and Statistics.
17. Garcia Coll CT, Meyer EC, Brillon L: Ethnic and minority parenting. In Bornstein MH, ed: *Handbook of parenting,* vol II, Mahwah, NJ, 1995, Lawrence Erlbaum Associates.
18. United States Bureau of Census: *US children and their families: current conditions and recent trends. Projections: 1988-2080.* Washington, DC, 1989, Government Printing Office.
19. United States Bureau of Census: US population estimates by age, sex, race and Hispanic origin, 1980-1988, *Current Population Reports,* Series P-25, No 1045. Washington, DC, 1990, US Government Printing Office.
20. Berger MM, ed: *Beyond the double bind: communication and family systems, theories, and techniques with schizophrenics,* New York, 1978, Brunner/Mazel.
21. von Bertalanffy L: *General systems theory,* New York, 1968, George Braziller.
22. Bowen M: *Family therapy in clinical practice,* New York, 1978, Jason Aronson.
23. Minuchin S: *Families and family therapy,* Cambridge, Mass, 1974, Harvard University Press.
24. Watzlawick P, Beavin JH, Jackson DD: *Pragmatics of human communication,* New York, 1967, WW Norton & Company.
25. Mahler MS, Pine F, Bergman A: *The psychological birth of the human infant,* New York, 1975, Basic Books.
26. Rothstein P: Psychological stress in families of children in the pediatric intensive care unit, *Pediatr Clin North Am* 27:613-620, 1980.
27. Miles MS: Impact of the intensive care unit on parents, *Issues Compr Pediatr Nurs* 3:72-90, 1979.
28. Youngblut JM, Jay SS: Emergent admission to the pediatric intensive care unit: parental concerns, *AACN Clin Issues Crit Care Nurs* 2:329-337, 1991.
29. Comoroff J, Maguire P: Ambiguity and the search for meaning: childhood leukaemia in the modern clinical context, *Soc Sci Med* 15B:115-123, 1981.
30. Mishel MH: Parent's perception of uncertainty concerning their hospitalized child, *Nurs Res* 32:324-330, 1983.
31. Turner MA, Tomlinson PS, Harbaugh BL: Parental uncertainty in critical care hospitalization of children, *MCN Am J Matern Child Nurs* 19:45-62, 1990.
32. Skipper JK, Leonard RC: Children, stress, and hospitalization, *J Health Soc Behav* 9:275-287, 1968.
33. Hebb DO: *Textbook of psychology,* ed 3, Philadelphia, 1972, WB Saunders.
34. Wolfer JA, Visintainer MA: Pediatric surgical patients' and parents' stress responses and adjustment, *Nurs Res* 24:244-255, 1975.
35. Mitchell PH, Johnson FB, Habermann Little B: Promoting physiologic stability: touch and ICP, *Communicat Nurs Res* 18:93, 1985.
36. Zeskind PS, Iacino R: Effects of maternal visitation to preterm infants in the neonatal intensive care unit, *Child Develop* 55:1887-1893, 1984.
37. Anderson GC: Current knowledge about skin-to-skin (kangaroo) care for preterm infants, *J Perinatol* 11:216-226, 1991.
38. Hill R: *Families under stress.* New York, 1949, Harper & Row.
39. Youngblut JM, Shiao SYP: Characteristics of a child's critical illness and parents' reactions: preliminary report of a pilot study, *Am J Crit Care* 1:80-84, 1992.
40. Broome ME: Working with the family of a critically ill child, *Heart Lung* 14:368-372, 1985.
41. McCubbin HI, Patterson JM: Family transitions: adaptation to stress. In McCubbin HI, Figley CR, eds: *Stress and the family: coping with normative transitions,* vol 1, New York, 1983, Brunner/Mazel.
42. Moos RH: *Coping with life crises: an integrated approach,* 1986, New York, 1986, Plenum Medical Books.
43. Lazarus RS, Folkman S: *Stress, appraisal, and coping,* New York, 1984, Springer.
44. Miles MS, Carter MC: Coping strategies used by parents during their child's hospitalization in an intensive care unit, *Child Health Care* 14:14-21, 1985.

45. LaMontagne LL, Pawlak R: Stress and coping of parents of children in a pediatric intensive care unit, *Heart Lung* 19:416-421, 1990.

46. LaMontagne LL, Hepworth JT, Pawlak R et al: Parental coping and activities during pediatric critical care, *Am J Crit Care* 1:76-80, 1992.

47. Philichi LM: Family adaptation during a pediatric intensive care hospitalization, *J Pediatr Nurs* 4:268-276, 1989.

48. Miles MS, Carter MC: Sources of parental stress in pediatric intensive care units, *Child Health Care* 11:65-69, 1982.

49. Carter MC, Miles MS, Buford TH et al: Parental environmental stress in pediatric intensive care units, *Dimens Crit Care Nurs* 4:180-188, 1985.

50. Eberly TW, Miles MS, Carter MC et al: Parental stress after the unexpected admission of a child to the intensive care unit, *Crit Care Q* 8:57-65, 1985.

51. Curley MAQ: Effects of the nursing mutual participation model of care and parental stress in the pediatric intensive care unit, unpublished master's thesis, New Haven, Conn, 1987, Yale University School of Nursing.

52. Curley MAQ, Wallace J: Effects of the nursing mutual participation model of care on parental stress in the pediatric intensive care unit: a replication, *J Pediatr Nurs* 7:377-385, 1992.

53. Miles MS, Carter MC, Spicher C et al: Maternal and paternal stress reactions when a child is hospitalized in a pediatric intensive care unit, *Issues Compr Pediatr Nurs* 7:333-342, 1984.

54. Seideman RY, Watson MA, Corff KE et al: Parent stress and coping in NICU and PICU, *J Pediatr Nurs* 12:169-177, 1997.

55. Rennick J: Reestablishing the parental role in a pediatric intensive care unit, *J Pediatr Nurs* 1:40-44, 1986.

56. Harrison H: *The premature baby book: a parent's guide to coping and caring in the first years,* New York, 1983, St Martin's Press.

57. Minde KK: The impact of prematurity on the later behavior of children and their families, *Clin Perinatol* 11:227-244, 1984.

58. Resnick MB, Eyler FD, Nelson RM et al: Developmental outcome for low birthweight infants: improved early developmental outcome, *Pediatrics* 80:68-74, 1987.

59. Jay SS: Pediatric intensive care involving parents in the care of their child, *MCN Am J Matern Child Nurs* 6:195-204, 1977.

60. Curley MAQ: Effects of the nursing mutual participation model of care and parental stress in the pediatric intensive care unit, *Heart Lung* 17:682-688, 1988.

61. Pass MD, Pass CM: Anticipatory guidance for parents of hospitalized children, *J Pediatr Nurs* 2:250-258, 1987.

62. Miles MS, Mathes M: Preparation of parents for the ICU experience: what are we missing, *Child Health Care* 20:132-137, 1991.

63. Lewandowski LA: Stressors and coping styles of parents of children undergoing open heart surgery, *Crit Care Q* 3:75-84, 1980.

64. Kirschbaum MS: *Needs of parents of critically ill children,* unpublished master's thesis, 1983, University of Illinois.

65. Kirschbaum MS: Needs of parents of critically ill children, *Dimens Crit Care Nurs* 9:344-352, 1990.

66. Melnyk BM, Alpert-Gillis L, Hensel PB et al: Helping mothers cope with a critically ill child: a pilot test of the COPE intervention, *Res Nurs Health* 20:3-14, 1997.

67. Melnyk BM, Alpert-Gillis LJ: The COPE program: a strategy to improve outcomes of critically ill young children and their parents, *Pediatr Nurs* 24:521-527, 1998.

68. Farrel MJ, Frost C: The most important needs of parents of critically ill children: parents' perceptions, *Intens Crit Care Nurs* 8:1-10, 1993.

69. Kasper J, Nyamathi A: Parents of children in the pediatric intensive care unit: what are their needs? *Heart Lung* 17, 574-581, 1988.

70. Jay SS, Youngblut JM: Parent stress associated with pediatric critical care nursing: linking research with practice, *AACN Clin Issues Crit Care Nurs* 2:276-284, 1991.

71. Tughan L: Visiting in the PICU: a study of the perceptions of patients, parents, and staff members, *Crit Care N Q* 15:57-68, 1992.

72. Proctor DL: Relationship between visitation policy in a pediatric intensive unit and parental anxiety, *Child Health Care* 16:13-17, 1987.

73. Carnevale FA: Striving to recapture our previous life: the experience of families with critically ill children, *Off J Can Assoc Crit Care Nurs* 10:16-22, 1999.

74. Wincek JM: Promoting family-centered visitation makes a difference, *AACN Clin Issues Crit Care Nurs* 2:293-298, 1991.

75. Miles MS: Vigilance as a parental coping strategy when a child is seriously ill. Abstract for poster presentation. Biennial meeting of the Society for Research in Child Development, Baltimore, Md, 1987.

76. Halm M: Effects of support groups on anxiety of family members during critical illness, *Heart Lung* 19:62-71, 1990.

77. Beckham JD: Andrew's not-so-excellent adventure, *Healthcare Forum J* 36:90-98, 1993.

78. Jacono J, Hicks G, Antonioni C et al: Comparison of perceived needs of family members between registered nurses and family members of critically ill patients in intensive care and neonatal intensive care unit, *Heart Lung* 19:72-78, 1990.

79. Johnson PA, Nelson GL, Brunnquell DJ: Parent and nurse perceptions of parental stress in the pediatric intensive care unit, *Child Health Care* 17:98-105, 1988.

80. Hayes VE, Knox JE: The experience of stress in parents of children hospitalized with long-term disabilities, *J Adv Nurs* 9:333-341, 1984.

81. Molter NC: Needs of relatives of critically ill patients: a descriptive study, *Heart Lung* 8:332-339, 1979.

82. Szasz TS, Hollender MH: A contribution to the philosophy of medicine, *Arch Intern Med* 97:585-592, 1956.

83. Brody DS: The patient's role in clinical decision making, *Ann Internal Med* 93:718-722, 1980.

84. Greeneich DS, Long CO: Using a model to assess family satisfaction, *Dimens Crit Care Nurs* 12:272-278, 1993.

85. Henneman EA, McKenzie JB, Dewa JB et al: An evaluation of interventions for meeting the informational needs of families of chronically ill patients, *Am J Crit Care* 1:85-93, 1992.

86. Fisher DH, Stanford G, Dorman DJ: Services for parental stress reduction in a pediatric ICU, *Crit Care Med* 12:504-507, 1984.

87. Hamilton DK: Design for flexibility in critical care, *New Horiz* 7:205-217, 1999.

88. McNamara ST, Meyer EC, Fraser KA et al: In the middle of the night: a psychosocial resource book for after hours, *J Emerg Nurs* 23:68-69, 1997.

89. Rubin R: Attainment of the maternal role, *Nurs Res* 16:83-91, 16:324-346, 1967.

90. Macnab AJ, Emerton-Downey J, Phillips N et al: Purpose of family photographs displayed in the pediatric intensive care unit, *Heart Lung* 26:68-75, 1997.

91. Vulcan BM, Nikulich-Barrett M: The effect of selected information on mothers' anxiety levels during their children's hospitalization, *J Pediatr Nurs* 3:97-102, 1988.

92. Rowe J: Making oneself at home? Examining the nurse-parent relationship, *Contemp Nurs* 5:101-106, 1996.

93. Sevedra M: Parental responses to a painful procedure performed on their child. In Azarnoff P, Hardgrove C, eds: *The family in child health care,* New York, 1981, John Wiley & Sons.

94. Shaw EG, Routh DK: Effect of mother's presence on children's reactions to aversive procedures, *J Pediatr Psychol* 7:33-42, 1982.

95. Robinson SM, Mackenzie-Ross S, Campbell Hewson GL et al: Psychological effect of witnessed resuscitation on bereaved relatives, *Lancet* 352:614-617, 1998.

96. Meyers TA, Erichhorn DJ, Guzzetta CE et al: Family presence during invasive procedures and resuscitation, *Am J Nurs* 100:32-42, 2000.

97. Gutstein SE, Tarnow JD: Parental facilitation of children's preparatory play behavior in a stressful situation, *J Abnormal Psychol* 11:181-191, 1983.

98. Scott LD: Perceived needs of parents of critically ill children. *J Soc Pediatr Nurs* 3:4-12, 1998.

99. Gilkerson L: Understanding institutional functioning style: a resource for hospital and early intervention collaboration, *Infants Young Children* 2:22-30, 1990.

100. Featherstone H: *A difference in the family: living with a disabled child,* New York, 1980, Basic Books.

101. Meyer EC, Zeanah CH, Boukydis CFZ et al: A clinical interview for parents of high-risk infants: concept and applications, *Infant Mental Health J* 14:192-207, 1993.

102. Doll-Speck L, Miller B, Rohrs K: Sibling education: implementing a program in the NICU, *Neonatal Netw* 12:49-52, 1993.

103. Maloney MJ, Ballard JL, Hollister L et al: A prospective, controlled study of scheduled sibling visits to a newborn intensive care unit, *J Am Acad Child Psychiatry* 22:565-570, 1983.

104. Lewandowski LA: Needs of children during the critical illness of a parent or sibling, *Crit Care Clin North Am* 4:573-585, 1992.

105. Newman CB, McSweeney M: A descriptive study of sibling visitation in the NICU, *Neonatal Netw* 9:27-31, 1990.

106. Titler M, Craft M, Cohen M: Impact of a critical care hospitalization: perceptions of patients, spouses, children, and nurses, *Heart Lung* 17:314-315, 1988.

107. Craft MT, Wyatt N: Effect of visitation upon siblings of hospitalized children, *MCN Am J Matern Child Nurs* 15:47-59, 1986.

108. Rushton CH, Booth P: The role of siblings during pediatric hospitalization. Presented at the 21st Annual Association for the Care of Children's Health Conference, San Francisco, Calif, 1986.

109. Nicholson AC, Titler MG, Montgomery LA et al: Effects of child visitation in adult critical care units: a pilot study, *Heart Lung* 22:36-45, 1993.

110. Barnsteiner J, Gillis-Donovan J: Being related and separate: a standard for therapeutic relationships, *MCN Am J Matern Child Nurs* 15:223-228, 1990.

111. McKlindon D, Barnsteiner JH: Therapeutic relationships: evolution of the Children's Hospital of Philadelphia model, *MCN Am J Matern Child Nurs* 24:237-243, 1999.

112. Barnsteiner JH, Gillis-Donovan J, Knox-Fischer C et al: Defining and implementing a standard for therapeutic relationships, *J Holistic Nurs* 12:35-49, 1994.

113. Gill KM: Health professionals' attitudes toward parent participation in hospitalized children's care, *Child Health Care* 22:257-271, 1993.

114. Hickey M, Lewandowski L: Critical care nurses' role with families: a descriptive study, *Heart Lung* 17:670-676, 1988.

115. Als H: Individualized, family focused developmental care for the very low birthweight preterm infant in the NICU. In Friedman SL, Sigman M, eds: *Advances in applied developmental psychology: the psychological development of low birthweight children,* Norwood, NJ, 1992, Ablex.

116. Appleyard ME, Gavaghan SR, Gonzalez C et al: Nurse-coached intervention for the families of patients in critical care units, *Crit Care Nurs* 20:40-48, 2000.

117. Harvey MA, Ninos NP, Adler D et al: Results of the consensus conference on fostering more humane critical care: creating a healing environment, *AACN Clin Issues Crit Care Nurs* 4:484-507, 1993.

118. Bouve LR, Rozmus CL, Giordano P: Preparing parents for their child's transfer from the PICU to the pediatric floor, *Appl Nurs Res* 12:114-120, 1999.

119. Bokinskie JC: Family conferences: a method to diminish transfer anxiety, *J Neurosci Nurs* 24:129-133, 1992.

120. Schiff HS: *The bereaved parent,* New York, 1977, Crown.

121. Miles MS, Perry K: Parental responses to sudden accidental death of a child, *Crit Care Q* 8:73-82, 1985.

122. Rando TA: *Parental loss of a child,* Champaign, Ill, 1986, Research Press Company.

123. Sanders CM: A comparison of adult bereavement in the death of a spouse, child, and parent, *Omega* 10:303-322, 1978-1980.

124. Fischoff J, O'Brien N: After the child dies, *J Pediatr* 88:140-146, 1976.

125. Jost KE, Haase JE: At the time of death: help for the child's parents, *Child Health Care* 18:146-152, 1989.

126. Strom-Paikin J: Our son is dead, *Nurs Life* 4:18-20, 1984.

127. Cauthorne CV: Coping with death in the emergency department, *J Emerg Nurs* 1:24-26, 1975.

128. Wortman CB, Silver RC: The myths of coping with loss. *J Consult Clin Psychol* 57:349-357, 1989.

129. Kubler-Ross E: *On death and dying,* New York, 1969, Macmillan.

130. Parkes CM: Bereavement and mental illness: a classification for bereavement reactions, *Br J Med Psychol* 38:13-26, 1965.

131. Miles MS: *The grief of parents when a child dies,* Oak Brook, Ill, 1980, Compassionate Friends.

132. Miles MS: Helping adults mourn the death of a child. In Wass H, Corr C, eds: *Children and death,* New York, 1984, Hemisphere.

133. Miles MS: Emotional symptoms and physical health in bereaved parents, *Nurs Res* 34:76-81, 1985.

134. Davies B, Eng B: Factors influencing nursing care of children who are terminally ill: a selective review, *Pediatr Nurs* 19:9-14, 1993.

135. Henneman E: Multidisciplinary care plan for the dying patient: a strategy to promote humane caring in ICU, *AACN Clin Issues Crit Care Nurs* 4:527, 1993.

136. Mendyka BE: The dying patient in the intensive care unit: assisting the family in crisis, *AACN Clin Issues Crit Care Nurs* 4:550-557, 1993.

137. Johnson L, Mattson S: Communication: the key to crisis intervention in pediatric death, *Crit Care Nurse* 12:23-27, 1992.

138. Johnson LC, Rincon B, Gober C et al: The development of a comprehensive bereavement program to assist families experiencing pediatric loss, *J Pediatr Nurs* 8:142-146, 1993.

139. McClelland ML: Our unit has a bereavement program, *Am J Nurs* 93:62-68, 1993.

140. Murphy SA: Preventive intervention following the accidental death of a child, *Image J Nurs Sch* 22:174-179, 1990.

141. Pazola K: Remembrance: a strategy to prevent bereavement overload, *Caring* 4, Winter 1988.

142. Richmond T, Craig M: Timeout: facing death in the ICU, *Dimens Critl Care Nurs* 4:41-45, 1985.

143. Vachon MLS: *Occupational stress in the care of the critically ill, the dying, and the bereaved,* New York, 1987, Hemisphere Publishing.

II

The Practice Environment

This section focuses on the milieu affecting nursing care delivery. The broadening professional responsibilities of the pediatric critical care nurse as leader, teacher, mentor, and advocate are acknowledged and supported.

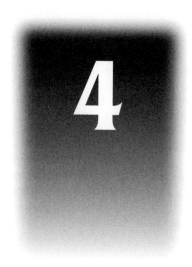

4 Leadership in Pediatric Critical Care

Mary J. Fagan

CURRENT CHALLENGES

EFFECTIVE LEADERSHIP
  Vision and Values
  Teamwork
  Conflict Resolution
  Empowerment and Accountability
  Coaching
  Assertive Communication
  Systems Thinking
  Listening to People
  Building Morale
  Stress Management
  Time Management
  Measuring Success

SUMMARY

A world-class pediatric intensive care unit—what does this mean and how is it achieved? Is it the technical skill of the staff? Is it the amount of research that is being done? Is it the physician talent? The answer is that none of these attributes, if taken in isolation, will create a world-class organization. Excellence is achieved through a combination of many factors, and it is highly dependent on effective leadership. The quality of the leadership is the most important component in determining whether a pediatric critical care unit (PICU) will stand out as being one of the best in the world, especially in this era of incredible change.

CURRENT CHALLENGES

The twenty-first century finds healthcare and nursing in a tumultuous state. Times have been tough, and they appear to be getting tougher. Never has the need for effective front-line leadership been more dramatic than it is today.

The 1990s presented an era of healthcare cost cutting to survive in the world of managed care. Organizations were forced to merge or reorganize and reengineer to drive out cost in the face of declining reimbursement. Turnaround efforts, largely led by outside consultants, engineered average cuts in clinical staff expenses by more than 60% and nursing department cuts by as much as 25% in an attempt to mend the bottom line.[1]

In the wake of these cutbacks, serious questions about quality of care in hospitals have been being raised. A New York State Nurses Association study found that 52% of the nurses responding believed that patient care was either minimally safe or not safe at all.[1] Responding to these concerns, many states passed legislation or were considering legislation creating mandatory nursing staff ratios. Nursing unionization activity was at an all-time high.

Nurses, physicians, and consumers all described inadequacies in care, while hospital administrators remained concerned with worsening margins. This left nurses feeling "beat up" by dissatisfied families and physicians and by the hospital's need to cut costs. Overall, stress levels were high, and morale was low. In fact, one study ranked posttraumatic stress disorder (PTSD) symptoms across disciplines and found intensive care unit (ICU) nurses to have the highest rate of all groups studied, ahead of Israeli soldiers and Vietnam veterans with PTSD.[2]

Lastly, a major nursing shortage looms. Nursing vacancy and turnover rates are on the rise, and open positions are being filled at alarming rates by inexperienced staff or new graduates. Vacancies are especially evident in areas that are highly specialized, such as Pediatric Critical Care. With the national average age of a registered nurse (RN) at 44.3 and rising, an even larger number of RNs will be leaving the profession in the coming years. This, coupled with the fact that nursing school enrollments in bachelor of science in nursing (BSN) programs are on the decline, has a lot of people worried.

Massive efforts have been instituted to recruit experienced nurses from one hospital to another. Sign-on bonuses and pay incentives have led to full-scale bidding wars for some positions.

Studies have demonstrated that improving manager leadership behaviors is more likely than any other intervention to improve retention of hospital nurses.[3] However, the dilemma is that most nurses who are promoted to leadership positions have exceptionally strong clinical skills. Their success at the bedside has led to promotion to a position of authority. Unfortunately, the skills that are required to be a great leader are not necessarily clinical in nature. This chapter describes some of the attributes and methods for developing strong leadership skills.

EFFECTIVE LEADERSHIP

Leadership is defined as "a relational process of bringing people together attempting to accomplish change or make a difference to benefit the common good."[4] It encompasses a broad spectrum of attributes, including those discussed next.

Vision and Values

The type of leadership necessary to support a world-class critical care department begins with a positive vision of the future. A vision is a clear mental picture of a desired future outcome. To emphasize the importance of a clear vision, Flaherty and Stark[5] describe the process of putting together a 1000-piece jigsaw puzzle. The picture on the top of the box is the end result or the vision of what is to be accomplished. It is much more difficult, if not impossible, to put a jigsaw puzzle together without ever looking at the picture. Trying to lead a group without a vision is like trying to put together a jigsaw puzzle without ever looking at the picture.

A good vision is clear and compelling. It works like a magnet, pulling people toward it. As the vision provides a clear picture of where to go, values provide the how. They provide the road map of how to achieve the vision. For example, the critical care unit at Children's Hospital in San Diego has articulated the following vision and values:

> We envision a critical care unit which is acknowledged as one of the world's premiere providers of pediatric critical care. Continuous learning and teamwork are the foundation upon which we develop our expertise. Our success is a result of the dedication and commitment of each member of our team to the work we do, the people we serve, and each other.

If an entire department shares the same vision and makes decisions on how to operationalize the vision based on the same set of consistent values, success will follow.

So how do leaders facilitate the process of establishing a shared vision? According to Senge,[6] shared visions emanate from personal visions. He encourages leaders to give up the traditional notion that visions must come from the top of an organization or that it is appropriate for the leaders to go off and write a "vision statement" that will then be shared with and adopted by others. Although shared visions may come from the top of an organization, Senge suggests visions that are truly shared take time to emerge and are most often the result of ongoing conversations, wherein people feel free to discuss their dreams and are inspired to truly listen to the dreams of others. People need not give up their personal visions; instead, over time and work, multiple visions begin to coexist, and shared visions are the result.

Senge[6] sees the development of a shared vision as one piece of a set of "governing ideas" that are necessary for organizations. These include the organization's vision, purpose or mission, and core values. A vision that is not consistent with the values people live from day to day will not be successful. The governing ideas are simply the answers to three basic questions: "What?" "Why?" and "How?" The vision is the "what," the purpose or mission is the "why," and the core values are the "how."

Teamwork

Aligning people into high-performing teams is an imperative to be a world-class department or organization. Common characteristics define these groups and set them apart from others. They demonstrate a participative leadership style that empowers members, a shared responsibility for group activities and their outcomes, an alignment of purpose with clearly delineated group goals, high levels of communication characterized by mutual trust and respect, a future focus, a task focus, encouragement and support of creative talents, and a penchant for rapid responses.

The landmark APACHE study demonstrated just how important teamwork is in overall critical care unit performance.[7] It studied adult critical care units that were stratified on the basis of severity-based outcomes. Significant variations in actual versus predicted mortality rates were apparent between the highest-performing units and the underachievers. Researchers evaluated many factors, including presence or absence of a board-certified attending physician, fellowship programs, size of departments, university affiliations, and percentage of RNs with CCRN status and found none to be significantly correlated with the results. The differences were largely explainable, however, by the level of teamwork between caregivers, especially nurses and physicians. The APACHE study demonstrated that effective teamwork saves lives and distinguishes those organizations that truly excel from the rest.

Perhaps the biggest barrier to teamwork is the absence of trust. Work groups in which little trust exists between members may go through the motions of teamwork but will not be effective. In *The 7 Habits of Highly Effective People*, Covey[8] describes the natural process of growth and development that groups must go through to establish trust and become high functioning. The process involves developing such principles as fairness, integrity, honesty, human dignity, service, excellence, potential, growth, patience, nurturance, and encouragement. Attempting to shortcut the process will result in disappointment and frustration. As a group leader, Covey states, "If you want to be trusted, be trustworthy." This process takes time and patience. Heider[9] has similar beliefs about the role of group leaders (Box 4-1).

Leaders can foster teamwork through systems that support collaboration and teamwork among all members.

Box 4-1
Doing Less and Being More

- Run an honest, open group.
- Your job is to facilitate and illuminate what is happening. Interfere as little as possible. Interference, however brilliant, creates dependency on the leader.
- The fewer the rules, the better. Rules reduce freedom and responsibility. Enforcement of rules is coercive and manipulative, which diminishes spontaneity and absorbs group energy.
- The more coercive you are, the more resistant the group will become. Your manipulations will only breed evasions. Every law creates an outlaw. This is no way to run a group.
- The wise leader establishes a wholesome climate in the group room. In the light of awareness, the group naturally acts in a wholesome manner.
- When the leader practices silence, the group remains focused. When the leader does not impose rules, the group discovers its own goodness. When the leader acts unselfishly, the group simply does what is to be done.
- Good leadership consists of doing less and being more.

From Heider J: *The Tao of leadership,* Atlanta, 1985, Humanics Publishing Group.

Sometimes, in organizations that have reputations for being world-class, a misconception is that success is a result of the skills of one superstar or perhaps a few individuals who really stand out. In fact, as demonstrated in the APACHE study, the level of collaboration among all team members, not just the skill of a superstar, makes an organization stand out. This phenomenon has been illustrated in the book *Sacred Hoops,* by previous Chicago Bulls coach, Phil Jackson.[10] In his book, Jackson describes his experience coaching a team that included the superstar Michael Jordan. In his early years with the team, even though Jordan was a clear superstar and crowd pleaser, the Bulls were not winning championships.

Then Jackson worked with Jordan and coached him to become more than an individual superstar. He learned to be a team leader, whose role was to elevate the level of play of *all* the Chicago Bulls players and to focus on the work of the team, not just his individual performance. This change in strategy is thought to be the number-one factor that led the Bulls to becoming more than "Michael Jordan's team." Instead, they became the most successful basketball team in history.

The Phil Jackson story has a lot of applicability to pediatric critical care units that are seeking to be the best. First, it outlines the importance of focusing on teamwork, as well as individual performance. Then, it emphasizes the role that the team's superstars should have in elevating the level of performance of every team member to be the best. An example of a situation in which this opportunity may arise is a change of shift in the PICU when a more experienced staff member takes over for a junior member. The more experienced individual may have some ideas about improvements in the plan of care. Here are some possible options: The senior staff member could wait until the junior member leaves, talk about how inexperienced the junior staff member was, and change the plan. Or, the senior staff member could discuss the possible care plan changes with the junior staff member, agree on any changes, and support the junior staff member in communicating the changes to the rest of the team. The second scenario is the one that will produce the winning team.

Conflict Resolution

Often, people will not take the approach outlined previously because they are afraid of conflict. A common problem for nurses in developing their leadership skills is dealing with difficult people and resolving conflict. Perhaps because of a desire to make things run smoothly or keep everyone happy, many nurses avoid dealing with these issues. There are several types of difficult people: the hostile aggressive, the complainer, the silent and unresponsive, the super agreeable, the negativist, the know-it-all expert, and the indecisive. To effectively deal with these types of people, Bramson[11] offers the following suggestions: (1) do not simply wish that the person were different, (2) consider reasons for the difficult person's behavior, (3) achieve distance from the difficult person, (4) develop a plan to cope with the individual, (5) implement the plan using support from others and principles from behavior modification, and (6) evaluate and update the plan as necessary. These suggestions are also valuable for management teams or groups of nursing staff. If an entire group sees a particular person as difficult, developing a plan to cope with the person that is implemented consistently with group support can be very powerful. Especially if the plan incorporates principles of behavior modification and is evaluated and updated regularly, positive results can be achieved.

Conflict is inevitable in organizations and in life. Certainly, in the emotionally charged atmosphere of the PICU, conflict is a daily occurrence. Conflict can be seen as a negative occurrence, or it can be seen as an opportunity for learning and growth. When conflict is resolved successfully, positive change has occurred. Five possible responses to conflict are competition, accommodation, avoidance, compromise, and collaboration. *Competition* is an aggressive and uncooperative approach to conflict. It creates a win-lose situation in which the loser is left feeling angry and antagonistic. *Accommodation* is cooperative but unassertive, and it creates a lose-win situation, leaving the accommodator feeling resentful and angry. *Avoidance* is unassertive and uncooperative, and it creates a lose-lose situation. Pretending that a conflict does not exist when it has surfaced serves no one well. *Compromise* has some aspects of cooperation and some of assertion. Each side makes concessions in a win-lose situation in which both sides win a little and lose a little. Compromise is preferable to competition, accommodation, and avoidance, but it is a weak conflict-resolution technique. Compromise results in decisions that both sides can live with but not necessarily the best solution that could have come from the interaction. *Collaboration* is both assertive and cooperative, creating a win-win situation. In this method, both sides work together to find the best solution to a problem.[12]

Empowerment and Accountability

Empowerment, a term that became an overused buzzword in the 1990s, still has applicability at the individual and organization level in the 2000s. When viewed from an individual perspective, empowerment means the ability to make a decision and take action responsibly. From an organizational position, empowerment is the process of increasing the power of others by allowing them to make decisions and take responsible actions.[5] Leaders support staff members by fostering empowerment on both an individual and an organizational level.

In the realm of individual empowerment, a model that illustrates 5 C's has been has been described by Flaherty and Stark.[5] The first *C,* and the foundation, is *choice*—the belief that everyone has choice in everything they do; next is *confidence*—believing that a positive outcome is possible; the third *C* is *courage*—the power to take action; the fourth is to *communicate* intentions; lastly, and at the top of the pyramid, is to *commit* to make it happen. Sharing these fundamentals with others can help to develop their personal sense of empowerment.

One cannot talk about empowerment without a clear definition and commitment to accountability. At risk of becoming the buzzword of the 2000s, *accountability* means accepting responsibility for one's actions and following through on commitments. Leaders can foster accountability by consistently maintaining and expecting high standards. This sounds simple, but in fact, it is an area in which many leaders struggle. *The Five Temptations of a CEO,* describes a "temptation" that many leaders have—to choose popularity over accountability.[13] It involves being more concerned with being popular with direct reports than in holding them accountable.

Organizational empowerment is based on trust and respect. Giving employees the power to make decisions and to take actions demonstrates trust in a dramatic way. Organizational systems such as Shared Governance are rooted in the belief that people, given the right information, will do the right thing. Again, it essential to build accountability measures into any system at the level in which decision making is done.

The first published reports of Shared Governance in hospital nursing departments came from Rose Medical Center in Denver and St. Joseph's Hospital in Atlanta in the early 1980s. These organizations described their experience with a model that employed a councilor structure, wherein responsibility and accountability rested with the same individuals or groups (Fig. 4-1). Their model included a council on practice, a council on management, a council on quality improvement, and a council on education. A coordinating council integrated and coordinated the governance structure.[14]

The major role of the council on nursing practice was the establishment of professional nursing practice standards. The council was composed of clinical specialists, educators, managers, and front-line staff, who represented the majority.

The council on quality assurance also had a staff nurse majority and included other nursing practitioners. This council's function was to review all nursing practices in the institution to ensure that the standards identified by the council on nursing practice were being carried out and to ensure their appropriateness.

The council on education had responsibility for ensuring that the educational needs of the staff are met and that the mechanisms to maintain high levels of competence are in place. This council has accountability at both the unit and the corporate level, and membership is broad, including all unit-level services.

Membership in the council on management consisted of the traditional management representatives, but the scope of responsibility changes dramatically from a traditional management role. This council is responsible for giving support to the nursing staff and allowing them to make decisions. Often, the role of the management council is to institute

NURSING OPERATIONAL FRAMEWORK
Organizational Structure

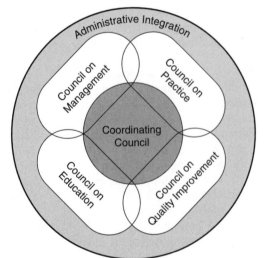

Fig. 4-1 Nursing operational framework— organizational structure. (From Porter-O'Grady T, Finnegan S: *Shared governance for nursing,* 1984, Copyright 1984 by Aspen Publishers.)

Functional Accountability
Practice
Governance
Quality Improvement
Nursing Professional
Development
Peer Behavior

measures to ensure that the decisions of the councils are carried out.

The coordinating council consists of chairpersons of each of the governance councils and the nursing administrator. This council focuses on all nursing activities, ensuring their congruence with the nursing department's philosophy, goals, and objectives.

In addition to the councils, Porter-O'Grady and Finnigan[14] describe a unit-based component to their model, the unit-level practice committees. These committees are subsets of the council on nursing practice and work under the leadership of the council. They are responsible for developing quality working relationships between physicians and nurses. These committees focus on the collaborative development of practice parameters, care plans, and intervention strategies.

Another form of shared governance, called *collaborative governance,* has been described by Jacoby and Terpstra.[15] This is a unit-based structure that has its roots in the 12 shared beliefs of the nursing department (Box 4-2).

These values provide the basis for consensual decision making in this structure and make bylaws unnecessary. The unit is the heart of collaborative governance, and a central structure ensures that unit activities are coordinated with departmental and hospital activities and goals.

Based on the philosophy that true professionalism means control over one's hours, as well as one's work, many hospitals have converted from hourly pay practices to salaried status. Most of the programs have been successful, with nurses reporting increases in professionalism, self-concept, and self-esteem.[16-18]

Box 4-2

Twelve Shared Beliefs of Collaborative Governance

1. Knowledge is power.
2. Given adequate information, people will make appropriate decisions.
3. Individuals are unique in their contributions.
4. A sense of purpose results when organization and personal values are congruent.
5. Maximum productivity results when organizational and personal goals are congruent.
6. Risk taking, with or without success, is growth.
7. People are honest and trustworthy and will work hard to achieve their full potential.
8. Individuals are accountable and responsible for their practice.
9. All problems identified are mutually owned, and responsibility for resolution begins with problem identification.
10. Weaknesses and strengths are the same characteristics used differently. (Weaknesses are strengths in excess.)
11. Our decisions will acknowledge federal and state regulations and reasonable economic restraints.
12. Full cooperation with other divisions must be maintained to fulfill the hospital's mission.

The pediatric critical care unit at University Children's Hospital in Hermann, Texas, devised a salaried status program that met the needs of the nursing staff and the hospital.[19] The plan, professional reimbursement for nurses (PRN), allowed each nursing staff member to be available for six 12-hour shifts with two on-call shifts in a 2-week period. The nurse's compensation was based on 84 hours of work and included usual shift differentials and overtime observed for the hours over 80. The nurse's salary, as a result, was based on 86 hours of work every 2 weeks. This schedule allowed the nurse to work a minimum of 72 hours per pay period or as many as 96 hours while receiving a salary based on 86.

Evaluation of the PRN program by staff and management was favorable. Ninety-one percent of the staff wanted to continue the plan. The staff cited reasons such as relief from floating, provision of reliable unit coverage with trained staff, more time off (actual hours worked often less than number paid), improved unit teamwork and professionalism, more suggestions from staff with regard to scheduling, and consistent quality care.

Management evaluation revealed many advantages: (1) unit coverage was more consistent for a variable census; (2) cost per patient day remained within the targeted goal (the salaried plan did not increase labor costs, a major concern of hospital administration); (3) individual nurses became more accountable for unit coverage, independently solving scheduling problems; and (4) staff participated more broadly in unit activities.

Turnover rate in the unit dropped 14% after initiation of the program, and as a result, orientation hours decreased. Overtime use decreased significantly, and sick leave use was reduced by 19 sick hours per employee per year. Overall, the plan was budget neutral, and patient care quality and unit morale were reported to be significantly improved. In becoming salaried employees, nurses must have the benefits and responsibilities attendant with being exempt employees. These include discussions on decision-making processes and scheduling practices.

Coaching

Being a good coach means seeing talent and potential in people that they may not presently see for themselves, providing honest feedback on performance, and presenting opportunities to learn and grow.

Feedback should be provided on an ongoing basis and also formally through the performance evaluation process. According to Covey,[8] the most successful method for evaluating performance is to have people evaluate themselves. If they participate in establishing the criteria by which they are evaluated, this method of evaluation can eliminate awkward and emotionally exhausting traditional methods. He conveyed experiences in self-evaluation with college students described as his best: He starts with a shared understanding of the goal up front: "This is what we are trying to accomplish. Here are the requirements for an A, B, or C grade. My goal is to help every one of you get an A. Now you take what we've talked about and analyze it and come up with your own understanding of what you want to accomplish that is unique to you. Then let's get together and agree on the grade you want and what you plan to do to get it." This type of evaluation is possible in nursing units. Specific criteria-based evaluation tools can be created in collaboration with those being evaluated and can still be tailored to meet the needs of each person. In addition, if leaders are committed to help each person achieve their agreed-on individual objectives, the evaluation process can be a very positive experience.

Feedback from others provides a powerful learning opportunity that may be incorporated into the evaluation process. Many institutions use peer review as a component of each team member's performance appraisal. Feedback of any type is most helpful if it is provided continuously, however, rather than only at the time of one's annual appraisal. Although most commonly referred to as either positive feedback or negative feedback, it is also most effective when it is not simply one way but circular and is incorporated into a "feedback loop" in which change and growth take place.

When leadership supports people to grow, learn, and be self-managing, the entire organization wins. The ultimate test for a leader is not whether he or she can make smart decisions and take decisive action, but whether he or she can teach others to be leaders and build an organization that remains successful even when he or she is not around.[20] It is this type of teaching and coaching that truly sets organizations apart from others.

Assertive Communication

An area in which many people in the healthcare field could benefit from coaching is in communicating assertively. Assertiveness is another learned skill that must be practiced. To be assertive is to be positive or confident in a persistent way. It is based on self-esteem and respect for self and others. Assertive behavior is standing up for one's rights to express one's feelings, reactions, or expectations without alienating the other person. Assertive communication is honest, direct, and appropriate. It is behavior-focused rather than personal criticism.

Assertion needs to be discussed in relation to its contrast to both passivity and aggression. Passive communicators do not stand up for themselves. They allow others to speak up for them or to push them around, and because of this, they may harbor resentment and anger. Aggressive people stand up for their individual rights but in a manner that infringes on the rights of others. Aggression allows a person to obtain what they desire but often alienates others in the process.

Baillie and co-workers[21] offer the following suggestions to assist in cultivating assertiveness skills.

Practice Positive Self-Communication.   Expressions of positive regard such as "I am confident," "I am an effective nurse and leader," and "I can do this" help us better deal with conflict and stressful situations that affect our self-worth.

Learn to Deal With Criticism.   People who have difficulty dealing with criticism are those who feel that it is essential to be liked and approved of by everyone or that they must never make a mistake. Many see criticism as a rejection of self instead of a rejection of an action. It is essential to separate the problem from one's integrity and then to respond to the criticism. Negative ways of responding to criticism include (1) apologizing more than is necessary, (2) becoming defensive, (3) attacking the critic, and (4) internalizing the stress and saying nothing. By contrast, one may deal with criticism in a productive and assertive manner. Options include (1) accepting it, (2) disagreeing with it, (3) setting limits for the critic, (4) fogging, and (5) delaying.

Accepting justified criticism from a respected individual is assertive as long as it is accepted without being considered an insult. Disagreeing with the critic is appropriate when the criticism is unjustified. It is important to back up a disagreement with a statement of self-affirmation. Setting limits with the critic is appropriate when the critic is behaving in an inappropriate manner, such as using foul language or yelling. In this situation, it is fitting to tell the individual to stop, to wait until a more suitable time for the interaction, or to leave the area. Fogging is a technique in which the individual acknowledges the critic but then immediately changes the subject. Delaying is simply responding to criticism with a statement that the person needs more time to gather information before responding.

Setting Limits and Saying "No."   In being assertive, it is important to set limits and say "no" when it is meant. Expectations must be made clear. Saying "no" and setting limits require allowing negative feelings to be expressed. With practice, one can learn to set limits and say "no" because it fits with one's values, and in this way people teach others how to treat them.

Making Requests and Expressing Initiative. Knowing what is wanted and asking for it are hallmarks of this strategy. It requires risk taking, a knowledge of self, and the ability to take "no" for an answer. Taking initiative and asking for what is wanted improves self-esteem and self-actualization, but it does not mean always getting what is asked.

Expressing Anger.   Expressing anger in an assertive manner requires being in touch with the feelings associated with anger and expressing them in a manner that allows further communication to occur. Using "I" instead of "you" statements allows the expression of anger without closing communication pathways.

Systems Thinking

One of the most important roles that leaders play is that of problem solver. Good problem solvers are typically people who approach issues with a can-do attitude and a willingness to make necessary changes. Often, leaders have been promoted within their institutions because they are good problem solvers. In a system such as a pediatric critical care unit within a healthcare organization, the best problem solvers are also systems thinkers. They understand that their area of focus is simply a piece of a larger puzzle, and they approach problem solving from the perspective of trying to understand the big picture.

All organizations are systems. Systems can be defined as a set of interdependent components that work together to achieve a common goal. Systems thinking describes a way of thinking about and a language for describing and understanding the forces and interrelationships that shape the behavior of systems.[6] It encompasses a large body of methods, tools, and principles all oriented at looking at the interrelatedness of forces—seeing them as a part of a common process. In pediatric critical care, this emphasizes the importance of seeing the work done in the ICU as part of the bigger picture of the organization.

Three main components of systems thinking are (1) studying and understanding processes that contribute to care, (2) measuring performance of processes and their outcomes using valid statistical methods, and (3) taking action to improve the way processes are designed and carried out.

An example of the use of systems thinking as a problem-solving tool in pediatric critical care follows: The problem was an increasing incidence of diverting trauma patients to other hospitals because of the unavailability of ICU beds or staff. Using a systems thinking approach to this problem, the first step was to *study and understand the processes that contribute to care.* Contributions were gathered from nursing staff, managers, staffing coordinators, physicians, and the trauma program manager, and a new data collection tool aimed at gathering information about why the hospital was refusing trauma admissions was devised and implemented. Next, performance was measured using *valid statistical method.* Concurrent data from the new tool were collected and presented using the actual numbers of trauma patients turned away (numerators) and the actual number of all trauma calls (denominators). Lastly, the group took *action to improve the way processes were carried out.* Based on the new data, it was evident that nursing staff members and bed availability were not the only reasons the hospital was referring trauma patients elsewhere. Other reasons included evaluating the appropriateness of the patients that were in the PICU, establishing systems to speed up the discharge process on the floors to open beds, and the inadequacy of the present per diem float pool. By improving the way these processes were carried out, more global improvements were possible.

Tools can be used in systems thinking to help understand the processes that are being studied and to clearly present the data that have been collected. Reliable data are essential to all systems improvement activities. Useful tools in understanding processes include brainstorming, the "fishbone" technique, and flowcharts. Brainstorming is a technique for generating ideas about an issue from a group. It involves defining the subject of the brainstorming session, allowing time for everyone to think about the issues, and setting a time limit. One way to implement brainstorming is for each group member to call out ideas with someone noting each idea. During this time, no one may comment or react to an idea. After all ideas have been shared, the group clarifies the ideas that were presented.

The fishbone technique is also known as a cause-and-effect diagram. This is a diagram showing a large number of possible causes for a problem, which, when constructed, looks something like a fishbone (Fig. 4-2). To construct a cause-and-effect diagram, a problem statement is placed to the right of a horizontal line with an arrow pointing to the problem. Major categories that contribute to the problem are then written on diagonal lines that point at the original horizontal line. If applicable, subcategories (or causes) may be listed that affect the main categories. The intent is to begin to understand the root causes of problems, and, once they are listed, the diagram can be used to determine obvious areas for improvement.

Flowcharts are graphic representations of the sequence of steps that are performed in a specific work process. They can be used to identify an actual path that a service follows to see if there are any redundancies, inefficiencies, or misunderstandings; to identify an ideal path for a product or service; or to create a common understanding of how a work process should be done. To implement a flowchart, it is necessary to decide on a starting and ending point for the process. Next, activities and decision points are arranged in the order of occurrence, and analysis of the flowchart serves to determine areas for improvement or explain the steps of a newly created process.

Tools that can be used to present data in an easily understandable fashion include histograms and run charts. Histograms are graphic representations of the frequency with which something occurs. They involve listing possible scores on one axis of a graph and the actual count for each category on the other axis (Fig. 4-3).

A run chart is a collection of points plotted on a graph in the order in which they became available over time. A graph is established with the horizontal axis representing time or sequence of the data and the vertical axis indicating increments of measure. Points are then plotted on the graph and connected with a line. The chart can be evaluated to identify meaningful trends or shifts in the average (Fig. 4-4).

These statistical tools are all incorporated to accomplish the goal of presenting accurate, understandable data. Without the use of statistical control measures, unsystematic data collection and subjective evaluation of care can render improvement activities futile.

Collaboration by departments and groups on problem-solving and systems improvement activities is crucial. For

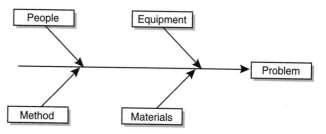

Fig. 4-2 Fishbone diagram. (Used with permission from *The memory jogger: a pocket guide of tools for continuous improvement.* Copyright 1988 by GOAL/QPC, 13 Branch Street, Methuen, MA 01844-1953. Tel: 508-685-3900.)

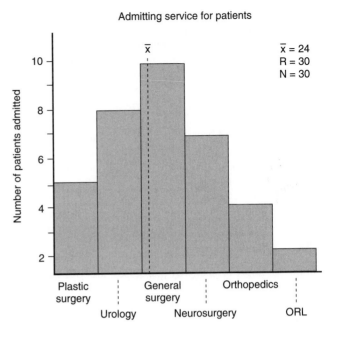

Fig. 4-3 Example of a histogram. (Used with permission from *The memory jogger: a pocket guide of tools for continuous improvement.* Copyright 1988 by GOAL/QPC, 13 Branch Street, Methuen, MA 01844-1953. Tel: 508-685-3900.)

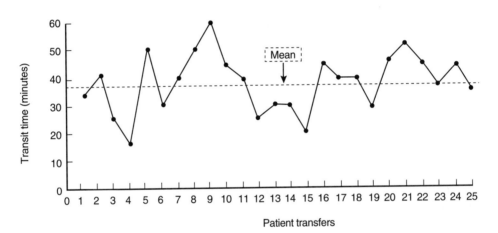

Fig. 4-4 Patient transfer process run chart. (Used with permission from *The memory jogger: a pocket guide of tools for continuous improvement.* Copyright 1988 by GOAL/QPC, 13 Branch Street, Methuen, MA 01844-1953. Tel: 508-685-3900.)

example, if a problem is identified that involves patient medications, it is essential that the pharmacy and nursing cooperate with other departments involved to study the processes that lead to medication administration and discover ways to improve current processes. A single department cannot conduct meaningful systems improvement activities in a vacuum.

Systems improvement must also be undertaken in a spirit of respect and support. This approach requires the belief that all people in the organization are committed to doing their best.

Listening to People

Visibility and a willingness to really listen are hallmarks of an excellent leader. The problem that many leaders face is how to find the time for these activities. The answer is very

simple—it just has to become an *absolute priority.* Leaders who could potentially be some of the busiest people in the world, such as Jack Welch, CEO of the General Electric, the world's largest corporation, and Roger Enrico, CEO of PepsiCo, say that they spend as much as 30% of their time interacting with and teaching others.[21] Being visible is essential to being an effective leader.

Listening may be the chief distinguisher between leaders who succeed and those who fail. Active, engaged listening is the goal. This kind of listening demonstrates respect for an individual, exhibits genuine concern, and encourages people to express their views in return. Developing active listening skills requires that one internalize what a speaker has said. This means that the time the person is speaking is not spent formulating a response. An excellent method to use in improving listening skills is to practice hearing what others mean to be saying. Repeating or validating a message is a useful tool. For those who are experiencing difficulty with listening skills, a helpful exercise is to have the listener repeat exactly what the speaker has said before responding. This is a time-consuming operation, but it serves to ensure active listening and can lead to the development of this important skill.

Building Morale

Leaders are never energy neutral. They either create positive energy by paying attention to spreading ideas and teaching values, or they sap energy by ignoring it. Positive energy creates positive morale. The most pivotal position in affecting the morale of a department is that of the front-line leader or manager. According to Taunton and colleagues,[3] improving managers' leadership behaviors will be more likely than any other intervention to improve retention of hospital nurses. Supportive management has been proven effective in the management of nursing professionals. Studies have demonstrated that supportive supervision has many positive effects, including decreasing job stress and burnout and increasing job satisfaction.[22-25]

A prime example of the effect of front-line management on morale is the landmark magnet hospital study originally conducted in 1982.[26] This study identified 41 hospitals across the United States that were known for their excellent nursing care, for being places where nurses wanted to work, and for having low turnover and vacancy rates.

In 1986, Kramer and Schmallenberg[27,28] conducted a follow-up study on a representative sample of 16 hospitals from this group. The results indicated that these hospitals were not experiencing problems from the nursing shortage that was occurring at that time and that they had remained institutions of excellence in the delivery of healthcare. A common thread was identified among the institutions—the hospitals and their nursing staffs were value driven. The values are highlighted in Box 4-3.

In 1989, Kramer[29] revisited the magnet hospitals and learned that they were still centers of nursing excellence. She found that these institutions had remained value driven and identified seven other common threads among these institutions.

Staff Mix: Still Moving Toward More RNs. These hospitals were increasing the percentage of RNs by decreasing the use of licensed vocational nurses (LVNs). They were also increasing the use of nursing assistants under various titles. The important component of the nursing assistant's role was that they were not assigned to patients; instead, they were assigned to a registered nurse. Their duties involved nonnursing patient care and environmental activities.

Organizational Structure: Middle Managers Had Been Removed From Clinical Decision Making. At these hospitals, the staff RNs were respected for their education, clinical competence, autonomy, and decision-making abilities. With a competent, autonomous RN staff, less supervision was needed, and the nurse manager role was redesigned. The role of the nurse manager was changed from that of controller to leader. The span of leadership

Box 4-3
Magnet Hospital Values

Quality care
Nurse autonomy
Informal, nonrigid communication
Innovation
Bringing out the best in each individual
Valuing education
Respect and caring for the individual
Striving for excellence

Data from Kramer M, Schmallenberg C: Magnet hospitals: institutions of excellence, *J Nurs Admin* 18:13-24, 1988.

responsibility was increased so that one person often had more than one unit to manage.

Salaried Status: Treating Nurses as Professionals. The trend toward having nurses become salaried employees was increasing. In 1986, nurses in 5 of the 16 magnet hospitals studied were on salaried status. In 1989, nurses in 9 hospitals were either salaried or moving toward salaried status.

Self-Governance: Minding Their Own Stores, but Participating in Department-Wide Issues. The trend toward self-governance in 1986 was continuing. The change noted was that at this time, many of the chief nurse executives were distinguishing between the concepts of shared and self-governance. Most of the magnet hospitals had a system of autonomous self-governed operation at the unit level and participative, representative involvement in department-wide issues.

Nursing Care Delivery Systems: More Flexibility According to Patient Needs. Probably the biggest difference seen in the years from 1982 until 1989 was in the delivery systems used. In 1982, almost all of the magnet hospitals were using the primary nursing model, but in 1986 the shift moved toward total patient care. As the patients' length of stay was decreasing and flexible scheduling (with 10- and 12-hour shifts) found nurses working fewer days, there was a push to individualize the delivery system to meet the needs of the patient population and the unit. Case management was gaining popularity as a delivery system, and primary nursing, for the most part, was on its way out. One chief nurse executive was quoted as saying, "Primary nursing has taken a real beating."[29] The hospitals were committed to the philosophy of primary nursing and wanted to continue to achieve the positive results that primary nursing brought about, but changes in the care delivery structure were needed.

Maximizing the Practice of Available Nurses. In the magnet hospitals, more than 50% of the RNs were BSN prepared. This mix provided the opportunity for nurses to work with other nurses who were clinically competent, experienced, and educated.

In addition, 12 of the 16 hospitals had a "no floating policy," which represents an increase from 10 of 16 in 1986. The hospitals were trying to stop or limit the use of agency nurses. There was a slight increase in the use of agency nurses in the magnet hospitals from 1986, but 11 used either none or fewer than four full-time equivalents (FTEs) per month.

The hospitals used RNs predominantly; they were committed to holding to selective hiring values and practices in the face of the nursing shortage. New graduate employment was also being limited. In nine hospitals, only 25% or less of the new hires were new graduates. Units were being self-managed. Nine of the 16 hospitals reported self-managed units.

Innovative New Programs. The hospitals were seeking to redesign or further develop new nursing care delivery systems. They were differentiating nurses' roles and setting up programs and activities to enable or empower staff. These institutions were focusing on strengthening nurse-physician practice relationships, flattening the organizational structure, and expanding computerization programs, particularly for documentation.

Stress Management

In the introduction, a study was referenced that described intensive care nurses as having higher levels of stress than even Vietnam war veterans with PTSD. Clearly, stress management is an area is which leaders of critical care should focus to support staff. Steinmetz and co-workers[30] describe a conceptual model that addresses the stressors that occur in the ICU. It includes three components: external stressors, internal stressors, and conflict avoidance. External stressors are those occurring as a result of crowded workplaces or confusing organizational policies. Internal stressors are created by role ambiguity, professional bureaucratic conflict, and situations such as dealing with angry people or believing that perfection is necessary. Conflict avoidance is a stressor brought on by failing to deal directly with conflicts or problematic situations.

In a study focusing on PICU nurses, Gilmer[31] identified the death of a child as the most stress-producing event. Other situations that were highly stressful to PICU nurses included dealing with families who were attempting to cope, problems involving interpersonal relationships, inefficient unit design, and the absence of necessary equipment.

Oehler and Davidson[32] measured the predictors and incidence of job stress and burnout in PICU and nonacute unit nurses and found that although burnout was more of a problem in critical care nurses, 22% of all pediatric nurses reported symptoms associated with burnout. Particularly troublesome was the high incidence of burnout associated with personal accomplishment. Thirty-nine percent of nonacute unit nurses and 59% of acute care nurses reported a low sense of personal accomplishment.

In relation to the contributors to burnout, results indicated that job stress makes the most significant contribution to feelings of burnout. The death of a child was the highest source of job stress, followed by workload. Conflict with physicians and uncertainty regarding treatment were the third and fourth factors. Oehler and Davidson[32] also found that state anxiety (the level of anxiety a person is experiencing at the present time) and trait anxiety (the amount of anxiety they usually experience) are powerful indicators of

burnout. Co-worker support was also a predictor of burnout, with groups perceiving low co-worker support demonstrating higher levels of burnout. In this study the amount of experience that the nurse had was the weakest predictor of burnout, with less experience being associated with higher rates of burnout.

To reduce stress and burnout, Oehler and Davidson[32] recommend programs to help all personnel cope with death, creative solutions to managing patient assignments and monitoring of individual workload, and work on strategies for improving nurse-physician communication (particularly on the issues of patient management). With respect to anxiety levels, they suggest referrals to personal assistance programs if available. In the area of co-worker support, work to develop a supportive work environment with group cohesiveness is recommended. They also suggest that less experienced nurses, because of their increased incidence of burnout, be targeted for special attention.

These findings were confirmed in a recent nationwide study that included over 1000 PICU RNs.[33] The report cited issues concerning families as the most frequently perceived stressor for PICU RNs, with staffing issues and concerns about death and dying completing the top three. Also reported was the finding that the amount of job stress perceived by PICU nurses was the most important predictor of both job satisfaction and organizational work satisfaction. The next most important predictor of job satisfaction was the quality of nursing leadership. The study concluded that retention efforts for PICU nurses should focus on management strategies that empower staff to provide quality care with specific interventions aimed at reducing the stress caused by nurse-family interactions.

Fein[34] has recommended strategies categorized as stress reducing, altering the perception of stress, managing physical well-being, and enhancing coping skills. Strategies to reduce stress include learning to say "no," distinguishing work from home activities, spending time efficiently, and developing friendship networks outside of work. In altering the perception of stress, Fein[34] recommends increasing self-awareness through introspection, reevaluating personal and professional goals, determining what is important, and accepting that which cannot be changed. Managing physical well-being includes taking time out, treating oneself with love and respect, learning to relax without drugs or alcohol, exercising regularly, and eating for health. In addition, organizational strategies aimed at managing stress and preventing burnout are described in Box 4-4.

Time Management

One of today's major stressors is the perception that there is not enough time to do everything that needs to get done. If there is one thing most people would say that they would like more of, it would probably be time. How do people find time? The answer is that they don't. Time management is really self-management. The challenge is not to manage time but to manage oneself. Covey[8] has identified four ways that time is spent involving the concepts of urgent and important. He has described a matrix with four quadrants in which *urgent* and *not urgent* are on the horizontal axis and *important* and *not important* are on the vertical axis. "Urgent" means that something requires immediate attention, and "importance" has to do with results—something that will contribute to accomplishing high-priority goals. Urgent matters are something to which people react, and important matters are those in which is it necessary to consciously act, to make things happen.

Activities that are both urgent and important are commonly referred to as "crises" or "problems." Everyone has some critical activities in their lives, but others seem to spend all of their time thrown from one crisis to another. They are often referred to as "crisis managers." As a relief from the stress of constantly solving crises, they sometimes seek relief in activities that are neither urgent nor important. They can thus run the risk of neglecting important yet not urgent activities, as well as those that are urgent but not important.

Covey[8] also describes people who spend much of their time dealing with urgent unimportant tasks. Although they may think they are dealing with the highest priority items, they are in fact reacting to the priorities of others, not their own.

People who deal primarily with unimportant issues, whether "urgent" or not, never address the highest priorities and basically lead irresponsible lives. Effective people avoid dealing with unimportant issues and spend most of their time on the important priorities.

Effective people spend most of their time dealing with issues that are important but not urgent. This is how they can reduce the amount of time spent with important-urgent issues ("crises")—by dealing with important issues before they become matters of critical urgency. Important, nonurgent concerns include such things as vision, building relationships, long-range planning, and exercising—things people know they need but often cannot seem to find the time to do.

To spend more time on the important nonurgent issues, it is necessary to spend less time on all the unimportant ones.

This will involve learning to say "no" to some activities, some of which may appear urgent. This means deciding what one's priorities are and sticking to them. It may then be necessary to kindly and courteously say "no" to some other things.

In organizing to spend as much time as possible dealing with important nonurgent issues, Covey[8] has found that four key activities are involved: identifying roles, selecting goals, scheduling, and daily adapting. As a method to understand his principles, he recommends that people try this experience by organizing 1 week.

Identifying roles is simply the practice of listing key roles. These include the role of being an individual and may include being a parent or a spouse, son or daughter, professional, manager, committee member, volunteer, neighbor, or church member, among others. After the roles have been identified, the next step is to think of two or three important results that should be accomplished during the next 7 days in each of the roles. These are listed as goals and should contain some quadrant II activities. For scheduling, the recommended process is to look ahead at the week and schedule time to achieve each of the listed goals. Previous commitments that are in line with established goals should then be added to the schedule, and those that are not in line should be rescheduled or canceled. Daily adapting is then the process of prioritizing activities and responding to unanticipated events in a meaningful way.

Covey[8] believes that this type of organizing allows people the freedom and flexibility to handle unanticipated events, to shift appointments if necessary, and to enjoy relationships and interactions with others while still knowing that their week has been organized to accomplish key goals in every area of their life.

One method to accomplish more in less time is to be an effective delegator. Delegation is used to get work done efficiently and with optimal use of human resources (Fig. 4-5). Effective delegation requires knowledge and skill. It is often said that it is easier to do a task oneself than to delegate, which may be true for those who have not acquired the knowledge and skill necessary to delegate effectively. Initially, the work to be done must be identified and defined. The individual to whom the work is being delegated must be aware of the definition and description of the work and the time frame in which it is to be accomplished. Helpful methods establish controls and checkpoints so that the work can be evaluated and maintain open lines of communication and mutually agreed-on goals.[35]

Stewardship delegation, as described by Covey,[8] is focused on results instead of methods. This type of delegation involves clear, direct mutual understanding and commitment regarding expectations in five areas. It takes more time in the beginning, but the time is well spent.

The five areas Covey is referring to are desired results, guidelines, resources, accountability, and consequences. With desired results, a clear, mutual understanding of what needs to be accomplished is important. This is not telling the person how to do the project, but rather stating what needs to be accomplished and the time frame that is involved. Guidelines refer to parameters within which the individual

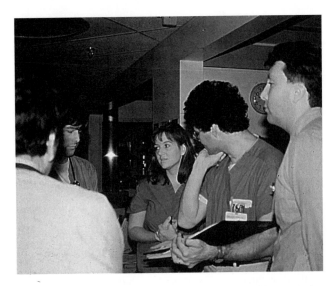

Fig. 4-5 Leadership role of the nurse is significant during multidisciplinary rounds.

should operate. These should not be overly restrictive but should provide assistance so that the person does not violate long-standing values or practices or have to re-create the wheel. Be honest—let the individual learn from previous mistakes and experiences. Do not tell people how to accomplish their objective, just give them a start. In the area of resources, Covey is referring to the human, financial, technical, or organizational resources people can use to accomplish their goals. Accountability means that specific standards of performance and time frames for evaluation should be determined in advance. Consequences are the specific things that will happen, good and bad, as a result of the evaluation. This could mean financial rewards, psychic rewards, promotions, or other consequences.

With a stewardship type of delegation, even when it takes more time initially, both parties benefit, and ultimately more work is done in less time. Stewards becomes their own boss, governed by agreed-on results, and they have the potential to use their own creative energies to achieve the desired results. In the words of Covey,[8] "Effective delegation is perhaps the best indicator of effective management because it is so basic to both personal and organizational growth."

Measuring Success

In *The Leadership Engine: How Winning Companies Build Leaders at Every Level*, Tichy and Cohen[20] offer the following question and answer: "How are you doing as a leader? The answer is, how are the people you lead doing? Do they visit customers? Do they manage conflict? Do they learn? Do they initiate change? Are they growing and getting promoted? When you retire, you won't remember what you did the in the first quarter or the third. What you'll remember is how many people you developed—how many people you helped have a better career because of your interest and dedication to their development. When confused about how you are doing as a leader, find out how the people you lead are doing. You'll know the answer."

What tools are available to measure the success of leadership? They are the same tools that measure the success of the product being delivered—patient outcomes, customer satisfaction, physician satisfaction, and staff satisfaction plus the measure offered by Tichy and Cohen[20]—how well the staff you lead are doing.

SUMMARY

In conclusion, this chapter has discussed the "essentialness" of leadership in creating a world-class pediatric critical care unit. Attributes and values such as teamwork and building morale have been addressed; however, perhaps the most essential ingredient to becoming a successful leader is having a solid sense of self-esteem. Self-esteem allows the leader to take risks and adapt to challenges and avoid the pitfalls that cause many leaders to fail. These pitfalls are so prevalent that they are the basis of the book *The Five Temptations of a CEO* (1998).[13] It depicts five behaviors that are essential for success in leadership and that if not adhered to will cause the leader to fail. The behaviors are described as temptations that must be rejected to succeed. All of the temptations are rooted in a need for a solid sense of self-esteem.

The first temptation is to focus on status rather than results. This occurs when the leader is more concerned with protecting career status and ego than in achieving results. The second was described as choosing popularity over accountability. This was discussed previously and is related to being more concerned with being popular with direct reports than with holding them accountable. The third temptation is to choose certainty over clarity. It is the temptation to ensure that all decisions are absolutely correct before proceeding and stems from a fear of being wrong. The fourth temptation is to choose harmony over conflict. In this scenario, the leader avoids heated discussions, disagreement, and conflict within the department for fear that someone will get hurt. The result is making decisions without the full benefit of everyone's ideas. Lastly, the fifth temptation is to choose invulnerability over trust. In this temptation, the leader is afraid to trust others, to be vulnerable, and to create an environment in which others trust him or her. It requires opening oneself to being burned.

The one area singled out as that which will make or break leaders in a changing environment is the establishment of trust. Trust is defined as the "firm belief or confidence in the honesty, integrity, reliability, and justice of another person."[36] Most of the struggles people encounter in providing effective leadership have to do with a lack of trust. This concept can be especially difficult for new nurse managers or those who have been recently promoted because the need to move forward at a rapid pace and make necessary changes is countered by the necessity to move slowly in establishing trust. A delicate balance must be achieved between spending time developing trusting relationships and spending time planning and acting on future goals. Most importantly, as Covey[8] has stated, "If you want to be trusted, be trustworthy."

REFERENCES

1. Health Care Advisory Board: *The journey begins: retaining nursing talent, reforming nursing costs in an era of lasting shortage.* Washington, DC, The Advisory Board Company, 1999.
2. Allen JJ: Intensive care nurses: Post traumatic stress disorder–like symptomatology [dissertation]. Loma Linda, Calif, 1999, Loma Linda University.
3. Taunton RL et al: Manager leadership and retention. *J Western Nursing Research* 19:205, 997
4. Komives SR, Lucas N, McMahon TR: *Exploring leadership,* San Francisco, 1998, Jossey-Bass.
5. Flaherty JS, Stark PB: *The competent leader: a powerful tool kit for managers and supervisors,* Amherst, Mass, 1999, HRD Press.
6. Senge PM: *The fifth discipline: the art and practice of the learning organization,* New York, 1990, Doubleday.
7. Knaus WA, Draper EA, Wagner DP et al: An evaluation of outcome from intensive care in major medical centers, *Ann Intern Med* 104:410-418, 1986.
8. Covey SR: *The 7 habits of highly effective people: powerful lessons in personal change,* New York, 1989, Simon & Schuster.
9. Heider J: *The Tao of leadership,* Atlanta, 1985, Humanics Publishing Group.
10. Jackson P: *Sacred hoops: spiritual lessons of a hardwood warrior,* New York, 1995, Hyperion.
11. Bramson R: *Coping with difficult people,* New York, 1981, Ballantine Books.
12. Todd SS: Coping with conflict, *Nursing* 19:100-106, 1989.
13. Lencioni P: *The five temptations of a CEO,* San Francisco, 1998, Jossey-Bass.
14. Porter-O'Grady T, Finnigan S: *Shared governance for nursing,* Rockville Md, 1984, Aspen.
15. Jacoby J, Terpstra M: Collaborative governance: Model for professional accountability, *Nurs Manag* 21:42-44, 1990.
16. Salaried status: a boost to professionalism? *OR Manag* 4:6-7, 1988.
17. Sills LR: Implementation of a salaried compensation program for registered nurses, *J Nurs Admin* 23:55-59, 1993.
18. Sierk TA: Implementation of a salary model for staff nurses, *Nurs Manage* 25:36-37, 1994.
19. Murphy CA, Walts L, Cavouras CA: The PRN plan: professional reimbursement for nurses, *Nurs Manage* 20:64Q-64X, 1989.
20. Tichy N, Cohen E: *The leadership engines: how winning companies build leaders at every level,* New York, 1997, HarperCollins.
21. Baillie VK, Trygstad L, Cordoni TI: *Effective nursing leadership: a practical guide,* Rockville, Md, 1989, Aspen.
22. Cronin-Stubbs D, Rooks CA: The stress, social support and burnout of critical care nurses: the results of research, *Heart Lung* 14:31-39, 1985.
23. Blegen MA, Mueller CW: Nurses' job satisfaction: a longitudinal analysis, *Res Nurs Health* 10:227-237, 1987.
24. Duxbury, ML, Armstrong GD, Drew DJ et al: Head nurse leadership style with staff nurse burnout and job satisfaction in neonatal intensive care units, *Nurs Res* 33:97-101, 1984.
25. Norbeck JS: Types and sources of social support for managing job stress in critical care nursing, *Nurs Res* 34:225-230, 1985.
26. Task Force on Nursing Practice in Hospitals: *Magnet hospitals: attraction and retention of professional nurses,* Kansas City, Mo, 1983, American Academy of Nursing.
27. Kramer M, Schmallenberg C: Magnet hospitals: institutions of excellence, part I, *J Nurs Admin* 18:13-24, 1988.
28. Kramer M, Schmallenberg C: Magnet hospitals: institutions of excellence, part II, *J Nurs Admin* 18:11-19, 1988.
29. Kramer M: Trends to watch at the magnet hospitals, *Nursing 90* 20(6):67-74, 1990.
30. Steinmetz J, Proctor S, Hall D et al: *Rx for stress: a nurse's guide,* Palo Alto, Calif, 1984, Bull Publishing.
31. Gilmer M: Nurses' perceptions of stresses in the pediatric intensive care unit. In Kramptitz S, Pavlovitch N, eds: *Readings in nursing research,* St Louis, 1981, Mosby.
32. Oehler JM, Davidson MG: Job stress and burnout in acute and nonacute pediatric nurses, *Am J Crit Care* 1:81-89, 1992.
33. Bratt MM, Broome M, Kelber S, Lostcocco L: Influence of stress and nursing leadership on job satisfaction of pediatric intensive care unit nurses. *Am J Crit Care* 9:307-317, 2000.
34. Fein SL: Burnout in nursing: prevention and management. In Fein IA, Strosberg MA, eds: *Managing the critical care unit,* Rockville, Md, 1987, Aspen Publishers.
35. McAlvanah MF: A guide to delegation, *Pediatr Nurs* 15:379, 1989.
36. *Webster's new twentieth century dictionary,* ed 2, 1983.

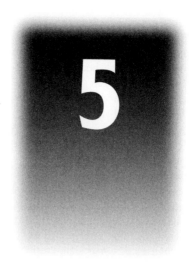

5 Facilitation of Learning

Sandra Czerwinski
Eugene D. Martin

The activity and process of staff development are a shared responsibility of the staff nurse, nurse manager, clinical nurse specialist, unit educator, and staff development department. Even though professional growth and development are facilitated by those in leadership positions, the ultimate responsibility is assumed by the individual staff nurse. Opportunities for professional development are best supported when the staff development plan for a unit is designed to support and enhance a well-defined clinical advancement program.

A successful critical care unit–based professional advancement program recognizes varying cognitive levels and staff nurses' knowledge and expertise and fosters advancement through a wide range of clinical learning and professional development experiences. Essential components of this program include an orientation program, a continuing education plan, an in-service education schedule, and an array of other opportunities for clinical and professional development. Unit-based advancement programs are most effective when they are linked to the nursing department's professional advancement program. In departments without central professional advancement programs, the philosophy and goals of a unit-based program should be congruent with the nursing department's stated philosophy and goals and mission of the organization.

This chapter describes how professional development in critical care nursing is facilitated through a staff development plan that supports a professional advancement model. Based on the understanding that novices in practice focus, interpret, and apply information differently than experts, a unit-based plan that recognizes developmental levels of practice best facilitates the professional advancement of all staff members.

A professional advancement program for the development, recognition, and reward of expertise contains elements of both clinical and professional development strategies. The Synergy Model, developed by the American Association of Critical-Care Nurses (AACN) Certification Corporation, reflects the values and philosophy of professional advancement.[1,2] The model's ability to describe a patient-nurse relationship that optimizes patient and family outcomes helps to clarify the various contributions of critical care nursing practice. The impact of these contributions can be measured based on the nurse's level of expertise, and professional development strategies can be focused to achieve the greatest influence on patient care. Therefore critical care education should include multiple opportunities for the promotion of both clinical and professional growth. Although many of these opportunities are ultimately interrelated for the advanced practitioner, planning a comprehensive unit-based program that fosters advancement necessitates separate consideration of these two areas.

To best accomplish this objective, levels of practice defined by Benner and supported within the framework of the Synergy Model[2,3] are used to illustrate aspects of clinical development. Implications for planning and implementing a program of professional advancement based on these levels are then discussed, and broad performance characteristics are described for each level. In addition, specific examples are given to illustrate critical care behaviors typical of each performance level.

RECOGNIZING CLINICAL DEVELOPMENT

Skill Acquisition Model

Dr. Patricia Benner applied a model of skill acquisition identified by Dreyfuss to nursing.[3] This model of skill acquisition serves as a useful framework for understanding how nurses integrate knowledge and skill over time and, with repeated experience, progress from a novice to an expert practitioner. Benner describes five levels of professional development: novice beginner, advanced beginner, competent, proficient, and expert practitioner.

Benner describes the novice and advanced beginner as a nurse who possesses little or no experience of situations in which they are expected to perform.[3] Behavior at these levels is governed by rules, and these practitioners are somewhat inflexible. The competent nurse has at least 2 to 3 years of experience in the same or similar clinical practice environment. This nurse is beginning to set long-term goals based on conscious, abstract, and analytical problem solving.[3] The proficient nurse conceptualizes more of the whole rather than individual parts. This practitioner learns from experience and demonstrates more sophisticated decision-making skills. The expert nurse has enormous breadth of experience and an intuitive grasp of each situation.

For each level of practice, Benner identifies clinical practice behaviors and teaching and learning needs.[3] Benner's work is particularly important in the design and implementation of a clinical practice program that differentiates practice, as well as specialized continuing education, because she connects specific aspects of clinical experience with the nurse's level of practice.

Thus clinical knowledge development can be enhanced by assisting the nurse at any particular level of practice to focus on the knowledge and experience associated with that level. Specific practice indicators for meeting advancement criteria can be developed to help staff identify examples of expected behaviors. It is important that staff understand these examples as one way, rather than the only way, to meet advancement criteria.

Synergy Model

Many problems are associated with recognizing and rewarding progressive clinical practice.[4] Historically, the most skilled nurses moved away from the bedside into management and educational roles to pursue professional advancement; expertise at the bedside failed to receive recognition and reward. In the current healthcare environment, nursing leadership is challenged to find innovative solutions that define, recognize, and reward expertise at the bedside. The Synergy Model achieves this by describing nurses' unique contributions to patients' outcomes and defining nursing's best practice and value-added services.[2]

The Synergy Model describes nursing practice based on the needs and characteristics of patients and the demands of the healthcare environment predicted for the future.[2] The model describes patients' characteristics that are of concern to nursing, nurse's competencies that are important to patients, and the outcomes that result when characteristics and competencies are mutually enhancing . The model is adaptable to all areas of nursing practice and is able to capture neonatal, pediatric, and adult patient care experiences. The patient exists within a variety of continua, not only reflecting the holistic and dynamic nature of the patient in a time of physiologic instability but also recognizing the family and community as essential components in determining a patient's outcome.[5]

Each patient and family possess unique personal characteristics that span the continuum of health and illness and affect essential nursing care. The Synergy Model describes eight patient characteristics that influence nursing care needs. These characteristics evolve over time and present a different picture as the individual's healthcare situation changes.[6]

The Synergy Model also defines nursing competencies.[2] The model articulates the wide variety of activities in which nurses are involved every day and reflects the behaviors that nurses often characterize as valuable to nursing practice. These competencies describe the unique contributions that nurses make. The competencies are clinical judgment, advocacy, moral agency, caring practices, facilitation of learning, collaboration, system thinking, response to diversity, and clinical inquiry. All of the competencies demonstrate the active combination of knowledge, skills, experience, and attitudes necessary to meet patients' needs and to optimize outcomes.[2] Nurses develop competency within each continuum so that they are able to meet the changing needs of their particular patient population. Each of these competencies is an essential part of nursing practice, but the degree of importance is determined by the patient's characteristics.

By combining the nurse competencies identified in the Synergy Model and the behaviors identified in Benner's levels of practice, a continuum of expertise can be developed that matches behavior with practice levels. It focuses recognition and reward on clinical practice. The impact of expert nurses on patient outcomes is presented in quantitative and financial parameters that can be understood throughout the healthcare system. The model provides the needed links between clinical competencies and patient outcomes.

The levels of clinical nursing practice can be used as the foundation for a clinical advancement program. As illustrated in Table 5-1, four levels of nursing practice are described using broad performance standards and specific behavioral characteristics associated with a selected competency of the Synergy Model.

RN I Practice

RN I practice is based on Benner's description of the novice and advanced beginners, those with little or no experience in the clinical area. The rule-governed behavior that is typical of this level practitioner is strict and limited. RN I staff nurses tend to apply rules equally to all situations with little or no ability to consider the context in which they are applied.[3] These factors significantly affect their ability to perform the competencies outlined in the Synergy Model.[2]

RN Is make clinical judgments based on policies, procedures, and textbook knowledge. At this level, they focus on one aspect of a situation and tend to weigh all assessment data equally because they lack prior experience. RN Is do not have a global perspective and will not be able to predict the patient's clinical course if it deviates from the norm. Collaboration is basic, which can be evidenced by their limited participation in multidisciplinary teams and their need to be coached through a situation. RN Is facilitate learning by knowing what resources are available and using them. They function as advocates simply by recognizing the need and securing help to meet the need. They demonstrate a basic awareness of the complex systems within the healthcare system but need assistance to integrate this knowledge into a meaningful plan of care. Clinical inquiry behaviors are evidenced through the RN I's use of unit resources and clinical experts. These nurses demonstrate empathetic, compassionate, and helpful hands-on caring practices.

New or relatively new graduates, nurses who have never practiced in critical care, and experienced critical care nurses new to pediatrics are considered RN I level practitioners. Orientation expectations are consistent for all new staff; though the rate at which orientation competencies are demonstrated varies between individuals, depending on past experience.

As RN Is complete orientation, learning experiences from actual situations that illustrate one aspect of care can be examined. These practitioners begin to see how the rules are influenced by the situation but require help to integrate the parts into the whole. RN Is benefit from repeated experiences with similar aspects of patient care and from mentors who can point out salient aspects of a patient's response to care. These beginners, although competent to provide safe care, benefit from assistance in interpreting assessments and in setting priorities. They require support in the clinical area so that important patient needs will not go unmet. If they are to care for complex unstable patients, close supervision and guidance are required.

As previously mentioned, RN Is respond to the situation according to rules, focus on only one aspect of the situation, and need help in setting priorities if the patient's response is not the one that is anticipated. For example, an RN I caring for a patient who requires emergency intubation can focus only on the airway during the crisis. This nurse performs bag-valve-mask ventilation with 100% oxygen, has suction available, and has the appropriate endotracheal tube and laryngoscope blade ready. The nurse requires additional support in this situation if the equipment malfunctions, if the patient's vital signs become unstable, or if the intubation is technically difficult. The RN I may be unable to recognize the need for additional resources or be unable to secure those that are obviously needed.

Educational opportunities, teaching methods, information, and content are provided in various forms to meet the needs of the individual learners at this level. Formalized lectures and presentations, unit in-services, self-study modules, computer-based learning modules, and bedside teaching are examples of learning activities that support the RN I. Historically, these skill-based, technical offerings have been the strength of unit- and hospital-based nursing education programs. Access to these programs is readily available through sources such as the Internet, professional organizations, medical libraries, texts, and professional literature. Costs for offering these basic classes to the RN I are predictable because many of these programs already exist. Evaluation of the effectiveness of these skill-based programs is measured by behavioral changes in the practice of the RN I. Successful integration of knowledge and skill will enable this nurse to care for increasingly complex critical care patients.

Support for this nurse is typically provided by the RN II, who functions in the preceptor role. Overall guidance for the development of the RN I is monitored by the clinical nurse specialist, unit educator, or nurse manager. Peer review processes, quality improvement activities, and exemplar writing are introduced to the RN I.

The overall expectations of RN Is are that they identify obvious patient care needs, provide safe care, and recognize the need for more experienced assistance. The RN I benefits from discussing the situation after the fact. Senior staff can identify areas for improvement, provide positive feedback, and allow RN Is to ask questions and practice skills.

RN II Practice

RN IIs, modeled after Benner's definition of competent nurses, are characterized by their organizational abilities in coping with the competing demands and shifting priorities of clinical practice.[3] These nurses gain efficiency and the ability to understand and react to a situation as a whole rather than in parts. RN IIs have developed the ability to recognize the unexpected turn of events and identify which aspects of a situation are more important than others. This increased knowledge and experience base enables them to demonstrate a higher level of competence within the synergy framework and have a greater impact on patient outcome than RN Is.

RN IIs use more sophisticated critical thinking skills as part of their clinical judgments. They question clinical practices, compare and contrast alternatives, and recognize that outcomes may vary. They collaborate more actively within the multidisciplinary team and recognize the need for patient and family participation in care decisions. These nurses assess the patient and family's readiness to learn and

Text continued on p. 94

Table 5-1 Performance Competency Documents: RN I to RN IV

Performance Competency Document

Position Title: RN I Entry Level

Position Summary: The RN I constantly demonstrates current, comprehensive, professional knowledge and skill in accordance with nursing standards and department policies when caring for patients and their families. The RN I develops individualized and collaborative plans of care using appropriate standards of care and practice and demonstrates effective communication to promote and maintain a professional environment.

Clinical Judgment: Clinical decision making, critical thinking, and global grasp of the situation coupled with nursing skills acquired by integrating formal and experiential knowledge

Performance Standard	Behavioral Characteristics	Performance Outcome Level	Outcome Measurement Tools
Recognizes the value of the nursing process.	Demonstrates application of the nursing process. Assesses, plans, implements, and evaluates patient care.	Patient/family/nurse interactions	Patient/family satisfaction Self-evaluation Director evaluation Peer review Clinical exemplar module
Performs physical, psychosocial, and developmental assessment of the patient and family. Identifies and documents deviations from the norm. Evaluates, documents, and communicates patient response to interventions and revises plan of care as indicated.	Demonstrates clinical thinking skills through early cognition of changing patient conditions, appropriately asking for assistance and timely follow-up with prioritized interventions. References unit-based resource materials. Documentation meets hospital standards. Assesses and anticipates patient needs from previous experiences. Identifies, establishes, documents, and communicates plan of care based on assessed patient characteristics. Patient characteristics are: Resiliency: capacity to return to or achieve a restorative or optimal level of functioning Vulnerability: susceptibility to stressors, which may impact the outcome Stability: risks associated with overall patient condition Complexity: interaction of multiple systems creating the patient's condition Resource availability: access to social, technical, emotional, or financial resources Participation in decision making and care: the patient/family's ability to collaborate in care Predictability: certainty of projected outcome		

Intervenes with safe, appropriate, and scientifically based nursing care.

Demonstrates the knowledge and skills necessary to assess and intervene appropriately based on developmental age of patients and families served on the assigned unit.

Performance Competency Document
Position Title: RN II Competent Level

Position Summary: The RN II consistently applies specialized knowledge and skills in the management of nursing care for specific types of patient populations and their families. The RN II recognizes the need for ongoing evaluation and inquiry to improve patient outcomes. The RN II develops patient-specific long-range goals and plans that are managed through organizing, prioritizing, and coping with multiple patient needs and skill requirements. At this level, expected performance outcomes are based on patient/family/nurse interactions.

Clinical Judgment: Clinical decision making, critical thinking, and global grasp of the situation, coupled with nursing skills acquired by integrating formal and experiential knowledge

Performance Standard	Behavioral Characteristics	Performance Outcome Level	Outcome Measurement Tools
Integrates the nursing process into the provision of safe patient care. Collects and interprets patient data. Evaluates, documents, and communicates patient response to interventions and revises plan of care as indicated.	Demonstrates application of the nursing process. Assesses, plans, implements, and evaluates patient care. Questions situations and recognizes variances in clinical outcomes. Demonstrates critical thinking skills through early recognition of changing patient conditions, appropriately asking for assistance and timely follow-up with prioritized interventions. Documentation meets hospital standards. Considers algorithms for treatment. Identifies, establishes, documents, and communicates plan of care based on assessed patient characteristics. Patient characteristics defined as: Resiliency: capacity to return to or achieve a restorative or optimal level of functioning Vulnerability: susceptibility to stressors, which may affect outcome Stability: risks associated with overall patient condition Complexity: interaction of multiple systems creating the patient's condition Resource availability: access to social, technical, emotional, or financial resources Participation in decision making and care: patient/family's ability to collaborate in care Predictability: certainty of projected outcome	Patient/family/nurse interactions	Patient/family satisfaction Self-evaluation Director evaluation Peer review Clinical exemplar Action plan

Continued

Table 5-1   Performance Competency Documents: RN I to RN IV—cont'd

Performs physical, psychosocial, and developmental assessment of the patient and family. Identifies, documents, and reports deviations from the norm.	Completes and uses age-specific assessment tools and individualizes to meet patient needs.
Intervenes with safe, appropriate, and scientifically based nursing care. Possesses mastery of technical skills that enable a response to the unique needs of the patient and family.	Anticipates and acts to prevent potential or preventable problems. Provides basic care for complex patients. Participates in unit-based quality assurance or quality improvement (QA/QI) activities.
Demonstrates competence in performaning nursing skills in stressful, complex, or unusual circumstances	
Recognizes limitations of own experience and knowledge.	Develops self-assessment skills to improve care delivery. Seeks new knowledge.

Performance Competency Document
Position Title: RN III Proficient Level

Position Summary: The RN III demonstrates advanced knowledge and skills in the management of nursing care for specific types of patient populations and their families. The RN III holistically views patient situations, anticipates exceptions, and implements a disease and treatment pathway in the planning of care and prevention of complications. The RN III leads to development and implementation of a interdisciplinary outcomes-oriented plan of care. The RN III collaboratively develops strategies to manage the care environment and negotiate the patient through the care experience. The RN III demonstrates commitment to nursing practice through unit-based leadership, educational interventions with outcomes analysis, and quality improvement activities to enhance the provision of optimal practice outcomes.

Clinical Judgment: Clinical decision making, critical thinking, and global grasp of the situation, coupled with nursing skills acquired by integrating formal and experiential knowledge

Performance Standard	Behavioral Characteristics	Performance Outcome Level	Outcome Measurement Tools
Considers patient as a whole person and anticipates exceptions in care. Anticipates a disease and treatment pathway in the planning of immediate care and in the prevention of complications. Recognizes subtle changes in patient assessments and intervenes with considerations toward multisystem interrelationships. Readily identifies the rapid state in which a patient's condition can change. Evaluates, documents, and communicates patient responses to interventions and revises plan of care as indicated.	Demonstrates and models application of the nursing process. Assesses, plans, implements, and evaluates patient care. Identifies, establishes, documents, and communicates plan of care based on assessed patient characteristics. Patient characteristics defined as: Resiliency: capacity to return to or achieve a restorative or optimal level of functioning Vulnerability: susceptibility to stressors, which may affect outcome Stability: risks associated with overall patient condition	Patient/family/nurse interactions Unit-based impact Outcome report to nursing division	Patient/family satisfaction Self-evaluation Director evaluation Peer review Clinical exemplar Action plan

Intervenes with safe, appropriate, well-planned, and scientifically based nursing care.

Demonstrates proficiency in performing nursing skills in stressful, complex, or unusual circumstances with minimal assistance in assessment of patient needs.

Demonstrates advanced knowledge of emergency care practices and intervenes appropriately.

Performs comprehensive physical, psycho-social, and developmental assessment of the patient and family.

Demonstrates the knowledge and skills necessary to assess and intervene appropriately based on the developmental age of the patients served on the assigned unit. Identifies, documents, and reports deviations from the norm.

Complexity: interaction of multiple systems creating the patient's condition

Resource availability: access to social, technical, emotional, or financial resources

Participation in decision making and care: patient/family's ability to collaborate in care

Predictability: certainty of projected outcome

Initiates, uses, and updates standards of care to support assessments and individualizes plan of care.

Documentation meets hospital standards.

Identifies problems and uses QA/QI projects to solve problems.

Anticipates and acts to prevent potential or preventable problems.

Demonstrates speed and flexibility in prioritizing, recognizing, and intervening in all aspects of care.

Maintains calm, professional demeanor during crisis situations.

Directs the care of multiple complex patients (charge nurse role).

Completes, revises, and individualizes age-specific assessment tools.

Continued

TABLE 5-1 Performance Competency Documents: RN I to RN IV—cont'd

Performance Competency Document

Position Title: RN IV Expert Level

Position Summary: The RN IV demonstrates a deep understanding of the unique meaning and imact of health and illness issues for the patient and family. Possessing a vast background of experience, the RN IV recognizes and responds to the dynamic situation by using past experiences to synthesize and interpret multiple, sometimes conflicting, sources of data. The RN IV models collaborative practice behaviors, provides mentorship, coaches, consults, and demonstrates professional commitment to the healthcare system. The RN IV engages in the development and implementation of research, quality improvement, leadership, publication, and community education programs for the advancement of clinical practice. The RN IV further performs analysis to demonstrate and support synergized, optimal patient, system, and professional outcomes.

Clinical Judgment: Clinical decision making, critical thinking, and global grasp of the situation, coupled with nursing skills acquired by integrating formal and experiential knowledge

Performance Standard	Behavioral Characteristics	Performance Outcome Level	Outcome Measurement Tools
Uses independent nursing action to meet unusual or stressful circumstances.	Demonstrates and supports peers in the application of the nursing process.	Patient/family/nurse interactions	Patient/family satisfaction
Recognizes and responds to the dynamic situation, using past experiences to anticipate problems.	Assesses, plans, implements, and evaluates patient care.	Unit-based impact	Self-evaluation
Fashions judgments based on an immediate grasp of the whole picture.	Incorporates long-range planning at onset of care.	Healthcare system impact	Director evaluation
Synthesizes and interprets multiple, sometimes conflicting sources of data.	Helps the family see the "big picture."	Outcome report to nursing division	Peer review
	Collaborates as clinical consultant.		Clinical exemplar
	Identifies, establishes, documents, and communicates plan of care based on assessed patient characteristics.		Action plan
	Patient characteristics defined as:		QA/QI activities
	Resiliency: capacity to return to or achieve a restorative or optimal level of functioning		
	Vulnerability: susceptibility to stressors, which may affect the outcome		
	Stability: risks associated with overall patient condition		

Complexity: interaction of multiple systems creating the patient's condition
Resource availability: assess to social, technical, emotional, or financial resources
Participation in decision making and care: patient/family's ability to collaborate in care
Predictability: certainty of projected outcome

Demonstrates critical thinking skills through early recognition of changing patient conditions, appropriately providing assistance and timely follow-up with prioritized interventions.
Recognizes subtle trends and intervenes before explicit diagnostic signs are evident.

Completes and revises age-specific assessment tools. Individualizes to meet patient needs. Models hospital standards for documentation.

Develops and teaches peers self-assessment skills to improve care delivery.
Interacts with community through inservices, presentations, and/or publication.
Serves as a role model for the standard and demonstrates professional practice based on academic or clinical experiences. Demonstrates independence by taking initiative, makes changes when appropriate, is self-directed and creative, and requires little or no supervision concerning standard.

Recognizes subtle changes in patient assessments and intervenes with consideration toward multisystem interrelationships.
Readily identifies the rapid state in which a child's or adult's condition can change.

Evaluates, documents, and communicates patient response to interventions and revises plan of care as indicated. Performs comprehensive physical, psychosocial, and developmental assessment of the patient and family. Identifies, documents, and communicates deviations from the norm.

Recognizes limitations of own experience and knowledge base.
Possesses mastery of technical skills that enable a response to the unique needs of patient and family.
Demonstrates expert skills in performing nursing care in stressful, complex, or unusual circumstances.

Adapted from Clinical Practice Program, All Children's Hospital, St. Petersburg, Fla.

can adapt available resources for learning. Many RN IIs are assuming mentor and preceptor roles for newer staff and are consulted about more complex patient care issues by inexperienced staff. RN II staff nurses recognize situations that may produce conflict and are active participants in the resolution of ethical dilemmas. Care is planned with input from the family, and decisions are based on this input when possible. RN IIs have a deeper understanding of the health system's effect on the patient and family and can anticipate the impact of the system on patient outcomes. They recognize resources and seek help when these resources are not available. Additional experience and knowledge allow the competent nurse to function more effectively and have a greater influence on the patient's safe passage through the healthcare system. These skills engender patient trust and improve satisfaction.

In the situation of the patient who requires emergency intubation mentioned earlier, the RN II responds in a more organized and proactive manner than the RN I. The RN II assists in airway management and has the appropriate equipment and drugs ready. The patient's response to therapy is anticipated, and the family is supported. This nurse demonstrates some mastery to cope with the potential emergency events that may be encountered. The RN II closely monitors for hemodynamic instability as an anticipated complication during intubation. The nurse recognizes the need to interrupt the intubation procedure if the patient requires bag-valve-mask ventilation.

RN IIs learn best from simulations that allow them to practice prioritizing, delegating, decision making, negotiating for resources, and problem solving in complex situations. They need to be challenged with increasing complex problems to maintain interest and identify areas for learning. Interactive case studies, journal clubs, and patient scenario simulations conducted at the unit level offer an excellent opportunity to challenge the critical thinking skills of this nurse. Integrating nursing research into practice is encouraged at this level. Learning activities offered through nursing education or staff development departments that support collaboration, diversity training, preceptorships, negotiation, self-assessment, and basic quality improvement skills are important to the maturation of this nurse. Cost management for these programs remains primarily at the unit level and can be incorporated in time allotted for staff meetings and unit-based in-service education. Personal responsibility for lifelong learning is an emphasis at this level and reflects the institutional culture as a learning organization. Networking with professional peers for improved practice options is encouraged. Evaluation of the effectiveness of these learning activities is measured in the ability to care for complex patients, effectively act in a preceptor role, participate in quality improvement activities, and safely manage care in a rapidly changing patient care environment.

Unit guidance for the RN II is provided by the RN III and RN IV. Clinical nurse specialists, unit educators, hospital educators, and nurse managers act in supportive coaching roles. The RN II participates in peer review activities that support practice improvements for colleagues. The RN II demonstrates individual nursing competency through written exemplars and a self-evaluation process. Goals and objectives developed by this nurse include plans for future learning activities, which have an affect on patient outcomes.

RN III Practice

RN IIIs practice at a level that Benner defines as proficient.[3] These nurses visualize the clinical situation as a whole. Judgment and decisions are based on experience and recent assessments. These nurses achieve an even greater degree of competency and can have a measurable impact on patient outcomes.

RN IIIs, who possess a minimum of 3 years of clinical nursing experience, demonstrate the ability to assess and evaluate the current clinical picture from a more global perspective.[3] Nursing practice reflects judgments and decisions based on accumulated knowledge and experience. RN IIIs sort out the nonessential aspects of a case, recognize subtleties, and intervene before they become a larger problem. Provision of care reflects an understanding of patients' needs as they progress across the healthcare continuum. RN IIIs are regarded as resources for specific care issues and use data to assist in decision making.

Proficient nurses know what to expect in a given situation and adjust plans in response to these changes. Because they recognize the difference between essential and nonessential, decision making is more efficient. Prioritization skills are well developed, and these nurses recognize subtle aspects of a situation that can significantly change the patient's outcome. RN IIIs function as clinical resources and preceptors, mentor new staff, and network throughout the healthcare system. They consistently integrate and formally and informally evaluate knowledge retention of their patients and fellow staff. Advocacy is highly visible in this level of practice. RN IIIs anticipate areas of potential conflict and work quickly to resolve issues. Cultural diversity issues are routinely integrated into an inclusive and holistic plan of care. RN IIIs' knowledge of the healthcare system enables patients to negotiate through the system more successfully. Their practice can have a significant impact on patient, family, and collegial relationships.

In the emergency intubation situation, the RN III responds in a controlled and organized manner and may be able to prevent the situation altogether. All resources are available, and less experienced staff are encouraged to learn from the experience. Communication with the family is a priority, and questions are anticipated. The situation is understood as a whole, and the response is accurate, influenced by past experience and recent changes. This situation is used as a learning opportunity for RN Is and RN IIs who are nearby.

RN IIIs learn best from case presentations and interactive situations that focus on realistic clinical events. These educational scenarios should have the same level of complexity and ambiguity as real clinical situations to stimulate thought and promote critical thinking. Encouraging this level of practitioner to learn in a way that makes sense is the best approach and encourages the advancement of the current practice level.

Educational experiences for RN IIIs are developed to reflect the assessed learning needs of the individual practitioner. Nursing competencies emphasized at this level include collaboration, systems thinking, clinical judgment, facilitation of learning, clinical inquiry, and advocacy and moral agency. Examples of learning activities that support this level of practice include development programs for presentation and communication skills, team-building activities, review and development of outcomes measurement tools, and unit-based leadership development, such as coaching and mentoring. RN IIIs are involved in teaching, coaching, and facilitating unit-based in-services, journal clubs, and case study discussions. They facilitate unit-based peer review processes and mentor RN Is and RN IIs in their practice. Accessing information from resources outside of the system and professional networking activities that improve patient care practices are expectations at this level.

RN IV Practice

RN IV staff or expert performers have broad experiences and do not rely solely on rules, guidelines, or other dogma to make decisions. The expert nurse focuses on the real issues without consideration of numerous unfruitful alternative diagnoses and solutions.[3] The expert takes the entire situation and past experience into account when responding to patient situations. This response is often characterized as intuitive and is an example of mastery: the ability to recognize a wide range of subtle cues, extract maximum information from those cues, and intervene decisively.[3,7] RN IVs are able to demonstrate the competencies of synergy most completely, and their practice has a significant impact on patients and implementation of cost-effective interventions.[8]

Staff at the RN IV level recognize subtle trends in their patients and can often intervene before the patient's decompensation. Itano[9] found evidence that highly skilled nurses make accurate judgments after only a few minutes of patient contact. They are adept at managing complex situations, and they manage intricate tasks considering the concerns of the family and other healthcare providers. These nurses are recognized as experts by physicians, and they can often impact medical decisions because of the level of respect that past performance has bestowed on them. Expertise at this level results from repeated similar experiences that prompt the nurse to begin to make predictions based on the patient's response.

These clinicians incorporate long-range planning at the onset of care and help the family understand the broader picture. They use creative approaches to empower patients and families. Knowledge of current clinical practice is based on both research and experience. Other clinical staff consults these nurses; they set the standard for the unit and practice specialty. They promote collaboration among cli-

nicians and seek opportunities to teach, coach, and mentor other staff. As expert clinicians, they educate less experienced staff. Facilitation of learning is a priority, and they anticipate the need to learn. These nurses are willing to share knowledge, and they often develop creative teaching methods. Leadership and role modeling are an expectation at this level. These nurses exhibit behaviors that are clearly recognized as expert practice, so other staff use them to guide and measure their own professional development.

When the situation is stable, RN IVs are in familiar territory. When they are not knowledgeable about a situation, RN IVs will do whatever is necessary to understand the situation.[10] These nurses care for patients holistically and incorporate cultural needs into the plan of care. RN IVs have a much broader understanding of the healthcare system and are able to procure necessary resources. Critical thinking skills are well developed, and the art of negotiation is practiced skillfully. Active participation in research and quality activities is an important component of the role. RN IVs encourage staff to question practice and use research and quality initiatives to evaluate effectiveness. They participate in professional activities, such as publishing and speaking. They maximize patient outcomes because they employ sophisticated assessment expertise, develop comprehensive plans of care, implement coordinated processes to accomplish the goals of the plan, and influence the success of the outcome.

In the emergency intubation situation, the RN IV may first recognize the need to electively intubate early and enlist a physician or colleague's assistance before the patient's condition further deteriorates. The RN IV is able to recognize a cluster of subtle cues as predictive and meaningful. Holden and Klinger[11] studied ways that expert nurses use critical thinking skills to differentiate cries in infants. These researchers support Benner's findings that expert nurses demonstrate increased problem-solving skills. Even if unsuccessful in convincing the physician to act, the RN IV is able to anticipate the patient's needs and responses.

Examples of learning activities for this level include opportunities to strengthen teaching skills, participation in quality improvement processes, and case management practices. Specific types of educational programs offered may include topics on research utilization, outcomes measurement tools and reporting, case management processes, legislative issues, and leadership and negotiation skills.

The clinical nurse specialist serves as the resource for nurses at all levels but provides important advanced practice learning opportunities for RN IVs. Educational opportunities that enable dialogue with other clinicians and pertain to realistic clinical situations are beneficial for nurses at this level. This is especially true if these case studies contain the many factors, subtle cues, and contextual meanings that nurses consider in their daily clinical decision making. Dealy and Bass[12] determined that expert nurses find it harder to leave the bedside to pursue professional development opportunities. These nurses typically choose to develop themselves by interacting with professional colleagues. As an important resource person, the clinical nurse specialist further pinpoints the subtle warning cues with which expert nurses identify and respond. Discussion of these cues is instructive for staff at many levels and may provide rich material for nursing research. RN IVs can participate in and offer unique contributions to clinical research.

Clinical Advancement Process

Clinical advancement programs were first developed in 1972 to recognize and reward increasingly effective nursing practice.[4] These programs continued to evolve and began to focus on recruitment and retention issues.[13-15] Although these programs had a solid theoretical foundation and acknowledged salary compensation issues, they did not clearly identify nursing behaviors that contribute to improved patient's outcome. They also did not adequately represent nursing satisfaction or fiscal responsibility.[10] Clinical advancement programs became increasingly difficult to defend in relation to return on investment to the healthcare system as a whole.

Financial resources to support clinical education and clinical advancement programs have been greatly reduced, yet these programs and services are directly linked to the retention of experienced expert nursing staff.[16] Nurses who possess certain expert skills are highly desirable and beneficial to the patient and organization. Researchers have quantified the financial impact of expert nurses in decreased medication costs, decreased patient falls, and increased quality of care.[10] A clinical advancement program that provides encouragement and guidance for the development of nurses and nursing practice can become an important tool in supporting organizational fiscal and quality objectives.

A structured, well-defined clinical advancement process can facilitate professional growth and personal feelings of value and worth in the staff nurse. The key to accomplishing these goals is implementing a model that links clinical competence with patient outcomes. The impact of practice evolution can only be recognized if clinical behaviors are identified within levels and core characteristics of the most expert clinicians are documented.[5] This process presents comprehensive methods to specify essential competencies and related skills that demonstrate advancement in diverse clinical settings. The process enables the recognition of the contributions of nursing to the patient and system. It encourages staff to see that what they value about nursing practice is reflected in the advancement process. They become capable of defining themselves within the concepts of nursing competence, patient characteristics, and outcome measures. The process assists in the articulation of the worth of clinical advancement from the perspective of patient and family satisfaction, market share, recruitment and retention cost offsets, cost benefit analysis or productivity, turnover, and unexpected time off.

Advancement of staff from one level to another is based on a variety of factors, including competent performance of characteristic behaviors that represent current level of practice, accomplishment of measurable outcomes, nurse manager support, peer review, self-evaluation, budgetary constraints, years of experience, and certification or academic qualifications at the expert level. This process should be clear and consistently applied to all applicants. A written guide to promotion at each level facilitates advancement and enhances understanding of the program as a whole. Table 5-2 outlines an example of advancement criteria.

The clinical advancement process can be completely centralized, completely unit based, or a combination of both. For example, the process may be unit based for advancement from RN I through RN III but centralized for RN IV so that a consistent description of expert practice throughout the nursing department exists and practice outcomes remain focused on system-wide issues. Clinical advancement can also be a centralized program built around core competencies that have distinct behavioral characteristics. These characteristics reflect the practice specialty and have outcome measures defined within the framework of that specialty practice. The competencies define discrete practice skills that can be adapted to fit a specific practice setting. Table 5-3 provides an overview of specific outcome examples developed for a pediatric intensive care unit.

Facilitating Clinical Learning

In the current healthcare environment, nurses are required to possess an extensive body of knowledge and meet the needs of the consumer and the organization. This responsibility requires a lifelong process of professional development targeted to specific levels of clinical practice. Professional development staff apply knowledge of instructional strategies appropriate to each practice level to facilitate clinical learning and promote job satisfaction. Benner[3] suggests that the way in which nurses approach problems is similar within each level of skill acquisition. She proposes that learning situations that pair a learner of one level with a preceptor closest to the learner's own skill level are the most successful.[3] Adult learning theory[17,18] supports this position because it involves the teacher's awareness of the learner's readiness to learn the information or skill being taught. Nurses can choose from many learning options, such as academic education, continuing education, participation in research, collaborative learning, case studies, and simulations.

Facilitation of professional advancement in a pediatric critical care setting can be realized through a well-designed, unit-based staff development program. This program is a key element in the advancement process and promotes the knowledge and skills necessary for continued professional development. Dealy and Bass[12] identified numerous factors that motivated nurses to seek professional development. Their work illustrated clinical advancement programs as strategies that promote professional growth.

A staff development program that reflects professional advancement criteria offers nurses the means to achieve professional advancement objectives. Furthermore, when these two important programs complement each other, nursing practice as a whole is strengthened.

TABLE 5-2 **Practice Differentiation Program Guidelines**

Practice Level Requirements

RN I: Entry Nurse	RN II: Competent Nurse	RN III: Proficient Nurse	RN IV: Expert Nurse
Entry level Maintains standards as described in RN I performance competency document (PCD) Completes the exemplar learning module before first year evaluation	**Maintenance of RN II** Maintains standards as described in RN II PCD Submits a clinical exemplar with annual self-evaluation Develops a plan with potential outcomes defined for patient/family/nurse Participates in peer review process Receives yearly merit increase as determined by performance	**Maintenance of RN III** Maintains standards as described in RN III PCD Submits clinical exemplar with annual self-evaluation Participates in peer review process Develops plan with potential defined outcomes for the patient/family/nurse/unit Receives yearly merit increase as determined by performance Reports goals and outcomes to the CAP Committee	**Maintenance of RN IV** Maintains standards as described in RN IV PCD Submits clinical exemplar with annual self-evaluation Participates in peer review process Develops a plan with potential outcomes for patient/family/nurse/hospital Maintains national certification, if applicable Receives yearly merit increase as determined by performance Reports goals and outcomes to the CAP Committee
Advancement to RN II Completes 1 year of RN experience Meets RN I performance competencies Participates in peer review process Develops a plan with potential outcomes defined for the patient/family/nurse Advances to RN II with title change, Clinical Advancement Program (CAP) incentive, and yearly merit increase as determined by performance	**Advancement to RN III** Has a minimum of 3 years of experience in nursing Meets RN II performance competencies RN III position vacant and posted Completes a request for transfer, if appropriate Interviews with respective department director to discuss possible advancement Develops plan or enhances RN II plan with potential defined outcomes for patient/family/nurse/unit Advances to RN III with title change, CAP incentive, and yearly merit increase as determined by performance, if applicable	**Advancement to RN IV** Has a minimum of 5 years of experience in nursing Must possess specialty national certification or bachelor's degree Meets RN III performance competencies RN IV position vacant and posted Completes a request for transfer, if appropriate Interviews with respective department director to discuss possible advancement Develops plan or enhances RN III plan with potential outcomes defined for patient/family/nurse/system Advances to RN IV with title change, CAP incentive, and yearly merit increase as determined by performance, if applicable	

Adapted from Clinical Practice Program, All Children's Hospital, St. Petersburg, Fla.

TABLE 5-3   Outcome Examples: Clinical Judgment–Infant Instability Assessment

RN I	RN II	RN III	RN IV
Recognizes child with signs of respiratory distress	Identifies early signs of respiratory distress	Functions as a preceptor for new staff; teaches assessment and communication skills	Functions as preceptor for new staff; tracks retention of staff
Notifies charge nurse and physician	Performs initial interventions (e.g., bag-valve-mask and cardiopulmonary resuscitation)	Serves as a peer consultant on the unit	Participates in the development of outcomes for the hospital Code Committee
Patient/family/nurse outcomes: practice demonstrates ability to assess changes in patient condition and communicate needs for assistance	Identifies respiratory distress as a frequent situation on the unit	Participates in hospital-wide mock codes	Develops an interdisciplinary protocol for the treatment of respiratory distress, tracks length of stay (LOS), or functional status on discharge
	Designs poster board and "pocket pal" for staff with references	Active member of the hospital Code Committee	Develops algorithm according to national standard and presents at conference
	Patient/family outcomes: life-threatening situation receives immediate intervention	Develops unit-specific protocol with respiratory therapy personnel	Patient/family outcomes: life-threatening situation receives immediate intervention
	Nurse outcomes: demonstrates ability to act effectively in an emergency situation	Patient/family outcomes: life-threatening situation receives immediate intervention	Nurse outcomes: demonstrates ability to lead others in effectively intervening in an emergency situation
		Nurse outcomes: demonstrates ability to act and support others in effectively intervening in an emergency situation	Unit outcomes: demonstrates changes in system practices that affect improvements in service, cost, or outcomes
		Unit outcomes: demonstrates changes in unit practices that affect improvements in service, cost, or outcomes	

Adapted from Clinical Practice Program, All Children's Hospital, St. Petersburg, Fla.

DESIGNING STAFF DEVELOPMENT PROGRAMS FOR PROFESSIONAL ADVANCEMENT

Multiple educational support components must be explored to support the development and maintenance of a clinical advancement program within the critical care setting. Learning activities, evaluation processes, and outcome measurement systems are aligned to meet the needs of the program. Learning activities become directly linked to improving patient outcomes, affecting system efficiencies, and influencing caregivers' satisfaction. A basic premise for staff development programs is that they support learning and nurture individuals to engage in lifelong learning activities.[19]

The fundamental aim of staff development programs for critical care nurses is safe, competent practice. Comprehensive programs for staff development provide the essential resources to support and promote this goal. Similarly, healthcare laws, regulations, and accreditation requirements focus on the basic importance of safe, competent patient care in an effort to protect the healthcare consumer. Professional nursing standards of practice likewise serve as guides for ensuring safe practice and consumer protection. To en-

sure that the institution meets all current standards, those responsible for designing critical care education programs must be familiar with all of these prerequisites. The establishment of a staff development program that is linked to clinical practice is key to the success of a professional advancement program.

The first step in establishing a staff development program is the acquisition of firm support from both nursing and hospital administration. This support requires a commitment to provide the human, financial, material, and environmental resources necessary to implement the program. Once this commitment is secured, the nurse educator may begin to structure the program.

Hospital-based critical care staff development programs may be centralized or decentralized. Centralized programs offer the advantage of maximizing resources within the entire nursing department and standardizing programs across units; whereas unit-based, or decentralized, programs maintain separate budgets to specifically respond to the needs of a particular unit.

Regardless of which option is chosen, the reporting relationship between the critical care nurse educator and nursing administration requires clarity. Once the administrative structure is in place, the program philosophy, goals, policies, and organizing framework may be developed.

Developing a Program Philosophy

A philosophy statement consists of a set of beliefs related to a specific issue. A comprehensive critical care staff development philosophy reflects the beliefs and values of the critical care area, the department of nursing, and the hospital. This consistency reinforces the program's integration within overall hospital and nursing programs and verifies a commitment to common goals. In addition, an essential component of the critical care staff development philosophy is a clearly stated philosophy of adult education that defines learning and the factors that distinguish both the role of the educator and the role of the learner. It is important that underlying beliefs about learning are clearly communicated.

Adult Learning Theory

Developing a philosophy statement that reflects adult educational principles requires a working knowledge of adult learning theory and the specific characteristics of adult learners. Fox[20] asserts that the purpose of adult learning is to enhance proficiency and improve performance. Pike[21] describes adults as "babies in big bodies," which implies that they expect much and like to play while they learn. As adult learners, nurses seek out learning experiences that meet personal needs or are interesting to them relative to their practice; they typically prefer to learn by doing rather than by observation.

Knowles[18] and other theorists of adult learning describe common characteristics of adult learners. They are self-directed, problem-oriented learners who are guided by their own values and come from a heterogeneous experience. Unlike children, adult learners hold an independent self-concept and value their personal time.[22] Principles of adult learning are derived from these characteristics.

The four principles of adult learning that are most applicable to critical care nurses are those concerning reinforcement, readiness to learn, goals, and the learning environment.[23] Reinforcement in the learning process may be positive or negative. If a newly learned behavior stimulates a positive response, the chances of the behavior recurring are increased. Likewise, if a behavior leads to the elimination of an undesirable response, that behavior will most likely be repeated. For example, an RN I who correctly manages a patient's slow cardiac rhythm by implementing a newly learned treatment protocol is likely to follow that protocol again.

Adults learn better if they perceive that an educational program meets their personal goals. If program content relates to their current concerns, they are more motivated to learn. For example, nurses interested in working with patients with a congenital diaphragmatic hernia will be more motivated to learn about extracorporeal membrane oxygenation (ECMO) than nurses with other interests. Self-directed learning promotes efficient self-management of learning,

enhances the decision-making process, and encourages continued learning.[24]

Organizing Framework for Staff Development

Nurses are part of a large group of "knowledge workers" currently in the workforce. Although nurses possess many technical skills, the real talent that each nurse demonstrates is the ability to assess and evaluate based on knowledge of various healthcare processes. The work is accomplished by making judgments based on the ability to gather information, identify problems, decide on an action, and accept accountability for the outcomes.

Critical care staff development programs can be designed to educate staff nurses within the competencies of the Synergy Model.[2] Each of these competencies comprises a tract in the overall staff development program design and serves as the link that connects the staff development program to the professional advancement program. The program is designed to build on the nurse's prior education and professional nursing experience, which facilitates attainment and maintenance of competence. Concepts inherent to the educational process and to critical care nursing are used as a framework around which educational programs and professional development opportunities are organized. Once defined, the organizing framework serves as the structure within which all development programs for critical care nursing staff are designed.

Skill education alone is no longer sufficient to meet the care delivery needs of the nurse in the critical care environment. Educational strategies that promote learning in the clinical unit and use experiential methods are incorporated into the educational plan. Critical care nurses require extensive knowledge and proficiency in areas such as communication, critical thinking, and collaboration.[25] They must acquire the diverse skills necessary to meet the complex needs of their patients and families.

Clinical narratives are used to teach the competencies of the Synergy Model.[2] Novice nurses learn and gain confidence by telling their stories and focusing on excellent practices identified in the narratives of expert staff. Focused group discussion and examination of the clinical stories add to each participant's knowledge base, can clarify issues, and redirect practice. For example, caring practices are taught and reinforced by using stories that highlight relationship building and the development of trust and support. According to Benner, Hooper-Kyriokidis, and Stannard,[26] critical care nurses disclose emotional responses in their clinical narratives. These emotional concerns and relationships direct clinical understanding and actions.[26] Much is learned about critical care nursing, the art of paying attention, and responding compassionately from reading these stories.

The theory and science of content necessary to meet the synergy competencies include topics such as disease processes, nursing procedures, cultural differences, moral and ethical principles and reasoning, research principles, and educational learning theories. This information is presented by lecture, written information, posters, self-studies, or computer-based technology. However, it is crucial that the information is related to realistic clinical situations. Clinical scenarios, case studies, and simulations representing the dynamic and ambiguous clinical situations that nurses encounter daily are most effective. These educational tools are focused to define behaviors associated with specific competencies.

Bedside teaching is particularly helpful in the development of clinical judgment and caring practice skills. Expert nurses, however, serve as tremendous role models for any of the competencies delineated by the Synergy Model. Novice nurses learn by observing these expert nurses and emulating behaviors. Clinical teaching also enables the novice practitioner to gain experience with unfamiliar interventions in a safe and protected environment. Open discussion and opportunities for questions about certain interventions impact learning for all staff. Communication and validation of clinical knowledge focus learning, positively affect patient outcomes, and add to the total body of nursing knowledge.

Information about research and research use builds clinical inquiry and system thinking skills. Demystifying the research, outcome, and quality processes significantly enhances these skills. Use of journal club formats and supporting staff involvement in research assist in developing clinical inquiry. Building knowledge in the areas of healthcare trends and political action assists nurses to expand their systems thinking skills. Attention to the development of critical thinking skills and problem-solving skills also assists with development of systems thinking.

Facilitation of learning skills are acquired by incorporating communication development into the professional development plan. Presenting clinical teaching strategies, assisting staff to determine learner readiness, and assessing understanding is also included. The importance of developing patience, flexibility, and a nonconfrontational style is reinforced.

Collaboration skills are developed by focusing on content such as negotiation, conflict resolution, time management, communication, and team building. Role-playing, role modeling, and clinical narratives are methods that have been used successfully. Expert nurses teach less experienced staff about the available resources that are helpful and how to access these resources.

Nurses learn technical skills and scientific knowledge in many ways, but the essential aspects of self-assurance, caring practices, and advocacy are only developed through relationships that evolve over time.[27] Nurturing, professional relationships with experienced staff are needed to facilitate the novice's integration into practice.[28] Experienced nurses who share their clinical knowledge and coach other nurses have a tremendous impact on collective learning.[29] Staff nurses who function as coaches are in their roles because they are able to clinically influence and guide situations. They demonstrate expert clinical and leadership skills and facilitate the ongoing clinical development of others.

Effective coaches are characterized by their ability to (1) acknowledge and reward individual strengths and accomplishments; (2) offer constructive, focused feedback; (3) support further growth; and (4) challenge people's proficiency with assignments that foster the individual's skills.[30] Coaching of individual staff is an evolving process that includes appraisal of current performance, mutual goal setting, development of a feedback mechanism, and implementation of an improvement plan.[31] The use of preceptors and mentors as teachers and coaches is linked to providing learning opportunities reflective of each level of practice.

Steps in Program Development

The steps in the process of program development for all types of nursing education programs are assessment, planning, implementation, and evaluation. Following these steps in an organized manner with specific time lines for each ensures quality programming.

Assessment. The first step in developing an educational program is conducting an assessment to identify staff nurses' educational needs, as well as those of the unit or institution as a whole. The method used may be simple or sophisticated, depending on the resources available. Five methods commonly used are (1) interviews with the leadership group, (2) nursing care audits, (3) quality improvement/risk management feedback, (4) Joint Commission on Accreditation of Healthcare Organizations (JCAHO) recommendations, and (5) staff surveys and interviews. Drawing the information from more than one source provides a broader perspective of needs and strengthens the validity of the data obtained. Key elements to consider when developing a needs assessment include patient population and nursing population characteristics. Knowledge and skills necessary to provide care to the patient population are identified to ensure that the specific needs of the units and nurse are addressed. Data are analyzed, and identified needs are ranked. Once the priorities are established, the appropriate educational delivery method, costs, and objectives are developed.

The needs assessment process is continuous to meet the changing needs of staff and the institution. This may be accomplished in part by incorporating needs assessment questions into individual program evaluation tools.

Planning. Once the data from the needs assessment are analyzed, program planning may begin. Overall goals for each program are established first, and outcome statements emerge from these. They serve as a framework for program design and guide the educator in selecting appropriate instructional methods. Outcome statements also provide a means for evaluating whether competencies were achieved and learning took place.

Outcome statements differ from traditional behavioral objectives because they require learners to become competent in skills used in practice.[32] Behavioral objectives typically focus on ways of learning and directions for learning content. Writing outcome statements involves the techniques of concisely stating what performance competence is expected, the extent to which it is expected, and how it will be demonstrated. The use of subjective terms such as *understand* or *know* should be avoided because it is unclear how to measure those behaviors. The use of action words such as *conduct, plan, integrate, provide,* and *engage* reflect practice-related abilities for which the content is learned. Box 5-1 provides some basic criteria for writing competency outcome statements.

Outcome statements provide the nurse educator with the basis for program format and design. The program content and time frame are related directly to the competency statements.

Implementation. Program implementation varies according to the teaching methods selected to meet program outcomes. The learners are encouraged to select the type of teaching methods that best match their learning style. A critical aspect of the educator's role is to ensure that the environment is conducive to learning both physically and psychologically.

Evaluation. Nursing education programs are evaluated in relation to the program goals, desired outcomes, and other predetermined criteria. All those involved in the program participate in the program evaluation. Nurse educators and managers evaluate the relevance of each offering to overall program goals, desired outcomes, and the current scope of practice. Learners evaluate the program content and teaching strategies relative to both the overall program and individual learner outcomes.

Abruzzese[33] developed a simple evaluation model that describes various levels of evaluation from simple to complex and is based on frequency of implementation and cost factors. The Roberta Straessle Abruzzese (RSA) model defines the first level as process evaluations. These evaluations are used for all educational programs and target the learner's general satisfaction with the program. If adult learners are not satisfied at this level, learning will be less effective. An evaluation form using a 3- to 5-point scale with qualitative descriptors such as agree/disagree or excellent/poor is often used for this level of evaluation. Questions focused on satisfaction with faculty, objectives, content, teaching methods, physical setting, and overall program management are often used.

The second level is content evaluation that occurs immediately after the learning experience. This level of

evaluation targets a change in knowledge, affect, skill, or a combination of these. Content evaluation can be assessed by using self-rating scales, pretests and posttests, simulations or case studies, return demonstration, or multiple-choice examinations. These criterion-referenced tools relate to the expected outcomes and are compared with preset criteria.

The third level is outcome evaluation, which is used to measure changes in clinical practice after a learning experience. These changes can be evidenced by integration of a new value or skill or creation of a new product or process. Outcome evaluation is generally performed 3 to 6 months after an extensive learning experience. The evaluation takes place on the clinical unit and can take the form of a questionnaire, observation of practice, audits of changes, or a system of self-report.

The fourth level is impact evaluation, which represents an institutional operational result such as a positive impact on quality, cost-benefit, cost effectiveness, decreased staff turnover, improved staff retention, or decreased risk management issues. These evaluations are developed for programs that can possibly influence changes at the unit, department, or institutional level. These tools are complex and resemble a formal research measurement process.

Every program does not need all four levels of evaluation. The third and fourth levels are reserved for more extensive and complex undertakings. The overall program evaluation focuses on the congruence of goals and accomplishments for the educational offerings. Measurement is accomplished through quarterly reports to administration, cost-benefit analysis, cost-effectiveness reports, and updates to a clinical advisory committee.

Developing valid and reliable evaluation tools is a difficult and time-consuming process. The type of tool used depends on the purpose and level of the evaluation; therefore an existing tool with established validity is often more desirable. Once the validity of the tool is established, the results may be considered with confidence.

COMPONENTS OF STAFF DEVELOPMENT

Staff development programs can be divided into three major categories: orientation, in-service, and continuing education programs. Each of these programs has its own scope, purpose, goals, and objectives. It is important that those responsible for nursing education programs distinguish and understand the difference between each category.

Orientation

The American Nurses Association (ANA) describes orientation as "the means by which new staff members are introduced to the philosophy, goals, policies, procedures, role expectations, physical facilities, and special services in a specific work setting."[34] This description implies that all nurses who begin employment in a critical care setting need to participate in some aspects of orientation regardless of their level of experience. For example, a nurse who transfers into a critical care area from another area in the same hospital needs to be oriented to the

---

Box 5-1
Basic Criteria for Writing Competency Outcome Statements

1. Use learner-oriented wording.
2. Describe the essential competency (psychomotor, cognitive, or affective) to be achieved.
3. Use clear, specific, and concise language.
4. Write measurable statements.
5. Use action-oriented words.
6. Be consistent with standards, practice, and real-world expectations for performance.

Adapted from Lenberg C: The framework, concepts, and methods of the competency, outcomes, and performance assessment (COPA), 1999, in *Online Journal of Issues in Nursing,* at http://wwwnursingworld.org/ojin/topic10-2.htm.

critical care nursing role expectations, special procedures, and services of the critical care unit. A nurse hired from outside the institution with previous experience in critical care also needs to be oriented to the new working environment. The challenge for the critical care educator is to design an orientation program that meets both the individual needs of nurses from a variety of backgrounds and unit-specific needs.

One way to accomplish this goal is to design a competency-based orientation program. "Competency-based education can be perceived as a very broad concept that is used as the conceptual framework for a total curriculum, or it can be interpreted in a very narrow way, as a framework for an individual unit of instruction such as a self-learning module."[35]

A competency-based orientation model has six characteristics: (1) an emphasis on outcomes, (2) use of self-directed learning activities, (3) flexibility and time allowed for achievement of outcomes, (4) use of the teacher as facilitator, (5) assessment of previous learning, and (6) assessment of learning styles.[36] A competency-based approach to orientation facilitates a more positive experience for the orientee through recognition of previously acquired knowledge and skills. For example, an experienced critical care nurse would be frustrated to participate in electrocardiogram recognition classes if that concept had been mastered. A competency-based program enables orientees to select those learning activities that meet their individual learning needs and demonstrate mastery of those required competencies.

As some of these needs are satisfied or reprioritized as a lesser need, others needs will be met in a "Maslowian" sequence.[37] A new nurse orientee first seeks safety in the environment and then progresses through stages to attain membership in the work team. At the end of a well-designed orientation, orientees should feel comfortable in the environment and integrated into the staff.

Critical care internship programs have been extensively used as a mechanism to recruit and train entry-level nurses. These programs are specifically designed to introduce nurses with little or no nursing experience into the complex critical care environment. They provide extended clinical support for novice nurses and introduce new knowledge more deliberately than traditional orientation programs. They focus on basic information and skill acquisition. This focus builds on the knowledge and skills that these nurses have previously acquired in their nursing school programs. Program development can be supported through the use of content outlines developed by AACN and can be individualized to address specific needs of staff, patients, and the institution. Teaching is characteristically under the direction of a clinical nurse specialist or hospital educator and usually involves the most senior staff as preceptors. Typically, competency development is focused on the delivery of safe care to the least complex patients. The program is designed to establish a foundation on which the novice can develop into a competent clinician. Critical care internship programs are developed to meet the needs of individual hospitals or health systems, so very little research

is available to measure the overall effectiveness of these programs. Internship programs can be costly, and outcomes require careful monitoring to ensure effectiveness.

Designing a Competency-Based Orientation Program

The steps to follow in designing a competency-based orientation are the same as those discussed earlier for program development, with emphasis on details specific to orientation.

Assessment. During the needs assessment phase, the competencies expected of an orientee in critical care are identified. "The competencies identified should represent realistic expectations of *general* categories of performance for a *beginning level* staff nurse on that unit."[38] The orientee should not be expected to function at the same level as senior staff by the end of the orientation period.

The process of identifying required competencies necessitates a comprehensive exploration of the specific field of practice. Resources to assist in identifying entry level competencies include (1) staff nurse position descriptions, (2) JCAHO requirements, (3) professional standards of practice (e.g., ANA and AACN), (4) review of the literature, (5) needs of the patient population on the specific unit, and (6) consensus of expert practitioners. Analysis of the information compiled from these resources provides the nurse educator with a foundation for formulating orientation competency statements. The greatest challenge in this process is to gain consensus from preceptors, staff, and managers regarding levels of competence to expect from orientees. Once this is achieved, the nurse educator ensures that these competencies are clearly stated and attainable by all orientees.

A competency statement is a broad sample of behavior that integrates knowledge, psychomotor skills, and attitudes. These broad competency statements are then separated into specific terminal performance criteria that are observable

---

Box 5-2
Sample Competency Statement With Related Performance Criteria

Competency
1. Provides safe nursing care for the patient who requires temporary cardiac pacing

Performance Criteria
1. Identifies clinical indications for temporary pacing
2. Labels wires *A* and *V*
3. Dresses insertion sites with occlusive dressing
4. Secures wires with 2-inch piece of tourniquet
5. Changes battery
6. Documents pacemaker function, settings, and patient response
7. Supports patient and family throughout the period of temporary cardiac pacing

and measurable examples of expected behaviors for demonstration of competency.

Competency statements and performance criteria are developed collaboratively with all those involved in orienting and evaluating new staff. This approach strengthens the validity of the competencies identified. Box 5-2 illustrates an example of a competency statement with its related performance criteria.

Planning. The next step in the orientation process is to consider which methods of evaluation are appropriate for determining attainment of performance criteria. The educator may choose among a written test, a skills laboratory inventory, a performance checklist, or a case study, depending on the nature of the criteria; sometimes a combination of two or more methods is preferable.

Prerequisites may exist for certain competencies before they can be achieved (e.g., knowledge of institutional policies or basic knowledge in critical care nursing). These prerequisites, along with the identified competencies, dictate the core content for critical care orientation.

The content outline for orientation is structured in an orderly manner that reflects the organizing framework of the staff development program. Performance criteria may be arranged according to knowledge, competence, and role and is integrated into the core content outline. The instructional methods for teaching this core content are then delineated.

Whenever possible, more than one instructional design is provided to enable orientees to select their own learning methods. Table 5-4 lists appropriate instructional techniques according to the type of behavioral outcome expected. The time frame for achievement of orientation competencies is also negotiated. Depending on the orientee's level of competence and the complexity of the unit, this may range from 6 weeks to 6 months. All these negotiated conditions may be written into a learning contract to serve as a guide for implementation and ongoing evaluation.

Implementation. A competency-based orientation program may be implemented using a variety of formats. The role of the nurse educator is to facilitate the acquisition of required competencies. This may involve some formal classes or skills-building workshops, depending on the orientee's needs and learning styles. A novice critical care nurse requires close supervision and continuous instruction.[3] An expert critical care nurse may demonstrate knowledge on written tests and validate current competence in performance of identified skills but may need instruction on role expectations specific to the institution. In each case, goals may be set for every day or week of orientation, which serve as guidelines for ongoing feedback for the orientee.

During the implementation phase of orientation, the expected level of competence must be clear to the orientee and educator. For example, competence in hemodynamic monitoring involves setting up equipment, assisting with insertion, identifying waveforms, troubleshooting, interpreting data, and analyzing the data concurrently with the clinical assessment of a specific patient. These tasks can be overwhelming to an orientee. A well-designed orientation program will allay some of a new orientee's anxiety by making specific expectations clear. Specific behaviors expected of an orientee relative to all competencies are stated explicitly.

Evaluation. Program elements (the program itself, the educator, and the orientee) are evaluated at the end of the orientation period. The orientee may be evaluated using

---

◆ TABLE 5-4 Behavioral Outcomes

Type of Behavioral Outcome	Most Appropriate Technique
Knowledge Generalizations about experience; internalization of information	Lecture, videotape, debate, dialogue, interview, symposium, panel, group discussion, book-based discussion, reading
Understanding Application of information and generalization	Audience participation, demonstration, dramatization, problem-solving, discussion, case study, games
Skills Incorporation of new ways of performing through practice	Role-playing, games, participative cases, skill labs
Attitudes Adoption of new feelings through experiencing greater success with them than with old	Experience-sharing discussion, group-centered discussion, role-playing, critical incident process, case method, games
Values Adoption and priority arrangement of beliefs	Videotape, lecture, debate, dialogue, symposium, dramatization, guided discussion, experience-sharing discussion, role-playing, critical incident process, games
Interests Satisfying exposure to new activities	Videotape, demonstration, dramatization, experience-sharing discussion, exhibits

the methods outlined in the planning phase of the program. An evaluation of overall job performance may also be included.

Orientees also evaluate how well the orientation program met their individual needs. The quality and appropriateness of instruction are part of that evaluation.

All those involved in the orientation process evaluate the program as a whole related to outcomes. This process should occur formally each year. The relationship of the orientation program outcomes to expected outcomes for the unit or the nursing department should be evident. Based on the evaluation data, recommendations for revisions may be made.

Preceptor Programs

For several years, preceptorship has been a popular approach to unit-based clinical orientation of critical care nurses. This person oversees the new staff nurse's orientation process in conjunction with the nurse manager, clinical nurse specialist, or nurse educator for the unit. The preceptor negotiates a learning contract with the orientee based on identified learning needs. During this process, the preceptor introduces the orientee to both written and unwritten policies and practices of the unit.

Preceptors act as role models, socializers, and educators.[39,40] They introduce the orientee to staff nurse role expectations by demonstrating clinical competence, good communication skills, and strong organizational skills. The preceptor socializes the new staff member into the work group through introductions to other nurses and by providing formal and informal opportunities for interactions with several members of the healthcare team during the orientation period.

The chief component of the preceptor role is that of educator. The preceptor assesses, plans, implements, and evaluates an individualized orientation plan with the orientee. The plan includes consideration of the orientee's previous experience and identified learning needs. At this point, the preceptor may clarify the expectation that the responsibility for meeting orientation requirements rests with the orientee. The preceptor acts as a resource and facilitates the orientee's accomplishment of program requirements. Clinical teachers consider the learner's level of practice and present information based on the individual's cognitive style. Selection criteria for preceptors are clearly defined before embarking on such a program. Common criteria include (1) clinical competence, (2) exemplary interpersonal skills, (3) teaching ability, (4) leadership ability, (5) conflict-resolution ability, (6) commitment to the program, and (7) a positive attitude.[41-43]

The role of the clinical nurse specialist or the nurse educator during the unit-based orientation is to establish ongoing communication and facilitate a trusting preceptor-orientee relationship. This goal may be achieved through weekly meetings with the preceptor and orientee to review accomplishments, set goals for the following week, and give feedback to the orientee. It also is an opportunity for the nurse educator to assess the preceptor-orientee relationship.

Many institutions require preceptor experience as one criterion for clinical advancement. Others consider it as professional recognition and responsibility without related promotional or financial reward. Whatever the institution's philosophy, some mechanism of positive reinforcement of the preceptor role must exist to avoid burnout. Alspach[44] proposed a preceptor's bill of rights, which includes the right to role preparation.[44] This is best accomplished by providing a preceptor development workshop. Workshop content includes (1) a description of the preceptor role, (2) an overview of adult learning principles, (3) steps in orientation needs assessment, (4) communication skills, (5) conflict-resolution strategies, and (6) evaluation strategies.

The workshop design should be highly interactive and provide participants opportunities in role-playing and clarifying expectations. A review of both central and unit-based orientation programs at the workshop is also essential. Preceptors need a clear understanding of the orientation program's goals and desired outcomes to maintain program consistency. This preceptor development workshop serves as a prerequisite to each preceptor's role in program evaluation and revision.

Follow-up sessions or "advanced" preceptor workshops are recommended to continue to support the development of expert preceptors. These sessions provide experienced preceptors with an opportunity to clarify issues and meet the changing needs of orientees, as well as recognize the preceptors' commitment to the program. Nurse managers and nurse recruiters may be invited to participate at these meetings to offer feedback to the preceptor group. These sessions should be continuous and responsive to the needs of preceptors if they are to support them in fulfilling role expectations. Moreover, this kind of support from the leadership group enhances retention of these vital staff members and promotes collaboration between educators and managers.

Critical Care Nursing In-service Education

In-service education programs, the most common type of staff development activity, involves learning experiences provided in the workplace to assist staff in the performance of assigned functions and maintenance of competency.[45] These programs are usually informal and narrow in scope. They are often unplanned, spontaneous sessions that arise from new situations on the unit in settings such as patient rounds or staff meetings. Examples of planned in-services are demonstrations of new equipment, procedure reviews, and patient care conferences.

These activities are the most unrecognized types of educational programs, and subsequently they often are not well documented. The astute nurse educator develops a mechanism for documenting these learning activities as part of the unit-based education program. The documentation substantiates ongoing efforts to ensure competence and compliance with JCAHO and other regulatory requirements.

In-service education, however, does not meet the criteria for continuing education credit in nursing. The scope of these programs is limited to the specific work setting and not necessarily to overall professional development of individual nurses. This distinction should be clarified with nursing staff who may be expecting continuing education credit from fire safety classes or other institution-specific in-services.

Continuing Education

The category of staff development activity that is in highest demand is continuing education. This need has been fueled by legislation, regulations, professional standards, and expectations of healthcare consumers. Continuing nursing education is an ongoing process that includes planned, organized learning experiences designed to expand knowledge and skills beyond the level of basic education.[46] The focus is on knowledge and skills that are not specific to one institution and build on previously acquired knowledge and skills. Examples of continuing education programs include formal conferences, seminars, workshops, and courses.

Limited financial and human resources, as well as evolving technologies, have encouraged the use of more creative educational strategies. Self-study, interactive computer-based programs, Internet options, case studies available on compact disk, and various distance learning opportunities have decreased classroom time and made education programs more accessible.

Accreditation of continuing education programs is the process by which an approving body recognizes that a program meets its required standards. The accreditation process in nursing is accomplished primarily through the ANA. The ANA Board on Accreditation has specific criteria that must be met for approval of continuing education credit. The ANA also has a mechanism for nursing associations to become accredited as approvers of continuing education so that an organization can approve the programs of its constituents. The AACN is one such accredited approver.

The measure by which continuing education credit is awarded is the 50-minute contact hour. For every 50 minutes of a planned, organized learning activity, 1 contact hour may be awarded. Partial credit may also be awarded. Three categories of continuing education may be approved for continuing education credit: an offering, program, or independent study. A summary of definitions and examples of each one is provided in Table 5-5.

The educational design criteria for all three categories of continuing education are similar. All of the defined criteria must be met to obtain continuing education credit. Each criterion is listed on the application for approval for continuing education credit.

The institution's provision of ongoing continuing education reflects two commitments to the nursing staff and to the public they serve. The first is to ensure that patients are cared for by nurses who are current in their practice. The second is a commitment to meet the changing learning needs of the nursing staff so that they are able to maintain competence.

The establishment of a comprehensive staff development program sustains varying levels of knowledge and skill in the educational preparation of nursing staff. It provides a climate that supports career development and fosters excellence in clinical practice. Nurses who practice in this type of environment are encouraged to accept new challenges in clinical and professional arenas and are supported through the growth process on the road to advancement.

Fostering Professional Advancement

Fostering professional advancement includes stimulating growth in clinical knowledge and skills, as well as promoting development of the nurse as an active participant in the profession of nursing. Supporting this type of growth and professional involvement requires that the educator be in touch with a variety of professional activities, opportunities, and resources appropriate for staff at all levels. These opportunities can and should be identified at the unit and institutional level (e.g., unit or interdepartmental councils, committees, or task forces), at the state level (e.g., state nurses associations, state political movements or organizations related to healthcare policy, healthcare program grants administered at the state level), and nationally (e.g., national nursing organizations, federal grants, and national policy agendas related to healthcare).

Formal and informal opportunities exist for staff to participate in professional development activities at the unit, institutional, local, state, or national level. These may include activities such as clinical role modeling, formal education, development of areas of expertise, certification, leadership role development, peer review, professional

◆ TABLE 5-5 Categories of Continuing Education

Category	Definition	Examples
Offering	A single educational activity that may be presented once or repeated	ECG Workshop Nursing Grand Rounds
Program	A series of offerings that have a common theme and common overall goal.	National Teaching Institute CCRN Core Review Program
Independent study module	Self-paced learning activity developed for use by an individual learner	Professional journal CEU articles Computer-assisted learning modules

presentations, writing for publication, and participation in nursing research related to critical care.

SUMMARY

Professional development activities are numerous in pediatric critical care and can serve to enhance and enrich clinical practice. They are supported at various levels of the organization and are directly linked to a professional advancement program that focuses on clinical support and educational development at the clinician's level of nursing practice. The concept of professional advancement reflects the institution's commitment to quality healthcare for consumers and to the protection of critically ill pediatric patients who are cared for by highly skilled and knowledgeable staff. A program that combines opportunities for professional growth and development with a professional advancement program that recognizes and supports nursing staff at all levels of practice can best meet these goals.

REFERENCES

1. Villaire M: The synergy model of certified practice: creating safe passage for patients, *Crit Care Nurs* 16:5-99, 1996.
2. Curley M: Patient-nurse synergy: optimizing patients' outcomes, *Am J Crit Care* 7:64-72, 1998.
3. Benner P: *From novice to expert,* Menlo Park, Calif, 1984, Addison Wesley.
4. Balasco E, Black A: Advancing nursing practice: description, recognition, and reward, *Nurs Admin Q* 12:52-57, 1988.
5. Czerwinski S, Blastic L, Rice B: The synergy model: building a clinical advancement program, *Crit Care Nurse* 19:72-77, 1999.
6. Biel M: *Reconceptualizing certified practice: envisioning critical care practice of the future,* Aliso Viejo, Calif, 1997, AACN Certification Corp.
7. Ruth-Sahd L: A modification of Benner's hierarchy of clinical practice: the development of clinical intuition in the novice trauma nurse, *Holis Nurs Pract* 7:8-14, 1993.
8. Lookinland S, Crenshaw J: Rewarding clinical competence in the ICU: using outcomes to reward practice, *Dimens Crit Care Nurs* 15:206-215, 1996.
9. Itano J: A comparison of the clinical judgement process in experienced registered nurses and student nurses, *J Nurs Educ* 28:120-126, 1998.
10. Shapiro M: A career ladder based on Benner's model: an analysis of expected outcomes, *J Nurs Adm* 28:13-19, 1998.
11. Holden G, Klinger A: Learning from experience: differences in how novice vs expert nurses diagnose why an infant is crying, *J Nurs Educ* 27:23-29, 1998.
12. Dealy M, Bass M: Professional development: factors that motivate staff, *Nurs Manage* 26:32f-32i, 1995.
13. Gassert C, Holt C, Pope K: Building a ladder, *Am J Nurs* 82:1527-1530, 1986.
14. Kleinknecht M, Hefferin E: Assisting nurses toward professional growth: a career development model, *J Nurs Adm* 12:30-36, 1982.
15. Weeks L, Vestal K: PACE: a unique career development program, *J Nurs Adm* 13:29-32, 1983.
16. Mark B, Sayler J, Smith C: A theoretical model for nursing systems outcome research, *Nurs Admin Q* 20(4):12-27, 1996.
17. Nielsen BB: Applying andragogy in nursing continuing education, *J Contin Educ Nurs* 20:86-90, 1989.
18. Knowles M: *The adult learner: a neglected species,* ed 4, Houston, 1990, Gulf Publishing.
19. Vail P: *Learning as a way of being,* San Francisco, 1996, Jossey-Bass.
20. Fox D: Career insurance for today's world, *Train Dev* 50:61-64, 1996.
21. Pike R: *Creative training techniques handbook,* Minneapolis, Minn, 1989, Lakewood Books.
22. Jiricka M: Principles of adult learning. In Jiricka MJ, ed: *Critical care orientation: a guide to the process,* Newport Beach, 1987, AACN.
23. Morrow KL: Principles of adult education. In Morrow KL, ed: *Preceptorships in nursing staff development,* Rockville, Md, 1984, Aspen.
24. Hammond M, Collins R: *Self-directed learning,* New York, 1991, Nichols/GP.
25. Dickerson P: A CQI approach to evaluating continuing education, *J Nurs Staff Dev* 16:34-40, 2000.
26. Benner P, Hooper-Kyriokidis P, Stannard D: *Clinical wisdom and interventions in critical care,* Philadelphia, 1999, WB Saunders.
27. Chamberlain S, Stengrevics S, Alpert H: Mentorship: a relationship for professional development. In Clifford J, Horvath K, eds: *Advancing professional nursing practice,* New York, 1990, Springer.
28. Trossman S: Mentoring leads to meaningful relationships, professional growth, *American Nurse,* 1998, at http://www.ana.org/tan/98marapr/feature3.htm.
29. Benner P, Tanner C, Cheslea C: *Expertise in nursing practice: caring, clinical judgement, and ethics,* New York, 1996, Springer.
30. Goleman D: *Working with emotional intelligence,* New York, 1998, Bantam.
31. Haas S: Coaching, developing key players, *J Nurs Adm* 22:54-58, 1992.
32. Lenburg C: The framework, concepts and methods of the competency, outcomes and performance assessment (COPA) model, *Online Journal of Issues in Nursing,* 1999, at http://wwwnursingworld.org/ojin/topic10_2.htm.
33. Abruzzese R: *Nursing staff development,* St Louis, 1992, Mosby.
34. American Nurses Association: *Guidelines for staff development,* Kansas City, 1978, American Nurses Association.
35. delBueno D: Competency based education, *Nurs Educ* 3:10-14, 1978.
36. delBueno D, Barker F, Christmyer C: Implementing a competency based orientation program, *J Nurs Adm* 11:24-29, 1981.
37. Buickus B: Orientation: we're with you all the way, *Nurs Manage* 15:40-45, 1984.
38. Alspach JG: Designing a competency based orientation for critical care nurses, *Heart Lung* 13:655-662, 1984.
39. Alspach JG: *Preceptor handbook,* Secaucus, NJ, 1988, Hospital Publications.
40. Goodman D: Application of the critical pathway and integrated teaching method to nursing, *J Contin Educ Nurs* 28:205-209, 1997.
41. Begle M: Developing senior staff nurses as preceptors, *Dimens Crit Care Nurs* 3:245-251, 1984.
42. Greipp ME: Nursing preceptors looking back, looking ahead, *J Nurs Staff Dev* 4:183185, 1989.
43. Hartline C: Preceptor selection and evaluation, *J Nurs Staff Dev* 9:188-192, 1993.
44. Alspach JG: The preceptor's bill of rights, *Crit Care Nurs* 7:1, 1987.
45. American Nurses Association: *Standards for nursing staff development,* Kansas City, 1990, American Nurses Association.
46. American Nurses Association: *Standards for nursing professional development: continuing education and staff development,* Washington, DC, 1994, American Nurses Association.

6

Advocacy and Moral Agency: A Road Map for Navigating Ethical Issues in Pediatric Critical Care

Cynda Hylton Rushton

Being a very ill child or the parent of a very ill child must test the outermost limits of human tolerance . . . being involved in the care of very ill children must be one of the most demanding responsibilities in the world, the failures more awful, the triumphs more rewarding than in almost any other kind of job. The stakes are so high: whole lifetimes.

Peggy Anderson[1]

Nurses accompany pediatric patients and their families on an uncertain journey from aggressive treatment aimed at cure, recovery, palliation, or—when cure is no longer possible—toward a peaceful death. Nurses assist patients and families in finding safe passage through the complex maze of decisions and treatment options. The situations that arise within pediatric critical care raise ethical questions concerning the rights of children to make their own treatment decisions, the status of parental rights, the obligations of nurses and other healthcare professionals to prevent and relieve suffering, and society's beliefs about how children should live and how they should die.

These questions arise in a context of increasingly scarce human and economic resources, health systems in disarray, and healthcare providers who are grieving the loss of their previous professional roles and relationships. These issues are often surrounded by confusion, ambivalence, and tension on the part of healthcare professionals, patients, and families. The emotional intensity that surrounds the care of critically ill children can magnify the ethical concerns.

The myriad ethical questions that surround the provision of pediatric critical care often arise from specific treatment choices such as do-not-attempt-resuscitation (DNAR) decisions, abatement of life-sustaining therapies including medically provided hydration and nutrition, use of innovative therapies, or pain management. Individuals may wonder, for example, whether it is morally justified under any circumstances to forgo life-sustaining therapy provided to a young child who has significant morbidity and a small chance of survival.

Ethical questions may also arise because there are genuine value conflicts about the right thing to do and the proper outcomes to pursue. For example, parents and professionals may disagree about which values ought to guide the treatment of a child with a life-threatening disease such as cancer or congenital heart disease. Evaluating the possible goals for the child involves important values about what makes life meaningful and what sorts of burdens are acceptable in order to achieve those goals. The parents may value the possibility, however small, to promote survival and therefore have a high threshold for the burdens they will tolerate in order to give the child a chance for life. The treatment team, in contrast, also values giving the child a chance for life but their threshold for reasonable burdens may instead be based on the possibility that survival may commit the child to a life of burden they believe is disproportionate in relation to the chance for survival now and into adulthood.

Nurses working in pediatric critical care may experience frustration and anguish as they watch children struggle against formidable odds and observe parents grapple with some of the most difficult decisions a family can ever confront. Nurses watch children bear the consequences of disease, injury, and technology. A nurse's perceived inability to minimize or eliminate tragic outcomes brings on feelings of powerlessness and helplessness. The demands of the critical care unit are hectic and at times unrelenting. Tasks are accomplished under high personal and professional tension. Ethical dilemmas grow as some children's lives end before potential is reached and other children's lives hang on too long. It is within this complex environment that nurses experience moral uncertainty, moral dilemmas, and moral distress.

Andrew Jameton sorts the moral problem nurses face into three categories[2]:

1. *Moral uncertainty*—When one is unsure of which principles or values apply, or even what the moral problem is.
2. *Moral dilemmas*—When two or more clear moral principles apply, but they support mutually inconsistent courses of action.
3. *Moral distress*—When one knows the right thing to do but is prevented by institutional or other constraints from pursuing the right course of action.

Moral uncertainty and moral dilemmas produce discomfort because of the nurse's inability to decide what is the right thing to do or the proper outcome to pursue. Moral distress, on the other hand, produces negative feelings because of the nurse's inability to maneuver through the environment, to do what he or she believes is right.

This chapter describes the specific moral issues that arise in the care of sick children and discusses the ethical principles of beneficence, nonmaleficence, autonomy, and veracity as they relate to pediatric critical care. The discussion of these principles along with a model for decision making will provide the nurse with practical assistance in sorting through the ethical dilemmas typically present in the pediatric critical care unit.

WHAT IS ETHICS?

Ethics is concerned with the behavior, choices, and character of individuals and groups. More specifically, ethics is the study of the process for determining the best course of action in the face of conflicting choices. Most people have a sense of what is right and what is wrong. These values are developed while growing up within a society that teaches specific social rules, expectations, and prohibitions. "Morality tells us not to harm others, not to kill, to be good persons, to keep promises, and to tell the truth."[3] Morality provides us with general rules of conduct; it tells us whether the consequences of actions are good or bad. Thus people form opinions about how one ought to act and what one ought to believe in certain situations.

Ethics, however, refers to the systematic study of principles and values. It is a discipline that looks at the way people act and asks whether their actions are good or harmful. The study of ethics goes beyond what *is* and asks what *ought to be*. In asking these questions, ethical inquiry helps form and change moral conduct. Ethical questions arise alongside, but differ from, fundamental social, legal, political, professional, and scientific questions. For example, public policies and laws surrounding end-of-life care set boundaries for human behavior but do not necessarily correspond to an individual's sense of what ought to be. Practically, ethical issues in the clinical arena primarily involve problem solving using a systematic process.[4]

Ethical deliberation involves a process of discernment, analysis, and articulation of ethically defensible positions, and then acting upon them. Ethical thinking helps give a reasoned account of an ethical position and move beyond intuition or emotions. The goal of ethical deliberations is not to achieve absolute certainty about what is right, but rather to achieve reliability and coherence in behavior, choices, character, process, and outcomes. This requires that participants make reasoned judgments about the justifications that are offered to support a particular course of action. Judgments should be grounded by ethical theories and principles to avoid making decisions based solely on individual opinions.[4]

ETHICAL PRINCIPLES FOR DECISION MAKING

Balancing Benefit and Harm

Based on the principles of beneficence and nonmaleficence, healthcare professionals seek to promote the well-being of their patients and to reduce or alleviate harm. The Code for Nurses of the American Nurses Association (ANA) stresses the alleviation of suffering as a nursing duty over saving life. The ANA Code for Nurses states: "Nursing encompasses the promotion and restoration of health, the prevention of illness and the alleviation of suffering."[5] When promoting "good" such as health, relief from pain and suffering, and the prevention of illness, nurses may seek answers to these difficult questions: How do you know what is good in a specific situation? Can circumstances alter the perception of what is good? When does doing good become harm? Who decides what is good? Is one doing good when one continues to treat a critically ill child for whom there is no hope? Is one doing good when a child in a persistent vegetative state continues to receive antibiotics, food, and fluids? Is one doing good when a 15-year-old child is forced to continue chemotherapy against his or her wishes?

Choices among treatments should benefit the infant or child, and clearly outweigh the associated burdens and harms. This "best interest" principle relies on subjective and objective weighing of the benefits and burdens of each therapy.[6] Weighing of benefits and burdens occurs within a framework of patient/family goals and preferences, treatment goals, and possible outcomes. The interests of infants and children are not limited to biologic interests and include developmental, emotional, social, spiritual, and other interests. A "best interest" standard recognizes the possibility that medically indicated treatment may result in a profoundly burdensome life for the child and that death may not be the "greatest evil to befall a person."[7] Thus, it presumes that prolongation of life may not always be in the child's best interest. Focusing on what is best for the child avoids morally dubious justification based preferentially on the interests of other involved parties such as the parents, siblings, healthcare professionals, or the institution.

When the best interest principle is applied to children, a "reasonable person" standard is generally used to evaluate benefits and burdens because children have frequently not expressed autonomous values or choices about treatment. A reasonable person standard relies on what most informed and reasonable persons would view as in the child's best interest. It is meant to reflect a social consensus about what would be the appropriate response for someone in a similar situation. However, in many instances a clear social consensus is lacking.[6,8]

A variety of criteria have been suggested to assess whether a treatment is in a child's best interest (Box 6-1).

Benefits and burdens may be understood based on the child's and/or parent's values and preferences for what constitutes a meaningful life and death. The following are commonly viewed as benefits to the critically ill child: (a) comfort or relief from suffering; (b) alertness; (c) unconsciousness of severe pain or anxiety; (d) awareness of one's condition, prognosis, or impending death (if cognitively able); (e) relating to friends and loved ones; (f) exercising authority over or participation in decisions; or (g) completing life tasks. These benefits must be weighed against the burdens associated with certain treatments such as: (a) repeated pain and suffering associated with invasive procedures and the underlying disease; (b) new, unrelieved, or exacerbated symptoms; (c) physical and emotional isolation; (d) anxiety; (e) lack of human contact; (f) loss of hope; (g) despair; (h) meaningless existence; (i) immobilization; (j) noninvolvement in decisions; (k) prolonged hospitalization; (l) developmental deprivation; or (m) lack of continuity by a consistent person of special significance.

Most medical interventions are not benign and are accompanied by some degree of pain, bodily invasion, and physical, psychologic, or spiritual burden. Hence the process of weighing benefits and burdens is ongoing and evolving over time. The threshold for tolerating the burdens of certain therapies may change as goals change in light of patient responses. For example, parents, children, and healthcare professionals may be willing to tolerate the side

---

Box 6-1

◆ **Assessment Criteria to Determine Whether Treatment Is in the Child's Best Interest**

1. The degree of pain and psychologic and spiritual suffering and the potential for relief.
2. The severity of the patient's medical condition. This may be assessed by: (a) verifying the diagnosis, (b) determining the accuracy of predicting prognosis, (c) determining the degree of certainty needed for diagnosis and prognosis, (d) determining the degree of major organ systems affected by the disease, and (e) the presence of severe neurologic impairment.
3. The potential for developing a capacity for self-determination.
4. The potential for personal satisfaction and enjoyment of life.
5. The potential for restoration of function, improvement in symptoms, or cure. Consider questions such as: Is this condition reversible? Will this treatment extend a meaningful life or prolong dying? Will the treatment change the disease trajectory or outcome? Will the therapy be effective in achieving an important goal? Is the treatment beneficial from the patient's perspective?
6. The goals that are possible for the patient and those desired by the patient, if competent, or by the surrogate. These goals may include restoration and cure, stabilization of functioning, or preparation for death.
7. The proportionality of treatment-related benefits and burdens.

Data from President's Commission for the Study of Ethics Problems in Medicine and Biomedical and Behavioral Research. *Deciding to forego life-sustaining treatment.* Washington, DC, 1983, US Government Printing Office; and Weil R, Bale J: Selective nontreatment of neurologically impaired neonates. *Neurol Clin North Am* 7:807-822, 1989.

---

effects of chemotherapy when cure is possible. However, after repeated relapses those same burdens may be viewed as unjustified.

Decision making is more complicated when the prospect of successful outcome is less certain, the outcome of the treatment is expected to be of marginal usefulness, or the degree of burden is high. This is most common during the terminal phases of many diseases. In these cases, the agony of certain treatments may be viewed as disproportionate in relation to the small statistical chance for survival, especially if the course of therapy is prolonged.[9]

Decisions regarding the treatment of critically ill children always occur under conditions of uncertainty. Determining the child's best interests can be particularly difficult when the precise diagnosis and/or prognosis is unclear or it is difficult to accurately predict the disease trajectory. As a consequence, it is more difficult to understand the benefits or burdens that will result from treatment or nontreatment. The unpredictability of a child's response to treatment may motivate caregivers or parents to try to reduce the uncertainty by pursuing additional diagnostic studies and innovative therapies. This creates ambiguity and controversy about whether the child's condition is reversible or whether it represents the terminal phase of the disease. Depending on how the uncertainty is viewed, either as threat or opportunity, caregivers or parents may be willing in some instances to accept a greater degree of burden in order to give the child an opportunity for a longer life and the possibility of future beneficial treatments.[10]

At times, however, the quest for absolute certainty may result in disproportionate burden by the patient. As uncertainty and the burdens associated with treatment escalate, other important moral considerations must be brought to bear on the decision. The prolongation of life cannot be considered exclusively. Priority must also be given to the comfort or ease with which a life is lived. Hence, as the benefits of medical interventions diminish, the focus of care necessarily shifts to relieving pain and promoting comfort, rather than on therapies to prolong life.

Assessing benefits and burdens in permanently unconscious children is particularly problematic. Presumably, a permanently unconscious child is not capable of experiencing benefits or burdens. In such instances, it has been argued that the child's interests are limited to the maintenance of biologic functions without an awareness of benefit or burden. For example, children who are permanently unconscious cannot interact with their environment or family nor can they derive satisfaction or pleasures associated with living. Similarly, these children cannot perceive the potential burdens associated with treatment. In such a state the child lacks the neurologic function to perceive pain. In this special circumstance, the best interest principle does not apply since it appears that the child's interests cannot be changed by enhancing benefits or reducing burdens. A vitalist argument based on sanctity of life may be used as justification for continuing treatment but does not rely on a benefit or burden for it's justification. Opponents may argue otherwise. Miller-Thiel and colleagues have suggested that consideration be given to whether the prolongation of the unconscious life of a child is an act of caring.[11] The Baby Doe regulations,[12] for example, regard permanent unconsciousness as a condition that does not require life-sustaining treatment; yet there are a wide range of views on the degree of neurologic impairment that justifies limiting or forgoing treatment.

Respect for Persons and the Role of Children in Decision Making

A second principle involved in decision making is respect for persons. In its broadest interpretation, respect for persons means recognizing another human being as sharing a common human destiny.[13] Each life, regardless of how diminished it may be, must be regarded with fundamental reverence and respect. There are opposing views about whether such respect for human life mandates that life must be sustained unconditionally. Despite this, the principle of respect for persons invites thoughtful consideration of the child's uniqueness and inherent worth.

Respect for persons requires that children be recognized as individuals whose thoughts, experiences, and opinions matter, despite their developmental immaturity and legal status as minors.[14] Even though children are not autonomous or self-determining, an element of respect is required because the lives of children have unique meaning. To treat children with respect is to acknowledge and value who they are outside of a medical context.[15] Even though a child may not be fully able to direct his or her own treatment, it is possible and desirable to involve even young children in decisions about their treatment. Many children with life-limiting conditions have an accelerated understanding of their condition and an intimate knowledge of the consequences of certain treatments. This profound personal knowledge should be given appropriate moral status in the decision-making process.

The degree of involvement of children and adolescents in treatment decisions varies depending upon their capacity and desire for involvement. The capacity to consent to medical treatment requires a person's ability to understand the treatment options and consequences, reason about them, and freely choose from various alternatives. Two factors that influence a child's level of participation in healthcare decisions are cognition and competence. As these aptitudes develop, a child is able to take on increased responsibility for treatment decisions. Children do not suddenly develop decision-making capacity when they reach 18 years of age. Children's ability to recognize their own best interest and to choose or refuse treatment follows a developmental process like any other normal path of growth and development. This ability develops gradually throughout childhood, at a pace that varies from one child to another.

How, then, does one weigh the child's ability to choose or refuse treatment? The normal childhood developmental processes have been fully explored by Erikson and Piaget.[16,17] They describe milestones or points at which a child masters certain tasks or processes. Although most children pass through these milestones at a steady pace, some children advance, stop, or even fall back as environmental conditions, such as their home life, limits in mental intelligence, and illness, interfere with normal progress. In particular, chronic or terminal illness often influences a child's developmental progress. Capacity for healthcare decision making is not an all-or-none concept and may be situational. For example, an individual child may be able to decide to discontinue chemotherapy but not have the capacity to decide to go home and die. Thus each child must be viewed individually, taking into account developmental, as well as chronologic, age and the particular characteristics of the situation.

Before the age of 11 or 12, children believe illness is caused by something external to their bodies or something they ingest.[18] Very young children who are sick are principally concerned with separation from their parents and the unpleasantness of the procedures that they must undergo. At about age 6 or 7 the child often believes that illness is retribution for bad thoughts or actions. By 12 years of age children develop the capacity to think abstractly. At this stage of development a child is able to consider multiple factors, hypothesize, and predict future consequences. The child is able to understand illness as a process caused by a malfunctioning of an internal organ system and is therefore able to understand the long-term risks of chronic disease, instead of just focusing on whether the disease will interfere with their immediate routine. By the time adolescents reach the age of 15, they are less likely to acquiesce to their parents' wishes. Thus the ability to freely assent to treatment or nontreatment has developed.

As children attain greater capacities to participate in decision making, they should be involved more fully in decisions about their care. McCabe and colleagues offer guidelines for determining the level of involvement of minors in treatment decisions. Involvement includes preparation of procedures and assent, shared decision making with parents, and autonomous decision making.[19] Generally, children who are not fully autonomous are asked to assent to treatment rather than consent, which requires decision-making capacity and autonomous decision making. Assent to treatment means that the child has agreed to proceed with a specific course of treatment or has decided to withhold or limit certain treatments, with the approval of the parent or surrogate. The process of obtaining assent confers respect for a child by encouraging involvement and understanding. Although it is important not to accept uncritically a child's reluctance to undergo painful and distressing interventions, it is essential to respect the wishes and self-defined goals of mature children, particularly when parents support making comfort the primary goal of management at the end of life.

When a child is incapable of forming and stating his or her own goals, respect is still required, but it is more difficult to determine the proper balance of benefits and harms. The nature of the consequences of the decision may be useful in determining the decision-making role of minors. Clearly, special caution should be exercised when death is a likely outcome of a decision. Confidence in assessing the child's decision-making capacity and the process for making decisions will be crucial for justified deference to his or her preferences and choices.[4]

At a minimum children should be granted the following: (a) informed in developmentally appropriate terms about the nature of their condition, proposed treatment, and expected outcomes; (b) informed about who is caring for them and performing procedures; (c) prepared for medications and treatments; (d) their views and preferences listened to and taken account of in decision making. Children with life-limiting conditions should, for instance, be involved in determining the how much, when, and to what extent they prefer to have information provided. Regardless of the child's level of participation in care planning, he or she should be given as much control over the treatment plan as possible.[19]

Children should not be deceived or misled about the scope of their authority in decisions.[9] If the child's preferences are not determinative of treatment, this should be openly acknowledged. For example, when decisions are made to forgo life-sustaining treatment, it is desirable to acknowledge how the child's preferences will be incorporated into the decision-making process and to determine whether or the extent to which the child's views will determine treatment.

Autonomy and Informed Consent

The ethical principle of autonomy, which is derived from respect for persons, refers to individual self-determination and freedom of choice. "It requires that we respect the rights of others to make autonomous decisions. To violate a person's autonomy is to treat that person merely as a means to an end that is in accordance with one's own beliefs and values."[20] An extension of the principle of respect for persons is the ethical standard for informed consent

Informed consent is also the legal standard by which permission is sought for medical treatment of an individual. The only acceptable legal exception to this law is that in which the need for medical treatment constitutes an emergency, that is, when the patient would suffer irreversible harm if not treated. Thus, when consent cannot be obtained because the patient is not competent and a surrogate decision maker is not immediately available, the treatment can proceed. However, in all other instances, the patient or the patient's surrogate must consent to or refuse treatment.

The Role of Minors. In caring for children, special ethical issues arise because children are not consenting adults. Since young children do not have the cognitive ability to provide informed consent or refusal, parents or legal guardians are usually responsible for treatment decisions for their children. As a child nears adolescence, parents' rights to make healthcare decisions may be limited by both the increase in the minor's cognitive ability and precepts of law.

The concept of "mature minor" has received increasing judicial approval. A mature minor statute recognizes that a young person (14 or 15 years of age or older) can understand the nature and consequences of certain proposed treatments. The treatment must not involve very serious risks and the physician must believe that the minor could give the same degree of informed consent as an adult.[21] Treatment for venereal disease, drug and alcohol abuse, pregnancy, and communicable diseases may fall into this area. In fact, California state law recommends that it may be appropriate to seek legal advice if a minor aged 14 or older objects when parental consent is given for a procedure that involves a significant risk of severe adverse consequences.[22]

Specific state statutory provisions "emancipate" minors for the purpose of making their own healthcare decisions. Generally, an emancipated minor is someone younger than 18 years of age who is not living at home and/or is self-supporting, married, in the military, or an unmarried mother. An emancipated minor statute reflects the judgment of a particular state that, when certain conditions are met, these minors are capable of consenting to their own healthcare. In particular, provisions that grant adult status to minor parents consenting to treatment for their own child have significant implications in the care and treatment of children.

State laws may need to be clarified in situations such as when a minor is in the custody of juvenile court or foster parents and when minors are suspected victims of child abuse. Legally, some minors have been given the authority to give consent for medical treatment in specific situations.

Although the federal Patient Self Determination Act of 1990 (PSDA) endorses adults making decisions for themselves and documents their choices, the spirit of the law reinforces the involvement of minors, especially adolescents, in their own treatment decisions and encourages the creation of an atmosphere in which children, with their parents, can make informed decisions.[23,24]

Ensuring Informedness. Although full informed consent has been said to be a theoretic ideal, reality must come as close as is possible to that ideal for parents to make decisions in the best interests of their child. Informed decisions are made with full knowledge of that which needs to be done and why. An atmosphere of open discussion must exist, free from fear of reprisal. Informing patients and their families is a dialogue, not a lecture, wherein the provision of information helps to clarify understanding.

To make a decision about medical treatment requires that the same information be provided to either an adult or a child. The physician must provide all the information necessary for the patient or the surrogate to make a reasoned, free choice about treatment. The risks of doing or not doing a procedure must be explained, as well as any alternative choices that are available. The information given should focus on the child and what life will be like with and without treatment. Parents should be asked questions about their goals and desires for the child; their values regarding disease, disability, and death; and their desire to be involved in healthcare decision making. It is within this fuller context of communication that informedness can be assured.

Information must be conveyed in a quiet atmosphere in which optimal communication can occur. The critical care unit can be a frightening place for parents and children alike. Constant artificial light, ceaseless activity, frequent emergencies, and the ever-present threat of death unnerves the sturdiest of families. Information should be provided in the language of the decision maker, minimizing the use of medical terminology. For example, "unconsciousness," "mental retardation," and "life support" are words that must be explained. Parents must be helped to understand that what they see as movement, for example, is actually involuntary motion indicating the child's level of neurologic damage. Whether a child has an 80% chance of survival or a 20% chance of dying has little meaning for many parents. Healthcare professionals must explain these serious discussion points in clear language and avoid using them to sway the parent's decision. Written materials should be offered to further clarify the circumstances whenever possible.

Obviously, no single information session ensures informedness, especially when decisions about life and death are involved. The nurse plays a vital role in ensuring informedness through ongoing discussion of the situation with the child and family, arranging to have medical specialists and social work professionals available for discussion, and by providing support, clarification, and understanding as decisions are reached. Davis[25] defined the role of nurses in the informed consent process as including: (1) monitoring informed consent, (2) advocating for patients to the physician, (3) providing patients with explanations and informa-

tion about alternatives, (4) coordinating consent processes with families and patients, and (5) negotiating between involved parties when there are differences of opinions. Clearly, the involvement of nurses is critical as parents and their children grapple with serious issues.

Truth Telling: The Ethical Principle of Veracity

Veracity, being truthful, is also derived from the principle of respect for persons. Whether to inform children about the seriousness of their illness and encourage their participation in treatment decisions is an issue with which both parents and healthcare professionals wrestle. The idea of having children actively participate in health-related decisions can be intimidating. Yet, when the child is able to reason and understand the consequences of actions, withholding information or lying is an act of paternalism and requires justification.

Parents and healthcare professionals who practice such deception do so because they believe that they are allaying fear and anxiety on the part of the child. "An overwhelming wish to protect the sick child from disturbing information, guilt feelings, or the emotional threat posed by the imminent death of their child may overshadow parental recognition or acceptance of the juveniles' autonomy or even his or her welfare."[26]

There is no certainty, however, that being honest, even when the situation is a difficult one, will cause a significant negative reaction. Knowing the full extent of the illness is often less anxiety provoking to the minor than receiving no or false information.[27]

Furthermore, withholding from children accurate and appropriate information denies them the opportunity to discuss their feelings and come to terms with what is happening to their bodies and minds. Family relationships may become strained at a time when both the child and the parents need each other. Talking and explaining helps children to see the reasons for medical treatment and understand the various treatment or nontreatment alternatives. In fact, researchers have demonstrated that children older than 5 years of age have an understanding of the finality of death and should be openly provided information and be involved in treatment decisions.[28]

Trust is at the foundation of the ethical principle of veracity. Veracity teaches us that truthfulness is fundamental to establishing trust between individuals. Sick children depend upon the trusting relationship they have with their parents and their healthcare providers, especially at a time when dependency needs are at their highest. Withholding information or lying threatens the trusting relationship and, consequently, children's ability to rely on the adults on whom they depend. As with adults, children may not want to hear certain information and may want their parents to make decisions. Such requests should be respected. However, it is necessary for ongoing dialogue to occur so that the children are certain that any information they request will be provided truthfully.

Justice

Justice pertains to fairness and equity in the treatment of others. It refers to an individual's access to an adequate level of healthcare and to the distribution of available healthcare resources. Justice demands that individual patients are treated fairly and decisions are not made based on criteria such as race, age, sex, diagnosis, religious beliefs, or socioeconomic status. Children, regardless of their life circumstances, should be availed of the same treatments and advantages as other children in a similar situation. Children with life-limiting conditions, for example, may be denied certain therapies or services because their life expectancy is shortened. Questions of justice arise when the reasons for denying such care is based on questionable criteria or criteria that is inherently discriminatory, such as ability to pay, social status, race, or age. In other instances, children who become wards of the state because their parents are unable or unwilling to act as their surrogate decision maker are at greater risk for discrimination, which could result in undertreatment or overtreatment.[4]

Questions of resource allocation and the proper limits of treatment often arise when the utilization and consumption of resources is high. An appeal to fairness compels healthcare professionals to create equitable systems for the distribution of scarce healthcare resources. Dying children, for example, may face unique threats to access to and reimbursement for end-of-life care. Regulatory criteria for access to hospice, for example, currently limit access to children because the criteria are based on an adult model of hospice that does not reflect the unique needs or trajectory of illness of children. Moreover, insurance criteria may create unjustified barriers to providing necessary services at the end of life based on inflexible interpretation of guidelines.[4]

Healthcare professionals have dual obligations for allocating resources at the individual and societal levels. Often these obligations create intense conflicts of interest and responsibility. The conventional wisdom is that decisions about what will benefit individual patients should generally be separated from decisions about how society will allocate its healthcare resources. Such decisions are not suited for the bedside, but belong within the context of a larger societal debate. Yet when marginally beneficial treatments or other scarce resources are considered, healthcare providers have a responsibility to allocate resources in a fair, fiscally responsible manner. A societal consensus about how to resolve these competing obligations is currently lacking, creating conflict for patients, families, providers, and other members of society.

An Ethic of Care

Traditional ethical reasoning requires providers to ascertain the rights of individuals and weigh the ethical principles in order to resolve conflicting obligations. Applying ethical principles alone cannot resolve the clinical quandaries that arise while caring for critically ill or dying children. When the rights of children are held in opposition to the rights of their parents, for example, an adversarial tension can be

established that may polarize discussion. This method of moral reasoning focuses on an ethic of rights that is achieved through a process of separation and individuation of the child from others including their family. In contrast, considering other aspects of the moral life, such as care, harmony, compassion, and responsibility for self and others, may reduce adversarial tensions between the rights of children and their parents. Such an approach allows for a more comprehensive appreciation of the attitudes, values, and moral commitments of decision makers within the context of their family and other significant relationships. This perspective is often referred to as an "ethic of care."[29]

From a care perspective, the resolution of ethical quandaries is focused on the child's needs in the context of the family, and the provider's corresponding responsibilities within the context of the professional-patient relationship. The professional is guided to focus on the special circumstances and context of the specific situation in which moral action occurs instead of merely considering the child's interests and preferences in isolation. In other words, the uniqueness of a child and the particular dynamics of his or her relationships are endorsed as essential components of moral decision making.[29] Such a model supports efforts to assist children and their families in finding unique meaning or purpose in their living or their dying and to assist them to realize goals that promote a meaningful life or death. AACN's Syngergy Model also supports attentiveness to these concerns.[30]

The values and expectations involved in certain roles and relationships are seen as primary from this vantage point. Therefore, being an advocate for a child with a critical illness or life-limiting condition involves appreciating the relationships significant to the child and understanding how those relationships affect care and decision making. Children develop an intricate web of relationships that support and sustain them throughout their lives. In keeping with a family-centered philosophy of care, families are viewed as essential partners in children's treatment and care. Professionals must recognize and respect these interconnections as central to the well-being of the child.[4]

A care perspective also emphasizes the interrelationships of the members of the healthcare team. It recognizes that nurses, physicians, and other caregivers work collaboratively to advance the interests and goals of children with life-limiting conditions. Threats to harmony and relationships are viewed as the essential nature of moral dilemmas from a care perspective. Therefore, when there is conflict or disharmony among caregivers or among caregivers and family members, relationships are threatened and the moral endeavor is undermined. The goal is to create connection, promote openness and dialogue, and engage in activities to promote healing of the fractured relationship.[4]

A care perspective also invites attention to the narrative dimensions of the case. The diagnosis and treatment of a child's disease evolves over time. The story of the process is an essential element of the context of ethical decision making. Focusing on the narrative dimensions of the process enables parents and professionals to negotiate meaning and to make sense of an often foreign and incomprehensible situation. The meaning that each person assigns to a particular situation is unique and is derived from his or her own social, cultural, familial, religious, political, and other influences. Understanding this context gives insight into how meaning is derived. The search for meaning often leads to understanding. Understanding adheres to meaning ascribed to a situation or set of values or behaviors, but it does not simply mean "knowing" certain facts or concepts. It requires an integration of the information into one's values, and requires cognitive activities that are not exclusively an act of reason. Within a care perspective, meaning and understanding are accessible and relevant to the decision-making process.

ETHICAL ISSUES IN PEDIATRIC CRITICAL CARE

Technologic achievements in critical care created unanticipated dilemmas as powerful diagnostic techniques, sophisticated surgical procedures, effective drugs, and expedient therapeutic interventions interrupted the usual course of illness and disability. Problems became magnified because life could be sustained for a significant period if the patient accepted dependence on a specific procedure or machine.

Medical technology can be a double-edged sword. It is usually beneficial in the care of sick or injured persons, sometimes dramatically so. However, since it is often intrusive, occasionally cruel, sometimes of little value, and almost always expensive, its use must be assessed critically, particularly in ICUs.[31]

The uncertainties and ambiguities that result from disease, injury, and the use of technology often force healthcare professionals to demand cure in the absence of otherwise compelling evidence to choose a different course. The inevitable conflicts that arise produce questions such as these: Can treatment be stopped once initiated? Who gives consent for medical treatment? Can patients be forced to go along with a recommended treatment plan? Do all patients have to be resuscitated? Who judges the quality of someone's life? When is a patient considered dead? The indecision that occurs reflects a growing uneasiness with the consequences of scientific advances, especially when death is not imminent but the quality of life is greatly impaired. In pediatric critical care, the problems are complicated further by the child's developmental stage, chronologic age, and family situation.

The ethical quandaries that arise in healthcare are not new. They have always been a part of clinical practice. Ethical considerations lie on or just below the surface of many clinical activities, yet are rarely noticed. It is only when decisions feel uncomfortable or when alternatives seem equally unsatisfactory that the finer issues of moral decision making are considered. Increasingly, a proactive process for addressing these issues using clinical guidelines has been advocated.[32] In the next section, prominent ethical issues that arise in pediatric critical care will be emphasized.

Forgoing Life-Sustaining Treatment

Numerous quandaries arise when treatment choices such as do-not-resuscitate (DNR) decisions, abatement of life-sustaining therapies including medically provided hydration and nutrition, and pain management are considered. There are many myths about forgoing life-sustaining treatment (Box 6-2) and terminology is often used inconsistently, leading to confusion about the justification and ethical propriety of certain acts that influence the timing and circumstances of death.

Forgoing life-sustaining treatment refers to discontinuing a therapy already begun or not starting a treatment. The reasons for forgoing life-sustaining treatment include: (1) cure is no longer possible, (2) the burdens of treatment outweigh the benefits, or (3) the quality of life is undesirable. In such instances questions may arise about whether current therapies ought to be continued or whether additional therapies should be added. Although it may be psychologically easier to withhold than to withdraw treatment, there is no ethical distinction between the reasons for stopping a therapy or not starting a therapy. Fear about stopping a treatment once started may lead clinicians to avoid a treatment with potential benefit. For example, parents or professionals may fear that trying mechanical ventilation in a child with pneumonia and multiple relapses of leukemia may result in chronic ventilator dependence. The American Academy of Pediatrics (AAP) recommends initiating potentially beneficial interventions and discontinuing them after a trial of therapy proves their ineffectiveness.[33] In this case it may be appropriate to institute a trial of mechanical ventilation to determine whether the pulmonary process is reversible. In the AAP's view, continuing nonbeneficial treatment causes children great burden and obviates professional responsibility.[33]

Resuscitation, mechanical ventilation, blood products, medications, medically provided hydration and nutrition, dialysis, and other therapies must be considered individually based on the goals for the patient. Clarifying goals of treatment is essential for determining an ethically justifiable course of treatment. It is unjustified, for instance, to assume

---

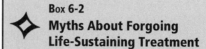

Box 6-2
Myths About Forgoing Life-Sustaining Treatment

- Anything that is not specifically permitted by law is prohibited.
- Termination of life support is murder or suicide.
- A patient must be terminally ill for life support to be stopped.
- It is permissible to terminate extraordinary treatments, not ordinary ones.
- Terminating tube feedings is legally different from stopping other treatments.
- Termination of life support requires going to court.

Data from Meisel A: Legal myths about terminating life support, *Arch Intern Med* 151:1497-1501.

that a decision not to resuscitate a dying child automatically means that all other aggressive measures will also be foregone. Cardiopulmonary resuscitation, for example, may not be desirable for a child dying with cancer but his or her parents may still desire that antibiotics, blood products, and other palliative interventions be continued.

Determining whether it is morally justifiable to forgo certain therapies depends upon the child's and the family's goals and preferences for certain therapies, weighing the benefits and burdens of each therapy in light of the goals, and the moral analysis. When a child is dying, for example, focusing on the comfort associated with dying rather than on therapies to prolong life may be justifiable.

Although it is difficult to determine what may count in determining a child's best interest, forgoing life-sustaining treatment is justifiable when a child experiences substantial and unrelievable suffering and when the child has suffered irreversible brain injury that precludes human or environmental interaction. When life is judged worse than death for a child, it is justified to choose death over continued suffering. The more severely burdened or damaged the child's condition and the greater the certainty of the nature, degree, and irreversibility of the child's condition, the greater the justification for not prolonging the dying process. When in good faith it is not possible to determine which is worse, the presumption for treatment that allows for a chance for life and greater certainty may be warranted. Those with decision-making authority must accept the responsibility of choosing the conditions that they believe be so dehumanized or dehumanizing as to justify terminating life-extending treatment. Based on the Baby Doe Regulations,[12] there appears to be consensus about terminal illness, permanent unconscious, medically futility, and disproportionate burdens of treatment over benefits as justifiable reasons to forgo life sustaining therapies.

In some cases, disagreement may arise about whether a particular intervention constitutes life prolonging treatment or comfort care. For example, when does suctioning of the pharynx merely prolong the dying process by preventing the patient from aspirating his secretions, and when is it an appropriate intervention that enhances the patient's comfort? A similar question may be asked about the use of antibiotics or supplemental oxygen. Again, each intervention must be assessed based on the goal of treatment and whether it contributes to the attainment of that goal. Establishing strict criteria for distinguishing life-prolonging interventions from those that are palliative and promote comfort are unlikely to resolve the controversy or ambiguity. Rather, clinicians and parents should openly discuss the use of interventions in the "gray zone" within the context of the child's condition, goals, and preferences.

Within this process, professionals should examine their own responses and reasoning in light of professional codes and guidelines and personal morality. Professionals may benefit from examining the extent to which the following factors may be influencing their view about forgoing life-sustaining treatment: (1) their own frustration of caring for an infant on a long-term basis, (2) the appearance of the infant, (3) lack of family involvement, (4) a biased impression of prognosis,[34] (5) their own threshold for balancing benefit and burden, and (6) the influence of personal social, economic, cultural, or religious values. The extent to which these factors can be illuminated will assist in clarifying the professional's moral obligations and defining ethically defensible boundaries for providing care.

Cardiopulmonary Resuscitation

Often the discussion about forgoing life sustaining treatments begins with a discussion about cardiopulmonary resuscitation (CPR). Valid and reliable data are essential to good decision making. When discussing resuscitation, it is essential that professionals accurately convey the likely outcomes of attempting CPR including the likelihood that the child will be restored to his or her current condition or sustain complications that may significantly alter their quality of life. When a child is dying, cardiac or respiratory arrest marks the terminal phase of the process. In this case, CPR disrupts the body's natural progression to death and may only prolong the dying process. When resuscitation will not change the course of the disease and will prolong dying, a DNAR order should be documented.[4]

Based on practice standards and ethical guidelines, slow codes are not ethically justifiable. If a patient does not have a DNAR documented, healthcare professional are obliged to resuscitate. This reality does not mean, however, that healthcare professionals are obliged to continue resuscitation beyond its usefulness. Like other interventions the application of CPR requires clinical judgment and knowledge of patient/family goals. DNAR orders do not imply that routine care, attention, and human presence are abandoned. Moreover, it does not necessarily mean that all other life-sustaining therapies should also be foregone. Each therapy must be evaluated individually to determine whether the initiation, continuation, or limitation is warranted.

Medically Provided Hydration and Nutrition

One of the most controversial areas of forgoing life-sustaining treatment involves medically provided hydration and nutrition (MPH&N). MPH&N includes the provision of fluids and/or nutrients via medical devices inserted into the gastrointestinal tract such as gastrostomy or nasogastric tubes or into blood vessels such as central venous lines and portable infusion devices.[35] Forgoing MPH&N in any circumstance remains controversial despite widespread consensus among professional groups, ethicists, and the courts that it is justifiable in some instances.[35-38] For a variety of psychologic, cultural, and societal reasons, the controversy intensifies when it is considered in children. These reasons may include the following: (1) the powerful symbolic significance of the act of feeding dependent children; (2) the view that providing hydration and nutrition is a basic care requirement to sustain life; (3) a child's incapacity for independent decision making, which creates a high threshold for continuing treatments until death is imminent; (4) diagnostic and prognostic uncertainty about determining a terminal condition; (5) the injustice of young children dying; and (6) fear of legal reprisal. Despite these reasons, Nelson and colleagues argue that decisions about forgoing medically provided hydration and nutrition should be guided by the presumption that it is medically and ethically appropriate in the majority of pediatric cases, and nutrition and fluids should always be offered by mouth, except in the unusual case when, for example, oral feedings unavoidably lead to recurrent direct aspiration.[35] They further argued that it is ethically permissible to forgo MPH&N in certain cases. These include neurologic devastation, irreversible total intestinal failure, and proximate death from any pathologic cause.[35]

When death is imminent, within days or weeks, it is ethically justified to stop those interventions that prolong the dying process.[11] The continuation of MPH&N can significantly lengthen the dying process by interfering with the natural dying process. In some instances, the provision of MPH&N can impose unnecessary burdens for the child and family. These include increased oral and pulmonary secretions, diarrhea, edema, increased urine output, abdominal distention, and discomfort.[11] A dying child is likely to have anorexia and decreased desire for eating or drinking. Forcing intake, either parenterally or enterally, may not promote the child's best interests at the end of life.

When MPH&N is considered as an option for forgoing life-sustaining treatment, it will be essential that the decision-making process allow for divergent views to be appreciated. Although many professionals and parents are comfortable with discontinuing mechanical ventilation, the issue of forgoing MPH&N may instigate intense emotional responses that will require vigilant attention and a fair and open process.

Pain Management

The ethical mandate to treat a child's pain is based on the principles of beneficence and nonmaleficence. Healthcare providers have an obligation to reduce or eliminate pain and suffering by assessing and managing it using their clinical knowledge and skill. Relieving the distress caused by pain is an inherently humanitarian act, embodying the ethical principle of beneficence—doing good for others. The American Nurses Association, the World Health Organization, and other organizations unequivocally endorse the professional's responsibility to assess and manage pain in children.[39,40] It is now indisputable that infants and children experience pain, and professionals have an unequivocal responsibility to assess and manage pain in children. Yet many infants and children continue to be undermedicated for pain despite efforts to enhance professional awareness of their needs. This is explained in part by philosophic and clinical barriers to providing analgesia that is commensurate with the intensity of the pain experienced by infants and children.

When the burdens of treatment outweigh the benefits of continued existence, the priority of care becomes the relief of pain and suffering. Making comfort the primary goal of

management may involve maximizing analgesic interventions despite hazards such as sedation and respiratory depression, or it may mean withdrawing or forgoing painful or invasive treatments such as CPR, ventilator, or diagnostic blood work. The benefits of the relief of pain and suffering include the following: (1) the child may feel more comfortable during the dying process; (2) the child may be more available for interaction with others, allowing the child and family to connect with each other and/or complete their life work together, thereby decreasing isolation and loneliness; (3) the child may experience an increased sense of control over his or her environment and treatment; (4) increased activity may allow the child and significant others to share important experiences together; and (5) the child's and family's perception of the treatment or the final stages of the child's life. These benefits must be weighed against the physical, psychologic, and spiritual burdens of unmanaged pain that include: (a) decreased interaction, isolation, or immobility, (b) real or perceived sense of abandonment, (c) anxiety and fear about being in pain without relief, (d) loss of trust in and fear of healthcare professionals, (e) irritability, (f) nightmares, and (g) decreased resources for coping and living. When pain occurs at the end of life, additional burdens include avoidance of the reality of death and decreased opportunities for child and family to complete their life work together.

Throughout treatment, healthcare professionals may need to discuss with the child and parents the plan for managing pain during treatment and, when appropriate, at the end of life. It is essential to note that intractable pain is uncommon in children because most diseases produce pain that is treatable with medications. For example, unlike adults, children with cancer overwhelmingly experience pain that is treatment related.[41,42] Clarification about the trade-offs that may be necessary to manage pain will be necessary. For example, some children may prefer to endure some pain in order to remain interactive and not be sedated. Others may prefer not to feel any pain and be drowsy and less responsive. Being clear about the goals of management and anticipating the various outcomes to different treatments may help to avoid conflicts. Moreover, in the spirit of full disclosure, a variety of pharmacologic and anesthetic options that are available to manage pain at the end of life that do not produce diminished awareness should also be explored.[32,43]

When children are dying, nurses and other healthcare providers often struggle to balance their obligation to relieve pain against the concern that their actions may cause the child's death. Although some philosophers have argued that there are no important differences between withdrawal of treatment and active euthanasia, many clinicians and ethicists have stressed the importance of maintaining a distinction between active killing and efforts to promote comfort at the end of life. Aggressive pain management at the end of life can be ethically justified based on several arguments. First, when a patient is dying, one may reason that the obligation to relieve pain and suffering overrides concerns about hastening death. In assessing risks and burdens, common side effects of analgesia such as sedation, nausea, and respiratory depression should be distinguished from rarer events such as the possibility of addiction.[40] Concerns about respiratory depression, addiction, or tolerance are insufficient reasons for inadequate pain management in the care of the dying.[40] Second, the intent of providing sufficient analgesia to the dying person is to relieve pain in order to enhance living until death occurs. In contrast, the intent of active euthanasia, which is the deliberate killing of the patient by lethal injections of toxic agents or overdoses of analgesics or sedatives, is to precipitate death.[41]

The means to achieving pain relief in the dying person are distinct from the means to achieving active euthanasia.[44] Generally analgesics are titrated in small increments with constant assessment and monitoring of the patient's response in an attempt to maximize comfort while minimizing undesirable side effects. Although death may occur secondary to the administration of the medication, it is in service to the goal of pain relief. In active euthanasia, large, sometimes massive doses that exceed the customary dosing parameters and intensity of the patient's pain are given with the intent of preventing any possibility that the person would survive the administration of the agent. In this instance the goal is irreversible cessation of heart rate and respiration. The difference in intent carries with it a corresponding difference in meaning for the patient, family, and caregivers.

Administering enough analgesia to relieve pain, even if death occurs secondarily, is morally permissible as long as the intent is to relieve suffering. Such an approach is consistent with American Nurses Association (ANA) "Code for Nurses."[45] The Code instructs nurses to promote health, relieve pain and suffering, or promote a peaceful death. An ANA position statement on pain relief at the end of life encourages nurses to aggressively advocate for and provide adequate pain relief in the dying patient even if it secondarily foreshortens life.[39] The pursuit of adequate pain relief is fully protected by laws and regulations governing the practice of medicine; however, active euthanasia is currently illegal in all 50 states. (One state [Oregon] has legalized assisted suicide but this deals exclusively with competent adults and therefore does not apply to children.)

To address concerns about pain management at the of life, it is prudent to use end-of-life pain management protocols that include a variety of safeguards, including incremental titration of medications, ongoing assessment, dosage parameters, and process guidelines. Careful attention and monitoring should be employed to minimize the risks associated with analgesia and to continually monitor the balance of benefits and burdens associated with various treatment regimens.[32]

Euthanasia

Strictly speaking, euthanasia means "good death." Although there is significant controversy about whether bright lines can be maintained between different categories of acts that lead to death, consensus among clinicians and some ethicists supports distinctions between killing and allowing to die. Many clinicians use the term *euthanasia* to refer to

acts that intentionally and deliberately cause a person's immediate death.[46] In this sense, euthanasia means killing the patient. *Allowing to die* is a term used to refer to the intentional avoidance of interventions that interfere with the natural progression of a disease or injury to death. Yet there is often confusion at the bedside on whether appropriate management of pain at the end of life (see previous discussion) or the forgoing of life-sustaining therapies constitutes active euthanasia. This is particularly problematic in intensive care settings where the availability and widespread use of complex technology blurs the distinctions between acts that are forestalling an inevitable death and those that are intended to end the patient's life. Moreover, there is considerable debate about the ethical justification of using pharmacologic paralytic agents during withdrawal of mechanical ventilation.[47,48]

As a practical matter, parents rarely request that professionals actively end their child's life. Yet parents may beg professionals to "do something" when their anguish at watching their child suffer becomes unbearable. Such requests do not necessarily imply that parent's are asking for euthanasia. Rather, such requests should invite further exploration of the feelings and the motivation behind such pleas. The request to intervene is insufficient justification for professionals to engage in acts that are outside their usual protocols for caring for dying children such as giving lethal injections in an effort to assuage parental and professional anguish.

Despite the confusion in terminology, it is clear that physicians and nurses have an obligation to respect life and not to kill patients. Decisions to forgo or limit life-sustaining treatment should always be subject to review and systematic scrutiny. Ethically justifiable end-of-life care can be enhanced when the process of decision making includes appropriate safeguards and clinical guidelines.[32]

DECISION-MAKING MODELS

In addition to an analysis of the ethical principles that apply to issues in pediatric critical care, elements of an ethical decision-making process should be taken into account. A shared decision-making model and AACN's Synergy Model are described below. Although not mutually exclusive, each offers a unique perspective on the ideal manner in which ethical issues may be resolved. In addition, the role of the critical care nurse in decision making is addressed.

Shared Decision Making

Historically, healthcare professionals did not consider a patient's or family's wishes, beliefs, and values. Wanting to protect patients from their own lack of knowledge and subsequent bad judgment, healthcare professionals did not involve patients or families in healthcare decisions. The norm that functioned promoted the belief that healthcare professionals knew what was best for patients. Patients were not to know too much about their diagnosis or prognosis and were not to interfere with treatment plans. This paternalistic attitude was often justified on the basis of doing no harm.

Duff called this attitude "ethical elitism" and noted that when paternalism thrives, the dictum of "do no harm" may be violated.[31] Caring for others requires consideration of *their* values and contributions.[49] Healthcare professionals who believe that they know best foster family dependency and increase feelings of loss of control. Healthcare professionals must remember that parental acceptance or rejection of recommended medical treatment is a moral decision and is not the healthcare professional's responsibility.

Despite our history, a moral framework based on a model of shared decision making has been endorsed as ideal.[15,33,50,51] The desired outcomes of shared decision making are summarized in Box 6-3. Shared decision making relies on establishing and nurturing a relationship that is synergistic and reciprocal among the child, family, and healthcare professionals. The relationship flourishes when honesty, openness, and trustworthy interactions prevail.

Endorsement of a model of shared decision making means that the outcome of the process of informed consent is evaluated based on the quality of the relationship rather than the amount or type of information shared. To accomplish this goal, parents must be respected and supported to engage fully in the process, be enabled to fully understand the range of possibilities for treatment and their consequences, and to share in meaningful ways in the dialogue about their goals, values, and aspirations for their child's life. Such a model goes beyond the legal requirements for disclosure, comprehension, and voluntary consent.[52] Although in theory professionals embrace the ideal of shared decision making as the desired model of parent-professional decision making, it is rarely accomplished in practice.[52]

One possible reason for the lack of success in achieving shared decision making is that professionals have focused primarily on the decision itself, rather than the process necessary to engage parents in a shared journey to realize their child's interests. A revised model of shared decision making would therefore focus more on the context of the situation, especially the relational dimensions, the parent's unique conception of good parenting, and the factors that mediate decision making, rather than the decision itself.

A broader conception of the process of shared decision making is necessary to account for the differences between approaches of parents and professionals. Professionals, for instance, must begin to appreciate the parental perspective

in decision making and not attempt to force parents to conform to the professional decision-making framework. Unlike the rational, scientific approach of professionals, the context for parents' attitudes and behaviors is derived from their unique conception of good parenting of which commitment to their child is a central feature.[53] Instead of asking parents whether they want their child to be resuscitated, professionals may find that focusing on the parent's commitments to their child's life and connecting with parents as human beings may be a more fruitful approach.

Professionals should carefully assess each parent's appraisals of their situation and their coping strategies in order to respect the myriad factors that may account for their diversity in their patterns of adjustment.[54] Box 6-4 describes some key questions to promote understanding and dialogue with parents. It must be acknowledged, however, that the way parents choose to participate in decisions and their need for control is varied. Some parents are accepting of and/or desire professional dominance[55]; others covet autonomous decision making on behalf of their child. Although many parents do not wish to abdicate their decision making authority to others, they struggle with their own ambivalence about what role they could play in a situation they view as largely out of their control.[53,56] Professionals may base their assessments of parental understanding on their own values about what is important and meaningful to the decision. Understanding each parent's conception of good parenting involves assessing and fostering decisional involvement for parents based on their particular style of decision making, coping strategies, and need for control. A supportive approach is to ask parents what role they desire regarding decisions for their child and what information is meaningful to their decision making.

The process of shared decision making is thwarted when parents and professionals fail to connect and achieve a shared meaning of values and value labels that guide decision making. This process can be undermined when professionals fail to understand the richness of the patient/family's life story and context, draw premature conclusions, or label

Box 6-3
Desired Outcomes of Shared Decision Making

- Mutual respect
- Preserved integrity
- Mutual participation, authority
- Understanding
- Shared meaning
- Hope balanced with honesty and realistic expectations
- Mutual satisfaction with the process regardless of the outcome

Box 6-4
Key Questions To Promote Understanding and Dialogue With Parents

- What is your understanding of your child's condition?
- Is there anything about your child's care that is worrying you?
- Do you feel you are being guided too much or too little?
- What would you find to be most helpful right now?
- Have you been able to consider that your child is in danger of not getting better or dying?
- What are you hoping for?
- What do you fear the most right now?
- What will this decision mean for your child's life?
- What will this decision mean for your family?

Adapted from Jellineck M, Catlin E, Todres D et al: Facing tragic decisions with parents in the neonatal intensive care unit: clinical perspectives. *Pediatrics* 89:119-122, 1992.

a parent or their behavior or actions without validating their interpretation of the action, behavior, or situation. For example, professionals may conclude that parents are denying the severity of their child's condition when they repeatedly ask when the child will go home. With clarification, professionals may learn that they parents understand their child's prognosis and their statement may be an expression of a deeply held desire to spend time with their child outside of the hospital, particularly if death is likely.

Increasingly a model of shared decision making has been challenged, particularly when parents request treatments that healthcare professionals perceive to be inappropriate or futile.[57,58] Unilateral decision making in certain situations has been suggested as a means for resolving conflicts. Such claims are based on the ethical integrity of the professionals and support the claim that professionals are not obligated to provide futile treatments. Unilateral decisions represent a significant departure from the usual model of shared decision making and should be subject to careful examination.

Parents may request treatments that are of questionable benefit for a variety of reasons. These include: (1) faulty reasoning about the efficacy or benefit of a therapy; (2) psychologic factors such as fear, anxiety, stress, or depression; (3) unrealistic expectations about the outcomes of certain treatments; (4) inability of the family to trust professionals to act in the child's best interest; (5) religious conviction that life must be preserved at all costs; and (6) an attitude that getting "everything" is an entitlement.[59] Understanding some of the reasons that may influence parental requests offers professionals avenues to explore as they work with parents to develop a mutually agreeable plan of care.

For shared decision making to be authentic, the parental perspective must be appreciated as legitimate and meaningful. Efforts should be undertaken to begin to bridge the gaps between the professional and parental perspectives. This means that the goals of the parent-professional relationship, the outcomes of the process, and the process itself must be closely scrutinized and evaluated.

Synergy Model

AACN's Synergy Model offers an additional framework for applying ethical principles to the care of critically ill children and their families and contributes to a process of ethical decision making.[30] Synergy, individuals working together in mutually enhancing ways toward a common goal, is one of the goals of the ethical decision-making process. Synergy derives from responsive interdependence, shared commonality, and equity within relationships congruent with an ethic of care (described previously). In the Synergy Model, the child's needs are considered within the individual family context, the community environment, and the child's unique personal characteristics. These factors can be incorporated into the assessment phase of the ethical decision-making process (see later section). By achieving the desired patient outcomes, integrity is promoted for the patient, family, healthcare professional, and broader community.[30]

Partners on the Journey: Critical Care Nurse Advocacy

Pediatric critical care nurses have a moral mandate to be involved in resolving the ethical issues that arise in the care of critically ill children and their families. Nurses bring a unique perspective to decision making for critically ill children because of their close proximity to patients and families and their professional orientation, knowledge, and skill. Their involvement is essential for the child and family's safe passage through the often tumultuous experience of critical illness. Simultaneously, they struggle to balance competing obligations to the patient, family, physician, institution, profession, colleagues, and society. It is within this context that their advocacy occurs.

Advocacy, acting to safeguard and advance the interests of another, is an essential dimension of critical care nursing practice.[5,30,60] The critical competencies described in AACN's Synergy Model are consistent with the moral obligations of nurses to advocate for the best interests of the child in the context of the family.[30] Nurses demonstrate their moral agency when they assume a leadership role in identifying and helping resolve ethical and clinical concerns. Effective advocacy requires clinical judgment, caring practices, collaboration, systems thinking, and a commitment to clinical inquiry. Clinical judgment, for example, is essential for understanding the child's disease trajectory and prognosis, assessing benefits and burdens, and participating in the development of goals and treatment plans, and responding to the unique needs of the child and family. Caring practices are how nurses express their moral commitments of compassion, beneficence, and nonmaleficence in promoting the child's best interests and well-being. Collaboration with the patient, family, and interdisciplinary team is the means for understanding the values and goals of the patient and family, communicating with others, and engaging members of the interdisciplinary team in achieving mutually determined goals. Systems thinking focuses on holistic interrelationships and the broader needs of the child and family in addition to an awareness of how to navigate effectively in the institution, healthcare system, and community. Such an orientation enables the nurse to nurture the child and family's inherent capacities and the resources of the healthcare system to promote the child's interests. Finally, a commitment to clinical inquiry involves an ongoing process of questioning and evaluating practice and providing practice based on available data. These key elements are essential for nurses to discharge their moral responsibilities on behalf of children and families.

PARENTS' AND CHILDREN'S RIGHTS

Based on the moral framework of shared decision making, it is necessary for someone to represent the interests of the child. In the United States there is presumption of parental moral and legal authority in matters of concern for their minor children. This is based on a belief that parents generally have a sincere concern to protect their child's life. Parents are obligated to protect their children from harm and to do as much good for them as possible. Parents are in the best position to know their child's wants and desires. They have a tendency to place their child's interests ahead of their own. As a result of a long-term specific relationship with their child, parents have a commitment to ongoing care. To respect a child is to respect the relationships that are central to the child's life. Thus, parents should have responsibility for their children's healthcare decisions. After all, they bear the financial, emotional, and medical consequences for those decisions. Long after well-meaning healthcare professionals have gone home, "the family will be remembering and incorporating this momentous decision into the fabric of their lives."[15]

Generally parents are considered to be competent decision makers when they put their child's interest as primary, appear to understand the essential components of their child's illness and prognosis, and demonstrate rational thinking processes.[61] This "reasonable parent standard" is consistent with the elements of adult decision making capacity. However, healthcare team members may question parental competency, particularly when their decisions are not congruent with professional recommendations. At times, assessment of parental competency is clouded by the parent's response to the crisis situation and grief. Under these circumstances, professionals often assume that parents are unable to participate in decision making because of lack of understanding emotional upheaval or because professionals believe they must protect the parent from future guilt. Professionals may also judge parental involvement, behavior, and visiting patterns without adequate information or verification of their perceptions.

Despite professional assumptions to the contrary, most parents in crisis are able to make sense out of the unexpected and uncertain situation they are thrust into by their child's illness. Their search for information, support, and meaning in the experience demonstrated their commitment to the life of their child. They demonstrated their commitment to their child's welfare by placing their own sense of self-worth and their emotional needs in abeyance. Parents make significant psychologic adjustments and major adjustments in interpersonal, family, financial, social, community, spiritual, and moral contexts. Rather than being incapacitated, parents demonstrate their advocacy by searching for acceptable resolutions to the issues and problems that they face.[53,54,62]

In practice, the issue of who decides is not usually raised to the surface. Only when disagreement arises over what measures will serve the child best does the question of who decides become a thorny one. For example, during the past two decades, the question of parents' rights to make medical decisions for their children has gained national attention. It began in 1975 with the case of Karen Ann Quinlan,[63] whose parents had to go to the New Jersey Supreme Court to be allowed to remove their comatose daughter from a ventilator. The Baby Doe cases in 1982 prompted an attempt by the federal government to take decision-making power away from parents who refused any medical intervention for seriously handicapped newborns.[12] Then in 1989 a father in a Chicago pediatric intensive care unit held hospital staff at bay with a shotgun while he unplugged the respirator from his son, who was diagnosed to be in a persistent vegetative state.[64]

Limits to Parental Authority

The social policy of the United States gives a great deal of discretion to parents and permits supplanting their authority only when the child's interests are clearly and severely threatened by parental action. Children exist and develop within the context of their families. As long as parents do not neglect those people under their care, society should not intervene. However, society has a responsibility to intervene when parents refuse to give care to children that would clearly benefit them or when parents subject children to clear harm. For example, parental rights do not include the right to abandon or endanger a child. However, when parents insist on undertreatment or overtreatment in situations in which the healthcare team is in disagreement, the responsibility for decision making is less certain.

Healthcare team members should use their knowledge of the child's health status to attempt to resolve disagreement with the family rather than supplant the family's decision-making authority. The physician and other team members must be certain that to withhold a specific treatment or a specific procedure would result in serious harm that would threaten the child's life. The process of informing parents often causes pain and anguish for them. Yet to avoid giving parents all the information available about their child's diagnosis and prognosis does not show respect for their right to make informed healthcare decisions and provide their child with needed support. Informed consent demands being given the information and then being allowed to make a choice.

The interests of parents and the family must take a high priority but do not override the fundamental respect for the best interest of the child. Accepting parental perceptions and actions does not imply that they must be blindly accepted or acted upon. Each person's conclusions are open to examination, reflection, and comparison to socially and politically determined norms of behavior. Parental decision must be assessed in light of the child's diagnosis, expected outcome with and without treatment, degree of uncertainty about the outcome, quality of the child's life, probability of benefits from treatment, and presumed burdens if treatment occurs or does not occur. However, parents' unique interpretations of their child's interests must be taken seriously. Based on an understanding of the parental perspective, it is, as Rhoden suggests, justified to begin the assessment with the assumption that parents are the best decision makers for their children and that their child's interests are primary in their decision making.[65] It is incumbent upon others who would challenge the parents' motives and commitments to prove that they should be disqualified as decision makers instead of parents having to prove their motives and commitments are authentic. Unless a child is in imminent danger of dying, the healthcare team has a duty to both the child and family to take the time and effort necessary to reach consensus on treatment decisions.

When assessing parents as decision makers, several key questions are recommended: (1) Do the parents meet the "reasonable parent" standard? (2) Is the parent's request within a morally acceptable range of options? (3) What evidence is there that the parents should be disqualified as the decision maker? (4) Are there actions that could be taken to enhance the parent's ability to act as their child's surrogate such as support and empathic listening, provisions for nourishment and sleep, transportation, counseling, child care, housing, or other resources?

Despite efforts to enable their participation, some parents may be unable or unwilling to function in their proper role as surrogate. In these relatively rare instances, healthcare professionals must seek an alternative surrogate decision maker who can represent the interests of the child. The issue of who will speak for a dying child is particularly poignant when an infant is unable to speak for himself or herself and does not have a parent advocate. Without a parent or surrogate to give meaning to the child's interests, to create opportunities to question, explore, accept, or reject the recommendations of caregivers, the child becomes voiceless. The balance of sharing in decision making can be tipped in favor of the interests of the healthcare providers or the bureaucracy of an overburdened state welfare system may jeopardize decision making. When morally appropriate surrogates are not present, caregivers must be more vigilant in adhering to and having in place stringent safeguards to protect the interest of the infant or child. When a parent surrogate is absent, additional safeguards are necessary to monitor how the balance of benefit and burden are interpreted to avoid using technology inappropriately or allowing treatment to continue beyond its usefulness.

Clearly there will always be cases in which assumptions about parental authority will be appropriately challenged; however, these will likely be few in number if a process of shared decision making is made a reality. Cases of abuse or neglect of the child (when a serious conflict of interest exists), or instances in which the parental decision maker lacks decision making capacity or refuses to serve as the decision maker are examples of the types of situations in which parental authority may be challenged. Safeguards to protect the interests of children, families, and healthcare providers will continue to be necessary and prudent.

The Courts

Although there is wide latitude given to families to practice various religions and lifestyles, courts have intervened to protect children and have not permitted refusal of standard medical treatment in life-threatening situations, for example, by parents who are Jehovah's Witnesses or Christian Scientists. The courts justify this interference by invoking the "parens patriae" doctrine; that is, the state's legitimate interest in the welfare of children and its right and duty to protect vulnerable people from harm. The "parens patriae" doctrine is often used in legislation and authorizes the state to intervene when parents fail to provide necessary medical care.[66]

Ultimately, a court must decide when parents will be disqualified as decision makers and another person designated to act in their stead. It is incumbent upon the healthcare team to show the court convincing evidence of why the parents should be removed as the child's decision maker. It has been argued that when parents appear unable to make decisions in the best interest of their child, a healthcare professional—usually the physician—ought to make the healthcare decisions. However, healthcare professionals are not necessarily unbiased participants. Personal feelings of defeat and helplessness become interwoven with their own individual beliefs about life and death. Conflicts among the various agendas of research, education, and treatment may slant their perspective.

A court may appoint a surrogate decision maker, who can be another family member or a person who is not a member of the healthcare team. The surrogate decision maker should have knowledge of the facts of the child's case and should be free of serious conflicts of interest. It is important that the healthcare team understand the circumstances under which the surrogate was appointed, which decisions the surrogate can make, and what other judicial action may be occurring.

If the state removed itself completely from such situations, the consequences could be devastating for many children. Yet, because of a primary belief that parents want to and do act in their child's best interest, the healthcare team should guard against reaching premature conclusions about parental intentions.

NAVAGATING THROUGH ETHICAL ISSUES

There are many ways of discerning the ethical dimensions of a situation or issue. The process of discernment is complex and is influenced by emotions, scientific facts, values, interpersonal relationships, culture, religion, the essence of who we are, and myriad situational factors. All of these elements converge to shape the way ethical questions are framed. The discernment process involves clarifying factual, conceptual, and ethical issues. For example, when a child is dying it is important to understand the diagnosis and prognosis and to clarify any factual issues related to medical care. Additionally, conceptual issues such as the meaning or quality of life or what constitutes a life worth living may also need clarification and discussion. Ethical issues such as the reasons for forgoing certain life-sustaining therapies will also require rigorous analysis and discernment.

When situations arise that precipitate feelings of ambiguity, conflict, or confusion, there is an occasion for reflection, analysis, and critique. A systematic process applying a moral framework for pediatric decision making can help to clarify and resolve the ethical tension. The first step is to assess and clarify what is at stake in the situation and the nature of the ambiguity, confusion, or conflict. Often important values of patients, families, and professionals such as patient self-determination, prevention of harm, or relief of pain and suffering may be in conflict. Responding to such conflicts involves clarifying and verifying the medical, psychosocial, and spiritual facts of the case. This includes ascertaining: (a) who is involved in the case; (b) who has decision-making authority—legally and morally—and the role of the child in decisions; (c) the patient's diagnosis, prognosis, and therapeutic options for treatment; (d) the context for the decision including a chronology of events and any factors that are influencing the decision making and implementation of actions; (e) goals of treatment and reasons to support various viewpoints; (f) application of clinical and moral criteria used in reaching a decision with particular attention to the degree of certainty needed or desired for decision making; and (g) determination of the healthcare professional's moral and professional obligations.[67]

Based on the Synergy Model, personal characteristics of the patient—stability, complexity, predictability, resiliency, vulnerability, participation in decision making and care and resource availability—offer a useful framework for illuminating the unique context for decision making.[30] For example, stability, complexity, predictability, resiliency, and vulnerability are key factors in assessing the child's clinical condition, prognosis, or morbidity associated with illness or injury. Assessing the child's and family's participation in decision making and care and the personal, psychologic, social, technical, and fiscal resources that the patient, the patient's family, and the community bring to the situation are essential for creating a comprehensive picture of the situation. Based on the model, patient characteristics must be evaluated on an ongoing basis as the situation evolves. This process invites healthcare professionals and parents to review these data regularly and continually assess goals, treatment plans, and prognosis.

Following the assessment and analysis stage, it is necessary to identify a range of reasonable options and the reasons to support each. This involves clarifying the above information, determining the effectiveness of the proposed treatments using a benefit-burden analysis for available treatment options, evaluating the relevance of factors such as age, quality of life, legal considerations, economics, cultural, and other patient/family factors, and examining the strengths and weaknesses of the moral arguments that support each option.[67] Again, the Synergy Model offers a useful framework for assessing these concerns.

The following questions may be helpful in this process[67]:

- Is the decision within a morally acceptable range of options?
- Does pursing a particular course of action violate other highly valued moral principles such as avoiding harm or self-determination?
- What competing personal or professional values might affect your willingness to take moral action in this case?
- What kinds of objections might be raised about the proposed decision? How can you explain your decision in a way that addresses those objections?

Once the analysis is complete the decision maker must choose the option that advances the child's interests best. The final step in the process is to implement the decision, evaluate the process and outcomes, and determine what you have learned that will be helpful in similar future

situations. Participants (parents and professionals) must engage in a disciplined decision-making process that includes procedural safeguards. Cassidy suggests a set of procedural checks to evaluate the quality of the ethical analysis (Box 6-5).[68]

Addressing Conflict

Providing care for critically children may result in controversy or conflict among patients, families, and healthcare professionals. When healthcare professionals, older children, and families disagree about the treatment plan or goals, a method for conflict resolution is necessary. During moments of conflict or confusion, individuals may experience vague feelings of unrest or a generalized feeling of distress or anxiety. At this stage such feelings may not be fully comprehensible and only partially articulated. Emotions are often heightened as participants attempt to interpret

---

Box 6-5
Procedural Check for Evaluating the Ethical Analysis

Clarity

Have participants been open and seen each factor as it is and incorporated it into the system without distortions? Have individuals projected their own views or values onto the meanings of others statements? Have assumptions been made or conclusions drawn without sufficient information or validation? Has a particular action or reason been labeled in a way that short-circuits the initiation or continuation of the moral work that is necessary to resolve quandaries and conflicts?

Consistency

Have key concepts such as *quality of life, euthanasia,* etc., been used consistently? Have terms or values been respected not only when they would serve individual purposes or interests, but also when they would inhibit them? Have the participants clarified the meanings of terms and concepts?

Coherence

Do all of the clear and consistent parts of a judgment truly fit together without contradictions or gaps? Are judgments sufficiently grounded in ethical theory, principles, and/or methodologies and lead to a rationally connected conclusion?

Comprehensiveness

Have all relevant views and factors been taken into account? Or, have the preferred elements such as facts, values, etc., been included while confounding views and factors been disregarded?

Conclusiveness

Have all countervailing views and arguments been openly recognized and honestly refuted? Have I fairly won the right to claim that my conclusion is conclusive?

Adapted from Cassidy R: From principles to practice. In Cassidy R, Fleishman A, eds: *Pediatric ethics—from principles to practice.* United Kingdom, 1996, Harwood Academic Publishers.

their "gut feeling" that something is amiss. Individuals often translate their intuitive and visceral signals into questions of "why are we doing this?" In response, individuals may either become quite determined in attempts to have their concerns acknowledged and discussed or become apathetic and retreat from the situation. Paying attention to one's intuitive signals can create an opportunity for further reflection and inquiry to identify and name the cause of the anxiety and moral distress. During this period there may be heightened levels of personal and professional hesitancy to act according to the proposed plan of care. Questions of "why are we doing this?" may become more intense. It is prudent that individuals share their concerns with colleagues and supervisors to avoid acting in isolation or implementing risky, unreflective, unethical, or illegal plans.[67]

For example, Sarah is a critical care nurse caring for Joshua, a 4-year-old with end-stage neuroblastoma. Joshua was transferred to the PICU 48 hours ago following a rapid deterioration in his condition in response to gram-negative sepsis. After initial stabilization with vasopressors, mechanical ventilation, neuromuscular blockade, antibiotics, and narcotics, Joshua's condition has steadily declined. Although Joshua's parents have been aware of the possibility of his death, they are clinging to the hope that he will be able to recover from the sepsis. The team caring for Joshua believes that it is unlikely that he will survive this episode of sepsis and that death in imminent.

A family meeting has been arranged to discuss the treatment plan. The physicians and nurses caring for Joshua convey their concern about his condition and prepare the family for the inevitability of his death. After appropriate grieving, the family states that they "do not want Joshua to suffer" and they agree that life-sustaining therapies should be discontinued. The team agrees to do everything possible to eliminate any distress during the process of treatment withdrawal.

An order is written to administer a combination of morphine sulfate at 10 times the current dose and a neuromuscular blocking agent. Following medication administration, vasopressors and mechanical ventilation are to be withdrawn. CPR is not to be initiated. Sarah calls the physician covering the case and questions the infusion regimen because it exceeds the unit standards for delivering analgesia at the end of life and violates standards governing the use of neuromuscular blockade. When Sarah questions the order, the physician becomes defensive, stating, "Just give the dose—he's dying anyway." When she returns to the bedside, his mother begs her to "do something to end this."

In this example, Sarah is experiencing conflicting obligations: first, to advance Joshua's well-being by promoting a humane death; to his mother who is begging her to end Joshua's suffering (and hers); to the physician who has ordered an inappropriate dose of medication; and to the employing institution to practice within institutional, professional, regulatory, and legal boundaries. Without systematic reflecting, Sarah could become confused about the moral justification for her actions.

First, Sarah must use her intuitive wisdom and her clinical expertise to identify what is at stake in this situation.

Second, it is useful to articulate and name the conflict using ethical terms and concepts. In this instance, she may reason that her primary goal is to relieve Joshua's pain and suffering. Administering a dose of narcotic that exceeds her assessment of his pain intensity combined with a neuromuscular blocking agent may threaten a moral boundary to avoid intentionally ending a patient's life. Third, it would be prudent to review the goals of treatment, the assessment data regarding Joshua's pain, his responses to dosage changes in the past, and to clarify the justification for using neuromuscular blocking agents with ventilator withdrawal, and to reiterate the moral foundation of pain relief at the end of life with the physician. Such clarification would also apply in response to the mother's request within a context of acknowledging and clarifying her fears and reassuring her about the nurse's continued presence and support throughout the process. Fourth, Sarah must use the chain of command to clarify issues and address concerns in a constructive manner. Nurses have an obligation to exercise their moral agency in situations that are illegal or unethical. Fifth, it would be helpful for Sarah to disclose the boundaries of ethical practice to both the physician and mother. Based on the ANA Code and End-of-Life Position Statements, she must convey to the physician and Joshua's mother whether she is willing to undertake any actions to intentionally end the life of any person. At the same time, it is important to reaffirm her commitment to providing humane care including aggressive treatment of pain, nonabandonment, continuing support, and presence. Sixth, Sarah may involve others in helping to resolve the issue (e.g., ethics consultants, palliative care specialists, or other advisors). Finally, Sarah must decide whether this situation warrants her conscientious refusal to participate in implementing the orders written for the patient. If she reasons that she cannot, she must ensure that the patient is not abandoned or compromised as a result of her refusal. In this case, following the institutional process for conscientious refusal, mandated by JCAHO, is essential.[69]

When approaching a questionable or controversial act or decision, special caution is advised as a response is formulated. Before acting upon the physician's order and the mother's request, further deliberation is warranted. The following questions can assist in clarifying issues and describing the nature of the ethical quandary[67]:

- Is the situation emotionally charged? Has the emotional nature of the situation changed over time? What is the emotional tenor of those involved in the case? Patient? Family? Healthcare professionals? Have relationships and interaction patterns changed?
- Has the patent's condition significantly changed? Is there confusion about the facts or values that surround the case? Is there explicit or overt conflict, disagreement, or questioning about the course of care? Is there some patient circumstance or characteristic (social, religious, economic, cultural, clinical, psychologic) that is unduly influencing decisions?
- Is there evidence of increased hesitancy about the right course of action? Is there increased resistance to

implementing the proposed plan of action? Is there evidence of intimidation, manipulation, coercion, or threats being leveraged by healthcare professionals, families, patients, or others?

- Is the proposed action a deviation from usual or customary practice? Does this action violate a practice standard or professional code of ethics?
- Is there a perceived need for secrecy around this action? Could a disinterested party interpret this action differently? Could you openly disclose the proposed action to the patient, family, colleagues, or the public? Would those involved be willing to be challenged, sanctioned, or punished for their actions by licensing boards, legal decision, professional organizations, or the public?

Answers to these questions may be helpful in articulating the nature of the ethical conflict, ambiguity, or confusion. Initiating this process of assessment and discernment may resolve the conflict. General strategies for resolving ethical conflicts are included in Box 6-6. In other instances, this process will be the beginning of a longer process that may involve ethics consultants or committees.

Environments That Support Ethical Practice

Critical care environments may be conducive and supportive of ethical thinking and decision making or may erect numerous formal or informal barriers to the process. Formal barriers may result, for example, from the development of

---

Box 6-6
Strategies for Addressing Conflicts

- Anticipate and address ethical concerns in a proactive manner.
- Be accessible and fully present in each encounter.
- Create an atmosphere of open communication
- Listen without problem solving.
- Engage in nonjudgmental listening.
- Acknowledge a common commitment to the child's well-being.
- Admit areas of uncertainty and the limits of prognostication.
- Communicate decisions and plan of care honestly and openly.
- Provide a forum for staff to discuss and understand the decision and the decision-making process that is not focused on convincing those who share different views.
- Develop policies regarding end-of-life care and decision making including do-not-resuscitate orders, forgoing life-sustaining treatment including medically provided hydration and nutrition, pain management, and terminal sedation.
- Honor healthcare providers' requests not to participate in morally objectionable situations based on hospital policy.
- When standard methods fail, involve outside parties such as ethics committees or ethics consultants.

---

end-of-life care institutional policies that are ambiguous, controversial, or ignored. Additionally the traditional hierarchy within medical institutions may effectively silence those who challenge the authority of physicians or administrators, or question the intent or substance of institutional policies.[70]

An ideal environment would bring into harmony ethical standards, the scientific basis for care, a holistic approach, and a family-centered focus. Pluralistic values and beliefs would not have to clash, but could be openly acknowledged and truthfully communicated in order for harmony to exist and for honorable decision making to occur. The following strategies may promote better care through the development of an environment that promotes ethical practice.

Clarify Personal and Professional Values.   Self-reflection and a process for clarifying personal and professional values that influence the provision of pediatric critical care is an essential first step in creating an ethical practice environment. Within this process, healthcare professionals must explore within themselves the boundaries of their commitment to accommodate values and commitments that are different from their own. For example, professionals who hold a strict sanctity of life view may find a request to forgo life-sustaining treatment morally objectionable. In such instances the person must ask what it would take to be able to accommodate and respect the conscience and integrity of another while preserving one's own. In the end, the person must determine whether integrity-preserving compromise is possible or whether the threat to one's deeply held values requires conscientious refusal to participate.

Specify Norms of Professional Behavior and Clinical Practice.   A key element in developing an ethical practice environment is to engage in a process of defining norms of professional behavior and clinical practice. Ideally, members of the community would be involved in developing the norms for end-of-life care, care of children with disabling or life-threatening conditions, etc., through participation in focus groups or institutional committees. Norms may include, for example, expectations about the process for decision making, advance care planning, pain and symptom management, end-of-life care, conflict resolution, professional communication, and collaboration. These norms become the "benchmarks" for evaluating quality of care and are the basis for professional accountability.[70]

Develop Processes to Monitor and Evaluate Ethical Performance.   Once norms are developed, it is essential that individuals are held accountable for upholding the norms of behavior and ethical performance. One mechanism for monitoring adherence to agreed-upon norms for clinical care is through quality improvement mechanisms. Through these mechanisms variances can be documented and strategies for recognizing excellence and addressing deficiencies developed.

Standards for ethical performance for the entire organization help to uphold the ethical values and behaviors. Structures to monitor ethical performance may include integration of ethical performance into quality improvement activities, and mechanisms for identifying and dealing with ethical violations, conscientious objection, and public accountability.

Develop a Culture of Integrity. The goal of monitoring and evaluating performance is not merely to determine whether compliance standards are met. Rather, the goal is toward a commitment to integrity in relationships, services, and decisions. If an institution is not clear about what it values, then decisions are likely to be guided by individual values and may result in incongruencies in clinical care or between the employees and the institution's leaders. Attitudes and actions of individuals at all levels of the organization are a tangible sign of their commitment to the values they espouse.[70]

Integrity is essential for maintaining a coherent professional identity that is based on compassion, caring, and trust and for preserving self-esteem. For professionals to see themselves as being trustworthy, they must believe that what they are doing is consistent with their personal or professional standards and moral guides. If professionals perceive that their personal or professional standards are being undermined or that there is inconsistency between what they believe and how they behave, their integrity is compromised. When integrity is threatened, professionals may be unable to convey confidence in their clinical practice to patients or others, their communication may be thwarted, their ability to respond compassionately to the needs of others may be eroded, and ultimately, the quality of patient care will be undermined.

Create or Refine Structures That Support Ethical Inquiry and Action. An ethical practice environment demands systems that support proactive identification and addressing of ethical issues. Participating in institutional ethics committees, creating and offering a curriculum for ethics education, developing forums such as ethics rounds for interdisciplinary discussion of ethical issues, and organizing ethics councils or interest groups are essential strategies to promote ethical inquiry and action. Each is described below.

Institutional Ethics Committees. Institutional ethics committees are an important tool for promoting individual and institutional sensitivity to the ethical issues faced at the bedside. When healthcare professionals, older children, and/or families disagree about the treatment plan or goals, a method for conflict resolution is necessary. Since the 1980s ethics committees have become a common institutional mechanism for clarifying, analyzing, and resolving difficult ethical issues. The Joint Commission on Accreditation of Healthcare Organizations (JCHAO) now requires healthcare institutions to have a mechanism for addressing ethical issues. In many cases, this involves a multidisciplinary ethics committee.[71] Most often ethics committees are used when standard approaches to decision making through collaboration are insufficient or are not successful in resolving the ethical tensions. Generally ethics committees function in an advisory capacity and in many cases provide education, mediation, support, and external review. Standards for ethics consultation have contributed to greater awareness of the need for consistency in approach,

specialized knowledge and skill, a systematic process, and ongoing education and evaluation.[72]

Ethics committees can assist parents and caregivers to reflect upon, analyze, and develop ethically sound responses to the ethical issues that may arise, particularly at the end of life. Ethics committees can provide a forum of impartiality to assist parents and healthcare professionals in the process of ethical decision making. Complex issues coupled with obvious disagreement about what the treatment should be or who should decide invite ethics committee consultation. Most ethics committees provide (1) education about ethical principles that guide decision making; (2) a forum for airing feelings and conflicts about dilemmas; (3) a system for emotional support for healthcare professionals and families; and (4) an interdisciplinary group to formulate policies that guide decision making. Generally, the actions of the committee are purely consultative and are not binding on any professional. However, submitting ethical dilemmas to uninvolved parties for consideration allows for objective discussion of various viewpoints.

The generic makeup of an ethics committee is not universally agreed upon. The consultation process is enhanced when committees include diverse representation including physician, nurses, social workers, chaplains, administrators, parents, and community members. A broad perspective enhances contributions on issues that may require knowledge about organizational systems and external resources that may aid decision making. Other committee members may include ethicists and/or attorneys, ideally ones without an institutional conflict of interest. It is most important that all committee members are willing to look beyond their own values and preferences and view issues from the patient's perspective. The members should have a desire to be informed about ethical theory and principles, as well as current issues. The members must be willing to listen to each other; accept ambiguity; and be reflective, critical thinkers.[20]

Access to ethics committees should be available to all members of the healthcare team, patients, and families. The committee should develop procedures to ensure timely and effective consultation. Written information that outlines the committee's roles should be provided to staff and families. Ideally parents and professionals are proactive in addressing ethical concerns. Professionals should anticipate decision points and potential sources of disagreement and conflict and regularly review and revise treatment goals based on patient/family preferences.

The involvement of the courts in resolving conflict should be reserved for cases of intractable conflict and only as a last resort. Professionals and parents must consider the limitations of the courts in resolving value conflicts and what the appropriate role the courts can play in resolving disputes. Pursuing court intervention necessarily alters the nature of the relationships and may serve to create or exacerbate adversarial tensions. It is prudent for ethics committees and attorneys to work collaboratively to appreciate both the ethical and legal context of troubling cases. The legal response may not necessarily be the best moral response. Therefore, the process of working through difficult cases must first focus on what is justifiable from an ethical perspective and how to address the legal concerns that accompany the best decision.

Ethics Education.   Healthcare professionals who work in critical care units have been expected to be experts in the moral issues that surround life and death. Unfortunately, most have received little education in ethics. Many professionals still practice with the belief that one's desire to do good is directly proportional to how much good is actually done. Thus, when called upon to buffer the powerful reality of disease and disability and to make sense out of alternative courses of action, healthcare professionals may not be successful.

Nurses can enhance their decision-making ability by taking advantage of educational opportunities that focus on ethical analysis and the specific moral issues faced by critical care nurses. Ethics education helps practitioners make moral choices based upon reason rather than intuition. Hospitals can provide a variety of educational opportunities for both nurses and physicians that enhance their knowledge of ethics and their collaboration. Grand rounds, unit-based rounds, and journal clubs are excellent additions to formal educational seminars.

Ethics Rounds.   Ethics rounds are similar to other formal case discussions. However, in ethics rounds the clinical aspects of the case become the backdrop for an organized discussion of the ethical dilemma and possible solutions. Ethics rounds can be multidisciplinary or confined to a homogeneous group such as nurses in the pediatric critical care unit. To be helpful, these rounds must be regularly scheduled and conducted by a skilled leader with knowledge in bioethics. It is helpful if this individual is also a nurse or is a person experienced in working with nurses on

resolving ethical issues so that nursing concerns are raised and discussed. Ethics rounds can be a discussion of retrospective or concurrent cases. They offer an opportunity to consider ethical concerns prospectively, rather than operating from a crisis position. The goal of these rounds is not to make clinical decisions, but to discuss moral problems confronting caregivers.

A commitment to ethical practice will incorporate a variety of these mechanisms, depending on the resources, priorities, and culture of the institution. Awareness of ethical principles and theories, a methodology for ethical analysis, and institutional support are key ingredients to support quality care and the integrity of parents and healthcare providers.

SUMMARY

Ethical reasoning and deliberation are essential for optimal care of critically ill children and their families. Understanding current ethical issues and a process for ethical decision making allows nurses to participate fully as a team member and patient advocate. Creating an ethical practice environment for professional practice and patient care involves establishing an environment in which communication and coordination of care are optimized, the focus is on the best interests of the child, and there are continual efforts to encourage the child's participation in decision making. Providing ongoing education through ethics rounds and participation in ethics committees will immeasurably enhance the ability of the healthcare team to support patients and families, as well as one another, when addressing the ethical issues that arise in pediatric critical care.

REFERENCES

1. Anderson P: *Children's hospital.* New York, 1985, Harper & Row.
2. Jameton A: *Nursing practice: the ethical issues,* Englewood Cliffs, NJ, 1984, Prentice-Hall.
3. Fowler D: Introduction to ethics and ethical theory: A road map to the discipline. In Fowler D, Levine-Ariff J, eds: *Ethics at the bedside: a source book for the critical care nurse.* Philadelphia, 1985, JB Lippincott.
4. Rushton C: Ethics and the child with a chronic condition. In Jackson PL, Vessey JA, eds: *Primary care of the child with a chronic condition.* St Louis, 1996, Mosby.
5. American Nurses Association: *Code for nurses.* Kansas City, Mo, 1976, The Association.
6. Buchanan A, Brock D: *Deciding for others: the ethics of surrogate decision making.* New York, 1989, Cambridge University Press.
7. Arras J: On the care of the imperiled newborn. *The Hastings Center Report* 14:27, 1984.
8. Boyle R: Decisions about treatment for newborns, infants, and children. In Fletcher J, Lombardo P, Marshall M et al, eds: *Introduction to clinical ethics.* Frederick, Md, 1997, University Publishing Group.
9. Fleishman A, Nolan K, Dubler N et al: Caring for gravely ill children. *Pediatrics* 94:433-439, 1994.
10. Mischel M: Uncertainty in illness. *Image J Nurs Sch* 20:225-232, 1988.
11. Miller-Thiel J, Glover J, Beliveau J: Caring for the dying child. *The Hospice Journal* 9:55-72, 1993.
12. Public Law 98-457. The child abuse amendments 42 US Code, 101, interpretative guidelines (45 CFR Part 1 1340.15 et eq.), Washington, DC, 1984, US Government Printing Office.
13. Curtin L: The nurse as advocate: a philosophical foundation for nursing. In Chinn P, ed: *Ethical issues in nursing,* Rockville, Md, 1986, Aspen Systems.
14. Midwest Bioethics Center Children's Rights Task Force: Healthcare treatment decision making guidelines for minors. *Bioethics Forum,* 11:A1-A16, 1995.
15. Rushton C, Glover J: Involving parents in decisions to forego life-sustaining treatments for critically ill infants and children. In Clochesy J et al, eds: *AACN clinical issues in critical care nursing.* Philadelphia, 1990, JB Lippincott.
16. Erickson E: *Childhood and society,* ed 2. New York, 1963, WW Norton.
17. Piaget J: *The language and thought of the child.* New York, 1926, Humanities Press.
18. Bibace R, Walsh M: Development of children's concept of illness. *Pediatrics* 66:912-917, 1980.
19. McCabe MA, Rushton C, Glover J, Murray M, Leikin S: Implications of the Patient Self-Determination Act: Guidelines for involving adolescents in medical decision making. *J Adolesc Health* 19(5):319-324.
20. Levine-Ariff J, Groh D: Creating an ethical environment. Baltimore, 1990, Williams & Wilkins.
21. Holder A: *Legal issues in pediatrics and adolescent medicine,* ed 2. New Haven, Conn, 1985, Yale University Press.
22. California Hospital Association: *California consent manual.* Sacramento, 1990, The Association.
23. Omnibus Reconciliation Act of 1990. Title IV, Section 4206. Congressional Record. October 26, 1990: h12456-h12457.
24. Rushton C, Lynch M: Dealing with advance directives for critically ill adolescents. *Critical Care Nurse* 12:31-37, 1992.

25. Davis A: Clinical nurses' ethical decision making in situations of informed consent, *Adv Nurs Sci* 12:63-69, 1989.

26. Leikin S: A proposal concerning decisions to forego life-sustaining treatment for young people. *J Pediatr* 115:18, 1989.

27. Chester M, Barbarin O: *Childhood cancer and the family: meeting the challenges of stress and support.* New York, 1987, Brunner/Mazel.

28. Nitschke R et al: Therapeutic choices made by patients with end-stage cancer. *J Pediatr* 101:471, 1982.

29. Carse A: The voice of care: implications for bioethical education. *J Med Philos* 16:5-28, 1991.

30. Curley, MAQ: Patient-nurse synergy: optimizing patient outcomes. *Am J Crit Care* 7:64-72, 1998.

31. Duff R: Guidelines on deciding care of critically ill or dying patients. *Pediatrics* 17:64, 1979.

32. Troug R, Cist A, Brackett S, Burns J et al: Practical guidelines for end-of-life care in the ICU. (Under review.)

33. American Academy of Pediatrics Committee on Bioethics: Guidelines for foregoing life-sustaining treatment. *Pediatrics* 3:532-536, 1994.

34. Cheswick M: Withdrawal of life support in babies: deceptive signals. *Arch Dis Child* 65:1096-1097, 1990.

35. Nelson L, Rushton C, Cranford R et al: Forgoing medically provided nutrition & hydration. *Journal of Law, Medicine, & Ethics* 23:33-46, 1995.

36. Coulter D: Is the vegetative state recognizable in infants? *Medical ethics for the physician,* 5:4-5, 10, 1990.

37. Paris J, Fletcher A: Infant Doe regulations and the absolute requirement to use nourishment and fluids for the dying infant, *Law, Medicine & Health Care* 11:210-213, 1983.

38. Frader J: (1986). Foregoing life-sustaining food and water: newborns. In Lynn J, ed: *By no extraordinary means.* Bloomington, Ind, 1986, University Press.

39. American Nurses Association: *Nurses' role in pain management at the end of life.* Washington, DC, 1994, The Association.

40. World Health Organization: *Cancer pain relief and palliative care in children.* Geneva, 1998, World Health Organization.

41. Miser A: Management of pain associated with childhood cancer. In Schecter N, Berde C, Yaster M, eds: *Pain in infants, children and adolescents.* Baltimore, 1993, Wilkins & Wilkins.

42. Wolfe J, Grier H, Klar N et al: Symptoms and suffering at the end of life in children with cancer. *N Engl J Med* 342:326-332, 2000.

43. Goldman A, Feret G, Bartolotta H, Weisman S: Pain in terminal illness. In Schecter N, Berde C, Yaster M, eds: *Pain in infants, children and adolescents.* Baltimore, 1993, Williams & Wilkins.

44. Sulmasy D, Pellegrino E: The rule of double effect: clearing up the double talk. *Arch Intern Med* 155:1250-1254, 1999.

45. American Nurses Association: *Code for nurses with interpretive statements.* Kansas City, Mo, 1985, American Nurses Association.

46. Reicheck W: Euthanasia: a contemporary moral quandary. *Lancet* 2:1321-1323, 1989.

47. Rushton C, Terry P: (1995) Neuromuscular blockade and ventilator withdrawal: ethical controversies. *Am J Crit Care* 4:112-115, 1995.

48. Troug RD, Burns JP, Mitchell C et al: Pharmacologic paralysis and withdrawal of mechanical ventilation at the end of life. *N Engl J Med* 342:508-511, 2000.

49. Mayeroff M: *On caring.* New York, 1971, Harper & Row.

50. President's Commission for the Study of Ethics Problems in Medicine and Biomedical and Behavioral Research: *Deciding to forego life-sustaining treatment.* Washington, DC, 1983, US Government Printing Office.

51. Zander R, Bliton M: Decisions in the NICU: the moral authority of parents. *Children's Health Care* 20:19-25, 1991.

52. King N: Transparency in neonatal intensive care. *Hastings Center Report* 22:18-25, 1992.

53. Rushton C (1994). Ethical decision making: the role of parents. *Capsules and Comments in Pediatric Nursing,* 1:1-10. 1994.

54. Affleck G, Tennen H (1991). The effect of newborn intensive care on parents' psychological well-being. *Children's Health Care* 20:6-14, 1991.

55. Pinch W, Spielman M: Ethical decision making for high risk infants: the parents' perspective. *Nurs Clin North Am* 24:1017-1023, 1989.

56. Able-Boone H, Dokecki P, Smith S: Parent and health care provider communication and decision making in the intensive care nursery. *Children's Health Care* 18:133-141, 1989.

57. Nelson L, Nelson R: Ethics and the provision of futile, harmful or burdensome treatment to children. *Crit Care Med* 20:427-433, 1992.

58. Fost N: Parents as decision makers for children. *Prim Care Clin North Am* 13:285-293, 1986.

59. Taylor C: Medical futility and nursing: *Image J Nurs Sch* 27:1-6, 1995.

60. American Association of Critical-Care Nurses: *The role of the critical care nurse as patient advocate.* Newport Beach, Calif, 1989, Association position statement.

61. Penticuff J: Neonatal intensive care: parent prerogatives, *J Perinatal, Neonatal Nursing* 2:77-86, 1988.

62. Rottman C: Ethics in neonatology: a parent's perspective. Unpublished dissertation. Case Western Reserve University, Michigan, 1985.

63. In re *Quinlan,* 70 N.J. 10, A.2d 647, 1976.

64. Lantos J, Miles M, Cassel ME et al: The Linares affair. *Law, Medicine, and Health Care* 17:308–315, 1989.

65. Rhoden N: Treating Baby Doe: the ethics of uncertainty, *Hastings Center Report* 16:34-42, 1986.

66. Larsen G: Child neglect in the exercise of religious freedom. *Kent Law Review* 32:83, 1954.

67. Rushton C, Scanlon C: A road map for navigating end-of-life care. *MEDSURG Nursing* 7:57-59, 1996.

68. Cassidy R: From principles to practice. In Cassidy R, Fleishman A, eds: *Pediatric ethics—from principles to practice.* London, United Kingdom, 1996, Harwood Academic Publishers.

69. Rushton C, Scanlon C: When values conflict with obligations: safeguards for nurses. *Pediatric Nursing* 21:260-261, 268, 1995.

70. Rushton C, Brooks-Brunn J: Environments that support ethical practice. *New Horizons* 5:20-29, 1997.

71. Joint Commission on Accreditation of Healthcare Organizations (JCAHO): Standards on patient rights and organizational ethics. Oakbrooke Terrace, Ill, 1998, JCAHO.

72. American Society for Bioethics and Humanities (ASHB) Task Force: Core competencies for health care ethics consultation. Glenview, Ill, 1998, ASHB.

III

Phenomena of Concern

Critical care nurses are concerned with tissue perfusion, oxygenation and ventilation, acid-base balance, intracranial dynamics, fluid and electrolyte regulation, nutrition, clinical pharmacology, thermal regulation, host defenses, skin integrity, and comfort in each critically ill infant and child for whom they provide care. These phenomena are the focus of the chapters in this section. Universal care needs, rather than specific primary problems, are examined where nurses play a major role in optimizing patient outcomes through a deliberate proactive process that integrates clinical knowledge and skillful assessment and intervention. Within each phenomenon of concern for critical care nurses, essential embryology, maturational anatomy and physiology, and instrumentation are discussed.

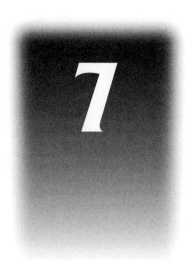

7

Tissue Perfusion

Janet Craig
Janis Bloedel Smith
Lori D. Fineman

Survival of cells, organ systems, and the individual depends on the maintenance of adequate tissue perfusion. The production of energy for the multitude of functions required for homeostasis is dependent on the delivery of sufficient oxygen and nutrients to cells throughout the body. Although cells in the human body vary widely in structure and function, mitochondria in all cells are responsible for the production of energy. In the presence of oxygen, the mitochondria synthesize significant quantities of adenosine triphosphate (ATP) from glucose. ATP forms adenosine diphosphate (ADP), releasing cellular energy in the process. Constant energy is available because ADP can recombine with a phosphate group to form another ATP. Without oxygen (that is, under anaerobic conditions) only a fraction of ATP normally synthesized from glucose is produced. All the processes that require energy can be disrupted if a pathophysiologic process interferes with the delivery of oxygen to cells.

The cardiovascular system is responsible for the delivery of oxygen and nutrients to tissues. Not only does the heart pump continuously to ensure that the billions of cells within the body are adequately perfused, but the cardiovascular system is responsive to demands for more or less blood to tissues.

This chapter provides a foundation for understanding the complex physiology of the cardiovascular system in infants and children. Fetal development of the heart is presented as a basis for understanding the structural abnormalities seen in congenital heart disease. Essential anatomy of the cardiovascular system is reviewed, and the physiology of cardiovascular performance is developed in greater detail, with attention to the maturational changes that are characteristic of infancy and childhood. Assessment of the cardiovascular system is related to the care of infants and children who are seriously ill and require intensive care. Pharmacologic support of cardiovascular function, pacemaker therapy, and mechanical support of circulation are discussed. Cardiovascular dysfunction is detailed in Chapter 18.

ESSENTIAL EMBRYOLOGY

Cardiac embryologic development begins just before the third week of gestation and is normally completed by the seventh week. The cardiovascular system is the first system to function in the embryo; its early development is most likely a response to the high metabolic demands of the rapidly developing fetus.

Development of the Heart

The origin of cardiac tissue is the mesoderm of the embryo. At day 18, during the third gestational week, a crescent, or arch, of mesoderm is formed from a pair of endothelial tubes. The endothelial tubes fuse and grow, establishing a single, straight "heart tube" at about day 20. A rhythmic ebb and flow of blood that precedes heartbeating characterize the primitive heart.

Continued cellular development around the cardiac tube results in the formation of distinct myocardium and endocardium. By day 22, contractile activity of the heart is evident, and forward blood flow is achieved. Between days 24 and 26, heartbeating is evident, as is the regulation of heart rate, vascular tone, and cardiac output through cardiac sympathetic nervous system innervation and action of circulating catecholamines.

Bulbus Cordis.   Because the anterior (arterial) and posterior (venous) ends of the cardiac tube are fixed in place, growth of cardiac tissue occurs in a confined space, causing torsion and flexion of the cardiac tube. At approximately 25 days' gestation, the straight tube has flexed into a loop with the rightward expansion forming the bulboventricular mass—the future right ventricle (Figure 7-1, *A*).

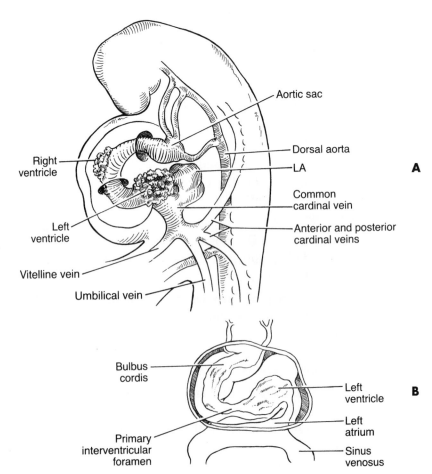

Fig. 7-1   **A** and **B,** Early embryonic heart. Straight tube has looped; ventricle is left and posterior; and bulbus cordis is right and anterior. Definitive right ventricle is noted to bud out of the bulbus cordis. Earliest connection between the primitive (left) ventricle and evolving right ventricle is the primary interventricular foramen (bulboventricular foramen). (From Holbrook PR: *Textbook of pediatric critical care,* Philadelphia, 1993, WB Saunders, p 243.)

Looping to the right is referred to as dextro- or D-looping and results in the right ventricle lying to the right of the primitive left ventricle. (Looping to the left is called levo- or L-looping, which results in ventricular inversion.)

Differentiation of the ventricles begins as continued hyperplasia of the cardiac tube (see Figure 7-1, *B*). Growth of the proximal bulbus cordis gives rise to the right ventricle. The midportion of the bulbus cordis, called the conus cordis, gives rise to the outflow portions of both ventricles. The distal portion of the bulbus cordis, the truncus arteriosus, divides into the aortic and pulmonary roots.

Septation of the Heart. The primitive ventricles are connected by the primary interventricular foramen, which is the only route for blood flow into the developing right ventricle because the atrioventricular (AV) canal is associated only with the left ventricle. As the ventricles enlarge, the muscular septum develops from the floor of the ventricles. The endocardial cushions, which initially appear as heaped up masses of endocardium, develop from the walls of the AV canal. The cushions grow toward each other, eventually fusing in a process that results in the origin of two AV valve orifices, each aligned with one ventricle. The tricuspid and mitral valves evolve from the processes, which divide and align the AV canal. A communication between the two ventricles, referred to as the secondary interventricular foramen, persists until the sixth week of gestation (Figure 7-2). The secondary interventricular foramen closes through contributions from the muscular septum, endocardial cushion tissue, and conus cordis.

The atria are separated by a series of partitions (Figure 7-3). The first to form is the septum primum, which grows toward the endocardial cushions. Communication between the atria persists through the ostium primum. As septum primum joins the AV septal portion of the AV canal, perforations of the septum primum join to give rise to the septum secundum. Growth of the septum secundum leads to the obliteration of any communication between the atria except for the foramen ovale. This flaplike valve is covered

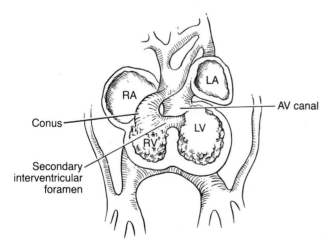

Fig. 7-2 Septation of the ventricles. Two ventricles are well formed and are connected by the secondary interventricular foramen. Outflow region of the heart is defined by the conus. (From Holbrook PR: *Textbook of pediatric critical care*, Philadelphia, 1993, WB Saunders, p 243.)

by a portion of septum primum and permits right-to-left blood flow across the atrial septum throughout gestation.

Conotruncal Development. The truncus arteriosus is the common outlet for blood flow from the heart. Ultimately it separates into an aortic and a pulmonary trunk. Ridges from the bulbus cordis form proximally as truncal ridges form distally. The ridges grow and fuse into the aorticopulmonary septum. Under the influence of streaming blood flow, the common truncus arteriosus spirals and divides into the great arteries around day 34 of gestation. Spiraling results in a right-to-left reversal of the aorta from above the right ventricle to the left ventricle. If the aorticopulmonary septum fails to align with the interventricular septum, a ventricular septal defect results. In addition, unequal partitioning or alignment can result in an undersized aorta or pulmonary artery. Persistence of the truncus arteriosus can also result, if aorticopulmonary septation fails, associated with ventricular septal defect, because the bulbar ridges contribute to ventricular septation as well.

The conus cordis, the midportion of the developing bulbus cordis, is important in right ventricular development, particularly in the development of the right ventricular outflow tract. The distal tissues of the conus also participate in septation of the truncus arteriosus. Development of the midportion of the conus results in the establishment of definitive continuity between the left ventricle and the aorta. The right side of the conus establishes the outflow tract or infundibulum of the right ventricle associated with the pulmonary trunk. If the conus is inverted, transposition of the great arteries results. Double-outlet right ventricle or Taussig-Bing malformation can result when the subaortic conus is not absorbed.

Pulmonary and Systemic Veins. The common pulmonary vein grows from the posterior atrial wall as atrial septation is developing (Figure 7-4). It forms connections with the splanchnic plexus, which is associated with both the developing lungs and the cardinal venous system, which in turn drains into the umbilical vein. Growth and expansion of the common pulmonary vein establishes four drainage channels from the lungs. As the four individual pulmonary veins enlarge, the left atrium enlarges as well, incorporating the pulmonary veins directly into its posterior wall. Connections of the systemic veins into the splanchnic plexus separate as the individual pulmonary veins develop. Subsequently, all pulmonary venous drainage from the splanchnic plexus flows to the left atrium via the pulmonary veins. Persistence of connections between the cardinal venous and pulmonary venous systems results in partial or total anomalous pulmonary venous connection or drainage.

The sinus venosus is the proximal end of the cardiac tube, the inlet chamber of the primitive heart. The right sinus horn ultimately forms the superior vena cava (SVC). The coronary sinus forms from the proximal left sinus horn and the connection of the two sinus horns. Development of the SVC and of pulmonary drainage of the splanchnic plexus results in involution of the left common cardinal vein and the distal portion of the left sinus horn by the end of the sixth week of gestation. The left innominate vein develops from the left common cardinal system. The right common cardinal system may persist as the azygous vein.

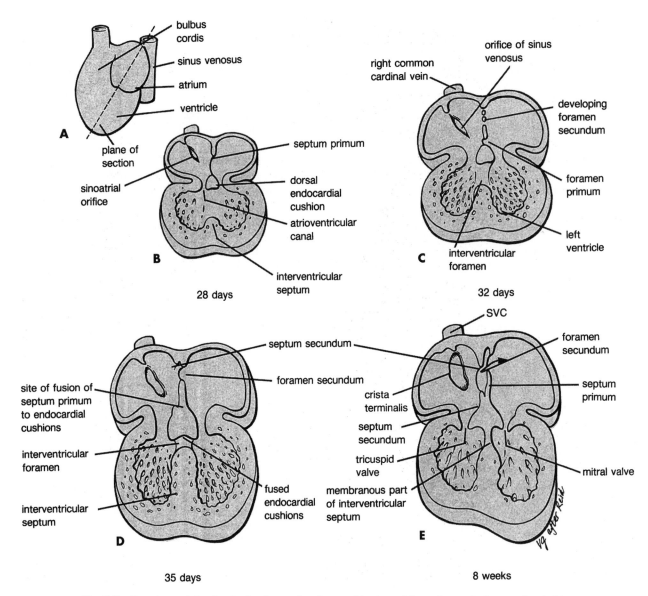

Fig. 7-3 Drawings of the developing heart, showing partitioning of the atrioventricular canal, primitive atrium, and ventricle. **A,** Sketch showing the plane of the coronal sections. **B,** During the fourth week (about 28 days), showing the early appearance of the septum primum, interventricular septum, and dorsal endocardial cushion. **C,** Section of the heart (about 32 days), showing perforations in the dorsal part of the septum. **D,** Section of the heart (about 35 days), showing the foramen secundum. **E,** About 8 weeks, showing the heart after it is partitioned into four chambers. (From Moore KL, Persaud TVN, Shiota K: *Color atlas of clinical embryology,* Philadelphia, 1994, WB Saunders, p 185.)

Atrioventricular Valves. The mitral and tricuspid valves develop primarily from the ventricles, with contributions to the anterior leaflets of both derived from the tissue that surrounds the developing AV valve orifices. Sheets of tissue form along ventricular trabeculations that subsequently create definitive valve leaflets with supporting tendons and muscles. The anterior leaflet of the mitral valve receives an important contribution from the superior endocardial cushion. The tricuspid valve develops almost exclusively from the right ventricle. Mitral valve development is complete before development of the tricuspid valve, which continues to 12 weeks of gestation.

Semilunar Valves. Partitioning of the truncus arteriosus into the aorta and pulmonary trunk has occurred by 33 days of gestation. Paired swellings of truncus cushion tissue form the primitive aortic and pulmonic valves. Blood flow through the valves results in evacuation and migration of the valves through 6 weeks of gestation.

Aortic Arch. Six pairs of aortic arches develop from the truncus arteriosus, giving rise to major arteries and the aortic arch itself. Head and neck arteries develop from the third and fourth pairs of arches. The fourth arch also develops into the aortic isthmus or the definitive aortic arch. The right and left sixth arches form the right and left

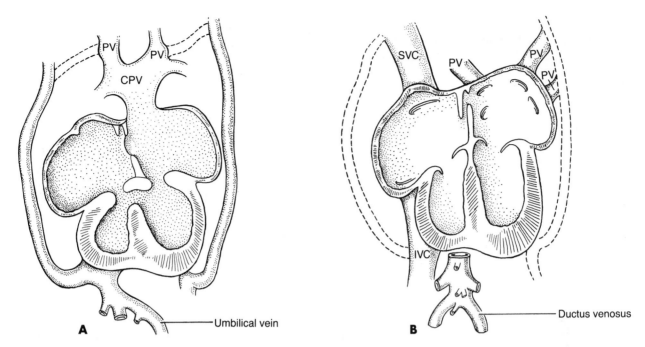

Fig. 7-4 **A,** Development of the common pulmonary vein *(CPV)*. As the individual pulmonary veins *(PV)* are defined, connections to the systemic veins are lost. During this time, ventricular and atrial septation are proceeding. **B,** Connection of the pulmonary veins. The common pulmonary vein becomes incorporated into the back of the left atrium, allowing connection of four individual veins. Septation is complete, and the cardinal system has atrophied. *SVC,* Superior vena cava; *IVC,* inferior vena cava. (From Holbrook PR: *Textbook of pediatric critical care,* Philadelphia, 1993, WB Saunders, p 244.)

pulmonary arteries. The distal portion of the left sixth arch persists as the ductus arteriosus. Incomplete involution of the aortic arch vessels can result in coarctation of the aorta, interrupted aortic arch, and other defects.

Congenital Cardiac Defects

No single classification system adequately organizes congenital cardiac malformations into major etiologic groups. One system divides congenital heart defects (CHDs) into four groups (Box 7-1): (1) anomalies of the three major cardiac segments, (2) defects of cardiac septation, (3) congenital defects of the arterial wall and intracardiac connective tissue, and (4) congenital abnormalities of the endomyocardium.[1] This system remains the most universally accepted.

Defects of Cardiac Segmentation. Van Praagh and Vlad[2] described the heart as consisting of three major segments: the visceroatrial situs, the ventricular loop, and the conotruncus. Variations of the visceroatrial situs include situs solitus (normal location of organs and vessels), situs inversus (mirror image of the normal location of organs and vessels) and heterotaxy (ambiguous location of organs). Heterotaxy infers an abnormal arrangement of body organs (situs ambiguous) with either duplication or absence of normally unilateral organs (spleen), hence the associated asplenia or polysplenia.

Ventricular looping refers to the position of the heart within the thorax. Dextrocardia denotes the heart is in the

right chest. In dextrocardia the heart may be structurally normal, or it may have structural defects. Levocardia denotes the heart is in the left chest. When levocardia occurs with situs inversus, it is almost always associated with complex structural heart disease.[3] Abnormal ventricular looping can also result in CHD such as corrected transposition of the great arteries, which is associated with defects in cardiac septation and abnormalities of the AV valves.

Many of the major cyanotic CHDs are most likely the result of anomalies of the developing conotruncus. Abnormal development of this vital area of the fetal heart may result in tetralogy of Fallot or transposition of the great arteries, the two most common cyanotic heart defects. Abnormal development of the conus almost invariably leads to secondary defects, including defects of the ventricular septum.

Defects of Cardiac Septation. Defects of the atrial septum are among the most common forms of structural heart disease. Most are compatible with multifactorial inheritance. Defects of the ventricular septum are even more common, probably because the ventricular septum closes over a longer period (as compared with other developmental occurrences in the fetal heart), leaving it susceptible to adverse environmental conditions.

The endocardial cushions play a role in both atrial and ventricular septation, as well as in the formation of the AV valves. Defects in their development result in severe CHD, including ostium primum atrial septal defect and complete AV canal defect. Infants with trisomy 21 have about a 40%

Box 7-1

Etiologic Classification of Congenital Heart Diseases

Defects of the Major Cardiac Segments

Dextrocardia
Levocardia with situs inversus
Corrected transposition
Tetralogy of Fallot
Transposition of the great arteries

Defects of Cardiac Septation

Atrial septal defect
Ventricular septal defect
Endocardial cushion defect
Aortic stenosis (valvar and subvalvar)
Pulmonic valve stenosis

Defects of the Arterial Wall and Cardiac Connective Tissue

Persistent ductus arteriosus
Coarctation of the aorta
Interrupted aortic arch
Peripheral pulmonary stenosis
Supravalvar aortic stenosis
Aortic, pulmonary, or mitral insufficiency

Defects of the Endomyocardium

Endocardial fibroelastosis
Glycogen storage disease
Hypertrophic obstructive cardiomyopathy
Cardiac conduction disorders

incidence of CHD; almost all are defects of atrial or ventricular septation and maldevelopment of the endocardial cushions. The precise reason for this association is unknown; the other major autosomal trisomies (15 and 18) also can have endocardial cushion anomalies or ventricular septal defects.

Defects of the Arterial Wall and Intracardiac Connective Tissue. Patency of the ductus arteriosus is likely the result of both prenatal and perinatal influences. Premature infants and those infants with congenital rubella syndrome have a higher incidence of patent ductus arteriosus. Perinatal hypoxia plays a role in persistent patency of the ductus, although the exact mechanism is unclear. An increased incidence of persistent patent ductus arteriosus is found among infants born at high altitude, and the ductus remains patent somewhat longer in infants with cyanotic heart disease than in the normal infant.

Coarctation of the aorta and interrupted aortic arch may be the result of reduced flow across the left ventricular outflow tract. Patients with interrupted aortic arch can also have an associated ventricular septal defect, transposition of the great arteries, or double-outlet right ventricle. These cases reflect complex events during cardiogenesis related to abnormal migration of neural crest cells, which contribute to the development of the aortic arch and the conotruncal region of the heart. Neural crest cells are also important in the development of the thymus. The association of conotruncal abnormalities (interrupted aortic arch, truncus arteriosus) and DiGeorge syndrome (hypoplasia to aplasia of thymus and parathyroids) may be related to neural crest abnormalities.

Coarctation of the aorta may occur as an isolated defect, suggesting that the events contributing to its development occur after development of the heart is complete. Coarctation usually involves a shelf of tissue that extends in the aortic wall around its circumference. The shelf may develop at the orifice of the left subclavian artery or the insertion of the ductus arteriosus.

Congenital rubella syndrome is associated with generalized hypoplasia of the pulmonary artery branches, which results in peripheral pulmonic stenosis. Supravalvular aortic stenosis is often a familial problem.

Abnormalities of intracardiac connective tissue may lead to aortic, pulmonary, or mitral valve insufficiency. Patients with Marfan's syndrome may have myxomatous degeneration of valve leaflets that most often affects the aortic and mitral valves.

Congenital Anomalies of the Myocardium, Endocardium, and Conducting System. Endocardial fibroelastosis (EFE) often is a sequela to perinatal viral infection. Glycogen storage disease is a metabolic disorder in which glycogen infiltrates the myocardium. An abnormal recessive gene results in the characteristic enzymatic abnormality. Prenatal diagnosis is possible. Hypertrophic obstructive cardiomyopathy (HOCM) is a progressive cardiomyopathy usually manifested in early adult life and is associated with left ventricular hypertrophy, left ventricular outflow tract obstruction, and rhythm disturbances. Multiple gene abnormalities have been identified as the cause, and at least 50% of affected individuals acquire this disease through an autosomal dominant trait.[4]

Several disorders of cardiac conduction, including Wolff-Parkinson-White (WPW) syndrome, are reported in families; however, the mode of inheritance of WPW syndrome is unclear. The congenital long QT syndrome is an inherited cardiac ion channel disorder in which five gene defects have been identified as the causative abnormality. This disorder is associated with syncope and torsade de pointes—a polymorphic form of ventricular tachycardia.

Fetal Circulation

Structure and function of the fetal cardiovascular system not only support fetal life and development but also permit nearly instantaneous transition to extrauterine life at birth. During fetal life, the placenta is the source of oxygenated blood, which flows from the placenta via the umbilical vein to the fetal liver (Figure 7-5). Here, flow divides. Some blood flows to the developing liver and abdominal viscera, while most is shunted through the ductus venosus to the fetal inferior vena cava (IVC). The most oxygen-rich blood passes up the IVC, where it preferentially streams across the foramen ovale to the left atrium and left ventricle, the aortic

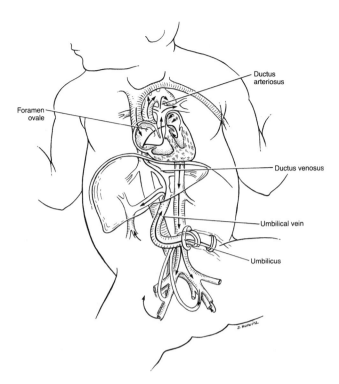

Fig. 7-5 Fetal circulation. Flow from the placenta is directed into the umbilical vein, through the liver via the ductus venosus, and into the right atrium. Streaming, aided by venous valves, carries the oxygenated blood through the foramen ovale to the systemic circulation. Smaller flows proceed through the right heart and ductus arteriosus to the descending aorta. (From Holbrook PR: *Textbook of pediatric critical care,* Philadelphia, 1993, WB Saunders, p 246.)

arch, and the developing heart (via the coronary circulation) and brain.

Blood from the coronary circulation, brain, and upper body of the fetus returns to the fetal heart via the SVC. Flow from the SVC, which has less oxygen than IVC blood, drains into the right ventricle and is ejected into the pulmonary artery. Flow here again divides. The majority flows across the ductus arteriosus to the descending aorta. All but 7% to 8% shunts away from the fetal lungs. SVC blood mixes with a smaller volume of blood descending from the aortic arch, supplies the lower body of the fetus, and returns to the placenta via the umbilical arteries.

Fetal oxygenation is unique. Blood from the placenta is 70% to 80% saturated with oxygen (Po_2, 32 to 35 mmHg). Blood ejected from the left ventricle, perfusing the heart, head, and brain, is 65% to 70% oxygenated (Po_2, 28 to 30 mmHg). Oxygen saturation in the descending aorta is 60% to 65% (Po_2, 20 to 22 mmHg). Blood returning to the placenta in the umbilical arteries is less than 60% saturated (Po_2, 14 to 21 mmHg). Polycythemia and fetal hemoglobin, which has an increased affinity for oxygen, permit compensation for the relative hypoxia of the fetal environment.

The largest volume of flow to the fetal heart is through the IVC. Therefore the hepatic circulation and the ductus venosus are significant regulators of the total venous return and ventricular preload. During periods of fetal stress or

hypoxia, the ductus venosus dilates to preserve delivery of oxygenated blood to the heart. Consequently, less blood flows through the hepatic veins. In addition, a larger percentage of SVC blood flows across the foramen ovale rather than streaming almost exclusively into the right ventricle. Both factors allow more efficient delivery of oxygen and nutrients to vital organs.[5]

Fetal Cardiac Output. During fetal life, mechanisms that are similar to those that function in the mature cardiovascular system regulate cardiac output. However, fetal response to regulatory mechanisms is different. As is true of the infant after birth, the capacity for change of stroke volume is limited. Thus the heart rate response to demands for increased cardiac output is especially important. Similarly, although the relationship between end-diastolic volume and stroke volume holds, the fetal heart, like that of the infant, functions near the top of the Frank-Starling curve. Because of fetal myocardial noncompliance, changes in filling volume often result in little change in cardiac output. Finally, as is also true in the infant, afterload is the primary regulator of cardiac output. When afterload is increased, cardiac output falls because of the limited capacity for increased contractility related to limited numbers of myofibrils and less efficient calcium exchange across the myocardial cell membrane.

Fetal Stress Response. Hypoxia is the major stress to the fetal heart. The mature cardiovascular system responds to hypoxia via neurohormonal and local vascular pathways, which result in tachycardia, vasoconstriction, increased cardiac output, and redistribution of blood flow to the brain and myocardium. However, in the fetus, hypoxia leads to bradycardia rather than tachycardia. Bradycardia results from both vagal action and decreased myocardial oxygenation. In addition, because hypoxia stimulates vasoconstriction in the fetus, afterload is increased, and both right and left ventricular output falls.

Circulatory Changes at Birth

At birth, as the neonate takes a first breath and the umbilical cord is clamped, rapid adaptation to extrauterine life occurs. The establishment of respiration is associated with increased Po_2. In addition, the onset of breathing stimulates synthesis of pulmonary vascular prostacyclin, which is undetectable in fetal life. Both prostacyclin and increased Po_2 have pulmonary vasodilatory effects. Consequently, pulmonary vascular resistance (PVR) falls acutely within 15 minutes, and pulmonary blood flow (PBF) increases. Pulmonary venous return to the left atrium is increased, raising left atrial pressure and forcing closure of the foramen ovale. Only functionally closed, the foramen ovale may open and permit right-to-left blood flow if PVR increases abruptly, as occurs with crying.

The ductus arteriosus, which diverts blood away from the pulmonary circuit during fetal life, may permit a persistent right-to-left shunt for up to 3 days in the normal newborn because of nearly equal pulmonary artery and aortic pressures. More commonly, PVR decreases rapidly, such that mean pulmonary artery pressure decreases from 60 to

30 mmHg during the first 10 hours of life. Right-to-left shunting is normal for about 6 hours after birth. Thereafter, flow across the ductus arteriosus reverses because systemic vascular resistance (SVR) and pressure are greater than that in the pulmonary circuit. Left-to-right shunting persists for an additional 9 hours. At about 15 hours, the ductus demonstrates physiologic (functional) closure. Ductal closure is partially a response to increased Po_2, which induces constriction of the duct. In addition, prostacyclin synthesis, responsible for pulmonary vasodilation, decreases significantly by 5 hours of life. Thrombosis and fibrosis of the ductus, which result in anatomic closure into the ligamentum arteriosum, take several more days and may extend into the first few weeks of life. During this time, the ductus may open and close physiologically.

Intravenous infusion of the potent vasodilator prostaglandin E_1 can reestablish or maintain ductal patency. Conversely, agents such as indomethacin inhibit prostacyclin and stimulate ductal closure.

Cardiac output increases steadily following birth as the right and left ventricles begin functioning in circular series and because of increased left ventricular end-diastolic volume. The increase in left ventricular volume is the result of several factors: decreased PVR and right ventricular afterload and increased PBF with subsequently increased pulmonary venous return to the left ventricle. The drop in PVR over time is exponential. By 6 weeks of age, resistance in the pulmonary circuit falls to levels near the normal adult range.

The normal adaptation of the cardiovascular system that occurs after birth may be delayed in sick newborns. Infants with hypoxemia, hypercarbia and acidosis, hypothermia, sepsis, low gestational age, hematologic abnormalities, and left-to-right cardiac shunting are at risk for delayed adaptation of the cardiovascular system to extrauterine life. Persistence of fetal circulation (i.e., the right-to-left shunt at the ductus arteriosus and foramen ovale) is related to continued elevated PVR.

ESSENTIAL ANATOMY AND PHYSIOLOGY

Structure and function of the cardiovascular system serve to deliver metabolic nutrients to cells and remove the end products of metabolism. The system is composed of the heart, divided into two coordinated pumps (the right ventricle and the left ventricle) and two circulations. The pulmonary circulation is between the right and left sides of the heart, and the systemic circulation is between the left and right sides of the heart.

The interatrial and interventricular septa divide the heart longitudinally. The right and left atria are thin-walled chambers that function primarily as reservoirs for blood returning to the heart. Atrial contraction at the end of ventricular diastole propels a small percentage of the end-diastolic volume into the ventricles. The AV valves separate the atria from the ventricles: the tricuspid valve on the right and the mitral valve on the left. During ventricular diastole, the AV valves are open, and blood flows through each into the relaxed muscular ventricles. During ventricular

systole, the ventricular muscle contracts and propels blood through the semilunar valves (the pulmonary valve on the right and the aortic valve on the left) into the pulmonary artery and the aorta.

Because the pulmonary circulation is short and broad, resistance to flow through it is low. In contrast, the systemic circulation is longer and has higher resistance to flow. Consequently, right heart and pulmonary pressures are low compared with left heart and systemic pressures. However, it is important to note that these characteristics are present in the mature cardiovascular system. The transition from fetal circulation to neonatal circulation includes changes in the resistance and pressure in the pulmonary circulation and the right side of the heart.

Ventricular contraction produces a pressure pulse that propels blood through the arteries. The arteries branch into arterioles and capillaries, which distribute blood to the microcirculation, deliver oxygen and nutrients to tissues, and remove metabolic waste products. The venules and veins coalesce as they return blood to the heart. The arterioles are the primary regulators of vascular resistance. The total cross-sectional area of the circulatory system increases as the arterioles branch, decreasing flow. The veins are capacitance vessels that serve as reservoirs for blood. The veins contain nearly two thirds of the total blood volume at any given time. As they coalesce, the cross-sectional area of circulation decreases, and flow increases as blood returns to the heart.

Blood moves from the arterial to the venous side of the circulation along a pressure gradient. Pressure steadily declines along the circulatory pathway. Mean arterial pressure in children is approximately 60 mmHg; central venous pressure, about 6 mmHg; and right ventricular end-diastolic pressure, 0 to 2 mmHg. The pulmonary system has similar arterial venous pressure differences, although the magnitude of the difference is less (Figure 7-6).

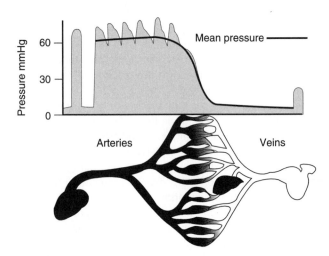

Fig. 7-6 Resistance and resulting loss of pressure within the circulation. Arterial pressure diminishes very rapidly in the small resistance vessels of the circulation. In the venous vessels the pressure gradient is very low. (Redrawn from Kinney MR et al: *AACN's clinical reference for critical care nursing,* ed 4, St Louis, 1998, Mosby.)

The Heart

The heart is located within the thoracic cavity in the mediastinal space, covered by the loosely fitting fibrous pericardium. The pericardium provides the heart with physical protection and a barrier to infection. It limits, somewhat, overdistension of the heart chambers. The pericardium consists of an inner serous layer and an outer fibrous layer. Between the layers is the pericardial space, a potential space that normally contains a small volume of serous fluid that acts as a lubricant during cardiac contraction and relaxation. The heart, suspended by the great vessels, is positioned obliquely so that the right atrium and ventricle are almost fully anterior to the left. Only a small portion of the lateral left ventricle is on the frontal plane of the heart.

Fibrous Skeleton. The cardiac skeleton consists of four interconnecting valve rings and surrounding connective tissues. It forms a rigid support for attachment of the heart valves and for insertion of cardiac muscle and separates the atria from the ventricles.

Cardiac Musculature. The walls of the heart are composed of two layers in the atria and three in the ventricles. Atrial muscle fibers originate in and insert on the fibrous cardiac skeleton. Deep muscle fibers within each atria propel blood through the AV valves with atrial contraction. Superficial muscle fibers pass through both atria and produce lateral constriction of the chambers and coordinated contraction between them.

The walls of the ventricle consist of three layers. The endocardium lines the ventricular chambers and is continuous with the lining of the blood vessels that leave the heart and with the myocardium. The myocardium is the middle layer, and the epicardium is the outermost layer. The muscle fibers of the ventricle arise from the fibrous skeleton and the roots of the aorta and pulmonary artery. The muscle fibers in each ventricle interlock and change orientation as they pass from the epicardium, through the myocardium, and to the endocardium. The interlocking arrangement of the fibers produces both circumferential and longitudinal compression of the ventricular chamber during cardiac contraction, which propels blood into the great arteries.

The Heart Valves. The heart valves provide unidirectional flow of blood through the heart and into the great arteries. The opening and closing motion of the valves is most likely the passive result of pressure changes between the heart chambers and between the ventricles and great arteries. During ventricular systole, the valve leaflets, valve annulus, papillary muscles, chordae tendineae, and atrial wall all function to ensure closure and competency of the AV valves. The valve leaflets begin to close when pressure in the ventricle exceeds atrial pressure. The valve annulus narrows as the ventricular chamber becomes smaller with contraction. Contraction of the papillary muscles exerts tension on the chordae tendineae to prevent eversion of the valve leaflets.

The aortic and pulmonic valves have three cusps, permitting them to open widely with ventricular ejection. During ventricular diastole, the cusps collect the retrograde flow of blood in the great arteries, ensuring complete closure of the valve.

There are no valves where blood enters the heart from the systemic and pulmonary veins. Venous congestion develops when outflow from either atrium is impeded.

The Coronary Circulation. The coronary arteries, which arise in the aortic root just above the aortic valve and traverse the heart's surface in the epicardium, provide the blood supply for the heart. The major epicardial vessels are the right coronary artery and the left main coronary artery, which divides near its origin to form the left anterior descending branch and the circumflex branch. The epicardial coronary arteries give off penetrating branches that perfuse the myocardium. Although the usual origin and course of the coronary arteries are well described, a number of variations are recognized to occur commonly. Figure 7-7 illustrates the usual route of the coronary arteries.

The right coronary artery runs laterally and posteriorly from its origin in the AV sulcus between the right atrium and right ventricle. The acute marginal branches perfuse the right ventricular free wall. The right coronary artery turns downward in the posterior right ventricular epicardium in the posterior interventricular sulcus and becomes the posterior descending coronary artery. The posterior descending artery perfuses the posterior aspect of the interventricular septum and a portion of the posterior left ventricle.

The left main coronary artery is very short and branches into the left anterior descending and the circumflex arteries. The left anterior descending artery runs in the anterior interventricular sulcus in an inferior direction, branching into septal perforates that perfuse most of both the interventricular septum and the conduction system. The diagonal branches perfuse the anterior and lateral walls of the left ventricle. The circumflex artery runs posterior in the AV sulcus and, with its major branches, perfuses the posterior wall of the left ventricle.

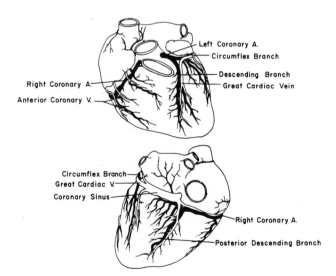

Fig. 7-7 Diagram showing location of major coronary arteries and veins on anterior *(top)* and posterior *(bottom)* surfaces of the heart. (From Little R, Little W: *Physiology of the heart and circulation,* St Louis, 1985, Mosby.)

After passing through the arteries and capillary beds, venous blood from the myocardium drains through the cardiac and coronary veins and the coronary sinus into the right atrium.

The metabolic needs of the myocardium regulate coronary artery blood flow. When cardiac work is increased, generalized coronary artery vasodilation occurs. The precise mediators of the vasodilation have not yet been fully determined; however, carbon dioxide, reduced oxygen tension, lactic acid, hydrogen ions, and other metabolites are suggested. The sympathetic nervous system (SNS) also plays a role in regulating coronary blood flow. Both α- and β-receptors are known to exist in the coronary arteries.

Cardiac contraction affects blood flow through the coronary arteries. Unlike flow in other arteries, coronary blood flow occurs during ventricular diastole rather than during systole. During systole, the muscular contraction compresses the coronary arteries and reduces flow.

Metabolic Needs of the Myocardium. Under normal conditions the heart extracts and consumes 60% to 80% of the oxygen delivered by the coronary arteries, compared with the approximately 25% consumed by skeletal muscle. Consequently, there is little oxygen reserve in coronary venous blood. Increased coronary flow is necessary to meet demands for increased oxygen. During strenuous exercise, coronary blood flow increases 4 to 5 times to meet the energy requirements of the heart.

The oxygen demands of the heart are a function of the ventricular wall tension generated to pump blood, stroke volume, the contractile state of the myocardium, and heart rate. When wall tension is greater, as occurs with ventricular dilation, the heart expends more energy to overcome the tension and decrease its size in contraction. Stroke work is the effort the heart expends to pump blood. The volume of blood ejected with each heartbeat and the pressure the ventricle must develop to eject blood against the resistances to flow determine stroke work. The contractile state of the myocardium refers to the heart's inherent ability to modulate its force of contraction without a change in end-diastolic volume, heart rate, or arterial pressure. Heart rate reflects the frequency with which the heart repeats the energy-consuming process of contraction. A higher heart rate increases oxygen demand.

The Conduction System. A unique rhythmic property of the heart allows it to beat independently of nervous system stimulation. Unlike skeletal muscle, the heart generates and conducts its own electrical impulses (action potentials). The conduction system of the heart is composed of modified myocardial tissue that forms the following:

1. Sinus (sinoatrial [SA]) node
2. Atrial internodal tracts
3. AV node
4. The His (common) bundle
5. Right and left bundle branches
6. Purkinje fibers (Figure 7-8)

These specialized tissues both generate and transmit electrical impulses more rapidly than other cardiac tissue, allowing control of heart rate and rhythm.

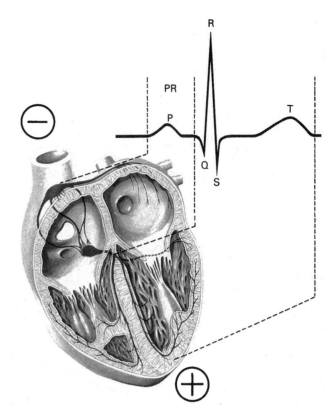

Fig. 7-8 Conduction system and corresponding normal waveforms using lead II. (From Curley MAQ: *Pediatric cardiac dysrhythmias,* Bowie, Md, 1985, Brady Communications, p 43.)

Normally, cells in the SA node initiate an electrical impulse that spreads to other cells via low-resistance pathways in the specialized conduction tissues throughout the atria to the AV node. Transmission of the impulse is slowed through the junctional fibers of the AV node to approximately one twenty-fifth the speed of conduction in other cardiac tissues. The delay in the transmission of electrical impulses at the AV node permits atrial contraction to occur before ventricular contraction begins. The impulse then spreads to the His bundle, bundle branches, Purkinje fibers, and, finally, from cell to cell in the ventricles. Transmission of the action potential in the ventricle is very rapid, allowing for nearly simultaneous excitation of the right and left ventricle and rapid ejection of blood from the heart.

Mechanisms of Contraction. A number of independent cylindrical elements called myofibrils compose cardiac muscle fibers. Each myofibril consists of smaller units that contain thin actin and thick myosin filaments. Each unit is a sarcomere, the functional unit of the contractile system in muscle. The actin and myosin filaments are embedded in the sarcoplasmic reticulum, an intracellular system of longitudinal tubules (T tubules) that conduct action potentials across the myofibrils and lateral sacs, which store calcium for release during muscle contraction.

When cardiac myofibrils are relaxed, regulatory proteins inhibit the active binding sites for myosin on actin. An action potential, propagated along the T tubule, triggers the release of calcium from the lateral sacs of the sarcoplasmic

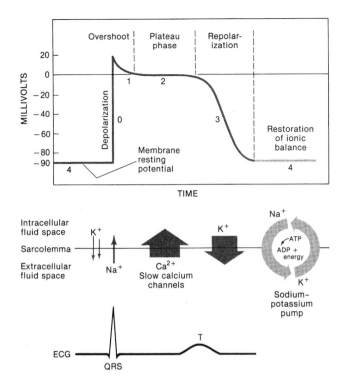

Fig. 7-9 Transmembrane potential in the resting, depolarized, and repolarized states. (Redrawn from Lipman BS, Dunn M, Massie E: *Clinical electrocardiography*, ed 7, St Louis, 1984, Mosby, p 35.)

reticulum and increases calcium diffusion from the interstitial fluid into the cytosol, the area of the actin and myosin filaments. The calcium ions bind with regulatory proteins in the myofibril, exposing the binding sites for myosin on actin. The myosin attaches to the actin, using energy from ATP. The binding, or crossbridging, of actin and myosin pulls the actin fiber past the myosin fiber toward the center of the sarcomere and results in fiber shortening. This process repeats many times during a single contraction, as long as calcium and ATP are available.

During muscle relaxation, calcium influx ceases, and active calcium pumps in the sarcoplasmic reticulum and T tubule remove calcium from the cytosol. The active binding sites on the actin filaments are again inhibited. Calcium is removed by means of the non–energy-dependent sodium-calcium exchange, in which two internal calcium ions are exchanged for one external sodium ion.

The strength and rate of contraction and the rate and degree of relaxation are all determined by intracellular calcium concentration, the rate of calcium exchange, and the resting myofibril length. Each of these factors influences the number of actin and myosin crossbridges that form. At rest, maximal crossbridge formation does not occur, and there is considerable systolic or contractile reserve. When SNS stimulation occurs, however, the amount of calcium that enters the cell and the rate of calcium exchange through energy-dependent channels are both increased. The strength of contraction and the rate of contraction and relaxation are greater. Medications that block calcium exchange channels decrease contractility and slow the rate of contraction and

relaxation. In addition, heart failure or intravascular volume overload with excessive myofibril stretch decreases crossbridge formation. Chronic heart failure results in depletion of endogenous catecholamine stores, which decreases calcium transport, further impairing contractile performance. Digitalis drugs, which block the sodium channels, increase the amount of calcium available and improve contractility. Myocardial ischemia and hypoxemia impair calcium transport out of the cytosol, diminishing ventricular relaxation and decreasing compliance.

The Heart's Electrical Activity

The electrical activity of myocardial cells depends primarily on changes in cell membrane permeability to the cations sodium, potassium, and calcium. Membrane permeability to these and other ions is dependent on the electrochemical gradient of the ions on each side of the membrane and the function of ionic pumps in the cell membrane. Movement of ions across the cell membrane occurs both passively along the electrochemical gradient and via energy-dependent ion pumps in the cell membrane, which actively transport ions against their electrochemical gradient.

Electrical activity or action potential in cardiac cells is divided into five phases, which are illustrated in Figure 7-9 and are summarized as follows:

Phase 0: depolarization, characterized by the rapid upstroke of the action potential
Phase 1: the brief period of repolarization
Phase 2: the plateau, which causes the action potential of cardiac muscle to persist far longer than in other muscle, resulting in a correspondingly increased period of contraction
Phase 3: the period of repolarization
Phase 4: the resting membrane potential

The cardiac cell membrane in a resting state is permeable to potassium and slightly permeable to sodium and calcium. Potassium slowly diffuses out of the intracellular compartment along its electrochemical concentration gradient, leaving the inside of the cell increasingly negative in charge. The resting membrane potential of the cell is −90 mV, which is established by the passive movement of potassium out of the cell and minimal influx of sodium and calcium ions. With electrical excitation of the membrane during phase 0, the cell membrane permeability to sodium increases rapidly as the voltage-regulated fast sodium channels open. There is rapid influx of sodium into the cell, as well as slowing of the efflux of potassium, so the membrane potential rises to +30 mV. In phase 1, the fast sodium channels close abruptly, decreasing membrane permeability to sodium. Slow efflux of potassium continues, bringing the membrane potential to near 0 mV.

Partial depolarization of the cell membrane results in the opening of the slow sodium and calcium channels in phase 2. The influx of calcium and sodium matches the efflux of potassium, and the cell membrane remains depolarized. The influx of calcium stimulates actin and myosin crossbridge formation, and mechanical contraction results. In the

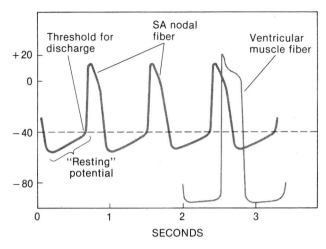

Fig. 7-10   Action potential of SA nodal fiber and ventricular muscle fiber. (Redrawn from Guyton AC: *Textbook of medical physiology,* ed 8, Philadelphia, 1991, WB Saunders, p 112.)

phase 3 repolarization period, the influx of sodium and calcium ceases as the slow channels close and membrane permeability to potassium rises sharply. The efflux of potassium from the cell restores the resting membrane potential at phase 4, which corresponds mechanically with ventricular diastole.

After an action potential there is a period during which the cell membrane is not polarized and cannot accept another electrical stimulus. During phases 0, 1, and 2, the cell is absolutely refractory or completely insensitive to stimulation. As the cell membrane potential is reestablished during phase 3, the cell is relatively refractory; that is, a more intense stimulus is required to initiate an action potential. At the end of phase 3, a supernormal period permits stimulation of an action potential by a weak stimulus. In cardiac muscle, the absolute refractory period is prolonged. Because this period is nearly as long as the heart's contraction, a second contraction cannot be stimulated until the first is over. The length of the absolute refractory period permits the alternating contraction and relaxation of cardiac muscle essential for its pumping action.

Sinus Node Action Potential.   Electrical activity in the sinus node differs from that described earlier (which is characteristic of the cells of the atria, ventricles, interatrial conducting fibers, and Purkinje fibers) in several important ways (Figure 7-10). In the sinus node, the resting membrane potential is −55 to −60 mV. The fast sodium channels are inactive at this membrane charge. During phase 0 of the sinus action potential, the rise is relatively slow because it is the result of opening of the slow calcium and sodium channels. There is no plateau phase (phase 2). Instead, when the slow calcium and sodium channels are inactivated and potassium efflux occurs, repolarization is permitted.

The third difference between the two cardiac action potentials is the spontaneous rise of phase 4 in the action potential of the sinus node. This rise is the basis of automaticity in the pacemaker cells of the heart, which produces an action potential without an outside stimulus such as that

required for skeletal muscle. During phase 4 in pacemaker cells, there is a slow decrease in the efflux of potassium (which limits the negativity of the cell's interior) or an increase in influx of sodium and calcium (which exerts the same effect) or both. Consequently, the cells automatically (or spontaneously) reach the threshold for depolarization and initiate depolarization of the entire heart.

The autonomic nervous system influences the slope of the rise in phase 4 of the pacemaker cells. Epinephrine and norepinephrine, released when the SNS is stimulated, increase the slope of phase 4 to firing threshold by increasing cell membrane permeability to calcium. Sinus node firing is increased. These neurotransmitters act along the entire length of the conduction system, increasing conduction velocity. Contractile cardiac cells are affected, as well.

Conversely, acetylcholine (which is released with parasympathetic nervous system stimulation) causes the resting membrane potential to be more negative and slows the rate of spontaneous depolarization in the SA node and the rate of conduction in the AV node. The increased negativity of the action potential is the result of slowed sodium influx in the face of persistent potassium efflux. Consequently, it takes longer for the cell membrane to reach firing threshold and longer for the electrical stimulus to be conducted through the AV node. Extreme vagal stimulation of the parasympathetic nervous system can produce complete conduction block at the AV node. Carotid massage may evoke such an extreme stimulus.

The action potentials of cardiac cells outside the SA and AV nodes can be converted to those of the specialized conduction nodes under certain abnormal circumstances. For example, myocardial ischemia and electrolyte imbalances predispose to premature ectopic beats and cardiac rhythm disturbances.

The Cardiac Cycle

The cardiac cycle is the relationship between the electrical events, mechanical events, and blood flow that occurs with each heartbeat (Figure 7-11). The electrocardiogram (ECG) records and permits evaluation of the electrical events of the heart. Measurement of atrial, ventricular, and aortic pressure and volume requires cardiac catheterization or echocardiography. However, atrial and arterial pressure can be monitored at the bedside and provide data that can be used in clinical evaluation of critically ill patients. The phonocardiogram records the heart sounds.

The cardiac cycle is divided into two parts: ventricular systole, the period during which the ventricles are contracting and blood is ejected from the heart, and ventricular diastole, the period when the ventricles are relaxed and are filled with blood. Atrial systole occurs late in ventricular diastole. During the cardiac cycle, electrical events precede mechanical events, and the mechanical events produce the heart sounds.

Ventricular Systole.   As a wave of depolarization passes through the ventricle, the ECG records the QRS complex. Mechanical contraction is stimulated and begins in

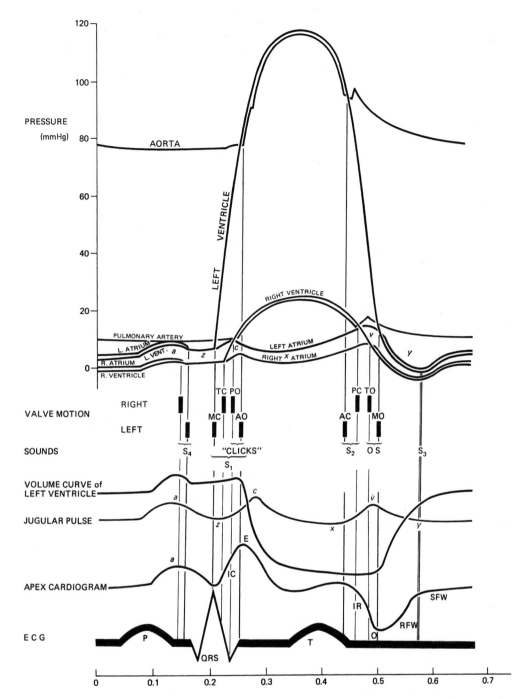

Fig. 7-11 Diagram of the cardiac cycle, showing the pressure curves of the great vessels and cardiac chambers, valvular events and heart sounds, left ventricular volume curve, jugular pulse wave, apex cardiogram (Sanborn piezo crystal), and the electrocardiogram. For illustrative purposes, the time intervals between the valvular events have been modified and the z point has been prolonged. Valve motion: *MC,* mitral component of the first heart sound; *MO,* mitral valve opening; *TC,* tricuspid component of the first heart sound; *TO,* tricuspid valve opening; *AC,* aortic component of the second heart sound; *AO,* aortic valve opening; *PC,* pulmonic valve component of the second heart sound; *PO,* pulmonic valve opening; *OS,* opening snap of atrioventricular valves. Apex cardiogram: *IC,* isovolumic or isovolumetric (isochoric) contraction wave; *IR,* isovolumic or isovolumetric (isochoric) relaxation wave; *O,* opening of mitral valve; *RFW,* rapid-filling wave; *SFW,* slow-filling wave. (From Hurst J et al, eds: *The heart, arteries and veins,* ed 7. Copyright 1978 by McGraw-Hill. Used by permission of McGraw-Hill Book Company.)

the middle of the QRS complex. As the ventricles begin to contract, ventricular pressure exceeds atrial pressure almost immediately, and the AV valves close, producing the first heart sound (S_1). The aortic and pulmonic valves remain closed because pressure in the ventricles is less than pressure in the aorta and pulmonary artery. The ventricles continue to contract, increasing the intraventricular pressure. Because all of the heart valves are closed, no change occurs in ventricular volume during this period—a condition called isovolumetric contraction. Ninety percent of myocardial oxygen consumption occurs during this phase of systole. The ventricle shortens from base to apex and becomes more spherical. The AV valves bulge into the atria, producing the *c* wave on the atrial pressure waveform. Continuing increases in ventricular tension pull the floor of each atrium downward, increasing their size and decreasing their pressure, as evidenced on the atrial waveform as the *x* descent.

When ventricular pressure exceeds pressure in the aorta and pulmonary artery, the semilunar valves open, and blood ejects rapidly from the heart. Ventricular contraction continues during ejection. The myofibrils shorten circumferentially and longitudinally, ventricular wall thickness increases, and chamber size decreases. Peak ejection produces systolic pressure in the aorta and pulmonary artery. More than 50% of the stroke volume is ejected in the first quarter of systole. The atria continue to fill with blood during ventricular systole. The subsequent increase in atrial pressure produces the *v* wave on the atrial pressure waveform.

As each ventricle empties, the volume of blood ejected decreases, and pressure in the ventricular chambers, aorta, and pulmonary artery falls. At the end of systole, intraventricular pressure falls suddenly as the ventricles relax. Retrograde flow in the aorta and pulmonary artery results, catching the cusps of the semilunar valves and closing them. Mechanical closure of the valves produces the second heart sound (S_2) and the dicrotic notch (or incisura) in the arterial pressure waveforms. Arterial pressure continues to decline to the diastolic level as blood runs off toward the periphery.

The ventricle does not empty completely with any contraction. Blood left in the heart at the end of systole is the residual or end-systolic volume (ESV). Stroke volume, the amount of blood ejected per beat, is the difference between end-diastolic volume (EDV) and ESV. The ejection fraction is the measure of the stroke volume as a percentage of the EDV. Normal ejection fraction is 65% to 70%. In the healthy heart, the ESV provides a reserve that can increase stroke volume and cardiac output with more vigorous contraction. In the failing myocardium, the ESV is typically elevated because of the poor contractile performance of the heart.

Ventricular Diastole. After closure of the aortic and pulmonic valves, the heart continues to relax with all the valves closed. Intraventricular volume does not change during this period of isovolumetric relaxation, and ventricular pressure falls below atrial pressure. The AV valves open, and blood that has filled the atria during systole pours into the ventricles, resulting in the *y* descent on the atrial pressure waveform. Ventricular relaxation continues; consequently, ventricular pressure continues to fall despite the

rapid filling of the chambers. A third heart sound (S_3) may be auscultated during the period of rapid ventricular filling if the ventricles are noncompliant or distended. In children an S_3 is not always indicative of a cardiac pathologic condition and can be a normal finding. Slow filling of the ventricle continues through the middle third of the diastolic period. The ventricular chambers do not relax further, but as the AV valves remain open, the ventricles continue to distend with blood that returns to the heart. The ventricular pressure waveform shows an increase in ventricular pressure.

The P wave on the ECG indicates atrial depolarization, which is followed by atrial contraction at end diastole. The final component of the ventricular EDV is delivered to the ventricles, marked by the *a* wave on the atrial pressure waveforms. In the normal, mature individual, atrial contraction contributes up to 20% of the EDV. The contribution is less in pediatric patients, who are less dependent on "atrial kick." However, in patients of any age with ventricular failure or excessively rapid heart rate, which limits the diastolic filling time, the atrial contribution to EDV is more significant. The propulsion of blood into the ventricle with atrial contraction may produce a fourth heart sound (S_4) if ventricular compliance is poor.

Regulation of Cardiac Performance

Cardiac output (CO) measures the efficiency or performance of the heart. CO is the volume of blood ejected from the heart in 1 minute. It is the product of heart rate (HR) and stroke volume (SV), the amount of blood pumped from the heart with each beat:

$$CO = HR \times SV$$

CO varies with body size; it is indexed to reflect that variation by dividing CO by body surface area (BSA). BSA is determined on a nomogram or calculated from the following equation:

$$0.007184 \times \text{weight (kg)} \times \text{height (cm)}$$
Normal cardiac index is 3.5 ± 0.7 L/min/m^2

Cardiac output varies with the physiologic demands of metabolizing tissues. The determinants of CO, HR, and SV are sensitive to a number of physiologic influences. In addition, maturation in growing infants and young children affects both. The sections that follow detail the impact of HR, heart rhythm, and the factors that control SV (i.e., preload, ventricular compliance, afterload, and ventricular contractility) on CO and describe the maturational factors that influence cardiac performance.

Determinants of Cardiac Output

Heart Rate. The expression "children are heart rate dependent" is often heard in pediatric critical care. In fact, HR is one half of the CO equation and is crucial to cardiac performance in all individuals. However, infants and young children are less able to vary SV when demand for CO is increased because myocardial performance in the young is near maximal under basal conditions. As a consequence, SV is less dynamic, and HR influences CO to a greater extent than in mature individuals.

When HR is normal for age, the systolic component of the cardiac cycle occupies about 30% of the time that elapses in the cycle, and the diastolic component occupies about 70%. When HR increases, the systolic component remains constant because ventricular contraction is an efficient process. However, the diastolic period of the cycle becomes progressively shorter. Figure 7-12 illustrates the shortening of the diastolic component of the cardiac cycle with elevation of HR to one and one-half and twice the normal.

The potential pathophysiologic consequences of the shortened diastolic period are twofold. First, the period during which the ventricles fill with blood is shorter. Ultimately, excessively rapid HR will diminish CO because preload is inadequate. Second, myocardial oxygen supply decreases during tachycardia because the coronary arteries fill and perfuse the myocardium during diastole. This decrease in supply occurs in the face of increased demand because a higher HR increases myocardial oxygen consumption. The consequences of prolonged tachyarrhythmias are myocardial failure and inadequate tissue perfusion.

Slow HR easily diminishes CO in infants and young children because SV is relatively fixed. In fact, clinically significant bradycardia necessitates active resuscitation in the infant. Infants are at risk for bradycardia because sympathetic innervation of the SA node and myocardium is incomplete at birth, whereas parasympathetic innervation is complete well before term. Consequently, vagal stimulation can result in bradycardia mediated by parasympathetic stimulation of the SA node, which is inadequately balanced by sympathetic impulses that would increase the HR.

Heart Rhythm. The sequential relationship between the electrical and the mechanical events of the cardiac cycle result from orderly electrical stimulation of the heart, which is followed by mechanical contraction and ejection of blood into the systemic and pulmonary circulations.

Whenever the electrical wave of depolarization that produces the mechanical contraction (excitation-contraction coupling) is disturbed, mechanical performance is influenced. When ventricular ejection occurs early (as with a premature ventricular contraction) or if it occurs without the preceding atrial contraction (as in a junctional rhythm), SV is diminished. Figure 7-13 demonstrates the altered SV as reflected in the arterial pressure waveform as a narrow pulse pressure that is the consequence of abnormal electrical stimulation of ventricular contraction.

Preload. Preload is the distending force or the stretch on myocardial muscle fibers just before electrical stimulation and ventricular contraction. As with skeletal muscle fibers, the force of myocardial muscle contraction is a function of the initial length of the muscle fibers. The well-known Frank-Starling law of the heart was defined at

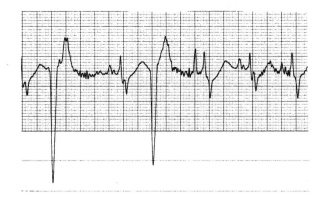

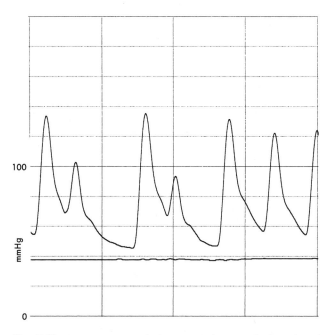

Fig. 7-13 Premature ventricular contractions producing altered stroke volume as reflected in the arterial pressure waveform. (From Daily, EK, Schroeder JS: *Techniques in bedside hemodynamic monitoring,* St Louis, 1989, Mosby.)

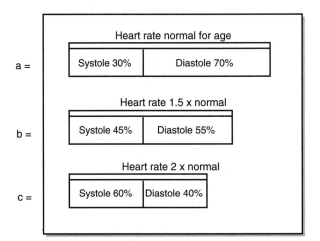

Fig. 7-12 Effect of tachycardia on the diastolic period of the cardiac cycle.

the end of the nineteenth century, when the length-tension relationship was first demonstrated by Frank and confirmed in later work by Starling. The law states that the more the diastolic volume or fiber stretch at end diastole, the greater the force of the next contraction during systole.

Preload determines the force and efficiency of ventricular contraction because it regulates the resting sarcomere's length, determining the number of actin and myosin crossbridges formed during systole. Most alterations in CO in the patient with a normal heart relate to the volume of venous return to the heart. Optimal stretch on the sarcomere facilitates crossbridge formation. The number of crossbridges formed directly relates to the muscular tension generated in the myocardium and therefore to the force of ventricular contraction. Modifications of venous return through volume administration contribute to relatively large changes in CO. Patients with heart failure have higher ventricular EDV and pressure for measured ventricular performance (Figure 7-14). Administration of additional volume in the face of myocardial failure is far less efficacious and may worsen the patient's clinical status.

Venous tone has a significant effect on venous return to the heart and therefore on CO. Vascular tone on the venous side of the circulation is dependent on a number of nervous system and hormonal factors. Venoconstriction results from SNS stimulation, muscular exercise, anxiety, and marked hypotension, as well as from medications, including the cardiac glycosides and sympathomimetic agents. Venous constriction has a profound effect on improving venous return and CO. However, even marked venous constriction does not adversely increase SVR because the venous system is normally highly compliant. Venous dilation can cause pooling of blood in the venous system outside the thorax. Generally, venodilation is the consequence of medications such as nitrates, β-blockers, or calcium channel blockers.

Total blood volume and blood distribution in the intravascular compartment affect ventricular EDV. Acute or massive reduction of the total blood volume causes SV to fall. However, gradual reduction or loss of less than 10% to 15% of the total blood volume does not result in perceptible decreases in CO.

Body position affects blood distribution. Blood pools in the lower extremities in the supine position. Trendelenburg position increases venous return and CO. Military antishock trousers (MAST) and intermittent liver compression improve CO by the same mechanism.

Normal respiration results in negative intrathoracic pressure during inspiration. This negative pressure pulls blood into the intrathoracic cavity, augmenting venous return. In addition, pulmonary artery pressure is lower during inspiration, enhancing PBF and left ventricular EDV. Positive pressure ventilation reverses both these phenomena, especially in combination with positive end-expiratory pressure.

Compliance. Compliance is the ability of the ventricle to relax and distend, that is, to fill, during diastole. The relationship between end-diastolic pressure and EDV defines compliance (Figure 7-15). The normal, mature ventricle is highly compliant, allowing it to accept large increases in EDV without a significant increase in pressure. However, as ventricular EDV increases, additions of more volume result in larger changes in end-diastolic pressure. In addition, if the ventricle is stiffer or less distensible (i.e., compliance is low), the pressure change is greater for any change in intracardiac volume.

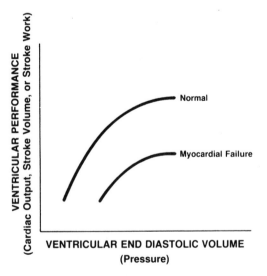

Fig. 7-14 Frank-Starling ventricular performance curves. In the normal ventricle when end-diastolic volume is increased, there is a concomitant increase in ventricular performance until a plateau is reached. Patients with myocardial dysfunction and heart failure demonstrate a shift of this curve downward and to the right. In heart failure, an increase in end-diastolic volume produces less of an increase in ventricular performance, and a "plateau" is reached at a much lower level of ventricular performance. (From Chernow B: *Pharmacologic approach to the critically ill patient,* Baltimore, 1988, Williams & Wilkins, p 347.)

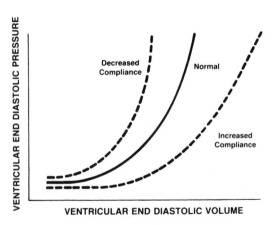

Fig. 7-15 Diastolic pressure-volume relationship of the left ventricle. At low ventricular volumes, substantial changes in volume produce little change in ventricular pressure. At higher ventricular volumes, small changes produce exponentially greater increases in pressure. Increasing ventricular compliance with vasodilator therapy shifts the curve to the right, allowing a greater end-diastolic volume at a lower pressure. (From Chernow B: *Pharmacologic approach to the critically ill patient,* Baltimore, 1988, Williams & Wilkins, p 347.)

At birth, infants have a greater proportion of noncontractile myocardial fibers than contractile elements. Consequently, the ventricle is relatively less compliant than is the case within several months. Reduced diastolic compliance limits diastolic reserve. In clinical practice, volume loading in the very young patient may achieve little improvement in cardiac performance, unless the patient is clearly hypovolemic. Instead, volume administration may produce an acute rise in ventricular end-diastolic pressure, resulting in possible myocardial failure. Ventricular interdependence also affects diastolic filling and subsequent CO. In the scenario of right ventricular volume overload, the ventricular septum will be displaced toward the left ventricle (LV). These phenomena will limit LV filling and obstruct the left ventricular outflow tract, subsequently decreasing LV output.

A number of clinical problems reduce ventricular compliance. Most common are myocardial hypoxemia and acidosis, which may be the consequence of a variety of pathophysiologic processes. Congestive heart failure (CHF), ventricular hypertrophy, and pericardial tamponade can all diminish compliance.

Unavoidable decreases in ventricular compliance are evidenced in patients who require the administration of positive inotropic agents or the application of high levels of positive end-expiratory pressure (PEEP). Conversely, ensuring adequate myocardial oxygenation and normal acid-base balance or administering afterload-reducing agents enhance compliance. Compliance is abnormally high in individuals with dilated cardiomyopathy.

Afterload. Afterload is the amount of resistance or impedance to ventricular ejection. The forces opposing ventricular fiber shortening include ventricular size and shape (the law of Laplace), aortic and pulmonary artery impedance, and systemic and pulmonary vascular resistance. SV is inversely proportional to afterload, whereas ventricular work and oxygen consumption are directly proportional to afterload.

EDV and the radius of the ventricle are the forces that oppose ventricular fiber shortening. When EDV is high, as it is in CHF or volume overload, fiber shortening must overcome a greater intraventricular pressure. The period of isovolumetric contraction is longer, and oxygen consumption is increased. Thus preload contributes to the force of ventricular afterload.

Before ejection of blood from the ventricles can occur, aortic and pulmonary artery impedance (the stiffness of the great arteries) and the inertia of the column of blood in each must be overcome. The more distensible the great arteries, the less the force that must be generated by the ventricles to eject their stroke volumes.

Vascular resistance is the major determinant of afterload and is a measure of the degree of constriction in the arterioles of either the systemic or the pulmonary circulation. SVR varies with tissue metabolic demands, the degree of autonomic nervous system stimulation, and the level of circulating catecholamines. In the mature cardiovascular system, *SVR* is the major determinant of afterload; however, in some pathophysiologic states and with some CHDs,

the *PVR* may be the factor that limits cardiovascular performance.

The pulmonary vascular bed is in a vasoconstricted state in the fetus by a mechanism or mechanisms that remain unknown despite many years of investigation. At birth, both oxygenation and expansion of the lungs are independently effective in decreasing PVR. Recruitment of peripheral arteries, which were closed in fetal life, for PBF, dilation of the normally muscular proximal arteries, and growth of peripheral vessels all contribute to decreased PVR from the first moments through several months of life.

PVR will not fall at birth, and persistent pulmonary artery hypertension will result as the consequence of several problems.[6] Maladaptation of the pulmonary vascular bed results if physiologic maturation has not occurred or the arteries are unresponsive to the mediators that decrease PVR at birth. A perinatal insult such as hypoxia may sustain the vasoconstricted state of the fetus, as does acute or chronic hypoxia in utero. Finally, structural maldevelopment of the pulmonary vascular bed and conditions that result in pulmonary hypoplasia, such as congenital diaphragmatic hernia, may also result in persistent pulmonary hypertension.

Pulmonary hypertension can also be induced by a number of factors.[6] High oxygen concentration used in the treatment of neonatal lung disease is associated with abnormal muscularization of the pulmonary arteries and hypertrophy of the medial layer of the proximal pulmonary arteries.

Heart defects such as ventricular or AV septal defects, which cause a left-to-right shunt as PVR begins to fall in the postnatal period, result in high pulmonary blood flow and pressure. If left unrepaired, subsequent structural changes in the pulmonary vascular bed result. These changes can be progressive and are associated with pulmonary hypertension and decreased reactivity of the pulmonary vascular bed to pulmonary vasodilators (i.e., nitric oxide or oxygen).

Pulmonary embolism, acute respiratory distress syndrome, upper airway obstruction, or chronic lung disease (bronchopulmonary dysplasia, cystic fibrosis) can lead to respiratory insufficiency and hypoxemia.[7] During these acute illnesses, PVR can increase sharply, resulting in right-sided heart failure and hemodynamic instability. Chronic conditions will result in pulmonary hypertension that can take months to years to develop.

If EDV (preload), contractility, and HR are held constant, an acute increase in pulmonary or systemic afterload decreases SV and CO or results in increased myocardial work to maintain SV. With normal cardiac function, the acute increase in afterload decreases SV, which increases ESV and thus the preload for the next cardiac contraction. Contractility increases for subsequent contractions and maintains CO, although at the expense of increased work.

Gradual increases in SVR or PVR, as occurs with chronic systemic or pulmonary hypertension, do not decrease SV or CO acutely (Figure 7-16). An increase in contractility maintains CO, overcoming the increased vascular resistance. However, malignant hypertension leads to heart failure.

When ventricular function is impaired and myocardial contractility is diminished, afterload is the most influential

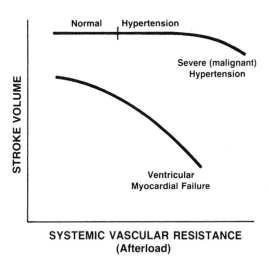

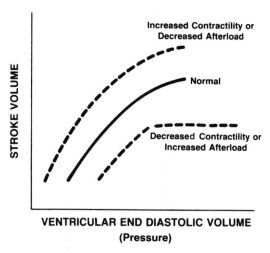

Fig. 7-16   Relationship of systemic vascular resistance to stroke volume in a normal and dysfunctional ventricle. Increases in afterload do not cause a decrease in stroke volume in a normal ventricle *(upper curve)* except at very high levels of afterload when severe hypertension caused ventricular decompensation. In a failing ventricle *(lower curve),* however, an increase in afterload causes a progressive depression of stroke volume and cardiac output. Thus vasodilator-induced reductions in afterload enhance stroke volume in patients with severe ventricular dysfunction. (From Chernow B: *Pharmacologic approach to the critically ill patient,* Baltimore, 1988, Williams & Wilkins, p 348.)

Fig. 7-17   Ventricular function curves demonstrating the effects of changes in contractility or afterload. If afterload is held constant, an increase in contractility of the ventricle will shift the functional curve upward and to the left, demonstrating improved ventricular performance at any given level of end-diastolic volume. If ventricle contractility is left unchanged, a decrease in afterload will produce a similar shift in the ventricular function curve. (From Chernow B: *Pharmacologic approach to the critically ill patient,* Baltimore, 1988, Williams & Wilkins, p 349.)

factor affecting SV and CO. Similarly, infants are exquisitely sensitive to increases in afterload because myocardial immaturity limits the ability of the heart to enhance contractile performance.

Contractility.   The inotropic capacity of the heart refers to the inherent capacity to modulate contractile performance (the rate and force of fiber shortening) independent of fiber length. Increased contractility results in increased CO independent of preload and afterload, although inverse changes in afterload produce very important clinical effects (Figure 7-17). SNS activity, circulating catecholamines, metabolic imbalances, exogenous pharmacologic agents, loss of contractile mass, and maturity influence contractility.

Sympathetic stimulation increases cardiac contractility because of direct release of norepinephrine in cardiac tissue. The adrenal medulla and extracardiac sympathetic ganglia also release catecholamines that circulate in the blood. Circulating catecholamines enhance contractility but do so more slowly than cardiac norepinephrine. However, depletion of the cardiac stores of catecholamine, as is the case with chronic severe CHF, increases the importance of circulating catecholamines. Catecholamines increase the rate of both calcium influx during stimulation and efflux during repolarization, increasing both the force and the rate of contraction and relaxation.

The physiologic milieu of the myocardium influences contractile performance. Hyponatremia slows depolarization and decreases contractility. Hyperkalemia decreases contractility, as does acidosis, hypoxia, and ischemia.

Pharmacologic agents can either augment or depress cardiac contractility. The cardiac glycosides, sympathomimetic agents, caffeine, and theophylline all have positive

inotropic effects. Conversely, β-adrenergic and calcium channel blockers, anesthetic agents, and barbiturates depress cardiac contractility.

Loss of functional cardiac muscle, as occurs with myocardial infarction, results in loss of contractile mass necessary for ventricular contraction. Myocardial infarction, although unusual in infants and children, does occur. This is most often secondary to abnormalities of coronary artery anatomy, Kawasaki disease, or familial hypercholesterolemia.

Relative immaturity is characteristic of the infant heart. Compared with that of the adult, the infant's heart differs in its mechanical properties, autonomic nervous system innervation, and the appearance of its ultrastructure. Myocardial cells in the very young are smaller in diameter and contain fewer contractile elements than later in life. Consequently, the force generated and the degree and velocity of fiber shortening are diminished. In conditions in which resistance to ventricular emptying (afterload) is increased, the functional capacity (systolic reserve) of the immature heart is limited. In addition, the newborn myocardium lacks complete development of sympathetic (adrenergic) innervation, whereas parasympathetic (cholinergic) innervation is complete at birth. Releasable stores of norepinephrine in ventricular myocardium are fewer, also decreasing the inotropic response that increases contractility in the mature heart. The infant heart may be functioning near capacity, limiting its ability to increase contractility.

Regulation of Tissue Perfusion

The volume of blood circulated to the various tissues of the body is dependent on the metabolic needs of each tissue. The cardiovascular system responds to differences among tissues and to changes in metabolic demand. Autoregulation, humoral factors, and the autonomic nervous system permit acute control of the circulation.

Autoregulation of Blood Flow. Factors not yet completely or precisely understood govern the autoregulation of tissue perfusion. Local metabolic needs control blood flow. When metabolic needs in a tissue are increased, vasodilation occurs and blood flow increases. The reverse is the case when metabolic needs are low. Decreased demand results in vasoconstriction and reduced flow.

Increased metabolic activity causes formation of substances including carbon dioxide, lactic acid, hydrogen ions, adenosine, and bradykinin, which are all vasodilators. Tissue hypoxia is responsible for the local release of these substances. Their release stimulates localized vasodilation and increased blood flow. Tissue oxygen deficiency may directly cause vasodilation. Oxygen is necessary to maintain normal vascular tone; thus hypoxia allows vascular smooth muscle to dilate.

Active hyperemia is the term that describes the increase in blood flow to an area at a time of increased demand. When flow to an abruptly obstructed area is reestablished, the surplus blood flow is reactive hyperemia. Reactive hyperemia may continue for minutes to hours after release of the obstruction. Hyperemia in both cases illustrates the relationship between metabolic demand and blood flow.

Changes in vascular tone may result from changes in arterial tone caused by increases or decreases in mean arterial pressure. When mean arterial pressure falls, arteriolar tone decreases and the vessel dilates, allowing increased flow to the area. Autoregulation may well be the result of a combination of all these factors.

Autonomic Nervous System Regulation of Blood Flow. The autonomic nervous system operates both globally and locally to regulate blood flow through sympathetic and parasympathetic functions. Sympathetic innervation of the heart and blood vessels arises from neurons located in the reticular formation of the brainstem. The axons of these neurons descend in the spinal cord. Cell bodies in the paravertebral ganglia and their postganglionic axons transmit impulses from the SNS to the cardiovascular system. The catecholamines released from the sympathetic nerve terminus (norepinephrine) and the adrenal medulla (epinephrine) mediate sympathetic control of cardiovascular function. Thus the catecholamines exert their effects locally at the receptor site and globally as a circulating hormone.[8]

Fibers of the SNS are widely distributed throughout the myocardium, the SA and AV nodes, and both arterial and venous smooth muscle. Their origin in the vasomotor center of the medulla is composed of three major areas: the vasoconstrictor area, the vasodilator area, and the cardioaccelerator area. The primary role of the vasodilator area is to inhibit vasoconstriction.

Stimulation of the cardioaccelerator and vasoconstrictor areas of the vasomotor system elicits SNS response. The results are increased cardiac inotropy and chronotropy, increased venous return by venous vasoconstriction, and increased SVR and blood pressure by generalized arteriolar constriction.

TABLE 7-1 Humoral Regulation of Blood Flow

Vasodilators	Vasoconstrictors
Systemic	**Systemic**
Carbon dioxide	Epinephrine
Lactic acid	Norepinephrine
Hydrogen ions	Angiotensin II
Adenosine	Vasopressin (antidiuretic hormone)
Bradykinin	
Histamine	
Serotonin	
Prostaglandins	
Pulmonary	**Pulmonary**
Nitric oxide	Carbon dioxide
Oxygen	Hypoxia
Prostaglandins	Hydrogen ions

Baroreceptors in the aortic arch, atria, large arteries, and veins stimulate the vasomotor centers of the medulla. Baroreceptors respond to decreased mean pressure or pulse pressure, which decreases their stretch by decreasing their rate of firing. The vasomotor center responds by increasing SNS output and decreasing the output from the parasympathetic nervous system (PNS). CO increases through the Starling mechanism as venoconstriction augments venous return to the heart, increasing EDV. Increased arteriolar tone maintains central blood pressure and diverts flow from the peripheral vascular beds to essential organs. Increased HR and force of contraction maintain CO despite the increase in SVR.

Parasympathetic innervation of the heart originates in the vagal nucleus in the medulla. The cardiac branches of the vagal nerve transmit impulses from the medulla to the heart itself. Parasympathetic stimulation inhibits SA node firing, slows conduction through the AV node, and decreases myocardial contractility. Normally, the PNS is tonically active and has a constraining effect on HR. Strong vagal stimulation can stop impulse formation at the SA node or block impulse transmission at the AV node. PNS effects on the vascular system are negligible.

Humoral Regulation of Blood Flow. The catecholamines and other substances described earlier, which influence local blood flow (carbon dioxide, hydrogen ions, lactic acid, etc.), are humoral factors that regulate blood flow. In addition, other hormones and vasoactive substances regulate blood flow and tissue perfusion (Table 7-1). It is important to note that some biologic modifiers that augment systemic vasodilation can have the reverse effect on the pulmonary vasculature. This circumstance has clear clinical implications in the management of patients with some forms of complex congenital heart disease. For example, acidosis and hypercarbia produce pulmonary vasoconstriction, but they vasodilate the systemic vascular bed.

Angiotensin II is a potent vasoconstricting substance that increases SVR and blood pressure. Decreased renal blood flow results in angiotensin II synthesis via the renin-angiotensin system (Figure 7-18). Decreased renal blood

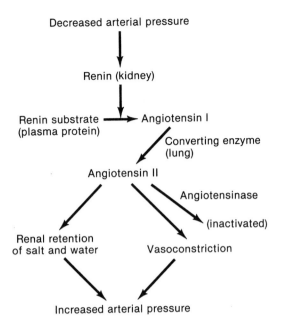

Fig. 7-18 Renin-angiotensin constrictor mechanisms for arterial pressure control. (From Guyton AC: *Textbook of medical physiology,* ed 8, Philadelphia, 1991, WB Saunders.)

flow, an early consequence of inadequate tissue perfusion, stimulates the release of renin from the juxtaglomerular cells of the kidney, where it is produced and stored. Renin acts on angiotensinogen to release angiotensin I, which, in the presence of a converting enzyme in the lung, results in the formation of angiotensin II. Angiotensin II has two major effects on blood flow and pressure. The first is a rapid and generalized arteriolar vasoconstriction; the second is a decrease in sodium and water excretion by the kidney. Water and sodium retention increases the blood volume, thereby increasing blood pressure as well. The renal effects of angiotensin II are not immediate but persist far longer than its vasoconstricting effects.

Vasopressin or antidiuretic hormone (ADH) is an even more potent vasoconstrictor than angiotensin II. However, the posterior pituitary gland releases it in such small quantities that it has little short-term impact on blood flow or blood pressure.

PHYSICAL EXAMINATION OF THE CARDIOVASCULAR SYSTEM

The stress of critical illness can impose significant physiologic demands on the cardiovascular system. In some cases, normal compensatory mechanisms may prevent the clinical recognition of the cardiovascular sequela of critical illness. In other cases, cardiac disease will be clearly evident. In either situation, expertise in pediatric cardiovascular assessment is necessary to ensure the timely recognition of aberrations in cardiac function.

General Health and Appearance

A child's general health and appearance often reflects cardiovascular status. However, any number of pathologic conditions can present with cardiac symptoms. For example, a child with growth retardation, poor appetite, frequent upper respiratory infections, and little energy may have a serious disorder that is not cardiac in etiology. On the other hand, poor weight gain in a child with known heart disease is a sign of concern, requiring intervention.

Accurate assessment of cardiovascular status cannot be established on the basis of general health and appearance alone. Careful review of past medical history and family history, as well as physical examination, may elicit information that leads to further investigation and determination of cardiac disease. Refer to Box 7-2 for review of areas of assessment that are closely related to cardiovascular function.

Vital Signs

Heart Rate. Heart rates in infants and children can be quite variable and are age dependent. Fever, dehydration, CHF, and sepsis can increase HR significantly. Cold, stress, sinus node disease, and heart block can lead to clinically significant bradycardia. A fixed HR, regardless of activity (asleep or awake), is cause for concern because this may represent atrial reentrant tachycardia or atrial flutter.

Blood Pressure. Indirect blood pressure (BP) measurement is best achieved by auscultation or through the use of noninvasive automatic equipment. These two techniques provide measurement of both systolic and diastolic pressures, allowing calculation of pulse pressure and mean arterial pressure. Palpation of the radial pulse while an arm BP cuff is deflated approximates only the systolic pressure.

Although a common maneuver for all nurses to perform, auscultation of BP can be fraught with error. Selection of an appropriately sized BP cuff is of critical importance. The cuff bladder width should be approximately 40% of the circumference of the arm, and when on, the cuff bladder must cover 80% to 100% of the circumference of the arm.[12] A cuff that is too narrow results in a falsely elevated measurement, and a large cuff may yield low measurements.[13]

Ideally, BP is measured in the right upper extremity. Although use of this site may not always be possible, it is preferred because arterial flow to the right arm is derived from the first vessels that branch from the aortic arch. In certain CHDs, such as interrupted aortic arch and coarctation of the aorta, it may be the only pressure that approximates proximal aortic pressure. Measurement of BP in all four extremities is indicated if hypertension is detected in the right arm measurement and in some children with CHD (i.e., those with an anatomic obstruction of the aorta). The systolic pressure in the thigh is equal to arm pressure in infants and young children. After the first year of life, the systolic pressure in the leg is 10 to 20 mmHg higher than the arm. Diastolic pressure in the upper and lower extremities is nearly equal.

Four factors are important in accurate and reproducible auscultation of indirect BP. They are (1) cuff placement, (2) rate of cuff deflation, (3) identification of systolic and diastolic pressure points, and (4) function of the auscultatory equipment.

Box 7-2
General Health Assessment

Physical growth: Height and weight are measured serially and plotted on a standard growth chart. Inadequate cardiac output and chronic cyanosis can impair growth.[18]

Nutritional status: Intake of food, caloric density of formula, dietary iron, and fluid are assessed. Infants should have caloric intake calculated as calories/kg/day. Anemia can contribute to exercise intolerance, limitations in oxygen delivery, hyperdynamic cardiac function, increased cardiac output, and worsening of ventricular outflow tract obstruction.

Activity: Feeding is the exercise of the infant. Therefore feeding difficulties, diaphoresis, or shortness of breath with feeding should be assessed. Squatting after exertion is a classic symptom of tetralogy of Fallot in children who are old enough to walk; however because of early surgical intervention, this phenomenon is rarely observed. School-age children and adolescents should be queried regarding exercise tolerance (both the child and parents should be questioned because perceptions can be quite dichotomous.)[9] Chest pain is a common complaint in children and adolescents; however, if it is associated with exercise, further investigation is required. Chest pain may be related to left ventricular outflow tract obstruction or myocardial ischemia.[10] Estimation of functional limitation

using the New York Heart Association (NYHA) grading system is helpful:
- *Class I:* Patients with heart disease who have no symptoms of any kind. Ordinary physical activity does not cause fatigue, palpitation, dyspnea, or anginal pain.
- *Class II:* Patients who are comfortable at rest but have symptoms with ordinary physical activity.
- *Class III:* Patients who are comfortable at rest but who have symptoms with less than ordinary effort.
- *Class IV:* Patients who have symptoms at rest.

Medications: Information regarding prescription and nonprescription medications should be obtained, as well as drug allergies.

Medical history: Prenatal, birth, and history of significant illness or hospitalizations may prove to be relevant. Frequent respiratory infections may be related to lesions with increased pulmonary blood flow.

Family history: Family history of congenital heart disease, sudden unexpected death in children or young adults, arrhythmias, or genetic diseases should be inquired about. The incidence of congenital heart disease in the general population is about 1%; this increases to 3% to 4% when a first-degree relative is affected.[11]

Cuff Placement. The inflatable bladder within the cuff is to be centered over the artery to be compressed. The measured pressure can be erroneous when the cuff is misplaced.

Deflation Rate. The cuff is to be deflated at a rate of 2 to 3 mmHg per heartbeat or per second. In patients with a slow HR, rapid cuff deflation can result in significant measurement error. The systolic pressure may be underestimated simply because the sounds are not heard at their true pressure reading but at a lower pressure because of rapid cuff deflation. Accurate assessment of diastolic BP is difficult if the cuff is deflated too rapidly.

Systolic and Diastolic Measurement Points. In BP auscultation the measurement points correlate with a series of sounds known as the Korotkoff sounds. Systolic pressure is determined by the onset of the audible tapping sound that occurs with cuff deflation. Measurement of diastolic pressure is more controversial. Previously it was thought that diastolic pressure in children should be recorded when a muffling of the Korotkoff sounds (rather than disappearance) occurred. However, in 1996 the Task Force on High Blood Pressure in Children and Adolescents reanalyzed the normative data on BP in pediatrics. Their findings determined that disappearance of the Korotkoff sound was a reliable measure of diastolic pressure and should now be the uniform designation for diastolic BP.[12]

Oscillometric Blood Pressure Monitoring. Oscillometric BP monitoring is a form of automated indirect BP monitoring often used in the critically ill child. It provides measurement of systolic, diastolic, and mean arterial pressure as long as the extremity is receiving adequate pulsatile flow. Units use two air bladders, one of which occludes

blood flow and the other measures arterial wall oscillations. The cuff deflates in a stepwise manner, measuring the amplitude of pulse oscillations. The first small, rhythmic oscillations correspond with systolic pressure. Maximal oscillations correspond with the mean arterial pressure. Subsequent recurrence of small oscillations generally corresponds with diastolic pressure. Stepwise deflation also allows time for the microprocessor in the unit to reject artifact, enhancing measurement accuracy.

In clinical practice, auscultatory systolic BP has been found to be less than and diastolic BP is greater than corresponding oscillometric measurements.[14] However, systolic BP obtained by auscultation is generally lower than the true physiologic systolic pressure. Generally, good correlation is found between direct and oscillometric measurement of BP in normotensive infants and children.

Reliability and accuracy can be questionable in hypotensive, vasoconstricted, or hemodynamically compromised critically ill children.[15,16] Clinical problems that can interfere with accurate measurement include muscular activity and patient movement. Some children find the tourniquet effect of the cuff uncomfortable. Frequent cuff inflation can contribute to skin breakdown with possible pressure necrosis; therefore frequent skin inspection is necessary. Ideally the cuff is not used on an extremity with an intravenous infusion distal to the cuff because frequent inflations may contribute to extravasation or clotting of the intravenous (IV) tubing.

Respiratory Assessment. The cardiovascular and respiratory systems are closely linked; therefore both must be assessed in the critically ill child. Cardiovascular pathologic conditions may be evidenced by respiratory symptoms, including retractions, increased work of breathing, and nasal flaring.

Physical Assessment

Inspection. Inspection is the first step in any physical examination and can be accomplished without disrupting the child. Initially the child is simply observed, preferably in a relaxed state or while being held by the parent. General appearance, body habitus, and level of comfort are evaluated. Physical abnormalities, such as dysmorphic features, skin color, edema, and chest wall deformities, are noted.

Color. Color is best assessed in natural lighting and at a comfortable temperature. Artificial lighting may create a blue or yellow cast to the skin. Environmental factors (temperature) can produce peripheral vasoconstriction with subsequent peripheral cyanosis, pallor, or mottling. However, vasoconstriction can also occur with low CO. In this situation, tachycardia, tachypnea, and cool extremities, along with other signs of physiologic distress, will be observed.

Color is best assessed in the highly vascularized areas of the head and neck, the earlobes, and the mucous membranes. Visual inspection is an indirect means of judging arterial oxygen saturation. Trends or acute changes alert caregivers to alterations in physical state when based on careful and continuous observation of the critically ill child. Continuous noninvasive pulse oximetry (Spo_2) provides more accurate evaluation of arterial desaturation.

Peripheral cyanosis is often observed in healthy children and is generally caused by environmental influences such as temperature. Central cyanosis is evident when 5 g/dl of hemoglobin is reduced, resulting in blueness of the tongue, mucous membranes, and nail beds. Visible cyanosis is dependent on arterial saturation and total hemoglobin. Therefore cyanosis may not be appreciated in anemic children (although they can be quite hypoxemic), and polycythemic patients can be cyanotic at a higher level of oxygen saturation.[17] Central cyanosis (and associated arterial desaturation) is secondary to intracardiac or intrapulmonary right-to-left shunt.[18] Cyanosis is difficult to detect in deeply pigmented skin. Chronic cyanosis results in other abnormalities, such as clubbing of the digits, dry skin, and polycythemia.

Clubbing. In the presence of chronic hypoxemia, proliferation and engorgement of the capillary bed occur at the base of the nail. This is a soft tissue deformity resulting in the loss of the normal angle between the nail and the nail bed. In severe cases the fingers and toes become broad and round. Clubbing from cyanotic heart disease rarely occurs before 3 months of age. Corrective surgery and removal of the chronic hypoxic stimulus can reverse this deformity.[18,19]

Edema. Generalized edema is rare in children, except in nephrotic syndrome. Periorbital edema and, more rarely, ankle, tibial, and sacral edema are detected in infants and children with CHF.

Visible Pulsations. The jugular veins are inspected for distension and abnormal pulsations. This maneuver is helpful in the child and adolescent, but the short neck of infants makes it difficult to assess the jugular veins.

When the child is supine, the jugular veins are normally distended and visible. When the head is elevated 35 to 45 degrees, the veins should no longer be visible. Neck vein distension indicates either elevated right atrial pressure or right ventricular volume overload. The typically rapid HR of infants and children often prevents visualization of the double pulsation in the jugular veins that are detected in the adult and correspond to the *a* and *v* waves. Carotid pulsations are normally visible in children in the supine position. They too are not visually detectable when the head is elevated. Visible, bounding carotid pulsations may occur with hypertension, hypoxia, anemia, or anxiety.

Chest Inspection. The chest is observed for symmetry, shape, contour, and pulsations. Obvious bulging over the precordium is caused by chronic cardiac enlargement. In young or thin children the apical pulse may be visible as a precordial impulse. This visible pulsation normally corresponds to the point of maximal impulse (PMI) and is usually the apex of the heart. An active precordium can be a normal finding; however, a heave is abnormal. A heave, or thrust, over the precordium will be noted in cardiac lesions that produce volume overload.

Palpation. Precordial palpation is performed to confirm and qualify visible findings and to detect normal and abnormal pulsations and thrills. A thrill indicates a loud murmur (at least grade 4) and is associated with turbulent blood flow. Use the palm of the hand to palpate in the areas outlined on Figure 7-19. Table 7-2 outlines cardiac defects associated with thrills. The PMI is normally located at the fourth left intercostal space in children less than 7 years old

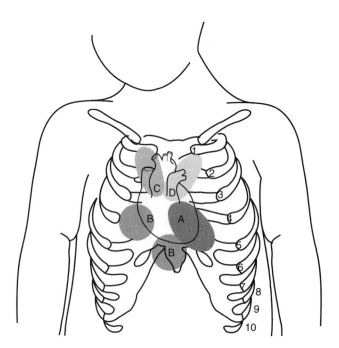

Fig. 7-19 Areas for auscultation and palpation of the heart. *A,* Mitral or apical area, where the first heart sound is loudest and where the third and fourth heart sounds may be heard. *B,* Tricuspid area, where a split in the first heart sound may be heard. *C,* Aortic area where the second heart sound is heard well. *D,* Pulmonic area, where a split in the second heart sound may be heard.

and moves to the fifth left intercostal space medial to the midclavicular line after 7 years. Lateral displacement of the PMI occurs with left ventricular hypertrophy (LVH). Medial displacement occurs with right ventricular hypertrophy.

Moving to the base of the heart, the aortic area is palpated for pulsations, thrills, or heaves. Palpation of the aortic area is enhanced when the patient sits up or leans forward. Pulsations in this area are not normal. A thrill in this area may indicate aortic stenosis.

In the pulmonic area, a single, slight, brief pulsation may be palpated simultaneously in timing with the PMI. This is a normal finding in the child with a thin chest wall, and it may be evident in children with fever or anemia or following exertion. A slow, sustained, forceful pulsation in this area may indicate pulmonary hypertension or mitral stenosis.

Palpation is continued over the parasternal area until the tricuspid or right ventricular area is reached. Pulsation in the tricuspid area may indicate right ventricle (RV) enlargement. A significant heave in this location indicates increased RV pressure or enlargement.

A pericardial friction rub may be palpated as a scratchy or grating sensation over the precordium. Unlike a pleural friction rub, it does not vary with respiration. It is always an abnormal finding. Subcutaneous air may be noted in postoperative patients, indicating a possible air leak.

Abdominal Palpation. Palpation of the abdomen is included in the cardiovascular examination because CHF in infants and young children is associated with hepatomegaly. The liver cannot usually be palpated in adolescents or adults because it is located well above the right costal margin. However, in the infant the liver edge is normally as much as 2 cm below the costal margin. The size of the liver relative to the child's size decreases with age: at age 1 year, the liver edge is palpable 2 cm below the costal margin, and by 4 or 5 years of age, it is located 1 cm below the costal margin. Palpation of a normal liver reveals a sharp edge, in contrast with the blunted edge of the liver distended in patients with CHF. In addition, the distended liver is usually tender. (Note that in abdominal situs inversus, the liver would be on the left.)

The epigastric area is palpated to detect pulsations present in that area. Pulsation of the aorta in children can often easily be detected and is not abnormal. Pulsation of the liver may be detected in the epigastric location, indicating CHF.

Pulses. Central and peripheral pulses are evaluated for their intensity and compared with one another in both timing and intensity. Intensity is graded on a scale from 0 to +4 (Box 7-3). The brachial and femoral pulses should be equal in intensity without pulse delay. Simultaneous palpation of upper and lower extremities pulses helps to evaluate for coarctation of the aorta.

Characteristics of the pulses provide important clinical data. Strong, bounding pulses are found in aortic regurgitation and patent ductus arteriosus. Weak, thready pulses are found in shock, severe aortic stenosis, and cardiac tamponade. Pulsus paradoxus is an exaggeration of the variation of arterial pulsation and BP with respiration. Normally, during inspiration the reduction in systolic BP is only a few millimeters of mercury. If the reduction is greater than 10 mmHg, then pulsus paradoxes exists. These phenomena can be appreciated on palpation of the pulses but are more accurately assessed with BP monitoring. Pulsus paradoxus occurs with pericardial effusion and cardiac tamponade.

Skin Temperature. Skin temperature assists in the assessment of peripheral perfusion. Normally the skin is warm and dry. In the presence of decreased perfusion temperature, demarcation assists in the determination of severity (i.e., cool to the knees, cool to the groin).

Capillary Refill Time. Capillary refill time is determined by compressing the skin on an extremity until it blanches and noting the time it takes to reperfuse the blanched area. Normal capillary refill is less than 3 seconds; prolonged capillary refill is associated with decreased CO.

Percussion. Percussion can be used to estimate heart and liver size and location. Chest radiograph and echocardiogram provide definitive data on cardiac size, shape, and position. Therefore percussion is generally reserved for evaluation of the liver.

Auscultation. The deceleration of blood flow and vibration of the valves produce normal heart sounds. The first heart sound (S_1) is produced by AV valve closure at the beginning of systole. Closure of the semilunar valves produces the second heart sound (S_2) at the beginning of diastole.

◆ TABLE 7-2	Palpable Cardiac Thrill
Defect	**Description of Associated Thrill**
Ductus arteriosus	Palpable throughout the cardiac cycle at the LSB; second and third ICS
Ventricular septal defect	Palpable during systole at the LSB; fourth, fifth, and sixth ICS; may radiate to axillary line
Aortic stenosis	Palpable during systole at RSB; second ICS and suprasternal notch; may radiate to right neck
Pulmonic stenosis	Palpable during systole at the LSB; second ICS; may radiate to left neck

LSB, Left sternal border; *ICS,* intercostal space; *RSB,* right sternal border.

Box 7-3
Pulse Intensity Scale

0 = absent
+1 = weak, easily obliterated
+2 = normal, easily palpated, cannot be obliterated
+3 = full
+4 = full, bounding

Auscultation of the chest requires a systematic approach that should be followed with each patient evaluation. The following is a recommendation; the most important caveat is that the examination is always consistent so that physical findings are not missed. Begin at the apex to best evaluate S_1. Then move the stethoscope to the left lower sternal border and move up the chest to the pulmonic region to best evaluate S_2. Systematically compare murmurs and heart sounds in the right and left sides of the chest, axilla, and posterior chest. Start with the diaphragm of the stethoscope for best auscultation of high-frequency sounds. Repeat the sequence with the bell to best evaluate low-frequency sounds. Refer to Figure 7-19 for areas of auscultation.

Split Heart Sounds. S_1 is usually heard as a single sound. In children, normal splitting of S_1 may be audible over the tricuspid area. It is not uncommon for systolic ejection clicks to be misinterpreted as splitting of S_1.[13]

Normal physiologic splitting of S_2 occurs with inspiration and is easily audible in children. A split S_2 is best heard at the second or third left intercostal space. S_2 is split on inspiration because of increased venous return that occurs during inspiration, resulting in delayed closure of the pulmonary valve. S_2 should become single with expiration. Normally the aortic valve (A_2) closes just before the pulmonary valve (P_2).[13,20]

Careful attention should be paid to physiologic splitting of the second heart sound because this can be quite diagnostic. If the second heart sound never becomes single with expiration (a "fixed" split), is always single (often difficult to determine in infants) or is wider on exhalation than on inspiration (a "paradoxical" split), the finding is considered pathologic and warrants further evaluation.[18] For example, a fixed split of S_2 occurs with atrial septal defect (ASD) and right bundle branch block (both of these phenomena delay pulmonary valve closure). A single S_2 is associated with pulmonary hypertension, pulmonary or aortic atresia, and dextro-transposition of the great arteries (D-TGA). Paradoxical splitting may occur when LV contraction is delayed because of a left bundle branch block, and the aortic valve closes after the pulmonic valve during exhalation.

Accentuated Heart Sounds. Each component of the second heart sound is also assessed for its intensity. An accentuated pulmonic (P_2) component of S_2 is a marker of pulmonary hypertension. P_2 may also be accentuated in heart failure and with an ASD. A_2 is accentuated with systemic hypertension. The aortic component of S_2 may be diminished when arterial pressure is low, as in hypovolemia or shock.

Extra Heart Sounds. Extra heart sounds include ejection clicks, S_3, and S_4. Ejection clicks can be heard in early, middle, or late systole and are associated with abnormalities of the cardiac valves. These crisp sounds are well localized to the valve areas. Pulmonic and aortic ejection clicks are heard in early systole just after S_1. A pulmonary ejection click may diminish in intensity during inspiration and is associated with pulmonary stenosis. An aortic ejection click does not vary with respiration and is associated with aortic valve stenosis or bicuspid aortic valve. Mitral valve prolapse produces a midsystolic click.

This is not an uncommon finding in the general population, and, although not a critical care problem, it may be detected in adolescents in the pediatric intensive care unit (PICU).

A third heart sound (S_3) occurs in early diastole during rapid filling of the ventricles. S_3 is a low-frequency sound best heard at the apex early in diastole, just after S_2. S_3 sounds like "ken-TUC-ky" and may be heard in normal children. A loud S_3 can occur as a result of resistance in ventricular filling from volume overload or decreased compliance and is sometimes referred to as a gallop rhythm. It is audible in mitral regurgitation, left-to-right shunts, CHF, and anemia.[21]

A fourth heart sound (S_4) is produced by atrial contraction, indicates altered ventricular compliance, and is almost never heard in normal children.[18,21] Like S_3, S_4 is a low-frequency sound best heard at the apex. S_4 is distinguished from S_3 by its timing in the cardiac cycle, occurring just before S_1. S_4 is often associated with systemic hypertension, hypertrophic cardiomyopathy, or CHF.

Summation gallop is noted when S_3 and S_4 occur simultaneously, producing a single sound. This heart sound is a pathologic finding associated with heart failure.

A pericardial friction rub is a transient scratching, grating, or squeaking sound that is high pitch. Indicative of pericarditis or postpericardiotomy syndrome, it is best heard between the apex of the heart and the left sternal border.

Cardiac Murmurs. Murmurs are the result of abnormal turbulent blood flow across septal defects, abnormal valves, or abnormal great vessels. The location and quality of the murmur are dependent on the defect that produces the abnormal blood flow. Murmurs are described in terms of timing, intensity, location, pitch, and quality.

The timing of a murmur is related to the cardiac cycle. Systolic murmurs occur between S_1 and S_2, during ventricular systole. They are best described as early, mid, or late systolic murmurs. Holosystolic murmurs are heard throughout systole. Diastolic murmurs occur after S_2 (early, mid, late), during ventricular diastole. Continuous murmurs occur throughout the cardiac cycle. Holosystolic and diastolic murmurs are never innocent.

The intensity of murmurs is graded on a scale from I to VI and is described in Table 7-3. Assigning a specific intensity to a murmur is subject to individual interpreta-

◆ TABLE 7-3   Intensity of Cardiac Murmurs

Grade	Description
I	Faintest murmur audible; often undiscovered initially
II	Faint, but heard without difficulty
III	Soft, but louder than II
IV	Loud, but not as loud as V; associated with a palpable thrill
V	Loud, still audible when stethoscope is lifted partially off the chest; associated with a palpable thrill
VI	Loudest murmur; remains audible when stethoscope is lifted away from the chest

tion, and discrepancies between examiners may exist. When the same examiner assesses a child with a murmur, trends and changes are appreciated in a timely manner.

Location is described as to where the murmur is best audible (left lower sternal border, midscapula, etc.) or according to the traditional landmarks, as illustrated in Figure 7-19. Pitch of heart murmurs is described as high, medium, or low. High-frequency (pitch) murmurs are best heard with the diaphragm of a stethoscope; low-frequency murmurs are best heard with the bell. The quality of the murmur is described with terms, including harsh, musical, blowing, or rumbling.

Heart murmurs that are produced by structural cardiac defects are called organic murmurs. Up to 50% of children have innocent murmurs, without structural or functional heart disease. Innocent murmurs are generally soft (grade I or II/VI), systolic, and of short duration, often with a characteristic vibratory quality. Children with innocent murmurs have no other symptoms and generally demonstrate normal growth. This diagnosis is usually made on physical examination without ancillary testing.[22]

NONINVASIVE EVALUATION AND DIAGNOSIS

Many noninvasive diagnostic tests are routinely used to evaluate infants and children with a potential for cardiac dysfunction. These tests include cardiac rhythm monitoring, radiographic evaluation of the heart, and echocardiography.

Monitoring and Evaluating Cardiac Rhythm

Patients at risk for the development of cardiac arrhythmias require careful monitoring, accurate diagnosis of the rhythm, and assessment of potential or real hemodynamic consequences. Primary cardiac arrhythmias, like primary cardiac arrest, are unusual among infants and children. Infants and children at risk for cardiac rhythm disturbance are those with congenital or acquired heart disease (particularly following cardiac surgical procedures), severe electrolyte imbalance, ingestion of a toxic substance, congenital complete heart block, and vagal sensitivity.

The clinical significance of an arrhythmia is determined by its affect on hemodynamics, CO, and the potential for degeneration to a lethal rhythm. Relative to adults, rhythm

abnormalities in children can degenerate quickly and have serious sequelae. Figure 7-20 illustrates the rapid (6-second) deterioration of supraventricular tachycardia (SVT) to ventricular tachycardia (VT) and ventricular fibrillation (VF) in a 9-month-old with viral myocarditis. Infants and small children do not tolerate persistent bradyarrhythmias and tachyarrhythmias; alterations in diastolic filling and decreased CO associated with rhythm disorders occur in the setting of a limited ability to adjust SV.

Accurate assessment of cardiac rhythm disturbances requires practice and understanding of four general principles. First, a systematic approach to ECG analysis must be adopted and applied consistently so that nothing is overlooked. Second, changes that are observed are followed for trends and clinical significance. Third, observed changes are compared with age-dependent normal values (Table 7-4). Finally, the rhythm disturbance is considered in terms of the patient's clinical situation (i.e., acid-base or electrolyte status, presence of structural defects, postoperative open-heart surgery). Of importance to note is that a child with heart disease can have a normal ECG, and conversely, a child without heart disease can have an abnormal ECG.

Monitoring Leads. Most PICUs use bedside cardiac monitors with three lead wires designated *RA* for right arm, *LA* for left arm, and *LL* for left leg. These bipolar leads monitor the leads I, II, and III via a positive, a negative, and a ground electrode. MCL_1 (modified chest lead) can also be monitored via three bipolar electrodes. The MCL_1 lead is more valuable than lead II in evaluating abnormal ventricular conduction. Figure 7-21, *A* and *B,* compares the position of the positive and negative electrodes in lead II and MCL_1.

Newer monitors provide multiple-lead monitoring (Figure 7-22) that allow real-time recording of both the bipolar leads (I, II, III, aV_F, aV_R, aV_L) and a chest lead (V), allowing full disclosure of cardiac rhythm. Depending on monitor configuration, one or more leads can be displayed, as well as a seven-lead ECG. Multiple-lead monitoring is particularly helpful in patients with structural or functional heart disease because these patients are prone to arrhythmias that can be difficult to identify with lead II alone (i.e., atrial ectopic tachycardia, junctional ectopic tachycardia, atrial flutter). In addition, analysis of multiple leads is helpful in differentiating SVT with aberrant conduction from VT. Lead selection is based on which lead gives the cleanest electrogram, as well as the patient's

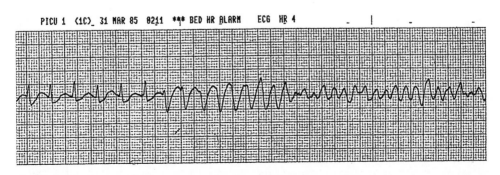

Fig. 7-20 Rapid (6-second) deterioration of supraventricular tachycardia (SVT) to ventricular tachycardia (VT) and ventricular fibrillation (VF) in a 9-month-old with viral myocarditis. (Courtesy MAQ Curley.)

TABLE 7-4   Normal Values in Pediatric Cardiac Rhythm Assessment

Age Group	Heart Rate (beats/min)*	Frontal Plane QRS Vector (degrees)	PR Interval (sec)	QRS Duration V5	Q III (mm)‡‡	Q V6 (mm)‡	RV1 (mm)	SV1 (mm)	R/SV1	RV6 (mm)	SV6 (mm)	R/SV6	SV1 + RV6 (mm)†	R + S V4 (mm)†
Less than 1 day	93-154 (123)	+59 to −163 (137)	0.08-0.16 (.11)	0.03-0.07 (.05)	4.5	2	5-26 (14)	0-23 (8)	.1-U (2.2)	0-11 (4)	0-9.5 (3)	.1-U (2.0)	28	52.5
1 to 2 days	91-159 (123)	+64 to −161 (134)	0.08-0.14 (.11)	0.03-0.07 (.05)	6.5	2.5	5-27 (14)	0-21 (9)	.1-U (2.0)	0-12 (4.5)	0-9.5 (3)	.1-U (2.5)	29	52
3 to 6 days	91-166 (129)	+77 to −163 (132)	0.07-0.14 (.10)	0.03-0.07 (.05)	5.5	3	3-24 (13)	0-17 (7)	.2-U (2.7)	.5-12 (5)	0-10 (3.5)	.1-U (2.2)	24.5	49
1 to 3 wk	107-182 (148)	+65 to +161 (110)	0.07-0.14 (.10)	0.03-0.08 (.05)	6	3	3-21 (11)	0-11 (4)	1.0-U (2.9)	2.5-16.5 (7.5)	0-10 (3.5)	.1-U (3.3)	21	49
1 to 2 mo	121-179 (149)	+31 to +113 (74)	0.07-0.13 (.10)	0.03-0.08 (.05)	7.5	3	3-18 (10)	0-12 (5)	.3-U (2.3)	5-21.5 (11.5)	0-6.5 (3)	.2-U (4.8)	29	53.5
3 to 5 mo	106-186 (141)	+7 to +104 (60)	0.07-0.15 (.11)	0.03-0.08 (.05)	6.5	3	3-20 (10)	0-17 (6)	.1-U (2.3)	6.5-22.5 (13)	0-10 (3)	.2-U (6.2)	35	61.5
6 to 11 mo	109-169 (134)	+6 to +99 (56)	0.07-0.16 (.11)	0.03-0.08 (.05)	8.5	3	1.5-20 (9.5)	.5-18 (4)	.1-3.9 (1.6)	6-22.5 (12.5)	0-7 (2)	.2-U (7.6)	32	53
1 to 2 yr	89-151 (119)	+7 to +101 (55)	0.08-0.15 (.11)	0.04-0.08 (.06)	6	3	2.5-17 (9)	.5-21 (8)	.05-4.3 (1.4)	6-22.5 (13)	0-6.5 (2)	.3-U (9.3)	39	49.5
3 to 4 yr	73-137 (108)	+6 to +104 (55)	0.09-0.16 (.12)	0.04-0.08 (.06)	5	3.5	1-18 (8)	.2-21 (10)	.03-2.8 (.9)	8-24.5 (15)	0-5 (1.5)	.6-U (10.8)	42	53.5
5 to 7 yr	65-133 (100)	+11 to +143 (65)	0.09-0.16 (.12)	0.04-0.08 (.06)	4	4.5	.5-14 (7)	.3-24 (12)	.02-2.0 (.7)	8.5-26.5 (16)	0-4 (1)	.9-U (11.5)	47	54
8 to 11 yr	62-130 (91)	+9 to +114 (61)	0.09-0.17 (.13)	0.04-0.09 (.06)	3	3	0-12 (5.5)	.3-25 (12)	0-1.8 (.5)	9-25.5 (16)	0-4 (1)	1.5-U (14.3)	45.5	53
12 to 15 yr	60-119 (85)	+11 to +130 (59)	0.09-0.18 (.14)	0.04-0.09 (.07)	3	.3	0-10 (4)	.3-21 (11)	0-1.7 (.5)	6.5-23 (14)	0-4 (1)	1.4-U (14.7)	41	50

From Garson A: Electrocardiography. In Garson A, Bricker JT, Fisher DJ et al, eds: *The science and practice of pediatric cardiology*, Philadelphia, 1998, Williams & Wilkins.
*2% to 98% (mean).
†Ninety-eighth percentile.
‡Millimeters at normal standardization.
U, Undefined.

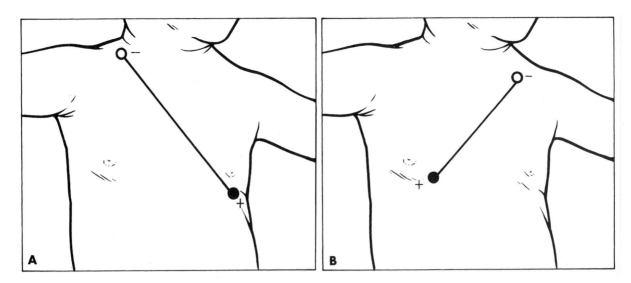

Fig. 7-21 **A,** Placement of the positive and negative electrodes for lead II monitoring. **B,** Electrode placement for MCL₁. (From Curley MAQ: *Pediatric cardiac dysrhythmias,* p 33, Bowie, Md. Copyright 1985 by Brady Communications Company.)

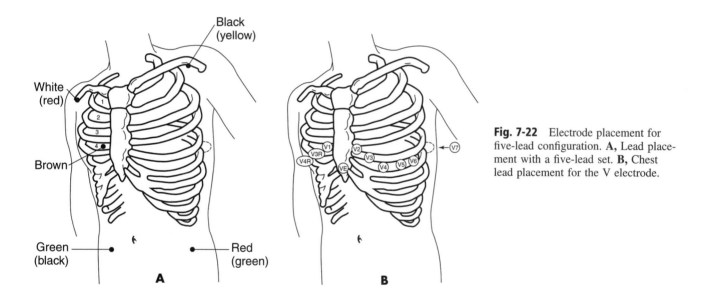

Fig. 7-22 Electrode placement for five-lead configuration. **A,** Lead placement with a five-lead set. **B,** Chest lead placement for the V electrode.

rhythm abnormality. Simultaneous monitoring of leads I, II, and aV$_F$ allow for evaluation of P wave axis and morphology, thus providing timely recognition of atrial arrhythmias. V$_1$ is used for the determination of right bundle branch block, and V$_6$ is used for the determination of left bundle branch block.[23,24]

Electrode Placement. Regardless of the lead that is monitored, accurate positioning of the electrodes in their precise anatomic locations improves the accuracy of the cardiac rhythm tracing. The exception to this principle is the placement of limb electrodes in the 12-lead ECG, which may be placed anywhere on the extremity. Moving a chest electrode a short distance from its designated location can alter the appearance of the cardiac rhythm tracing dramatically. The RA and LA electrodes should be placed at the respective shoulder and the LL electrode placed on the left lower torso. Often, surgical incisions, dressings, transthoracic intracardiac lines, or chest tubes preclude the accurate placement of chest leads. Therefore monitoring of the anterior chest leads may have to be forgone rather than placing the leads in an inappropriate position that could alter waveform configuration.

Cardiac Rhythm Assessment. Ten factors are systematically assessed when evaluating cardiac rhythm. Applying this approach permits accurate detection and diagnosis of rhythm disturbances.

The first parameter to evaluate is HR. Metabolic demands, age, and clinical status determine HR. There is a gradual increase in average HR during the first month of life, followed by an even more gradual decrease across childhood and adolescence. Table 7-4 gives the normal age-dependent ranges for HR.

Sinus bradycardia is a HR that is lower than normal, and sinus tachycardia is a rate that is faster than normal. They are evaluated relative to the child's level of activity and clinical status. For example, a sinus tachycardia of 200 beats/min is not an unexpected or abnormal finding in a stressed, febrile, anemic infant. Conversely, a sinus bradycardia of 90 beats/min can also be observed in a sleeping infant. Most often, clinically significant bradycardia is the result of hypoxia, acidosis, or vagal stimulation.

Faster inherent rates are present in all of the potential pacemaker cells located throughout the myocardium. As a consequence, infants and children have faster escape rhythms than those seen in adults. Therefore accurately diagnosing an ectopic rhythm on the basis of HR alone is not possible. When rapid heart rhythms are detected, the first element in accurate interpretation of the rhythm is consideration of the patient's history and current clinical situation. For example, sinus tachycardia (ST) is most often associated with fever, anemia, or hypovolemia. Infants with SVT can present with a several-day history of poor feeding, lethargy, and CHF.[25] Incisional atrial reentrant tachycardia (IART), historically known as atrial flutter, generally presents in patients after atrial surgery (i.e., Fontan, Mustard, and Senning procedures). VT is most often seen in patients with history of severe metabolic or electrolyte imbalance, toxic ingestion, cardiomyopathy, or cardiac surgery.[26]

Sinus tachycardia is a secondary rhythm disturbance that reflects the need for more CO in patients with increased metabolic demands. Tachycardias such as SVT, AF (atrial flutter), and VT, can produce signs of cardiac dysfunction. Inadequate tissue perfusion, if present, is the consequence of the rhythm disturbance, not the result of increased metabolic demands.

Mechanism of onset is an important factor in the diagnosis of tachycardia. ST is characterized by a gradual acceleration of the HR. SVT and AF are tachyarrhythmias with abrupt onset to rates of 230 to 320 beats/min. These are most often the result of a reentry mechanism.

Two distinct pathways form a reentry mechanism (Figure 7-23) with unidirectional block in one limb. After a premature contraction the electrical impulse is blocked in the first limb of the circuit but is conducted antegrade (forward) through the second limb. The impulse then can "reenter" the first limb and be conducted retrograde, or in the other direction, with subsequent antegrade propagation down the first limb. As a result of perfect reciprocal timing of both limbs of the circuit, perpetuation of very rapid heart rates occurs. Pacing terminates reentrant rhythms.[27] AV node block with adenosine terminates most SVT because the AV node serves as one limb of the reentrant circuit.

The second parameter for evaluation of a rhythm strip is the regularity of the rhythm, as well as the presence of grouped beats. Sinus rhythm is fairly regular, but some variability is normal because of changes in vagal tone. Sinus arrhythmia is common in children and reflects normal HR variation with respiration. HR will increase with inspiration and decrease with expiration.

SVT and AF are regular rhythms that generally do not vary with patient activity or sleep. These phenomena can be

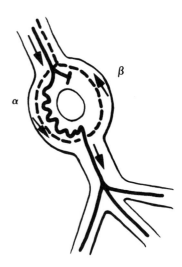

Fig. 7-23 Reentry circuit. (From Holbrook PR: *Textbook of pediatric critical care,* Philadelphia, 1993, WB Saunders, p 386.)

easily identified using the trend recordings of HR available on some cardiac monitors. Group beating (i.e., clustering of QRS complexes identified by examination of a long rhythm strip) can be observed with sinus arrhythmia and type I and type II second-degree heart block.

The third parameter to assess is the P wave. The P wave is evaluated for amplitude (height), duration, and morphology. P wave size and duration correspond to the relative size of the atria. Normally P wave amplitude is no greater than 3 mm, and maximal P wave duration is 0.10 seconds in children over 1 year old (0.08 seconds in infants less than 1 year old).[23] Tall P waves may indicate right atrial enlargement, and wide P waves may indicate left atrial enlargement. Bilateral atrial enlargement is indicated by P waves that are both wide and tall.[24] Figure 7-24, *A,* illustrates altered P wave morphology reflective of right and left atrial enlargement.

P waves should be upright and consistent in appearance in lead II. If they are not, an ectopic rhythm is suspected. "Flutter" waves replace normal P waves during AF (Figure 7-24, *B*). However, this can be easily missed in patients who have low-amplitude P waves after extensive atrial surgery. With premature atrial contractions, low atrial rhythm, or atrial ectopic tachycardia, P wave morphology or axis will be different from the P wave in sinus rhythm.[27,28] This can be manifest as a negative P wave in aV_F, lead I, or lead II. In junctional rhythms, the P waves are dissociated, absent, or inverted after the QRS complex (Figure 7-24, *C*).[29]

The fourth parameter for evaluation is the PR interval. The length of the PR interval varies both with age and HR. (See Table 7-4 for age-dependent norms.) First-degree heart block is defined as a PR interval longer than the norm for age. It can be a normal variant caused by increased vagal tone, and in this situation, it is a benign condition.[30] Digoxin can increase the PR interval at therapeutic doses; however, first-degree AV block may be a sign of toxicity. PR prolongation can also be seen in myocarditis, hyperkalemia,

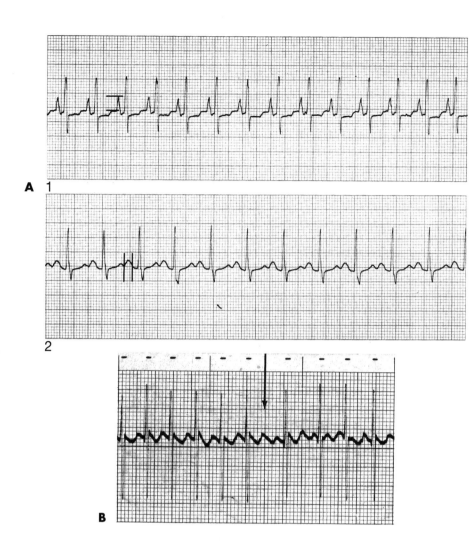

Fig. 7-24 **A,** Abnormal P waves in a pediatric patient. *1,* Right atrial enlargement; P waves measure 5 mm. *2,* Left atrial enlargement; P wave duration measures 0.12 second. **B,** Normal P waves replaced by flutter waves in atrial flutter. (From Curley MAQ: *Pediatric cardiac dysrhythmias,* pp 59, 88, 101, 102. Bowie, Md. Copyright 1985 by Brady Communications Company.) *Continued*

Kawasaki disease, acute rheumatic fever, and corrected (levo) transposition of the great arteries (L-TGA).[23]

Short PR intervals occur in rhythms with AV dissociation, such as complete heart block or junctional ectopic tachycardia (JET). Although no association exists between atrial and ventricular contraction in these rhythms, occasionally the P wave appears just before the QRS with a very short PR interval.

In ventricular preexcitation (WPW syndrome) the PR interval is short on ECG. This condition is due to a manifest accessory connection that allows rapid antegrade (forward) conduction of a sinus beat to the ventricles at the same time there is ventricular depolarization by the AV node. As a result of the early activation of the ventricles, the PR interval is short. Ventricular preexcitation is apparent on ECG by the presence of a delta wave (Figure 7-25).

The fifth parameter for assessment is the P-QRS relationship. Every P wave should be conducted to the ventricles and produce ventricular depolarization and a QRS complex. If a one-to-one P-QRS relationship does not exist, heart block or AV dissociation is suspected. See Figure 7-26 for an illustration of various forms of AV block.

In patients with second-degree heart block, the rhythm strip reveals more than one P wave for each QRS complex. Second-degree heart block is classified in two groups: Mobitz type I (Wenckebach) or Mobitz type II. In Mobitz type I, there is progressive prolongation of the PR interval with eventual failure to conduct an atrial impulse to the ventricles. The rhythm strip reveals progressive lengthening of the PR interval and concomitant shortening of the RR interval until a QRS complex does not follow a P wave. Characteristic grouping of complexes is evident. Mobitz type I second-degree heart block may reflect AV node dysfunction in patients following intracardiac surgical procedures near the AV node or in those with digoxin, β-blocker, calcium channel blocker, or quinidine toxicity. It can be detected in people without pathophysiologic conditions, especially during sleep. Mobitz type I second-degree heart block does not usually progress to third-degree (complete) heart block. No treatment is indicated unless the ventricular rate is excessively slow and CO is compromised as a consequence. Permanent pacing is indicated in those children with symptomatic Mobitz type I block, although this is infrequent.[30]

Mobitz type II second-degree heart block results in either normal AV conduction or completely blocked conduction. The atrial rate is normal (regular P waves), but the ventricular rate (QRS) depends on the number of normally conducted beats. On a rhythm strip, this is manifest by occasional or a patterned block of AV conduction. A QRS complex does not follow each P wave. This type of heart block is at the bundle or lower and can progress to

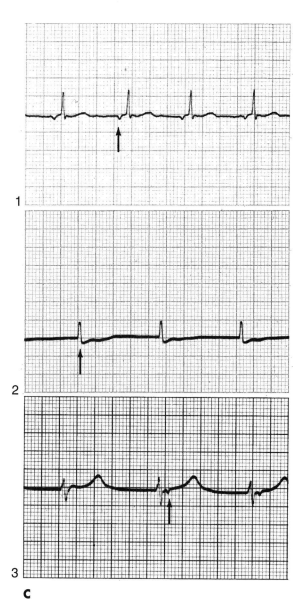

Fig. 7-24—cont'd **C,** Altered P wave morphology and location. *1,* Inverted P waves before the QRS complex characteristic of low atrial rhythm. *2,* Buried P wave within the QRS complex, atrial and ventricular depolarization occur at the same time (junctional rhythm). *3,* Inverted P wave after the QRS complex ventricular depolarization first, then atrial depolarization (junctional rhythm). (From Curley MAQ: *Pediatric cardiac dysrhythmias,* pp 59, 88, 101, 102. Bowie, Md. Copyright 1985 by Brady Communications Company.)

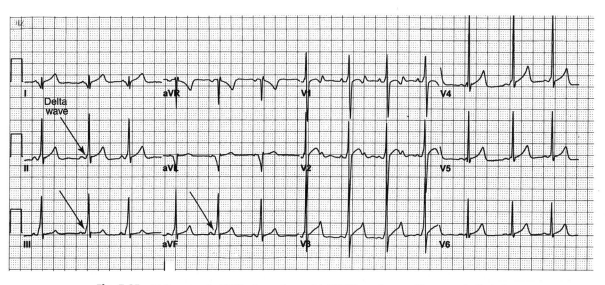

Fig. 7-25 Delta wave in ECG of a patient with WPW syndrome. (Courtesy J. Craig.)

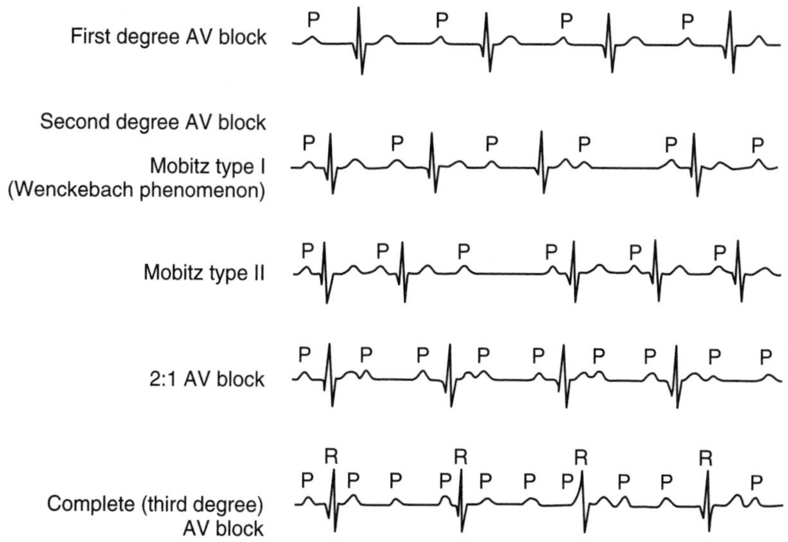

Fig. 7-26 Disturbances of atrioventricular *(AV)* conduction. (From Park PK: *How to read pediatric ECGs,* ed 3, St. Louis, 1992, Mosby.)

third-degree heart block.[23] If the patient is unstable with this rhythm, intravenous isoproterenol, atropine, or epinephrine may be helpful in increasing ventricular rate until pacemaker therapy is available.

Occasionally 2:1 AV block is noted; this occurs when a QRS follows every second P wave. Without conducting an electrophysiology study, it is difficult to determine if 2:1 AV block is Mobitz type I or type II because the AV node can develop a Wenckebach after every other sinus beat.

Third-degree, or complete heart, block (CHB) can either be congenital or acquired. Regardless of the cause, the SA node paces the atria, and either a junctional or ventricular escape rhythm paces the ventricles. On ECG the atrial rate is regular and faster than the ventricular rate, and no relationship exists between the P waves and QRS.

Acquired CHB may result from severe metabolic derangement, such as hypoxia, acidosis, hypothermia, hypoglycemia, electrolyte imbalance (especially of potassium or calcium), drug toxicity, acquired myocardial disease (including myocarditis), or as a consequence of open heart surgery. In most cases, acquired CHB is transient, requiring only temporary support. Administration of intravenous isoproterenol or epinephrine (0.05-0.1 µg/kg/min) to increase the ventricular rate is usually necessary. Temporary pacing is accomplished via transvenous or transcutaneous epicardial approach. However, esophageal atrial pacing is **not** of benefit in CHB because atrial impulses cannot be conducted to the ventricles. Permanent pacing is necessitated if acquired CHB persists for longer than 14 days because the ventricular rate is too slow to support CO and does not increase significantly to support metabolic demands.[30,31]

Congenital CHB is often associated with maternal collagen vascular diseases, such as systemic lupus erythematosus. In addition, some 30% of infants with congenital CHB have CHDs, including L-transposition, univentricular heart, AV canal, and tricuspid atresia.[32] Infants with congenital CHB are often diagnosed prenatally on fetal echocardiogram. In some, the HR is so slow that severe CHF is present at birth, and mortality is high in this group.

Infants who are asymptomatic at birth, except for the slow HR, generally have an escape rhythm of 60 to 70 beats/min. A mean awake HR of less than 55 beats/min is a poor prognostic indicator.[32-34]

In the symptomatic infant, administration of isoproterenol or epinephrine may be necessary to increase HR until placement of a permanent pacemaker. In the asymptomatic infant, close observation with frequent Holter monitoring is necessary to evaluate for rate response with exercise, ventricular escape rhythm, or mean HR. If CHF, syncope, inability to increase HR, a long QT interval, VT, or wide-complex escape rhythm develops, then placement of a permanent pacemaker is indicated.

The P-QRS relationship may also be useful in diagnosis of tachyarrhythmias (although it is often difficult to detect P waves on ECG at very high heart rates). SVT can have P waves conducted retrograde that follow the QRS. In JET or VT, AV dissociation is present.

Many diagnostic tools are available to assist in the assessment of the AV relationship during tachycardia. First, AV dissociation can be assessed from the RA hemodynamic waveform. On atrial pressure lines (central venous pressure, left atrial pressure), cannon *a* waves are present in AV dissociation, occurring when the atria contract against a closed tricuspid or mitral valve (Figure 7-27). Second, assessing the P-QRS relationship in more than one lead is often useful. Figure 7-28 is a 12-lead ECG in a 9-year-old with wide-complex tachycardia. In V_1, AV dissociation is evident, aiding the diagnosis of VT.

Finally, an atrial electrogram can be recorded using a transesophageal electrode or an existing transthoracic atrial wire placed during cardiac surgery. These maneuvers are helpful in the diagnosis of atrial tachyarrhythmias or JET. Atrial activity is detected with the transesophageal lead because the lower esophagus lies posterior to the left atrium (LA). An atrial esophageal lead is placed like a nasogastric tube and slowly withdrawn to provide optimal visualization of atrial waves (Figure 7-29). An epicardial atrial electrogram allows the direct recording of atrial activity. When obtained simultaneously with a rhythm strip, atrial activation and AV association can be clearly identified (Figure 7-30). In addition, atrial overdrive pacing to terminate reentrant arrhythmias can be accomplished via either transesophageal or atrial epicardial wires. Less traumatic than traditional cardioversion, atrial overdrive pacing is useful when the patient is hemodynamically unstable or is refractory to drug therapy.

The sixth assessment parameter is duration of the QRS complex. QRS duration correlates with ventricular mass and becomes wider as the infant or child grows (see Table 7-4).

Wider than expected QRS complexes occur when ventricular impulse conduction is delayed or aberrant. For example, premature ventricular contractions (PVCs) and bundle branch block (BBB) result in abnormally long conduction pathways. PVCs are often benign; however, multiform PVCs, couplets, or triplets warrant further investigation. Electrolyte, acid-base status, and hemodynamic function should be evaluated in critically ill children with PVCs.

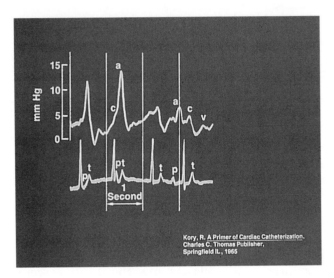

Fig. 7-27 Cannon *a* waves in AV dissociation as the atria contract against a closed tricuspid valve.

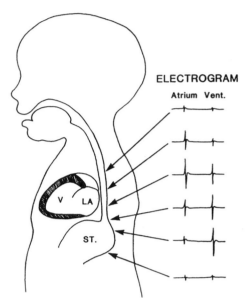

Fig. 7-29 Anatomic relationship between the esophagus and the cardiac chambers in infants. The ideal electrogram at midesophagus has an atrial spike that is equal to, or larger than, the ventricular signal. *V,* Ventricle; *LA,* left atrium; *ST,* stomach. (From Walsh EP: Electrocardiography and introduction to electrophysiological techniques. In Fyler DC, ed: *Nadas' pediatric cardiology,* Philadelphia, 1992, Hanley & Belfus, p 147.)

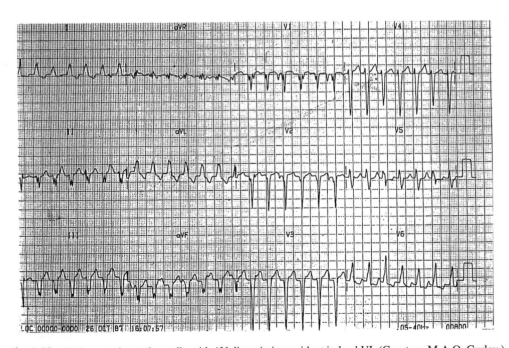

Fig. 7-28 Wide-complex tachycardia with AV dissociation evident in lead VI. (Courtesy M.A.Q. Curley.)

Intraventricular conduction blocks can occur in either the right or the left bundle branch because of CHDs or myocardial inflammation. Right BBB is common after surgical repairs that involve the ventricular septum. The type of intraventricular block (that is, partial or complete BBB) is monitored with serial ECGs but is not usually of clinical significance for most pediatric patients.

Wide QRS complex tachyarrhythmias pose a significant problem to caregivers in the PICU. Differentiating between SVT with aberrant conduction and VT is critically important because treatment of these two arrhythmias is quite differ-

ent. The following factors are considered in making the distinction between the two:

1. Rate. The rate of SVT is age dependent. The normal rate of the SA node is 220 minus the patient's age; anything faster than this is usually considered an abnormal tachyarrhythmia. SVT and VT rates range from 150 to 300 beats/min.[35]
2. Rhythm. VT is generally a regular rhythm; SVT is monotonously regular.
3. P-QRS relationship. In SVT the relationship is one to one (1:1), whereas AV dissociation exists in VT. In VT the ventricular rate is greater than the atrial rate.[35] (At rapid heart rates, this can be difficult to determine using a surface ECG.)
4. QRS duration. Generally, wide-complex tachycardia is considered VT until proven otherwise. In VT the QRS duration is different than the sinus QRS and wide at 120 to 140 milliseconds. In the majority of patients with SVT, the QRS complex is normal and narrow complex. However, up to 15% to 30% of patients with SVT can have rate-dependent BBB,[27] which is most often a right BBB best identified in V_1.
5. Fusion complexes. Fusion complexes are created in part by a normally conducted supraventricular impulse and in part by an ectopic ventricular impulse. The result is in normalization of the QRS complex.[23]

Figure 7-31 shows rhythm strips in which wide-complex tachycardia is noted. The most crucial assessment in each case is the impact of the rhythm disturbance on hemodynamics and patient condition.

Evaluation of QRS duration is helpful in monitoring critically ill children with electrolyte imbalances or over-

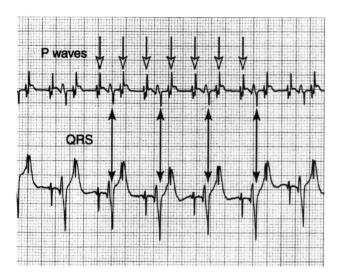

Fig. 7-30   Atrial electrocardiogram; note the atrial rate in the top lead is faster than the ventricular rate (QRS) in the bottom lead.

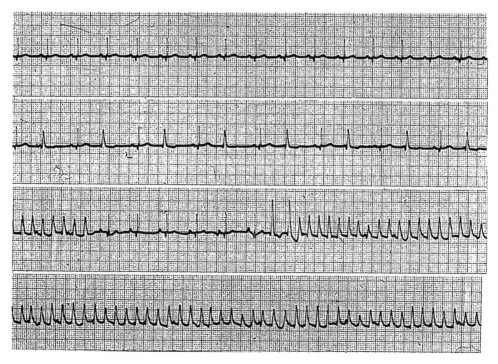

Fig. 7-31   Wide-complex tachycardia. (Courtesy M.A.Q. Curley.)

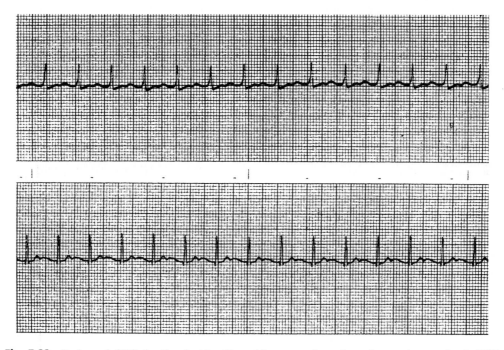

Fig. 7-32 Prolonged QRS duration in tricyclic antidepressant ingestion; changes in a patient's ECG over 8 hours. (From Kelley SJ: *Pediatric emergency nursing,* ed 2, Norwalk, Conn, 1994, Appleton & Lange, p 234.)

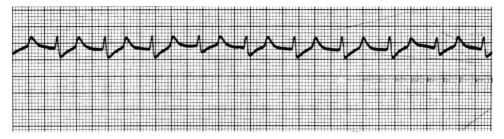

Fig. 7-33 Hyperkalemia prolongs cardiac conduction: the QRS duration and PR interval are prolonged, and the P wave is broad. (From Curley MAQ: *Pediatric cardiac dysrhythmias,* p 153. Bowie, Md. Copyright 1985 by Brady Communications Company.)

dose. Tricyclic ingestion results in prolongation of the QRS complex and provides a bedside guide to predict which patients are at risk for significant complications (i.e., seizures, ventricular arrhythmias, and death) (Figure 7-32).

In patients with hyperkalemia, peaked T waves are noted initially; however, this is a nonspecific sign because many normal children can have peaked T waves. As the serum potassium level continues to rise, cardiac conductivity is decreased, resulting in bizarre wide QRS complexes.[24] Figure 7-33 represents the rhythm strip of a patient with hyperkalemia.

The seventh assessment parameter is the ST segment. The ST segment is evaluated from the J point (the junction of the QRS complex and the ST segment) and compared with the isoelectric line or baseline of the rhythm strip. Normally the ST segment is not elevated more than 1 mm or depressed more than 0.5 mm in children. An exception to this is early repolarization syndrome in adolescents that is a benign condition resulting in ST segment elevation of up to

4 mm.[24] Abnormal ST segments are associated with myocarditis, pericarditis, myocardial ischemia, potassium abnormalities, severe ventricular hypertrophy, and intracranial pathologic conditions (Figure 7-34).

The eighth parameter for assessment is the T wave. The T wave is normally asymmetric, and measurement of amplitude is difficult because of normal variability in children. Low-voltage or flat T waves in multiple leads may indicate ischemia. T waves should be upright in leads I and II after 48 hours of age. T waves are normally inverted in V_1 after 5 days of age until adolescence, at which point they become upright.[24] Abnormalities in the T wave are the result of abnormal depolarization (such as that which occurs with PVC) or when repolarization is abnormal (as in patients with myocarditis).

Tall, peaked T waves are apparent in hyperkalemia, LVH with volume overload, and intracranial hemorrhage. Flattened T waves are apparent in hypothyroidism, hypokalemia, myocarditis, ischemia, or digoxin toxicity.[23]

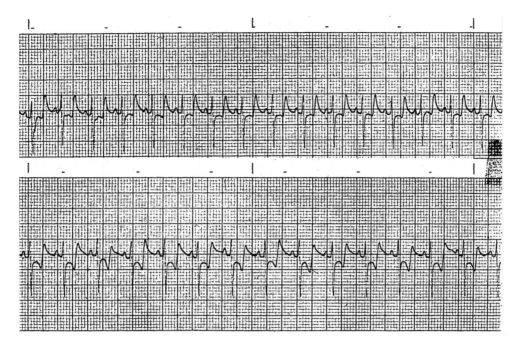

Fig. 7-34 Depression of the ST segment with tachycardia. (Courtesy M.A.Q. Curley.)

Figure 7-35 shows T wave changes associated with changes in serum potassium levels.

The ninth parameter evaluated is the QT interval. The QT interval represents ventricular repolarization and varies with HR, increasing with slower rates and decreasing with rapid rates. Bazett's formula is widely accepted for calculation of the QT interval. However, the data in support of Bazett's formula is from adults and has been extrapolated to children. The QT interval has been found to be influenced by gender and age. Adolescent girls have the longest QT intervals.[36] The QT interval is corrected for HR; however, validity is questioned at very slow heart rates (<50 beats/min) and in bigeminal rhythms. This measurement must be made using the QT following three consecutive sinus beats.

QTc = measured QT interval ÷ square root of the RR interval
(expressed in seconds)

The QT interval ends at the end of the T wave. If a U wave (see next section) is present and the U wave amplitude is 50% or less of the T wave amplitude, then the QT interval ends at the extrapolated downslope of the T wave. The corrected QT should be less than or equal to 0.44 second, except in newborns where it may be up to 0.47 second.

Shortening of the QT interval is detected in patients receiving digoxin and in those with hypercalcemia. Prolonged QT interval occurs with hypocalcemia, myocarditis, hypomagnesemia, hypokalemia, hypothermia, organophosphorous insecticide poisoning, medication toxicity (i.e., haloperidol [Haldol], tricyclic antidepressants, cisapride, erythromycin, procainamide, and amiodarone among others), and long QT syndrome (Figure 7-36).

Long QT syndrome is a genetic mutation of one of the voltage-activated channels altering normal ionic flow, resulting in ventricular repolarization abnormalities. These patients are predisposed to ventricular arrhythmias and torsades de pointes.[37] Long QT syndrome should be suspected in children with QTc prolongation, syncope, palpitations, and family history of sudden death.

The tenth parameter assessed is the presence of U waves. U waves are small positive deflections that occur at the end of the T wave. Prominent U waves are apparent in hypokalemia and myocardial ischemia.

Radiographic Evaluation

Chest radiographs (CXR) of the seriously ill pediatric patient provide important information about heart size, chamber enlargement, and PBF. Most of these data are obtained from a standard anteroposterior (AP) and lateral chest film. Oblique films may be helpful in the detection of specific changes in cardiac shape and size.

Detection of cardiac enlargement is an important goal of chest radiography. Heart size is determined by the cardiothoracic ratio. The largest transverse dimension of the heart is compared with the widest intercostal diameter of the chest. (The presence of a thymic shadow can make this measurement difficult in infants.) Cardiomegaly is present when the heart size is greater than one-half the width of the thorax. The film should be taken during peak inspiration because an expiratory film will falsely enlarge the cardiac silhouette.[38] In the AP film, the right cardiac border is the right atrium, and the lower left border is the left ventricle. The aorta should arch to the left and slightly displace the trachea to the right. In the lateral film, the lower anterior

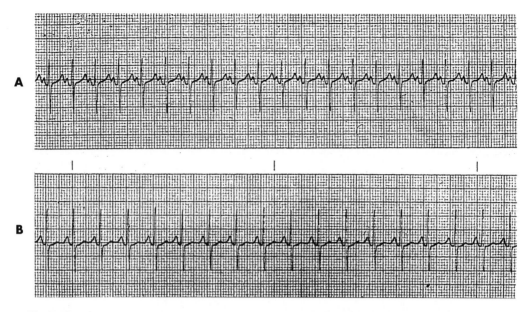

Fig. 7-35 T wave changes that resulted when the serum potassium fell from 7.9 to 2.1 mEq/L in a patient with diabetic ketoacidosis. **A,** Serum potassium 7.9 mEq/L. **B,** Serum potassium 2.1 mEq/L. (Courtesy MAQ Curley.)

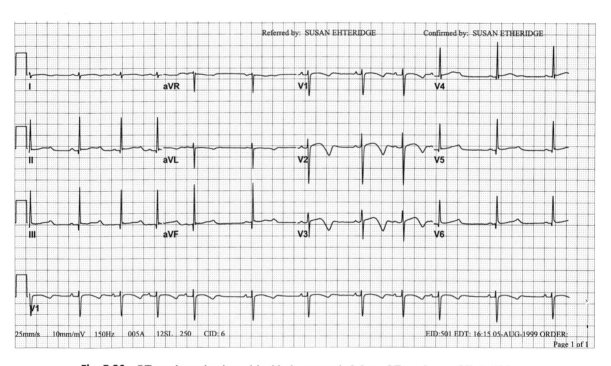

Fig. 7-36 QTc prolongation in a girl with the congenital, long QT syndrome. QTc is 485 ms.

border is the right ventricle, and the posterior border is the left atrium (upper) and left ventricle (lower).[39] Serial changes in heart size should be monitored.

Assessment of the vascular markings on the CXR detects alterations in PBF. With a large left-to-right shunt, PBF is increased, resulting in increased size and prominence of the pulmonary blood vessels well into the peripheral lung fields. Patients with heart defects that result in decreased PBF have diminished pulmonary vascular markings.

The skeletal aspects of the CXR are examined because of the association between CHDs and congenital anomalies (many of which have bony abnormalities). The pulmonary parenchyma is inspected because pneumonia and/or atelectasis can be a problem in the postoperative period and in children with increased PBF.

Magnetic resonance imaging (MRI) adds substantially to the cardiac evaluation. Historically, barium swallow esophagrams were used for the detection of atrial enlargement and coarctation of the aorta. However, MRI has largely replaced the use of barium swallow for these indications.

MRI can complement echocardiography if findings on the echocardiogram are equivocal. In some situations (coarctation of the aorta in older children, thoracic vascular abnormalities, or pulmonary vascular abnormalities), MRI has replaced cardiac catheterization as the primary diagnostic tool.[40] The accuracy and quality of MRI images require patient cooperation and limitation of movement. Many children require sedation, particularly infants and small children. The presence of metal near the heart may degrade the quality of the image, so a careful history should be obtained to determine the presence of permanent pacemakers, vascular clips, shrapnel, or other magnetic metal. MRI should be avoided in children with permanent pacemakers or defibrillators because these can pose a significant hazard to the patient (i.e., reprogramming of generator, inappropriate function, ventricular fibrillation).

Echocardiography

Echocardiography provides the most complete noninvasive assessment of cardiac structure, function, blood flow patterns, and pressure gradients. Echocardiography uses transthoracic ultrasound imaging. A pulse generator sends electrical pulses to a transducer that emits short bursts of sound energy through the chest wall. The transducer then receives the sound energy returning from the tissues and converts it into an electrical signal that can be viewed on an image processor. Transthoracic two-dimensional and Doppler echocardiography have become the primary diagnostic tools in the evaluation of children with congenital heart disease. The ability of echocardiography to provide a detailed assessment of cardiac structure has allowed most children with major CHDs to undergo primary complete surgical repair without the need for cardiac catheterization.[41]

M-mode echocardiography provides one-dimensional imaging of the heart. With this technique, the transducer emits a thin beam of ultrasound energy directed to a specific area of the heart. Cardiac structures that lie along that beam are viewed on a strip recording that shows the motion of the structures over time. With this limited view, M-mode cannot provide diagnosis of structural cardiac defects and is primarily used in the evaluation of LV size and function.

Two-dimensional echocardiography provides a cross-sectional view of the heart. This is accomplished by aiming the ultrasound beam across an angle, viewing the structures of the heart within that area. This produces a sector or image of the structures within the area of the ultrasound beam. The result is a detailed two-dimensional image of the entire heart and associated structures, making it the primary tool for the diagnosis of structural cardiac defects.

Doppler ultrasound adds information to the two-dimensional picture by evaluating the blood flow through the heart. In this technique, sound waves are bounced off moving blood, making it possible to measure the velocity of its flow. Color Doppler uses computer technology to assign a color to the various blood flow velocities, making it useful in the evaluation of intracardiac shunts and valve regurgitation. Spectral Doppler displays the blood flow velocity and pattern directly on the screen and is most useful in the evaluation of intracardiac valve obstructions.

The primary indications for echocardiography in the PICU include diagnosis of CHDs, identification of residual cardiac lesions after cardiac surgery, presence of pericardial effusion and/or cardiac tamponade, evaluation of cardiac chamber volume and function, identification of intracardiac thrombi or vegetations, and possibly the evaluation of diaphragm movement (Figure 7-37). In addition, echocardiography is utilized to guide pericardiocentesis in the setting of pericardial effusion or cardiac tamponade.

Echocardiography can be used to evaluate ventricular function by measuring shortening fraction or ejection fraction. Shortening fraction is the percent change in ventricular diameter during systole and diastole, and ejection fraction is the percent of volume change. Normal shortening fraction is $32 \pm 4\%$, and a normal ejection fraction is $65 \pm 10\%$. Shortening fraction is calculated by measuring the transverse diameter of the ventricle in diastole and systole, where LV diastolic diameter minus LV systolic diameter divided by LV diastolic diameter gives shortening fraction. Ejection fraction is best measured by obtaining biplane measurements of the ventricle from the apex. The entire wall of the ventricle is traced, measuring the volume during diastole and systole, where the LV diastolic volume minus the LV systolic volume divided by the LV diastolic volume gives the ejection fraction. These data can only be accurately applied to the morphologic left ventricle. Evaluation of a systemic right ventricle (Mustard or Senning for TGA) or morphologic single right ventricle (hypoplastic left heart syndrome) is generally performed subjectively by the echocardiographer.

Both methods of evaluating ventricular function have limitations. Shortening fraction depends on normal wall movement and is only applicable to a structurally normal left ventricle. Conditions that produce RV volume overload (atrial septal defect, or severe tricuspid or pulmonary valve insufficiency), wall motion abnormalities (myocardial infarction, synthetic septal patch), and paradoxical septal wall motion can make shortening fraction inaccurate. Ejection fraction requires biplane measurements from either the apical or subcostal views and therefore are often difficult to obtain. If the entire wall is not visualized, errors in tracing can lead to inaccurate measurements.

Echocardiographic techniques using Doppler flow measurements to estimate CO are also available. These techniques are often inaccurate and not as reliable as invasive measurements of CO using the Fick or thermodilution methods.

Transesophageal Echocardiography. Although transthoracic echocardiography has become the primary

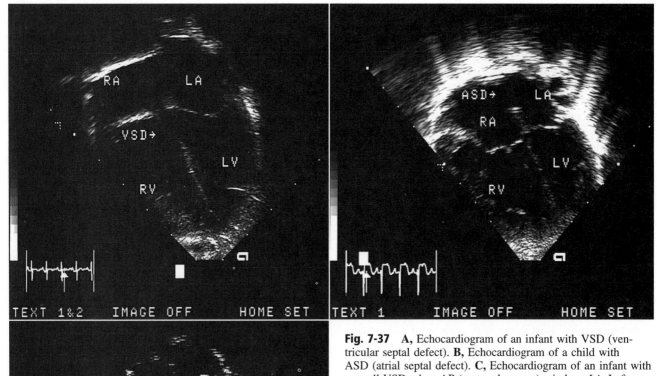

Fig. 7-37   **A,** Echocardiogram of an infant with VSD (ventricular septal defect). **B,** Echocardiogram of a child with ASD (atrial septal defect). **C,** Echocardiogram of an infant with a small VSD ad an AP (aortopulmonary) window. *LA,* Left atrium; *LV,* left ventricle; *RA,* right atrium; *RV,* right ventricle.

diagnostic tool in the evaluation of children with congenital heart disease, specific circumstances may limit its use. For example, the presence of multiple chest tubes, invasive monitoring lines, and an open sternum may limit the accessibility necessary to achieve adequate images for diagnosis. In these circumstances, transesophageal echocardiography (TEE) may be indicated. TEE uses a flexible ultrasound probe with a high-resolution ultrasonic transducer at the tip. With the patient deeply sedated (and possibly intubated), the probe is passed orally into the esophagus and placed in the retrocardiac position, where two-dimensional imaging and Doppler analysis provide high-quality evaluation of cardiac structure and blood flow. When placed into the stomach, subcostal views of the heart can be obtained from below the diaphragm, providing a better image for measuring flow velocities through the ventricular outflow tracts.

In the operating room, TEE is used before the initiation of cardiopulmonary bypass to confirm the diagnosis, identify any additional diagnostic information that may alter the surgical approach, evaluate AV valve insufficiency, and assess cardiac function. Immediately following the separation from cardiopulmonary bypass, TEE is used to identify postoperative structural abnormalities that require additional surgical procedures and to evaluate postoperative cardiac function that may impact medical management. In approximately 6% of pediatric cardiac surgery patients, TEE findings prompt a return to cardiopulmonary bypass for further surgery or for revision of the surgery.[42,43] In 75% of these patients, the problem identified by TEE was corrected, and the patients had a good outcome. The most common cardiac lesions requiring return to cardiopulmonary bypass are tetralogy of Fallot and AV canal defects.

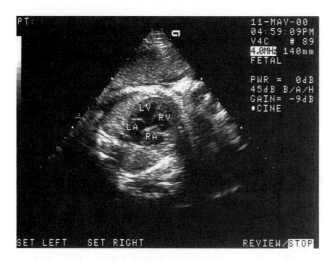

Fig. 7-38 Fetal echo.

TEE is used in the catheterization laboratory during device closure procedures to ensure proper placement of the device and to evaluate adequate closure of the defect. Occasionally it may be used during electrophysiology studies for electrode placement, particularly in single-ventricle patients.

TEE is also the best method to diagnose intracardiac thrombi, particularly in the left atrium. This should be performed in patients who have been in atrial fibrillation/flutter for protracted periods to rule out systemic heart thrombi before cardioversion because the risk for embolization is significant.[44,45]

Limitations of TEE include its use in small infants and previous esophageal surgery, making passage of the probe difficult. Cardiac lesions that are not well visualized with this method include partial anomalous pulmonary venous drainage, left superior vena cava to left atria connection, and distal branch pulmonary artery stenosis. Although no significant morbidity or mortality has been reported with the use of TEE, care must be taken on removal of the probe in intubated patients to prevent accidental endotracheal extubation.

Fetal Echocardiography. The development of high-resolution ultrasound scanners, along with the evolution of Doppler and color Doppler capabilities, has led to the use of ultrasonography in the prenatal diagnosis of fetal cardiac anomalies (Figure 7-38). Fetal echocardiography is successful in the diagnosis of structural cardiac abnormalities, arrhythmias, and abnormal cardiac function in fetuses as early as 16 to 18 weeks' gestation. An elective evaluation, however, is preferred between 18 to 20 weeks' gestation when the cardiac valves are well developed and the heart is an adequate size for study.

A primary indication for fetal echocardiography is the presence of an abnormal four-chamber view of the fetal heart on an obstetric ultrasound. When referred for this reason, the occurrence of congenital heart disease is 50% to 80%.[46,47] The presence of fetal risk factors for congenital heart disease is another indication for detailed fetal echocardiography. These include the following: (1) previous occurrence of congenital heart disease in siblings or parents;

(2) maternal diseases known to affect the fetus, such as diabetes mellitus and connective tissue disease; (3) maternal drug use, such as alcohol and lithium; (4) abnormalities of other fetal systems, such as chromosomal abnormalities, diaphragmatic hernia, omphalocele, and polyhydramnios, or oligohydramnios; (5) nonimmune hydrops; and (6) abnormalities of fetal heart rhythm. In this setting, structural cardiac defects have been found in 9% of the cases and rhythm abnormalities identified in 17% of the cases.[48]

A primary benefit of fetal echocardiography is the ability to provide the family with diagnostic and prognostic information to facilitate planning and decision making. The diagnosis of severe structural heart defects, such as ductal-dependant lesions, may determine the site of delivery to optimize surgical and medical management during the newborn period. For example, fetal diagnosis of hypoplastic left heart syndrome is associated with improved postnatal outcome.[49] When the likelihood of fetal demise related to congenital heart disease is high, termination of the pregnancy may be considered. In the case of fetal arrhythmias, early management with antiarrhythmic agents, along with echocardiographic monitoring, may decrease the development of fetal hydrops and improve clinical outcome. In the future, fetal diagnosis of structural cardiac defects, along with the possibility of fetal cardiac intervention and/or surgery, may improve the outcome of specific high-risk defects.

INVASIVE EVALUATION AND DIAGNOSIS

Definitive diagnosis of cardiac structure and function may require invasive diagnostic techniques. In the intensive care unit, hemodynamic monitoring provides valuable information regarding cardiovascular function. Definitive structural and functional information about the heart is obtained, in some instances only by cardiac catheterization.

Hemodynamic Monitoring

Invasive hemodynamic monitoring of infants and children in the PICU is routinely performed. Although the ability to measure, monitor, and calculate many physiologic parameters related to cardiovascular performance is valuable in the care of critically ill pediatric patients, numeric hemodynamic data alone is inadequate for clinical decision making. The sections that follow focus on the measurement of hemodynamic parameters and the calculation of derived hemodynamic data. The correlation of hemodynamic data with clinical assessment information and the effects of various modes of therapy are integrated. Accurate clinical decision making is based on the integration of hemodynamic monitoring data and sound clinical evaluation.

Fundamentals of Hemodynamic Monitoring. Invasive hemodynamic monitoring systems use a transducer to convert one energy form to another. The physical energy of BP is converted to an electrical signal that is amplified and displayed. Disposable transducer systems are routinely used and preferred to reusable systems. Disposable transducers have an improved dynamic frequency response, have less pressure drift with changes in temperature, are cost effective, and may decrease the risk of infection.

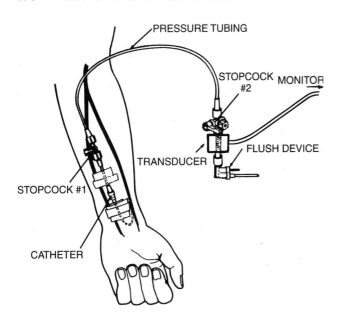

Fig. 7-39 Arterial blood pressure–monitoring system. (From Gardner RM, Hujcs M: Fundamentals of physiologic monitoring, *AACN Clin Issues Crit Care Nurs* 4:19, 1993.)

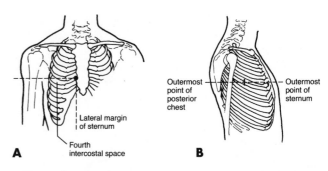

Fig. 7-40 Phlebostatic axis. Crossing of two imaginary lines defines the assumed position of the monitoring catheter tip within the body (i.e., right atrial level). **A,** Line that passes from the fourth intercostal space at the lateral margin of the sternum down the side of the body beneath the axilla. **B,** Line that runs horizontally at a point midway between the outermost portion of the anterior and posterior surfaces of the chest. (From Darovic GO: *Hemodynamic monitoring: invasive and non-invasive clinical applications,* Philadelphia, 1987, WB Saunders, p 126.)

Figure 7-39 illustrates one example of an arterial BP monitoring system. A radial artery catheter is connected through a short piece of pressure tubing to a stopcock. The stopcock near the insertion site is connected to a second stopcock at the transducer with a longer pressure tube. The transducer is connected to an infusion pump that delivers a continuous infusion at a controlled rate. The transducer is also connected to the monitor that displays the pressure waveform and the numeric measurement of the BP. Basic transducer setups vary among institutions. With the implementation of needleless access systems, most pressure setups use methods for avoiding needles.

Setting the Zero Point for the Monitoring System.
All systemic arterial catheter transducers must be leveled to an anatomically consistent point and zeroed to eliminate the effects of hydrostatic and atmospheric pressure. The proper technique for setting the zero point for a pressure monitoring system is illustrated in Figure 7-40. The transducer must be carefully positioned at the phlebostatic reference point, which is the fourth intercostal space–midaxillary line. Inaccurate transducer position can result in large errors in pressure measurement, especially when pressures are low, as when central venous or pulmonary artery wedge pressures are monitored. For example, a transducer positioned 15 cm above the phlebostatic reference point will result in a venous pressure reading 11 mmHg lower than is actually the case; a transducer located 15 cm below the midaxillary line will result in a venous pressure reading 11 mmHg above the actual pressure. These inaccuracies are the consequence of the effects of hydrostatic pressure on the BP reading. When more than one pressure is monitored, all transducers are placed in one holder to ensure accuracy when correlating data.

When the transducer is accurately positioned, either the stopcock at the patient's end of the system or the stopcock

at the transducer is opened to air and the monitor zeroed. Care must be taken to ensure that excessively long lengths of tubing between the patient and the transducer are avoided and that the tubing does not hang below the transducer.

Unusual pressure readings should always prompt reassessment of the system position and rezeroing of the monitoring system, especially if treatment changes are anticipated based on the pressure measured. Changes in the transducer or amplifier related to time and temperature and changes in the patient's position relative to the transducer can produce zero changes.

System Calibration. Transducer manufacturers calibrate the system sensitivity to within ±1%. Thus only zeroing is required when using standardized, disposable transducers. Checking the calibration with a column of air or mercury is unnecessary and may introduce risk of system contamination or embolism.

Optimizing System Accuracy. Hemodynamic pressure waveforms are dynamic, not static. The accuracy and reliability of the system's transmission of a pressure waveform to the transducer are crucial. To ensure accuracy of invasive pressure monitoring, the following procedures are necessary, in addition to the zeroing procedure described earlier.[50,51]

1. All air bubbles in the system are eliminated. Air bubbles result in underestimation of the systolic pressure and overestimation of the diastolic pressure. Air bubbles often are located in stopcocks when all the ports have not been filled with fluid and at connection points between tubings and between tubings and stopcocks.
2. Blood clots are prevented by the continuous infusion of flush solution. Thrombus formation on the catheter has the same effects described when air bubbles are present in the system.
3. Only noncompliant pressure tubing, in the shortest lengths possible (no longer than 3 to 4 feet), is used. Venous tubing, which is excessively compliant, or

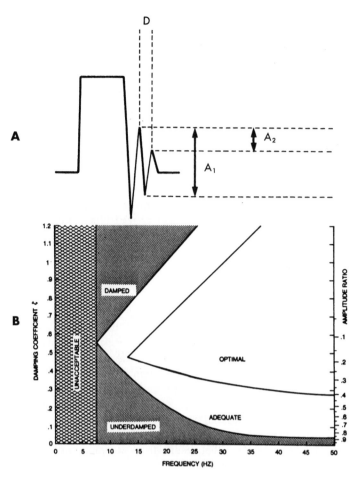

Fig. 7-41 **A,** Schematic illustration of a fast flush test. The natural frequency is determined by measuring the distance *(D)* between two consecutive oscillating peaks. This interval (millimeters) is divided by the paper speed (usually 25 mm/sec). Damping coefficient is determined by calculating the ratio between the amplitude of two consecutive peaks (A_1/A_2). This ratio is then plotted on the scale illustrated to obtain the damping coefficient. **B,** Scale for determining damping coefficient. Amplitude ratio on the right is referenced across to the damping coefficient on the left. Optimal systems have a high natural frequency (20 to 25 Hz) and a damping coefficient between 0.5 and 0.75). (**A** from Daily EK, Schroeder JS: *Techniques in bedside hemodynamic monitoring,* St Louis, 1989, Mosby; **B** from Gardner RM: Direct BP measurement: dynamic response requirements, *Anesthesiology* 54:227-236, 1981.)

long lengths of tubing result in the same errors described earlier.
4. The number of tubing connections is minimized. All loose-fitting connections are corrected.

Ensuring that pressure monitoring equipment is properly set up and maintained provides accurate and valuable data to critical care personnel. Attention to detail ensures the acquisition of accurate physiologic data.

Dynamic Response Validation. The ability of the hemodynamic monitoring system to accurately transmit a pressure waveform is a function of both the system's "natural frequency" (analogous to a car tire bouncing on a highway) and its "damping coefficient" (how quickly the car stabilizes after each bounce).[52] The fast flush test stimulates the hemodynamic monitoring system with high pressure so that the natural frequency and damping coefficient can be observed. Opening and quickly closing the fast flush device to temporarily interrupt the physiologic pressure waveform performs the fast flush test. A "square wave" pressure, followed by oscillations that revert to the pressure waveform being monitored, is observed (Figure 7-41, *A* and *B*). Daily and Schroeder[53] detail the fast flush test procedure.

Performing the fast flush test necessitates brief but rapid infusion of flush solution into the vascular catheter. Small arteries in patients with inadequate tissue perfusion may

spasm in response to rapid flushing. In this circumstance, it is impossible to perform the fast flush test. However, natural frequency is maximized in every patient's monitoring system by meticulous attention to the factors listed earlier that enhance system accuracy.

Arterial Blood Pressure Monitoring. Continuous invasive monitoring of systemic arterial BP is frequently necessary in the pediatric intensive care setting to ensure accurate evaluation of changes in patient status and the effects of therapies prescribed. Direct BP measurement is preferred in patients with circulatory dysfunction because impaired peripheral circulation and vasoconstriction render indirect measurement inaccurate or impossible to obtain. In addition, arterial cannulation for direct BP measurement provides reliable access for blood sampling when frequent laboratory evaluation, such as of arterial blood gases, is required.

Arterial Cannulation Sites. The choice of an arterial pressure monitoring site is based on the identification of an artery that is large enough to accurately reflect systemic BP and has adequate collateral circulation. The Allen test is performed when the radial artery is selected for cannulation to determine the adequacy of collateral circulation to the hand. To do this, both the radial and ulnar arteries are compressed until the hand blanches. The ulnar artery only is released, and the hand is assessed for return of color in 5 to 7 seconds. Color returning within 7 to 15 seconds is suggestive of slowed filling. If perfusion is delayed for more than 15 seconds, collateral circulation is considered inadequate, and another arterial site is selected for cannulation.[54,55] Similar technique for evaluating other arterial sites is necessary. For example, the posterior tibial and dorsalis pedis artery combination is assessed when either is considered for cannulation.

Other considerations in the selection of an arterial pressure monitoring site include easy access for blood sampling, care of the line, and assessment of the insertion site; avoidance of areas likely to be contaminated or where wounds exist; and selection of an artery large enough to permit blood flow around the catheter.[56] Arterial catheters are not placed in extremities with vascular prostheses such as those used for hemodialysis.

Possible sites for arterial cannulation and continuous monitoring include the radial, dorsalis pedis, posterior tibial, femoral, axillary, and umbilical arteries. The brachial artery is generally avoided because it is an artery without sufficient collateral circulation. Brachial artery occlusion with a catheter has been associated with the loss of the entire distal forearm. Temporal arteries are also avoided for cannulation. Flushing of this vessel can result in retrograde infusion of air or clot into the internal carotid artery and has been associated with brain infarction.

The umbilical arteries can be cannulated for the first several days of life before they become obliterated. In the young infant, they provide reliable and safe arterial access. Verified by radiographs, optimal position of the distal catheter is either high, above the diaphragm at T4 to T10, or low, at L3 to L4. These positions avoid the renal and mesenteric arteries. In either position, perfusion of the lower extremities is carefully assessed.

The radial artery is the most common and preferred site for arterial cannulation because it is easy to access and has good collateral blood flow via the ulnar artery. The arteries of the foot may be used, but access is often more difficult to obtain in small children. In addition, maintaining the catheter in either the dorsalis pedis or posterior tibial artery in position for proper functioning may be more difficult. Often the foot cannot be positioned comfortably.

The femoral artery is also an artery with minimal collateral circulation. However, this vessel is large enough to provide adequate blood flow around a small catheter and is therefore used for cannulation and monitoring. Careful assessment of the distal extremity pulses and perfusion should be evaluated frequently to observe for signs of thrombosis and ischemia. When low CO states exist, there may be an increased risk for distal ischemia, necessitating careful monitoring. Cannulation of the femoral artery should be avoided in the presence of occlusive vascular disease involving the leg. In addition, care should be provided to keep the site dressing free of urine or fecal contamination to prevent catheter infection.

The axillary artery is a large artery with good collateral circulation; therefore thrombosis with distal ischemia is rarely seen. Retrograde embolism, however, is a potential complication because of the proximity of the axillary vessel to the aortic arch and cerebral vessels. Careful attention

must be given to avoid rapid flushing and the presence of air or clot.

Arterial Pressure Analysis. Invasive BP measurement provides a moment-to-moment picture and a visual display of systolic, diastolic, and mean arterial pressure. Systolic arterial pressure (SAP) is the pressure exerted within the systemic arterial vasculature during ventricular contraction. Diastolic arterial pressure (DAP) reflects the pressure of the systemic arterial vasculature during ventricular relaxation. Pulse pressure (PP) is the arithmetic difference between the systolic and diastolic measurements and is a function of SV and arterial capacitance. For example, PP is typically decreased or narrowed when intravascular volume is inadequate. Mean arterial blood pressure (MAP) is the average pressure throughout the cardiac cycle. It is calculated by one of two formulas (all measures are in millimeters of mercury):

$$MAP = SAP + 2(DAP) \div 3 \text{ or } MAP = DAP + PP \div 3$$

MAP is not the mathematical mean of the systolic and diastolic BPs because diastole normally persists for approximately two thirds of the cardiac cycle. Electronic monitoring equipment performs the calculation of MAP automatically and provides a visual display of SAP, DAP, and the mean pressure. MAP is dependent on blood volume and the elasticity of the arterial walls and is representative of the perfusion pressure throughout the capillaries.

The pressure wave that results from contraction of the ventricle begins in the aorta. Arterial systole begins with the opening of the aortic valve and rapid ejection of blood into the aorta. Runoff of blood from the proximal aorta to the peripheral arteries follows. The arterial pressure waveform shows these events as a sharp rise in pressure that is followed by a decline in pressure. As the ventricles relax and the aortic valve closes, a small rise in arterial pressure occurs, resulting in the dicrotic notch on the downstroke of the arterial pressure waveform. Figure 7-42 shows a normal arterial waveform.

The arterial pressure differs both in contour and in measured value in various arterial locations. Impedance increases as the pressure wave travels toward the periphery, causing an increase in amplitude. The height of the pressure wave and the measured systolic pressure are greater distally than centrally. In addition, the more distal the location of the arterial catheter, the sharper the systolic upstroke and the less defined the dicrotic notch. The normally higher systolic pressure in the lower extremities that is normal in older children results in higher systolic pressures in the femoral artery than in the arteries of the upper extremities.

The systolic arterial pressure rises immediately after ventricular depolarization, that is, after the QRS complex on the rhythm strip. Delay is related to the catheter location and the length of tubing between the catheter and transducer. The dicrotic notch occurs after the T wave of the rhythm strip.

A decrease in the slope of the arterial pressure upstroke reflects a decrease in the velocity with which blood is ejected from the left ventricle, which is consistent with a decrease in ventricular contractility. Ventricular outflow

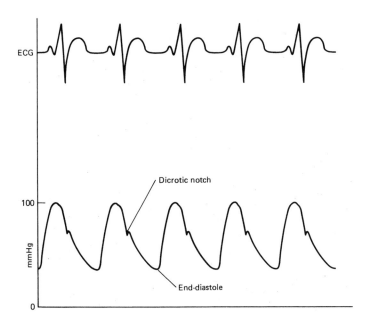

Fig. 7-42 Normal arterial pressure tracing. *ECG,* Electrocardiogram. (From Smith JB: *Pediatric critical care,* Albany, NY, 1985, Delmar, p 111.)

obstruction, produced by aortic stenosis or pericardial tamponade, also decreases the slope of the arterial pressure upstroke. A rapid, exaggerated upstroke and little area under the pulse contour correspond to decreased SV and increased vascular resistance, even when systolic BP is "normal" for age. Decreased CO and increased SVR also elevate the diastolic BP and narrow the PP. In the normally compliant lung, excessive positive pressure may restrict venous return to the heart. Therefore patients who are intravascularly volume depleted or who require excessive positive pressure may demonstrate a decrease in arterial pressure with mechanical inspiration or high levels of positive end-expiratory pressure (PEEP).

Dampened waveforms occur when obstacles prevent the pressure wave from being transmitted freely along the system. Dampened waveforms have a characteristic smoothed out appearance and are identified by a gradual upstroke, rounded-out peak systole, poor dicrotic notch, and narrow PP. Troubleshooting includes assessment of the entire system from cannula to solution for catheter obstruction, clot formation, air in the system, and arterial spasm. Overzealous flushing is avoided because it has been associated with complications such as cerebral emboli.

Overshoot, resulting from high flow within a narrow artery or high resonance within the catheter system, produces a more than 20 mmHg pressure gradient. In this case, dP/dT (the rate of the pressure rise over the time interval) is high. This may be caused by rapid HRs, excessive length of pressure tubing from the patient to the transducer, use of compliant tubing, and air that amplifies the wave. Overshoot can be avoided by using only noncompliant tubing of the shortest possible length.

Arterial spasms may occur with catheter manipulation, especially if peripheral perfusion is poor. Spasms are usually self-limiting. During cannula insertion, lidocaine without epinephrine may be used to flood the area, for example, up to 1 ml of 20% (20 mg/ml) lidocaine or 1 mg/kg—whichever is less—may be injected.

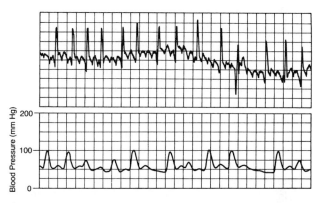

Fig. 7-43 Effect of altered cardiac rhythm on the arterial pressure waveform. (From Darovic GO: *Hemodynamic monitoring: invasive and non-invasive clinical applications,* Philadelphia, 1987, WB Saunders, p 111.)

Cardiac rhythm abnormalities alter the arterial pressure waveform. For example, in atrial fibrillation the arterial pressure varies considerably depending on the RR intervals and the corresponding time in any one cardiac cycle for ventricular filling (Figure 7-43). When a PVC occurs, ventricular contraction is initiated early. The result is diminished SV, reflected in a lowered arterial systolic pressure. Isolated occasional PVCs are usually well tolerated because of the increased SV and arterial pressure with the subsequent ventricular contraction.

Complications. Neurologic and vascular function of the extremity can be compromised in the extremity with an arterial catheter in place. Necrosis of the overlying skin is characterized by skin that blanches during catheter flushing progressing to skin that remains blanched. Small offshoots of the radial artery that lack collateral circulation perfuse the distal forearm. The tip of the cannula or the thrombus that forms around the cannula within 48 hours may occlude these vessels. Repositioning or removal of the cannula may be necessary.

Ischemia and necrosis of digits have occurred. Assessments of pain, blanched or pale areas beyond the cannulation site, pulselessness distal to the catheter, numbness and tingling, or motor impairment are essential to avoid or minimize these complications.

Local and systemic infection is a potential complication of any invasive monitoring system. However, peripheral arterial catheters may be associated with a substantially lower risk of local catheter-related infection than in other venous locations for comparable lengths of time. Although the reasons for this are not completely understood, the higher vascular pressures and increased flows at arterial cannulation sites may contribute to this decreased risk. Factors that predispose patients with arterial catheters to increased risk of infection include inflammation at the catheter insertion site, catheterization for more than 4 days, or catheter insertion by cutdown.[57,58] Unlike central venous catheters, peripheral arterial catheters in the femoral area are not associated with a greater risk of infection.[59]

Although the pathogenesis of catheter-related infections is multifactorial, evidence shows that they may result from the migration of skin bacteria from the insertion site along the catheter, resulting in catheter colonization and potential systemic infection. Therefore skin cleansing of the insertion site and dressing regimens play a critical role in the prevention of infection. Cutaneous antiseptics and antimicrobial ointments have been examined in numerous studies. The use of 2% aqueous chlorhexidine has been shown to be superior to either 10% povidone-iodine or 70% alcohol in preventing central venous and arterial catheter-related infections.[60] Recently, sustained-release chlorhexidine patches have been used on various invasive monitoring sites; however, the efficacy has yet to be determined. The application of antimicrobial ointments to the catheter site is generally avoided because its use has not been proven to decrease catheter infections. In addition, polyantibiotic ointments may increase the risk of fungal catheter colonization and fungal sepsis. Transparent, semipermeable, polyurethane dressings have become popular because they secure vascular devices well, and they provide direct visualization of the catheter insertion site. However, their use in the prevention of infection in arterial lines is unknown. When transparent dressings are used, the dressing is generally changed every 72 hours. When gauze is used, the dressing should be changed every 24 hours to evaluate the condition of the insertion site.

Arterial catheter infection is also prevented by maintenance of a sterile, closed system and use of heparinized normal saline solution for catheter flushing to prevent thrombus formation. The flush solution is changed every 24 hours, and the tubing system, every 48 to 72 hours.[61] The Centers for Disease Control also recommend that if the vascular catheter is suspected as a source of infection, it should be removed and, if necessary, placed at another site. The patient is assessed for unexplained fever and other signs of infection.

Thrombosis of an artery can develop while an invasive arterial pressure monitoring catheter is in place, after the catheter has been removed, or as a consequence of multiple arterial punctures, either to establish invasive monitoring or sample arterial blood. Multiple arterial punctures increase the risk of thrombosis, as does catheterization beyond 4 days, intermittent (versus continuous) flushing of the catheter, and catheter size larger than 20 gauge. Patients who experience hematoma formation at the arterial catheterization site and those with inadequate tissue perfusion, particularly if the administration of vasoactive medications is required, are at increased risk to develop thrombosis. After an artery has been cannulated for invasive monitoring, recannulation of the vessel can extend from days to several weeks.[56]

Thrombosis of an artery or at the catheter tip interferes with accurate BP measurement and blood sampling. Thrombosis can be minimized by avoiding the problems that are recognized to increase the incidence of thrombosis when possible and by the use of tapered-tipped, Teflon-coated catheters. When thrombosis is suspected, gentle aspiration of the catheter is indicated. Forceful flushing can result in embolization of the thrombus. If the catheter cannot be aspirated, it is discontinued.

Air embolism can develop from air in the flush system or when the system is opened to sample blood. Care in preparation and maintenance of the system can prevent the problem. Flushing of all arterial catheters should be done slowly to avoid retrograde infusion and arterial spasm.

Catheter Removal. When the arterial catheter is removed, pressure is applied at the insertion site for as long as necessary to achieve complete hemostasis; this is followed by application of a pressure dressing. Some recommend that a syringe be attached to the catheter and negative pressure applied while removing the catheter to minimize the risks of leaving thrombus on the catheter tip within the blood vessel.[56] Peripheral neurovascular function is assessed. The insertion site is assessed for signs of infection, ecchymosis, and local ischemia and necrosis. The catheter tip may be sent for culture if infection is suspected.

Central Venous Pressure Monitoring. Catheterization of the central venous circulation is frequently undertaken in critically ill infants and children for hemodynamic monitoring, infusion of parenteral nutrition, infusion of vasoactive medications, infusions of fluid and electrolytes, and intravenous access when peripheral veins are inaccessible. Hemodynamic monitoring of central venous pressure (CVP) reflects intravascular volume status and RV function. Low CVP measurements indicate hypovolemia, whereas high CVP measurements indicate either hypervolemia or elevated right ventricular end-diastolic pressure (RVEDP). Elevations of RVEDP are suggestive of RV dysfunction. In healthy individuals, CVP may also be used to monitor LV preload and function because RVEDP and LV end-diastolic pressure (LVEDP) correlate well. However, in patients who display a difference in right and left ventricular function, CVP cannot be used to evaluate LV preload or function. Severe respiratory disease and the use of positive pressure ventilation at high pressures, hypothermia, massive blood transfusion, and CHDs alter the relationship between CVP and LVEDP. Pathophysiologic factors that increase

PVR, such as hypoxemia and acidosis, also alter the relationship. Use of pulmonary artery catheters or direct LA catheters (e.g., in the postoperative cardiac surgery patient) for evaluation of LVEDP and left heart function is necessary in these situations.

Central Venous Cannulation. Central venous access in pediatric patients is obtained either by cutdown or percutaneous technique after the administration of sedation. The most commonly used sites are the internal jugular, femoral, subclavian, and antecubital veins. Ideally, the catheter is advanced to the caval-atrial junction. In this position, there is little motion of the catheter with respect to the heart, improving the accuracy of hemodynamic monitoring; less chance of inducing arrhythmias than when the catheter is advanced within the right atrium; less chance of cardiac perforation; and less thrombus formation because blood flow is rapid and the vessel caliber is large.[62] Central venous catheters can be placed in the umbilical vein of the newborn infant.

In patients younger than 1 year and weighing less than 6 kg, the internal and external jugular veins are often considered for venous access because they enter the superior vena cava with a straight course. The subclavian veins enter the central venous circulation at acute angles, which become less acute as the child grows.[63] The infraclavicular approach to the subclavian vein is sometimes preferred for long-term central venous catheterization in children, although risks of pneumothorax, hydrothorax, and hemothorax exist.

The femoral vein provides a large vessel that is easily identified and cannulated in both infants and children. The basilic vein in the antecubital space is also easily palpable, but the success rate in reaching the central venous circulation is limited in small children. This site provides successful central venous placement more often in children weighing more than 20 kg.[63]

Monitoring of intravascular volume status and RV function can also be accomplished via a transthoracic right atrial (RA) catheter inserted, most commonly, at cardiac surgery. The RA line is used exclusively for hemodynamic monitoring rather than for infusion of fluids or medications, unless other venous access is unobtainable or in the case of an emergency.

Venous Pressure Waveform Analysis. The normal central venous waveform is diagrammed in Figure 7-44. The pressure changes within the right atrium are small, consisting of three positive deflections—the *a, c,* and *v* waves—each followed by a descent in pressure. The *a* wave is the pressure rise produced by atrial contraction. The *c* wave may appear as a distinct positive deflection, as a notch on the *a* wave, or may be absent altogether. The *c* wave reflects the slight increase in intraatrial pressure that occurs with closure of the AV valve leaflets. It may be absent in pediatric patients because the atria are very distensible in youngsters. The *v* wave is produced by increased atrial pressure resulting from contraction of the ventricles, which causes the AV valve leaflets to bulge into the atria with concomitant atrial filling.

The descents that follow the *a* and *c* waves (the *x* and *x'* descents) are produced by the decrease in pressure during atrial relaxation and the downward pulling of the floor of the atrium at the onset of ventricular systole. The descent following the *v* wave (the *y* descent) is produced by the opening of the AV valve leaflets and emptying of the atria into the relaxed ventricles.

The pressure rises during atrial systole (the *a* wave) and atrial diastole (the *v* wave) are nearly the same. As a consequence, atrial pressure is monitored as the average or mean of both pressure rises. However, RA pressure waveforms are characterized by a dominant or larger *a* wave, compared with the *v* wave, whereas the reverse is true of the LA waveform. The *v* wave is dominant on the LA pres-

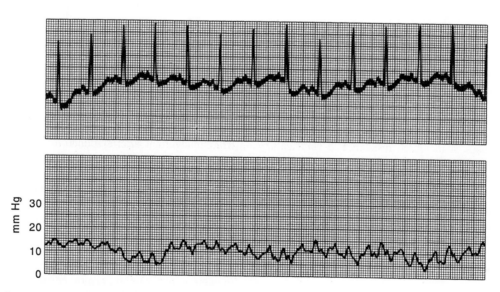

Fig. 7-44 Normal central venous pressure waveform. Central venous pressure waveform with simultaneous electrocardiogram. (From Clochesy JM, Breu C, Cardin S et al, eds: *Critical care nursing,* Philadelphia, 1993, WB Saunders, p 159.)

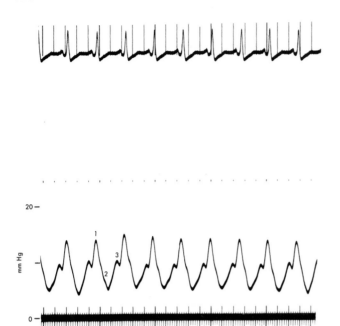

Fig. 7-45 Elevated right atrial pressure with exaggerated *a* wave *(1)* in a patient with right ventricle failure and increased resistance to ventricular filling *(2, x* descent; *3, v* wave). (From Daily EK, Schroeder JS: *Techniques in bedside hemodynamic monitoring,* St Louis, 1989, Mosby, p 102.)

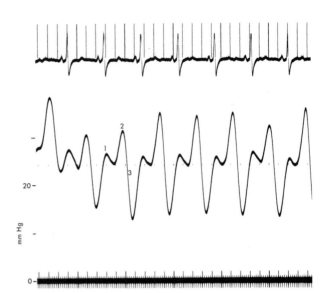

Fig. 7-46 Elevated right atrial pressure with exaggerated *v* wave *(2)* and rapid *y* descent *(3)* in a patient with tricuspid regurgitation as a result of acute right ventricle (RV) failure. The *a* wave *(1)* of approximately 26 mmHg reflects an elevated RVEDP and RV failure. (From Daily EK, Schroeder JS: *Techniques in bedside hemodynamic monitoring,* St Louis, 1989, Mosby, p 103.)

sure tracing, and higher mean pressure is found in the left atrium (4 to 12 mmHg) compared with that of the right (3 to 7 mmHg).

Correlation of the atrial pressure tracing with the ECG is helpful in differentiating the positive pressure deflections. The *a* wave immediately follows the P wave on the ECG, generally occurring in the PR interval. The *c* wave corresponds to the RS-T junction of the ECG. The *v* wave occurs during the TP interval.

Atrial fibrillation results in the absence of uniform atrial contraction, and consequently, no *a* wave is visible on the atrial pressure tracing. Only the *v* wave produces a distinct positive deflection. If the atria contract while the AV valves are closed (AV dissociation), a large or cannon *a* wave results.

Increased atrial pressure and elevation of the *a* wave are also seen with ventricular dysfunction and hypertrophy. Other causes of increased resistance to ventricular filling, such as AV valve stenosis or pulmonary hypertension, also exaggerate and elevate the *a* wave (Figure 7-45). Severe AV valve regurgitation, which may occur with severe ventricular failure or structural valve incompetence, produces marked elevation of the atrial *v* wave (Figure 7-46). In addition, atrial septal defects, which increase flow into the right atrium during ventricular systole, increase the size of the *v* wave. Both the *a* and *v* waves are elevated in cardiac tamponade.

Changes in intrathoracic pressure with ventilation are readily transmitted through the relatively thin-walled atria and great veins and are reflected in the CVP and atrial

pressure. During spontaneous and negative pressure ventilation, inspiration lowers the CVP (Figure 7-47). Positive pressure ventilation increases the CVP during inspiration, as does coughing and Valsalva maneuver. The application of PEEP to a patient's airway can also be transmitted to the central vasculature and increase right atrial pressure (RAP) and CVP. These circumstances can make the interpretation of high venous pressure difficult in isolation. Other clinical findings regarding the adequacy of venous return, intravascular volume, and cardiac function are key to accurate interpretation of numeric data.

Complications. During insertion of a central venous catheter, there is potential for local tissue injury of adjacent tissues and blood vessels. Inadvertent arterial puncture is the most common injury, which is usually not significant if the needle is immediately withdrawn and local pressure applied. Localized hematoma formation may develop from inadvertent arterial puncture or some venous punctures. This problem is minimized by use of a small-gauge needle to locate the central vein, by attention to proper technique, and by experience with central venous catheterization procedure.

Pneumothorax or hemothorax may be associated with needle puncture of the pleura during central venous catheter insertion. The subclavian approach is associated with risks of injury to mediastinal structures as well, resulting in pneumomediastinum, hemomediastinum, pneumopericardium, and pericardial tamponade.

Air embolism is a potentially fatal complication of central venous catheterization, which can occur during insertion

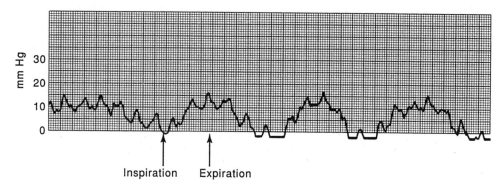

Fig. 7-47 Effect of spontaneous breathing on the central venous pressure waveform. (From Clochesy JM, Breu C, Cardin S et al, eds: *Critical care nursing,* Philadelphia, 1993, WB Saunders, p 159.)

of the catheter if the needle is not capped with a syringe. It can also occur when IV tubings are changed or if they are inadvertently disconnected. Proper attention to detail at insertion and meticulous care of central venous catheters and associated IV or hemodynamic monitoring tubings prevent air embolism.

Complications that may occur after insertion of a central venous catheter include infection and thrombosis. Perforation of vascular or cardiac structures is a potential risk but is extremely rare.

All central venous lines are potential sources for local infection and sepsis. Contamination can occur at the time of insertion if sterile technique is breached. Contamination can also occur from downward migration of normal skin flora after catheter placement. In addition, catheter colonization can result from contaminated tubing, pressure transducers, or IV flush solutions. Once the central venous catheter is colonized, it may become a source for disseminated infection, particularly in critically ill and immunocompromised patients. The risk of catheter-related bloodstream infections is approximately 4% when central venous catheters are used, compared with a 1% risk for peripheral IV catheters.[64] Organisms most commonly associated with central line infections include *Staphylococcus aureus, Staphylococcus epidermidis,* gram-negative bacilli, and enterococcus.

Risk factors for infection include multilumen catheters, internal jugular vein insertion, repeated catheterization, presence of an infectious focus elsewhere in the body, exposure of the catheter to bacteremia, absence of systemic antimicrobial therapy, duration of catheterization, type of dressing, and the experience of the personnel inserting the device. Most bloodstream infections related to IV catheters originate from either the patient's bacterial flora or from organisms on the hands of caregivers. Scrupulous attention to aseptic technique at the time of catheter insertion and during dressing changes is necessary to prevent the invasion of organisms. Careful maintenance of sterile IV solutions, tubings, and transducers is necessary. Sterile technique is mandatory when dressing changes are made. The dressing should be changed every 48 to 72 hours and when dressings are soiled, wet, or not intact. Current recommendations include cleansing with 2% aqueous chlor-

hexidine and covering the site with a transparent, semipermeable dressing. When gauze is used to cover the insertion site, the dressing should be changed every 24 hours to evaluate the site. To avoid infection, the catheter should be manipulated as little as possible and should be removed as soon as it is no longer needed.

Catheter-associated bacteremia can be identified while the infection is localized. Generally, a positive result on culture of blood drawn through the catheter with more than 15 colonies denotes infection, even if a peripheral blood culture result is negative. The patient then is at clear risk for catheter-related septicemia. Most often the catheter is withdrawn and replaced, if necessary.

Venous thrombosis and thrombophlebitis are associated with the presence of a central venous catheter. Most patients with thrombosis demonstrate edema of the arm, neck, and face, which is localized to the involved side. When central venous thrombosis is present, microembolization and pulmonary embolism can occur. If the patient's clinical situation indicates pulmonary embolism, thrombosis of the central veins is suspected. A venogram may be necessary to confirm thrombosis, although treatment may be initiated without radiographic confirmation. Treatment requires removal of the catheter and consideration of IV heparin or thrombolytic therapy.

Superior vena cava syndrome is a potential complication from central venous catheters placed in the superior vena cava. When thrombus formation occurs around the catheter, or the catheter itself obstructs the superior vena cava, inadequate venous return from the head can occur, resulting in head and neck swelling and discoloration. If this happens, the catheter should be removed, and the vessel should be evaluated for thrombus formation.

Catheter occlusion can result from blood clot or precipitant formation within the catheter. When blood clot formation is suspected, a fibrinolytic drug can be infused into the catheter in attempt to restore patency. With the current unavailability of urokinase, tissue plasminogen activator (t-PA) is being used for declotting central venous lines. t-PA is a naturally occurring protein secreted by vascular endothelial cells that converts inactive plasminogen to active plasmin. Synthetic t-PA binds plasminogen at the site of a clot and converts plasminogen to plasmin, producing local fibrinolysis. For catheter declotting, a small amount of t-PA is slowly injected into the catheter port, avoiding excessive pressure. Approximately 2 ml of a 1 mg/ml concentration of t-PA may be used for this procedure. Once instilled, t-PA is allowed to dwell in the catheter for 2 hours, at which time the port is gently aspirated to evaluate the effectiveness of the therapy. A second instillation may be necessary to fully dissolve the clot.

Catheter Removal. The central venous catheter is removed when the hemodynamic data obtained from it is no longer necessary for clinical decision making and the patient's condition permits administration of necessary IV fluids via a peripheral catheter. Aseptic technique and universal precautions must be ensured when the catheter is removed. Having patients perform a Valsalva maneuver prevents air entry into the central vein, if they are able to cooperate and the maneuver is not contraindicated (e.g., by increased intracranial pressure). In all patients, the catheter is most safely removed at the end of inspiration, when intrathoracic pressure is highest. The catheter is clamped and withdrawn with a steady motion. After removal, manual pressure is applied to the insertion site until hemostasis is ensured. The insertion site is assessed for signs of inflammation or infection, and the catheter is inspected to check that it has been removed in its entirety. The tip of the catheter may be sent for culture if line sepsis is suspected.

Peripherally Inserted Central Venous Catheters. Peripherally inserted central venous catheters (PICCs) provide an alternative to other central venous catheters. These catheters are typically inserted into the superior vena cava by way of the cephalic and basilar veins of the antecubital space. PICCs are associated with fewer mechanical complications, cost less than other central venous catheters, are easier to maintain than short peripheral catheters, and are associated with a lower rate of infection than other central venous catheters.[58,65] Indications for the use of PICCs in the PICU include the need for long-term access, typically for antibiotic therapy, and the administration of parenteral nutrition. Blood products may be administered through larger PICCs.

Catheter site care is similar to that of other central venous catheters. Dressing changes are performed every 72 hours to once a week. When a gauze is used to cover the insertion site, the dressing should be changed every day to evaluate the site for signs of infection. Heparin flush protocols are similar to those followed for other central venous catheters.

Pulmonary Artery Pressure Monitoring. Pulmonary artery (PA) catheters were first introduced in 1970 and were used enthusiastically in critically ill adults during the 1970s and early 1980s. Recognition of serious potential complications has resulted in more conservative use; that is, a PA catheter is indicated only when the data obtained will improve clinical decision making.

The PA catheter is valuable in the diagnosis and treatment of critically ill patients with cardiopulmonary failure. It measures RAP; pulmonary artery systolic, diastolic, and mean pressures; and the pulmonary artery wedge pressure. The PA catheter can be used for rapid determination of CO

using the thermodilution technique. Other parameters, such as cardiac index, SVR, PVR, and ventricular contractility indicators, can be derived from these data. The catheter can be used to sample mixed venous blood for intermittent analysis or, if equipped with a fiberoptic lumen, to continuously monitor mixed venous oxygen saturation.

PA Catheter Description. The multiple lumens of the PA catheter provide the means to assess a variety of physiologic characteristics of the cardiovascular system (Figure 7-48). The standard quadruple lumen PA catheter is available in three sizes: 5, 7, and 7.5 French (Fr). The 5 Fr size is suitable for children weighing less than 18 kg; the 7 and 7.5 Fr catheters are used for larger children and adults. The distal tip of the PA catheter is open and associated with a lumen that runs the entire length of the catheter. The inflatable balloon is positioned just proximal to the tip of the catheter. When the balloon is inflated through its lumen, it encompasses the tip of the catheter, reducing irritation of the endocardium during insertion. In general, the thermistor is 4 cm from the tip of the catheter; however, thermistor position can vary in custom-made thermodilution catheters. Insulated wires run through a third lumen to the thermistor hub,

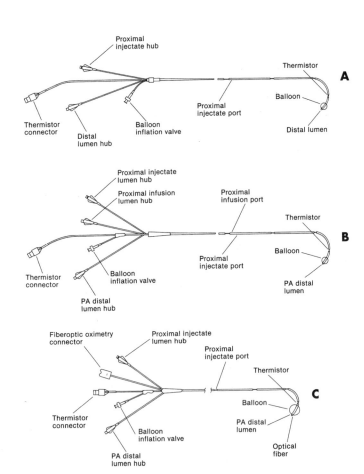

Fig. 7-48 Types of pulmonary artery catheters. **A,** Triple-lumen catheter. **B,** Quadruple lumen catheter. **C,** Oximetry catheter. (Redrawn from Baxter Healthcare Corporation, Edwards Critical-Care Division. All rights reserved. In Clochesy JM, Breu C, Cardin S et al, eds: *Critical care nursing,* Philadelphia, 1993, WB Saunders, p 164.)

and these connect to the CO computer. The proximal lumen of the PA catheter is located 15 to 30 cm from the catheter tip. The catheter size and specifications determine the position of the proximal lumen. (Specifications of custom-designed catheters can vary; the reader is referred to the package insert provided by the manufacturer.) Ideally the proximal port will be located in the RA when the distal port is in the PA.

Pulmonary Artery Cannulation. Before inserting the PA catheter, the patient's serum electrolyte (especially potassium, calcium, and magnesium), acid-base, and coagulation study results are evaluated. Hypoxemia, acidosis, hypokalemia, hypocalcemia, and hypomagnesemia place the patient at increased risk for the development of serious arrhythmias. Abnormal coagulation can result in hemorrhage or extensive hematoma formation.[66] In anticipation of possible ventricular arrhythmias, a lidocaine bolus (1 mg/kg) is prepared, and the defibrillator should be readily available.

Catheterization of the pulmonary artery is most often accomplished from the internal jugular vein, although the subclavian, femoral, or external jugular veins may be selected. The internal jugular is preferred because of a lower incidence of pneumothorax associated with this approach and because the catheter is easily secured in the neck area. Before catheter insertion, each catheter lumen is flushed with heparinized solution, inflating and inspecting the balloon assess balloon integrity, and connecting the thermistor hub to the CO machine and watching for a temperature assess thermistor integrity. Two pressure transducers are prepared, leveled with the patient's phlebostatic axis, connected to the monitor, and zeroed. The distal lumen of the catheter is connected to the transducer to permit waveform assessment during catheter insertion.

Insertion of the catheter is usually performed through an introducer (dilator) sheath that remains in place with the catheter. A sterile sleeve is placed over the catheter and attached to the introducer, permitting positioning and manipulation of the catheter without contamination.

The catheter is advanced from the internal jugular vein to the right atrium. When location within the right atrium is identified from the pressure waveform, the balloon is inflated to its full volume (about 0.5 to 1.5 ml; refer to manufacturer specifications). With continuous waveform monitoring (Figure 7-49), the catheter is carefully advanced through the right ventricle and into the pulmonary artery. Ultimately the PA catheter wedges, or is in the occlusion pressure position, in a pulmonary artery branch. The balloon is then deflated and the PA systolic and diastolic pressures are continuously monitored. The pressures and waveforms assessed during catheter insertion are documented as baseline data. Documentation of the length of catheter inserted and the external markings at the exit site are helpful in assessing and ensuring maintenance of the desired catheter position.

Waveform Analysis. Measurement of the RA mean pressure and analysis of the RA waveform during PA catheterization is the same as previously described. As the catheter passes through the tricuspid valve, the peak systolic RV pressure and the RVEDP are measured. The characteristic RV pressure waveform reflects the dynamic pumping action of that chamber. Figure 7-50 depicts the normal RV pressure waveform and illustrates the specific events that occur during ventricular systole and diastole. The normal peak RV systolic pressure range is 20 to 30 mmHg. RVEDP is measured after atrial systole (the *a* wave on the pressure waveform) and normally ranges from 2 to 8 mmHg. The systolic portion of the RV pressure waveform corresponds to ventricular depolarization and occurs during the QT interval of the ECG. The diastolic portion of the waveform occurs in the TQ period of the ECG.

Although RV pressure is not routinely monitored at the bedside, the initial pressures and waveforms should be documented as a reference. The RA pressure should be equal to the RVEDP (in the absence of tricuspid valve disease). The PA systolic and RV systolic pressures are also normally equal (in the absence of pulmonary valve disease). As a result, the RV pressure is monitored indirectly via these two pressures. If the RV pressure waveform were noted on the monitor subsequent to final catheter placement, it would indicate catheter migration. If detected, withdrawal of the catheter into the right atrium is indicated. From the right atrium, the balloon can be reinflated and the catheter can be refloated back to the pulmonary artery.

RV systolic pressure may be increased by a number of clinical problems. Any condition that increases PVR results in increased RV pressure, including pulmonary artery hypertension (PAH), hypoxemia, adult respiratory distress syndrome, pulmonary embolism, obstructive pulmonary disease, or pulmonary venous hypertension. RV systolic pressure may also be elevated by pulmonic stenosis (because of increased resistance to ventricular ejection) or ventricular septal defect (caused by left-to-right shunting of blood under high pressure). Increased RV diastolic pressure is the consequence of the same factors that increase the atrial pressure. Most often, increased RVEDP is the consequence of the ventricular dysfunction characteristic of heart failure.

PA Pressure. The pressure waveform in the pulmonary artery is divided into three phases: systolic, diastolic, and mean. Systolic pressure is representative of the rapid ejection of blood into the pulmonary artery after RV contraction and opening of the pulmonic valve. This is depicted as a sharp rise in pressure on the waveform, followed by a decline in pressure as the volume of blood ejected declines (Figure 7-51). Normal PA systolic pressure is the same as RV systolic pressure.

When RV pressure falls below the pressure in the pulmonary artery, the pulmonic valve closes, creating the dicrotic notch on the downslope of the waveform. Diastole follows closure of the pulmonic valve, as runoff of blood into the pulmonary vascular system occurs without any further blood flow from the RV. The PA diastolic pressure is measured immediately before the next systole and corresponds closely to the LVEDP, in the absence of pulmonary vascular and mitral valve disease. The normal PA diastolic pressure is 4 to 12 mmHg. Pulmonary artery mean pressure (PAM) is calculated, as is mean systemic arterial pressure. Normally the PAM pressure is 7 to 18 mmHg.

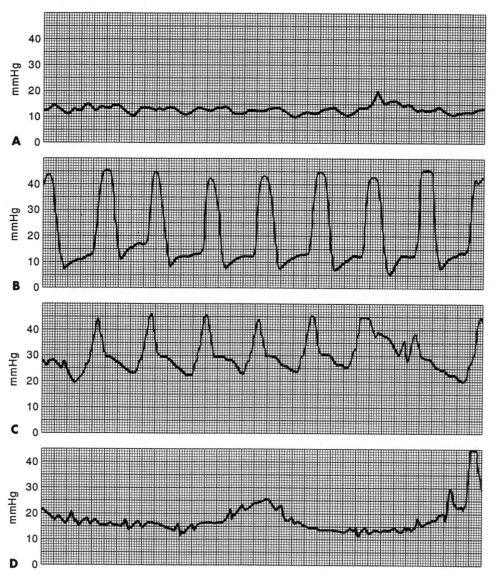

Fig. 7-49 Waveforms observed during insertion of a pulmonary artery catheter. **A,** Right atrial pressure. **B,** Right ventricular pressure. **C,** Pulmonary artery pressure. **D,** Pulmonary artery wedge pressure. (From Clochesy JM, Breu C, Cardin S et al, eds: *Critical care nursing,* Philadelphia, 1993, WB Saunders, p 165.)

Fig. 7-50 Normal right ventricular pressure waveform (*1,* isovolumetric contraction; *2,* rapid ejection; *3,* reduced ejection; *4,* isovolumetric relaxation; *5,* early diastole; *6,* atrial systole; *7,* end diastole). (From Daily EK, Schroeder JS: *Techniques in bedside hemodynamic monitoring,* St Louis, 1989, Mosby, p 108.)

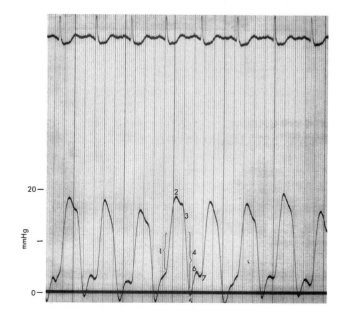

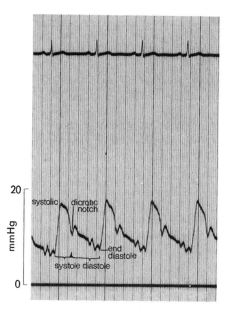

Fig. 7-51 Pulmonary artery (PA) pressure waveform showing phases of systole, dicrotic notch (pulmonic valve closure), and end diastole. Normally, PA end diastole closely represents LVEDP. (From Daily EK, Schroeder JS: *Techniques in bedside hemodynamic monitoring,* St Louis, 1989, Mosby, p 110.)

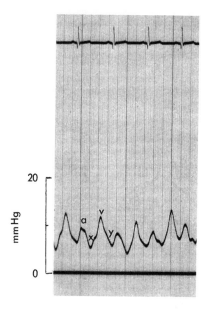

Fig. 7-52 Normal pulmonary artery wedge pressure waveform showing *a* and *v* waves and *x* and *y* descents. (From Daily EK, Schroeder JS: *Techniques in bedside hemodynamic monitoring,* St Louis, 1989, Mosby, p 116.)

The systolic pressure in the PA corresponds with ventricular depolarization. However, the length of the PA catheter and monitoring tubing delay the signal somewhat. PA systole occurs in the QT interval of the ECG.

High systolic PA pressures are the consequence of either increased PBF, as with a left-to-right intracardiac shunt, or increased PVR. Increased PVR is often observed in pulmonary disease, pulmonary artery hypertension, pulmonary embolism, and severe heart failure. The pulmonary artery diastolic (PAD) pressure may not accurately reflect the LVEDP in patients with pulmonary disease or pulmonary embolism. Tachycardias, which shorten the diastolic period of the cardiac cycle, falsely elevate the PAD pressure.

PA Wedge Pressure. When a PA catheter is properly positioned, inflation of the balloon results in movement of the catheter to a small branch of the pulmonary artery. The balloon then occludes the vessel and obstructs forward blood flow. The pressure measurement that is obtained is referred to as the PA wedge (PAW) pressure or PA occlusion pressure (PAOP). This pressure, transmitted across the pulmonary veins to the catheter tip, is approximately the same as LA pressure, and indicates LV filling pressure. The PAW pressure waveform is similar to the RA or LA waveform (*a* and *v* waves; most often the *c* wave cannot be seen) because the pressure is produced by the same physiologic events (Figure 7-52). Normal, resting PAW pressure is the same as LA pressure (i.e., 4 to 12 mmHg) and is measured as a mean pressure because the *a* and *v* waves normally are of the same amplitude.

As with atrial pressure monitoring, the *a* wave follows the PR interval on the ECG and the *v* wave follows the QRST interval. However, in PAW pressure monitoring, a longer delay occurs between electrical and mechanical

events because of the time lag between cardiac contraction and retrograde measurement in the pulmonary artery. In addition, the length of the catheter and tubing contribute to this lag time. The effects of rhythm disturbances on the PAW pressure measurement are the same as described with atrial pressure monitoring.

Abnormal PAW pressure occurs with a number of clinical problems. The *a* wave may be elevated (cannon *a* waves) with LV failure or mitral stenosis because these conditions increase the resistance to LV filling. In addition, any arrhythmia that interferes with AV synchrony (JET) will result in cannon *a* waves because the atria is contracting against a closed AV valve. The *v* wave is elevated with mitral regurgitation, which may be the consequence of either structural abnormality or severe LV failure (Figure 7-53). Elevated PAW pressure may also be the result of intravascular volume overload, cardiac tamponade, or pericardial effusion. Decreased PAW pressure is seen in patients with hypovolemia.

The PA diastolic pressure and the PAW pressure are usually within 1 to 5 mmHg of each other when PVR is low, pulmonary function is normal, and the mitral valve is competent. An increase in the PA diastolic pressure to the point that the gradient between it and the PAW pressure is greater than 5 mmHg can result from tachycardia, pulmonary artery hypertension, cor pulmonale, or pulmonary embolus. PAW pressure exceeds the PAD pressure only in patients with mitral regurgitation.

Technical Problems in PA Monitoring. Mechanical problems may interfere with accurate PA pressure monitoring. Dampening of the pressure waveform is the most common problem. The overdampened waveform loses sharp definition and appears rounded, the dicrotic notch is absent or poorly defined, the systolic pressure is measured falsely low, and the diastolic pressure is overestimated. Overdampening may be the result of technical problems that can be easily corrected. These include the use of an excessive number of stopcocks (no more than three are recommended[50]) and the presence of air bubbles, blood, loose connections, or kinked tubing. Excessively long or compliant pressure tubing may overdamp the system as well.

Overdampened pressure waveforms are also the consequence of problems with the catheter itself. Kinking of the catheter can occur at the insertion site or internally, the catheter can be wedged against the vessel wall, or fibrin can be deposited on the tip of the catheter. Problems with

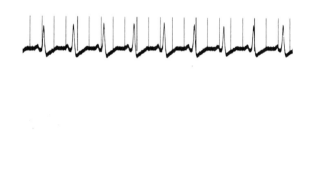

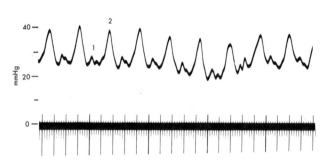

Fig. 7-53 Elevated pulmonary artery wedge pressure with a dominant and elevated *v* wave *(2)* as a result of mitral regurgitation. The *a* wave *(1)* is also elevated, indicating left ventricle (LV) failure. In this case, the mitral regurgitation is most likely functional secondary to LV failure and dilation. (From Daily EK, Schroeder JS: *Techniques in bedside hemodynamic monitoring,* St Louis, 1989, Mosby, p 119.)

catheter kinking or position may be resolved by repositioning the catheter. However, if fibrin or clot deposition is suspected, urokinase or t-PA can be used to clear the catheter or it will have to be replaced.

Exaggerated oscillations of the pressure waveform, referred to as catheter "fling" or "whip," can occur when blood flow is turbulent (Figure 7-54). This may occur if the catheter is located near the pulmonic valve or coiled in the RV or in patients with PAH or dilated pulmonary arteries.[53] Catheter repositioning will correct the problem if its location was the source of the difficulty. In the latter situations, accurate PA pressure monitoring is difficult at best and may be impossible. When catheter fling does not resolve, only the PAM pressure is measured (the PAD continues to be monitored for catheter migration into the RV).

Catheter migration can result in several technical problems during PA pressure monitoring. The catheter may spontaneously or accidentally migrate into the RV. The usual signs of this are the detection of the lower diastolic pressure (characteristic of the RV), presence of RV waveform on the monitor, and ventricular arrhythmias (usually PVCs). The catheter can most often be repositioned by withdrawing the catheter into the RA and reinflating the balloon, floating it out into the PA. Balloon inflation while the catheter is in the RV may damage RV trabecula.

Catheter migration into small pulmonary vessels can result in spontaneous wedging of the catheter. In spontaneous wedging, there is potential for loss of blood supply to a PA branch vessel with subsequent infarction. Overwedging of the PA catheter, caused by overinflation or uneven inflation of the balloon of the catheter, may result in PA rupture. Overwedging is avoided by careful assessment of the PA waveform as the balloon is inflated. The balloon is inflated only until the morphology of the atrial waveform is clearly appreciated (i.e., the appearance of *a* and *v* waves). Overinflation results in loss of the waveform characteristics and a linear increase or decrease in the pressure (Figure 7-55). If the catheter wedges at an unexpectedly low inflation volume or if spontaneous wedging occurs, prompt repositioning of the catheter is necessary.

Accurate pressure measurement is dependent on maintenance of the monitoring system. It is crucial that the phlebostatic axis be accurately determined and that the transducer be accurately leveled at this reference point. Changes in hemodynamic data may be the result from a

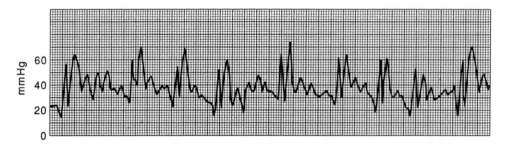

Fig. 7-54 Pulmonary artery pressure waveform with catheter "whip" or "fling." (From Clochesy JM, Breu C, Cardin S et al, eds: *Critical care nursing,* Philadelphia, 1993, WB Saunders, p 171.)

change in the patient's condition; however, before treatment measures are undertaken, it is important to assess the system for potential sources of error. A rapid assessment of the transducer position, and rezeroing of the system, as well as reassessment of the pressure waveform morphology, ensures that the data is accurate.

Clinical Factors in PA Monitoring. A number of physiologic and clinical factors affect PA pressure measurement. The first is *PBF.* Three physiologic zones of blood flow have been identified in the lungs.[67] These zones are not anatomic divisions but correspond to the interaction among pulmonary alveolar, arterial, and venous pressures and gravitational forces in each zone that affect resulting blood flow (Figure 7-56). Accurate PA pressure determination necessitates that the catheter be positioned where PBF is continuous (zone 3) and not affected by alveolar pressure. Only in this position does the PA reflect LA pressure. In zones 1 or 2, where alveolar pressure affects pulmonary flow, the PA pressure reflects alveolar pressure and not the downstream LA pressure.

Location of the catheter in zone 3 is confirmed by waveform analysis and chest radiograph. Lateral chest radiography, most accurately reveals that the tip of the PA catheter is below the level of the left atrium. Catheter location in zone 3 is also verified by the appearance of the characteristic atrial waveform when the PA catheter is wedged. If the catheter is located in zone 1 or 2, wedging produces marked respiratory variation and loss of the characteristic atrial pressure waveform.[16]

Pulmonary artery pressure (PAP) varies with both *spontaneous and mechanical ventilation.* During spontaneous breathing, the pressure in the pulmonary artery follows intrathoracic pressure (i.e., both the PA and PAW pressures fall during inspiration and rise with exhalation). All hemodynamic pressures are read at one point in the respiratory cycle, traditionally at end exhalation.

PEEP may be transmitted from the airways to the pulmonary blood vessels and alters all intrathoracic pressure readings. Note that this phenomenon is dependent on lung compliance; if the lungs are stiff and noncompliant, there may be little or no transmission of PEEP to the intrathorax. Discontinuing PEEP is not recommended to obtain pressure readings. First, if pressure readings are obtained without PEEP, the patient's clinical situation is not accurately depicted. Second, discontinuing PEEP can result in alveolar collapse, rapid movement of interstitial fluid into the alveoli, and deterioration in the patient's condition.[68] An estimation of the effects of PEEP can be calculated: every 5 cm of PEEP results in a 1.5-mmHg increase in PAW pressure (Figure 7-57). In general it is better to disregard the

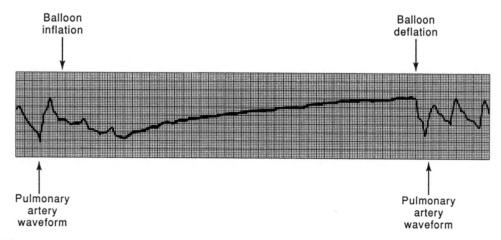

Fig. 7-55 Overwedging of the pulmonary artery catheter during balloon inflation. (From Clochesy JM, Breu C, Cardin S et al, eds: *Critical care nursing,* Philadelphia, 1993, WB Saunders, p 172.)

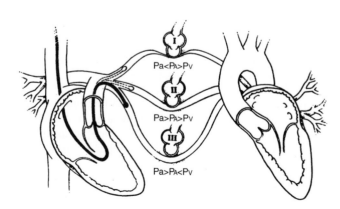

Fig. 7-56 Lung zones. Pulmonary artery wedge pressure estimates left atrial pressure (LAP) only when the catheter is in lung zone 3 (capillaries below left atrium level), allowing for a continuous column of blood to exist from catheter tip to left atrium. *Pa,* Pulmonary arterial pressure; *PA,* pulmonary alveolar pressure; *Pv,* pulmonary venous pressure. (Reprinted with permission from O'Quin R, Marini JJ: Pulmonary artery occlusion pressure: clinical physiology, measurement and interpretation, *Am Rev Respir Dis* 128:319-326, 1983.)

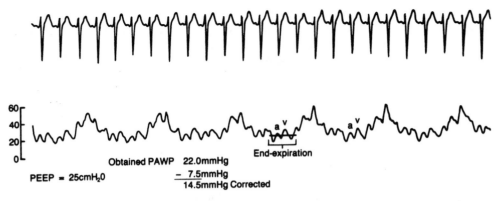

Fig. 7-57 Effects of positive end-expiratory pressure *(PEEP)* on measured pulmonary artery wedge pressure *(PAWP)*. (From Gardner RM: Pressure monitoring, *AACN Clin Issues Crit Care Nurs* 4:113, 1993.)

mathematical effects of PEEP on PA pressures and follow the data for trends. If a correction is made for the effect of PEEP on the PA pressure, it is important that all caregivers be consistent in the practice so that hemodynamic data is not misinterpreted.

Complications. Because central venous access is achieved for insertion of a PA catheter, the potential complications of adjacent tissue damage are present during PA catheterization. In addition, during flotation of the PA catheter, arrhythmias, heart valve damage, and intracardiac knotting of the catheter can occur. Intracardiac knotting requires manipulation of the catheter under fluoroscopy, withdrawal of the catheter, or, occasionally, surgical intervention. Tricuspid and pulmonary valve damage has been associated with prolonged PA catheterization.

Cardiac rhythm disturbances that occur during insertion of the PA catheter are usually self-limited. PVCs most often cease when the catheter has exited the right ventricle. If PVCs are sustained or if they progress to VT, the catheter is withdrawn into the right atrium until the ectopy subsides. Ectopy can reoccur following insertion and is usually associated with either looping of the catheter in the heart or migration into the ventricle. Rarely, a continuous infusion of lidocaine is necessary to prevent ectopy and increase patient tolerance of the PA catheter. Repositioning or removal of the catheter may be necessary if the rhythm disturbance is resistant to lidocaine.

Improper position of the PA catheter places the patient at risk for pulmonary infarction and PA rupture. Pulmonary infarction is most often the result of persistent wedging of the catheter in a peripheral pulmonary arteriole or obstruction of a more central artery by an inflated balloon. Prolonged balloon inflation is avoided and the catheter is repositioned if spontaneous wedging occurs.

PA rupture leads to massive hemorrhage and death. Risk factors for serious PA injury include PAH and hypothermia.[69] Imminent rupture may be preceded by only a small amount of pulmonary bleeding evidenced by hemoptysis or bloody endotracheal tube secretions. Fatal hemorrhage may occur without PA rupture in patients receiving anticoagulants. Usually PA bleeding and rupture are associated with distal migration of the catheter and subsequent balloon inflation. Children with PAH require extreme caution during balloon inflation and measurements of PAW pressure. The balloon should be inflated for only two to three respiratory cycles and for no longer than 10 to 15 seconds. If the PAD and PAW pressures correlate well, the PAD pressure is substituted for the PAW pressure and balloon inflation is limited.

Local and systemic infection can develop in patients with PA catheters. The risk for bacteremia increases when the catheter is in place for more than 72 hours or the insertion site is infected.[16] Diagnosis and treatment of the child with a catheter-related infection are the same as for any child with infection related to a central venous catheter.

Catheter Removal. The PA catheter is removed once the data obtained with it are no longer needed to guide clinical decision making and patient care. The catheter is removed in the same manner as a central venous catheter. In addition, as the catheter is withdrawn using a steady motion, the patient's ECG is observed for the presence of transient arrhythmias that can occur while the catheter is in the RV. If any resistance is encountered during removal, the procedure is discontinued until the patient can be assessed under fluoroscopy for catheter knotting or kinking. A knotted catheter may ensnare or perforate intracardiac structures with forced removal. When the catheter is completely withdrawn, hemostasis is achieved, and the insertion site is assessed and dressed with a dry, sterile dressing. The catheter is assessed to ascertain that it was removed in its entirety. The PA catheter is often exchanged for a multilumen central venous catheter placed over a wire to maintain central venous access.

Left Atrial Pressure Monitoring. Direct measurement of left atrial pressure (LAP) is reserved for cardiac surgical patients in whom a transthoracic catheter is placed at the time of operation. These catheters are used for continuous, accurate assessment of LV filling pressure and function during weaning and discontinuation of cardiopulmonary bypass, as well as during the acute postoperative period. RA and PA pressures may also be directly monitored after cardiac surgery.

LA Waveform Analysis. Analysis of the LA waveform is the same as that described for monitoring venous pressures. Given the proximity of the catheter to the mechanical events produced by the heart's electrical activity, the correlation between the ECG and the pressure waveform is close.

Complications and Catheter Removal. Transthoracic intracardiac monitoring of RAP and LAP has been associated with arrhythmias secondary to catheter dislodgment into the ventricle, difficult removal, and tamponade after catheter removal.[69] Although the incidence of complications is low, their potential risk is high and necessitates special caution at the time of catheter removal.

Ventricular arrhythmias (PVCs) or an abrupt change in the pressure and waveform indicates malposition of the catheter. If these conditions become manifest, the catheter must be repositioned or removed. LA lines are removed when the data is no longer necessary for patient management, before chest tube removal, and when coagulation profiles are normal. Mediastinal drainage with a chest tube must be ensured, and blood should be readily available if tamponade occurs.

Cardiac Output Determination. In the intensive care setting, CO is measured by techniques that are based on the Fick principle. The Fick principle uses the following relationships to determine CO:

$$CO = \dot{V}o_2 \div [Cao_2 - C\bar{v}o_2]$$

Under normal conditions, and in the absence of intracardiac or intrapulmonary shunt, the amount of blood ejected from the right ventricle equals the amount of blood ejected from the left ventricle.

The Fick principle states that the difference between the mixed venous and arterial oxygen content reflects oxygen uptake by the blood as it flows through the lungs. In the preceding equation, CO (the amount of blood flowing through the lungs) is equal to oxygen consumption divided by the difference between the oxygen saturations of mixed venous blood (flowing into the lungs) and arterial blood (leaving the lungs).

Calculation of CO with the Fick method requires collection and measurement of exhaled gas volume and oxygen content to determine $\dot{V}o_2$; or $\dot{V}o_2$ can be assumed by using predetermined tables, taking into consideration body surface area, age, sex, and HR. This measurement is considered the gold standard against which all other measurements of CO are made.[70] Until recently, this method was only used during cardiac catheterization. With the advent of continuous Spo_2 and Svo_2 monitoring, along with bedside metabolic monitoring, this method is used in some centers for continuous CO evaluation.[71] Inaccurate measurements are related to sampling errors of mixed venous blood or exhaled gases, the length of the time over which the measurements are made, and the presence of cardiac or pulmonary shunts.[72]

Indicator-Dilution Method. The indicator-dilution method of CO determination is based on the principle that if a known amount of indicator is added to an unknown quantity of blood flow, and the concentration of the indicator is measured downstream, this concentration, along with the timing of delivery, gives a measurement of flow.

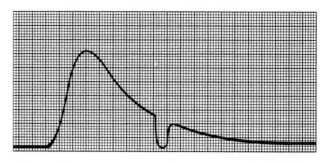

Fig. 7-58 Time-temperature cardiac output curve (From Clochesy JM, Breu C, Cardin S et al, eds: *Critical care nursing,* Philadelphia, 1993, WB Saunders, p 172.)

The usual indicator for CO determination is a nontoxic dye, indocyanine green, which is measured with a photodensitometer. A bolus of the dye is injected into the venous circulation, and blood is sampled from an artery through the densitometer to determine concentration. Use of the indicator-dilution method for determining CO has been refined to use a thermal indicator rather than dye. Dye dilution is rarely used in the critical care setting.

Thermodilution Method. The use of a thermal indicator was first introduced by Fegler in 1954 and further refined by Swan and Ganz in 1971.[73,74] This technique has become known as thermodilution and has been shown to be simple, rapid, accurate, and safe. Thermodilution uses a balloon-tipped PA catheter; therefore it measures blood flow through the pulmonary bed. In the absence of an intracardiac shunt, PBF equals systemic flow.

Thermodilution is a modification of the indicator-dilution technique, whereby a known volume at a known temperature of either 5% dextrose or normal saline is injected into the right atrium or one of the venae cavae through the proximal lumen of a PA catheter. The thermistor at the distal end of the PA catheter measures the temperature decrease of the blood as the cool solution (either room temperature or previously iced) passes through the heart, and a time-temperature curve is produced (Figure 7-58). A computer calculates the area beneath the curve and displays the CO in a measurement of liters per minute. The values obtained using thermodilution correlate well with the Fick method.[71] However, as with other CO measurement techniques, there are a number of potential sources of error in thermodilution CO determination (Table 7-5).

In addition, structural heart disease may alter CO data obtained by thermodilution. The presence of a left-to-right shunt will increase PBF and overestimate systemic CO. Conversely, obstruction to pulmonary flow will decrease PBF and underestimate systemic CO. Therefore structural heart disease may preclude the use of bedside thermodilution or at least prompt careful scrutiny of the obtained data.

Technical Consideration. Accurate CO measurement by thermodilution requires that the PA catheter be properly positioned to ensure that the thermistor can measure the temperature change occurring when the injectate is instilled. The PA waveform is assessed for damping or wedging caused by catheter migration.

TABLE 7-5   Potential Sources of Error in Thermodilution CO Measurement

Source of Error	Resulting Problem/Error
Faulty computer or cables	Wide discrepancy in CO measurements
Cable connection not secure	No readings
	PA or injectate temperature does not register
PA Catheter	
Clotted proximal lumen	Difficulty injecting solution; may be impossible to inject
Catheter malposition	Thermistor lying against small vessel wall because of catheter migration; CO curve has low amplitude
	Tip of catheter not in zone 3 lung; measured CO affected by ventilation
Catheter kinking at entrance site or within the heart	Difficulty injecting solution
Fibrin growth on catheter	Difficulty injecting solution; variations in core temperature measurements
Technique Related	
Incorrect injectate volume	CO values do not correspond to the patient's clinical condition
Incorrect computation constant entered in computer	
Injectate temperature outside specified range	
Uneven, prolonged injectate delivery	
Patient Related	
Patient movement during measurement	Variation in serial CO measurements
Cardiac arrhythmias	Oscillations of the baseline
Mechanical ventilation	
Low CO states	Recirculation of thermal indicator; prolonged baseline drift
Hypothermia	Low-amplitude CO curve because of small temperature difference between blood and injectate

CO, Cardiac output; *PA,* pulmonary artery.

The computation constant (specific to the catheter size, volume, and temperature of the injectate) and the patient's blood temperature, if not automatically measured and recorded, are entered into the CO computer. These values are incorporated into the computer's calculations to adjust for the expected warming of the injectate as it travels downstream. The connections between the injectate probe cable, the thermistor coupling, the catheter-connecting cable, and the computer are secured.

The patient is usually positioned supine with conservative elevations in the head of the bed (0 to 20 degrees). Flat positioning is not necessary because measurements taken in both the supine and modest head elevation positions have been found to correlate.[16]

Rapid, even injection within 2 to 4 seconds is essential to ensure a smooth time-temperature curve.[69] Injectate volumes are determined by patient and catheter size. Generally 5 or 10 ml are used; small thermodilution catheters used in infants have the capability to use 3-ml injectate volumes (if there is a corresponding computation constant on the package insert). Hemodynamically unstable infants may not tolerate frequent large injectate volumes because of volume overload; therefore, 3- to 5-ml volumes can be employed.[71] Both iced and room temperature injectate can be used. Iced injectate produces a larger thermal signal than solution kept at room temperature and (given the lack of pediatric data) should be used when injectate volumes are less than 10 ml.

Timing of the injection with end expiration produces less variable results because the effects of the phase of respira-tion on PA temperature are eliminated. End-expiration is judged most convenient and is most often used.

The CO computer displays the calculated CO approximately 15 seconds after the injection. A second and a third determination of CO are made, separated by 45 to 90 seconds. The three measurements are averaged, unless a measurement falls outside 10% of the middle value. In a series, a CO value that falls outside the standard error of the estimate (10%) is discarded, and the remaining two are averaged or a fourth measurement is made.

Accuracy of the measurement is also assessed by inspection of the thermodilution curve. The configuration should be smooth with a rapid upslope to peak and a gradual downslope to the baseline (see Figure 7-58).

Hemodynamic Calculations. CO, calculated in liters per minute (L/min), is the basis for calculation of a number of additional, derived hemodynamic indices (Box 7-4). The first is cardiac index, which is the most accurate expression of CO in children because of variability in patient size. Calculations are performed automatically by the CO computer, necessitating that data entry be accurate.

SV is equal to CO divided by the HR during the CO determination. Normal SV depends on the patient's size and activity level. SV index is obtained by dividing SV by the patient's body surface area. As with cardiac index, this normalizes the measurement to the patient's size.

The stroke work of the ventricle is a measure of the ventricle's work during any one cardiac contraction, as well

Box 7-4
Derived Hemodynamic Parameters

Cardiac Index (CI)

Normal = 2.5 to 5 L/min/m^2

CI = Cardiac output/Body surface area

Stroke Index (SI)

Normal = 30 to 60 ml/beat/m^2

SI = Cardiac index/Heart rate

Stroke Work Index (SWI)

LVSWI Normal = 56 ± 6 g-m/m^2

LVSWI = (MAP − PAWP) × SI × 0.0136

RVSWI Normal = 6 ± 0.9 g-m/m^2

RVSW = (PAM − CVP) × SI × 0.0136

Where:

LV = left ventricular

RV = right ventricular

CVP = central venous pressure

MAP = mean arterial pressure

PAM = pulmonary artery mean (pressure)

PAWP = pulmonary artery wedge pressure

SI = stroke index

0.0136 = conversion factor for pressure to work (measured in grams)

Systemic Vascular Resistance Index (SVRI)*

SVRI = MAP − CVP/CI × 80

Normal = 800-1600 dynes/sec/cm^{-5} or

       10-15 Woods units/m^2 infants;

15-20 Woods units/m^2 1-2 years;

15-30 Woods units/m^2 child/adolescent

Where:

MAP = mean arterial pressure

CVP = central venous pressure

CI = cardiac index

Pulmonary Vascular Resistance Index (PVRI)

PVRI = PAM − PAWP(or LAP)/CI × 80

Normal = 80-240 dynes/sec/cm^{-5} or

       1-3 Woods units/m^2 over 8 weeks of age;

8-10 Woods units/m^2 under 8 weeks of age

Where:

PAM = pulmonary artery mean (pressure)

PAWP = pulmonary artery wedge pressure

CI = cardiac index

LAP = left atrial pressure

*Vascular resistance can be expressed as dynes/sec/cm^{-5} or Woods units. Dynes/sec/cm^{-5} are primarily used in the ICU and Woods units in the cardiac catheterization laboratory. Dynes/sec/cm^{-5} can be converted to Woods units by dividing by 80.

Box 7-5
Indications for Cardiac Catheterization

Define cardiovascular anatomy: The morphology, position, relations, and connections of the:
    Systemic and pulmonary veins
    Atria
    Atrioventricular valves
    Ventricles and outflow tracts
    Proximal pulmonary and systemic arteries
    Peripheral pulmonary and systemic arteries
Measure and calculate central and peripheral hemodynamics:
    Blood pressure in the systemic and pulmonary arteries and veins
    Blood flow in the systemic and pulmonary circulation
    Calculate shunts
    Calculate vascular resistance in the pulmonary and systemic beds
    Calculate valve areas
Evaluate cardiac pump function
Evaluate cardiac muscle function
Monitor changes in hemodynamics and cardiac function in response to drug, respirator, or surgical interventions
Electrophysiologic studies and therapy
Myocardial biopsy

work is decreased with poor myocardial contractility, as is seen in patients with CHF or shock.

Vascular resistance is another index of ventricular work, representative of the force a ventricle must overcome to eject its contents. To calculate SVR, the difference between the MAP and CVP is divided by the CO. To calculate PVR, the difference between the MAP and LA (or wedge) pressure is divided by the CO. Both SVR and PVR measurements are also indexed to the patient's size using CI as the denominator.

Cardiac Catheterization

Cardiac catheterization provides complete evaluation of cardiac anatomy and hemodynamic function. Angiography provides detailed information on coronary artery anatomy, pulmonary collaterals, size and continuity of the branch pulmonary arteries, cardiac chamber size, valvar size, ventricular function, and ventricular septal defect (VSD) size and location, to name a few. Measurement of intracardiac and peripheral hemodynamics aid in the assessment of physiologic sequelae of heart disease. Because of technologic refinements in echocardiography, diagnostic catheterization and angiography are generally only necessary in patients with unusual anatomy or inadequate echocardiographic windows. Not all patients with heart disease require a cardiac catheterization (Box 7-5). The decision to perform a catheterization should be carefully made based on patient need. If the procedure or data obtained will not alter patient care, then it may not be necessary.

Currently, interventional procedures for palliation or treatment of congenital heart disease are performed during

as an indicator of the effectiveness of the heart's pumping function or functional capacity. Stroke work is the product of the average pressure generated by the ventricle during contraction multiplied by the SV ejected with that beat. Stroke work is also indexed to the size of the patient. Hypertension or increased vascular resistance, as well as hypervolemia, increases the ventricle's stroke work. Stroke

TABLE 7-6   Normal Hemodynamic Values Obtained at Cardiac Catheterization

	a Wave	v Wave	Mean	Systolic	End Diastolic	Mean
Pressures (mmHg)						
Right atrium	2-10	2-10	0-8			
Right ventricle				15-30	0-8	
Pulmonary artery				15-30	3-12	9-16
PAW, left atrium	3-15	3-12	1-10			
Left ventricle				100-140	3-12	
Systemic arteries				100-140	60-90	70-105

Oxygen consumption index	110-150 (ml/min/m^2) at rest
Arteriovenous oxygen difference	30-50 ml/L or 3-5 ml/dl
Cardiac index	2.5-5 (L/min/m^2)

Resistances (Woods units/m^2)

Pulmonary vascular:	Under 8 weeks of age	8-10
	Over 8 weeks of age	1-3
Systemic vascular:	Infant	10-15
	1-2 years	15-20
	Child/adolescent	15-30

PAW, Pulmonary artery wedge.

catheterization. Therefore although diagnostic procedures are performed often, interventional procedures continue to keep most pediatric catheterization laboratories very busy.

Precatheterization assessment is critically important to define the goals of the procedure and to prevent any potential complications. A history, physical, and pertinent laboratory investigations should be performed. Laboratory data include a complete blood count because the hemoglobin and hematocrit values are used in hemodynamic calculations. Acid-base, electrolyte, and glucose abnormalities should be corrected beforehand. A two-dimensional echocardiogram should be obtained on all children before cardiac catheterization to evaluate basic cardiac and venous anatomy. These data assist in planning for vascular access and help to minimize the use of contrast. Neonates, critically ill patients, or those undergoing prolonged or interventional procedures require deep sedation and intubation to provide stabilization and prevent movement at inopportune times.[75] It is possible to transport patients supported by extracorporeal membrane oxygenation (ECMO) or ventricular assist devices (VADs) to the catheterization laboratory if it is believed that the data obtained will elucidate the nature of the patient's problem or determine future therapeutic intervention.

The right side of the heart, the left side, or both may be accessed according to the patient's anatomy or therapeutic need. Right-sided heart catheterization is accomplished by cannulation of the femoral vein, although the axillary, umbilical (in neonates), or brachial can also be used. The catheter is then passed antegrade in to the right side of the heart.[76] Many children with complex congenital heart disease have had multiple vascular procedures that adversely affect venous access. In these patients, percutaneous

transhepatic puncture is advocated. For this procedure, a puncture is made in the lower margin of the liver, and a sheath is placed under fluoroscopic guidance. A needle and guidewire can then be advanced through the liver into the hepatic vein and toward the right atrium.[77] The left side of the heart can be accessed retrograde via the femoral artery. If the foramen ovale is patent or in the presence of an ASD, the left side of the heart is accessed from the right atrium; or a transeptal puncture across the atrial septum is used to gain access to the left side of the heart. Any time the left side of the heart is entered, the patient should be systemically anticoagulated (usually with heparin).

Hemodynamic measurements can be obtained during cardiac catheterization. Hemodynamic indices include intracardiac pressures and waveforms, pressure gradients across the valves, cardiac index, shunt determinations, and calculation of vascular resistances (Table 7-6). In addition, changes in hemodynamics can be monitored following intervention with drugs, oxygen, nitric oxide, or changes in modes of ventilation. Blood sampling from different chambers in the heart allows measurement of oxygen saturation (Figure 7-59). Intracardiac differences in oxygen saturation aid in the calculation of shunt and CO indices.

Interventional catheterization is used to palliate or treat congenital defects. Specific procedures include atrial septostomy, balloon valvuloplasty, balloon dilation, and coil or stent placement. Atrial septostomy is often performed under echocardiographic guidance to palliate transposition of the great arteries, tricuspid atresia, or pulmonary atresia with intact ventricular septum. However, in those patients with a thick atrial septum, this procedure is aided by fluoroscopy in the catheterization laboratory. Balloon valvuloplasty, or dilation, is an attractive option that can delay or prevent

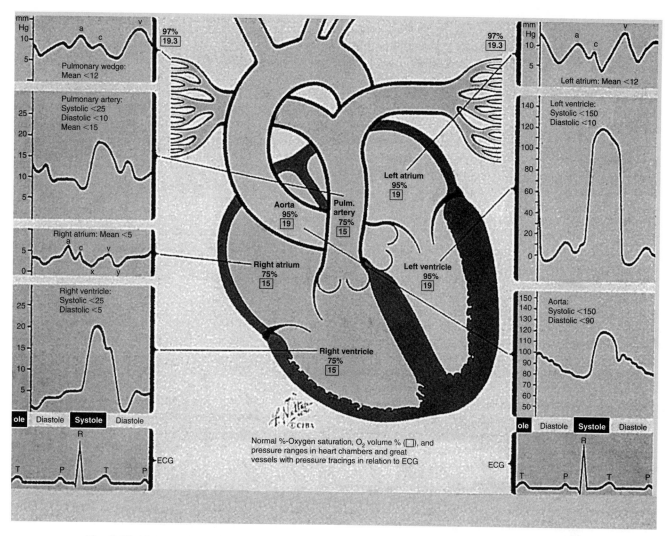

Fig. 7-59 Hemodynamic indices and oxygen saturation normal values measured at cardiac catheterization. (© Copyright 1996. CIBA-GEIGY Corporation. Reprinted with permission from the Ciba Collection of Medical Illustrations, illustrated by Frank Netter, M.D. All rights reserved.)

surgical intervention for pulmonary or aortic stenosis. Indeed, this procedure is the treatment of choice for valvar pulmonary stenosis (PS), including critical PS in the newborn.[75,78] Aortic valve dilation is best accomplished if the valve is trileaflet or bicuspid. Unicuspid or severely dysplastic valves do not respond as well and can be left with severe aortic regurgitation after the procedure.[78,79] Coil embolization is used to occlude patent ductus arteriosus (PDA), unwanted systemic or venous collaterals, and coronary artery fistulas. In some centers, PDA embolization is the treatment of choice, avoiding surgery[80]; The exception to this is the very small premature infant, whose size precludes coil embolization. Collateral vessels are embolized if they contribute to persistent cyanosis or if they interfere with PBF. Intravascular stents are used in a number of conditions, including peripheral pulmonary stenosis that is distal to the hilum of the lung, recurrent coarctation of the aorta, conduit, and postoperative vessel stenosis.[75,81] This intervention has replaced surgery in many instances. In

addition, a number of stents respond to repeat balloon dilation if stenosis subsequently occurs.[82] Device closure for ASD and VSD is currently under Food and Drug Administration (FDA) investigation at select centers.

Electrophysiology (EP) study is the evaluation of normal and abnormal impulse conduction performed in the catheterization laboratory. Often a special EP laboratory is designed specifically for this procedure. EP study can either be an intracardiac evaluation (using catheters with monitoring and pacing electrodes) or a transesophageal evaluation (using a transesophageal electrode and pacing catheter). Indications include but are not limited to evaluation of mechanisms and characteristics of abnormal tachycardia, determination of response to therapy (pharmacologic, ablative, or surgical), determination of risk for sudden death in WPW syndrome, evaluation of sinus node function in patients with sinus node disease, and identification of arrhythmia focus. The most common reason for radiofrequency catheter ablation in pediatrics is the treatment of

SVT.[83] Once an arrhythmogenic focus or accessory connection is identified, radiofrequency catheter ablation can be used to generate thermal injury, creating a localized lesion that results in arrhythmia eradication. Currently a multicenter study is under way to evaluate the long-term outcomes and complications in pediatric patients undergoing radiofrequency catheter ablation.

Complications associated with cardiac catheterization include bleeding, vessel thrombosis, arrhythmia, and cardiac tamponade, and vessel perforation. The independent risk of complication increases with young age (<2 years), critical illness, and during interventional procedures, for example, devices or stents. Rarely, cerebral embolism or death can occur.[84]

PHARMACOLOGIC SUPPORT OF CARDIOVASCULAR FUNCTION

Management of acute cardiovascular dysfunction is multifaceted. It may require (1) restoration of adequate, but not excessive, intravascular fluid volume; (2) improvement of myocardial contractility; (3) treatment of abnormal vascular capacitance and resistance; or (4) correction of abnormal cardiac rate or rhythm. Chronic cardiovascular dysfunction is managed from these same perspectives; inotropes are administered to improve contractility, with diuretics given to decrease volume load. New guidelines for care of adults with chronic heart failure emphasize control of the underlying neurohormonal response to inadequate tissue perfusion. The SNS, renin-angiotensin system, and endocrine system individually and in combination influence cardiovascular performance in patients with chronic heart failure. Angiotensin-converting enzyme (ACE) inhibitors, β-blockers, aldosterone antagonists, angiotensin-receptor blockers, and digoxin are used for the purpose of "resetting" neurohormonal balance.[85] Appropriate long-term pediatric studies of heart failure are needed. Chronic cardiac rhythm disturbances are currently managed with pharmacotherapy or radiofrequency catheter ablation of the arrhythmogenic substrate. Heart failure and arrhythmias are discussed further in Chapter 18.

Compared with adults, immature animals and humans respond differently to many medications. The response of neonates to inotropes is attenuated.[86] This may be the consequence of developmental differences in the concentration of adrenergic receptors in a variety of target organs.[87,88] Differences including reduced ventricular compliance, greater ventricular interdependence, and reduced myocardial contractile protein in the immature heart point to structural and ultrastructural differences that are clinically important. As a related consequence, when compared with older infants and adults, the young infant's heart does not tolerate or respond well to volume loading. Care of critically ill infants and children necessitates that caregivers appreciate both the limited response to augmented preload and the reduced sensitivity of the heart and vasculature to adrenergic agents, characteristic of some patients in the PICU. An important caveat to efficacy is that infants and children are subject to maturational factors and adults are not.

The practical consequences of these differences have not all been established; consequently, a precise age-based paradigm for pharmacotherapy is not yet possible. Most new drugs have not been adequately tested in pediatric patients because of real and perceived barriers. Insufficient pediatric sample size is an impediment to adequate clinical trials. Many medications approved for use with adult patients and used in children do not have FDA-approved labeling. The pediatric dose of these medications is extrapolated from the usual adult dose. The National Institutes of Health have established a unit for pediatric pharmacology research, and the FDA now requires expanded information about pediatric use for all prescription medications.[89] Scientific, randomized clinical trials, as opposed to anecdotal reports, will provide the data necessary to determine pediatric safety, efficacy, and dosing.[90] Pharmacologic management of all critically ill patients requires vigilant assessment of drug effect and side effect. However, special considerations are necessary when dosing medications for pediatric patients: infants and children continue to lack access to safety and effectiveness data.

Intravascular Volume Restoration

Volume expansion to restore preload and ventricular filling is essential in circumstances involving either absolute (abnormal fluid losses) or relative (maldistributed fluid volume) hypovolemia. Vascular access is of primary importance, followed by the timing and volume of fluid administered. It is critical to restore adequate perfusion before irreversible tissue ischemia occurs. Aliquots of normal saline (10 to 20 ml/kg) or 5% albumin (5 to 10 ml/kg) can be safely administered to pediatric patients over 1 to 15 minutes and repeated in 15 minutes. Two important exceptions to the practice of fluid resuscitation in pediatric practice are patients in cardiogenic shock and premature infants at risk for intraventricular hemorrhage.

Important initial physiologic responses to fluid administration are a decrease in HR, broadening of the pulse pressure or increase in BP (if hypotension was detected), and improvement in the quality of peripheral pulses. Fluid administration continues until perfusion of the skin, kidneys, and central nervous system (CNS) improves, as evidenced by brisk capillary refill and warm extremities, adequate urine output, and appropriate level of consciousness. Infusion of 60 to 100 ml/kg of fluid may be required over a brief period for patients with marked intravascular volume depletion.

Diuretic Therapy.   The kidneys respond to inadequate renal perfusion by increasing sodium reabsorption. Volume expansion follows, leading to systemic and pulmonary circulatory congestion and elevated end-diastolic volume and pressure. The fundamental aim is improving renal perfusion with inotropic or vasodilating agents. However, managing the relative fluid volume overload is critical. Diuretic therapy interferes with sodium reabsorption at various sites along the nephron and increases excretion of water. An integral part of treating CHF, diuretic therapy decreases ventricular dilation and improves diastolic function by lessening the hemodynamic load and producing a more efficient volume-pressure relationship. Pulmonary and peripheral edema are decreased, and the work of breathing is eased.[91,92]

Three classes of diuretics are commonly used to lessen the congestion caused by heart failure in infants and children.[85] Loop diuretics, primarily furosemide, are potent medications that have a rapid onset and provoke brisk diuresis, especially when administered parenterally. Thiazides, such as chlorothiazide, act in the distal tubules. Thiazides are less potent than loop diuretics and are more affected by low CO and reduced glomerular filtration rate. Potassium-sparing diuretics, spironolactone for example, also act in the distal tubule. They are weak diuretics most often added to therapy to counteract the potassium depletion, which occurs with either loop diuretics or thiazides.

Furosemide. Furosemide is a potent loop diuretic that inhibits the reabsorption of sodium and chloride in the ascending loop of Henle and the distal renal tubule by interfering with the chloride binding transport system. Consequently, excretion of water, sodium, chloride, magnesium, and calcium is increased. Its primary use is to decrease the congestion and edema associated with heart failure and hepatic or renal disease in infants and children.

Furosemide is administered intravenously to patients with acute or decompensated heart failure. The usual dose is 1 to 2 mg/kg IV, and the dose can be repeated every 6 to 12 hours. The onset of action occurs within 5 minutes of IV administration; duration of action is 2 hours. Furosemide can be administered undiluted, direct IV, at a maximum rate of 0.5 mg/kg/min. When large doses (greater than 120 mg) are required, the rate of administration should not exceed 4 mg/min. It can also be diluted to a concentration of 1 to 2 mg/ml and infused over 10 to 15 minutes. Continuous infusion of 0.05 mg/kg/hr is titrated for clinical effectiveness. Most often reserved for patients with refractory edema, continuous infusion maintains a constant blood level of diuretic and elicits diuresis by limiting any opportunity for the kidneys to retain sodium.[85]

The oral dose of furosemide is 1 to 6 mg/kg/day divided every 6 to 12 hours. It may be administered with milk or food to decrease the gastrointestinal distress associated with the oral solution. Onset of action is within 30 to 60 minutes following oral administration, and duration of action is 6 to 8 hours.

Loop diuretics are potent; profound diuresis with excessive volume and/or electrolyte loss can occur. The cardiovascular effects include hypovolemia and hypotension. Orthostatic hypotension can persist with dizziness, vertigo, and headache accompanying it. Dehydration, hypokalemia, hyponatremia, hypochloremia, and metabolic alkalosis can develop. The oral solutions are manufactured with sorbitol, which may cause diarrhea. Anorexia, vomiting, constipation, and abdominal cramping are other gastrointestinal adverse reactions. Ototoxicity associated with furosemide may be transient or permanent. The risk for ototoxicity is increased in the preterm infant and when other ototoxic medications are administered concurrently (aminoglycosides). The risk for ototoxicity may be minimized through the use of continuous rather than bolus infusion to prevent peak serum levels.[93]

Ethacrynic Acid. Ethacrynic acid is a potent loop diuretic with actions and adverse reactions like those of furosemide. Most often, it is used in hospitalized patients with critical, acute cardiac failure or those with refractory CHF. An oral preparation for long-term administration is available.

Ethacrynic acid is diluted with 5% dextrose or normal saline to a concentration of 1 mg/ml and injected over several minutes or infused over 20 to 30 minutes. It is a tissue irritant; extravasation is avoided, and intramuscular or subcutaneous injection is contraindicated. The usual intravenous or oral dose is 1 mg/kg/dose. Repeat intravenous doses are not routinely recommended; however, if indicated, repeat doses are administered every 8 to 12 hours. The oral dose can be increased at intervals of 2 or 3 days to a maximum of 3 mg/kg/day.[94]

Acute cardiovascular, fluid, and electrolyte adverse reactions are like those of furosemide. Potassium depletion can be pronounced. Oral preparations are administered with food or milk to minimize gastrointestinal irritation, which is also more pronounced than with furosemide. Ototoxicity and tinnitus can occur.

Bumetanide. Bumetanide is a potent loop diuretic that inhibits reabsorption of sodium and chloride in the ascending loop of Henle, resulting in subsequent excretion of water, sodium, chloride, magnesium, calcium, and phosphate. Primary indications for use are treatment of refractory edema secondary to CHF, hepatic disease, or renal disease.

Bumetanide can be administered intravenously, intramuscularly, or orally. Doses are equivalent regardless of the administrative route. Usual dose in neonates is 0.01 to 0.05 mg/kg/dose every 24 to 48 hours. Infants and children require 0.015 to 0.1 mg/kg/dose every 6 to 24 hours, with a maximum dose of 10 mg/day. Oral preparations should be administered with food to prevent gastrointestinal upset. IV preparations are administered without additional dilution over 1 to 2 minutes.

Contraindications include anuria and hypersensitivity. Adverse reactions include profound diuresis with excessive water and electrolyte loss, hypotension, nausea, muscle weakness, and increased liver enzymes. The risk for hypotension increases if given concurrently with other hypertensive agents or ACE inhibitors.

Chorothiazide. Chlorothiazide is used in the management of edema associated with CHF or nephrotic syndrome. It inhibits sodium reabsorption in the distal tubules, causing increased excretion of sodium, chloride, potassium, bicarbonate, magnesium, phosphate, and water. Because it acts at the distal tubule, chlorothiazide is less potent and less effective than the loop diuretics in low-CO states when the glomerular filtration rate is decreased.

The oral dose of chlorothiazide is 20 mg/kg/day in two divided doses. Infants less than 6 months of age may require up to 40 mg/kg/day. It is available in tablet and oral suspension; both are administered with food. The IV dose for infants and children has not been established. Doses are extrapolated from the oral doses and have been used safely.[94] The IV dose is 4 mg/kg/day in two divided doses; infants younger than 6 months receive doses of 2 to 8 mg/kg/day. IV doses are administered by direct infusion over several minutes or infused in dextrose or normal saline over 30 minutes. Extravasation of the parenteral solution is avoided because the drug is irritating to tissue. The solution must not be injected intramuscularly or subcutaneously.

Adverse reactions are similar to those associated with the loop diuretics. Hypotension, hypokalemia, and hypochloremic alkalosis can occur, as can similar gastrointestinal side effects. There are rare instances of prerenal azotemia, intrahepatic cholestasis, and blood dyscrasias.

Metolazone. Metolazone is thiazide diuretic that inhibits sodium reabsorption in the distal tubules, producing increased excretion of water and sodium. It is used to manage the edema associated with CHF and renal impairment. The most common indications for use in children are the treatment of postoperative edema and/or CHF that is not responsive to loop diuretics. Metolazone is administered orally. The usual dosage in children is 0.2 to 0.4 mg/kg/day divided every 12 to 24 hours, and it should be administered with food to prevent gastrointestinal upset.

Contraindications to use include anuria, hepatic coma, and hypersensitivity to metolazone, sulfa drugs, or thiazide diuretics. Adverse reactions include orthostatic hypotension, vertigo, headache, electrolyte abnormalities, nausea, and blood dyscrasias. If given concurrently with digoxin, there is an increased risk for digoxin toxicity secondary to potassium and magnesium depletion.[94]

Spironolactone. Spironolactone is a potassium-sparing diuretic used to manage edema seen with excessive aldosterone excretion (which may occur with chronic heart failure or primary hyperaldosteronism), hypokalemia, and hypertension. It competes with aldosterone for receptor binding sites in the distal renal tubule. It may also block aldosterone's effect on arterial smooth muscle. At the kidney, it increases sodium, chloride, and water excretion while conserving potassium and hydrogen ions. Spironolactone is a weak diuretic most often added to therapy to counteract the potassium-depleting effect of loop diuretics and thiazides.

Spironolactone is administered orally in doses of 1 to 3 mg/kg/day (or 60 mg/m^2/day). It may be administered in a single dose or divided 2 to 4 times.

Spironolactone can cause lethargy and drowsiness. Gastrointestinal effects are like those of other diuretic agents. Azotemia can develop. Spironolactone is tumorigenic in rats treated with 25 to 250 times the usual human dose.[94]

Inotropic Therapy

Increased intracellular calcium concentration is the central cellular event that enhances the contractility of the myocardium. Drugs that improve the inotropic performance of the myocardium act at one of several steps in the sequence of events that couple electrical excitation and mechanical contraction. Cyclic adenosine monophosphate (cAMP) is a pivotal mediator in many of the reactions that produce myocardial contraction. Increased intracellular cAMP ultimately increases intracellular calcium concentration, which affects myocardial systolic and diastolic function and HR. The catecholamines augment cardiac contractility by action that simulates the SNS receptors to increase cAMP concentration within the cell. Phosphodiesterase (PDE) inhibitors also increase intracellular cAMP. Digitalis glycosides enhance contractility by a route not dependent on cAMP.

Sympathetic Nervous System (Adrenergic) Stimulation. Sympathomimetic agents interact with cell surface adrenergic receptors. Adrenergic receptors are glycoproteins with genetically related structure. They extend between the internal and external surfaces of the cell membrane and are transducers of signals or information across the cell membrane; that is, stimulation of an adrenergic receptor elicits an intracellular response. Table 7-7 is a classification of the adrenergic receptors and indicates the physiologic responses to stimulation of each. The medications listed (in order of their potency) are receptor agonists. With the exception of the α_1 receptor, adrenergic receptors affect cell function by increasing the intracellular concentration of cAMP.

Adrenergic receptors' sensitivity to stimulation changes with a number of factors. Exposure of the receptors to sympathomimetic agents causes receptor desensitization. Endotoxin, tumor necrosis factor, and CHF also cause receptor desensitization.

Phosphodiesterase Inhibition. The methylxanthines (theophylline) and the bipyridines (amrinone, milrinone) inhibit the PDE that inactivates cAMP, thereby increasing cAMP concentration and leading to higher intracellular calcium and enhanced contractility. The PDE inhibitors are called *inodilators* because of their additional vasodilatory effect. The bipyridines selectively inhibit only PDE III, whereas the methylxanthines inhibit all three known types of PDE. Consequently, the inotropic action of amrinone and milrinone is more selective, compared with the limited inotropic and marked chronotropic actions of theophylline.[95]

Digitalis Glycosides. The digitalis glycosides act on the heart through a mechanism independent of cAMP, but the final outcome, increased intracellular calcium, is similar.[85,96] Digoxin inhibits the sodium-potassium pump, thereby increasing intracellular sodium concentration. The secondary consequence is a shift in the sodium and calcium exchange in favor of retaining more calcium within the cell. The increase in intracellular calcium concentration translates into a positive inotropic effect.

Digoxin has been shown to exert a favorable neurohormonal effect, which occurs before and is separate from its inotropic effect in adult patients. Through a mechanism not yet clear, it potentiates parasympathetic discharge, which decreases sympathetic outflow. Inhibition of sympathetic discharge is likely accomplished by inhibition of the baroreceptor sodium-potassium pump. The neurohormonal effects of digoxin have not yet been studied in children. In

TABLE 7-7   Adrenergic Receptors, Physiologic Responses, and Sympathomimetic Agonists

Receptor	Physiologic Responses	Agonist
α_1	Increase intracellular Ca, muscle contraction, vasoconstriction, inhibit insulin secretion	Epinephrine Norepinephrine Dopamine
α_2	Decrease cAMP, inhibit NE release, vasodilation, negative chronotropy	Epinephrine Norepinephrine
β_1	Increase cAMP, inotropy, chronotropy, enhance renin secretion	Isoproterenol Epinephrine Dopamine Norepinephrine
β_2	Increase cAMP, smooth muscle relaxation, vasodilation, bronchodilation, enhance glucagon secretion, hypokalemia	Isoproterenol Epinephrine Dopamine Norepinephrine
D_1	Increase cAMP, smooth muscle relaxation	Dopamine
D_2	Decrease cAMP, inhibit prolactin and β-endorphin	Dopamine

Modified from Notterman DA: Pharmacologic support of the failing circulation: an approach for infants and children, *Probl Anesth* 3:288-294, 1989.
Ca, Calcium; *cAMP*, cyclic adenosine monophosphate; *NE*, norepinephrine; *D*, dopamine.

 TABLE 7-8   Recommended Digoxin Doses for Pediatric Patients

Intravenous Digitalization	Enteral Digitalization
Total digitalizing dose = 30 µg/kg/24 hours Maximum dose = 800 µg IV First dose: Digoxin 15 µg/kg IV Digoxin 7.5 µg/kg IV 8 hours after first dose Digoxin 7.5 µg/kg IV 8 hours after second dose Begin maintenance digoxin (7.5 µg/kg/day) 12 hours after third dose	Total digitalizing dose = 40 µg/kg/24 hours Maximum dose = 1 mg PO/NG First dose: Digoxin 20 µg/kg PO/NG Digoxin 10 µg/kg PO/NG 8 hours after first dose Digoxin 10 µg/kg PO/NG 8 hours after second dose Begin maintenance digoxin (10 µg/kg/day) 12 hours after third dose

NG, Nasogastric (tube).

those with heart failure from a large left-to-right shunt, contractility is often normal. The ameliorative effects of digoxin in this group of pediatric patients suggest that modulation of the autonomic nervous system may be valuable.[85]

Cardiac glycosides are prescribed for patients in whom poor myocardial contractility is expected to persist beyond a few days. The elevated HR associated with CHF is reduced by digoxin. In patients with chronic CHF, digoxin remains a mainstay of pharmacologic therapy.

Digoxin increases myocardial contractility in normal and diseased hearts. When CHF is present, digoxin increases SV and reduces elevated ventricular filling pressures. When digoxin is administered to infants, contractility increases, as judged by echocardiographic examination. Adult patients with acute heart failure who were given a single dose of digoxin experienced a 69% increase in LV stroke work index, a 25% reduction in PAW pressure, and a 16% to 28% increase in cardiac index.[97] Similar invasive hemodynamic measurements have not been made in infants or children.

The kidney eliminates digoxin. Renal dysfunction that impairs glomerular filtration interferes with elimination. Hypokalemia increases digoxin binding to cell receptor sites, accounting in part for digoxin-induced cardiac rhythm disturbances during hypokalemia.

Dosage and Administration.   Infants and young children eliminate digoxin rapidly and have a large volume of distribution for the drug. Consequently, they require higher doses of digoxin than do adults to achieve a therapeutic plasma level of 0.8 to 2 ng/ml. Dosage is based on the age of the patient, the indication for therapy, the route of administration, and the presumed sensitivity of the myocardium to potential toxicity.[96] There is substantial individual variation in response to "usual" doses.[94] Table 7-8 indicates the recommended digoxin doses for pediatric patients. It is important to note that inadequate renal function, electrolyte imbalance, or evidence of myocardial irritability (i.e., arrhythmia) necessitates that the doses be reduced and, during digitalization, the pace of digitalizing be slowed. Not all patients require a digitalizing dose during drug initiation.

The need for digitalization is determined by the child's clinical condition and physician preference.

Serum digoxin levels are of limited benefit as a guide to therapeutic response because there is wide variability in the serum concentration required to achieve the desired response. However, serum digoxin levels are of benefit to ensure that the dose given is sufficient to achieve a measurable blood concentration and to confirm the clinical suspicion of toxicity. Serum levels are obtained 8 to 12 hours after a dose of digoxin, preferably just before the next scheduled dose. HR, rhythm, and the ECG; serum potassium, magnesium, and calcium; and blood urea nitrogen (BUN) are closely monitored to avoid toxicity. Serum drug concentration, in combination with clinical symptoms and ECG confirmation, is used for monitoring digoxin toxicity.

Digoxin Toxicity. Toxic levels of digoxin are capable of producing virtually every cardiac rhythm disturbance known. Infants and children are most likely to develop bradycardia and AV conduction delay. Sinus bradycardia is produced by digoxin suppression of sinus node discharge. All degrees of AV block can occur, sometimes associated with ectopic atrial beats or JET. Ectopy and tachyarrhythmias are more common in adult patients, probably because of myocardial irritability from ischemia. However, the myocardium of infants and children is not less sensitive to digoxin than that of older patients.

Digoxin toxicity can occur because of accidental or intentional ingestion. One study reported fatal digoxin overdose in one half of the cases of acute ingestion.[98] Toxicity can also occur because of dosing error or because of a change in the patient's sensitivity to the drug or in its pharmacokinetics. Assessment of the patient for predisposing factors (hypokalemia, renal dysfunction) is an important initial step in treatment. Hypomagnesemia, hypoxemia, myocarditis, and coadministration of catecholamines or calcium all exacerbate digoxin toxicity. In patients receiving constant digoxin doses with stable serum concentration, digoxin toxicity can still develop if cardiac status deteriorates or metabolic disturbances develop.[96]

Digoxin immune Fab (Digibind) is the antidote used to treat life-threatening digoxin toxicity. It binds with free molecules of digoxin and is then excreted by the kidney. It should be reconstituted with normal saline and administered intravenously over 15 to 30 minutes. Dosing is complex, so the reader is referred to a pediatric drug reference book for further information.[94] Serum digoxin levels rise precipitously after administration of digoxin immune Fab; however, this reflects digoxin bound to Digibind, so results will be clinically misleading. Hypokalemia can occur after administration, so potassium levels must be monitored.

Catecholamines and Other Inotropes

Epinephrine. Epinephrine is an endogenous catecholamine that is produced and released from the adrenal gland in response to stress. Its direct cardiac effects are the result of stimulation of the β-adrenergic receptors. Epinephrine shortens systole by improving contractility and speeding conduction through the AV node and Purkinje system. It accelerates SA node firing. Epinephrine increases coronary blood flow but also increases myocardial oxygen demand, so the potential for a mismatch exists. It also decreases the refractory period of ventricular muscle, causing a predisposition to arrhythmias.

The clinical effects of epinephrine vary with the rate of infusion. At a low dose (0.05 to 0.2 μg/kg/min), peripheral vasodilation and increased HR and contractility are the consequence of β_1- and β_2-adrenergic stimulation. The pulse pressure is widened, SVR and PVR decrease, and SV and CO increase if the patient's intravascular volume is adequate.

Increasing infusion rates result in stimulation of the α-adrenergic receptors. Increased SVR and elevated BP occur. Afterload increases and may ultimately affect CO if the myocardium is unable to maintain SV. Epinephrine is a potent renal artery vasoconstrictor, potentially reducing renal blood flow and urine output. However, the improvement in CO achieved with epinephrine may increase renal blood flow.

Dosage and Administration. In pediatric patients, infusion rates of 0.05 to 0.3 μg/kg/min are recommended in treatment of shock associated with myocardial dysfunction. Epinephrine may be most useful when combined with a vasodilator for afterload reduction. When catecholamine stores are depleted, epinephrine may be the inotrope of choice. In asystole or pulseless arrest, the continuous infusion dose is 0.01 to 1 μg/kg/min. The use of epinephrine in Pediatric Advanced Life Support (PALS) is detailed in Chapter 31.

Epinephrine is best administered through a central venous line because infiltration from peripheral venous administration can cause local tissue ulceration. Infusion rate is controlled with a constant infusion pump. Epinephrine is compatible with both dextrose and normal saline solutions; alkaline solutions are not used because catecholamines are inactivated at a higher pH.

Side Effects. Epinephrine may induce CNS excitation marked by restlessness, fear, anxiety, or dread and a throbbing vascular type headache. Tachycardia is always produced, and atrial and ventricular ectopy and tachyarrhythmias are risks with increasing infusion rates. Severe hypertension and anginal pain can occur. Severe mismatching of myocardial oxygen delivery with oxygen consumption and subsequent ischemia may be detected on ECG. Local tissue injury from extravasation is reviewed in Chapter 16.

Norepinephrine. Norepinephrine is the hormone precursor of epinephrine and is the neurotransmitter of the SNS. Norepinephrine raises BP and improves tissue perfusion in hypotensive patients who have normal or elevated cardiac index. Although norepinephrine possesses α-and β-adrenergic receptor activity, its α-adrenergic effects predominate at all but the lowest infusion rates. SVR rises sharply because of α-adrenergic mediated vasoconstriction. The peripheral, renal, splanchnic, and hepatic vascular beds are constricted, as is the pulmonary vasculature. Cardiac contractility is augmented, and SV and cardiac index rise, if the increase in afterload can be tolerated. Chronotropy is opposed by reflex vagal activity, which slows the rate of sinus node discharge.

The hemodynamic effects of norepinephrine limit its use in pediatric critical care almost exclusively to treatment of patients with septic shock. It is most often used to augment vascular tone when shock persists after volume repletion and administration of other inotropes.[8,96]

Dosage and Administration. Initial infusion rates are 0.05 to 0.1 µg/kg/min. Successful treatment results in improved perfusion pressure, which maintains vital organ function. The lowest possible dose that achieves improved skin color and temperature, normalization of pH, and urine output is used. Invasive monitoring is useful to evaluate both SVR and PVR. The rate of infusion is titrated to a maximum 1 to 2 µg/kg/min.

Side Effects. Careful monitoring is necessary during norepinephrine administration to prevent excessive increases in ventricular afterload and organ ischemia. If norepinephrine elevates BP but does not improve clinical evidence of tissue perfusion, continuing its infusion may lead to ischemic injury of the extremities, widespread organ failure, and death.[96] Profound hypertension can result from inadvertent boluses or excessive infusion rates, resulting in myocardial infarction or cerebral hemorrhage. In patients with coronary artery thrombosis the area of infarct may be extended. As is true with epinephrine, local extravasation can cause ischemic necrosis and sloughing of superficial tissues. Local tissue injury from extravasation is reviewed in Chapter 16.

Isoproterenol. Isoproterenol is a synthetic catecholamine structurally related to epinephrine and norepinephrine. It has beta (β_1 and β) specificity and does not affect α-adrenergic receptors. Its potent effects on the heart include an increase in cardiac contractility, HR, and conduction velocity. Stimulation of peripheral β_2-receptors results in vascular smooth muscle relaxation, decreased SVR, and a fall in diastolic BP. Widened pulse pressure is detected because the systolic BP increases. Tachycardia may be extreme because the decline in diastolic pressure augments the chronotropic effect of the drug. In the face of hypovolemia, hypotension may develop when isoproterenol therapy is initiated. An increase in CO is ensured only if circulating blood volume is adequate. Because HR and contractility are increased, isoproterenol increases myocardial oxygen consumption. Simultaneous decreases in both diastolic filling time and diastolic perfusion pressure may impair myocardial oxygen supply and result in myocardial ischemia. Myocardial ischemia, myocardial infarction, and fatal myocardial necrosis have been reported in adolescents receiving continuous isoproterenol infusion.

Isoproterenol also relaxes pulmonary vascular and bronchial airway smooth muscle. Historically, isoproterenol was used in severe refractory status asthmaticus; however, newer β_2-selective intravenous agents have all but supplanted the use of isoproterenol in this population. Once used to treat a variety of shock states, newer drugs and an improved understanding of the pathophysiology of shock have made isoproterenol obsolete for this purpose. It is, however, still employed to treat hemodynamically significant or atropine-resistant bradycardias. In addition, it is the chronotrope of choice in the postoperative heart transplant patient to augment HR in the denervated heart. In heart block resistant to atropine, isoproterenol may be used until definitive treatment with pacemaker placement occurs. Low-dose epinephrine infusion may be better tolerated, however, because it maintains diastolic coronary perfusion pressure better than isoproterenol.

Dosage and Administration. Isoproterenol infusion is initiated at a rate of 0.01 µg/kg/min and adjusted to a rate of 0.05 to 0.1 µg/kg/min until the desired chronotropic or hemodynamic effect is achieved.

Side Effects. Sustained tachycardia, vasodilation, and the risk of myocardial ischemia limit isoproterenol's utility in all but a select group of patients.[96] HR, ECG, and BP are closely monitored. ST segment changes or T wave flattening are evidence of myocardial ischemia. Cardiac enzymes can be followed to monitor for myocardial ischemia in those patients receiving high doses. Isoproterenol can be safely administered via a peripheral vein because extravasation of the drug does not produce tissue necrosis.

Dopamine. Dopamine is a neurotransmitter in the central and sympathetic nervous systems and is found in the adrenal medulla, where it is the immediate precursor of norepinephrine. Dopamine stimulates dopamine (DA) receptors (D_1 and D_2) in the vascular beds of the kidney, mesentery, and coronary arteries at low doses, producing vasodilation. As the dose of dopamine increases, β- and then α-adrenergic receptors are activated. In addition to these direct sympathomimetic effects, dopamine stimulates release of norepinephrine from sympathetic nerve terminals, resulting in indirect sympathetic stimulation.

Renal blood flow and urine output increase with infusion of dopamine at 0.5 to 2 µg/kg/min because of the selective action at DA receptors that occurs at this dose. Low-dose dopamine augments renal function, inhibiting tubular reabsorption of sodium and promoting sodium excretion via increased renal blood flow. Low-dose dopamine reduces renal and SVR, suppresses aldosterone secretion, and interacts with atrial natriuretic factor. Renal effects are enhanced by the combination of low-dose dopamine with furosemide or prostaglandin.[99] Infusion of dopamine at 2 to 5 µg/kg/min increases cardiac contractility and CO, with little change in HR or vascular resistance. At doses of 5 to 6 µg/kg/min, both BP and HR increase, although the tachycardia is less than that seen with isoproterenol. Doses up to 10 µg/kg/min further increase CO. At doses of more than 10 µg/kg/min, increasing α-adrenergic effects are seen with beginning increases in SVR and tachycardia. The salutary effect on the renal vascular bed may be lost when α-adrenergic effects predominate at doses greater than 15 µg/kg/min.

There are data suggesting that infants have reduced sensitivity to dopamine; however, the evidence is not strong.[100] Notterman, DeBruin, and Metakis[100] also note, importantly, that dopamine crosses the blood-brain barrier in preterm neonates and warn against its use for trivial indications in this age-group. Although low-dose infusion of dopamine is often administered to augment renal function among critically ill patients, there is no evidence of the influence of this practice on the incidence of renal failure resulting from poor perfusion.

Although dopamine is used widely in pediatric critical care practice, little systematically collected data exist regarding its use. Dopamine has both inotropic and vasopressor properties, as well as the potential to enhance renal blood flow. Shock with cardiovascular dysfunction and mild to moderate hypotension are improved with dopamine infusion. At moderate infusion rates, it is unlikely to produce excessive tachycardia or arrhythmias, compared with either epinephrine or isoproterenol. When hypotension is marked and cardiac index is very low, epinephrine is the drug of choice. Dopamine is not the agent of choice in distributive shock when cardiac index is high and vascular resistance is low. If BP is normal but cardiac contractility is abnormal, a pure inotrope, such as dobutamine or amrinone, is preferable.[101]

Dosage and Administration. As with other catecholamines, dopamine is not mixed with alkaline IV solutions and is administered into a central vein using a continuous infusion device. Significant skin injury from extravasation is a risk with peripheral administration. Dextrose and normal saline solutions are compatible.

Infusion rates of 0.5 to 2 μg/kg/min result in selective DA actions on vascular beds. Infusion rates between 5 and 10 μg/kg/min produce dominant β-adrenergic effects; doses between 10 and 20 μg/kg/min have mixed α- and β-adrenergic effects. α-Adrenergic effects begin to dominate at infusion doses greater than 15 μg/kg/min and are predominant with doses greater than 20 μg/kg/min.

Side Effects. Limb ischemia, gangrene, and extensive loss of skin are associated with dopamine infusion in peripheral veins and with extravasation because dopamine both releases norepinephrine from synaptic terminals and is converted to norepinephrine when metabolized. Local tissue injury from extravasation is reviewed in Chapter 16.

Dopamine increases myocardial oxygen demand as increased contractility increases myocardial work. It is likely to produce less myocardial oxygen supply and demand mismatch than epinephrine or isoproterenol because it is associated with less tachycardia; however, it is more likely to do so than dobutamine or amrinone.

Dobutamine. Dobutamine is synthesized to model a catecholamine that has specific, selective inotropic action with limited chronotropic or vasopressor activity. Infusion of dobutamine produces prompt improvement in cardiac performance. With improved contractility, a decrease in atrial filling pressures follows. A decrease in SVR and PVR is associated with dobutamine. Tachycardia is unusual. Improved CO, along with direct stimulation of the renal dopaminergic receptors, improves renal blood flow and urine output.

Dobutamine is most useful when the primary disturbance impairing tissue perfusion is cardiac. Typical indications include viral myocarditis, cardiomyopathies, or myocardial infarction (Kawasaki disease). Dobutamine has been used as a bridge for patients awaiting heart transplantation. Positive inotropic effect and little increase in HR have been

demonstrated in children given dobutamine for a variety of shock states. Dobutamine is less effective in septic shock than in cardiogenic shock. In postoperative cardiac surgery patients, results have been uneven; children with some CHDs had a positive inotropic response, whereas others did not. Others demonstrated improved CO only because HR increased. It has been postulated that those who did not demonstrate improvement in inotropic response may not have had significant impairment of contractility (as is the case in many children undergoing surgery for CHDs).[96]

In adults with CHF, dobutamine increased myocardial oxygen demand. However, in the absence of coronary obstruction, coronary blood flow and oxygen supply also increased, favorably affecting oxygen balance.[102] A similar response can reasonably be expected in children with depressed contractility and patent coronary arteries. Because HR increases only modestly with dobutamine, the metabolic demand anticipated is less than with inotropes associated with significant tachycardia. Dobutamine is also less likely to produce atrial and ventricular arrhythmias than other inotropes, although these problems can occur.

Dosage and Administration. Dobutamine therapy is initiated with a continuous IV infusion at 2 to 5 μg/kg/min. Maximal effects are generally seen at doses of 10 to 15 μg/kg/min. The maximal therapeutic dose is not known. Infusion is generally recommended via a central venous line, although dobutamine does not have significant vasoconstricting effects.

Side Effects. Side effects include excessive HR and arrhythmias, although both are less common than is the case with other inotropes. Headaches, anxiety, tremors, and excessive fluctuations in BP have been reported.

Amrinone. Amrinone produces positive inotropic actions on the heart and has both systemic and pulmonary vasodilating effects. It is the first bipyridine to be widely used in the United States for infants, children, and adults with impaired myocardial contractility. Amrinone is a selective PDE inhibitor that increases myocardial cAMP content and provides a positive inotropic effect. It has profound vasodilating action, also via increased cAMP. At the heart, intracellular calcium is increased; it is blocked at the level of the vascular smooth muscle.[103] Unlike other inotropes, PDE inhibitors improve cardiac performance in the failing heart with unchanged or reduced oxygen demand. This is possible in part because systemic vasodilation reduces ventricular wall stress. In addition, myocardial perfusion is increased because coronary resistance is decreased. PDE inhibitors act synergistically with other catecholamines. They may be particularly useful for patients whose symptoms are refractory to catecholamine therapy because of excessive SNS activation or adrenergic receptor down-regulation from lengthy exposure to catecholamines.[103]

For patients with CHF, amrinone increases SV and cardiac index while simultaneously decreasing SVR, CVP, and LVEDP. Tachycardia is not observed, and both systolic myocardial contractility and diastolic relaxation are improved.[103-106] In children with a cardiac left-to-right shunt, amrinone's pulmonary vasodilator effects appear to be selective. In those with normal PAP and resistance, the hemodynamic effect was beneficial. In those with elevated PAP and PVR, pressure and resistance were significantly reduced, without causing systemic hypotension.[107] Amrinone effectively increases CO in children who have undergone cardiac operations, including the Fontan procedure, arterial switch, and repair of complete AV septal defect.[108-110] Amrinone is useful in the treatment of both acute myocardial failure and chronic CHF and has been employed for patients with end-stage heart disease awaiting cardiac transplantation.[111]

Dosage and Administration. Amrinone is mixed in normal saline (glucose solutions are *not* used) and is administered by continuous IV infusion following a bolus IV dose administered over 10 minutes. Critically ill pediatric patients have a large volume of distribution for the drug and require a loading dose of at least 3 mg/kg. The recommended loading dose for adults is 0.75 to 1.5 mg/kg. The higher dose is necessary to achieve serum concentrations similar to the therapeutic level for adults.[105,106,112] The loading dose is 0.75 mg/kg, administered by IV bolus over 3 to 5 minutes and followed by continuous infusion. When followed by a constant infusion, steady state is obtained within 1 hour of initiating therapy, but the loading dose may need to be repeated every 15 to 30 minutes.[94,106] The usual infusion dose is 5 to 10 μg/kg/min. Daily dose should not exceed 10 mg/kg/24 hours.

Side Effects. Hypotension is the principal concern, particularly during administration of the loading dose. Hypotension is more likely when patients have low CVP. It is important to note that ventricular filling pressures may be high in patients with heart failure, but when SVR is reduced a relative hypovolemia may ensue. If hypotension occurs, fluid therapy corrects the problem. Hypotension is avoided by slow administration of the loading dose and by ensuring adequate intravascular volume.

Amrinone may cause cardiac rhythm disturbances. In adult patients, ventricular ectopy and brief episodes of VT were seen in approximately 10% of patients, and sustained VT or ventricular fibrillation was seen in 1%.[113] The incidence of supraventricular and ventricular arrhythmias in pediatric patients is 3%.[94] Arrhythmias may be related to the patient's underlying pathophysiologic condition or to the infusion rate.

Thrombocytopenia is a common adverse effect of amrinone when it is administered orally. With IV therapy, the incidence of thrombocytopenia is far lower. When amrinone is discontinued, the platelet count returns to normal within several days.

Milrinone. Milrinone is a slightly newer member of the bipyridine, inodilating agents with PDE inhibiting action. Its actions and indications for use are like those of amrinone. Milrinone demonstrated potent inotropic effects and a greater effect on both right- and left-sided heart filling pressures (consistent with greater vasodilation) when compared with both dobutamine and nitroprusside in adult patients with severe heart failure.[104] Milrinone administered in pediatric patients with septic shock improved cardiac index and decreased SVR.[114,115] Pediatric and neonatal patients demonstrated increased cardiac index and lowered

SVR and PVR with milrinone infusion after surgery for congenital cardiac defects.[116,117]

Dosage and Administration. Milrinone is administered with a loading dose of 50 μg/kg infused over 10 minutes and followed by a continuous IV infusion of 0.375 to 0.75 μg/kg/min. The volume of distribution of milrinone may be different in pediatric patients, as it is for amrinone, but this has not yet been systematically investigated and reported. Milrinone is administered in normal saline or 5% dextrose solutions.

Side Effects. Hypotension and cardiac rhythm disturbances occur with milrinone administration, as is the case with amrinone. The incidence of thrombocytopenia with milrinone is less than that seen with patients receiving amrinone.

Vasodilating Agents

Myocardial failure results in activation of a number of compensatory mechanisms designed to maintain systemic BP and perfusion of vital organs. Regardless of the cause of myocardial failure, attempts at compensation are the same in all. First, the ventricle dilates to increase EDV. Increased EDV eventually exceeds the optimal level and is inappropriately elevated, as is end-diastolic pressure. Second is an increase in adrenergic stimulation of the heart, augmenting cardiac contractility and HR. Finally, SVR increases in response to low SV, increased renin-angiotensin activity, and other factors. In many patients with heart failure, SVR is inappropriately elevated and will decrease SV.

For patients with reduced SV and systemic vasoconstriction, inotropic support alone may be ineffective in restoring adequate CO. In addition, inotropes (with the exception of the new PDE inhibitors) may exact a significant penalty by increasing myocardial oxygen consumption. Vasodilating agents in these patients are highly effective, augmenting CO by changing preload or afterload conditions through relaxation of vascular smooth muscle.[84,91,92] Venous vasodilators increase the capacitance of the venous system, reducing elevations in ventricular end-diastolic volume and pressure. By reducing arterial vasoconstriction and afterload, arterial vasodilators increase SV and CO. HR does not increase in most patients treated with vasodilators. BP decreases only slightly or not at all, as a result of increased SV.

Vasodilators exert their positive effects on cardiac performance while also decreasing myocardial oxygen consumption. By decreasing preload and reducing ventricular size, in addition to decreasing ventricular systolic pressure, myocardial oxygen needs are also reduced. Although the mechanism of action is not clearly known, vasodilators also enhance ventricular compliance. Vasodilators shift the volume pressure curve to the right, where there is a greater increase in EDV at a lower end-diastolic pressure.

Vasodilators are classified based on their primary site of action on either the arterial or venous or both (balanced) sides of the systemic vascular bed (Table 7-9). Of note is that all vasodilators, regardless of classification, exert some effect on both the venous and arterial circuits. The selection of an appropriate vasodilator in children with cardiac shunts is important (Table 7-10). Hemodynamic deterioration can occur with balanced or venous vasodilators in the infant with a large left-to-right shunt, whereas arterial vasodilators improve systemic output.[85]

PDE inhibitors are often used as vasodilators because their inotropic effect can be equally as beneficial. However, when close and rapid titration of drug effect is needed, medications with a short half-life (such as nitroprusside or nitroglycerin) remain the vasodilators of choice.[85] When long-term afterload or BP reduction is required, ACE inhibitors and third-generation β-blockers have become the agents of choice. Their additional neurohormonal modulation and ventricular remodeling effects are beneficial.[85]

Sodium Nitroprusside. Sodium nitroprusside is a balanced vasodilator, with approximately equal actions on the venous and arterial circuits. It is useful to treat acute, severe hypertension but is used more often as adjunctive therapy in severe CHF or cardiogenic shock. Its role in pediatric critical care may be modified as experience with the PDE inhibitors expands.

Infusion of nitroprusside results in rapid, widespread, and marked vasodilation affecting both the arterial and venous systems. If SVR is not elevated, SV and cardiac index decline and BP is reduced. HR increases reflexively. However, when SVR is high and contractility is depressed,

as seen in patients with severe ventricular failure, the reduction in afterload and preload that is achieved with nitroprusside results in increased SV and cardiac index. The increase in SV is proportional to the decrease in SVR. HR declines and BP is unchanged. Nitroprusside is useful for treating CHF and cardiogenic shock and as adjunctive therapy for impaired ventricular performance in the immediate postoperative period following cardiac surgery.

Dosage and Administration. Nitroprusside has an extremely rapid onset and short duration of action. Peak effects are noted within 2 minutes, and effects dissipate within 3 minutes of stopping an infusion. Administered by continuous IV infusion, the beginning dose is 0.5 µg/kg/min. SVR is generally reduced with doses between 1.5 and 2 µg/kg/min. Occasionally, doses as high as 5 to 10 µg/kg/min are required if vasoconstriction is profound.

Nitroprusside is administered in 5% dextrose solution with an infusion pump. The solution is light sensitive, requiring that solutions be used within 24 hours and that the administration container and tubing be opaque or covered.

Side Effects. Hypotension is the most common problem encountered with nitroprusside administration. It is rapidly corrected by a reduction in the infusion rate but should always prompt a reevaluation of the patient's intravascular volume status as well.

Toxicity. Nitroprusside undergoes intravascular metabolism into both nitric oxide, the agent responsible for its vasodilating effects, and cyanide. Cyanide is metabolized in the liver to thiocyanate, which is then excreted by the kidney. Accumulation of thiocyanate can develop in patients with inadequate renal function, resulting in CNS excitation evidenced by confusion, delirium, and seizures. Blood thiocyanate levels are determined in patients with poor renal function and in those who receive nitroprusside for longer than 72 to 96 hours. Thiocyanate is cleared by dialysis.

Cyanide poisoning is the cause of death in animals given massive doses of nitroprusside and has been reported in humans. However, concern for cyanide accumulation has probably been overstated.[96] Because an early sign of

TABLE 7-9 Classification of Vasodilators Based on Predominant Site of Action

Venous	Arterial	Balanced
Nitroglycerin	Diazoxide	Nitroprusside
	Nifedipine	Phentolamine
	Tolazoline	Captopril
	Hydralazine	Enalapril
		Prazosin

TABLE 7-10 Hemodynamic Effects of Vasodilating Agents

	CO	HR	PAP	RAP	SVR	PVR	BP
Captopril	0	0	0	0	↓↓	0-↓	↓
Diazoxide	↑	↑	0	0	↓↓	↓	↓
Hydralazine	↑	↑	0	0	↓↓	↓	↓
Nifedipine	0-↑	0-↑	↓↓	↑	↓↓	↓	↓↓
Nitroglycerin	0-↑	0	↓↓	↓	0-↓	↓↓	↓
Nitroprusside	0-↑↑	↑	↓	↓	↓↓	↓↓	0-↓
Phentolamine	↑	↑	0-↓	?	0-↓	0-↓	0-↓
Tolazoline	↑	↑	0-↓	?	0-↓	0-↓	0-↓
Prazosin	0-↑	0	↓	0-↓	↓↓	↓	↓↓
Enalapril	0	0	0	0	↓↓	0-↓	↓

Data from Packer M: Vasodilator therapy for primary pulmonary artery hypertension: limitations and hazards, *Ann Intern Med* 103:258, 1985; Taketomo CK, Hodding JH, Kraus DM: *Pediatric dosage handbook*, Cleveland, 1998-1999, Lexicomp.
CO, Cardiac output; *HR,* heart rate; *PAP,* pulmonary artery pressure; *RAP,* right atrial pressure; *SVR,* systemic vascular resistance; *PVR,* pulmonary vascular resistance; *BP,* blood pressure.

cyanide poisoning is lactic acidosis, serum lactate levels should be monitored in patients receiving high dosages or prolonged infusions of nitroprusside.

Nitroglycerin. Nitroglycerin is a venous vasodilator employed extensively in the critical care of adult patients. Its major indication for use is myocardial ischemia from coronary artery disease. Only in the last 10 to 15 years has nitroglycerin been used to treat patients with CHF and pulmonary edema. Another occasional indication is PAH.

The primary effect of nitroglycerin for patients with heart failure is to reduce ventricular filling pressures by dilation of systemic and pulmonary veins. Enlarging the venous capacitance decreases filling pressures and ventricular volume load, thus improving ventricular compliance. In general, central venous, atrial, and PAW pressures are reduced, without systemic hypotension. For patients with acute CHF and pulmonary edema, nitroglycerin may be the drug of choice, particularly if systemic BP is marginal. Nitroglycerin does decrease arterial vascular resistance, but to a lesser extent than does nitroprusside.

Nitroglycerin has been used in children with PAH secondary to CHDs with increased PBF. Some children with preoperative PAH experience a decrease in PVR and an increase in CO in response to nitroglycerin. The use of nitroglycerin for treatment of idiopathic or primary PAH is uncertain.

Dosage and Administration. Nitroglycerin migrates into many plastics, resulting in substantial loss of medication potency when conventional polyvinyl chloride IV administration sets are used. Dosage recommendations for pediatric patients also are difficult to make because investigators have not reported whether special non–polyvinyl chloride infusion sets were used. Experience with adult patients leads to a suggested starting dose of 0.1 μg/kg/min, increasing the dose by 0.1 to 0.2 μg/kg/min until the desired effect is achieved. Administration of nitroglycerin with non–polyvinyl chloride infusion sets is recommended to minimize variation in dosage and the potential for error.

The nitrate pastes used among adult patients with coronary artery disease have not been systematically investigated in pediatric patients.

Side Effects. Nitroglycerin administration increases intracranial pressure; adults report severe headache that persists for several days with continued therapy. Cautious use is necessary with patients in whom increased intracranial pressure is a potential problem. More commonly, as with nitroprusside, hypotension complicates nitroglycerin administration. Temporary cessation of the infusion or reduction in the infusion dosage restores BP because the duration of action of nitroglycerin is short. Adequate intravascular volume is ensured, as well.

Nifedipine. Nifedipine is a vasodilator that blocks the calcium channels in vascular smooth muscle and inhibits contraction. Systemic and coronary artery relaxation and vasodilation result; myocardial oxygen delivery is increased. Limited data are available regarding its efficacy in acute heart failure in pediatric patients, but it has been used in adults with cardiogenic pulmonary edema, chronic CHF, vasospastic angina, and hypertension. In pediatric critical care, nifedipine has been used in hypertensive emergencies,[118] to treat patients with primary PAH,[119] and in children and adolescents with hypertrophic cardiomyopathy. Truttmann and colleagues[120] cautioned against the use of sublingual nifedipine in pediatric patients because its BP-lowering effect is not predictable and excessive hypotension might occur.

Dosage and Administration. Nifedipine administered sublingually, orally, or via a "bite and swallow" capsule has a rapid onset of action. Effects are seen in 10 to 15 minutes, with peak action at 60 to 90 minutes. Patients with hypertensive emergencies are administered a dose of 0.25 to 0.5 mg/kg, which can be repeated if needed every 4 to 6 hours. For patients with hypertrophic cardiomyopathy, the dose is 0.6 to 0.9 mg/kg/day in three or four divided doses. The maximum daily dose is 1 to 2 mg/kg/day.[94]

Toxicity. Calcium channel blockers have a direct depressant effect on the myocardium and must be used with caution for patients with heart failure. However, nifedipine has more profound vasodilating effects than myocardial depression. Patients given nifedipine may experience headache and other symptoms and signs of vasodilation: sweating, flushing, and feelings of warmth. Hypotension, tachycardia, palpitations, and syncope can occur.

Diltiazem. Diltiazem is a calcium channel blocker used for patients with angina from coronary vasospasm, chronic stable angina, or hypertension. Recently it has emerged as an effective agent for the termination of paroxysmal SVT and atrial fibrillation or flutter. When used for its vasodilating effects, a dose 1.5 to 3.5 mg/kg/day is administered in three or four divided doses.

Angiotensin-Converting Enzyme Inhibitors. Moderate to severe heart failure results in activation of the renin-angiotensin-aldosterone system (RAAS), causing compensatory fluid retention to maintain BP. However, the vasoconstrictor substance angiotensin II contributes to inappropriately elevated afterload in advanced heart failure. It also stimulates catecholamine release at adrenal and sympathetic nerve terminals. Catecholamines stimulate release of renin at the juxtaglomerular apparatus, perpetuating a vicious cycle of excessive and continuous activity. Inhibition of the renin-angiotensin system reduces afterload and improves cardiac performance. The ACE inhibitors (ACEIs) have become practical agents for chronic afterload reduction for patients with heart failure secondary to hypertension, myocardial dysfunction, and intracardiac left-to-right shunt.[85,91,92]

ACEIs produce their effects through a number of mechanisms. Angiotensin II production from angiotensin I is inhibited, and norepinephrine release from sympathetic nerve endings is inhibited. Also, ACEIs block the enzyme that degrades bradykinin, and circulating levels of this potent vasodilator are increased. In addition, cardiac remodeling, a compensatory response to heart failure, is affected. Cardiac remodeling involves compensatory hypertrophy. Adaptive hypertrophy maintains the normal proportion of myocytes (contractile elements) to nonmyocytes (noncontractile elements, specifically, collagen fibers) in the myocardium to preserve compliance and contractility. Aldosterone and angiotensin II play a role in collagen synthesis.[85] ACEIs prevent this development and actually reverse maladaptive fibrosis. ACEIs produce clinical improvement and reduce mortality for adult heart failure patients.[121,122] This may be the consequence of their salutary effects on the myocardium and the down-regulation of overstimulated compensatory mechanisms.

Captopril and Enalapril. Captopril and enalapril are ACEIs available as oral suspensions for infants and young children. In patients with chronic heart failure, ACEIs provide reduction in both afterload and preload. The hemodynamic effect produced is similar to that seen with nitroprusside: CO increases proportionately to the decrease in afterload achieved. Because angiotensin II is inhibited, aldosterone release is not stimulated, and potassium is spared from renal excretion. Use in pediatric patients with heart failure includes those with Kawasaki disease, dilated cardiomyopathy, myocarditis, CHDs, and those with end-stage heart disease awaiting transplantation. The hemodynamic improvement seen with ACEIs can be evidenced shortly after the initiation of therapy. Adequate afterload reduction is obtained, and CO is augmented as myocardial function improves. However, cardiovascular remodeling is a slower process, occurring over 6 to 12 weeks.[85]

ACEIs are also useful in renovascular hypertension and in treating patients with hypertension related to immunosuppression following organ transplantation. BP is reduced without postural hypotension or a reflex increase in sympathetic nervous system activity. HR is usually not affected.

Dosage and Administration. Captopril is administered in a dose of 0.05 to 0.1 mg/kg every 8 to 24 hours to neonates. Infants are prescribed 0.15 to 0.3 mg/kg/dose and children receive 0.3 to 0.5 mg/kg/dose every 6 to 24 hours. The maximum dose is 6 mg/kg/day; 2.5 to 6 mg/kg/day is usually an effective dose.[94] Enalapril is dosed at 0.1 mg/kg/day in one or two divided doses to a maximum of 0.5 mg/kg/day. Captopril is administered 1 hour before or 2 hours after meals, on an empty stomach. Enalapril may be administered without regard to food. Enalapril is available for IV administration for patients with severe hypertension or acute CHF; 5 to 10 μg/kg/dose is administered every 8 to 24 hours.

Side Effects. First-dose hypotension can occur in volume-depleted patients or those who are receiving intense diuretic therapy. Tachycardia often accompanies hypotension. Lower initial doses, carefully titrated to the maximally tolerated dose, are recommended. These effects can also occur following a first higher dose. ACEIs can cause immunologic side effects; the most common is a pruritic rash, which is sometimes accompanied by fever. Neutropenia occurs in some patients and may be severe, necessitating that therapy be discontinued. Occasionally, because ACEIs impair the breakdown of bradykinin, life-threatening angioedema develops. Increased levels of bradykinin in the circulation may result in chronic cough. Renal side effects include proteinuria. Potassium levels should be monitored because hyperkalemia can occur with potas-

sium supplements, or potassium-sparing diuretics are given concurrently.

β-Adrenergic Blocking Agents. β-Blockers (esmolol) have been described for the management of pediatric hypertension after surgical repair of coarctation of the aorta and other cardiac operations.[123] Historically β-blocking agents were considered to be contraindicated in patients with heart failure because of their negative inotropic effects. Recently attempts to modulate the neurohormonal responses in heart failure have led to the inclusion of β-blockers in therapy. These agents increase LV ejection fraction, improve contractility, reduce ventricular EDVs, decrease symptoms, and increase survival in adults with cardiomyopathy.[124] Initially, clinical symptoms may worsen as a result of negative inotropic effects. However, the newest β-blockers (the third-generation medications such as carvedilol) have added vasodilatory properties that improve their hemodynamic profile.[85] The exact mechanisms through which the β-blockers improve cardiac performance in CHF are not known. Likely, one of the important beneficial effects is suppression of the deleterious effects of the catecholamines on the failing myocardium. Increased SNS activity is characteristic of heart failure in infants and children from congenital and acquired causes. β-Blockers can acutely worsen heart failure. Precautions are necessary when therapy is initiated. Therapy is contraindicated in patients with significant bronchospasm, symptomatic bradycardia or hypotension, heart block, and decompensated heart failure.[125] Initiation of therapy with the lowest doses of medication can minimize clinical deterioration. Worsening of clinical status is treated with diuretics. Only a few studies report the use of β-blockers in children with heart failure.[126-129] Clinical and ventricular function improvement was reported for some patients awaiting heart transplantation.[127,129] Low-dose β-blocker therapy combined with digoxin and diuretics improved heart failure scores in six infants with large left-to-right shunts.[128] Which children may benefit most from β-blocker therapy and which β-blockers are most effective have not yet been determined.

Other New Agents. Angiotensin II receptor antagonists (AIIRA) have been approved for the treatment of adults with hypertension.[125] Because they have a mechanism of action similar to the ACEIs, they are anticipated to be effective in the treatment of heart failure. They offer more complete blockade of the RAAS, and patients tolerated the medication better than the ACEIs. The incidence of cough was decreased, and no episodes of angioedema occurred.[130]

Spironolactone, an aldosterone receptor antagonist, decreases ventricular fibrosis in cardiac remodeling, which occurs with effective heart failure treatment. A new study with adults combined spironolactone with conventional therapy for heart failure, including ACEIs. Morbidity and mortality were reduced.[131] No formal studies with children have been conducted, although spironolactone is used routinely as a diuretic for children because of its potassium-sparing effect.

Antiarrhythmic Agents

Recent advances in the understanding of cardiac electrophysiology have led to improved management of cardiac rhythm abnormalities. Newer, more specific antiarrhythmic agents are being developed, and older, more traditional agents continue to undergo scrutiny in multicenter drug trials. As this evolution continues to take place, some agents are withdrawn from use (e.g., encainide), mechanisms of action are redefined, and indications for use are revised.[132] Although most drug trials are performed in adults, pediatric indications for antiarrhythmic agents continue to evolve.

With the advent of radiofrequency ablation for treatment of many abnormal rhythms, drug therapy is often short term and is based on efficacy rates, safety, and natural history of the arrhythmia. Pharmacologic management can become complex in patients who have resistant arrhythmias or when ablation is not an option.

The Vaughan-Williams classification system for antiarrhythmics groups medications according to their predominant electrophysiologic effects. The system allows grouping of agents with similar mechanisms of action and potential clinical use but (like all classification systems) cannot predict the efficacy of a given drug in an individual patient (Table 7-11).

Class I Agents. Class I agents are "local anesthetics" that block the sodium cell membrane channels, delay repolarization, and have some antivagal effects.

Class IA Agents. Quinidine, procainamide, and disopyramide are the class IA agents. Quinidine is infrequently used in children because of side effects (see later text), procainamide is the most commonly used class IA antiarrhythmic in pediatrics, and disopyramide is rarely used.

Quinidine. Quinidine is the oldest of these agents and is occasionally used for treatment of VT or VF (although newer agents have replaced quinidine). It is a potent sodium and potassium channel blocker with low-level effects on α-receptors.

Quinidine is given in a dose of 30 to 60 mg/kg/day in three to four divided doses. A test dose (2 mg/kg) is recommended to evaluate for idiosyncratic reactions or syncope. IV administration is avoided.[94] In-hospital initiation is indicated because of proarrhythmic side effects. Quinidine is metabolized by the liver, and elimination half-life is 6 to 8 hours. This drug is extensively protein bound, so hypoalbuminemia will increase serum levels. Therapeutic levels range from 2 to 7 μg/ml, and toxic levels are those exceeding 8 μg/ml.

Side effects are common and are experienced by at least one third of patients.[133] These include gastrointestinal disturbances, headache, tinnitus, thrombocytopenia, impaired vision or hearing, syncope, and hypotension. The most significant side effects are cardiac, leading to potential proarrhythmia. ECG effects commonly observed are PR, QRS, and QT interval prolongation. Bradycardia and AV block may be seen as well. Drug-induced torsade de pointes

◆ TABLE 7-11 Vaughan-Williams Classification of Antiarrhythmic Drugs

Class	Major Action	ECG Effects	Examples
I	Sodium channel blockade	Ia: moderate decrease in conductivity, moderate increase in repolarization	Quinidine Procainamide Disopyramide
		Ib: mild increase in conductivity, shortened effective refractory period	Lidocaine Mexiletine Tocainide Moricizine
		Ic: marked decrease in conductivity, little effect on repolarization	Flecainide Propafenone
II	β-Adrenergic blockade	Antagonizes endogenous catecholamines	Propranolol Metoprolol Nadolol Atenolol Esmolol
III	Potassium channel blockade	Prolongs action potential and repolarization	Amiodarone Sotalol Bretylium
IV	Calcium channel blockade	Slows conduction at AV node, decreases SA, AV nodal automaticity	Verapamil Diltiazem
Other	Digitalis glycosides	Slows conduction at AV node, decreases SA node discharge rate	Digoxin
	9-β-D-ribofuranosyladenine	Decreases automaticity, slows conduction in AV node	Adenosine

AV, Atrioventricular; *SA,* sinoatrial.

is the most serious proarrhythmic effect that can lead to sudden death.

Procainamide. Procainamide is commonly used in the acute management of many tachyarrhythmias (SVT, JET, atrial ectopic tachycardia) and is given as a continuous IV infusion.[134,135] Frequent dosing intervals make this a difficult enteral drug for long-term use in infants and small children. The sustained-release enteral form can be used in older children and adolescents for long-term therapy. Procainamide is a potent sodium channel blocker with no alpha or beta effects.

An IV loading dose of procainamide is given at 5 to 15 mg/kg over 5 to 30 minutes; in the presence of severe hemodynamic compromise, it must be given more slowly. A continuous infusion at 20 to 60 μg/kg/min is titrated to keep the procainamide blood level 4 to 10 μg/ml. Plasma levels are obtained 4 hours after initiation of therapy or after an increase in dosage.[94]

Long-term oral therapy is dosed in the range of 15 to 50 mg/kg/day. This must be divided so that it is given every 4 to 6 hours, and older children may take a sustained-release preparation.

Procainamide is metabolized by the liver and excreted by the kidney. In patients with hepatic or renal disease, dosing is adjusted accordingly. The liver metabolizes procainamide to *N*-acetyl procainamide (NAPA), an active metabolite with some mild antiarrhythmic effects. NAPA levels are monitored during IV therapy and maintained at less than 30 μg/ml. There is minimal protein binding.

With intravenous use, procainamide side effects are dependent on plasma levels. Hypotension and negative inotropy are associated with IV administration. Adverse reactions include tachycardia, QRS and QT prolongation, gastrointestinal disturbances, confusion, and AV block. In children with atrial tachycardia and 2:1 AV conduction, procainamide may actually increase AV node conduction, resulting in 1:1 conduction and increased ventricular rate. Chronic oral therapy is associated with a lupuslike syndrome; 20% of patients may become symptomatic and develop a positive antinuclear antibody (ANA).[135] Procainamide may potentiate skeletal muscle relaxants. Cimetidine, ranitidine, amiodarone, and β-blockers can increase procainamide and NAPA levels.

Class IB Agents. Lidocaine, mexiletine, tocainide, and moricizine are class IB agents. Lidocaine is the most commonly used class IB agent prescribed in the pediatric critical care setting. Mexiletine is not widely used in children, although it is emerging as a therapeutic modality for the treatment of congenital long QT syndrome caused by sodium channel defects.[136] Tocainide and moricizine are infrequently used in pediatrics.

Lidocaine. Lidocaine blocks the fast sodium channel and shortens repolarization in abnormal cells, thus improving the overall homogeneity of repolarization with resultant blockade of conduction. It also suppresses automaticity and spontaneous depolarization. It is primarily used to control symptomatic ventricular ectopy.

Lidocaine is administered as a continuous IV infusion following a loading dose of 1 to 3 mg/kg; the typical infusion rate is 20 to 50 μg/kg/min. It is metabolized by the liver, so the dose is decreased in the face of low CO or hepatic disease. Active metabolites can accumulate and cause CNS toxicity. Toxicity develops when serum levels exceed 7 μg/ml.[135]

Major adverse reactions of lidocaine include disorientation, changes in level of consciousness, seizures, or apnea. Nausea, vomiting, and blurred vision are less severe side effects. Cardiac adverse reactions include bradycardia, hypotension, heart block, or arrhythmia.

Mexiletine. Mexiletine is an oral agent structurally related to lidocaine. Its primary effects are on the fast sodium channels. No loading dose is required. Usual dosing begins at 2 mg/kg per dose every 8 hours, and this can be increased to 5 mg/kg/dose. The liver metabolizes mexiletine, so dosing is adjusted accordingly in patients with hepatic dysfunction. Adverse reactions are common, occurring in 20% to 70% of patients.[135] The most common reactions are rash, gastrointestinal upset, and dizziness.

Class IC Agents. Class IC agents are potent sodium channel blockers with variable effect on repolarization. Flecainide and propafenone are class IC agents. They are used for the chronic treatment of SVT and VT.[137]

Flecainide. Flecainide is a potent inhibitor of the rapid sodium channel, slowing conduction in the atria, AV node, ventricles, and Purkinje fibers. Flecainide dosing is based on body surface area (rather than weight) and has been found to correlate best with serum trough levels.[137] Starting doses are 80 to 100 mg/m^2, with no loading dose. Milk inhibits absorption, so dietary changes can markedly affect serum levels. A trough level of 200 to 1000 ng/ml is therapeutic. Flecainide is excreted unchanged by the kidney because it is not extensively metabolized by the liver. Half-life can be up to 27 hours in infants and 6 to 8 hours in older children.[135]

Flecainide is not given to patients with structural or functional heart disease because the incidence of sudden death is increased in this group. Flecainide is generally safe in those with a normal heart.[138] The exception to this would be the infant in incessant SVT who has CHF; once the rhythm is controlled, heart failure is reversed. Blurred vision can occur with overdose.

Propafenone. Propafenone has effects similar to flecainide; in addition, it has clinically significant β-blocking activity. The β-blockade effects seem to vary with dose and metabolism,[132] and it is particularly efficacious in the management of ectopic arrhythmias. Oral dosing begins at 150 to 200 mg/m^2; the maximum dose is 600 mg/m^2, divided every 8 hours. The IV dose is 0.2 to 1.0 mg/kg given over 10 minutes as a loading dose, and the maximum loading dose is 2 mg/kg. Continuous infusions of 4 to 10 μg/kg/min are used. IV propafenone is associated with significant hypotension, so concurrent IV fluid administration may be necessary. Propafenone should be used with caution in children with structural heart disease because sudden death has been reported in this group of patients.[139] Other side effects are similar to flecainide, including blurred vision, paresthesias, and nausea.

Class II Agents. The class II agents are the β-adrenergic blockers and are some of the most frequently used antiarrhythmics in pediatrics. The commonly used agents are propranolol, atenolol, metoprolol, nadolol, and esmolol. These agents differ in their β-receptor "selectivity," half-life, and side effects. β-Blockers inhibit catecholamine binding at the β-receptor sites, resulting in a decrease in HR, myocardial contractility, AV node conduction, and BP.

β-Blockers are used as a single agent or in combination with other antiarrhythmics to control SVT or to slow the ventricular response to atrial fibrillation or flutter.[132,140] They are also the mainstays of therapy for congenital long QT syndrome to help prevent the occurrence of torsades de pointes associated with increased sympathetic activity.

Propranolol is a nonselective β-blocker that is most commonly used to treat SVT in infants. **Atenolol** is the second most commonly used β-blocker in older children and adolescents; it is long acting and is selective for β$_1$-receptors in the heart. **Metoprolol** is a selective β$_1$-agent that is gaining favor in pediatric use. **Nadolol** is nonselective and long acting. **Esmolol** is an IV β-blocker that is short acting and is useful in the acute treatment of tachyarrhythmias in the PICU.

Dosage and Administration. Atenolol, metoprolol, and nadolol are oral agents only. Esmolol is administered intravenously only. Propranolol can be administered both orally and intravenously. However, IV administration, particularly in infants less that 1 year old, is associated with significant bradycardia and hypotension. It is most often avoided in this age-group because newer and safer intravenous agents are currently available.

Propranolol oral dosing begins at 1 mg/kg/day every 6 hours and can be adjusted upward to 4 mg/kg/day as clinically indicated. The IV dose is 0.1 to 0.2 mg/dose over 5 minutes and necessitates vigilant monitoring for hypotension and bradycardia.

Atenolol is dosed at 1 to 3 mg/kg/day, given as a single dose or divided twice a day. Metoprolol is used in adolescents, beginning at 50 mg twice a day and increasing to 150 to 200 mg twice a day as indicated. Nadolol dosing begins at 0.5 to 1 mg/kg once daily, increasing to a maximum of 2.5 mg/kg/day.[94,134]

Esmolol requires a loading dose of 100 to 500 μg/kg given over 5 minutes. A continuous infusion is titrated to therapeutic effect, at 50 to 200 μg/kg/min. Esmolol is an ultrashort-acting β-blocker; onset of action occurs in 2 to 10 minutes, elimination half-life is 7 to 10 minutes, and duration of effect is up to 30 minutes.

Side Effects. β-Blockers are negative inotropes, may impair ventricular function, and worsen heart failure in some patients. Acute negative inotropic effects are most common with IV administration of propranolol. AV block, severe bradycardia, hypotension, and asystole can occur. An isoproterenol infusion or a temporary external pacemaker is readied when IV propranolol is required. Hypotension can also occur with esmolol at high doses (>200 μg/kg/min).

β-Adrenergic receptors in other organs can also be blocked with class II agents, resulting in significant systemic affects. Worsening of bronchospasm may occur in patients with reactive airway disease. The signs and symptoms of hypoglycemia may be masked with β-blockers; therefore these agents are used cautiously in diabetics, and fasting in all patients is to be avoided. Other side effects observed with long-term therapy are fatigue, hypotension, mood changes, lethargy, depression, vivid dreams, and nightmares. However, these effects are less common in the β$_1$-selective agents. Slowing of the sinus node, with resultant bradycardia, can occur as well.

Class III Agents. The class III agents include amiodarone, sotalol, and bretylium. The primary mode of action is prolongation of the refractory period. There are also diverse drug-dependent effects on receptor and ion channel blockade.

Amiodarone. Amiodarone prolongs the refractory period by delaying the outward potassium channels and prolonging repolarization. It is also a sodium channel blocker with concurrent noncompetitive α- and β-adrenergic blockade and inhibition of presynaptic norepinephrine release.

Amiodarone is effective as a single agent or in combination with β-blockers in the acute and chronic control of SVT, atrial flutter, JET, and ventricular arrhythmias.[140-142] Amiodarone is useful in patients with structural and functional heart disease because it is less of a negative inotrope than other antiarrhythmics.

Dosage and Administration. Hospitalization for initiation of oral amiodarone is recommended to monitor for proarrhythmic side effects (ventricular tachycardia, torsade de pointes) during medication loading. The oral loading dose is 10 mg/kg/day administered every 12 hours for 3 to 10 days. Neonates and infants may require loading doses as high as 20 mg/kg/day because of erratic absorption in this age-group.[25,141] Chronic oral therapy is 5 to 10 mg/kg/day in a single dose. It may take several days to see clinical effect with initiation of therapy because of the slow and incomplete absorption. Amiodarone is highly lipid soluble and metabolized in the liver to an active agent, desethylamiodarone. Both amiodarone and desethylamiodarone are stored in a large volume of distribution in the body. Therefore drug levels continue to be therapeutic for several months after discontinuation of use. Half-life ranges from 26 to 100 days.[94] Serum levels are not useful as a guide to therapy because they correlate poorly with clinical effect. Monitoring of blood levels may be helpful to assess if absorption is occurring at all, particularly in infants with resistant SVT.

Intravenous amiodarone has been shown to be clinically effective in the treatment of resistant life-threatening tachyarrhythmias. The drug has a rapid onset of action (30 to 45 minutes), with arrhythmia suppression sometimes occurring with the first dose.[143] In a randomized, double-blinded comparison trial between IV amiodarone and bretylium for the treatment of VT and VF, amiodarone was found to be more efficacious in preventing recurrences and had fewer side effects than bretylium.[144] IV loading doses begin at 5 mg/kg/dose administered over 1 hour, incrementally increased every 30 minutes to a maximum of 15 mg/kg as clinically indicated. A continuous infusion of 10 to

15 mg/kg/day may be necessary in some patients if needed for sustained arrhythmia suppression.[142]

Side Effects. The most common adverse reaction with IV amiodarone is significant hypotension during the loading dose. Hypotension is managed with administration of IV volume and calcium. Clinically significant bradycardia or AV block may occur, necessitating temporary ventricular pacing.

The electrophysiologic effects of both oral and intravenous amiodarone include PR, QRS, and QT prolongation; bradycardia; proarrhythmia; and AV block. ECGs are monitored daily during drug initiation for QTc prolongation because QTc prolongation can predispose patients to torsades de pointes.

Common noncardiac side effects include photosensitivity, chemical hepatitis, hypothyroidism or hyperthyroidism, and corneal microdeposits. All patients taking amiodarone should use high-grade sun screen (SPF >15). Liver function and thyroid function tests should be monitored every 6 months. Elevation of liver transaminases or hyperthyroidism may necessitate discontinuation of the medication. Patients who have hypothyroidism benefit from thyroid replacement therapy.[132] Pulmonary fibrosis has been reported in adults receiving long-term amiodarone therapy. This condition has been reported infrequently in infants and children but can be identified on a CXR or pulmonary function test.[145] Therefore all children receiving long-term amiodarone therapy require periodic CXRs or (if applicable) pulmonary function tests.

Amiodarone has a number of drug interactions. It inhibits P-450 enzymes, so it may increase plasma concentrations of digoxin, cyclosporine, flecainide, procainamide, warfarin, and phenytoin. Dosage adjustment and monitoring of serum levels of these drugs are warranted.

Sotalol. Sotalol has class III effects, as well as being a nonselective β-blocker. At lower doses, β-blockade effects predominate; at higher doses, sodium and potassium channels are affected to prolong the refractory period. Sotalol is used for the treatment of refractory SVT and VT, often in children with congenital heart disease.[146,147] The starting dose is 90 to 100 mg/m²/day, incrementally increasing to 200 mg/m²/day given in two to three divided doses. The drug is excreted in the urine, and there are no active metabolites. Serum levels are not helpful. Adverse effects include headache, nausea, dizziness, fatigue, depression, bradycardia, and proarrhythmia. The most serious side effect is torsade de pointes, associated with QTc prolongation, although this is more commonly seen in adult patients at higher drug doses.[147,148]

Bretylium. Bretylium has limited use in pediatrics and is reserved for ventricular tachycardia that is refractory to other therapeutic interventions. With the advent of IV amiodarone, its efficacy has been called into question.[144] Bretylium prolongs the action potential and refractory period. Initially it causes release of norepinephrine, then it subsequently prevents additional release and reuptake. For life-threatening VT, the dose is 5 mg/kg IV push, repeated every 10 to 30 minutes to a maximum dose of 30 mg/kg. Continuous infusion rates are 15 to

30 μg/kg/min.[94] The primary adverse effect is hypotension resulting from peripheral α-adrenergic blocking. Other effects include flushing, bradycardia, syncope, confusion, nausea, and vomiting.[135]

Class IV Agents. Class IV drugs are the calcium channel blockers. The predominant agents in use for arrhythmia control are verapamil and diltiazem.

Verapamil. Verapamil is a calcium channel blocker with its greatest effect on the SA and AV nodes. It is effective in suppressing enhanced automaticity and has some α-adrenergic blocking effects. Initially it was used for acute and chronic treatment of SVT. However, with the advent of newer agents (particularly adenosine for acute treatment), it is now primarily used as a second or third agent in resistant SVT or in patients with hypertrophic cardiomyopathy.[149] Verapamil can increase the ventricular response rate in patients with WPW syndrome who are in atrial fibrillation, so it should be avoided in this patient subset.

Dosage and Administration. Intravenous verapamil should not be administered in infants younger than 1 year of age because it can precipitate asystole and cardiovascular collapse. In older children the dose is 0.1 to 0.3 mg/kg/dose, and the maximum dose is 5 mg. Oral dosing ranges from 4 to 17 mg/kg/day in three or four divided doses. Elimination half-life is 4 to 7 hours, and it is metabolized in the liver. Low CO and hepatic dysfunction can increase half-life.

Side Effects. With oral therapy the most common adverse effects are constipation, headaches, dizziness, and rashes. Cardiac adverse effects include bradycardia, AV block, and worsening of CHF resulting from its negative inotropic effects. Coadministration of verapamil with β-blockers is contraindicated because of synergistic negative inotropic effects. Intravenous administration in infancy is contraindicated.

Diltiazem. Diltiazem was initially used for afterload reduction in pediatrics; however, it is emerging as an effective antiarrhythmic for the control of SVT and atrial flutter. It is a moderately potent calcium channel blocker with no alpha effects.[150] Initial IV dose is 0.25 mg/kg as a bolus over 2 minutes. A second bolus of 0.35 mg/kg can be administered if necessary; this is followed by a continuous infusion of 0.003 mg/kg/min.[135,151] Oral dosing for children has not been described. The usual dose for adolescents is 30 to 120 mg 3 or 4 times a day. This amount is adjusted upward as needed to a maintenance dose of 180 to 360 mg/day. Adverse reactions include headache, postural hypotension, bradycardia, and AV block.

Other Agents. Two additional medications are often used in the management of pediatric arrhythmias. Digoxin is probably the most widely prescribed antiarrhythmic in children. Adenosine is an antiarrhythmic that is currently the mainstay in emergency treatment of SVT.

Digoxin. Digoxin has both direct and indirect actions on the myocardium. The indirect actions are due to autonomic effects mediated by the PNS. The direct actions are due to intracellular increase of calcium ions secondary to inhibition of the Na-K membrane pump, resulting in increased force of contraction. It also slows conduction through the SA and AV node.

Because digoxin has been used for so long, scientific clinical efficacy trials have been limited to support its use as an antiarrhythmic. Although digoxin is known to slow AV node conduction, this effect is not maintained during periods of increased sympathetic activity (exercise, stress, CHF).[152] Many children with CHF develop tachyarrhythmias and are prescribed digoxin. Improved hemodynamics can contribute to conversion to normal sinus rhythm; hence it is difficult to know if digoxin prevailed as a positive inotrope or as an antiarrhythmic. In addition, in patients with WPW syndrome, digoxin can increase impulse conduction antegrade across the accessory tract, resulting in a rapid ventricular response during atrial fibrillation and sudden death.[153] Nevertheless, digoxin continues to be prescribed by many practitioners for control of SVT, atrial fibrillation, and atrial arrhythmias. See Table 7-8 for digitalizing and maintenance doses. When digoxin is administered intravenously, its effects occur in 5 to 30 minutes, with peak effects in 1 to 4 hours. Coadministration of verapamil, propafenone, and amiodarone increase serum digoxin levels. Digoxin doses are adjusted to maintain therapeutic levels and avoid toxicity.

Adenosine. Adenosine increases potassium channel conduction and depresses the slow inward calcium current, resulting in transient sinus bradycardia and AV block. Adenosine is the drug of choice for the acute termination of SVT by temporarily blocking the AV node. It can also be helpful in the diagnosis of atrial ectopic tachycardia or atrial flutter because it will block the AV node and slow the ventricular response, allowing the identification of the atrial arrhythmia.

Dosage and Administration. Adenosine can only be given by rapid IV push (followed quickly with a 3- to 10-ml flush); otherwise, it is ineffective as a result of rapid systemic metabolism. Its onset of action is nearly immediate, and its half-life is less than 10 seconds; this is beneficial in the ICU because multiple doses can be administered close together, and side effects, if they occur, are short lived. The initial dose is 100 µg/kg, followed by incremental increases of 100 to 300 µg/kg/dose; maximum dose is 12 mg. Adenosine is administered using a venous port closest to the heart; a central line is preferable. Umbilical arterial catheter administration is ineffective because the drug is metabolized before reaching the heart.

Side Effects. Adenosine may produce transient shortness of breath and dyspnea as a result of bronchospasm. Cardiovascular side effects include AV block, marked sinus bradycardia, flushing, and hypotension. Generally, these effects are short lived. Rarely, ventricular ectopy or atrial fibrillation occurs.

MANIPULATION OF DUCTAL PATENCY AND PULMONARY VASCULAR RESISTANCE

The first hours and days after birth are characterized by stabilization of the respiratory and cardiovascular systems. Closure of the ductus arteriosus and the dramatic fall in PVR are two of the most important events during the transition to

establish normal postnatal blood flow patterns. Failure of these events may result in excessive PBF or persistent pulmonary hypertension of the newborn, respectively. However, infants with some complex CHDs depend on patency of the ductus arteriosus for survival after birth. For example, neonates with decreased PBF may require a patent ductus arteriosus to maintain adequate PBF, and neonates with left-sided obstructive lesions may require a patent ductus arteriosus to maintain adequate systemic blood flow. In addition, the status of the pulmonary circulation is crucial in the perioperative management of many children with congenital heart disease.

Developmental Physiology of the Pulmonary Vasculature

Fetal pulmonary vascular development parallels development of the lungs. From the sixteenth week of gestation, the pulmonary arteries and the preacinar arteries that accompany the terminal bronchioles are present. Throughout the remainder of gestation, respiratory units develop from the terminal bronchioles and are accompanied by developing intraacinar arteries and pulmonary capillaries. The preacinar arteries have a muscular wall, as do the arteries at the level of the terminal bronchioles. The intraacinar arteries are largely nonmuscular.[6,154]

In the fetus, normal gas exchange occurs in the placenta, and PBF is low, supplying only nutritional requirements for lung growth and performing some metabolic functions. Only about 8% of the CO from both the right and left ventricles perfuse the fetal lungs because of high PVR. Conversely, SVR is low owing to the low-pressure placenta.

After birth, with initiation of ventilation by the lungs and the subsequent increase in pulmonary and systemic arterial blood O_2 tensions, PVR decreases, and PBF increases by eightfold to tenfold to match systemic blood flow. The decrease in PVR with ventilation and oxygenation at birth is regulated by a complex and incompletely understood interplay between metabolic and mechanical factors. Oxygenation and expansion of the lungs are independently effective at decreasing PVR, and other factors, such as nitric oxide and prostacyclin, have been identified as instrumental in the drop in pressure. Previously closed peripheral arteries are recruited for circulation; there is dilation of the proximal, muscular arteries; and the peripheral vessels continue to grow and branch. Although dilation of the smallest and most distal vessels occurs across months and muscle extension into the walls of the peripheral arteries takes years,[6,154] PVR decreases by 80% in the first hour after birth and reaches adult levels during the first months of life. Simultaneously, SVR increases owing to separation of the newborn from the placenta. The consequences of the resistance changes at birth (and other factors) are increased PBF, improved oxygenation, and eventual closure of the fetal shunts at the foramen ovale and ductus arteriosus.

Normal pulmonary vascular development can be disrupted by a number of problems. Abnormal structure and function may be the consequence of maladaptation (the fetal lung does not mature appropriately), maldevelopment (increased muscularization may be the consequence of intrauterine insult or a CHD that obstructs pulmonary venous drainage), or underdevelopment (pulmonary hypoplasia resulting from a condition such as diaphragmatic hernia).[6] Either acute or chronic fetal or postnatal hypoxia prevents the anticipated fall in PVR after birth. Hypoxia sustains the vasoconstricted state, and PVR and pulmonary artery pressures remain high. CHD associated with decreased PBF may result in hypoplasia of the pulmonary vascular bed and may increase PVR as a consequence. High oxygen concentrations used in the treatment of neonatal lung disease may be detrimental to both alveolar and arterial growth and development.

Manipulating the Ductus Arteriosus

In the fetus, the ductus arteriosus is a large vascular structure that diverts RV output away from the lungs and into the descending aorta to be used for gas exchange in the placenta. The vasodilating prostaglandins, PGE_2 in particular, play a significant role in maintaining ductal patency in the fetus. After birth, functional closure of the ductus occurs over the first 12 to 15 hours, with complete closure occurring in 50% of newborns by 18 hours and in 100% by 48 hours of life. The cessation of blood flow leads to necrosis of the ductus smooth muscle and subsequent fibrosis, resulting in permanent anatomic closure at 2 to 3 weeks of age.[155] Kennedy and Clark[156] first demonstrated in 1942 that oxygen is responsible for constriction of the ductus after birth. However, the biochemical basis for this response remains incompletely understood.

Maintaining Ductal Patency: PGE_1. In newborns with CHDs that are dependent on patency of the ductus for pulmonary or systemic blood flow, exogenous administration of PGE_1 may restore or maintain ductal patency. This can improve arterial oxygen saturation, enhance tissue perfusion, correct tissue hypoxia and acidosis, and maintain systemic BP.[157-159] Table 7-12 lists CHD types in

TABLE 7-12 Congenital Heart Defects in Which PGE_1 Is Recommended

To Improve Pulmonary Blood Flow or Arteriovenous Mixing	To Maintain Systemic Perfusion
Pulmonary atresia	Interrupted aortic arch
Critical pulmonary stenosis	Critical coarctation of the
Tricuspid atresia	aorta
Transposition of the great	Hypoplastic left heart
arteries with intact	syndrome
ventricular septum	Critical aortic stenosis
Tetralogy of Fallot with	
pulmonary atresia or	
pulmonary artery hypoplasia	

Adapted from Rikard DH: Nursing care of the neonate receiving prostaglandin E₁ therapy, *Neonatal Network*, 12:17-22, 1993.

which PGE_1 is indicated. Undoubtedly, since the FDA approved PGE_1 for use in neonates with CHD in 1981, the morbidity and mortality of these newborns have significantly decreased.

Infants with pulmonary atresia, tricuspid atresia, and severe pulmonary stenosis can be better oxygenated after initiation of PGE_1; improvement is generally seen within 30 minutes. Lack of dramatic improvement may indicate that the ductus has maximally dilated, but pulmonary vasodilation with PGE_1 often enhances PBF and provides at least a modest increase in arterial oxygen saturation.[157] Infants with other cyanotic CHDs, such as transposition of the great arteries, may benefit from PGE_1 infusion by improving arteriovenous mixing.

Infants with left-sided obstructive lesions may develop cardiovascular collapse because ductal closure prevents systemic perfusion. In those with interrupted aortic arch (IAA), severe coarctation of the aorta, hypoplastic left heart syndrome, and severe aortic stenosis, PGE_1 maintains ductal patency with subsequent reversal of tissue hypoxia and acidosis. Infants with these obstructive CHDs may not respond as rapidly to PGE_1 as do cyanotic infants. Freed and co-workers[157] found that infants with IAA had maximal response in 90 minutes, whereas those with severe coarctation did not respond for up to 3 hours. In the case of a critically ill newborn in whom either a cyanotic or obstructive heart lesion is suspected, PGE_1 is instituted quickly. The infusion is maintained while definitive echocardiographic diagnosis is obtained, and surgery is performed.

Dosage and Administration. PGE_1 can be administered via central or peripheral IV or via an umbilical artery catheter. Intravenous therapy is preferred because cutaneous vasodilation may be more pronounced with intraarterial administration.[160] The initial recommended infusion rate is 0.05 to 0.1 μg/kg/min. When improvement in arterial oxygenation or systemic perfusion has been achieved, the lowest dose that maintains the response is administered. Typically, 0.05 to 0.2 μg/kg/min achieves the desired clinical effect. The infusion is continued until surgical intervention is provided or until further assessment shows no need to maintain ductal patency.

Side effects. Side effects to PGE_1 infusion are fairly common. Respiratory depression, evidenced by apnea or hypoventilation, is very common. Cardiovascular side effects, most likely related to vasodilation, include bradycardia, tachycardia, and hypotension. Infants weighing less than 2 kg at birth experience the most significant respiratory and cardiovascular side effects.[160] Less frequently observed side effects include seizures, jitteriness, hypoglycemia, hypocalcemia, diarrhea, renal failure, and clotting abnormalities.[160]

Manipulating Pulmonary Vascular Resistance

Determinants of Pulmonary Vascular Resistance.
PVR is related to several factors and can be estimated by applying the hydraulic equivalent of Ohm's law and Poiseuille's law.[161] The hydraulic equivalent of Ohm's law

states that the resistance to flow between two points along a tube equals the pressure drop between these points divided by the flow. For the pulmonary vascular bed, where Rp is resistance and Qp is PBF, the pressure drop occurs from the pulmonary artery *(Ppa)* to the pulmonary vein *(Ppv)*, as follows:

$$Rp = (Ppa − Ppv)/Qp$$

If the pressure in the pulmonary vein is substituted by left atrial pressure *(LAP)* or pulmonary capillary wedge pressure *(Pcwp)*, then the equation is simplified as follows:

$$Rp = (Ppa − LAP)/Qp \text{ or } Rp = (Ppa − Pcwp)/Qp$$

An increase in pulmonary artery pressure caused by large communications at the ventricular or great vessel level or pulmonary vasoconstriction secondary to alveolar hypoxia or other noxious stimuli increases PVR. An increase in pulmonary venous pressure caused by left-sided inflow obstruction or LV dysfunction also increases PVR. To maintain the driving pressure across the lungs, this increase in pulmonary venous pressure also increases pulmonary arterial pressure, resulting in pulmonary edema, alveolar hypoxia, and further pulmonary vasoconstriction.

Other factors that affect PVR can be defined by Poiseuille's law, which describes the resistance to flow of a Newtonian fluid through a straight glass tube of round cross-section. When modified for the pulmonary circulation to take into account the number of pulmonary arteries, the following applies:

$$Rp = 8(l)(\eta)/n\pi r^4$$

where l is the length of the pulmonary arteries, η is the viscosity of blood, n is the number of arteries, and r is the radius. As seen in this equation, changes in viscosity, the number of small pulmonary arteries, or the radius of these arteries affect PVR. Increasing the viscosity of blood perfusing the lungs or decreasing the number of the small pulmonary arteries (cross-sectional area of the pulmonary vascular bed [$n\pi r^4$]) increases PVR. Blood viscosity is related to red cell number, fibrinogen concentration, and red cell deformability. PVR increases logarithmically with an increase in hematocrit, and this relationship becomes important with hematocrits above 55%. A decreased number of small pulmonary arteries is seen in underdeveloped pulmonary circulation, such as congenital diaphragmatic hernia. As seen in the equation, small changes in the radius of the small pulmonary arteries will have a dramatic affect on PVR (r^4); decreases in the radius increase resistance, and increases in the radius decrease resistance. The two determinants of the internal radius are the amount of smooth muscle present and active vasoconstriction and vasodilation. The amount of smooth muscle found in the small pulmonary arteries can be increased over time when the pulmonary circulation is exposed to increased flow or pressure. After surgical correction of the offending heart defects, these changes in smooth muscle will slowly regress and normalize over months. However, pulmonary vasoconstriction and vasodilation are very acute processes and are paramount in regulating the pulmonary circulation in the perioperative period.

Pulmonary Vasoconstriction and Vasodilation. Hypoxia, acidosis, and α_1-adrenergic stimulation are the most important mediators of pulmonary vasoconstriction.[162] The ability of the pulmonary vasculature to constrict in response to alveolar hypoxia is unique to the pulmonary circulation and adaptive; it limits PBF in poorly ventilated lung regions, thereby preserving ventilation/perfusion matching. Conversely, oxygen is a potent pulmonary vasodilator, selective to the pulmonary circulation with no systemic effects. Although the effects of the oxygen environment on the pulmonary circulation have been extensively studied, their mechanisms remain poorly understood. Clinically, manipulating the amount of oxygen delivered to the pulmonary circulation is crucial to the perioperative management of children undergoing cardiac surgery. A change in systemic arterial pH is also a potent regulator of the pulmonary circulation. Acidosis produces vasoconstriction, and alkalosis produces vasodilation. These effects are independent of the source (metabolic vs. respiratory) and solely dependent on the pH.[163] The pulmonary vasodilating effects of alkalosis are predominantly selective to the pulmonary circulation. Lastly α_1-adrenergic stimulation produces nonselective vasoconstriction, both pulmonary and systemic. This may occur via the release of endogenous catecholamines, secondary to pain or agitation, or the administration of exogenous catecholamines.

Hyperoxia and alkalosis most commonly induce pulmonary vasodilation. As previously discussed, these agents induce selective pulmonary vasodilation. β_2-Receptor stimulation induces nonselective pulmonary vasodilation via increased intracellular cAMP concentrations. Vasoactive agents such as dobutamine and isoproterenol induce vasodilation via β_2-receptors.

Nitric Oxide. Nitric oxide (NO) is a labile humoral factor that is locally produced in the pulmonary vascular endothelium. It is a potent vasodilator, and its continuous basal production is a very important regulator of normal pulmonary vascular tone. In fact, aberrations in NO production have been implicated in the pathophysiology of pulmonary hypertensive disorders.[164] Nitrovasodilators (i.e., sodium nitroprusside, nitroglycerin) are a class of vasodilators whose clinical effects are secondary to the stimulated release of NO. When administered, they produce nonselective pulmonary and systemic vasodilation. When NO is delivered directly into the airways (inhaled NO [iNO]), it diffuses through the alveolar wall, crosses the epithelial cell membrane, and reaches small pulmonary arteries. Then, NO diffuses across the adventitia and enters the vascular smooth muscle cell, where it initiates a cascade, resulting in pulmonary vasodilation via increased intracellular cyclic guanosine monophosphate (cGMP). With entry into the bloodstream, NO rapidly binds to hemoglobin and is inactivated, resulting in potent selective pulmonary vasodilation.[165] Large, randomized controlled studies have demonstrated that iNO (5 to 80 ppm) improves oxygenation and decreases the need for ECMO in newborns with persistent pulmonary hypertension.[166-168] In addition, noncontrolled studies have demonstrated that iNO does produce potent, selective pulmonary vasodilation in many children with postoperative pulmonary hypertension.[169] Case reports also suggest that iNO administration during cardiac catheterization may aid in the evaluation of the vasoreactivity of the pulmonary vascular bed, thereby distinguishing between reactive, reversible pulmonary vasoconstriction versus residual anatomic pulmonary obstruction.[170,171] Its efficacy to improve oxygenation, CO, or both in patients following pulmonary-caval anastomosis or Fontan procedures is not well documented. Optimal dosing of inhaled NO remains unclear. The pulmonary vasodilating effects are dose dependent, whereas the improvement in oxygenation appears dose independent. Doses of 80 ppm produce maximal vasodilation but may increase potential toxicities (see later text). Currently, maximal doses of 40 ppm are recommended for prolonged periods of administration, with a decreasing dosing strategy that weans to the lowest dose that maintains its beneficial effects (2 to 5 ppm).

When iNO combines with oxygen, it is oxidized to nitrogen dioxide (NO_2).[172] Inhalation of gas mixtures containing high levels of NO_2 produces severe, acute pulmonary injury with pulmonary edema. However, recent advances in iNO delivery and monitoring systems have significantly reduced the risk of NO_2-induced lung injury during iNO therapy.[173] During inflammation, NO may combine with superoxide anions to form peroxynitrate, another potential lung toxin.[174] To date, this remains theoretical, with no clear clinical evidence. NO that diffuses into the intravascular space combines with hemoglobin to produce methemoglobin.[175] At higher concentrations of NO, clinically significant reductions of arterial oxygen content may result (5% to 10%). At low concentrations, methemoglobin levels may increase but not to a level that interferes with tissue oxygenation (2% to 5%). Methemoglobin levels should be routinely monitored during iNO therapy. One of the most important issues regarding iNO therapy is the safety of acute withdrawal. Several studies have noted a potentially life-threatening increase in PVR on acute withdrawal of iNO.[176] This rebound pulmonary hypertension is manifested by an increase in PVR, compromised CO, or severe hypoxemia. It can occur within hours after therapy is discontinued and is independent of the patient's initial response; patients with no initial pulmonary vasodilatory response can have life-threatening pulmonary vasoconstriction on withdrawal. Therefore acute interruption of iNO therapy must be avoided during suctioning, and the dose must be slowly weaned before termination. Current FDA approval for iNO is limited to neonates with hypoxemic respiratory failure.

Increasing Pulmonary Vascular Resistance

Infants with single ventricle physiology (HLHS) or with defects that result in parallel pulmonary and systemic circulation (truncus arteriosus) require a balance between pulmonary and systemic blood flow for support of optimal hemodynamics. The former also frequently depend on a PDA or surgically created shunt for pulmonary blood flow. The balance of pulmonary (Qp) and systemic (Qs) blood flow is critically important for survival and is ideally maintained at 1. A Qp/Qs of greater than one occurs with excessive pulmonary blood flow and results in systemic hypoperfusion and metabolic acidosis. A Qp/Qs of less than one results from pulmonary undercirculation and results in systemic hypoxemia. Due to the parallel relationship of the pulmonary and systemic circulation in this population, changes in the relative vascular resistance can result in hemodynamic instability and death.

If pulmonary vascular resistance falls significantly, then pulmonary blood flow will increase at the expense of systemic flow. The administration of oxygen, hyperventilation, alkalosis, and systemic vasoconstriction may potentiate pulmonary vasodilation and are avoided. Nonetheless some infants continue to demonstrate pulmonary overcirculation requiring additional therapeutic interventions.

Maneuvers to increase pulmonary vascular resistance include hypoventilation, ventilation with hypoxic gas mixture (subambient oxygen) or added carbon dioxide (CO_2).[177] To monitor clinical effect, Sao_2 and Svo_2 measurements provide an estimate of adequate Qp/Qs. Excessively low Svo_2 suggests pulmonary overcirculation with subsequent low systemic blood flow. Clinical indicators of perfusion (skin temperature, pulses, skin color) and blood gases are monitored closely as well. Poor perfusion and metabolic acidosis suggests decreased systemic blood flow.

Controlled mechanical hypoventilation will result in CO_2 elevation, increased PVR, and decreased pulmonary blood flow. To prevent atelectasis, the rate is gradually decreased while maintaining the same tidal volume.[178] This intervention requires neuromuscular paralysis to prevent the normal physiologic increase in respiratory rate that occurs with hypercarbia.

Hypoxic Gas Ventilation.   Ventilation with subambient oxygen involves the addition of nitrogen (N_2) to room air to achieve an Fio_2 of 15% to 20%. This has been shown to increase pulmonary vascular tone, increase PVR and PAP, and decrease pulmonary blood flow.[178a,178b] Ideally systemic blood flow will improve as a consequence.

Dosage and Administration.   Pure N_2 (0% oxygen) is blended into room air; as the N_2 flow increases, the downstream Fio_2 will fall. Usually the nitrogen can be administered at low flows (<2 L/min) and is titrated to therapeutic response. An oxygen-analyzing port is inserted downstream for continuous monitoring and adjustment of the desired Fio_2. This intervention can be used with cannulae, hoods, manual ventilation bags, and ventilators. Careful monitoring of gas mixture and Fio_2 is imperative; if bulk gas flow is turned off, the consequence will be delivery of 0% oxygen.

Toxicity.   Toxicity from N_2 administration is secondary to the sequelae of subambient oxygen and not to direct delivery. As previously discussed, high flows of N_2 will significantly decrease inspired oxygen concentration; therefore careful monitoring is critically important. Chronic hypoxia contributes to morphologic changes in the pulmonary bed with subsequent arterial medial thickening.[178b] Hence long-term therapy should be avoided.

Carbon Dioxide. Carbon dioxide is a potent pulmonary vasoconstrictor. The administration of CO_2 gas in increasing increments of 1% $FICO_2$ has been shown to augment pulmonary vasoconstriction, increase PVR and PAP, decrease pulmonary blood flow, and increase systemic blood flow.[178c,178d]

Dosage and Administration. The usual concentration of CO_2 in room air is 0.03%. The addition of CO_2 to the inspired gas mixture is titrated to clinical effect; usually an $FICO_2$ of 1% to 4% is sufficient and does not result in a subambient gas mix. Different concentrations of CO_2 have different magnitudes of effect on PVR.[178e] In general the $PaCO_2$ is kept between 40 and 50 mmHg. Inspired CO_2 gas can be used with hoods, manual ventilation bags, or ventilators.

Toxicity. Toxicity is generally the result of the sequela of CO_2 administration. The lowest possible $FICO_2$ should be administered to prevent excessive pulmonary vasoconstriction. Monitoring of inspired gas mix and arterial blood gases will prevent complications. Significant elevation of $PaCO_2$ will produce cerebral vasoconstriction and an ensuing fall in cerebral perfusion. Careful monitoring of neurologic status, anterior fontanel, and head circumference is important in these critically ill infants.

PACEMAKER THERAPY

Technologic advances in pacemaker therapy and a greater understanding of the electrophysiologic mechanisms of cardiac rhythm abnormalities have contributed to the safety and efficacy of temporary and permanent pacing in children. In the PICU the most common indication for temporary pacing is transient heart block associated with congenital heart surgery. In addition, many nonsurgical patients may require temporary pacing to support CO in the presence of symptomatic bradycardia. Overdrive pacing can be effective in the termination of tachyarrhythmias, such as atrial flutter and SVT. It is also implemented as an adjunctive therapy to establish AV synchrony in postoperative JET. Temporary pacing can be accomplished through the use of epicardial, transvenous, esophageal, and transthoracic noninvasive pacing electrodes. Permanent pacing is not discussed because this therapy rarely warrants ICU management.

Indications

Bradyarrhythmias. Sinus or AV node dysfunction after surgical repair of congenital heart disease is the most common cause of symptomatic bradycardia in infants and children. Transient AV block is thought to be the result of surgical manipulation or suturing near the conduction system, but it can also be secondary to acid-base or electrolyte abnormalities. Depending on the surgical procedure performed, temporary atrial or ventricular epicardial pacing wires are placed in the operating room for use if indicated. Atrial epicardial pacing wires can also be used to obtain an atrial electrogram to assist in the diagnosis

of tachyarrhythmias. Postoperative heart block usually resolves within 7 to 14 days, with subsequent restoration of sinus rhythm.[31] When AV node recovery does not occur and temporary external pacing is required for longer than 10 days, permanent pacemaker implantation is recommended.[179]

Congenital CHB can occur in infants with and without structurally normal hearts. The risk for heart failure, syncope, and sudden death exists in both groups; however, those with structural heart disease have greater morbidity and mortality rates associated with CHB. Pacing is indicated for one or more of the following: CHF, ventricular rate less than 55 in infants and less than 40 in adolescents, QTc prolongation, syncope, or frequent ventricular escape beats.[34]

Conduction disturbances, heart block, and subsequent bradycardia can occur secondary to infection. Although rare, viral myocarditis is associated with AV node block and ventricular arrhythmias.[180] Often this phenomena is transient; however, the rare patient will require temporary supportive or permanent pacing.

Other Rhythm Disturbances. Although less common than bradyarrhythmias in infants and children, other rhythm disturbances may be treated with temporary or permanent cardiac pacing. SVT, atrial flutter, and JET can be pace terminated with both temporary or permanent devices. Newer innovative indications for pacing include hypertrophic cardiomyopathy, congenital long QT syndrome, and cardioinhibitory neurally mediated syncope. Generally, these children undergo implantation of a permanent pacemaker without the need for temporary pacing.

Temporary External Cardiac Pacing

A temporary pacing system consists of a generator, connecting cable(s), and pacing leads. Lead and generator selection is determined by clinical indication and institution preference. PICU nurses should be familiar with the specific device used in their unit.

Temporary Pacing Leads

Epicardial Leads. These leads are routinely placed after most cardiac surgeries. Epicardial pacing leads vary somewhat among manufacturers, but in general, they are an insulated multifilament stainless steel wire with the pacing end consisting of a solid electrode that fixates to the heart. A needle is connected to the proximal end to bring the lead out through the chest wall, the needle is then broken away, and the remaining end functions as the contact pin to connect to the cable. Physician preference and clinical indication determine lead placement. Two pairs may be placed on the free wall of both the right atrial and ventricular epicardium; or one epicardial lead is placed on the respective chamber, and the second of the pair is secured to the sternum or subcutaneous tissue. Either method of lead placement results in a bipolar configuration. The epicardial lead is always the negative (−) pole, and the skin is the positive (+) pole.[181,182] If there are two functional epicardial leads, they can be used as either (+ or −) pole. Atrial leads can be used to pace the atrium and provide AV synchrony in the presence of sinus node disease or JET. However, the presence of complete AV node block precludes the use of single-chamber atrial pacing. In this situation a dual-chamber system, using atrial and ventricular leads, provides the best physiologic support. Occasionally only ventricular leads are placed for backup support in the event of acute bradycardia. When both atrial and ventricular leads are placed, the atrial leads are brought out through the chest to the right of the sternum, and the ventricular leads are brought out to the left of the sternum. To aid in easy, rapid identification of the pacing leads, it is helpful to label them accordingly as soon as the patient arrives to the PICU from the operating room.

Ideally, epicardial leads will sense the underlying rhythm and pace reliably. However, these leads are made for short-term use, so sensing and pacing abilities usually decrease with time.[182] In addition, in children who have undergone previous cardiac surgeries that result in epicardial adhesions and scar tissue, myocardial pacing thresholds (minimum amount of current to consistently pace the heart) may be high. Scarring (that occurs over days in the immediate post-operative period) around the lead also elevates pacing and sensing thresholds. This must be monitored closely and pacemaker settings adjusted accordingly.

Temporary Transvenous Leads. Transvenous pacing leads are placed percutaneously through the femoral, jugular, or subclavian veins into the right atria or ventricle. The pacing catheter is a self-contained bipolar system with two pins at the proximal end for placement into the connecting cable or generator. The most common indication for this type of pacing is temporary support of the child with congenital CHB or to support children with temporary heart block secondary to myocarditis or infection.[183,184]

This form of pacing has several limitations in children. First and foremost, ventricular perforation can occur because these pacing leads are rather stiff, and for best results the catheter tip should be positioned into the RV apex. Ventricular perforation can result in loss of capture, pericardial effusion, and cardiac tamponade. Second, lead dislodgment with subsequent loss of capture can occur in up to 25% of temporary transvenous pacing systems.[185] Finally, the risk of infection increases if the catheter is in place for greater than 72 hours because it is placed like a central line. These pacing catheters should be cared for in the same manner as a central line, performing sterile dressing changes according to unit or hospital protocol.[186]

Transesophageal Leads. Bipolar pacing catheters designed for positioning in the esophagus just behind the left atrium permit temporary atrial pacing, as well as recording of an atrial electrogram. Generally, this system is used for the diagnosis (transesophageal electrophysiology study) and termination of SVT. Occasionally it is used for treating symptomatic bradycardia when the AV node is intact (because esophageal pacing is ineffective in the presence of AV node block). For consistent capture of the atrium, high-energy outputs are required. This stimulus can be quite painful for the child, so sedation and analgesia is necessary.

Temporary Pulse Generator. The pulse generator is battery powered and contains the internal software to both sense the patient's native rhythm and to provide the electrical stimulus (output) to depolarize (capture) the myocardium. These devices can vary slightly among manufacturers, but in general, they allow rapid manipulation of HR, mode of pacing, timing intervals, electrical output, and sensitivity.

Many devices include the manually operated ability to temporarily provide rapid atrial pacing (rates of 200 to 800 beats/min) for burst atrial pacing in an effort to terminate SVT or JET. Although lifesaving, operation of this mode requires close patient monitoring and personnel skilled in burst atrial pacing.

Pacing Modes. Modern pacemakers offer a number of features in an effort to replicate physiologic cardiac rhythm and provide rhythm modulation as clinically indicated. To facilitate common understanding among healthcare providers, the North American Society of Pacing and Electrophysiology (NASPE) and the British Pacing and Electrophysiology Group (BPEG) devised a generic pacemaker code (NBG code) to describe the types and function of different devices (Table 7-13). The five-position code is for permanent pacemakers; temporary devices use the first three codes. In practice the pacing mode is described as the three letter acronym that corresponds to the NBG code.

The first letter corresponds to the chamber paced (*A,* atrium; *V,* ventricle; *D,* dual or both). The second letter corresponds to the chamber sensed (*A,* atrium; *V,* ventricle; *D,* dual or both). The third letter corresponds to the generator activity in response to sensing (*O,* none; *T,* triggered; *I,* inhibited; *D,* dual, both inhibited and triggered).

◆ TABLE 7-13 **NASPE/BPEG Generic Pacemaker (NBG) Code**

I Chamber(s) Paced	II Chamber(s) Sensed	III Response to Sensing	IV Programmable Functions	V Antitachyarrhythmia Function
	O = none	O = none	O = none	O = none
A = atrium	A = atrium	I = inhibited	P = simple programmable	P = pacing (antiarrhythmia)
V = ventricle	V = ventricle	T = triggered	M = multiprogrammable	S = shock
D = dual	D = dual	D = triggered and inhibited	C = communicating	D = dual
				R = rate modulated

For example: AAI mode indicates that the atrium is paced, the atrium is sensed, and the generator is inhibited if it senses native atrial electrical activity (a P wave). As expected, this mode of pacing is contraindicated in the presence of complete AV node block. VVI mode provides single-chamber pacing and sensing in the ventricle only, and pacing is inhibited in the presence of native ventricular electrical activity (R wave). This mode provides HR support, but it does not provide for AV synchrony because it has no pacing or sensing function in the atrium. AOO, VOO, and DOO pacing provide asynchronous pacing in the atrium, ventricle, or both chambers, respectively. These modes are to be avoided (except in emergencies where VOO is best) because intrinsic activity is not sensed and competition can occur. Competition is when the generator continually paces without regard for the patient's intrinsic rhythm. If left unchecked, it can result in "R on T" phenomena, with possible development of ventricular tachycardia or fibrillation.

The best physiologic mode of pacing is DDD. This mode paces and senses both atrium and ventricle. In addition, it provides triggered and inhibited activity in response to sensed native electrical activity. If the sinus rate is sufficient and heart block is present, the generator will sense the P wave, wait the preset AV interval (corresponds to PR interval on surface ECG), and then begin "looking" for a native R wave. If AV conduction does not occur and there is no native R wave, the generator will pace the ventricle. This behavior can occur over a range of operator preset atrial rates and is referred to as "tracking." So if a patient has a physiologic increase in sinus rate, the pacemaker can respond accordingly, increasing the ventricular pacing rate to increase CO and meet metabolic demands.

Pacemaker Settings.   The newer generators allow the setting of the mode, pacing rates, timing intervals, output, and sensing to best facilitate support of cardiac rhythm and hemodynamics. Figure 7-60 shows one type of temporary generator.

In single-chamber pacing (AAI, VVI) the rate determines how low the patient's HR must fall to activate pacing. For example: If the low rate is set at 100, the generator is inhibited (will not pace) as long as the intrinsic HR is above 100 beats/min. If the intrinsic HR falls below 100 beats/min, the pacemaker will begin pacing. In the DDD mode, there are two rate settings—low and high rate. The low rate indicates how low the intrinsic sinus rate must fall before the generator paces the atrium. The high rate determines the tracking rate of the ventricle in response to an increase in the sinus rate. If the sinus rate *exceeds* the high rate, the generator will exhibit Wenckebach or 2:1 AV blocking behavior (the P wave is sensed, but there is not corresponding ventricular pace) to prevent rapid ventricular pacing in response to atrial tachycardia or flutter. The high rate set is dependent on the preset timing intervals.

The timing intervals that can be manipulated on temporary generators include AV interval and postventricular atrial refractory period (PVARP). The AV interval corresponds to the PR interval on ECG and is the time between atrial sense or pace and ventricular sense or pace. This interval is not available for programming in single-chamber pacing. The duration of the AV interval should be long enough to allow physiologic atrial contraction with subsequent diastolic filling. In the DDD mode, this interval will adjust automatically (to a certain extent) according to changes in the patient's HR. The PVARP is the time interval during which the atrial lead does not sense or respond to intrinsic atrial activity. This is protective in two ways. First, it can prevent ventricular pacing in response to premature atrial contractions. Second (and more importantly), it prevents sensing of retrograde P waves that can follow ventricular pacing if the AV node is capable of retrograde conduction. The phenomenon of atrial sensing of retrograde P waves with subsequent ventricular tracking and pacing is responsible for pacer-mediated tachycardia (PMT). Therefore the PVARP should be long enough to prevent PMT but short enough to allow sensing of increased sinus rates (usually about 275 milliseconds).

Output is the electrical current that depolarizes the myocardium. This is programmed as milliampere (mA); the higher the mA the higher the output. The minimum amount of output required to consistently capture the chamber being paced is the *capture threshold*. Capture can be determined by the consistent presence of a P wave after atrial pace and a QRS after ventricular pace. Usually the output is set 2 to 3 times higher than the capture threshold to allow a margin of safety.

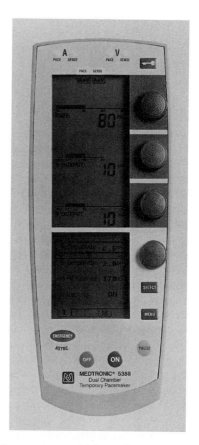

Fig. 7-60   Temporary external demand, dual chamber pacemaker. (Copyright 1998 by Medtronic, Inc. Reprinted with permission.)

Sensing behavior of the generator implies the ability to recognize intrinsic atrial or ventricular depolarization. Sensing in the atrium is determined by the amplitude of the P wave and in the ventricle, by the amplitude of the R wave. This is programmed as millivolts (mV); lowering the mV setting *increases* sensitivity, and increasing the mV setting *decreases* sensitivity. For example: If the ventricular sensitivity is set at 10 mV, the intrinsic R wave amplitude must be greater than or equal to 10 mV to be sensed appropriately. If the intrinsic R wave amplitude drops to 5 mV (less than 10 mV), it will not be sensed. So decreasing the programmed setting to 5 mV will increase the sensitivity because now the R wave will be sensed if it is 5 or 10 mV. The level at which the generator consistently senses intrinsic activity is termed the *sensing threshold*. Generally, the programmed sensing setting should be half the sensing threshold (e.g., if threshold is 8, sensing should be set at 4); this provides a margin of safety and ensures appropriate sensing as P and R wave amplitudes vary.

Nursing Care of Patients With Temporary External Pacemakers

Nurses who care for patients supported by temporary pacing should be thoroughly familiar with the specific devices used in their units and with the unit's policies and procedures regarding temporary pacing. All of these children require continuous ECG monitoring and close observation. In addition, a number of nursing interventions should be followed to prevent complications.

The pacing leads can deliver extraneous electrical current to the heart, producing microshock and the subsequent development of lethal arrhythmias. The PICU environment is replete with electrical equipment (IV pumps, electric beds, ventilators, lamps, etc.) that are capable of current leakage. All electrical equipment must be serviced regularly, and all plugs must have a ground prong. Patients vulnerable to microshock should not use electric hair dryers, fans, razors, and curling irons. Low humidity and carpeted floors increase the occurrence of static electricity, both of which can contribute to microshock. Care should be taken to prevent exposure of uninsulated pacing leads or cables. When in use the entire system should be kept intact. If the leads are not being used, they should be isolated and protected by placing in a glove, finger cot, or dry glass phlebotomy tube. If the leads remain attached to the connecting cable, then the end of the cable should be isolated or placed in the generator. Some centers recommend using gloves when handling transvenous or epicardial leads.[187]

Infection is always a nosocomial risk of any invasive intervention. Transvenous pacing catheters should be treated like central lines, with dressing changes carried out according to unit policy. The care of epicardial leads is less well defined. The site should be cleansed daily and kept clean and dry. The type of agent used for site cleaning, the type of dressing, and frequency of dressing change vary greatly among centers.[186] Site care is often difficult because of the proximity of epicardial leads to chest tube sites. The care of epicardial pacing leads is an area that would benefit greatly from nursing research to help delineate practice.

Another challenging aspect of care in this population is the prevention of inadvertent pacemaker adjustment by inquisitive, mobile infants and toddlers (or siblings). Many of the newer devices have a lockout setting to prevent such an occurrence. Older devices have a plastic shield that should be kept on at all times.

Although nursing practices vary among institutions, every effort should be made to determine capture and sensing thresholds on a daily basis. Frequently in the postoperative period, thresholds increase, and daily assessment will allow settings to be adjusted accordingly. See Box 7-6 for guidelines for the systemic assessment of capture and sensing thresholds.

Timely recognition and intervention of pacemaker dysfunction are critically important. Always evaluate the patient first. In emergencies, cardiopulmonary resuscitation (CPR) should be instituted while someone else simultaneously troubleshoots the pacing system. If the patient is hemodynamically stable, then one can proceed with troubleshooting, as described next. Pacemaker-dependent patients should have a fresh battery or extra generator at their bedside in the event of battery depletion.

Troubleshooting

Pacemaker Dysfunction. The most common reasons for abnormal pacer function are undersensing, oversensing, and noncapture (Table 7-14). Fusion beats do not denote abnormal pacemaker function but should be corrected to prevent competition.

Undersensing occurs when the pacemaker fails to detect intrinsic cardiac depolarization and continues to pace regardless of the native rate of rhythm. This can result in competition or R on T phenomena with the possible development of lethal arrhythmias. Possible causes are lead fracture or disconnection from the heart or generator, sensitivity set too low (higher mV number on generator), or low battery. To correct this problem, make sure that all connections are tight, replace the battery, change leads and/or increase the sensitivity setting by adjusting the sensitivity control to a *smaller* number.

Oversensing occurs when the device detects noncardiac electrical events (extraneous electrical sources, muscle movement) and interprets them as cardiac depolarization. The pacemaker is then inhibited when it should not be, which can produce significant bradycardia or asystole in pacemaker-dependent patients. Causes of oversensing are shivering, chest wall fasciculation caused by emergence from depolarizing neuromuscular blocking agents, or ungrounded electrical equipment. Measures to prevent this problem include decreasing sensitivity (adjust sensing level to higher number) and removing all ungrounded equipment.

Loss of capture occurs when the output stimulus from the pacemaker fails to depolarize (capture) the myocardium. This can result in loss of atrial kick in the case of atrial pacing, or it can result in clinically significant bradycardia in pacemaker-dependent patients. Causes include lead disconnection or fracture, low battery, output set too low, or an increase in the pacing threshold caused by edema or scarring. Interventions include ensuring all connections are

---

Box 7-6
Guide to Pacemaker Checks

Note: This should not be done if the patient is pacemaker dependent with an unstable underlying rhythm.

1. Patient is connected to the pulse generator and is monitored continuously on ECG.
2. Set pulse generator's rate 10 beats/min slower than patient's intrinsic rate. (The "sense indicator" will flash regularly.) Do not continue if the patient becomes hemodynamically unstable.
3. Reduce output (mA) to the minimum value of 0.1. (Doing this avoids risk of competitive pacing.)
4. Increase the sensitivity value until the ECG indicates that the pulse generator is delivering its output pulses asynchronously. (The sense indicator will stop flashing, indicating a loss of sensing. The "pace indicator" will start flashing. Capture is not likely to occur at the minimum output [mA] value.)
5. Decrease the sensitivity value until the ECG indicates that asynchronous pacing is no longer occurring. The sense indicator light will start flashing, indicating that sensing has been restored. (The pace indicator will stop flashing.) The value when this occurs is the sensing threshold for the chamber being sensed.
6. Set sensitivity value to half (½) the sensitivity threshold value. This provides a margin of safety, allowing for continued sensing during threshold variation.
Example: Sensitivity threshold = 5 mV
Set sensitivity = 2.5 mV
7. Ensure mA is at lowest value.
8. Set pulse generator at least 10 beats/min faster than the patient's intrinsic heart rate. (The pace indicator will be flashing regularly at the set rate.)
9. Increase the output (mA) to gain 1:1 capture. This value is the stimulation threshold for the chamber being paced. (The pace indicator will be flashing, and the sense indicator will not flash.) If the patient does not tolerate pacing, turn down the rate or mA (remember the threshold) until the patient's native rate is present.
10. Set the output value 2 to 3 times higher than the threshold value. This safety margin will allow threshold variation while maintaining capture.
Example: Stimulation threshold = 2.5 mA
Set output = 5 to 7.5 mA
11. For continuous pacing, set the pulse generator rate appropriate for age and clinical condition. For backup pacing, set the generator rate at an age-appropriate lower level.

---

tight, changing leads, replacing the battery and/or increasing the output in the noncaptured chamber.

Fusion beats are noted when an atrial pacing spike occurs simultaneously with a native P wave, or a ventricular pacing spike occurs simultaneously with a native QRS. In the case of atrial fusion, decreasing the rate is helpful so that the pacemaker will be inhibited; also, atrial sensing can be increased. In the case of ventricular fusion, either the rate can be decreased (VVI mode), the AV interval can be prolonged (DDD mode), or ventricular sensing can be increased.

Noninvasive Transthoracic Pacing

Temporary transthoracic cardiac pacing is used primarily during emergency situations for the treatment of hemodynamically significant bradycardia that does not respond to oxygen, hand ventilation, epinephrine, or atropine. The primary advantage of this mode is that application can be achieved without interruption of CPR.

Most modern defibrillators have multifunction pads that allow both defibrillation and noninvasive transthoracic pacing (NTP). Therefore a single set of pads can be used for both emergent interventions. NTP can be used in the single-chamber (VVI) demand mode if the patient is connected to the ECG on the defibrillator, or it can be used asynchronously. Unfortunately a high output current (40 to 60 mA) is usually required to consistently capture the ventricle secondary to chest wall impedance.[185]

Implementation of NTP. The posterior multifunction electrode is applied on the patient's back to the left of the spine and below the scapula (Figure 7-61). Positioning the electrode over large bony areas is best to be avoided because bone increases the impedance to pacing. The anterior electrode is placed in the V_2 to V_5 position on the precordium. In the vernacular, a "heart sandwich" is made with the pacing electrodes. If the electrodes are used for a prolonged period, they should be changed every 24 hours. Prolonged use decreases the effectiveness of the contact gel.

The pacemaker is turned on, the rate is set at an age-appropriate level, and the output is increased until consistent ventricular capture is demonstrated on the monitor. As with any emergency cardiac maneuver, a pulse should be palpated to ensure adequate CO.

Troubleshooting Common NTP Problems. The most common clinical problems encountered with NTP are painful stimulation, undersensing, and loss of capture.

Painful Stimulation. NTP is quite painful because high outputs are required to pace the heart; this also produces chest muscle contractions. Sometimes the contractions are so severe that the patient appears to be levitated off the bed. Pain is minimized if the pacing threshold is set at the lowest effective level. Almost uniformly, conscious patients require sedation.

Undersensing. Unnecessary pacing may occur when the pacemaker does not sense the patient's intrinsic HR. Most often, contact between the electrode and the patient's skin is inadequate. Adherence may lessen across time, especially in the presence of diaphoresis, and should be checked regularly. When the multifunction electrodes are changed, it is important to remember to turn off all pacemaker controls or turn the function control knob to "monitor only" to avoid accidental electrical shock.

Table 7-14 Demonstration of Abnormal Pacemaker Function Related to Undersensing, Oversensing, or Noncapture

Sample ECG Appearance	Some Possible Clinical Consequences	Some Possible Causes	Corrective Measures
Undersensing Device fails to detect existing cardiac depolarizations, therefore competes with the native rhythm These native R waves are not detected… …therefore the pacer emits these unneeded spikes	Competition with a native rhythm Stimulation of dysrhythmias ("R-on-T")	Lead disconnected from pacer or from viable myocardium Sensitivity set too low Lead fracture Low battery	Check connection of lead to pacer Increase sensitivity (turn sensing control to a SMALLER number) Sensitivity (mV) Reposition or change lead Change battery
Oversensing Device detects noncardiac electrical events and interprets them as cardiac depolarizations, therefore is wrongly inhibited from pacing Pacing should occur as indicated by the arrows but is inhibited by oversensed non-cardiac electrical noise When the noise ceases, pacing resumes	Pacemaker-dependent patients receive no stimuli from the pacemaker, producing a pause in rhythm and reduction in cardiac output	Electrical potential caused by noncardiac muscle contraction (especially pectorals) is detected and misinterpreted by the device Interference from electrical sources (ungrounded equipment, short circuits) is detected and misinterpreted by the device Sensitivity set too high	Decrease sensitivity (turn sensing control to a LARGER number) Sensitivity (mV) Remove all ungrounded electrical equipment or have it evaluated by hospital engineers
Noncapture Device emits stimuli, which fail to depolarize the myocardium This dual chamber device paces and captures in the atrium and ventricle for the first two beats. Ventricular capture is then lost; the ventricular pacing spikes are not followed by depolarizations. Fortunately, ventricular escape begins.	Pacemaker-dependent patients receive no stimuli from the pacemaker, producing a pause in rhythm and reduction in cardiac output	Lead disconnected from pacer or from viable myocardium Output set too low in the noncaptured chamber Lead fracture High pacing threshold resulting from medication or metabolic changes Low battery	Check connection of lead to pacer Increase output in the noncaptured chamber Reposition or change lead Change battery Alter medication regimen, correct metabolic changes

From Witherall CL: Cardiac rhythm control devices, *Crit Care Nurs Clin North Am* 6:95-102, 1994.

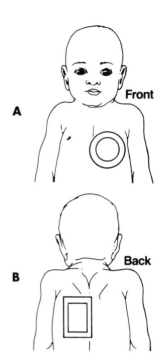

A   Front

B   Back

Fig. 7-61   Positions of the multifunction electrodes for noninvasive transcutaneous pacing. **A,** "Heart sandwich" is made with the pacing electrodes. **B,** Posterior electrode is applied to the back left of the spine and below the scapula. (Courtesy Zoll Medical Corporation, Burlington, Mass.)

Loss of Capture.   Loss of capture can occur because of changes in patient position, which may decrease adherence of the electrode or loosen pacer connections. Measures to prevent poor contact between the electrode and the patient's skin are crucial.

Changes in the patient's physiologic status can influence pacemaker capture. With all types of cardiac pacing, the pacing threshold may change with electrolyte imbalance, acid-base imbalance, myocardial ischemia, hypoxia, and new drug therapy. Reassessment of the pacing threshold with any of these changes is necessary to avoid loss of capture.

MECHANICAL SUPPORT OF CARDIOVASCULAR FUNCTION

Mechanical circulatory support after the failure of conventional medical management is now an established treatment option for infants and children with reversible cardiac dysfunction. The modalities available for support, however, are limited because of small patient size and available technology. In adults with LV failure secondary to cardiac surgery or myocardial ischemia, the intraaortic balloon pump (IABP) has been widely used with high success rates and is the primary method for mechanical circulatory support. In children, the success of ECMO in neonates with pulmonary dysfunction has led to its application as the primary method for mechanical circulatory support in infants and children. With the introduction of pediatric centrifugal pumps, however, the VAD has also become a

Box 7-7
Clinical Indications for Intraaortic Balloon Pumping in Children

Postoperative Left Ventricular Dysfunction
Failure to wean from cardiopulmonary bypass
Refractory left ventricular dysfunction in the intensive care unit

Preoperative Left Ventricular Support
Anomalous left coronary artery
Pretransplant bridge

Medical Support
Myocarditis
Kawasaki disease
Sepsis with ventricular dysfunction
Persistent ventricular arrhythmias

From Hawkins JA, Minich LL: Intra-aortic balloon counterpulsation in pediatric cardiac patients. in Duncan BW, ed: *Mechanical circulatory support for pediatric cardiac patients,* Washington DC, Marcell Decker (in press).

successful option in the management of pediatric patients with reversible cardiac dysfunction.

Indications for Mechanical Circulatory Support

The primary indication for mechanical circulatory support is persistent low CO despite maximal medical therapy. Before the decision is made to provide mechanical support, cardiac dysfunction should be deemed reversible. Whenever possible, a neurologic examination should be performed to evaluate for the presence of a neurologic insult that would exclude a reasonable recovery. In cardiac surgery patients who are not able to be weaned from cardiopulmonary bypass or who demonstrate postoperative low CO, residual structural lesions should be ruled out before the initiation of mechanical support. The definition of maximal medical therapy and the threshold for initiating mechanical support may be individualized. For example, mechanical support may be initiated earlier in postoperative neonates with single-ventricle physiology because their ability to compensate is limited. Finally, providing support for persistent low CO early avoids prolonged end-organ ischemia and worse clinical outcomes.

The choice of mechanical support method is largely dependent on institutional experience and support. Specific indications for IABP in children include poor peripheral perfusion, persistent metabolic acidosis, mixed venous Po_2 persistently less than 25 torr, urine output less than 1 ml/kg/hr, and LA pressure greater than 20 mmHg.[188] Cardiac arrhythmias secondary to inadequate coronary blood flow may also be an indication for IABP therapy. Clinical situations that may warrant the use of IABP therapy are listed in Box 7-7. Contraindications in children include the presence of a patent ductus arteriosus, recent coarctation of the aortic arch repair, significant aortic valve insufficiency, severe LV dysfunction, and irreversible myocardial dysfunction. Coagulation disorders are a relative contraindication, potentially leading to uncontrolled bleeding at the insertion site.

With the limited cardiac support from the IABP, many institutions provide VAD or ECMO support for patients with cardiac dysfunction. Although ECMO was more commonly used in the past, the introduction and success with centrifugal VADs have made this a reasonable option in children who do not require pulmonary support. Indications for the use of ECMO and VAD for cardiac support are noted in Box 7-8.

Although the choice between VAD or ECMO for cardiac support may largely depend on institutional experience and preference, specific clinical criteria in addition to understanding the advantages and disadvantages of each modality, may assist in the selection of the appropriate mode of support for a particular clinical situation. When pulmonary support is required in addition to cardiac support, ECMO is preferred. However, many children with hypoxemia secondary to LV dysfunction and pulmonary edema may no longer require pulmonary support after the decompression of the left ventricle with an assist device. When cardiac support alone is required, either left ventricular or right ventricular, a VAD is sufficient for support. If biventricular support is required, a biventricular assist device (BVAD) (one VAD for the right ventricle and one for the left ventricle, used in series) or ECMO may be used. Some institutions prefer ECMO in this situation because it requires only two cannulation sites compared with four cannulation sites required for BVAD. This factor may be particularly impor-

tant when BVAD is indicated in neonates. In the clinical situation where a VAD is used to support one ventricle, the dysfunction of the other ventricle may be unmasked, making it necessary to transition the child to BVAD or ECMO.

Some authors suggest that small patient size is an indication for ECMO for cardiac support; however, recent success with the VAD in young infants has been reported.[189-191] In one series, 38 of 53 patients supported with a VAD weighed less than 6 kg, and the probability of weaning was similar to that for the older patients. This included the successful VAD support of a 1.9-kg baby with Taussig-Bing anomaly and arch obstruction who was placed on a VAD after a postoperative cardiac arrest.[189]

The presence of an intracardiac communication (patent foramen ovale or atrial septal defect) may be a contraindication for a VAD. In this case, the use of a left ventricular assist device (LVAD) would result in a right-to-left atrial shunt and systemic arterial oxygen desaturation. A right ventricular assist device (RVAD) would result in a left-to-right atrial shunt and decreased systemic CO. ECMO may be the therapy of choice in this situation. Contraindications for both ECMO and VAD may include severe dysfunction of other organ systems (specifically, CNS) before support initiation and extreme prematurity.[191]

ECMO and VAD systems can be used to resuscitate children having cardiac arrest in the PICU after cardiac surgery. The advantage of the VAD system for resuscitation is the short time it takes to assemble and prime the extracorporeal circuit (approximately 10 minutes). In this case, CPR is initiated, the chest is opened, and the cannulas are placed. At this point the VAD circuit is primed and ready to implement, resulting in shorter resuscitation times. The recent use of rapid-deployment ECMO systems, however, has demonstrated success with ECMO as a method of support during cardiac arrest.[192] Modified ECMO circuits that are vacuum and carbon dioxide primed are available to initiate support within 15 minutes of notification of their need.

Advantages and disadvantages of each system exist. The primary advantage of ECMO is that it is more widely available in pediatric centers because of its use for pulmonary support in neonates. In addition, ECMO can use peripheral neck or groin cannulation, whereas VAD cannulation requires a sternotomy with direct access to the atria and aorta or pulmonary artery. The primary advantage of the VAD is the simplicity of the circuit, making it easy to assemble, prime, and maintain. In addition, the absence of an oxygenator in the VAD circuit results in less anticoagulation requirement, less blood trauma, and less bedside nursing support. ECMO traditionally uses two nurses at the bedside, one for patient care and one for circuit maintenance and monitoring, whereas the VAD circuit uses one nurse for both the patient care and circuit monitoring. Circuit monitoring for the VAD is usually a shared responsibility among the nurse, physician, and perfusionist. Finally, the VAD or BVAD more effectively performs LV decompression. With ECMO support the presence of LV distension often requires LA venting with an additional cannula or balloon atrial septostomy.

Box 7-8

Indications for the Use of ECMO and VAD for Cardiac Support

Inability to wean from cardiopulmonary bypass
  Postoperative
  Low cardiac output
Cardiac arrest
Intractable arrhythmias: intractable ventricular tachycardia
  (VT) or junctional ectopic tachycardia (JET) with hemodynamic compromise
Pulmonary hypertension not responsive to medical therapy
  and nitric oxide
Nonsurgical reversible myocardial injury
  Acute myocarditis or cardiomyopathy
Bridge to transplantation
Preoperative or postoperative pulmonary dysfunction
  Persistent pulmonary hypertension in neonates
  Pulmonary hemorrhage
  Postbypass pulmonary dysfunction
Neonatal respiratory distress or meconium aspiration in a
  neonate with congenital heart disease

From Reddy VM, Hanley FL: Mechanical support of the myocardium. In Chang AC et al, eds: *Pediatric cardiac intensive care*, Baltimore, 1998, Williams & Wilkins.

ECMO, Extracorporeal membrane oxygenation; *VAD*, ventricular assist device.

Intraaortic Balloon Counterpulsation

The IABP uses the principle of counterpulsation. With the balloon placed in the upper thoracic aorta, it inflates at the onset of diastole with aortic valve closure and deflates at the onset of systole with aortic valve opening. Inflation of the balloon results in displacement of blood volume, thereby augmenting diastolic pressure and coronary artery blood flow. Deflation of the balloon results in aortic afterload reduction and reduction in aortic impedance to LV ejection, thereby decreasing myocardial work and increasing CO. Additional benefits seen in adults include a reduction in LAP, LVEDP, and PA pressure.[188] RV function has also been shown to improve in adults receiving IABP therapy for cardiogenic shock.[193]

Despite its widespread use in adults, the application of IABP in pediatric patients has been limited. Historically, the unavailability of small balloon catheters has been the primary limitation for its use in infants and children. Currently, however, the use of IABP has increased in some centers with the development of smaller balloons that can be used in infants. The relative small size of the femoral artery in comparison with the size of the catheter, the increased compliance of the immature aorta, and the limited improvements in CO continue to limit its use in pediatric patients. In addition, higher heart rates in children make it difficult to synchronize the IABP, and there is no direct support of the right ventricle. The increased compliance and distensibility of the immature aorta have been suggested to reduce both the afterload benefits and the diastolic augmentation in children younger than 5 years of age.[194] Other investigators, however, have demonstrated clinical improvements in diastolic augmentation in even young infants.[195] Finally, increases in CO have not been quantified in pediatrics and presumably do not exceed the 10% gains reported for adult patients.[196] Therefore IABP must be used in adjunct with pharmacologic support to optimize CO. The use of inotropic support may not allow sufficient rest of the sick ventricle. For severe myocardial dysfunction, mechanical support modalities that can maximize CO and provide ventricular rest may be warranted.

Equipment and Insertion. The balloon pump consists of two components: the balloon catheter itself and the console that regulates balloon inflation and deflation.

Pediatric balloons range from 2.5- to 20-ml inflation volumes, mounted on catheters from 4.5 to 7 Fr. These catheters, unlike the adult-size balloons, do not contain an arterial pressure lumen for monitoring the central aortic pressure. The guidelines for choosing an appropriate-size catheter are delineated in Table 7-15.

The IABP console regulates the pumping of helium gas into the balloon chamber. The light weight of helium allows the gas to be displaced rapidly in and out of the balloon. The console controls allow operator regulation of the IABP triggering and timing of balloon inflation and deflation. A variety of ECG or arterial pressure signals can be used to regulate the balloon triggers, or what the pump should recognize as systole and diastole. The operator can then fine-tune the balloon timing, including both inflation and deflation points, to optimize hemodynamic parameters.

The balloon may be inserted in the intensive care unit, cardiac catheterization laboratory, emergency room, or operating room. The femoral artery is the most common site for insertion. Although percutaneous insertion is used in adults, catheter placement in infants and children requires surgical exposure of the common femoral artery, a 4- to 5-cm longitudinal arteriotomy, and placement of a sidearm synthetic graft around the artery and catheter. Once in the vessel, the catheter is advanced to the thoracic aorta and positioned with the tip of the balloon 1 to 2 cm distal to the left subclavian artery. The catheter is then sutured in place and covered with a sterile occlusive dressing. When hemostasis is achieved, a heparin infusion is initiated to maintain a partial thromboplastin time (PTT) of 40 to 60 seconds.

The catheter is then connected to the gas line of the IABP console, and pumping is started. If femoral artery cannulation is impossible, the catheter may be inserted via sternotomy directly into the aortic arch or possibly into the external iliac artery through an anterior flank incision.

Balloon Timing. Optimal timing of balloon inflation during diastole and deflation before systole is crucial (Figure 7-62). With a second set of ECG electrodes attached to the patient and the IABP console, initial timing is obtained from the R wave of the ECG tracing while monitoring the arterial pressure waveform. In this mode the IABP uses ECG signals to determine systole and diastole,

TABLE 7-15 Guidelines for Sizing Intraaortic Balloon Pump Catheters in Children

Age (yr)	Weight (kg)	Balloon Volume (ml)	Catheter Size (Fr)	Balloon Length (cm)	Balloon Diameter (mm)
<1	<8	2.5	4.5	10.7	6
1-2.5	8-13	5.0	5.5	12.8	8
2.5-5	13-18	7.0	5.5	14.2	9
5-12	18-40	12.0	7.0	17.8	10
>12	>40	20.0	7.0	19.4	19.4

From Hawkins JA, Minich LL: Intra-aortic balloon counterpulsation in pediatric cardiac patients. in Duncan BW, ed: *Mechanical circulatory support for pediatric cardiac patients,* Washington DC, Marcell Decker (in press).

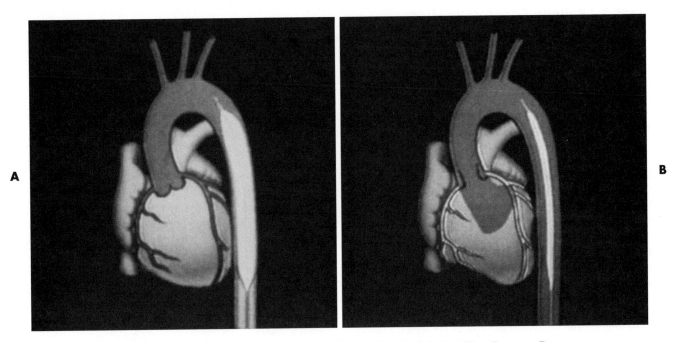

Fig. 7-62   Intraaortic balloon position during inflation **(A)** and deflation **(B)**. (Courtesy Datascope Corporation.)

automatically deflating with R wave sensing to avoid balloon inflation during systole. Balloon inflation is timed to occur with the midpoint of the T wave, which coincides with the onset of diastole.[197]

Once initiated, timing is adjusted manually to obtain maximal diastolic augmentation and a maximal decrease in peak systolic pressure. This can be achieved through the comparison of augmented (balloon-assisted) and nonaugmented beats on the arterial waveform when the IABP is inflated every other beat (1:2 augmentation). Timing of balloon inflation just before the dicrotic notch (before the onset of diastole) has been advocated to increase the duration of assisted diastolic perfusion.[198] Use of the arterial waveform, however, may not be accurate because of the delay between the central aortic pressure and the peripheral arterial pressure that is frequently monitored in children. In this case, the observed dicrotic notch may not accurately reflect diastole; therefore, if the balloon is inflated during this time, it may actually be during late diastole, and deflation may not occur until after systole has begun. Some investigators believe the best timing can be obtained when initial triggering is obtained from the ECG in combination with M-mode echocardiography. With this method, echocardiography provides simultaneous images of the balloon and the aortic valve, allowing precise adjustments to be made so that balloon inflation and deflation coincide with aortic valve closure and opening.[199]

Rapid heart rates in children may require special timing considerations. In the past, 1:2 balloon assistance was advocated when the HR exceeded 160 beats/min.[200] Recent improvements in compressor response time and the use of echocardiographic timing, however, have allowed better tracking ability at very high heart rates, allowing 1:1 balloon assistance. In this situation, the gas is shuttled back and forth quickly, causing more rapid diffusion of the helium, which

results in the need for manual filling of the balloon every 1 to 2 hours.

When optimal timing has been achieved, hemodynamic benefits are evident both clinically and on the arterial BP tracing. Diastolic augmentation should reach suprasystolic levels, meaning the balloon-assisted diastolic pressure becomes the highest point on the waveform. Afterload reduction is evidenced by a decreased systolic pressure following balloon inflation, as well as by lowered aortic end-diastolic pressures (Figure 7-63). In reality, these "ideal" tracing landmarks are not always evident, despite clinical improvements in CO and tissue perfusion. Additional indications, such as decreased HR, and improvements in urine output, mixed venous oxygen saturation, and peripheral perfusion should be monitored to evaluate the effectiveness of the balloon pump.

Continuous hemodynamic and HR monitoring provides evidence of the need for IABP timing adjustments, which should be made for signs of deteriorating clinical status, a change in cardiac rhythm, or HR changes greater than 10 beats/min.[201] Improper IABP timing can result in suboptimal cardiac support or severely compromised cardiac ejection.

Nursing Care.   Care of the child receiving IABP therapy requires expert nursing knowledge of cardiac physiology, as well as knowledge and skill of the IABP device. The potential infrequent use of this therapy makes it difficult to maintain nursing competency and experience. Typically, nursing care is provided by two nurses: one to care for the patient and one to monitor and manipulate the balloon pump. Nursing care responsibilities include manipulating the pump, monitoring hemodynamics, evaluating the effectiveness of the therapy, assessing the progression of cardiac failure, monitoring for complications of the therapy, and providing family education and support. Nursing care

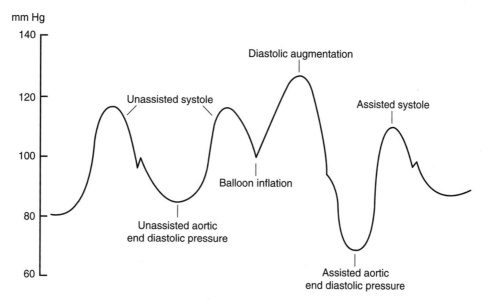

Fig. 7-63 Arterial pressure waveform characteristics during intraaortic balloon counterpulsation therapy.

may be more complex than in adults because of the challenges of timing requiring frequent manual timing and the difficulty in the interpretation of IABP waveforms.[202]

Once IABP therapy is initiated and minor adjustments in balloon timing are complete, an hourly assessment is performed that includes recording of IABP parameters, evaluation of hemodynamic parameters, assessment of leg perfusion distal to the catheter, urine output, and laboratory results.[202] The ECG tracing and the IABP waveforms are constantly monitored to interpret the effectiveness of balloon pumping. Timing is evaluated every 1 to 2 hours along with the manual filling of the balloon.

Continuous monitoring and evaluation of the effectiveness of IABP support are crucial. Frequent assessment of hemodynamic parameters should reveal the anticipated benefits of IABP counterpulsation, including signs of increased CO, decreased SVR and filling pressures, and improved end-organ perfusion. Failure to achieve these parameters may be the result of improper IABP timing, arrhythmias, catheter dislodgment or damage, or worsening ventricular function.

Catheter migration may result in decreased perfusion of either the kidneys or left arm. An abrupt cessation of urine output may indicate downward balloon migration with obstruction of the renal arteries. Upward balloon displacement can result in obstruction of the left subclavian artery, resulting in impaired left arm perfusion. Correct IABP position should be evaluated with a daily chest radiograph.

Careful assessment of the cannulated lower extremity is also important. The quality of peripheral pulses should be assessed before and after balloon placement to note changes from baseline. Asymptomatic loss of palpable distal pulses occurs commonly after IABP insertion and often does not progress to severe limb ischemia. If systemic output is improved after balloon placement, tissue perfusion to the cannulated leg may improve despite diminished distal pulses. Signs of more severe obstruction to blood flow, including pain, pallor, or mottling, and decreased sensation or loss of motor function should be aggressively evaluated.

Weaning From IABP. Weaning from IABP can be initiated when hemodynamics are stable, pharmacologic support has been significantly reduced, and improvements in cardiac function are evident. Echocardiography is often used to evaluate LV shortening fraction and ejection fraction to document improvements in ventricular function before weaning from IABP.

Weaning to discontinuation of support is usually performed over a 24- to 48-hour period. Weaning is achieved by decreasing the frequency of augmentation from every beat (1:1) to every second, fourth, or eighth beat (1:2, 1:4, 1:8). During this process the nurse monitors and evaluates the patient for signs of failure to wean, including signs of decreased CO and tissue perfusion, increased filling pressures, and cardiac arrhythmias. Pharmacologic support may be increased at this time to optimize cardiac function. If weaning is tolerated, the catheter is removed surgically, and the incision is closed. Embolectomy catheters may be used immediately after catheter removal to remove any clot trapped in the femoral artery.[188] Careful assessment of distal extremity pulses and perfusion following the discontinuation of therapy is critical to identify thrombus formation or distal embolization of clot.

Outcomes. In 1980, Pollock and co-workers[194] reported the use of IABP in 14 children between 1.5 and 18 years of age following cardiac surgery. Although six children (43%) were long-term survivors, no child under the age of 5 years survived. They concluded that young children with minimal CO and immature aortas could not be adequately augmented with the IABP. Later, this same series was reported with additional patients. With the improvements in equipment, they reported the successful augmentation of CO in a 2-kg infant with LV failure of unknown cause. The total number of patients over a 10-year period was 38 with a 37% survival. In this group, the patients with the highest mortality were those who were postoperative Fontan patients.

The largest series to date reports the use of IABP in 43 patients over a 15-year period. This series included both postsurgical and medical patients ranging in age from 5 days to 18 years, weighing 4.2 to 40 kg; 19 of the patients were less than 3 years of age. In this series, 51% of the patients were weaned from the IABP, and 42% were long-term survivors. With increased experience over the 15 years, improvements in technology, and the implementation of echocardiographic timing, the more recent survival in this group has improved. Since 1994, reported survival has been 78%.[188]

Complications reported with the use of IABP include limb ischemia, renal failure, mesenteric ischemia, balloon rupture, vessel perforation, hematoma, and wound infection. The increased experience and improved technology, however, have shown a decrease in these complications. Pollock and colleagues[194] reported that 14% of the patients suffered severe leg ischemia, 14% experienced renal failure, and 7% had abdominal distension. More recently, Hawkins and Minich[188] reported that over the last 10 years, complications related to IABP therapy have been few. In 22 patients, 1 patient had limb ischemia and 1 developed sepsis; however, neither complication required removal of the IABP.

Ventricular Assist Devices

A VAD is an extracorporeal pump that takes over a variable percent of left or right ventricular output. It is used in situations of life-threatening ventricular dysfunction. Although several types of VADs exist, the centrifugal pump is most commonly used for temporary cardiac support in children. The primary advantage of the VAD is its ability to support 100% of the CO, thereby allowing the inotropes to be weaned and the heart to sufficiently rest and recover. In addition, the VAD is a simple extracorporeal circuit and pump that requires little manipulation once support has been initiated.

Pneumatic VADs can be used in adult-size children, usually in the setting of bridge to transplantation. They consist of a paracorporeal air-driven blood pump, and an electropneumatic driving system that provides pulsatile blood flow. The blood pump circuit consists of short segments of tubing that connect directly to the intracardiac cannulas, artificial ventricles that house a blood chamber, and an air chamber separated by a polyurethane membrane. The console allows adjustments of HR, drive pressure, and percentage of systole to optimize hemodynamics. The system can be operated in an asynchronous mode or triggered by the ECG for cardiac synchrony. Although there are case reports of their use in small children, pneumatic VADs are currently limited secondary to size constraints, flow requirements, and the need for multiple pumps, with

different stroke volumes to accommodate a wide range of pediatric sizes.

The centrifugal VAD pump transports blood through an extracorporeal circuit by imparting kinetic energy to it (Figure 7-64). Power is applied to a magnetic pump head that rotates a magnet in a cone-shaped impeller that, in turn, rotates the blood inside the cone, creating a centrifugal force that transports the blood through the circuit. There is no obligatory volume displacement by the pump, and the flow through the circuit is both preload and afterload sensitive. Venous return to the pump is active and not dependent on gravity. The revolutions per minute (rpm) are set to achieve a desired flow (CO) through the circuit. Blood flow through this extracorporeal circuit is continuous and nonpulsatile. There is no reservoir, oxygenator, or heat exchanger present; therefore, it is a completely closed system.

When a LVAD is indicated, the extracorporeal circuit consists of a LA cannula connected by a short segment of tubing to the cone segment of the pump. The cone segment is connected by another short segment of tubing to an aortic cannula. When RV assist is indicated, RA and PA cannulas are connected to the pump tubing and pump. When biventricular support is indicated, the left atrium and aorta are connected to one pump, and the right atrium and pulmonary artery are connected to a second pump. When a VAD is indicated for a single-ventricle heart, the cannulas are place in the common atria and the aorta. In all cases, a flow probe is present on the inflow (aortic/pulmonary artery) tubing. This measures the flow, or CO, provide by the VAD.

Equipment and Insertion.   The Bio-Medicus (Medtronic) system is the most common VAD used in children who require mechanical cardiac support. This system consists of a Bio-Console, the Bio-Probe monitoring system, a disposable Bio-Pump circuit, and an emergency handcrank. The Bio-Console contains the operator controls, monitors, and alarms, as well as the pump receptacle. It operates on standard line voltage or battery power. Two pump sizes are available for support: the BP-50 Bio-Pump is used for patients weighing less than 10 kg, and the BP-80 Bio-Pump is used for patients weighing more than 10 kg. The ¼-inch tubing fits the BP-50 with a complete priming volume of approximately 180 ml, and ⅜-inch tubing fits the BP-80 with a priming volume of 350 ml. Both pump sizes fit the same drive unit. The pump is equipped with an internal battery that will maintain pump function when there is not AC power. The battery, when charged, lasts approximately 45 minutes at a 3500-RPM pump speed. The cannulas used for standard cardiopulmonary bypass are used for the VAD.

The initiation of VAD support can occur in the PICU or in the operating room. When initiated in the operating room, every effort is made to control the surgical bleeding before initiating mechanical support. When possible, the patient is weaned from cardiopulmonary bypass, the heparin is reversed, and clotting factors are administered. Following this, VAD support is initiated with limited and controlled anticoagulation.

The cannulas are placed via open sternotomy and connected to the extracorporeal circuit that has been primed

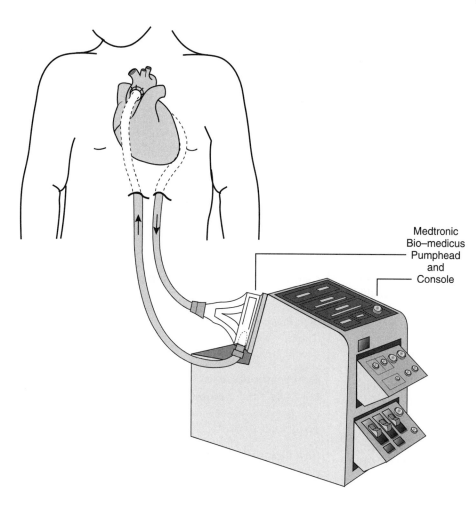

Medtronic
Bio–medicus
Pumphead
and
Console

Fig. 7-64 Left ventricular assist device support with Medtronic Bio-Medicus centrifugal device. (Copyright 1990 by Medtronic, Inc. Reprinted with permission.)

with 5% albumin or whole blood. The pump head is placed into the console, and blood flow through the circuit is initiated by increasing the RPMs to achieve a desired extracorporeal flow (CO). The percentage of CO provided by the VAD depends on the degree of myocardial dysfunction. Generally, flow is increased until desired mean systemic arterial pressure and atrial pressures are achieved. Hemodynamic parameters, peripheral perfusion, color, urine output, and systemic arterial blood gases are immediately evaluated for signs of improved oxygen delivery.

The cannulas are securely sutured in place, and the mediastinum is left open and covered with a Silastic patch. Occasionally in older children, the sternum is left open, and the skin is closed. A continuous infusion of heparin is initiated to maintain an activated clotting time (ACT) of 160 to 200 seconds, depending on VAD flow rates.

Management. Care of the patient requiring centrifugal VAD support requires a highly skilled, multidisciplinary approach to provide a safe environment, minimize complications, and promote optimal recovery. Hemodynamic parameters are monitored and evaluated continuously. Mean systemic arterial pressure is usually maintained at 40 mmHg or greater in neonates and 60 mmHg in older children.[203] The arterial line will have variable pulsatility depending on the amount of nonpulsatile flow provided by the VAD. Therefore the MAP is monitored as a measure of

CO. As ventricular function improves and VAD support is decreased, pulsatility on the arterial waveform should improve. Pulse oximetry may also be difficult to monitor because of the absence of distal pulses. In this case, blood gas analysis should be used to evaluate systemic arterial oxygenation.

The pump RPM is adjusted to provide a CO that results in an atrial pressure (RA or LA) of 6 to 10 mmHg. When an isolated LVAD is used, RA pressure is used to monitor volume status and is maintained between 5 to 10 mmHg. When RA pressure is elevated, RV dysfunction should be suspected. With an isolated RVAD, LA pressure is used to monitor volume status, assuming the left ventricle is working adequately. In any case, atrial pressures are always maintained over 5 mmHg to prevent any air from being entrained into the circuit. This is especially important when an LVAD is used because the entry of air could result in cerebral or coronary air embolism.

A systemic continuous infusion of heparin is provided to avoid clot formation in the cannulas and extracorporeal circuit. When a full CO is provided by the VAD, ACT is titrated to about 150 to 180 seconds. When pump support is less than 50% of CO, ACT is titrated to about 180 to 200 seconds. Lower ACT (160 to 180 seconds) may be maintained if tubing coated with the Carmeda BioActive Surface is used.[191] The patient's hematocrit should be maintained at about 40%, depending on the patient's physiology, to optimize oxygen delivery. Inotropic support will vary, depending on the phase of the assist device period. During the early support phase (initial 48 hours) when nearly 100% support is provided, inotropic support should be minimal and used to support the non–pump-assisted ventricle (5 µg/kg/min of dopamine, no epinephrine), allowing optimal rest of the sick ventricle. During the weaning phase, inotropic support will need to be increased to achieve acceptable biventricular function.

Because the centrifugal VAD has no obligatory volume displacement, the flow through the circuit is both preload and afterload sensitive. Changes in the patient's preload and systemic and pulmonary vascular resistances will alter the flow through the circuit. For example, if the patient loses blood volume, flow through the VAD will decrease. If SVR increases on a patient receiving LVAD therapy, this will also result in a decreasing flow through the circuit and potentially increasing the volume load on the left ventricle. VAD flow alarms must be monitoring closely to detect changes in circuit flow.

During VAD support, it is crucial that all hemodynamic parameters are monitored and evaluated continuously to recognize changes in VAD flow, ventricular function, volume status, and VAD complications. Specific troubleshooting for hemodynamic parameters and complications are listed in Box 7-9.

Nursing Care. Specific nursing responsibilities when caring for patients on a centrifugal VAD include the following: (1) maintaining the safety and security of the extracorporeal circuit; (2) hourly monitoring of the circuit for air and clot formation; (3) monitoring hemodynamic parameters, VAD flow, and signs of adequate oxygen delivery; (4) thermoregulation; (5) skin care; (6) assessment and management of comfort; (7) observing for complications; and (8) support and education of the family. Collaborative responsibilities include troubleshooting, treatment of complications, and management of emergencies.

Nurses have a primary responsibility to ensure the safety of the patient's environment and to prevent complications of therapy. Specific safety interventions for the VAD include the following: (1) securing the cannula(s) to the patient; (2) securing the circuit tubing to the patient and the bed; (3) maintaining system security during procedures, such as radiographic examinations, and position changes; (4) ensuring that emergency electrical power is maintained; (5) appropriately setting hemodynamic and VAD alarm limits; and (6) carefully observing for air or thrombus formation in the circuit. Although thrombus formation can occur at any location in the circuit, it is more likely to occur where connections exist, for example, in the connectors between the cannulas and the circuit tubing. The surgeons should be alerted of any thrombus formation. When thrombus is removed, the patient is temporarily removed from VAD support while the thrombus is evacuated; therefore interventions must be implemented to support the heart during this time. Air can enter the circuit if the atrial pressure falls below 5 mmHg. For small amount of static air, the surgeons should be alerted and plans made to remove it. If large amounts of air have entered and are moving toward the

---

Box 7-9
Troubleshooting Patients on the Centrifugal Ventricular Assist Device

Left Ventricular Assist Device (LVAD)
Low Left Atrial (LA) Pressure
Consider: hypovolemia, right ventricle (RV) failure, excessive pump support, LA line in the pericardial space, malfunctioning LA line

High Left Atrial Pressure
Consider: volume overload, worsening left ventricle (LV) failure, inadequate pump support, LA line near the mitral valve or wedged in the atria or pulmonary vein

Low Right Atrial (RA) Pressure
Consider: hypovolemia, PFO or ASD, RA line in the pericardial space

High Right Atrial Pressure
Consider: volume overload, RV failure, RA line in the RV or wedged in the atria, PHT

Right Ventricular Assist Device (RVAD)
Low Right Atrial Pressure
Consider: hypovolemia, excessive pump support, RA line in the pericardial space

High Right Atrial Pressure
Consider: worsening RV failure, inadequate pump support, volume overload, RA line near the tricuspid valve or wedged in the atria

Low Left Atrial Pressure
Consider: hypovolemia, malpositioned LA line, PFO, or ASD

High Left Atrial Pressure
Consider: LV failure, malpositioned LA line, volume overload, increased afterload in systemic circulation

RVAD or LVAD
Deteriorating Blood Gases
Consider: worsening heart failure, primary pulmonary problem, ASD, or PFO

Inability to Maintain Adequate Flow
Consider: hypovolemia, malpositioned cannulas, thrombosis of cannulas or circuit, kink in the circuit tubing, increased afterload

Excessive Mediastinal Hemorrhage
Consider: overheparinization, consumptive coagulopathy, cannula dislodgment, surgical bleeding

PFO, Patent foramen ovale; *ASD,* atrial septal defect.

---

patient, it may be necessary for the nurse to emergently clamp the aortic/pulmonary artery cannulas to prevent air entry to the patient. When the cannulas or tubing are clamped, the patient will be acutely removed from VAD support and resuscitative measures should be implemented.

Maintaining the patient's temperature is also crucial. Without a heat exchanger in the centrifugal VAD circuit, pediatric patients, especially neonates and infants, may quickly become hypothermic. Every effort should be made before the initiation of therapy to warm the patient. Such interventions include increasing the ambient room temperature, placing a warming device under or over the patient, and placing a warming blanket under the extracorporal circuit tubing. In addition, the patient's temperature should be monitored continuously to avoid sudden drops in temperature. Cooling from the extracorporeal circuit may mask the presence of a fever. Other signs of infection should be monitored closely.

Careful monitoring of hemodynamic parameters, along with VAD flow, will provide information regarding adequacy of oxygen delivery and recovery of ventricular function. Atrial alarm limits should be set at 5 mmHg so that the nurse is immediately alerted immediately to low atrial pressures. Interventions must be implemented to prevent the entry of air into the circuit. These include volume administration or lowering of the VAD flow until atrial pressure increases to 6 to 10 mmHg. Changes in atrial pressure, BP, and VAD flow may indicate changes in preload or afterload and should be evaluated immediately.

Interventions to maintain skin integrity and prevent other complications of immobility must be implemented. Patients can safely be turned side to side even small amounts to assess the skin and prevent breakdown on pressure points. When doing so, one nurse should hold the cannulas and circuit tubing to prevent accidental kinking or disconnection. When possible, the use of a pressure-reducing air mattress should be considered before implementation of VAD therapy. Typically these patients receive continuous infusions of analgesics and sedatives and intermittent neuromuscular blocking agents.

Bleeding is the most common complication associated with VAD use and therefore must be carefully assessed and managed by the PICU team. Common causes include surgical bleeding, anticoagulation, and coagulopathy. Assessment for bleeding complications includes strict monitoring of chest tube output, evaluation of hematocrit and coagulation studies, monitoring for signs of cardiac tamponade, and observing the open chest for accumulation of blood. Packed red blood cells, fresh frozen plasma, and platelets may be administered to maintain hemostasis. Careful attention must be made, however, to the risk of thrombus formation in the extracorporeal circuit when fresh frozen plasma and platelets are administered. Cryoprecipitate and vitamin K are generally avoided because of the potential for acute thrombus formation.[204]

Potential emergency situations include cardiac arrest, circuit disruption, and pump malfunction. Box 7-10 outlines general guidelines for the management of these emergencies. Specific measures for resuscitation should be established in each institution and for individual clinical situations. Emergency resuscitation with open chest cardiac compressions poses a risk of cannula disruption; however, the exact risk is unknown and may not necessitate the avoidance of compressions. Clamps are kept at the bedside

---

Box 7-10

General Guidelines for the Management of VAD Emergencies

In the event of a cardiac arrest:

BiVAD:	Turn pumps to full cardiac support
RVAD or LVAD:	CPR to resuscitate the heart
	Defibrillation for ventricular fibrillation

In the event of a circuit disruption:

Outside the chest:	Clamp the circuit tubing or cannulaes
Inside the chest:	Notify surgeons immediately—CPR

In the event of pump malfunction:

Hand crank for power failure
Notify surgeons and perfusionists immediately
Evaluate cardiovascular status—CPR

VAD, Ventricular assist device; *CPR,* cardiopulmonary resuscitation.

---

for prevention of hemorrhage with circuit disruption and to prevent air entry into the aorta. Clamps can be placed onto the circuit tubing while the pump is running. The centrifugal nature of the VAD flow prevents increases in circuit pressure and leak when clamped.

Weaning From VAD. Weaning from the VAD is accomplished when the patient's hemodynamics have improved and there is echocardiographic evidence that ventricular function has recovered. Typically, recovery can be observed when there is a return of a pulsatile waveform on the peripheral arterial trace on high levels of device support (80% of the CO provided by the VAD).[191] Weaning to discontinuation of therapy can take place in the operating room or the PICU and usually occurs over several hours. Once inotropic support is optimized, the VAD flow is gradually decreased while carefully evaluating the patient's hemodynamics. When the VAD flow is at a minimum, HR, systemic arterial BP, atrial pressure, and arterial blood gases are evaluated for signs of adequate oxygen delivery. In addition, transesophageal echocardiography is performed to evaluate ventricular function. When medical therapy is optimized, mechanical support is completely withdrawn. After discontinuation, the patient should be closely monitored for signs of low CO. The chest may be left open until adequate ventricular function and hemodynamic stability have been ensured.

Outcomes. Several small series report the use of centrifugal ventricular assist devices in children.[189-191,205-208] The most common indications for VAD support were the failure to wean from cardiopulmonary bypass and postoperative low CO. In these series, duration of support ranged from 1 to 8 days (mean of approximately 43 hours), and survival ranged from 31% to 70%. Thuys and colleagues[189] reported VAD use in 34 postoperative infants weighing under 6 kg, with the most common diagnosis being hypoplastic left heart syndrome. Sixty-four percent of these infants were weaned from VAD, and 31% survived to hospital discharge. Del Nido and associates[190] reported 70% survival in children receiving VAD support after repair of anomalous origin of the left coronary artery from the pulmonary artery (AL-CAPA). These demonstrate the role that diagnosis may have on survival.

In a larger series, Duncan and co-workers[191] reported the use of VAD support in 29 children with cardiac disease. Survival in this group was 41%, with the most common causes of death being ventricular failure and multiple organ system failure. Patients who did not demonstrate return of ventricular function within 48 to 72 hours of the institution of support either died or required cardiac transplantation. Costa and colleagues[208] reported the highest mortality to be in patients requiring support for postoperative low CO, emphasizing the importance of early institution of therapy to avoid multiple organ system failure.

Potential complications of VAD therapy include bleeding, circuit thrombus formation, infection, air emboli, neurologic damage, hemolysis, and mechanical problems. Bleeding secondary to anticoagulation, surgical bleeding, or coagulopathy is the most common complication of VAD support. Duncan and co-workers[191] reported that 44% of VAD patients experienced excessive bleeding. Risk factors included chest cannulation and need for initiation of support in the operating room. Thuys and associates[189] reported thrombus formation in the VAD circuit to be the most common complication, occurring in 38% of patients. Of these patients, four required pump head changes, one required circuit change, and eight required no intervention.

In the series listed previously, serious infections, including mediastinitis, pneumonia, and positive blood cultures, have been reported in up to 30% of patients requiring VAD support. Potential predisposing factors may include preoperative infection, delayed sternal closure, use of invasive monitoring lines and catheters, mediastinal exploration for bleeding, and prolonged ventilatory support. Measures to decrease infection include frequent handwashing, strict aseptic technique during contact with invasive lines, prompt removal of nonessential lines and catheters, aggressive pulmonary hygiene measures, and use of sterile technique during open sternal dressing changes. Additional reported complications, such as hemolysis and mechanical problems, are less common but must be carefully assessed in all VAD patients.

Extracorporeal Membrane Oxygenation for Cardiac Support

ECMO consists of an extracorporeal circuit that contains an oxygen membrane, a pump, and a heat exchanger. Like the VAD, ECMO can support a variable amount of the CO. The primary advantage over the VAD is its ability to provide both oxygenation and cardiac support. The disadvantage compared with the VAD is the complexity of the circuit and the increased need for anticoagulation. ECMO for cardiac support is used primarily in postoperative cardiac surgery patients who suffer from low CO in addition to hypoxemia or pulmonary hypertension. Its use in children with cardiomyopathy or myocarditis has also been described. The use of ECMO for the resuscitation of pediatric patients with

heart disease following cardiac arrest has also been reported with successful outcomes.[192,209]

Equipment and Insertion. Techniques and systems used for ECMO support are well described in Chapter 8. In brief, a servoregulated flow system driven by a pump with a membrane oxygenator and a heat exchanger is used. Blood is drained by gravity through the venous cannulas into the servoregulated system. Although a roller pump is commonly used in the ECMO circuit, a centrifugal pump can be used in its place. Premembrane and postmembrane pressures are monitored. Venoarterial support is used in the majority of patients; however, in cardiac patients suffering isolated pulmonary dysfunction, venovenous ECMO may be used.

Initiation of support can occur in the PICU or the operating room. For cardiac patients, the site of cannulation will vary depending on surgical preference and the clinical situation. Patients who require immediate postoperative support or those who require support during resuscitation usually have transthoracic cannulas placed directly into the RA appendage and the aorta. Peripheral cannulation via the neck or femoral vessels may be used in patients who require support later in their postoperative period. In general, large venous cannulas are required secondary to the high flow rates used for cardiac support. In addition to the RA and aortic cannulas, the placement of an LA cannula is often necessary. Blood return to the left atrium, along with the increased LV afterload resulting from the high flow rates to the ascending aorta, can cause increases in LVEDP and LAP. To adequately rest the left ventricle and prevent pulmonary edema, a LA cannula is placed to decompress the left ventricle. This cannula is connected to the venous tubing of the ECMO circuit with a Y connection. When transthoracic cannulas are used, the chest is usually left open and covered with a Silastic patch.

Management. The ECMO procedure for cardiac support is similar to that required for acute respiratory failure in children; however, the goals of support are different. In the patients requiring ECMO for acute respiratory failure, pump flows are adjusted to achieve satisfactory arterial oxygenation. In patients with low CO after cardiac operations, the goal is to maintain adequate tissue perfusion while providing complete or nearly complete cardiac bypass to prevent cardiac distension, minimize myocardial energy expenditure, and maximize the chance of cardiac recovery. Once support is initiated, flow rates are adjusted to provide a systemic MAP of approximately 40 mmHg in neonates and 60 mmHg in children and atrial pressures of 4 to 8 mmHg. Patients are assessed for a reversal in their shock state, including improvements in peripheral perfusion, increases in urine output, reversal of metabolic acidosis, and improvements in systemic and mixed venous oxygen saturations. Generally, flow rates of 100 to 200 ml/kg/min are required to support perfusion and allow ventricular rest. Once stabilized, inotropic infusions are minimized to reduce their adverse effects on the heart and allow ventricular rest. Mechanical ventilator settings can be minimized to prevent barotrauma and allow pulmonary recovery. Nonpulsatile flow provided by the ECMO circuit results in a dampened arterial waveform and the inability to use pulse oximetry.

Children on ECMO usually receive prophylactic antibiotic therapy; however, broad-spectrum coverage is generally avoided. Antibiotic coverage is individualized when specific organisms are cultured. Anticoagulation is provided by a continuous infusion of heparin administered via the ECMO circuit. Heparin is titrated to achieve an activated clotting time of 180 to 220 seconds. Parenteral nutrition is initiated within 24 to 48 hours. Enteral nutrition is avoided until full recovery of the hypoperfusion state has occurred. Typically, continuous infusions of analgesics and sedatives along with intermittent doses of neuromuscular blocking agents are administered.

Patients who are oliguric or anuric can receive renal replacement therapy through peritoneal dialysis or hemofiltration. A hemofilter can be placed from the arterial tubing to the venous tubing, essentially providing continuous arteriovenous hemofiltration. This can provide both solute clearance and fluid removal until renal function improves. Countercurrent dialysate flow can be provided when additional solute clearance is required.

Weaning From ECMO Support. In general, patients are maintained on full ECMO support for 48 to 72 hours before any attempt to wean. The duration of ECMO when used for cardiac support is less than when used for acute respiratory failure. The technique for weaning is also different. When weaning for respiratory failure, pump flow is decreased as pulmonary function improves. When used for cardiac failure, pump flow is gradually turned down while maintaining adequate filling pressures and systemic BP. Pump flow is gradually reduced in small increments over a 12- to 24-hour period. During this time, ventilator settings are increased to achieve adequate oxygenation, ventilation, and acid-base status. Inotropic support is also increased to optimize myocardial function. The pulse contour on the systemic arterial tracing is closely observed, along with other signs of adequate systemic perfusion. Atrial pressures usually rise to normal or elevated levels, augmented by volume administration as indicated. Transesophageal echocardiography may be performed during the weaning phase to assess myocardial contractility and ventricular ejection in relation to systolic BP as blood flow pump is decreased. Once optimal CO and pulmonary function are achieved, the patient is tried off ECMO for a brief period, followed by decannulation. The chest is often left open after the discontinuation of ECMO until optimal hemodynamics and oxygen saturation have been achieved.

Nursing Care. Caring for the patient receiving ECMO for cardiac support requires two nurses. One nurse provides direct patient care while the second nurse provides the monitoring and manipulation of the ECMO circuit. Nursing care for the ECMO patient is well described in Chapter 8. Specific nursing considerations are made for the patient receiving ECMO after cardiac surgery. These are related to the assessment and management of cardiac function and the recognition and management of complications secondary to the use of cardiac ECMO.

Monitoring Cardiac Function. MAP, RA pressure, and LA pressure are continuously monitored. Increases in atrial pressures may indicate worsening cardiac function or volume overload, whereas decreases in atrial pressures may indicate improving ventricular function, excessive ECMO support, or hypovolemia. Isolated increases in LA pressure may indicate inadequate LV decompression and should be addressed. When a LA cannula is present for LV decompression, flow through it may be sluggish and should be carefully monitored. When thrombus forms in the LA vent, the tubing should be changed to avoid left atrial and ventricular distension. HR and rhythm must also be supported to optimize hemodynamics. Cardiac arrhythmias should be promptly treated with antiarrhythmic medications or pacemaker therapy to maintain a normal sinus rhythm. Additional signs of adequate oxygen delivery should be monitored closely to ensure adequate extracorporeal support. Systemic arterial pulsatility should improve when cardiac function has recovered, despite high levels of ECMO support. Some patients experience systemic hypertension when receiving cardiopulmonary bypass from ECMO and may require afterload reduction. This may be related to the renin-angiotensin response to nonpulsatile flow.

Assessment and Management of Complications. Bleeding is a major complication of ECMO when used for cardiac support and may require multiple exploration of the mediastinum to remove blood and to evaluate for surgical bleeding. Multiple suture lines, the use of cardiopulmonary bypass, the need for systemic heparinization, delayed sternal closure, and the use of multiple drainage tubes and monitoring lines result in generalized chest bleeding. In addition to chest bleeding, significant gastrointestinal, pulmonary, and intraabdominal bleeding has been reported. Nursing interventions include careful monitoring of blood loss, specifically through the chest tubes. Assessment of the mediastinum under the Silastic patch is crucial to evaluate the accumulation of mediastinal blood and the possible development of cardiac tamponade. Replacement of blood in addition to platelets and fresh frozen plasma is often necessary. Although bleeding can be treated with transfusions, massive transfusions can result in pulmonary impairment that may impact morbidity and mortality. Ionized calcium levels may fall when large amounts of blood transfusions are administered. Adequate replacement of calcium must be given to prevent negative inotrope associated with hypocalcemia.

The nursing team must provide the prevention, assessment, and management of other potential complications. Most commonly these include neurologic complications, infection, and renal failure. Although the patients typically receive continuous infusions of analgesics and sedatives, the intermittent use of neuromuscular blocking agents allows periods when a neurologic examination can be performed. Clinical evidence of seizures must be reported and managed aggressively. Neonates should receive head ultrasounds when abnormal neurologic examinations are present. The prevention of infection and the early identification of infection are crucial. Prevention strategies include meticulous dressing and wound care, sterile technique and maintenance of a sterile environment for mediastinal explorations, limited entry into the ECMO circuit and invasive catheters, and meticulous handwashing. Although signs of infection must be monitored, it should be remembered that fever may be masked by the heat exchanger and changes in platelet count may be altered by the use of the extracorporeal circuit. Elevations in white blood cell counts and positive cultures must be aggressively treated. The presence of renal failure may be managed by hemofiltration through the ECMO circuit. Strict monitoring of intake and output and frequent evaluation of laboratory data are critical to avoid complications related to hypovolemia, hypervolemia, or electrolyte disturbance.

The stress of ECMO therapy after cardiac surgery affects family coping. The severity of illness, sight of the extracorporeal circuit, and increased risk for morbidity and mortality are particularly stressful to families.[210] Preparation for visiting, regular communication, and providing accurate information is important. As with any critically ill child, families must be supported in their attempts to be involved in their child's care, regardless of their acuity.

Outcomes. Over the last decade, several centers have reported the use of ECMO for cardiac support.[191,211-218] In these series, success with weaning from ECMO support was reported in 52% to 75% of patients, and survival to hospital discharge has occurred in 33% to 58% of patients. In a recent larger series, Duncan and colleagues[191] reported the use of ECMO for cardiac support in 67 patients, with an overall survival of 40.3%.

Several authors have attempted to determine outcome-associated factors for pediatric cardiac ECMO.[191,216-218] In these series, factors associated with mortality included the presence of residual cardiac defects, the presence of single-ventricle physiology, the need to initiate ECMO support in the operating room immediately following cardiopulmonary bypass, renal failure, and the lack of return of ventricular function after 72 hours of ECMO support. Black and co-workers[216] reported the maximum time required for ventricular recovery among 31 postcardiotomy patients was 6 days; all children supported longer than 6 days died. Duncan and colleagues[191] concluded that there were no ECMO survivors with a serum pH below 7.38 or serum bicarbonate below 22 mmol/dl at 24 hours of ECMO support. This finding presumably reflected the impact of significant hypoperfusion before the initiation of ECMO support.

The use of ECMO to resuscitate children having cardiac arrest after cardiac surgery has demonstrated better results than in other patient populations.[192,209,215] In one series in which eleven cardiac patients were resuscitated with ECMO, 91% were weaned from ECMO, and 64% were discharged from the hospital. The reasons for better outcomes in pediatric patients with cardiac disease may be related to witnessed arrests in the PICU, the use of open chest CPR, the degree of core cooling, and the possible acute yet reversible cause of the arrest, such as cardiac arrhythmias.

Complications reported with cardiac ECMO include bleeding, infection, renal failure, neurologic complications, multiple system organ failure, and mechanical problems. When comparing ECMO and VAD therapy for cardiac support, all complications occurred more often in ECMO patients.[191] In one series, survival was low (<22%) in patients who had any complication.[218] Bleeding is the most common complication associated with cardiac ECMO, occurring in approximately 40% of patients. Excessive blood loss has been shown to be a risk factor for death in ECMO-supported patients.[191] In this series, risk factors for excessive bleeding included chest cannulation and the need for ECMO support in the operating room.

Neurologic complications include seizures, intracranial hemorrhage, embolus or thrombus, and anoxic encephalopathy. Although these complications may not result in death, they have a significant impact on morbidity. Other than intracranial hemorrhage, it may be difficult to determine if the neurologic complications result from the ECMO or the pre-ECMO condition.

Infection occurs in approximately 25% of patients receiving cardiac ECMO support.[191,217] Most often these infections include mediastinitis, pneumonia, and sepsis. Renal failure occurs in approximately 20% of patients and often requires hemofiltration.[191,218]

Mechanical problems occur more often in ECMO support than VAD support; however, they may not be associated with a significantly higher mortality. The increased mechanical problems are presumably related to the increased complexity of the ECMO circuit. The presence of the oxygenator is a significant source of morbidity, resulting in trauma to blood elements and activation of systemic inflammatory and coagulation cascades.

SUMMARY

This chapter has provided a review of fetal development of the heart and fetal circulation and the circulatory changes that occur at birth. Normal fetal cardiovascular development provided a mechanism to introduce congenital heart disease. The physical properties of the cardiovascular system were reviewed next; including an overview of essential anatomy, the function of the heart's electrical system, the cardiac cycle, and regulation of CO. Attention was directed at the effects of maturation on cardiovascular function.

The second major focus of the chapter was assessment of the cardiovascular system. Both physical assessment and noninvasive evaluation were reviewed. Discussion of intensive care unit monitoring of cardiovascular function and cardiac catheterization followed.

Sections that detailed cardiovascular support to maintain adequate tissue perfusion concluded the chapter. Pharmacologic support, pacemaker therapy, and mechanical support were discussed. Because cardiovascular failure and inadequate tissue perfusion are the final common pathophysiologic pathways in a variety of critical illnesses and injuries in infants and children, critical care nurses must master complex therapies and technologies aimed at restoring health to this patient population.

Chapter 7 Tissue Perfusion 227

REFERENCES

1. Neill CA: Etiology of congenital heart disease, *Cardiovasc Clin* 4:137-148, 1972.
2. Van Praagh R, Vlad P: Dextrocardia, mesocardia and levocardia. In Keith JD, Rowe RD, Vlad P, eds: *Heart disease in infancy and childhood,* New York, 1967, Macmillan.
3. Gutgesell HP: Cardiac malposition and heterotaxy. In Garson A, Bricker JT, Fisher DJ et al, eds: *The science and practice of pediatric cardiology,* Philadelphia, 1998, Williams & Wilkins.
4. Towbin JA: Pediatric myocardial disease, *Pediatr Clin North Am* 46:289-312, 1999.
5. Ruckman RN: Development and maturation of the cardiovascular system. In Holbrook PR, ed: *Textbook of pediatric critical care,* Philadelphia, 1993, WB Saunders.
6. Rabinovitch M: Structure and function of the pulmonary vascular bed: an update, *Cardiol Clin* 7:227-238, 1989.
7. Reed LJ, Keegan MJ: Fat embolism syndrome: a complication of trauma, *Crit Care Nurse* 13:33-38, 1993.
8. Zaritsky A, Chernow B: Use of catecholamines in pediatrics, *J Pediatr* 105:341-350, 1984.
9. Paridon SM: Congenital heart disease: cardiac performance and adaptations to exercise, *Pediatr Exercise Sci* 9:308-323, 1997.
10. Kocis KC: Chest pain in pediatrics, *Pediatr Clin North Am* 46:189-203, 1999.
11. Strauss AW, Johnson MC: The genetic basis of pediatric cardiovascular disease, *Semin Perinatol* 20:564-576, 1996.
12. National High Blood Pressure Education Program Working Group on Hypertension Control in Children and Adolescents: Update on the 1987 Task Force on High Blood Pressure in Children and Adolescents: a working group report from the National High Blood Pressure Education Program, *Pediatrics* 98:649-657, 1996.
13. Lehrer S: *Understanding pediatric heart sounds,* Philadelphia, 1992, WB Saunders.
14. Weaver MG, Park MK, Lee DH: Differences in blood pressure levels obtained by auscultatory and oscillometric methods, *Am J Dis Child* 144:911-914, 1990.
15. Gevers M, van Genderingen HR, Lafeber HN et al: Accuracy of oscillometric blood pressure measurement in critically ill neonates with reference to the arterial pressure wave shape, *Intensive Care Med* 22:242-248, 1996.
16. Darovic GO: Hemodynamic monitoring: invasive and noninvasive clinical application, Philadelphia, 1995, WB Saunders.
17. Devine S, Anisman PC, Robinson BW: A basic guide to cyanotic congenital heart disease, *Contemp Pediatr* 15:133-163, 1998.
18. Duff DF, McNamara DG: History and physical examination of the cardiovascular system. In Garson A, Bricker JT, Fisher DJ et al, eds: *The science and practice of pediatric cardiology,* Philadelphia, 1998, Williams & Wilkins.
19. Veasy LG: History and physical examination. In Emmanouilides GC, Allen HG, Riemenschneider TA et al, eds: *Heart disease in infants, children, and adolescents,* ed 5, Philadelphia, 1995, Williams & Wilkins.
20. Moody LY: Pediatric cardiovascular assessment and referral in the primary care setting, *Nurse Pract* 22:120-134, 1997.
21. Callow L, Suddaby EC, Slota MC: Cardiovascular system. In Slota MC, ed: *Core curriculum for pediatric critical care nursing,* Philadelphia, 1998, WB Saunders
22. Driscoll D, Allen HD, Atkins DL et al: Guidelines for evaluation and management of common congenital cardiac problems in infants, children, and adolescents, American Heart Association, 1994, at www.americanheart.org/scientific/statements/1994/109402.html.
23. Park MK: *How to read pediatric ECGs,* St Louis, 1992, Mosby.
24. Garson A: Electrocardiography. In Garson A, Bricker JT, Fisher DJ et al, eds: *The science and practice of pediatric cardiology,* Philadelphia, 1998, Williams & Wilkins.
25. Etheridge SP, Judd VE: Supraventricular tachycardia in infancy: evaluation, management and follow-up, *Arch Pediatr Adolesc Med* 153:267-271, 1999.
26. Zeigler VL: Care of adolescents and young adults with cardiac arrhythmias, *Prog Cardiovasc Nurs* 10:13-21, 1995.
27. Deal BJ: Supraventricular tachycardia mechanisms and natural history. In Deal BJ, Wolff GA, Gelband H, eds: *Current concepts in diagnosis and management of arrhythmias in infants and children,* Armonk, NY, 1998, Futura Publishing.
28. Case CL, Gillette PC: Automatic atrial and junctional tachycardias in the pediatric patient: strategies for diagnosis and management, *Pacing Clin Electrophysiol* 16:1323-1335, 1993.
29. Kugler JD: Benign arrhythmias: neonate throughout childhood. In Deal BJ, Wolff GA, Gelband H, eds: *Current concepts in diagnosis and management of arrhythmias in infants and children,* Armonk, NY, 1998, Futura Publishing.
30. Friedman RA: Sinus and atrioventricular conduction disorders. In Deal BJ, Wolff GA, Gelband H, eds: *Current concepts in diagnosis and management of arrhythmias in infants and children,* Armonk NY, 1998, Futura Publishing.
31. Friedman RA, Collins E, Fenrich AL: Pacing in children: indications and techniques, *Prog Pediatr Cardiol* 4:21-29, 1995.
32. Michaelsson M: Congenital complete atrioventricular block, *Prog Pediatr Cardiol* 4:1-10, 1995.
33. Odemuyiwa O, Camm AJ: Prophylactic pacing for prevention of sudden death in congenital complete heart block? *Pacing Clin Electrophysiol* 15:1526-1530, 1992.
34. Michaelsson M, Riesenfeld T, Jonzon A: Natural history of congenital complete atrioventricular block, *Pacing Clin Electrophysiol* 20:2098-2101, 1997.
35. Dick M, Russell MW: Ventricular tachycardia. In Deal BJ, Wolff GA, Gelband H, eds: *Current concepts in diagnosis and management of arrhythmias in infants and children,* Armonk NY, 1998, Futura Publishing.
36. Eberle T, Hessling G, Ulmer HE et al: Prediction of normal QT intervals in children, *J Electrocardiol* 31:121-125, 1998.
37. Vizgirda VM: The genetic basis for cardiac dysrhythmias and the long QT syndrome, *J Cardiovasc Nurs* 13:34-45, 1999.
38. Strife JL, Sze RW: Radiographic evaluation of the neonate with congenital heart disease, *Radiol Clin North Am* 37:1093-1107, 1999.
39. Singleton EB, Morriss MJH: Plain radiographic diagnosis congenital heart disease. In Garson A, Bricker JT, Fisher DJ et al, eds: *The science and practice of pediatric cardiology,* Philadelphia, 1998, Williams & Wilkins.
40. Choe YH, Kim YM, Han BK et al: MR imaging in the morphologic diagnosis of congenital heart disease, *Radiographics* 17:403-422, 1997.
41. Tworetzky W, McElhinney DB, Brook MM et al: Echocardiographic diagnosis alone for the complete repair of major congenital heart defects, *J Am Coll Cardiol* 33:228-233, 1999.
42. Muhiudeen, IA, Roberson, DA, Silverman NH et al: Intraoperative echocardiography for evaluation of congenital heart defects in infants and children, *Anesthesiology* 76:165-172, 1992.
43. Stevenson JG: Role of intraoperative transesophageal echocardiography during repair of congenital cardiac defects, *Acta Paediatrica* 410:23-33, 1995.
44. Leung DY, Davidson RM, Cranney GB et al: Thromboembolic risks of left atrial thrombus detected by transesophageal echocardiogram, *Am J Cardiol* 79:626-629, 1997.
45. Lanzarotti CJ, Olshansky B: Thromboembolism in chronic atrial flutter: is the risk underestimated? *J Am Coll Cardiol* 30:1506-1511, 1997.
46. Friedman AH, Copel JA, Kleinman CS: Fetal echocardiography and fetal cardiology: indications, diagnosis and management, *Semin Perinatol* 17:76-82, 1993.
47. Frommelt MA, Frommelt PC: Advances in echocardiographic diagnostic modalities for the pediatrician. In Berger S, ed: *The pediatric clinics of North America,* Philadelphia, 1999, WB Saunders.
48. Brook MM, Silverman NH, Villegas M: Cardiac ultrasonography in structural abnormalities and arrhythmias, *West J Med* 159:286-300, 1993.
49. Tworetzky W, McElhinney DB, Reddy VM et al: Does prenatal diagnosis of hypoplastic left heart syndrome lead to improved surgical outcome? *J Am Coll Cardiol* 31(suppl A):71A, 1998.
50. Gardner RM, Hujcs M: Fundamentals of physiologic monitoring, *AACN Clin Issues Crit Care Nurs* 4:11-24, 1993.
51. Quaal SJ: Quality assurance in hemodynamic monitoring, *AACN Clin Issues Crit Care Nurs* 4:197-206, 1993.
52. Gardner RM, Hollingsworth KW: Optimizing the electrocardiogram and pressure monitoring, *Crit Care Med* 14:651-658, 1986.

53. Daily EK, Schroeder JS: (1989). *Techniques in bedside hemodynamic monitoring,* St Louis, 1989, Mosby.

54. Fuhrman TM, Pippin WD, Talmage LA et al: Evaluation of collateral circulation of the hand, *J Clin Monit* 8:28-32, 1992.

55. VanRiper S, VanRiper J: Arterial pressure monitoring. In Darovic GO, ed: *Hemodynamic monitoring: invasive and noninvasive clinical methods,* Philadelphia, 1987, WB Saunders.

56. Gorny DA: Arterial blood pressure measurement technique, *AACN Clin Issues Crit Care Nurs* 4:66-80, 1993.

57. Band JD, Maki DG: Infections caused by arterial catheters used for hemodynamic monitoring, *Am J Med* 67:735-741, 1979.

58. Raad I, Umphrey J, Khan A et al: The duration of placement as a predictor of peripheral and pulmonary arterial catheter infections, *J Hosp Infect* 23:17-26, 1993.

59. Thomas F, Burke JP, Parker J: The risk of infection related to radial vs femoral sites for arterial catheterization, *Crit Care Med* 11:807-812, 1983.

60. Maki DG, Ringer M, Alvarado CJ: Prospective randomized trial of povidone-iodine, alcohol, and chlorhexidine for prevention of infection associated with central venous and arterial catheters, *Lancet* 338:339-343, 1991.

61. Simmons BP: CDC guidelines for the prevention of nosocomial infections: guidelines for prevention of intravascular infections. *Am J Infect Control* 11:183-193, 1983.

62. Martin GR, Holley DG: Cardiovascular monitoring and evaluation. In Holbrook PR, ed: *Textbook of pediatric critical care,* Philadelphia, 1993, WB Saunders.

63. Schwenzer KJ: Venous and pulmonary pressures. In Lake CL, ed: *Clinical monitoring,* Philadelphia, 1990, WB Saunders.

64. Maki DG: Infections associated with intravascular lines. In Schwatrz M, Remintion J, eds: *Current topics in clinical infectious disease,* New York, 1982, McGraw-Hill.

65. Ryder MA: Peripheral access options, *Surg Oncol Clin North Am* 4:395-427, 1995.

66. Gardner PE: Pulmonary artery pressure monitoring, *AACN Clin Issues Crit Care Nurs* 4:98-119, 1993.

67. West JB: *Respiratory physiology,* Baltimore, 1990, Williams & Wilkins.

68. Lookinland S: Comparison of pulmonary vascular pressures based on blood volume and ventilator status, *Nurs Res* 38:68-72, 1989.

69. Roth SJ: Postoperative care. In Chang AC, Hanley FL, Wernovsky G et al, eds: *Pediatric cardiac intensive care,* Baltimore, 1998, Williams & Wilkins.

70. Visscher MD, Johnson JA: The Fick principle: analysis of potential errors in its conventional application, *J Appl Physiol* 5:635-638, 1953.

71. Wippermann CF, Huth RG, Schmidt FX et al: Continuous measurement of cardiac output by the Fick principle in infants and children: comparison with the thermodilution technique, *Intensive Care Med* 22:467-471, 1996.

72. Vargo TA: Cardiac catheterization: hemodynamic measurements. In Garson A, JT Bricker, Fisher DJ et al, eds: *The science and practice of pediatric cardiology,* Philadelphia, 1998, Williams & Wilkins.

73. Fegler G: Measurement of cardiac output in anesthetized animals by thermodilution method, *Q J Exp Psychol* 39:153-164, 1954.

74. Ganz W, Donoso R, Marcus HS et al: A new technique for measurement of cardiac output by thermodilution in man, *Am J Cardiol* 27:392-396, 1971.

75. Mandell VS: Interventional procedures for congenital heart disease, *Radiol Clin North Am* 37:439-461, 1999.

76. Nihill MR: Catheterization and angiography. In Garson A, Bricker JT, Fisher DJ et al, eds: *The science and practice of pediatric cardiology,* Philadelphia, 1998, Williams & Wilkins.

77. Shim D, Lloyd TR, Cho KJ et al: Transhepatic cardiac catheterization in children: evaluation of efficacy and safety, *Circulation* 92:1526-1530, 1995.

78. Gatzoulis MA, Rigby ML, Redington AN: Interventional catheterization in paediatric cardiology, *Eur Heart J* 16:1767-1772, 1995.

79. Moore P, Egito E, Mowrey H et al: Midterm results of balloon dilation of congenital aortic stenosis: predictors of success, *J Am Coll Cardiol* 27:1257-1263, 1996.

80. Ing FF, Sommer RJ: The snare-assisted technique for transcatheter coil occlusion of moderate to large patent ductus arteriosus: immediate and intermediate results, *J Am Coll Cardiol* 33:1710-1718, 1999.

81. Fogelman R, Nykanen D, Smallhorn JF et al: Endovascular stents in the pulmonary circulation: clinical impact on management and medium term follow-up, *Circulation* 92:881-885, 1995.

82. Ing JJ, Grifka RG, Nihill MR et al: Repeat dilation of intravascular stents in congenital heart defects, *Circulation* 92:893-897, 1995.

83. Kugler JD, Danford DA, Houston K et al: Radiofrequency catheter ablation for paroxysmal supraventricular tachycardia in children and adolescents without structural heart disease, *Am J Cardiol* 80:1438-1443, 1997.

84. Vitiello R, McCrindle BW, Nykanen D et al: Complications associated with pediatric cardiac catheterization, *J Am Coll Cardiol* 32:1433-1440, 1998.

85. Balaguru D, Artman M, Auslender M: Management of heart failure in children, *Curr Probl Pediatr* 30:1-35, 2000.

86. Driscoll DJ, Gillette PC, Ezrailson EG et al: Inotropic response of the neonatal canine myocardium to dopamine, *Pediatr Res* 12:42-47, 1978.

87. Whitsett JA, Noguchi A, Moore JJ: Developmental aspects of alpha and beta adrenergic receptors, *Semin Perinatol* 6:125-131, 1982.

88. Boreus LO, Hjemdahl P, Lagercrantz H: β adrenoceptor function in white blood cells from human infants: no relation to plasma catecholamine levels, *Pediatr Res* 20:1152-1158, 1986.

89. Pediatric Patients: regulations requiring manufacturers to assess the safety and effectiveness of new drugs and biological products. Washington DC, Department of Health and Human Services, Food and Drug Administration, 21 CFR Parts 201, 312, 314, 601. 62(158), 43899-916, 1997.

90. Schreiner MS: Safety and effectiveness data: will children gain access? *Am Heart J* 136:4-5, 1998.

91. Kohr LM, O'Brien P: Current management of congestive heart failure in infants and children, *Nurs Clin North Am* 30:261-290, 1995.

92. O'Laughlin MP: Congestive heart failure in children, *Pediatr Clin North Am* 46:263-273, 1999.

93. Eades SK, Christensen ML: The clinical pharmacology of loop diuretics in the pediatric patient. *Pediatr Nephrol* 12:603-616, 1998.

94. Taketomo CK, Hodding JH, Kraus DM: *Pediatric dosage handbook,* Hudson, Ohio, 1998-1999, Lexi-Comp.

95. Lawless ST, Orr R: Axillary arterial pressure monitoring in pediatric patients, *Pediatrics* 84:273-275, 1989.

96. Notterman DA: Cardiovascular support: pharmacologic. In Holbrook PR, ed: *Textbook of pediatric critical care,* Philadelphia, 1993, WB Saunders.

97. Rackow EC, Packman MI, Weil MH: Hemodynamic effects of digoxin during acute cardiac failure, *Crit Care Med* 12:1001-1007, 1987.

98. Ordog GI, Beneron S: Serum digoxin levels and mortality in 5,100 patients, *Ann Emerg Med* 16:32-36, 1987.

99. Carcoana H, Hines RL: Is renal dose dopamine protective or therapeutic? Yes, *Crit Care Clin* 12:677-685, 1996.

100. Notterman DA, DeBruin W, Metakis L: Plasma catecholamine levels in critically ill children: evidence of early β-adrenergic receptor desensitization, *Pediatr Res* 25:42-44A, 1989.

101. Notterman DA: Pharmacologic support of the failing circulation: an approach for infants and children, *Probl Anesthesia* 3:288-294, 1989.

102. Marjerus TC, Dasta JF, Bauman JL et al: Dobutamine: ten years later, *Pharmacotherapy* 9:245-250, 1989.

103. Skoyles JR, Sherry KM: Pharmacology, mechanisms of action and uses of selective phosphodiesterase inhibitors, *Br J Anaesth* 68:293-302, 1992.

104. Colucci WS, Wright RF, Braunwald E: New inotropic agents in the treatment of congestive heart failure, *New Engl J Med* 314:290-299, 1986.

105. Lawless ST, Burckart G, Diven W et al: Pharmacokinetics of amrinone in neonates and infants, *J Clin Pharmacol* 28:283-284, 1988.

106. Lawless ST, Zaritsky A, Miles M: The acute pharmacokinetics and pharmacodynamics of amrinone in pediatric patients, *J Clin Pharmacol* 31:800-803, 1991.

107. Robinson BW, Gelband H, Mas MS: Selective pulmonary and systemic vasodilator effects of amrinone in children: new therapeutic implications, *J Am Coll Cardiol* 21:1461-1465, 1993.

108. Sorenson GK, Ramamoorthy C, Lynn AM et al: Hemodynamic effects of amrinone in children after Fontan surgery, *Anesth Analg* 82:241-246, 1996.

109. Laitinen P, Happonen JM, Sairanen H et al: Amrinone vs. dopamine-nitroglycerin after arterial switch operation for transposition of the great arteries, *J Cardiothorac Vasc Anesth* 13:186-190, 1999.

110. Laitinen P, Happonen JM, Sairanen H et al: Amrinone vs. dopamine-nitroglycerin after reconstructive surgery for complete atrioventricular septal defect, *J Cardiothorac Vasc Anesth* 11:870-874, 1997.

111. Watson DM, Sherry KM, Weston GA: Milrinone: a bridge to heart transplantation, *Anaesthesia* 46:285-288, 1990.

112. Allen-Webb EM, Ross MP, Pappas JB et al: Age-related amrinone pharmacokinetics in a pediatric population, *Crit Care Med* 22:1016-1024, 1994.

113. Naccarelli GV, Gray EL, Dougherty AH: Amrinone: acute electrophysiologic and hemodynamic effects in patients with congestive heart failure, *Am Heart J* 54:600-604, 1984.

114. Lindsey CA, Barton P, Lawless S et al: Pharmacokinetics and pharmacodynamics of milrinone lactate in pediatric patients with septic shock, *J Pediatr* 132:329-334, 1998.

115. Barton P, Garcia J, Kouatli A et al: Hemodynamic effects of IV milrinone lactate in pediatric patients with septic shock, *Chest* 109:1302-1312, 1996.

116. Chang AC, Atz AM, Wernovsky G et al: Milrinone: sytemic and pulmonary hemodynamic effects in neonates after cardiac surgery, *Crit Care Med* 23:1907-1914, 1995.

117. Bailey JM, Miller BE, Lu W et al: The pharmacokinetics of milrinone in pediatric patients after cardiac surgery, *Anesthesiology* 90:1012-1018, 1999.

118. Ruley EJ: Hypertension. In Holbrook PJ, ed: *Textbook of pediatric critical care,* Philadelphia, 1993, WB Saunders.

119. Rich S, Brundage BH: High dose calcium channel blocking therapy for primary pulmonary hypertension: evidence for long-term reduction in pulmonary arterial pressure and regression of right ventricular hypertrophy, *Circulation* 76:135-143, 1987.

120. Truttmann AC, Zehnder-Schlapbach S, Blanchetti MG: A moratorium should be placed on the use of short-acting nifedipine for hypertensive crises, *Pediatr Nephrol* 12:259-261, 1998.

121. Abramowicz M: Drugs for chronic heart failure, *Medical Letter* 8:40-42, 1993.

122. Pfeffer MA, Braunwald E, Moye LA et al: Effect of captopril on mortality and morbidity in patients with left ventricular dysfunction after myocardial infarction, *New Engl J Med* 327:669-677, 1992.

123. Wiest DB, Garner SS, Uber WE et al: Esmolol for the management of pediatric hypertension after cardiac operations, *J Thorac Cardiovasc Surg* 115:890-897, 1998.

124. Waagstein F: Efficacy of beta blockers in idiopathic dilated cardiomyopathy and ischemic cardiomyopathy, *Am J Cardiol* 80:45J-49J, 1997.

125. Havranek EP, Weinberger J: Update on the treatment of heart failure, *Prog Cardiovasc Nurs* 11:111-113, 1999.

126. Shaddy RE, Olsen SL, Bristow MR et al: Efficacy and safety of metoprolol in the treatment of doxorubicin-induced cardiomyopathy in pediatric patients, *Am Heart J* 129:197-199, 1995.

127. Shaddy RE: β-Blocker therapy in young children with congestive heart failure under consideration for heart transplantation, *Am Heart J* 136:19-21, 1998.

128. Buchhorn, R, Bartmus D, Sickmeyer W et al: Beta-blocker therapy of severe congestive heart failure in infants with left to right shunts, *Am J Cardiol* 81:1366-1368, 1998.

129. Shaddy RE, Tani LY, Gidding SS et al: Beta-blocker treatment of dilated radiomyopathy with congestive heart failure in children: a multi-institutional experience, *J Heart Lung Transplant* 18:269-274, 1999.

130. Brunner-La Rocca H, Vaddadi G, Esler MD: Recent insight into therapy of congestive heart failure: focus on ACE inhibitors and angiotensin II antagonism, *J Am Coll Cardiol* 33:1163-1173, 1999.

131. Pitt B, Zannad F, Remme WJ et al: The effect of spironolactone on morbidity and mortality in patients with severe heart failure, *N Engl J Med* 341:709-717, 1999.

132. Reiffel JA, Estes NAM, Waldo AL et al: A consensus report on antiarrhythmic drug use, *Clin Cardiol* 17:103-116, 1994.

133. Perry JC: Pharmacologic therapy of arrhythmias. In Deal BJ, Wolff GA, Gelband H, eds: *Current concepts in diagnosis and management of arrhythmias in infants and children,* Armonk, NY, 1998, Futura Publishing.

134. Walsh EP, Saul JP, Sholler GF et al: Evaluation of a staged treatment protocol for rapid automatic junctional tachycardia after operation for congenital heart disease, *J Am Coll Cardiol* 29:1046-1053, 1997.

135. Luedtke SA, Kuhn RJ, McCaffrey FM: Pharmacologic management of supraventricular tachycardias in children. Part 2. Atrial flutter, atrial fibrillation, and junctional and atrial ectopic tachycardia, *Ann Pharmacother* 31:1347-1359, 1997.

136. Roden DM, Lazzara R, Rosen M et al: Multiple mechanism in the long QT syndrome: current knowledge, gaps, and future directions, *Circulation* 94:1996-2012, 1996.

137. Perry JC, Garson A: Flecainide acetate for treatment of tachyarrhythmias in children: review of world literature on efficacy, safety, and dosing, *Am Heart J* 6:1614-1621, 1992.

138. Fish FA, Gillette PC, Benson DW: Proarrhythmia, cardiac arrest and death in young patients receiving encainide and fecainide, *J Am Coll Cardiol* 18:356-365, 1991.

139. Erickson C, Perry J, Marlow D et al: Sudden death during propafenone therapy for atrial flutter in young post-operative heart patients, *Pacing Clin Electrophysiol* 16:939, 1993.

140. Etheridge SP, Craig J: Amiodarone is safe and highly effective as primary therapy for tachycardia in infancy, *Pediatrics* 104:657, 1999.

141. Drago F, Mazza A, Guccione P et al: Amiodarone used alone or in combination with propranolol: a very effective therapy for tachyarrhythmias in infants and children, *Pediatr Cardiol* 19:445-449, 1998.

142. Perry JC, Fenrich AL, Hulse E et al: Pediatric use of intravenous amiodarone: efficacy and safety in critically ill patients from a multicenter protocol, *J Am Coll Cardiol* 27:1246-1250, 1996.

143. Figa FH, Gow RM, Hamilton RM et al: Clinical efficacy and safety of intravenous amiodarone in infants and children, *Am J Cardiol* 74:573-577, 1994.

144. Kowey PR, Levine JH, Herre JM et al: Randomized, double blind comparison of intravenous amiodarone and bretylium in the treatment of patients with recurrent, hemodynamically destabilizing ventricular tachycardia or fibrillation, *Circulation* 92:3255-3263, 1995.

145. Bowers PN, Fields J, Schwartz D et al: Amiodarone induced pulmonary fibrosis in infancy, *Pacing Clin Electrophysiol* 21:1665-1667, 1998.

146. Tanel RE, Walsh EP, Lulu JA et al: Sotalol for refractory arrhythmias in pediatric and young adult patients: initial efficacy and long-term outcome, *Am Heart J* 130:791-797, 1995.

147. Beaufort-Krol GCM, Bink-Boelkens MTE: Sotalol for atrial tachycardias after surgery for congenital heart disease, *Pacing Clin Electrophysiol* 20:2125-2129, 1997.

148. Hohnloser SH, Arendts W, Quart B: Incidence, type and dose-dependence of proarrhythmic events during sotalol therapy in patients treated for sustained VT/VF, *Pacing Clin Electrophysiol* 15:173-175, 1992.

149. Chameides L, Hazinski MF, eds: *Pediatric advanced life support,* Dallas, 1997, American Heart Association.

150. Ellenbogen KA, Dias VC, Cardello FP et al: Safety and efficacy of intravenous diltiazem in atrial fibrillation and atrial flutter, *Am J Cardiol* 75:45-49, 1995.

151. Dougherty AH, Jackman WM, Naccarelli GV et al: Acute conversion of paroxysmal supraventricular tachycardia with intravenous diltiazem, *Am J Cardiol* 70:587-592, 1992.

152. Falk RH, Leavitt JI: Digoxin for atrial fibrillation: a drug whose time has gone, *Ann Intern Med* 114:573-575, 1991.

153. Sarter BH, Marchlinski FE: Redefining the role of digoxin in the treatment of atrial fibrillation, *Am J Cardiol* 69:71G-81G, 1992.

154. Rabinovitch M: Developmental biology of the pulmonary vascular bed. In Freddom R, Benson L, Smallhorn J, eds: *Neonatal heart disease,* London, 1992, Springer-Verlag.

155. Gentile R, Stevenson G, Dooley T et al: Pulsed Doppler echocardiographic determination of time of ductal closure in normal newborn infants, *J Pediatr* 98:443, 1981.

156. Kennedy JA, Clark SL: Observation on the physiologic reactions of the ductus arteriosus, *Am J Physiol* 136:140, 1942.

157. Freed MD, Heymann MA, Lewis AB et al: Prostaglandin E-1 in infants with ductus arteriosus-dependent congenital heart disease, *Circulation* 64:899-905, 1981.

158. Schneeweiss A: Prostaglandin E. In *Drug therapy in infants and children with cardiovascular diseases*, Philadelphia, 1986, Lea & Febiger.

159. Noerr B: Prostaglandin E-1, *Neonatal Netw* 9:66-67, 1991.

160. Lewis AB, Freed MD, Heymann MA et al: Side effects of therapy with prostaglandin E-1 in infants with critical congenital heart disease, *Circulation* 64:893-897, 1981.

161. Roos A: Poiseuille's law and its limitations in vascular systems, *Med Thorac* 19:224-238, 1962.

162. Rudolph AM, Yuan S: Response of the pulmonary vasculature to hypoxia and H^+ ion concentration changes, *J Clin Invest* 45:399-411, 1966.

163. Schreiber MD, Heymann MA, Soifer SJ: Increased arterial pH, not decreased $PaCO_2$, attenuates hypoxia-induced pulmonary vasoconstriction in newborn lambs, *Pediatr Res* 20:113-117, 1986.

164. Fineman JR, Soifer SJ, Heymann MA: Regulation of pulmonary vascular tone in the perinatal period, *Annu Rev Physiol* 57:115-134, 1995.

165. Frostell C, Blomquist H, Hedenstierna H et al: Inhaled nitric oxide selectively reverses human hypoxic pulmonary vasoconstriction without causing systemic vasodilation, *Anesthesiology* 78:427-435, 1993.

166. Roberts JD Jr, Fineman JR, Morin FC et al: Inhaled nitric oxide and persistent pulmonary hypertension of the newborn: results of a randomized controlled trial, *N Engl J Med* 336:605-610, 1997.

167. Canadian Inhaled Nitric Oxide Study Group and the NICHD Neonatal Research Network: The neonatal inhaled nitric oxide study in the term and near-term infant with hypoxic respiratory failure: a multicenter randomized trial, *N Engl J Med* 336:597-604, 1997.

168. Clark RH, Kueser TJ, Walker MW et al: Low-dose nitric oxide therapy for persistent pulmonary hypertension of the newborn, *New Engl J Med* 342:469-474, 2000.

169. Roberts JP, Lang P, Bigatello L et al: Inhaled nitric oxide in congenital heart disease, *Circulation* 87:447-453, 1993.

170. Berner M, Beghetti M, Spahr-Schopfer I et al: Inhaled nitric oxide to test the vasodilator capacity of the pulmonary vascular bed in children with long-standing pulmonary hypertension and congenital heart disease, *Am J Cardiol* 77:532-535, 1996.

171. Adatia I, Atz AM, Jonas RA et al: Diagnostic use of inhaled nitric oxide after neonatal cardiac operations, *J Thorac Cardiovasc Surg* 112:1403-1405, 1996.

172. Oda H, Nogami H, Nakajima T: Reaction of hemoglobin with nitric oxide and nitrogen dioxides in mice, *J Toxicol Environ Health* 6:673-678, 1980.

173. Wessel DL, Adatia I, Thompson JE et al: Delivery and monitoring of inhaled nitric oxide in patients with pulmonary hypertension, *Crit Care Med* 22:930-938, 1994.

174. Radi R, Beckman JS, Bush KM et al: Peroxynitrite-induced membrane lipid peroxidation: the cytotoxic potential of superoxide and nitric oxide, *Arch Biochem Biophys* 288:481-487, 1991.

175. Oda H, Kusumoto S, Kakajimia T: Nitrosylhemoglobin formation in the blood of animals exposed to nitric oxide, *Arch Environ Health* 30:453-465, 1975.

176. Atz A, Adatia I, Wessel D: Rebound pulmonary hypertension after inhalation of nitric oxide, *Ann Thorac Surg* 62:1759-1764, 1996.

177. Wessel DL: Commentary: Simple gases and complex single ventricles, *J Thora Cardiovasc Surg* 112:655-657, 1996.

178. Chang AC, Zucker HA, Hickey PR, Wessel DL: Pulmonary vascular resistance in infants after cardiac surgery: role of carbon dioxide and hydrogen ion, *Critical Care Medicine* 23:568-574, 1995.

178a. Reddy VM, Liddicoat JR, Fineman JR et al: Fetal model of single ventricle physiology: hemodynamic effects of oxygen, nitric oxide, carbon dioxide, and hypoxia in the early postnatal period, *Cardiovasc Surg* 112:437-449, 1996.

178b. Fike CD, Kaplowitz MR: Effect of chronic hypoxia on pulmonary vascular pressures in isolated lungs of newborn pigs, *J Appl Physiol* 77(6):2853-2862, 1994.

178c. Jobes DR, Nicolson SC, Steven JM et al: Carbon dioxide prevents pulmonary overcirculation in hypoplastic left heart syndrome, *Ann Thorac Surg* 54:150-151, 1992.

178d. Mora GA, Pizarro C, Jacobs ML, Norwood WI: Experimental model of single ventricle: influence of carbon dioxide on pulmonary vascular dynamics, *Circulation* 90(part 2): II-43-II-46, 1994.

178e. Riordan CJ, Randsback F, Storey JH et al: Effects of oxygen, positive end-expiratory pressure, and carbon dioxide on oxygen delivery in an animal model of the univentricular heart, *J Thorac Cardiovasc Surg* 112:644-654, 1996.

179. Gregoratos G, Cheitlin MD, Conill A et al: ACC/AHA guidelines for implantation of cardiac pacemakers and antiarrhythmia devices: executive summary, *Circulation* 97: 1325-1335, 1998.

180. Gajarski RJ, Towbin JA: Recent advances in the etiology, diagnosis, and treatment of myocarditis and cardiomyopathies in children, *Curr Opin Pediatr* 7:587-594, 1995.

181. Ohm OJ, Breivik K, Segadal L et al: New temporary atrial and ventricular pacing leads for patients after cardiac operations, *J Thorac Cardiovasc Surg* 110:1725-1731, 1995.

182. Halldorsson AO, Vigneswaran WT, Podbielski FJ et al: Electrophysiological and clinical comparison of two temporary pacing leads following cardiac surgery, *Pacing Clin Electrophysiol* 22:1221-1225, 1999.

183. Bennie RE, Dierdorf SF, Hubbard JE: Perioperative management of children with third degree heart block undergoing pacemaker placement: a ten year review, *Paediatr Anaesth* 7:301-304, 1997.

184. Conway SP: Pediatric pacemakers for patients with complete heart block, *Dimens Crit Care Nurs* 16:29-39, 1997.

185. Silka EP: Emergency management of arrhythmias. In Deal BJ, Wolff GA, Gelband H, eds: *Current concepts in diagnosis and management of arrhythmias in infants and children*, Armonk, NY, 1998, Futura Publishing.

186. Berry TA, Baas LS, Hickey CS: Infection precautions with temporary pacing leads: a descriptive study, *Heart Lung* 25:182-189, 1996.

187. Baas LS, Beery TA, Hickey CS: Care and safety of pacemaker electrodes in intensive care and telemetry nursing units, *Am J Crit Care* 6:302-311, 1997.

188. Hawkins JA, Minich LL: Intra-aortic balloon counterpulsation in pediatric cardiac patients. In Duncan BW, ed: *Mechanical circulatory support for pediatric cardiac patients*, New York, Marcell Decker (in press).

189. Thuys CA, Mullaly RJ, Horton SB et al: Centrifugal ventricular assist in children under 6 kg, *Eur J Cardiothorac Surg* 13: 130-134, 1998.

190. del Nido PJ, Duncan BW, Mayer JE et al: Left ventricular assist device improves survival in children with left ventricular dysfunction after repair of anomalous origin of the left coronary artery from the pulmonary artery, *Ann Thorac Surg* 67:169-172, 1999.

191. Duncan BW, Hraska V, Jonas RA et al: Mechanical circulatory support in children with cardiac disease, *J Thorac Cardiovasc Surg* 117:529-542, 1999.

192. Duncan BW, Ibrahim AE, Hraska V et al: Use of rapid-deployment extracorporeal membrane oxygenation for the resuscitation of pediatric patients with heart disease after cardiac arrest, *J Thorac Cardiovasc Surg* 116:305-311, 1998.

193. Holub DA, Ido SR, Johnson MD et al: Changes in right ventricular function associated with intraaortic balloon pumping (IABP) in the cardiogenic shock patient, *Clin Res* 25:553A, 1977.

194. Pollock JC, Charlton MC, Williams WG et al: Intraaortic balloon pumping in children, *Ann Thorac Surg* 29:522-528, 1980.

195. Veasy LG, Blalock RC, Orth JL et al: Intra-aortic balloon pumping in infants and children, *Circulation* 68:1095-1100, 1983.

196. Smith RG, Cleavinger M: Current perspectives on the use of circulatory assist devices, *AACN Clin Issues Crit Care Nurs* 2:488-499, 1991.

197. Quaal SJ: *Comprehensive intra-aortic balloon counterpulsation*, St Louis, 1993, Mosby.

198. Veasy LG: Pediatric adaptation in balloon pumping. In Quaal SJ, ed: *Comprehensive intraaortic balloon counterpulsation,* ed 2, St Louis: Mosby, 1993.
199. Minich LL, Tani LY, McGough EC et al: A novel approach to pediatric intraaortic balloon pump timing using m-mode echocardiography, *Am J Cardiol* 80:367-369, 1997.
200. Dunn JM: The use of intra-aortic balloon pumping in pediatric patients, *Cardiac Assists* 5:2-4, 1989.
201. Anella J, McCloskey A, Vieweg C: Nursing dynamics of pediatric intraaortic balloon pumping, *Crit Care Nurse* 10:24-36, 1990.
202. Geiger J, Hall T, Breeze E et al: Intra-aortic balloon pumps in children: a small nursing team approach, *Crit Care Nurse* 17:79-86, 1997.
203. Reddy VM, Hanley FL: Mechanical support of the myocardium. In Chang AC et al, eds: *Pediatric cardiac intensive care,* Baltimore, 1998, Williams & Wilkins.
204. Reedy JE, Ruzevich SA, Noedel NR et al: Nursing care of the ambulatory patient with a mechanical assist device, *J Heart Transplant* 9:97-105, 1990.
205. Karl TR, Sano S, Horton S et al: Centrifugal pump left heart assist in pediatric cardiac operations, *J Thorac Cardiovasc Surg* 102:624-630, 1991.
206. Scheinin SA, Radovancevic B, Parnis SM et al: Mechanical circulatory support in children, *Eur J Cardiothorac Surg* 8(10):537-540, 1994.
207. Ashton RC, Oz MC, Michler RE: Left ventricular assist device options in pediatric patients, *ASAIO Journal* 41:M277-M280, 1995.
208. Costa RJ, Chard RB, Nunn GR, Cartmill TB: Ventricular assist devices in pediatric cardiac surgery, *Ann Thorac Surg* 60:S536-538, 1995.
209. del Nido PJ, Dalton HJ, Thompson AE et al: Extracorporeal membrane oxygenator rescue in children during cardiac arrest after cardiac surgery, *Circulation* 86:II-300-304, 1992.
210. Suddaby EC, O'Brien AM: ECMO for cardiac support in children, *Heart Lung* 22:401-407, 1993.
211. Klein MD, Shaleen KW, Whittlesey GC et al: Extracorporeal membrane oxygenation for the circulatory support of children after repair of congenital heart disease, *J Thorac Cardiovasc Surg* 100:498-505, 1990.
212. Delius RE, Bove EL, Meliones JN et al: Use of extracorporeal life support in patients with congenital heart disease, *Crit Care Med* 20:1216-1222, 1992.
213. Raithel SC, Pennington DG, Boegner E et al: Extracorporeal membrane oxygenation in children after cardiac surgery, *Circulation* 86:II305-310, 1992.
214. Ziomek S, Harrell J, Fasules J et al: Extracorporeal membrane oxygenation for cardiac failure after congenital heart operation, *Ann Thorac Surg* 54:861-868, 1992.
215. Dalton HJ, Siewers RD, Fuhrman BP et al: Extracorporeal membrane oxygenation for cardiac rescue in children with severe myocardial dysfunction, *Crit Care Med* 21:1020-1028, 1993.
216. Black MD, Coles JG, Williams WG et al: Determinants of success in pediatric cardiac patients undergoing extracorporeal membrane oxygenation, *Ann Thorac Surg* 60:133-138, 1995.
217. Walters HL, Hakimi M, Rice MD et al: Pediatric cardiac surgical ECMO: multivariant analysis of risk factors for hospital death, *Ann Thorac Surg* 60:329-337, 1995.
218. Kulik TJ, Moler FW, Palmisano JM et al: Outcome-associated factors in pediatric patients treated with extracorporeal membrane oxygenator after cardiac surgery, *Circulation* 94:II63-68, 1996.

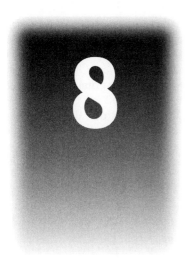

8

Oxygenation and Ventilation

Martha A.Q. Curley
John E. Thompson

Support of oxygenation or ventilation is integral to the practice of pediatric critical care nursing because the majority of critically ill infants and children require interventions to stabilize the pulmonary system.[1,2] Although general principles of care are similar within all age groups, striking differences do exist among them.

Pulmonary system functioning continues to mature throughout childhood. Developmental immaturity of the pulmonary system places the infant and young child at risk for organ system dysfunction. Respiratory failure is the number one factor contributing to cardiopulmonary arrest in the pediatric population.[3]

This chapter discusses principles of oxygenation and ventilation as they pertain to critically ill or injured children.

Essential embryology, anatomy, and physiology are reviewed. Pulmonary assessment is presented, followed by a discussion of pulmonary intensive care monitoring, diagnostic testing, and mechanical support of ventilation. The chapter concludes with a discussion of nursing care issues related to infants and children who require alternative modes of pulmonary support.

ESSENTIAL EMBRYOLOGY

The human lung is designed for the single purpose of gas exchange across an intact alveolar-pulmonary capillary membrane. The lungs enrich blood with oxygen and eliminate carbon dioxide. Pulmonary function is immediately essential to extrauterine life. Embryonic development is detailed next (Fig. 8-1).

Pulmonary development is divided into five stages, named to reflect histologic maturation of the lung.[4] The duration of each stage can only be approximated because fetal growth is somewhat individualized. The lung first appears as a ventral outpouching of the primitive foregut in the *embryonic period,* days 26 to 52 of gestation. The foregut is eventually divided into a dorsal portion, the esophagus, and a ventral portion, the trachea and the lung buds. The primary bronchial buds split into two buds on the left and three buds on the right, thus giving shape to the developing bronchial tree.[5] The left lung bud develops into two main bronchi and two lobes. The right bud forms three main bronchi and three lobes. This early developing bronchial tree is nourished by the main pulmonary artery.

The *pseudoglandular period* follows the embryonic period from day 52 to week 16 of gestation. During

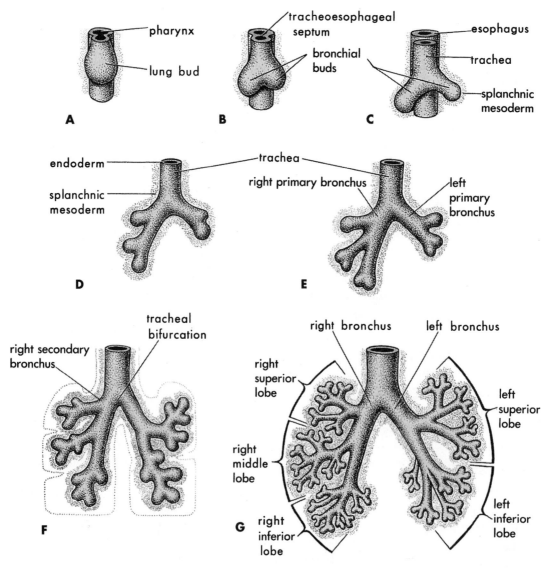

Fig. 8-1 Successive stages in the development of bronchi and lungs. **A** to **C,** 4 weeks; **D** and **E,** 5 weeks; **F,** 6 weeks; **G,** 8 weeks. (From Moore KL, Persaud TVN: *The developing human,* ed 5, Philadelphia, 1993, WB Saunders, p 230.)

this period, all major conducting airways including terminal bronchioles are formed. Arterial supply throughout the bronchial tree becomes more evident. The diaphragm, derived from the fusion of the pleuroperitoneal folds, is formed during the eighth to tenth week of gestation.[6]

Development of respiratory bronchioles characterizes the *canalicular period,* weeks 17 to 24 of gestation. Each bronchiole ends in two or three thin-walled dilations called terminal sacs or primitive alveoli.[7] The rich pulmonary vascular bed continues to develop as capillaries proliferate around the terminal bronchioles.

The *saccular period,* characterized by intense vascularization of the lung and loss of its glandular appearance, occurs during the weeks 28 to 36 of gestation. Elastic fibers, important in true alveolar development, begin to develop. For the first time, close contact between the air spaces and the pulmonary capillaries is established. There is concurrent active development of the lymphatic capillaries. The first true alveoli are present at 34 weeks; gas exchange is possible but not optimal.

The final period of development is the *alveolar period,* week 36 to term. Here, further refinement of the terminal sacs and formation of the walls of the true alveoli occur (Fig. 8-2). Columnar cells within the alveolar wall differentiate into type I and type II cells. Type I cells provide the alveolar surface area necessary for gas exchange. Type II cells secrete surfactant, a complex lipid substance that forms a monomolecular film over the walls of alveoli and is responsible for lowering alveolar surface tension. Surfactant is necessary for sustained inflation of the lung. Surfactant production increases during the later stages of pregnancy, especially during the last 2 weeks of gestation. Infants born prematurely are at risk for surfactant deficiency, which results in respiratory distress syndrome (RDS).

An important note is that the pulmonary system continues to mature after birth. Postnatal maturation continues until at least the eighth year of life and perhaps into early adolescence. Although alveoli increase in size after birth, pulmonary maturation is primarily due to an increase in the number of respiratory bronchioles and primitive alveoli—alveoli that have the potential for forming additional alveoli

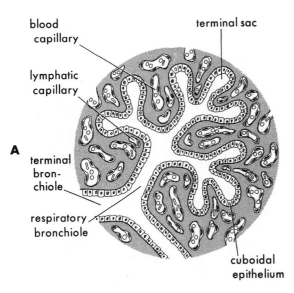

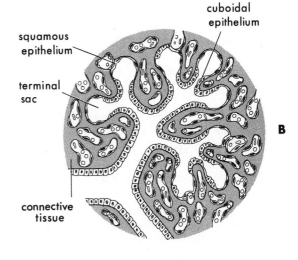

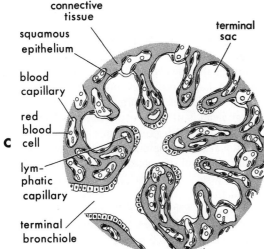

Fig. 8-2 Diagrammatic sketches of histologic sections, illustrating progressive stages of lung development. **A,** Late canalicular period (about 24 weeks). **B,** Early terminal sac period (about 26 weeks). **C,** Newborn infant (early alveolar period). Note that the alveolar-pulmonary capillary membrane is thin and that some of the capillaries have begun to bulge into the terminal sacs (future alveoli). (From Moore KL, Persaud TVN: *The developing human,* ed 5, Philadelphia, 1993, WB Saunders, p 231)

◆ **TABLE 8-1   Changes in Respiratory System Dimensions With Growth**

	Newborn to 1 Month	Infant	1-5 Yr	6-8 Yr	12-14 Yr	Adult
Chest diameter (cm)						
Transverse	10	14	15.5	19	25	28
Anteroposterior	7.5	9	10.5	11.5	14.5	16.5-18.5
Trachea length (mm)	40/57	42/67	45/81	57	64	90-150
Diameter (mm)	4	5	8.5	10	11	15-16
CSA (mm²)	26	34	50.5	79	112	200-250
Mainstem bronchi diameter (mm)	4	4	6.5	8	—	12
CSA, right/left	—	20/13	38/20	65/44	81/56	138/116
Bronchioles, diameter (mm)	0.3	0.4	0.5	—	—	0.7
CSA	0.07	0.12	0.2	—	—	0.4
Terminal bronchioles, diameter (mm)	0.2	0.3	0.3	—	—	0.5-0.6
Internal diameter (mm)	0.1	0.12	0.14	0.15	0.17	0.2
CSA	0.03	0.07	0.07	—	—	0.2
Alveoli, diameter (mm)	0.05	0.06-0.07	0.08-0.10	0.10-0.20	0.15-0.25	0.3
Surface area (M²)	2.8	6.5	12.5	32	—	64-75
Body length (cm)	50	—	—	123	—	175
Weight (kg)	3.4	—	—	24	—	70
Surface area (M²)	0.21	0.3	0.46	0.56	—	1.8

From Polgar G, Weng TR: The functional development of the respiratory system, *Am Rev Respir Dis* 120:677, 1979.
CSA, Cross-sectional area.

(Table 8-1). During the postnatal period, tracheal diameter triples, alveolar dimensions increase fourfold, and alveoli numbers increase tenfold, resulting in 24 million alveoli present at birth and 200 to 600×10^6 alveoli present in the adult.[8]

Congenital anomalies or malformations of the lower respiratory tract are relatively rare. Congenital diaphragmatic hernia occurs in approximately 1 in 2000 births, whereas tracheoesophageal fistula occurs in 1 in 2500 births.[7] A congenital diaphragmatic hernia occurs when the diaphragm fails to completely separate the pleuroperitoneal cavity into the abdominal and thoracic cavities. As the herniated abdominal viscera continue to grow and develop within the chest throughout gestation, pulmonary development is compromised. A tracheoesophageal fistula or communication between the trachea and esophagus results from incomplete division of the foregut into the respiratory and digestive systems. Pulmonary agenesis or absence of one lung results from the failure of a lung bud to develop. Congenital cysts of the lung form by dilation of the terminal or larger bronchi.[9] If multiple cysts are present, the lung may have a honeycomb appearance on x-ray film.

ESSENTIAL ANATOMY AND PHYSIOLOGY

Airways

The airway can be divided into three major areas: the supraglottic airway, the glottis, and the intrathoracic airway. The supraglottic airway includes the nose, the naso-oropharynx, and the epiglottis. The glottis includes the vocal cords, subglottic area, and cervical trachea. The intrathoracic airway includes the thoracic trachea, the mainstem bronchi, and the lungs. Each of these areas has unique features in the infant and young child.

Supraglottic Airway.   The nose, lined with ciliated mucous epithelium, serves as the passageway for air. The nasal structures are protective in that they heat, humidify, and filter inspired air. The nasal passages are narrow, and any factor that further decreases the diameter, for example, secretions, edema, or bleeding, will increase airways resistance and compromise ventilation. The newborn is considered an obligate nose breather for at least the first few months of life. Some infants do not mouth breathe until 5 to 6 months of life. Therefore any obstruction to the infant's nares causes respiratory distress, for example, choanal atresia. The area from the nasal cavity to the nasopharynx is abundantly lined with lymphoid tissue, the adenoids or pharyngeal tonsils, which can also obstruct the upper airway.

The mouth of the young child is small, and the tongue is large in relation to the mandible. The palatine tonsils are located at the junction of the mouth and oropharynx. Although the tonsils are thought to prevent upper airway infection, large tonsils can potentially obstruct the airway. In addition to the small mouth and large tongue, the infant has a large head, soft neck, and weak shoulder girdle. In total, these factors predispose infants to airway obstruction by position alone. To maintain an open airway in an infant with an altered level of consciousness, the head is placed in a neutral position, and a small roll is placed under the shoulders.

Glottis.   The infant's epiglottis is omega shaped and floppy. The epiglottis enters the anterior pharyngeal wall at a 45-degree angle and projects more posteriorly than in the older child. These factors make visualization of the glottis

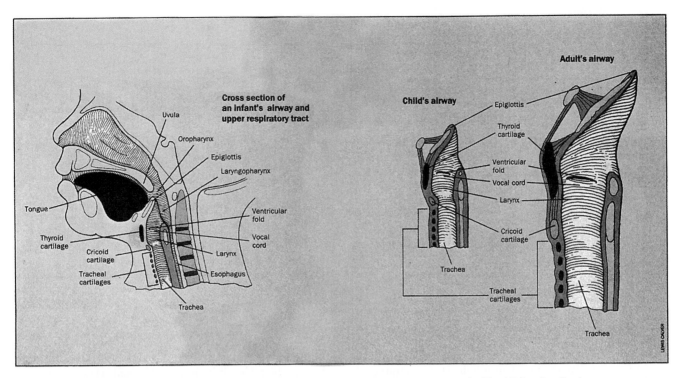

Fig. 8-3 Comparative anatomy of adult and infant airways. (From Thomas DO: The ABCs of pediatric emergencies, *RN* 49:34-41, 48, 1986.)

difficult in the infant and young child.[10] The epiglottis is also very susceptible to trauma and infection, which may cause edema and airway obstruction.

The larynx of the infant is more cephalad than in the older child. The glottis, the area between the vocal cords, is located between the second and third vertebrae in infants and descends to the fourth and fifth cervical vertebrae in adults. The infant's vocal cords are approximately 50% cartilage and thus are less distensible than in the older child. The cricoid ring, the only complete ring of cartilage in the pediatric airway, is the most narrow portion of the upper airway in infants and children, whereas the glottis is the most narrow portion of the adult upper airway (Fig. 8-3). In the newborn, the cricoid ring is approximately 6 mm in diameter, which places infants at particular risk for airway obstruction in this area.

Thoracic Airway. From the larynx, air passes through the trachea, which is short in the infant—approximately 4 to 5 cm long from the cricoid to the carina. The trachea is approximately 7 cm long in the young adolescent. The bifurcation of the trachea at the carina forms the right and left mainstem bronchi. Because the right mainstem angles down more vertically and is somewhat larger that the left, objects aspirated into the airway commonly lodge in the right mainstem bronchus.

The lower airways are smaller and less developed than in the adult. Airway obstruction results in increased airways resistance. Factors that impact airways resistance include the length and radius of the airway. Critically important in infants and children is airway radius. According to Poiseuille's law, resistance to airflow is inversely proportional

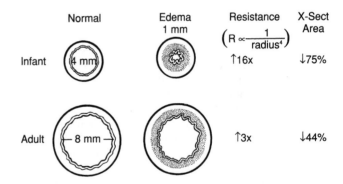

Fig. 8-4 Effects of edema on airways resistance in the infant versus the adult. Normal airways are represented on the left and edematous airways (1-mm circumferential edema) on the right. Resistance to flow is inversely proportional to the radius of the lumen to the fourth power for laminar flow and the fifth power for turbulent flow. The net result is a 75% decrease in cross-sectional area and a sixteenfold increase in resistance in the infant versus 44% and threefold, respectively, in the adult. (From Coté C, Todres ID: The pediatric airway. In Ryan JF, Todres ID, Coté C et al, eds: *A practice of anesthesia for infants and children,* New York, 1986, Grune & Stratton, p 39.)

to the fourth power of the radius for laminar flow ($1/r^4$) and to the fifth power for turbulent flow ($1/r^5$). Thus a reduction in diameter by half reduces laminar flow to one sixteenth of its former level. To maintain the same flow requires a sixteenfold increase in pressure, which significantly increases the work of breathing.[11] As noted in Fig. 8-4, minor reductions in the already small-diameter pediatric airway result in a large reduction in the cross-sectional area.

The walls of the tracheobronchial tree are composed of smooth muscle. The airways of the newborn contain little smooth muscle; however, by 4 to 5 months of life, enough smooth muscle is present to cause airway narrowing in response to an irritating stimulus. Smooth muscle development by 1 year of age is comparable with that of an adult.

Developmental changes also take place in the alveoli and the terminal bronchioles. The terminal bronchioles continue branching during the first year of life. The number and size of alveoli continue to increase until at least 8 years of age. These changes are responsible for the increased respiratory surface area available for gas exchange in the older child and adult. At birth, the interstitium of the lung contains little collagen and elastin. This may explain the frequency of alveolar rupture in the premature infant. Collagen and elastin production increases in the postnatal period.[12]

Little collateral ventilation exists in infants and young children. Pores of Kohn, which allow interalveolar communication, first appear between the first and second years of life.[13] Canals of Lambert, which allow bronchiole-alveolar communication, start to form after age 6.[14] With age, both structures allow ventilation of alveoli distal to an obstructed airway. Absence of collateral pathways contributes to patchy atelectasis when airways disease is present in infants and young children.[12]

Thoracic Cavity

The ribs, vertebrae, and sternum provide the bony framework of the thoracic cavity. Within the thoracic cavity lie three lobes of lung on the right, two lobes of lung on the left, and the mediastinum, which is off center to the left containing the heart, great vessels, esophagus, and trachea. The entire thoracic cavity is lined with parietal pleura, whereas the lungs are encased by visceral pleura. In health, the potential space between the pleura is filled with just enough fluid to allow the two pleura to glide over each other during ventilation. In illness states, the pleural space may fill with air (pneumothorax), fluid (pleural effusion), blood (hemothorax), lymph (chylothorax), or pus (empyema).

The contour of the thoracic cavity changes shape over time. The infant's thorax is round at birth with the anteroposterior diameter equal to the transverse diameter (1:1). This gradually changes, so that by 6 years of age the thorax reaches the adult diameter (1:2). In infancy, the chest wall is thin, with little musculature, and is highly compliant. The muscles of respiration include the diaphragm, intercostal, accessory, and abdominal muscles. The diaphragm is the most important muscle of respiration because it is responsible for most of the inspiratory effort. The phrenic nerve, formed by components of the third, fourth, and fifth cervical spinal nerves, supplies the diaphragm with both motor and sensory innervation. The intercostal and accessory muscles are poorly developed in infants, so they contribute little toward respiratory effort. The infant uses abdominal muscles to assist with ventilation. This combination of muscle use gives the appearance of seesaw breathing—that

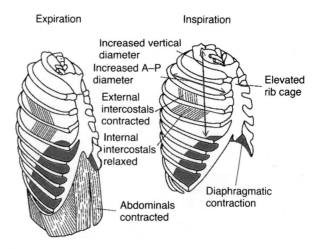

Fig. 8-5 Expansion and contraction of the thoracic cage during expiration and inspiration, illustrating especially diaphragmatic contraction, elevation of rib cage, and function of intercostals. (From Guyton AC: *Textbook of medical physiology,* ed 8, Philadelphia, 1991, WB Saunders.)

is, a paradoxical movement of the chest and abdomen. Seesaw breathing becomes exaggerated when intrapulmonary compliance decreases.

The infant's chest wall is very compliant, which allows (1) passage through the birth canal and (2) removal of intrapulmonary fluid before the first breath. In the presence of respiratory disease, the diaphragm contracts, and the chest wall moves inward on inspiration. In the older child or adolescent, the chest wall is rigid. When the diaphragm contracts, the rib cage is elevated, and the chest wall moves outward (Fig. 8-5). The soft, flexible rib cage of the infant makes retractions a prominent feature in respiratory distress and prevents the generation of high intrathoracic pressures needed to reexpand collapsed alveoli.

Pulmonary Circulation

The lungs receive blood from both ventricles. Unoxygenated blood flow from the right ventricle reaches the lungs by way of the pulmonary arteries. The pulmonary arteries divide into two systems: the conventional and the supernumerary. Conventional arteries travel with the airways, dividing as the airways divide. Supernumerary arteries, which exceed the conventional arteries in number, provide blood supply directly to the gas-exchanging units. Pulmonary vessels, similar to airways, develop with growth. (See Chapter 7 for an in-depth discussion of pulmonary vascular development and resistance.)

The left ventricle provides oxygenated blood to the lungs by way of three bronchial arteries. The bronchial arteries perfuse the bronchi, bronchioles, lymph nodes, and visceral pleura. Pulmonary venous drainage returns to the right and left atria. The right atrium receives blood via the bronchial veins, and the left atrium receives blood via the pulmonary veins. Bronchial arteries do hypertrophy in the presence of pulmonary infection. Hemoptysis may begin in these bronchial vessels in disorders such as cystic fibrosis.[4]

Lymphatic System

The major function of the lymphatic system is to return interstitial fluid to the systemic circulation. As blood flows through the pulmonary capillaries, plasma is filtered into the interstitium, where it collects in lymphatic channels and is returned to the circulation by the lymphatic system. Lymphatic drainage can significantly increase in certain disease states, for example, in patients with pulmonary edema. Most fluid is returned to the systemic circulation by the lymphatic system scattered throughout the lung parenchyma, whereas another set of lymphatic vessels returns lymphatic drainage over the surface of the lung within the pleura. In conditions in which the major lymphatic drainage through the thoracic duct is blocked, lymph may back up to form a chylous effusion.

Pulmonary Metabolism

The lungs have the only capillary bed in which the entire blood volume passes. Considering this, the pulmonary capillary circulation is uniquely suited for exercising a controlling influence on a number of circulating vasoactive agents. These include activation of angiotensin I to angiotensin II; inactivation of bradykinin, serotonin, prostaglandin E (PGE), and PGF_2; and partial inactivation of norepinephrine and perhaps histamine. In addition to modulating bronchial and pulmonary vascular diameter, the systemic effects of these agents include increased capillary permeability, platelet aggregation, and peripheral vasodilation.

Control of Respiration

The neural and chemical control of respiration involves an intricate balance of numerous factors that serve to maintain Pao_2, $Paco_2$, and pH at levels that promote cellular functioning. Nervous system control of breathing includes the cerebral cortex through the corticospinal tracts to the respiratory muscles and autonomic control through the medulla and pons of the brainstem.

Expansion of the thoracic cavity on inspiration occurs by stimulation of the phrenic nerve, which innervates the diaphragm, and stimulation of the spinal nerves, which innervate the external intercostal muscles. If expiration must be facilitated, stimulation through the spinal nerves causes contraction of the internal intercostal and abdominal muscles.

Rhythmic discharge of neurons in the medulla oblongata produces spontaneous respiration. Although specific pacemaker cells that drive respiration have not been identified, two groups of respiratory neurons in the medulla influence respiration: the dorsal respiratory group (DRG) and the ventral respiratory group (VRG). The DRG is the source of rhythmic drive to the contralateral phrenic motor neurons, and the VRG innervates ipsilateral accessory muscles and provides inspiratory and expiratory input to the intercostal muscles. Rhythmic discharge of the medullary neurons is modified by centers in the pons and by afferent information from the vagus nerve stretch receptors in the chest.

The pneumotaxic center is located in the rostral section of the pons. Stimulation of the expiratory neurons inhibits the inspiratory center in the medulla; thus the pneumotaxic center works with the medulla to generate regular cyclical respirations. The apneustic center is located in the middle and caudal pons. Stimulation of this center along with a vagotomy produces apneustic respiration, a respiratory pattern characterized by extremely prolonged inspiratory periods.

Scattered throughout the upper airway, trachea, and lungs are mechanoreceptors that provide information to the respiratory center via the vagus nerve. These receptors include slowly adapting stretch receptors, rapidly adapting stretch receptors, and C fibers. Slowly adapting receptors (SARs) are activated by increases in lung volume; when stimulated, the SARs are responsible for prolonging expiratory time. Rapidly adapting receptors (RARs) are activated by lung inflation and a variety of chemical substances (histamine and prostaglandin) and cause an increase in respiratory rate (RR). C fibers are also activated by chemical substances (histamine, prostaglandin, bradykinin, and serotonin) and cause apnea, followed by rapid, shallow breathing.

Central chemoreceptors, responsible for the dramatic increase in minute ventilation ($\dot{V}_E$) when $Paco_2$ levels are elevated, are located in the medulla. Medullary chemoreceptors monitor H^+ ion concentration of cerebrospinal fluid and brainstem interstitial fluid. Although H^+ and HCO_3^- ions are unable to cross the blood-brain barrier easily, CO_2 readily penetrates and immediately hydrates to form carbonic acid (H_2CO_3), which dissipates into H^+ and HCO_3^-. The concentration of H^+ ions in the brain's interstitial fluid parallels $Paco_2$ and acts as a stimulus to increase respirations.

The peripheral chemoreceptors include the carotid body located near the bifurcation of the internal and external carotid arteries and the aortic bodies located near the arch of the aorta. The carotid bodies are sensitive to Pao_2 and potentiated by H^+ ion and $Paco_2$ concentration; aortic bodies are sensitive to circulatory changes. Afferent nerve fibers from the carotid and aortic bodies ascend to the medulla to increase ventilation as necessary. Chronic sustained hypoxia decreases the carotid bodies' response to low Pao_2.

Oxygen Transport

"Adequate" oxygenation can only be defined when tissue oxygen supply matches tissue oxygen demand. Essential factors to be considered include (1) alveolar-pulmonary capillary oxygen transport, (2) oxygen transport in the blood, and (3) cellular respiration. Table 8-2 provides a summary of oxygenation profile parameters.

Alveolar-Pulmonary Capillary Oxygen Transport. Between the extremely thin alveoli walls is an almost solid network of interconnecting capillaries. Gas exchange occurs throughout the alveolar-pulmonary capillary membrane of all the terminal portions of the lungs. Oxygen and CO_2 move across the seven-layer alveolar-pulmonary capillary membrane by passive diffusion from an area of high partial pressure to an area of low partial pressure (Fig. 8-6). Diffusion is directly proportional to the gradient of partial

<table>
<tr><th colspan="3">◆ TABLE 8-2   Normal Oxygenation Profile Values</th></tr>
</table>

Parameter	Calculation	Norms
Cao_2	$Cao_2 = (Hgb \times 1.34 \times Sao_2) + (Pao_2 \times 0.003)$	20 ml/dl
$C\bar{v}o_2$	$C\bar{v}o_2 = (Hgb \times 1.34 \times S\bar{v}o_2) + (P\bar{v}o_2 \times 0.003)$	15 ml/dl
a-vDo_2	$Cao_2 - C\bar{v}o_2$	3.5-5 ml/dl
$\dot{D}o_2$	$\dot{D}o_2 = Cao_2 \times CI \times 10$	620 ± 50 ml/min/M^2
$\dot{V}o_2$	$\dot{V}o_2 = (Cao_2 - C\bar{v}o_2) \times CI \times 10$	120-200 ml/min/M^2
O_2ER	$(Cao_2 - C\bar{v}o_2)/Cao_2 \times 100$	$25 \pm 2\%$
$S\bar{v}o_2$		75% (60-80%)

Cao_2, Arterial oxygen content; *Hgb*, hemoglobin; *Sao_2*, arterial oxygen saturation; *CI*, cardiac index; *$\dot{D}o_2$*, oxygen delivery; *Pao_2*, arterial partial pressure of oxygen; *$C\bar{v}o_2$*, venous oxygen content; *$S\bar{v}o_2$*, venous oxygen saturation; *$P\bar{v}o_2$*, venous partial pressure of oxygen; *a-$\bar{v}Do_2$*, arteriovenous oxygen difference; *$\dot{V}o_2$*, oxygen consumption; *O_2ER*, oxygen extraction ratio.

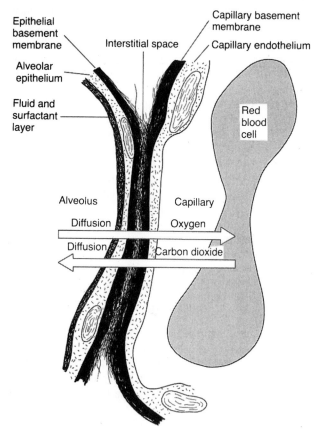

Fig. 8-6 Cross-section of pulmonary capillary membrane. (From Guyton AC: *Textbook of medical physiology*, ed 8, Philadelphia, 1991, WB Saunders.)

pressure across the alveolar-pulmonary capillary membrane, the alveolar-pulmonary capillary surface area, and the gas solubility. Diffusion is inversely proportional to the thickness of the alveolar-pulmonary capillary membrane and the molecular weight of the gas.

According to Dalton's law of partial pressures, the total pressure of a mixture of gases is equal to the sum of the pressures of the individual gases. The total pressure of gas in the atmosphere, the atmospheric pressure, is 760 mmHg at sea level. Thus partial pressures of a component gas depend on the fraction of the total mixture occupied by that gas. Room air contains 21% oxygen; thus oxygen exerts a partial pressure of 21% of 760 mmHg, which is 160 mmHg. At high altitudes, the percent concentration of oxygen does not change, but the absolute number of molecules in a given volume does. For example, at 5000 feet, atmospheric pressure is 632 mmHg; 21% of 632 mmHg is 133 mmHg.

As gases are inhaled into the upper airway, they are warmed and humidified. The pressure of water vapor depends on the temperature of atmospheric gas. At high temperatures, atmospheric gas has more water in vapor form, whereas the opposite is true with low temperatures. Water vapor exerts a pressure of 47 mmHg at 30° C. Water vapor reduces the partial pressure of inspired oxygen; 760 − 47 = 713; 21% of 713 is 149.7 mmHg.

Alveolar ventilation refers to the portion of ventilation that undergoes gas exchange. Inspired gas is mixed in the alveoli with gas that contains water vapor and CO_2. Alveolar partial pressure of oxygen (Pao_2) is calculated using the *alveolar gas equation:* $Pao_2 = Pio_2 − Paco_2/RQ$. The inspired partial pressure of oxygen (Pio_2) is corrected for water vapor (47 mmHg) and is $Pio_2 = (Pb − 47) \times Fio_2$. The value of CO_2 is corrected by the respiratory quotient (RQ), which takes into consideration that more O_2 is consumed than CO_2 is produced. In room air, at normal barometric pressure (Pb) and normal $Paco_2$, with an RQ of 0.8, the Pao_2 is equal to 99.7 mmHg; $Pao_2 = (760 − 47) \times 0.21 = 149.7$ mmHg − 40/0.8.

The partial pressures of alveolar gases equal atmospheric pressure; any increase in one alveolar gas is associated with a decrease in another. Decreases in pulmonary uptake of oxygen are related to either diffusion or ventilation-perfusion deficits. For example, diffusion defects occur secondary to problems affecting the diffusion of gases over the alveolar-pulmonary capillary membrane (interstitial edema), whereas ventilation-perfusion deficits occur secondary to problems affecting alveolar ventilation (atelectasis) or alveolar perfusion (cardiovascular collapse).

Considering that the Pao_2 is close to 100 mmHg and the normal venous partial pressure of oxygen ($P\bar{v}o_2$) is 40 mmHg, the alveolar-capillary diffusion gradient for oxygen is about 60 mmHg. The capillary-alveolar diffusion gradient for CO_2 is significantly less (46 − 40 mmHg = 6 mmHg); but CO_2 is 24 times more soluble than oxygen, and its molecular weight is greater than oxygen. Differences in solubility and size make CO_2 20 times more diffusible than oxygen. Pao_2 better reflects ventilation to perfusion matching, whereas $Paco_2$ better reflects the adequacy of alveolar ventilation.

Oxygen Transport in the Blood. Oxygen is carried in the blood in two forms: in combination with hemoglobin and dissolved in plasma. Oxygen binds rapidly and reversibly with hemoglobin to form oxyhemoglobin (Hbo_2). Almost all oxygen is carried as oxyhemoglobin.

The *arterial oxygen content* (Cao_2) describes the total amount of oxygen carried by arterial blood. Cao_2 (ml/dl) = ($Hgb \times 1.34 \times Sao_2$) + ($Pao_2 \times 0.003$). For example: with a hemoglobin (Hgb) concentration of 15 g/dl of blood, arterial saturation (Sao_2) of 98%, and a Pao_2 of 100 mmHg, Cao_2 (ml/dl) = ($15 \times 1.34 \times 98\%$) + ($100 \times 0.003$); Cao_2 = 19.7 + 0.3; Cao_2 = 20 ml/dl. When fully saturated, 1 g of hemoglobin carries 1.34 ml of oxygen; plasma carries only 0.003 ml of oxygen per mmHg O_2 per deciliter. The Pao_2 gives excellent information regarding lung function, whereas Pao_2 assumes an insignificant role in oxygen transport. The Cao_2 clearly demonstrates the highly significant role of hemoglobin in oxygen transport. Alternative shortened formulas for Cao_2 calculation eliminate the Pao_2 portion of the equation. Note that once hemoglobin is fully saturated at 100%, the only way to dramatically improve Cao_2 is through erythrocyte administration, increasing hemoglobin concentration.

Oxygen-Hemoglobin Affinity: Oxyhemoglobin Dissociation Curve (ODC). The oxygen-carrying capacity of blood is directly related to hemoglobin concentration and the affinity of oxygen for hemoglobin. Although Pao_2 contributes little to Cao_2, Pao_2 plays a major role in determining the affinity of oxygen for hemoglobin as described by the sigmoid-shaped ODC (Fig. 8-7, *A*).

The S-shaped curve facilitates alveolar capillary uptake of oxygen (the association process) and tissue release of oxygen (the dissociation process). Over the upper flat portion of the curve (>70 mmHg → ∞), hemoglobin bond to oxygen is favored. A large change in oxygen tension results in a small change in oxygen saturation/content. Hemoglobin remains fully saturated, providing a consistent oxygen content/saturation over a wide range of oxygen tensions commonly found in the alveolar capillary bed. Over the steep portion of the curve (Po_2 of 10 to 40 mmHg), hemoglobin release of oxygen is favored. A small drop in oxygen tension results in a large drop in oxygen saturation/content. This ensures delivery of large quantities of oxygen to the tissue capillary beds.

The affinity of oxygen for hemoglobin may change and shift the position of the ODC to the right or left. The Po_2 at which hemoglobin is 50% saturated, the P_{50}, is used as a marker for the relative position of the ODC. At a pH of 7.4 and temperature of 37° C, P_{50} for hemoglobin A is 27 mmHg. A *shift to the left* (decreased P_{50}) means that oxygen is more tightly bound to hemoglobin; a *shift to the right* (increased P_{50}) means that oxygen is readily released from hemoglobin (see Fig. 8-7, *A*). A shift to the right has little effect on the association process, but the dissociation process is enhanced. For example, at the upper flat portion of the curve, slightly less than 100% saturation occurs; but at the steep portion of the curve, significantly more oxygen is unloaded to the

tissues. The opposite is true of a shift to the left; the association process is enhanced, whereas the dissociation process is diminished.

Principal modulators of oxygen-hemoglobin affinity include temperature, Pco_2/pH, and the concentration of red blood cell 2,3-diphosphoglycerate (DPG) (an enzyme that accumulates in response to sustained periods of impaired oxygen delivery).

Hyperthermia results in a decreased oxygen affinity (right shift), whereas hypothermia results in a increased oxygen affinity (left shift). Clinically, oxygen becomes more available to the tissues when there is an increased metabolic need marked by hyperthermia.

Known as the Bohr effect, increased H^+ ion concentration shifts the ODC to the right. Associated with the hydration of CO_2 to carbonic acid (HCO_3), acidosis results in decreased oxygen affinity. Clinically, a shift to the right favors the release of oxygen for aerobic metabolism in the more acidotic CO_2-rich environment of tissue capillary beds.

The organic phosphate 2,3-DPG decreases oxygen affinity for hemoglobin, resulting in an increased oxygen release to the tissues. Increased levels of 2,3-DPG are associated with chronic anemic and hypoxic states, for example, in patients with cyanotic heart disease and chronic lung disease; decreased levels are found with inorganic phosphate deficiency and in sepsis. Also, 2,3-DPG concentrations decrease with advanced red blood cell age, for example, in banked blood.

In infants and children, a cluster of ODCs exist (see Fig. 8-7, *B*). As mentioned, at a pH of 7.4 and temperature of 37° C, the P_{50} for hemoglobin A is 27 mmHg. Hemoglobin A, adult type hemoglobin, consists of two α-chains and two β-chains, with each containing a heme group with iron. Fetal hemoglobin, hemoglobin F, consists of two α-chain and two γ-chain units. The transition from fetal to adult hemoglobin starts to occur just before birth in full-term infants and is complete by 6 months of age. Term newborns have approximately 70% hemoglobin A and 30% hemoglobin F. Compared with hemoglobin A, hemoglobin F has an increased oxygen affinity. Under similar conditions, P_{50} at birth for hemoglobin F is 19.4 mmHg. P_{50} then shifts to approximately 30 mmHg by 11 months of age. The left shift of fetal hemoglobin allows higher oxygen saturation at lower oxygen tensions. This is crucial for adequate oxygenation of the fetus because placental blood normally provides a Po_2 of 35 to 40 mmHg.

Oxygen delivery ($\dot{D}o_2$), the amount of oxygen delivered to the tissues, is equal to $Cao_2 \times$ cardiac index (CI) $\times$ a conversion factor of 10, which changes the Cao_2 measurement from deciliters to liters; $\dot{D}o_2 = Cao_2 \times CI \times 10$. Normal $\dot{D}o_2$ is 620 ± 50 ml/min/M^2. Barcoft[15] identified three separate causes of inadequate $\dot{D}o_2$: hypoxia, anemia, or stagnant flow. Hypoxia occurs secondary to a low arterial oxygen saturation, for example, hypoxia associated with ventilation-perfusion mismatch. Anemia occurs secondary to low hemoglobin concentration, for example, anemia after hemorrhage. Stagnant flow occurs secondary to low cardiac output, for example, shock states. The clinical significance of alterations in the determinates of $\dot{D}o_2$ are reviewed in

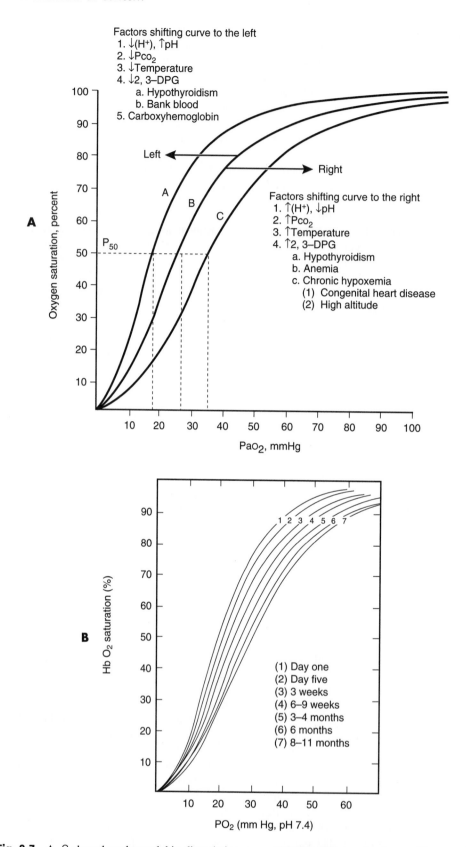

Fig. 8-7 **A,** S-shaped oxyhemoglobin dissociation curve (ODC) facilitates alveolar capillary uptake of oxygen (association process) and tissue release of oxygen (dissociation process). **B,** Age-dependent ODCs. (**A** redrawn from Kinney MR, Dunbar SB, Brooks-Brunn JA et al, eds: *AACN clinical reference for critical care nursing,* ed 4, St Louis, 1998, Mosby; **B** from Oski FA: The unique fetal red cell and its function. E. Mead Johnson Award address, *Pediatrics* 51:494, 1973.)

TABLE 8-3 Clinical Significance of Alterations in the Determinates of $\dot{D}o_2$

$\dot{D}o_2 = Cao_2 \times CI \times 10$, where Cao_2 (ml/dl) = (Hgb $\times$ 1.34 $\times$ Sao_2) + ($Pao_2 \times 0.003$)

State	Hgb(g/dl)	Sao_2 (%)	Pao_2 (mmHg)	Cao_2 (ml/dl)	CI (L/min/M²)	$\dot{D}o_2$ (ml/min/M²)
Normal	12-15	95-100	80-100	20	3.5-5.5	620 ± 50
Hypoxia	15	**85**	**50**	17	4	680
Anemia	**8**	100	100	11	4	440
Stagnant flow	15	100	100	20	**2**	400

$\dot{D}o_2$, Oxygen delivery; Cao_2, arterial oxygen content; *CI*, cardiac index; *Hgb*, hemoglobin; Sao_2, arterial oxygen saturation; Pao_2, arterial partial pressure of oxygen. Bold numbers represent abnormal values.

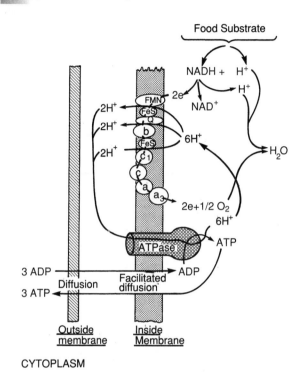

Fig. 8-8 Oxidative phosphorylation produces massive quantities of ATP. (From Guyton AC: *Textbook of medical physiology,* ed 8, Philadelphia, 1991, WB Saunders.)

Table 8-3. Deficits occur in isolation or in combination. Also, parameters compensate for the other; for example, tachycardia increases after hemorrhage. Clinical management strategies are directed toward correction of the primary problem and supporting compensatory mechanisms.

Cellular Respiration. Tissue oxygenation is dependent on microcirculation regulated by arteriolar and precapillary sphincter tone and $\dot{D}o_2$. Capillary oxygen moves from erythrocytes, through plasma, and into tissue by diffusion.

Adjustments in microcirculation can enhance oxygen extraction and preserve organ metabolism. Precapillary sphincters, located at the arterial end of each capillary, maintain capillaries open or closed depending on the metabolic requirements of the specific tissue bed. A local increase in H^+ ion concentration shifts the ODC to the right to augment hemoglobin release of oxygen.

All cells are dependent on a continuous supply of oxygen to support aerobic metabolism necessary for the synthesis of high-energy compounds (adenosine triphos-

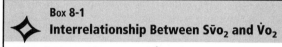

Box 8-1
Interrelationship Between $S\bar{v}o_2$ and $\dot{V}o_2$

Normal $S\bar{v}o_2$ and Increased $\dot{V}o_2$

Compensation effective—increased supply ($\dot{D}o_2$) to preserve venous reserve

Decreased $S\bar{v}o_2$ and Increased $\dot{V}o_2$

Compensation ineffective or impossible—patient using venous reserve

Increased $S\bar{v}o_2$ and Decreased $\dot{V}o_2$

Decreased need
Increased supply
Decreased use (sepsis, left shift to ODC, cyanide toxicity)
Left-to-right shunting (CHD, AV malformations, AV fistulas, loss of autoregulation of blood flow, vasodilated states)

AV, Arteriovenous; *CHD,* congenital heart disease; $\dot{D}o_2$, oxygen delivery; *ODC,* oxyhemoglobin dissociation curve; $S\bar{v}o_2$, venous oxygen saturation; $\dot{V}o_2$, oxygen consumption.

phate [ATP]) essential for cell life and function. Most cellular oxygen is consumed by the mitochondria to drive oxidative phosphorylation (Fig. 8-8). In the absence of oxygen, electron transport activity decreases, and cells start to produce ATP anaerobically from the conversion of pyruvate to lactate. Not only is this process less efficient (20 times less ATP is produced), but also lactic acid lowers tissue pH and depletes cellular nicotinamide adenine dinucleotide (oxidized [NAD^+]) necessary for aerobic glycolysis.

Oxygen delivery does not provide information about the adequacy of tissue oxygenation. For example, in septic shock $\dot{D}o_2$ is high, but blood is shunted across tissue-capillary beds without unloading oxygen. Indirect methods of assessing the adequacy of tissue oxygenation include monitoring mixed venous oxygenation, oxygen consumption, and oxygen extraction ratio.

Blood returning from various regions of the body becomes well mixed in the right ventricle. To avoid regional contamination, true mixed venous oxygenation is monitored from the pulmonary artery. Pulmonary artery catheters, designed specifically for continuous $S\bar{v}o_2$ monitoring, are available in sizes designed specifically for the pediatric population. The interrelationship between $S\bar{v}o_2$ values and $\dot{V}o_2$ is noted in Box 8-1.

Reflecting metabolic requirements, *oxygen consumption* ($\dot{V}o_2$) is the amount of oxygen used by tissues. $\dot{V}o_2$ is assessed as the net oxygen difference between the amount of oxygen entering tissue and the amount of oxygen leaving tissue. $\dot{V}o_2$ can be approximated by using a modified version of the Fick equation: $\dot{V}o_2 = (Cao_2 - C\bar{v}o_2) \times CI \times 10$, where $C\bar{v}o_2 = (Hgb \times 1.36 \times S\bar{v}o_2) + (p\bar{v}o_2 \times 0.003)$; $C\bar{v}o_2$ norm is 15 ml/dl or vol%. The conversion factor of 10 is necessary to change deciliters to liters. Resting $\dot{V}o_2$ in infants and young children is almost twice that of an adult. The significantly higher $\dot{V}o_2$ reflects the metabolic requirements of continued growth, that is, growth adds a metabolic burden. Factors that affect $\dot{V}o_2$ are noted in Table 8-4.

Oxygen extraction ratio, O_2ER, is a ratio of $\dot{V}o_2$ to $\dot{D}o_2$ (oxygen consumption to oxygen delivery or availability). The O_2ER represents the proportion of $\dot{D}o_2$ that is actually used by the tissues. O_2ER is calculated as follows: $O_2ER = (Cao_2 - C\bar{v}o_2)/Cao_2 \times 100$. The O_2ER is normally 25%. This means that only 25% of the oxygen delivered to the tissues is actually utilized. This apparently low O_2ER is

protective in that significantly more O_2 can be extracted if necessary to maintain adequate tissue delivery when $\dot{V}o_2$ increases or $\dot{D}o_2$ decreases. The O_2ER increases when the demand for O_2 increases (fever, pain) or the supply of O_2 decreases (decreased hemoglobin, Sao_2, or cardiac index); the O_2ER decreases when demand for O_2 decreases (hypothermia, adequate sedation, and chemical paralysis) or when supply, relative to demand, increases. The O_2ER is not a valid measure when the $C\bar{v}o_2$ is contaminated with right-to-left blood shunted across anatomic cardiac defects.

Physiologic oxygen supply dependency describes the *normal* biphasic relationship between $\dot{D}o_2$ and $\dot{V}o_2$ (Fig. 8-9). Initially when $\dot{D}o_2$ falls, oxygen extraction increases to

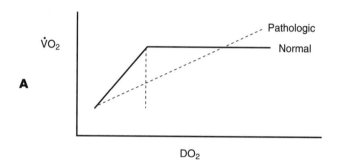

TABLE 8-4	**Factors That Affect Tissue Oxygen Consumption ($\dot{V}o_2$)**

% Increase $\dot{V}o_2$	
138	Head injury, nonsedated
100	Burns
50-100	Sepsis
50-100	Shivering
89	Head injury, sedated
20-80	Multiple system organ dysfunction
60	Chest trauma
40	Work of breathing
25-40	Nasal ETT intubation
36	Patient weight
35	Bronchial hygiene
31	Position change
10-30	Orthopedic injuries
27	ETT suctioning
25	Chest x-ray film
23	Bath
20	Physical examination
18	Agitation
16	Electrocardiogram
10	Fever (increase for each °C)
10	Dressing change
7	Routine postoperative procedures
% Decrease $\dot{V}o_2$	
50	Anesthesia in burned patients
25	Anesthesia
25-50	Sleep, relaxation, pain relief, paralysis, hypothermia

Data from White KM, Winslow EH, Clark AP et al: The physiologic basis for continuous mixed venous oxygen saturation monitoring, *Heart Lung* 19:548-551, 1990.
ETT, Endotracheal tube.

Fig. 8-9 A, Normal and pathologic relationships of oxygen consumption *($\dot{V}o_2$)* and oxygen delivery *($\dot{D}o_2$).* The normal critical $\dot{D}o_2$ is shown as the vertical line separating the independent and dependent portions of the normal $\dot{V}o_2$ and $\dot{D}o_2$ relationship. The pathologic relationship is characterized by greater critical $\dot{D}o_2$ compared with the normal relationship. In animal models, the pathologic relationship has a plateau of $\dot{V}o_2$, and increased critical $\dot{D}o_2$ is clearly identified. However, clinical studies have not shown a plateau of $\dot{V}o_2$ in individual patients who have pathologic dependence of $\dot{V}o_2$ on $\dot{D}o_2$. **B,** Normal and pathologic relationships of oxygen extraction ratio *(ER)* and $\dot{D}o_2$. The critical oxygen ER is the extraction ratio at the critical $\dot{D}o_2$ shown as the vertical line corresponding to the critical $\dot{D}o_2$ determined by the $\dot{D}o_2/\dot{V}o_2$ relationship above. In the normal relationship, oxygen ER continues to increase below critical oxygen ER, but not enough to maintain $\dot{V}o_2$ constant. In the pathologic relationship, oxygen ER remains relatively constant, and therefore $\dot{V}o_2$ is dependent on $\dot{D}o_2$. In animal models, pathologic dependence of $\dot{V}o_2$ on $\dot{D}o_2$ is characterized by lower critical oxygen ER than normal. (Adapted from Russell JA, Phang PT: The oxygen delivery/consumption controversy: approaches to management of the critically ill, *Am J Respir Crit Care Med* 149:533-537, 1994.)

maintain $\dot{V}_{O_2}$ until a critical level of $\dot{D}_{O_2}$ is reached. At this critical level of $\dot{D}_{O_2}$, referred to as critical oxygen transport, $\dot{V}_{O_2}$ progressively decreases and becomes linearly dependent on $\dot{D}_{O_2}$. Metabolic demands are met on the flat portion of the curve as long as the O_2ER can increase to meet tissue demands for oxygen.

In contrast, *pathologic oxygen supply dependency* describes an *abnormal* relationship between $\dot{D}_{O_2}$ and $\dot{V}_{O_2}$; O_2ER remains low, and $\dot{V}_{O_2}$ is linearly dependent on $\dot{D}_{O_2}$ over a wide range of values (see Fig. 8-9). This abnormal $\dot{V}_{O_2}$-$\dot{D}_{O_2}$ relationship is thought to occur in several disease states, for example, adult respiratory distress syndrome (ARDS) and sepsis.[16]

Under normal circumstances, organ blood flow (oxygen supply) is distributed to match organ metabolic need (oxygen demand). Control of oxygen flow to match metabolism is regulated by the resistance of capillary vessels. This event, along with alterations in hemoglobin affinity, enhances peripheral oxygen extraction to sustain tissue metabolism. When $\dot{D}_{O_2}$ decreases or if $\dot{V}_{O_2}$ increases *and* systemic blood flow is distributed to match metabolic need, the O_2ER (an average of each individual organ oxygen extraction) should increase. If systemic blood flow is not distributed to match metabolic need, hypoxia and a low O_2ER result.

Pulmonary Ventilation

Ventilation, the process of inspiration followed by expiration, is accomplished when the diaphragm functions to move air in and out of the lungs. When the thoracic cavity changes in size, pressure gradients are created between the intrapleural space, intraalveolar space, and the atmosphere. The external pressure exerted on the thorax is atmospheric at 760 mmHg. Intraalveolar pressure, which is in direct communication with the atmosphere, is also 760 mmHg. Intrapleural pressure, the pressure between the visceral and parietal pleura, is subatmospheric at 757.5 mmHg or at −2.5 mmHg.

Inspiration is an active process in that energy is required for the contraction of inspiratory muscles that expand the thoracic cavity. As the thoracic cavity expands, intrapleural pressure becomes increasingly subatmospheric at −6 mmHg. Intraalveolar pressure also becomes subatmospheric, and air moves in bulk flow from the atmosphere to alveoli, where diffusion can occur.

Expiration is a passive process in that the muscles of respiration relax and the size of the intrathoracic cavity decreases. When the muscles relax, the elastic properties of the lung followed by the elastic properties of the chest wall pull the thoracic cavity back to a resting position. As the size of the intrathoracic cavity decreases, intraalveolar pressure becomes supraatmospheric, and air moves in bulk flow from the alveoli to the atmosphere. Because of normal increased airways resistance during expiration, passive expiration requires more time than inspiration.

Compliance. Compliance refers to the stretchability, distensibility, or elasticity of the lungs and thoracic structures. The elastic properties of the lungs and chest wall

allow the thoracic cavity to return to a resting state after inspiration. Compliance describes the relationship between volume (V) and pressure (P) ($\Delta V/\Delta P$) and is an indicator of elastic recoil and surface tension of the lung. Total compliance is the product of lung compliance and chest wall compliance. Clinically, total compliance is approximated by dividing the plateau pressure minus the positive end-expiratory pressure (PEEP) into measured tidal volume (V_T): $\Delta V/\Delta P = V_T \div P_{plat} - PEEP$. (The plateau pressure is a pause pressure obtained at end inspiration.) For example, if the V_T/plateau pressure − PEEP were 60 ml ÷ 15 cm H_2O, the total lung compliance is approximately 4 ml/cm H_2O.

Lung compliance is measured in either a dynamic or static state. *Dynamic compliance* is equal to V_T divided by the transpulmonary pressure. The transpulmonary pressure (PL) is the difference between the alveolar pressure and the intrapleural pressure. Because dynamic compliance is measured during breathing, airways resistance and respiratory rate influence it. *Static compliance* (Cst) is equal to V_T divided by PL at the cessation of airflow. Because Cst is measured under zero-flow conditions, it reflects the elastic properties of the lungs.[17] Clinically, PL can be approximated by subtracting intraesophageal pressure (as measured by an esophageal catheter or balloon placed in the lower third of the esophagus) from proximal airway pressures (using an adapter placed on the endotracheal tube) at the same point in a single breath. Similar results can also be achieved by measuring volume and flow by respiratory inductance plethysmography. A curve relating ΔV to ΔPL is constructed; the slope of the curve describes lung compliance (Fig. 8-10). Shifts to the right indicate decreased lung compliance.

The pressure/volume characteristics of the lungs are not linear; at very high and very low lung volumes, changes in pressure produce little change in volume (the flatter the

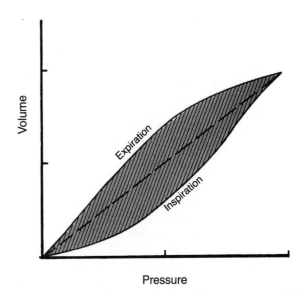

Fig. 8-10 Pressure (P)/volume (V) curve relating ΔP to ΔV is constructed; slope of curve describes lung compliance. (From Guyton AC: *Textbook of medical physiology,* ed 8, Philadelphia, 1991, WB Saunders.)

curve, the stiffer the lungs). The lower inflection point (P_{flex}) on the P/V curve reflects a sudden increase in compliance—specifically, the point at which small increases in transpulmonary pressure produce large increases in pulmonary volume. The upper inflection point reflects a sudden decrease in compliance—specifically, the point at which small increases in transpulmonary pressure produce small increases in pulmonary volume. Volume/pressure relationships also differ during inspiration and exhalation; more pressure is required to increase volume during inspiration than the reciprocal during exhalation.

Lung compliance changes with age, normally decreasing with increasing age and changes with disease, for example, surfactant-deficient ARDS. Thoracic compliance can be significantly reduced in many clinical states, for example, in patients with scoliosis, muscular dystrophy, or obesity and in the postoperative patient with surgical splinting.

Airways Resistance. Total pulmonary resistance is affected by (1) radius, length, and number of divisions of bronchi; (2) diameter and length of the endotracheal tube; (3) gas flow; and (4) character of gas flow. Airways resistance, or the rigidity of the bronchioles and thoracic structures, refers to the ease of air movement through conducting airways. Airways resistance is the pressure required to move a volume of gas at a given flow rate. Airways resistance is the product of the peak inspiratory pressure *(PIP)* minus the plateau pressure divided by the gas flow ($R_{aw} = PIP - P_{plat} \div V$).

The volume of gas that is pulled into the lungs and forced out of the lungs is inversely related to airways resistance. Until 5 or 6 years of age, small peripheral airways contribute up to 50% of total airways resistance compared with only 20% in adults.[18] Diseases that affect the small airways, for example, bronchiolitis and asthma, can cause a significant increase in airways resistance and work of breathing in the younger, more vulnerable age group.

During normal spontaneous ventilation, the airways widen during inspiration and become narrow on exhalation. Autonomic nervous system regulation of bronchiolar smooth muscle can decrease (sympathetic) or increase (parasympathetic) airways resistance. Bronchiolar smooth muscle is also very sensitive to chemicals, such as histamine and low CO_2 levels, causing bronchoconstriction, whereas high CO_2 levels cause bronchodilation.

Time Constants. The tidal flow of gas into and out of the lung depends on the compliance of the alveoli and the resistance of the airways. The relationship between compliance and resistance determines the actual rate of alveolar filling and emptying. The relationship between these two properties can be expressed mathematically as the time constant (Fig. 8-11; time constant = resistance × compliance). The time constant is expressed in seconds as the product of compliance and resistance. One time constant is the measure of the time necessary for the alveolar pressure to reach 63% of the total change in airway pressure. About 99% of pressure equilibration occurs within three to five time constants. The longer the time constant, the longer alveolar filling and emptying will take (Fig. 8-12).

Increased airways resistance prolongs the time necessary to fill alveoli with air; likewise, a region of low compliance takes more time to fill with air than an area of high compliance. Pulmonary disease affecting either airways resistance or lung compliance exhibits nonhomogeneous time constants, that is, areas with both prolonged and normal time constants. Alveoli with normal time constants fill with air first, followed by alveoli with prolonged time constants. As respiratory rates increase, alveoli with normal time constants may overfill and compress alveoli with prolonged time constants. Overdistended alveoli become less compliant because they have reached their elastic limit.

An appreciation of time constants is especially important when managing the infant or child who requires mechanical ventilation because a wide range of ventilator settings can be employed to manage clinical conditions with dif-

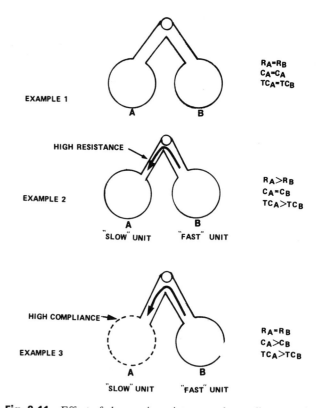

Fig. 8-11 Effect of changes in resistance and compliance on the distribution of gas between lung units. In example 1, resistances *(R)* and compliances *(C)* and thus time constants *(TC)* between lung units *A* and *B* are equal, and no redistribution of gas occurs if inspiration ends before the lung units are filled to maximal capacity. In example 2, TC of *A* is lengthened by increasing its resistance. Both will eventually attain the same volume because the compliances are the same, but unit *A* will take longer to fill. If inspiration ends prematurely, gas will be redistributed from *B* to *A*. In example 3, TC of *A* is lengthened by increasing its compliance relative to *B* while the resistances of both remain equal. The less compliant unit *B* will never inflate to as great a volume as *A*. If inspiration ends prematurely, gas will be redistributed from *B* to *A*. (From Helfaer MA, Nichols DG, Rogers MC: Developmental physiology of the respiratory system. In Rogers MC, ed: *Textbook of pediatric intensive care*, ed 2, Baltimore, 1992, Williams & Wilkins, p 112.)

ferent combinations of resistance and compliance states (Table 8-5).

Pulmonary Volumes. Pulmonary volumes and capacities are defined and illustrated in Fig. 8-13. Changes in body position can affect pulmonary volumes and capacities. In a prone position, values may decrease if abdominal contents exert pressure on the diaphragm, and to a lesser extent, increased pulmonary blood volumes may decrease available space for pulmonary air.

Dead space is the volume of inhaled air that does not participate in gas exchange. *Anatomic dead space* includes the volume of conducting air that fills the nose, mouth, pharynx, larynx, trachea, bronchi, and the distal bronchial branching that does not participate in gas exchange (Fig. 8-14). Normal anatomic dead space is approximately 2 ml/kg. *Alveolar dead space* refers to the volume of gas that fills alveoli whose perfusion is abnormally reduced or absent. Factors that contribute to alveolar dead space include hypotension, compression of the alveolar capillary

bed, and pulmonary embolus. Physiologic dead space is the sum of both anatomic and alveolar dead space. *Dead space ventilation* (V_D) refers to the amount of gas ventilating physiologic dead space per minute. Physiologic dead space is usually expressed as a fraction of tidal volume (V_D/V_T). The normal V_D/V_T ratio is 0.3, that is, 30% of the volume of each breath does not participate in gas exchange.

Minute ventilation ($\dot{V}_E$) is the volume of air that moves in or out of the lungs per minute. Minute ventilation is the product of tidal volume and respiratory rate. *Alveolar*

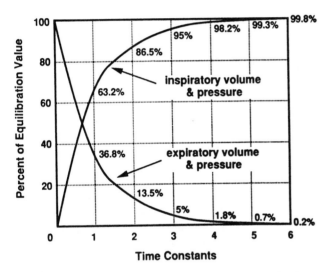

Fig. 8-12 Exponential rise and fall of lung pressures and volumes during inspiration and expiration in terms of time constants. (From Chatburn RL: Principles and practice of neonatal and pediatric mechanical ventilation, *Respir Care* 36:578, 1991.)

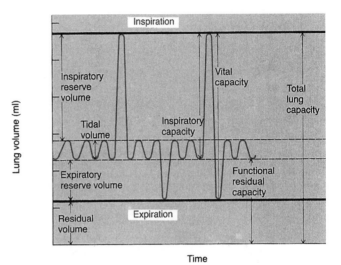

Fig. 8-13 Pulmonary volumes and capacities. *Tidal volume (V_T):* volume of air entering and leaving lungs during a single breath in a resting state, 6 to 8 ml/kg. *Inspiratory reserve volume (IRV):* amount of air that can be inspired over and above resting tidal volume. *Expiratory reserve volume (ERV):* air remaining in lungs at the end of a normal expiration that can be exhaled by active contraction of expiratory muscles. *Residual volume (RV):* amount of air remaining in lungs after maximal expiration. *Vital capacity (VC):* sum of normal V_T, IRV, and ERV; infants, 33 to 40 ml/kg; adults, 52 ml/kg. *Inspiratory capacity (IC):* sum of IRV and V_T. *Functional residual capacity (FRC):* sum of ERV and RV; infants, 30 ml/kg; adults, 34 ml/kg. *Total lung capacity (TLC):* amount of air in lungs after a maximal inspiration; infants, 63 ml/kg; adults, 86 ml/kg. (From Guyton AC: *Textbook of medical physiology,* ed 8, Philadelphia, 1991, WB Saunders, p 285.)

 TABLE 8-5 Effect of Varying Compliance and Resistance States on Time Constant and Associated Conditions

Compliance	Resistance	Time Constant	Clinical Conditions
Decrease	Normal	Short	Pneumonia Pneumothorax Atelectasis
Increase	Normal	Long	Neuromuscular disease
Normal	Decrease	Short	Postbronchodilator
Normal	Increase	Long	Airway obstructions Intubated patient
Increase	Increase	Long	BPD, COPD
Decrease	Increase	Long/short	Bronchiolitis

BPD, Bronchopulmonary dysplasia; *COPD,* chronic obstructive pulmonary disease.

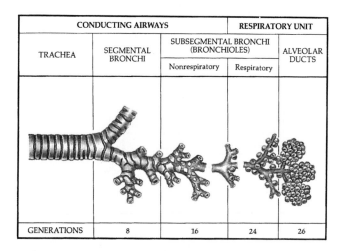

CONDUCTING AIRWAYS				RESPIRATORY UNIT
TRACHEA	SEGMENTAL BRONCHI	SUBSEGMENTAL BRONCHI (BRONCHIOLES)		ALVEOLAR DUCTS
		Nonrespiratory	Respiratory	
GENERATIONS	8	16	24	26

Fig. 8-14   Dead space ventilation continues down to the respiratory unit. (From Thompson JM, McFarland GK, Hirsh JE et al, eds: *Mosby's clinical nursing,* ed 4, St Louis, 1997, Mosby, p 125.)

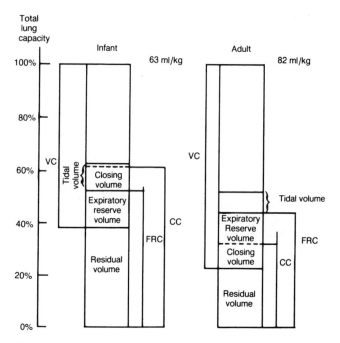

Fig. 8-15   Lung volumes in infants and adults. Note that tidal breathing in the infant takes place in the range of closing capacity *(CC)* of the lung. *VC,* Vital capacity; *FRC,* functional residual capacity. (From Smith CA, Nelson, NM: *The physiology of the newborn infant,* ed 4, Springfield, Ill, 1976, Charles C Thomas, p 207.)

ventilation ($\dot{V}_A$) is the volume per minute that ventilates all perfused alveoli and is the difference between minute ventilation and dead space ventilation ($\dot{V}_A = \dot{V}_E - V_D$). CO_2 production is dependent on metabolic rate, whereas CO_2 elimination from the lungs is determined by the effectiveness of $\dot{V}_A$ (V_T, RR, V_D). Adequate alveolar ventilation is present when the $Paco_2$ is maintained less than 40 mmHg with a normal $\dot{V}_E$. With hyperventilation, $\dot{V}_E$ is high, driving down the $Paco_2$; whereas with hypoventilation, $\dot{V}_E$ is low, driving up the $Paco_2$.

Forced vital capacity (FVC) is the volume of air forcibly exhaled after inhaling to total lung capacity. The volume of gas exhaled over time is usually plotted out to include the volume exhaled in 1 second (FEV_1) and the volume exhaled in 3 seconds (FEV_3). Patients with airway obstruction show a reduced rate of airflow on exhalation. The smaller the ratio of FEV_1 to FVC, the more difficult it is to exhale. Preexpiratory and postexpiratory FVC measurements are used to assess the effectiveness of bronchodilating drugs in patients with obstructive airways disease.

Functional residual capacity (FRC) is the amount of air remaining in the lungs at the end of normal expiration. With atelectasis, FRC falls as the number of alveoli that participate in gas exchange decreases. Airway closure occurs in dependent areas of the lung at low volumes. The lung volume at which airway closure occurs is called *closing capacity.* In adults, closing capacity is usually at residual volume (amount of air remaining in the lungs after maximal expiration). In infants, closing capacity is at FRC as a result of reduced elastic tissue, so closing capacity may be present during normal tidal breathing (Fig. 8-15). Pulmonary diseases that affect the relationship between tidal volume, FRC, and closing capacity contribute significantly to

ventilation-perfusion mismatch and hypoxemia. PEEP, which increases FRC above closing capacity, helps to limit alveolar collapse.

Work of Breathing.   Work of breathing, defined as the pressure generated by the respiratory muscles to move a volume of gas, can be divided into three components: (1) compliance work—required to expand the elastic forces of the lung; (2) resistance work—required to overcome the viscosity of the lung and thoracic cage; and (3) airways resistance—work required to overcome resistance to gas flow (Fig. 8-16). Under normal situations, most of the work of breathing is expended during inspiration to overcome the elastic properties of the lung.

Pulmonary disease can increase the work of breathing of any or all of the three components. Rapid respirations and increased airways resistance can cause expiratory work to surpass inspiratory work. Small changes in the work of breathing can significantly increase the metabolic rate and oxygen demand, resulting in respiratory muscle fatigue.

Ventilation/Perfusion Ratio

Gas exchange becomes optimal when both ventilation and pulmonary blood flow are equally matched. Under normal conditions, the *ventilation-to-perfusion ratio* ($\dot{V}/\dot{Q}$) is not equal to 1.0. This discrepancy is due to gravitational forces that create regional differences in intrapleural pressures and pulmonary vascular pressures.

During spontaneous breathing, a greater proportion of air and perfusion is directed toward dependent areas of the

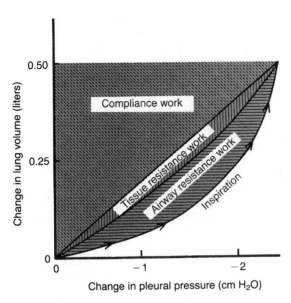

Fig. 8-16 Graphic representation of three different types of work accomplished during inspiration. (From Guyton AC: *Textbook of medical physiology,* ed 8, Philadelphia, 1991, WB Saunders.)

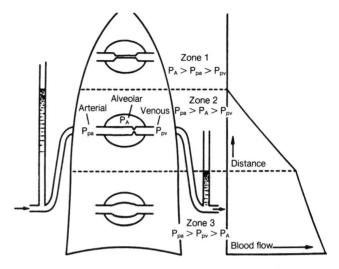

Fig. 8-17 Zones of perfusion in the lung. (From West JB, Dollery CT, Naimark A: Distribution of blood flow in isolated lung: relation to vascular and alveolar pressures, *J Appl Physiol* 19:713, 1964.)

lung. In the upright patient at rest between breaths, intrapleural pressures at the top of the lung are more negative than at the base of the lung, creating larger alveoli at the apex and smaller, more compliant alveoli at the base. During spontaneous inspiration, ventilation is preferentially distributed to the more compliant alveoli at the base rather than the apex. Similarly, gravitational forces distribute perfusion of the lung greatest in the base and lowest in the apex. However, in total, ventilation is greater than perfusion at the apex, and perfusion is greater than ventilation at the base. This results in an overall $\dot{V}/\dot{Q}$ of 0.8.

West and colleagues[19] described regional differences in lung perfusion in upright adults (Fig. 8-17). West's zone I conditions occur when the mean pulmonary artery pressure is less than or equal to alveolar pressure (PA > Ppa > Ppv). Zone I conditions are present in the apices of an upright adult and are characterized by a lack of pulmonary blood flow and gas exchange. West's zone II conditions are characterized by pulmonary artery pressures greater than alveoli pressure (Ppa > PA > Ppv). Zone II conditions are present in the midportion of the lung, and blood flow is determined by a balance of arterial and alveolar pressures not influenced by venous pressures. West's zone III conditions are characterized by pulmonary artery and venous pressures that exceed alveolar pressures (Ppa > Ppv > PA). Zone III conditions are located at the base of the lung, and blood flow is a function of the two vascular pressures. Although similar research in the pediatric population does not exist, it is reasonable to assume that zone II and III conditions are similar in younger age groups. Because the height of the lung is reduced when lying flat, zone I conditions probably do not exist in the supine position, especially in the infant population.[20]

Ventilation-Perfusion Abnormalities. Intrapulmonary shunting is the major cause of clinical hypoxemia. Characterized by a low $\dot{V}/\dot{Q}$ ratio, a *shunt* refers to venous blood that travels from the right to left side of the circulation without ever coming in contact with ventilated lung. Two categories of shunts exist: an anatomic shunt and a capillary shunt. An *anatomic shunt* refers to normal or abnormal right-to-left connections, for example, bronchial, pleural, and thebesian veins (the pulmonary circulation) or right-to-left congenital heart defects. A *capillary shunt* occurs when alveolar-capillary blood flow comes in contact with nonventilating alveoli, for example, atelectasis, pneumonia, and pneumothorax. As expected, mixing oxygenated and unoxygenated blood significantly impacts oxygenation, and hypoxemia results (Fig. 8-18).

Normally, an almost immediate diffusion of gases occurs over the alveolar-capillary membrane, so arterial and alveolar gas concentrations are similar. Venous blood passing nonfunctional alveoli creates an admixture of venous and arterial blood, decreasing Pao_2. *Venous admixture* represents the ratio of shunted blood ($\dot{Q}s$) to total pulmonary blood flow ($\dot{Q}t$). The $\dot{Q}s/\dot{Q}t$ ratio is calculated using the shunt equation: $\dot{Q}s/\dot{Q}t = (Cpco_2 - Cao_2)/(Cpco_2 - C\bar{v}o_2)$, where $Cpco_2$, Cao_2, and $C\bar{v}o_2$ are the pulmonary capillary, arterial, and mixed venous oxygen contents, respectively. The $Cpco_2$ is computed using the alveolar gas equation ($Pao_2 = Pio_2 - Paco_2/RQ$, where $Pio_2 = [760 - 47] \times Fio_2$, and $RQ = 0.8$). The $\dot{Q}s/\dot{Q}t$ normally ranges from 3% to 7%; changes greater than 5% are considered significant. Work of breathing significantly increases when $\dot{Q}s/\dot{Q}t$ is greater than 15%.

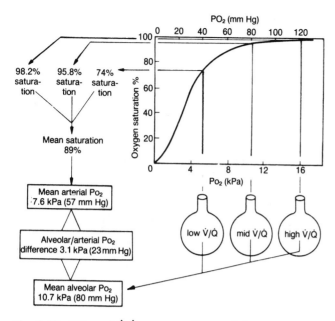

Fig. 8-18 Effect of $\dot{V}/\dot{Q}$ scatter on Pao_2 and Sao_2. Three lung units with low, mid, and high $\dot{V}/\dot{Q}$ ratios and PAO_2 of 40, 80, and 120 mmHg. Because of the shape of the ODC, the mean Pao_2 is only 57 mmHg, and the mean saturation is only 89%. (From Nunn JF: *Applied respiratory physiology,* ed 2, London, 1977, Butterworths, p 284.)

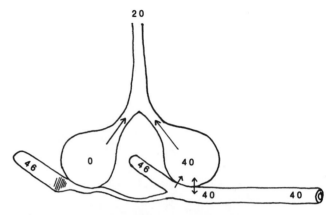

Fig. 8-19 Dead space unit. (From Swedlow DB: Capnometry and capnography: the anesthesia disaster early warning system, *Semin Anesthesia* V[3]:194-205, 1986.)

When a pulmonary artery catheter is not available to provide the mixed venous blood specimen necessary for calculating an intrapulmonary shunt, an alveolar-arterial Po_2 difference (A-aDo_2) or Pao_2/Fio_2 ratio can be used to estimate the percent shunt. The alveolar partial pressure of oxygen (PAO_2) is again calculated using the alveolar gas equation: $PAO_2 = Pio_2 - PaCo_2/RQ$, and the Pao_2 is obtained from a standard arterial blood gas (ABG) report. To obtain an A-aDo_2, the Pao_2 is subtracted from the calculated PAO_2. Normally, the A-aDo_2 should be less than 20 mmHg. The Pao_2/Fio_2 ratio calculation is straightforward; the norm is greater than 286.

The magnitude of the shunt helps to determine what effect increasing the Fio_2 might have on the Pao_2. If the shunt is insignificant, changes in the Pao_2 will occur in direct proportion to changes in Fio_2. If the shunt is significant, increases in Fio_2 will not impact Pao_2. PEEP is used to increase FRC, which potentially decreases $\dot{Q}s/\dot{Q}t$ and the risk of oxygen toxicity associated with the use of high Fio_2. Continuous assessment of the entire oxygenation profile is required to balance excessive PEEP, which may contribute to cardiac depression, and inadequate PEEP, which may contribute to progressive pulmonary hypoxemia.

In addition to the actual amount of shunted blood, the $C\bar{v}o_2$ of shunted blood also impacts Cao_2. The Cao_2 will fall if the shunted blood ($C\bar{v}o_2$) is more hypoxic secondary to increases in $\dot{V}o_2$ or decreases in $\dot{D}o_2$.

Characterized by a high $\dot{V}/\dot{Q}$ ratio, *dead space* refers to alveoli that are ventilated but not perfused (Fig. 8-19). As discussed, $Paco_2$ is determined by alveolar ventilation in relation to CO_2 production. Alveolar ventilation is compromised by increased dead space ventilation.

Physiologic dead space is calculated by the physiologic dead space/tidal volume ratio: $V_D/V_T = (Paco_2 - Peco_2) \div Paco_2$. This is measured by drawing an arterial sample to obtain a $Paco_2$ and by collecting the patient's expired air in a Douglas bag or similar device for several minutes to obtain a P_Eco_2 (partial pressure of carbon dioxide in the mixed expired air).

Calculating an end-tidal CO_2-$Paco_2$ gradient, the A-aDco_2 can also approximate dead space ventilation. In dead space units, mixed venous CO_2 is approximately 46 mmHg; alveolar CO_2 is 40 mmHg in the perfused unit, as is the pulmonary vein draining that unit. The alveolar CO_2 in the unperfused lung is zero because no blood has supplied it with CO_2. Down-line, the arterial CO_2 is an average of only the units perfused (40/1 = 40 mmHg), and $ETco_2$ is an average of all units ventilated (40/2 = 20 mmHg). Thus with 50% dead space ventilation, the A-aDco_2 will be 20 mmHg.

To compensate for increasing V_D/V_T, $\dot{V}_E$ must increase. Increases in $\dot{V}_E$ increase the work of breathing in direct proportion to increasing V_D/V_T. Thus assessment of $\dot{V}_E$ (respiratory rate and tidal volume) and $Paco_2$ levels are helpful tools in assessing dead space. If $\dot{V}_E$ increases, $Paco_2$ levels should decrease if V_D/V_T is normal; if $\dot{V}_E$ increases and $Paco_2$ remains the same, V_D/V_T is probably increased, or pulmonary blood flow is decreased. The $Paco_2$ is maintained at normal levels as long as the $\dot{V}_A$ can be maintained.

Various pulmonary diseases accentuate ventilation-perfusion abnormalities resulting in significant alterations in oxygenation and CO_2 removal. In fact, positive pressure ventilation alone immediately contributes to $\dot{V}/\dot{Q}$ mismatching; preferential ventilation is switched to nondependent areas, while preferential perfusion continues to dependent areas. Various physiologic mechanisms attempt to match ventilation to perfusion. For example, ventilation is altered by high CO_2 levels, which result in bronchodilation, whereas low CO_2 levels result in bronchoconstriction. Pulmonary arteriolar smooth muscle is very sensitive to the partial pressure of oxygen; increased alveolar oxygen results in vasodilation, and decreased alveolar oxygen results in vasoconstriction. This mechanism, known as *hypoxic pul-*

monary vasoconstriction (HPV), attempts to enhance perfusion of well-ventilated alveoli and limit perfusion to unventilated alveoli. Many drugs used in the intensive care unit (ICU) can attenuate HPV. Propranolol and dopamine enhance HPV, whereas nitric oxide, calcium channel blockers, vasodilators, β-agonists, and anesthetic agents diminish HPV. Pulmonary arteriolar smooth muscle is also very sensitive to H^+ ion concentration, which is directly related to CO_2 concentration. An increase in H^+ ion concentration results in vasoconstriction and shunting of blood away from poorly ventilated alveoli, with high alveolar CO_2 levels to better-ventilated alveoli.

ASSESSMENT OF PULMONARY FUNCTIONING

History

Patient assessment begins with data collection to describe the scope of the patient's problem, to identify the progression of illness, and to help delineate the initial management plan. Especially in patients with chronic respiratory illnesses, parents provide excellent data, particularly regarding the success of past management strategies.

When obtaining a medical history, interview depth and content are individualized to the age of the patient, the relevancy of information as it relates to the present illness, and the urgency of the current problem. For example, prenatal, natal, and postnatal history is relevant for infants admitted with a respiratory illness within the first year of life. If a perinatal history were significant, knowledge of whether the infant ever required assisted ventilation is important. Extensive questions about medication and environmental allergies are critical in patients with reactive airways disease. Questions related to fever are important if infection is suspected. Questions related to dietary intake, exercise tolerance, and schoolwork may give clues related to the chronicity of the illness. As a general rule, infants and young children should not experience more than five uncomplicated upper respiratory infections per year. In patients with chronic respiratory illness, activity tolerance, oxygen dependency, home ventilator settings, and successful coping strategies provide meaningful baseline information.

Questions related to the onset of the present illness are also important. Acute-onset illnesses include asthma, pneumonia, and upper airway obstruction. Aspiration of a foreign body is suggested when the onset of distress is acute, especially in the inquisitive toddler. Chronic or recurrent illnesses suggest infection or an unresolved foreign body but also allergic or immunologic problems, late-presentation congenital anomalies, or extrapulmonary problems, such as heart disease or cancer.

Physical Assessment

Inspection. When first approaching an infant or young child, note the child's position of comfort. Infants and children normally assume a wide variety of positions to enable ventilation and limit the work of breathing. Classic (yet rarely seen) positions include that of a drooling 3-year-old with epiglottitis whose survival depends on maintaining an upright position, usually tripod, with neck extended. Also classic is the older child with cystic fibrosis who while exhaling through pursed lips prefers to sit forward with arms supported on an overbed table. As a general rule, support the patient's attempts to find and maintain his or her own position of comfort.

Note the patient's facial expression; even young infants appear tense, tired, and anxious when gas exchange is inadequate. Integrate the patient's level of consciousness into the examination; hypoxia is reflected as anxious, restless, and irritable behavior, whereas hypercapnia produces drowsy and obtunded behavior. Note the presence of pallor or cyanosis. Skin color should be consistent with the individual's race. Cyanosis, a late sign of respiratory distress, is evident when more than 5 g of reduced hemoglobin is present per deciliter of blood. Patients who are chronically cyanotic exhibit clubbing of their distal phalanges.

Assess the rate, rhythm, and effort of breathing. Breathing is usually quiet and effortless; inspiration should be the only active phase of respiration. Respiratory rates in infants and children are highly variable, depending on age, medical history of lung disease, activity, anxiety level, and temperature. Respiratory rates are determined while the patient is at rest. Normal breaths per minute range from 30 to 60 in newborns, 20 to 40 in early childhood, and 15 to 25 during late childhood, reaching adult levels by age 15. Tachypnea is often the first sign of respiratory distress. With time, infants especially will fatigue and decrease their respiratory rates. The pattern of tachypnea followed by bradypnea with intermittent periods of apnea is a ominous sign.

Abnormal respiratory patterns are described in terms of rate, depth, and pattern (Table 8-6). Respiratory patterns vary considerably during the first year of life; that is, 1 minute the infant breathes slowly, but then the next minute, the infant breathes more rapidly. Apnea lasting greater than 15 seconds accompanied by duskiness, cyanosis, or respiratory rates greater than 60 breaths per minute is considered significant in the newborn.[21]

Normal inspiratory/expiratory (I:E) ratio is 1:2. Prolonged inspiration occurs with upper airway obstruction, whereas prolonged expiration occurs with lower airway obstruction. Inspiratory stridor may also be present with upper airways disease, whereas expiratory wheezing is present with lower airways disease. Grunting, forced expiration against a partially closed glottis accomplishes the same effect as pursed-lip breathing in older children. Both occur in an attempt to maintain FRC, thus oxygenation. When present, consider oxygen administration if not already in place.

Note the shape of the chest. Chest deformities can limit vital capacity. Scoliosis is a lateral curvature of the spine at the extreme, resulting in an S-shaped configuration. Kyphosis is an exaggeration of the normal posterior convexity of the thoracic spine. In pectus carinatum, the sternum is displaced in an anterior position; in pectus excavatum, the sternum is displaced posteriorly.

TABLE 8-6 Abnormal Respiratory Patterns

Type	Description	Potential Etiologic Conditions
Apnea	Absent	Central neurologic depression Obstructive sleep apnea
Bradypnea	Slow for age	Hypothermia Drug-induced respiratory depression Increased intracranial pressure Metabolic alkalosis (intestinal obstruction)
Dyspnea	Difficult or labored breathing	Acute distress (pneumothorax) Chronic distress (cystic fibrosis) Intermittent distress (asthma)
Hyperpnea	Deep and rapid for age	Central neurogenic hyperventilation
Kussmaul	Deep (fast or slow)	Diabetic ketoacidosis
Orthopnea	Intolerant of supine position	Asthma Pulmonary edema
Tachypnea (with respiratory distress)	Rapid for age	Pulmonary disease
Tachypnea (without respiratory distress)	Rapid for age	Nonpulmonary disease Metabolic acidosis Increased metabolic need Anxiety Severe diarrhea Salicylate toxicity Chronic renal insufficiency Inborn errors in metabolism
Apneustic	Extremely prolonged inspiratory periods	Stimulation of the apneustic center (located in the middle and lower pons) along with vagotomy
Ataxic	Unpredictable, irregular	Cerebral dysfunction at level of medulla
Central neurogenic hyperventilation	Rapid, deep	Cerebral dysfunction at midbrain level
Cheyne-Stokes	Cyclic hyperpnea-apnea pattern	Bilateral diencephalon dysfunction
Cluster	Irregular cluster	Cerebral dysfunction at the level of the pons

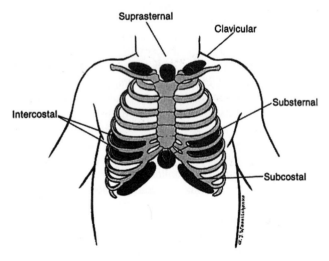

Fig. 8-20 Locations of retractions. (From Whaley LF, Wong DL: *Nursing care of infants and children,* ed 5, St Louis, 1995, Mosby, p 1340.)

Note how the chest moves. Early in infancy, diaphragmatic breathing is predominant and thoracic excursion is minimal; this reverses by 7 years of age. Diaphragmatic breathing produces a paradoxical breathing pattern: on inspiration, the lower ribs are pulled in while the abdomen is pushed out; the opposite is true on expiration. Paradoxic breathing becomes exaggerated—that is, it takes on a seesaw appearance—when pulmonary compliance is decreased. If paradoxic breathing is replaced by thoracic breathing in an infant, diaphragmatic dysfunction is suspected; if thoracic breathing is replaced by abdominal breathing in a child, parenchymal disease is suspected.

During a patient's deep breath, confirm symmetric chest excursion. Unequal chest excursion is associated with atelectasis, pneumonia, thoracic trauma, or pneumothorax.

When respirations are labored, accessory muscles are recruited to support ventilation. The sternomastoid, scaleni, pectorals, internal and external intercostals, and abdominal muscles may contract visibly. Head bobbing, or extension of the neck on inspiration, indicates the use of neck accessory muscles. Nasal flaring on inspiration is often observed with labored respirations. Suprasternal, substernal, supraclavicular, and intercostal retractions may occur (Fig. 8-20).

TABLE 8-7	Normal Breath Sounds			
Breath Sound	**I:E Ratio**	**Pitch**	**Intensity**	**Location**
Bronchial	$I \leq E$	High	Loud	Large airways
Bronchovesicular	$I = E$	Moderate	Moderate	Midairway and peripheral lung fields
Vesicular	$I > E$	Low	Soft	Peripheral lung fields

I:E, Inspiratory-to-expiratory.

Retractions of the upper chest are associated with upper airways disease, whereas retractions of the lower chest usually suggest lower airways disease. As the work of breathing increases, so do oxygen requirements. Metabolic acidosis follows respiratory acidosis when the work of breathing exceeds the ability to provide adequate tissue oxygenation.[3]

Assess for the presence of a characteristic cough: for example, gradual or sudden onset, productive or nonproductive, dry or congested, associated with decreased or increased activity, able or unable to sleep, and associated with a febrile or afebrile state. A barking or croupy cough is present with laryngotracheobronchitis or epiglottitis. A progressive cough—that is, from dry to wet—is characteristic of congestive heart failure. Coughs caused by bronchitis or pneumonia are congested. If a cough is productive, the sputum is described in terms of color, consistency, and odor. The significance of sputum color is as follows: white or clear with bronchitis or viral infections; yellow or green with bacterial infections; pink or frothy with pulmonary edema; and rust color with tuberculosis.

Palpation and Percussion. The entire chest wall is palpated for tactile fremitus, that is, palpable vibrations transmitted from the lung to the chest wall when the patient speaks or cries. Fremitus should be symmetric. Increased transmission is noted over areas of consolidation, for example, pneumonia or atelectasis. Decreased or absent transmission is noted over areas of decreased airflow, for example, in asthma, pneumothorax, or pleural effusion.

Percussion helps to determine whether the underlying tissue is air filled, fluid filled, or solid. The infant's round chest normally produces a hyperresonant pitch. A resonant pitch, indicating healthy lung, is present by age 6. After age 6, hyperresonance may indicate the pathologic presence of air, for example, with a pneumothorax. A resonant pitch before 6 years of age or a dull pitch thereafter indicates consolidation, for example, atelectasis, pneumonia, or pleural effusion.

Crepitus, or subcutaneous emphysema, occurs when free air enters subcutaneous tissue. When palpated, crepitus feels crunchy, creating a crackling sensation over the skin surface. Subcutaneous air may follow tracheotomy or any disruption in the larynx or trachea. Crepitus may also occur after a thoracentesis around the wound site or dissect large surface areas, as in patients with severe air-leak syndrome. Crepitus is usually self-limiting and does not require treatment; resolution occurs by reabsorption after resolution of the primary problem. On rare occasions, tracheal compression may require surgical intervention.

Auscultation. Three types of breath sounds can be auscultated in infants and children: bronchial, bronchovesicular, and vesicular (Table 8-7). Symmetry, comparing right and left sides, allows patients to serve as their own control. Progressing systematically from top to bottom, assess the pitch, intensity, and duration of each breath sound. Assess for (1) the presence and location of normal breath sounds, (2) the presence of normal breath sounds heard over abnormal locations, and (3) the presence of adventitious breath sounds.

Breath sounds are usually louder in infants and young children because the thinner chest wall brings the stethoscope closer to the origin of the sounds. Bronchovesicular sounds are usually auscultated throughout the lung periphery. Although seldom heard in infants, displaced bronchial breath sounds may indicate consolidation. Because breath sounds are easily transmitted throughout the small thoracic cavity, referred breath sounds are prevalent in infants and young children. Even when a significant pneumothorax is present, breath sounds can be auscultated over collapsed areas. Decreased breath sounds do occur in older children with obstructed bronchi, hyperinflated lungs, pneumothorax, or pleural effusion.

Three types of adventitious breath sounds can be identified: crackles, wheezes, and pleural rubs.[22] Crackles are discrete, noncontinuous sounds that can be simulated by rolling a lock of hair between the fingers near an ear. End-inspiratory crackles (previously termed *crepitant rales*) result from the reopening of previously collapsed alveoli, for example, during pneumonia and congestive heart failure. Early inspiratory crackles (previously termed *rhonchi*) may be heard in the airway of patients with obstructive airways disease. Loud inspiratory and expiratory crackles may be heard with bronchiectasis.

Wheezes are musical sounds produced by the rapid passage of air through narrowed airways. Wheezing occurs more commonly in infants because of the size of their airways. Although wheezes are typically expiratory, they may be heard on both inspiration and expiration. During normal spontaneous ventilation, intrathoracic airways widen during inspiration and narrow on exhalation, whereas the opposite is true of extrathoracic airways. Because maximum resistance to airflow occurs during expiration in intrathoracic airways and during inspiration in extrathoracic airways, expiratory wheezes usually indicate lower airway problems, and inspiratory wheezes usually indicate upper airway problems. The disappearance of wheezing in a severe asthmatic may be disconcerting because it may indicate that the patient is no longer moving air through narrowed airways.

Pleural rubs result from the friction generated by the movement of inflamed pleural surfaces over one another. Pleural rubs are usually painful, loud yet low pitched, synchronous with respiration, and confined to a small surface area.

When assessing adventitious sounds, the location and timing—that is, when in the respiratory cycle they are auscultated—are noted.

Assessment of the Intubated Infant or Child

When caring for an infant or child with an endotracheal tube (ETT), assessment priorities include patient safety and comfort. Assess the security of the ETT, and ensure that the tape securing the ETT is adherent to the skin *and* ETT. Compare the ETT exit markings at the lip or naris line with those noted immediately after intubation or after the ETT was last repositioned. Assess for the potential of ETT-induced pressure necrosis to the naris or corner of the mouth. If present, reposition and retape the ETT as soon as possible.

Once ETT security has been addressed, determine whether the ETT itself is causing respiratory distress. Inadequate ETT size will precipitate signs and symptoms of upper airway obstruction. Determine whether excessive ETT length may contribute dead space. If the patient is hypercapnic, consider shortening the ETT to a reasonable length (approximately 5 mm) after confirming correct ETT placement on chest x-ray film with the patient's head in neutral position.

Assess the comfort level of the infant or child. Provide a level of sedation necessary to ensure airway maintenance. This is highly individual because patient tolerance may be high or extremely low. Freedom sleeves or limb restraints are essential to prevent unintentional extubation. Ensure that the ETT and tubing are supported to allow head movements but prevent accidental extubation, especially in the active infant and child. Drain oxygen delivery tubing of condensation on a regular basis to prevent inadvertent water entry into the patient's airway and unnecessary weight on the patient's ETT. All equipment necessary to reintubate the individual infant or child, as well as an emergency tracheostomy tray, should be readily available in the unit.

Patients with oral and nasal ETTs are assessed in a similar manner. Awake children with oral ETTs may require a bite block to prevent biting down on the ETT. Children with an altered level of consciousness and oral ETT may require an oral airway. In addition, nasal ETTs can obstruct eustachian tubes, which empty into the nasopharynx. There should be a high index of suspicion for middle ear infections and sinusitis whenever caring for patients with nasal ETTs.

In general, intubated patients should be positioned with their head of the bed elevated to decrease the incidence of nosocomial pneumonia. Although similar pediatric data do not exist, the supine body position is a well-established risk

factor for nosocomial pneumonia in adult patients supported on mechanical ventilation.[23] Nosocomial pneumonia results from the microaspiration of colonized oropharyngeal secretions. Factors influencing oropharyngeal colonization include enteral nutrition, antacids, and gastrointestinal reflux.

When caring for an infant or child with a new tracheostomy tube (TT), priorities again include patient safety and comfort. Tracheostomy holders are assessed for security, and the entire neck is assessed for skin breakdown under the tracheostomy holder. The character of the tracheostomy site is assessed for infection, and dressings or sponges are examined for drainage. If the patient is connected to a ventilator, potential pressure points created by the TT adapter should be cushioned. Finally, an extra same-size tracheostomy tube should be positioned in clear view at the bedside in case of an emergency.

Intubated patients require instruction on how best to establish and maintain communication with family and caregivers. The inability to communicate, no matter how temporary, has been consistently identified as a major source of ICU-related stress. Costello[24] reviewed current options to establish and maintain communication in cognitively appropriate pediatric ICU patients. These interventions include the use of an unaided yes/no response, picture and alphabet boards for pointing, magic slates or felt-tip pens for writing, and small typing and communication systems using prerecorded voice for pressing. Whichever system is used, it seems reasonable to prepare the patient (if possible) for the loss of voice and offer a range of options that would be reasonable in the sedated intubated pediatric patient.

Assessment of the Ventilated Infant or Child

Assessment of the infant or child supported on mechanical ventilation includes (1) assessing patient-ventilator synchrony, (2) validating the ventilator settings and alarm systems, and (3) assessing for the presence of air leaks around uncuffed endotracheal or tracheostomy tubes.

Start by assessing the patient's level of comfort. Does the infant or child appear anxious? Is chest expansion adequate during a delivered breath? Is the I:E ratio normal? Is the inspiratory time too short? Does the patient have enough time to exhale before receiving another breath? Is the patient able to generate a sufficient number of adequate spontaneous breaths? Is the patient tachypneic?

Next check the ventilator settings to ensure that the patient is supported on the intended settings. Ensure that alarm settings are activated and are within a tight range to call immediate attention to problems.

Assess for the presence of an air leak on end inspiration. Air leaks are not uncommon in infants or children with uncuffed ETTs, especially when pulmonary compliance is low. Air leaks should be quantified. When measured tidal volumes are significantly compromised, air leaks can be addressed by ventilator or patient manipulations. Ventilator manipulations include those that result in increasing the delivered tidal volume to compensate for the air leak. Patient manipulations range from simply changing head position to reintubating the patient with a larger ETT or TT.

If a cuffed ETT or TT is in place and delivered tidal volumes are compromised, consider inflating the cuff with just enough volume to eliminate the air leak. This *minimal occlusion volume* (MOV) technique is accomplished by placing a stethoscope over the larynx and slowly inflating the cuff until sounds cease over the larynx. Once the air leak is eliminated, cuff pressures are obtained to ensure that the cuff pressure is less than 20 mmHg. Most tubes will seal at pressures between 14 and 20 mmHg. The amount of pressure and volume to obtain a seal and prevent mucosal pressure depends on tube size and design, cuff configuration, mode of ventilation, and the individual's airway and arterial pressure. Mucosal ischemia occurs when lateral wall pressure exceeds capillary perfusion pressure, resulting in decreasing mucosal blood flow.[25] Iatrogenic complications from cuff inflation include tracheal stenosis, necrosis, tracheoesophageal fistula, and tracheomalacia.

If cuff total occlusion is unnecessary, consider the *minimal leak volume* (MLV) technique. Here a stethoscope is again placed over the larynx. The cuff is inflated then slowly deflated until a small air leak is heard at end inspiration. Check to ensure that the air leak is occurring at less than 20 mmHg inflating pressure or directly measure the cuff pressure.

When patients are chemically paralyzed, assessments include the adequacy of the paralysis. This may be assessed by one of two methods: "daily honeymoon" or train-of-four monitoring. With a "daily honeymoon" technique, continuously administered neuromuscular blockade is temporary discontinued until the patient is observed to move. Initial movements often include abdominal fasciculations. Train-of-four monitoring is used when spontaneous breathing would potentially cause the patient harm, for example, when the patient is receiving maximal ventilatory support and patient effort/asynchrony would cause barotrauma or desaturation. In train-of-four monitoring, two electrodes are placed in line along the distal ulna and then connected to a nerve stimulator that delivers four electrical stimuli at preset intervals.[26] Ordinarily, stimulation of the ulnar nerve produces four serial thumb adductions (Fig. 8-21). With neuromuscular blockade (induced by nondepolarization agents), this response fades; that is, each successive twitch becomes weaker. As blockade increases, the last twitch is obliterated, then the third, and so on. When train-of-four

TOF Suppression and Degree of Neuromuscular Blockade

TOF Suppression					Approximate Percentage of Block
Four responses					0–75
Three responses					75–80
Two responses					80–90
One response					90
No response					100

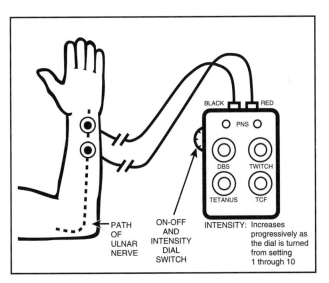

Clinically Relevant Levels of Neuromuscular Blockade

Percentage of Blockade	Clinical Interpretation
90–95	Conditions may be suitable for endotracheal intubation and long-term mechanical ventilation
80–90	Block may be adequate for short-term relaxation and long-term mechanical ventilation
75	Maintenance doses may be needed to extend duration of relaxation
≤75	Patient may be susceptible to rapid reversal with cholinesterase antagonists
<75	Patient's spontaneous recovery is probably satisfactory

Fig. 8-21 Train-of-four (TOF) monitoring.

TABLE 8-8   Assessment of the Ventilated Patient

Primary Survey

General Appearance
Skin color
Airway—endotracheal tube size, cuffed or uncuffed, amount
   of dead space
Spontaneous respiratory effort
Respiratory excursion—ventilator and spontaneous breaths
Abdominal distension
Level of responsiveness or comfort
Muscle tone
Respiratory rate
   Ventilator + spontaneous = total
 	
Presence of subcutaneous air
	Breath sounds
	Equality
	Normal and adventitious
	Quality of spontaneous and ventilator breaths
	
	Air leak
	   Endotracheal tube
	   Chest tubes
	Noninvasive gas monitoring
	   Spo_2, $ETco_2$, tidal volume

Secondary Survey

Ventilator settings and safety check
Blood studies
   Arterial blood gases
   Hemoglobin
	Chest x-ray films
	Hemodynamic and oxygenation profiles

stimulation elicits only one twitch, spontaneous respirations are suppressed. Continuous infusion rates are titrated or additional boluses of chemical muscle relaxants are administered to maintain a single twitch in the train-of-four response. Table 8-8 provides a summary of the primary and secondary assessment parameters for the ventilated infant or child.

NONINVASIVE PULMONARY INTENSIVE CARE MONITORING

With the recognition of technical difficulties and associated risks of invasive pediatric monitoring, an explosion in the use noninvasive monitoring techniques has occurred. As alternative monitoring techniques become available in the pediatric population, it is essential that they be valid and reliable. Pediatric monitors must not only accommodate the wide range of sizes but also be sensitive enough to detect both the rapid and small quantitative physiologic changes that often hallmark states of pediatric crisis. Low arterial pressures, cardiac outputs, and oxygen reserves matched with high oxygen requirements offer little buffer and require rapid detection.

Effective clinical use of any technology requires an understanding of what is actually measured, how it is measured, and the patient care requirements for applying that technology. This section focuses on these issues as they relate to noninvasive monitoring of pulmonary function.

Pulse Oximetry

Continuous monitoring of oxygen saturation has made a significant impact on patient assessment. Unlike measuring ABGs, pulse oximetry provides *continuous* arterial hemo-

globin saturation (Spo_2) data and almost immediate detection of hypoxemic events.

Because oxygen is primarily transported in blood chemically attached to hemoglobin, Spo_2 monitoring provides a more complete picture of the patient's oxygenation status. Saturation monitoring also provides a more reliable indicator of hypoxemia during extreme shifts of the ODC: inadequate oxygenation despite a Pao_2 greater than 50 mmHg during a shift of the ODC to the right or adequate oxygenation despite a Pao_2 less than 50 mmHg during a shift of the ODC to the left. In the upper part of the ODC, small changes in Sao_2 correspond to very large and potentially toxic levels of Pao_2. Bucher and co-workers[27] reported that when Spo_2 was maintained at less than 96%, the Pao_2 was never higher than 100 mmHg. The researchers proposed that maintaining the patient's Spo_2 around 96% would prevent hyperoxia. Manufacturers claim an error factor of less than 3% at a Spo_2 greater than 70%.

Mechanism of Measurement. Pulse oximeters measure the absorption of two wavelengths of light passed through pulsating tissue (Fig. 8-22). Oxyhemoglobin and reduced hemoglobin absorb varying degrees of light. For a given site, the light absorption of bone, tissue, venous blood, and arterial blood remains constant except for the absorption from the added blood volume associated with arterial pulsation. The varying absorption is translated into two waveforms, and the ratio between the amplitude of these waveforms is used to calculate the Spo_2.

Pulse oximeters update Spo_2 with each heartbeat. They provide accurate data to heart rates of 250 beats/min. A high correlation between heart rates obtained from a cardiac monitor and Spo_2 monitor helps to establish the reliability of Spo_2 data. Qualitative analysis of perfusion is also available by assessment of the perfusion bar, which pulsates with each

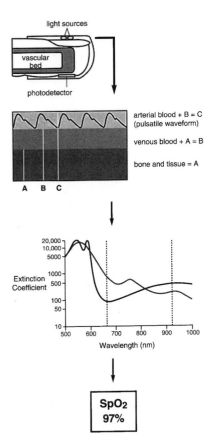

Fig. 8-22 Pulse oximeters measure absorption of two wavelengths of light passed through pulsating tissue. Oxyhemoglobin and reduced hemoglobin absorb varying degrees of light. For a given site, light absorption of bone, tissue, venous blood, and arterial blood remains constant except for absorption from the added blood volume associated with arterial pulsation. Varying absorption is translated into two waveforms, and the ratio between the amplitude of these waveforms is used to calculate Spo_2. (Reprinted by permission of Nellcor Puritan Bennett, Pleasanton, Calif.)

heartbeat. An audible tone varies in pitch according to saturation. This feature is very important during procedures that may affect Sao_2; attention can be paid to the procedure while listening for changes in the tone of the pulse oximeter, indicating changes in saturation.

Sensors contain three optical components: two light sources (red and infrared) and one light receiver. To function properly, the sensor must be positioned so that the light source and photodetector oppose one another (see Fig. 8-22). Sensors are available in various shapes and sizes to facilitate monitoring at different locations and with varying patient sizes. If the patient is sensitive to adhesive, it can be removed with adhesive remover. The sensor is then attached using a gauze dressing. All sensor sites are assessed frequently for skin abrasion and circulatory impairment. Pressure necrosis may occur when a sensor is placed too tightly or for prolonged period.

To enhance performance, the appropriate probe for the size of infant should be used. In infants with right-to-left shunting, the right hand is used for preductal Spo_2, and the left hand or either foot is used for postductal Spo_2.

Troubleshooting. Interference with Spo_2 readings typically result from problems related to the signal-to-noise ratio. Too little signal may result from poor perfusion or improper probe placement; too much noise may result from excessive motion, ambient light, electrocautery, or a venous pressure wave.

Sensors incorporate ambient light protection, but strong light sources—for example, fluorescent, procedural, and bilirubin lights—may interfere with Spo_2 measurement. Problems with ambient light are easily resolved by covering the sensors with a blanket. Patient motion may also affect system performance. Occasionally, a large dicrotic notch may be sensed as a separate arterial pulse, resulting in twice the actual heart rate. Any event that significantly reduces arterial pulsation will affect Spo_2 readings. Although accurate to extremely low mean arterial pressures, pulsations may be lost with severe hypotension, with low cardiac output states, or in patients receiving venoarterial extracorporeal membrane oxygenation. Oximetry may also fail in patients with severe anemia or hemodilution, for example, when the hemoglobin is less than 5 g/dl. High bilirubin levels do not affect Spo_2 readings. To help eliminate this problem, newer pulse oximetry models have incorporated an algorithm to help identify motion and poor perfusion artifact.[28]

Significant venous pulsations can also lead to inaccurate low Spo_2 readings. This occurs when a sensor is wrapped too tightly; when the sensor is placed on a dependent limb; or during decreased venous return states, such as increased intrathoracic pressure or congestive heart failure or during a Valsalva maneuver. Falsely low readings can also occur if the finger probe is malpositioned beyond the fingertip.[29]

Because of the different ways saturation is measured, pulse oximetry data cannot be validated by other saturation measures. Pulse oximeters are calibrated to read functional hemoglobin or the percentage of hemoglobin available to bind with oxygen. Saturation readings obtained with ABG reports are calculated from Pao_2 values and thus may be invalid because of shifts in the ODC. Specific requests for a measured Sao_2 with a co-oximeter in the laboratory will provide fractional Sao_2 readings, for example, carboxyhemoglobin and methemoglobin. All carboxyhemoglobin will be counted as oxyhemoglobin by the pulse oximeter, so the Spo_2 may be misleadingly normal in carbon monoxide poisoning. When methemoglobin levels are less than 20%, the pulse oximeter will add half the actual percent to the Spo_2 reading. When methemoglobin levels are greater than 20%, the pulse oximeter will always read 85%. The impact of methemoglobin levels on pulse oximeter values is important when medications that increase these levels are prescribed (dapsone and nitric oxide). Lastly, when high concentrations of fetal hemoglobin are present, because of absorption differences, the laboratory co-oximeter reports erroneously high carboxyhemoglobin and low oxyhemoglobin fractions.

Clinical Applications. Saturation monitoring is considered a standard in most pediatric ICUs. Spo_2 readings are particularly helpful as a continuous monitor of intrapulmonary shunt ($\dot{Q}s/\dot{Q}t$) and during pulmonary care and titration

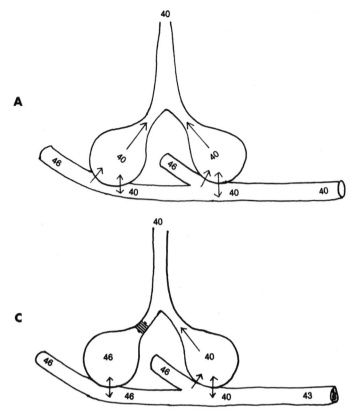

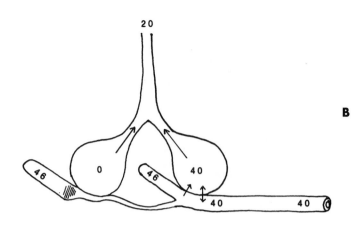

Fig. 8-23 **A,** Normal $\dot{V}/\dot{Q}$ ratio. **B,** Dead space units—high $\dot{V}/\dot{Q}$ ratio. **C,** Shunt units—low $\dot{V}/\dot{Q}$ ratio. (From Swedlow DB: Capnometry and capnography: the anesthesia disaster early warning system, *Semin Anesthesia* V[3]:194-205, 1986.)

of oxygen therapy. Continuous monitoring of Spo_2 levels during ventilator weaning eliminates the need for repeated blood gases.

End-Tidal CO₂ Monitoring

Until recently, the only method to quantify the adequacy of ventilation was through assessment of ABGs. End-tidal CO_2 monitoring provides a noninvasive, continuous real-time measurement of end-exhaled CO_2 gases. Normally, if ventilation and perfusion are well matched, the $ETco_2$ closely approximates the $Paco_2$ (Fig. 8-23, *A*). As illustrated, mixed venous CO_2 (blood returning from the systemic circulation) is approximately 46 mmHg. Carbon dioxide rapidly diffuses into the alveolar space until the alveolar pulmonary-capillary CO_2 and the alveolar CO_2 become equal at 40 mmHg. Thus down-line at the sampling points, arterial and $ETco_2$ should be approximately equal at 40 mmHg. In those with normal lungs, the $A\text{-}aDco_2$ gradient (difference between alveolar and arterial CO_2) is usually less that 2 to 3 mmHg with $ETco_2$ lower than arterial Pco_2. Changes in the noninvasive $ETco_2$ will continuously reflect changes in the invasive $Paco_2$ or the $A\text{-}aDco_2$ gradient.

Mechanism of Measurement. The most common device used to measure CO_2 concentration in exhaled gases is the infrared analyzer or capnometer. The analyzer makes use of the fact that gaseous CO_2 absorbs infrared light within a specific wavelength range, specifically waves about 4.3 μm in length. As this narrow band of light is projected through a gas sample, an attenuation of the light beam results, and the intensity of attenuated light is measured. The

greater the concentration of CO_2, the greater the absorption and less infrared detection by the sample detector cell.

The two basic types of sampling techniques are sidestream and mainstream. With the sidestream capnometer, the gas sample is continuously aspirated from the respiratory circuit through a small-bore tube leading to a sensing chamber within a monitor. With the mainstream capnometer, the sensor is incorporated between the ventilator circuit and an artificial airway.

An advantage to the sidestream monitor is that it can be used in the intubated or nonintubated patient. In the nonintubated patient, the aspirating tube is placed at or a few centimeters into the naris. The patient may not tolerate this technique, or the results may not be acceptable if mouth breathing is present. Also, if the monitor entrains room air, the readings will be falsely low, providing a false sense of security when alveolar hypoventilation is present. Further disadvantages to the sidestream capnometer include a total delay time,[30] a falsely low $ETco_2$ created by high aspirating flow rates, and potential for analyzer contamination if water and mucus is drawn back into the monitor. An airway adapter with water trap has been designed to address the last problem.

Mainstream capnometers require intubation and have two main advantages. First, delay time is less, and second, water or moisture is less apt to affect sensor function. Also, the mainstream capnometers have been reported to more accurately reflect $ETco_2$ data in pediatrics.[30] A disadvantage, especially in pediatrics, is that some sensors are heavy and require support to avoid tension on the ETT and the size may add excessive dead space.

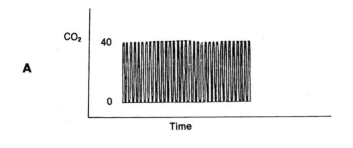

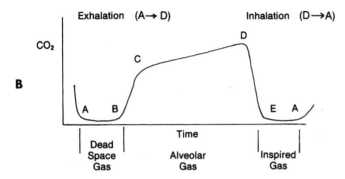

Fig. 8-24 **A,** Slow-speed capnogram recorded at 12.5 mm/sec. **B,** Fast-speed capnogram recorded at 25 mm/sec. (From Curley MA, Thompson JE: End-tidal CO_2 monitoring in critically ill infants and children, *Pediatr Nurs* 16:397, 1990.)

Capnometers used in the pediatric population must be able to rapidly respond to changes in CO_2, respond to the small exhaled volumes, and be sensitive to track small changes in CO_2.

Clinical Applications. Capnography is the recording and analysis of waveforms produced by changes in the level of exhaled CO_2. Capnograms can be recorded at a slow (12.5 mm/sec) or fast (25 mm/sec) speed (Fig. 8-24). The vertical axis represents CO_2 concentration, whereas the horizontal axis represents time. Slow recordings are suitable for trending baseline and $ETco_2$ levels. Fast recordings allow individual waveform analysis. Any factor that alters CO_2 production, CO_2 transport to the lungs, alveolar ventilation, $\dot{V}/\dot{Q}$ ratio, and CO_2 transport to the sampling site will affect the $ETco_2$.

Capnogram Analysis: Slow Speed. Changes in CO_2 production are usually matched by changes in minute ventilation, so $ETco_2$ levels should remain constant. In those unable to alter their tidal volumes or respiratory rates sufficiently, increased production will be manifested by increased $ETco_2$ whereas decreased production will be manifested by decreased $ETco_2$. Fever, pain, stress, increased muscle activity (seizures and shivering), sodium bicarbonate infusion, increased carbohydrate intake, malignant hyperthermia, and hyperthyroidism all increase CO_2 production. Hypothermia and increased fat intake decrease CO_2 production.

As discussed, alveoli can only eliminate CO_2 that is presented by the pulmonary capillary membrane, so changes

in lung perfusion will be reflected in the capnogram (see Fig. 8-23, *B*). The $ETco_2$ will fall in shock states, when excessive positive end-expiratory pressure (PEEP) is used, or in those with a pulmonary embolus. These states are characterized by a high ventilation/perfusion ($\dot{V}/\dot{Q}$) ratio or dead space units (see previous discussion). The A-aDco_2 gradient can be followed to detect insidious shock and evaluate response to treatment.

During a cardiac arrest, the $ETco_2$ acutely disappears, reappearing only when circulation is restored by effective cardiac resuscitation. The extent to which advanced life support measures maintain cardiac output can be rapidly assessed by $ETco_2$ monitoring (Fig. 8-25, *A*).

With alveolar hypoventilation, the arterial and $ETco_2$ both increase. Hypoventilation may occur in those with central nervous system depression, with neuromuscular disease, and in the chemically paralyzed patient with inadequate ventilator parameters.

When hypoventilation is severe (where air only in the conducting airways is moved), the $ETco_2$ will decrease. With apnea, the $ETco_2$ disappears completely because CO_2 is no longer transported from the lungs to the gas-sampling point (see Fig. 8-25, *B*). Capnography is thus a good apnea alarm because periods of apnea can be confirmed, timed, and documented. The $ETco_2$ reappears after ventilation is restored and usually overshoots previous readings.

Alveolar hyperventilation decreases $ETco_2$ and arterial CO_2. An important application of $ETco_2$ monitoring is in the cerebral hypertensive patient in whom CO_2 retention produces pronounced cerebral vasodilation and further compromises intracranial pressure.

The pathophysiologic effects of shunting, characterized by a low $\dot{V}/\dot{Q}$ ratio, are seen in many pulmonary disease states (see Fig. 8-23, *C*). In shunt units, those that are perfused but not ventilated, mixed venous CO_2 is approximately 46 mmHg. The alveolar CO_2 is 40 mmHg in the ventilated unit, as is the pulmonary vein draining that unit. The alveolar CO_2 in the unventilated unit is 46 mmHg because it is in equilibrium with its pulmonary capillary membrane. Down-line, the arterial CO_2 is an average of all the lung units perfused ($46 + 40/2 = 43$ mmHg), and $ETco_2$ is an average of all units ventilated ($40/1 = 40$ mmHg). Thus with a 50% shunt, the A-aDco_2 will be only 3 mmHg. An undramatic A-aDco_2 gradient but a dramatic decrease in arterial saturation characterizes shunt units.

$ETco_2$ monitoring of unstable, intubated, chemically paralyzed patients helps to reduce iatrogenic injury.[31] $ETco_2$ monitoring helps to determine correct ETT placement because little or no CO_2 reading can be gained from the esophagus. $ETco_2$ monitoring also allows rapid detection of ETT displacement (see Fig. 8-25, *C*).

$ETco_2$ monitoring can be an effective, noninvasive way to monitor alveolar ventilation in patients who are being weaned from mechanical ventilation. Ventilator rates can be gradually decreased to the lowest point at which the patient can comfortably maintain effective alveolar ventilation. If the $ETco_2$ rises or if the patient appears to be working too hard, as evidenced by rapid spontaneous respiratory rates,

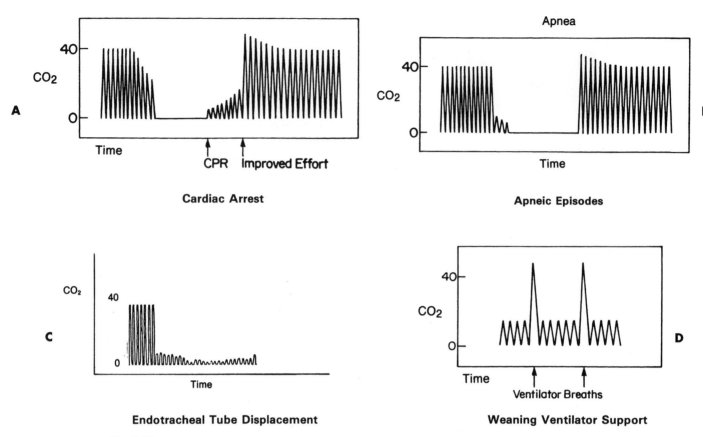

Fig. 8-25 Slow-speed capnograms. **A,** Cardiac arrest. Decreased perfusion to the pulmonary vascular bed will gradually decrease the $ETco_2$. **B,** Apneic episodes. $ETco_2$ disappears during apneic episodes, then overshoots previous readings. **C,** Endotracheal tube (ETT) displacement. $ETco_2$ will fall to zero when ETT is displaced. **D,** Weaning ventilator support. Note that $ETco_2$ is lower during spontaneous breaths than during ventilator breaths. (From Curley MA, Thompson JE: End-tidal CO_2 monitoring in critically ill infants and children, *Pediatr Nurs* 16:397, 1990.)

ventilator rates can be returned to previously acceptable settings.

In patients with chronic pulmonary disease, the $ETco_2$ of spontaneous breaths may be much lower than the $ETco_2$ of larger ventilator-initiated breaths (see Fig. 8-25, *D*). Generally, stability of the $ETco_2$ during spontaneous and ventilator breaths indicates the patient's readiness for weaning ventilator breaths. Use of this assessment parameter is especially helpful in weaning patients when there is uncertainty as to whether they can physiologically resume the work of breathing. Noninvasive gas monitoring is less traumatic for the patient in relation to the pain and anxiety of ABGs.

Capnogram Analysis: Fast Speed. The normal capnogram, recorded at a fast speed, is illustrated in Fig. 8-24, *B.* At the beginning of exhalation, the CO_2 concentration is zero as primarily dead space of the conducting airways empties of its CO_2-free gas *(A-B)*. As exhalation continues, there is a steep rise in CO_2 tension when dead space gas mixes with CO_2-rich alveolar gas *(B-C)*. Levels quickly reach a near-constant horizontal plateau representing CO_2-rich alveolar gas that has been in equilibrium with the pulmonary capillary membrane *(C-D)*. The end point of this segment, the highest value of CO_2 concentration at the end

of normal exhalation in the upper right corner of the waveform, is the $ETco_2$ *(D)*. Immediately following $ETco_2$, the CO_2 concentration falls, indicating dilution of CO_2-rich gas with CO_2-free inspired gas *(D-E)*. Finally, only inspired gas is present at the gas-sampling port, producing the inspiratory baseline. Capnographic characteristics vary and can be diagnostic of certain disease states.

First assess the baseline CO_2 level. Baseline CO_2 should be zero because it primarily represents previously inspired dead space, CO_2-free gas. Any increase in baseline indicates that rebreathing is occurring (Fig. 8-26, *A*).

Next assess the slope where dead space gas mixes with CO_2-rich alveolar gas. The slope should be nearly vertical to the plateau phase. Occasionally, the slope is significant to the point at which the plateau disappears (see Fig. 8-26, *B*). This is caused by lung units emptying at different rates, prolonged exhalation secondary to small airway obstruction (asthma) or a partially kinked ETT. A good alveolar plateau ensures that the $ETco_2$ is a reliable estimate of mixed alveolar gas.

Capnograms can be useful in assessing the effectiveness of bronchodilator treatments in the asthmatic patient or racemic epinephrine treatments in the patient with laryngotracheobronchitis. A decrease in the slope, less peaking of

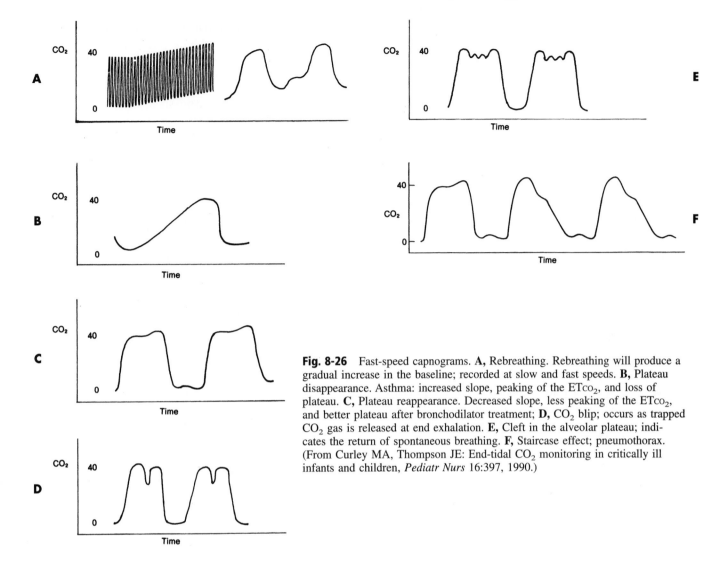

Fig. 8-26 Fast-speed capnograms. **A,** Rebreathing. Rebreathing will produce a gradual increase in the baseline; recorded at slow and fast speeds. **B,** Plateau disappearance. Asthma: increased slope, peaking of the $ETco_2$, and loss of plateau. **C,** Plateau reappearance. Decreased slope, less peaking of the $ETco_2$, and better plateau after bronchodilator treatment; **D,** CO_2 blip; occurs as trapped CO_2 gas is released at end exhalation. **E,** Cleft in the alveolar plateau; indicates the return of spontaneous breathing. **F,** Staircase effect; pneumothorax. (From Curley MA, Thompson JE: End-tidal CO_2 monitoring in critically ill infants and children, *Pediatr Nurs* 16:397, 1990.)

the $ETco_2$, and an increase in plateauing all correlate with a positive response to treatment in the patient with severe obstruction (see Fig. 8-26, *C*).

With atelectasis, a CO_2 blip followed by a sharp terminal rise in $ETco_2$ appears as trapped air at end exhalation is released (see Fig. 8-26, *D*). These blips and peaks can be smoothed out when adequate PEEP is applied. Capnography provides rapid feedback on the effects of changing ventilator settings that control minute ventilation, tidal volume, and respiratory rates. The necessity for frequent ABGs can be avoided.

Partial neuromuscular blockade or return of voluntary function is first seen in capnograms as a cleft in the alveolar plateau (see Fig. 8-26, *E*). This is caused by the rush of CO_2-free gas as the diaphragm contracts. Capnograms can provide early information that more chemical-paralyzing agent is needed.

Descending limb analysis also provides information. A staircase effect on the descending limb is seen when a pneumothorax is present (see Fig. 8-26, *F*). When chest tubes are in place, a staircase effect may indicate chest tube obstruction.

$ETco_2$ monitoring provides a continuous real-time monitor, thus closer surveillance of the adequacy of ventilation. $ETco_2$ does not completely replace ABGs because the $ETco_2$ measure is not the same as the $Paco_2$ in many clinical situations. $ETco_2$ monitoring also provides information that is not derivable from ABGs alone. The A-aDco_2 gradient can render a $ETco_2$ useful rather than being a limitation. Presence of an appreciable gradient indicates a serious $\dot{V}/\dot{Q}$ disturbance, whereas closure of the gradient indicates effective treatment or improvement of lung disease. Capnography provides a useful adjunct to the more frequently used methods of respiratory system assessment and provides early detection of potentially dangerous trends that can be reversed before crises result.

Pedi-CAP. Pedi-CAP (Nellcor, Hayward, Calif.) is a disposable pediatric end-tidal CO_2 detector that is useful when correct ETT position is in question.[32] Specifically, when attached to an ETT, the nontoxic indicator located within the cap responds to exhaled CO_2 by changing color from purple to yellow. The pediatric size limits dead space to 3 ml and is recommended for patients weighing 1 to 15 kg.

Single-Breath CO_2 Monitoring

Single-breath CO_2 ($SBco_2$) monitoring integrates $ETco_2$ and V_T measurement. $SBco_2$ allows the accurate measurement of airway and alveolar dead space and CO_2 production. The V_D/V_T ratio is used to assess minute ventilation and wasted ventilation. CO_2 production is used to evaluate changes in metabolism and CO_2 elimination. $SBco_2$ analysis offers the precision to differentiate the alveolar dead space from airway dead space; quantification of alveolar dead space may be directly related to effective pulmonary perfusion.[33,34]

INVASIVE PULMONARY INTENSIVE CARE MONITORING

Critically ill patients require rapid titration of therapy based on astute and accurate assessments of hemodynamic and oxygenation data. The instruments that provide data have evolved significantly in recent years. What has also developed is how we use hemodynamic and oxygenation profile data to optimize care. For example, the cardiovascular and respiratory systems are interrelated. Alterations in one system often elicit a change in the other. Achieving and maintaining optimal functioning of both systems are fundamental objectives in critical care. This section reviews invasive monitoring of cardiopulmonary function in critically ill pediatric patients, including the clinical significance of direct and derived data and the importance of trending the determinates of $\dot{D}o_2$ and O_2 use.

Blood Gas Analysis

Blood gases are analyzed for two major reasons: (1) to directly assess the patient's oxygenation and ventilation status and (2) to provide information regarding the patient's acid-base status. Blood gas analysis can be performed using arterial, venous, or capillary blood. *Arterial blood gas* (ABG) analysis provides primary information about the adequacy of the lungs to oxygenate blood. *Venous blood gas* (VBG) analysis provides indirect information regarding tissue perfusion and $\dot{V}o_2$. *Capillary blood gas* (CBG) analysis provides limited information that can be trended over time when arterial and venous blood gases are unavailable.

Limitations associated with blood gas analysis include the procedure. Unless vascular access is available, a painful and perhaps time-consuming procedure is performed. Blood gases are expensive, require the removal of oxygen-carrying cells from the patient, and provide only intermittent data. Blood gases are also not infallible. They can be altered by the amount of air left in the syringe, the amount of heparin in the syringe, the amount of time the specimen sits before analysis, and hyperventilation or breath holding if the patient cries during the procedure.[35]

Arterial Blood Gases.   ABGs are obtained through an existing arterial line or by arterial puncture. The sites most commonly used for arterial puncture include the radial, dorsalis pedis, posterior tibial, and femoral arteries. The femoral artery is the last choice because hemorrhage and hematomas are difficult to control in this area and because of the high potential for limb ischemia if artery damage occurs.

To perform an arterial puncture, a setup typically consisting of a 23- or 25-gauge butterfly needle attached to a 1- to 3-ml heparinized syringe is prepared. Preheparinized syringes are now available and should be used to save pharmacy expense, by avoiding the waste of discarding partially used vials of heparin (1 : 1000 U/ml concentration); nursing expense, in the time it takes to prepare a heparinized syringe; and laboratory expense, in having to repeat an ABG with an erroneously low pH linked to having too much heparin in the syringe.

Before attempting arterial puncture, the adequacy of collateral circulation is assessed. The Allen test is used to assess the adequacy of ulnar collateral flow when the radial artery is considered for arterial puncture. Here the hand is elevated above the heart, and while compressing both ulnar and radial arteries, the hand is passively opened and closed. When the hand appears pale, ulnar compression is released while radial compression is maintained. If the hand flushes or if the pulse oximeter Spo_2 on any of the fingers of the hand returns to normal, ulnar competency is considered adequate. A similar evaluation of the foot is accomplished before dorsalis pedis puncture. The dorsalis pedis is compressed, and the big toe is blanched by compressing the toenail. Collateral flow is considered adequate if the toenail flushes when pressure is released.

Under controlled circumstances, EMLA cream should be used to ease the patient's discomfort. The pain and anxiety associated with arterial puncture will alter the infant's or child's breathing pattern and obscure results. After removing all air from the syringe and capping it with an occlusive barrier, ABGs are immediately sent to the laboratory on ice. Excessive air will distort the gas results, and ice will slow metabolism in the blood sample. Apply firm pressure to the puncture site for 5 minutes or until bleeding stops. Once bleeding stops, apply a pressure dressing. Because of patient discomfort and the potential for vasospasm, hematoma formation, and neurovascular compromise, arterial cannulation should be performed if frequent sampling is required to manage the patient's condition.

Venous Blood Gases.   To obtain a representation of systemic perfusion and $\dot{V}o_2$, a true mixed venous blood sample is obtained from the distal port of a pulmonary artery catheter. Venous blood gases obtained from more peripheral sites vary considerably, depending on the $\dot{V}o_2$ of nearby organ systems. This is especially true during shock or septic states. When obtaining a mixed venous sample, the mixed flush/blood discard and blood specimen is drawn slowly over 2 minutes from the distal port of a pulmonary artery catheter. This time frame is necessary to prevent "arterialization" of the specimen (i.e., pulling blood over the alveolar pulmonary-capillary membrane) that would produce erroneously high mixed venous oxygenation data. The $P\bar{v}co_2$ should always be higher than a simultaneous drawn $Paco_2$; if not, the mixed venous specimen is probably arterialized. After drawing the mixed venous sample, care is taken to adequately flush the lumen to prevent clot formation, especially in the smaller PA catheters.

Capillary Blood Gases. If peripheral perfusion is adequate, CBG data will correlate with arterial pH, $Paco_2$, and HCO_3. Because adequate peripheral perfusion is necessary for arterial correlation, capillary blood gases are usually not an option in critical care. To maximize CBG-ABG correlation, an "arterialized" CBG is obtained. This is accomplished by collecting a free-flowing blood specimen from a site that had been wrapped in a warm (45° C) wet cloth for 5 to 7 minutes. Skin-puncturing devices designed for blood glucose monitoring can be used for CBGs. CBGs are usually drawn from the medial or lateral surface of the heel in infants or from one of the digits in older infants and children.

Interpretation. Blood gas analyses typically report the pH, Po_2, Pco_2, So_2, HCO_3, and base excess (BE)/base deficit (BD). Normal ranges are noted in Table 8-9. According to Dalton's law of partial pressures, the total pressure of a group of gases is equal to the sum of the partial pressures of the individual gases in a mixture. When oxygen and carbon dioxide dissolve in blood, they exert a pressure. The Po_2 and Pco_2 reflect the partial pressures of dissolved oxygen and carbon dioxide in blood. The So_2 is the percent hemoglobin saturation with oxygen; when 100% saturated, each gram of hemoglobin carries 1.34 ml of oxygen. The Pao_2 and Sao_2 reflect the adequacy of oxygenation, whereas the $Paco_2$ reflects the adequacy of ventilation.

The $Paco_2$ level can only be influenced by pulmonary function. Two abnormal conditions are associated with changes in $Paco_2$: respiratory acidosis and respiratory alkalosis. A decreased pH and increased $Paco_2$ evidence respiratory acidosis. Respiratory acidosis is caused by decreased CO_2 elimination, that is, hypoventilation. Respiratory alkalosis is evidenced by an increased pH and decreased $Paco_2$. Respiratory alkalosis is caused by an increase in CO_2 elimination, that is, hyperventilation.

The pH is inversely proportional to H^+ concentration. As H^+ concentration increases in the blood, the pH falls; when H^+ ion concentration decreases in the blood, the pH rises. Bicarbonate (HCO_3^-) is a base that buffers H^+ concentration. The BE/BD mainly reflects an excess/deficit concentration of bicarbonate that can only be influenced by nonpulmonary function.

Donlen[36] described a three-step method that is helpful in interpreting blood gases. First, the pH is evaluated for acidosis or alkalosis. Next, analyzing HCO_3, BE/BD, and Pco_2 levels identifies the origin of the disorder. This step is followed by an assessment of compensation. See Chapter 9 for interpretation of acid-base imbalances.

Oxygenation Profile Monitoring

Invasive oxygenation profile monitoring is extremely helpful in patients with acute respiratory failure to help manage Fio_2 and mechanical ventilation. Patient management is directed toward resolution of the primary problem while titrating therapy to achieve an optimal physiologic, oxygenation, and hemodynamic state and limiting the potential for iatrogenic injury. Normal parameters may not be optimal in these patients. The most challenging aspect of care is to identify and support optimal parameters (which change almost constantly) for an individual patient. Another important factor is to trend the parameters over time and assess whether they make clinical sense and correlate with changes in the physical examination.

Monitoring Oxygen Supply and Demand. The goal in managing critically ill patients is to ensure adequate O_2 supply with respect to demand. Each phase of oxygenation is monitored: (1) gas exchange over the pulmonary capillary membrane, (2) oxygen transport in the blood, and (3) oxygen consumption. All three parameters are interrelated in that changes affecting one phase affect the others.

Gas exchange over the pulmonary capillary membrane is assessed by calculating the alveolar-arterial Po_2 difference (A-aDo_2). To obtain an A-aDo_2, the Pao_2 (obtained from an ABG report) is subtracted from the Pao_2 (calculated using the alveolar air equation: $Pao_2 = Pio_2 - Paco_2/RQ$). Normally, the A-a$Do_2$ should be less than 20 mmHg.

When mixed venous gases are available, the $\dot{Q}s/\dot{Q}t$ ratio, the ratio of shunted blood ($\dot{Q}s$) to total pulmonary blood flow ($\dot{Q}t$), is calculated using the shunt equation: $\dot{Q}s/\dot{Q}t = (Cpco_2 - Cao_2)/(Cpco_2 - C\bar{v}o_2)$, where $Cpco_2$, Cao_2, and $C\bar{v}o_2$ are the pulmonary capillary, arterial, and mixed venous oxygen contents, respectively. The alveolar air equation is used to provide data for the $Cpco_2$. The $\dot{Q}s/\dot{Q}t$ normally ranges from 3% to 7%. Shunt fractions greater than 50% are not uncommon in patients with severe ARDS.

Oxygen transport in the blood refers to the amount of arterial O_2 available for tissue use. $\dot{D}o_2$ is the amount of O_2

◆ TABLE 8-9 Normal Blood Gas Values

Parameter	Arterial	Mixed Venous	Capillary*
pH	7.35-7.45	7.31-7.41	7.35-7.45
O_2 saturation	95%-97%	60%-80%	Less than arterial
Po_2	80-100 mmHg	36-42 mmHg	Less than arterial
Pco_2	35-45 mmHg	40-50 mmHg	Same as arterial
HCO_3	22-26 mEq/L	Same as arterial	Same as arterial
Total CO_2 content	23-27 mEq/L	Same as arterial	Same as arterial
Base excess/deficit	+2 to -2	Same as arterial	Same as arterial

*Capillary Po_2 is approximately 10 mmHg less than arterial except when decreased tissue perfusion is present, that is, cardiovascular collapse or hypothermia. In these states, samples will not accurately reflect Pao_2. Total CO_2 content equals HCO_3 plus Pco_2 (0.03 to convert mmHg to mEq/L).

leaving the heart to be delivered to tissues. Oxygen delivery is calculated by $\dot{D}o_2 = Cao_2 \times CI \times 10$. Normal $\dot{D}o_2$ is 620 ± 50 ml/min/M^2.

Oxygen reserve is the amount of oxygen returned to the venous side of the circulation not used by the tissues. Oxygen reserve is calculated in a similar manner to $\dot{D}o_2$ but includes the $C\bar{v}o_2$. The oxygen reserve $= C\bar{v}o_2 \times CI \times 10$. The high oxygen reserve, more than 400 ml/min/M^2, serves as a protective mechanism to prevent tissue hypoxia during periods of hypermetabolic need.

Oxygen consumption ($\dot{V}o_2$), the total amount of oxygen consumed by the body per minute, is calculated as the difference between the $\dot{D}o_2$ and oxygen reserve; that is, $(Cao_2 - C\bar{v}o_2) \times CI \times 10$. Normal resting $\dot{V}o_2$ in infants and young children is twice that of adults; varying with age, the $\dot{V}o_2$ ranges from 120 to 200 ml/min/M^2. The higher $\dot{V}o_2$ in the younger age group (approximately 175 ml/min/M^2) is due to the additional metabolic burden of growth. "Adequate" $\dot{D}o_2$ is considered to be 4 times $\dot{V}o_2$.

The arterial-venous oxygen difference ($a\text{-}\bar{v}Do_2 = Cao_2 - C\bar{v}o_2$) reflects tissue O_2 uptake. Normally, only a 3 to 5.5 ml/dl difference exists between the Cao_2 and the $C\bar{v}o_2$, again reflecting 25% oxygen use.

The O_2ER represents the percent of oxygen delivered to tissues that is actually used. The O_2ER indicates adequacy of $\dot{D}o_2$ with respect to $\dot{V}o_2$. The rate of oxygen consumption/availability is calculated by: $a\text{-}\bar{v}Do_2/Cao_2 \times 10$. Normal O_2ER is $25 \pm 2\%$.

$S\bar{v}o_2$ Monitoring

Pediatric-size oximetry pulmonary artery catheters allow continuous monitoring of mixed venous oxygen saturation ($S\bar{v}o_2$). The technology is very similar to pulse oximetry except that the sensor sits at the end of a pulmonary artery catheter and continuously monitors $S\bar{v}o_2$. Mixed venous oxygen saturation continuously reflects the interaction among all variables impacting $\dot{D}o_2$ and $\dot{V}o_2$.

As $\dot{V}o_2$ increases, the body compensates by increasing oxygen supply in an effort to preserve venous reserve. Sympathetic stimulation increases both cardiac output and minute ventilation, so $S\bar{v}o_2$ remains unchanged.

If compensation starts to deteriorate or is ineffective or impossible (e.g., the cardiac output, Sao_2, or hemoglobin is or cannot be further maximized), threefold increases in tissue extraction can occur to prevent hypoxemia. A decreased $S\bar{v}o_2$ indicates that the patient is using venous reserve; alterations of more than 5% lasting for more than 5 minutes are considered significant.

Decreased $S\bar{v}o_2$ can result from increased $\dot{V}o_2$ or decreased $\dot{D}o_2$. Factors that impact $\dot{V}o_2$ are noted in Table 8-4. Factors that decrease $\dot{D}o_2$ include a myriad of problems affecting cardiac output, hemoglobin concentration, and saturation. Primary interventions are always focused to correct the primary problem, followed by interventions focused to support compensatory mechanisms.

Although $S\bar{v}o_2$ trends are critically important in patient care management, one of the greatest benefits of continuous $S\bar{v}o_2$ monitoring is assessment of patient tolerance to care procedures. Patients with little oxygen reserve have negligible tolerance to basic care activities, such as repositioning and physical care. In addition, these extremely vulnerable patients may undergo desaturation with suctioning, no matter how cautiously the procedure is performed. Trending the patient's ability to recover from necessary procedures is helpful in determining how best to administer care, for example, separating or clustering care.

Increased $S\bar{v}o_2$ can result from decreased $\dot{V}o_2$ or improved $\dot{D}o_2$. Factors that decrease $\dot{V}o_2$ include sleep, adequate sedation and pain relief, normothermia, chemical paralysis, and anesthesia. Pathologic issues that decrease $\dot{V}o_2$ include right-to-left shunting associated with sepsis and cyanide toxicity associated with nitroprusside administration. Factors that improve $\dot{D}o_2$ include interventions that optimize cardiac output, hemoglobin concentration, and saturation.

Convergent oximetry—that is, decreasing Sao_2 and increasing $S\bar{v}o_2$—equates with cell death, whereas divergent oximetry—that is, increasing Sao_2 and decreasing $S\bar{v}o_2$—equates with cell life.

PULMONARY DIAGNOSTIC STUDIES

Radiologic Procedures

Serial chest x-ray films are used to monitor the progression of disease and response to therapy and to confirm various tube placements preventing iatrogenic injury. Although the quality of portable films varies, they are often performed in ICU settings. Fundamental skills in x-ray interpretation are necessary because critical care nurses are often the first individuals to assess the chest x-ray film and are responsible for manipulating various tubes into position. Access to films is even more prevalent, given the increased use of computerized systems that directly image films in the ICU.

Just before obtaining a chest x-ray film, it is important to ensure the best quality film possible by removing anything from the patient's chest that would obscure the image. The head and neck are placed in alignment, and the head is positioned in a neutral position. Neck flexion or extension would displace the ETT. Radiation precautions for patients include gonad shielding.

When evaluating a film, one interprets the characteristics of and relationships between structures of varying density ranging from air, fat, and water to bone. If the structure is not dense (air-filled alveoli, pneumothorax, air in the stomach), the x-ray beam passes through the tissue, resulting in a dark gray or black image on the film. A very dense structure (bone) will block most of the x-ray beam, preventing it from reaching the film and resulting in a light gray or white image. Usually, lung is translucent, whereas the heart, blood vessels, liver, spleen, and muscle appear opaque on x-ray.

As illustrated in Fig. 8-27, the trachea has a tubelike appearance and is visible in the midline of the anterior mediastinal cavity. The trachea bifurcates into the right and left mainstem bronchi at approximately the level of the fourth rib. The bronchi are usually not clearly visible but have a tubelike appearance if surrounded by consolidated lung. The heart is visible in the anterior left mediastinal

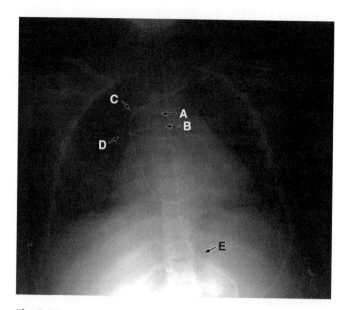

Fig. 8-27 Chest x-ray film with landmarks. *A,* Endotracheal tube 1 cm above the carina. *B,* Carina. *C,* Left subclavian introducer tip. *D,* Pulmonary artery catheter tip in the RUL. *E,* Nasogastric tube tip off film in region of duodenum. (Courtesy Robert Cleveland, MD. Radiology Department, Children's Hospital, Boston, Mass.)

cavity and should occupy less than one half of the thoracic cavity. The clavicle and ribs are evaluated for continuity. The lung parenchyma is usually not visible throughout the lung fields except for white lines radiating from the hilum, which represent the pulmonary vascular tree. Pulmonary vascular markings are usually visible in the proximal two thirds of the lung. If the density of the lung changes, for example, with atelectasis, pneumonia, pulmonary edema, or hemorrhage, the lung will appear more opaque. When structures of similar density, for example, the heart and atelectatic lung, are positioned side by side, they cannot be differentiated from each other, so the heart border disappears. The heights of the right and left diaphragm are compared for symmetry. The costophrenic angles should be well defined and taper into points. The dark gastric bubble is seen under the left diaphragm.

Major problems such as a pneumothorax, or a displaced airway, central line, or feeding tube, should be identified so that immediate interventions can occur.[37] The patient's ETT should be visualized within the trachea midway between the carina and clavicles. The radiopaque markings on the ETT should end 2 to 3 cm above the carina—the point at which the right and left mainstem bronchi bifurcate. When assessing ETT position, head position is first assessed to ensure a neutral position. If the neck were flexed, the ETT would be displaced downward; if the neck were extended, the ETT would be displaced upward. When the ETT is "too high," the tip is positioned at the level of the clavicles. When the ETT is "too low," the tip is positioned near the carina or down either mainstem bronchi—most often the right because it is more vertical than the left. When the ETT intubates either bronchus, hyperinflation of the affected lung occurs along with hypoinflation and atelectasis of the unintubated lung.

Lung tissue normally fills the chest, so pulmonary markings should be equal and visible out to the rib margins. If the pulmonary markings are replaced with a dark edge, consider a pneumothorax. When significant, the trachea may deviate away from the collapsed lung. If a dark line encircles the mediastinum, consider a pneumomediastinum.

The patient's central line should sit high within the right atrium. The patient's pulmonary artery catheter should sit within the main pulmonary artery or proximal within the right or left pulmonary artery. The patient's nasogastric tube should sit within the stomach. Landmarks include the right atrium (RA), which is located to the right of the sternum and extends down to the diaphragm. Above the RA is the superior vena cava (SVC). The left ventricle (LV) is to the left of the sternum and rests on the diaphragm. Above the LV is the left atrium (LA), and above that are the pulmonary arteries (PAs). The stomach sits under the left diaphragm.

Other radiologic procedures of the pulmonary system include fluoroscopy, angiography, and $\dot{V}/\dot{Q}$ and computed tomography (CT) scanning. Fluoroscopy images the dynamic process of ventilation and thus is very useful during pulmonary artery catheter insertion in a small infant and in assessing diaphragmatic function. Pulmonary angiography is a radiologic study of the pulmonary vessels used to delineate pulmonary arteriovenous malformations and pulmonary embolus. $\dot{V}/\dot{Q}$ scanning includes two complementary tests involving the inhalation and IV injection of necular material for the purpose of determining the match of ventilation to perfusion. $\dot{V}/\dot{Q}$ scanning provides valuable information in the lung transplant patient. Before sequential single-lung transplant, a $\dot{V}/\dot{Q}$ scan is used to help determine the better lung to maintain ventilation while the other lung is being transplanted. CT scan images correlate closely with macroscopic appearances of the lung, so in the context of diffuse lung injury, they represent a substantial improvement over chest x-ray films.

Bronchoscopy

Technologic advances have provided the opportunity for even the smallest of neonates to benefit from bronchoscopy. Two types of bronchoscopic examinations are available: rigid and flexible. Rigid bronchoscopy is often performed in the operating room under general anesthesia, whereas flexible bronchoscopy is often performed within the ICU environment. Bronchoscopes have all or some of the following features: fiberoptics for visualization and ports for ventilation, suction, retrieval of objects, or collection of specimens.

Box 8-2 provides a summary of the potential indications for bronchoscopy. Rigid bronchoscopy offers a large channel, so it is used predominately for the retrieval of a foreign body and control of bleeding in the presence of massive hemoptysis. The three most common techniques employed through flexible bronchoscopy include bronchoalveolar lavage, transbronchial biopsy, and bronchial brushing.

Nursing care during a bedside bronchoscopic examination is generally supportive; the priority is ensuring a safe environment. Anesthesia, if indicated, is provided by an anesthesiologist. Conscious sedation and coaching the patient through the procedure are nursing responsibilities. Emergency medications should be prepared before the procedure and access to a vascular line maintained during the procedure. Potential complications include laryngospasm, hypoxia, cardiac dysrhythmias secondary to hypoxia or vagal stimulation, bronchial tears, pneumothoraces, pulmonary hemorrhage, epistaxis, subglottic edema, contamination of the lower airway with upper airway flora, and oversedation.

Box 8-2
◆ **Potential Indications for Bronchoscopy**

Rigid Scope

Foreign body removal
Tissue mass removal
Massive hemoptysis
Establishment of an airway in patients with an upper airway obstruction

Flexible Scope

Evaluation of stridor
Persistent or recurrent atelectasis
Identification of infectious organisms
Hemoptysis
Difficult intubation
Abnormal cry or hoarseness
Vocal cord paralysis
Evaluation of a mass lesion

From Behnke M, Koff PB: Patient assessment. In Koff PB, Eitzman D, Neu J, eds: *Neonatal and pediatric respiratory care,* ed 2, St Louis, 1993, Mosby, p 45.

RESPIRATORY SUPPORT

Oxygen Therapy

The goal of oxygen therapy is to relieve hypoxemia, decrease the work of breathing, and reduce myocardial stress.[38] Oxygen, considered a medication, is administered in the lowest possible concentration to support life while avoiding toxicity. Pulmonary toxic effects of oxygen are progressive and include diminished mucociliary clearance, capillary endothelial damage, interstitial edema, and destruction of type I pneumocytes. Subsequent progression includes hyperplasia of the type II pneumocytes, interstitial fibrosis, and then death.[39]

Environmental gases are warmed and humidified to 100% relative humidity. Proper humidification of inspired gas prevents drying of the tracheobronchial tree, which may cause impaired ciliary activity, inflammatory changes, and retention of thick secretions.[38] Providing warmed humidified gas is particularly important in infants who are sensitive to heat loss and in patients with a bypassed upper airway, as in those who are intubated.

When the airway is secure and the patient is spontaneously breathing, oxygen can be delivered as needed by several modalities. These include simple mask, partial or nonrebreathing mask, face tent, nasal cannula, oxygen hood, hut tent, and mist tent. Any of these delivery devices can be regulated to achieve desired oxygen concentrations. Table 8-10 summarizes the advantages and disadvantages of several commonly used oxygen delivery devices.

Oxygen Delivery Devices

Simple Face Mask. The most common type of oxygen delivery device is the simple face mask. Available in a wide variety of sizes, these masks are designed to deliver oxygen through a cone-shaped face piece with open

---

◆ **TABLE 8-10   Oxygen Delivery Devices**

Device	F_{IO_2}	Flow Rate (L/min)	Advantages	Disadvantages
Simple face mask	0.35-0.55	Child: 3-5 Adolescent: 5-10	Easy to use	Patient may overbreathe flow rate and entrain room air CO_2 retention at low flow rates Patient intolerance
Rebreathing mask	To 0.60	Variable—adjust to keep reservoir partially filled	Delivers higher F_{IO_2}	Same as for simple face masks
Nonrebreathing mask	To 1.0	Variable—adjust to keep reservoir partially filled	Delivers higher F_{IO_2} Can be used to administer other gases (HeO_2)	Same as for simple face masks
Nasal cannula	Variable	25 ml/min to 6 L/min	Ease of use Patient tolerance	F_{IO_2} varies Gastric inflation at high flow rates May occlude with nasal secretions
Oxygen hood Hut tent	To 1.0	10-15	Patient tolerance Patient access	Noise level Limited to infants younger than 1 year
Mist tent	To 0.5	10-15	Provides cool mist	Limited and variable F_{IO_2} Cumbersome

Data from Wilson BG, Desautels DA: Oxygen therapy. In Koff PB, Eitzman D, Neu J, eds: *Neonatal and pediatric respiratory care,* ed 2, St Louis, 1993, Mosby.

exhalation ports. The F_{IO_2} is influenced by the size of the mask, the patient's ventilatory pattern and tidal volume, and oxygen flow. As tidal volume increases, F_{IO_2} is decreased as more environmental air is pulled in (entrained) through the exhalation ports. Too small of a mask will decrease inspired F_{IO_2}; a mask too large will add excessive dead space. An F_{IO_2} of 0.35 to 0.55 can be achieved when oxygen flow rates of 3 to 5 L/min in a child and 5 to 10 L/min in the adolescent are used.[40]

Face masks are not usually tolerated by infants and small children. This age group does not understand the benefit of a tight-fitting mask blowing moist air on their face. If the patient struggles, hypoxemia will worsen as $\dot{V}_{O_2}$ increases while $\dot{D}_{O_2}$ remains unchanged. There is also an increased risk of aspiration if the infant or child vomits into the mask.

Partial Rebreathing Mask. A partial rebreathing mask is similar to a simple face mask with an added reservoir bag. The purpose of the reservoir bag is to collect the first third of the patient's exhaled gas, dead space gas that is high in oxygen and low in carbon dioxide. Allowing rebreathing of this gas mixed with a fresh oxygen source will allow an F_{IO_2} as high as 0.6.[40] Entrainment of room air is reduced, and rebreathing of carbon dioxide from the mask is prevented by maintaining an oxygen flow rate into the bag that is greater than the patient's minute ventilation. This is determined by adjusting the flow rate high enough to keep the bag from completely deflating during inspiration; generally, gas flows at 10 to 12 L/min are required.[3]

Nonrebreathing Mask. A nonrebreathing mask is similar to the partial rebreathing mask except that one-way exhalation valves are incorporated into the sides of the mask to prevent entrainment of room air and a valve is placed at the reservoir bag to prevent gas flow back into the bag during exhalation. The patient can only draw gas from the oxygen-rich reservoir bag and displace gas through the exhalation valves. To achieve maximum oxygen concentration, the mask must fit snugly. When the mask fits properly and the reservoir is inflated, this device can provide an F_{IO_2} close to 1.0.[40]

Most disposable nonrebreathing masks are manufactured with one exhalation valve removed. This safety mechanism allows the patient to breathe room air if gas flow into the mask is interrupted. This type of nonrebreathing mask (manufactured with only one exhalation valve) is only slightly more effective in delivering high F_{IO_2} than a partial rebreathing mask.

Face Tent. Sometimes referred to as a shovel or scoop, a face tent is a soft plastic mask that fits close to the chin but is completely open around the patient's face. This device is better tolerated by infants and children because the face is accessible, allowing the patient to use a pacifier, eat, or talk.[3] The downside of this device is that even at high flow rates, an F_{IO_2} in excess of 0.4 is difficult to achieve.

Nasal Cannula. A nasal cannula provides a light-weight, less restrictive system for oxygen delivery. The device consists of either soft plastic prongs that are inserted into the nares or slits within soft plastic tubing that direct oxygen toward the posterior naso-oropharynx. It is difficult to predict and control the F_{IO_2} using these devices. The F_{IO_2} depends on the flow rate of oxygen, the patient's spontane-

ous minute ventilation, peak inspiratory flow, the volume of environmental air inhaled by the patient, cannula position, the proportion of nose to mouth breathing, and the size of the upper airway, which provides an anatomic oxygen reservoir.[38] Changes in any of these parameters result in changes in the F_{IO_2}.

In infants, low-flow flowmeters are used to allow more precise titration of gas flow. Titrations in flow rates are made based on the desired S_{PO_2} and blood gas. Oxygen flow (L/min) should not exceed the patient's predicted minute ventilation ($V_T \times RR$). Excessive flow rates may cause gastric distension and vomiting.[41]

Nasal cannulas are useful in clinical situations in which the infant or child requires less precise and low F_{IO_2} concentrations for extended periods. Nasal cannulas allow the patient to use a pacifier, eat, or talk while receiving a continuous flow of oxygen. To maintain skin integrity, cannulas can be taped to small pieces of Duoderm Extra Thin (Convatec, Princeton, N.J.) placed directly on the maxilla. Potential problems include otitis media, sinusitis, and a local reaction to the plastic prongs.

Oxyhood and Hut Tents. An oxyhood is a clear plastic enclosure that fits over the infant's entire head and neck. A hut tent is a small tent frame with canopy that fits over the infant's upper body. Capable of delivering an F_{IO_2} of 1.0, both require a flow rate of 10 to 15 L/min to flush out exhaled CO_2. Oxygen may layer within the hood or hut, producing a higher oxygen concentration at the bottom of the device. Oxygen concentrations are continuously monitored close to the infant's head with high and low alarm limits set on the oxygen analyzer.[38]

Oxyhoods are well tolerated by infants because free head movement is allowed, in addition to the use of pacifiers and other comfort measures. Hut tents allow the infant hand-mouth self-stimulation. One potential problem is the noise level produced by incoming gas. Also, the delivery of cold gas can result in considerable stress to small infants; therefore heating and humidification must be provided.

Mist Tent. Mist tents are clear plastic enclosures that fit over the patient's entire body, providing cool aerosol and low to moderate concentrations of oxygen. The F_{IO_2} varies, depending on total gas flow, tent volume, and the tightness of seal around the bottom of the tent. Again, higher levels of oxygen are found lower in the tent. An F_{IO_2} of up to 0.5 can be achieved at flow rates of 10 to 15 L/min if patients are left undisturbed. However, leaving a critically ill patient undisturbed is usually not an option within the ICU environment. In addition to limited patient access, the mist may also compromise caregiver observation of the patient. For comfort, frequent linen changes are necessary. For fire safety, patients are instructed not to play with any electrical or friction toys within the tent.

Resuscitation Bag-Valve-Masks. Bag-valve-mask ventilation provides a method of ventilating a patient with ineffective or absent respirations. Resuscitation bags and face masks are available in a wide variety of sizes to accommodate the wide range in pediatric size. Correctly sized masks provide an airtight seal around the patient's face from the bridge of the nose to the cleft of the chin. Round masks function well in small infants, whereas anatomically correct masks reduce the potential for ocular pressure that precipitates vagal stimulation and tend to provide a better seal in older children. Masks should have a small undermask volume to decrease dead space and prevent rebreathing. Clear masks are preferred because continuous assessment of the patient's color and early identification of regurgitation are possible.[3]

Bag size is selected to accommodate patient lung volume. Two types of resuscitation bags are available: self-inflating and anesthesia.

Self-Inflating Bags. Self-inflating bags consist of a standard 15/22-mm connector for mask or endotracheal tube connection, a nonrebreathing valve assembly that also regulates inspiratory and expiratory pressures, a pressure release valve, and a self-inflating bag with distal ports for oxygen and a reservoir to entrain room air. The oxygen gas inlet has a one-way valve that fills the bag with oxygen. At 10 L/min of oxygen flow, the self-inflating bag will deliver an FiO_2 of 0.3 to 0.8; higher concentrations can be achieved if an oxygen reservoir is attached to the room air port. The bag automatically fills independently of gas flow.

During bag inflation, the gas valve opens, entraining room air or oxygen from the reservoir. During bag compression, the gas intake valve closes, and the patient valve is opened. During patient exhalation, the nonrebreathing valve closes, and exhaled volumes are displaced into the environment.

To avoid barotrauma, most self-inflating bags are equipped with a preset (or adjustable) pop-off valve that allows a maximum peak inspiratory pressure of 30 to 35 cm H_2O. Although appropriate in the intubated patient, preset valved bag-valve-masks have limited use in extubated patients with poor lung compliance who require high inflating pressures for adequate tidal volume. Also, because of the bag-valve assembly, self-inflating bags cannot be used to provide supplemental oxygen to a spontaneously breathing patient. Even if the pediatric patient could generate sufficient negative pressure to open the valve, the added work of breathing is not optimal. Also, some self-inflating bags are designed to deliver volume only when the bag is actually compressed.

Anesthesia Bags. Sometimes called flow-inflating or "Mapleson" bags, anesthesia bags inflate when a gas is delivered into the bag. These bags consist of a standard 15/22-mm connector for mask or endotracheal tube connec-

tion, a gas inlet port, pressure gauge port with manometer, a corrugated reservoir tube, a non–self-inflating reservoir bag, and a distal adjustable gas escape port or pop-off valve. Careful adjustment of flow is required to maintain volume in the reservoir tube and bag while also flushing out exhaled gases. When the reservoir bag is compressed, the patient receives tidal volume from the oxygen source and corrugated reservoir tube. Flow rates 2 to 3 times the patient's $\dot{V}_E$ are usually adequate to keep the bag half inflated between breaths.

Careful adjustment to gas escape is required to provide adequate tidal volume, peak inflating time and pressure, and end-expiratory pressure. High inflation pressures, continuous positive airway pressure (CPAP), and ventilatory rates are matched by high flow rates to adequately inflate the bag. Improper use may result in pulmonary barotrauma (high flow, low escape), insufficient washout of exhaled gases (low flow, low escape), or insufficient tidal volumes (high or low flow, high escape). To prevent barotrauma, an in-line manometer should be used to monitor and deliver appropriate levels of peak inspiratory and end-expiratory pressures. Because of the continuous flow, anesthesia bags can be used to provide oxygen and CPAP in the spontaneously breathing patient.

Airway Adjuncts

The goals of airway management include recognition and treatment of obstruction, prevention of aspiration of gastric contents, and promotion of adequate gas exchange.[42] Repositioning the patient using a chin lift or jaw thrust may relieve upper airway obstruction. Although endotracheal intubation may be required, nasopharyngeal or oropharyngeal airways are simpler devices when assisted ventilation is unnecessary.

Nasopharyngeal Airways. A nasopharyngeal airway is a soft rubber tube that, when properly positioned, extends below the base of the tongue. Nasopharyngeal airways rarely induce vomiting, so they can be used in both the conscious and obtunded patient. Available in sizes 12 to 36 Fr, the size chosen should fit snugly within the naris without causing sustained blanching.[3] The 12 Fr size usually accommodates an infant. Appropriate length is determined by measuring the distance from the tip of the nose to the tragus of the ear (Fig. 8-28, *A*).

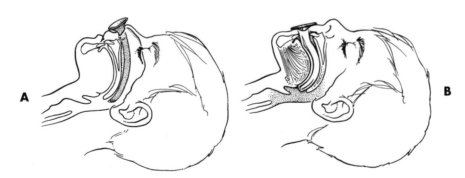

Fig. 8-28 **A,** Placement of nasopharyngeal airway. **B,** Oropharyngeal airway. (Adapted from Cote CJ, Todres ID: The pediatric airway. In Cote CJ, Ryan JF, Todres ID et al, eds: *A practice of anesthesia in infants and children,* ed 3, Philadelphia, 1999, WB Saunders.)

Care measures include maintaining skin integrity and tube patency. Potential complications from nasopharyngeal airways include epistaxis and ulceration of the tip of the nose. Laryngospasm may occur if the airway is too long and impinges on the epiglottis. Nasopharyngeal airways should not be placed in those at high risk for uncontrolled bleeding (e.g., anticoagulated patients) and in those with head or facial trauma at high risk for cribriform plate fracture.

Oropharyngeal Airways. An oropharyngeal airway is a rigid plastic device that curves over the base of the tongue, pulling it forward away from the pharyngeal wall. Because of the potential for induced vomiting and laryngospasm, oropharyngeal airways are placed only in unconscious patients. Oropharyngeal airways are used to (1) relieve airway obstruction caused by the tongue, (2) facilitate oropharyngeal suctioning, and (3) facilitate endotracheal suctioning and ventilation when the patient is biting down on an oral ETT. The correct size for an oropharyngeal airway is determined by placing the airway next to the patient's face with the phalange next to the teeth. The tip of the airway should reach the angle of the jaw (see Fig. 8-28, *B*). The airway is inserted by depressing the tongue with a blade and inserting the airway to follow the natural curve of the tongue. Inserting the airway upside down then rotating it 180 degrees may cause damage to fragile oral mucosa.

Care measures include maintaining skin integrity of the lips, tongue, and mouth. A misplaced oropharyngeal airway will result in airway obstruction by pushing the tongue back in the oropharynx. Complications of oropharyngeal airways include trauma to the lips, teeth, tongue, and surrounding soft tissue.[42]

Endotracheal Tubes. ETTs are constructed of soft plastic (polyvinyl chloride). The proximal end is fitted with a standard 15-mm male adapter. The tip is beveled to allow smooth passage through the nares, and a side hole ("Murphy eye") provides ventilation in the event of distal obstruction. ETT labeling includes the size of the ETT, a radiopaque line down the entire length of the ETT, and distance hatch markings (in centimeters) that provide reference points to facilitate tube placement. A distal vocal cord marker is placed at the level of the glottic opening to ensure that the tip of the ETT is in a midtracheal position.[3]

Uncuffed ETTs are typically used in children younger than 8 years of age because the cricoid cartilage serves as a physiologic cuff. When air leaks around ETTs become unmanageable, cuffed ETTs may be used. Soft cuffs, low-pressure high-volume cuffs, exert low and equal lateral tracheal wall pressure to minimize the potential for tracheal injury. The inflating tube is constructed with a distal one-way valve and a "pilot" balloon that indicates the presence of air within the cuff.

Approximate ETT size can be calculated using the following formula: ID = 16 + age in years ÷ 4 (where *ID* is the internal diameter in mm). Usually, a 3- to 3.5-mm ETT will accommodate term newborns, whereas a 4-mm ETT can be used in infants younger than 1 year of age. A quick check can be made by comparing the outside diameter of an ETT with the patient's little finger. Table 8-11 lists recommended sizes per age of the patient.

Endotracheal Intubation. Indications for endotracheal intubation include establishment of a secure airway in patients with a diminished gag or cough reflex and the need for controlled ventilation. Before endotracheal intubation, the patient is positioned in a sniffing position, and equipment is prepared (Box 8-3). An adequate cardiac and pulse oximetry tracing is ensured. A suction source and Yankauer are made available to clear the oropharynx of thick

TABLE 8-11 ETT and Suction Catheter Sizes

Age	ETT Size (mm)	Suction Catheter Size
Newborn	3-3.5 uncuffed	6-8 Fr
6 months	3.5-4 uncuffed	8 Fr
1 year	4-4.5 uncuffed	8-10 Fr
2 years	4.5 uncuffed	8-10 Fr
4 years	5 uncuffed	10 Fr
6 years	5.5 uncuffed	10-12 Fr
8 years	6 cuffed or uncuffed	12 Fr
12 years	6.5 cuffed or uncuffed	12-14 Fr
Adolescent	7-8 cuffed	14 Fr
Adult	7.5-8 cuffed	14-16 Fr

Box 8-3
Intubation Equipment Checklist

Patient

Monitoring equipment
  Good cardiac tracing
  Strong Spo$_2$ pulse indicator
  Good A-line tracing or operational blood pressure cuff
Medications
  Sedation
  Muscle relaxant

Equipment

Oxygen
  Adequately sized mask
  Resuscitation bag to provide Fio$_2$ of 1.0
Suction
  Large-bore Yankauer or tonsil-tip suction
  Sterile suction catheters that will fit the selected endotracheal tube (ETT)
Laryngoscope
  Handle, correct size and shape of blade, strong light source
ETTs
  Calculated size—one size larger and smaller than calculated
  Stylet to fit the selected ETT
  Water-soluble lubricant for nasotracheal intubation
  Magill forceps for nasotracheal intubation
Adhesive tape and skin protector
Appropriately sized nasogastric tube with attached catheter tip syringe
Gloves and goggles—per universal precautions

TABLE 8-12 **Intubation Medications**

Drug	Dose (duration)	Comment
Sedatives and Narcotics		
Midazolam (Versed)	0.05-0.1 mg/kg IV (1-2 hr)	May cause respiratory depression
Fentanyl	1-5 μg/kg IV (0.5-1.5 hr)	Respiratory depression; large doses given rapidly may cause bradycardia and chest wall rigidity
Morphine	0.1-0.2 mg/kg IV (2-4 hr)	Respiratory depression; histamine release producing bronchospasm and hypotension
Anesthetic Agents		
Ketamine	0.5-2 mg/kg IV (10-15 min) Intubation: administer with glycopyrrolate	Useful in hypotensive patients because of catecholamine release (increases HR and BP); potent bronchodilator; increases ICP; spontaneous respirations maintained but may cause laryngospasm; copious secretions
Etomidate	0.3 mg/kg IV	Minimal cardiovascular effects; decreases cerebral metabolic rate, cerebral blood flow, intracranial pressure.
Propofol	2-3 mg/kg (4-8 min)	Short acting; less sedation on awakening; dose-dependent cardiovascular depression; pain on injection
Thiopental (Pentothal) Methohexital (Brevital)	2-4 mg/kg IV (5-10 min) 1-2 mg/kg	Potent myocardial depressant; decreases peripheral vascular resistance and may precipitate CV collapse in the patient with MC dysfunction and hypovolemia; will produce apnea in doses greater than 4 mg/kg; decreases cerebral metabolic rate, cerebral blood flow, intracranial pressure
Neuromuscular Blocking Agents *Depolarizing*		
Succinylcholine (Anectine)	Infants: 2 mg/kg Children: 1-2 mg/kg Adolescents: 1-1.5 mg/kg (3-12 min) Administer with atropine	Decrease HR; may increase intracranial, intraocular, and intragastric pressure; arrhythmias common with second dose; may cause massive elevation in serum potassium in patients with severe burns, crush injuries, spinal cord injury, and neuromuscular disease; known trigger for malignant hyperthermia; myoglobinuria in healthy children

HR, Heart rate; *BP,* blood pressure; *ICP,* intracranial pressure; *CV,* cardiovascular; *MC,* myocardial. *Continued*

secretions, vomit, or blood. An appropriately sized resuscitation bag and mask are needed to pre/reoxygenate the patient with an F$_{IO_2}$ of 1.0. To visualize the vocal cords, the large floppy epiglottis in infants and children is raised using a straight Miller laryngoscope blade.

The sedatives, narcotics, anesthetics, and neuromuscular blocking agents commonly used to facilitate intubation are noted in Table 8-12. Neuromuscular blocking agents are divided into two groups: depolarizing and nondepolarizing agents. Depolarizing agents mimic the action of acetylcholine but produce prolonged depolarization of the neuromuscular junction. Nondepolarization agents bind to acetylcholine receptor sites, preventing depolarization of the neuromuscular junction. Use of neuromuscular blocking agents are contraindicated when the ability to establish an artificial airway is in question or difficulty in maintaining adequate ventilation is anticipated.[43] Only time will reverse the effects of a depolarizing agent, whereas pharmacologic reversal of nondepolarizing agents can be obtained by increasing the concentration of acetylcholine at the neuromuscular junction. Administration of an anticholinesterase inhibitor plus muscarinic antagonist will accomplish this effect (see Table 8-12).

Unless contraindicated, the depolarizing agent succinylcholine is recommended for intubation because of its rapid onset (45 to 60 seconds) and short duration (5 to 10 minutes). For intubation, succinylcholine is usually administered with an anticholinergic agent (atropine) to prevent excessive vagal effects related to the initial release of acetylcholine. If succinylcholine is contraindicated, a rapid-acting nondepolarizing agent, for example, either atracurium or vecuronium, can be used. To produce a more rapid effect, a priming dose (one-tenth the intubating dose) is administered 5 minutes before the intubating dose.

The technique of endotracheal intubation depends on the indication for intubation and the condition of the patient.

TABLE 8-12 Intubation Medications—cont'd

Drug	Dose (duration)	Comment
Neuromuscular Blocking Agents—cont'd		
Nondepolarizing		
Cisatracurium besylate (Nimbex)	0.1-0.2 mg/kg IV (15-20 min) 0.1-0.2 mg/kg/hr infusion	Mild histamine release; hypotension; neither renal nor hepatic function necessary for excretion; active metabolites
Vecuronium bromide (Norcuron)	0.1-0.15 mg/kg/dose IV (children: 35 min; infants: 70 min) 0.06-0.1 mg/kg/hr infusion	Minimal CV effect Elimination: liver
Pancuronium bromide (Pavulon)	0.1-0.15 mg/kg IV (30-90 min)	Vagolytic effect increases HR; may increase BP Elimination: liver and kidney (repeated doses contraindicated in renal failure)
Rocuronium (Zemuron)	0.6-1.2 mg/kg IV (20-30 min; 45-60 min)	Minimal cardiovascular effect; rapid onset of action using larger dose; possible alternative to succinylcholine for rapid-sequence induction; hepatic clearance
Rapacuronium (Raplon)	1.5 mg/kg (10-15 min)	Onset 60-90 sec—alternative to succinylcholine for rapid-sequence induction
Reversal Agents		
Anticholinesterase Inhibitors		
Neostigmine	0.06 mg/kg; max 2.5 mg	Reverses the effects of nondepolarizing neuromuscular blockade; always precede with atropine
Pyridostigmine	0.1-0.25 mg/kg; max 10 mg	
Muscarinic Anticholinergics		
Atropine	0.02-0.03 mg/kg; min 0.1 mg/max 2 mg	Used to prevent bradycardia, salivation, bronchospasm, and gastrointestinal hypermotility
Glycopyrrolate	0.01 mg/kg	
Miscellaneous		
Lidocaine	1-2 mg/kg IV qh	Given 2 min before suctioning may prevent elevations in ICP

There are many accepted techniques for ETT placement. ETTs may be placed nasally or orally, patients may be fully awake or receive some combination of sedation and analgesia, and patients may be pharmacologically paralyzed or breathing spontaneously. Common approaches in the intensive care setting include nasal, rapid sequence, awake oral, unconscious oral, and fiberoptic bronchoscopy. Whatever approach is used, the patient's vital signs and oxygen saturation are continuously assessed. The intubation procedure is immediately interrupted and the patient receives hand ventilation with a bag-valve-mask if desaturation occurs.

Nasotracheal intubation is preferred if intubation is anticipated for a long period. Nasotracheal ETTs are more comfortable for the patient, allow continued oral stimulation, are easier to secure, and are less apt to be displaced. Complications associated with nasotracheal intubation include epistaxis, trauma to adenoids, pressure necrosis to the naris, obstruction of the eustachian tube, and sinusitis.

If nasotracheal intubation is performed, the ETT is lubricated, inserted nasally, and gently advanced until the tip is visualized in the pharynx. The laryngoscope is then used to visualize the cords, and the Magill forceps are used to direct the tip of the tube through the vocal cords. Contraindications of nasotracheal intubation include fracture of the cribriform plate with a cerebrospinal leak, bleeding disorders, and nasal deformities.

Orotracheal intubation can be performed rapidly and is associated with minimal complications. A curved Macintosh laryngoscope blade is inserted into the vallecula above the epiglottis, whereas a straight Miller blade is passed over the epiglottis to rest above the glottic opening. Once the vocal cords are visualized, the ETT is advanced. Stylets are used to stiffen and shape ETTs to facilitate insertion. When used, stylets are positioned proximal to the side hole and should not protrude through the end of the ETT because this may cause vocal cord damage.

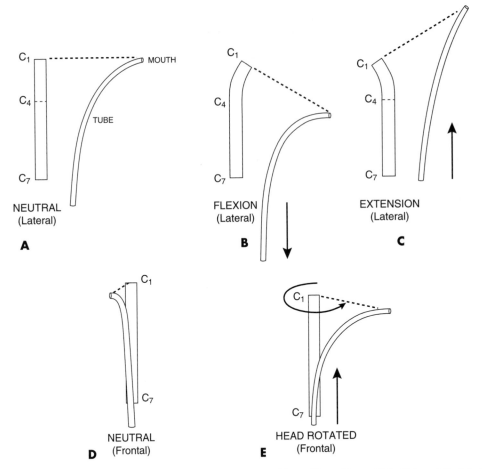

Fig. 8-29 **A** to **E,** Effect of head position on ETT position. (From Donn SM, Kuhns LR: Mechanism of endotracheal tube movement with change of head position in the neonate, *Pediatr Radiol* 9:37-40, 1980.)

Rapid-sequence intubation is used to decrease the risk of aspiration of gastric contents. Patients at high risk for aspiration include those with a full stomach caused by prior oral intake or decreased gastric emptying, resulting from pain, shock, or increased abdominal pressure. The procedure is accomplished by an IV infusion of a rapid-acting anesthetic or sedative, for example, some combination of thiopental sodium (Pentothal), methohexital sodium (Brevital), ketamine, or midazolam with a muscle relaxant, usually succinylcholine. Cricoid pressure is applied to prevent passive regurgitation, and the ETT is inserted orally. If the patient's gag and cough reflex is intact, gastric decompression occurs before intubation. This technique should not be attempted if anatomic abnormalities that potentially may prevent rapid intubation are present.

Fiberoptic bronchoscopy is used if endotracheal intubation is expected to be difficult. Here, an ETT is threaded over a fiberoptic bronchoscope. Once the scope passes through the vocal cords, the previously threaded ETT is advanced forward into position. The flexible fiberoptic scope is also useful in evaluating vocal cord movement before extubation.[10]

Intubating a patient with *increased intracranial pressure* (ICP) is specifically challenging. The goal is airway access

while averting cerebral hypertension associated with increased mean arterial pressure and hypercapnia. Intubation is accomplished by anesthetizing the patient in an effort to blunt expected cardiovascular responses. After preparing the equipment, an anesthetic dose of thiopental sodium (4 mg/kg) is administered, followed by vecuronium (0.1-0.2 mg/kg). Thiopental decreases cerebral oxygen consumption and thereby lowers cerebral blood flow and ICP. Vecuronium is a nondepolarizing neuromuscular blocking agent chosen to avoid histamine release and sympathetic stimulation. Lidocaine (1.5 mg/kg IV) is also administered to diminish cardiovascular reflexes activated with intubation. The patient is then hyperventilated to decrease $Paco_2$ and then intubated.

Also challenging is intubating the patient with a compromised airway secondary to a *large mediastinal mass.* These patients are able to stent their airways open through spontaneous chest movement. If respiratory muscle function becomes impaired (through sedation, anesthesia, or neuromuscular blockade) a large mediastinal mass can collapse the airway, leading to sudden and complete airway obstruction despite positive pressure ventilation. The goal is to keep the patient breathing spontaneously until radiation or chemotherapy can reduce the size of the mass.

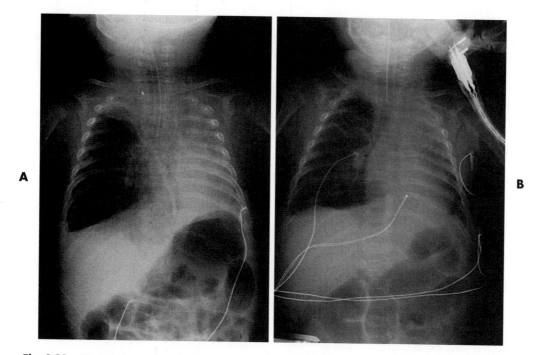

Fig. 8-30   Chest radiographs demonstrating impact of small movements of ETT. In the first radiograph (**A**), right mainstem bronchus is intubated and left lung has collapsed. After withdrawing ETT just 1 cm (**B**), left lung is partially reinflated.

Correct Placement.   Once the ETT is placed, the patient receives hand ventilation, which is done cautiously with a resuscitation bag while ETT position is evaluated. Correct ETT positioning is marked by observation of condensation within the ETT, bilateral chest excursion, symmetric breath sounds, normal ETco$_2$/capnogram, and adequate oxygenation. Auscultation of breath sounds is best accomplished at the apex of each axilla; auscultation over the stomach rules out esophageal intubation. Unilateral chest excursion marks mainstem bronchus intubation, whereas breath sounds will not be heard with esophageal intubation. End-tidal CO$_2$ monitoring helps confirm correct ETT placement; a capnogram is possible only with endotracheal intubation.

After securing the ETT, a chest radiograph (with the head in a neutral position) is obtained to confirm proper tube position in the trachea midway between the carina and clavicles. Once correct placement is established, continued assessment of ETT position can be accomplished by noting the depth of its insertion at regular intervals, that is, documenting the mark on the tube that appears at the child's lip or nares and carefully monitoring bilateral breath sounds. Care is taken whenever moving an intubated infant or child. Neck flexion shortens the mouth-to-carina distance, thus displacing the uncuffed ETT tip downward and increasing the danger of endobronchial intubation (Fig. 8-29). Neck extension increases this distance, promoting accidental extubation. Increased respiratory distress, grunting, crying, or vocalization indicating air movement through the glottis hallmarks inadvertent extubation.

Securing the ETT.   Once ETT position appears satisfactory, the ETT is secured. To prevent inadvertent extuba-

tion, two people perform the procedure of taping or retaping an ETT. One person is responsible for immobilizing the head and holding the tube with the specific ETT markings at the naris or lip line, while the other person is responsible for the actual taping procedure. Breath sounds are auscultated before and after taping. ETT position is changed from one side of the mouth to the other during a tape change to prevent pressure necrosis.

Numerous methods to secure ETTs in the pediatric population have been described. Benjamin, Thompson, and O'Rourke[44] reported a relatively low 3% incidence of accidental extubation with the use of white cloth adhesive tape slit down the middle, resulting in a Y configuration. For an *oral ETT,* the skin of the upper lip and ETT are prepped with tincture of benzoin and then allowed to dry. The ETT is positioned so that it will be attached to the least mobile area of the mouth, that is, the upper lip away from the corner of the mouth. One arm of the Y is attached to the upper lip, and the other arm of the Y is wrapped around the ETT. A second piece, mirroring the first but started from the opposite side of the mouth, can be placed for added security. For a *nasal ETT,* the nose, upper lip, and ETT are prepped with tincture of benzoin and then allowed to dry. The untorn piece of tape is applied to the nose; one arm of the Y is applied to the upper lip, and the other arm is wrapped around the ETT. A second Y can be applied, positioning the untorn arm on the cheek; one arm of the Y layers is placed over the first piece on the upper lip, and the other is wrapped over the first piece on the ETT. While taping a nasal ETT, care is taken to avoid excessive pressure to the skin at the nasal septum and outer upper ridge of the naris. Care is also taken to avoid gaps in the tape when wrapping the ETT. Gaps fill with secretions, which eventually loosen the tape. First applying Duoderm (Convatec, Princeton, N.J.) to the face and then attaching the tape to the Duoderm may protect sensitive skin.

Complications from endotracheal intubation can occur during laryngoscopy, any time during the intubation period, or after extubation. Complications occurring during the intubation procedure include dental and soft tissue trauma, aspiration of gastric contents, esophageal intubation, right mainstem intubation, and cardiac dysrhythmias from hypoxia. Obstruction of the ETT from secretions, kinking, or biting; accidental extubation; and increased resistance to breathing are the common complications during the intubation period.[42] Later complications include laryngeal and tracheal edema or damage, acquired subglottic stenosis, and the inability to extubate.

Extubation. The reported incidence of inadvertent extubation in pediatric intensive care units (PICUs) ranges from 3% to 13%.[45] Although whether this variability is related to differences in patients or in patient care practices is unclear, several risk factors for accidental extubation have been identified. Infants may be at particular risk because their tracheas are shorter and head movement alone can dislocate the ETT.[46] Scott and associates[45] found that spontaneous extubation was more likely to occur in a patient who is younger, has a large amount of secretions and ETT slippage, and a higher level of consciousness. In this particular study, 29% of those patients reintubated after an accidental extubation had at least one subsequent unplanned extubation, and 88% of the patients who had spontaneous extubation did so despite restraints. In another study,[47] level of sedation, lack of two-point or more restraints, and the performance of a patient procedure at the bedside were identified as critical factors contributing to accidental extubation. Various methods are employed to secure the ETT, but to avoid spontaneous extubation or inadvertent advancement of the tube, frequent assessment of the patient and the position and stability of the ETT are required. To rule out right mainstem bronchus intubation (Fig. 8-30), auscultation compares bilateral air movement at the third intercostal space midaxillary line—a point at which referred breath sounds from the opposite lung are less likely to be heard. Restraints, which are necessary to prevent the child from removing the ETT, are not used in isolation. Measures to reduce anxiety should also be taken, including the use of anxiolytics or sedatives, decreasing noxious or threatening stimuli, and encouraging family presence and participation in care.

Once the indications for intubation have been resolved, extubation may be considered. Enteral feedings are stopped for 2 to 4 hours before extubation is attempted. Sedation is avoided before extubation so that the patient's cough and gag reflexes are intact and active. The ETT is suctioned, as well as the oropharynx. Care is taken to remove secretions above the ETT cuff; the cuff is then deflated on exhalation. The ETT is removed on exhalation, followed by delivery of humidified oxygen by mask or hood.

Symptoms of hoarseness and croupy cough may occur after extubation. Those at high risk include patients younger than 4 years of age and those with a cuffed ETT. Also

prevalent are patients who have experienced traumatic or repeated intubations, excessive movement of the ETT, or airway abnormalities or infection. Postextubation croup usually resolves with cool mist or humidity, as well as the use of racemic epinephrine. The action of racemic epinephrine is unclear; however, benefit may be related to its topical mucosal vasoconstriction effect. Until a wellness trajectory can be predicted, feedings and deep suctioning are withheld and familiar sources of comfort are provided to avoid vigorous crying. If reintubation is necessary, management of second or subsequent extubation attempts include dexamethasone (Decadron), 0.5 mg/kg up to a maximum of 4 mg, 6 hours before extubation, at the time of extubation, and 6 to 12 hours after extubation.[48]

Cricothyrotomy. In an emergency, when other methods of gaining airway access have failed, a cricothyrotomy can be performed. The cricothyroid membrane is a relatively avascular membrane that extends from the cricoid to thyroid cartilage. It is palpated as an anterior and midline transverse indentation between the two cartilages. The membrane can be punctured and the underlying trachea entered percutaneously using a large-bore cannula. The 14-gauge cannula is directed in the midline caudally and posteriorly at a 45-degree angle. A cricothyrotomy can also be accomplished surgically with a short horizontal incision. After incision, a 3-mm ETT can then be threaded into the tracheal opening.

Tracheostomy Tube. Similar to ETTs, TTs are available in a wide variety of sizes and styles. Variations in TT specifications are found among manufacturers (Table 8-13). For example, a standard 3.5-mm ETT is comparable with a Shiley pediatric 0 and a Portex pediatric 1 TT. Companies also provide custom TT lengths on request. As with ETTs, low-pressure, high-volume cuffed TTs are used when air leaks become unmanageable. Larger sizes may have an inner cannula that can be removed for cleaning. No data support the necessary frequency of cleaning inner cannulas, thus this should be determined by individual patient need.

Indications for tracheostomy include an acute upper airway obstruction, prolonged need for mechanical ventilation, and prevention of aspiration. TTs are inserted into an incision made below the cricoid cartilage through the second to fourth tracheal rings. Elective tracheostomy is performed in the operating room. When performed within the ICU environment, nursing care and responsibility are similar to those followed for any sterile invasive procedure. Priorities include continued patient monitoring and safety.

Postoperative tracheostomy holders are left intact for the first 3 days after surgery and are not changed. For added security, the outer phalange of the TT is often sutured to the skin to avoid inadvertent decannulation. Until the stoma is secure, reinsertion of a TT could be quite difficult. Routine care includes (1) assessing the TT holders for security, (2) assessing the character of the skin under the TT and holders, and (3) stoma care.

Tracheostomy holders should be secure enough to hold the TT in place but not too tight as to cause pressure necrosis of the neck. When assessing skin integrity, the entire circumference of the neck is assessed with particular attention given to the infant's skin folds. Available in a wide

TABLE 8-13   Tracheostomy Tube Specifications

Size	Shiley Inner Diameter (mm)	Portex Inner Diameter (mm)	Shiley Outer Diameter (mm)	Portex Outer Diameter (mm)	Shiley Length (mm)	Portex Length (mm)
Neonatal 00	3.1	2.5	4.5	Same	30	Same
0	3.4	3.0	5.0	5.2	32	Same
1	3.7	3.5	5.5	5.8	34	Same
Pediatric 00	3.1	2.5	4.5	Same	39	30
0	3.4	3.0	5.0	5.2	40	36
1	3.7	3.5	5.5	5.8	41	40
2	4.1	4.0	6.0	6.5	42	44
2.5	—	4.5	—	7.1	—	48
3	4.8	5.0	7.0	7.7	44	50
4	5.5	Same	8.0	8.3	46	52

Adapted from Scott AA, Koff PB: Airway care and chest physiotherapy. In Koff PB, Eitzman D, Neu J, eds: *Neonatal and pediatric respiratory care,* ed 2, St Louis, 1993, Mosby, pp 285-302.

variety of sizes, soft foam Velcro tracheostomy holders are used because they are less traumatic to the skin.

Traditional stoma care includes cleansing the skin with one-half strength H_2O_2 and applying antibacterial water-soluble gel and a dry, sterile split-gauze tracheostomy dressing. Care is taken to avoid displacing the TT with multilayered tracheostomy dressings. Once the stoma is healed, sterile dressings are replaced with sponges to collect secretions as necessary.

Skin surrounding the stoma and chin is assessed for pressure ulcers secondary to the TT phalange or TT connector. The phalange of the TT may need to be shaved down to eliminate pressure points. Skin around the tracheostomy site and chin can be protected using Duoderm or moleskin.

Tracheostomy masks provide humidified gases to the airway. General principles are similar to those of face masks, except that tracheostomy masks are secured gently to avoid decannulation in the active patient. Various styles of trachea-to-ventilator or resuscitation bag connections are available. The ideal connector provides little dead space and the greatest range of motion to the head and neck.

Changing a TT may be necessary after inadvertent decannulation, when secretions compromise the inside diameter, or routinely per institutional norm. The surgeon who originally placed the TT usually performs the first TT change. Any individual variance is noted for future reference. Subsequent TT changes are accomplished by the nurse. If the infant or child is going home with the TT, parents are invited to participate in the procedure. If not for education, the parents' presence can provide a source of comfort for their infant or child. The patient is held NPO for 2 to 4 hours. Sedation is considered according to the individual infant or child. All equipment, including a correctly sized face mask and one size smaller TT, is prepared. The new same-size TT is examined, the obturator is removed and replaced, the balloon is tested (if appropriate), and the TT is lubricated with a water-soluble gel. The patient's TT is suctioned, followed by vigilant removal of upper airway secretions. The patient is positioned supine with a small roll placed behind the shoulders. The patient is

preoxygenated with an F_{IO_2} of 1.0. On exhalation, the existing TT is removed following the natural curve of the tube, then the new TT is immediately inserted in a similar manner. Slight tension should be expected. If the TT cannot be reinserted, the patient is reoxygenated using a face mask and resuscitation bag while the stoma is gently occluded with a gloved finger(s). When the patient is adequately reoxygenated, reinsertion of the same size or one size smaller TT is reattempted.

Consideration of the patient's need for and ability to communicate may affect the choice of replacement TT. Several fenestrated "talking" TTs are currently available and have been used in small pediatric patients with variable success.

If none of the specialized TTs are appropriate, the Passy-Muir Speaking Valve (PMSV; Passy-Muir Inc., Irvine, Calif.) may be used. The PMSV is a one-way, positive closure, Silastic membrane valve that attaches to the universal adapter (15 mm) of the TT. During inhalation the valve is opened, allowing air into the lungs. At exhalation the valve closes, forcing air through the vocal cords, nose, and mouth. Engleman and Turnage-Carrier[49] described the use of PMSV in infants and children younger than 2 years of age when infant tracheostomy may lead to later difficulties in language acquisition and articulation. Of the 29 children in the trial, 24 (83%) tolerated the PMSV on the first trial, and another 21% produced vocalizations on a subsequent trial.

Absolute contraindications for PMSV use include the lack of air leak around a tracheostomy tube or upper airway obstruction; relative contraindications include frequent aspiration and thick, unmanageable secretions.[50,51] Nursing care centers on patient teaching and assessment. Initial trials are usually limited to a few minutes and slowly increased with patient tolerance. Ventilator volumes, pressures, and F_{IO_2} are adjusted to compensate for losses. PEEP may need to be decreased to compensate for auto-PEEP.

Decannulation of the tracheostomy patient usually occurs as a planned admission to the ICU. In preparation for decannulation, the child's TT may be replaced with a progressively smaller TT. Because of the size of the pediatric airway, this maneuver may not be an option in infants and small children. Removal occurs as per TT change (see preceding text), but the patient is usually held in an upright position on the parent's lap. Sterile gauze is placed over the stoma after TT removal. Supplemental humidified oxygen may be administered. The patient is assessed for increased work of breathing, stridor, and desaturation. Length of ICU observation after decannulation depends on the patient, family, and system. The stoma will close in 48 to 72 hours postdecannulation.

Suction Catheters. Numerous types of suction catheters are available in various distal tip configurations. Common features include measured distance markings in centimeters, a blunt tip (beveled or straight), and side holes (one to four). In pediatrics, comparing the actual size of the distal opening is especially important when comparing manufacturers. Outside diameters of suction catheters are similar, whereas the size of distal openings may vary. Because smaller catheters are used in the pediatric population, smaller distal openings further compromise the ability to suction thick secretions. The amount of suction applied is regulated to prevent hypoxia and mucosal damage. Appropriate negative pressure includes 60 to 80 mmHg in infants under 1 year of age, 80 to 120 mmHg in children 1 to 8 years of age, and 120 to 150 mmHg in children over 8 years of age.

Airway Management

Nasopharyngeal and oropharyngeal suctioning is indicated in patients who cannot clear secretions in their upper airway or to elicit deep breathing and a cough. The nasopharynx is suctioned first because it is considered cleaner than the oropharynx. Catheter size should fit comfortably into the naris using water-soluble lubricant. Appropriate insertion length is determined by measuring the distance from the tip of the nose to the tragus of the ear. To minimize mucosal injury, the catheter is inserted next to the nasal septum and advanced caudally. After inserting to appropriate length, suction is applied, and the catheter is slowly withdrawn in a rotating manner.

Endotracheal Suctioning. Because endotracheal intubation prevents an effective cough and both bypasses and impairs normal mucociliary clearing mechanisms, endotracheal suctioning is an important intervention for intubated patients. Endotracheal suctioning is not, however, a benign procedure. Suctioning has been associated with a host of negative side effects and complications, including hypoxia, pulmonary artery hypertension,[52] dysrhythmias, atelectasis, trauma to the trachea and bronchi, and increased ICP. It seems reasonable that one of the most commonly performed procedures in the PICU, which is associated with serious risks, should be guided by sound clinical research data. Unfortunately, much of what constitutes "routine suctioning technique" is guided more by ritual than scientific rationale.[53,54] Many suctioning practices of concern to pediatric critical care nurses, including hyperoxygenation, hyperinflation or hyperventilation, depth of suctioning, endotracheal instillation of normal saline, and the frequency of

endotracheal suctioning, have been examined. Devices intended to minimize suction-induced hypoxemia have also been considered. Each will be discussed in the following section.

When suctioning an artificial airway, although ideal, using a catheter size of no more than one half of the inside diameter of the tube is impractical in the pediatric population. In reality, the largest suction catheter that can comfortably fit down the ETT or TT is used (see Table 8-11).

Hyperoxygenation is a maneuver designed to reduce hypoxemia associated with suctioning. This step is accomplished in children by increasing the F_{IO_2} to 1.0 before (30 seconds), during, and after (at least 1 minute) the suctioning procedure. The F_{IO_2} can be delivered via the ventilator or manually using a resuscitation bag. Because hyperoxia should be avoided, the amount of supplemental O_2 administered during suctioning is determined by the patient's arterial oxygenation. Oxygen saturation, monitored continuously by pulse oximeter, can generally be maintained between 92% to 94% by increasing F_{IO_2} 10% to 20% over baseline requirements, but the actual F_{IO_2} used is based on each individual patient's needs.[55]

Hyperinflation and hyperventilation are additional techniques used during suctioning to lessen hypoxemia, presumably by reinflating collapsed lung segments. However, no uniform definition exists for either maneuver. Generally, hyperinflation entails delivering several breaths before suctioning (and after each pass of the suction catheter) using either a manual resuscitation bag or the ventilator circuit. Each of these breaths is approximately 1.5 times the patient's usual tidal volume. Alternatively, peak inspiratory pressure (PIP) is increased approximately 10 cm H_2O above the patient's usual requirements. Using PIP to guide hyperinflation may be more appropriate in pediatrics because children are usually intubated with uncuffed ETTs and have a variably sized leak around the tube. In clinical practice, however, hyperinflation is often accomplished by a brief period of hand ventilation with the tidal volume or PIP determined by "feel," chest wall movement, and values shown on noninvasive monitors during the maneuver (e.g., pulse oximetry and end-tidal CO_2). Similarly, hyperventilation is often not standardized but consists of some increase in ventilatory frequency over the patient's respiratory rate.

Considerable research has focused on the efficacy of hyperoxygenation, hyperinflation, or hyperventilation in reducing suction-induced hypoxemia. Some combination of the three techniques probably provides the best protection from arterial oxygen desaturation.[55] However, that combination has yet to be clearly defined, especially in infants and children. Until consensus is reached, guidelines should be flexible enough to encourage clinicians to design procedures tailored to the individual needs of the patient.

In contrast, research data already exist to direct the *depth of ETT suctioning*. Deep endotracheal suctioning has been routinely performed in PICUs. However, evidence associating that practice with bronchial perforation[56,57] and acute histologic changes in the tracheobronchial tree should change that technique. Using an animal model, Kleiber, Krutzfield, and Rose[58] have demonstrated that merely

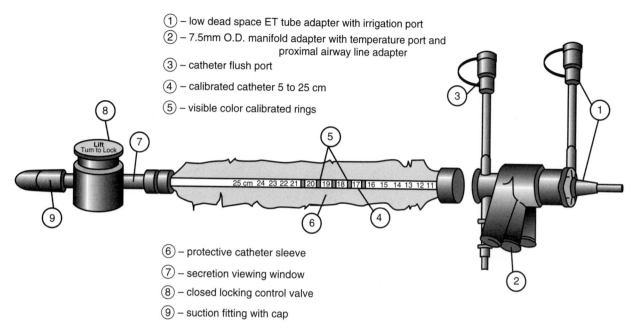

① – low dead space ET tube adapter with irrigation port
② – 7.5mm O.D. manifold adapter with temperature port and
      proximal airway line adapter
③ – catheter flush port
④ – calibrated catheter 5 to 25 cm
⑤ – visible color calibrated rings

Lift
Turn to Lock

25 cm 24 23 22 21 20 19 18 17 16 15 14 13 12 11

⑥ – protective catheter sleeve
⑦ – secretion viewing window
⑧ – closed locking control valve
⑨ – suction fitting with cap

Fig. 8-31   Ballard's Trach Care closed-system suction catheter. (Courtesy Ballard Medical Products, Draper, Utah.)

inserting a suction catheter into the ETT until resistance is met (i.e., to the carina or mainstem bronchus) causes as much tissue damage as insertion to resistance with the subsequent application of suction.[58] Because of the alignment of the right middle lobe with the trachea, this type of chronic irritation of the bronchial mucosa can lead to persistent right middle lobe atelectasis (resulting from airway narrowing because of inflammation or stenosis), especially in infants. For these reasons, catheter insertion should stop short of the carina. An appropriate depth for endotracheal suctioning can be ensured by premeasuring and marking the suction catheter or using a numerically calibrated catheter marked in centimeter increments and inserted 1 cm past the corresponding markings of the ETT.[58]

Once the catheter is inserted to the proper depth, suction is applied, and the catheter is withdrawn. Sterile technique should be employed. Each pass of the catheter is considered a suction event that should not exceed 10 to 15 seconds in duration.[59]

The *endotracheal instillation of normal saline* is an example of a widely practiced nursing routine that is not supported by research.[60,61] Normal saline has been used for the purpose of loosening or thinning tenacious secretions, but because mucus does not readily mix with saline, the effect is probably more that of a lavage.[62] As such, it may enhance secretion clearance through cough stimulation[63] but may also cause mucosal irritation with little effect on mucous clearance.[60] Bostick and Wendelgass[64] found that the use of normal saline neither improved postsuctioning Pao_2 nor increased the amount of secretions retrieved. Other studies suggest that providing adequate systemic hydration[65] and warming and humidifying inspired gases[66] are more appropriate interventions for thinning secretions.

Furthermore, saline instillation may dislodge viable bacteria from a colonized ETT into the lower airway, contributing to the development of nosocomial pneumonia.[67] In total, although the pediatric research is scarce, routine use of normal saline with ETT suctioning should be avoided.

The *frequency of endotracheal suctioning* is determined by careful patient assessment. Endotracheal suctioning should not be performed on a routine basis. Assessment of the need for endotracheal suctioning includes coarse breath sounds, increased PIPs during volume-controlled mechanical ventilation or decreased V_T during pressure-controlled ventilation, patient's inability to generate an effective spontaneous cough, visible secretions in the airway, changes in monitored flow and pressure graphics, suspected aspiration of gastric or upper airway secretions, clinically apparent increased work of breathing, deterioration in arterial blood gases, and radiologic changes consistent with retention of pulmonary secretions, specifically, pulmonary atelectasis or consolidation.[59] Evaluating a patient over time and documenting assessments permit early detection of clinical changes and recognition of individual patient responses that will guide subsequent interventions. Clinical outcomes to evaluate after endotracheal suctioning include improvement of breath sounds, decreased PIP with narrowing PIP-$P_{Plateau}$, decreased airway resistance or increased dynamic compliance, increased V_T during pressure-limited ventilation, and improvement in ABGs or SpO_2.[59]

Several devices have been designed to ameliorate suction-induced hypoxemia. Two such devices, oxygen insufflation catheters and closed tracheal suction systems, may be especially useful when high levels of Fio_2 and PEEP are required. *Oxygen insufflation catheters* can increase Pao_2 during suctioning by permitting simultaneous delivery of O_2 during the procedure or alternate delivery of oxygen

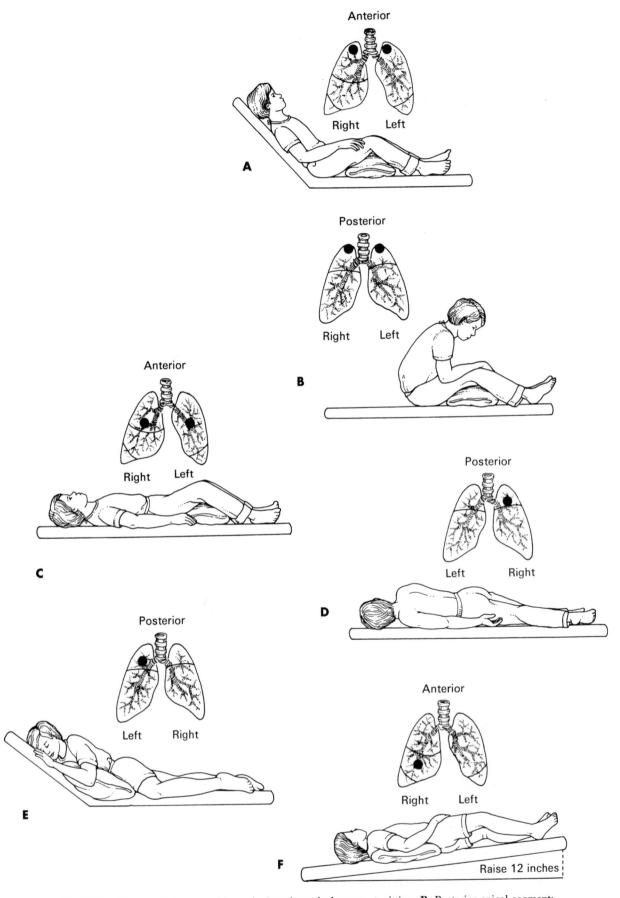

Fig. 8-32 Postural drainage positions. **A,** Anterior apical segment; sitting. **B,** Posterior apical segment; sitting. **C,** Anterior segment; lying flat on back. **D,** Right posterior segment; lying on left side. **E,** Left posterior segment; lying on right side. **F,** Right middle lobe; lying on left side. (From Thompson JM, McFarland GK, Hirsh JE et al, eds: *Mosby's clinical nursing,* ed 4, 1997, pp 201-202.)

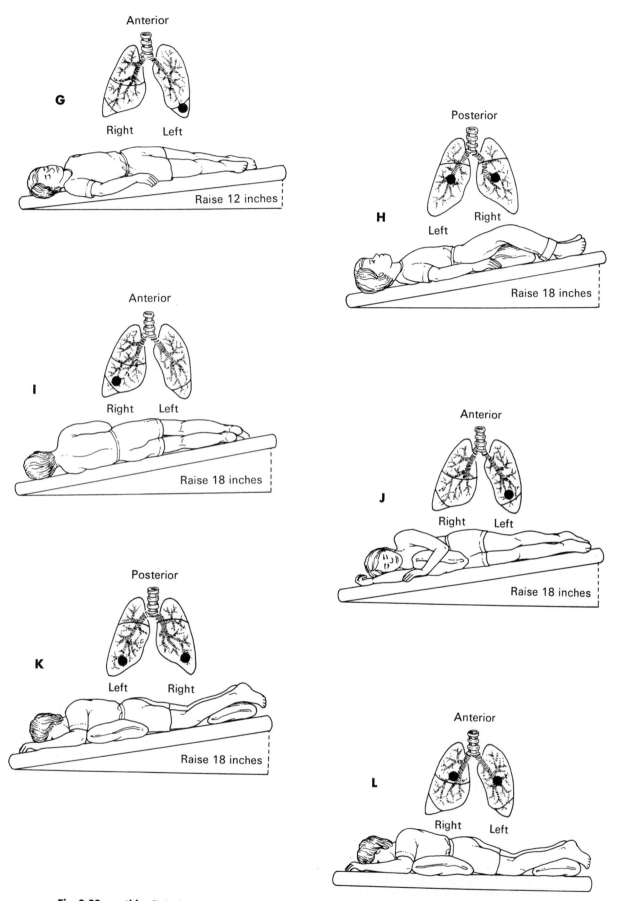

Fig. 8-32, cont'd **G,** Left lingula; lying on right side. **H,** Anterior segments; lying on back. **I,** Right lateral segment; lying on left side. **J,** Left lateral segment; lying on right side. **K,** Posterior segments; lying on stomach. **L,** Superior segments; lying on stomach. (From Thompson JM, McFarland GK, Hirsh JE et al, eds: *Mosby's clinical nursing,* ed 4, 1997, pp 201-202.)

or suction. Unfortunately, their use is limited in infants and children because of the smaller ETT size.

One factor contributing to suction-induced hypoxemia is the necessity of interrupting the patient's regular ventilatory cycle during the procedure. A *closed tracheal suction system* (CTSS), however, permits mechanical ventilation (including PEEP) to continue during suctioning.[68] One type of CTSS consists of a suction catheter in a plastic sheath that remains attached to the ventilator circuit with an adapter, a suction control device, and an irrigation port for tracheal lavage and rinsing of the catheter (Fig. 8-31). While stabilizing the adapter with one hand, the nurse uses the thumb and forefinger of the other hand to advance the catheter the desired depth into the ETT through the protective sheath; the procedure can easily be performed by one caregiver. Because the CTSS is left in place for 24 hours, suctioning can be accomplished quickly and immediately, without taking time to assemble supplies.[69] Hyperoxygenation, hyperinflation, and hyperventilation are still provided using the ventilator.[70] CTSS is reported to be as effective as conventional open suction techniques in maintaining oxygenation[71] and in clearing secretions,[72] and it may have added benefits of preventing nosocomial lower respiratory tract infections[73] and avoiding aerosolization of contaminated secretions.

Concerns about CTSS include decreased effectiveness of suctioning, excessive negative pressure, and autocontamination.[74] Because of the smaller ETTs used in the pediatric population, the concern over the accumulation of secretions within the ETT and its affect on internal ETT diameter, increased airway resistance, and impaired gas flow is of special concern. Glass, Grap, and Sessler[74] recently reported that ETTs in adult patients were markedly narrowed (mean internal diameter of 0.64 mm) by the buildup of secretions after CTSS.[74] The duration of intubation (not ETT size or amount of secretions) was associated with the degree of narrowing.

Suction catheters as small as 6 Fr are available. Mosca and colleagues[75] compared closed with open ETT suctioning in 11 preterm infants. Significant reductions in heart rate and Spo$_2$ were observed after open suctioning; the magnitude and duration of these negative effects were significantly reduced with closed suctioning.

Chest Physiotherapy

Chest physiotherapy (CPT) consists of many procedures, including postural drainage, percussion, vibration, and coughing. The goals of these interventions are to improve mucociliary clearance, to increase the volume of sputum expectorated, and to improve airway function.[76] Kirilloff and co-workers[77] reviewed the literature with regard to the efficacy of CPT in acute and chronic illness in adults. They concluded that CPT appeared beneficial in patients with large amounts of secretions and those with lobar atelectasis as well. Patients with chronic illnesses associated with increased mucous production (e.g., cystic fibrosis) clearly benefited from CPT. In contrast, CPT did not help patients in status asthmaticus and caused bronchospasm and hypoxemia in some acutely ill patients. The component activities of CPT were not uniformly associated with positive results. Postural drainage was usually effective, although directed coughing (teaching the patient cough techniques) may be as efficacious. No data have shown a beneficial effect of percussion or vibration. Because these studies were of adult patients, caution should be used in generalizing the results to infants and children. The mixed findings suggest, however, that CPT is not uniformly effective in pediatric disorders, and further research is certainly needed.[78]

Postural drainage uses gravity to move lung secretions from smaller peripheral lung segments into larger, more central airways where coughing or suctioning clears the secretions. A variety of positions are employed to drain different lung segments (Fig. 8-32). The chest x-ray film guides the intervention, and the patient is positioned to drain areas identified as needing improvement. The patient is kept in a position for 15 minutes or 5 minutes if combined with percussion and vibration. Patient tolerance often controls the variety of positions used during postural drainage. Also, several positions are contraindicated in some patients, for example, Trendelenburg in the cerebral hypertensive patient or in the patient with gastric reflux.

In conjunction with postural drainage, *chest percussion and vibration* help mobilize secretions from nondependent lung segments to central airways for removal. Chest percussion and vibration may improve the effectiveness of postural drainage. Percussion is performed using a cupped hand or percussion cup and rhythmically "clapping" the chest wall. Chest percussion is performed only over the rib cage and not over a bony prominence, for example, the clavicle, scapula, vertebrae, and sternum. Vibration is accomplished by shaking the chest on exhalation using the hands in tremorlike movements. Mechanical vibrators can be used in small infants. Gentle chest vibration is used apart from chest percussion in patients with thrombocytopenia or in those at risk for bone injuries or fractures, for example, patients with osteogenesis imperfecta. Both maneuvers are useful in conditions in which large amounts of sputum are produced, for example, cystic fibrosis, bronchiectasis, retained secretions, and lobar atelectasis.

Deep breathing and coughing are useful only in the alert cooperative patient. Games, such as bubble blowing and incentive spirometers, also increase the depth of inspiration in patients who may not take deep breaths on their own. Deep inspiration prevents atelectasis, promotes lung expansion, improves oxygenation, and provides an opportunity for patients to actively participate in their own care.[79] Forced exhalation helps to clear secretions. If patients are unable to cough spontaneously, naso-oropharyngeal or tracheal suctioning may be necessary to stimulate a cough to help remove mobilized pulmonary secretions.

Bronchial hygiene is not a benign procedure. The benefits of selected maneuvers—specifically, percussion and postural drainage—have been challenged.[80] Transient, yet significant, decreases in Pao$_2$ may follow chest physiotherapy. Also, the presence of a focal abscess theoretically presents a risk to the contralateral lung for contamination during postural drainage.[39] Individualized care is warranted.

Box 8-4

✦ **Troubleshooting Triple-Chamber Chest Tube Drainage Systems**

Drainage tubing: Tight connections; no kinks, compressions, or dependent loops
Fluid-filled dependent loop or kink impedes drainage:
Straighten tubing and anchor to the bed linen
Collection chamber: Positioned below the patient's chest; assess volume and character of drainage
No change in drainage:
None if drainage is stopped
Check for patency of tubing
Consider milking chest tube if obvious clots are present
Large volume of drainage accumulated in a short time:
Assess for signs and symptoms of hypovolemia—report drainage
Collection chamber is full:
Change the unit—once prepared, switch units without clamping chest tube
Water-seal chamber: Filled to appropriate level; bubbling present; fluctuations if to gravity
Water seal is underfilled (so no effective seal is present):
Fill the water seal to the 2-cm level with sterile water or saline
Water seal is overfilled (creating more resistance for air escape from the pleural space):
Using the self-sealing diaphragm, remove enough fluid to return the water seal to 2 cm
Continuous bubbling in the water-seal chamber (air leak between the patient and system):
Locate the source by systemically and momentarily clamping the system from the chest wall to unit
Bubbling will stop when a clamp is placed between the air leak and unit
If the bubbling never stops, the unit may be cracked, so change the unit

Tighten/reband loose connections
Report if new bubbling occurs
Intermittent bubbling in water-seal chamber:
Expect bubbling when suction first applied
Patient may have a small air leak
No fluctuations or bubbling in the water-seal chamber of a patient with gravity drainage, and the solution has crept up to a fixed position:
Lung has reexpanded—expect equal breath sounds and easy respirations
Tubing is obstructed—check for dependent loops or kinks
Large fluctuations in the water-seal chamber of a patient with gravity drainage:
High intrapleural negative pressure on inspiration indicative of increased work of breathing
Suction control chamber: Filled to appropriate level; gentle continuous bubbling; if suction is off, tubing detracted from suction source and open to air
Suction control chamber is underfilled to prescribed level:
Fill to prescribed level with sterile water or saline, then turn on the suction until gentle bubbling occurs
Suction control chamber is overfilled from prescribed level:
Using the self-sealing diaphragm, remove enough fluid to obtain the prescribed level, then turn on the suction until gentle bubbling occurs
Bubbling in the suction control chamber is too vigorous:
Wall suction is set higher than needed—turn down
No bubbling in the suction control chamber
Reconnect wall suction
Turn up wall suction until gentle bubbling occurs

Data from Erickson RS: Mastering the ins and outs of chest drainage, part 1, *Nursing 89* May, 37-43; Part 2, June, 46-49, 1989.

Chest Tubes

The primary purpose of a chest tube is to reestablish full expansion of the lung and evacuate air, fluid, or blood from the pleural space as rapidly and simply as possible. Chest tubes vary in size from 10 to 36 Fr and 10 to 18 inches long, and they consist of vinyl, silicone, or latex nonthrombogenic material. The distal end that sits within the pleura has a number of drainage holes to prevent occlusion; the proximal end is connected to the chest drainage system.

Chest tubes are inserted at the bedside under sterile conditions and while the patient is under local anesthesia. The insertion site depends on the problem. A chest tube inserted for a pneumothorax is placed at the second intercostal space at the midclavicular line because air will rise to the apex. Alternative sites, especially in female patients, include a more lateral position in the third to fifth intercostal space with the chest tube threaded up into the apex. A chest tube inserted for any type of fluid collection is placed at the fifth to seventh intercostal space at the midaxillary line because gravity will pool fluid to the base

of the lung. Once in place, the chest tube is sutured to the skin to prevent displacement and taped to prevent lateral movement. An occlusive dressing consisting of petrolatum gauge and a dry, sterile, split gauze is applied. Placement is confirmed on chest x-ray film.

The chest drainage system removes air or fluid from the pleural space and prevents the backflow of air and fluid into the pleural space. All connection points are banded to ensure that the system remains airtight. Chest tube milking or stripping is not advised because transient high negative pressures cause patient discomfort, inflict tissue trauma, and may cause bleeding. Special circumstances may necessitate chest tube stripping; for example, to keep a chest tube patent in a patient who is hemorrhaging while blood component therapy is administered to enhance patient clotting. Clamping chest tubes is also not advised. Once clamped, trapped air and fluid accumulate in the pleural space, and a tension pneumothorax may result. If clamping is necessary to precisely identify the location of an air leak, clamps are left on only for several breaths per test site location.

TABLE 8-14 Drugs Used for Aerosol Therapy

Drug	Dose	Peak Onset Duration	Comments
β-Sympathomimetic (Side effects common to class include muscle tremor, tachycardia, hypokalemia, dysrhythmia, hypertension, anxiety, headache, and dizziness)			
Albuterol (Proventil 5%, Ventolin)	0.25-0.5 ml in 2.5 ml* Continuous nebulization: 0.3 mg/kg/hr to a maximum of 15 mg/hr	0.5-1 hr 6-8 hr	Bronchodilation β_2-Selective
Isoetharine (Bronkosol 1%)	0.2-0.5 ml in 2.5 ml*	15-60 min 1-2 hr	Bronchodilation Less cardiac effect than isoproterenol
Metaproterenol (Alupent 5%)	0.1-0.3 ml in 2.5 ml*	0.5-1 hr 4-6 hr	Bronchodilation Less cardiac effect than isoproterenol
Terbutaline (Brethine 1 mg/ 1 ml)	0.25 mg in 2 ml* Continuous nebulization: 0.3 mg/kg/hr to a maximum of 15 mg/hr	5-20 min 6-8 hr	Bronchodilation β_2-Selective
α-Sympathomimetic			
Racemic epinephrine (Micronefrin, Vaponefrin)	0.25-0.5 ml in 2.5 ml*	2-4 min 1-2 hr	Reduces mucosal swelling by vasoconstriction
Parasympathomimetic			
Atropine	0.05 mg/kg (max 2.5 mg)	1 hr 3-4 hr	Synergistic with β_2-agents; more effective in large airway bronchospasm; may cause mucous plugging, tachycardia, hypertension
Ipratropium (Atrovent)	0.25-1 mg	1.5 hr 6 hr	
Mucolytic			
Acetylcysteine (Mucomyst 20%)	1-2 ml in 2.5 ml* q6h		Enhanced mobilization of secretions Foul smelling—may cause nausea May cause bronchospasm—administer with a bronchodilator
Antimicrobial			
Gentamicin	20-125 mg in 4 ml*; twice daily		Gram-negative bacteria
Tobramycin	80-240 mg in 4 ml*; twice daily		Cystic fibrosis; use preservative-free solution
Ribavirin	Nonintubated: 2 g in 33 ml* over 2 hours, 3 times/day for 3-5 days Intubated: 6 g in 100 ml* over 16 hours for 3-5 days		Respiratory syncytial virus Caregiver precautions are essential
Pentamidine	300 mg in 6 ml* (daily for treatment; monthly for prophylaxis)		Prophylaxis against *Pneumocystis carinii* Caregiver precautions are essential

Data from Lough M: Medicated aerosol therapy. In Blummer JL, ed: *A practical guide to pediatric intensive care,* St Louis, 1990, Mosby, pp 978-980.
*Normal saline is used as the diluent.

Closed chest tube drainage systems use gravity or suction to restore intrapleural negative pressure. Chest tubes are connected to an underwater seal drainage system so that air can only escape from and not enter the pleural space. A Heimlich flutter valve or bottle of saline can be used as a temporary measure until a chest tube drainage system is available. The early bottle systems have been replaced by disposable triple-chamber chest drainage systems. Basic principles are exactly the same whatever system is used.

The triple-chamber systems consist of (1) a drainage collection chamber connected to (2) a water-seal chamber connected to (3) a vacuum-control chamber. All three are positioned side by side in a molded plastic disposable unit. Step-by-step instructions for setting up these disposable systems vary and are included in the package inset or printed on the unit itself. The units can be hung below the level of the chest on the crib using the attached hanger hooks or are positioned on the floor using the built-in stand.

The first chamber is graduated so that chest drainage can be accurately measured. The second chamber (directly connected to the first) provides the water-seal chamber that prevents air from reentering the chest. When the system is placed on gravity drainage, respiratory fluctuations in the water-seal chamber reflect normal fluctuations in intrapleural pressure and thus indicate an intact system. Bubbling in this chamber indicates a air leak within the system. When all connection points are occlusive, the air leak can come only from the patient. To verify the source of an air leak, the chest tube and connecting tubes are systemically clamped at various levels. Once a clamp is located between the air leak and the water seal, the bubbling will stop. The third chamber controls the amount of suction applied to the chest tube when wall suction is connected to the system. Suction is necessary for rapid pulmonary reexpansion. The fluid level within the unit determines the amount of suction applied to the chest tube; usually a negative 15 to 20 cm H_2O is adequate. Wall suction is adjusted to produce continuous bubbling within the suction chamber. Turning up the wall suction only causes more bubbling within the suction chamber as more air is pulled into the system. Vigorous bubbling creates more noise that can be distracting to the patient and hastens fluid evaporation. Safety features vary but usually include both high negativity and positive pressure release valves. See Box 8-4 for troubleshooting triple-chamber chest drainage systems.

Removal of a chest tube is performed when the lung has reexpanded, the air leak has resolved, and drainage has ceased. After providing adequate analgesia, stay sutures are removed, and the chest tube is pulled on exhalation. An occlusive dressing consisting of petrolatum gauge and a dry, sterile gauze is then applied.

Inhaled Medications

Inhalation is commonly the most optimal method of delivery of medications into the respiratory tract. Aerosolization of medication is often better-tolerated, safer, and more effective than systemic administration. Aerosols consist of particulate water suspended in gas. Theoretically, the smaller the size of the aerosol particle, the more distal the particles are deposited into the bronchial tree. Airway resistance and breathing pattern also influence the amount of medication reaching the airways.[81] In the adult population, approximately 10% of nebulized medication reaches the lung periphery in nonintubated patients,[82] whereas 1.2% to 4.8% of the nebulized medication reaches the lung periphery in intubated patients.[83]

A small-volume nebulizer (SVN) is commonly used to aerosolize medications. Particles are generated by passage of a high-velocity gas stream (usually oxygen) across a tube, creating a Bernoulli effect; the medication is pulled from the reservoir and becomes nebulized. A baffle in front of the gas stream removes larger particles, returning them for renebulization, while smaller particles (1 to 5 μm in diameter) are delivered to the patient's airway. Flow rates of 6 to 8 L/min are necessary to achieve an adequate particle size to reach the conducting airways. If possible, the patient is instructed to take slow, deep breaths through the mouth and hold at end inspiration.[84]

Ultrasonic nebulizers generate ultrasonic sound waves directed at the air-liquid surface, producing a cloud of fine particles whose diameter varies depending on the frequency of the sound used. The small-particle aerosol generator (SPAG) unit is a pneumatically operated nebulizer used for ribavirin therapy. Aerosol therapy for the intubated patient is accomplished by either hand bagging the medication or by placing the nebulizer in the ventilator circuit.[85]

Table 8-14 lists some of the more common agents used for nebulization. Clinical responses to aerosol therapy are closely assessed because of the varying amount of medication reaching the distal airways. Because of variable delivery, optimal dosages are determined by the clinical responsiveness of the individual patient. An important note is that aerosol therapy also delivers free water to the patient and a mode of bacterial transmission to the lower respiratory tract.

Bronchodilators, affecting sympathetic and parasympathetic airway receptors, are by far the most common. Inhaled sympathetic agents stimulate β2-receptors producing bronchodilation. In addition, sympathomimetics inhibit mast cell degranulation, reduce mucous gland secretion, augment mucociliary clearance, and improve respiratory muscle contractility. Sympathomimetics vary in their peak onset and duration of action. Newer agents are β2-selective, limiting β1 cardiovascular side effects. Continuous nebulized bronchodilator therapy is popular in the ICU setting.[86] Continuous nebulization of albuterol[87] and terbutaline[88] is safe, provides more rapid clinical improvement, and is cost effective.

MECHANICAL SUPPORT OF VENTILATION

The primary objective of mechanical ventilation is to improve the balance of ventilation to perfusion, the most common cause of impairment of oxygenation and CO_2 removal.[89] In the presence of disease, ventilation often exceeds the level of perfusion (high $\dot{V}/\dot{Q}$), or perfusion may exceed the level of ventilation (low $\dot{V}/\dot{Q}$). Overventilation results in dead space ventilation (wasted ventilation) and an increased $Paco_2$. On the other hand, underventilation results in a physiologic shunt and a decreased Pao_2. When mechanical ventilation is instituted, perfusion to well-ventilated regions may decrease from the effects of positive pressure, which may necessitate delivery of larger than physiologic minute volumes to maintain an acceptable $Paco_2$. Any ventilator maneuver that has the potential to increase intrathoracic pressure may impair cardiac output and tissue perfusion and ultimately impair cellular gas exchange. Fig. 8-33 summarizes the physiologic differences in thoracic pressure under conditions of spontaneous versus positive pressure ventilation.

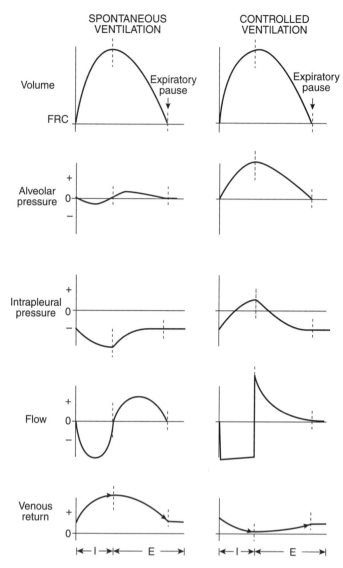

Fig. 8-33 Physiologic differences in thoracic pressures under conditions of spontaneous versus positive pressure ventilation. *FRC,* Functional residual capacity; *I,* inspiration; *E,* expiration; *flow,* pulmonary blood flow. (From Dupuis YG: *Ventilators: theory and clinical application,* ed 2, St Louis, 1992, Mosby.)

Managing the pediatric patient supported on mechanical ventilation presents a particular challenge because this group of patients require a wide variety of interventions that technology can now offer. To uniquely separate pediatric mechanical ventilation from that of neonates and adults is difficult because the practical applications are similar. What is essential to safe and effective ventilation of this population is knowledge of time constants, $\dot{V}/\dot{Q}$ relationships, and ventilator options and strategies. Having previously discussed time constants and $\dot{V}/\dot{Q}$ relationships, this section discusses ventilator options and strategies in terms relevant to the pediatric patient.

Indications for Initiating Assisted Ventilation

The indications for mechanical ventilation in the pediatric population are mainly subjective. The younger the patient, the more subjective the indications become. Standard spirometry is seldom used in pediatrics as an indication for mechanical ventilation. Vital capacity requires an alert and cooperative patient not affected by pain, characteristics rarely found in critically ill patients under 6 years of age. Muscle function, chest wall disorders, and parenchymal disease affect vital capacity. Acute muscle weakness only slightly affects vital capacity.

Physiologic measurements define respiratory or ventilatory failure. Respiratory failure is described as Pao_2/Fio_2 ratio less than 200. Ventilatory failure is described as an acutely elevated or rising $Paco_2$ greater than 60 mmHg with respiratory acidosis. Other physiologic parameters include increased work of breathing, which is described as a respiratory rate twice baseline with the use of accessory muscles.

Types of Ventilators

Technologic advances continue to provide numerous options to support the patient in acute respiratory failure. Ventilators are described according to which ventilation variable is controlled in the inspiratory phase of each cycle.[90]

Pressure Controlled. Most infant ventilators are pressure controlled so that peak pressure remains constant, but tidal volumes change as compliance and resistance vary. A continuous gas flow provides the patient a source of fresh gas for spontaneous breathing. Infants weighing less than 10 kg often receive ventilation from pressure-limited time-cycled ventilators.

Volume Controlled. Most adult ventilators are designed to deliver a preset tidal volume. Flow is the variable controlled by the ventilator to deliver a consistent volume. Because flow and volume are functions of each other, these machines are called volume controllers. Airway pressure varies with resistance and compliance during a volume-controlled breath.

Pressure Controlled and Volume Controlled. The newest generation of ventilators offer several modes in which pressure or volume can be the control variable. It is the actual operational mode that is most relevant to clinical management because it best describes the interaction between patient and machine.

Modes of Ventilation

Pressure, volume, flow, and time are used as phase variables that determine the parameters for each ventilatory cycle.[90] The *trigger* variable describes the variable used to initiate inspiration. The *limit* variable describes the variable in which a preset value cannot be exceeded during inspiration. The *cycle* variable describes the variable used to end inspiration. *Baseline* variables describe the variables that are controlled during expiration. Combinations of these four phase variables describe the various modes of ventilation.

TABLE 8-15   Indications and Special Considerations for Commonly Used Ventilator Modes

Mode	Indications	Special Considerations
Controlled ventilation (CV)	Chest wall instability Central nervous system dysfunction Respiratory muscle paralysis	Dynamic patient needs not accounted for Respiratory muscle inactivity leads to muscle atrophy
SIMV pressure controlled	Infants approximately less than 10 kg where pressure is desired control variable	V_T will vary with patient compliance and resistance V_T delivery may be limited in larger patients Continuous flow available for spontaneous breaths
SIMV volume controlled	Older infants or where volume is the desired control variable	The smaller the patient, the more relative V_T lost to the compressible volume of the ventilator tubing V_T may vary in presence of ETT leaks and changes in compliance and resistance Demand valve spontaneous flow systems may have poor response to high respiratory rates. Addition of continuous flow (2-5 L/min) may help
Pressure control ventilation (PCV)	Patients with low compliance or high resistance states ARDS Unilateral lung disease Large ETT leaks	V_T should be closely monitored PIP should be lower than in volume-limited modes Mean airway pressure may be higher than in volume-limited modes
Pressure support ventilation (PSV)	Failure to wean Muscle reconditioning Asynchrony	Backup SIMV rate may be provided Patients with ETT less than 4 mm may prematurely cycle breath Patients with large ETT leaks may not cycle off breath appropriately Patient must be able to trigger pressure support (PS) breath with ease
Flow synchronization PSV	Weaning Muscle conditioning Asynchrony	Patient triggered Premature termination prevented with ETT less then 4 mm Patients with large leaks may not cycle off breath
Continuous positive airway pressure (CPAP)	Conditions with decreased functional residual capacity	Should provide continuous flow Patient must be spontaneously breathing

ETT, Endotracheal tube; *ARDS*, adult respiratory distress syndrome; V_T, tidal volume; *SIMV*, synchronized intermittent mandatory ventilation; *PIP*, peak inspiratory pressure.

The major indications and special considerations for commonly used ventilator modes are summarized in Table 8-15.

Controlled Ventilation. Controlled ventilation (CV) generally refers to a volume-controlled mode whereby all breaths are determined by the preset machine parameters and are completely independent of the patient's respiratory efforts or breathing pattern. This mode is poorly tolerated in spontaneously breathing patients and offers no benefit over other modes that allow the patient to initiate a ventilator breath on demand or to breathe in between mechanical breaths. This mode of ventilation is used in chemically paralyzed patients when spontaneous breathing can be potentially detrimental, for example, in the patient with a flail chest.

Intermittent Mandatory Ventilation. Intermittent mandatory ventilation (IMV) allows a patient to breathe spontaneously from a continuous flow or demand valve in between preset mandatory breaths that are either pressure controlled or volume controlled. The patient is thereby able to breathe at his or her own rate and comfort level. $\dot{V}/\dot{Q}$ matching is mixed because the spontaneous breaths result in increased ventilation to dependent lung regions, whereas the mechanical breaths result in increased ventilation to nondependent lung regions. This mode is thought to be beneficial for weaning because the patient is able to maintain the use of his or her respiratory muscles and provide increasing spontaneous support as the IMV or mandatory rate is gradually decreased. The clinician should be aware that the work of breathing may increase as the patient assumes responsibility for more of the ventilatory load.

Synchronized IMV. The synchronized IMV (SIMV) mode, as with IMV, offers preset mandatory breaths but synchronizes these breaths with a patient effort that is generally detected by a circuit change in pressure or flow. The theoretical advantages are that the patient will not have a mechanical breath superimposed on a spontaneous one and that patient's work will be more synchronous.

Pressure Control Ventilation. Pressure control ventilation (PCV) is a mode that is comparable with pressure-controlled SIMV, in that a preset pressure is reached with every breath. However, in PCV a very high initial flow rate allows an almost immediate rise to the preset PIP. This PIP is then sustained throughout the preset inspiratory time. One theoretical advantage of this mode is that gas distribution is enhanced during the sustained PIP plateau.

Pressure Support Ventilation. The pressure support ventilation (PSV) mode of mechanical ventilation augments only the patient's spontaneous efforts with a preset level of airway pressure. In PSV, the inspiratory pressure plateau is reached early in inspiration and is maintained until inspiratory flow decreases to approximately 25% (may be clinician set) of initial peak flow. At this point, inspiration ends, affording the patient control of inspiration and expiration. PSV can be used alone or in conjunction with a mandatory mode, such as SIMV and PCV. Pressures of 5 to 30 cm H_2O are typically set; pressures of 5 to 15 cm H_2O are ideal. V_T can be variable as the patient's pulmonary mechanics change.

The pediatric patient unable to tolerate weaning will demonstrate decreased spontaneous tidal volumes leading to atelectasis, increased work of breathing, and an increased respiratory rate. In such patients, PSV may reverse this spiral and decrease patient work. Although the benefits of PSV are untested in pediatrics, the authors have found this mode to be useful in achieving patient comfort during a protracted weaning process. Generally, the authors judge PSV to be beneficial if the patient's respiratory rate drops and work of breathing decreases.

A few unique problems are encountered when PSV is used in infants and small children. First, the increased airway resistance posed by smaller ETTs (less than 4 mm) may precipitate premature termination of PSV; that is, inspiration ends because of the high resistance created by the airway and not because of the patient's respiratory effort. This will reduce the effectiveness of PSV in augmenting V_T. Modern ventilators allow adjustments to the inspiratory flow or rise time to help prevent this termination. Second, if a significant ETT or TT air leak is present, the ventilator may be unable to sense the decrease in flow that normally occurs at end inspiration. When this happens, the patient loses control over end inspiration because the ventilator automatically uses a built-in time limit to end inspiration.

Flow-Synchronized Pressure Support Ventilation. Microprocessors and the evolution of sensor technology have made possible patient-synchronized ventilation in infants and small children. A number of systems are available that allow the patient's spontaneous breathing effort to trigger positive pressure breaths.

Ventilator breaths can be triggered by a drop in patient airway pressure, the detection of a set inspiratory volume, and even the chest or abdominal movement preceding a spontaneous breath. However, the measurement of inspiratory flow is one of the most sensitive methods of patient triggering. Flow triggering requires the use of a flow sensor to detect a spontaneous breathing effort. This sensor generates a flow signal that the ventilator uses to detect a spontaneous breath. A machine-assisted breath is initiated when the ventilator senses an inspiratory flow rate equal to the set trigger sensitivity.

The availability to patient-trigger ventilator breaths provides the option of two patient-triggered modes of mechanical ventilation—SIMV and assist/control (A/C). SIMV delivers a fixed number of mandatory breaths that are synchronized with the patient's spontaneous breathing efforts and allows unassisted spontaneous breathing between mandatory breaths. With A/C, every patient effort that meets the trigger sensitivity criteria initiates a machine-assisted breath.

Although the term *flow synchronization* has generally been applied to the use of flow to trigger ventilator breaths, the inspiratory flow signal can also be used to cycle (terminate) the inspiratory phase of ventilator breaths. The VIP Bird with flow synchronization uses the inspiratory flow signal to both trigger and cycle ventilator breaths. With flow cycling, the inspiratory phase is terminated when the inspiratory flow rate falls to a preset percentage of the peak inspiratory flow rate for that breath. Thus ventilator rate and inspiratory time are primarily a function of the patient's ventilatory drive and respiratory mechanics. However, manipulating the flow cycling threshold, which is adjustable from 5% to 25% of peak flow rate, can also influence inspiratory time. The ability to flow trigger and flow cycle provides a high level of patient regulation of ventilation.

The potential benefits of flow-synchronized ventilation (and patient-synchronized ventilation in general) include enhanced gas exchange (particularly oxygenation), decreased incidence of barotrauma, decreased incidence of intraventricular hemorrhage, decreased need for heavy sedation and paralysis, and a decrease in the duration of mechanical ventilation.

Continuous Positive Airway Pressure. CPAP is a spontaneous mode that provides a constant preset distending pressure. This constant pressure increases FRC and prevents atelectasis. Increased lung volume increases pulmonary compliance and thus decreases the work of breathing. Low levels of CPAP are considered "physiologic" whenever the upper airway is bypassed with an ETT or TT. When these low levels—for example, a CPAP of 3 to 5 cm H_2O—are reached, extubation is usually considered. On CPAP, the resistance imposed by smaller pediatric ETTs may result in a higher work of breathing than the patient might experience extubated. Therefore it is common to extubate from low rates of 4 or 6 breaths per minute.

Pressure-Controlled Inverse Ratio Ventilation. This mode of ventilation describes the delivery of volume at a preset PIP, whereby the time spent in inspiration exceeds that of expiration. In pressure-controlled inverse ratio ventilation (PCIRV), PIPs are reached early in inspiration, creating a decelerating flow wave pattern and square pressure wave pattern. V_T depends on inspiratory time, PIP, and the patient's pulmonary mechanics. The square pressure plateau wave facilitates alveolar recruitment and allows a more even distribution of gases within the lung in patients with nonhomogeneous lung disease.[91] Prolonged inspiratory times allow higher mean airway pressures (MAPs) while limiting PIPs and PEEPs and maintaining Pao_2. Shorter expiratory times deter alveoli from falling below their closing capacity.

Patients supported on PCIRV require nursing assessment of alterations in cardiac output and pulmonary barotrauma occurring secondary to an inadequate expiratory phase, hyperinflation, and the development of auto-PEEP.[92] The altered breathing pattern may also give patients a feeling of fullness that can be uncomfortable, making them anxious and restless, increasing their work of breathing and increasing $\dot{V}o_2$.[93] Analgesia, sedation, and chemical paralysis are required for patient comfort and compliance.

Airway Pressure Release Ventilation. In this mode of ventilation, the patient breathes spontaneously at a positive baseline (CPAP). Periodically, this baseline is released to a lower pressure level for 1 to 2 seconds, allowing CO_2 to be exhaled. Airway pressure release ventilation (APRV) is an alternative mode to improve oxygenation with lower mean airway pressures.

Mandatory Minute Ventilation. Mandatory minute ventilation (MMV) is a mode of computer-generated ventilation that ensures the delivery of a predetermined minute ventilation distributed between spontaneous and ventilator breaths. If the patient's $\dot{V}_E$ is calculated to be low, additional breaths are delivered to the patient. One disadvantage of this mode is that the quality of the patient's spontaneous breaths is not considered. A rapid, shallow pattern is not distinguished from a slow, deep pattern because the $\dot{V}_E$ is the same. Altered respiratory patterns can lead to acid-base disturbances and atelectasis.[94]

Ventilation Parameters

Tidal Volume. In a volume-limited mode, V_T is set directly in cubic centimeters (cc). In a pressure-limited mode, V_T is determined by the difference between PIP and PEEP; this is referred to as delta P ($\Delta P = PIP - PEEP$).

Frequency. Frequency (F) is the ventilator rate adjustable in breaths per minute.

Inspiratory Time. Inspiratory time (Ti) together with F determines the I:E ratio. Prolonging Ti generally improves oxygenation by increasing the time the alveoli remain distended participating in gas exchange. Faster Ti and longer expiratory times are used to prevent hyperinflation in patients with airways disease. Some ventilators offer an inspiratory hold or pause that prolongs Ti.

Positive End-Expiratory Pressure. PEEP is the pressure that is sustained at the end of expiration. PEEP improves oxygenation by increasing FRC, preventing alveolar collapse, and enhancing the ratio of ventilation to perfusion. Excessive levels of PEEP cause hyperinflation

and CO_2 retention by adding unnecessary dead space. Excessive PEEP also impedes venous return to the chest, which will eventually decrease the patient's cardiac output and oxygen delivery.

Peak Inspiratory Pressure. PIP is the pressure that is reached and sustained during inspiration. PIP is directly adjusted in the pressure-limited modes but varies with compliance and resistance in the volume-limited modes.

Mean Airway Pressure. Measured in cm H_2O, MAP is the average airway pressure over a respiratory cycle.[95] Factors that increase MAP during pressure-controlled ventilation include increased inspiratory flow, increased PIP, increased Ti, increased PEEP, and increased F. MAPs over 12 cm H_2O are considered significant. This parameter is a monitored value on most ventilators.

Fraction of Inspired Oxygen. FIO_2 is the inspired oxygen concentration. FIO_2 levels less than 0.6 are generally considered safe.[91]

Flow Rate. Flow rate is the continuous flow of ventilator gas adjusted in liters per minute. Pressure-controlled ventilators require adequate flow rates for the delivery of PIP, for optimal V_T, and for a continuous source of gas for spontaneous breaths. Flow rates determine the time it takes to reach PIP during inspiration. When flow rates are low, PIP is reached at the end of inspiration, decreasing the plateau phase; if flow rates are high, PIP is reached early in inspiration, increasing the plateau phase.[91] The inspiratory plateau affects gas distribution; the longer the plateau, the better the distribution of gas throughout the lung (Fig. 8-34).

Alarm Systems. For patient safety, ventilator alarms remain activated within a tight range at all times. Most ventilators are equipped with an inspiratory line pressure alarm to detect a sudden loss in pressure (disconnect) and a sudden increase in pressure (obstruction). Other alarms include gas supply, FIO_2, gas humidity and temperature, and electricity failure. Ventilator alarms that allow a 10- to 15-second automatic reset are safer for the patient because the human factor is eliminated.

Initiation of Mechanical Ventilation

Before initiating mechanical ventilation, the clinician evaluates the patient's pulmonary mechanics by "feel" during manual hand ventilation using an anesthesia bag and attached manometer. Initial ventilator settings are then matched to those identified as optimal during hand ventilation.

An alternative strategy is to begin with the suggested ventilator settings listed in Table-8-16, which take into consideration anticipated time constants. Faster rates without stacking of breaths can be used in patients with lung disease states characterized by short time constants (lungs quickly fill and empty). Slower rates and longer expiratory times are used in patients with lung disease characterized by long time constants (lungs take a long time to fill and empty). Once the patient is receiving mechanical support, ventilator settings are fine-tuned within established ABG parameters and measured pulmonary mechanics.

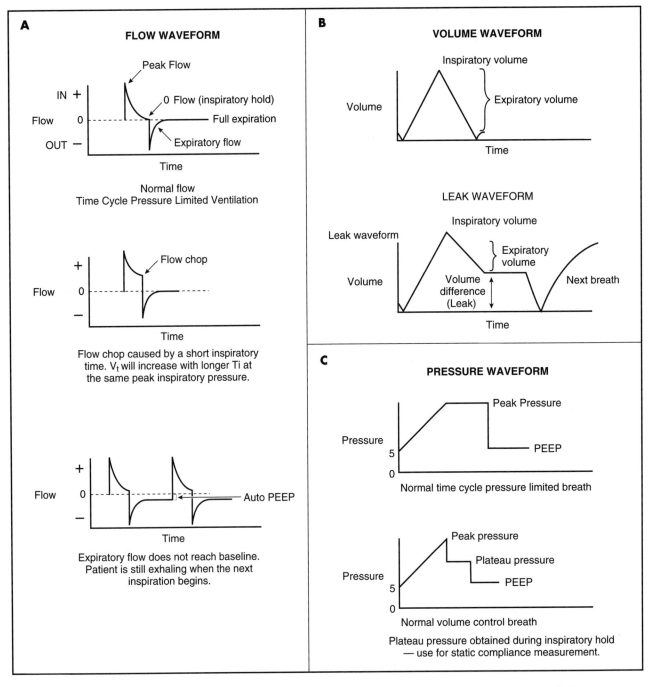

Fig. 8-34   Examples of **A,** flow waveform; **B,** volume waveform; **C,** pressure waveform. V_T, Tidal volume; *Ti*, inspiratory time; *PEEP*, positive end-expiratory pressure.

Ventilator Strategies

Mechanical ventilation has two goals: to maintain mean lung volume and to maintain alveolar ventilation. As mentioned, reduction in $\dot{V}/\dot{Q}$ imbalance must also be a consideration, and although ventilator manipulations may optimize ventilation, the $\dot{V}/\dot{Q}$ relationship is best viewed as a dynamic phenomenon. The clinician's challenge is to achieve acceptable minute ventilation with respect to perfusion in the presence of an adequate mean lung volume. Factors to assess on initiation of mechanical ventilation are

included in Box 8-5. Some newer ventilators have automated modes to initiate or wean the ventilator.

The Hamilton Galileo ventilator (Hamilton Medical Inc., Reno, Nev.) uses a complex algorithm to assess the patient's respiratory mechanics. The ventilator then chooses the amount of pressure support to achieve a clinician and ventilator set goal. This mode is a rules-based strategy called adaptive support ventilation (ASV). The Servo 300 (Siemens, Danvers, Mass.) has automode, which automatically switches the patient from a control mode to a

Table 8-16 Suggested Initial Ventilator Settings for Various Time Constants

Ventilator Setting	Long Time Constant	Normal Time Constant	Short Time Constant
V_T	8-10 ml/kg	6-10 ml/kg	6-8 ml/kg
F (breaths/min)	8-15	10-20	15-30
I:E ratio	>1:4	1:2	1:1
PEEP	0-5	3-5	>5

V_T, Tidal volume; *F*, frequency; *I:E*, inspiratory/expiratory; *PEEP*, positive end-expiratory pressure.

Box 8-5

Factors to Assess on Initiation of Mechanical Ventilation

1. Baseline breath sounds (quality, adequate expiratory time)
2. Decreased work of breathing (decreased respiratory rate, severity of retractions, nasal flaring, grunting, etc.)
3. Chest excursion and symmetry
4. Chest x-ray film (ETT position, improved lung volume, pathologic condition)
5. Pulmonary mechanics (decreased airways resistance, increased compliance, and FRC [time constants, auto-PEEP])
6. Arterial blood gases (improved oxygenation, decreased $Paco_2$, and improved pH)
7. Need for noninvasive monitoring
8. Need for muscle relaxants, sedation (chemical restraint)
9. Need for pulmonary hygiene
10. Need for aerosolized or systemic bronchodilator therapy

spontaneous mode when the ventilator senses a patient's spontaneous breath. These modes continue to grow in popularity, but little pediatric data exists.

Making the Right Maneuver

Paco₂. $Paco_2$ is inversely related to minute ventilation ($\dot{V}_E$) ($\dot{V}_E = V_T \times F$). A portion of V_T is composed of dead space volume (V_D) and therefore will not participate in gas exchange. V_D is related to body surface area and normally accounts for 30% of V_T. In patients supported on mechanical ventilation, V_D may be as high as 50% to 60% from the effects of positive pressure on the airways. Accordingly, changes in ventilator parameters can alter V_D. Any tubing or adapters distal to the patient ventilator will add mechanical dead space because this volume acts as an extension of the patient's airway. Mechanical V_D should be kept to a minimum.

Pao₂. The most basic control of Pao_2 is Fio_2. The relationship between Fio_2 and Pao_2 is not as straightforward as that between $Paco_2$ and $\dot{V}_E$. This is due to the effects of water vapor pressure in the lung and oxygen diffusibility relative to the (diseased) alveolar-pulmonary capillary

membrane. The degree and pattern of ventilation and $\dot{V}/\dot{Q}$ ratio also affect Pao_2. The MAP is a very useful index of the overall effect of changes in ventilation variables and is directly related to Pao_2. Any maneuver that alters MAP has the potential to change Pao_2. The five factors that affect the MAP include (1) PIP, (2) PEEP, (3) inspiratory time, (4) inspiratory flow, and (5) increased respiratory rate with same inspiratory time. Optimal MAP is found when gas exchange is efficient and beyond which alveolar overdistension occurs.[96]

Chest X-ray Film. In general, there should be radiologic evidence of improved lung volume. The ninth anterior rib above the dome of the diaphragm evidences adequate lung volume, although aeration is relative to surrounding structures. Assuming the film is taken during inspiration, the diaphragm should be neither elevated nor flattened. Hypoaeration is managed by increasing PEEP or Ti.

Auto-PEEP. In situations in which the F is high or the patient has long time constants, the clinician should check for the presence of auto-PEEP or intrinsic PEEP. Auto-PEEP refers to the spontaneous development of PEEP at the alveolar level as a result of insufficient expiratory time.[97] Auto-PEEP can be detected in a noncontinuous flow ventilator system and is checked by occluding the expiratory limb of the ventilator at end expiration. If auto-PEEP is present, the baseline pressure (PEEP) will rise as expiratory flow continues from the patient. The level of auto-PEEP is clinically important because its presence may contribute to enhanced oxygenation or CO_2 retention. Although the presence of 1 to 3 cm H_2O of auto-PEEP may not be clinically deleterious, this number should be monitored in appropriate patients because it is a dynamic number (unlike set PEEP) and can change rapidly.

Blood Gas Monitoring. Whenever possible, ABGs should be obtained in the newly ventilated patient to assess for improved gas exchange. If arterial access is not immediately possible, a venous blood gas may be helpful in assessing acid-base status. Pulse oximeters continuously and noninvasively assess oxygenation. $ETco_2$ monitoring is useful; however, the presence of large ETT leaks can result in inaccurate low readings, and some monitors will not read accurately at high (>30) respiratory rates.

Bronchial Hygiene. Adequate suctioning is essential in the pediatric patient. Smaller ETT diameters predispose these patients to airway obstruction. The relative small size of the conducting airways places the child at increased risk for significant compromise from the effects of infection, edema, and secretions. Partial or complete obstruction of the bronchioles and bronchi can result in air trapping and atelectasis. What may seem like an insignificant amount of secretions may have a significant impact on airways resistance.

Sedation. Ensuring an adequate level of comfort for the patient receiving mechanical ventilation is fundamental to humane care. Artificial airways and imposed breaths are poorly tolerated by an alert child. Because of developmental immaturity, one cannot depend on patient cooperation. In fact, if a toddler, for example, cooperates with a stranger when the parents are not present, one would question the child's level of consciousness. In addition to parents, analgesics and sedatives are often used to help the patient tolerate both the ICU environment and the treatments involved. Chemical restraints should be used in combination with physical restraints. In assessing agitation, it is important to determine what comes first—hypoxia or agitation. A distressed intubated patient may be trying to indicate inadequate ventilator settings, an obstructed ETT, a pneumothorax, pain, or the need for a more quiet environment. The use of neuromuscular blocking agents may be indicated in the sedated patient in acute respiratory failure when ventilator support is escalating and the child is asynchronous with or fighting the ventilator. These agents are not used indiscriminately because they remove critically important assessment signs, such as activity and comfort levels.

Positioning. The supine position and the length of time an intubated patient is kept supine are potential risk factors for aspiration of gastric contents.[23,98] Unless contraindicated, all intubated patients should be positioned in a semirecumbent position.

Special Considerations in Ventilating Pediatric Patients

Endotracheal Tube Leaks. Because of the use of uncuffed ETTs in young children, leaks are often present and can compromise ventilation if they are excessive. An ETT leak detected above an inspiratory pressure of 20 cm H_2O is generally desirable because this may help reduce the occurrence of airway trauma and postextubation swelling, yet this may in turn limit the ability to deliver an adequate V_T in patients who require higher PIP. Very large ETT leaks may cause autotriggering of mechanical breaths on some ventilators where loss of PEEP may be sensed as the patient's inspiratory effort. It is therefore important to assess ETT leaks periodically by hand ventilating the patient with a manometer in-line to note at what pressure the leak begins. A volume-monitoring device can further quantify leaks. Many of the newest ventilators have the capability to measure volume at the patient airway, which can accurately quantify an ETT leak. Leaks are notoriously variable and can vary with ETT position, head position, and fluid balance. If a leak is thought to be compromising ventilation, reintubation may be necessary with a larger tube.

ETT Resistance. Reducing the diameter of a tube by one half results in a sixteenfold decrease in flow through that tube. The small ETT diameters used in children cause a substantial increase in flow resistance and therefore a significant increase in the work of breathing. For this reason, children are usually not extubated from ventilator rates less than 4 to 6 breaths/min. The work imposed by the pediatric ETT is often compared with "breathing through a straw." Attentiveness to this phenomenon is especially important in the child with a history of significant respiratory failure.

Compressible Volume. The compressible volume of a ventilator circuit refers to the amount of the tidal volume that is lost with each breath to displacement and compression of the volume of the ventilator tubing. This portion of the breath never enters the patient's lungs. Ventilator tubing has a measurable compliance or distensibility that can be used to distinguish the actual delivered tidal volume from the lost compressible volume. This is the compressible volume factor. The loss of compressible volume is particularly important in volume-limited ventilation when small tidal volumes are used. For example, in a situation in which tubing has a compressible volume factor of 3 ml/cm H_2O and peak inspiratory pressure is 40, the set tidal volume would be reduced by 120 ml (3×40). The loss of volume is quite relevant in pediatric mechanical ventilation because of the small volumes used. For instance, if a tidal volume of 200 ml were set in the previous situation, the delivered volume would be approximately 80 ml.

Ventilator Limitations. Infants and small children may have difficulty using the assist-control mode of ventilation because they need to inhale a greater proportion of their V_T before creating enough negative pressure to trigger the ventilator's sensing mechanism. Once triggered, the response time may be too slow to support the faster pediatric respiratory rate. An inadequate response time can lead to an increased work of breathing. A similar problem occurs during spontaneous ventilation; usually gas flow is delivered to the circuit when a demand valve is activated by negative airway pressure. This demand valve may be too difficult for the pediatric patient, so a continuous-flow reservoir is typically added to the circuit in patients weighing less than 15 kg. Providing a low level of added continuous flow may alleviate the problem, allowing the child to spontaneously breathe without triggering the demand valve system.

Volume Monitoring. Monitoring of V_T should be considered in the patient for whom one of the aforementioned variables might compromise the delivery of a consistent tidal volume. This may involve intermittent checks to note changes after setting changes or continuous monitoring in patients with large or variable ETT leaks. V_T monitoring is now easily accomplished with equipment specifically designed for the pediatric population, including Bournes Neonatal Volume Monitor-NVM (Bear Medical System, Riverside, Calif.), Bicore (Bear Medical System, Riverside, Calif.), Ventrak (Novametric Medical Systems, Wallingford, Conn.), and Partner IIi (Bird Medical Corp, Palm Springs, Calif.). Ventilator settings can be adjusted to deliver a specific V_T (ml/kg). A constant V_T will stabilize the FRC and allow immediate corrective action for acute changes. Computers, used in conjunction with volume monitors, allow calculation of respiratory mechanics, for example, compliance, resistance, time constants, work of breathing, flow/volume loops, and pressure/volume curve. Scalar tracings of flow, pressure, and volume of each breath allow bedside graphic interpretation (see Fig. 8-34).

Complications of Mechanical Ventilation

Rapid deterioration in the pediatric patient is often attributable to one of the factors listed in Box 8-6. The incidence of pneumothorax in pediatrics has been reported to be between 4.5% and 8% and in some studies has been correlated with

Box 8-6
Common Respiratory Causes of Rapid Clinical Deterioration

1. ETT position change
2. Large or positional ETT leak
3. Excessive secretions
4. Bronchospasm
5. Development of auto-PEEP
6. Pneumothorax

TABLE 8-17   Complications of Mechanical Ventilation

Air leak	Pneumothorax
	Pneumomediastinum
	Pneumopericardium
	Pneumoperitoneum
	Subcutaneous emphysema
Infection	Pneumonia
	Septicemia
Airway	Dislodgment
	Occlusion
	Accidental extubation
	Erosion
	Stenosis
Hyperinflation	Air trapping (auto-PEEP)
Cardiovascular	Decreased venous return
	Decreased cardiac output
	Increased pulmonary vascular resistance
Extrathoracic organs	Decreased urine output
	Increased antidiuretic hormone
	Decreased hepatic blood flow
	Increased intracranial pressure
Mechanical	Ventilator malfunction
	Disconnection

mortality.[44] Certainly, this complication must be recognized promptly and treated. In patients with reactive airways disease, sudden development of bronchospasm may occur in the absence of a precipitating event and result in significant compromise. As previously mentioned, auto-PEEP is a dynamic phenomenon that can have adverse effects and should be periodically checked if the clinical picture is suggestive of its presence. Acute ETT obstruction is common in pediatrics, and if it is suspected, the patient should be reintubated if an attempt to clear the tube is unsuccessful. The instrumented pediatric airway is difficult to maintain because of patient size and lack of cooperation. Slight changes in ETT position can result in right mainstem intubation or accidental extubation. Finally, an increasing ETT leak can occur from resolving airway edema or diuresis resulting in decreased $\dot{V}_E$ or failure to hold PEEP.

General complications of mechanical ventilation are listed in Table 8-17. The major side effects of CPAP and PEEP include hemodynamic complications and pulmonary barotrauma. Increased intrathoracic pressure leads to decreased systemic venous return resulting in decreased cardiac output. These hemodynamic effects can be easily monitored with a pulmonary artery catheter. Esophageal pressure monitoring can also approximate optimal levels of CPAP and PEEP. Esophageal pressure should increase slightly with each increase of CPAP and PEEP until optimal levels are reached. After that, esophageal pressures will increase exponentially with only slight increases in CPAP and PEEP. In addition to producing pulmonary barotrauma, overdistension increases V_D and results in a rising $Paco_2$. When faced with progressively worsening ABGs, one strategy is to cautiously decrease inflating pressures when the possibility of overinflation is present.

Guidelines for the Weaning Process

Weaning from mechanical ventilation accounts for approximately 40% of the time that critically ill children with respiratory failure are supported on mechanical ventilation.[99] Weaning patients from mechanical ventilation involves assessing the patient's readiness to wean, optimizing factors that can facilitate weaning, selecting the appropriate weaning method, and continually assessing the patient's progress.[100] Studies have shown that on average, objective measures based on frequent testing of the patient's ability to tolerate decreases in ventilator support result in earlier initiation of weaning.[101] For example, using a preweaning CPAP trial may help determine if a patient is ready for extubation, avoiding the weaning process altogether.

The picture of weaning readiness is a collective assessment of improving lung function; sepsis in control; decreasing heart rate, weight and central venous pressure (CVP); improving cardiovascular performance; good tissue perfusion; less noisy breathing; nutritional balance; and normal serum albumin and total calcium.[99] Patient response to weaning includes increasing respiratory rates, decreasing $Paco_2$, and increasing arterial pH.[99]

In the adolescent, adult criteria can be used as guidelines: a vital capacity of 15 to 20 ml/kg, negative inspiratory force (NIF) of −20 cm H_2O, tidal volume of 6 to 10 ml/kg, and a maximum voluntary ventilation (MVV) of greater than twice the minute ventilation.[102] For pediatric patients, the best indication for weaning is respiratory rate. Pediatric patients respond to respiratory compromise by decreasing tidal volume and increasing respiratory rate. During weaning, regardless of the strategy, the respiratory rate should be below 2 times the baseline.

The modes most commonly used to wean patients include CPAP, SIMV, and PSV. Mechanical support is gradually decreased one parameter at a time until a minimal amount of support is reached. Usually, the longer a patient has been supported on mechanical ventilation, the longer the weaning process. Because of respiratory muscle atrophy, a period of muscle reconditioning is required before extubation. This is accomplished by progressively exercising the respiratory muscles to rebuild endurance. Chronically ventilated patients are not weaned at night because adequate rest is critically important to success.

Starting with the most potentially toxic parameter, settings can be gradually weaned or the patient can be switched to PSV. Generally, Ti is returned to normal; the F_{IO_2} is decreased by 2% to 10% to maintain a Spo_2 greater than 90%; PIPs are decreased by 2 to 5 cm H_2O to the low 20s to maintain V_T in the 5 to 7 ml/kg range; PEEP is decreased to 3 to 5 cm H_2O, provided that oxygenation is adequate on low F_{IO_2}; and rate is decreased by 1 to 2 breaths slowly over hours to days (depending on tolerance) to maintain a $Paco_2$ within normal limits for the patient and to allow spontaneous breaths without excessive work of breathing.

When ventilatory rates are weaned to a low rate of 6 breaths per minute in an infant or 4 breaths/min in a child, or successful trial of 3 to 5 cm H_2O of CPAP has been accomplished, extubation is considered if criteria are reached—that is, good gases on an F_{IO_2} less than 0.5, adequate cough and gag, and thin or moderate consistency in the character of secretions. Note that infants are extubated from higher rates because of the increased airways resistance created by the smaller ETT.

The major benefit of PSV is that it reestablishes the patient's control over breathing, improves patient-ventilator synchrony, decreases diaphragmatic muscle fatigue, and reduces the work of breathing. PSV eliminates the shallow ineffective spontaneous V_T associated with progressive tachypnea and atelectasis that may occur during more traditional weaning methods.

Curley and Fackler[99] identified three patterns of progress when weaning pediatric patients with acute respiratory failure from mechanical ventilation—specifically, the sprint, consistent, and inconsistent patterns: the sprint subset, weaned in 1 day; the consistent subset, weaned every day; and the inconsistent subset, did not wean every day. Patients at risk for inconsistent weaning are those admitted with a sepsis/shock ARDS trigger; those discharged with more functional disability; and those who experienced more days of mechanical ventilation and had a higher oxygenation index during weaning.

Although no pediatric protocols currently exist, Kollef and colleagues[103] showed that protocol-directed weaning from mechanical ventilation, performed by nurses and respiratory therapists, was safe and resulted in shorter duration of mechanical ventilation when compared with a traditional practice of physician-directed weaning. Protocol-directed weaning resulted in the earlier initiation of weaning and more rapid progression of weaning to extubation. Key features include developing a unit-based protocol, strict entry and exit criteria, nurse and therapist education, and on-site clinical support.

After extubation, the patient may benefit from a 20% increase in F_{IO_2} or nasal/facial CPAP or noninvasive positive pressure ventilation (bilevel positive airway pressure [BIPAP]) if lung volume is a problem. Nasal/facial CPAP or BIPAP may help prevent alveolar collapse and is weaned as tolerated—usually, if the patient struggles more when it is on, it is time to take it off. The patient is observed for long-term endurance failure.

Box 8-7
Indications for NPPV Support

1. Acute respiratory failure (early intervention to prevent deterioration as an alternative to endotracheal intubation in patients who can control their airway)
2. Following endotracheal extubation as a bridge to complete separation from ventilatory support
3. Obstructive sleep apnea
4. Hypoventilation syndromes
5. Progressive neuromuscular disease
6. Chronic respiratory failure in which tracheostomy may not be an option (e.g., cystic fibrosis)
7. Thoracic cage abnormalities
8. High-level paraplegic trauma

NPPV, Noninvasive positive pressure ventilation.

Nasal/Facial Continuous Positive Airway Pressure. Relatively low levels of CPAP can be administered to spontaneously breathing extubated patients using specialty nasal prongs or masks. The success of this strategy is variable but may be used as either a continuous or intermittent bridge to extubation in the chronically ventilated patient. The success of nasal CPAP in infants depends on the degree of mouth breathing and crying present. The success of facial CPAP in the child depends on patient tolerance and a mask that adequately fits the patient. Side effects include gastric distension; a nasogastric tube can be used to continuously vent the stomach.

Noninvasive Positive Pressure Ventilation

Commonly referred to as BIPAP, noninvasive positive pressure ventilation (NPPV) provides ventilatory support by nasal mask, pillows, or facial mask. Box 8-7 outlines the still-evolving multifaceted indications for NPPV in the pediatric population.[104] Generally, NPPV can be used (1) early in patients with acute respiratory failure to help stabilize deterioration, (2) as a bridge to unassisted breathing in difficult-to-wean patients, (3) as a treatment option in patients who require only intermittent ventilatory support, or (4) as a temporizing agent in patients with end-stage disease in whom the trajectory of illness is unclear. NPPV candidates should have a patent natural airway and an adequate respiratory drive. Patients can continue to eat and speak and are free of the discomfort and complications associated with an artificial airway.

The NPPV system may be totally patient triggered, or a ventilator rate may be set. The mode is pressure controlled with continuous flow that compensates for the leak that occurs around the mask. Two levels of positive pressure are set: one for inspiration (IPAP) and one for expiration (EPAP). This mode allows the ventilator to cycle between baseline pressure (EPAP) and pressure support (IPAP). NPPV augments V_T in response to a spontaneously breathing patient's inspiratory effort. The degree of support is determined by a clinician-selected inspiratory pressure and expiratory or baseline pressure.

The American Respiratory Care Foundation's consensus statement on NPPV recognizes two levels of support. Type I support is defined as providing life-sustaining support that if terminated could be life threatening.[105] Type II support is beneficial, but interruption is not life threatening. Patient placement (ICU/non-ICU) is determined on an individual case-by-case basis. NPPV can be safely provided out of an ICU environment when system supports are available, when the patient's trajectory of illness is clear, when the patient can easily call for help when necessary, and when the patient is able to maintain spontaneous ventilation without NPPV.

Complications of NPPV are the same as positive pressure ventilation (e.g., barotrauma or decreased cardiac output) but also include facial skin breakdown and the inability to determine the exact concentration of oxygen delivered. Nursing care for patients receiving NPPV includes selecting the appropriate face mask and headgear and then helping the patient breathe comfortably with NPPV support. The mask should fit snugly along the lateral boarder of the nose and rest on the upper lip but not extend more than two thirds up the bridge of the nose. Inserting pressure-relieving material (e.g., hydrogels [Spenco Medical Corp., Waco, TX]) between the face mask and bridge of the nose and alternating different facial appliances may help decrease the severity of pressure ulcers in this high-risk area.

The patient should be monitored for air leaks around the mask. Headgear is adjusted to ensure that pressure targets are achieved, and a chin strap may be needed during sleep to minimize mouth leaks. The patient should also be monitored for gastric distension. With NPPV, air may be swallowed or forced down the esophagus. To manage this, IPAPs can be decreased (if tolerated), or an NGT can be used to decompress the stomach. SpO_2 monitoring is used to adjust oxygen concentration.

Negative Pressure Ventilators

Iron lungs, cuirasses, and raincoats create negative abdominal pressure, allowing the diaphragm to distend and draw air into the lungs (Fig. 8-35). A negative pressure ventilator (NPV) is pressure controlled; tidal volumes are dependent on the patient's transthoracic pressure and thoracic compliance. Increased transthoracic pressures augment FRC, limit intrapulmonary shunting, and improve systemic oxygenation. Tidal volumes can be measured at the patient airway using a spirometer.

NPVs are generally used for nontracheotomized patients who cannot tolerate noninvasive positive pressure ventilation. NPVs may be used continuously, intermittently, or at night to permit the patient to rest. Patients with hypercapnic respiratory failure secondary to alveolar hypoventilation syndromes or neuromuscular or chest wall mechanical problems may benefit from NPVs. NPVs may also benefit the postoperative cardiovascular surgery patient who requires assisted ventilation but would benefit from lower

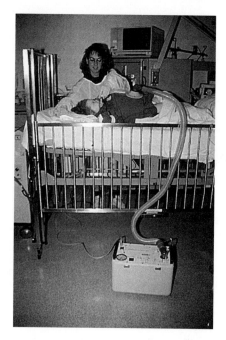

Fig. 8-35 Raincoat negative pressure ventilator.

pulmonary artery pressures and enhanced pulmonary and central venous return.

Blaufuss and Wallace[106] delineated the nursing care issues involved in caring for patients supported on NPVs. These patients are at risk for airway obstruction and pulmonary aspiration. Nasojejunal tubes are recommended for enteral feedings. Hypothermia secondary to convective cooling as air is pulled through the collar may become an issue. Maintaining skin integrity and vascular access requires proactive interventions. Patients commonly experience claustrophobia, helplessness, and sleep deprivation, so diversional therapy is also very important.

ALTERNATIVE THERAPIES

High-Frequency Ventilation

High-frequency ventilation (HFV) has become increasingly popular in supporting infants and children with acute respiratory failure (ARF) who cannot receive ventilation by traditional means. Conventional mechanical ventilation (CMV) is not without risk; the delivery of normal V_T to a patient with sick, noncompliant lungs necessitates high inflating pressures. However, decreased compliance is not a global phenomenon, and regions of high compliance become overdistended.[107] These extreme swings in airway pressure, from PIP to PEEP, contribute to the incidence of pulmonary barotrauma and associated air leak syndrome, for example, pneumothorax, pneumomediastinum, pneumopericardium, pneumoperitoneum, and pulmonary interstitial edema (PIE).

With HFV, small V_T (equal to or less than V_D) delivered at high frequencies maintains constant lung volumes at airway pressures just above alveolar closing pressure. The

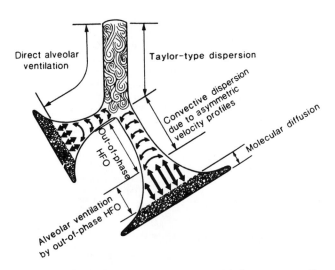

Fig. 8-36 Modes of gas transport during high-frequency ventilation. *HFO,* High-frequency oscillation. (From Villar J et al: Non-conventional techniques of ventilatory support, *Crit Care Clin* 6:579, 1990.)

lungs stay inflated while both volume and pressure peaks and valleys associated with continuous forced opening and passive closing of alveoli are avoided. One potential, but unsupported, benefit of HFV is the reduction of iatrogenic ventilator injury while maintaining adequate gas exchange using similar MAPs but lower PIPs associated with CMV.

Definition. HFV is a broad term used to describe numerous techniques of ventilation that deliver V_T less than the patient's dead space at supraphysiologic rates. In adults, HFV is operationally defined as 60 or more breaths/min or 1 hertz (Hz). This definition has obvious limitations in sick infants and children, who normally have respiratory rates within this range. A better definition for the pediatric population is the use of ventilatory rates greater than 150 breaths/min at V_T that approaches anatomic V_D.

Mechanism of Gas Transport in HFV. CMV attempts to simulate spontaneous ventilation by delivering gas in bulk volume that approximates V_T at physiologic respiratory rates. Gas transport in the larger airways occurs primarily by bulk convection of 3 times V_D, whereas diffusion is important in the terminal airways and alveoli.

Traditional physiology, based on bulk flow, cannot explain the mechanism of gas exchange in HFV. In 1915, Henderson and others noted that when smoke was blown down a tube, it formed a thin spike; the quicker the puff, the thinner and sharper the spike. Correlating their observation to panting dogs, they believed that gas exchange, sufficient to support life, was possible when V_T was less than V_D. Chang and Harf[108] identified five mechanisms of gas transport thought to be important in HFV: (1) convection, (2) pendelluft flow, (3) Taylor dispersion, (4) asymmetric velocity, and (5) molecular diffusion (Fig. 8-36).

Convection refers to the bulk flow of inspired gas to the level of the alveoli. Unlike CMV, HFV delivers V_T equal to at least one half to three quarters of anatomic V_D. Direct alveolar ventilation becomes less pronounced as V_T approaches V_D.[109] *Pendelluft flow* refers to interregional gas mixing or the movement of gas between neighboring lung units dependent on time constants. Pendelluft flow is enhanced during HFV and facilitates interregional gas mixing of adjacent lung units. *Taylor dispersion* describes the distribution of gas moving in a column: axial dispersion and radial diffusion. Gas flowing through a straight tube forms a parabolic (bullet-tipped) velocity profile, with the highest velocity occurring at the center. This effect disperses gas across the front of the moving column of gas (axial dispersion) and facilitates molecular diffusion around its periphery (radial diffusion). *Asymmetric velocity* is the mixing of inspiratory and expiratory gases in the airway. Inspiratory gas (O_2) moves toward the alveoli in the center of the airway, and expiratory gas (CO_2) moves away from the alveolus along the periphery. *Molecular diffusion,* the process of gas transport across the alveolar pulmonary-capillary membrane, is the primary mechanism of gas transfer between the alveolus and blood. The literal shaking of the chest during HFV probably enhances molecular diffusion.

Although gas transport during HFV is thought to be a function of all five mechanisms, observations made in the laboratory setting using rigid uniform cylinders cannot be applied to humans with a complex tracheobronchial tree. The exact mechanisms of gas exchange in HFV are controversial but probably vary in different areas of the lung, in different disease states, and with different techniques employed.

Classification. The early days of HFV were characterized by device confusion, that is, a technology in search of a disease.[110] Since that time, a variety of HFV techniques have been used in clinical trials. Four techniques are in clinical use today: high-frequency positive-pressure ventilation (HFPPV), high-frequency jet ventilation (HFJV), high-frequency flow interruption (HFFI), and high-frequency oscillation ventilation (HFOV). Table 8-18 provides an overview of these techniques. When analyzing research related to HFV, the method of HFV, as well as the ventilation strategy, is important.

HFPPV, considered by many to be an extension of CMV, employs a standard ventilator modified with low-compliance tubing so that adequate V_T can be delivered using short Ti.[109] Flow is intermittently delivered to the patient through a pneumatic valve located at the airway. Effective ventilation can occur within an open or closed system. When closed, the system allows an accurate determination of V_T because environmental air entrainment does not occur. Tidal volume is delivered via a standard ETT with the inspiratory phase the only active phase of the respiratory cycle. Expiration is achieved by passive lung recoil. Ventilation frequency, V_T, FIO_2, and Ti can be controlled. Starting frequencies are usually in the range of 60 to 120 breaths/min (1 to 2 Hz), V_T of 3 to 4 ml/kg, and Ti of 20% to 33%.[111] Heijman and co-workers[112] cautioned that high frequencies may limit V_T and compromise actual alveolar ventilation despite an increase in minute ventilation.

TABLE 8-18 *Overview of High-Frequency Ventilation Techniques*

	HFPPV	HFJV	HFFI	HFOV
Flow generator	High-pressure gas source	High-pressure gas source	High-pressure gas source	Piston pump
Fresh gas delivery system	Continuous or valved fresh gas flow	Jet catheter with continuous fresh gas bias flow	Valved flow interrupter	Continuous fresh gas flow
V_T	$>V_D$	$><V_D$	$><V_D$	$<V_D$
Expiration	Passive	Passive	Passive	Active
Airway pressure waveform	Variable	Triangular	Triangular	Sine wave
Entrainment	None	Yes	None	None
Frequency	60-120 (1-2 Hz)	60-600 (1-10 Hz)	300-1200 (5-20 Hz)	60-3600 (1-60 Hz)
Ventilator	Siemens	Bunnell Universal	Emerson Infant Star	Hummingbird Sensormedics

Data from Coghill CH, Haywood JL, Chatburn RL et al: Neonatal and pediatric high-frequency ventilation: principles and practice, *Respir Care* 36:596-609, 1991; Martin LD, Rafferty JF, Walker LK et al: Principles of respiratory support and mechanical ventilation. In Rogers MC, ed: *Textbook of pediatric intensive care,* Baltimore, 1992, Williams & Wilkins, pp 134-203.
HFPPV, High-frequency positive-pressure ventilation; *HFJV,* high-frequency jet ventilation; *HFFI,* high-frequency flow interruption; *HFOV,* high-frequency oscillation ventilation.

HFJV delivers small bursts of gas from a high-pressure source into the patient's trachea through an injector port of an ETT designed specifically for jet ventilation (Fig. 8-37, *A*). The burst of gas, representing inspiration, is the only active phase of the ventilatory cycle; expiration depends on passive lung recoil. Tidal volumes are generated by the jet volume plus varying volumes entrained by a Venturi effect from a parallel continuous low-pressure flow circuit. Entrainment occurs when the jet burst entering the airway under high pressure creates an area of low pressure behind the entry point. Gas from the upper airway is pulled into the low-pressure area, giving additional V_T to each jet pulse. The volume delivered depends on ventilator settings and pulmonary mechanics, such as airway resistance. The presence of a large back-pressure may impede gas entrainment and jet flow. Frequencies range from 4 to 10 Hz. Concerns with this mode of HFV include providing adequate humidification and the need to reintubate a critically ill patient with the special ETT.

HFFI, considered a hybrid of HFJV, provides small bursts of gas at high frequencies into the ventilator circuit rather than the patient's trachea. Ventilation occurs through the interruption of high-pressure gas flow by either a shutter system or rotating ball device (see Fig. 8-37, *B*). Compared with HFJV, humidification is better, a special ETT is unnecessary, and gas entrainment does not occur.[113] Frequencies can be adjusted to 20 Hz.

HFOV uses a piston acting across a low-bias flow circuit to deliver small volumes of gas through a standard ETT (see Fig. 8-37, *C*). Gas is pushed in, and as the direction of the piston reverses, similar volumes are extracted from the lung. The primary difference between HFOV and other modes of HVF is that exhalation is active, not entirely dependent on passive lung recoil. Active exhalation not only enhances CO_2 removal but also reduces the incidence of stacking of breaths causing inadvertent increases in lung volume.[114]

Because of the active exhalation phase, very fast rates from 60 to 3600/min or 1 to 60 Hz can be used.

Equal power is applied to both inspiratory and expiratory phases. As long as the inspiratory and expiratory time constants of the lungs are equivalent, equal volumes of gas are delivered and extracted. Time constants are rarely equal, and at 50% Ti at high frequency, air trapping can occur, resulting in an increase in lung volume. As long as Ti is less than 40% of the respiratory cycle, mean alveolar pressure will not exceed mean proximal airway pressure.[115]

Oscillatory ventilation holds lung volume constant, which not only eliminates potential mechanical damage from the opening and closing of the delicate small airways and alveoli but also eliminates the need for high peak pressure breaths needed to reopen closed alveoli. Lung volume is held relatively constant to enhance alveolar recruitment.

Clinical Issues. Coghill and colleagues[109] noted that regardless of the technique used, the most consistent observation in HFV is that CO_2 elimination is usually easily accomplished. CO_2 elimination is related to both V_T and frequency; but unlike CMV, V_T appears to be more important in HFV.

Delivered V_T increases with ETT size and decreases with frequency.[113] In HFPPV and HFJV, $Paco_2$ increases when the frequency passes a threshold level as a result of decreased delivered V_T. Insufficient expiratory time (<66%) will cause an increased lung volume and impedance to lung inflation at higher frequencies. During HFOV, increasing the frequency will decrease the $Paco_2$ until a plateau is reached. HFOV eliminates CO_2 faster than expiratory-passive forms of HFV. In HFJV, the position of the jet cannula tip in the airway is also an important factor; the closer the tip is to the carina, the better the CO_2 elimination.

As in CMV, MAP and its correlate—lung volume— largely determine oxygenation. Compared with CMV, some proponents of HFV believe that oxygenation can be

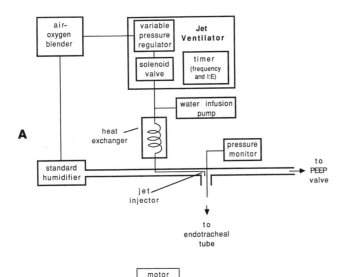

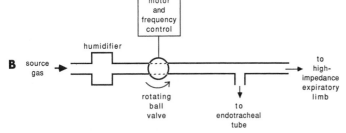

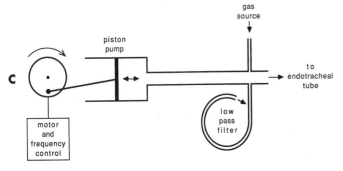

Fig. 8-37 A, Schema of high-frequency jet ventilation system. **B,** Schema of high-frequency flow interruption system. **C,** Schema of high-frequency oscillatory ventilation system. (From Chatburn RL: High-frequency ventilation. In Blummer JL, ed: *A practical guide to pediatric intensive care,* ed 3, St Louis, 1990, Mosby, pp 957-958.)

accomplished using lower MAPs. However, MAPs measured at the proximal airway are probably different than alveoli pressure.[116] Comparisons of oxygenation between CMV and HFV at similar proximal airway pressures have not necessarily ensured equivalence of mean alveolar pressure and lung volumes.[111] PIPs are lower with HFV because of smaller delivered V_T.

During CMV, there is a gradual increase in alveolar pressure during inspiration. At end inspiration, alveolar pressure may become supraatmospheric and restrain pulmonary capillary blood flow. Increased intrathoracic pressure

associated with positive pressure ventilation also decreases venous return, stroke volume, and cardiac output. Attempts to limit these adverse circulatory effects prompted enthusiasm for HFV. However, studies comparing cardiac output and other hemodynamic variables during HFV and CMV at equal mean alveolar pressures in animals have failed to reveal significant differences.[111]

The effects of HFV on the pulmonary circulation and $\dot{V}/\dot{Q}$ matching have not been adequately defined. Humorally mediated attenuation of the hypoxemic pulmonary vasomotor response during HFV may contribute to pulmonary venous admixture and arterial desaturation.[111]

In the setting of intracranial hypertension, the negative impact of high intrathoracic pressure on cerebral circulation is well documented. Decreased respiratory variation in intrathoracic and central vascular pressures during HFV should diminish phasic swings in ICP. Total and regional blood flow does not appear to be different during HFV and CMV.

The early use of HFJV was complicated by necrotizing tracheobronchitis (NTB) characterized by epithelial erosion, loss of ciliated cells, squamous cell metaplasia, and infiltration of the mucosa by neutrophils.[107] Symptoms of NTB include acute airway obstruction and aspiration of necrotic debris from the airway. Possible pathogenesis of NTB includes inadequate humidification of delivered gas and extremely high-velocity jet flows.[113] Although data conflict regarding the effect of HFV on mucociliary transport, without adequate humidification, mucous clearance becomes a problem.

Studies investigating the effects of HFV on lung water and edema formation have produced contradictory findings. Pulmonary compliance and surfactant activity have been studied and suggest that mechanical pressure-volume relationships and surfactant activity of the lung are not negatively influenced during HFV.[111]

Eucapnic apnea has been observed with HFV. This apneic state associated with HFV is mediated by chest wall receptors and vagal afferent fibers and appears to be independent of chemical respiratory drive and lung volume changes.

Clinical Applications.   Compared with the neonatal population, the use of HFV in infants and young children has received less attention. Although the benefits of HFV in pediatrics are unproved, pediatric applications include major pulmonary air leaks, interstitial pneumonia, ARDS, and congenital diaphragmatic hernia.[110] Research is needed to determine when, if, and what type of HFV can improve patient outcome. Using HFOV and an aggressive volume recruitment strategy, Arnold and co-workers[117] demonstrated an improvement in oxygenation and a lower frequency of barotrauma compared with conventional ventilation.

The most persuasive indication for HFV is pulmonary air leak. Bronchopleural fistulas, major airway disruptions, and pneumothoraces respond favorably to HFV.[118] Healing of disrupted airways occurs more rapidly in the presence of lower tidal swings in airway pressure associated with HFV.[111]

HFPPV and HFJV have been used in short-term support of ventilation during airway procedures such as bronchoscopy and laryngoscopy. Airway visualization is enhanced and ventilatory motion is decreased with these techniques of HFV.

Nursing Care of a Patient Supported on HFOV. Nursing care of the patient supported on HFOV centers around vigilance in monitoring and in preventing complications.[119] Although monitoring is critical, constant vibration of the child's body and noise from the ventilator limit traditional assessment methods. Auscultation of heart, breath, and bowel sounds is difficult if not impossible. The only time auscultation is possible is during a suctioning procedure when the patient is being hand ventilated. Most patients on HFOV are chemically paralyzed and sedated. Because it is difficult to detect fine movements that hallmark the need for additional chemical paralyzing agent, continuous infusions guided by peripheral nerve stimulation provide a more reasonable approach to the use of chemical paralysis in this population. Electroencephalograms (EEGs) cannot be used to assess for the presence of seizure activity. Possible autonomic symptoms of seizure activity include cyclic increases in heart rate and blood pressure, dilated pupils, and, possibly, worsening blood gases.

Impaired Gas Exchange: Hypoxemia and Hypercapnia. The goal of HFOV is to reduce or eliminate hypoxemia and hypercapnia using similar MAPs but lower PIPs than used with CMV while minimizing the risk of barotrauma and oxygen toxicity. Frequent ABGs are necessary with the initiation of therapy but should be delayed because changes in ventilator settings may take up to an hour to be reflected in the patient's ABGs. Baseline ABGs are individualized; lower Pao_2 (<50 mmHg) and higher $Paco_2$ (>70 mmHg) may be tolerated as long as the pH remains greater than 7.25. Acidosis is managed with tromethamine (THAM), a non–CO_2-generating buffer. Spo_2 monitoring provides an ongoing trend in oxygenation. Oxygenation profiles provide data regarding the adequacy of Do_2 compared with Vo_2.

Improved Oxygenation: Optimize Lung Volume. To ensure adequate alveolar recruitment, the MAP is initially set 5 to 8 cm H_2O higher than that required on CMV.[120] The MAP is increased in 1- to 2-cm H_2O increments until the Spo_2 is greater than 90% with a baseline Fio_2 of 0.6 or until overinflation is evidenced on chest x-ray film. Appropriate MAPs will increase alveolar recruitment and lung volume and thus oxygenation, whereas excessive MAPs will cause overdistension, air trapping, and $\dot{V}/\dot{Q}$ mismatch and impair oxygenation.

Ventilation strategy for the manipulation of MAP varies among disease categories.[110] The goal in a patient with diffuse alveolar disease (DAD) characterized by a noncompliant, surfactant-deficient lung is *high volume*. Alveolar recruitment to maintain optimal lung volume is a priority; thus high MAPs are used while the Fio_2 is maintained less than 0.6. The goal in air leak syndrome (ALS) is *low volume,* to promote lung healing and recovery. Attempts are made to decrease or maintain MAPs until air leak is resolved tolerating higher Fio_2.

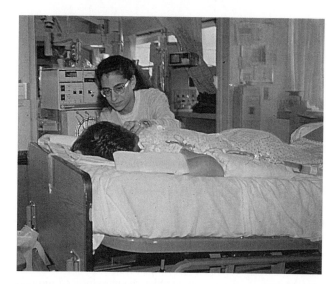

Fig. 8-38   Patient supported on high-frequency oscillation ventilation in prone position.

Other factors to be considered include improving $\dot{D}o_2$, limiting $\dot{V}o_2$, and altering pulmonary mechanics; for example, sedation, muscle relaxants, repositioning, suctioning, and managing bronchospasm. If chest wall vibration suddenly decreases, decreasing lung compliance, pneumothorax, additional atelectasis, ETT obstruction or malposition, and hyperinflation with $\dot{V}/\dot{Q}$ mismatch are considered. Prone position may improve $\dot{V}/\dot{Q}$ matching (Fig. 8-38). "Best" positioning is reevaluated daily as patient tolerance permits.

Improve CO_2 Elimination: Frequency and Tidal Volume. As discussed, alterations in V_T will have a much greater effect on CO_2 elimination than changes in frequency. Adjusting the oscillatory amplitude, which is the power control, controls CO_2 elimination. Power is responsible for the volume of air exchanges with each oscillatory cycle. The power is adjusted until adequate chest wiggle, that is, ΔP, V_T, is achieved. Given the attenuation of airway pressure from the proximal airway to the distal airways, predicting exactly how much pressure is transmitted to the lungs is very difficult. Presumably, the larger the ETT, the greater the pressure transmission.

Starting frequencies employed with HFOV (which approximate the resonant frequency of lung) are 15 Hz in neonates and 5 to 10 Hz in older children. If maximum ΔP is unable to improve ventilation in older children, a secondary strategy includes decreasing frequency and increasing power to increase V_T and expiratory time. If an elevated $Paco_2$ persists, a 10% increase in V_T can be obtained by increasing the Ti toward 50% of the cycle. This maneuver is used with caution because higher frequencies and Ti close to 50% may result in increased lung volume and stacking of breaths. Follow-up chest x-ray films are used to assess for overinflation.

Weaning. The patient's lung compliance often improves rapidly and requires aggressive weaning of the airway pressure to avoid overdistension and development of pneumothoraces. Signs of improvement are often subtle, that is, increase in the percent piston displacement using the same power, improved tolerance to hand ventilation and procedures, improving Spo_2 with an Fio_2 less than 0.6, and resolving air leaks. Frequency is not weaned even in the event of an improved patient condition. Airway pressure is decreased by 1- to 2-cm increments every 12 to 24 hours, followed by close observation. In the event of decreasing Spo_2 and lower Pao_2, a chest x-ray film is justified to assess for atelectasis from the decrease in MAP. Increasing the MAPs back to the original settings or perhaps 1 to 2 cm higher helps reexpand collapsed alveoli.

No guidelines help determine the best time to return to CMV. CMV may be reinitiated when MAPs are weaned to 15 to 20 cm H_2O with an Fio_2 of less than 0.6, air leaks are resolved, chest x-ray film has improved, and the patient is able to tolerate suctioning without prolonged periods of desaturation.[121] Some patients have been extubated directly from HFOV without returning to CMV.

Potential for Injury. *Pulmonary toilet* for the patient on HFOV is challenging for several reasons; in addition to the lack of indicators (breath sounds cannot be auscultated, and high peak pressure ventilatory alarms do not exist), patient tolerance is extremely low as demonstrated by prolonged periods of recovery after suctioning. Although the patient receiving HFV does not seem to require more frequent suctioning than the patient receiving CMV, the effectiveness of HFV is extremely sensitive to a buildup of secretions in the ETT.[114]

Frequency of suctioning depends on the disease, fluid balance, recent chest x-ray film findings, ABGs, and Sao_2. Initially, patients with alveolar disease may require suctioning once daily and then progress to every 12 hours as tolerated; patients with ALS may need suctioning as little as every 24 to 36 hours.

Because most patients are intolerant of suctioning, the procedure may include premedication with lidocaine and preoxygenation with the ventilator by increasing the Fio_2 to 1.0 and MAPs 2 to 4 cm H_2O 15 to 20 minutes before suctioning. Because it is impossible to mimic the ventilatory pattern or rate of HFOV, the oscillator is turned off, and the MAP is maintained during the suctioning procedure. A minimal number of suction passes are made using an in-line suctioning device. Vibrations are used if the patient's platelet count is greater than 50,000 and the patient is hemodynamically stable.

Because oxygenation is critically dependent on lung volume, rerecruitment procedures may be necessary after the suctioning procedure. After the patient reaches presuctioning Spo_2, the Fio_2 and MAPs are returned to baseline as tolerated.

Patients supported on HVOF are at high risk for *alterations in skin integrity* secondary to immobility. Eggcrates are used, whereas air mattresses are avoided because they may affect the resonant frequency of the chest. The ventilator is moved from one side of the bed to the other every 12 to 24 hours so that the patient's head can be fully repositioned. Lastly, these patients also experience an increased number of radiologic procedures and require strict maintenance of shielding techniques.

Optimal Sensory Perception. The loud cadence of HFOV, along with other ICU monitoring devices, often results in an altered sleep and rest pattern. Earshields, earplugs, and music are used in a therapeutic manner to hallmark "safe times."

Altered Coping: Child and Family. Stress precautions are taken to help control the environment for these liable infants and children. In addition to the stress related to having their child require an extraordinary level of care, parents require support in understanding the apparently unnatural breathing pattern. Data regarding the memories of children supported by this ventilatory strategy are nonexistent.

Extracorporeal Membrane Oxygenation

Despite significant advances in ventilator therapy, some patients with ARF will fail to respond and die unless alternative therapy is available.[122] Extracorporeal membrane oxygenation (ECMO) is prolonged cardiopulmonary bypass performed at the bedside. It is an alternative intervention for patients in profound respiratory or cardiopulmonary failure who are refractory to maximal conventional therapies. ECMO supports the cardiopulmonary system so that toxic high positive airway pressures and levels of oxygen can be avoided while permitting resolution of a *reversible* pathologic condition.

ECMO is considered "standard rescue therapy" in supporting critically ill neonates in ARF. Based on its success in the neonatal population, some centers have extended the use of ECMO to a carefully selected group of pediatric patients.[123] However, some very important differences exist between these two patient populations: pulmonary vascular reactivity significantly decreases after 2 weeks of age; diseases that cause pediatric ARF are not as homogeneous as those that cause neonatal ARF; and most causes of pediatric ARF involve pulmonary parenchymal dysfunction. In the pediatric population, ECMO is not considered "rescue" therapy but a supportive intervention that may prevent iatrogenic injury related to oxygen and ventilator support.[124]

Current Application. There are no precise indications for ECMO in the pediatric population. ECMO may be helpful in a pediatric patient with reversible disease that can be resolved within the feasible time limit for maintaining ECMO. A typical pediatric ECMO course for pulmonary support is usually much longer than a pediatric ECMO course for cardiac support—2 to 4 weeks compared with 4 to 5 days. ECMO may be considered when the disease trajectory is directed toward the patient's demise, the patient is refractory to maximal conventional therapy, and there is still potential for good neurologic outcome. Maximal conventional therapy, ill defined and controversial among centers, includes optimal ventilator, pharmacologic, or surgical therapy. In describing maximal conventional ventilation, the "process of care" becomes important. Some centers derive excellent results from alternative ventilator management techniques—some with high-frequency ventilation, and others with ECMO. The success of any one therapy at a

Box 8-8
Guidelines for ECMO in the Pulmonary Patient

Evidence of a significant intrapulmonary right-to-left shunting; >30% during maximal conventional therapy

Static compliance <0.5 ml/cm H_2O/kg

Pao_2 <50 mmHg; $Paco_2$ >50 mmHg with MAPs >18 cm H_2O, barotrauma, hypotension/arrest

Alveolar-arterial O_2 gradient (A-aDo_2) >580 with PIPs >40 cm H_2O will predict 81% mortality in children

Oxygenation index (OI) >0.4 predicts 77% mortality in children

Present twice more than 30 minutes apart despite maximal conventional therapy

ECMO, Extracorporeal membrane oxygenation; *MAPs,* mean airway pressures.

Box 8-9
Contraindications of ECMO Support

Multisystem organ failure

Severe neurologic damage

Irreversible lung damage

Greater than 7-10 days on high ventilator pressures and Fio_2

Prolonged period since injury occurred

Slow escalation of therapy

Bronchoalveolar lavage and biopsy: increased macrophages

Prolonged shock (base deficit −5; oliguria; decreased MAP for >12 hours)

Current or prior cardiac arrest with unknown neurologic status

Condition incompatible with normal healthy childhood (institutional care, incurable disease, metastatic cancer)

ECMO, Extracorporeal membrane oxygenation; *MAP,* mean airway pressure.

Box 8-10
Comparisons of VA and VV ECMO

VA ECMO

Provides cardiac and pulmonary support

Decompresses the pulmonary vascular bed

Carotid artery is used

Potential lethality of emboli

Coronary artery blood flow is derived from the left ventricle (<Pao_2)

VV ECMO

Provides only pulmonary support—does not support cardiac function

Normal pulmonary circulation is maintained

Can still assess pulmonary artery pressures—cannot use thermodilution cardiac output

Provides higher $S\bar{v}o_2$ saturations to the pulmonary vascular bed, so it may help decrease PVR and heal the lung

May require a 20% increase in flow to compensate for "pump recirculation"

Requires standard ventilator management

Selective perfusion is not a problem—myocardial circulation maintained

Normal pulsatile pulse contour is maintained

Carotid artery is spared

May develop problems with the femoral vein related to chronic venous insufficiency or edema

Longer cannulation time—two sites

Less concern over emboli—returning blood to the venous system

ECMO, Extracorporeal membrane oxygenation; *PVR,* pulmonary vascular resistance; *VA,* venoarterial; *VV,* venovenous.

particular institution may not be able to be replicated in another.

Pediatric ECMO has been used successfully to support patients with *reversible single-organ failure,* that is, ARF before iatrogenic lung injury or multisystem organ failure (MSOF) develops or to support patients after cardiovascular surgery for congenital heart disease (see Chapter 7). Criteria for patients with pulmonary dysfunction are difficult to establish because the specificity of various measures is not exact; most criteria are unit dependent (Box 8-8). One common theme is that the patient will die of reversible ARF unless ECMO is offered.

Compared with indications, contraindications of ECMO support are easier to identify. Factors include those that preclude a quality outcome or a successful ECMO run (Box 8-9). Identifying reversible pulmonary disease is difficult. In children, diseases that cause respiratory failure leading to interstitial inflammation may result in pulmonary fibrosis and necrosis. Lung biopsy or documentation of fixed pulmonary vascular resistance may be necessary to rule out irreversible lung damage. The extent of pulmonary fibrosis is related to the severity and duration of the interstitial inflammation, as well as to the duration of high positive airway pressures from mechanical ventilation. Typically, a patient's primary problem will shift from respiratory failure to ventilatory failure when fibrosis becomes significant.

ECMO Circuit. There are two options when providing ECMO support: venoarterial (VA) and venovenous (VV). In VA ECMO, blood is drained from the venous circulation via a cannula placed in the right atrium, and oxygenated blood is returned to the arterial circulation through a cannula placed in the aortic arch. In VV ECMO, blood is drained in a similar manner, but oxygenated blood is returned to the venous circulation through a cannula commonly placed in one of the common femoral veins. A double-lumen cannula (DLC) (Kendall Healthcare Products, Mansfield, Mass.) placed in the right internal jugular vein has been used successfully to provide VV support.[125] Use of the DLC is currently limited by the 14 Fr cannula size, which can only accommodate neonates of up to 4 kg. Larger and smaller cannula sizes are under development.

Although VA ECMO is currently more widely used, VV

ECMO is gaining popularity. Box 8-10 contrasts the major differences between VA and VV ECMO support. Contraindications to VV ECMO include the patient in cardiac failure and the patient with inadequate venous access. An advantage of VV ECMO is that it may limit the physiologic consequences of microemboli. Most children receiving long-term VA ECMO support die of MSOF, probably related to microemboli from the ECMO circuit.

Regardless of whether VA or VV ECMO is used, the ECMO circuit remains the same (Fig. 8-39). Blood is drained by gravity from the venous cannula in the right atrium down to a 30- to 50-ml polyethylene bladder that is servoregulating the hemopump. This venous reservoir is in direct contact with a microswitch that can sense a decrease in bladder size, indicating a diminished venous blood supply. Insufficient drainage into the bladder causes the bladder to collapse, which automatically shuts off the pump. Known as "bladder chatter," this may be a result of hypovolemia; excessive flow; or a kinked, malpositioned, or inadequately sized drainage cannula. Failure of the pump to shut off in response to a loss of venous blood supply could result in air emboli or right atrial suction.

From the bladder, blood is drawn into a hemopump, where either a centrifuge or roller pump propels the blood forward. Pump flow regulates the volume of blood sent through the oxygenator; as a result, the pump flow also regulates the patient's Pao_2. The flow is usually maintained at 70 to 120 ml/kg/min. The blood is pumped into the membrane oxygenator for oxygenation and CO_2 removal. The membrane oxygenator is a flat silicone envelope tightly wound into a coil that divides the membrane into two compartments; ventilating gas flows down on one side, and blood is pumped up on the other. Oxygen, measured in liters per minute, is administered via a sweep gas. Because the membrane is 6 to 7 times more permeable to carbon dioxide than oxygen, carbogen (5% carbon dioxide and 95% oxygen) is usually added to prevent or correct hypocapnia. Premembrane and postmembrane pressures are monitored for the early detection of circuit malfunction. Premembrane pressures are kept below 300 mmHg to avoid red cell and platelet destruction; postmembrane pressures should be between 200 and 300 mmHg. A rise in postmembrane pressures indicates occlusion or kinking of the return cannula.

Arterialized, the blood leaves the oxygenator and flows into the heat exchanger, which in the pediatric patient may be housed within the oxygenator. Blood flows through seven stainless steel rods that are surrounded by a water bath warmed to 39° C. This temperature allows ambient cooling as the blood returns to the patient through the return cannula placed in the right common carotid artery (aorta) in VA ECMO or through the selected venovenous cannula in VV ECMO.

The "bridge" links the drainage and return lines. This connection allows the patient to be excluded from the ECMO circuit without fear of blood stasis and associated clot formation. Clamped during ECMO support, the bridge is opened during elective or emergent isolation from ECMO.

Cannulation.   ECMO cannulation is a surgical procedure performed in the PICU. The patient is chemically paralyzed to avoid respiratory movement, which may precipitate an air embolus during venous cannulation. Fentanyl (20 μg/kg) is used for anesthesia, keeping the heart rate and blood pressure within a tight 10- to 20-point range.[126] The surgical team, including scrub nurse, controls the sterile environment, which includes the surgical space, instrument tables, suction, and electrocautery; all personnel within 6 feet of the operative field wear caps and masks. The bed is raised to facilitate venous drainage, and the patient is positioned with a roll under the shoulders and the head turned to the left for neck cannulation. Routine prepping and draping are performed.

The critical care nurse maintains access to the patient, including the airway and preferably a large-gauge central IV line to administer emergency medications, platelets, and heparin. Access to the arterial line is desirable but is not always possible. Concentrated platelets (amounts varies with circuit size) is administered as the sternocleidomastoid incision is opened. The carotid sheath is exposed, and the vessels are isolated. The largest possible venous cannula (16 to 28 Fr) is selected and inserted into the right internal jugular vein. The large cannula size and multiple side ports usually allow venous drainage equivalent to the normal resting cardiac output of most patients. The arterial cannula (12 to 22 Fr) has one large distal opening and is inserted into the right common carotid artery. Heparin, 30 U/kg, is

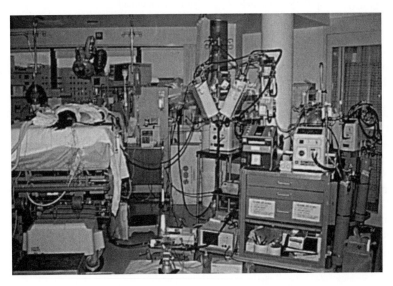

Fig. 8-39   ECMO circuit: from the right atrium, blood drains by gravity to a blood reservoir, is pumped to the membrane oxygenator, heated, and then returned to the patient.

administered intravenously as the cannulas are inserted. In VV ECMO, a separate surgical team cannulates the femoral vein. An alternate cannulation site in the cardiac surgical patient includes a transthoracic approach. Another unit of concentrated platelets is administered as the incision(s) is(are) closed.

When cannulation is complete, the patient is connected to the ECMO circuit, the clamps are released, and the ECMO flow is started at 100 ml/min. ECMO flow is gradually increased over 5 to 10 minutes to a rate of 80 to 120 ml/kg/min while the adequacy of venous return and Spo_2 are assessed.

As VA ECMO flow increases, inotropic support can be gradually weaned. By increasing the nonpulsatile flow in VA ECMO, it is possible to assume approximately 80% of the patient's cardiac output, which is evidenced by a narrowing of the arterial pulse pressure (Fig. 8-40). Hypertension and bradycardia may result from a too rapid increase in VA ECMO flow or too slow an inotropic wean. Time may resolve these effects, but antihypertensive medications, for example, hydralazine 0.1 to 0.4 mg/kg IV, may be necessary.

In VV ECMO, no change should occur in the patient's pulse pressure. Inotropic agents usually cannot be immediately weaned, and continuous mixed venous saturation monitoring ($S\bar{v}o_2$) of the drainage line is used to assess for pump recirculation. The goal is less than an 80% $S\bar{v}o_2$ in the drainage line. Pump recirculation is suspected when the $S\bar{v}o_2$ of the drainage line is equal to or greater than Spo_2.

After the incisions are dressed, the patient is repositioned. The patient's head is placed in a midline position.

Nursing Care of a Patient Supported on ECMO. Care of the patient requires the ability to rapidly assess a complex critically ill patient and intervene appropriately using clinical practice guidelines. Throughout the ECMO course, the nurse works in collaboration with other members of the team and side by side with the ECMO specialist.

The bedside nurse is responsible for the overall care of the patient. The ECMO specialist performs all circuit

manipulations, adjusts the level of anticoagulation, and regulates pump flow within the parameters set by the physician.[127] Although the ECMO specialist administers medications through the circuit, the nurse is responsible for preparing the correct drug dose, properly diluted and correctly labeled, before giving it to the ECMO specialist for administration.

Impaired Gas Exchange. The patient remains intubated and ventilated while supported on VA ECMO, but minimal ventilator settings are used to avoid further barotrauma. These settings are individualized but usually include PIPs of less than 35 cm H_2O, PEEP of 8 to 12 cm H_2O, and Fio_2 of 0.21 to 0.40. The ventilator rate may be set at 5 to 10 breaths/min with a tidal volume of less than or equal to 8 ml/kg. Patients are not routinely chemically paralyzed, so normocapnia will continue to stimulate respiratory efforts and help to maintain respiratory muscle tone and coordination.

The underlying disease, the patient's immediate condition, and progress dictate individualized pulmonary toilet and airway care. Suctioning may be needed as often as every 3 hours or may be therapeutically delayed to once every 12 hours. Manual deep inflation breaths help to maintain alveolar volume. Lung compliance and aeration are assessed with every pulmonary intervention. Aggressive bronchial hygiene is often limited because of systemic heparinization, but with adequate platelet counts, it may be safely accomplished. Bronchoscopy and bronchoalveolar lavage can be helpful if persistent areas of atelectasis and consolidation are present. Bronchodilators—for example, albuterol and terbutaline—may be helpful in the bronchospastic patient.

Arterial and mixed venous blood gases are closely monitored. With an ECMO flow rate of 100 ml/kg/min, arterial blood saturation should be greater than 95%. The mixed venous blood gases should have a normal pH, a $P\bar{v}o_2$ greater than 37 mmHg, and $S\bar{v}o_2$ of 70%. In VA ECMO, adequate Pao_2 levels are accomplished through manipulating the ECMO flow rate. The higher the rate, the more blood that interfaces with the membrane oxygenator, resulting in a higher Pao_2. Adjustments for $Paco_2$ levels are made through the addition and manipulations of carbogen. With the inclusion or increase of carbogen, there is also an infusion of additional oxygen, so the oxygen sweep gas may need to be decreased. In summary, to increase the Pao_2, the blood flow is increased; to decrease the $Paco_2$, the gas flow is increased.

Care of the patient supported on VV ECMO is similar to the care of the patient supported on VA ECMO. With normal pulmonary blood flow, the lungs contribute significantly to gas exchange. Ventilator settings are maintained at settings that avoid iatrogenic injury. Pulmonary toilet is aggressive; arterial and venous blood gases dictate changes in ventilator management. There are fewer manipulations of the ECMO flows and sweep gases than on VA ECMO.

Daily chest x-ray films reflect the disease process and document patient progress. Complete opacification, or "white out," is common for the ECMO patient. This phenomenon is thought to be related to the sudden withdrawal of distending airway pressure on conversion to ECMO and to the blood-circuit surface interaction that

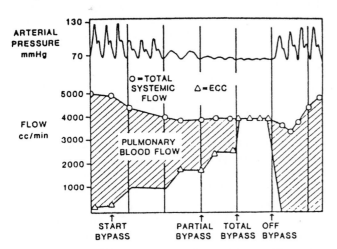

Fig. 8-40 Pulse pressure changes on VA ECMO. *ECC,* Extracorporeal circulation. (From Bartlett RH et al: *Extracorporeal membrane oxygenation technical specialist manual,* ed 7, Ann Arbor, 1984, The University of Michigan Department of Surgery, p 28.)

initially causes the release of vasoactive substances.[128] Both changes are associated with generalized capillary leak and interstitial pulmonary fluid shifts. This condition may further compromise the pulmonary status during the first 24 to 48 hours of ECMO support.

Iatrogenic complications of maximal mechanical ventilation before ECMO—that is, pneumothoraces—are not uncommon. If a pneumothorax were to develop while the patient was supported on VA ECMO, signs and symptoms would include an increase in Pao_2 and a decrease in peripheral perfusion, followed by a decrease in venous drainage and progressive hemodynamic deterioration. The presence or absence of air leaks is documented. Persistent pulmonary air leaks may be managed by decreasing the mean airway pressure to just under the pressure associated with an air leak. Chest tube patency is maintained with water-seal drainage or suction set at 20 cm H_2O. Stripping of chest tubes is controversial, especially in the heparinized patient. All chest tube drainage is documented and may require colloid replacement.

Alterations in Cardiac Output. The ECMO circuit contains approximately twice the blood volume of the patient. VA ECMO flow overrides the patient's inherent cardiac output, which significantly narrows the pulse pressure. Once the pulse pressure is lost, the mean arterial pressure guides nursing interventions, inotropic support, and fluid administration. Normal mean arterial pressure is age dependent, but a value greater than 60 mmHg is considered baseline. Even though resuscitative events before ECMO often leave the patient in a positive fluid balance, equilibration between the patient's own circulation and the ECMO circuit often requires additional colloid.

Hypotension may result from hypovolemia, an insufficient flow rate, and sepsis-related vasodilation, or oversedation. Associated clinical signs include pallor; prolonged capillary refill; cool, mottled extremities; and decreased urinary output.

Persistent hypovolemia, evidenced by a decreased mean arterial pressure, frequent "bladder chatter," and S$\bar{v}o_2$ less than 70%, requires volume administration. Packed red cells (PRCs), fresh frozen plasma (FFP), or 5% albumin 10 to 20 ml/kg may be given to maintain the mean arterial pressure and hematologic parameters. After volume expansion, the use of vasopressors, such as dopamine, may be considered.

Hypervolemia, inadequate sedation, or excessive environmental stimuli may be primary or secondary causes of hypertension. Diuretics, antihypertensives, or sedatives are used; stress precautions are enforced; and the underlying cause for hypertension is investigated and managed.

Hypervolemia may result from pre-ECMO resuscitative efforts, fluid retention caused by prerenal oliguric states, or third spacing from capillary leakage resulting from sepsis. A diuretic regimen, sometimes accompanied by the use of 25% albumin, may be employed.

Idiopathic hypertension is common in the pediatric ECMO patient. The nonpulsatile flow, characteristic of VA ECMO, downloads baroreceptors. The kidneys may also interpret the nonpulsatile flow as a low-flow or hypotensive state, stimulating renin release and activation of the renin-angiotensin and aldosterone system. The net result is vasoconstriction and sodium and water retention. With normal pulmonary vascular resistance, overriding the patient's inherent cardiac output with VA ECMO may be impossible. Hypertension may result from the two cardiac outputs existing within a single circulatory system. Because oxygenation is determined by the ECMO flow rate, lowering the flow to treat hypertension will compromise oxygenation.

Hypertension exacerbates bleeding, so it is aggressively managed in the ECMO patient. Antihypertensive drugs, such as hydralazine, may be used for blood pressure control. In addition, nitroprusside, nitroglycerin, phentolamine, and diazoxide have been used in refractory situations. Short-acting β-blockers, which depress the patient's native cardiac output, are used cautiously because if an unexpected interruption of ECMO support occurs, cardiac output would be significantly reduced.

VV ECMO provides no cardiac override. The native cardiac output remains fully pulsatile; thus a normal arterial pulse pressure is maintained. Cardiac output is augmented as with any critically ill patient.

Environmental stimuli, anxiety, and pain contribute to patient stress. Controlling the environment and clustering nursing care to allow periods of uninterrupted sleep become a nursing priority. Effective nursing intervention requires coordinating respiratory therapists, physicians, and other staff in providing their care in a sequence that maximizes a calm, quiet atmosphere. In addition, minimizing the numbers of bedside personnel and providing adequate sedation aid in reducing anxiety.

Alteration in Fluid and Electrolyte Balance. The goal of fluid management is to promote diuresis while maintaining adequate tissue perfusion, nutrition, and hematologic values.[126] This goal requires astute assessment of hypotension, tachycardia, decreased urine output, poor capillary refill, and "bladder chatter." Administration of fluids and drugs is easily accomplished via the ECMO circuit. A multiple-port manifold is used to deliver maintenance intravenous (IV) fluid, parenteral nutrition and 10% intralipids, and numerous medications through a bladder port. The heparin drip is infused through a separate port that allows minuscule changes in dosage to be recognized immediately, independent of the rates of the other solutions.

The patient's total hourly IV rate is usually restricted to three-quarters maintenance to avoid fluid overload, which can compromise ventilation and weaning from ECMO. As with normal ventilation, there is an insensible water loss over the ECMO membrane. The daily volume of this loss is dependent on the size of the membrane and gas flow.

Prerenal oliguric states may be related to hypotensive insults before ECMO support, the dehydrating regimen while on ECMO, or the primarily nonpulsatile VA ECMO blood flow. Blood urea nitrogen (BUN) values frequently increase during ECMO support. Aggressive diuretic therapy with furosemide is administered to return patients to their dry weight. Low-dose dopamine (2.5 µg/kg/min) is often used to augment renal perfusion.

For patients who are resistant to diuretics, ultrafiltration can be incorporated within the ECMO circuit and used for fluid removal. Heparinization and access are nonissues in ECMO. Priming the hemofilter requires approximately 50 ml of blood; therefore additional colloid is kept available to compensate for this diversion. Blood is diverted from the oxygenator, ultrafiltrated, and then returned to the bladder. The volume of ultrafiltrate removed is determined by the patient's condition, dry weight, and estimated volume of fluid excess. The use of the hemofilter has little impact on serum electrolytes. However, rapid removal of excess fluid may result in dehydration with attendant elevations in BUN. The clinical signs of dehydration—that is, sunken eyes, dry mucous membranes, dry skin with poor turgor, and a depressed anterior fontanelle in the infant—are monitored. Accurate documentation of fluid balance is maintained, and the use of an ongoing cumulative balance sheet over the entire ECMO course is helpful in evaluating the total fluid status of the patient. Acute renal failure, as evidenced by anuria, progressive hyperkalemia, and increased BUN and creatinine, is managed with hemodialysis placed similarly within the ECMO circuit.

Alteration in Hemostasis. Activated clotting times (ACTs) are closely monitored to guide the degree of heparinization necessary to avoid clot formation within the circuit and prevent untoward systemic bleeding. When the initial postcannulation ACT is 300 seconds, a heparin drip is started at 10 U/kg/hr. ACTs are performed hourly at the bedside, and the heparin drip is titrated to maintain the ACT between 180 and 220 seconds. Several factors, such as low flow rates, bleeding, renal function, or platelet administration, may alter this range. A low flow rate caused by bladder chatter may require higher ACTs; the slower the flow, the greater the chance of clot formation within the circuit. Diuresis and platelet administration both require an increase in heparin dosage. The kidneys excrete heparin, so a lower ACT can be expected after a large diuresis; the opposite is true in renal failure. Platelets contain heparinase, an enzyme that metabolizes heparin; therefore the heparin dose is increased when platelets are administered. Before platelet administration, a baseline ACT is performed, and if it is less than 200 seconds, a heparin bolus equal to one half of the hourly infusion dose is administered. When half of the platelets have been infused, a repeat ACT is performed and treated. In addition to a bolus dose, the heparin drip rate may need to be increased by 10 to 20 U/hr at this time. Another ACT is checked at the end of the platelet transfusion and is treated if necessary.

Because the membrane and the pump both contribute to platelet destruction, daily platelet transfusions may be necessary to maintain a platelet count greater than 100,000. If fluid volume is an issue, the platelets may be concentrated or "spun," which in itself destroys some platelets. Thus a greater increase is seen in the posttransfusion platelet count if the platelets are administered in their unconcentrated form. Platelets can be given directly to the patient via a peripheral or central IV line or infused through the circuit postmembrane. Infusion into the circuit premembrane results in platelet aggregation within the membrane, which

diminishes platelet effectiveness and increases the possibility of clot formation in the membrane.

Prothrombin time is kept below 17 seconds. An elevation of 3 seconds over control will require FFP of 10 to 20 ml/kg. Partial thromboplastin times (PTTs) are not followed because they will always be greater than 100 as a result of heparinization. Large volumes of chest tube drainage may require replacement of FFP at the rate of 0.5 ml per milliliter of drainage.

Fibrinogen levels are maintained at 200%. One to three units of cryoprecipitate are given to correct low fibrinogen levels but cannot be infused through the circuit because the factors are destroyed by the heat exchanger.

As with any systemically heparinized patient, precautions are necessary to avoid bleeding. Insertion of all vascular lines, nasogastric tube, bladder catheter, or other indwelling tubes should be accomplished before the initiation of ECMO. No intramuscular medications should be given, nor should finger or heel sticks be performed. Should manipulation or replacement of an indwelling catheter be necessary during ECMO, a platelet transfusion before the event helps avoid or minimize bleeding. All large catheters should remain in place for the duration of ECMO support to avoid hemorrhage on removal. The topical administration of a microfibrillar collagen hemostat (Avitene) and absorbable gelatin (Gelfoam) may control cannula site oozing with a pressure dressing. Uncontrollable bleeding may require surgical exploration of the wound, and all site bleeding should be measured and counted as output.

Unlike the neonatal population, spontaneous intracranial bleeding is rare in the pediatric population. In the United States, a 20% incidence of extracranial bleeding in seen in neonates; the incidence more than doubles to 50% in the pediatric population. Assessment of fluids, vasopressors, antihypertensives, diuretics, and blood product replacement requires constant vigilance. Persistent hypovolemia, especially increasing red blood cell requirements, is a warning sign of occult bleeding. Subtle clinical signs include increased pallor, agitation, increased respiratory rate, and decreased capillary refill. All bodily secretions are checked for the presence of blood. Pulmonary hemorrhage is obvious by bright red blood endotracheal secretions or massive chest tube drainage. Mucous membrane bleeding, most often involving the oronasopharynx, may require packing. Gastric bleeding becomes evident through nasogastric tube drainage or melena. Abdominal girths are monitored; abdominal x-ray and ultrasound studies may confirm any abdominal bleeding.

Maintaining an adequate platelet count and a lower ACT can minimize most bleeding. Unfortunately, the progression of almost any bleeding process during ECMO is almost inevitable.

A continuous infusion of aminocaproic acid (Amicar; Lederle Parenterals, Carolina, Puerto Rico) has been helpful in controlling bleeding in high-risk patients.[129] Amicar stabilizes clot formation through inhibition of thrombolysis. Amicar inhibits both plasminogen activator substances and, to a lesser degree, antiplasmin activity. It also slows the production of plasmin, which lyses fibrin and fibrinogen.

After cannulation, Amicar, 100 mg/kg, is administered diluted in equal volumes of 5% dextrose in water or normal saline through a peripheral IV over 5 to 10 minutes. A constant infusion of 30 mg/kg/hr is then infused via the ECMO circuit. Therapeutic dosage is achieved when a daily plasminogen activator time is greater than 120 seconds. ACTs remain in the 180- to 200-second range. Amicar is discontinued if bleeding is not a problem after 72 hours.

Potential Alterations in Nutrition. Transpyloric enteral or parenteral nutrition provides the child with the necessary 80 to 100 kcal/kg for healing to occur. If the patient is fluid restricted, then ultrafiltration can be used to permit earlier initiation of full nutrition. Pettignano and colleagues[130] reported that full enteral nutrition in patients supported on either VV or VA ECMO was well tolerated, provided adequate nutrition, was cost effective, and was without complications. Otherwise, the ECMO circuit is limited to 10% intralipids at 1 g/kg/day because the fat may interfere with membrane function. Any additional or more concentrated intralipid solution is delivered through a peripheral or central IV. Usually patients initially are given ranitidine (Zantac) to inhibit gastric acid secretion. Gastric pH is monitored routinely. The nutritional status may be evaluated by following serum albumin and total protein levels, by stringently monitoring fluid balances, and by clinical observation.

Alteration in Comfort. With rare exceptions, the pediatric ECMO patient is a previously healthy child who perceives and reacts to pain and is subject to fear and anxiety. The pediatric patient supported on ECMO for ARF lives prone for at least 3 weeks in an overstimulating environment with little opportunity for long periods of undisturbed rest. Constant infusions and bolus doses of morphine sulfate are used to alleviate discomfort.[131] Fentanyl is avoided because of membrane binding and patient tolerance. The ECMO circuit continuously binds close to 1000 μg of fentanyl, and tolerance, achieved at different times, increases approximately 10% per day.[132]

The ECMO patient is at risk for cannula displacement with excessive head or shoulder movement. The head is supported in an optimal position, but sedation *must* be sufficient for patient safety. Benzodiazepines such as lorazepam (Ativan) or midazolam (Versed) are used for sedation and amnesia. The goal is to provide the patient with a comfortable ECMO course while still allowing neurologic evaluation and periodic social interaction. Depending on the level of sedation achieved, the patient may require premedication with a narcotic or sedative for suctioning, dressing changes, or other noxious procedures.

Maintaining skin integrity can be a particularly challenging when caring for the pediatric ECMO patient. Hypervigilance is essential. A low air-loss bed and gel pillow placed under the occiput are often used. It is not impossible to slightly turn the patient on a routine basis to minimize pressure points, visualize the back, and provide skin care. Other nursing comfort measures include, but are not limited to, passive range of motion and repositioning of the extremities, hand rolls, and skin and mouth care.

With organization of nursing and medical procedures, the patient should have periods to simply rest undisturbed. During these times, listening to favorite music or television programs may be relaxing. Radios and tape decks may be used; headphones may be carefully placed on the older child. The presence of the child's family often provides the most comfort.

Preventing Iatrogenic Injury
Sepsis. Although the potential for sepsis increases with ECMO support, it is very difficult to detect. The usual first sign of sepsis is fever, but temperature instability is blunted by the heat exchanger. A consistently low platelet count, often an indicator of sepsis, is unreliable because of the degree of platelet consumption by the circuit. A persistent elevation in white blood cells, with or without a significant shift in the differential, or positive cultures may be the only dependable sign. Blood, urine, and tracheal aspiration cultures are obtained every other day. Prophylactic antibiotics (ampicillin, oxacillin, cefotaxime) are administered throughout the ECMO course. Gentamicin levels are closely monitored. Because of slow gentamicin excretion, higher trough levels result, necessitating the extension of dose intervals to every 18 hours.

Accidental Decannulation. In a properly sedated, carefully monitored ECMO patient, accidental decannulation is rare. The patient becomes most vulnerable during any examination or exploration of the insertion site, being moved for procedures or linen change, or during patient transport. Accidental decannulation can result in death by exsanguination. Emergency action includes applying very firm pressure to the cannulation site and clamping the remaining cannula. There may be no chance for recannulation without entering the thoracic cavity.

Cardiac Arrest. In the event of a cardiac arrest, cardiac compressions are unnecessary in patients supported on VA ECMO because pump flow can be increased to provide optimal cardiac output for organ perfusion. Compressions with ventilations are still necessary in the patient supported on VV ECMO.

Mechanical Failure. Occasionally a portion of the ECMO circuit will malfunction, requiring the patient to be immediately isolated from the system. There is a specific sequence of clamping the ECMO circuit when coming off ECMO: (1) clamp the venous cannula, (2) unclamp the bridge, and then (3) clamp the arterial cannula. Clamping in this sequence allows the venous drainage to stop before the arterial return is clamped, increases the patient's blood volume, and helps prevent hypotension. The patient's ventilator settings are increased, and colloid and drugs, including chemical paralyzing agents, are administered as needed. The gas source is removed from the membrane to prevent air emboli; system repairs are performed by the ECMO specialist, and therapy is resumed as soon as possible.

Normally, the rapid, high-volume blood flow through the circuit inhibits clot formation. However, treating hemorrhage in the pediatric ECMO patient requires lower heparin doses, which may result in an increase in clot formation. The bridge is one portion of the system that has the potential for blood stagnation. Periodic opening of the bridge provides a flush of blood that remixes pooled blood and reduces the potential for clot formation. Small clots that form on the membrane may decrease its overall efficiency but may not be life threatening. Occasionally, a clot will form and enlarge in a portion of the circuit that will require replacement of that section of the circuit or, in some cases, changing the entire ECMO circuit.

The multiple access ports and connectors increase the potential for air emboli. Air on the venous side is allowed to drift down to the bladder, where it may be aspirated from a bladder port. Air on the arterial side is a life-threatening emergency. Here, air can be forced across the bridge into the venous side of the circuit and then aspirated out.

The maximum efficiency of the membrane is often limited to approximately 2 weeks but may be further restricted in the presence of low flow rates or ACT ranges. The premembrane pressure should be less than 300 mmHg to avoid red blood cell and platelet destruction. A rise in this pressure, especially when accompanied with a change in ABGs, indicates a failing membrane. Because CO_2 transfer is dependent on gas flow and the surface area of the membrane, a rising $Paco_2$ can be a sensitive indicator of loss of functioning membrane. If the sum of both premembrane and postmembrane pressures is greater than 700 mmHg, a very real danger of membrane rupture exists.

The area where the ECMO tubing is compressed by the pump's rollers is called the "raceway." The raceway is advanced several times during the ECMO course to avoid constant pressure on the same portion of tubing. Areas of wear could eventually rupture, causing rapid blood loss. All caretakers must use eye protection, as delineated by universal precautions, at ECMO bedspaces.

In the event of a pump failure, a hand crank may be used to propel blood manually. A fully charged backup generator should be located at the bedside at all times.

A failure or improper setting of the thermostat of the heater can result in the exchanger's water bath either cooling to room temperature or overheating to unacceptable limits. A cooled water bath will result in a hypothermic, mottled, bradycardiac, and hypotensive child. The patient will become feverish, tachycardiac, and hypertensive if the heater temperature becomes excessive.

Alteration in Parental Role. In rapid succession, parents are faced with a PICU admission, information of a grave illness and possible death, and requests for permission to use life-supporting technologies that have no guarantees for outcome and a long list of potential complications. Often, the child must be transported to an ECMO center, separating the parents from home, family, and support systems.

Meeting the parents either before cannulation or soon after to explain what they will see and hear in the ECMO bedspace is necessary. The high-technology environment is taken to the extreme with ECMO. Seeing the child connected to so many machines with his or blood circulating outside the body is frightening. Parent-oriented ECMO literature may be helpful in reinforcing explanations.

Time is allotted for the patient's team to talk with the parents and answer their questions. Honest, pertinent information is the base on which the parents will make future decisions regarding changes in life support. Given the potential complications of pediatric ECMO, predictors are unreliable. Hope is always supported by acknowledging the positive or neutral aspects of the child's condition, accepting the parents' future plans that include the child, and displaying guarded optimism. Only when the decision is made to terminate all support is hope tempered with reality.

Although nursing plays an enormous role in parental support, talking with another parent whose child was supported on ECMO may be invaluable. Several regional ECMO parent support groups are available with parents of ECMO survivors providing telephone contact with new ECMO parents. The parent support groups provide a supportive forum for the intimate exchange of feelings and ideas.

Coming off ECMO. It may take as little as 5 days or as long as 6 weeks for indicators of improved pulmonary function to occur. These include a clearing chest x-ray film, increasing lung compliance, and normalizing blood gases. On VA ECMO, the child's Pao_2 represents a mixture of pump blood and the blood that traverses his or her native cardiopulmonary circuit. With flows held constant, any decrease in Pao_2 represents an increase in patient contribution. Early in the course of ECMO, the patient contributes little, so pump flows are maintained at high levels. As the patient's pulmonary status improves, ECMO support can be titrated in one of two ways.

Weaning. In concert with improved lung function, pump flows are gradually decreased and ventilator settings are increased. Vital signs, pulse oximetry, and ABGs are monitored. The pump flow is weaned down to 20% to 30% of the original rate, and, if tolerated, the patient is clamped off ECMO. With this method, the patient is continuously challenged over many hours or days.

Cycling. Cycling is a time-limited method of trailing off ECMO. The patient is chemically paralyzed and sedated, all ventilator settings are increased, and the flows are gradually turned down until total flow is decreased to 30 ml/kg/min. If these steps are tolerated, the patient is clamped off ECMO. Following vital signs, pulse oximetry, and ABGs, the ventilator support is gradually decreased. If the patient can realize a Pao_2 greater than 60 mmHg and a $Paco_2$ less than 45 mmHg on reasonable ventilator settings, the decision is usually made to decannulate. If these parameters cannot be met, the patient is cycled again at a later time, with modified ventilator settings to promote alveolar recruitment, after aggressive pulmonary care to mobilize secretions, or with inotropic support. The goal is to minimize O_2 toxicity and barotrauma but to wean ECMO support as soon as possible. With this method, the patient is challenged only once or twice a day for a short time, and the low flow rates that are associated with thromboemboli can be avoided. After cycling, flows are gradually increased, and the patient is observed for rebound hypertension.

In either case, once the patient is excluded from the ECMO circuit, the bridge between the arterial and venous tubing is opened, and ECMO circulation continues. When weaning or cycling is completed, the patient is placed back on ECMO while the decision to continue or stop ECMO support is made. This is unnecessary when weaning or cycling from VV ECMO. In VV ECMO, the ventilator settings are increased as in VA ECMO, but the oxygen source to the membrane is capped. The ECMO blood flow continues to circulate through the patient, as well as the system.

Nursing responsibilities during cycling include reassuring the patient and parents that all the additional activity is controlled and assessing the patient's tolerance to weaning. Accurate documentation of vital signs, pulse oximetry, ventilator settings, and laboratory results is also necessary. If it is likely that the patient will be isolated from the ECMO circuit, all infusions are transferred to a peripheral or central IV. The heparin infusion remains in the circuit, but the dose is reduced by 50% until the patient is again supported on ECMO and an ACT is rechecked.

Decannulation. Decannulation is a surgical procedure performed in the PICU. The patient is anesthetized and paralyzed, all infusions are transferred to a peripheral or central IV, and the heparin drip is discontinued. The patient is prepped and draped, with the nurse maintaining access to a patent IV for any necessary drug administration. Two units of platelets are given postdecannulation. If cannulation and the ECMO course have done minimal damage to the vessels, the surgeon may attempt reconstruction. Otherwise, both are ligated. Advances in cannulas and technique allow vessel repair.[133] If the carotid artery is ligated, collateral flow to the right cerebral hemisphere is maintained by the external carotid and vertebral arteries. Complications and long-term problems related specifically to ligation or repair of the carotid artery are unknown.

Postdecannulation, patient movement is limited until all clotting factors have returned to baseline. Narcotics are slowly weaned; the patient is assessed for iatrogenic physical withdrawal. A smooth transition can be accomplished by switching the patient over to longer-acting narcotics, for example, methadone in equal analgesic doses.

SUMMARY

Caring for an infant or child who requires support of oxygenation or ventilation is inherent to the practice of pediatric critical care nursing. Even so, there is not a significant amount of nursing research to help guide it. This chapter presents selected principles of oxygenation and ventilation as they pertain to critically ill or injured infants and children. As discussed, pulmonary system functioning is essential for life and because of developmental immaturity, the pediatric patient is at high risk for system dysfunction.

The next decade brings hope for primary prevention to avoid pediatric critical illness involving the pulmonary system. The next decade also brings new therapies, for example, intratracheal pulmonary ventilation and liquid perfluorocarbon ventilation.[134,135] As new therapies become available, what constitutes conventional and unconventional support of the pulmonary system will be redefined.

REFERENCES

1. AACN Certification Corporation: *Pediatric examination: a blueprint for study,* Aliso Viejo, Calif, 1999, AACN Certification Corporation.
2. Biel M, Eastwood JA, Muenzen P et al: Evolving trends in critical care nursing practice: results of a certification role delineation study, *Am J Crit Care* 8:285-290, 1999.
3. Chameides L, Hazinski MF, eds: *Textbook of pediatric advanced life support,* Dallas, 1997, American Heart Association.
4. O'Brodovich HM, Haddad GG: The functional basis of respiratory pathology. In Chernick V, ed: *Kendig's disorders of the respiratory tract in children,* Philadelphia, 1990, WB Saunders.
5. Charnock EL, Doershuk CF: Developmental aspects of the human lung, *Pediatr Clin North Am* 20:275-292, 1973.
6. Sadler TW: *Langman's medical embryology,* Baltimore, 1990, Williams & Wilkins.
7. Moore KL, Persaud TVN: *The respiratory system: the developing human,* Philadelphia, 1993, WB Saunders.
8. Polgar, G, Weng TR: The functional development of the respiratory system, *Am Rev Respir Dis* 120:625-695, 1979.
9. Salzberg AM: Congenital malformations of the lower respiratory tract. In Kendig EL Jr, Chernick V, eds: *Disorders of the respiratory tract in children,* vol 1, Philadelphia, 1977, WB Saunders.

10. Backofen JE, Rogers MC: Emergency management of the airway. In Rogers MC, ed: *Textbook of pediatric intensive care,* vol 1, Baltimore, 1992, Williams & Wilkins.
11. Thompson JE, Farrell E, McManus M: Neonatal and pediatric airway emergencies, *Respir Care* 37:582-599, 1992.
12. Wohl ME, Mead J: Age as a factor in respiratory distress. In Chernick V, ed: *Kendig's disorders of the respiratory tract in children,* Philadelphia, 1990, WB Saunders.
13. Macklem PT: Airway obstruction and collateral ventilation, *Physiol Rev* 51:368, 1971.
14. Boyden EA: Development and growth of the airways. In Hodson WA, ed: *Development of the lung,* New York, 1977, Marcel Dekker.
15. Barcoft J: On anoxaemia, *Lancet* 2:485, 1920.
16. Lister G: Oxygen supply/demand in the critically ill. In Taylor R, ed: *Critical care: state of the art,* vol 12, Fullerton, Calif, 1991, Society of Critical Care Medicine.
17. Behnke M, Koff PB: Patient assessment. In Koff PB, Eitzman D, Neu J, eds: *Neonatal and pediatric respiratory care,* ed 2, St Louis, 1993, Mosby.
18. Hogg JC, Williams J, Richardson JB et al: Age as a factors in the distribution of lower airway conductance and in the pathologic anatomy of obstructive lung disease, *N Engl J Med* 282:1283, 1970.

19. West JB, Dollery CT, Naimark A: Distribution of blood flow in isolated lung: relation to vascular and alveolar pressures, *J Appl Physiol* 19:713, 1964.
20. Helfaer MA, Nichols DG, Rogers MC: Developmental physiology of the respiratory system. In Rogers MC, ed: *Textbook of pediatric intensive care,* ed 2, Baltimore, 1992, Williams & Wilkins.
21. Endo AS, Nishioka E: Neonatal assessment. In Kenner C, Brueggemeyer A, Gunderson LP, eds: *Comprehensive neonatal nursing,* Philadelphia, 1993, WB Saunders.
22. Forgacs P: The functional basis of pulmonary sounds, *Chest* 73:399, 1978.
23. Drakulovic MB, Torres A, Bauer TT et al: Supine body position as a risk factor for nosocomial pneumonia in mechanically ventilated patients: a randomised trial, *Lancet* 354:1851-1858, 1999.
24. Costello JM: AAC Intervention in the intensive care unit: The Children's Hospital, Boston model, *AAC Augmentative and Alternative Communication* 16 (September) (in press).
25. Boggs RL: Airway management. In Boggs RL, Wooldridge-King M, eds: *AACN procedure manual for critical care,* ed 3, Philadelphia, 1993, WB Saunders.
26. Henneman EA, Bellamy P, Togashi C: Peripheral nerve stimulators in the critical care setting: a policy for monitoring neuro-

muscular blockade, *Crit Care Nurs* 15:82-88, 1995.

27. Bucher H, Fanconi S, Baeckert P et al: Hyperoxemia in newborn infants, *Pediatrics* 84:226-230, 1989.

28. Barker SJ, Shah NK: The effects of motion on performance of oximeters in volunteers, *Anesthesiology* 86:101-108, 1997.

29. Kellehen JF, Ruff RH: The penumbra effect: vasomotion-dependent pulse oximeter artifact due to probe malposition, *Anesthesiology* 71:787-791, 1989.

30. Pascucci RC, Schena JA, Thompson JE: Comparison of a sidestream and mainstream capnometer in infants, *Crit Care Med* 17:560-562, 1989.

31. Eichhorn JH, Cooper JB, Cullen DJ et al: Standards for patient monitoring during anesthesia at Harvard Medical School. *JAMA* 256:1017-1020, 1986.

32. Bhende MS, Thompson AE: Evaluation of an end-tidal CO_2 detector during pediatric cardiopulmonary resuscitation, *Pediatrics* 95:395-400, 1995.

33. Arnold JH, Thompson JE, Arnold LW: Single breath CO_2 analysis: description and validation of a method, *Crit Care Med* 24:96-102, 1996.

34. Arnold JH, Stenz RI, Grenier B et al: Single-breath CO_2 analysis as a predictor of lung volume change in a model of acute lung injury, *Crit Care Med* 28:760-764, 2000.

35. Szaflarski N: Preanalytic error associated with blood gas/pH measurement, *Crit Care Nurs* 16:89-100, 1996.

36. Donlen J: Interpreting acid-base problems through arterial blood gases, *Crit Care Nurs* 3:34-38, 1983.

37. Kelly-Heidenthal P, O'Connor M: Nursing assessment of portable AP chest X-rays, *Dimens Crit Care Nurs* 13:127-132, 1994.

38. Wilson BG, Desautels DA: Oxygen therapy. In Koff PB, Eitzman D, Neu J, eds: *Neonatal and pediatric respiratory care,* ed 2, St Louis, 1993, Mosby.

39. Martin LD, Rafferty FF, Gioia FR: Principles of respiratory support and mechanical ventilation. In Rogers MC, ed: *Textbook of pediatric intensive care,* vol 1, Baltimore, 1992, Williams & Wilkins.

40. McPherson SP: *Respiratory therapy equipment,* St Louis, 1990, Mosby.

41. Lough MD, Doershuk CF, Stern RC: *Pediatric respiratory therapy,* St Louis, 1985, Mosby.

42. Yaster M: Airway management. In Nicholes DG et al, eds: *Golden hour: the handbook of advanced pediatric life support,* St Louis, 1991, Mosby.

43. Arnold J, Castro C: Endotracheal intubation. In Blummer JL, ed: *A practical guide to pediatric intensive care,* ed 3, St Louis, 1990, Mosby.

44. Benjamin PK, Thompson JE, O'Rourke PP: Complications of mechanical ventilation in a children's hospital multidisciplinary intensive care unit, *Respir Care* 35:873-878, 1990.

45. Scott PH, Eigen H, Moye LA et al: Predictability and consequences of spontaneous extubation in a pediatric ICU, *Crit Care Med* 13:228-232, 1985.

46. Franck LS, Vaughn B, Wallace J: Extubation reintubation in the NICU: identifying opportunities to improve care, *Pediatr Nurs* 18:267-270, 1992.

47. Little LA, Koenig JC Jr, Newth CJL: Factors affecting accidental extubations in neonatal and pediatric intensive care patients, *Crit Care Med* 18:163-165, 1990.

48. Manning SC, Brown OE: Sequelae of intubation. In Levin DL, Morris FC, eds: *Essentials of pediatric intensive care,* St Louis, 1990, Quality Medical Publishing.

49. Engleman SG, Turnage-Carrier C: Tolerance of the Passy-Muir speaking valve in infants and children less than 2 years of age, *Pediatr Nurs* 23:571-573, 1997.

50. Jackson D, Albamonte S: Enhancing communication with the Passy-Muir valve, *Pediatr Nurs* 20:149-153, 1994.

51. Kaut K, Turcott JC, Lavery M: Passy-Muir speaking valve, *Dimens Crit Care Nurs* 15:298-306, 1996.

52. Daicoff BB, Langham MR Jr, Mullet TW et al: Physiologic response to two endotracheal suctioning techniques in newborn lambs with and without acute pulmonary hypertension, *Am J Crit Care* 4:453-459, 1995.

53. Swartz K, Noonan DM, Edwards-Beckett J: A national survey of endotracheal suctioning techniques in the pediatric population, *Heart Lung* 25:52-60, 1996.

54. Copnell B, Fergusson D: Endotracheal suctioning: time-worn ritual or timely intervention, *Am J Crit Care* 4:100-105, 1995.

55. Turner B: Maintaining the artificial airway: current concepts, *Pediatr Nurs* 16:487-493, 1990.

56. Alpan G, Glick B, Peleg O et al: Pneumothorax due to endotracheal tube suction, *Am J Perinatol* 1, 345-348, 1984.

57. Anderson KD, Chandra R: Pneumothorax secondary to perforation of sequential bronchi by suction catheters, *J Pediatr Surg* 11:687-693, 1976.

58. Kleiber C, Krutzfield N, Rose E: Acute histologic changes in the tracheobronchial tree associated with different suction catheter insertion techniques, *Heart Lung* 17:10-14, 1988.

59. AARC—American Association for Respiratory Care: Clinical practice guideline: endotracheal suctioning of mechanically ventilated adults and children with artificial airways, *Respir Care* 38:500-504, 1993.

60. Ackerman MH, Ecklund MM, Abu-Jumah M: A review of normal saline instillation: implications for practice, *Dimens Crit Care Nurs* 15:31-38, 1996.

61. Raymond SJ: Normal saline instillation before suctioning: helpful or harmful? A review of the literature, *Am J Crit Care* 4:267-271, 1995.

62. Shekleton ME, Nield M: Ineffective airway clearance related to artificial airway, *Nurs Clin North Am* 22:161-177, 1987.

63. Gray JE, MacIntyre NR, Kronenberger WG: The effects of bolus normal-saline instillation in conjunction with endotracheal suctioning, *Respir Care* 35:785-790, 1990.

64. Bostick J, Wendelgass ST: Normal saline instillation as part of the suction procedure: effects on paO_2 and amount of secretions, *Heart Lung* 16:532-537, 1987.

65. Chopra SG, Taplin V, Simmons DH et al: Effects of hydration and physical therapy on tracheal transport velocity, *Am Rev Respir Dis* 115:1009-1014, 1977.

66. Kahn RC: Humidification of the airways: adequate for function and integrity, *Chest* 84:510-511, 1983.

67. Hagler DA, Traver GA: Endotracheal saline and suction catheters: sources of lower airway contamination, *Am J Crit Care* 3:444-447, 1994.

68. Ochsenreither JM: Closed tracheal suctioning advantages, drawbacks, and research recommendations, *The Online Journal of Knowledge Synthesis for Nursing,* 1995, vol 2, Document no 2; online number 14.

69. Noll MA, Hix CD, Scott G: Closed tracheal suction systems: effectiveness and nursing implications. *AACN Clin Issues Crit Care Nurs* 1:318-326, 1990.

70. Paul-Allen J, Ostrow CL: Survey of nursing practices with closed-system suctioning, *Am J Crit Care* 9:9-17, 2000.

71. Carlon GC, Fox SJ, Ackerman NJ: Evaluation of a closed-tracheal suction system, *Crit Care Med* 15:522-525, 1987.

72. Witmer MT, Hess D, Simmons M: An evaluation of the effectiveness of secretion removal with a closed-circuit suction catheter, *Respir Care* 35:1117, 1990.

73. Baker T, Taylor M, Wilson M et al: Evaluation of a closed system endotracheal suction catheter, *Am J Infect Control* 17:97, 1989.

74. Glass C, Grap MJ, Sessler CN: Endotracheal tube narrowing after closed-system suctioning: prevalence and risk factors, *Am J Crit Care* 8:93-100, 1999.

75. Mosca FA, Colnaghi M, Lattanzio et al: Closed versus open endotracheal suctioning in preterm infants: effects on cerebral oxygenation and blood volume, *Biol Neonate* 72:9-14, 1997.

76. Scott AA, Koff PB: Airway care and chest physiotherapy. In Koff PB, Eitzman D, Neu J, eds: *Neonatal and pediatric respiratory care,* ed 2, St Louis, 1993, Mosby.

77. Kirilloff L, Owens G, Rogers R et al: Does chest physical therapy work? *Chest* 88:436-444, 1985.

78. Krause MF, Hoehn T: Chest physiotherapy in mechanically ventilated children: a review, *Crit Care Med* 28:1648-1651, 2000.

79. Wigal DT, Will MW: Incentive spirometry treatments. In Boggs RL, Wooldridge-King M, eds: *AACN procedure manual for critical care,* ed 3, Philadelphia, 1993, WB Saunders.

80. Anderson JB, Falk M: Chest physiotherapy in the pediatric age group, *Respir Care* 36:546-552, 1991.

81. Lough M: Medicated aerosol therapy. In Blummer JL ed: *A practical guide to pediatric intensive care,* St Louis, 1990, Mosby.

82. MacIntyre NR, Silver RM, Miller CW et al: Aerosol delivery in intubated mechanically ventilated patients, *Crit Care Med* 13:81-84, 1985.

83. Fuller HD, Dolovich MB, Posmituck G et al: Pressurized aerosol versus jet aerosol delivery to mechanically ventilated patients: comparison of dose to the lungs, *Am Rev Respir Dis* 141:440-444, 1990.

84. Koff PB, Durmowicz AG: Pharmacology. In Koff PB, Eitzman D, Neu J, eds: *Neonatal and pediatric respiratory care,* ed 2, St Louis, 1993, Mosby.

85. Salyer JW, Chatburn RL: Patterns of practice in neonatal and pediatric respiratory care, *Respir Care* 35:879-888, 1990.

86. Portnoy J, Nadel G, Amado M et al: Continuous nebulization for status asthmaticus, *Ann Allergy* 69:71-79, 1992.

87. Papo MC, Frank J, Thompson AE: A prospective, randomized study of continuous versus intermittent nebulized albuterol for severe status asthmaticus in children, *Crit Care Med* 21:1479-1486, 1993.

88. Kelly HW, Williams BC, Katz R et al: Safety of frequent high dose nebulized terbutaline in children with acute severe asthma. *Ann Allergy* 64:229-233, 1990.

89. Chatburn RL: A new system for understanding mechanical ventilators, *Respir Care* 36:1123-1155, 1991.

90. Chatburn RL: Principles and practice of neonatal and pediatric mechanical ventilation, *Respir Care* 36:569-595, 1991.

91. Betit P, Thompson JE, Benjamin PK: Mechanical ventilation. In Koff PB, Eitzman D, Neu J, eds: *Neonatal and pediatric respiratory care,* ed 2, St Louis, 1993, Mosby.

92. Juarez P: Mechanical ventilation for the patient with severe ARDS: PC-IRV, *Crit Care Nurs* 12:34-39, 1992.

93. Briones TL: Pressure controlled inverse ration ventilation in respiratory failure, *Dimens Crit Care Nurs* 10:254-261, 1991.

94. Boegner E: Pediatric ventilatory support and weaning parameters, *AACN Clin Issues Crit Care Nurs* 1:378-386, 1990.

95. AARC—American Association for Respiratory Care: Consensus statement on the essentials of mechanical ventilators—1992, *Respir Care* 37:1000-1008, 1992.

96. Oakes D: *Neonatal/pediatric respiratory care,* Old Towne, Me, 1990, Health Educator Publications.

97. Benson MS, Pierson DJ: Autopeep during mechanical ventilation of adults, *Respir Care* 33:557-568, 1988.

98. Torres A, Serra-Batlles J, Ros E et al: Pulmonary aspiration of gastric contents in patients receiving mechanical ventilation: the effect of body position, *Ann Intern Med* 116:540-543, 1992.

99. Curley MAQ, Fackler JC: Weaning from mechanical ventilation: patterns in young children recovering from acute hypoxemic respiratory failure, *Am J Crit Care* 7:335-345, 1998.

100. Weilitz, PB: Weaning a patient from mechanical ventilation, *Crit Care Nurs* 13:33-41, 1993.

101. Randolph A: Weaning from mechanical ventilation, *New Horiz* 7:374-385, 1999.

102. Henneman EA: The art and science of weaning from mechanical ventilation, *Focus Crit Care* 18:490-500, 1991.

103. Kollef MH, Shapiro SD, Silver P et al: A randomized, controlled trial of protocol-directed versus physician-directed weaning from mechanical ventilation, *Crit Care Med* 25:567-574, 1997.

104. O'Neill N: Improving ventilation in children using bilevel positive airway pressure, *Pediatr Nurs* 24:377-382, 1998.

105. American Respiratory Care Foundation Consensus Statement: Non-invasive positive pressure ventilation, *Respir Care* 42:365-369, 1997.

106. Blaufuss JA, Wallace CJ: Two negative pressure ventilators: current clinical application and nursing care, *Crit Care Nurs Q* 9:14-30, 1987.

107. Chatburn RL: High-frequency ventilation. In Blummer JL, ed: *A practical guide to pediatric intensive care,* ed 3, Philadelphia, 1990, Mosby.

108. Chang HK, Harf A: High frequency ventilation: a review. *Respir Physiol* 157:135-152.

109. Coghill CH, Haywood JL, Chatburn RL et al: Neonatal and pediatric high-frequency ventilation: principles and practice, *Respir Care* 36:596-609, 1991.

110. Arnold JH, Truog RD, Thompson JE et al: High frequency oscillatory ventilation in pediatric respiratory failure, *Crit Care Med* 21:272-278, 1993.

111. Wetzel RC, Gioia FR: High frequency ventilation, *Pediatr Clin North Am* 34:15-37, 1987.

112. Heijman K, Heijman L, Jonzon A et al: High frequency positive pressure ventilation during anaesthesia and routine surgery in man, *Acta Anaesthesiol Scand* 16:172, 1972.

113. Tsuzaki K: High-frequency ventilation in neonates, *J Clin Anesth* 2:387-392, 1990.

114. Weber KR, Asselin JM: High frequency oscillatory ventilation, *Neonatal Intensive Care* 3:20-23, 1990.

115. Venegas D: Abstract: effects of HFV on distribution of ventilation, *Sixth conference of HFV in infants,* Snowbird, Utah, 1989.

116. Froese A, Bryan C: State of the art: high frequency ventilation, *Am Rev Respir Dis* 135:1363-1374, 1987.

117. Arnold JH, Hanson JH, Toro-Figuero LO et al: Prospective, randomized comparison of high-frequency oscillatory ventilation and conventional mechanical ventilation in pediatric respiratory failure, *Crit Care Med* 22:1530-1539, 1994.

118. Gonzalez F, Harris T, Black P et al: Decreased gas flow through pneumothoraces in neonates receiving high-frequency jet ventilation versus conventional ventilation, *J Pediatr* 110:464-466, 1987.

119. Curley MAQ, Molengraft JA: Care of the child supported on high frequency oscillatory ventilation, *AACN Clin Issues Crit Care Nurs* 5:49-58, 1994.

120. Arnold J: High-frequency ventilation in pediatric ARDS, *Respir Care* 43:961-965, 1998.

121. Grenier B, Thompson J: High-frequency oscillatory ventilation in pediatric patients, *Respir Care Clin N Am* 2:545-557, 1996.

122. Redmond CR, Loe, WA, Bartlett RH et al: Extracorporeal membrane oxygenation. In Goldsmith JP, Karotkin EH: *Assisted ventilation of the neonate,* Philadelphia, 1988, WB Saunders.

123. Fuhrman BP, Dalton HJ: Progress in pediatric extracorporeal membrane oxygenation, *Crit Care Clin* 8:191-202, 1992.

124. Dalton HJ, Heulitt MJ: Extracorporeal life support and pediatric respiratory failure: past, present, and future, *Respir Care* 43:966-977, 1998.

125. Anderson HL, Otsu T, Chapman RA et al: Venovenous extracorporeal life support in neonates using a double lumen catheter, *ASAIO Transactions* 35:650-653, 1989.

126. McDermott BK, Curley, MAQ: ECMO: current use and future directions, *AACN Clin Issues Crit Care Nurs* 1:348-364, 1990.

127. Chapman RA, Bartlett RH: *Extracorporeal life support for adult and pediatric patients,* Ann Arbor, Mich, 1990, ELSO & University of Michigan ECMO Team.

128. Keszler M, Subramanian S, Smith YA, et al: Pulmonary management during extracorporeal membrane oxygenation, *Crit Care Med* 17:495-500, 1989.

129. Wilson JM, Bower LK, Fackler JC et al: Aminocaproic acid decreases the incidence of intracranial hemorrhage and other bleeding complications of ECMO, *J Pediatr Surg* 28:536-540, 1993.

130. Pettignano R, Hears M, Davis R et al: Total enteral nutrition versus total parenteral nutrition during pediatric extracorporeal membrane oxygenation, *Crit Care Med* 26:358-363, 1998.

131. Caron E, Maguire DP: Narcotic dependency of the infant on ECMO, *J Perinat Neonatal Nurs* 4:63-74, 1990.

132. Arnold JH, Truog RD, Scavone JM et al: Changes in the pharmacodynamic response to fentanyl in neonates during continuous infusion, *J Pediatr* 119:639-643, 1991.

133. Adolph V, Bonis S, Falteman K et al: Carotid artery repair after pediatric extracorporeal membrane oxygenation, *J Pediatr Surg* 25:867-869, 1990.

134. Fuhrman BT, Paczan PR, Defrancisis M: Perfluorocarbon-associated gas exchange, *Crit Care Med* 19:712-722, 1991.

135. Greenspan JS: Liquid ventilation: a developing technology, *Neonatal Netw* 12:23-32, 1993.

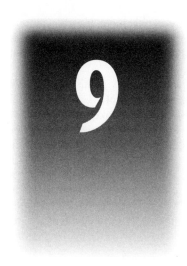

Acid-Base Balance

Ann Powers

All patients who are admitted to the pediatric critical care unit are at risk for acid-base disturbances that may complicate their underlying disorder and further compromise their overall status. Acid-base balance is maintained through a variety of physiologic processes, which may be disrupted with serious illness or injury. Knowledge of acid-base balance is essential to the practice of pediatric critical care nursing so that appropriate assessment, monitoring, and intervention can be provided in a timely manner to optimize the child's outcome.

DEFINITION OF ACID-BASE BALANCE

Normal metabolism results in the production of acids. An acid is a proton or hydrogen ion (H^+) donor, and a base is a proton or hydrogen ion acceptor. A large number of potential hydrogen ions exist in the body, most of which are buffered and therefore not in free form. The normal concentration of free H^+ in the extracellular fluid (ECF) is extremely small, approximately 40 nmEq/L, which is equivalent to one millionth of a mEq/L concentration of sodium. The term *pH* expresses the negative logarithm of free H^+ concentration. The relationship is inversely proportional in that as free H^+ concentration increases, pH decreases, and vice versa. A normal arterial pH of 7.40 correlates with a free H^+ concentration of 40 nmEq/L. For each 0.01-unit (U) change in pH from 7.40, H^+ concentration changes 1 nmEq/L in the opposite direction, provided that the pH range is between 7.20 and 7.50.

Normal metabolism produces hydrogen in the form of volatile and fixed acids. To maintain pH within its normal narrow range of 7.35 to 7.45, acids must be buffered or excreted. A buffer is defined as a substance that reduces the change in a solution's free H^+ concentration when an acid or base is added to it. In other words, the presence of a buffer in a solution increases the amount of acid or base that must be added to change the pH.

The largest amount of acid load in the body is in the form of carbonic acid (H_2CO_3), which is a volatile acid. Carbonic acid is formed, or dissociated, into either hydrogen and bicarbonate or carbon dioxide and water. This is illustrated by the following equation:

$$H^+ + HCO_3^- \rightleftharpoons H_2CO_3 \rightleftharpoons CO_2 + H_2O$$

Carbonic acid
H_2CO_3

H^+ + HCO_3^- CO_2 + H_2O
Hydrogen   Bicarbonate   Carbon dioxide   Water

The specific reaction (dissociation or formation of carbonic acid) is determined by the underlying acid-base environment.

Hydrogen that is generated in the form of a fixed acid includes lactic acid, ketoacid, phosphoric acid, and sulfuric

---

Box 9-1

◆ **Physiologic Effects of Alterations in pH**

Increase pH

Increase

Insulin-induced glycolysis
Responsiveness to catecholamines
Lactate production

Decrease

Krebs cycle oxidations in muscles and renal cortex
Gluconeogenesis in the renal cortex
2,3-Diphosphoglycerate concentration with a corresponding
   left shift in the oxyhemoglobin dissociation curve
Vascular tone and resistance

Decrease pH

Increase

Glycolysis
Lipolysis
Krebs cycle oxidations in muscles and renal cortex
Gluconeogenesis in the renal cortex
2,3-Diphosphoglycerate concentration with a correspond-
   ing right shift in the oxyhemoglobin dissociation curve
Pulmonary vascular resistance

Decrease

Quantities of liver glycogen
Lactate production
Insulin secretion and binding to receptors
Pancreatic amylase secretion
Threshold for ventricular fibrillation
Responsiveness to catecholamines
Peripheral vascular resistance
Mesenteric blood flow
Pulmonary macrophage function
Granulocyte function
Immune response

Data from Czekaj L: Promoting acid base balance. In Kinney MR et al, eds: *AACN's clinical reference for critical care nursing,* St Louis, 1998, Mosby, pp 135-144.

---

acid. These are buffered by extracellular bicarbonate and eventually excreted by the kidneys. Dietary intake of acids and alkali are also metabolized and buffered to prevent changes in pH balance.

Biochemical processes are extremely sensitive to minute changes (0.1 to 0.2 U) in body fluid pH. Cardiac, central nervous system, and metabolic function may be significantly altered by changes in pH. Box 9-1 summarizes the physiologic effects of alterations in pH. An interval of 1 pH unit (6.8 to 7.8) is the widest range compatible with human life.

REGULATION OF ACID-BASE BALANCE

Three systems function interdependently to regulate and maintain acid-base balance. They are the buffer, respiratory, and renal systems.

Buffer System

The buffer system can be activated within seconds and thus is considered the first line of defense against changes in pH (Table 9-1). The most important of these buffers is the bicarbonate–carbonic acid (HCO_3^--H_2CO_3) pair, which is responsible for buffering ECF. This buffer pair consists of a weak acid (H_2CO_3), which is activated when the pH is threatened by a strong base, and a weak base (HCO_3^-), which is activated when the pH is threatened by a strong acid. Whenever a buffering reaction occurs, the concentration of one member of the pair increases while the other decreases. The bicarbonate–carbonic acid system is assessed clinically by arterial blood gas pH, Pco_2, and HCO_3^-. In clinical settings where arterial plasma HCO_3^- measurement is unavailable, it can be estimated as being approximately 1 mEq/L less than the venous serum total CO_2 content as measured with electrolytes. Therefore an elevated total CO_2 would suggest buffering of a strong base. Arterial blood gas analysis also reveals whether other systems (respiratory or renal) are involved in maintaining or attempting to restore acid-base balance.

A simple and clinically relevant way of relating pH to alterations in the acid-base ratio is:

$$pH = Base/Acid = HCO_3^-/H_2CO_3 = 20/1$$

The second most abundant buffer pair is hemoglobin and oxyhemoglobin, an important buffer of carbonic acid. As

---

◆ **TABLE 9-1   Buffer System Pairs**

Weak Acid	Weak Base	% Total Buffer Action
Carbonic acid (H_2CO_3)	Sodium bicarbonate ($NaHCO_3$)	53
Hemoglobin (Hb)	Potassium hemoglobinate (KHb)	35
Oxyhemoglobin (Hbo_2)	Potassium oxyhemoglobinate ($KHbo_2$)	35
Plasma protein (HPr)	Proteinate (NaPr)	7
Acid organic phosphate ($NaRHPO_4$)	Alkaline organic phosphate (Na_2PO_4)	3
Acid inorganic phosphate (NaH_2PO_4)	Alkaline inorganic phosphate ($NaHPO_4$)	2

From Baer CL: Regulation and assessment of acid base balance. In Kinney MR et al, eds: *AACN's clinical reference for critical care nursing,* ed 3, New York, 1993, McGraw-Hill.

blood passes from the arterial to the venous end of a capillary, cellular CO_2 enters erythrocytes and combines with water to form carbonic acid. At the same time, oxyhemoglobin gives up its oxygen to the cells, some of which becomes reduced hemoglobin carrying a negative charge. The hemoglobin ion then attracts the H^+ from carbonic acid, resulting in a weaker acid than carbonic acid. When this system is active, the exchange demonstrates why erythrocytes tend to give up oxygen more rapidly when Pco_2

is elevated (as in respiratory acidosis), resulting in a shift to the right of the oxyhemoglobin dissociation curve. Erythrocytes hold on to oxygen when Pco_2 is decreased (as in respiratory alkalosis), resulting in a shift to the left in the oxyhemoglobin dissociation curve (Fig. 9-1). This is termed the Bohr effect.[1]

The protein buffer pair is the most abundant intracellular and ECF buffer. Proteins are composed of amino acids, which contain at least one carboxyl and one amine group. The carboxyl group tends to function like an acid, whereas the amine group tends to act like a base. Thus proteins can act as both acid and base buffers.

The phosphate buffer pair, which works in the same manner as the bicarbonate–carbonic acid pair, is an important regulator of both erythrocyte and renal tubular pH. This buffer pair consists of acid-alkaline organic and inorganic sodium phosphate.

Respiratory System

Ventilation also plays a major role in maintaining pH balance. The respiratory system can activate changes in pH within 1 to 3 minutes and can eliminate or conserve CO_2 (which directly affects acid-base status) more quickly and efficiently than all the buffer systems combined.

As discussed, when a strong acid is present in the body, the bicarbonate–carbonic acid buffer pair is activated to buffer the acid. This results in a net increase of carbonic acid, which dissociates into CO_2 and H_2O. Carbon dioxide is then eliminated by the lungs (Fig. 9-2). An increase in H^+ concentration in the blood stimulates the breathing center in the medulla to increase the respiratory rate, which facilitates CO_2 elimination. If, on the other hand, pH is elevated secondary to an increase in HCO_3^-, the respiratory center is inhibited, and the respiratory rate decreases. This results in

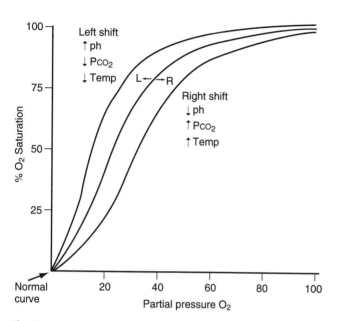

Fig. 9-1 pH effect on oxyhemoglobin dissociation curve. (Modified from Shapiro B: *Clinical application of blood gases,* ed 5, St Louis, 1994, Mosby.)

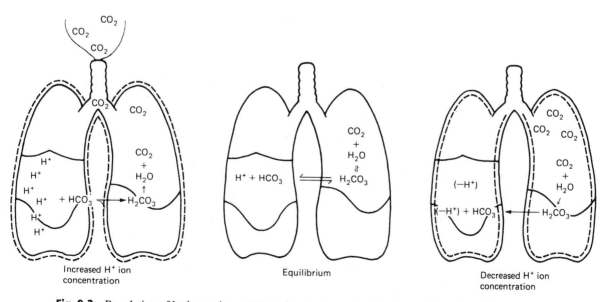

Fig. 9-2 Regulation of hydrogen ion concentration by the respiratory system. (From Baer CL: Acid-base balance. In Kinney MR et al, eds: *AACN's clinical reference for critical care nursing,* ed 3, St Louis, 1993, Mosby, p 211.)

CO_2 retention, which then becomes available to form carbonic acid, which buffers the excess bicarbonate. The respiratory system is thus able to compensate for changes in pH related to metabolic disorders (e.g., diabetic ketoacidosis) by regulating Pco_2, which alters the bicarbonate–carbonic acid ratio. The respiratory system cannot, however, produce any loss or gain of hydrogen ions. Respiratory compensation is activated within minutes and is usually fully functional within 1 to 2 days.

Renal System

Compared with the respiratory system, which operates by passive CO_2 diffusion, the kidneys control acid-base balance through several highly developed active transport processes. Renal compensation is a slower process, requir-

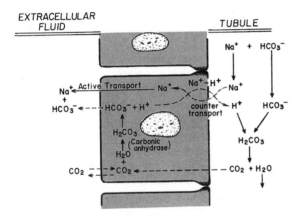

Fig. 9-3 Chemical reactions for (1) secondary active secretion of hydrogen ions into the tubule, (2) sodium ion reabsorption in exchange for the hydrogen ions secreted, and (3) combination of hydrogen ions with bicarbonate ions in the tubules to form carbon dioxide and water. (From Guyton AC: *Human physiology and mechanisms of disease,* ed 6, San Diego, 1996, Harcourt, Brace.)

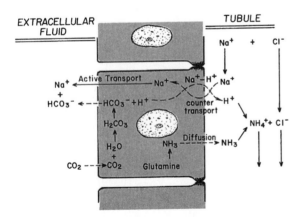

Fig. 9-4 Primary active transport of hydrogen ions through the luminal membrane of the tubular epithelial cell. Note that one bicarbonate ion is absorbed for each hydrogen ion secreted, and a chloride ion is secreted passively along with the hydrogen ion. (From Guyton AC: *Human physiology and mechanisms of disease,* ed 6, San Diego, 1996, Harcourt, Brace.)

ing 1 to 2 days for complete activation, with disorders resulting in respiratory alkalosis, and 3 to 5 days to be fully functional, with disorders resulting in respiratory acidosis. The length of time a primary acid-base disturbance has been present is an important factor in determining the expected degree of renal compensation.

The kidneys react to changes in pH by regulating the excretion or conservation of H^+ and HCO_3^- (Fig. 9-3). A low pH stimulates excretion of H^+ into the urine. As H^+ enters the urine, it displaces another positive ion, usually Na^+. At the same time, HCO_3^- is reabsorbed in exchange for the H^+. The Na^+ is then reabsorbed into the tubule cell, where it combines with HCO_3^- to form $NaHCO_3$, which is then available to buffer other H^+ in the blood. The rate of H^+ excretion, and therefore the rate of HCO_3^- reabsorption, is proportionate to arterial Pco_2. This reaction is reversed for increases in pH.

The transport of H^+ in the renal tubules is facilitated by the buffer's phosphate (as previously discussed) and ammonia, which is classified as a base. Most ammonia is converted to urea by the liver and is eliminated from the body in urine. The remaining ammonia combines with H^+ to form the ammonium ion (NH_4^+) in the renal tubules (Fig. 9-4). NH_4^+ also displaces Na^+ and is eliminated in the urine. The Na^+ is then reabsorbed into the tubule cells, where it combines with HCO_3^- to form $NaHCO_3$, which is absorbed into the blood to buffer excess H^+.

The amount of H^+ excreted in the urine can be measured by determining the amount of alkali required to neutralize the urine and is called *titratable acidity.* As a result of H^+ and NH_4^+ excretion, urine usually has an acidic pH of 6. In the clinical setting, checking urine pH can be a useful indicator of the degree of renal compensation when assessing acid-base status. For example, a low or acidic blood pH will be accompanied a few days later by a low or acidic urine pH when renal compensatory mechanisms are active. The reverse is true in alkalotic states.

ELECTROLYTES AND ACID-BASE BALANCE

In the clinical setting, recognizing how H^+ interacts with other ions is extremely important so that metabolic and electrolyte imbalances can be anticipated and managed in a timely and appropriate manner. Fig. 9-5 illustrates the location of the major concentrations of electrolytes that are affected by acid-base balance. As discussed, an increase in plasma CO_2 results in an increased renal excretion of H^+ and reabsorption of HCO_3^-, which then buffers excess H^+ in the body. This is a very important compensatory mechanism that can stabilize pH.

Potassium (K^+) also interacts in very important ways with H^+; the two share a reciprocal relationship. When H^+ concentration is elevated in the ECF, as occurs in metabolic acidosis, H^+ moves into the cell, and K^+ moves out. This exchange allows H^+ access to the intracellular protein buffers, which can minimize changes in pH. However, during this process, the shift in K^+ from the intracellular fluid (ICF) to the ECF results in hyperkalemia. A shift in a very small amount of the ICF K^+ will produce a significant increase in ECF K⁺ concentration and may lead to the potentially lethal cardiac dysrhythmias associated with hyperkalemia (see Chapter 11). When H⁺ concentration is decreased (as in metabolic alkalosis), H⁺ moves out of the cell, and K⁺ moves in, which can result in a hypokalemic state. Cardiac dysrhythmias are also possible with hypokalemia but are usually not life threatening.

Sodium is affected by H⁺ balance, as previously discussed. When H⁺ concentration is elevated, Na⁺ is displaced in the renal tubules so that excess H⁺ can be eliminated in the urine. The displaced Na⁺ is reabsorbed, which tends to increase HCO₃⁻ reabsorption. Normally, this process alone does not affect pH. However, if tubular Na⁺ reabsorption is significantly elevated (as in prolonged sodium deprivation), a metabolic alkalosis with hyponatremia may result.

The chloride ion (Cl⁻) can also contribute to acid-base imbalance because it usually follows Na⁺ passively. An increase in Cl⁻ results in a decreased reabsorption of HCO₃⁻

with Na⁺ in the renal tubules, which can result in a metabolic acidosis associated with hyperchloremia. The reverse of this (increase in HCO₃⁻ resulting in a decreased reabsorption of Cl⁻ with Na⁺) can result in a hypochloremic metabolic alkalosis.

Calcium (Ca⁺) is another ion that is affected by acid-base balance. Maintaining Ca⁺ levels within their normally narrow range is critical to normal neuromuscular and cardiac function. When pH is normal, 40% of the total plasma Ca⁺ is bound to protein (mostly albumin) and 60% is present as ionized calcium in the plasma. Changes in pH alter the amount of Ca⁺ bound by proteins, which, in turn, alters ionized Ca⁺ levels. A change in pH of 0.1 U will effect a corresponding change in protein-bound calcium of 0.12 mg/dl. When metabolic alkalosis is present in a child with a low serum Ca⁺, the ionized Ca⁺ is likely to be very low and can lead to neuromuscular and cardiac dysfunction. In a child with a metabolic acidosis and a low Ca⁺ level, the

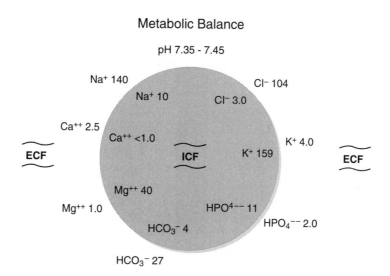

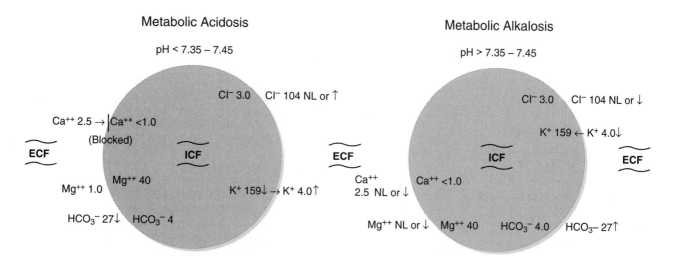

Fig. 9-5 Location of major concentrations of electrolytes that affect acid-base balance (in mEq/L). *ECF,* Extracellular fluid; *ICF,* intracellular fluid. (Redrawn from Mathewson-Kuhn M: *Pharmacotherapeutics: a nursing process approach,* ed 3, Philadelphia, 1994, FA Davis.)

ionized Ca^+ may be within normal limits. Chronic metabolic acidosis increases renal clearance of Ca^+. $NaHCO_3$ administration reestablishes normal calcium reabsorption.

MATURATIONAL FACTORS

The systems that regulate and maintain acid-base balance become fully operational at different developmental periods. The buffer systems are functional in utero. Respiratory system control of acid-base balance is mature in newborns, provided that pulmonary function is adequate. Any respiratory, neuromuscular, or neurologic disorder that alters CO_2 elimination can result in an acid-base disturbance.

Renal system control of acid-base balance is not fully functional at birth. Newborns have a limited ability to excrete hydrogen and ammonium ions. Because H^+ excretion matures rapidly, the ability of the kidney to excrete a maximal acid load is achieved by 2 months of age in both term and preterm infants. Ammonium production may not fully mature until age 2. Newborns also have a low serum bicarbonate level, which is secondary to a lower renal threshold for bicarbonate. The mechanism for this is unknown, but it may be related to an expanded ECF volume and immaturity in the transport capacity for bicarbonate reabsorption. Because of these immature renal functions, infants have a diminished renal capacity for dealing with acid-base disturbances.

ANALYZING ACID-BASE BALANCE

Before discussing specific acid-base disturbances, a review of terminology and guidelines for analyzing acid-base balance are presented. The terms *base excess* and *base deficit* are often used in the clinical setting in relation to acid-base balance. Base excess describes the presence of an excessive amount of base (HCO_3^-) or a deficit in the amount of fixed acid (not including H_2CO_3).

Base excess or deficit can be determined clinically by application of three *rules*.[2] These rules assist in determining if a disorder is respiratory, metabolic, or mixed. *Rule I* states that an acute change in Pco_2 of 10 torr is associated with an increase or decrease in pH of 0.08 U. Normally, if pH is 7.40, the Pco_2 would be 40 torr in the absence of metabolic acidosis. Application of rule I would reveal the following:

$$Pco_2\ 50\ (40+10)=pH\ 7.32\ (7.40-0.08)$$
$$Pco_2\ 30\ (40-10)=pH\ 7.48\ (7.40+0.08)$$

Rule II states that for every 0.01-U change in pH not caused by a change in Pco_2, there is a $\frac{2}{3}$ mEq/L change in the base. For example, if the pH is 7.26 and the Pco_2 is 50 torr, the increase in Pco_2 would indicate respiratory acidosis. The calculated pH would be 7.32 (according to rule I). Because the measured pH is 7.26, there is a pH difference of 0.06 U By applying rule II ($6\times\frac{2}{3}$), the calculated base deficit would be 4 mEq/L. Thus a metabolic and respiratory acidosis are both present.

Rule III states the following:

Total body bicarbonate deficit =
Base deficit (mEq/L) × Patient's weight (kg) × 0.3

HCO_3^- is located primarily in ECF, which is equal to 30% of body weight; thus total base deficit can be determined by multiplying base deficit by body weight by 0.3. In a 10-kg child with a Pco_2 of 50 and a pH of 7.24, the Pco_2 is 10 torr above normal, suggesting that the pH would be 7.32 if the child had a respiratory acidosis. The unexplained pH difference of 0.08 U must therefore be attributed to a metabolic acidosis with a base deficit of 6 mEq/L (according to rule II). Application of the preceding equation would reveal the following:

$$\text{Total bicarbonate deficit}=\text{Base deficit}\times\text{Weight (kg)}\times0.3$$
$$18=6\times10\times0.3$$

To avoid overcorrection and a rebound metabolic alkalosis, total bicarbonate correction is not recommended. One quarter to one half of the calculated dose is most often used. Note that the usual recommended dose of $NaHCO_3$ for correction of moderate metabolic acidosis, 1 mEq/kg, (which is approximately one fourth of the calculated dose), is very close to the more complicated calculation using rule III. Therefore a standard dose of 1 mEq/kg is acceptable for quick determination of bicarbonate replacement.

ACID-BASE DISTURBANCES

The buffer, respiratory, and renal compensatory mechanisms function interdependently at specific time intervals to restore acid-base balance. Signs and symptoms and the clinical significance of acid-base disturbances are directly related to the rate at which the pH changes. Disorders that develop slowly, such as chronic renal or respiratory failure, allow time for maximum compensation to occur and thus are accompanied by minimal changes in pH. Rapidly progressing or sudden insults, such as a cardiac arrest, allow little or no time for compensation to occur, resulting in profound alterations in pH that may be fatal if immediate and effective intervention is not initiated. The arterial blood gas (ABG) is the most useful diagnostic tool in determining acid-base imbalances in the clinical setting. Normal blood gas values are listed in Table 9-2. The steps used to analyze arterial blood gases to determine the acid-base imbalance are illustrated in Fig. 9-6.

Respiratory Acidosis

Respiratory acidosis is an excess of ECF carbonic acid that is caused by conditions resulting in hypoventilation and CO_2 retention. These conditions are summarized in Box 9-2. Buffer response to hypercapnia occurs immediately and is complete within 10 to 15 minutes. Renal compensatory mechanisms are activated within 2 to 5 hours but take 3 to 5 days to function at maximum capacity.

Signs and symptoms depend on the severity of the

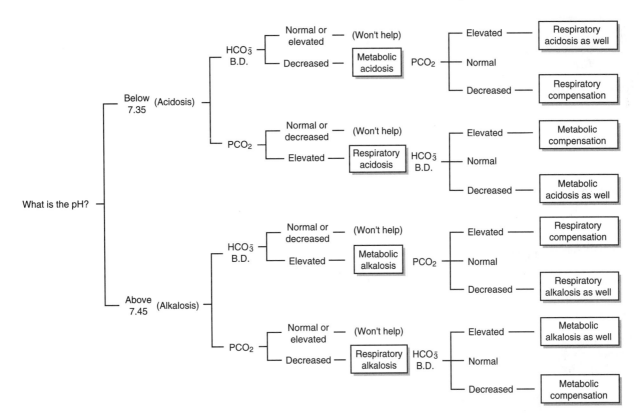

Fig. 9-6   Arterial blood gas analysis to determine acid-base imbalance. *B.D.,* Base deficits. (From Donlen J: Interpreting acid-base problems through arterial blood gases. Reprinted with permission of *Crit Care Nurs* 3:38, 1983.)

◆ **TABLE 9-2   Normal Blood Gas Values**

Parameter	Arterial	Mixed Venous	Capillary
pH	7.35-7.45	7.31-7.41	7.35-7.45
Po_2	80-100 mmHg	35-40 mmHg	Less than arterial*
O_2 saturation	95%-97%	70%-75%	Less than arterial
Pco_2	35-45 mmHg	40-50 mmHg	35-45 mmHg
HCO_3	22-26 mEq/L	22-26 mEq/L	22-26 mEq/L
Total CO_2 content	20-27 mEq/L	20-27 mEq/L	20-27 mEq/L
Base excess	+2 to –2	+2 to –2	+2 to –2

*Capillary Po_2 is approximately 10 mmHg less than arterial Po_2 except when decreased tissue perfusion is present, that is, cardiovascular collapse or hypothermia. In these states, capillary samples will not accurately reflect arterial Po_2.

respiratory acidosis (Table 9-3). Changes in respiratory function, such as decreased respiratory rate and shallow breathing, occur secondary to the underlying problem that has triggered the alveolar hypoventilation. Dyspnea is caused by stimulation of the respiratory center in the medulla and peripheral chemoreceptors that are triggered by a decrease in blood pH. Cardiovascular effects such as tachycardia, increased cardiac output, and increased blood pressure occur secondary to sympathetic stimulation and epinephrine release from the adrenal medulla. This mechanism is stimulated by hypercapnia and a low pH. Although receptor response to catecholamines is blunted in acidosis, this is initially offset by a surge in catechol-amine release. Acute hypercapnia has opposing effects on peripheral vasculature. Vasodilation occurs by its direct effect on vascular smooth muscles. Vasoconstriction is simultaneously produced by catecholamine release. This usually results in either a mild vasoconstriction or vasodilation.

Important exceptions to this occur in the pulmonary and cerebral vessels. Cerebral vascular resistance decreases and cerebral blood flow increases proportionately with an increase in Pco_2, whereas the opposite occurs in the pulmonary vascular bed. Increased cerebral blood flow precipitates the headache associated with hypercapnia and respiratory acidosis. An acute increase

Box 9-2
Disorders Associated With Respiratory Acidosis

Acute Obstructive Airway Disorders
Croup
Epiglottitis
Foreign body
Asthma
Bronchiolitis

Chronic Obstructive Airway Disorders
Bronchopulmonary dysplasia
Cystic fibrosis

Pulmonary Restrictive Disorders
Pneumonia
Aspiration
Adult respiratory distress syndrome
Pulmonary edema
Interstitial lung disease
Pleural effusion
Pneumothorax
Flail chest
Kyphoscoliosis
Pierre Robin syndrome

Neuromuscular Disorders
Muscular dystrophy
Multiple sclerosis
Spinal muscular atrophy
Guillain-Barré syndrome
Brainstem injury or tumor
Botulism
Spinal cord injury or tumor
Myasthenia gravis
Diaphragmatic paralysis
Pickwickian syndrome
Poliomyelitis

Central Nervous System Depressants
Narcotics
General anesthesia
Sedatives
Cerebral trauma or infection
Brain tumor
Circulatory crises
Cardiac arrest
Severe pulmonary edema
Massive pulmonary embolism

Iatrogenic Causes
Inadequate mechanical ventilation
Hyperalimentation with high carbohydrate content
Sorbent regenerative hemodialysis

in Pco_2 may precipitate pulmonary vasospasm, resulting in an abrupt increase in pulmonary vascular resistance and decreased pulmonary blood flow. Any increase in pulmonary vascular resistance may worsen the underlying disorder responsible for the respiratory acidosis.

The pathophysiologic effects on the central nervous system (CNS) are unclear. Cerebrospinal fluid (CSF) pH changes in relation to blood pH. CO_2 permeates the blood-brain barrier, so increases in arterial Pco_2 are seen immediately in the CSF. However, the CSF contains fewer buffers than the blood, so CSF pH falls more dramatically, which may contribute to the CNS symptoms that occur with respiratory acidosis. CNS symptoms can vary greatly in different individuals. For example, similar increases in Pco_2 cause some children to become somnolent and others to become apprehensive and agitated.

In respiratory acidosis, the arterial pH is less than 7.35, the Pco_2 is greater than 45 torr, and the HCO_3^- is normal or elevated (depending on the degree of renal compensation). It is important to note that hypoxemia may be a very late sign of respiratory acidosis; therefore cyanosis may not be present until the child progresses to respiratory failure. Serum potassium increases 0.1 mEq/L for each 0.1-U decrease in blood pH and therefore would be normal to slightly elevated with respiratory acidosis. Blood lactate levels fall slightly, and phosphorus becomes mildly elevated. Urine pH may be decreased, again depending on the degree of renal compensation.

Clinical management of respiratory acidosis is directed toward reestablishing effective ventilation and treating the underlying problem. The child may require intubation, mechanical ventilation, or a change in the ventilation plan while the primary problem is being treated. Oxygen and $NaHCO_3$ may be given based on the ABG results. Although hypoxemia does not usually affect acid-base balance, a Po_2 of less than 35 torr may induce a lactic (metabolic) acidosis. $NaHCO_3$ is administered only to correct severe metabolic acidosis. Effective ventilation must be established before the administration of $NaHCO_3$; otherwise, the acidosis will worsen.

The *clinical significance* of respiratory acidosis depends on the child's general health and the physiologic effects of the acidosis and hypoxemia. Nursing assessment parameters include vital signs, noting heart and respiratory rate, rhythm, character, and pattern; blood pressure, perfusion status, peripheral and distal pulses, level of consciousness, and urine output; muscle strength and movement; oxygenation status, noting color of nail beds and mucous membranes, and Sao_2; gastrointestinal function; degree of comfort; and laboratory data.

Nursing interventions include positioning the child to optimize ventilation, administering oxygen, and suctioning to clear the airways and enhance CO_2 elimination. Care is directed to minimize O_2 consumption by providing an environment with minimal stimulation and uninterrupted periods of rest. Inherently important is providing the child and family with appropriate explanations, support, and reassurance.

TABLE 9-3   Signs and Symptoms Associated With Acid-Base Imbalance

Respiratory Acidosis	Respiratory Alkalosis	Metabolic Acidosis	Metabolic Alkalosis
Decreased respiratory rate	Hyperventilation	Tachypnea → Kussmaul respirations	Hypoventilation
Shallow breathing	Breathlessness	Tachycardia → bradycardia	Cardiac dysrhythmias
Dyspnea	Cardiac dysrhythmias	Cardiac dysrhythmias	Decreased perfusion
Tachycardia	Hypotension	Hypotension	Hypotension
Headache	Extremity and perioral paresthesias	Poor perfusion with a grayish pallor	Confusion
Decreased responsiveness			Lethargy
Disorientation	Vertigo	Decreased peripheral pulses	Unresponsiveness
Restlessness	Syncope	Increased capillary refill time	Hyperreflexia
Apprehension	Anxiety	Decreased urine output	Muscle cramps
Agitation	Nervousness	Decreased level of consciousness	Twitching
Fatigue	Confusion		Tetany
Weakness	Decreased level of consciousness	Congestive heart failure	Seizures
Diminished reflexes		Fatigue	Nausea, vomiting, and diarrhea
Seizures	Decreased psychomotor performance	Drowsiness	
Nausea and vomiting		Confusion	
	Hyperreflexia	Apathy	
	Muscle cramps	Unresponsiveness	
	Twitching	Seizures	
	Tetany	Nausea and vomiting	
	Seizures	Abdominal distension and pain	

Respiratory Alkalosis

Respiratory alkalosis is an ECF deficit of carbonic acid caused by conditions resulting in alveolar hyperventilation and CO_2 deficit. Rare as a primary problem, disorders associated with respiratory alkalosis in children are summarized in Box 9-3. Buffer response to hypocapnia begins immediately and is complete within 10 to 15 minutes. Renal compensatory mechanisms are activated within 2 to 5 hours in respiratory alkalosis and take 1 to 2 days to be fully functional.

Hyperventilation results from stimulation of the respiratory center in the medulla and stimulation of peripheral chemoreceptors and nociceptive receptors in the lungs. Hyperventilation may also occur when signals from the cerebral cortex override the chemoreceptors, as in voluntary hyperventilation.

Heart rate increases secondary to sympathetic stimulation and the resultant catecholamine release from the adrenal medulla. This response can cause atrial and ventricular tachydysrhythmias. There is usually no major change in cardiac output and blood pressure in awake children. Cardiovascular response to hypocapnia differs in anesthetized children. Although tachycardia may not develop, cardiac output and perfusion may decrease. This response occurs secondary to increased intrathoracic pressures associated with passive hyperventilation, resulting in decreased venous return. Pulmonary vasodilation occurs with hypocapnia; however, peripheral vasoconstriction also occurs. This results in decreased blood flow to the skin and contributes to paresthesias. Cerebral blood flow (CBF) is

also drastically reduced secondary to cerebral vasoconstriction. This vasoconstriction decreases intracranial and intraocular hydrostatic pressure. Cerebral oxygen consumption does not decrease when blood flow is reduced, so cerebral hypoxemia and hypoxia may develop, leading to lightheadedness, syncope, anxiety, altered levels of consciousness, and seizures.

Calcium binding, resulting in hypocalcemia, occurs with alkalemia. This condition also contributes to the development of seizures, as well as neuromuscular irritability, hyperreflexia, muscle cramps, twitching, and tetany.

In respiratory alkalosis, the arterial pH is greater than 7.45, the Pco_2 is less than 35 torr, and the HCO_3^- is normal or decreased (less than 25 mEq/L). Potassium concentration decreases 0.1 mEq/L for each 0.1-U increase in pH and therefore should be normal or slightly decreased. Urine pH is normal to increased, depending on the degree of renal compensation.

The *clinical management* of respiratory alkalosis is directed toward restoring effective ventilation and treating the underlying cause. Sedation, breathing exercises, and relaxation with controlled breathing can correct the imbalance (if the child is developmentally capable of participating in such activities). Administration of 3% to 5% CO_2 and neuromuscular paralysis with intubation and mechanical ventilation may also be necessary if respiratory alkalosis is severe and other measures are ineffective.

The *clinical significance* of respiratory alkalosis depends on the presence and extent of neuromuscular effects. Seizures from respiratory alkalosis can be life threatening.

Box 9-3
Disorders Associated With Respiratory Alkalosis

Intoxications

Alcohol
Salicylate
Paraldehyde
Xanthine

Increased Intracranial Pressure

Meningitis
Encephalitis
Head trauma
Vascular accidents
Brain lesions

Pulmonary Disorders

Pneumonia
Pulmonary edema
Pulmonary emboli

Increased Metabolic Rate

Fever
Hyperthyroidism
Exercise
Anemia
Gram-negative sepsis
Interstitial lung disease

Miscellaneous

High altitude
Voluntary hyperventilation
Anxiety
Hysteria
Hepatic failure
Congestive heart failure with hypoxemia
Mechanical ventilation

Box 9-4
Disorders Associated With Metabolic Acidosis

Increased Anion Gap (Normochloremic)

Cardiovascular collapse
Diabetic ketoacidosis
Lactic acidosis (tissue hypoxia)
Starvation
Drugs/toxins (methanol, ethanol, salicylate, fructose, sorbitol, cyanide, carbon monoxide, paraldehyde)
Organic acid metabolism (pyruvate)
Hepatic failure
Renal failure
Congenital enzymatic defects
Glucose 6-phosphate deficiency
Fructose 1,6-diphosphatase deficiency
Pyruvate carboxylase deficiency
Methylmalonic aciduria

Normal Anion Gap (Hyperchloremic)

Diarrhea
Intake of chloride-containing compounds (HCl, NH_4Cl, $CaCl_2$, $MgCl_2$, arginine HCl, cholestyramine)
Hyperalimentation
Pancreatic, small bowel, or biliary tubes or fistulas
Ureterosigmoidostomy, ileal conduit
Carbonic anhydrase inhibitors (acetazolamide)
Extracellular fluid volume expansion
Mineralocorticoid deficiency (adrenal disorders)
Renal tubular acidosis
Early uremic acidosis

Nursing assessment parameters include vital signs, noting heart and respiratory rate, rhythm, character, and pattern, blood pressure, perfusion status, peripheral and central pulses, level of consciousness, and urine output; muscle movement and strength; sensation in the extremities and around the perioral area; and seizure activity.

Nursing interventions with respiratory alkalosis include maintaining seizure precautions. If age and clinical condition indicate, interventions may include assisting with relaxation and slow breathing techniques or having the child breathe through a paper bag. Care is directed toward providing a safe environment with age- and condition-appropriate activities, minimal stimulation, and uninterrupted periods of rest.

Metabolic Acidosis

Metabolic acidosis is an ECF deficit of bicarbonate caused by conditions that result in a loss of bicarbonate or an increase in fixed acids. These conditions are summarized in Box 9-4. Note that the most common cause of metabolic acidosis in the pediatric population is insufficient tissue perfusion. Situations that produce an increase in fixed acids result in a normochloremic acidosis with an increased anion gap. Situations that cause a bicarbonate loss result in a hyperchloremic acidosis with a normal anion gap. The normal range for the anion gap is 8 to 16 mEq/L and is calculated using the following formula:

$$\text{Anion gap} = Na^+ - (Cl^- + HCO_3^-)$$

Buffer and respiratory compensatory mechanisms are activated within minutes with metabolic acidosis. Respiratory compensation results in an increased respiratory rate to eliminate excess CO_2; however, it is not usually effective in correcting the imbalance.

Signs and symptoms depend on the severity of the metabolic acidosis (see Box 9-4). Tachycardia results from sympathetic stimulation and the subsequent release of epinephrine from the adrenal medulla, which is stimulated by acidosis. As pH falls below 7.10, heart rate progressively slows. This reaction is most likely related to the inhibitory effect that acidosis has on the action of catecholamines or accumulation of acetylcholine caused by the inhibition of acetylcholinesterase. Ventricular dysrhythmias are usually related to the electrolyte imbalances seen with acidosis, particularly hyperkalemia. Acidosis also decreases the fibrillation threshold, so the child is at greater risk for ventricular fibrillation. As pH falls from 7.40 to 7.20, the negative inotropic effect of acidosis and the positive inotropic effect of catecholamine release offset each other so that effective myocardial contraction is maintained. However, as pH falls below 7.20, the negative inotropic effect dominates, which results in poor perfusion and hypotension. Calcium entry into the cell is also inhibited at this point, which further decreases effective myocardial contraction. Although epinephrine facilitates calcium entry into the cells in early acidosis, this becomes inhibited as H^+ concentration increases. Infants and children who are receiving β-adrenergic antagonists or calcium channel blocking agents, as well as those who are chronically stressed and have limited endogenous catecholamine stores, are more susceptible to the negative inotropic effects of acidosis. A pH of less than 7.20 also effects arterial and venous tone. The arterial system dilates while the venous system constricts, which forces blood to flow centrally. This increases the workload of the heart and can result in congestive heart failure.

Tachypnea results from stimulation of the respiratory center in the medulla. Kussmaul respirations develop with acute severe metabolic acidosis as the child increases tidal volume and respiratory rate to improve oxygenation and eliminate CO_2. Oxygen delivery to the tissues is enhanced by metabolic acidosis as the oxyhemoglobin dissociation curve shifts to the right (see Fig. 9-1). However, if acidosis progresses, glycolysis slows, and red blood cell 2,3-diphosphoglycerate (DPG) is depleted, which eliminates the beneficial Bohr effect as previously described. Hypoxemia and tissue hypoxia then progress. Neurologic changes are related to decreased perfusion to the brain, hypoxemia, hypoxia, and metabolic and electrolyte imbalances.

The gastrointestinal symptoms associated with metabolic acidosis are likely related to either ketogenesis or electrolyte and biochemical changes that accompany acidosis. Normal tone and contraction of the gastrointestinal tract are altered, resulting in abdominal pain, distension, nausea, and vomiting.

In metabolic acidosis, the arterial pH is less than 7.35, the Pco_2 is decreased (a normal or elevated Pco_2 would indicate failing respiratory compensation and the development of respiratory acidosis), and HCO_3^- is less than 25 mEq/L. Serum potassium is elevated 0.1 mEq/L for each 0.01 U decrease in pH; chloride is normal or elevated (depending on the cause); and urine pH is normal or decreased, again depending on the cause of the acidosis.

Clinical management of metabolic acidosis is directed toward identifying and treating the underlying problem and would include restoring fluid and electrolyte imbalance, preventing or treating a catabolic state, and providing adequate ventilation. Bicarbonate losses should be replaced in severe acidosis. $NaHCO_3$ is now used conservatively, most often indicated for a pH below 7.20, when there is depressed myocardial function, and when compensatory respiratory efforts cannot be maintained and respiratory failure is imminent. $NaHCO_3$ should be administered to achieve a slight undercorrection and thus prevent a rebound metabolic alkalosis from occurring. A recommended dose of 1 mEq/kg will provide approximately one fourth to one half

of calculated bicarbonate losses (see previous discussion under Analyzing Acid-Base Balance). Adverse effects associated with $NaHCO_3$ administration include a transient increase in Pco_2, which may further compromise cellular function, myocardial contractility, and cerebral acidosis. Hyperosmolarity, hypernatremia, and iatrogenic metabolic alkalosis may also occur. The alkalosis may decrease ionized calcium and potassium levels, shift the oxyhemoglobin dissociation curve to the left (inhibiting O_2 release to the tissues), and predispose the patient to life-threatening dysrhythmias. The potential risks and benefits must be carefully considered in individual clinical situations when deciding if $NaHCO_3$ is indicated. It is critical to remember that to maintain the buffering capacity of $NaHCO_3$, effective ventilation or mild hyperventilation must be present.

The *clinical significance* of metabolic acidosis depends on the severity of the disorder. The body does not tolerate changes in H^+ concentration well. Without appropriate intervention, metabolic acidosis will progress to life-threatening alterations in cardiac, neurologic, and metabolic function. Nursing assessment parameters include vital signs, noting heart and respiratory rate, rhythm, character, and pattern, blood pressure, perfusion status, peripheral and central pulses, level of consciousness, and urine output; seizure activity; gastrointestinal function; intake and output; muscle strength; signs of hyperkalemia; the child's level of comfort; and appropriate laboratory data.

Nursing interventions include administering medications and fluids, positioning the child to optimize ventilation, maintaining seizure precautions, and providing comfort measures for gastrointestinal upset. Care is directed toward providing a safe environment with age- and condition-appropriate activities, minimal stimulation, and uninterrupted periods of rest.

Metabolic Alkalosis

Metabolic alkalosis is an ECF excess of HCO_3^- caused by conditions resulting in excess base because of loss of H^+, reabsorption of HCO_3^-, or loss of other ions (i.e., chloride, sodium). These conditions are summarized in Box 9-5. Buffer and respiratory compensatory mechanisms are activated immediately with metabolic alkalosis. Respiratory compensation results in a decreased respiratory rate to conserve CO_2; however, this response is ineffective and does not correct the imbalance.

Hypoventilation results from stimulation of the respiratory center in the medulla, which attempts to conserve Pco_2 by decreasing alveolar ventilation. This condition may result in hypoxemia, which can further compromise the child's status. Cardiac dysrhythmias with a subsequent decrease in cardiac output and blood pressure usually occur secondary to hypoxemia or hypokalemia.

Changes in level of consciousness occur secondary to decreased CBF, which results from the cerebral vasoconstriction that is associated with alkalosis. Seizures can develop secondary to hypoxemia, hypocalcemia, or hypomagnesemia. Calcium binding increases with alkalemia, resulting in hypocalcemia. Magnesium levels decrease in relation to calcium. Hypocalcemia also contributes to the

Box 9-5
Disorders Associated With Metabolic Alkalosis

Vomiting
Gastrointestinal suctioning
Cl^--wasting diarrhea
Cl^--deficient formula
Diuretics
Hypokalemia
Hypocalcemia
Hypochloremia
Exogenous alkali intake: HCO_3^-, citrate, lactate, acetate
Excessive steroid use
Renal failure
Extracellular fluid volume depletion
Cystic fibrosis
Excess mineralocorticoid
Hyperaldosteronism, Cushing's syndrome, adrenogenital syndrome
Laxative, licorice abuse
Excessive tobacco chewing
Bartter's syndrome

development of neuromuscular irritability, muscle cramps, and tetany. Gastrointestinal effects are usually associated with the underlying problem, which results in nausea, vomiting, and diarrhea.

In metabolic alkalosis, the arterial pH is greater than 7.45, HCO_3^- is greater than 30 mEq/L, base excess is greater than +2, and Pco_2 is normal or elevated. Serum electrolytes usually reveal a hypokalemia, with a 0.1 mEq/L decrease in potassium for each 0.01 U increase in blood pH. Hypocalcemia and hypochloremia may also be present. Urine chloride is usually decreased, and urine pH is normal or increased; the degree depends on the cause.

The *clinical management* of metabolic alkalosis is directed toward identifying and treating the underlying cause of the imbalance. This approach usually involves expanding ECF volume with saline, administering chloride (arginine or ammonium chloride if the NaCl is insufficient to replace the lost ion), correcting hypokalemia with potassium chloride, and facilitating excretion of HCO_3^- with carbonic anhydrase–inhibiting diuretics (e.g., acetazolamide) or dialysis if renal impairment is present.

The *clinical significance* of metabolic alkalosis depends on the severity of the disorder and the accompanying neuromuscular and respiratory effects. Nursing assessment parameters include vital signs, noting heart and respiratory rate, rhythm, character, and pattern, blood pressure, perfusion status, peripheral and central pulses, level of consciousness, and urine output; neuromuscular function; muscle movement and strength; Chvostek's and Trousseau's signs for hypocalcemia; strict intake and output; stooling pattern and characteristics; and laboratory data.

Nursing interventions with metabolic alkalosis include administering medications and fluids, maintaining seizure precautions, and providing comfort measures for gastroin-

testinal upset. Care is directed toward providing a safe environment with age- and condition-appropriate activities, minimal stimulation, and uninterrupted periods of rest.

MIXED ACID-BASE DISORDERS

Mixed acid-base disturbances often occur in infants and children with a variety of multisystem problems. Mixed disturbances can result in excessive or diminished compensation. The clinical significance of the imbalances depends on the net change in pH.

In general, mixed disorders that drive the pH in opposite directions (respiratory acidosis with metabolic alkalosis) are better tolerated because each compensates for the other to keep the pH near or within normal limits. Mixed disorders that drive the pH in the same direction (respiratory and metabolic acidosis) have profound effects on pH because compensation is impossible. Because the body is unable to tolerate significant changes in pH, mixed disorders can significantly alter cardiac, neurologic, and metabolic function and be life threatening without appropriate intervention. Treating each component of the mixed disorder simultaneously is important to avoid exacerbating one while correcting the other. Accurate interpretation of ABGs and monitoring of the child's clinical response to therapy are critical nursing interventions because the patient's response to therapy may be asynchronous.

Respiratory Acidosis With Metabolic Alkalosis

Respiratory acidosis and metabolic alkalosis can occur in children with obstructive pulmonary disease (e.g., bronchopulmonary dysplasia, or cystic fibrosis) who are receiving diuretics as part of their management plan. Such children usually live in a state of compensated respiratory acidosis secondary to CO_2 retention related to their pulmonary disease. Chronic diuretic therapy with potassium-wasting drugs (such as furosemide) can lead to hypokalemia and metabolic alkalosis. A similar scenario also occurs in children with congestive heart failure and chronic respiratory acidosis who are receiving long-term diuretic therapy. The pH with this mixed imbalance is usually near or within normal limits because of compensation. If, however, the pH rises with the metabolic alkalosis, respiratory drive may be depressed in the medulla, resulting in a decrease in Po_2 and an increase in Pco_2, which can progress to respiratory failure.

Clinical management of this mixed imbalance is directed toward correcting the metabolic alkalosis, which is accomplished by administering sodium and potassium chloride to facilitate renal excretion of HCO_3^-. This must be done cautiously to avoid inducing or exacerbating congestive heart failure. Although pH may fall to acidemic levels, this will stimulate respiration and subsequently increase Po_2 and decrease Pco_2 levels. Oxygen must be administered carefully because increasing the Po_2 above the patient's normal threshold may depress the respiratory drive in the medulla. Knowing the baseline ABG status for the patient with chronic lung disease is extremely helpful in establishing appropriate treatment goals.

Nursing assessment and interventions would be the same as those listed under each disorder. Consideration must be given to these children's underlying disease process and to the degree that they are compromised when planning, implementing, and evaluating clinical management.

Respiratory and Metabolic Acidosis

Respiratory and metabolic acidosis may develop in infants and children with chronic obstructive pulmonary disease who are in shock, who have any type of metabolic acidosis and develop respiratory failure, and in those who suffer cardiopulmonary arrest. Compensation is not possible with this mixed disorder, and the pH falls dramatically, even when changes in Pco_2 and HCO_3^- are moderate. The clinical significance is related to the fall in pH and can result in cardiac, neurologic, and metabolic dysfunction.

Clinical management of this imbalance is directed toward careful correction of both the respiratory and metabolic component to normalize pH. Knowing the baseline status of the patient with chronic lung disease is helpful, as previously discussed. Special consideration must be given to the care of these children because the goal will be to return them to their baseline compromised status, which will include normalizing pH but not necessarily other ABG parameters. Mechanical ventilation may be necessary to eliminate excess CO_2 and return these children to their baseline status. $NaHCO_3$ is usually administered after adequate ventilation is established. Nursing assessment and intervention are as discussed under each disorder.

Respiratory Alkalosis With Metabolic Acidosis

The mixed imbalance of respiratory alkalosis with metabolic acidosis may be seen in children with hepatic failure. The respiratory alkalosis is due to hyperventilation (secondary to restrictive lung capacity with liver enlargement), and the metabolic acidosis is due to hepatic failure with lactic acidosis, renal failure, or renal tubular acidosis. This imbalance can also occur in children with chronic renal failure and acute sepsis. The respiratory alkalosis develops secondary to the hyperventilation that accompanies sepsis, and the metabolic acidosis is associated with the renal failure. Salicylate intoxication also results in a respiratory alkalosis, which is related to stimulation of the breathing center in the medulla, and metabolic acidosis, which occurs secondary to disruption of the Krebs cycle with accumulation of lactic and other organic acids.

Clinical management of the child with this mixed imbalance is directed toward correction of the underlying problem. The pH is usually close to or within normal limits because of effective or excessive compensation and may not require specific treatment. Nursing assessment and interventions are as discussed under each disorder.

Respiratory and Metabolic Alkalosis

The combination of respiratory and metabolic alkalosis is seen in children with chronic hepatic failure who are receiving diuretics or who develop vomiting. The respiratory alkalosis is due to hyperventilation from restrictive lung disease related to hepatic enlargement, and the metabolic alkalosis is due to potassium or fixed acid loss related to diuretic therapy or vomiting (respectively). This condition is also seen in children with chronic respiratory acidosis (from chronic lung disease) with appropriately elevated HCO_3^- levels who are supported on mechanical ventilation and are overventilated, resulting in a drastic fall in Pco_2 leading to respiratory alkalosis. Neither disorder is able to compensate for the other, and pH rises dramatically.

Clinical management of this imbalance is directed toward treating the underlying problem and normalizing the pH. The respiratory component is managed by treating the cause of hyperventilation or adjusting the ventilator. The metabolic component is corrected with sodium and potassium chloride. Fluids must be administered cautiously to avoid inducing congestive heart failure or pulmonary edema. Nursing assessments and interventions are as listed under each disorder.

Triple Acid-Base Disorders

Triple acid-base disorders may occur in children with disorders affecting more than one body system, such as those with chronic liver failure. Hyperventilation and respiratory alkalosis result from restrictive lung capacity related to the enlarged abdomen. Metabolic alkalosis occurs if the child is receiving diuretics, develops vomiting, or requires nasogastric suctioning. Finally, metabolic acidosis may develop secondary to renal tubular acidosis, diarrhea, uremic acidosis, and lactic acidosis. Clinical management of such a complicated disorder involves careful assessment and correction of each component simultaneously to normalize pH. Nursing assessment and intervention would include those listed under each disorder.

SUMMARY

Acid-base disturbances are associated with many disorders and diseases seen in the pediatric critical care unit. The nurse must be able to accurately assess the child's acid-base status, to recognize imbalances, and to anticipate the potentially life-threatening complications that may result from them. Appropriate interventions can then be implemented to prevent or minimize these complications and thus improve the patient's outcome.

REFERENCES

1. Antonini E, Brunori M: Hemoglobin, *Ann Rev Biochem* 39:977-1042, 1970.
2. Chameides L, Hazinski MF: Fluid and medication therapy. In *Pediatric advanced life support,* ed 3, Dallas, 1997, American Heart Association.

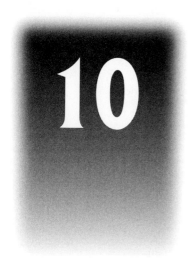

10

Intracranial Dynamics

Paula Vernon-Levett

Unlike in other organ systems, functional immaturity of the neurologic system is extremely obvious when approaching the infant and young child in the pediatric intensive care unit (ICU). Neurologic developmental immaturity affects every aspect of care: nurses' approach to patients, assessment strategies, and management priorities.

Neurologic dysfunction may be primary or may occur secondarily from other major organ system dysfunction, for example, cardiovascular collapse or acute respiratory failure. Compared with other organ systems, the neurologic system is unforgiving. Cells within the central nervous system cannot regenerate; short periods of inadequate perfusion may result in long-term devastating outcomes. Although infants may compensate for significant neurologic deficits, older children and adolescents may require extensive rehabilitation.

Based on the Role Delineation Study implemented by the American Association of Critical-Care Nurses (AACN) Certification Corporation, approximately 10% of pediatric critical care practice involves caring for patients with neurologic dysfunction.[1] Because of the pervasiveness of neurologic alterations in critical care patients, requisite knowledge of the neurologic system is essential. This chapter reviews essential neurologic embryology, anatomy, and associated physiology. Neurologic assessment is presented, followed by a discussion of neurologic intensive care monitoring and diagnostic testing.

ESSENTIAL EMBRYOLOGY

The third week of human development is a period of rapid embryonic development with differentiation of the three primitive germ layers: ectoderm, mesoderm, and endoderm. The ectoderm layer gives rise to the central nervous system (CNS), consisting of the brain, spinal cord, and other structures, for example, the skin.

The notochord, a cellular rod, develops during the third week of gestation, defining the primitive axis of the embryo and giving it some rigidity. The embryonic ectoderm over the notochord (neuroectoderm) thickens to form the neural plate. On approximately the eighteenth

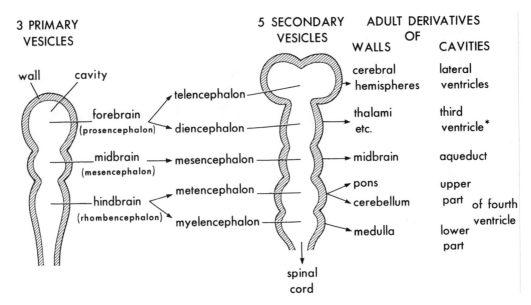

Fig. 10-1 Diagrammatic sketches of the brain vesicles indicating the adult derivatives of their walls and cavities. *The rostral (anterior) part of the third ventricle forms from the cavity of the telencephalon; most of the third ventricle is derived from the cavity of the diencephalon. (From Moore KL, Persaud TVN: *The developing human: clinically oriented embryology,* ed 5, Philadelphia, 1993, WB Saunders, p 401.)

day of embryonic development, the neural plate invaginates to form the longitudinal neural groove with two adjacent neural folds. At the end of the third week, the neural folds move together and begin to fuse to form the neural tube. Fusion of the two neural folds begins centrally and expands toward the future brain (rostrally) and the sacral area (caudally). The rostral end closes first, followed 2 days later by closure of the caudal end. The cranial two thirds of the neural tube develops further to form the future brain, and the caudal one third becomes the spinal cord. The neural tube canal becomes the ventricular system of the brain and the central canal of the spinal cord. The process of embryonic development from neural plate formation to neural tube development is referred to as neurulation and is complete by the fourth week of gestation.

As the neural folds fuse, the neural tube separates from the surface ectoderm. During this fusion, groups of neuroectoderm cells lying on the crest of each neural fold separate from the neural tube. These neuroectoderm cells, collectively called the neural crest, form a mass between the surface ectoderm and neuroectoderm. The neural crest cells differentiate into a number of cells in the peripheral nervous system, autonomic nervous system, cranial and skeletal nerves, and some skeletal nerves and muscular components of the head.

During the fourth week and before closure of the caudal and rostral neuropores, three primary brain vesicles begin to appear that later develop into the brain (Fig. 10-1). The most rostral vesicle is the forebrain, or prosencephalon, the middle vesicle is the midbrain, or mesencephalon, and the most caudal vesicle is the hindbrain, or rhombencephalon.

During the fifth week, with further development, two of the primary vesicles subdivide to form secondary vesicles. The prosencephalon develops into the telencephalon and the diencephalon, and the rhombencephalon develops into the metencephalon and the myelencephalon. The mesencephalon remains unchanged.

A longitudinal groove, called the sulcus limitans, forms along the lateral surface of the neural tube canal during the fourth week. This groove subdivides the dorsal part (alar plate) of the spinal cord from the ventral part (basal plate). These plates form longitudinal bulges that extend most of the length of the spinal cord. This regional separation is important in terms of spinal cord function. The alar plate is later associated with afferent function, and the basal plate is associated with efferent function.

Most abnormal development of the CNS results from failure of the neural tube to close properly during the fourth week of development. Defective closure of the caudal opening of the neural tube (caudal neuropore) produces malformations of the spinal cord and the overlying tissue. These malformations, collectively referred to as spina bifida, range in severity from minor, clinically insignificant defects (spina bifida occulta) to severe defects with neurologic deficits (myelomeningocele). Defective closure of the rostral opening of the neural tube (rostral neuropore) results in severe malformations of the brain, for example, anencephaly or exencephaly. Other CNS malformations may result from faulty histogenesis of the cerebral cortex, interference with cerebrospinal fluid (CSF) circulation and absorption, and defective formation of the cranium. Table 10-1 summarizes congenital malformations of the CNS.

TABLE 10-1   Congenital Malformations of the Central Nervous System

Name	Description
Neural Tube Defects	
Anencephaly	Absence of most of cerebral hemispheres and calvaria
Exencephaly	Herniation or protrusion of brain and meninges through a defect in the skull
Meningocele	Protrusion of saclike cyst containing meninges and spinal fluid through a defect in the vertebral arch
Myelomeningocele	Protrusion of saclike cyst containing meninges, spinal fluid, and portion of the spinal cord with its nerves through a defect in the vertebral arch
Arnold-Chiari malformation*	Downward displacement of brainstem and cerebellum through the foramen magnum and into spinal canal. Hydrocephalus from CSF obstruction occurs in majority of cases
Cranial Deformities	
Acrania	Almost complete absence of cranial vault. Often associated with vertebral column defect
Craniosynostosis	Premature closure of one or more of the cranial sutures
Microcephaly	Small calvaria and brain with normal-sized face
Miscellaneous	
Agenesis of corpus callosum	Complete or partial absence of corpus callosum

*Does not result from defective closure of the neural tube but is often associated with a myelomeningocele.
CSF, Cerebrospinal fluid.

ESSENTIAL ANATOMY AND PHYSIOLOGY

The nervous system is divided into the peripheral nervous system (PNS) and the CNS. The PNS is composed of the cranial and spinal nerves, and the CNS is composed of the brain and spinal cord. The basic unit of the nervous system is the neuron. The following section briefly discusses each of the microscopic and macroscopic structures of the nervous system, as well as the CNS coverings, the ventricular system, and cerebral circulation.

Microscopic Structures

The two basic cellular elements of the nervous system are neurons and glial cells. The neuron is the primary cell of the CNS and is responsible for detecting environmental changes and initiating body responses. Neuroglial cells of the CNS and PNS provide nutrition and structural support to the neurons.

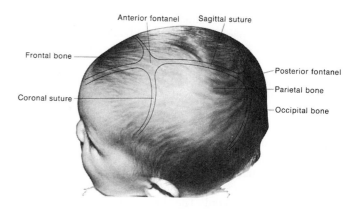

Fig. 10-2   Location of the anterior and posterior fontanelles. (From Betz CL, Hunsberger M, Wright S: *Family-centered nursing care of children,* ed 2, Philadelphia, 1994, WB Saunders, p 124.)

Neurons come in a variety of sizes and shapes with a number of different functions. Most neurons have three components: a cell body, dendrites, and an axon. The cell body contains a nucleus but lacks the ability to reproduce itself. The dendrites carry nerve impulses to the cell body, and the axon(s) conducts impulses away from the body. Numerous descriptive terminology exists to classify neurons, based on their location, morphology, and function.

Glial cells (neuroglia) compose approximately 50% of CNS tissue volume and outnumber neurons by a factor of 10. There are different types of glial cells with different functions. Oligodendroglia in the CNS and Schwann cells in the PNS form myelin sheaths around axons to increase the speed of conduction of an impulse. Other types of glial cells assist with metabolic functions, remove cellular debris, and form special contacts between neuronal surfaces and the circulation.

Extracranial Structures

The skull (cranial vault) consists of two components: neurocranium and viscerocranium. The neurocranium is a protective covering of the brain, and the viscerocranium is the skeleton of the jaw. At birth, the newborn's skull is cartilaginous and consists of eight bones: one frontal, one ethmoid, one sphenoid, two temporal, two parietal, and one occipital. The flat bones are separated by dense, white, fibrous connective tissue membranes called sutures. These sutures accommodate the rapid growth of brain tissue, which is greatest during the first 2 years of life. Several sutures join together at six areas to form fontanelles (Fig. 10-2). The posterolateral fontanelles and the anterior fontanelle close during the first and second years of life, respectively, from growth of surrounding bone.

Meninges is the term given to describe the three membranous connective tissue layers that cover and protect the brain and spinal cord (Fig. 10-3, *A*). The outermost layer is the dura mater (dura) and consists of two thick, membranous layers. The outer (periosteum) layer adheres to the inner surface of the skull and the vertebral column. The inner layer of the dura divides the two cerebral hemispheres along the median longitudinal fissure (falx cerebri), the cerebral hemispheres from the cerebellum and brainstem (tentorium cerebelli), and the two cerebellar hemispheres (falx cerebelli) (Fig. 10-3, *B*).

The middle covering is named after the Greek word *arachne,* which means "spider web." This arachnoid layer is a transparent avascular covering with many thin strands of collagen called trabeculars. The trabeculae are believed to help suspend the brain within the meninges.[2]

The pia mater (pia) is the innermost meningeal layer. It is a very delicate, clear membrane that directly adheres to the surface of the brain, following all of the contours of the brain and spinal cord. The arachnoid and pia layers are collectively called the leptomeninges and are sometimes referred to as the same entity.

The outer layer of the dura normally adheres closely to the inner table of the skull, especially in the infant. A potential space (epidural or extradural) may develop from bleeding that causes separation of the dura from the skull. The space between the dura and arachnoid layers is the subdural space. It is narrow and contains a small amount of serous fluid that prevents adhesions from forming between the two layers. The subarachnoid space is between the arachnoid and pia layers. This space is relatively large and contains circulating CSF.

Brain

The brain is divided into three gross anatomic units: the cerebrum, the brainstem, and the cerebellum. The cerebrum

is further subdivided into the telencephalon and the diencephalon, and the brainstem is subdivided into the mesencephalon (midbrain), the metencephalon (pons), and the myelencephalon (medulla).

Telencephalon. The telencephalon is composed of the right and left cerebral hemispheres and the basal ganglia. The cerebral hemispheres are mirror images divided from each other by the median longitudinal fissure. The surfaces of the cerebral hemispheres have convolutions, and each of these ridges is known as a gyrus. Each gyrus is separated by a shallow groove (sulcus) or a deep groove (fissure). The outer layer of the cerebral hemispheres or cortex is gray and consists primarily of cell bodies. The inner layer is white and consists of myelinated axons. Axons that pass from one lobe to another in the same hemisphere are known as associative fibers. Axons that pass between hemispheres, such as the corpus callosum, are known as commissural fibers. Axons that pass from a cerebral hemisphere to other areas of the CNS are known as projection fibers.

The basal ganglia, including the caudate nucleus, putamen, globus pallidus, claustrum, and amygdala, is a collection of gray matter nuclei located deep in the white matter of the cerebral hemispheres on either side of the midline. General function of the basal ganglia includes unconscious control of lower motor centers. Damage or dysfunction of the basal ganglia may produce disturbances of muscle tone and various abnormal involuntary movements.

Anatomic fissures divide each of the cerebral hemispheres into four lobes: the temporal, parietal, frontal, and occipital (Fig. 10-4). These lobes have some distinct

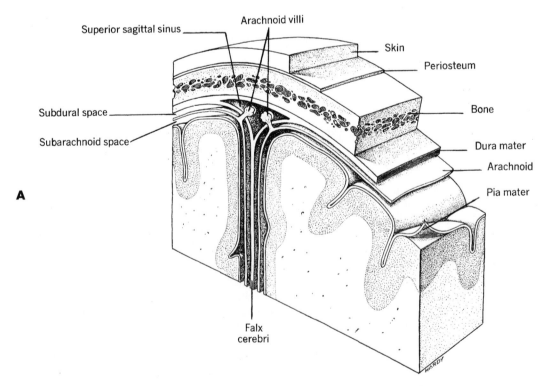

Fig. 10-3 **A,** Cranial meninges. Arachnoid villi shown within superior sagittal sinus are one site of passage of cerebrospinal fluid into the blood. (From Chaffee EE, Lytle IM: *Basic physiology and anatomy,* Philadelphia, 1980, JB Lippincott.) *Continued*

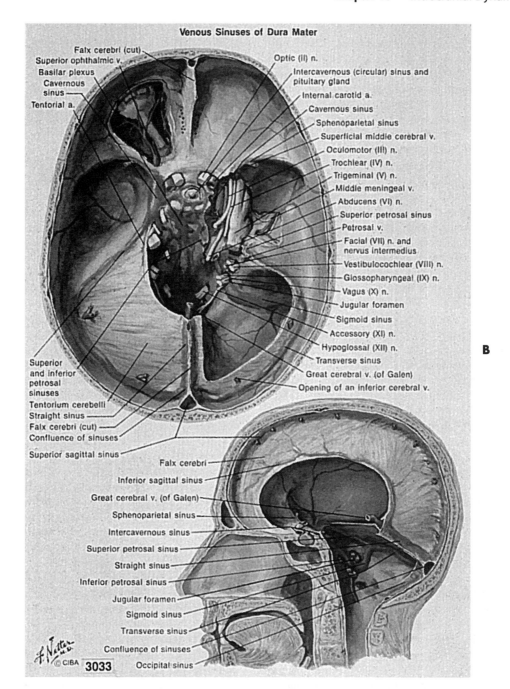

Venous Sinuses of Dura Mater

Falx cerebri (cut)
Superior ophthalmic v.
Basilar plexus
Cavernous sinus
Tentorial a.

Optic (II) n.
Intercavernous (circular) sinus and pituitary gland
Internal carotid a.
Cavernous sinus
Sphenoparietal sinus
Superficial middle cerebral v.
Oculomotor (III) n.
Trochlear (IV) n.
Trigeminal (V) n.
Middle meningeal v.
Abducens (VI) n.
Superior petrosal sinus
Petrosal v.
Facial (VII) n. and nervus intermedius
Vestibulocochlear (VIII) n.
Glossopharyngeal (IX) n.
Vagus (X) n.
Jugular foramen
Sigmoid sinus
Accessory (XI) n.
Hypoglossal (XII) n.
Transverse sinus
Great cerebral v. (of Galen)
Opening of an inferior cerebral v.

B

Superior and inferior petrosal sinuses
Tentorium cerebelli
Straight sinus
Falx cerebri (cut)
Confluence of sinuses
Superior sagittal sinus

Falx cerebri
Inferior sagittal sinus
Great cerebral v. (of Galen)
Sphenoparietal sinus
Intercavernous sinus
Superior petrosal sinus
Straight sinus
Inferior petrosal sinus
Jugular foramen
Sigmoid sinus
Transverse sinus
Confluence of sinuses
Occipital sinus

Fig. 10-3, cont'd **B,** Dural folds and venous sinuses. (Copyright 1996 by CIBA-GEIGY Corporation. Reprinted with permission from the Ciba Collection of Medical Illustrations, illustrated by Frank Netter, MD. All rights reserved.)

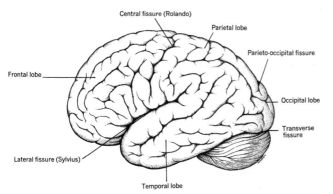

Central fissure (Rolando)
Parietal lobe
Parieto-occipital fissure
Occipital lobe
Transverse fissure
Frontal lobe
Lateral fissure (Sylvius)
Temporal lobe

Fig. 10-4 Lateral aspect of the left cerebral and cerebellar hemispheres. (From Hickey JV: *The clinical practice of neurological and neurosurgical nursing,* ed 2, Philadelphia, 1986, JB Lippincott, p 32.)

functions; however, they are not precise, and considerable functional overlap is found among lobes. Some neuroanatomy texts consider a fifth lobe, called the insula, which is buried deep in the lateral sulcus and has no known function in humans. Although oversimplified, functional descriptions of the four lobes are given for purposes of general orientation. (Refer to neuroanatomy references at the end of this chapter for a more detailed discussion of cortical function.)

The frontal lobe is the largest lobe of the cerebral hemispheres. The central sulcus (fissure of Rolando) divides the frontal lobe from the parietal lobe, and the lateral cerebral fissure (fissure of Sylvius) divides the frontal lobe from the temporal lobe. The frontal lobe has four general functional areas: the primary motor cortex and premotor areas are involved in the initiation of voluntary movements, Broca's area is involved with written and spoken language, and the prefrontal cortex is the origin of "personality." Injury or impairment of the frontal lobe may cause personality changes, altered intellectual functioning, memory deficits, language deficits, or impaired body movements.

The temporal lobe is separated superiorly from the frontal lobe by the lateral cerebral fissure. Posteriorly, it is divided from the occipital lobe by an imaginary line from the parieto-occipital fissure. General functions of the temporal lobe include reception and interpretation of auditory information, expression of emotional and visceral responses, and retention of recent memory. Injury or impairment of the temporal lobe may cause an inability to interpret sensory experiences.

The parietal lobe is separated from the frontal lobe by the central sulcus and from the temporal and occipital lobe by the parieto-occipital fissure. The parietal lobe is associated with three general functions: initial processing of tactile and proprioceptive information, comprehension of language (together with the temporal lobe), and orientation of spatial relationships and time. Injury or impairment of the parietal lobe may result in language dysfunction, aphasia, and motor and sensory loss in the lower extremities.

The occipital lobe is relatively small and sits on the tentorium cerebelli. The rostral border is the parieto-occipital sulcus. The lateral surface is poorly delineated from the parietal lobe and is composed of a number of irregularly shaped lateral occipital gyri. The major function of the occipital lobe is reception and interpretation of visual stimuli. Injury or impairment of the occipital lobe may impair vision.

Diencephalon. The diencephalon is a paired structure on each side of the third ventricle between the cerebral hemispheres (Fig. 10-5). It protrudes over the most rostral end of the brainstem, and some consider it a part of the brainstem. It is divided into the thalamus, the hypothalamus, and the epithalamus.

The thalamus is the largest subdivision of the diencephalon. It is an egg-shaped nuclear mass, part of which surrounds the third ventricle. The enlarged lateral and caudal portions of the thalamus overlie the midbrain structures. A very simplistic description of its function is that of a relay station. However, it also performs complex, interrelated

functions; it transfers sensory input to the cerebral cortex, controls electrocortical activity, and assists to modulate motor functions. Damage or dysfunction of the thalamus may result in impaired consciousness.

The hypothalamus, as its name indicates, lies below and anterior to the thalamus forming the floor and walls of the third ventricle (see Fig. 10-5, *B*). Although small, it has many vital functions. It plays an important role in physiologic homeostasis by regulating visceral, endocrine, and metabolic activity. It also regulates such functions as temperature control, sleep, hunger, and emotion. Damage or dysfunction of the hypothalamus may cause alterations in vegetative, endocrine, and metabolic functions, for example, coma and diabetes insipidus (see Chapter 23).

The epithalamus is made up of the pineal gland and some small neural structures. The pineal gland or epiphysis is a small, cone-shaped body attached to a stalk. It is attached midline to the roof of the third ventricle (see Fig. 10-5, *C*). The exact function of this gland is not well understood. However, apparently it may function as a biologic clock regulating both physiologic and behavioral processes.

Mesencephalon (Midbrain). The mesencephalon is one of three structures that compose the wedge-shaped brainstem. The mesencephalon is the smallest of all of the five divisions of the brain and is located rostrally on the brainstem between the diencephalon and the metencephalon (Fig. 10-6). The mesencephalon is further divided into three areas: the tectum, the tegmentum, and the paired cerebral peduncles. The tectum is made up of two upper rounded projections (superior colliculi) and two lower rounded projections (inferior colliculi). These four projections are associated with visual and auditory functions. The body of the mesencephalon where fiber tracts pass is referred to as the tegmentum. Also situated in the tegmentum are the nuclei from the oculomotor nerve and the trochlear nerve. At the base of the mesencephalon are a pair of fiber bundles (cerebral peduncles) that are continuations of descending fibers. Damage or dysfunction of the mesencephalon may cause impaired consciousness, decerebrate posturing, and neurologic hyperventilation.

Metencephalon (Pons). The metencephalon is located between the midbrain and the medulla. It is ventral (anterior) to the cerebellum, separated from it by the fourth ventricle (see Fig. 10-6). The ventral portion of the metencephalon is called the basis pontis. It contains longitudinal descending fiber bundles, pontine nuclei, and transverse fibers that connect with the cerebellum. Dorsal to the basis pontis is the tegmental portion of the metencephalon. The tegmentum contains collections of cells and fibers that form the reticular formation that is continuous with the medulla and midbrain. Also within the tegmentum are cranial nerve (CN) nuclei V, VI, VII, and VIII and ascending and descending fiber tracts. Damage or dysfunction of the metencephalon may cause impaired consciousness; deep, rapid, periodic breathing; and impaired muscle function innervated by CN V through VIII.

Myelencephalon (Medulla). The myelencephalon is also called the medulla or medulla oblongata. It is located below the pons ventral to the cerebellum (see Fig. 10-6).

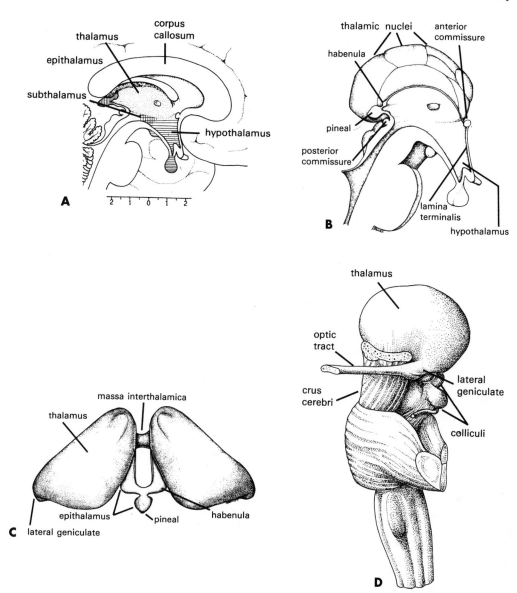

Fig. 10-5   Different views of the diencephalon. **A,** Left midsagittal surface. **B,** Midsagittal surface dissected exposes dorsal surface of thalamus. **C,** Dorsal view of thalamus. **D,** Lateral view of brainstem and diencephalon. (From Romero-Sierra C: *Neuroanatomy: a conceptual approach,* New York, 1986, Churchill Livingstone.)

The fourth ventricle is located in the dorsal midline of the myelencephalon. Like the pons and midbrain, the myelencephalon contains ascending and descending fiber tracts. It also contains CN nuclei IX through XII. The reticular formation originates from the medulla containing cardiac, respiratory, and arousability centers. Damage or dysfunction to the myelencephalon may cause impaired vital functions, alteration in consciousness, ataxic breathing, and loss of gag and corneal reflexes.

Cerebellum.   The cerebellum is a wedge-shaped structure that lies in the posterior fossa dorsal to most of the brainstem and inferior to the tentorium. It is divided into two lobes or hemispheres by a midline structure, the vermis, and is anchored to the brainstem via three pairs of fiber bundles called the cerebellar peduncles. The dorsal surface is arranged in multiple small folds, giving it a banded external appearance and increasing its surface area. The cerebellum is primarily concerned with coordination of voluntary movements, control of muscle tone, and maintenance of equilibrium. Damage or dysfunction of the cerebellum may cause a variety of problems with coordination, gait, and general motor function.

Cerebrospinal Fluid and the Ventricular System

Deep within the brain is the ventricular system, which consists of four interconnecting chambers that produce and circulate CSF (Fig. 10-7). The two paired lateral ventricles are the largest of the four chambers and are contained within

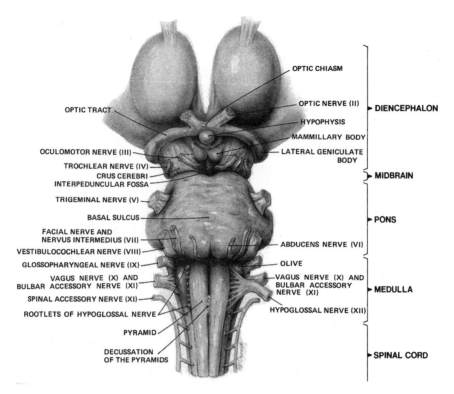

Fig. 10-6 Ventral surface of the human brainstem and diencephalon. (From Gilman S, Winans SS: *Manter & Gatz's essentials of clinical neuroanatomy and neurophysiology,* ed 6, Philadelphia, 1982, FA Davis.)

the cerebral hemispheres. Each lateral ventricle is divided into five parts: an anterior horn, a body, an atrium, a posterior horn, and an inferior horn.

The lateral ventricles communicate with each other and the third ventricle through the interventricular foramen (foramen of Monro). The third ventricle is a small, narrow slit that connects with the fourth ventricle through the aqueduct of Sylvius. Unlike the lateral and third ventricles, which communicate only with other parts of the ventricular system, the fourth ventricle also communicates with the subarachnoid space. Circulation of CSF occurs between the ventricular system and the subarachnoid space around the brain and spinal cord via three openings: the paired foramina of Luschka (lateral) and the midline foramen of Magendie.

CSF is produced primarily by the choroid plexus, present in all four ventricles, and to a lesser degree by the brain parenchyma. Its primary functions are protection, nutrition, and fluid and electrolyte balance of the CNS tissue. The microscopic structure of the choroid plexus is a three-layer membrane: choroid capillary endothelium, pial cells, and choroid epithelium. CSF is formed by active transport. CSF is a colorless liquid that has an ionic composition similar to that of plasma, but it is low in proteins and cells (Table 10-2). The rate of production of CSF is relatively constant at 0.35 ml/kg/min and is unaffected by systemic blood pressure or intraventricular pressure.

After CSF circulates in the subarachnoid space over the cerebral hemispheres and around the spinal cord, it travels back to the superior sagittal sinus, where it is reabsorbed by the arachnoid villi (see Fig. 10-7). These villi are small arachnoid projections that function as one-way valves between the subarachnoid space and the sagittal sinus. They allow CSF to enter the dural venous blood but prevent blood from entering the subarachnoid space.

Disturbances may occur in CSF production and circulation that may result in dilation of the ventricular system with an excessive increase in head size in the infant (hydrocephalus). The three conditions that produce hydrocephalus are obstruction of CSF circulatory pathways, diminished reabsorption of CSF, and overproduction of CSF. The most common of these causes is obstruction of the CSF pathways from either congenital or acquired conditions. Malabsorption of CSF is rare; it is occasionally seen with a subarachnoid hemorrhage when the arachnoid villi are obstructed from debris. Overproduction of CSF may be caused by a choroid plexus papilloma.

Spinal Cord

The spinal cord is a long, cylindric structure, encased within the vertebral column. Rostrally, it begins at the foramen magnum and extends caudally to the level of the second lumbar vertebra (L2), where it becomes cone shaped (conus medullaris). The spinal cord is covered with the same three meningeal layers as on the brain.

A cross-sectional view of the cord reveals a centrally located H-shaped area of gray matter that consists of

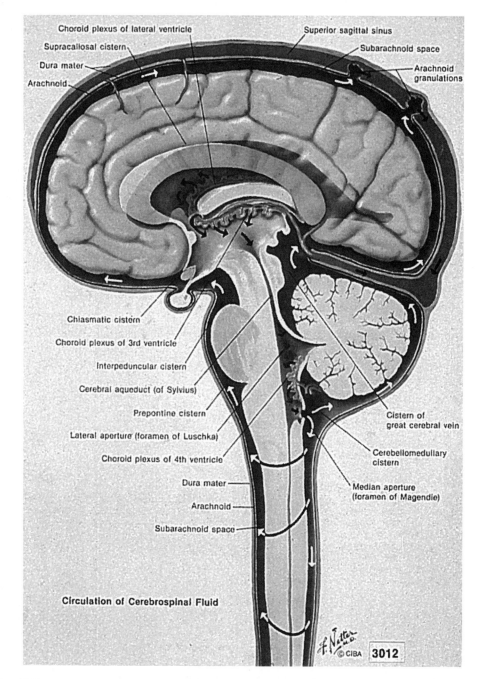

Choroid plexus of lateral ventricle
Supracallosal cistern
Dura mater
Arachnoid
Superior sagittal sinus
Subarachnoid space
Arachnoid granulations

Chiasmatic cistern
Choroid plexus of 3rd ventricle
Interpeduncular cistern
Cerebral aqueduct (of Sylvius)
Prepontine cistern
Lateral aperture (foramen of Luschka)
Choroid plexus of 4th ventricle
Dura mater
Arachnoid
Subarachnoid space
Cistern of great cerebral vein
Cerebellomedullary cistern
Median aperture (foramen of Magendie)

Circulation of Cerebrospinal Fluid

© CIBA 3012

Fig. 10-7 Ventricular system. (Copyright 1996 by CIBA-GEIGY Corporation. Reprinted with permission from the Ciba Collection of Medical Illustrations, illustrated by Frank Netter, MD. All rights reserved.)

neuronal cell bodies and their processes (Fig. 10-8). The gray matter has two anterior (ventral) horns and two posterior (dorsal) horns. The anterior horns contain motor neurons (lower motor neurons) that supply skeletal muscles, and the posterior horns contain neurons that are associated with sensory input to the spinal cord. The size of the gray matter varies, depending on the number of structures innervated at a particular spinal cord level. For example, the gray matter is larger in the cervical and lumbosacral areas because innervation of the extremities occurs from these areas of the cord.

Surrounding the gray matter is white matter composed of

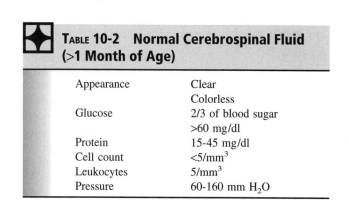

TABLE 10-2 Normal Cerebrospinal Fluid (>1 Month of Age)

Appearance	Clear Colorless
Glucose	2/3 of blood sugar >60 mg/dl
Protein	15-45 mg/dl
Cell count	<5/mm^3
Leukocytes	5/mm^3
Pressure	60-160 mm H$_2$O

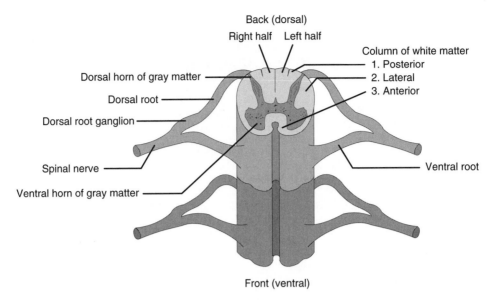

Fig. 10-8 Cross-section of the spinal cord.

Table 10-3 Common Ascending and Descending Spinal Tracts

Tract Name	Function
Ascending (Sensory)	
Dorsal (posterior) spino-cerebellar	Proprioception
Ventral (anterior) spino-cerebellar	Proprioception
Lateral spinothalamic	Pain, temperature
Ventral (anterior) spinothalamic	Touch, pressure
Descending (Motor)	
Corticospinal (pyramidal tracts)	
Ventral (anterior) corticospinal	Skilled voluntary movements
Lateral corticospinal	Skilled voluntary movements
Rubrospinal	Fine movements, muscle tone
Vestibulospinal	Aids equilibrium, extensor muscle tone
Reticulospinal	Posture, muscle tone
Tectospinal	Mediates optic and auditory reflex movement

Peripheral Nervous System

Spinal Nerves. Within the PNS are 31 pairs of spinal nerves with related branches and ganglia. They form from the convergence of the ventral (motor) efferent and dorsal (sensory) afferent rootlets that exit the spinal cord through the intervertebral foramen. The paired spinal nerves are divided into five segments: cervical (8), thoracic (12), lumbar (5), sacral (5), and coccygeal (1). Spinal nerves are numbered after the vertebral level from which they exit. Because there are eight cervical spinal nerves, they take their number from the vertebral level below their exit. The remaining spinal nerves are numbered to correspond to the vertebral level above their exit.

Cranial Nerves. There are 12 pairs of cranial nerves, with their nuclei originating from the CNS. Because they connect the CNS with peripheral structures, they are generally classified as belonging to the PNS. Most of the cranial nerves have both sensory and motor functions, although some have purely sensory or motor functions. Damage directly to cranial nerves or to surrounding structures can often be determined by assessing cranial nerve function. Fig. 10-9 illustrates the cephalocaudal location of CN nuclei I through XII. Table 10-4 outlines CN function, how each is tested according to age, and the clinical significance of abnormal findings.

Autonomic Nervous System

The autonomic nervous system (ANS) has structures that are located in both the CNS and the PNS; however, most consider it part of the efferent division of the PNS. The ANS unconsciously regulates three types of body tissue: cardiac muscle, smooth muscle, and most glands. The ANS is divided structurally and functionally into two parts: the sympathetic and parasympathetic nervous system. Both systems are based on a two-neuron pathway. The first neuron is referred to as a preganglionic neuron and the second, a

myelinated nerve fibers. The nerve fibers consist of one of three types: long ascending fibers from the spinal cord to the brainstem, cerebellum, or brainstem nuclei; long descending fibers from the cerebral cortex or brainstem nuclei to the spinal cord gray matter; and short fibers that interconnect various segments of the spinal cord. Descending and ascending fibers that have similar functions tend to travel together and are called spinal tracts. Numerous tracts are arranged together to form a funiculus. Table 10-3 summarizes the most common ascending and descending tracts.

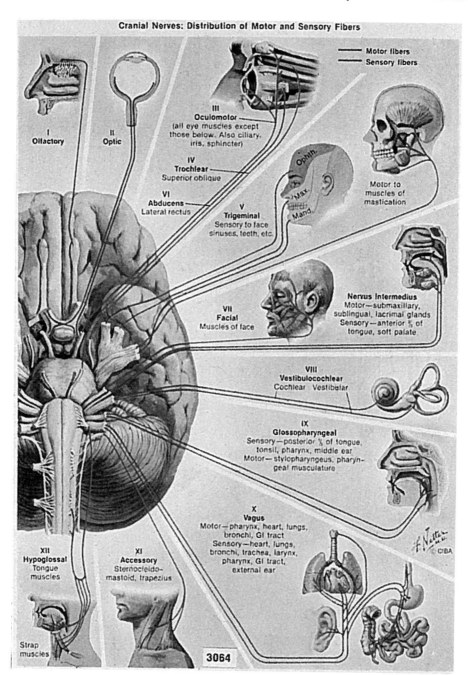

Fig. 10-9 Cranial nerves (Copyright 1996 by CIBA-GEIGY Corporation. Reprinted with permission from the Ciba Collection of Medical Illustrations, illustrated by Frank Netter, MD. All rights reserved.)

postganglionic neuron. With few exceptions, these two systems have neurons that stimulate and control the same organs (Fig. 10-10). Because the parasympathetic and sympathetic systems have antagonistic functions, they are usually maintained in balance. An imbalance can occur between the two systems in one of two ways: by increasing the stimulus from one system or by decreasing the stimulus from the other system.

Parasympathetic System. The parasympathetic system is the division of the ANS that usually dominates when a person is resting. The neurotransmitter acetylcholine is released in the synapse between the parasympa-

thetic postganglionic neurons and the effector organ. Activation of the parasympathetic system produces responses such as increased peristalsis, decreased heart rate, and secretion of intestinal enzymes. Administration of exogenous sources of acetylcholine or stimulation of a nerve that contains many parasympathetic nerve fibers (e.g., the vagus nerve) produces a characteristic parasympathetic response.

Sympathetic System. The sympathetic nervous system is responsible for increasing the overall energy level of the body when necessary to overcome a stressful situation, whether it is physical or psychologic. Unlike the parasym-

TABLE 10-4	Assessment of Cranial Nerve Function			
		Testing		
Cranial Nerve	**Function**	**Infant**	**Child**	**Altered Level of Consciousness**	**Clinical Significance**
I—Olfactory	Smell	Usually not assessed, young infant responds to strong odors with generalized movement, but testing is unreliable	Assess each nostril separately using common odors (e.g., soap, mints, orange). Testing is unreliable in very young children	Not tested	Must have patient cooperation. Damage to the nerve or olfactory bulbs can alter or result in loss of smell
II—Optic	Vision	Introduce a bright light and observe for a blink response in the newborn. Observe older infants' ability to pick up small objects	Visual acuity tested in young child through recognition of familiar objects at various distances. The older child can be tested with Snellen chart or measuring tape with numbers. Ophthalmoscopic examination performed at end of session in young child. The child is instructed to fixate on a distant object	Assess pupillary response to light	Any abnormality requires further investigation. Lesions in the optic chiasm generally produce bilateral but nonhomonomous defects. Lesions behind chiasm produce homonomous field defects in both fields of vision. Lesion of the eye and optic tract produce visual defects in the visual field of one eye only. Papilledema may indicate elevated intracranial pressure. The optic disc is pale, gray, and poorly developed in the infant. The child's retina is lighter than the adult's. Failure of pupil constriction to light may indicate optic nerve damage or oculomotor nerve paralysis

Cranial Nerve	Function	Assessment Technique: Older Child	Assessment Technique: Toddler	Assessment Technique: Infant	Comments
III—Oculomotor	Pupillary constriction, extraocular movements, elevation of upper eyelid	Assess pupillary response; shine a bright light in each eye starting from the outer periphery of the visual field. Assess consensual response by shining a bright light in one eye and observing for constriction in the other eye. Assess accommodation by noting convergence and constriction as a bright light is brought toward the nose. Assess eyelids for ptosis (drooping). Extraocular movements are tested with cranial nerves III, IV, and VI (see below)	Same as infant	Assess pupillary response to light	Elevated intracranial pressure may produce unequal pupils; unreactive or sluggish pupillary response to light; or dilated pupil(s). Roving eye movements may be present in the comatose patient with intact nerve
III—Oculomotor IV—Trochlear VI—Abducens	IV—Downward and inward movement of the eye VI—Lateral movement of the eye III—All other extracellular movements	Assess the six fields of gaze; note conjugate movement of the eyes as a bright object is moved from the midline into each of the six fields of gaze	Assess the six fields of gaze with the infant	Tested with efferent portion of oculocephalic and oculovestibular responses	Binocular fixation usually present by 3 months of age. Nystagmus normal in premature infants and neonates. Damage to cranial nerve IV can cause diplopia and altered downward movement. Dysconjugate gaze after 6 months of age may indicate blindness. A paralysis of gaze may indicate a lesion or dysfunction of various parts of the brain. Be prepared to protect airway if oculocephalic or oculovestibular responses absent (negative)
V—Trigeminal	Motor division: muscles of mastication Sensory division: innervation of the face with three branches (ophthalmic, maxillary, mandibular)	Palpate the temporal and masseter muscles while the child is clenching; assess for strength and symmetry. Observe jaw movement for symmetry while talking, laughing, crying. Test the three regions of the face (eyes closed) for sensation. Test the corneal reflex as in the infant	Assess corneal reflex	Test strength of muscles by assessing the infant sucking on a finger or nipple. Test rooting reflex. Test corneal reflex by lightly touching the cornea with a cotton wisp. Observe for blinking and tearing	Damage to the motor division can result in impaired mastication. Damage to the sensory division may impair facial sensation or cause pain. Tears are usually not present in infants less than 2-3 months of age. Use of contact lenses may diminish or abolish corneal reflex

Modified from Slota MC: Neurological assessment of the infant and toddler, *Crit Care Nurs* 3:87, 1983; Slota MC: Pediatric neurological assessment, *Crit Care Nurs* 3:106, 1983.

Continued

TABLE 10-4   Assessment of Cranial Nerve Function—cont'd

Cranial Nerve	Function	Testing — Infant	Testing — Child	Altered Level of Consciousness	Clinical Significance
VII—Facial	Motor division: motor innervation of facial muscles and mouth. Sensory division: taste in anterior two thirds of tongue	Facial tone can best be observed during crying and smiling. Movement should be symmetric. Testing for discrimination of taste not possible	Motor innervation of the face can be tested by asking the child to make a "mad" face and observe facial tone while smiling or crying. Ask the child to "puff out" his or her cheeks. Sensation tested by applying various substances to the anterior tongue	Not tested	Damage to the nerve can produce facial paralysis or weakness and loss of taste sensation to the anterior tongue
VIII—Acoustic	Cochlear division: hearing. Vestibular division: balance	Hearing can be assessed in newborns by testing the acoustic blink reflex: a loud noise by the infant will produce a blink response. Older infants will stop moving when listening to sound or move head in direction of sound. Vestibular function is not routinely tested. Oculovestibular response may be tested in patient with altered mental status	Hearing is tested using a variety of high- and low-pitched sounds. Vestibular function not routinely tested. Oculovestibular response (caloric testing) may be tested for complaints of tinnitus or vertigo. May also be tested in patient with altered mental status	Tested with afferent portion of oculocephalic and oculovestibular responses	Damage to the nerve can result in impairment of hearing, deafness, vertigo, tinnitus, and nystagmus. A normal response to caloric testing in the awake patient is jerk nystagmus, nausea, and/or vomiting. Caloric testing in the comatose patient with brainstem damage produces no response (i.e., eyes are fixed)
IX—Glossopharyngeal	Sensory innervation to the pharynx and posterior one third of the tongue	Assess together with cranial nerve X. Stimulate a gag reflex by touching posterior portion of the tongue. Note hoarse or stridorous crying	Assess together with cranial nerve X. Instruct the child to say "ah" and note movement of the soft palate. Movement should be upward. Stimulate a gag reflex. Observe child's ability to swallow without pain or choking. Note excess drooling or coughing	Assess gag reflex	Damage to the nerve can result in dysphagia, dysarthria, impaired sensation, excessive drooling, stridor, and autonomic nervous system changes related to the vagus nerve

Cranial Nerve	Function	Assessment		Clinical Significance
X—Vagus	Sensory division: innervation to the larynx and pharynx. Motor division: innervation to the palate and pharynx and parasympathetic functions			
XI—Spinal accessory	Motor innervation of the sternocleidomastoid muscle and the upper portion of the trapezius muscle	Observe for normal side-to-side head movement	Ask the child to shrug his or her shoulders against the pressure of your hands. Ask the child to turn his or her head side to side against the pressure of your hand. Observe for strength and symmetry	Not tested
XII—Hypoglossal	Motor innervation to the tongue	Observe the tongue or fasciculations, asymmetric movement or atrophy	Same as the infant	Not tested

Fasciculation is occasionally seen in denervating diseases. Damage to this nerve can result in asymmetric shoulder posture, impaired strength, and difficulty moving the head from side to side

In pyramidal disorders, the tongue may be spastic. Unilateral damage to the nerve or its nucleus can cause deviation of the tongue toward the side of the lesion. Damage to this nerve can cause paresis, paralysis, fasciculations, or atrophy

Modified from Slota MC: Neurological assessment of the infant and toddler, *Crit Care Nurs* 3:87, 1983; Slota MC: Pediatric neurological assessment, *Crit Care Nurs* 3:106, 1983.

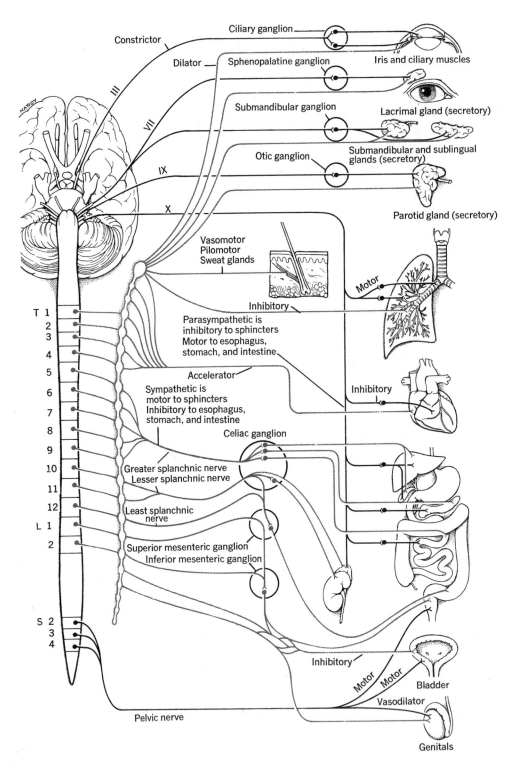

Fig. 10-10 Diagram of the autonomic nervous system, including parasympathetic or craniosacral fibers and sympathetic or thoracolumbar fibers. Note that most organs have a double nerve supply. (From Chaffee EE, Lytle IM: *Basic physiology and anatomy,* Philadelphia, 1980, JB Lippincott.)

pathetic system, whose postganglionic neurons secrete acetylcholine, sympathetic postganglionic neurons secrete norepinephrine. Activation of the sympathetic system with release of norepinephrine produces a characteristic response: bronchiolar dilation, increased heart rate and contractility, vasodilation of blood vessels to vital organs, and pupillary dilation. Similarly, if a person is administered an exogenous source of epinephrine or if the parasympathetic system is blocked, the body mimics responses that directly result from sympathetic activation.

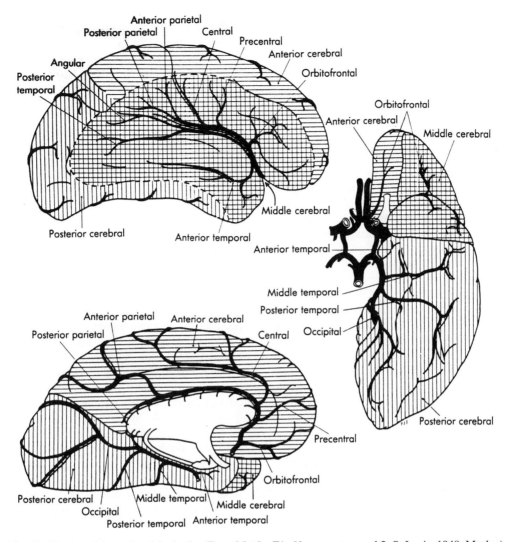

Fig. 10-11   Arterial supply of the brain. (From Mettler FA: *Neuroanatomy,* ed 2, St Louis, 1948, Mosby.)

Central Nervous System Circulation

In comparison with other organs of the body, the brain's metabolic demands for glucose and oxygen are very high. The amount of glucose and oxygen required by the brain per minute is referred to as the cerebral metabolic rate of glucose (CMR glucose) and the cerebral metabolic rate of oxygen ($CMRO_2$). The CMR glucose is approximately 4.5 to 5.5 mg/100 g/min, and the $CMRO_2$ is approximately 3 to 3.5 ml/100 g/min. To meet these metabolic demands, approximately 20% of the body's cardiac output must be continuously delivered to the brain.[3]

Arterial System.   The predominant arterial flow to the brain is from two systems: the paired carotid arteries anteriorly and the paired vertebral arteries posteriorly (Fig. 10-11). The majority of cerebral blood flow (CBF) is supplied by the internal carotid arteries, which originate from the common carotid arteries. The internal carotid arteries further subdivide into the anterior and middle cerebral arteries. The anterior cerebral artery supplies blood to the basal ganglia of the corpus callosum, the medial surface of the cerebral hemispheres, and the superior surface of the frontal and parietal lobes. The middle cerebral artery supplies blood to the frontal lobe, the parietal lobe, and the cortical surfaces of the temporal lobe. Occlusion of the anterior cerebral artery may lead to weakness or hemiplegia on the contralateral side of the body. Occlusion of the middle cerebral artery may cause aphasia and contralateral hemiplegia.

The paired vertebral arteries originate at the subclavian arteries. They join to form the basilar artery on the ventral surface of the brainstem at the junction of the pons and medulla. The basilar artery proceeds rostrally, and at the level of the midbrain, it divides to form the paired posterior cerebral arteries. The vertebral-basilar arteries supply blood to the posterior sections of the cerebral hemispheres, the cerebellum, and the brainstem. Occlusion of the vertebral-basilar arteries may cause a variety disorders, such as sensory loss, visual loss, and contralateral hemiplegia.

At the base of the brain, the posterior cerebral arteries, the posterior communicating arteries, the internal carotid arteries, the anterior cerebral arteries, and the anterior communicating artery fuse to form the circle of Willis. As these large conducting arteries leave the circle of Willis, their diameter becomes smaller to form arterioles and pial arteries. These smaller arterioles branch off at 90-degree angles into the brain parenchyma and are called penetrating or nutrient arteries.

Venous System.   The two systems of venous drainage in the brain consist of superficial and deep veins, all of which are valveless (see Fig. 10-3, *B*). In general, the superficial veins drain venous blood from the cerebral hemispheres and empty into the dural venous sinuses. The deep veins drain internal structures and empty centrally into the great cerebral vein (of Galen), which eventually empties into the straight sinus. All venous drainage ultimately exits at the base of the skull via the internal jugular veins. Obstruction of venous outflow may cause headaches, cerebral edema, or cerebral hypertension.

Blood-Brain Barrier.   Blood-brain barrier is the term used to describe the anatomic structures and physiologic processes that separate the brain and CSF compartments from the blood compartment. Anatomic barriers include the arachnoid layer, the blood-CSF barrier, and the cerebral capillary barrier. All barrier sites are characterized by cells with tight junctions between them. These tightly connected cells function as a single layer of cells, allowing precise regulation of chemicals among the brain, CSF, and plasma.

The blood-brain barrier protects the CNS by preventing passage of potentially harmful molecules from the blood to the brain. However, this barrier is equally effective in preventing the passage of many antibiotic and chemotherapeutic medications. Consequently, a reduced number of therapeutic agents are available to treat CNS disorders. The blood-brain barrier may be altered from a number of CNS insults, for example, chemical, physical, biologic, or infective insults.

Spinal Cord.   The arterial supply of the spinal cord originates from the vertebral arteries and radicular arteries. At the base of the skull, the vertebral arteries give rise to the posterior spinal arteries and the anterior spinal artery, which descend alongside the spinal cord. Radicular arteries originate from the thoracic and abdominal aorta and enter the spinal canal through the intervertebral foramen. The radicular arteries and the spinal arteries eventually connect. Venous drainage of the spinal cord is via a series of plexiform channels, which in turn drain into the radicular veins. There are no valves in the spinal venous network.

INTRACRANIAL PRESSURE DYNAMICS

Modified Monro-Kellie Doctrine

The Monro-Kellie doctrine, which has been modified over the years, provides the basis for understanding the determinants of intracranial pressure (ICP). This doctrine states that the skull and relatively inelastic dural sheath provide a rigid container filled to capacity with nearly noncompressible contents. The three volume components of the intracranial space are brain tissue, CSF, and blood. The most important concept of this doctrine is that if there is a change in any one of the volume compartments, there must be a reciprocal

TABLE 10-5   Normal ICP in Infants and Children

Age Group	Normal ICP (mmHg)
Newborn	0.7-1.5
Infants	1.5-6.0
Children	3.0-7.5
Adults	<10

Data from Welch K: The intracranial pressure in infants, *J Neurosurg* 52:693-699, 1980.

change in one or more of the other volume compartments to maintain equilibrium. With reciprocal changes in volume, abnormal increases in ICP can be diverted.

Brain tissue represents the largest volume component of the intracranial space, composing approximately 80% to 90% of the total. This volume may be increased by the presence of neuropathologic conditions such as cerebral edema or a brain tumor. The cerebral blood and CSF compartments each represent 5% to 10% of intracranial volume. The total cerebral blood volume may be altered in the same way that CBF is controlled, for example, by arterial carbon dioxide tension ($Paco_2$) and arterial oxygen tension (Pao_2), or by local pH. CSF volume may also be increased by mechanisms described earlier (see Cerebrospinal Fluid and the Ventricular System).

Because the skull is not rigid until closure of the fontanelles and fusion of the cranial sutures (which occurs around 5 years of age), the Monro-Kellie hypothesis is often thought not to apply in the infant and young child. Although in the first 3 years of life, *slow* increases in intracranial volume are accommodated by increasing head circumference, rapid or unabated increases in intracranial volume overburden this adaptive mechanism. Studies also suggest that expansion of the skull evidenced by increased head circumference occurs only after critical ICPs have been reached.[4] At best, the nonrigid container in the young child tends to make the signs and symptoms of cerebral hypertension less striking. Astute nursing assessment to detect subtle changes in neurologic status is therefore necessary to avoid secondary neurologic injury.

Volume/Pressure Relationships

Normal ICP varies in different age groups (Table 10-5). Derived from the age-dependent norms, increased ICP is also age dependent. Clinically, pressures greater than 15 mmHg are considered elevated, pressures between 20 and 40 mmHg are considered moderately elevated, and ICPs greater than 40 mmHg indicate cerebral hypertension.

ICP is dynamic and fluctuates with each heartbeat and respiration. ICP increases momentarily with certain activities and physiologic responses, including coughing or sneezing and during Valsalva maneuvers and rapid eye movement (REM) sleep. Temporary increases in intracranial volume and subsequent ICP are normally well tolerated.

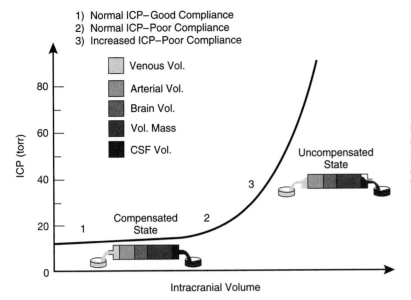

1) Normal ICP– Good Compliance
2) Normal ICP– Poor Compliance
3) Increased ICP– Poor Compliance

Fig. 10-12 Intracranial volume/pressure curve. (Adapted from Becker DP, Mickell J, Keenan R: In Shoemaker WC, Thomson WL, eds: *Critical care: state of the art,* Fullerton, Calif, 1981, Society of Critical Care Medicine, p 1.)

CSF volume manipulation is a major adaptive mechanism when the subarachnoid space and ventricular outflow tracts are patent. Along with decreased production and increased reabsorption, CSF is translocated from the brain to the distensible spinal subarachnoid space. When compensation is maximized, slit ventricles and absence of sulci are viewed on computed tomography scan. To a lesser degree, reducing total cerebral blood volume or brain mass may also offset an increase in ICP.

The patient's adaptive capacity is dependent on the volume of the mass lesion, its rate of expansion, the total volume of the intracranial cavity, and the relative volume of blood and CSF that is available for displacement. When adaptive mechanisms are obliterated, ICP will increase rapidly, often with minor changes in cerebral blood volume.

The intracranial volume/pressure relationship curve describes how much intracranial volume produces how great a change in ICP (Fig. 10-12). Elastance is the term used to describe the change in pressure that occurs with a change in volume into the intracranial space; elastance = $\Delta P/\Delta V$. Compliance is the inverse of elastance and is used to describe the same volume/pressure relationship when pressure changes are induced; compliance = $\Delta V/\Delta P$.

The relationship between intracranial volume and ICP is not linear. The intracranial volume/pressure (V/P) curve has three distinct phases: flat, exponential, and increased ICP. Phase 1, the flat portion of the curve, illustrates normal ICP with good compliance. At this point, compensation is effective in that the volume added is equal to the volume removed from the intracranial compartment. Phase 2, the exponential portion of the curve, illustrates normal ICP with poor compliance. Here, the intracranial compartment is described as "tight," adaptive capacity is reached, and any further small increase in volume produces disproportionately large increases in ICP that may not return to baseline. Phase 3 illustrates increased ICP with poor compliance. Compensatory mechanisms have been exhausted. The exponential relationship of the V/P curve explains the

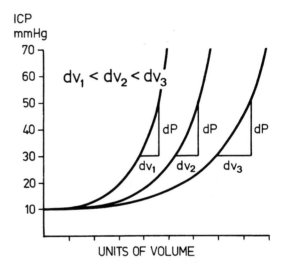

Fig. 10-13 Variation in the volume/pressure curve. Diagram to illustrate how changes in the gradient of the pressure/volume curve mean that different volumetric changes are needed to produce a given pressure change: less where the curve is steep and more where the curve is flatter. Alternatively, the same volume change will produce greater and lesser changes in pressure. *dP,* Change in pressure; *dV,* change in volume. (From Miller JD: Increased intracranial pressure: theoretical considerations. In Pellock JM, Myer EC, eds: *Neurological emergencies in infants and children,* Philadelphia, 1984, Harper & Row, p 65.)

variability in ICP response among individuals and also in the same individual at different times.

The critical point when compensation is lost varies and depends on such factors as the rate of volumetric change, systemic arterial pressure, and osmotic therapy. Age has also been found to be a variable, with the younger child having less buffering capacity.[5,6] Thus when speaking of intracranial compliance, a series of compliance curves exist rather than a single curve (Fig. 10-13). For example, the first V/P curve (dv_1) may represent the acute increase in ICP that occurs within 24 to 48 hours after head trauma. The second V/P curve (dv$_2$) may represent the 48- to 72-hour delay in increased ICP after a hypoxic-ischemic episode. The last V/P curve (dv$_3$) may represent the slow increase in ICP that occurs in a patient with a brain tumor. The collaborative management goal is to shift the patient's ICP *down to the right of one curve* or, better yet, to improve intracranial compliance and shift the patient's ICP *to a new V/P curve on the left of the curve.*

Cerebral Blood Flow

The normal rate of CBF is approximately 40 ml/100 g/min in newborns and 53 ml/100 g/min in older children.[7] A severe and prolonged increase in ICP may cause a lethal reduction in CBF. A progressive increase in intracranial volume may cause obstruction of the CSF pathways, eliminating the primary means of buffering increased ICP. In addition, increased ICP may cause venous outflow obstruction and compensatory arterial hypertension. As a consequence, capillary pressure increases, predisposing the brain to cerebral edema. The end result is a further increase in intracranial volume that ultimately may precipitate herniation of brain structures and a reduction in CBF.

As mentioned earlier, the brain requires constant and consistent delivery of blood flow to meet its high metabolic demands. The determinants of CBF are arteriolar radius, blood viscosity, perfusion pressure, and length of the vascular bed. Practically speaking, the length of the vascular bed and blood viscosity remain constant. Therefore the important variables of CBF are cerebral perfusion pressure and arteriolar radius.

Cerebral Perfusion Pressure. Cerebral perfusion pressure (CPP) represents the pressure drop between the inflow (arterial) pressure and outflow (venous) pressure. Traystman[8] identified three separate conditions that require consideration (Fig. 10-14). In condition I, the ICP is greater than the mean arterial pressure (MAP), and both are greater than the central venous pressure (CVP). When these conditions are present, CBF is impossible. In condition II, the MAP is greater than the ICP, and both are greater than the CVP. Here, the CPP is calculated as MAP minus the ICP. In condition III, the MAP is greater than the CVP, and both are greater than the ICP. Here, the CPP is calculated as MAP minus the CVP. Clinically, the CPP = MAP−ICP unless the CVP is significantly elevated; then the CPP = MAP−CVP. Because it is possible to have a normal ICP but no blood flow (thus no oxygen extraction) through damaged areas of the brain, some research centers trend cross-brain oxygen consumption and metabolic rates with ICP and CPP.

Normal CPP is unknown in the pediatric population, but it is thought that a CPP greater than 50 mmHg is necessary for adequate cerebral perfusion. CPPs less than 40 mmHg, because of cerebral hypertension or systemic hypotension, are thought to be the cutoff point between good-quality survival and poor outcomes. This critical point is much less in the neonate. In this age group, normal CPP is thought to depend on weight and be about 30 mmHg.[9]

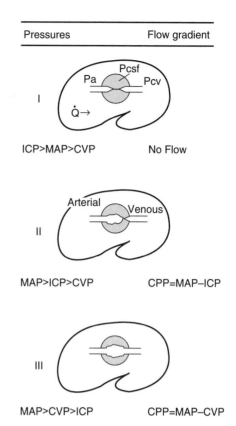

Fig. 10-14 Three separate conditions that require evaluation when calculating cerebral perfusion pressure. *CVP,* Central venous pressure; *ICP,* intracranial pressure; *MAP,* mean arterial pressure; *Pa,* arterial pressure; *Pcsf,* cerebrospinal fluid pressure; *Pcv,* central venous pressure; *Q,* flow. (Adapted from Mortillaro NA: *The physiology and pharmacology of the microcirculation,* New York, 1983, Academic Press, pp 237-238.)

Cerebral Autoregulation. Normally, CBF matches the cerebral metabolic rate (CMR). For example, when the CMR increases, there is a concomitant increase in CBF; when CMR decreases, there is a concomitant decrease in CBF. This compensatory process, known as autoregulation, matches CBF with CMR and is accomplished by either cerebral vasoconstriction or vasodilation. This mechanism is believed to occur from a myogenic mechanism located in the muscular arterioles.[10] Changes in arteriolar transmural pressure produce changes in arteriolar radius by vasoconstriction or vasodilation.

Under normal circumstances, autoregulation is maintained when the CPP ranges from approximately 60 to 160 mmHg.[11] If these limits are exceeded, CBF is passively dependent on CPP. The upper limit of CPP may be higher in individuals with chronic hypertension. Furthermore, autoregulation may be altered locally or globally with CNS insult. If CBF is greater than the CMR, hyperemia occurs, which is a common finding after pediatric head trauma. When CBF is less than the CMR, cerebral hypoxia ensues, which is a common finding during pediatric resuscitation.

Chemical Regulation. In addition to pressure autoregulation, CBF is also affected by chemical autoregulation. Both Paco$_2$ and Pao$_2$ affect CBF and cerebral blood volume by altering cerebral arteriolar radius. High levels of Pa_{CO_2} cause vasodilation of the cerebral vasculature with an increase in CBF and therefore an increase in cerebral blood volume. Conversely, a decrease in Pa_{CO_2} produces a decrease in CBF. Thus lowering Pa_{CO_2} with hyperventilation is a clinically useful tool for emergent management of intracranial hypertension.

In contrast to Pa_{CO_2}, the cerebral vasculature seems to be somewhat less sensitive to Pa_{O_2}. Hypoxia, Pa_{O_2} less than 50 mmHg, increases CBF by producing a vasodilatory response. Conversely, hyperoxia produces a mild vasoconstrictive response with only a modest decrease in CBF. The critical lower limit of Pa_{O_2} that causes a increase in CBF may be lower in the neonate.[8] Newborns are relatively hypoxic (normal Pa_{O_2} range of 65 to 70 mmHg) compared with infants and young children, and the actual delivery of oxygen to the tissues is affected by the percentage of fetal hemoglobin.[12]

NEUROLOGIC ASSESSMENT

CNS development is incomplete at birth, maturing over the first several years of life. Maturation reflects myelinization, dendritic arborization, increases in synaptic connections, increases in glial cell population, and changes in neurochemical properties. As a result, the infant has incomplete cortical integrative function and has immature neuromuscular control. Therefore neurologic assessment of the infant and young child requires a developmental approach that reflects the age and temperament of the child.

The neurologic examination not only requires developmental adaptation, but the condition of the patient must be considered. Consequently, the focus of the examination occurs on two levels. The first level involves a comprehensive assessment of both the central and peripheral nervous systems. It is usually performed in an outpatient or nonacute setting and is intended to diagnose or rule out neurologic dysfunction. The second level of a neurologic examination is usually performed in an acute care setting. It is conducted at prescribed intervals and focuses on significant deterioration (often life threatening) or improvement of the nervous system. The following section describes the components of neurologic assessment in the infant and young child. The critical care nurse is challenged with adapting these components to the age, temperament, and condition of the child.

History

The neurologic history provides the framework for guiding the neurologic examination. The data obtained from the history assist the critical care nurse in formulating preliminary nursing diagnoses that are either supported or rejected by the physical examination. The length of the interview, the specific questions, and the timing depend on whether the child has a static, a progressive, or an acute condition. Taking of history may need to be delayed if the parents are not present and the child is preverbal or if the child's physical status is life threatening.

The first component of the neurologic history is the *chief complaint.* Whenever possible, the school-age child should be asked questions directly. Preschool children are less reliable and, like the preverbal child, often require their parents to describe the problem.

Once the chief problem has been stated, questions are asked to obtain information leading up to the *present illness.* Questions should be formulated so that the nurse can determine whether the patient's condition is progressive or static, focal or generalized, and acute or insidious.

Specific questions that must be addressed regarding the patient's history depend in part on the patient's age and present illness. For the infant and young child, a summary of the antenatal, perinatal, and postnatal courses should be obtained. This includes but does not exhaust questions regarding maternal infections, drug intake during pregnancy, gestational age, and Apgar scores. A history of meconium staining, neonatal seizure activity, or oxygen use necessitates further investigation. Medical history should also include a chronologic list of the child's developmental milestones, which is then compared against established norms (see Chapter 2).

For the older child who was previously healthy, questions should be asked to differentiate between metabolic and structural causes of neurologic dysfunction. For example, has the child had a recent fall or been exposed to chemical toxins, or does he or she have an endocrine disorder such as diabetes?

The *family history* should include questions regarding neurologic illnesses in family members, as well as specific signs and symptoms that may have a neurologic basis. Most neurodegenerative disorders are transmitted as a recessive gene, and some epilepsies are transmitted as a dominant trait.[13]

Physical Examination

For the awake, stable child, vital signs, height, and weight should be measured. The general appearance of the child should be observed—in particular, dysmorphic features, asymmetries, cutaneous lesions (e.g., café au lait spots, angiomas), condition of scalp and hair, palmar creases, and unusual odors.

Skull Examination. For infants, the neurologic assessment includes a skull examination. Head circumference should be measured on admission and repeated at regular intervals as determined by the patient's condition. The largest circumference (occipitofrontal) should be consistently measured and plotted on a head growth chart. Because head growth reflects brain growth, a significantly small head circumference may indicate impaired brain growth. In contrast, an unusually large head may be a manifestation of hydrocephalus or some other abnormal fluid accumulation or tissue growth. The normal rate of head growth in the first 12 months of life is 2 cm per month for the first 3 months, 1 cm per month for the fourth through sixth months, and 0.5 cm per month for the remaining 6 months.[14]

The cranial sutures and associated fontanelles should be palpated gently. The posterior fontanelle usually closes within the first few months of life, and the anterior fontanelle remains open until approximately 12 to 18 months of life. In a U. S. study,[15] the average diameter of the anterior fontanelle at birth was found to be 2.1 cm. However, an unusually small or large fontanelle may not, by itself, reflect an abnormality in the infant. Its presence should be correlated with other clinical findings. Ideally, the fontanelle should be palpated while the infant is sitting upright and in a quiet state. Normally, the fontanelle feels soft and flat or slightly depressed compared with the surrounding skull.

The cranial sutures should be palpated to determine if they are overriding or widely separated. Overriding sutures from head molding in the birth canal may be a normal finding in the newborn. However, it may also represent premature closure of the sutures (craniosynostosis) or inadequate brain growth. Widely separated sutures may suggest hydrocephalus.

Transillumination is a simple, noninvasive technique used to detect abnormal fluid collection within the scalp and beneath the calvaria. Its use is restricted to the first 9 to 12 months of age because of the thickness of the skull beyond this age. Many commercial instruments are available, but a battery flashlight with a rubber adapter (fits close to the skull) is very reliable. The light source is placed on the infant's skull, usually starting at the anterior fontanelle. In the normal full-term newborn, the frontal area has a larger rim of transillumination (as much as 3 cm) compared with the occipital area.[16] An area of increased or asymmetric transillumination should be noted.

If time and the patient's condition permit, the calvaria should be auscultated for bruits. Although the presence of a bruit in young infants may be normal, a particularly loud or asymmetric bruit may be heard with an intracranial vascular malformation. An extreme downward rotation of the eyes at rest and paralysis of upward gaze are known as the "setting-sun" sign. It may be intermittent and is seen in some children with increased ICP. It is a common clinical characteristic of hydrocephalus. A similar appearance may be seen with abnormal retraction of the upper eyelids (Collier's sign) from lesions affecting the costal midbrain and third ventricle. When the cranial sutures are separated because of increased ICP, Macewen's sign or a "cracked pot" sound maybe heard during percussion of the skull.

Level of Consciousness. Consciousness is a state of awareness of self and environment. There are two physiologic components of consciousness: content and arousal. Content is controlled by cerebral function, and arousal is controlled by physiologic mechanisms that originate in the reticular formation. Dysfunction of the cerebral hemispheres or the reticular activating system (RAS) of the upper brainstem, hypothalamus, and thalamus will produce an alteration in consciousness.[17] Altered states of consciousness are on a continuum ranging from the extremes of complete consciousness to coma. For the patient with minimal alteration in consciousness, mental status is assessed. For more severely altered states, coma scales may be required to assess level of consciousness.

Mental Status. Cortical growth occurs both quantitatively and qualitatively within the first 2 years of life.

Consequently, the mental status (cerebral function) portion of the neurologic examination is individualized according to the infant and young child's age. Specific areas to assess in the infant and young child include alertness and level of activity, quality of cry, feeding patterns, language development, and presence or absence of primitive reflexes.

Ideally, the young infant's state of alertness is assessed during a period when stress is at a minimum. Usual patterns of sleep and wakefulness are assessed and evaluated based on the infant's age, nutritional state, and quality of sleep within the previous 24 hours. In general, extreme states of agitation or lethargy are noted.

Normally, the infant's cry is loud and energetic. Abnormal cries include ones that are difficult to elicit, associated with cyanosis, high pitched, weak, monotonous, or moaning.[18]

Normal feeding behavior includes a strong suck and good suck-swallowing coordination. Therefore if the young child cannot finish a bottle without tiring or becomes cyanotic, or if the child has excessive gagging and choking, these reactions should be noted.

Normal speech and language skills develop over several years. These skills depend on normal development of motor control of the oral musculature. Therefore if the child deviates significantly from established norms, the gag reflex and tongue movements are tested for coordination and strength.

In the older awake child, a comprehensive evaluation of mental status includes attention, alertness, orientation, cognition, memory, affect, and perception. Most of the assessment can take place during normal conversation with the child. Care should be taken when determining which questions to ask the child. Questions are individualized according to the child's age and temperament.

Motor Function. Assessment of motor function is adapted to the age of the child. A variety of primitive reflexes are normally present in the infant, and determining their presence or absence is an important component of the neurologic examination. The disappearance of primitive reflexes reflects increasing maturation of the cortex. As myelinization progresses, higher cortical centers become functional and gradually suppress these reflexes. Abnormal findings include the persistence of a primitive reflex significantly beyond the normal time of disappearance or the reappearance of a primitive reflex.

Normal motor development proceeds cephalocaudally and proximodistally. Early in life, movements are more generalized and reflexive. Fine motor control follows development of gross motor control. The infant's extremities are assessed for muscle symmetry, mass, and tone. When examining the young infant, the head is maintained in a midline position to prevent an asymmetric tonic neck reflex. In infants less than 3 months of age, increased flexor tone is normal.[19] The newborn's hands are usually closed; however, they may open and close spontaneously while sleeping or when very quiet. Hands that are always closed after 2 months of age represent an abnormal finding, which is correlated with other neurologic findings to determine its significance.[18] Definite hand dominance is usually not present until the second or third year of life. Hand preference in infants younger than 24 months may indicate weakness or spasticity of the other hand.[20]

Reflexes

Deep Tendon Reflexes. Testing deep tendon reflexes helps to evaluate both the lower motor neurons and the motor and sensory fibers within a particular spinal level. In the older child, deep tendon reflexes are readily tested and graded narratively or by using a stick figure. The most common reflexes examined are the biceps, triceps, brachioradialis, patellar, and Achilles reflex. Hyperreflexia may indicate corticospinal dysfunction or may be a response from an abnormal "spread" of responses, that is, abnormal contraction of muscle groups that usually do not contract when a reflex is being tested.[21] Hyporeflexia may be seen with lower motor unit dysfunction.

In infants, some deep tendon responses are not present at birth and when present are less reliable because of the immaturity of its corticospinal tracts. In general, responses in the infant that require further investigation include reflexes that are very brisk, are asymmetric, or deviate from previous assessments.[19,20] Ankle clonus is often present in the newborn period, but it is rarely sustained and usually disappears by 2 months of age.

Superficial Reflexes. A positive Babinski reflex, that is, dorsiflexion of the foot and fanning of the toes after stroking the sole laterally from heel to toe, is normally present in the infant. This response disappears in the second year of life at approximately 18 to 24 months of age. Persistence or reoccurrence of this response is pathologic, indicative of dysfunction of the corticospinal tracts or the motor area of the cerebrum. Abdominal and cremasteric responses are present at birth. The abdominal response is elicited by stroking the abdomen from a lateral position moving to the umbilicus in all four quadrants. A normal response is slight muscle contraction and movement of the umbilicus toward the stimulus. The cremasteric response is elicited in males by stroking downward on the inner aspects of the upper thigh. The scrotum should contract and elevate. Unilateral absence of the abdominal response and absence or asymmetry of the cremasteric response may indicate corticospinal dysfunction.

Sensory Function. Responses to sensory testing in the infant are more variable and less reliable than in the older child. However, the infant should respond to light stroking of the extremities. With normal sensory function, the infant will usually withdraw the limb being tested. Vibration sense may be tested by placing a tuning fork over bony areas. In response, the infant will usually stop all movement and display a look of surprise. Proprioception cannot be tested at this age. Pain sensation is tested at the end of the examination by nail bed pressure.

In the older child, sensory function can be tested in the usual fashion. For initial screening, light touch and superficial pain are tested in all four extremities. If abnormalities are suspected or detected, more thorough segmental sensory testing is indicated, including temperature, vibration, pres-

sure, and position sensations. Fig. 10-15 is a drawing of segmental sensory innervation of the body.

Cerebellar Function. Cerebellar function of the older child and adolescent can be evaluated in much the same way as in the adult. Rapid alternating movements, as well as finger-to-nose, finger-to-finger, and heel-shin testing, is possible. Maneuvers to evaluate the young child and infant are less precise. Much information can be obtained by observing the young child in play, noting tremors, dysmetria, and truncal swaying. Once again, familiarity with age-dependent motor skills when determining the adequacy in which a child performs a maneuver is important.

Cranial Nerve Function. With the exception of the olfactory nerve, all of the cranial nerves originate in the brainstem. An evaluation of their function provides valuable diagnostic evaluative information about the child's neurologic status. The specific cranial nerves that should be tested and the order in which they are tested depend on the age and condition of the child. A complete cranial nerve assessment is usually not needed for routine screening. Table 10-4 lists the 12 cranial nerves, how they are tested according to age, and the clinical significance of abnormal findings.

Funduscopic Examination. Normally, the funduscopic examination reveals a red reflex that is orange-red and fairly uniform in color, a creamy pink optic disc with an indented center (physiologic depression) and smooth margins, and veins (slightly wider than arteries) that have no light reflex and manifest slight pulsations. Papilledema, represented as blurring of the nasal and upper edges of the optic disc, is commonly seen with increased ICP in the older child. Papilledema is an unusual finding during infancy because the cranial sutures usually spread and the head enlarges in response to chronic increases in ICP. Retinal hemorrhages may be present with significant head injury and subarachnoid hemorrhage (commonly associated with "shaken baby syndrome" in child abuse). Decreased peripheral retinal vascularity is seen in infants with retrolental fibroplasia.

Assessment of the Neurologically Impaired Child

The child with an altered level of arousal requires frequent clinical assessment of neurologic function. Patterns of pathophysiologic responses and their evolution provide valuable information about the location, extent, and progression of neurologic dysfunction. Five assessment parameters are critical to the neurologic evaluation: level of consciousness, motor function, respiratory patterns, cranial nerve response, and vital signs. The neurologic assessment of the child begins with assessment of level of consciousness. Cerebral hemispheric function is determined by assessing motor function. As neurologic dysfunction progresses caudally, characteristic respiratory patterns may occur. In late stages with lower brainstem dysfunction, abnormal cranial nerve responses occur, followed by abnormal vital signs.

Level of Consciousness. Consciousness is described as the state of awareness of self and environment.[17] Level of

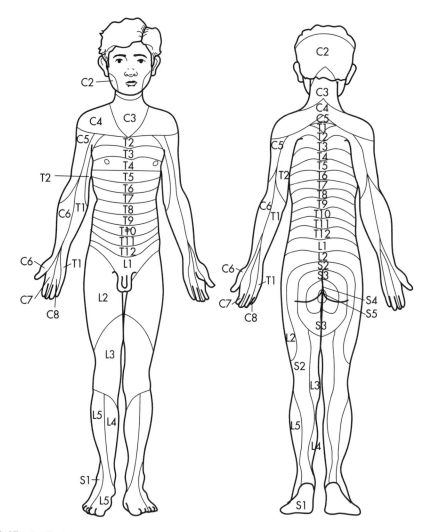

Fig. 10-15 Radicular cutaneous fields. (From Swaiman KF: Neurologic examination of the older child. In Swaiman KF, Ashwal S, eds: *Pediatric neurology: principles and practice,* ed 3, St Louis, 1999, Mosby, pp 14-30.)

◆ TABLE 10-6 Altered States of Consciousness	
Clouding of consciousness	Reduced wakefulness: reduced attention, confused, drowsiness alternating with hyperexcitability
Delirium	Disorientation, fear, irritability, visual hallucinations, agitation; patients may be loud, offensive, and suspicious
Obtundation	Mild to moderate reduction in alertness, reduced interest in environment, increased periods of sleep
Stupor	Unresponsive except to vigorous and repeated stimuli
Coma	No motor or verbal response to environment

Data from Plum F, Posner JB: *The diagnosis of stupor and coma,* ed 3, Philadelphia, 1982, FA Davis.

consciousness is the most important initial assessment and it is fundamental to understanding higher cortical functioning. All neurologic findings must be interpreted based on state of consciousness and awareness. Accurate and consistent assessment of level of consciousness can indicate if the patient's condition is improving, deteriorating, or remaining static. There is a range of altered states of consciousness and a number of ways to label and define these states. Table 10-6 defines commonly used terms to describe various states of consciousness. More important than labels are the patient's actual behaviors and responses.

Numerous coma scales have been developed, most notably the Glasgow coma scale (GCS; Table 10-7). Originally developed as a prognostic tool for patients with head injury, the GCS also helps to identify the depth of coma by standardizing assessments.[22] It allows serial reassessment that reflects the patient's condition at a specific point in time. Despite its widespread application, the GCS has limited use with preverbal infants and intubated patients. As a result, a number of modifications have been developed.

TABLE 10-7   Glasgow Coma Scale

	Score
Eye Opening	
Spontaneous	4
To speech	3
To pain	2
None	1
Best Verbal Response (If Patient Intubated, Give Best Estimate)	
Oriented	5
Confused conversation	4
Inappropriate words	3
Incomprehensible sounds	2
None	1
Best Motor Response (Extremities of Best Side)	
Obeys	6
Localizes	5
Withdraws	4
Abnormal flexion	3
Extends	2
None	1
TOTAL SCORE	

From Jennett B, Bond M: Assessment of outcome after severe brain damage: a practical scale, *Lancet* 1:480-485, 1975. Copyright by The Lancet, Ltd, 1975.

TABLE 10-8   Modified Coma Scale for Infants

	Score
Eye Opening	
Spontaneous	4
To speech	3
To pain	2
None	1
Best Verbal Response	
Coos and babbles	5
Irritable cries	4
Cries to pain	3
Moans to pain	2
None	1
Best Motor Response	
Normal spontaneous movements	6
Withdraws to touch	5
Withdraws to pain	4
Abnormal flexion	3
Abnormal extension	2
None	1
TOTAL SCORE	3-15

From Rogers MC: *Textbook of pediatric intensive care,* Baltimore, 1992, Williams & Wilkins.

Tables 10-8 and 10-9 are examples of coma scales adapted for infants and neonates.

The GCS yields a score of 3 to 15 based on the best response to stimuli in three categories: eye opening, verbal response, and motor response. When using a stimulus to assess level of consciousness, the least noxious stimuli is used first. For example, start with a voice stimulus, then progress to touch; if the patient is still unresponsive, apply a painful stimulus. Care is taken to avoid harming the patient, especially when coagulation factors are abnormal. Nail bed pressure is a reliable stimulus because it can be consistently reproduced by numerous individuals. The exact stimulus that provides a minimal response is documented so that progression of neurologic defects can be easily identified. Careful assessment is necessary to differentiate between appropriate withdrawal to stimuli, which involves cortical activity, and a spinal cord stretch reflex, which does not.

Motor Function. In addition to assessing motor response with the GCS, motor function is also evaluated in terms of symmetry of response and the presence of pathologic signs. Normally, posture is controlled by the interaction between higher inhibiting brain centers and lower exciting brain centers. In the comatose patient, some degree of cortical control over motor function may be lost, allowing primitive postural reflexes to emerge. Spontaneous motor movement may occur in the unconscious patient. Localization represents movement of an extremity across the midline of the body toward the opposite extremity receiving a pain-

TABLE 10-9   Neonatal Arousal Scale

	Score
Best Response to Bell	
Facial and extremity movements	5
Grimaces/blinks	4
Increase in RR/HR	3
Seizures/extensor posturing	2
No response	1
Best Response to Light	
Blink and facial/extremity movements	4
Blink	3
Seizures/extensor posturing	2
No response	1
Best Motor Response	
Spontaneous	6
Periods of activity alternating with sleep	5
Occasional spontaneous movements	
Sternal rub	4
Extremity movements	3
Grimace/facial movements	2
Seizures/extensor posturing	1
No response	
TOTAL SCORE	3-15

From Duncan CC, Ment LR, Smith B et al: A scale for the assessment of neonatal neurologic status, *Child's Brain* 8:299-306, 1981.
RR, Respiratory rate; *HR,* heart rate.

ful stimulus. In the comatose patient, both localization and spontaneous movement are favorable prognostic signs.

When there is severe dysfunction of the cortex and subcortical white matter and preservation of the brainstem, decorticate posturing emerges. Typically, decorticate posturing includes flexion of the upper extremities and extension of the lower extremities. Decerebrate posturing represents dysfunction of the cortex and brainstem at the level of the pons. It is manifested by extension of the upper and lower extremities with rigidity. No motor response to noxious stimuli (bilateral flaccidity) in all four extremities is an ominous sign and is one criterion for brain death determination. Care must be taken to rule out other causes of flaccidity, such as stroke or spinal cord injury. Fig. 10-16 schematically illustrates decorticate and decerebrate posturing.

Respiratory Patterns. Alteration in respiratory pattern is an early and reliable sign of neurologic dysfunction. Breathing is primarily regulated by metabolism in the so-called respiratory centers of the brainstem and by behavior in the forebrain. The presence of two major breathing centers at different levels of the brain sometimes produces characteristic breathing patterns that reflect the location of the neuropathology. Table 10-10 describes the most common pathologic respiratory patterns and their neuropathologic location.[17] Even though the presence of characteristic breathing patterns is well described, overlap in patterns may occur, or patterns may change very rapidly. The most ominous breathing pattern is one that is irregular and slow progressing to apnea (ataxic).

Cranial Nerve Response

Pupil Size and Reactivity. Pupillary size and reactivity are regulated by the autonomic nervous system, an intact afferent connection of CN II and CN III nucleus. Pupillary size changes almost continuously because of the interaction of parasympathetic and sympathetic fibers. Stimulation of parasympathetic fibers causes the pupil to constrict (miosis), and stimulation of sympathetic fibers causes the pupil to dilate (mydriasis). Because the brainstem contains adjacent areas that control both pupillary reactivity

and arousal, testing pupillary response provides valuable information regarding the presence and location of brainstem dysfunction producing coma. Fig. 10-17 illustrates autonomic and cranial nerve control of pupillary response.

Both pupils should first be observed and the exact size noted. The usual range in size varies between 2 and 6 mm. The size of the pupil changes with age, being the smallest during infancy and the largest during adolescence.[23,24] Most

◆ TABLE 10-10 Pathologic Respiratory Patterns and Their Neuropathologic Location

Name	Location	Description
Cheyne-Stokes	Bilateral Hemispheric Diencephalon	Periodic breathing; phases of hyperpnea alternating with apnea
Central neurogenic hyperventilation	Rostral Brainstem Tegmentum	Sustained, rapid, and deep hyperpnea
Apneustic	Mid- or caudal-pontine level	Prolonged inspiration with a pause at full inspiration
Ataxic	Medulla	Irregular pattern; deep and shallow breaths occur randomly

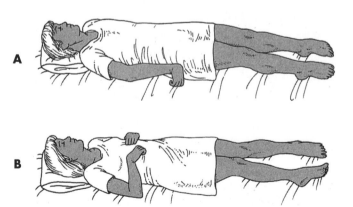

Fig. 10-16 Pathologic posturing occurring in severe brain injury. **A,** Extension posturing (decerebrate rigidity). **B,** Abnormal flexion (decorticate rigidity). (From Betz CL, Hunsberger M, Wright S: *Family-centered nursing care of children,* ed 2, Philadelphia, 1994, WB Saunders, p 1726.)

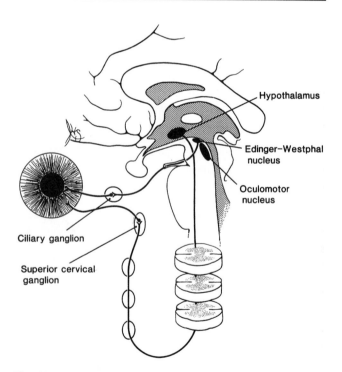

Fig. 10-17 Pupillary responses to light stimulation in differentiating ocular or optic nerve disease from oculomotor nerve dysfunction. (From Vannucci RC, Young RSK: Diagnosis and management of coma in children. In Pellock JM, Myer EC, eds: *Neurological emergencies in infants and children,* Philadelphia, 1984, Harper & Row.)

children have equal-sized pupils, but a 1-mm discrepancy between pupils (anisocoria) may be normal (i.e., for patients with a known discrepancy). Extremely small pupils may indicate opiate effects, pontine hemorrhage, metabolic encephalopathy, or lower brainstem compression. Pupils that are widely dilated and unresponsive result from CN III compression commonly seen with transtentorial herniation or from the midbrain lesion in the area of the Edinger-Westphal nucleus.[23] The acute appearance of this pupillary finding is an ominous and late sign requiring immediate attention. Other common causes of dilated and unreactive pupils include severe hypothermia, anoxia, ischemia, and ingestion of atropine-like substances.

After observing the pupils for size and equality, reactivity to light is tested. To test the pupils' reaction to direct light, use a light with a narrow, bright beam. Test each eye independently by covering or closing one eye while testing the other. Approach the eye from the periphery to avoid constriction of the pupil by accommodation. Once the eye is exposed to the direct light, the pupil should constrict briskly. Document the pupils' response and grade how briskly the pupil constricts using consistent labels or a numerical scale. For example, "both pupils are 3 mm in size and react to light briskly."

Consensual or indirect light response refers to the pupillary constriction that occurs in the eye opposite the eye being stimulated with light. The normal consensual pupillary response represents transmission of light to the brainstem where the Edinger-Westphal nucleus activates the parasympathetic efferent fibers of both pupils.[23] Abnormalities in the direct light response or the consensual response can help determine whether damage has occurred to the optic nerve (CN II) or to the oculomotor nerve (CN III).

Ocular Movements.   Eye movements are controlled by both voluntary cerebral hemispheric centers and involuntary control centers in the brainstem. These areas interact with three paired cranial nerves (III, IV, and VI) that innervate the extraocular muscles that control ocular movement (Fig. 10-18). Normally, the eyes move together synchronously, that is, conjugate eye movements.

Abnormal eye movements include nystagmus, dysconjugate eye movements, and extraocular palsies. Nystagmus refers to a repetitive, involuntary oscillation of one or both eyes. The usual planes of nystagmus are horizontal, vertical, and rotary. Horizontal nystagmus is seen normally with extreme lateral gaze, with the use of certain drugs (e.g., anticonvulsants, barbiturates, alcohol), and sometimes with cerebellar dysfunction.[25,26]

Conjugate eye movement is controlled by several different areas of the brain: frontal gaze center, occipital gaze center, and medial longitudinal fasciculus (MLF). Thus damage to several parts of the brain can cause dysconjugate eye movements.

Extraocular palsies of cranial nerves III, IV, and VI can also cause abnormal eye movements. However, their presence is less precise in identifying a specific area of brainstem dysfunction because they may also result from increased ICP.

Oculocephalic Response (Fig. 10-19, *A*).   In the comatose patient, the integrity of the brainstem can also be assessed by testing the oculocephalic response (doll's eye maneuver). This maneuver determines the integrity of cranial nerves III, VI, and VIII. It can only be performed in the unconscious patient or in an infant younger than 2 months of age.[27] After clearing the cervical spine for injury, the test is performed by briskly turning the head from side to side. With an intact brainstem, the eyes will deviate to the opposite side the head is turned and then slowly turn in the direction the head is rotated.[28] With severe brainstem injury, the patient's eyes remain midpositioned or fixed while the head is turned.

Oculovestibular Response (see Fig. 12-19, *B*).   Like the oculocephalic response, the oculovestibular response (cold calorics) can be used to assess the integrity of the brainstem. This test is performed by first elevating the head of the bed 30 degrees, confirming an intact tympanic membrane and dura, and removing cerumen from the external canal. The reflex is elicited by injecting water (usually 30° C) into the external canal. With an intact brainstem in the unconscious patient, there is slow conjugate

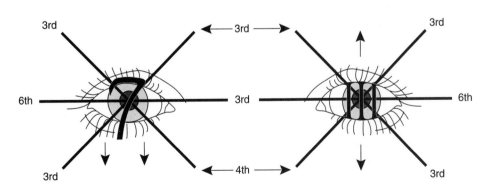

Fig. 10-18   Three paired cranial nerves—III, IV, and VI—control ocular movement. Cranial nerve VII closes the eyelid; cranial nerve III elevates the eyelid. (Modified from Goldberg: *Clinical neuroanatomy made ridiculously simple,* Miami, 1995, MedMaster.)

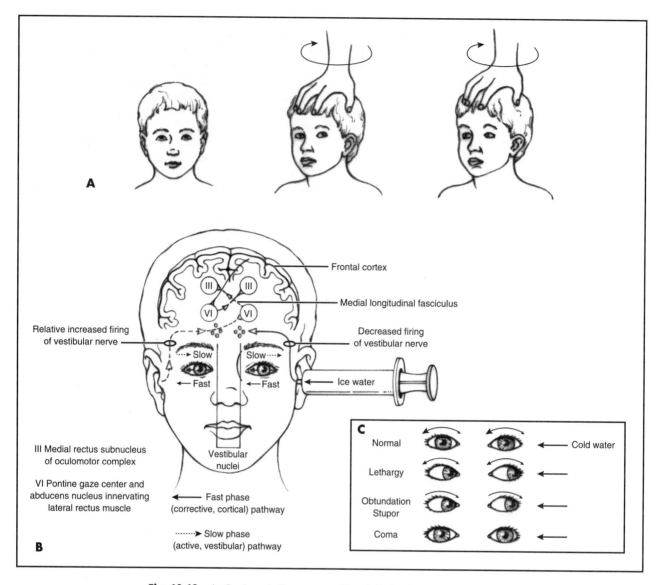

Fig. 10-19   **A,** Oculocephalic response. **B** and **C,** Oculovestibular response.

movement of the eyes toward the stimulus followed by fast return to the midline. A patient with a low brainstem lesion would have eyes that remain at midposition and fixed.

Vital Signs.   Changes in vital signs, indicative of brainstem dysfunction, occur before cardiopulmonary arrest. Cushing's triad includes the classic signs of increased systolic pressure, widened pulse pressure, and bradycardia.

Neurologic Assessment of the Chemically Paralyzed Child

Neuromuscular blocking agents are commonly used as adjunctive therapy in critically ill infants and children. These agents cause skeletal muscle relaxation by altering the response of acetylcholine at the neuromuscular junction.[29] After an appropriate dose of a neuromuscular agent is injected, the onset of effects is rapid. Motor weakness progresses to flaccid paralysis in the following sequence: eyes and fingers; limbs, neck, and trunk; intercostal

muscles; and, finally, the diaphragm. Recovery of muscles occurs in the reverse order. The most common indications for use in children are to (1) improve controlled ventilation, (2) stabilize or maintain ICP, and (3) decrease oxygen consumption.

Despite the advantages of neuromuscular blocking agents, their use precludes most of the neurologic assessment. Because peripheral skeletal muscle paralysis is present, the patient will be unable to respond to commands and is unresponsive to standard tests of motor function, reflexes, and sensation. However, because these agents are unable to cross the blood-brain barrier, consciousness and normal sleep-wake cycles are preserved. These patients are able to hear and feel pain. Consequently, sedatives and analgesics are always administered concurrently. Pupillary reflexes can be tested, and abnormal responses indicate the same clinical significance as in the nonparalyzed patient. Normal oculovestibular and oculocephalic responses are blocked with neuromuscular blocking agents.

Autonomic function is preserved; thus changes in vital signs can be used to assess the patient's responsiveness. An increase in the baseline heart rate may indicate the patient is responding to parents or experiencing pain, anxiety, or a seizure. Pain or anxiety is usually accompanied by a sympathetic response with diaphoresis (sweaty brow). The only clue of a seizure may be an abrupt increase in heart rate and blood pressure. An electroencephalogram (EEG) is used to determine cerebral electrical activity.

If the patient's condition permits, intermittent withdrawal or reversal of the agent allows determination of the neurologic status. Recovery from neuromuscular blockade may be prolonged because of certain physiologic states or concurrent administration with other medications. More precise monitoring of neuromuscular activity, as well as confirmation of patient flaccidity, may be determined by a peripheral nerve stimulator (see Chapter 8).[29]

NEUROLOGIC INTENSIVE CARE MONITORING

Caring for the pediatric patient at risk for neurologic deterioration is uniquely challenging. The collaborative goal is to preserve cerebral functioning. Although clinical examination provides invaluable information, it is often lost in the critically ill child. Bedside neurologic monitoring augments the clinical examination and provides continuous insight into the CNS environment. The following section focuses on major monitoring modalities, presenting general principles, current devices, and essential elements of nursing care.

INTRACRANIAL PRESSURE MONITORING

Only when the ICP is known can therapy to manage cerebral hypertension be rationally directed. ICP monitoring is considered in comatose patients with a known potential for developing intracranial hypertension. ICP monitoring has several clinical benefits. First, it assists in the detection of increasing ICP and compromised CPP before changes seen in the neurologic examination. This is especially true when the neurologic examination is diminished by therapy, such as administration of anesthetics or chemical paralysis. Second, it assists clinical evaluation of intracranial compliance, for example, V/P response testing. Third, ICP monitoring evaluates the effectiveness of therapeutic interventions. Finally, it provides prognostic data of the patient's clinical status.

Knowledge of ICP and CPP allows precise titration of therapy intended to prevent secondary neurologic injury from cerebral ischemia or herniation. Successful control of ICP and CPP after hypoxic-encephalopathic injury does not ensure intact neurologic survival. Sustained late increases in ICP indicate a profound primary neurologic insult.[30] ICP monitoring in this patient population is used more for prognostication than to avert further neurologic injury.[31,32]

Although an ICP greater than 15 indicates reduced adaptive capacity, a normal ICP does not reliably reflect normal intracranial compliance or adequate adaptive capacity. To determine intracranial compliance or identify the patient on the V/P curve, direct or indirect V/P response testing is helpful.

With direct compliance testing, an intensivist injects 0.1 to 1 ml of sterile normal saline without preservative into an intraventricular catheter (IVC) and notes the resultant change in ICP. Although unreliable with enlarged ventricles, the value derived is the ratio of change in ICP to the amount of volume introduced. Miller[33] noted that reduced cerebral adaptive capacity was present when an injection of approximately 7% of the intracranial volume into an IVC caused a increase in the mean ICP of greater than 4 mmHg/ml. Similar information can be obtained by removing CSF. Currently, indirect methods of testing intracranial compliance are more common because of the potential risks of adding volume into a tight intracranial compartment and infection related to opening the system.

Indirect compliance testing involves trending the patient's response to procedures known to increase ICP. All nursing interventions to some extent affect ICP in the patient with reduced adaptive capacity. A significant response is defined as a 10-mmHg increase in ICP lasting more than 3 minutes. The intensivist may also elect to apply unilateral or bilateral internal jugular compression or abdominal pressure to provide a rapidly reversible unquantified volume challenge to the intracranial space.

ICP Monitoring Systems

ICP monitoring has evolved over the last three decades. Pioneered in the 1970s, fluid-coupled systems first became available for patient use.[34] Approximately 10 years later, fiberoptic-tipped catheters were introduced, followed by microsensor-tipped catheters in the 1990s. Depending on the system, a variety of intra- and extracranial locations can be monitored. Although technologic improvements in ICP monitoring have been made, all of the monitoring systems have advantages and disadvantages. The ideal ICP monitoring system is accurate and reliable, free of complications, and inexpensive.

Fluid-coupled systems are similar to traditional hemodynamic monitoring systems but do not contain a slow continuous-infusion device. They have an external straingauge transducer that is coupled to the patient's intracranial space via a fluid-filled line. IVCs have traditionally been the gold standard for ICP monitoring because they are reliable and accurate, relatively inexpensive, and can be recalibrated.

Disadvantages of fluid-coupled systems include obstruction of the catheter tip with tissue or blood and inaccuracies in readings resulting from system problems with fluid-filled tubing (e.g., air bubbles, kinks, and loose connections). In addition, CSF fluid drainage and ICP monitoring cannot occur simultaneously. Furthermore, the external transducer must be maintained at a fixed reference point. Typically, this reference point is institution specific, determined by the preference of the neurosurgical team, that is, at the head (lateral ventricle) or at the heart (right atrium). The lateral ventricle is approximated by positioning the transducer at the level of external auditory meatus or at the top of a triangle formed by the external auditory meatus, the outer canthus of the eye, and behind the hairline. Positioning the transducer at the fourth intercostal space at the midaxillary line approximates the right atrium. Regarding the reference point that is chosen, it must be consistently used, and the monitored data must be used as trend data and not as independent decision points. Consistency in readings can be enhanced if the ICP transducer, when referenced to the head, is attached to the head dressing or secured to an arm board resting on the patient's shoulder. The combination of disadvantages and significant improvements in other ICP monitoring technology has all but eliminated fluid-coupled systems in many centers.

Fiberoptic systems use catheters that are light-sending and light-receiving systems that respond to the movement of a mirror-diaphragm located at the tip. Light is analyzed by a microcomputer and converted to an analog signal that displays the mean ICP. The Camino fiberoptic system (Camino Laboratories, San Diego, Calif.) has been available since the 1980s and is widely used in most institutions. It consists of a disposable 4 Fr catheter with a miniaturized fiberoptic transducer at the tip (Fig. 10-20). The portable Camino monitor interfaces with a conventional monitoring system for waveform display. The Camino catheter can be placed at any number of locations: intraventricular, intraparenchymal, subarachnoid, epidural, or the fontanelle. Unlike fluid-coupled systems, the Camino catheter allows direct intraparenchymal monitoring, providing extremely clear recordings of ICP waveforms.[35]

Like all ICP monitoring systems, advantages and disadvantages exist and vary according to fiberoptic placement. Fiberoptic systems eliminate the need for a fluid path, which typically requires frequent intervention that may place the patient at a higher risk of infection. Because the transducer is located in the tip of the catheter, there is no concern about where to level the transducer. Another advantage is that the fiberoptic catheter slips through the IVC, so CSF can be drained while also obtaining ICP measurements.

Each Camino catheter is calibrated by the manufacturer and is not adjustable. Before insertion, the catheter's zero is matched to the Camino monitor by turning a screw at the hub of the catheter. Anytime afterward, the Camino monitor's zero and calibration are matched to the bedside monitor by depressing the "CAL" button on the Camino monitor and simultaneously adjusting the bedside monitor. Once inserted, the catheter cannot be rezeroed; 24-hour drift is reported as less than 1 mmHg.[36,37]

One disadvantage of fiberoptic catheters is that they require gentle handling, especially during insertion and manipulation. Fiberoptic breakage requires replacement at an increased risk and cost to the patient.[35,38] The rigid catheter cannot be tunneled and stands straight up from the point of insertion, so it must be protected (Fig. 10-21). Another disadvantage is the cost of purchasing an additional monitor. However, the cost may be justified by the other advantages of the system and because the monitor is portable, allowing continuous ICP monitoring during high-risk patient transport.

Catheter-tip strain-gauge catheters were approved for use in the 1990s. The Codman Microsensor ICP system (Codman, Johnson & Johnson, Raynham, Mass.) is an example of this type of monitoring system and consists of a miniature strain-gauge pressure sensor positioned at the tip of a 100-cm flexible nylon tube. Like the fiberoptic-tipped catheter, several locations can be monitored, including subdural, parenchymal (with or without a bolt), and intraventricular. The microsensor transducer is also calibrated before insertion, and unlike fluid-coupled systems, if drift presents, it cannot be corrected. It is used with a pressure monitor that interfaces with a wide variety of patient bedside monitors.

Accuracy and stability of this system have been documented when compared with standard ventricular fluid pressure as measured with an external transducer.[39] One study monitored this system for stability and found maximal drift of 1 mmHg over 9 days.[40] If these results can be replicated, the microsensor offers a distinct advantage over other systems.

Similar to the fiberoptic-tipped catheter, the microsensor transducer can monitor a variety of intracranial locations

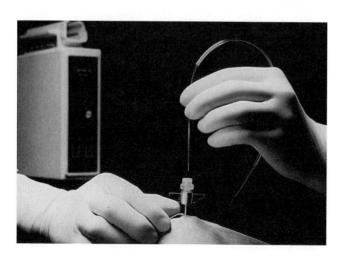

Fig. 10-20 Camino fiberoptic system. (Courtesy Camino Laboratories, San Diego, Calif.)

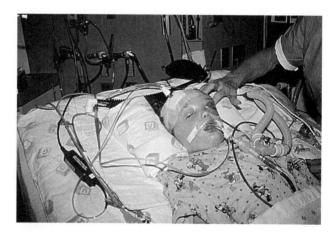

Fig. 10-21 Patient monitoring with a Camino fiberoptic system.

and can drain CSF while monitoring ICP. It also eliminates the need for repeated alignment of the transducer to the patient's head and rezeroing. False readings caused by fluid tubing obstructions are eliminated. One advantage over fiberoptic-tipped catheters is that the microsensor transducer is housed in flexible nylon tubing, which is resistant to costly breakage and allows tunneling under the scalp. Assuming replication studies can confirm the reliability and stability of the microsensor transducer, disadvantages are few. The major concern is cost, especially if institutions have made prior investments in other expensive systems.

Intracranial Catheter Locations.   As stated previously, ICP monitoring systems can be placed in a variety of locations. However, the most accurate and reliable locations for monitoring are the lateral ventricles followed by the parenchyma. Currently, subarachnoid, subdural, and epidural locations are less reliable and are used less often.[41]

An **intraventricular catheter** is a radiopaque catheter placed within a lateral ventricle for purposes of ICP monitoring, CSF drainage and sampling, intrathecal medication administration, and direct compliance testing. The IVC provides high-quality waveforms and is considered the "gold standard" of ICP monitoring unless error is introduced through the measurement system.

While the patient is under local anesthesia, an IVC is inserted through a burr hole on the nondominant side at the intersection of the level of the pupil and external auditory meatus in the area of the coronal suture. The right side is usually chosen until hand dominance can be identified after 3 years of age. During insertion, the head is steadied; the patient will feel pressure and hear the sound of the turning drill. The IVC is inserted into the frontal horn of the lateral ventricle using a stylet. This area is chosen because it has little or no choroid plexus, which may obstruct the IVC, and also avoids penetration of vital brain areas. When the ventricles are compressed or shifted, it may be difficult to place the IVC. However, collapsed ventricles are not considered a contraindication to catheter placement because pressures may be adequately monitored as long as waveforms remain distinct.

Location is verified when CSF is returned. If fluid-coupled or microsensor transducer systems are used, the IVC is tunneled 2 to 3 cm under the scalp and brought out through a separate incision. The separate incision allows the natural defenses of the skin to prevent organisms from gaining access to the CNS. This level of protection is not possible with a Camino IVC. The Camino fiberoptic system is secured directly into the bolt attachment, which is screwed into the skull.

Controlled CSF Venting.   A distinct advantage of IVCs is a reduction of CSF volume accomplished through controlled continuous or intermittent CSF drainage. To avoid ventricular collapse, drainage is accomplished against a positive pressure gradient of at least 15 mmHg. To accomplish this, the intraventricular drainage system drip chamber is placed approximately 27 cm above the reference point of the external auditory meatus. In this position, CSF will automatically drain when the ICP is greater than 20 mmHg. (Because mercury is 13.6 times heavier than

H_2O, 1 mmHg is equal to 1.36 cm H_2O.) Care is taken to avoid the risk of uncontrolled CSF loss with incorrect stopcock position or drainage position.

Intermittent CSF venting follows preset guidelines that include (1) the level of ICP at which to initiate drainage, usually greater than 15 mmHg after nursing measures to decrease ICP are unsuccessful (see Chapter 20); (2) the frequency of drainage, usually every hour; (3) the time interval for drainage, usually 5 minutes; and (4) the maximal amount of CSF, which depends on CSF production and degree of obstruction. Some institutions prescribe CSF drainage at a rate that matches the rate of CSF production. This is approximately 0.35 ml/min or 21 ml/hr in an adolescent and 0.30 ml/min or 18 ml/hr in a young child. A regimen such as this may avoid ventricular collapse with ICP spikes. Drainage also provides a check for IVC patency. Because the amount of drainage reflects the degree of ventricular obstruction, the amount and character of CSF drainage are trended over time. Care is taken to clamp the drainage system before changes in the patient's head position in relation to the drainage device.[42]

Intraparenchymal monitoring is possible with fiberoptic-tipped catheter and microsensor transducer catheter systems. Both systems provide high-fidelity ICP waveforms that are transmitted through brain tissue. Catheter insertion with the Camino fiberoptic catheter is similar to that of a subarachnoid bolt. Once the bolt is placed, the fiberoptic catheter is inserted through the bolt into the brain parenchyma approximately 0.5 to 1 cm beyond the surface of the dura. To prevent kinking or dislocation, the catheter is looped and attached to the head dressing. With the Codman microsensor, two insertion options are available with parenchymal placement: catheter insertion through a subarachnoid bolt or catheter tunneling without a bolt. Intraparenchymal monitoring has replaced fluid-coupled subarachnoid bolts and epidural monitoring in many centers.

Patient Complications.   ICP catheters not only have technical problems but also potential patient-related complications. The two most commonly cited complications are infection and intraparenchymal hemorrhage. Although long-term morbidity and mortality are rare complications of ICP devices, increased costs may be associated with catheter replacement or additional medical treatment.

Infection.   Defining infection associated with ICP devices varies among studies, depending on the methodology. Some studies define infection as a positive CSF culture, whereas other studies use a positive culture of the actual ICP device as their operational definition. Clinically, Mayhall and colleagues[43] found that CSF pleocytosis was more significantly related to the diagnosis of ventriculitis or meningitis than were fever and leukocytosis.

Based on an extensive review of the literature, bacterial colonization of an ICP device was reported as 5% for IVCs, 5% for subarachnoid bolts, 4% for subdural, and 14% for intraparenchymal catheters.[43] Colonization of ICP devices increases significantly after 5 days.[43-45] Even though there is a rising risk of colonization the longer an IVC is in place, Halloway and others found no advantage in prophylactically exchanging catheters for prolonged monitoring (>5 days).[45a]

Despite widely reported colonization of devices, clinically significant infection is rarely associated with ICP monitoring devices.[35,46,47] Furthermore, research does not support using prophylactic antibiotics either systemically, in line, or at the incisional area.[43,48,49]

Hemorrhage and Hematoma. Similar to infection, significant bleeding from ICP monitoring is rare. The incidence of hematoma with all ICP devices is 1.4%. When bleeding does occur, parenchymally placed catheters are the usual cause, with a reported incidence of 1% to 5%.[35,44,47,50,51] Although parenchymal catheters are generally considered safe, alternative monitoring sites are considered in patients with coagulopathies.

ICP Waveform Analysis

ICP waveforms mimic in shape but are of lower amplitude than the arterial waveform (Fig. 10-22). Respiratory fluctuations alter the baseline through transference of

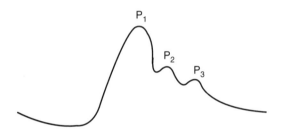

Fig. 10-22 ICP waveforms. (From McQuillan KA: Intracranial pressure monitoring: technical imperatives, *AACN Clin Issues Crit Care Nurs* 2:623-636, 1991.)

pressure through the venous system. Waveform clarity depends on the location of the device and the monitoring system used. Because of narrow intracranial pulse pressures, ICP is monitored in the mean mode. The scale that permits adequate waveform definition, usually 20 to 40 mmHg, is used.

The ICP waveform has three or more descending sawtooth peaks. The first three components are always present. Additional peaks vary and are thought to be caused by retrograde venous pulsations. Their clinical significance has not been established. P_1, the percussion wave, is a sharp, fairly consistent peak generated primarily by the arterial pulsations of the choroid plexus that are modified by the viscoelastic properties of the brain. P_2, the rebound or tidal wave, is variable in shape, ending on the dicrotic notch. P_3, the dicrotic wave, immediately follows the notch, tapering down to the diastolic portion unless retrograde pulsations add a few more peaks.

Waveform changes have been associated with decreased adaptive capacity.[52,53] With cerebral vasodilation, the pulse wave becomes less restrained by the arterioles and is allowed to pass to the compliant capillaries and veins. Signs of decreased adaptive capacity include a P_2 equal to or higher than P_1, followed by an increase in the waveform pulse pressure (Fig. 10-23). If compliance continues to decrease, the diastolic component will elevate, and the waveform will become rounder; then, at higher ICPs, it will assume a triangular shape.[54] Given the predictable, evolving waveform pattern that indicates decreased intracranial compliance,[55] rapid therapeutic interventions and environmental adjustment should be possible. Additional nursing research is necessary to confirm this.

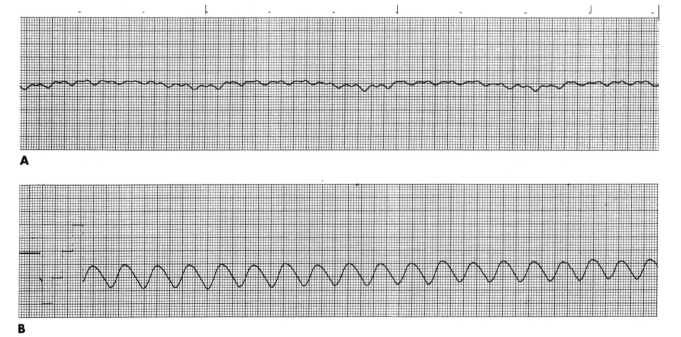

Fig. 10-23 Signs of decreased adaptive capacity include a P_2 equal to or higher than P_1, followed by an increase in the waveform pulse pressure. Two-year, 9-month toddler with decreased cerebral compliance. Note waveform change from **A** to **B**. (Courtesy MAQ Curley.)

ICP Trend Recordings

In addition to continuous ICP waveform assessment, trend recordings (25 mm/min) allow detection of baseline elevations over time. They can also correlate ICP with therapeutic interventions. Last, they can identify Lundberg A, B, and C waves (Fig. 10-24), which are not true waves but are graphically displayed ICP waveforms that are trended over minutes or hours.

A waves or plateau waves are spontaneous, rapid, irregular increases in ICP 50 to 100 mmHg over baseline lasting 5 to 20 minutes per wave, followed by a rapid decrease in ICP. A waves progress through four phases generated by a complex interaction between systemic arterial pressure, intracranial compliance, and cerebrovascular autoregulation.[56] The A wave begins with the *drift phase,* which is characterized by a progressive decrease in MAP. The *plateau phase* follows as hypotension decreases the CPP, stimulating autoregulatory cerebral vasodilation and resulting in an increase in cerebral blood volume and ICP. The *ischemic phase* ensues when progressive cerebral hypertension produces brainstem ischemia and activates the Cushing's response to increase both MAP then CPP. The *resolution phase* terminates the A wave when cerebral perfusion improves, decreasing cerebral vasodilation, cerebral blood volume, and ICP. In summary,

plateau waves are observed in patients with preserved cerebral autoregulation but reduced pressure-volume compensatory reserve.[57]

A waves are clinically significant, reliably signaling reduced intracranial compliance. The more square the shape of the wave, the greater the reduction in intracranial compliance. *A* waves are associated with impaired CBF. Patients with cerebral hypertension die of diminished cerebral perfusion during plateau waves. A waves may be accompanied by transient neurologic deficits, for example, pupil dilation, headache, and vegetative responses, which include sweating, flushing, and bradycardia.

B waves are sharp rhythmic increases in ICP to 50 mmHg lasting 30 seconds to 2 minutes. B waves may precede A waves, indicating a progressive loss of cerebral compliance. B waves may occur before a seizure; during headache, posturing, or isometric movement; or accompany respiratory compromise and decreased level of consciousness.

C waves are normal rhythmic ICP fluctuations associated with respirations. They are considered benign but may indicate an increase in venous pressure or a decrease in venous outflow.

Monitoring ICP trends allows a proactive management of cerebral hypertension. Anticipating care by using an individualized protocol to decrease ICP may prevent secondary neuronal injury. Pressure waves greater than 20 mmHg and lasting for more than a few minutes, especially if associated with a change in neurologic status or the inability to maintain CPP greater than 50 mmHg or ICP less than 15 mmHg, require *immediate* intervention. Occult seizure activity should be considered a potential problem when increased ICP is unresponsive to standard management.

Nursing Implications

Priorities for nursing care of patients who require ICP monitoring include (1) keeping the ICP monitoring system intact and operational, (2) ensuring the accuracy of the data, and (3) limiting iatrogenic injury. Both ICP and CPP are constantly assessed throughout any intervention to evaluate the patient's response to therapy. Trends in patient tolerance of care are noted over time.

The accuracy of data obtained from ICP monitoring is assessed from waveform analysis. Good-quality tracings correspond with good measurements, unless the transducer is leveled inaccurately when using fluid-coupled systems. As with hemodynamic monitoring transducers, 1 inch out of position will produce a 2-mmHg deviation in measurement, higher readings with the transducer too low, or lower readings with the transducer is too high. ICP measurements should always correlate with the neurologic examination and reflect clinical interventions.

Because the cranium is compartmentalized, Weaver, Winn, and Jane[58] found significant differences in ICP measurements (using a fluid-coupled subarachnoid bolt) between the ipsilateral and contralateral side of a focal supratentorial lesion. They recommend that supratentorial subarachnoid pressure be measured ipsilateral to the site of the focal lesion. Pressure increases in nonpathogenic

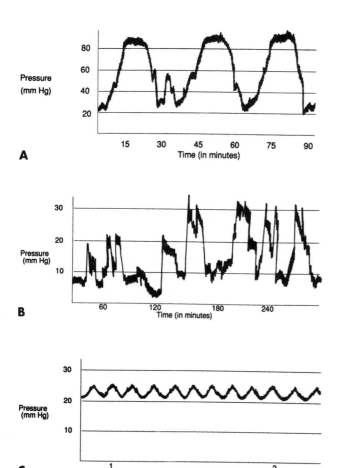

Fig. 10-24 A to **C,** Lundberg A, B, and C waves (From McQuillan KA: Intracranial pressure monitoring: technical imperatives, *AACN Clin Issues Crit Care Nurs* 2:623-636, 1991.)

compartments occur only after herniation. Note that with the fiberoptic system, intraparenchymal pressures more accurately reflect ipsilateral and contralateral pressures.[59] IVCs and bolts measure supratentorial pressure. Patients with a posterior fossa mass or infratentorial lesion must be observed carefully for the development of respiratory and cardiovascular distress even when normal or low supratentorial ICP is present.

When calculating CPP, controversy exists over where it is best to reference fluid-coupled transducers. The basis of the controversy is that two different reference points are created when the head of the bed is elevated in a patient with a ventriculostomy referenced at the lateral ventricle and arterial line referenced at the right atrium. In this scenario, ICP may be underestimated, and CPP may be overestimated. Some try to remedy this problem by referencing both transducers at either the head or the heart. Whichever method is used, it is imperative that it be used consistently to allow CPP trending over time.

Currently, there is lack of nursing research to guide clinical practice in the care of patients with ICP devices. Protocols usually reflect central line protocols. It seems reasonable that ICP devices function under different principles because they exist within a system protected by the blood-brain barrier. This natural barrier limits high antibiotic and immunoglobulin concentration, so theoretically, risk of infection may be increased.

Until nursing research is available, some recommendations can be made. Site care includes use of an occlusive dry sterile dressing. Dressings are changed every 72 hours to inspect the insertion site for signs and symptoms of infection and CSF leakage.

Even though fluid-coupled ICP monitoring is being used less often, infection control practices must be enforced. Currently, no data suggest that ICP monitor tubing should be changed with the same frequency as arterial and venous pressure lines.[60] Strict aseptic technique is used whenever the system is opened. Before insertion, the monitoring system is prepared in a nontraveled area while masks and gloves are worn. All systems should be maintained as closed systems and left intact unless contaminated.

MONITORING CEREBRAL FUNCTION

Neurophysiologic studies are an important component of the diagnostic evaluation in the infant and child with suspected neurologic dysfunction. Although ICP monitoring provides information about the neurologic environment, EEG and evoked potential monitoring provide information about actual neurologic functioning. The goal of continuous neurologic monitoring is to detect a decline in a patient's condition before physical signs and symptoms present. This approach is particularly critical in patients in which the physical examination has been eliminated; for example, chemically induced paralysis to control ventilation.

Continuous EEG Monitoring

Continuous bedside EEG monitoring provides information about the spontaneous electrical activity produced by the outer 20% or 6-mm surface of cerebral cortex located near the electrodes. The EEG does not provide information on white matter or brainstem function. It is useful for detecting status epilepticus, nonconvulsive seizures, metabolic disorders, intracerebral tumors, and coma. It is also used to monitor patients who may experience a decline in CBF or other ischemic events.

EEG monitoring is used most often in the pediatric intensive care unit (PICU) for identification of seizure activity (Fig. 10-25, *A*). Undetected and untreated seizure activity can result in neuronal death.[61] Continuous EEG monitoring is also essential when managing therapeutic barbiturate coma.[62,63] Barbiturate coma is used to suppress CMR and requirements. The goal of barbiturate coma is burst suppression—electrical activity progressing to an isoelectric line, then resumption of electrical activity (see Fig. 10-25, *B*). Length of burst suppression depends on drug levels; the higher the level, the longer the isoelectric line. When barbiturate coma is used to manage intractable seizures, abnormal cerebral electrical activity is suppressed completely to permit the return of normal activity.[64] If inadequate barbiturate doses are used, the therapeutic benefit may not be realized; whereas if excessive doses are used, cardiovascular instability may result.

EEG monitoring also permits indirect visualization of the effects of compromised CBF associated with significant episodes of cerebral hypertension. When CBF is compromised, normal EEG rhythms are reduced in both amplitude and frequency.[65] An isoelectric EEG results when CBF is less than 12 to 15 ml/100 g/min (see Fig. 12-25, *C*).[66]

EEGs also provide a prognostic tool to predict return of cognitive function after an hypoxic-ischemic injury. Poor neurologic outcomes have been correlated with slower frequencies, amplitude suppression, and a static EEG frequency spectrum over time.[67] In the absence of barbiturates, burst suppression is an ominous finding after a major hypoxic-ischemic injury to the brain.[68] Although not absolute in drug overdose or hypothermia, cerebral silence (as evidenced by an isoelectric EEG) has been used as a criterion for confirming brain death. EEG activity may persist in some patients with cortical necrosis; survival is possible because EEGs do not assess brainstem activity.

Waveform Analysis. EEG waveforms are described in terms of frequency, amplitude, velocity, distribution, regularity, and specific pattern (Table 10-11). The EEG traditionally records voltage over time from 16 channels. Waveform frequency is described in hertz (Hz) or cycles per second. Waveform amplitude, measured from peak to peak, is described in microvolts (μV). Waveform velocity describes the rate of climb and descent of waves; for example, a spike has a duration less than 80 milliseconds (ms), whereas a sharp wave has a longer duration.

As noted in Table 10-11, waveforms correlate with level of consciousness and range from high frequency–low amplitude to low frequency–high amplitude. Background alpha activity is regulated by brainstem neurons known as "pacemaker" cells. Right and left hemispheric symmetry is analyzed by assessing lead pairs clustered down the EEG page.

EEG interpretation is complex, especially in the pediatric

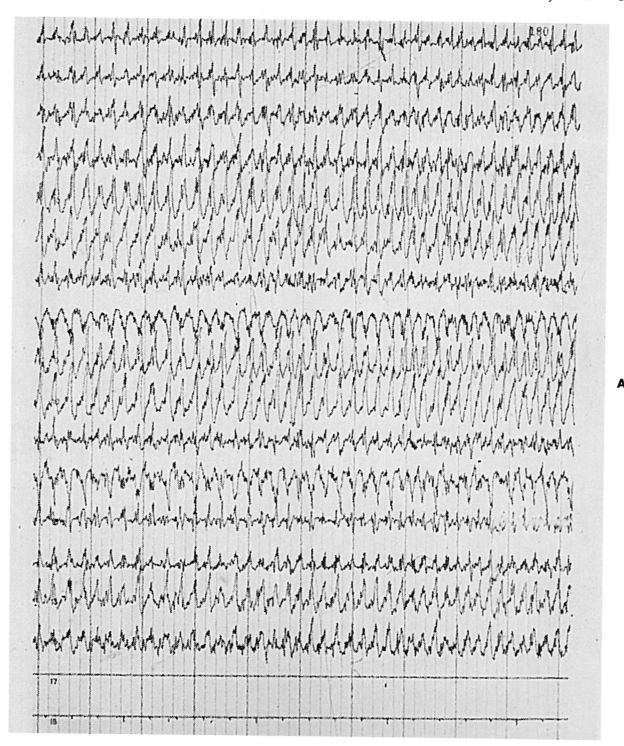

Fig. 10-25 **A,** Seizure activity. (Courtesy MAQ Curley.)   *Continued*

population, where individual maturational factors complicate EEG interpretation. For example, in the newborn, cortical activity is irregular in frequency and incidence. Asymmetry and asynchrony may be normal throughout infancy. Alpha rhythms are slow to develop and may not reach adult range until 10 to 12 years of age.[66]

Seizure activity begins with a change in background activity, followed by generalized low-voltage fast activity, which increases in amplitude and slows in frequency. This pattern progresses to generalized polyspikes and wave patterns from 1 to 4 Hz.[69] Different seizure classes generate specific spike and wave patterns. As expected, focal seizures are asymmetric. Focal seizures with secondary generalization can be identified and tracked on the EEG. Postictal activity can be identified as diffuse depression of background activity.

EEG analysis depends on pattern recognition placed in the context of the patient's changing clinical picture.

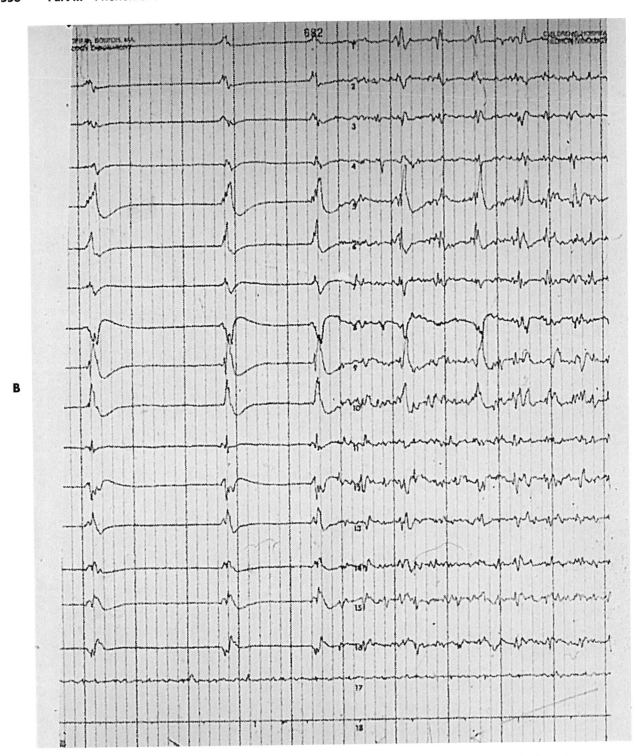

Fig. 10-25, cont'd **B,** Burst suppression: electrical activity progressing to an isoelectric line, then resumption of electrical activity. (Courtesy MAQ Curley.)

Continued

Accurate interpretation requires years of experience and analysis of enormous amounts of data.

Two-lead bipolar (pairs) systems can screen for seizure activity (Fig. 10-26). These single-channel systems use five electrodes: two placed over each mastoid process, two placed over each temporal area, and one ground electrode placed over the middle of the forehead. Esposito and Westgate[70] describe using the Siemens EEG cassette in a

PICU setting. This system reflects EEG activity only within close proximity of the electrode pairs, one set at a time.

Computerized EEG Recordings. Computerized EEG (CEEG) recordings are useful for continuous monitoring in the critical care setting. They facilitate recognition of neurologic alterations before the development of clinical signs. A variety of CEEG devices and monitoring techniques are available in graphic form for use at

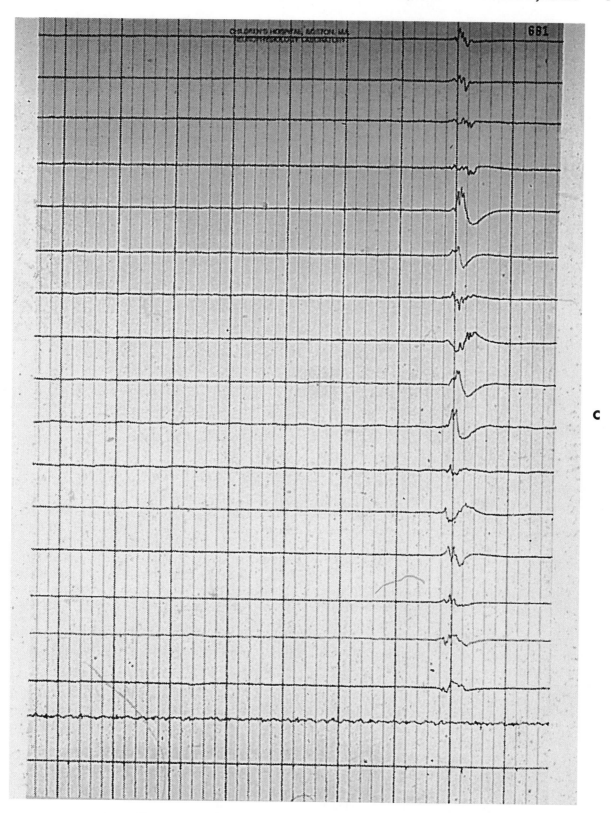

Fig. 10-25, cont'd C, Isoelectric EEG. (Courtesy MAQ Curley.)

the bedside. The common feature among them is their ability to compress hours of data into useful graphics.[71] Used only as a trending device, processed EEG recordings do not replace the need for periodic 16-channel EEG assessment.

First-generation processed EEG monitors include the *Cerebral Function Monitor* (CFM; Criticon Inc., Tampa, Fla.). This system is a single-channel, single-lead bipolar trend recording of EEG amplitude and variability. Three electrodes are used: one placed over each parietal area and

TABLE 10-11 EEG Waveforms

Rhythm	Frequency (Cycle/sec)	Amplitude (Peak-Peak)	Area	State	Waveform
Beta	13-30Hz	10-20 μV Intermittent	Frontal and central	Awake Eyes open	
Alpha	8-13Hz	Infant: 20 μV Child: 75 μV Adult: 50 μV	Dominant rhythm of occipital and parietal	Awake Eyes closed	
Theta	4-7Hz	Child: 50 μV Adult: 10 μV	Temporal or central area in children to age 3	Drowsiness Encephalopathies	
Delta	1-4Hz	100 μV	Frontal	4th-stage sleep–coma Structural lesions Normal in young children	

one ground electrode placed over the frontal area. The lower printout records amplitude: 0 to 10 μV, then 10 to 100 μV. The upper printout records frequency: top, 0 Hz, and bottom, 16 Hz. The paper speed condenses about 2 minutes of EEG activity into a 1-cm tracing. Two characteristics are assessed: the overall amplitude, reflecting the average of cortical activity, and the width, reflecting the degree of variability in cortical activity. High, wide tracings indicate high EEG voltages with considerable variability in peak-peak amplitude. Conversely, a low, narrow tracing results from low voltage with little variability in amplitude. The limitation of this system is that it cannot assess regional activity because only two leads are used.

The CFM is helpful in the PICU to assess EEG trends and identify classic EEG patterns.[72] For example, episodic high-voltage activity suggests the presence of seizure activity. Progressive increase in EEG amplitude correlates with improved neurologic outcome following a hypoxic-ischemic event; the opposite is associated with a poor neurologic outcome. Presence of EEG activity during periods of increased ICP suggests that adequate CPP is maintained.[65] Finally, a "comb" pattern indicates burst suppression.[73]

Another first-generation processed EEG recorder is *compressed spectral array* (CSA). Here, raw EEG data are rearranged from voltages versus time to amplitude versus frequency during a sampling period (Fig. 10-27). Frequency is on the horizontal axis with delta waves on the left and beta waves on the right. The power spectrum is then plotted and stacked vertically into a three-dimensional representation for trend analysis.

Because CSA compresses a significant amount of data, critical events may be smoothed together, including, for example, burst suppression and seizure activity. Like the CFM, CSA is helpful in the assessment of EEG trends and identification of classic patterns. CSA is particularly helpful

in the prediction of outcome from coma. A fluctuating frequency spectrum carries a more favorable prognosis than an invariable type.[74]

Aperiodic analysis, *Lifescan* (Neurometrics, Inc., San Diego, Calif.), is considered a second-generation processed EEG recorder. Aperiodic analysis assesses each wave vector and displays it in a three-dimensional glass box. Two sets of leads are used; the negative electrode is placed behind the ears; the positive electrode, in the frontal area; and ground electrode, in the center of the forehead. Frequency bands are positioned from left to right: 0.5 Hz to the left and 30 Hz to the right. To enhance visualization, waves are color coded; beta waves are yellow, alpha waves are green, subalpha are magenta, theta are light blue, and delta waves are dark blue. Waveform amplitude is approximated by vector height. Time is expressed on the diagonal. The activity edge, a white line on the top of the each box, trends changes in both frequency and amplitude over time (Fig. 10-28).

The acronym SAFE can be used to systematically assess the Lifescan recording. *S* represents symmetry between the left and right cerebral hemispheres, *A* represents vector amplitude, *F* represents vector frequency, and *E* represents activity edge. Vector height should vary over time and from one frequency to another. Vector distribution should also vary over time. The activity edge should reflect symmetry between the left and right hemisphere and vary symmetrically over time.

Narcotics produce a gradual shift of the activity edge to the left, reflecting an increase in delta activity. Cerebral ischemia also produces a left shift of the activity edge, with a reduction in amplitude at all frequencies. Unilateral ischemia produces an asymmetric shift to the left, whereas bilateral ischemia produces a symmetric shift to the left. Burst suppression decreases alpha/beta activity and

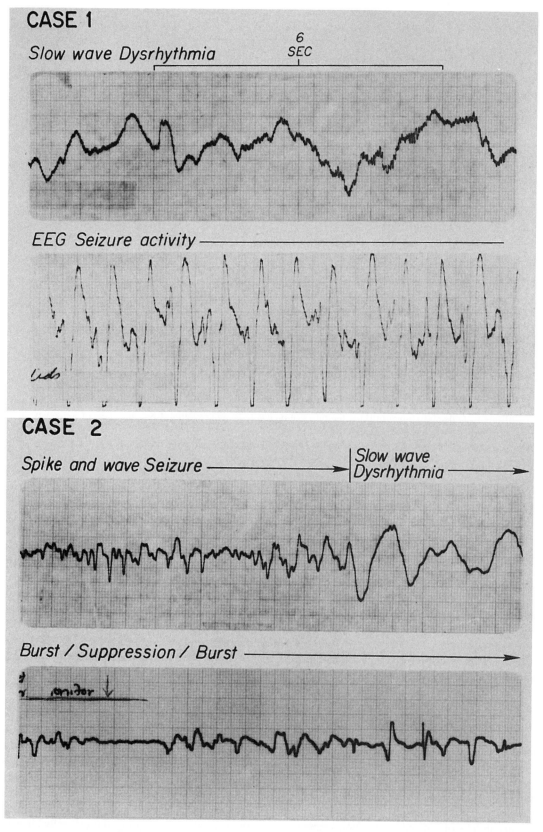

Fig. 10-26   Two-lead bipolar (pairs) systems. (From Esposito N, Westgate P: Continuous EEG monitoring in the PICU, *J Pediatr Nurs* 2:272-277, 1987.)

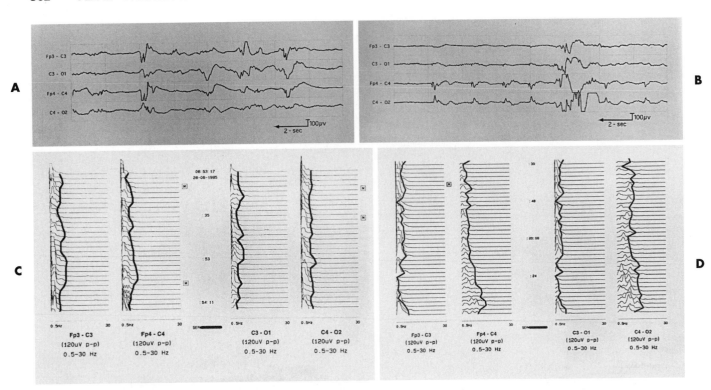

Fig. 10-27 **A** to **D,** Cerebral function monitor. **C,** Compressed spectral array (CSA) of raw EEG display shown in **A.** CSA represents a 2-second update rate with a frequency band of 0.5 to 30 Hz. **D** presents CSA of raw EEG display shown in **B.** At the onset of an electrographic seizure, CSA increases in frequency as the spike and wave activity occurs.

increases delta/theta activity. The activity edge shifts far to the left and then back to the right. Alterations in temperature produce high or low activity at all levels; the edge shifts bilaterally to the right or left.

Evoked Potential Monitoring

Evoked potential (EP) monitoring provides a computerized summation of the electrical potentials produced by specific neural pathways in response to an external stimulus. EP monitoring is useful because the nerve pathways tested are less sensitive to drug effects. In addition, the waveforms correlate to the anatomy of the sensory tracts. EP monitoring offers the possibility of assessing structures not seen with EEG (Fig. 10-29).

Each EP is a series of waves plotted as voltage versus time. The amplitude (voltage) and latencies (time) reflect conduction and processing of sensory information through the CNS. The EP is assessed for changes in the presence and absence of waves, individual latencies, interwave latencies, and relative amplitudes. Again, maturational factors are important because development affects interwave latencies in children less than 2 years of age.[75]

Loss of transmission or slowed conduction (increased latency) indicates functional injury related to cerebral hypoxia, compression, or other factors that affect cerebral metabolism. Decreased amplitudes are related to decreased CBF. Loss of transmission after a particular wave identifies the specific level of dysfunction (Table 10-12).

The three EP modes are visual, somatosensory, and auditory. Multimodal EPs (MEPs) assess several different tracts to provide specific information regarding various components of the CNS.

Generated by a flashing light, **visual evoked potentials** (VEPs) assess the integrity of the retinal-occipital pathway. York and associates[76] found that increases in ICP secondary to either cerebral edema or hydrocephalus produced characteristic alteration in VEPs (increased latency of wave N_2) through compression of intercerebral visual pathways. The relationship establishes a reliable noninvasive method of estimating ICP.[77]

Somatosensory evoked potentials (SEPs) assess the integrity of the sensory pathways from the peripheral nerve to the sensory cortex from either the median nerve in the wrist or the posterior tibial nerve in the ankle to the cerebral hemispheres. SEP is useful in identifying the level of spinal cord injury. An absent waveform below the region of spinal injury indicates a complete injury, whereas the presence of the wave indicates an incomplete lesion. Presence or return of SEPs often precedes clinical improvement and offers a favorable prognosis.

Brainstem auditory evoked responses (BAERs) are often used in monitoring the critically ill patient. BAERs measure the change in EP in the auditory pathways to the brainstem in response to a noise (click). Electrodes are placed on top of the head and in the external auditory meatus. After ensuring patency of the auditory canal and an intact tympanic membrane, repeated clicks are delivered

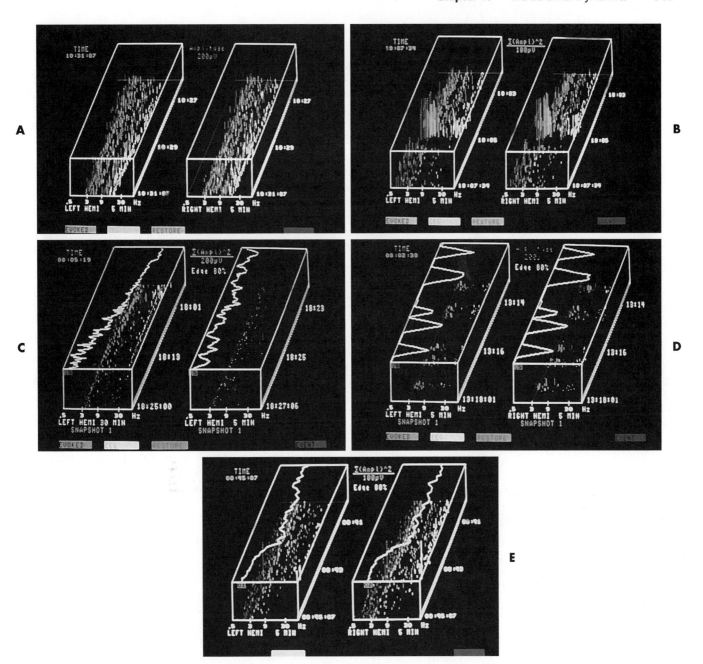

Fig. 10-28 Lifescan Brain Activity Monitor. **A,** Normal display. **B,** Seizure activity. **C,** Barbiturate coma. **D,** Burst suppression. **E,** Bilateral ischemic event. (Courtesy Diatek Neurometrics, San Diego, Calif.)

through an earpiece at about 10 Hz while "white noise" masks stimulation to the other ear. Click intensity is increased about 60 decibels above minimal hearing threshold. The signal is amplified 50,000 times, and averaging is performed over a 10-ms sweep after each click. Usually, over 2000 clicks are averaged.

The time measured from peak to peak, known as the interpeak latency, is unaffected by changes in the intensity of the stimulus and peripheral hearing apparatus. Normal BAERs suggest the absence of lesions when toxic or metabolic comas or a diffuse cortical process is present. BAERs are unaffected by barbiturates, so they are useful to monitor brainstem integrity during therapeutic coma. If

BAERs are normal in the comatose patient, nursing care can be planned to provide appropriate auditory stimulation. Decreasing amplitude or increased latency of wave V indicates brainstem compression secondary to increased ICP. Loss of wave V indicates severe brainstem dysfunction and suggests central herniation. In brain death, BAERs are not conducted past wave I. Brain death may also include wave I, but the integrity of the peripheral auditory apparatus cannot be validated.

MEPs combine the use of several EPs for localization of defects and prognostic evaluation.[78] With brainstem dysfunction, SEPs and BAERs are abnormal, whereas VEPs are normal. With hemispheric dysfunction, VEPs and BAER

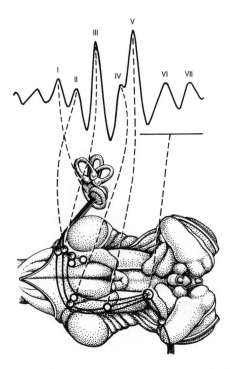

Fig. 10-29 Brainstem auditory evoked potentials (BAEPs). Neural generations of the BAEPs. It is most likely that each wave has components arising from different generators that include brainstem nuclei and white matter tracts. *I* to *VII*, waveforms. (From Wiznitzer M: In Blumer JL, ed: *A practical guide to pediatric intensive care,* St Louis, 1990, Mosby.)

Wave	Location	Level of Pathway
I	Acoustic nerve (CN VIII)	Peripheral receptor
II	Cochlear nuclei	Medulla
III	Superior olivary complex	Pons
IV	Lateral lemniscus	Mid to upper pons
V	Inferior colliculus	Midbrain
VI	Medial geniculate	Thalamus
VII	Auditory radiations	Thalamocortical

◆ **TABLE 10-12 Brainstem Auditory Evoked Potentials**

and SEP *cortical* EPs are abnormal, but BAER and SEP *subcortical* EPs are normal (Fig. 10-30). If all EPs are dysfunctional, global dysfunction is probably present.

As a prognostic indicator in coma, 80% of patients with mild abnormalities in MEP awaken within 30 days, and 90% of patients with mild EP abnormalities at 14 days make a good neurologic recovery.[65] Goodwin, Friedman, and Bellefleur[79] studied BAERs and SEPs in 41 children ranging in age from 6 weeks to 18 years. When assessing survivor outcome, determined both at discharge and by follow-up examination conducted 1 to 3 years later, no false pessimistic predictions had been made, and only two were falsely optimistic.

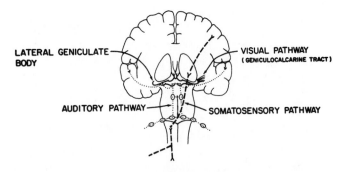

Fig. 10-30 Schematic view of sensory pathways involved in the generation of multimodality evoked potentials. Sensory input generating somatosensory and auditory evoked potentials traverses more caudal regions of the brainstem than does sensory input for visual evoked potentials. (From *J Neurosurg,* vol 56, Jan 1982.)

EP limitations are present when ocular, auditory, or peripheral nerve disease is present. Also, EPs test only specific nerve tracts. The frontal lobes, cerebellum, and cognitive function are not tested.

Computerized processing of multilead EEG and EP allows total *brain mapping.* Moment-to-moment variations in the brain's spontaneous or evoked electrical activity are displayed on a computer monitor in the form of multicolored maps. Different colors and color shades are used to indicate the magnitude of positive and negative EEG voltages simultaneously measured from various scalp locations. Mapping techniques can be useful in identifying functional abnormalities not distinguished by anatomic or metabolic studies.

NEURODIAGNOSTIC STUDIES

Under nonemergent circumstances, patient and family preparation precedes *all* procedures. Nursing responsibility includes augmenting the primary information provided by the attending physician. Specific concerns that are often addressed by nurses include how the procedure is performed, what the expectations of the patient will be during the procedure, what the patient will experience during the procedure, the anticipated response of the patient to the procedure, and how the parents might help the patient through the procedure.

A **lumbar puncture** involves the insertion of a spinal needle into the subarachnoid space for the purposes of measuring spinal fluid pressure and obtaining CSF for laboratory analysis (see Table 10-2 for normal CSF characteristics). During the procedure, the nurse continuously monitors the patient while helping the patient maintain a side-lying position with hips and neck flexed. Under local anesthesia, the spinal needle is inserted into the L3-4 or L4-5 vertebral interspace. A manometer is used to measure opening and closing spinal pressures. CSF samples are collected in tubes to allow visualization and laboratory analysis. Usually, CSF cell count and Gram stain are obtained first, followed by CSF chemistries and then CSF culture.

A lumbar puncture should not be performed in patients at high risk for bleeding or in those with increased ICP. In patients with increased ICP, withdrawing CSF from the spinal compartment may create a significant pressure differential between the cerebral and spinal compartments. This disequilibrium results in further compression and herniation of thalamus and midbrain through the tentorial notch and may eventually cause infarction of these structures. Consequently, the fundi are checked for papilledema before performing a lumbar puncture.[63]

CBF measurements are very important when monitoring the balance between cerebral oxygen supply and demand, especially when autoregulation is lost. Modifications of the Fick principle (the uptake of a substance by an organ is equal to the amount of the substance that enters it minus the amount that leaves it) can be used to approximate the CMR. Cross-brain concentration gradients of glucose (CMR/glu), lactate (CMRL), and oxygen ($CMRO_2$) have been used. For example, the $CMRO_2$ is equal to the CBF multiplied by the difference between the cerebral arterial and venous oxygen difference ($avDo_2$).

Normally, CBF matches the $CMRO_2$. When autoregulation is intact, changes in the $CMRO_2$ will be matched by reciprocal changes in CBF, and cerebral $avDo_2$ will remain constant. The $CMRO_2$ and CBF are often modulated by alterations in temperature, seizure activity, and certain medications—for example, narcotics, sedatives, and analgesics. When autoregulation is lost, changes in $CMRO_2$ do not produce reciprocal alterations in CBF, and the $avDo_2$ can serve as an indicator of the adequacy of CBF.[80]

Although cerebral arterial blood can be sampled from any artery, cerebral venous blood should not be contaminated by extracerebral blood. To accomplish this, Goetting and Preston[81] described a method of percutaneous cannulation of the jugular venous bulb by retrograde advancement of a catheter placed into the jugular vein (Fig. 10-31).

Oximetric catheters placed in the jugular venous bulb have been used to continuously monitor cerebral venous saturation. The ratio of $CMRO_2$ to CBF can be expressed as the cerebral extraction of oxygen (CEO_2), which is the difference between arterial saturation (Sao_2) and jugular bulb saturation (Sjo_2).[80,82] The CEO_2 can serve as a continuous trend monitor of cerebral oxygen supply and demand. Increased CEO_2 indicates either decreased extraction or increased delivery. Decreased CEO_2 indicates either increased extraction or decreased delivery.

Similar to pulse oximetry, cerebral oxygen saturation can be noninvasively evaluated with **near infrared spectroscopy** (NIRS) examination of cytochrome *c* oxidase and hemoglobin (INVOS 3100; Somanetics, Troy, NY).[83] Infrared light (650-1100 nm) can penetrate extracerebral tissue and return with valuable information about the attenuation of that light. Intracerebral cells capable of attenuating light include oxyhemoglobin, deoxyhemoglobin, and oxidized cytochrome *c* oxidase, all of which are important in oxygen delivery.

Inhalation or injection of xenon-133, a radioisotope, is also used to assess CBF. [133]Xe study is based on the principle that the rate of uptake of an inert diffusible gas is

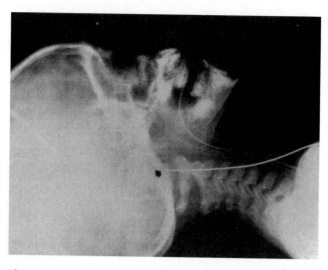

Fig. 10-31 Jugular venous bulb SVo_2 monitoring. Skull x-ray demonstrating proper catheter tip position. Arrow indicates jugular bulb (From Goetting MG, Preston G: Jugular bulb catheterization: experience with 123 patients, *Crit Care Med*, 18:1220-1223, 1990. Copyright by Williams & Wilkins, 1990.)

dependent on blood flow.[68] This study can be accomplished rapidly and provides useful information when cerebral hypoperfusion associated with stroke, massive cerebral hypertension, or brain death is suspected.

Cranial ultrasound uses sound waves to identify cranial structures of different densities. In infants with open fontanelles, serial cranial ultrasound can assist in accurate identification of the ventricular system and is helpful in the rapid identification and management of intraventricular hemorrhage. Ultrasound technology has also been used to monitor CBF by **Doppler ultrasonography.**[84] The velocity of CBF is measured by sound waves reflecting back from moving red blood cells through the anterior cerebral artery. After closure of the anterior fontanel, the circle of Willis is insonated via the temporal bones. Direction of flow can also be identified with color imaging. Although an isolated number is of little significance, serial numbers are valuable in trending the course of a patient.

Skull and spine x-rays are the most common radiologic tests performed on the neurologic system. A variety of skull and spine views are selected to identify fractures, abnormal calcification, and tissue densities. Suture lines may appear widened in the patient with cerebral hypertension. In the multiple-trauma patient, spinal cord immobilization is essential until spinal x-rays are read as negative by a radiologist.

Computed tomography (CT) and **magnetic resonance imaging** (MRI) have revolutionized neurodiagnostic imaging. These noninvasive studies provide clear visualization of neuroanatomy. CT differentiates tissues by x-ray density. Areas of low density (air) appear dark, and areas of high density (bone) appear white. CT with contrast is used to enhance visualization of blood vessels, well-vascularized lesions, and localized alteration in the blood-brain barrier. The use of contrast media is contraindicated in patients with acute renal failure and in those with a positive history of allergy to contrast media. CT scan uses about the same amount of radiation as a standard skull series.

The MRI image is formed by the tissue-specific realignment of protons when short radio frequencies are applied from a strong external magnetic field to move them out of uniform alignment. When moved, the atoms resonate and emit signals based on nuclear density and realignment time. The signals are tracked on an image revealed on a high-resolution screen.

CT scans are selected when global neuroanatomic information is needed, for example, ventricular size, shift, and distortion of brain tissue in the patient with cerebral hypertension. MRI delineates between tissue structure (e.g., white and gray matter differentiation); thus MRI can be helpful in evaluating brain tumors, especially when located in the posterior fossa, where x-ray artifact from adjacent bone obstructs the CT view. Because personnel and metal objects cannot be in immediate proximity to the patient during MRI, its use in critical care is extremely limited.

Transporting the critically ill patient to radiology for either CT or MRI places the patient in an extremely vulnerable position. Transport requires forethought and teamwork, and planning for potential emergencies is key. Patients and personnel with implanted magnetic devices should not be near an MRI because the magnetic field may dislodge or interfere with the function of the device. Expecting infants and young children to cooperate by holding still during the examination, especially during the loud knocking MRI sounds, is unrealistic. Sedation in this age group is often used to accomplish both CT scan and MRI.

During **cerebral angiography,** radiopaque contrast medium is injected into the carotid artery, and sequential skull x-rays films are taken to track medium flow throughout the cerebral vasculature. Cerebral angiography is used to delineate arteriovenous malformations or to assess the circulation to a brain tumor. Common to any angiographic procedure is a potential for arterial spasm, embolism, and thrombosis. Allergic reaction to the contrast medium may occur. Hematoma formation at the injection site is another potential risk. Patients may report a burning or warm sensation for about 20 to 30 seconds when the medium is injected.

Positron emission tomography (PET) scans provide information regarding cerebral metabolic function. Positron-emitting isotopes, which readily cross the blood-brain barrier, are either inhaled or injected. When the positrons (positive electron charge) come in contact with electrons (negative electron charge), gamma rays are released. The intensity of the gamma rays is then measured by a computerized detector that creates an image indicating the pattern of metabolic activity. The half-life of the nuclides is extremely short, so there is no risk of radiation exposure to either patients or caregivers. Although use in critical care is limited, PET scanning has been found to be valuable in locating epileptic foci in infants and young children before excision.

SUMMARY

In summary, care of the patient at risk for neurologic compromise is inherent to the practice of critical care nursing. The astute neurologic examination, repeated at frequent intervals by an expert clinician, is the most reliable monitor of neurologic functioning. When neurophysiologic monitoring and studies are used in combination with history and physical examination, the diagnostic process is complete, and clinical judgment is optimized.

REFERENCES

1. AACN Certification Corporation: *Pediatric examination: a blueprint for study,* Aliso Viejo, Calif, 1998, AACN Certification Corporation.
2. Nolte J: *The human brain: an introduction to its functional anatomy,* ed 2, St Louis, 1988, Mosby.
3. Sundt TM: Blood flow regulation in normal and ischemic brain, *Current concepts,* Peapack, NJ, 1979, Pharmacia & Upjohn.
4. Vidyasugar D, Raju TNK: A simple noninvasive technique of releasing intracranial pressure in the newborn, *Pediatrics* 59:957-961, 1977.
5. Shapiro K, Marmarou A, Shulman K: Characterization of clinical CSF dynamics and neural axis compliance using the pressure-volume index. I, The normal pressure-volume index, *Ann Neurol* 7:508-514, 1980.
6. Shapiro K, Marmarou A, Shulman K: A method for predicting PVI in normal patients. In Shulman K, Marmarou A, Miller JD et al, eds: *Intracranial pressure IV,* New York, 1980, Springer-Verlag.

7. Shapiro KF, Morris WJ, Teo C: Intracranial hypertension: mechanisms and management. In Cheek WR, Marlin AE, McLone DJ et al, eds: *Pediatric neurosurgery: surgery of the developing nervous system,* Philadelphia, 1994, WB Saunders.
8. Traystman RJ: Microcirculation of the brain. In Mortillaro NA, ed: *The physiology and pharmacology of the microcirculation,* New York, 1983, Academic Press.
9. Raju TNK, Vidyasagar D, Papazafiratou C: Cerebral perfusion pressure and abnormal intracranial pressure wave forms: their relation to outcome in birth asphyxia, *Crit Care Med* 9:449-453, 1981.
10. Folkow B: Description of the myogenic hypothesis, *Circ Res* 14, 15(suppl 1):I279-I287, 1964.
11. Rogers MC, Nugent SK, Traystman RJ: Control of cerebral circulation in the neonate and infant, *Crit Care Med* 8:570-574, 1980.
12. Duc G: Assessment of hypoxia in the newborn: suggestions for a practical approach, *Pediatrics* 48:469-481, 1971.

13. Menkes JH, Till K, Gabriel RS: Malformations of the central nervous system. In Menkes JH, ed: *Textbook of child neurology,* Philadelphia, 1990, Lea & Febiger.
14. Jacobson RI: Congenital structural defects. In Swaiman KF, ed: *Pediatric neurology: principles and practice,* vol 1, St Louis, 1989, Mosby.
15. Popich GA, Smith DW: Fontanels: range of normal size, *J Pediatr* 80:749-752, 1972.
16. Haller JS: Skull transillumination. In Coleman M, ed: *Neonatal neurology,* Baltimore, 1981, University Park Press.
17. Plum R, Posner JB: *The diagnosis of stupor and coma,* ed 3, Philadelphia, 1982, FA Davis.
18. Amiel-Tison C: A method for neurologic evaluation within the first year of life, *Curr Probl Pediatr* 7:9-31, 1976.
19. Slota MC: Pediatric neurological assessment, *Crit Care Nurs* 8:106-112, 1983.
20. Swaiman KF: Neurologic examination after the newborn period until 2 years of age.

In Swaiman KF, Ashwal S, eds: *Pediatric neurology: principles and practice,* ed 3, St Louis, 1999, Mosby.

21. Swaiman KF: Neurologic examination in the older child. In Swaiman KF, Ashwal S, eds: *Pediatric neurology: principles and practice,* ed 3, St Louis, 1999, Mosby.

22. Jennett B, Bond M: Assessment of outcome after severe brain damage: a practical scale, *Lancet* 1:480-485, 1975.

23. March K: Look into my eyes, *J Neurosurg Nurs* 15:213-221, 1983.

24. Norman S: The pupil check, *Am J Nurs* 82:588-591, 1982.

25. Bishop BS: Pathologic pupillary signs: self-learning module. II, *Crit Care Nurs* 11:58-67, 1991.

26. Eviatar L: Vertigo. In Swaiman KF, Ashwal S, eds: *Pediatric neurology: principles and practice,* ed 3, St Louis, 1999, Mosby.

27. Moore PC: When you have to think small for a neurological exam, *RN* 51:38-44, 1988.

28. Taylor DA, Ashwal S: Impairment of consciousness and coma. In Swaiman KF, Ashwal S, eds: *Pediatric neurology: principles and practice,* ed 3, St Louis, 1999, Mosby.

29. Grehn LS: Adverse responses to analgesia, sedation, and neuromuscular blocking agents in infants and children, *AACN Clin Issues Crit Care Nurs* 9:36-48, 1998.

30. Dearden NM: Mechanisms and prevention of secondary brain damage during intensive care, *Clin Neuropathol* 17:221-228, 1998.

31. Dean JM, McComb JG: Intracranial pressure monitoring in severe pediatric near-drowning, *Neurosurgery* 9:627-630, 1981.

32. Nussbaum E, Galant SP: Intracranial pressure monitoring as a guide to prognosis in the nearly drowned, severely comatose child, *J Pediatr* 102:215-218, 1983.

33. Miller JD: Intracranial pressure-volume relationships in pathological conditions, *J Neurosurg Sci* 20:203, 1976.

34. Crippen DW: Neurologic monitoring in the intensive care unit, *New Horiz* 2:107-120, 1994.

35. Shapiro S, Bowman R, Callahan J et al: The fiberoptic intraparenchymal cerebral pressure monitor in 244 patients, *Surg Neurol* 45:278-282, 1996.

36. Morgalla MH, Mettenleiter H, Bitzer M et al: ICP measurement control: laboratory test of 7 types of intracranial pressure transducers, *J Med Eng Technol* 23:144-151, 1999.

37. Schurer L, Munch E, Piepgras A et al: Assessment of the Camino intracranial pressure device in clinical practice, *Acta Neurochir (Wien)* 70:296-298, 1997.

38. Stewart-Amidei C: Neurologic monitoring in the ICU, *Crit Care Nurs Q* 21:47-60, 1998.

39. Marmarou A, Tsuji O, Dunbar J: Experimental evaluation of new solid state ICP monitor. In *Proceedings of the Ninth International Symposium on Intracranial Pressure: ICP IX: IP and its related problems,* New York, 1994, Springer-Verlag.

40. Gopinath SP, Cherian L, Robertson CS et al: Evaluation of a microsensor intracranial pressure transducer, *J Neurosci Methods* 49:11-15, 1993.

41. Brain Trauma Foundation: Recommendations for intracranial pressure monitoring technology, *J Neurotrauma* 13:685-692, 1996.

42. Tilem D, Greenberg CS: Nursing care of the child with a ventriculostomy, *J Pediatr Nurs* 3:188-193, 1988.

43. Mayhall CG, Archer NH, Lamb VA et al: Ventriculostomy related infections: a prospective epidemiologic study, *N Engl J Med* 310:533-559, 1984.

44. Bekar A, Goren S, Korfali E et al: Complications of brain tissue pressure monitoring with a fiberoptic device, *Neurosurg Rev* 21:254-259, 1998.

45. Paramore CG, Turner DA: Relative risks of ventriculostomy infection and morbidity, *Acta Neurochir (Wien)* 127:79-84, 1994.

45a. Halloway KL, Barnes T, Choi S et al: Ventriculostomy infections: the effect of monitoring duration and catheter exchange in 584 patients, *J Neurosurg* 85:419-424, 1996.

46. Kanter RK, Weiner LB, Patti AM et al: Infectious complications and duration of intracranial pressure monitoring, *Crit Care Med* 13:837-839, 1985.

47. Rozzi S, Buzzi R, Paparella A et al: Complications and safety associated with ICP monitoring: a study of 542 patients, *Acta Neurochir Suppl (Wien)* 71:91-93, 1998.

48. Aucoin PJ, Kotilainen HR, Gantz NM et al: Intracranial pressure monitors, epidemiologic study of risk factors and infections, *Am J Med* 80:369-376, 1986.

49. Prabhu VC, Kaufman HH, Voelker JL et al: Prophylactic antibiotics with intracranial pressure monitors and external ventricular drains: a review of the evidence, *Surg Neurol* 52:226-236, 1999.

50. Ghajar J: Intracranial pressure monitoring techniques, *New Horiz* 3:395-399, 1995.

51. Munch E, Weigel R, Schmiedek P et al: The Camino intracranial pressure device in clinical practice: reliability, handling characteristics and complications, *Acta Neurochir (Wien)* 140:1113-1119, 1998.

52. Germon K: Intracranial pressure monitoring in the 1990s, *Crit Care Nurs Q* 17:21-32, 1994.

53. Price MP: Significance of intracranial pressure waveform, *J Neurosurg Nurs* 13:202-206, 1981.

54. Cardoso ER, Rowan JO, Galbraith S: Analysis of the cerebrospinal fluid pulse wave in intracranial pressure, *J Neurosurg* 59:817-821, 1983.

55. Germon K: Interpretation of ICP pulse waves to determine intracerebral compliance, *J Neurosci Nurs* 20:344-349, 1988.

56. Bergman I: Pediatric neurological assessment and monitoring. In Fuhrman BP, Zimmerman JJ, eds: *Pediatric critical care,* St Louis, 1992, Mosby.

57. Czosnyka M, Smielewski P, Piechnik S et al: Hemodynamic characterization of intracranial pressure plateau waves in head-injury patients, *J Neurosurg* 91:9-11, 1999.

58. Weaver DD, Winn HR, Jane JA: Differential intracranial pressure in patients with unilateral mass lesions, *J Neurosurg* 56:660-665, 1982.

59. Crutchfield JS, Narayan RK, Robertson CS et al: Evaluation of a fiberoptic intracranial pressure monitor, *J Neurosurg* 72:482-487, 1990.

60. Hickman KM, Mayer BL, Muwaswes M: Intracranial pressure monitoring: review of risk factors associated with infection, *Heart Lung* 19:84-92, 1990.

61. Pellock JM: Status epilepticus. In Swaiman KF, Ashwal S, eds: *Pediatric neurology: principles and practice,* ed 3, St Louis, 1999, Mosby.

62. Brain Trauma Foundation: The use of barbiturates in the control of intracranial hypertension, *J Neurotrauma* 13:711-714, 1996.

63. Kotagal S: Increased intracranial pressure. In Swaiman KF, Ashwal S, eds: *Pediatric neurology: principles and practice,* ed 3, St Louis, 1999, Mosby.

64. Orlowski JP, Erenberg G, Lueders H et al: Hypothermia and barbiturate coma for refractory status epilepticus, *Crit Care Med* 12:367-372, 1989.

65. Sloan TB: Neurologic monitoring, *Crit Care Clin* 4:543-557, 1988.

66. Wiznitzer M: Neuroelectrophysiologic monitoring. In Blumer JL, ed: *A practical guide to pediatric intensive care,* ed 3, St Louis, 1990, Mosby.

67. Filloux F, Dean JM, Kirsch JR: Monitoring the central nervous system. In Rogers MC, ed: *Textbook of pediatric intensive care,* ed 2, Baltimore, 1992, Williams & Wilkins.

68. Johnston MV: Development, structure, and function of the brain and neuromuscular systems. In Fuhrman BP, Zimmerman JF, eds: *Pediatric critical care,* St Louis, 1992, Mosby.

69. Orlowski MP, Rothner AD: Diagnosis and treatment of status epilepticus. In Fuhrman BP, Zimmerman JJ, eds: *Pediatric critical care,* St Louis, 1992, Mosby.

70. Esposito N, Westgate P: Continuous EEG monitoring in the PICU, *J Pediatr Nurs* 2:272-277, 1987.

71. Buzea CE: Understanding computerized EEG monitoring in the intensive care unit, *J Neurosci Nurs* 27:292-297, 1995.

72. Stidham GL, Nugent SK, Rogers MC: Monitoring cerebral electrical function in the ICU, *Crit Care Med* 8:519-522, 1980.

73. Talwar D, Torres F: Continuous electrophysiologic monitoring of cerebral function in the pediatric intensive care unit, *Pediatr Neurol* 4:137-147, 1988.

74. Cant BR, Shaw NA: Monitoring by compressed spectral array in prolonged coma, *Neurology* 34:35-39, 1984.

75. Mizrahi EM, Dorfman LJ: Sensory evoked potentials: clinical applications in pediatrics, *J Pediatr* 97:1-10, 1980.

76. York DH, Pulliam MW, Rosenfeld JG et al: Relationship between visual evoked potentials and intracranial pressure, *J Neurosurg* 55:909-916, 1981.

77. York D, Legan M, Benner S et al: Further studies with a noninvasive method of intracranial pressure estimation, *Neurosurgery* 14:456-461, 1984.

78. Greenberg RP, Ducker TB: Evoked potentials in the clinical neurosciences, *J Neurosurg* 56:1-18, 1982.

79. Goodwin SR, Friedman WA, Bellefleur M: Is it time to use evoked potentials to predict outcome in comatose children and adults, *Crit Care Med* 19:518-524, 1991.

80. Robertson CS, Narayan RM, Gokaslan ZK et al: Cerebral arteriovenous oxygen difference as an estimate of cerebral blood flow in comatose patients, *J Neurosurg* 70:222-230, 1989.

81. Goetting MG, Preston G: Jugular bulb catheterization: experience with 123 patients, *Crit Care Med* 18:1220-1223, 1990.

82. Cruz J, Miner ME, Allen SJ et al: Continuous monitoring of cerebral oxygenation in acute brain injury: injection of mannitol during hyperventilation, *J Neurosurg* 73:725-730, 1990.

83. McCormick PW, Stewart M, Goetting MG et al: Noninvasive cerebral optical spectroscopy for monitoring cerebral oxygen delivery and hemodynamics, *Crit Care Med* 19:89-97, 1991.

84. Hassler W, Steinmetz H, Gawlowski J: Transcranial Doppler ultrasonography in raised intracranial pressure and in intracranial circulatory arrest, *J Neurosurg* 68:745-751, 1988.

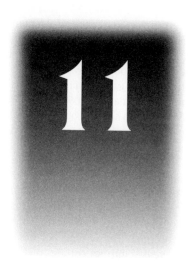

11

Fluid and Electrolyte Regulation

Kathryn E. Roberts

The concepts of fluid and electrolyte balance apply to a broad spectrum of pediatric critically ill children. Many disease states alter the intake and elimination of fluids and electrolytes, but physiologic immaturity places infants and children at higher risk for the consequences of imbalance. Fluid and electrolyte regulation is dependent on renal function. The kidney provides for the maintenance of the body's internal environment that supports cellular processes. Although the immature kidneys are well

suited to meet their homeostatic requirements, critical illness often overburdens them. A disturbance in fluid and electrolyte balance affects the ability of the kidney to regulate water and many hormones (see Chapter 21). This, in turn, affects regulation in a number of body systems, including the cardiac and respiratory systems. For these reasons, a major goal of critical care management is to prevent major fluctuations in electrolyte concentrations and to stabilize fluid in the correct compartment. When critical imbalances occur, astute assessment and rapid intervention can determine a successful outcome. The nurse's responsibility is to observe for insidious changes and to initiate interventions that will correct imbalances. An awareness of fluid and electrolyte regulation guides the nurse in anticipating potential problems and ensuring that appropriate interventions take place.

MATURATIONAL IMPACT OF FLUID AND ELECTROLYTE REGULATION

Composition of Body Fluids

Fluid and electrolyte homeostasis occurs when fluid and electrolyte balance is maintained within narrow limits despite a wide variation in dietary intake, metabolic rate, and kidney function. Body fluids are composed primarily of water and electrolytes.

An electrolyte is a substance that develops an electrical charge (ion) when dissolved in water. Those substances that develop a positive electrical charge are called cations (i.e., potassium, K^+; sodium, Na^+; calcium, Ca^{++}; and magnesium, Mg^{++}). Electrolytes that develop a negative charge are called anions (i.e., chloride, Cl^-, and bicarbonate, HCO_3^-). Electrolytes are regulated by intake, output, acid-base balance, hormonal influence, and cellular integrity. Nonelectrolytes are small solute particles that do not carry an electrical charge when dissolved in water. Examples are simple sugars (i.e., glucose), proteins, oxygen, carbon dioxide, and organic acids.

Total Body Water

Water constitutes approximately 65% to 80% of body weight. Total body water (TBW) varies from person to person and is dependent on several factors: age, gender, skeletal muscle mass, and fat content. The water content of adipose tissue is approximately 10% as compared with a water content of 73% in lean body tissues.[1] Thus the amount of fat in the body determines, to a major degree, the amount of water.

As the infant and child mature, TBW, as a percentage of body weight, changes. During the first year of life, the total body fluid percentage decreases, with the most rapid change occurring in the first 6 months.[2] TBW accounts for 75% 80% of body weight in the newborn, 70% at 6 months, and 65% at 1 year of age. In children, the percentage of total weight as body water decreases steadily until the adult percentage (55% to 60%) is reached at about 8 years of age[3] (Table 11-1). On the average, obese children and women generally have lower percentages of TBW as water. TBW is distributed in two separate compartments: the intracellular fluid (ICF) compartment and the extracellular fluid (ECF) compartment (Fig. 11-1).

In addition to the changes in the percentage of TBW as body weight, infants and young children have a relatively higher percentage of ECF compartment compared with adults. More than half of the infant's body weight is ECF compartment. This decreases quickly over the first 6 to 8 weeks of life, and by 3 years of age, body fluid components more closely resemble those of the adult with an ECF compartment of approximately 20% to 23% and an ICF compartment of 40% to 50%.[1,2]

Intracellular Compartment. ICF consists of all liquid within the cell membranes of the body and is the largest fluid compartment, accounting for 40% of the body weight of the child by 1 year of age (see Table 11-1). Much of the ICF compartment is found within muscle cells. The primary electrolytes of the ICF compartment are potassium and phosphate. The ICF compartment contains only small quantities of sodium and chloride ions and almost no calcium ions. The cells contain 4 times as much protein as the plasma.

Extracellular Compartment. The extracellular compartment is not a homogenous compartment. It is composed of interstitial fluid (ISF), plasma, and transcellular water (TSW). The ISF bathes all of the body cells and includes lymph fluid, the largest component of ECF compartment. ISF volume accounts for approximately 20% of TBW. Plasma is the liquid component of whole blood, contained within the vascular system. Although plasma accounts for only 8% of TBW, it is essential to the functioning of the cardiovascular system. TSW is composed of the fluids found in pleural, pericardial, synovial, peritoneal, and joint spaces. In addition, TSW includes the secretions of the salivary glands and pancreas and fluid in the respiratory and gastrointestinal tracts. The function of TSW is to either lubricate or cushion. TSW accounts for a small portion of TBW; however, it can increase during certain disease states.[4]

The serum or plasma portion of the extracellular compartment contains the electrolytes found in the ECF compartment and a large amount of protein. The plasma proteins determine colloid osmotic (oncotic) pressure, with the most abundant plasma protein being albumin. Albumin, because of its size, remains in the vascular space and exerts a differential osmotic force or oncotic pressure between the capillary lumen and the interstitial space. The consequence is maintenance of volume in the intravascular space. Oncotic pressure is also important in the kidney, influencing filtration and reabsorption of water and solutes.

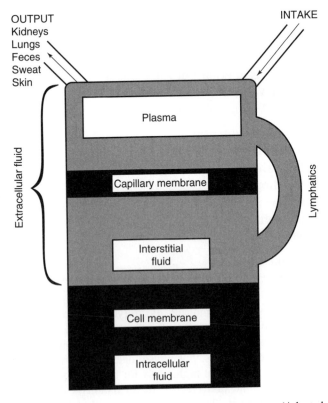

Fig. 11-1 Fluid distribution—body compartments. (Adapted from Guyton AC, Hall JE: *Textbook of medical physiology,* ed 9, Philadelphia, 1996, WB Saunders, p 298.)

◆ **TABLE 11-1   Changes in Total Body Water (TBW) and Body Compartments During Development**

Age	TBW (% Body Weight)	Extracellular Fluid (% Body Weight)	Intracellular Fluid (% Body Weight)
Newborn	72-79	32-44	35-40
1-2 years	59	25	33
3-5 years	62	21	41
10-16 years	58	18	39

From Finberg L, Kravath R, Hellerstein S et al, eds: *Water and electrolytes in pediatrics: physiology, pathophysiology, and treatment,* Philadelphia, 1993, WB Saunders, pp 13-15.

The ECF compartment contains large quantities of sodium and chloride ions; reasonably large quantities of bicarbonate ion; and small quantities of potassium, calcium, magnesium, phosphate, sulfate, and organic acid ions. The ECF compartment makes up just 20% of body weight in the adult but 50% in full-term infants.[1] The infant's entire ECF compartment volume is replaced every 3 days. By the age of 1 year, ECF compartment decreases by one half and declines very slowly thereafter (see Table 11-1).

Regulation of Water and Electrolyte Balance

A dynamic relationship exists between the extracellular and intracellular fluid compartments. This relationship maintains cellular homeostasis through the exchange of fluids and electrolytes. The compartments are kept separate by the structural and functional integrity of cell membranes. Both passive and active processes regulate the movement of water and solutes across the cell membrane. The selective permeability of the cell membrane and the specific active transport activity of the cell determine the characteristics of intracellular and extracellular fluid compartments. A profound alteration in any one of the fluid compartments can disrupt cellular health and may result in a fatal systemic response.

Homeostatic maintenance of fluid balance ensures that TBW remains constant. The aim is to have intake equal output plus insensible water loss. Intake is composed of water from enteral or intravenous solutions and fluid metabolically produced through oxidative metabolism (300 ml/24 hours). Intake is regulated mainly through the mechanism of thirst. This mechanism cannot be relied on to obtain adequate intake in critically ill infants and children because they may not be able to demonstrate or respond to thirst.

Output of fluids and electrolytes is regulated by the integumentary, respiratory, digestive, and renal systems. All of these systems work together to protect adequate elimination and retention of body water. Several factors, such as humidity and ambient temperatures, affect the amount of

---

TABLE 11-2   Factors Known to Influence Insensible (Evaporative) Fluid Losses

Increased Insensible Loss	Decreased Insensible Loss
Hyperthermia*	Hypothermia
Increased activity	Decreased activity
Hyperventilation	Sedation
Radiant warmers†	Humidified air
Phototherapy‡	

From Besunder JB: Abnormalities in fluids, minerals, and glucose. In Blumer JL, ed: *A practical guide to pediatric intensive care*, ed 3, St Louis, 1990, Mosby, p 546.
*Increases sensible losses by 12% per Celsius degree above 38° C.
†Increases insensible losses by 40% to 50% in infants less than 1500 g; percentage may be higher in larger infants.
‡Increases insensible losses by approximately 40% in infants less than 1500 g; percentage may be higher in larger infants.

---

water lost. Factors affecting insensible water loss are presented in Table 11-2.

ASSESSMENT OF FLUID AND ELECTROLYTE BALANCE

The kidneys, in conjunction with the endocrine system, are responsible for maintaining the body's fluid and electrolyte balance. The regulation of fluid and electrolytes in designated compartments (intracellular and extracellular) is dependent on the osmotic pressure, colloid osmotic pressure, hydrostatic pressure (pressure exerted by a liquid) in the vascular spaces, and capillary permeability. Hydrostatic pressure is produced through the action of the cardiovascular and lymphatic systems. The force of cardiac contractions generates capillary hydrostatic pressure.

The term *colloid osmotic pressure* (COP) is used to distinguish the osmotic effects of the colloid from those of dissolved crystalloids such as sodium. COP is a pulling force generated by plasma proteins that opposes fluid filtration from the capillaries. The plasma proteins are large colloid molecules that disperse in the blood and sometimes escape into the tissue spaces. Both the intravascular and interstitial compartments contain plasma proteins, including albumin, the globulins, and fibrinogen. Albumin, the smallest and most abundant of the plasma proteins, accounts for about 70% of the total osmotic pressure. Albumin provides for the return of fluid to the vascular compartment from the tissue spaces. When plasma protein concentration falls acutely, plasma oncotic pressure falls, and fluid may leave the vascular space, resulting in third spacing of fluid.

Movement of Fluids and Electrolytes

For water and electrolytes to function effectively in the body, a regulatory process that controls fluid movement is required. The regulatory process is dependent on the concentration of the specific fluid or electrolyte (osmolality) and on the functioning capacity of the renal system. Fluids move constantly from one body compartment to another and then remain in specific compartments until an inequality in concentration of electrolytes develops. Then, movement once again occurs. Movement is through one of four transport mechanisms: osmosis, diffusion, filtration, and active transport.

Osmosis is the movement of water through a semipermeable membrane from an area of lower solute content to an area of higher solute activity (with lower activity of water molecules) (Fig. 11-2). Osmosis occurs only when the membrane is more permeable to water than solutes. The force of the movement, or shift, of water depends on serum osmolality, which controls distribution and movement of water between compartments.

Osmolality refers to the concentration of particles (proteins and electrolytes) per liter of water. The osmolality of a solution does not depend on the size, molecular weight, or electrical charge of the molecules. Osmotic pressure of a solution is described by the terms *osmole* and *milliosmole*.

The osmolar concentration of a solution is called the osmolality when the concentration is expressed as osmoles per kilogram of water. The terms *tonicity* and *osmolality* are used interchangeably.

Serum osmolality can be estimated by the following formula:

$$\text{Serum osmolality} = 2(\text{Serum Na}) + \text{Glucose}/18 + \text{BUN}/2.8$$

where *BUN* is blood urea nitrogen.

Normally, the amount of water that diffuses in and out of the cell is balanced, and the volumes within the extracellular and intracellular fluid compartments remain constant. Because water moves freely between the blood, ISF, and tissues, changes in the osmolality of one body compartment

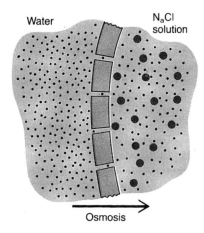

Fig. 11-2 Osmosis at cell membrane when sodium chloride solution is placed on one side of the membrane and water on the other side. (From Guyton AC: *Textbook of medical physiology,* ed 8, Philadelphia, 1991, WB Saunders, p 45.)

produce a shift in all other compartments. Consequently, in most cases, the osmolality of the plasma is equal to the osmolality of other compartments.

Water moves from the ECF compartment to the ICF compartment if the ICF compartment osmolality increases (Fig. 11-3). Conversely, if the ECF compartment osmolality increases, water will shift from the ICF compartment into the ECF compartment (see Fig. 11-3). When the movement of water causes a concentration difference, the cells either shrink or swell, depending on the direction of the net movement. Isotonic solutions (0.9% saline) do not cause cells to either shrink or swell. Hypertonic solutions (one with greater than 0.9% saline) cause cells to shrink by moving water from within the cell to the ECF compartment, which has less sodium than the cell. Hypotonic solutions (such as 5% dextrose and 0.2% normal saline) cause cells to swell.

Diffusion is the movement of a substance (electrolytes and nonelectrolytes) from an area of higher concentration to one of lower concentration through a solution or gas (Fig. 11-4). Diffusion ceases when equilibrium occurs. Electrical potential differences and pressure differences across the pores of a semipermeable membrane also influence diffusion, although the most important factor determining the rate of diffusion is the concentration difference. The greater the concentration difference, the greater the rate of diffusion.

Molecules moving via simple diffusion must possess one of two capabilities: lipid solubility or a negative charge. The lipid-soluble molecules, such as oxygen, carbon dioxide, and alcohol, are able to diffuse readily through the lipid component of the cell membrane. Chloride is an example of a negatively charged particle able to pass easily through the membrane pores.

Filtration is the transfer of water and dissolved substances through a semipermeable membrane from a region

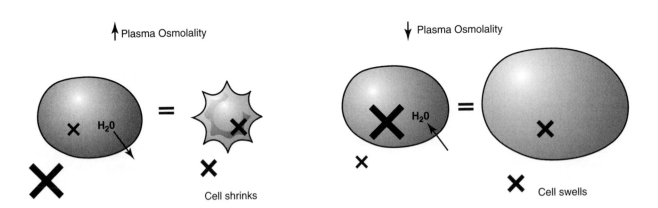

Fig. 11-3 Fluid movement with changes in osmolality. (From Toto KH: Regulation of plasma osmolality: thirst and vasopressin, *Crit Care Nurs Clin North Am* 6:662, 1994.)

of high pressure to a region of low pressure. The force causing filtration is hydrostatic pressure. An example of filtration is the passage of water and electrolytes from the arterial capillary bed to the ISF in response to blood pressure. The pumping action of the heart causes the hydrostatic pressure.[2]

Movement against a concentration or electrochemical gradient is known as **active transport,** and energy, in the form of adenosine triphosphatase (ATPase), is required for the activity (Fig. 11-5). The transport occurs somewhat like a "pump" in the membrane of the cell, driven by the energy

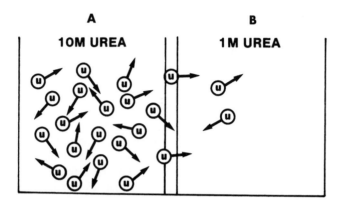

A 10M UREA   B 1M UREA

Fig. 11-4 Simple diffusion. A membrane permeable to urea separates two solutions. Side **A** contains a tenfold greater concentration of urea than side **B**. Random motion of individual solute molecules results in net movement of urea from **A** to **B**. (From Wright E, Schulman G: Dynamics of body water: principles of epithelial transport. In Maxwell MH, Kleeman CR, Narins RG, eds: *Clinical disorders of fluid and electrolyte metabolism,* New York, 1985, McGraw-Hill, p 17.)

generated by cellular respiration. Regulation and distribution of sodium and potassium within the interstitial and the intracellular fluid compartments are via the sodium-potassium pump. Active transport is necessary to move sodium from the cells to the ECF compartment. The active process of pumping sodium out of the cells forces potassium into the cell.

An example of the effects of the sodium-potassium pump is seen in children with severe burns. The injury causes more sodium than water to be drawn into the interstitial spaces. This decreases the efficiency of the sodium pump, which allows more water and sodium to enter the intracellular space. The increased osmotic pressure gradient drives potassium out of the cell. The loss of water and sodium from the intravascular space results in the increased secretion of aldosterone and antidiuretic hormone (ADH) as compensatory mechanisms, which contributes to the retention of sodium and water.

Not only is energy required to move substances against a concentration gradient, but a carrier substance is required for the transport of sodium, potassium, chloride, sugars, and amino acids. Carrier substances are either a protein or a lipoprotein. The protein carriers function by providing an attachment site for the specific substance to be transported. The lipoprotein facilitates the solubility of the substance in the lipid portion of the cell membrane.

Fluid Volume Regulation

Water is the most abundant component of the body. Although serving a vital role in the regulation of body heat through insulation or evaporation, water further serves as the diluent for cell solids and as a message carrier among the

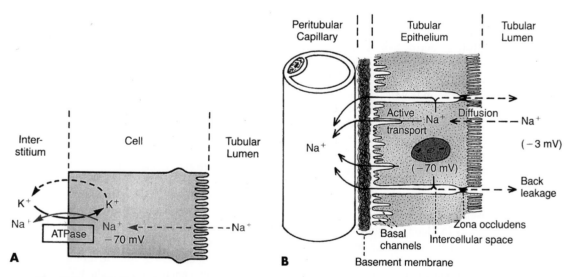

Fig. 11-5 **A,** Basic mechanism for active transport of sodium through a layer of cell. This figure shows active transport by the sodium potassium pump, which pumps sodium out of the basolateral membrane of the cell and simultaneously creates a very low intracellular sodium concentration, as well as a negative intracellular potential. The low intracellular sodium concentration and the negative potential then cause sodium ions to diffuse from the tubular lumen into the cell through the brush border. **B,** Net mechanism for active transport of sodium from the tubular lumen all the way into the peritubular capillary. (From Guyton AC: *Textbook of medical physiology,* ed 9, Philadelphia, 1996, WB Saunders, p 54.)

cells, tissues, and organs of the body. Water also provides the body with form and structure.

Renal regulation of water and sodium is the most important mechanism of volume regulation. This occurs through normal functioning of the nephron in conjunction with certain hormonal factors, including ADH, aldosterone, and natriuretic factors.[4]

Nephron.   Sodium is filtered at the glomerulus and is reabsorbed by the renal tubules. In the normally functioning nephron, 99% of the filtered load of sodium is reabsorbed. However, changes in the glomerular filtration rate (GFR) affect the amount of sodium that is reabsorbed or excreted. The GFR increases over the first 2 years of life, stabilizing in a range between 30% to 50% of adult levels by the end of the first year and reaching adult levels by the age of 2 years.[5] During times of volume expansion, the GFR increases, and sodium and water excretion are increased in an attempt to return intravascular volume to normal levels. In contrast, in times of volume depletion, the GFR decreases, and more sodium and water are retained in an attempt to restore intravascular volume.[1]

Antidiuretic Hormone.   ADH, or vasopressin, is manufactured in the hypothalamus of the brain and is released by the posterior pituitary gland. ADH acts on the cells of the renal collecting ducts to increase their permeability to water, promoting a simultaneous increase in ECF compartment volume and decrease in urinary output through selective reabsorption of water without sodium.

Three major stimuli for the regulation of ADH secretion are (1) plasma osmolality, (2) changes in the ECF compartment volume, and (3) changes in arterial blood pressure. When sufficient water is not being taken in or excessive loss occurs, serum osmolality rises. A small increase in serum osmolality of 1% to 2% is sufficient to cause ADH release, which acts at the nephrons, signaling them to conserve water and produce a more concentrated urine. ADH is released when the osmotic pressure of the ECF compartment is greater than that of the cells (e.g., during hyperglycemic and hypernatremic states). When osmotic pressure of the ECF compartment is less than that of the cells, ADH is inhibited, causing renal excretion of water.[2] When the blood pressure falls or blood volume decreases, ADH is also released.

ADH has a direct vasoconstrictor effect on the blood vessels, resulting in elevation of blood pressure. Other stimuli affecting ADH secretion are angiotensin II, drugs (opiates, nicotine, barbiturates, alcohol), stress, and severe pain. Release of angiotensin II, stress reaction, and severe pain cause release of ADH and thus increase blood pressure. Opiates, barbiturates, and alcohol reduce ADH secretion and are associated with decreases in blood pressure.

Aldosterone.   The adrenal cortex secretes aldosterone, which is a mineralocorticoid and a primary influence in fluid homeostasis. Sodium depletion, increases in potassium concentration, angiotensin II, and adrenocorticotropic hormone (ACTH) stimulate aldosterone release. The distal renal tubules, sweat glands, salivary glands, and intestines are the receptors of aldosterone activity.

Aldosterone causes the renal retention of sodium and water in exchange for the excretion of potassium and hydrogen. When the serum level of sodium falls, aldosterone is secreted. This leads to sodium and water retention in the renal tubules. Potassium is then given up by the renal tubules in a further effort to increase sodium levels. When aldosterone secretion is inhibited, potassium is retained, and sodium and water are excreted. Aldosterone helps regulate blood volume by regulating sodium retention.

Natriuretic Factors.   Natriuretic factors are salt-losing hormones that influence blood pressure and blood volume. These factors are produced by the hypothalamus and by the left and right atrial walls of the heart. The natriuretic hormone produced by the heart is atrial natriuretic factor (ANF). ANF is released when the atria are stretched, as in volume overload. Once released, ANF acts on the kidneys, where sodium reabsorption is inhibited, and a salt diuresis results.

MONITORING FLUID AND ELECTROLYTE BALANCE

A significant focus in the management of fluid and electrolyte balance involves monitoring for the occurrence or worsening of imbalances. Monitoring for fluid and electrolyte imbalances requires an understanding of the physiologic mechanisms behind the imbalances in addition to the clinical signs.

Clinical Assessment

Clinical assessment of the critically ill infant or child is a critical component in monitoring fluid and electrolyte balance. Suspicious findings often precipitate validation with invasive monitoring or diagnostic testing. Table 11-3 summarizes the clinical signs and symptoms associated with the most common fluid volume and electrolyte imbalances.

Key components of the cardiovascular system include the assessment of the patient's cardiac output and perfusion: heart rate, blood pressure, strength and quality of central and peripheral pulses, capillary refill time, color of the mucous membranes, and perfusion of extremities.[6] The presence of edema or hepatomegaly is assessed. A gallop rhythm, indicative of volume overload, may be noted on cardiac auscultation. Changes in the patient's electrocardiogram (ECG) may indicate various electrolyte imbalances. Table 11-4 summarizes the ECG abnormalities associated with various electrolyte imbalances.

Respiratory system examination includes an assessment of the patient's respiratory effort, an increase or decrease in respiratory rate and depth, and work of breathing. The presence of rales on auscultation, indicating fluid volume excess, is observed.

Key components of the neurologic examination include an assessment of the patient's level of consciousness (i.e., confusion, lethargy, orientation) and presence of seizures. In addition, the patient is assessed for hyporeflexia or hyperreflexia, muscle cramps, paresthesias, tetany, and Chvostek's or Trousseau's sign. Chvostek's sign is twitching of the facial muscle in response to gentle percussion at the top of the cheek just below the

TABLE 11-3   Clinical Signs and Symptoms Associated With Common Fluid and Electrolyte Imbalances

Imbalance	Clinical Signs and Symptoms
Fluid volume deficit	Acute weight loss, ↓ urine output, ↓ central venous pressure, altered level of consciousness, dry skin and mucous membranes
Fluid volume excess	Acute weight gain, edema, ↑ central venous pressure, tachypnea, hepatomegaly
Hyponatremia Na <135 mEq/L	Lethargy, disorientation (may progress to seizures or coma), muscle cramps, nausea/vomiting
Hypernatremia Na >145 mEq/L	Irritability, lethargy, ↑ muscle tone, coma
Hypokalemia K <3.5 mEq/L	Muscle weakness, abdominal distension, paralytic ileus, lethargy, irritability, hyperreflexia, tetany, nausea/vomiting
Hyperkalemia K >5.5 mEq/L	Muscle weakness, confusion, ascending paralysis, altered cardiac function, nausea, diarrhea, hyperactive bowel sounds
Hypocalcemia Ca <8 mg/dl	Tingling around the mouth or in fingertips/hands, Chvostek's or Trousseau's signs, muscle cramps, lethargy, seizures, hypotension
Hypercalcemia Ca >10.5 mg/dl	Lethargy, stupor (can progress to coma), seizures, anorexia, nausea/vomiting
Hypochloremia Cl <95 mEq/L	Hyperirritability; agitation; muscle weakness; tetany; slow, shallow respirations
Hyperchloremia Cl >108 mEq/L	Muscle weakness; decreased level of consciousness; deep, rapid respirations
Hypophosphatemia PO$_4$ <3 mg/dl	Irritability, disorientation, tremors, seizures, hemolytic anemia, ↓ myocardial function, potential respiratory failure, potential coma
Hyperphosphatemia PO$_4$ >4.5 mg/dl	Tachycardia, hyperreflexia, abdominal cramps, nausea, diarrhea, muscle tetany
Hypomagnesemia Mg <1.4 mEq/L	Neuromuscular excitability, vertigo, ataxia, nystagmus, tetany, respiratory depression, tachycardia, hypertension, confusion, dizziness, headache, hallucinations, seizures, coma
Hypermagnesemia Mg >2.5 mEq/L	Lethargy, muscle weakness, inability to swallow, ↓ gag reflex, bradycardia, hypotension, hyporeflexia

 TABLE 11-4   Common ECG Abnormalities Associated With Electrolyte Imbalances

Electrolyte Imbalance	ECG Findings
Hypokalemia	Flattened, inverted T waves; presence of U waves
Hyperkalemia	Tall, peaked T waves, followed by widened QRS and prolonged PR interval; can progress to ventricular arrhythmias and cardiac arrest
Hypocalcemia	Prolonged QT interval
Hypercalcemia	Shortened QT interval
Hypophosphatemia	Premature ectopic beats
Hypomagnesemia	Premature ventricular contractions, ventricular tachycardia, ventricular fibrillation
Hypermagnesemia	Prolonged PR, QRS, and QT intervals; AV block

zygomatic bone. Trousseau's sign is carpopedal spasm produced by prolonged blood pressure cuff inflation (>3 minutes). Both of these signs are clinical manifestations of hypocalcemia.

The renal examination provides important information regarding fluid volume status. This examination includes an assessment of the patient's urine output and urine specific gravity, hourly assessment of intake and output, and patient weight. Trends in weight gain or weight loss are assessed using the same scale with notations of any items weighed with the child (i.e., arm board, dressings). The severity of alterations in fluid volume is estimated by changes in body weight (1 liter of water is equivalent to 1 kg of body weight). Significant increases in weight gains are 50 g/24 hours in the infant, 200 g/24 hours in the child, and 500 g/24 hours in the adolescent.

The skin and mucous membranes are examined for moisture and elasticity. The skin in a patient with a fluid volume deficit is typically dry and warm. Mucous membranes may also be dry.

Laboratory Tests

Urea is measured in the blood as blood urea nitrogen (BUN) (normal level: 8 to 25 mg/dl). Urea is produced as the end product of protein metabolism and occurs as the result of the breakdown of ammonia in the liver. An elevated BUN may be associated with reduced renal blood flow secondary to fluid volume depletion. However, it may also be elevated as the result of increased protein intake. A decreased BUN is associated with fluid volume excess and with malnutrition or liver failure.[2]

Creatinine (normal level: 0.6 to 1.2 mg/dl) is an end product of protein metabolism synthesized in muscle cells and excreted by the kidney. An elevated creatinine usually indicates volume depletion or impaired renal function. A decrease in creatinine may be seen with fluid volume excess. Creatinine is a more specific indicator of kidney function than BUN because nonrenal causes of creatinine elevation are minimal. However, creatine may also rise in instances of muscle injury (crushing injuries, burns, etc.) independent of renal function.[4] Therefore the BUN/creatinine ratio is a more accurate indicator of fluid volume status than either value alone.

The **BUN/creatinine ratio** (normal value: 10:1 to 15:1) is useful in evaluating hydration status. An elevation in the BUN/creatinine ratio is associated with a decrease in renal perfusion or increased protein metabolism. A decrease in this ratio may be due to low protein intake, hepatic insufficiency, or repeated dialysis. The patient with an increase in both BUN and creatinine who maintains a ratio of 10:1 may have intrinsic renal disease.[7]

Serum sodium levels (normal value: 135 to 145 mEq/L) are closely related to fluid volume status. However, this value alone is not an indicator of volume status. Both fluid volume depletion and excess can be associated with a normal, decreased, or elevated serum sodium. As a result, serum sodium must be evaluated in light of the physical findings, water balance, and other laboratory values.

The **serum osmolality** (normal value: 280 to 295 mOsm/L) is determined mainly by serum sodium concentration. An elevated osmolality may indicate hypernatremic dehydration, hyperglycemia, or an elevated BUN. A decreased osmolality is seen in patients who are hyponatremic and may be seen with euvolemia, hypovolemia, hypervolemia.

Hematocrit (normal values: males, 40% to 52%; females, 37% to 46%) is the percentage of red blood cells in plasma. Plasma volume is ECF and red cell volume is ICF. Changes in plasma volume may result in changes in the hematocrit. An elevated hematocrit is seen in fluid volume depletion, and a decreased hematocrit is seen in fluid volume excess. However, these changes may only be interpreted in terms of fluid balance in the absence of changes of red cell mass (i.e., bleeding or hemolysis).

Total protein values (normal level: 6.3 to 8.2 g/dl) are affected by changes in volume status in a similar manner to hematocrit values. An elevation in total protein reflects a volume-depleted state. A decrease in total protein is the result of the dilutional effect of a volume-overloaded state.

Urine specific gravity (USG) (1.010 to 1.030) and **urine osmolality** (50 to 1200 mOsm/kg) are a reflection of the kidney's ability to concentrate and dilute. In states of volume depletion associated with normal kidney function, both the USG and the osmolality are typically elevated. The urine volume is usually diminished except in the instance of an osmotic diuresis. In volume-overloaded states, the urine is typically dilute with a decreased USG and osmolality and an increased volume. However, infant kidneys have a limited ability to concentrate urine,[2] and USG values may not be as helpful in the assessment of fluid volume status in this population.

Urine sodium values tend to vary with changes in volume status in much the same manner as USG and osmolality values do. Urine sodium is typically decreased in volume-depleted states and increased in volume-overloaded states. In volume-depleted states, the kidneys attempt to hold onto water and sodium in an effort to restore and maintain intravascular volume. In volume-overloaded states, the kidneys attempt to excrete water and sodium. Exceptions to this occur in renal failure in which the kidney loses its ability to concentrate urine. As a result, urine in renal failure may be dilute, and urine sodium values will not change, regardless of volume status.[4]

SUPPORT OF FLUID AND ELECTROLYTE BALANCE

Intravenous (IV) therapy is the most common type of therapy used to support the balance of fluids and electrolytes. It allows more rapid replacement of fluids and electrolytes than oral administration.[6] In addition, oral administration is not always the most practical method in the critically ill infant or child. Table 11-5 describes the most commonly used IV solutions in critically ill children.

Diuretics are commonly used to increase the urine output and excretion of sodium and chloride. These agents act by decreasing the rate of sodium reabsorption by the kidney tubules, which in turn leads to natriuresis and diuresis.[8] Diuretics are most commonly used to decrease extracellular volume. For the most part, diuretics can be grouped into three major classes: loop diuretics, thiazide-type diuretics, and potassium-sparing diuretics. Table 11-6 provides an overview of some commonly used diuretics.

IV administration of electrolyte supplements is another therapy in the management of fluid and electrolyte imbalances. Table 11-7 presents suggested guidelines for the administration of these solutions.

ALTERATIONS IN FLUID VOLUME BALANCE

Fluid Volume Deficit

Etiology. Fluid volume deficit is defined as negative body fluid or water balance. When extracellular volume depletion is present, hypovolemia exists, and circulatory collapse can result. In infants and children, *fluid volume deficit* and *dehydration* are terms often used interchange-

TABLE 11-5 Composition of Common Parenteral Fluid Solutions

Solution	Solute	Concentration (g/dl)	pH	Na⁺	K⁺	Ca²⁺	Cl⁻	Lactate	Calculated Osm (mOsm/L)
Dextrose in Water									
5%	Glucose	5	4.7	—	—	—	—	—	250
10%	Glucose	10	4.6	—	—	—	—	—	505
Saline									
0.45% (hypotonic)	NaCl	0.45	5.3	77	—	—	77	—	155
0.90% (isotonic)	NaCl	0.9	5.3	154	—	—	154	—	310
Dextrose in Saline									
2.5% in 0.45%	Glucose	2.5							
	NaCl	0.45	4.9	77	—	—	77	—	280
5% in 0.20%	Glucose	5							
	NaCl	0.20	4.6	34	—	—	34	—	320
5% in 0.45%	Glucose	5							
	NaCl	0.45	4.6	77	—	—	77	—	405
5% in 0.90%	Glucose	5							
	NaCl	0.90	4.6	154	—	—	154	—	560
Polyionic									
Ringer's lactate (RL)	Lactate	0.31							
	NaCl	0.60	6.3	130	4	3	109	28	275
	KCl	0.03							
	CaCl₂	0.02							
Dextrose in Polyionic									
2.5% in ½ RL	Glucose	2.5							
	Lactate	0.155	5.1	65	2	.015	54	14	265
	NaCl	0.30							
	KCl	0.015							
	CaCl₂	0.01							
4% in modified RL	Glucose	4							
	Lactate	0.062	5.0	26	0.8	0.5	22	5.5	280
	NaCl	0.12							
	KCl	0.006							
	CaCl₂	0.004							
5% in RL	Glucose	5							
	Lactate	0.31	4.7	130	4	3	109	28	515
	NaCl	0.60							
	KCl	0.03							
	CaCl₂	0.02							
5% albumin (Plasmanate)	Albumin	5	6.9	154	1		154	—	310
	NaCl	0.9							

From Krau SD: Selecting and managing fluid therapy: colloids versus crystalloids, *Crit Care Nurs Clin North Am* 10:401-410, 1998; Perkin RM, Levin DL: Common fluid and electrolyte problems in the pediatric intensive care unit, *Pediatr Clin North Am* 27:567-586, 1980.

ably. Fluid volume deficit is a common problem in critically ill infants and children. Negative water balance occurs from (1) excess loss of fluids and electrolytes, which can result from diarrhea or vomiting; (2) shifts of fluids and electrolytes into nonaccessible third spaces, such as in the severely burned child or following abdominal surgery; and (3) decreased intake of fluid and electrolytes, such as in the child who has nothing by mouth (is NPO).[9]

Excessive fluid volume loss and loss of electrolytes are major contributing factors to dehydration in infants and children. Increased insensible water loss may occur with burns, hyperventilation, fever, renal or gastrointestinal disease, increased ambient temperature, diaphoresis, and cystic fibrosis. As much as 400 to 2000 ml/m² of water may be lost each day in children losing fluid as a result of diaphoresis.[10] In cystic fibrosis, not only is excessive fluid lost, but sodium losses in sweat may vary between 50 and 130 mEq/L.[11] Increased renal water loss occurs as a result of osmotic diuresis, central diabetes insipidus, impaired tubular response to ADH, renal tubular dysfunction, and

TABLE 11-6   Diuretic Overview

Diuretics	Diuretic Mechanism of Action	Dose	Complications
Loop	↑ excretion of Na and Cl by inhibiting reabsorption		↓ serum K, Na, Mg Volume depletion Ototoxicity Metabolic alkalosis
Furosemide (Lasix)		1-2 mg/kg/dose IV 2-4 mg/kg/dose PO	
Bumetanide (Bumex)		0.25-0.5 mg/dose IV 0.01-0.02 mg/kg/dose PO	
Thiazide	↓ NaCl entry into cell		Volume depletion ↓ serum K, Na Metabolic alkalosis
Chlorothiazide (Diuril)		10-20 mg/kg/day PO	
Metolazone (Zaroxolyn)		0.1-0.4 mg/kg/day PO	
Potassium-Sparing	Depresses reabsorption of Na Depresses excretion of K		↑ serum K Metabolic acidosis
Spironalactone (Aldactone)		1.3-3 mg/kg/day PO	
Osmotic	↓ osmotic pressure		Volume depletion ↓ serum K, Na Metabolic acidosis
Mannitol		0.25-2 g/kg/dose IV	

Data from Sherbotie JR, Kaplan BS: Diuretics. In Yaffe SJ, Aranda JV, eds: *Pediatric pharmacology: therapeutic principles in practice*, Philadelphia, 1992, WB Saunders, pp 524-534.

TABLE 11-7   Suggested Guidelines for Administration of Electrolyte Solutions

Electrolyte	Administration Guidelines	Monitoring
Sodium (chloride)	Hypertonic saline (3%) may be given for severe hyponatremia (<120 mEq/L) when the patient is symptomatic. The amount of hypertonic saline solution needed can be calculated by the following formula: mEq Na = (0.60) (body weight in kg) (125 − Na). Discontinue infusion when serum Na reaches 120-125 mEq/L and begin water restriction.	Monitor serum sodium frequently. Administer through large vein. Maximum rate: 1 mEq/kg/hr.
Potassium (chloride)	IV push or undiluted potassium is never administered. Recommended maximum dose is 0.5 mEq/kg/hr in children, although dosages of 0.25-1 mEq/kg/hr may be used for severe depletion. Recommended maximum concentration for solution for peripheral lines is 40 mEq/L to prevent local irritation at infusion site. Recommended maximum concentration for infusion for central lines is 1 mEq/2 ml. Infusion rates of less than 0.3 mEq/kg/hr and concentrations of less than 60 mEq/L are usually adequate for replacement and maintenance of potassium.	Continuous ECG monitoring is necessary during KCl intermittent infusion (0.5 mEq/kg/hr). Monitor serum potassium levels frequently. Use with caution in patients with renal impairment (avoid use if patient is anuric or severely oliguric).

Continued

TABLE 11-7   Suggested Guidelines for Administration of Electrolyte Solutions—cont'd

Electrolyte	Administration Guidelines	Monitoring
Calcium (chloride, gluconate)	Administer slowly (no faster than 50 mg/min for $CaCl_2$; 100 mg/min for Ca gluconate) into a central line (in an emergent situation, may be given into a peripheral line if no central access is available). May be administered by continuous infusion via peripheral intravenous line. Maximum concentration should not exceed 20 mg/ml. Administer boluses in a dextrose or saline solution with no additives. Calcium is incompatible with many medications. Boluses are not administered in parenteral nutrition solutions or with intralipids.	Monitor intravenous site closely. Necrosis and sloughing will occur with extravasation. Monitor patients taking digoxin who are receiving calcium supplements closely because elevated calcium levels precipitate digoxin-related arrhythmias. (Monitor for bradycardia, hypotension, and cardiac arrhythmias.)
Phosphorus	Potassium or sodium phosphate can be diluted in IV maintenance fluids; infusion rate should not exceed 0.05 mmol/kg/hr. The usual dose for both is 0.15-0.33 mmol/kg/dose IV over 6 hours.	Side effects associated with rapid administration include hypotension.
381Magnesium (sulfate)	Administration by IV push is not recommended but in emergent situations may be diluted to 10 mg/ml and given slowly over 3-5 min. Dose should not exceed 150 mg/min. ECG should be monitored during administration. Infusions are recommended to be diluted to <10 mg/ml and infused over at least 15-30 min. Maximum concentration is 200 mg/ml.	Monitor patient closely for signs of hypermagnesemia. Cardiac arrest may occur with magnesium levels of 12-15 mEq/L.

sodium wasting conditions.[12] Gastrointestinal water loss from diarrheal disease is ordinarily the most common cause of excess fluid volume loss in infants and children.

In the critically ill child, fluid volume loss through "third spacing" is a common cause of fluid volume deficit. Third spacing occurs when extracellular fluid compartment volume is shifted into cavities, where it accumulates and is physiologically inaccessible for use by the body. Third spacing develops in ascites, pancreatitis, burns, peritonitis, sepsis, and intestinal obstruction.

Fluid deficit produced by inadequate intake is primarily caused by unreplaced normal insensible water loss. Examples of underlying clinical problems that contribute to decreased intake are coma, dysphagia, debilitation, impaired thirst, or anorexia. In addition, intake may not be adequate if ongoing losses are undetected or excessive.

Pathophysiology. Dehydration is usually classified on the basis of the serum sodium level because the level in dehydrated patients may be low, normal, or high, depending on electrolyte losses. Dehydration is classified as hyponatremic when serum sodium levels are less than 130 mEq/L, isonatremic when serum sodium levels are 130 to 150 mEq/L, and hypernatremic when serum sodium levels are above 150 mEq/L.[13] These forms of dehydration are also hypotonic, isotonic, and hypertonic, respectively, because plasma osmolality reflects sodium concentration. However, the two sets of terms cannot be used interchangeably because changes in tonicity do not always indicate sodium concentration.

Hyponatremic dehydration occurs when there is a proportionately greater loss of sodium compared with fluid loss. This often results when a child who is experiencing diarrhea or vomiting at home is given a hypotonic fluid such as water. An osmolar gradient results and produces a fluid shift from the hyponatremic extracellular space into the intracellular space, increasing the ECF compartment loss.

Isonatremic dehydration occurs when equal amounts of fluid and electrolytes are lost. When there is no osmolar gradient and isotonicity exists, the resultant fluid volume depletion is primarily extracellular.

Hypernatremic dehydration is characterized by an increased osmolality of the ECF compartment, which results in a shift of fluid from within the cells to maintain osmolar equilibrium.[9] ICF compartment volume is depleted, and ECF compartment loss is less than expected.

Critical Care Management. In addition to the previously discussed components of the physical examination, an estimate of the degree of dehydration is made, based on the child's physical examination and weight loss (Tables 11-8 and 11-9). An estimate of fluid loss is made by considering that 1 g of weight is equal to 1 ml of fluid. Adelman and Solhaug[13] also note that fluid loss can be approximated by capillary refill time. Specifically, a capillary refill of less than 2 seconds is associated with a fluid loss of less than 50 ml/kg; capillary refill time of 2 to 3 seconds is associated with losses of 50 to 90 ml/kg; and capillary refill time greater than 3 seconds occurs with losses of 100 ml/kg or more.

◆ **TABLE 11-8** **Clinical Assessment of Severity of Dehydration**

Signs and Symptoms	Mild Dehydration	Moderate Dehydration	Severe Dehydration
General Appearance and Condition			
Infants and young children	Thirsty, alert, restless	Thirsty, restless or lethargic but irritable to touch or drowsy	Drowsy, limp, cold, sweaty, cyanotic extremities, may be comatose
Older children and adults	Thirsty, alert, restless	Thirsty, alert, postural hypotension	Usually conscious, apprehensive, cold, sweaty, cyanotic extremities, wrinkled skin of fingers and toes, muscle cramps
Radial pulse	Normal rate and strength	Rapid and weak	Rapid, feeble, sometimes impalpable
Respiration	Normal	Deep, may be rapid	Deep and rapid
Anterior fontanelle	Normal	Sunken	Very sunken
Systolic blood pressure	Normal	Normal or low Orthostatic hypotension	Low, may be unrecordable
Skin elasticity	Pinch retracts immediately	Pinch retracts slowly	Pinch retracts very slowly (>2 seconds)
Eyes	Normal	Sunken (detectable)	Grossly sunken
Tears	Present	Absent	Absent
Mucous membranes	Moist	Dry	Very dry
Urine output	Normal	Reduced amount and dark	None passed for several hours, empty bladder
Body weight loss	3%-5%	6%-9%	≥10%
Estimated fluid deficit	30-50 ml/kg	60-90 ml/kg	≥100 ml/kg

Data from Adelman RD, Solhaug MJ: Pathophysiology of body fluids and fluid therapy. In Behrman RE, ed: *Nelson textbook of pediatrics,* ed 15, Philadelphia, 1996, WB Saunders, pp 185-222.

◆ **TABLE 11-9** **Effects of Type of Dehydration on Physical Signs**

Parameter	Isonatremic Dehydration (Proportionate Loss of Water and Sodium)	Hyponatremic Dehydration (Loss of Sodium in Excess of Water)	Hypernatremic Dehydration (Loss of Water in Excess of Sodium)
ECF volume	Markedly decreased	Severely decreased	Decreased
ICF volume	Maintained	Increased	Decreased
Physical signs			
Skin color*	Gray	Gray	Gray
Temperature	Cold	Cold	Cold or hot
Turgor†	Poor	Very poor	Fair
Feel	Dry	Clammy	Thickened, doughy
Mucous membranes	Dry	Slightly moist	Parched‡
Eyeball	Sunken and Soft	Sunken and soft	Sunken
Fontanelle	Sunken	Sunken	Sunken
Psyche	Lethargic	Coma	Hyperirritable
Pulse*	Rapid	Rapid	Moderately rapid
Blood pressure*	Low	Very low	Moderately low

Data from McCarthy PL: General considerations in the care of sick children. In Behrman RE, ed: *Nelson textbook of pediatrics,* ed 14, Philadelphia, 1992, WB Saunders, pp 171-211.
*Signs of shock rather than of dehydration itself.
†Reflects magnitude of fluid loss from ECF.
‡Tongue often has shriveled appearance because of loss of cellular fluid.
ECF, Extracellular fluid; *ICF,* Intracellular fluid.

Initial therapy for the child with a fluid volume deficit is directed toward quickly expanding ECF compartment volume to treat or prevent shock. Repeated boluses of 10 to 20 ml/kg of Ringer's lactate or normal saline (NS) is usually administered. For the child with severe dehydration, rapid fluid resuscitation with up to 60 ml/kg may be necessary. Peripheral perfusion, heart rate, urine output, and blood pressure are monitored to determine the child's response to therapy.

Once initial resuscitation has been accomplished, therapy is directed toward definitive water and electrolyte replacement. For isotonic or hypotonic dehydration, one half of the calculated fluid loss is replaced along with maintenance fluids over the next 8 hours, usually with 5% dextrose and 0.45% NS.[14] The calculated fluid loss can be determined by multiplying the assessed percentage of dehydration by the child's body weight. For example, a 10-kg child who is 10% dehydrated has lost 10% of his or her body weight, or 100 ml/kg, for a total fluid loss of 1000 ml.[14] Calculation of maintenance fluid is presented in Table

11-10. Potassium chloride (20 mEq/L) may be added once urine output has been established. Ongoing losses may be replaced concurrently with Ringer's lactate. The other half of the calculated loss along with maintenance fluid is replaced over the next 16 hours, usually with 5% dextrose and 0.45% NS with 20 mEq/L of potassium. The resuscitation bolus of Ringer's lactate or NS is not included in the calculation to determine deficit and maintenance needs.[14] An example of fluid replacement in a dehydrated child is presented in Table 11-11.

Fluid resuscitation as described earlier is the initial treatment, if appropriate, for moderate to severe dehydration. After initial therapy, further replacement is calculated as maintenance plus estimated fluid deficit given evenly over the next 48 to 72 hours, with 5% dextrose and 0.2% NS being the fluid of choice. Fluid replacement that occurs too rapidly can precipitate neurologic complications hallmarked by seizure activity.

An additional early consideration for the child with hyponatremic dehydration is sodium replacement. If the child is severely hyponatremic (serum sodium <120 mEq/L), a 3% solution of sodium chloride (NaCl) can be rapidly given. Four ml/kg is usually given over 10 minutes to return the serum sodium level to 125 mEq/L.[14]

The extent of hypernatremic dehydration is more difficult to assess because water moves from the intracellular to the extracellular space, thus preserving the circulating volume. Seizures may develop before or during replacement therapy and are thought to be the result of intracellular dehydration. Long-term neurologic sequelae and death may result.

Serum Na correction in hypernatremia takes place no faster than 0.5 to 1 mEq/L/hr because rapid correction of serum sodium can lead to cerebral edema. During replacement therapy, serum sodium levels are monitored every 4 hours. If serum sodium levels decrease too rapidly, the rate of hydration is decreased or the sodium content in the replacement fluid is increased. If levels decrease too slowly, the rate of hydration is increased. If the child demonstrates neurologic symptoms, cerebral edema is suspected and treated.

TABLE 11-10 Calculation of Maintenance Fluid

Per Day Body Weight (kg)	Fluid Requirements/Day
<10	100 ml/kg
10-20	1000 ml + 50 ml/kg for each kg above 10
>20	1500 ml + 20 ml/kg for each kg above 20

Per Hour Body Weight (kg)	Fluid Requirements/Hr
<10	4 ml/kg
10-20	2 ml/kg for each kg above 10
>20	1 ml/kg for each kg above 20

TABLE 11-11 Fluid Replacement in Dehydration

To calculate the fluid requirements for a 20-kg child who is 10% dehydrated (serum sodium level of 132 mEq/L).

Deficit	20 kg ×10% (or 100 ml/kg) = 2000 ml
Maintenance	(10 kg × 4 ml/kg/hr) + (10 kg × 2 ml/kg/hr) = 60 ml/hr

Time	Administered Fluid
0-30 minutes	20 ml/kg Ringer's lactate
30 min-8 hours	1/2 the deficit (1000 ml)/8 hours = 125 ml/hr + maintenance fluids (60 ml/hr) or 185 ml/hr of D₅ .45 NS + 20 mEq/L potassium
9-24 hours	1/2 the deficit (1000 ml)/16 hours = 63 ml/hr + maintenance fluids (60 ml/hr) or 123 ml/hr of D₅ .45 NS + 20 mEq/L potassium

From Wetzel RC: Shock and fluid resuscitation. In Nichols DG et al, eds: *Golden hour: the handbook of advanced pediatric life support*, St Louis, 1996, Mosby.
NS, Normal saline.

Fluid Volume Excess

Etiology. Fluid volume excess or fluid volume overload is defined as the actual excess of total body fluid or a relative excess in one or more fluid compartments.[6] It occurs when there is (1) increased sodium concentration and water volume because of retention and/or excessive intake, (2) decreased renal excretion of water and sodium, and (3) decreased mobilization of fluid within the intracellular space.[6] The major causes of excess fluid volume in critically ill infants and children are cardiorespiratory dysfunction, renal dysfunction, and inappropriate secretion of ADH, in which serum sodium levels are decreased in the presence of fluid overload.

Pathophysiology. As with dehydration, fluid volume overload may be classified as isotonic, hypotonic, or hypertonic. The most commonly occurring types of fluid volume overload are isotonic and hypotonic.[6]

Isotonic fluid excess or hypervolemia occurs when excess fluid is in the ECF compartment in both the intravascular and interstitial spaces. Common causes of isotonic fluid excess include excessive fluid administration or the use of hypotonic fluids to replace isotonic losses. The hypervolemia causes an increase in blood pressure, which results in an increased venous return to the heart or increased preload. This increased preload causes stretching of the myocardium and an increase in cardiac output. This response stimulates an increase in the GFR, which results in increased excretion of water and sodium.

Hypotonic fluid excess is also known as water intoxication. Common causes include syndrome of inappropriate antidiuretic hormone (SIADH) (see Chapter 23), excessive water intake, and congestive heart failure. This condition occurs when the excess fluid is hypotonic to other body fluids, resulting in a decrease in plasma osmolality. The resulting osmotic gradient causes ECF compartment to shift into the ICF compartment. Overexpansion of all body fluid compartments and dilutional electrolyte deficits then occur.

Critical Care Management. The goal of management is to restore fluid balance, correct any electrolyte imbalances that may be present, and eliminate or control the cause of the fluid volume excess. The critically ill infant or child with fluid volume excess has the potential to develop heart failure and pulmonary or cerebral edema, which are potentially life-threatening complications. Excessive ECF compartment volume is usually treated by eradicating the underlying causes, as well as reducing the excessive volume. General fluid volume excess is treated with fluid restriction and the use of diuretics (if renal function is adequate). Low-dose dopamine may be useful to increase renal blood flow and promote sodium and water excretion. Sodium restriction may be used to indirectly decrease fluid retention.

Children with certain conditions, such as septic shock, may manifest signs and symptoms of pulmonary edema, despite the presence of hypovolemia. This occurs because of increased capillary permeability, which results in capillary "leak." Therefore interventions may be required to treat the pulmonary edema, increase the ECF compartment volume, and treat the underlying shock.

ELECTROLYTE DISORDERS

Sodium

Sodium is the major cation of the extracellular compartment. It regulates the voltage of action potentials in skeletal muscles, nerves, and the myocardium. The action or diffusion potential of the cell membrane occurs in response to the sodium and potassium concentration in the ECF compartment and the ICF compartment. Sodium plays a significant role in the maintenance of acid-base balance through combining with anions such as chloride and bicarbonate. Sodium is also responsible for the maintenance of water balance (volume) in the ECF compartment through maintenance of the osmotic pressure (osmolality). Consequently, imbalances in water and sodium often occur together and are equated with alteration in serum osmolality. Extracellular sodium concentration is normally 135 to 145 mEq/L. The intracellular sodium concentration is usually 3 to 5 mEq/L.

Sodium is actively absorbed by the intestines and excreted by the kidneys and skin. The kidneys regulate sodium excretion primarily under the influence of the renin-angiotensin-aldosterone system. Renin is released by the kidneys in response to sodium concentration changes in the tubular fluid. The major factors that influence sodium excretion are GFR and aldosterone. Alterations in the sodium levels in the body are often the result of clinical conditions involving fluid volume excess or deficit.

Hyponatremia

Etiology. Hyponatremia is defined as a serum sodium concentration below 135 mEq/L. It is usually a secondary manifestation of another disease state. In the critically ill child, hyponatremia may occur as the result of excess water retention in the ECF compartment, sodium loss from the ECF compartment, or both. Hyponatremia may occur in conjunction with hypovolemia, euvolemia, or hypervolemia. However, true hyponatremia must be differentiated from pseudohyponatremia. Pseudohyponatremia is a falsely low serum sodium value that may occur in patients with hyperlipidemia, hyperproteinemia, or both. In children, diabetes mellitus is the most common cause of pseudohyponatremia.

Pathophysiology. Decreases in serum sodium cause a shift in water from the ECF compartment to the ICF compartment, resulting in generalized cellular swelling or edema. In the brain, where there is limited capacity for expansion, the development of cerebral edema can have catastrophic consequences (i.e., cerebral herniation and death). The severity of the sodium deficit and the speed with which it occurs have the most impact on the severity of the clinical symptoms. Serum sodium levels of less than 120 mEq/L are associated with seizures and coma. This is related to the development of cerebral edema, resulting from cellular swelling, and may be severe enough to cause cerebral herniation and death. Children who develop hyponatremia less acutely (over several days to weeks) may be asymptomatic or may develop only lethargy, nausea, and vomiting.

Hyponatremia occurs most often with hypervolemia in situations when the retention of water exceeds that of sodium. Causes include water intoxication, nephrotic syndrome, cardiac failure, cirrhosis, renal failure, and SIADH. In this situation, the hyponatremia is usually dilutional, so true total body sodium is normal or even elevated.

Hyponatremia in conjunction with hypovolemia is less common but may occur with renal or extrarenal losses. Losses may occur through diarrhea and vomiting, third spacing, or other disorders such as burns. Other causes include excessive use of diuretics, osmotic diuresis, and adrenal insufficiency.

Critical Care Management. The management of a child with hyponatremia varies depending on the relationship to fluid volume. In severe symptomatic hyponatremia with hypovolemia, serum sodium levels are rapidly elevated to 120 to 125 mEq/L by infusion of a hypertonic 3% saline solution. The amount of 3% saline necessary to raise the serum sodium level is judged to be 4 ml/kg or is calculated by the formula[15]:

$$(125 \text{ mEq/L} - \text{Observed Na}^+ \text{ zmEq/L}) \times \text{Body weight (kg)} \times 0.6 \text{ L/kg}$$

A solution of 3% saline contains approximately 0.5 mEq Na/mL and is given at a rate of 1 mEq/kg/hr (see Table 11-7). Serum sodium levels are monitored closely. If shock is present because of hypovolemia, 0.9% NS is given rapidly. Ongoing losses are replaced, and specific treatment of the underlying cause is given.

Correction of hyponatremia with hypervolemia is directed toward treatment of the underlying cause. Administration of saline to increase sodium levels is not recommended because total body sodium may be normal and saline infusion may expand the ECF compartment, worsening the situation. TBW may be decreased by fluid restriction up to as much as 50% maintenance.

Hypernatremia

Etiology. Hypernatremia is defined as an excess of sodium in the ECF compartment. It exists when serum sodium levels exceed 145 mEq/L. Hypernatremia may occur as the result of pure sodium excess or of water deficit. Pure sodium excess is unusual but has been reported as a result of feeding improperly mixed high-sodium rehydration solutions or formulas to infants or to older children who cannot gain water by themselves.[16] Sodium excess may also occur as the result of excessive administration of sodium bicarbonate during resuscitation endeavors.

In addition to an actual increase in sodium, hypernatremia can result from losses of water or from water deficit in excess of sodium deficit.[17] Conditions that produce fluid deficit and hypernatremia include diabetes insipidus, diabetes mellitus, excess sweating, increased insensible water loss, diarrhea, dehydration, and lack of thirst.[16]

Pathophysiology. Typically, when serum sodium begins to rise, the body responds with the release of ADH and stimulation of the thirst mechanism in an attempt to retain water and decrease serum sodium. However, in the critically ill infant and child, this response may not be sufficient to prevent the serum sodium from continuing to rise.

Hypernatremia initially causes a generalized shrinking of cells as fluid moves from the ICF compartment to the ECF compartment. Central nervous system (CNS) dysfunction often accompanies serum sodium concentrations over 158 mEq/L.[9] The CNS changes are thought to be the result of several mechanisms, including intracellular dehydration; shift of fluid from brain cells to cerebral vessels leading to subdural, subarachnoid, and intracerebral bleeding; decreased microvascular perfusion related to increased blood viscosity caused by increased plasma osmolarity; and intracranial bleeding caused by damage to the bridging veins as brain content contracts away from the skull.[15] Symptoms progress from restlessness and irritability through ataxia and tremulousness, tonic jerks, seizures, and eventually to death if uncorrected.[16] Although the severity of the symptoms is directly related to the level of excess sodium, recovery from the CNS dysfunction appears unrelated, and neurologic sequelae are common.[2]

Critical Care Management. Hypernatremia may produce serious problems related to CNS dysfunction (see Table 11-3). The severity of the initial clinical signs is not predictive of the degree of residual neurologic impairment. Therefore although careful attention must be directed at monitoring the child with hypernatremia, evaluating children at risk for hypernatremia is also important to prevent neurologic dysfunction from occurring. Frequent assessments of the child's neurologic status, fluid gains and losses, and serum sodium levels are done throughout the treatment of hypernatremia.

Treatment of hypernatremia is directed toward removal of excess sodium, if present, and correction of the underlying disorder. If fluid volume deficit is severe and shock is present or imminent, volume expansion must be undertaken, regardless of sodium levels. Isotonic solutions such as NS or Ringer's lactate solution are used in initial treatment. After initial stabilization and blood pressure recovery, hypotonic fluids may be administered to bring sodium levels down at the rate of 0.5 mEq/L/hr.[16] More rapid reduction is associated with neurologic morbidity and mortality. Administration of fluid without sodium is never indicated, even during correction.

Children with hypernatremia and fluid volume deficit are at significant risk for cerebral edema and seizures with rapid correction of fluid deficit. Volume deficits are replaced over 48 to 72 hours after initial intervention to prevent shock.

For children with increased total body sodium and overhydration, excess sodium may be removed through the use of diuretics and decreased sodium administration if renal function is intact. If renal function is not intact, dialysis may be required.[18]

Potassium

Potassium has four major roles in the body. As the primary intracellular cation, potassium plays an important role in the action potentials in the nervous system, skin and smooth muscles, and the cardiac conduction system. Acid-base balance is enhanced through the maintenance of electroneutrality of the body fluids. In cell anabolism, potassium is released from cells when the body relies on cell catabolism for energy. The biochemical reactions related to carbohydrate metabolism and synthesis of proteins also require potassium. Maintenance of intracellular osmolarity is accomplished through the sodium-potassium (active transport) pump (see Fig. 11-5). The normal range of serum potassium is 3.5 to 5.5 mEq/L, with a concentration of 160 mEq/L inside the cell.

Potassium excretion is enhanced by aldosterone, an increase in cellular potassium, and increased activity of the distal portion of the nephron. Aldosterone is the primary controller of potassium secretion by the kidneys.

Hypokalemia

Etiology. Hypokalemia is defined as a potassium deficit in the ECF compartment, with a serum potassium concentration of less than 3.5 mEq/L. Hypokalemia occurs as the result of either a true deficit of potassium or a shift in potassium out of the intravascular space into the intracellular space. Excessive renal secretion, excessive gastrointestinal losses, and excessive sweating or decreased intake of potassium (rare)[19] can cause a true deficit of potassium. A shift of potassium out of the intravascular space into the intracellular space can be caused by an increased cellular uptake of potassium, which occurs with alkalosis or as the result of excessive secretion or administration of insulin, or in relation to increased cell production.

Pathophysiology. Serum potassium levels may not always provide an accurate representation of total body stores of potassium. Intracellular stores of potassium are quite high, and when a deficit in extracellular stores occurs, small quantities of intracellular potassium can be exchanged into the extracellular space. As a result, serum levels of potassium may remain within normal limits even though body stores are somewhat depleted. However, once this quantity of exchanged potassium is depleted, decreased serum potassium levels will indicate a decrease in total body potassium.[19] In addition, a decrease in serum potassium may be seen even though total body stores are adequate, as is seen when alkalosis is present, because alkalosis causes a shift of intravascular potassium into the cells.

Increased renal excretion of potassium typically occurs as a result of increased mineralocorticoid activity, acid-base disturbances, or increased sodium delivery to the nephron. Hyperaldosteronism increases renal wasting of potassium and can cause severe hypokalemia. Primary hyperaldosteronism occurs as the result of adrenal adenomas and adrenal hyperplasia. Secondary hyperaldosteronism is seen in patients with nephrotic syndrome, congestive heart failure, or malignant hypertension.[2]

Acid-base disturbances can cause deficits in potassium stores and hypokalemia as the result of increased potassium loss via the kidneys.[23] A decline in serum potassium accompanies respiratory and metabolic alkalosis because potassium ions move into the cells to maintain the transmembrane electrical potential. However, the most severe potassium deficiencies occur with metabolic alkalosis. In patients who are alkalotic, potassium is taken up by the cells from the ECF in exchange for hydrogen ions. In the initial stages of alkalosis, the serum hypokalemia that occurs is not reflective of body stores. However, as the alkalosis progresses, a marked depletion of body stores occurs as the result of increased exchange of potassium for hydrogen ions. The direction of the change in pH is opposite the change in serum potassium values.

The use of potassium-losing diuretics, such as thiazides or furosemide, results in increased sodium delivery to the distal nephrons. When this occurs in the presence of increased aldosterone concentrations, an increased amount of potassium is secreted into the tubular fluid and then lost in the urine.[19]

Gastrointestinal (GI) losses are a common cause of potassium depletion. The potassium concentration of gastric fluids is higher than that of serum concentration. Excessive losses of these fluids (i.e., through vomiting or nasogastric suctioning) can result in hypokalemia. This condition occurs because of an actual loss of potassium and as the result of the metabolic alkalosis associated with the GI losses.

Critical Care Management. Patients at risk for hypokalemia are monitored for ECG changes and alterations in their neuromuscular assessment (see Tables 11-3 and 11-4). The most significant problems caused by hypokalemia are related to cardiac dysfunction and muscle paralysis, including paralytic ileus. Treatment of hypokalemia is indicated whenever the serum potassium level falls below 3 mEq/L or the child exhibits symptoms related to hypokalemia.[15] Oral replacement is preferred if time and the child's condition permit. A dose of 0.5 to 1 mEq/kg (maximum, 20 mEq) usually corrects the hypokalemia if ongoing losses are controlled.[15] This dose may be repeated every 4 to 8 hours. If IV replacement is required, concentrations up to 40 mEq/L are considered safe. The underlying cause of the hypokalemia is considered and treated.

In severe cases of potassium depletion, in which serum potassium levels are below 2.5 mEq/L, IV potassium replacement is used. Dosages of 0.25 to 1 mEq/kg/hr may be given to correct severe depletion. The correction of hypokalemia is not an emergency and should be accomplished slowly because too rapid a correction may cause lethal hyperkalemia. Table 11-7 provides additional recommendations for administration. Continuous ECG monitoring for T wave assessments and frequent determination of serum potassium levels are critical to avoid complications associated with hyperkalemia.

If the child is alkalotic, potassium is replaced as the chloride salt because chloride depletion often accompanies hypokalemia.[20] If the child is hypokalemic and acidotic, serum potassium levels at a normal pH are lower. Thus correcting the pH before the hypokalemia can make the serum potassium level dangerously low.[20]

Hyperkalemia

Etiology. Hyperkalemia is an excess of potassium in the ECF, existing when the plasma potassium level exceeds 5.5 mEq/L.[21] The four general categories of causes are altered renal excretion, impaired extrarenal regulation, shift from the intracellular to extracellular fluid, and increased potassium intake.[22] Pseudohyperkalemia is relatively common and may be produced by conditions such as an increased white blood cell count above 100,000/mm^3 or a platelet count greater than 750,000/mm^3.[9] A release of intracellular potassium during the clotting process results in the abnormal serum potassium level seen in that circumstance.

Pathophysiology. Alterations in renal excretion of potassium may result from either a decrease in the GFR or a decrease in potassium secretion by the renal tubules.[21] Conditions associated with altered renal excretion include renal dysfunction and the administration of potassium-sparing diuretics such as spironolactone and triamterene.[22] Children with long-standing or congenital urologic abnormalities are likely to demonstrate subtly impaired renal potassium excretion. Reflux nephropathy, prune-belly syndrome, and obstructions associated with bilateral hydronephrosis are likely to be associated with dysfunction of tubular epithelium leading to abnormalities of potassium excretion.[22]

Impaired extrarenal regulation may be produced by such conditions as diabetes mellitus and adrenocortical insufficiencies or administration of drugs such as heparin, β-blocking agents, and angiotensin-converting enzyme (ACE) inhibitors. The absence of insulin limits the uptake of potassium from the ECF compartment.[12] Decreased mineralocorticoid activity impairs excretion of potassium by the kidney and colon, whereas drugs such as heparin or ACE inhibitors limit aldosterone release from the adrenal gland.[22]

The shift of potassium from intracellular to extracellular fluid may be produced by rapid cell breakdown, which can accompany cancer chemotherapy, burns or trauma, metabolic acidosis, hyperosmolar states, rhabdomyolysis, or the administration of succinylcholine.[22] In these cases, normal body stores of potassium may be available despite abnormal serum levels.

Hyperkalemia may also be produced by excessive intake of potassium, usually in the form of IV fluids or the oral ingestion of medications or food substances high in potassium. Although hyperkalemia may occur in young children by this mechanism, hyperkalemia related to excessive intake is most often linked with impaired renal function.

Critical Care Management. Hyperkalemia is one of the most dangerous electrolyte imbalances because of the potential to cause sudden death.[1] Hyperkalemia can eventually result in ventricular arrhythmias and cardiac arrest.[21]

Treatment of hyperkalemia depends on the clinical presentation. Potassium levels less than 6.5 mEq/L may require only discontinuation of fluids containing potassium along with close monitoring of serum potassium levels. Increasing potassium excretion with sodium polystyrene sulfonate (Kayexalate), especially in patients with diminished renal function, also helps to decrease potassium levels. Kayexalate, 1 to 2 g/kg, is given orally (PO), by nasogastric (NG) tube, or preferably, by rectum in a dextrose or sorbitol solution. Sorbitol precipitates diarrhea, which aids in potassium excretion. Kayexalate can be given every 6 hours orally or nasogastrically or every 2 to 6 hours rectally. Because Kayexalate may bind calcium and magnesium, symptoms related to deficiencies in these electrolytes may occur.

Potassium levels higher than 6.5 mEq/L or those producing ECG changes are treated immediately. In the presence of life-threatening arrhythmias, calcium gluconate at 100 mg/kg or calcium chloride at 20 mg/kg may be given to reduce the cardiac toxicity associated with hyperkalemia.[24] Calcium increases the cardiac threshold potential, thereby reducing membrane depolarization and reestablishing a more normal relationship between resting membrane potential and firing threshold.[24] The onset of action of calcium is within minutes, and the effects last for about 30 minutes.

Redistribution of potassium from the ECF compartment to ICF compartment decreases the elevated serum potassium level. This is accomplished by the administration of sodium bicarbonate, 1 to 2 mEq/kg, injected intravenously over 3 to 5 minutes. Sodium bicarbonate lowers the serum potassium level within 30 to 60 minutes, with the effects lasting several hours. Blood pH is monitored in children receiving this therapy. Children with respiratory failure are carefully evaluated because sodium bicarbonate increases carbon dioxide (CO_2) production and may worsen respiratory acidosis if CO_2 cannot be excreted by the lungs.

Glucose, 0.5 g/kg, accompanied by regular insulin, 0.1 U/kg, may also be used to shift potassium into the ICF compartment. Cellular uptake of potassium from the ECF compartment is enhanced with combined glucose and insulin administration. The decrease in serum potassium level associated with glucose and insulin therapy may last several hours.[24]

Albuterol, a β$_2$-adrenergic agonist, causes an acute decrease in plasma potassium and is another treatment option for hyperkalemia. Albuterol activates the sodium-potassium pump and stimulates the β$_2$-receptors of the pancreas to release insulin, thereby shifting potassium into the cells.[21] It is administered via inhalation or IV infusion. The recommendation is that albuterol be administered in conjunction with insulin because of the additive effect of the two drugs.[21]

The diuretic furosemide (Lasix) may also be used to aid in children with adequate renal function. However, the amount of potassium removed is unpredictable. Therefore diuretics are used only as an additional treatment modality.

The most rapid mechanism for potassium removal is renal replacement therapy (see Chapter 21). Although peritoneal dialysis may be used, it must be started early to be effective. Continuous venovenous filtration or hemodialysis is used when potassium levels are lethal and emergency life-saving treatment is necessary.

Calcium

Calcium, along with phosphorus and magnesium, plays a critical role in nerve transmission, bone composition, and regulation of enzymatic processes. Balance of these three electrolytes is maintained through intestinal absorption and renal excretion. The majority of calcium (98% to 99%) is stored in the skeleton and teeth, and the remainder is found in soft tissue and serum. Approximately 50% of serum calcium is ionized; the rest is bound to protein or anions. Only ionized calcium is used by the body for essential processes such as cardiac function, muscular contraction, nerve impulse transmission, and clotting. Therefore the ionized calcium level is of greatest physiologic significance. Because ionized calcium level has little relationship to total serum calcium, direct measurement of ionized calcium is critical whenever a clinically important situation exists in which calcium levels may play a role. Total serum calcium levels range between 9 and 11 mg/dl; ionized calcium levels range between 4.4 and 5.4 mg/dl (1.14 to 1.29 mmol/L).

The roles of calcium in the body are conduction of electrical impulses in cardiac and skeletal muscles, activation of clotting mechanisms, involvement in the coagulation process, formation of bones and teeth, and mediation of hormonal production. Calcium also activates serum complement, a major factor in the function of the immune system. Calcium lines the pores of all cells and, with its positive charge, controls the ability of sodium to enter during depolarization because like charges repel each other. Consequently, calcium aids in the maintenance of cellular permeability.

Calcium regulation takes place through many different factors. Vitamin D-1,25 controls the intestinal absorption of calcium. Parathyroid hormone (PTH) regulates renal excretion of calcium. PTH secretion varies inversely with ionized calcium levels and is inhibited by hypomagnesemia and vitamin $D_{1,25}$.[25] Vitamin D, PTH, and serum phosphate levels control bone deposition and resorption of calcium.

Normally, because of the constant activity of bone deposition and resorption, there is little net change in serum calcium. However, when this activity is disturbed, bone is a reservoir to balance serum calcium levels. PTH, along with vitamin D-1,25 can change the degree of bone resorption. With increased levels of PTH, release of calcium from the bone is increased.

As mentioned earlier, PTH controls renal calcium regulation in the distal nephron. Renal calcium reabsorption increases with increases in serum PTH.

Hypocalcemia

Etiology. Hypocalcemia is a decrease of calcium in the ECF and exists when serum calcium levels are below 8 mg/dl in full-term infants and older children and when ionized calcium levels are below 4 mg/dl. Hypocalcemia in children may be related to protein malnutrition because decreased albumin for binding leads to decreased calcium levels. Other causes are listed in Box 11-1. Alterations in acid-base balance may also result in hypocalcemia.

Pathophysiology. Though the definition of hypocalcemia reflects a deficit in ECF concentration, the majority of calcium is bound either to bone or to protein. Because serum stores are replaced through the action of PTH, most discussions of hypocalcemia are related to parathyroid function. In addition, absorption of calcium from the intestinal tract, excretion from the kidneys, and bone rebuilding help regulate the available stores.

Approximately 40% of the total serum calcium is bound to protein. Changes in plasma protein levels affect total serum calcium levels. Hypoalbuminemia decreases total serum calcium, and increased levels have the opposite effect. Changes in serum albumin levels affect calcium. For every 1 mg/dl change in albumin from the normal value, a corresponding 0.8 mg/dl change occurs in ionized calcium.[26] The binding of calcium to protein is affected by pH. If the pH is normal, approximately 40% of the total plasma calcium is bound to the serum albumin. An increase in pH as seen with alkalosis increases binding and decreases ionized calcium. Even though the ionized calcium level is changed, total serum calcium levels may be unchanged.

Critical Care Management. The child with hypocalcemia may be asymptomatic but requires monitoring for clinical signs and symptoms (see Table 11-3), with particular attention paid to neurologic, neuromuscular, and cardiac examinations. In addition, these children are monitored for changes in their ECG (see Table 11-4).

The total serum calcium, magnesium and phosphate levels, and serum ionized calcium are useful laboratory tests in managing hypocalcemia. Arterial blood gases may demonstrate respiratory alkalosis as a cause of hypocalcemia. Because hypocalcemia may be linked to parathyroid dysfunction, complete evaluation may include analysis of PTH levels. In addition, because hypocalcemia is associated

---

Box 11-1

◆ Causes of Hypocalcemia

Hypoparathyroidism (primary or surgically induced)	Nephrotic syndrome
Hypomagnesemia	Renal failure
Hyperphosphatemia	Acute pancreatitis
Inadequate vitamin D	Burns
Decreased intake	Gram-negative sepsis
Malabsorption syndromes	Chemotherapy
Protein malnutrition	Transfusion with citrate-preserved blood
Parenchymal liver disease	Certain medications: aminoglycosides, glucagon, phenobarbital, phenytoin
Anticonvulsant therapy	

Data from Metheny NM: *Fluid and electrolyte balance: nursing considerations,* ed 2, Philadelphia, 1992, JB Lippincott, pp 98-100.

with hypoproteinemia, plasma protein levels may be evaluated (Table 11-12).

Two major areas of concern in the child experiencing hypocalcemia are neuromuscular dysfunction and altered cardiac function. Treatment of hypocalcemia is directed at both identification of the underlying cause and correction of the alteration. Treatment of underlying conditions that are causing hypocalcemia is considered. Respiratory alkalosis is readily treatable. If hyperphosphatemia exists, correction is necessary because administration of calcium may cause deposition of calcium-phosphate salts. A calcium-phosphate product in a dose higher (*total serum calcium × phosphate*) than 80 mg/dl is avoided.[15] Because hypomagnesemia affects PTH release and correction of hypocalcemia, this complication is considered and treated if hypocalcemia is severe or persistent. Any other underlying conditions, such as renal disease or hypoproteinemia, are also treated.

Acute hypocalcemia, especially in the child with impending neuromuscular or cardiovascular collapse, requires restoration of the serum ionized calcium level. Treatment is provided by IV administration of either calcium gluconate (9 mg elemental calcium/ml) or calcium chloride (36 mg elemental calcium/ml). The dosage for calcium gluconate is 100 mg/kg; the dose for calcium chloride is 10 to 20 mg/kg. Less thrombophlebitis and tissue necrosis with extravasation is noted with calcium gluconate, although all solutions with calcium salts are capable of causing tissue damage with extravasation. For this reason, calcium salts are administered through a central vein. Calcium is used cautiously in the digitalized child because calcium may potentiate digoxin toxicity. Rapid administration of calcium may cause bradycardia and asystole, and thus ECG monitoring and slow administration (50 mg/min for $CaCl_2$; 100 mg/min for Ca gluconate) are indicated (see Table 11-7).

Hypercalcemia

Etiology. Hypercalcemia is an excess of calcium in the ECF compartment and exists when the total serum calcium level exceeds 10.5 to 11 mg/dl.[6] However, symptoms are not usually noted until the serum calcium level is higher than 12 mg/dl. Levels higher than 15 mg/dl may be life threatening. Hypercalcemia is not a common occurrence. In general, it is caused by excessive amounts of calcium moving from the bones and intestines into the ECF compartment. A pseudohypercalcemia may be seen in children with a fluid volume deficit when an increase in serum calcium levels is caused by a concentrational effect. Specific conditions associated with hypercalcemia may include iatrogenic overtreatment of hypocalcemia, malignancies or neoplasms, immobility, hypophosphatemia, hyperparathyroidism, vitamin D intoxication, use of thiazide diuretics, hypophosphatasia, and familial hypercalcemia. It is seen most commonly in the critically ill child concurrently with hyponatremia and hyperkalemia and as chronic renal failure resolves.

Pathophysiology. Hypercalcemia occurs when calcium influx into the ECF compartment overwhelms the calcium regulatory hormones (PTH and vitamin D) and renal excretion mechanisms or when an abnormality of one or both of these hormones exists.[27] As discussed earlier, protein and pH also affect calcium levels. Increased albumin levels result in increased serum calcium levels. A decrease in serum pH as seen with acidosis increases ionized calcium. In this situation, more calcium is removed from protein-binding sites and is available for participation in chemical reactions.

Critical Care Management. Patients who are at risk for and those with hypercalcemia are identified and monitored for the clinical manifestations of hypercalcemia (see Table 11-3), with emphasis placed on the neurologic and GI examinations. The ECG is monitored for changes (see Table 11-4). Laboratory values are monitored and may include serum calcium, ionized calcium, and plasma protein levels and parathyroid hormone concentration (see Table 11-12).

Because serum calcium levels above 15 mg/dl may be life threatening, immediate attention is directed at reducing the amount of calcium in the ECF compartment in addition to treating the underlying disorder. This is accomplished by administration of IV fluids to dilute the calcium in the ECF compartment. Loop diuretics, such as furosemide, may also be used to enhance calcium excretion.[17] These therapies can also produce losses of sodium, potassium, magnesium, and phosphate.[25] Thiazide diuretics restrict calcium excretion and are therefore contraindicated in the management of hypercalcemia.[28] Vitamin D and antacids with calcium are not administered.

Additional therapies may be used to treat the underlying disorder. If excessive bone resorption because of malignancy or immobility is a problem, calcitonin (10 U/kg IV every 4 to 6 hours), mithramycin (25 μg/kg IV over 4 hours), prednisone (1 to 2 mg/kg/day IV divided into four doses), and indomethacin (1 mg/kg/day) may inhibit the process.[25] Calcitonin is the least toxic and works by impeding PTH-induced bone resorption. It peaks at about 1 hour after administration.

Mithramycin is a toxic antibiotic that inhibits osteoclastic activity, but it depresses liver, kidney, and bone marrow function. Prednisone inhibits osteoclastic activity and intestinal absorption of calcium. Indomethacin acts only when bone resorption is the result of prostaglandin-secreting tumors, which are rare. IV or oral phosphorus preparations may be used to increase bone deposition of calcium,

TABLE 11-12 **Normal Laboratory Values in Assessment of Calcium Alterations**

Test	Normal Values
Calcium (total)	
Infant	7.0-12.0 mg/dl
Child	8.0-11.0 mg/dl
Adolescent	8.5-11.0 mg/dl
Calcium (ionized)	4.4-5.4 mg/dl
Plasma protein (total)	
Infant (1-3 mo)	4.7-7.4 g/dl
Infant (3-12 mo)	5-7.5 g/dl
Child (1-15 yr)	6.5-8.6 g/dl
Serum parathyroid hormone	
C-terminal	400-900 pg/ml
N-terminal	200-600 pg/ml

although they are not used in patients with hyperphosphatemia or renal failure because of the risk of calcification in the soft tissues.

Chloride

Chloride is the most abundant anion found in the ECF compartment. Its major role is as a buffer in the maintenance of acid-base balance. Chloride, with sodium, also maintains serum osmolality. Chloride competes with bicarbonate for the cations in ECF compartment to establish electrical neutrality. Passively attracted to positively charged cations, chloride ions balance the positively charged electrolytes in ECF compartment and create sodium chloride (NaCl), hydrochloric acid (HCl), potassium chloride (KCl), and calcium chloride ($CaCl_2$). Because chloride is usually combined with one of the major cations in the body, changes in serum chloride levels usually indicate changes in other electrolytes or in acid-base balance.[17]

Chloride ions are highly concentrated in gastric secretions and perspiration. Factors influencing excretion are acidosis and alkalosis because as serum levels of bicarbonate change from the secretion of hydrogen ions, reciprocal changes in the serum chloride commonly occur.[13] Normal serum chloride levels in children are 95 to 108 mEq/L.

Hypochloremia

Etiology. Hypochloremia is a deficit of chloride in the ECF compartment, which exists when serum chloride levels are below 95 mEq/L. The most common causes of hypochloremia include GI losses, renal losses, and loss of chloride through excessive sweating.[6]

Pathophysiology. Hypochloremia may occur in conjunction with metabolic alkalosis. When chloride decreases, bicarbonate increases in an effort to maintain the electrical neutrality of the ECF compartment. Thus as the chloride decreases, the kidneys retain extra bicarbonate ions to balance the sodium ions. This in turn results in a hypochloremic metabolic alkalosis. Chronic lung disease (respiratory acidosis) may also be associated with hypochloremia. This condition results from the renal compensation and reabsorption of bicarbonate, which occurs in response to the respiratory acidosis.

Hypochloremia may also occur when the loss of chloride from the body exceeds sodium losses. It may be caused by excessive loss of gastric secretions or prolonged diarrhea or as a consequence of excessive use of potent diuretics. Urinary losses of chloride may exceed sodium losses during correction of metabolic acidosis and during potassium deficiency. Hypochloremia may occur as the result of limitation of chloride intake, which might accompany salt-restricted diets, and excessive sweating, such as that seen with the febrile child.

Critical Care Management. Table 11-3 lists the clinical findings seen in a child with chloride loss that is disproportionate to sodium loss. When there has been proportionate loss of sodium and chloride, clinical findings are characteristic of those found in hyponatremia and fluid volume deficit. Laboratory values are monitored and may

include serum chloride, serum sodium, and bicarbonate levels and pH. The pattern characteristic of hypochloremia is a decreased serum chloride, decreased serum sodium, and increased pH and bicarbonate levels.[13]

Prevention of chloride deficit is an important goal of management. The use of IV solutions containing chloride as opposed to water will help to prevent such a deficit.

Treatment for hypochloremia includes treating the primary underlying cause while correcting the imbalance. The imbalance is usually corrected through the administration of sodium chloride, potassium chloride, or ammonium chloride. Three fourths of the imbalance is often replaced with sodium chloride, and the remaining one fourth is replaced with potassium chloride. Ammonium chloride is used instead of potassium chloride if serum potassium levels are elevated.[26] A 0.9% solution of sodium chloride is used to correct chloride imbalance. The dose varies, based on the child's normal fluid volume requirements. Usually potassium chloride is given in a dose of 0.5 to 1 mEq/kg over a 1- to 2-hour period. The dosage of ammonium chloride is calculated by multiplying the serum chloride deficit by the ECF compartment volume (approximately 20% of body weight in kilograms).[29]

Hyperchloremia

Etiology. Hyperchloremia is an excess of chloride in the ECF compartment and exists when serum chloride levels exceed 108 mEq/L. Causes of hyperchloremia include excessive chloride intake, usually associated with medication administration, and conditions that lead to metabolic acidosis with excessive loss of bicarbonate ions, such as diarrhea, renal failure, and administration of isotonic saline solution.[17]

Pathophysiology. Hyperchloremia may present as a metabolic acidosis. The metabolic acidosis occurs as the result of a decrease in bicarbonate, which results in an increase in chloride, or as the result of an accumulation of hydrogen ions.

Hyperchloremia may also result from an excess of chloride ions being ingested or retained. Excess intake causes bicarbonate ions to be released in the kidney tubules, resulting in decreased serum bicarbonate levels. Chloride excess also occurs as the result of administration of cortisone preparations, which cause sodium retention; severe diarrhea, which results in a loss of bicarbonate ions; head injury and sodium retention; and acute renal failure.[6] A pseudo-hyperchloremia may be seen in fluid volume deficit as the result of a concentrational effect on serum chloride values.

Critical Care Management. When chloride excess occurs proportionately to sodium excess, the signs and symptoms associated with hypernatremia or fluid volume deficit predominate. Laboratory values including serum chloride, sodium, and bicarbonate levels and pH are monitored. The pattern of laboratory values seen in hyperchloremia includes elevated serum chloride and sodium and decreased bicarbonate and pH levels. The changes in pH and bicarbonate levels reflect the acid-base disturbance that accompanies hyperchloremia rather than the hyperchloremia itself.

Treatment of hyperchloremia includes identification of the underlying cause and correction of acid-base disturbances and electrolyte and fluid imbalances. Fluids (either oral or IV) may be increased to dilute the excess chloride. In an emergency, sodium bicarbonate may be administered to correct the underlying metabolic acidosis. Diuretics may be used to eliminate chloride, as well as sodium.

Phosphate

Phosphate, like calcium, is present in large quantities in bone. Eighty-five percent of phosphorus is held in the bone with calcium. Ten percent of phosphorus is found in the ECF compartment. Phosphorus is also found in the teeth and soft tissues, and 5% of the total level is in the ICF compartment. Phosphorus, the primary intracellular anion, exists in a variety of forms as phosphate and elemental phosphorus. Phosphates (components of phosphoproteins and phospholipids) play a significant role in intracellular energy-producing reactions. In addition, phosphates influence tissue oxygenation, CNS function, carbohydrate use, and leukocyte function. Tissue oxygenation is dependent on the ability of red blood cells (RBCs) to transport oxygen to the tissues and on 2,3-diphosphoglycerate (2,3-DPG), an organic phosphate in RBCs that binds hemoglobin and decreases its affinity for oxygen. The kidney plays the major role in phosphorus homeostasis. More than 90% of plasma phosphate is filtered at the kidney, and most reabsorption occurs in the proximal tubule.

Serum phosphorus levels are higher in the pediatric population because of the high rate of skeletal growth. The normal serum phosphate level may be as high as 6 mg/dl in infants and children, compared with levels of 2.5 to 4.5 mg/dl in adults.

Hypophosphatemia

Etiology. Hypophosphatemia is defined as an abnormally low concentration of inorganic phosphorus in serum. In children, levels below 3 mg/dl are usually defined as hypophosphatemia, although symptoms may not be present until the level is below 2 mg/dl.[12] Levels lower than 1 mg/dl may be life threatening. Hypophosphatemia may occur as the result of a total body deficit or may be a reflection of a shift of phosphorus into the cells. The major causes of phosphate deficiency are severely limited intake, shift of phosphate from the ECF compartment into the cell, decreased absorption from the GI tract, and increased renal phosphate excretion.[30]

Pathophysiology. Because phosphorus is abundant in normally consumed foods and beverages, limited intake of phosphate is related to vomiting or long-term starvation. Cellular shifts of phosphorus may occur during rapid cellular growth or hypermetabolic states. Intestinal malabsorption of phosphate may occur because of excessive use of antacids, which bind phosphorus in the GI tract, and malabsorption syndromes in which watery stools result, such as Crohn's disease or ulcerative colitis.[31] Malabsorption of phosphate also occurs in the presence of increased calcium levels. Increased renal phosphate losses occur with rapid catabolism and destruction of body tissue. Metabolic acidosis is the predominant finding when this mechanism of phosphate loss is present. In children, burns may also produce hypophosphatemia as a result of renal wasting.[32] In addition, diuretic administration may lead to renal tubular leaks.

Hypophosphatemia is also seen in children with diabetic ketoacidosis (because of renal wasting), as a concurrent finding with administration of cytotoxic agents for treatment of tumors, with phosphate-poor parenteral hyperalimentation, and when low-phosphate diets are used to treat renal failure.[17]

Hematologic changes are commonly encountered with hypophosphatemia. Hemolytic anemia may result from inadequate ATP for maintenance of the red cell membrane. Oxygen-hemoglobin binding capacity drops as a result of reduced availability of 2,3-DPG.[6] Leukocytes demonstrate decreased phagocytosis, and platelet abnormalities are also seen. The platelet abnormalities may account for increased epistaxis and GI bleeding in children with hypophosphatemia.[13]

Critical Care Management. Patients with or at risk for hypophosphatemia are assessed carefully for the clinical manifestations of this electrolyte imbalance (see Tables 11-3 and 11-4). Severe hypophosphatemia can affect multiple body systems and may result in coma and respiratory failure. Serum phosphorus, pH, and bicarbonate levels are monitored.

As with all electrolyte imbalances, the first step in the treatment process is to identify the underlying cause and take steps to correct it. Then, replacement of phosphorus is undertaken. Replacement is generally done very slowly because the actual serum level may not reflect a deficit in the intracellular compartment. Unless acute symptoms are present, phosphate depletion is treated by enteral administration of phosphorus 10 to 20 mg/kg/day divided into several doses to minimize diarrhea.[15] Parenteral administration of phosphates is usually restricted to children with levels below 1 mg/dl.[30] The dose generally recommended is 0.15 to 0.33 mmol/kg given as a continuous infusion over at least 6 hours (see Table 11-7). Subsequent dosages are based on the response to the initial dose. Either potassium or sodium phosphate may be used, with the potential complications associated with hyperkalemia or hypernatremia. Other adverse effects of phosphate administration include hyperphosphatemia, which may result in hypocalcemia, and hypotension. Care must be exercised in the administration of parenteral phosphorus. It must be well diluted to avoid irritation of the blood vessels, extravasation, or infiltration leading to tissue necrosis. Administration of large quantities of phosphorus may lead to precipitation with calcium if levels are not carefully monitored.[17]

Hyperphosphatemia

Etiology. Hyperphosphatemia is defined as an excess of phosphate in the ECF compartment and exists when phosphate levels exceed 4.5 mg/dl. Hyperphosphatemia may be produced by chronic renal failure, rapid cell catabolism, excessive intake of phosphates, neoplastic diseases, hypoparathyroidism, and excess consumption of vitamin D metabolites.[6,17] Elevated phosphate levels seldom become a concern unless renal excretion of phosphorus is impaired.

Pathophysiology. In chronic renal failure the renal tubules no longer excrete phosphorus, despite continued uptake in the GI system. The disruption in renal function accompanied by a decreased GFR leads to impaired phosphate elimination.

Rapid cell catabolism leads to the release of the cellular phosphorus stores into the ECF compartment. Children being treated with chemotherapy for neoplastic disease of lymphatic origin may also develop hyperphosphatemia because of leakage of phosphates into the circulation as a result of cytolysis.[2]

Hyperphosphatemia may also be seen in children at times of rapid growth because serum phosphate levels may reach 6 mg/dl during these periods. Vitamin D, which increases absorption of phosphorus in the GI tract, may be helpful in providing phosphorus for bone growth and cellular function.

Critical Care Management. Patients with hyperphosphatemia are monitored for the clinical manifestations of hyperphosphatemia and hypocalcemia (see Table 11-3). An inverse relationship exists between phosphorus and calcium in the ECF compartment. Therefore in conditions producing hyperphosphatemia, hypocalcemia also exists. The relationship between these two imbalances accounts for the fact that the clinical signs and symptoms associated with hyperphosphatemia are the same as those found in the child experiencing hypocalcemia. If the hyperphosphatemia is not associated with a hypocalcemia, phosphorus may precipitate into body tissues as phosphate salts, and conjunctivitis, pruritus, or renal deposits may occur.[6]

Serum phosphate and calcium levels are monitored. An elevated phosphate level is seen in conjunction with a clinically significant decreased serum calcium value.

Treatment should be directed both at determining the underlying cause and correcting the imbalance. Hyperphosphatemia may be treated using dietary restrictions of phosphorus. If this diet does not result in lowered phosphate levels, aluminum antacids may be used. The antacids bind with the phosphate in the intestines and thus facilitate elimination. Adequate hydration and correction of hypocalcemia also enhance phosphate elimination. If increased phosphorus is not the result of an influx of phosphorus related to renal failure, the administration of sodium bicarbonate may be used to enhance renal excretion of phosphorus.[6] For the child with life-threatening symptoms, fluids to increase renal phosphate losses, treatment of hypocalcemia, or dialysis may be indicated.

Magnesium

Magnesium is the fourth most abundant cation in the body and the second most abundant intracellular cation. The distribution of magnesium is similar to that of potassium and is approximately 60% in the mineral component of bone, 40% in the body cells, and less than 1% in the ECF compartment. The major roles of magnesium can be divided into three areas: enzyme and biochemical activation, mediation of skeletal muscle tension, and inhibition of electrical activity at the neuromuscular junction. Magnesium serves as a cofactor in numerous enzyme reactions that involve transfer of a phosphate group: metabolism of glucose, pyruvic acid, and ATP. Magnesium has a similar role to calcium as an inhibitor of electrical activity in neuromuscular function. Magnesium acts directly on the myoneural junction, affecting neuromuscular irritability and contractility of cardiac and skeletal smooth muscle.[3]

The serum magnesium concentration is regulated by the kidney, GI tract, and bones. However, the kidneys are the primary regulators. The kidneys have an extraordinary ability to conserve magnesium and with decreased intake of magnesium excrete less than 1 mEq/day. When the concentration of magnesium in the glomerular filtrate exceeds certain limits, large quantities of magnesium are lost in the urine.[33] Reabsorption occurs in the ascending limb of the loop of Henle and is modulated by the serum concentration of ionized magnesium.

Serum magnesium levels are a poor indicator of total body stores because less than 1% of total body magnesium exists in the serum. Normal magnesium levels in the child are 1.5 to 2.5 mEq/L. Magnesium levels show small variations, correlating directly with changes in serum calcium and inversely with phosphorus.[27] About 35% of the available magnesium is bound to protein.

Hypomagnesemia

Etiology. Hypomagnesemia generally exists when the serum magnesium level is less than 1.4 mEq/L. However, a decrease in serum magnesium is not always synonymous with a decrease in body stores. Two principal causes of decreased magnesium in the ECF compartment are decreased absorption or increased excretion.[30]

Pathophysiology. Decreased intestinal absorption of magnesium may occur intrinsically or may be drug induced (i.e., laxatives). Conditions that may be associated with decreased absorption include pancreatitis, chronic or severe diarrhea, prolonged nasogastric suctioning, prolonged vomiting, intestinal and biliary fistulas, and malabsorption syndromes.[33]

Increased renal excretion of magnesium can occur with the use of diuretics, in particular, loop diuretics and thiazides. Patients with conditions causing a rapid diuresis (i.e., diabetic ketoacidosis and hyperosmolar, hyperglycemic, nonketotic coma) also demonstrate an increased excretion of magnesium. Aminoglycoside antibiotics and antineoplastic agents may induce hypomagnesemia in children because these drugs cause renal magnesium wasting.[34] Hypomagnesemia may also be related to lack of magnesium administration during the time the child is NPO or caused by malnutrition.

Other imbalances seen with hypomagnesemia are hyponatremia, hypokalemia, hypophosphatemia, and distal renal tubular acidosis. Hypomagnesemia may damage the ATP-dependent sodium, potassium, phosphate, and hydrogen pumps, which would cause excess urinary losses of these electrolytes.[35]

Critical Care Management.   The infant or child with a decreased serum magnesium level is monitored closely for the clinical manifestations of hypomagnesemia (see Table 11-3). Despite generalized neuromuscular excitability, respiratory muscle depression and hypoventilation may occur, creating a need for mechanical ventilation.[30] Continuous ECG monitoring is indicated to assess for arrhythmias (see Table 11-4).

In addition, the child may present with many of the same clinical signs that are found with hypocalcemia. The signs and symptoms of hypomagnesemia are often compounded by the coexistence of hypocalcemia and hypokalemia. When these electrolyte disturbances are persistent, hypomagnesemia may also exist.

Serum magnesium, potassium, and calcium levels are monitored. Decreased serum magnesium levels are accompanied by decreased potassium levels in 50% of children evaluated.[34] Urine magnesium levels are also decreased and may be monitored.

Treatment of hypomagnesemia is directed at identification of the underlying cause and correction of the imbalance. With severe magnesium deficiency resulting in symptoms such as ventricular arrhythmias or seizures, IV magnesium sulfate may be diluted to 10 mg/ml and given slowly over 3 to 5 minutes. Subsequent doses may be repeated if necessary, based on the child's response and serum magnesium levels. Adequate renal function is ensured before treatment is undertaken because if function is diminished, hypermagnesemia results.[17] Other complications of parenteral magnesium administration include neuromuscular and respiratory depression, hypotension, and malignant arrhythmias.

Although oral and intramuscular magnesium administration may be more easily accomplished, neither can be relied on to correct a serious deficit. Intramuscular magnesium absorption is erratic, based on the amount of subcutaneous fat tissue. Intestinal absorption of oral magnesium is extremely variable. If either intramuscular or oral replacement is chosen, careful attention must be directed at monitoring serum levels.

Hypermagnesemia

Etiology.   Hypermagnesemia is defined as an excess of magnesium in the ECF compartment. Hypermagnesemia exists when the serum magnesium level exceeds 2.5 mEq/L.

Hypermagnesemia occurs far less often than hypomagnesemia. This condition most commonly occurs as the result of underlying chronic renal disease. Transient increases in serum magnesium levels may accompany ECF compartment deficit or excessive administration of magnesium-containing drugs.[2]

Pathophysiology.   Hypermagnesemia may occur as the result of an increase in magnesium load or a decrease in GFR. An increase in magnesium load is rare but may occur with the administration of large doses of magnesium-containing electrolyte supplements, laxatives, or antacids in the patient with compromised renal function. A decrease in GFR is typically associated with chronic renal disease, acute renal failure, or hypovolemia.[27] The result is inadequate filtration and excretion of magnesium.

Critical Care Management.   Because hypermagnesemia is a rare occurrence, the nurse must maintain a high index of suspicion in those patients who are at high risk (see Table 11-3). In addition, the child is monitored for ECG changes. Severe hypermagnesemia may lead to coma or cardiac arrest. Laboratory values are obtained and may include serum magnesium level and renal function tests, including BUN and serum creatinine.

Treatment of hypermagnesemia is directed at both correction of the imbalance and identification and treatment of the underlying cause. Calcium gluconate or other calcium salts may be administered because calcium is an antagonist to magnesium and often reverses the cardiac manifestations of hypermagnesemia. IV hydration facilitates renal excretion of excess magnesium in the presence of normal renal function. If renal dysfunction is apparent, dialysis may be indicated.

SUMMARY

This chapter has presented the regulation and assessment of fluid and electrolyte balance in the critically ill child. Care of the critically ill child depends on accurate assessment and complete understanding of the unique interrelationships of these substances. Minor deviations in electrolyte and fluid balance may produce profound complications in children. Therefore careful attention to signs and symptoms and appropriate intervention to alleviate the abnormality and correct the underlying cause may reduce the severity and length of time of critical illness.

REFERENCES

1. Hellerstein S: Fluids and electrolytes: physiology, *Pediatr Rev* 14:70-79, 1993.
2. Metheny N: *Fluid and electrolyte balance: nursing considerations,* ed 2, Philadelphia, 1992, JB Lippincott.
3. Innerarity S, Stark J: *Fluid and electrolytes,* Springhouse, Pa, 1990, Springhouse.
4. Toto KH: Fluid balance assessment: the total perspective, *Crit Care Nurs Clin North Am* 10:383-400, 1998.
5. Andrews M, Mooney K: Alteration of renal and urinary tract function in children. In McCance K, Huether S, eds: *Pathophysi-*
ology: the biologic basis for disease in adults and children, St Louis, 1990, Mosby, pp 1160-1171.
6. Lee C, Barrett C, Ignatavicius D: *Fluids and electrolytes: a practical approach,* Philadelphia, 1996, FA Davis.
7. Stark J: Interpretation of BUN and serum creatinine: an interactive exercise, *Crit Care Nurs Clin North Am* 10:491-496, 1998.
8. Guyton A, Hall J: *Textbook of medical physiology,* ed 9, Philadelphia, 1996, WB Saunders.
9. Jospe N, Forbes G: Fluids and electrolytes: clinical aspects, *Pediatr Rev* 17:395-403, 1996.
10. Goldberger E: *Primer of water, electrolyte and acid-base syndromes,* Philadelphia, 1986, Lea & Febiger.
11. Kravath R: Cystic Fibrosis. In Finberg L, Kravath R, Hellerstein S, eds: *Water and electrolytes in pediatrics: physiology, pathophysiology, and treatment,* ed 2, Philadelphia, 1993, WB Saunders.
12. Finberg L: Isotonic and hyponatremic dehydration. In Finberg L, Kravath R, Hellerstein

S, eds: *Water and electrolytes in pediatrics: physiology, pathophysiology, and treatment,* ed 2, Philadelphia, 1993, WB Saunders.

13. Adelman RD, Solhaug MJ: Pathophysiology of body fluids and fluid therapy. In RE Behrman, ed: *Nelson textbook of pediatrics,* ed 15, Philadelphia, 1996, WB Saunders.

14. Wetzel RC: Shock and fluid resuscitation. In Nichols DG et al, eds: *Golden hour: the handbook of advanced pediatric life support,* St Louis, 1996, Mosby.

15. Paschall JA, Melvin T: Fluid and electrolyte therapy. In Holbrook PR, ed: *Textbook of pediatric critical care,* Philadelphia, 1993, WB Saunders.

16. Conley S: Hypernatremia, *Pediatr Clin North Am* 37:365-372, 1990.

17. Thelan L, Davie J, Urden L: *Textbook of critical care nursing: diagnosis and management,* St Louis, 1990, Mosby.

18. Wood EG, Lynch RE: Fluid and electrolyte balance. In Fuhrman BP, Zimmerman JJ, eds: *Pediatric critical care,* St Louis, 1992, Mosby.

19. Bräxmeyer DL, Keyes JL: The pathophysiology of potassium balance, *Crit Care Nurs* 16:59-71, 1996.

20. Perkin RM, Levin DL: Mineral and glucose requirements and abnormalities. In Levin DL, Morriss FC, eds: *Essentials of pediatric intensive care,* St Louis, 1990, Quality Medical Publishing.

21. Chmielewski CM: Hyperkalemic emergencies: mechanisms, manifestations, and management, *Crit Care Nurs Clin North Am* 10:449-458, 1998.

22. Brem, A: Disorders of potassium homeostasis, *Pediatr Clin North Am* 37:419-427, 1990.

23. Finberg L: Sodium, potassium, and chloride ions: metabolism and regulation. In Finberg L, Kravath R, Hellerstein, S, eds: *Water and electrolytes in pediatrics: physiology, pathophysiology, and treatment,* ed 2, Philadelphia, 1993, WB Saunders.

24. Farrington E: Treatment of hyperkalemia, *Pediatr Nurs* 17:190-192, 1991.

25. Allen DB: Disorders of the endocrine system relevant to pediatric critical illness. In Fuhrman BP, Zimmerman JJ, eds: *Pediatric critical care,* St Louis, 1992, Mosby.

26. Baer C: Regulation and assessment of fluid and electrolyte balance. In Kinney M, Packa D, Dunbar S, eds: *AACN's Clinical reference for critical-care nursing,* ed 2, New York, 1988, McGraw-Hill.

27. Cogan M: *Fluids and electrolytes: physiology and pathophysiology,* Norwalk, Conn, 1991, Appleton & Lange.

28. Miekley TF: A patient-focused approach to managing diuretic therapy, *Crit Care Nurs Clin North Am* 10:421-431, 1998.

29. Alfaro-LeFevre R et al: *Drug handbook: a nursing process approach,* Redwood City, Calif, 1992, Addison-Wesley Nursing, The Benjamin/Cummings Publishing.

30. Workman ML: Magnesium and phosphorus: the neglected electrolytes, *AACN Clin Issues Crit Care Nurs* 3:655-663, 1992.

31. Graves L: Disorders of calcium, phosphorus, and magnesium, *Crit Care Nurs Q* 13:3-13, 1990.

32. Baker W: Hypophosphatemia, *Am J Nurs* 22:999, 1985.

33. Toto KH, Yucha CB: Magnesium: homeostasis, imbalances, and therapeutic uses, *Crit Care Nurs Clin North Am* 6:767-781, 1994.

34. Innerarity S: Electrolyte emergencies in the critically ill renal patient, *Crit Care Nurs Clin North Am* 2:89-99, 1990.

35. Kohane DS, Tobin JR, Kohane IS: Endocrine, mineral, and metabolic disease in pediatric intensive care. In Rogers MC, ed: *Textbook of pediatric intensive care,* ed 3, Baltimore, 1996, Williams & Wilkins.

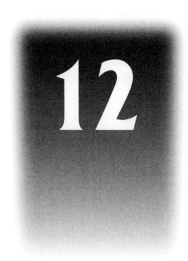

Nutrition Support

Judy Verger
Greg Schears

Nutrition is an essential component of caring for critically ill children. Nutritional interventions can improve patient recovery and survival.[1] Both an acquired and a preexisting tendency toward protein-energy malnutrition (PEM) has been documented in hospitalized children.[2,3] In the 1980s, Pollack and associates[2,3] found that 16% to 19% of pediatric intensive care unit (PICU) patients were malnourished. Those children at risk for serious nutritional deficiencies were younger than 2 years of age and had medical problems rather than surgical problems. Acute PEM has been linked to higher mortality and increased physiologic instability.[4] The value of nutrition in health and disease is now being established. In today's healthcare environment, early nutritional assessment is considered best practice. Nutrition support started within 24 to 48 hours of admission to the critical care unit is the current standard of care. Designer formulas with specific additives that are thought to enhance immune function show promise. A variety of delivery methods, including postpyloric enteral tube placement, supports the value and safety of early nutrition.

The risk of malnutrition for critically ill children is increased by their higher metabolic needs and by other associated conditions common to the pediatric intensive care population. Congenital heart disease, bronchopulmonary dysplasia, gastrointestinal reflux, and other chronic conditions commonly lead to feeding difficulties and can predispose critically ill children to undernutrition and growth failure.[5] Compared with adults, children have proportionately larger obligate energy needs. The major metabolic organs make up a larger proportion of body weight. These higher energy requirements combined with lower macronutrient stores result in children being less able to withstand nutritional deprivation.

Protein-calorie malnutrition is a deficiency of both protein and energy and has a detrimental effect on a number of major body systems. Malnutrition causes mobilization of muscle protein stores and negative nitrogen balance. Malnutrition may be a cofactor in morbidity and death in patients with hypermetabolism and organ dysfunction.[6,7] Protein and calorie depletion dramatically compromises immunocompetence, resulting in an increased risk of infection with a reduction in the number of T lymphocytes, a decrease in B-cell function, changing cytokine activity, diminished interleukin-2 response, and impaired wound healing.[8-10] Protein, carbohydrates, fats, and various vitamins and minerals are responsible for synthesis and collagen strength and therefore wound integrity.

The heart and lung muscles, like other muscles in the body, require sufficient protein and calories to perform their physiologic activities.[11] Without adequate protein and energy support, the patient can experience a decrease in ventilatory drive and respiratory efficiency; decrease in surfactant, resulting in a change in pulmonary compliance; decrease in diaphragm mass and muscle atrophy; decrease in vital capacity; and decrease in clearance of bacteria by the lungs.[12,13] Weaning from mechanical ventilation may be inhibited. Hypomagnesemia and hypophosphatemia may specifically contribute to respiratory muscle depletion.[14,15] Structural and functional effects on the cardiac muscle have been demonstrated as a response to malnutrition.[16] Vitamin and trace element deficiencies may affect cardiac performance. Other physiologic conditions associated with malnutrition include the gastrointestinal changes of gut mucosal atrophy, decreased intestinal motility, bacterial translocation, malabsorption, and decreased pancreatic function.[17,18]

PATIENT RESPONSE TO STARVATION AND CRITICAL ILLNESS

An understanding of the dramatic differences of the body's response to starvation and the catabolic effects of stress is important for safe and effective nutritional support of critically ill children (Table 12-1). Unlike critical illness, which results in rapid PEM, starvation produces malnutrition in days to weeks. The process of starvation results from a decrease of nutrient intake with normal nutrient use. This phenomenon essentially represents no stress to the body. Carbohydrate stores are usually consumed within 24 hours. The breakdown of amino acids from protein (gluconeogenesis) is initiated to supply glucose. If starvation continues for several weeks, the body adapts to lack of glucose. Protein use is reduced, nutrients are conserved, and body fat becomes the major energy source. Starvation causes a decrease in the child's metabolic rate and total energy expenditure. Little or no activation of metabolic mediators occurs, and no increase in insulin resistance exists.

The metabolic response of critical illness is very different from that of simple starvation.[19,20] Hypermetabolism is characterized by hyperglycemia, and normal use of nutrients is altered. This response is coordinated by catecholamines, cortisol, glucagon, and growth hormone and characterized by use of nutrients from all sources.[21] Interleukin-6 is an integral mediator for the physiologic response to injury.[22] Interleukin-1 and tumor necrosis factor also participate as mediators for the stress response.

Catecholamines released in response to the stress of injury or illness create a diabetic-like response by increasing the mobilization of glucose and resistance to insulin. Epinephrine suppresses insulin, leaving additional glucose available for energy needs. Glucagon antagonizes the anabolic effect of insulin, leading to more hyperglycemia and protein breakdown. Glucocorticoids trigger gluconeogenesis, converting amino acids to glucose. Endogenous protein breakdown is accelerated to provide glucose to meet energy needs. Much of protein degradation comes from the wasting of skeletal muscle and results in an increased loss of nitrogen through the urine. Amino acids may supply up to 25% of the energy in the stressed patient, resulting in a higher respiratory quotient (RQ) than with starvation.[23] Fat mobilization, use, and depletion are also increased. Cortisol acts to enhance the catecholamine effect by breaking down fat into free fatty acids.

The metabolic response to critical illness is not preventable; however, nutrition support can minimize protein loss.[21,24] The catabolic effect of breaking down cellular materials, which occurs during critical illness, precludes growth and organ development. When catabolism exceeds anabolism, the synthesis of cellular materials, body tissues

TABLE 12-1   Metabolic Response of Stress Versus Starvation

Characteristics	Critical Illness	Starvation
Metabolic rate	+ to +++	−
Energy requirements	+ to +++	−
Primary fuels	Mixed	Fat
Protein breakdown	+++	+
Amino acid oxidation	+++	+
Urinary nitrogen excretion	+++	+
Hepatic protein synthesis	+++	+
Total body protein synthesis	−	−
Gluconeogenesis	+++	+
Ketone production	+	++++
Rate of malnutrition development	+++	+

Adapted from Pollack M: Nutritional support of children in the intensive care unit. In Suskind R, Lewinter-Suskind L, eds: *Textbook of pediatric nutrition*, ed 2, New York, 1993, Raven Press, p 209; Cerra F: Nutrition in trauma, stress and sepsis. In Shoemaker W, Ayers S, Grevnik A et al, eds: *Textbook of critical care*, ed 2, Philadelphia, 1989, WB Saunders, p 1118.
+, Increased; −, decreased.

are lost and weight decreases. Catabolism and anabolism cannot occur simultaneously. The degree of increase in energy expenditure and protein catabolism is proportionate to the severity of illness and previous nutritional status of the child.[25] For example, a child with a minor infection does not have as much energy expenditure and protein breakdown as a child with sepsis. This increase in energy expenditure plays a major role in the development of PEM in the intensive care unit (ICU).

NUTRITION ASSESSMENT

The nutritional assessment of a critically ill child requires various methods and tests. No single clinical, biochemical, or growth measurement gives a complete picture of a child's nutrition status. The process of nutritional assessment is dynamic and must allow selection of varying assessment methods throughout the child's ICU stay.

The purpose of the nutritional assessment is to identify the presence or absence of malnutrition, determine the child's nutritional requirements and preferred alimentation method, and assess the effects of any nutrition intervention. A systematic review of the child's history and physical examination combined with accurate anthropometric and laboratory measurements are required.

Patient History

A reliable and complete history is the first step in accomplishing a nutritional assessment (Box 12-1). These data aid in providing a basis for subsequent assessment parameters. Valuable information can be gathered from watching the parent feed the child. Review of the child's medications is also helpful because of the possible effect of these

Data from Hobenbrink K: The pediatric patient. In Lang C, ed: *Nutritional support in critical illness,* Gaithersburg, Md, 1987, Aspen Publication, pp 33-59.

medications on the gastrointestinal tract and their potential for causing nutritional disturbances.

Dietary History

The child's dietary history and an analysis of the child's current diet to determine nutritional composition and quantity are important. Knowledge of the child's preadmission intake may be particularly helpful for the chronically ill child in the ICU. To collect information regarding the child's preadmission diet, parents can be asked to recall the child's intake in the past 24 to 48 hours. Calorie count is the best method to document a child's current diet. The child's enteral and intravenous intake for a 24-hour period can be recorded and analyzed.

Physical Assessment

A careful physical examination is performed with a specific interest in uncovering subtle signs of deficiencies in macronutrients (protein, energy) and micronutrients (vitamins, minerals, and trace elements) (Table 12-2). The goal of the physical examination is to corroborate and add to findings of the history. Among the clinical signs that may provide evidence suggesting nutritional deficiencies are the child's general appearance; subcutaneous fat and muscle

wasting; neuromuscular irritability; and skeletal structure, including signs of bone disease and bone tenderness. A decrease in muscle strength precedes a reduction in nitrogen and protein levels in malnutrition.[26] The condition of the gums, teeth, hair, skin, and eyes are assessed for signs of nutritional depletion. The child may also have diarrhea, constipation, or vomiting. Because the origin of these signs may not be nutritional, further testing is necessary to determine the cause.

Anthropometric Measurements

Assessment of growth is a vital component in the care of critically ill children. Anthropometric measurements including weight, length, height, head circumference, triceps skin fold, and midarm circumference are noninvasive and easily taken. Weight, length, height, and head circumference are traditionally considered convenient clinical measurements and can serve as minimum standards for the average ICU patient.

Plotting weight, stature, head circumference, and body mass index (BMI) on growth charts is essential to identifying growth patterns that are indicative of acute or chronic malnutrition. Weight for age, height for age, head circumference, weight for stature, and BMI can be plotted using National Center for Health Statistics (NCHS) charts.[27] Standard growth charts can be found in Appendix II. Special growth charts are also available for children with special health problems such as trisomy 21 and prematurity.

Weight is used as a gross indicator of body fat and protein stores. For the typical pediatric patient in the ICU, weight is measured on a calibrated pan or sling scale. The scale is accurately calibrated with whatever gown, sheet, diaper, or equipment is needed for the child. Arm boards, casts, and other heavy items are estimated and then subtracted from the total weight. Ideally the child is weighed with the same scale and at the same time each day.

The child is weighed on admission as a baseline and daily as the child's acuity permits and until the child's growth pattern has stabilized. Weekly weight trends are more relevant than daily fluctuations in assessing a critically ill child's growth. An unexplained weight loss of greater than 10% of the child's admission weight places the child nutritionally at risk.[28] The frequent changes in body water content from the occurrence of capillary leak syndrome with edema reduce the effectiveness of weight as an indicator of changes in body mass and therefore nutritional status.

Obtaining the child's length and height assists in estimating ideal body weight and monitoring length and height variations over time. After 1 to 2 years of age, a healthy infant's height and weight normally proceed along the same percentile. Length and height are affected when undernutrition occurs chronically. Recumbent length measurement is typically obtained on children from birth to 2 years of age. Standing height is obtained on ambulatory children who are 2 to 18 years of age. Because most critically ill children cannot stand, limited options are available. Direct measurement of a child with a tape measure will sacrifice accuracy. For children up to 36 months of age, a

TABLE 12-2	Selected Clinical Findings Associated With Nutritional Deficiencies/Excesses	
Organ	**Finding**	**Nutritional Deficiency/Excesses to Consider**
General	Underweight, short stature	Calories
	Overweight	Excess calories
	Edematous, decreased activity level	Protein
Subcutaneous tissue	Decreased fat fold	Calories
	Increased fat fold	Excess calories
	Edema	Protein, thiamine
Face	Moon face, diffuse depigmentation	Protein
Mucous membranes	Pale	Anemia
Hair	Lack of curl, dull altered texture, depigmented, easily plucked, thin	Protein
	Hair loss	Zinc, biotin, essential fatty acids
	Coiled, corkscrew-like	Vitamin A, ascorbic acid
Lips	Angular stomatitis	Riboflavin
Gums	Swollen, bleeding	Ascorbic acid
Teeth	Caries	Fluoride
	Mottled, pitted enamel	Excess fluoride
Tongue	Smooth, pale, atrophic	Anemia, B complex
	Red, painful, denuded, edema	Niacin, riboflavin, vitamin B_{12}
Nails	Spoon-shaped, koilonychia	Iron
Muscles	Decreased muscle mass (wasting)	Protein, calories
Neurologic	Ataxia, sensory loss, motor weakness	Vitamin B_{12}, vitamin E, chromium
	Psychomotor change, confusion, irritable	Protein, chromium
	Loss of vibratory sense, deep tendon reflexes	Thiamine, vitamin B_{12}
	Sensory loss, motor weakness	Thiamine
	Peripheral neuropathy	Pyridoxine
Skin	Generalized dermatitis	Zinc, biotin, essential fatty acids, tryptophan
	Symmetric dermatitis of skin exposed to sunlight, thickened pressure points, trauma	Niacin
	Petechiae, purpura, ecchymosis	Ascorbic acid, vitamin K
	Scrotal, vulval dermatitis	Riboflavin
Eyes	Dry (xerosis) conjunctiva	Vitamin A
	Photophobia	Zinc
	Conjunctival pallor	Anemia
Skeletal	Costochondral beading, pigeon chest	Vitamin D
	Harrison's groove, knock-kneed or bowed legs, craniotabes, frontal and parietal bossing, open anterior fontanelle	
	Epiphyseal enlargement	Vitamin D, ascorbic acid
	Bone tenderness, hemorrhages	Ascorbic acid, copper
Gastrointestinal	Hepatomegaly (fatty infiltration)	Protein
Cardiovascular	Tachycardia, cardiomegaly, congestive heart failure	Thiamine
	Cardiomyopathy	Selenium
Endocrine	Hypothyroidism, goiter	Iodine
	Glucose intolerance	Chromium
Other	Altered taste	Zinc
	Delayed wound healing	Zinc, ascorbic acid, protein
	Parotid enlargement	Protein

Adapted from Figueroa-Colon R: Clinical and laboratory assessment of the malnourished child. In Suskind R, Lewinter-Suskind L, eds: *Textbook of pediatric nutrition,* ed 2, New York, 1993, Raven Press, p 195.

length board can be used. The recumbent measurement may result in approximately 1 to 2 cm greater length than an upright height measurement. The length of a nonambulatory child of age 3 to 18 years can be estimated by measuring lower leg or upper arm length and comparing the measurement to a standard.[29] This technique is an estimate of linear growth in children when height and length cannot be reliably assessed using traditional means. Upper arm length is measured from the acromion to the head of the radius. Lower leg length is measured from the superior medial border of the tibia to the inferior border of the medial malleolus with the child sitting and one leg crossed over the other horizontally.

BMI for age is calculated in children greater than 2 years of age from the child's weight and height measurements. BMI assists the clinician in making a judgment of whether the child's weight is appropriate for his or her age. In older children and adolescents, BMI closely relates to body fat. A child with a measurement of less than the 5th percentile may have growth failure, and further nutritional assessment is warranted. A measurement of greater than the 95th percentile may be considered overnourished.

Head circumference measurement also contributes to a complete nutritional assessment. Head circumference changes with chronic malnutrition. The brain is often preferentially spared for growth during malnutrition and only slows its growth with long-term chronic malnutrition. Reductions in weight and height precede a nutrition-related change in head circumference. Serious malnourishment during critical stages of brain development may cause diminished brain and head growth and impaired developmental and intellectual potentials. Measurements are obtained in children of up to 36 months of age using a flexible, nonstretchable tape measure. The head is measured at the greatest circumference around the frontal bones, superior to the supraorbital ridge and over the occipital prominence. The recommendation is that infants age 1 week to 15 months have a head circumference measurement each week and children age 15 months to 3 years have their head circumference measured every 3 to 4 weeks.

Triceps skinfold (TSF) and midarm circumference (MAC) assist in the assessment of muscle mass and subcutaneous fat content, respectively. These measurements require the use of constant tension calipers such as Lange or Holtain skinfold calipers and a nonstretchable tape measure. Because approximately 50% of the body's adipose tissue is located in the subcutaneous tissue, TSF provides an estimate of body fat stores. Skinfold calipers pinch the skin and its underlying subcutaneous tissue over the triceps midway between the shoulder (acromion) and the elbow (olecranon). To ensure accuracy, this process is repeated three times using established techniques. Midarm circumference is used in combination with TSF to estimate skeletal muscle mass and somatic protein reserves. To measure MAC the diameter of the arm is determined by using a tape measure over the same area of the arm used when measuring TSF. These measurements are then compared with age- and sex-specific standards.

The child's measurements are compared with standards established by the Ten State Nutrition Study.[30] Excessive fat stores and muscle mass are indicated by a greater than 95th percentile, and depletion in fat stores and muscle mass is indicated by less than the 5th percentile. The accuracy of both TSF and MAC may be affected by fluid shifts and edema.

Biochemical Indices

Laboratory data can be used to evaluate biologic functions dependent on nutrition. Of equal importance to assessing protein and calorie deficits is assessment of micronutrients. Serum and urine assays provide objective information to support dietary assessments, physical findings, and anthropometric measurements. Cholesterol levels below normal are seen in malnourished patients and correlate with mortality.[31] Biochemical measurements serve to identify nutritional deficiencies that are not found clinically (Table 12-3).

Plasma Proteins.   As a means of quantifying a child's body protein stores, certain proteins that circulate in the body can be measured.[28,32] Protein measurements, however, reflect body stores with varying degrees of precision. Many physiologic and pathologic factors seen in critically ill children, such as liver disease, renal failure, trauma, infection, and inflammation, also affect body protein and make the interpretation of these measurements difficult.

Prealbumin is sensitive to acute visceral protein changes and may be the most helpful protein measurement in the critically ill patient.[33] Prealbumin closely correlates to nitrogen balance. Prealbumin levels are significantly decreased in the flow phase of injury.[34,35] Prealbumin has a relatively short half-life (2 days) and smaller body pool than albumin. Prealbumin decreases rapidly with lower than normal protein or energy intake and produces a significant rise with adequate protein and calorie replacement. Prealbumin is partially catabolized by the kidneys and increases with renal insufficiency.[35] Prealbumin aids in the transport of thyroxin and is also affected by infection and trauma.

Serum albumin, the major protein synthesized by the liver, was one of the first biochemical markers identified for malnutrition. A low level of serum albumin has been associated with a decrease in dietary protein intake and an increase in morbidity and mortality.[36] Once released into the plasma, albumin has a half-life of 20 days and reacts very slowly to changes in protein intake. Albumin levels are affected by hepatic disease, as well as infection, injury, hydration of the child, renal failure, intestinal disease, ongoing protein losses from drainage tubes or wounds, and exogenous infusion of albumin. Short-term reductions in intake may decrease albumin synthesis but have little effect on albumin levels because of the low turnover rate and large pool size of albumin within the body. In children older than age 1 year, serum albumin levels of 2.8 to 3.5 g/dl may indicate mild protein depletion, whereas severe depletion may be indicated by serum albumin levels less than 2.1 g/dl. The nonsensitivity and nonspecificity of albumin make it a poor indicator of acute malnutrition in a critically ill child. Its major role is in the assessment of the severity of chronic malnutrition.

Transferrin is also used to reflect protein status in the hospitalized child. This plasma protein is synthesized by the liver. Transferrin is used to transport the majority of the iron

TABLE 12-3   Biochemical Indices

	Age				
Test	Neonate Birth-1 mo	Infant 1-12 mo	Child 1-4 yr	Child 5-8 yr	Child 9-18 yr
Protein					
Blood					
Serum albumin (g/dl)	≥2.5	≥3	≥3.5	≥3.5	≥3.5
Retinol binding protein (mg/dl)	2-3	2-3	2-3	2-3	3-6
Blood urea nitrogen (mg/dl)	7-22	7-22	7-22	7-22	7-22
Prealbumin (mg/dl)	20-50	20-50	20-50	20-50	20-50/60
Transferrin (mg/dl)	170-250	170-250	170-250	170-250	170-250
Fibronectin (mg/dl)	30-40	30-40	30-40	30-40	30-40
Urine					
Creatinine/height index	>0.9	>0.9	>0.9	>0.9	>0.9
Vitamin A					
Plasma retinol (g/dl)	≥30	≥30	≥30	≥30	≥30
Vitamin D					
25-OH-D_3 (ng/ml)	≥20	≥20	≥20	≥20	≥20
Riboflavin					
Red cell glutathione reductase stimulation effect (%)	<20	<20	<20	<20	<20
Folacin					
Serum folate (ng/ml)	>6	>6	>6	>6	>6
Red blood cell folate (ng/dl)	>160	>160	>160	>160	>160
Vitamin K					
Prothrombin time (seconds)	11-15	11-15	11-15	11-15	11-15
Vitamin E					
Red blood cell hemolysis test (%)	≤10	≤10	≤10	≤10	≤10
Vitamin C					
Plasma (mg/dl)	>0.2	>0.2	>0.2	>0.2	>0.2
Thiamine					
Red blood cell transketolase stimulation effect (%)	<15	<15	<15	<15	<15
Vitamin B_{12}					
Serum vitamin B_{12} (pg/ml)	≥200	≥200	≥200	≥200	≥200
Iron					
Hematocrit (%)	31	33	36	39	36
Hemoglobin (g/dl)	12	12	13	14	13
Serum ferritin (ng/ml)	>10	>10	>10	>10	>10
Serum iron (g/dl)	>30	>40	>50	>60	>60
Serum total iron-binding capacity (g/dl)	350-400	350-400	350-400	350-400	350-400
Zinc					
Serum zinc (g/dl)	80-120	80-120	80-120	80-120	80-120

Adapted from Klish W: Nutritional assessment. In Wyllie R, Hyams J, eds: *Pediatric gastrointestinal disease,* Philadelphia, 1993, WB Saunders, p 1108.

in the plasma. Transferrin has a half-life of approximately 8 days and therefore is more sensitive than albumin to protein deficiency. A transferrin level of 100 to 170 mg/dl may reflect moderate malnutrition, and a level of less than 100 mg/dl may indicate severe malnutrition. Transferrin is known to rise rapidly during iron deficiency and may be affected by other nonnutritional factors, including nephrotic syndrome, neoplastic disease, and liver disorders.

Retinol-binding protein levels also vary with protein-energy status. Relative to the other visceral proteins, retinol-binding protein has a very short half-life (10 to 12 hours). However, retinol-binding protein is not used often for diagnosis of malnutrition because it is present only in very small concentrations. Serum levels may rise in liver disease and renal insufficiency and be lowered in vitamin A deficiency.

Urine Screening for Somatic Proteins. Although urine is sometimes difficult to collect, urine screening for creatinine and urea nitrogen can be valuable in assessing the nutrition status of the critically ill child. Creatinine height index (CHI) reflects muscle mass, assuming that renal function is normal. Creatinine, the metabolic product of creatine, is stored in muscle and excreted by the kidney at a relatively constant rate. Creatinine excretion is measured in a 24-hour urine collection. The 24-hour creatinine excretion of the patient is divided by a 24-hour creatinine excretion of the same-height child and multiplied by 100 to obtain an index:

$$\frac{\text{24-Hour urine creatinine excretion (mg)}}{\substack{\text{24-Hour urine creatinine excretion of} \\ \text{same–height child (mg)}}} \times 100$$

In the well-nourished child the CHI is 90% to 100%. Severe protein-calorie malnutrition is indicated by a CHI under 40%, moderate depletion is indicated by a CHI of 40% to 60%, and mild depletion is indicated by a CHI of 60% to 80%.[32] Creatinine excretion can be affected by hydration state and catabolic states. Patients taking diuretics and those with renal disease are likely to have low excretions of creatinine.[28]

Urea nitrogen excretion also requires 24-hour urine collection and can be used to estimate nitrogen balance and assess catabolic state. Nitrogen balance determines the state of metabolic balance or protein turnover by subtracting nitrogen excretion from nitrogen intake. Nitrogen balance is calculated as follows:

(Protein intake [g/24 hours]/6.25) –
(Urine urea nitrogen [g/24 hours] + 4)

Protein intake is divided by 6.25 to determine the intake of nitrogen. This factor is the average nitrogen intake in 1 g of dietary protein. A constant of 4 is added to urine urea nitrogen to account for the other body nitrogen losses (stool, skin, etc.). If the answer to this equation is above zero, the patient is adding lean body mass and is in an anabolic state. This result indicates growth or recovery from an illness. If the number is negative or below zero, the child is catabolic and losing protein or lean body mass. This state suggests the need to add protein alone or a combination of protein and calories to the diet. In addition to malnutrition, a negative nitrogen balance may also be caused by hypoperfusion, fever, sepsis, shock, and steroid therapy.

Other Methods of Assessment

Body Composition. Measurement of body composition is currently being used in some settings for nutritional analysis and involves the estimation of body components. Different methods exist with varying accuracy, technique, and applicability to the child in the ICU. For the majority of these tests, their relationship to patient outcome has not yet been demonstrated.[28,32]

Two methods of measuring body composition include dual-energy x-ray analysis (DEXA) and total body water (TBW). Bone mineral content (BMC), fat free mass (FFM), and percentage of body fat (%BF) can be determined by x-ray examination. This noninvasive method is especially helpful in detecting bone loss in children. TBW uses isotopes to measure FFB and %BF. Small amounts of isotopes are administered to the patient. The concentration of the isotopes is then measured in the urine to estimate TBW.

Indirect Calorimetry. Calorimetry is the process of measuring energy expenditure and is based on the premise that energy is produced by thermal reactions. Energy expenditure was initially measured in a laboratory setting by directly quantifying heat dissipating from a subject. With the advent of indirect calorimetry, measuring energy expenditure can now be done at a patient's bedside.[37] Indirect calorimetry is now the reference standard for energy expenditure. Indirect calorimeters assist in evaluating caloric needs and measuring the use of various nutrients in critically ill children.[38-40]

Metabolic carts brought to the bedside measure the rate of pulmonary gas exchange. Using a sophisticated analyzer, carbon dioxide and oxygen levels in inspired and expired air are measured and compared to determine energy expenditure.[41,42] Oxygen consumption and carbon dioxide production represent valid measurements of intracellular metabolism. The amount of oxygen absorbed across the lung is assumed to be equal to the amount of oxygen consumed for metabolic processes.

Metabolic carts are capable of calculating a child's respiratory quotient (RQ) or ratio of carbon dioxide molecules produced to molecules of oxygen consumed.[43] The determination of RQ assists in evaluating overfeeding and substrate use. The RQ varies from 0.7 to 1.2 depending on the metabolite.[44] An RQ of 1 reflects pure carbohydrate metabolism; whereas an RQ of 0.82 suggests protein metabolism, and an RQ of 0.71 suggests fat use.[45] The administration of large glucose concentrations has been associated with increased carbon dioxide production, which may lead to an increased RQ.[42] Edes, Walk, and Austin[44] suggest when RQ is greater than 1, total calories may be decreased. When RQ is less than 1 but greater than 0.85, carbohydrates are being converted to fat.[7] Fat calories can be substituted for carbohydrate calories when further reduction of the RQ is seen as beneficial to the child. Simply adding fat calories, however, may not benefit the child if total calories are in excess of his or her needs. Edes, Walk, and Austin[44] also suggest that those patients receiving long-term ventilatory support or patients who will not undergo weaning for several days may not benefit from a reduction in RQ or a change in the diet to high-fat feedings. The goal is to keep the child, once fed, at an RQ of equal to or slightly lower than 0.85 to 0.9.[7,35]

Although indirect calorimetry predicts energy expenditure with much higher confidence than the traditional formulas, this method has some limitations.[42] Measurements are affected by oxygen concentrations of greater than 40% to 60%. Higher oxygen concentrations broaden the margin for error. The reproducibility of the measurements is also affected by loss of exhaled volume from a leak in the system. The expense of the necessary equipment, the importance of an experienced technician, and the continued need to standardize equipment in the pediatric population have limited the use of indirect calorimetry in many PICUs.

NUTRITION MANAGEMENT

Nutrition management of the child in the ICU involves providing protein and calories sufficient to address the child's stress-related needs while enhancing protein and calories for growth and supplementing vitamins and minerals. Preventing malnutrition is easier than recovering from the effects of undernutrition. Specialized nutrition support is initiated with specific therapeutic goals. Various organ systems and disease entities may benefit from tailored interventions.[46] During the beginning phase of critical illness, the goal of therapy is to stabilize lean body mass. After the initial hypermetabolic period, nutritional goals broaden to include improvement of visceral protein, replenishment of muscle glycogen and mineral stores, and provision of positive anabolic growth. The correction of the organ system dysfunction associated with malnutrition may take days to weeks. The ultimate plan for nutritional support depends on the basal metabolic needs, the nutritional condition of the child, the metabolic response and nutrient requirements of critical illness, the child's age, and the ability to provide parenteral and enteral therapy. Although brief nutritional inadequacies may have limited consequences if adequate oral intake is not expected, children admitted to ICUs should receive nutrition support within 24 to 48 hours after their admission. Those children with injury or sepsis or those who are admitted to the PICU in a malnourished state are particularly vulnerable and require the highest priority.

Determining Energy Needs

Estimation of the child's energy needs is essential for providing nutrition support. The energy requirements of a critically ill child are highly individualized and may vary widely. Some researchers have found a trend of increasing energy needs during the first week after injury or sepsis with a peak during the second week of admission.[47] Others have reported total energy expenditure close to resting energy expenditure for trauma patients who are deeply sedated[48] and no significant difference between preoperative and postoperative needs.[49,50] Ventilated patients with little work of breathing may only minimally increase their energy expenditure.

Because metabolism affects energy needs, whatever changes metabolic response affects caloric and nutrient needs of the child. More than 60% of the child's energy needs are necessary for daily function of the heart, kidneys, and brain. These body organs make up 16% to 17% of the body weight of a child, compared with 5% to 6% of the body weight for adults. Basal metabolic rate (BMR) is the energy required to maintain functional cellular activities at complete rest in a fasting state. Infants have a higher metabolic demand per kilogram, requiring a larger percentage of calories for growth. During infancy, BMR is approximately 50 kcal/kg/day; by adolescence the caloric needs of the child have decreased by 50% to 20 kcal/kg/day.[5] BMR is at its highest level per kilogram up to the age of 24 months. BMR is affected by a variety of factors other than age. In both starvation and obesity, BMR decreases. For every 1° increase in temperature, there is a 10% to 14% increase in metabolic rate. Drugs such as caffeine, β-blockers, and catecholamines increase BMR. Pathologic states, such as respiratory failure, increase BMR.

Establishing caloric needs of critically ill children is

TABLE 12-4 Stress Factors	
Representative Stress State	**Stress Factor**
Simple starvation	0.9
Sepsis (moderate)	1.3
Sepsis (severe)	1.5-1.6
Trauma: central nervous system (sedated)	1.3
Trauma: moderate to severe	1.5
Burns (proportionate to burn size)	Up to 2
Catch up growth	1.5-2.0

Pollack M: Nutritional support of children in the intensive care unit. In Suskind R, Lewinter-Suskind L, eds: *Textbook of pediatric nutrition,* ed 2, New York, 1993, Raven Press, p 214; Jew R: *The Children's Hospital of Philadelphia pharmacy handbook and formulary,* Ohio, 1998, Lexi-Comp.

challenging. Although the recommended daily allowance (RDA) guidelines are standard for estimating the energy needs of healthy children, these recommendations exceed basic energy expenditure by approximately 20% to 50% and are not reliable estimates of for critically ill children.[51] More accurately, caloric needs for critically ill children are approximated by calculating resting energy expenditure (REE) and multiplying by activity and injury stress factor (Table 12-4). Although REE and BMR are often used interchangeably, REE is approximately 10% higher than BMR, reflecting a measurement time closer to the consumption of food. The World Health Organization (WHO) REE recommendations have been proven relatively accurate for children older than 1 year of age.[29,52] Activity and stress factors are used to adjust for increases in energy expenditure as they relate to illness and activity. For obese children (those greater 120% of ideal body weight), the Schofield height/weight equations may be more useful.[53-55] Indirect calorimetry, as previously discussed, may also be used to estimate caloric needs, especially in cases when multiple processes are occurring simultaneously.

Once determined, REE is multiplied by a stress and activity factor. Cerra[56-58] initially quantified the metabolic effect of various types of activities and degrees of stress. Routine activities common to the ICU were found to affect oxygen consumption and energy expenditure[59] (see Chapter 8). A decrease in energy expenditure may occur with paralysis (58%) and with sedation and pain relief (5% to 10%).[60,61] In the late 1990s, many authors contested the initial stress factor guidelines suggested by Cerra.[38,62] Studies done using indirect calorimetry to measure REE found energy expenditure to be lower than previous research using other methods to estimate increased caloric needs.

Results from pediatric studies examining measured energy expenditure in the critically ill child have confirmed energy expenditure above REE.[49,50,63] In practice, for the majority of critically ill children with moderate stress from trauma, sepsis, or surgery, REE can be multiplied by a factor of 1.5 to 1.6 or a 50% to 60% increase above REE.[35] Otherwise, the well-nourished child on bed rest with moderate stress, for example, skeletal trauma, may require REE times 1.2 to 1.3 or 20% to 30% above REE. Long-term growth failure may require an increase of 50% to 100%

TABLE 12-5 Comparisons of Macronutrient Needs

Age	Total Calories (kcal/kg/day)	Protein (g/kg/day)	Carbohydrates (%)	Fat (%)
Preterm	100-120	2.5-3.5	34-39	39-43
Infant (<12 months)	80-110	2.0-3.0	35-65	30-55
Toddler (1-2 years)	85-95	1.5-2.0	50-55	30
Preschool (3-5 years)	80-90	1.2-2.0	55-60	30
School (7-12 years)	70-80	1.0	55-60	30
Adolescent (13-18 years)	40-65	1.0	55-60	30

Adapted from Huddleston K, Ferraro-McDuffie A, Wolff-Small T: Nutritional support of the critically ill child, *Crit Care Nurs Clin North Am* 5:68, 1993; data from Hobenbrink K, Oddlesitson N: Pediatric nutrition support. In Shronts E, ed: *Nutrition support dietetics,* Gaithersburg, Md, 1989, Aspen Publications, p 231; Pereira G, Barbosa N: Controversies in neonatal nutrition, *Pediatr Clin North Am* 33:1, 1986; Jew R: *The Children's Hospital of Philadelphia pharmacy handbook and formulary,* Ohio, 1998, Lexi-comp, p 375.

above REE. Stress factors of over 2 are commonly reserved for children with burns.

Although adequate nutrition is essential for the critically ill child, overnutrition cannot be overlooked as a potential complication.[37,64] Overfeeding with excessive calories may cause hyperglycemia, added nosocomial infections, hepatic dysfunction, and congestive heart failure; may worsen respiratory insufficiency; and may increase metabolic rate.[13,65-67] Altered body weight changes energy expenditure.[64] The work of breathing may be affected by an increase in adipose tissue throughout the abdomen and chest. Increases in oxygen consumption and hypercapnia, which may result from overfeeding, can interfere with weaning.[68] Storage of fuels such as glycogen and adipose are associated with significant increases in energy expenditure.[69] Elevations in the RQ can be attributed to the metabolism of an increased carbohydrate load. Some have even recommended permissive underfeeding in the adult population, providing a hypocaloric, hypoprotein diet in the first days after injury or sepsis.[70,71]

Despite the reported overestimation of energy expenditure, formulas continue to be standard for determining caloric needs of critically ill children.[72] Some speculate that because of improvements in the treatments and procedures, these equations are no longer predictive.[73] In practice, clinical response to feeding is the best indicator of caloric adequacy.

Nutrient Distribution

Once a child's total caloric needs are estimated, macronutrient distribution of kilocalories is determined. Appropriate amounts of vitamins, minerals, and trace elements are also added. Providing a mixed fuel source for patients is recommended[74] (Table 12-5).

Macronutrient Needs. Protein provides amino acids for continuous tissue synthesis and repair, transport of nutrients, and maintenance of immune function. Protein requirements change, as does metabolic rate.[75,76] Dietary protein is an important determinant of postinjury nitrogen balance. As a child gets older and metabolic needs decrease, so will the need for protein. The RDA provides guidelines for protein intake. These recommendations are based on minimum protein intake necessary to maintain nitrogen balance.[51] One gram of protein equals 4 calories. Infants require 10% to

20% protein, and children older than 2 years require 10% to 15% protein in the diet.[29] Nitrogen balance is possible at levels of nitrogen intake exceeding the rate of protein catabolism. In patients with head injury, however, protein catabolism was not reduced despite an intake of twice the calculated requirements.[77] Early feeding of ICU patients with small peptide-based protein has improved nitrogen balance and returned prealbumin to normal levels.[78]

Nonprotein calories are provided to the body by carbohydrates and fat. Carbohydrates ingested primarily as disaccharides, starches, and polysaccharides are the major source of energy for the body. Depending on the source, 1 g of carbohydrate equals approximately 4 calories. A high glucose load may also cause hyperglycemia and hepatic steatosis.[66] Carbohydrates often supply approximately 35% to 65% of the infant diet and 55% to 60% of the diet for children older than 2 years of age.[29] Fat is essential to cell integrity and provides a high caloric content. Fat has the highest caloric density of any nutrient, with 1 g of fat equal to approximately 9 calories. In general, to avoid essential fatty acid deficiency, 4% to 8% of the total calories ingested should be from a lipid source.[18] The recommendation is for approximately 30% to 55% of the full-term infant's diet and 30% of the diet for children older than 2 years of age be provided by fat.[29] Infant metabolism requires a greater dependence on fat for energy.[5]

To ensure maximum use of protein, calculating the ratio of nonprotein calories to nitrogen may be useful. The amount of nitrogen reflects protein in the diet. One gram of nitrogen is equal to 6.25 g of protein. In the typical American diet, the ratio of nonprotein calories, those from carbohydrates and fat, to grams of nitrogen is approximately 200 to 300 calories to 1 g of nitrogen. The inefficient use of amino acids, along with an increase in excretion of urinary urea nitrogen by the critically ill, suggests the need for higher protein intake.[34] Providing nonprotein-to-nitrogen ratios of approximately 80:1 to 100:1 for highly stressed patients may maximize nutritional support. Lowering the ratio of nonprotein calories to nitrogen may benefit children with high protein needs caused by burns, continuing losses through chest tube drainage, nasogastric suctioning, intractable diarrhea, and substantial blood loss.[7] For critically ill patients, increasing the fat portion of the nonprotein energy requirement by shifting away from the carbohydrate

TABLE 12-6 Vitamins, Minerals, and Trace Elements

		Fat-Soluble Vitamins				Water-Soluble Vitamins						
Age* (yr)		Vit. A (μg)	Vit. D (μg)	Vit. E (mg)	Vit. K (μg)	Vit. C (mg)	Thamine (mg)	Riboflavin (mg)	Niacin (mg NE)	Vit. B$_6$ (mg)	Folate (μg)	Vit. B$_{12}$ (mg)
Infants	0.0-0.5	375	7.5	3	5	30	0.3	0.4	5	0.3	25	0.3
	0.5-1	375	10	4	10	35	0.4	0.5	6	0.6	35	0.5
	1-3	400	10	6	15	40	0.7	0.8	9	1.0	50	0.7
	4-6	500	10	7	20	45	0.9	1.1	12	1.1	75	1.0
	7-10	700	10	7	30	45	1.0	1.2	13	1.4	100	1.4
Males	11-14	1000	10	10	45	50	1.3	1.5	17	1.7	150	2.0
	15-18	1000	10	10	65	60	1.5	1.8	20	2.0	200	2.0
	19-24	1000	10	10	70	60	1.5	1.7	19	2.0	200	2.0
Females	11-14	800	10	8	45	50	1.1	1.3	15	1.4	150	2.0
	15-18	800	10	8	55	60	1.1	1.3	15	1.5	180	2.0
	19-24	800	10	8	60	60	1.1	1.3	15	1.6	180	2.0

Adapted with permission from *Recommended dietary allowances: 10th edition.* Copyright 1989 by the National Academy of Sciences. Courtesy of the National Academy Press, Washington, D.C.
*Normal height and weight for age.

portion may decrease hyperglycemia and prevent respiratory failure.[79]

Micronutrient Needs. Micronutrients are an essential part of the critically ill child's diet. Children have increased requirements of calcium and phosphorus. Guidelines established by the RDA for vitamins, minerals, and trace elements are used as recommendations for providing micronutrients (Table 12-6). For the critically ill child, individually calculated amounts of vitamins and electrolytes are often necessary. Replacement of these elements is guided by monitoring appropriate serum levels. These deficiencies may affect the metabolic processes that are necessary for recovery. Deficiencies may have occurred before the child's critical illness or from inadequate replacement of current needs. If deficiencies exist, supplementation is necessary. Trace elements such as zinc, copper, chromium, manganese, selenium, iodine, molybdenum, and iron are important for growth and development. Small infants also have a reduced capacity to store minerals.[5]

Immune-Enhancing Additives

Amino acids such as glutamine, arginine and others; nucleotides; ω-3 fatty acids; recombinant growth hormone; and antioxidant vitamins have a role in maintaining the structure and function of the gut and in treating the stressed, hypermetabolic patient.[23,80-82] Glutamine is important in protein synthesis and may be the principal means of nitrogen transfer from the muscle to visceral organs.[83] During hypermetabolic states, glutamine is consumed at higher concentrations by the gastrointestinal tract and may reflect an increase in metabolic need. The addition of glutamine to enteral and parenteral nutrition may improve nitrogen balance, enhance intestinal mucosal repair, minimize villous atrophy, and reduce bacterial translocation.[84,85] Arginine may reduce protein breakdown, which may have a potent effect on depressed immunity and also enhance the body's

wound healing ability.[86,87] Although the evidence is inconclusive, adjusting the protein source to include branched-chain amino acids (valine, isoleucine, and leucine) has also been identified by some to benefit patients during injury or sepsis.[88] Nucleotides have also been added to various formulas to influence immunocompetence.[80] An increase in ω-3 fatty acids potentiates the immunoregulatory properties of fat emulsion.[89] An ω-6 to ω-3 fatty acid ratio of 2:1 may benefit the critically ill child. By reducing triglyceride level in the plasma and thereby decreasing the risk of coronary heart disease, ω-3 fatty acids make a valuable addition to the diet. The ω-3 fatty acids may also have a positive effect on atherosclerosis, hypertension, inflammatory disease, and ventricular dysrthymias.[90-92] Administration of growth hormone has been shown to decrease RQ and to contribute to a positive nitrogen balance.[93-95] However, in septic patients, no improvement in protein status was noted.[96,97] Diets with arginine, ω-3 fatty acids, and ribonucleic acid may increase muscle protein levels, improve nitrogen balance, reduce weight loss, and improve immune function.[98] However, immune-enhancing formulas have not proven advantageous to all patient populations.[99,100] Vitamin C, vitamin A, riboflavin, and pantothenic acid are indicated for wound healing.[101] Zinc loss is directly related to severity of illness. It is sequestered in the liver during stress and is used in essential metabolic pathways.[35]

Collaborative Interventions

Delivery of nutrients to a critically ill child is often challenging. If oral intake is inadequate or not feasible, nourishment by another delivery method is necessary.

Enteral Feeding. When oral intake is insufficient in a child with adequate digestive and absorptive capacity, enteral tube feedings are initiated. Increasing evidence confirms that enteral feeding is superior to parenteral nutrition with regard to gut structure and function.[102,103] However,

Age* (yr)		Minerals			Trace Elements			
		Calcium (mg)	Phosphorus (mg)	Magnesium (mg)	Iron (mg)	Zinc (mg)	Iodine (mg)	Selenium (mg)
Infants	0.0-0.5	400	300	40	6	5	40	10
	0.5-1	600	500	60	10	5	50	15
	1-3	800	800	80	10	10	70	20
	4-6	800	800	120	10	10	90	20
	7-10	800	800	170	10	10	120	30
Males	11-14	1200	1200	270	12	15	150	40
	15-18	1200	1200	400	12	15	150	70
	19-24	1200	1200	350	10	15	150	70
Females	11-14	1200	1200	280	15	12	150	45
	15-18	1200	1200	300	15	12	150	50
	19-24	1200	1200	280	15	12	150	55

controversy remains regarding whether parenteral nutrition alone or overfeeding itself is the cause of the perceived inferiority of parenteral nutrition.[104] The enteral mode of therapy preserves the normal sequence of nutrient delivery. In addition, this mode is safer and less costly. Enteral nutrition is associated with reduced morbidity and mortality, decreased potential for bacterial translocation into mesenteric lymph nodes, improved host response, higher pancreatic enzymes and disaccharidase activities, and enhanced nutrient use, compared with parenteral therapy.[105-108] Enteral support may be essential for continued production of immunoglobulin A (IgA).[101] Reduced IgA may allow introduction of foreign substances into the lymphatic system via the gut.[109]

Despite the common practice during the initial phase of critical illness of withholding enteral nutrition to prevent feeding intolerances and avoid gut malfunction, early enteral feedings have significant benefits.[110-116] Seemingly small amounts of nutrients administered enterally benefit the integrity and function of the GI tract. Therefore, when it is not possible to provide full nutrition support with enteral feedings, trophic feedings should be initiated to provide gut protection (see Appendix VII). Although use of parenteral nutrition for up to 2 weeks may not cause mucosal atrophy, evidence does indicate that impairment of absorptive capacity may occur when nutrients are not supplied directly to the gastrointestinal tract.[117-119]

Few contraindications to the exclusive use of enteral feedings exist, the most significant of which include GI obstruction involving the entire small intestine, caloric requirements beyond those which safe enteral feedings can provide, and active upper GI bleeding[120] (see Appendix VII). Withholding enteral feedings is also considered for patients who require endotracheal intubation or extubations within 4 hours, hemodynamically unstable patients with escalating therapy, and patients with significant graft versus host disease. In addition, an infant at risk for developing necrotizing enterocolitis may need a delay in enteral feedings for 1 to 2 weeks. Enteral feedings in the past have been avoided in the initial phases of critical illness because of the potential for gastric stasis. Although hemodynamic instability is a contraindication for some, complications may be avoided by placing the feeding tube in the child's duodenum or jejunum.

Selection of Formulas. Human breast milk, along with a variety of formulas, is available for the enteral nutrition of infants (Table 12-7). The selection of these enteral products is based on the child's age-related nutritional needs, underlying physiologic and pathophysiologic conditions, clinical status, and GI function.

Breast milk has long been recommended as the ideal food for infants and is given strong consideration for the critically ill infant.[121] Human milk provides essential immunologic benefits, growth-stimulating properties, and a balance of nutrients and digestive substances.[122-125] Human milk proteins provide amino acids for growth, as well as for digestion, host defense, and possibly tissue maturation.[126] For infants at greater risk of infection, breast milk may be especially beneficial. The decreased infection rate in breast-fed infants has been attributed by some to IgA and other antimicrobial properties found in human milk. The fat in human breast milk is thought to be more absorbable because of the positioning of the fatty acids. Iron, zinc, and other nutrients, except chloride, tend to be more bioavailable in human milk. While the infant is in the intensive care unit, breast-feeding mothers require support.[127-129] Providing staff support to the mother at regular intervals, as well as continued staff education, has been found to improve the duration of breast-feeding.[130] Mothers offered a quiet place in a private room can use manual or electric breast pumps to express milk for their infant. Breast milk can then be stored in glass or plastic containers in the refrigerator for 24 to 48 hours, in the freezer compartment of refrigerators for 2 to 3 weeks, or in a

TABLE 12-7 **Breast Milk and Selected Infant Formulas**

	Kcal/ml	Carbohydrate (g/dl)	Fat (g/dl)	Protein (g/dl)	Components
Breast Milk	0.67	7.2	4	1.05	
Cow's Milk					
Term Protein Formulas					
Similac	0.67	7.2	3.6	1.5	Lactose; soy, coconut oil; nonfat milk
Enfamil	0.67	6.9	3.8	1.4	Lactose; coconut oil, soy; nonfat milk, demineralized whey
Carnation Good Start	0.67	7.2	3.4	1.6	Hydrolyzed whey, whey protein concentrate; lactose maltodextrins; palm oil, safflower oil, soy oil
Similac PM 60/40	0.67	6.9	3.8	1.6	Lactalbumin; coconut, corn oil; lactose; reduced sodium
MCT-Containing Formulas					
Portagen	0.67	7.8	3.2	2.3	Corn syrup solids, lactose; MCT oil and corn oil; sodium caseinate
Lacto-free	.67	6.9	3.8	1.5	Corn syrup solids; milk protein isolate; palm, soy, coconut, sunflower oil
Soy-Based Formulas					
Isomil	0.67	6.8	3.6	2.0	Corn syrup solids, sucrose; soy and coconut oil; soy protein isolate, L-methionine
ProSobee	0.67	6.9	3.6	2.0	Corn syrup solids, soy and coconut oil; soy protein isolate, L-methionine
Preterm Infant Formulas					
Similac Special Care (24 cal/oz)	0.81	8.6	4.4	2.2	Corn syrup solids, lactose; MCT oil, corn and coconut oil; nonfat milk, demineralized whey
Enfamil Premature	0.81	8.9	4.1	2.4	Same as above
Neosure	0.75	7.7	4.1	1.9	Nonfat milk with whey protein; sunflower, soy, MCT and coconut oil; corn syrup
Amino Acid–Based: Elemental Formulas					
Neocate	0.67	7.9	3.0	2.1	
Peptide-Based Formulas					
Nutramigen	0.67	8.8	2.6	2.2	Sucrose, modified tapioca starch; corn oil; casein hydrolysate
Pregestimil	0.67	9.1	2.7	1.9	Corn syrup solids, modified tapioca starch; corn oil and MCT oil; casein hydrolysate with amino acids
Alimentum	0.67	6.8	3.7	1.8	Tapioca starch, sucrose; MCT oil, safflower oil, soy oil, casein hydrolysate with amino acids

Adapted from Abad-Sinden A, Sutphen J: The practical use of infant formulas. In Wyllie R, Hyams J, eds: *Pediatric gastrointestinal disease,* Philadelphia, 1993, WB Saunders, p 1084; data from American Academy of Pediatrics. Committee on Nutrition: *Pediatric nutrition handbook,* ed 3, Elk Grove Village, Ill., 1993, American Academy of Pediatrics; Jew R, ed: *Pharmacy handbook and formulary,* The Children's Hospital of Philadelphia, Ohio, 1998, Lexi-Comp, p 375.
MCT, Medium-chain triglyceride.

deep freeze of −20° C for 3 to 6 months and given to the infant as needed.[131] Frozen milk is thawed quickly under running water. Once the milk is defrosted, it can be refrigerated for 24 hours.

If breast milk is not available, a variety of commercially prepared formulas can be given. For most patients, resuming their previously established diet is most appropriate. Otherwise, evaluation of the child's age and nutritional needs is

necessary to determine the most appropriate formula. Standard formulas for infants younger than 12 months of age contain whole protein and require intact biliary, pancreatic, and intestinal function. Although based on breast milk, formulas tend to have higher levels of polyunsaturated fat and lower levels of monounsaturated fat. Formulas also lack the range of complex carbohydrates found in breast milk. Infant formulas tend to have higher concentrations of some nutri-

TABLE 12-8   Selection of Infant Formulas (<1 Year of Age)

	Formula Description	Example of Formulas
Healthy term infant	60:40 whey/casein or casein formula	Enfamil Similac
	Whey hydrolyzed; hypoallergenic	Carnation Good Start
<34 Weeks' gestation	Premature infant formula	Similac Special Care Neosure Enfamil Premature
Uncomplicated lactose intolerance; casein sensitive	Lactose-free soy protein Isolate formula (sucrose and corn-free also available)	Lacto-free Prosobee Isomil
Organ dysfunction (e.g., renal, cardiac)	Low renal solute load	Similac PM 60/40 Good Start
Diarrhea management	Soy protein containing fiber	Isomil DF
Severe steatorrhea associated with bile acid deficiency, ileal resection, or lymphatic anomalies; fat malabsorption	Infant formula with MCT oil	Portagen Pregestimil Alimentum
Allergy to cow's milk (casein) and soy protein	Hypoallergenic casein hydrolysate; peptide based	Nutramigen Pregestimil Alimentum
Abnormal nutrient absorption, digestion, and transport; generalized malabsorption; severe intractable diarrhea; protein calorie malnutrition	Hydrolyzed casein with part of fat from MCT oil (lactose-free); peptide based	Pregestimil Alimentum
Abnormal nutrient absorption and transport; malabsorption of protein and fat; intractable diarrhea; protein calorie malnutrition	Hydrolyzed casein with percentage of fat from MCT oil (lactose-free and sucrose-free); peptide based; 100% Amino acid based	Pregestimil Neocate

Adapted from Wilson SE, Dietz WH Jr, Grand RJ et al: An algorithm for pediatric enteral alimentation, *Pediatr Ann* 16:233, 1987; Hendricks K, Walker W: *Manual of pediatric nutrition,* ed 2, St Louis, 1990, Mosby.
MCT, Medium-chain triglyceride.

ents compared with breast milk because the bioavailability of the nutrients contained in formula is lower. For children younger than 1 year of age, standard formulas have the same caloric densities, are of nearly identical osmolalities (250 to 320 mOsm), and provide similar calories (20 calories/ounce [cal/oz] or 0.67 calorie/ml). The type of infant formula can be selected based on the child's needs (Table 12-8) (see Appendix VII). Cow's milk–based formulas for healthy full-term infants (e.g., Similac, Enfamil with Fe) contain lactose as the major carbohydrate. Soy and coconut oil blends provide fat for the majority of these formulas. Lactose-free cow's milk–based formulas (e.g., Lacto-free) are also available for infants with suspected lactose intolerance. Soy-based formulas (e.g., Isomil, Prosobee) may also be recommended for infants exhibiting a primary or secondary lactose intolerance. Specialized formulas (Pregestimil, Alimentum, and Neosure) are available for infants who have malabsorption problems or are intolerant of the carbohydrates, fats, or protein contained in standard infant formulas. When fortified breast milk is not available, preterm infants require nutrient dense formulas (e.g., Similac Special Care). Formulas are prepared and refrigerated when opened for no longer than 24 hours.

For children older than 1 year of age, various formula options are available (Table 12-9) (see Appendix VII).

Pediatric formulas (e.g., Pediasure, Nutren Jr.) are specifically designed for children 1 to 10 years of age. These formulas provide a higher caloric value with an increase in grams of protein and carbohydrate and a decrease in fat content, compared with infant formulas. Higher amounts of calcium, phosphorus, and vitamin D with similar osmolarity to infant formulas (325 mOsm/kg) are also characteristic of pediatric formulas. Peptide-based formulas (e.g., Peptamin Jr.) are available for children with malabsorption problems. Elemental formulas such as Pediatric Vivonex may also be necessary for some children with severe problems. Pediasure with Fiber and Nutren Jr. are also available with fiber and are considered for children with diarrhea, constipation, neuromuscular disease, and immobility.

Adult formulations are generally used in children older than 10 years of age. These products range in caloric density from 1 to 2 kcal/ml and in general have a higher osmolarity (450 to 810 mOsm/L). Standard adult formulas require the patient to have normal digestive capacity. These formulas are isotonic, providing 1 cal/ml with a relatively high carbohydrate-to-fat ratio and intact or almost intact protein. Selection of these formulas is based on standards similar to those of infant formulas (Table 12-10) (see Appendix VII). Complete or standard lactose-free formulas (e.g., Isocal, Ensure) are adequate for the majority of patients. Fiber-

TABLE 12-9 Selected Pediatric and Adult Formulas

	Calories (kcal/ml)	Protein (g/L)	Fat (g/L)	Carbohydrate (g/L)
Standard Formulas (1-10 years)				
Nutren Jr.	1	21	42	127
Pediasure	1	30	50	110
Fiber Formula				
Pediasure with Fiber	1	30	50	110
Peptide-Based Formula Peptamin Jr.	1	30	38.5	137.5
Elemental Formula Neocate one plus	6.7	20.9	30	79
Standard Formulas (>10 years)				
Ensure	1.06	54.9	37.2	145
Ensure Plus	1.5	34	53	200
Isocal	1.06	44	44	133
Jevity	1.06	70	36.8	151.7
Magnacal	2	70	80	250
Osmolite	2	57	37	145
Isosource	1.06			
MCT-Containing Formula				
Lipisorb	1.35	57	57	161
Impact	1	56	28	132
Oxcepa	1.5	62.5	93.7	105.5
Amino Acid–Based Formulas				
Amin-Aid	1.96	19.4	46	366
Vivonex TEN	1.8	38	3	206
Fiber-Enriched Formulas				
Peptide Based With MCT				
Peptamin	1	40	39	127
Crucial	1.5	94	68	135
Hepatic Aid	1.78	44	36	169
Pulmocare	1.5	63	92	106
TraumaCal	1.5	82	68	142

Adapted from Committee on Nutrition, American Academy of Pediatrics: *Pediatric nutrition handbook,* ed 3, Elk Grove Village, Ill, 1993, pp 380-384; data from Jew R, ed: *Pharmacy handbook and formulary,* The Children's Hospital of Philadelphia, Ohio, 1998, Lexi-Comp, pp 425-438.
MCT, Medium-chain triglyceride.

TABLE 12-10 Selection of Older Child and Adolescent Formulas

	Formula Description	Suggested Formulas
Normal GI tract (child 1-10 yr)	Nutritionally complete for age group	Pediasure Nutren Jr.
Requiring Fiber	Nutritionally complete with fiber	Pediasure with Fiber
Abnormal GI tract	Peptide based	Peptamin Jr.
	MCT containing	Neocate plus one
	Elemental	Vivonex Pediatric
Normal GI tract (>10 yr)	Nutritionally complete	Ensure
Standard meal replacement		Osmolite
		Isocal
Higher protein/calorie needs (e.g., burns)	Nutritionally complete with high protein/calorie formula	Ensure Plus Magnacal
Significant pulmonary compromise	High-fat formulation	Oxcepa Pulmocare
Significant trauma requiring very high protein needs	High-protein formulation	TraumaCal Crucial
Abnormal GI tract functioning	Peptide based	Peptamen Vivonex TEN Amin-Aid Lipisorb

Adapted from Hendricks K, Walker W: *Manual of pediatric nutrition,* ed 2, St Louis, 1990, Mosby, pp 91-92.
MCT, Medium-chain triglyceride; *GI,* gastrointestinal.

◆ TABLE 12-11   Methods for Increasing Caloric Density of Infant Formulas

Method	Advantages	Disadvantages	Recommendations
Add less water to powdered/liquid concentrate formulas	Simple, easy Maintains standard ratio of protein, fat, and carbohydrate	Increases solute load May prolong gastric emptying, especially if >24 kcal/oz May cause diarrhea May precipitate dehydration in patients at risk for excessive losses	Monitor renal status Monitor for symptoms of reflux, abdominal distension Monitor for symptoms of dehydration
Add protein (e.g., Casec)	Relatively easy	May increase solute load High caloric density	See recommendation for other additives
Add carbohydrate (e.g., Polycose, Moducal)	Relatively easy to obtain and add to formula Relatively inexpensive Provides readily available source of energy Polycose and Moducal are easily digested Does not delay gastric emptying	When used in excess, may increase work of breathing May cause osmotic diarrhea Base formula may fall short of RDA for protein Overall vitamin and mineral content may be below RDA	Monitor respiratory status Monitor stool output; check stool for reducing substances Monitor total daily protein Supplement vitamins and minerals as required
Add fat (i.e., long-chain triglycerides [LCT], vegetable oils, microlipids, medium-chain triglycerides [MCT], MCT oil)	LCT easy to obtain and inexpensive MCT more rapidly digested, more readily absorbed Microlipids are emulsified MCT are not emulsified	LCT slow gastric emptying May aggravate reflux MCT very expensive MCT will adhere to tubing May cause diarrhea Aspiration of fat can be dangerous Base formula may fall short of RDA for protein Overall vitamins and minerals may fall short of RDA	Monitor for reflux, abdominal distension Reserve MCT for fat malabsorption, or delayed gastric emptying Combination of LCT and MCT may improve tolerance Monitor tolerance, stool output, serum triglycerides Monitor daily protein Do not exceed 60% of total calories from fat Supplement vitamins and minerals

Adapted from Huddleston K, Ferraro-McDuffie A, Wolff-Small T: Nutritional support of the critically ill child, *Crit Care Nurs Clin North Am* 5:75, 1993. *RDA,* Recommended daily allowance.

enriched formulas (e.g., Ensure and Sustacal with Fiber) may be useful for patients receiving tube feedings on a long-term basis or for those patients with diarrhea or constipation. Vivonex and Peptamen may be considered for older children with impaired gut perfusion. These formulas are usually isotonic to slightly hypertonic and provide 1 kcal/ml. Fiber-containing formulas may be beneficial in normalizing bowel pattern and maintaining a healthy gut mucosa.

Predigested or elemental formulas are usually hyperosmolar solutions that contain oligopeptides or amino acids as protein and oligosaccharides or disaccharides as carbohydrate. These formulas are appropriate for older children and adolescents with malabsorption problems because they require minimal digestion and are almost completely absorbed. Predigested or elemental formulas typically provide 1 cal/ml. Elemental formulas reduce bile acid excretion, which is one of the reasons that they are useful for malabsorption problems.

Specialized formulas vary in amino acid and nutrition distribution. Higher visceral protein levels have been demonstrated in patients receiving peptide-based formulas instead of those containing intact protein.[78] Formulas are now available that have been designed specifically with the needs of patients with adult respiratory distress syndrome (e.g., Oxcepa) and stress-induced hypermetabolism (e.g., Crucial, Impact).[80,114] Increased dietary component such as glutamine, arginine and ω-3 fatty acids when supplied in large quantities appear to have beneficial affects on burn patients.[133] A diet supplemented with arginine, ω-3 fatty acids, and ribonucleic acid (Impact) has also shown a positive immunologic effect.[98]

Formula Enhancement.   There are several methods of providing increased caloric density of formula above standard (Table 12-11). Calorically enhanced infant and adult formulas are available. These formulas may be used for patients who require fluid restriction or those who require a higher caloric intake. Many infant formulas are now commercially available in concentrations of 24 cal/oz (0.8 cal/ml) and 27 cal/oz (0.9 cal/ml). Also, when reconstituting infant formulas, calories can be increased above the formula's standard caloric concentration by using less free water. High-calorie adult formulas usually contain 1.5 to 2 cal/ml. When providing concentrated formulas to an infant or child, being conscious of the increasing renal solute load is important.

Single modular components can also be added to standard formula in the form of protein, fats, or carbohydrates. Protein can be added to the diet to increase protein density. Fat modules, such as medium-chain triglyceride (MCT) oil (7.7 cal/ml) and microlipids (4.5 cal/ml), can be added in small volumes to existing formulas to increase caloric density. Smaller volumes avoid separation of fat in the formula and reduce the chance of overwhelming the absorptive capacity of the intestine, which may occur with a large bolus of lipid. MCTs are more easily absorbed, better utilized, and smaller and have greater water solubility. Carbohydrate modules like Moducal (19 kcal/tbsp) and Polycose (2 cal/ml) provide supplemental carbohydrates. Protein modules such as Casec (4 g/tbsp) can also be added to the diet. A human milk fortifier can also be used to increase the caloric content of breast milk. Two packets per 50 ml provide 24 cal/oz. Protein, calcium, phosphorus, and vitamin concentrations are also increased with human milk fortifier. A higher risk of nutrient imbalances can occur when modular units are added to the diet, and therefore extra care must be taken to adhere to the recommended nutrient distribution guidelines.

Implementing and Advancing Feedings. Establishing a goal of therapy improves the implementation process of any feeding regimen. Feeding into the gut can meet the child's nutritional needs or be instituted to stimulate gut mucosal integrity and function. Using a systemic approach to the initiation of feeding is helpful (see Appendix VII).

Delivery Methods. Adequate delivery of enteral feedings can be accomplished by several methods[134] (Table 12-12). The route chosen for enteral nutrition depends on the level of GI function, the expected duration of tube feeding, and the child's potential for aspiration. Feeding the child into the stomach allows gastric acid and other hormones to respond normally in the digestive process. Typically, gastric feedings enable the child to tolerate a larger osmotic load with a lower incidence of dumping syndrome, allow more flexibility in feeding schedule, and have greater mobility between feedings. Gastric feedings also incur less administrative expense.[135] The gastric feeding site is recommended when there is minimal risk of aspiration. Enteral tubes may be inserted into the duodenum or jejunum in children with the potential for difficulties in tolerating feeding from inadequate gastric motility or with an unacceptable risk of aspiration from a depressed gag reflex and gastroesophageal reflux (GER). Placing the tube past the pyloric sphincter reduces the risk of aspiration and is recommended with increasing regularity as the method of enteral feeding administration for critically ill children.[1,134,136] Montecalvo and associates[137] found that for patients administered nasojejunal feedings, a higher prealbumin level and a higher percentage of their caloric goal was met. When tubes are placed past the pylorus, a gastric decompression tube may be necessary.

An orogastric, nasogastric (NG), or intestinal tube can be placed for temporary enteral feedings (see Appendix VII). Orogastric tubes are appropriate for infants younger than 4 weeks of age. The oropharynx is used to avoid potential airway obstruction in these obligate nose breathers. Nasoenteric tubes are commonly placed in older infants and children. Tubes composed of soft, nonreactive materials, such as silicone or polyurethane, are desirable. These tubes are long-lasting, pliable, and less likely to cause nose irritation.[135] Decompression tubes are never used for feeding children because of the risk of aspiration. With feeding, aspiration becomes more likely because the side holes of decompression tubes often lie proximal to the stomach.

Although the method of placement for gastric tubes is a standard nursing procedure, various methods for transpyloric placement of feeding tubes have been reported in the literature.[138-143] At the bedside, Chellis and colleagues[138] placed postpyloric enteral tubes using nonweighted silicone 6 Fr and 8 Fr 36-inch tubes in critically ill children with a 93% success rate using air insufflation, a prokinetic agent (e.g., metoclopramide [Reglan]), and positioning. To use this method of tube placement, the operator first marks the tube at the gastroesophageal junction (measured from mouth to ear to xiphoid process) and then the pylorus (measured by continuing the tube to left or right costal margin) (Fig. 12-1, *A*). Initially, the child is placed supine with the head of the bed elevated 15 to 30 degrees. The stomach is decompressed, and the tube is inserted to the gastroesophageal junction. If no signs of coiling or tracheal intubation are evident, the patient is turned to the right lateral oblique position, and the tube is advanced at 1- to 2-cm intervals until air is auscultated over the right upper quadrant (RUQ). Reglan 0.1 mg/kg is given intravenously, and while instilling 5 to 10 ml of air and auscultating the abdomen, the tube is advanced 1 cm at a time. Placement occurs when sounds change from resonant low-pitched gurgles to high-pitched propagating crackles near the RUQ and the operator is unable to withdraw air (see Fig. 12-1, *B*). The tube is then advanced 5 to 10 cm to ensure placement in the distal duodenum or jejunum.[138] The inability to aspirate insufflated air was 99% predictive of correct tube placement in critically ill children using the technique documented by Chellis and associates.[144] Another technique using feeding tubes with a pH sensor predicted greater than a 95% success rate when the pH was measured.[139,145] The use of ranitidine (Zantac) may invalidate the use of pH as an indicator of tube placement.

Checking tube placement is an essential component of delivering enteral feedings. The traditional method of air insufflation into the tube and auscultation of a "whooshing" sound can no longer be recommended. This method may be misleading and dangerous to the patient.[146-149] Metheny and associates[150] demonstrated that sounds generated by air insufflation through small-bore feeding tubes are unreliable for indicating tube placement. In addition, these tubes often migrate from the intended location. Also, aspiration can contribute information that may help identify tube location[151]; however, fluid alone does not ensure that the tube is

TABLE 12-12   Enteral Feeding Sites and Routes

Site	Route	Advantage	Disadvantage	Indications	Contraindications
Stomach		Allows for normal digestive processes and hormonal responses Tolerance of larger osmotic loads Decreased incidence of dumping syndrome Greater mobility between feedings Greater flexibility in feeding schedule and formula choice		Usually first consideration for enteral nutrition	Delayed gastric emptying Pulmonary aspiration Gastroesophageal reflux Intractable vomiting Impaired or absent gag reflex
	Orogastric	Does not obstruct nasal passage	May increase salivary flow and make clearance more difficult	Infants <4 weeks of age Nasal passage obstruction Basilar skull fracture	Older infant or child with gag reflex
	Nasogastric	Easy intubation	Nasal, esophageal, or tracheal irritation Easily dislodged by an uncooperative child Easily dislodged by a forceful cough May stimulate gag Caretaker must be trained Limited long-term compliance in the home care setting	For short-term use	Same as for the stomach
	Gastrostomy	Allows patient greater mobility Feedings are generally well tolerated Larger-diameter feeding tube lessens chances of tube obstruction Does not obstruct the airway	May require a surgical procedure for placement May result in increased gastroesophageal reflux Occasional leakage around the insertion site Skin irritation and infection Risk of intraabdominal leak with peritonitis	Prolonged enteral nutritional support	Same as for the stomach
Small intestine		Feed enterally despite poor gastric motility and persistent high gastric residuals Lessens the chances of gastric distension, gastroesophageal reflux, pulmonary aspiration	Less mixing of formula with pancreatic enzymes Limited choices of feeding schedule and formula selection Greater risk of bacterial overgrowth Greater risk of bowel perforation Changes small bowel intestinal flora	Congenital upper gastrointestinal (GI) anomalies Inadequate gastric motility Following upper GI surgery Patients with increased risk of aspiration	Nonfunctioning GI tract
	Nasojejunal/ nasoduodenal		More complicated placement; tube may be more easily displaced during peristalsis	For intermediate-term nutritional support	
	Jejunostomy		Technically difficult to place	Jejunal feedings for >6 mo For postoperative nutritional management of abdominal surgery while a paralytic ileus exists	Patients at operative risk

Adapted from Hendricks R, Walker W: *Manual of pediatric nutrition*, ed 2, St Louis, 1990, Mosby, pp 74-75.

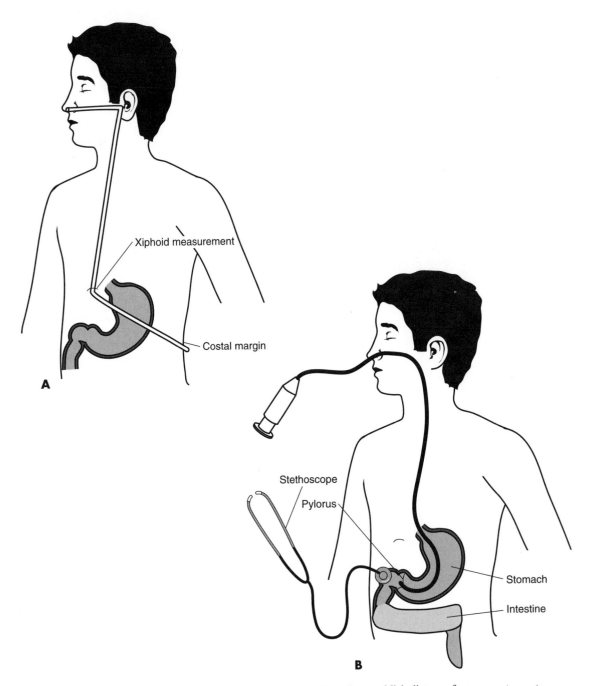

Fig. 12-1 After pyloric tube placement. **A,** Measure feeding tube: establish distance from nares to ear to xiphoid, make first mark; continue tube to right or left lateral costal margin, make second mark. **B,** Insert tube, auscultate over right upper quadrant, passing tube at 1- to 2-cm intervals. (From Chellis MJ, Sanders SV, Dean JM et al: Bedside transpyloric tube placement in the pediatric intensive care unit, *JPEN J Parenter Enteral Nutr* 20:88-90, 1996.)

in the correct position.[152] Fluid may be inadvertently aspirated from the pleural space or lung. The aspirate's pH must be checked with pH paper to ensure correct placement.[153,154] An acidic pH of less than 4 indicates that the tube is in the stomach when gastric acid inhibitors are not used, and a highly alkaline pH of greater than 7 indicates intestinal fluid.[155] Because of questions regarding the reliability of traditional methods for checking tube placement, an abdominal radiograph is the definitive method for confirming correct tube placement.[134,154]

For those children requiring a prolonged enteral delivery system, a gastrostomy or jejunostomy is indicated.[156-158] Traditionally, gastrostomy tubes have been placed surgically. For these children, GER becomes a common problem. Gastrostomy tubes can cause skin breakdown and reduced gastric capacity. Traditional gastrostomies do not provide stabilization of the tube at the stoma and therefore tend to migrate in and out of the abdominal cavity, causing enlargement of the stoma and inadvertent removal of the tube.

With the advent of percutaneous endoscopic gastrostomy (PEG) tubes, a safe nonsurgical option can now be offered to children requiring this delivery method.[159-161] Under endoscopic guidance, a feeding tube is placed through a wall puncture.[162] The placement of a PEG tube may be done at the bedside or in the endoscopy suite with intravenous sedation or, in the case of young uncooperative children, in the operating room under general anesthesia. The PEG tube is stabilized by crossbars internally and externally in a subcutaneous fistula created between the gastric mucosa and abdominal wall. When anesthesia is not used, the intraoperative and postoperative complications are avoided. Feedings can usually be introduced within 24 hours.

Skin level profile and nonreflux devices, such as the Button, Gastroport, and Mic-Key, are an option for children requiring long-term feeding tubes.[163-165] The Button is a type of gastrostomy device that has a mushroom dome with a one-way antireflux valve in the stomach. The Button sits flush against the skin, reducing migration along the GI tract and the risk of accidental removal. A well-developed gastrostomy stoma is needed before placement of a Button. The Mic-Key can be used for both feeding and decompression.[166] This device operates like a Foley catheter and is held in place with a balloon.

A jejunostomy can also be placed in a child with long-term nutrition support needs. This route is employed in those children who are at increased risk for gastric aspiration or who have undergone extensive gastric or duodenal surgery.[167] Endoscopic jejunostomy requires a similar placement method to a PEG, although it is technically more difficult.[156]

Intermittent and continuous feedings are two techniques of administering enteral feeding. Intermittent tube feedings mimic normal eating patterns by allowing the gut to rest. Intermittent bolus feedings are often preferred for older children or those children with no history of or potential for feeding intolerance. These feedings are typically administered via gastric tubes because the stomach is needed as a reservoir for the large volumes of formula administered. Gastrostomy tube feedings are commonly given by the bolus method. Bolus feedings do not require a feeding pump and therefore are typically less expensive and increase patient mobility. A suggested feeding schedule for infants 1 to 3 months of age is five to seven feedings per day, decreasing the frequency to three to four feedings per day by the time the child is 6 months old.

In the acute phase of critical illness, continuous feedings may be better tolerated than bolus feedings.[168] Continuous feedings typically decrease the risk of aspiration and are indicated for children with a significant risk of respiratory distress. Infants with smaller gastric capacity and those children with the potential for GER especially benefit from continuous feedings. Continuous feedings can be delivered throughout the day or while the child is asleep. Transpyloric and continuous feedings are preferred in head-injured patients to prevent aspiration and achieve maximum caloric intake.[143] Feedings via the duodenum or jejunum require formula to be infused continuously to avoid distension of the bowel, fluid and electrolyte shifts, and diarrhea. A potential risk of formula contamination exists with continuous feedings because of the longer amount of time that formula is at room temperature.

The common practice is to start with clear liquids if the child has a questionable ability to protect the airway and to dilute formulas to one-half strength at the onset of enteral feedings. Formula dilution, however, is often unnecessary unless the child is receiving hypertonic feeds, has been given nothing by mouth for greater than 2 weeks, is at risk for gut ischemia, or is malnourished before admission (see Appendix VII). If graded feedings are preferred for nutritional support, it is reasonable to start with 50% of the therapeutic goal of the appropriate formula and then increase each feeding by 25% as tolerated. If the goal of feeding is to provide trophic feedings to protect the gut, advancement is slow. In this case, half-strength formula is maintained at 0.5 ml/kg/hr for 2 to 3 days. Increasing the infusion rate 2 ml/hr every 12 hours has been recommended.[169] Use of free water should be considered, especially for patients who are receiving calorically dense formula or if constipation is an issue.

Monitoring Enteral Therapy.   Monitoring enteral feeding and evaluating tolerance are important aspects of caring for the child with enteral feedings (Table 12-13). When caring for critically ill children, evaluating complications, taking preventative steps, and intervening when appropriate are important responsibilities for the healthcare provider (Table 12-14).

GI complications, including diarrhea, constipation, nausea, and vomiting, with or without subsequent aspiration has been reported in the enterally fed patients.[134] Smith and colleagues[170] reported that 63% of critically ill mechanically ventilated patients who were tube fed had associated diarrhea. Hypertonic formula, excessive volumes, and rapid infusion rates are often blamed as the cause of diarrhea. Edes, Walk, and Austin,[44] however, concluded that formula is often not responsible for diarrhea in tube-fed patients. Hyperosmolar electrolyte replacement and medications, especially when infused undiluted into the intestinal tract, can contribute to diarrhea.[171] Sorbitol, an ingredient in many drug preparations, is often linked to diarrhea.[44]

Treatment for diarrhea depends on its cause. Diarrhea is significant when it affects growth. Reducing substances of the stool are checked to evaluate the source of the diarrhea. Eliminating or reducing problem nutrients, such as fat or lactose, may manage diarrhea. Changing the delivery rate or the administration method from intermittent to continuous or adding dietary fiber to the feeding may also be useful. The addition of some antidiarrheal agents to the formula has been noted to decrease loose stool.

Constipation may occur as a result of a low-fiber diet or inadequate fluid intake. Adding fiber or choosing a high-fiber formula may eliminate constipation in the critically ill child. Constipation may also be avoided by increasing dietary free water.

Vomiting and nausea occur in patients who are tube fed. Vomiting may have its origin in esophageal tube placement or as a consequence of delayed gastric emptying. Lower esophageal sphincter incompetence with gastric reflux and pulmonary aspiration may occur. Large volumes, fast rates of infusion, hyperosmolar formulas, and hypertonic medi-

| | | | | | |

Table 12-13　Enteral Feedings: Patient-Monitoring Guidelines

Parameter	Intermittent Feedings	Continuous Feedings	Possible Complications	Therapy	Comments
Gastrointestinal					
Stool frequency	Check each stool	Check each stool	Diarrhea	Reduce the rate of feed, change formula, or use continuous feeds	
			Constipation	Adequate hydration; use fiber-containing formulas; use stool softeners, if indicated	
Hemetest	Daily until 48 hours if negative results; prn thereafter	Daily until 48 hours if negative results; prn thereafter	Gastrointestinal irritation	Evaluate cause	
Reducing substance	Daily during advancement; prn thereafter	Daily during advancement; prn thereafter	Carbohydrate intolerance	Dilute feed, change formula	
pH	Daily until 48 hours; thereafter prn if pH greater than 60	Daily until 48 hours; thereafter prn if pH greater than 6.0	Carbohydrate intolerance, bacterial overgrowth	Dilute feed, change formula	
Abdominal girth	As necessary	q12h and prn	Feeding intolerance	Evaluate cause; Adjust feeds prn	
Metabolic					
Urine specific gravity	q4-8h then daily	q4-8h then daily	Fluid imbalance	Adjust fluid intake, adjust concentration of formula	
Sugar/acetone	Daily during advancement; thereafter prn	Daily during advancement; thereafter prn	Glucose intolerance	Reduce feeds, give insulin, continuous feeds	

Parameter			Complication	Intervention	Comments
Serum electrolytes	q24-48h during advancement; thereafter prn	q24-48h during advancement; thereafter prn	Electrolyte imbalance	Readjust formula as needed	Electrolyte imbalances in tube-fed patients are usually associated with underlying medical conditions
Complete nutrition assessment	Weekly	Weekly			
Mechanical/Technical					
Skin	Every feed	q4-8h		Reinsert tube in contra-lateral nares with changes; Use skin barrier; Avoid angulation when taping	
Tube occlusion	Every feed	q4-8h		Flush tube with warm water; Flush after medications; If occlusion persists, flush with Viokase enzyme solution	
Tube placement	Every feed	q3-4h	Tube displacement	Reposition tube	Secure tube independent of position
Position patient	Every feed	q3h	Aspiration	Maintain upper body position of 30 degrees during feeds and for 30-45 min thereafter	Especially important for children with gastro-esophageal reflux and altered gastric motility

Adapted from Hendricks R, Walker WA: *Manual of pediatric nutrition*, ed 2, St Louis, 1990, Mosby, pp 104-105.

TABLE 12-14 Common Complications of Enteral Feedings

Problem	Causes	Prevention/Intervention
Gastrointestinal		
Diarrhea/dumping syndrome	Medications Rapidly delivered formula Hypertonic formula Hypertonic medications Substrate intolerance Bacterial contamination of formula Lack of fiber Concomitant antibiotic therapy Mucosal atrophy and malnutrition Impaction	Decrease delivery rate Alter formula carbohydrate and electrolyte content Recognize or avoid if possible drugs that result in diarrhea Use parenteral nutrition or elemental formula Recognize and eliminate the source of the contamination Avoid lactose-containing products
Constipation	Low fiber intake Inadequate fluid intake	Add fiber or choose a high-fiber formula Increase free water intake Add prune juice
Vomiting, nausea, GER, pulmonary aspiration	Fat intolerance Bowel ileus Swallowing excess air Improper tube placement Infusion rate too rapid Large residuals Hyperosmolar formula Hypertonic medications Gastroesophageal reflux Gastric hypomotility	Reevaluate tube placement Consider continuous or transpyloric feedings Metoclopramide may be given to enhance motility Reduce carbohydrate content of formula Reduce rate and/or concentration as indicated Aspirate air from feeding tube before feedings Position patient on the right side
Technical		
Clogged feeding tube	Failure to irrigate feeding tube regularly Formula too viscous for diameter of feeding tube Administration of medications via feeding tube	Flush tubing with water Enzyme solution Replace tubing Follow manufacturer's recommendations for tube size
GI tract perforation	Improper tube placement	Stop feedings, confirm placement by chest x-ray film
Nasal, pharyngeal, esophageal irritation	Improper skin care Extended use of polyvinyl tubes	Evaluate appropriateness of tube size Periodically change naris used for feeding tube
Metabolic Disturbances		
Fluid and electrolyte imbalance	Cardiac and/or renal insufficiency Hypertonic medications Severe protein-calorie malnutrition Malabsorption Inadequate fluid intake	Evaluate cause and treat Increase fluid intake as indicated Decrease formula concentration
Hyperglycemia	Insufficient insulin production or use Trauma or sepsis Excessive carbohydrate intake	Give insulin Reduce flow rate Reduce carbohydrate content of formula Avoid abrupt cessation of feedings Monitor glucose levels
Azotemia	High protein intake Renal immaturity or dysfunction Liver disease Metabolic dysfunction (e.g., inborn errors of metabolism)	Decrease protein content of the feeding
Infection	Inadequate mouth care Improper formula-mixing technique Use of contaminated equipment or supplies Long hang time of formula	Routine mouth care Use clean technique when mixing formula Change delivery setups every 24-48 hours Hang formula for 4-8 hours only
Oral aversion	Negative oral experiences (e.g., traumatic tube intubation) No positive oral experiences (e.g., thumb sucking, nipple feeding)	Provide pacifier for non-nutritive sucking Implement oral stimulation program

Adapted from Hendricks K, Walker W: *Manual of pediatric nutrition*, ed 2, St Louis, 1990, Mosby, pp 106-107.

cations may contribute to the risk of nausea and vomiting. Excessive air in the stomach from air spillage of positive pressure ventilation and air flushing of feeding tubes also may lead to vomiting. Checking abdominal girth every 12 hours may help to identify feeding intolerance in jejunal feedings.

Pulmonary aspiration may be the most serious common complication of enteral tube feeding.[13,167] A high incidence of GER exists in patients with both orotracheal and NG tubes.[172] To reduce vomiting and the risk of aspiration, administering formula continuously rather than by the bolus method, and placing the tube past the pylorus may be useful. Also recommended to reduce (but not eliminate) GER is elevating the head of the bed 30 to 40 degrees during feeding and for a period after feeding. While advancing the diet and when abdominal distension or vomiting occurs, a routine of checking and refeeding residual gastric contents before each feeding is recommended.[173] If half the feeding or 2 hours of continuous feedings are aspirated, jejunal feeding should be considered (see Appendix VII).

To detect silent aspiration, pulmonary secretions may be checked for the presence of glucose with oxidant reagent strips or by placing a small quantity of blue food coloring in the formula. Respiratory distress may indicate aspiration or stomach distension. For those children with cuffed endotracheal tubes, inflation of the cuff may reduce the likelihood of aspiration.[174] A gastric emptying agent such as metoclopramide (Reglan) or erythromycin may be given to assist in gastric motility and to improve gastric emptying.[175,176]

Nasal and pharyngeal irritation and tube occlusions are among the common technical complications of feeding tubes. Maintaining skin integrity is critical to preventing nasopharyngeal erosion. Polyurethane and Silastic pediatric tubes allow longer use of each tube and reduced rate of tissue irritation and erosion.[1] Frequent assessment of the naris is essential to identify skin breakdown, and routine skin care of the area is recommended. Replacing feeding tubes once per month will rotate pressure areas and may help to reduce tube occlusions. When enteral tubes are changed, using the contralateral naris is recommended. Clogging of the feeding tube may occur, especially when using tubes with small diameters. Thick formula remaining in the tube and highly viscous medications increase the likelihood of this type of complication. Aspiration of residuals also has been identified as a contributing factor in tube occlusion.[177] Checking tube placement only when dislodgment is suspected may reduce this complication. Continuous feedings are 3 times more likely to obstruct the feeding tube.[178] To ensure enteral tube patency and prevent tube occlusion, water or saline may be flushed through the tube routinely before and after checking residuals. For bolus feedings, the tube may be flushed after each feeding, and for continuous feedings, the tube may be flushed every 8 hours. To relieve an obstruction, warm water alternating with air has been suggested.[134] Also, an enzymatic solution containing pancrelipase (Viokase) has been found to be helpful (see Appendix VII). Preventing infection related to enteral feeding is a necessary aspect of the care of a tube-fed child. A child who is receiving enteral feedings and nothing by mouth needs routine mouth care with saline or an antimi-

crobial mouthwash. This important aspect of care provides comfort and prevents infection in the oral cavity. Tube feeding is an almost perfect medium for bacterial growth. Contamination can occur while the feeding is mixed or during administration of the formula. To reduce the risk of infection and prevent formula contamination, feeding bags and delivery sets are changed every 24 to 48 hours. A supply of formula lasting no more than 4 to 8 hours is to be hung at one time. Adding new formula to remaining formula is to be avoided.

Metabolic monitoring to prevent electrolyte and other nutrient imbalances is key for patients on nutritional support. Children receiving high-caloric formulas require frequent testing of urine specific gravity, sugar, and acetone. Monitoring serum electrolytes, liver function tests, triglycerides, complete blood count, and serum proteins, such as prealbumin, may be necessary. Use of high-caloric formulas can lead to increased renal solute load and potential dehydration.

Enterostomy tubes carry the additional potential complications of wound infection or dehiscence, skin irritation from leakage of gastric contents around the tube site, inadvertent traumatic removal of the tube, obstruction of the pylorus, and small intestine adhesion.[134] The gastrostomy site is inspected daily for redness, swelling, and drainage, and the site is cleaned with soap and water. Bacitracin ointment may be applied and the site dressed.[162] A stoma adhesive or skin barrier can be used to protect the skin. For the child with a gastric Button, the device is rotated in a full circle during cleaning.[165]

Enterally administered medications and drug-nutrient interactions can cause difficulty for the enterally fed critically ill child.[171,179] Food can have a significant effect on drug absorption (Table 12-15). Administration of hypertonic medications may cause gastric distension, nausea, vomiting, and diarrhea.[44] Tube placement can affect absorption and bioavailability of medications. Hypertonic preparations (e.g., potassium chloride elixir, hyperosmolar antibiotic suspension) must be administered in the stomach to avoid GI intolerance. High-fat diets can alter the release of theophylline and result in toxic serum concentrations of the drug.[171] Absorption of phenytoin, phenobarbital, and aspirin may be impaired when mixed with enteral products.[180,181] Apparently an interaction between phenytoin and the sodium, calcium caseinates, and calcium chloride is found in many formulas. A decrease in absorption of many antibiotics in the presence of food has been demonstrated.[171] Also, ingesting vitamin C may inhibit the therapeutic effect of warfarin sodium (Coumadin).

General recommendations for administering medications through a feeding tube include flushing the feeding tube with a bolus of water before and after administering the drug, preventing the mixing of drugs before administration, diluting hyperosmolar or irritant medications, giving liquid medications when possible, and crushing tablets to a fine powder before administration[182] (see Appendix VII).

Transitioning to Oral Feeding. A critical component in the care of any infant who is not fed by mouth is the promotion of the suck-swallow reflex. Transitioning tube feedings to oral feedings can be a challenge. Children who

◆ TABLE 12-15 Effects of Nutrients on Absorption of Selected Drugs

Decreased Drug Absorption With Food in the Stomach	Delayed Drug Absorption With Food in the Stomach	Enhanced Drug Absorption With Food in the Stomach
Ampicillin	Acetaminophen	Chlorothiazide
Aspirin	Aspirin	Diazepam
Captopril	Cephalexin	Erythromycin estolate
Cephalexin suspension	Sulfonamides	Erythromycin ethylsuccinate
Tetracycline	Cimetidine	Hydralazine
Erythromycin stearate	Digoxin	Propranolol
Hydrochlorothiazide	Furosemide	Spironolactone
Nafcillin	Quinidine	Theophylline
Penicillins	Ciprofloxacin	Griseofulvin
Phenobarbital		Macrodantin
Rifampin		

Adapted from Miller M: Nutrient-drug interactions in children. In Suskind R, Lewinter-Suskind L, eds: *Textbook of pediatric nutrition,* New York, 1993, Raven Press, p 254.

have had few positive oral experiences often develop an oral aversion. This problem is particularly common in the medically fragile patients who are technology dependent. Nonnutritive sucking appears to enhance physical growth and assist the child in the transition from tube feedings to oral feedings. Nonnutritive sucking is believed to increase nutrient absorption from the gut.[183,184] Studies involving premature infants demonstrated earlier weaning from gavage feeding when the infant was provided with opportunities for nonnutritive sucking. To encourage the transition to oral feedings, these early pleasurable feeding experiences assist in reducing the risk of food aversions.[185] For the child receiving chronic enteral feedings, an oromotor stimulation program is an especially important adjunct to tube feeding. Referral to an occupational therapist is considered for infants not accepting nonnutritive sucking. Although it may take months to years for some children to achieve the transition, it is important to always keep in mind the goal of weaning the child from tube feedings to oral feedings.

Parenteral Nutrition. Parenteral nutrition (PN) is composed of a hypertonic solution of water, glucose, amino acids, vitamins, minerals, trace elements, and an isotonic lipid emulsion. PN is a lifesaving technology for some patients. When the critically ill child's GI tract is unable to absorb nutrients or when the enteral route cannot be used for a prolonged period, PN can greatly benefit the child. PN is also considered for patients with intractable vomiting from acute pancreatitis and with severe diarrhea from disorders such as inflammatory bowel disease, paralytic ileus, and small bowel obstruction.[173,186] In children, PN is delivered over 24 hours and via continuous infusion pump.

Selection of Route. PN may be given via the peripheral or central route.[187,188] The hypertonic fluids of PN require a large-diameter, high-flow vein, with a dedicated port. The choice between peripheral and central routes is based on the child's nutritional needs, clinical condition, and expected duration of illness. The peripheral route is designed to supplement oral intake or to meet short-term nutritional needs (less than 7 days) without high nutritional

requirements. The peripheral route is limited by the glucose content of the fluid and is restricted to 10% to 12.5% dextrose solutions.

The central route provides a larger, more stable vein that can tolerate higher intravenous glucose concentrations.[189] To administer PN centrally for relatively short periods, a catheter is typically placed in the distal superior vena cava, via the internal or external jugular or subclavian vein with the catheter tip just above the right atrium. The inferior vena cava via the femoral vein may also be used. The femoral vein is usually avoided because of the increased risk of contamination.

Another alternative to percutaneous central line access is a peripherally inserted central catheter (PICC).[190-192] A PICC is a long, flexible silicone catheter designed to be inserted into the median basilic or cephalic vein via the antecubital space. The catheter is threaded until it reaches the inferior vena cava or the superior vena cava. This type of catheter may also be placed in the large saphenous vein and advanced to the inferior vena cava, particularly in neonates.

For those patients who require long-term PN, catheters can be placed surgically. The Broviac catheter was the first long-term, small-lumen, flexible catheter. The Hickman catheter was introduced shortly thereafter, followed by the development of various other single-lumen and multilumen long-term catheters.[187,193] Implantable ports are also considered for long-term access and may offer less risk of infection. A subcutaneous pocket, usually on the chest, is created to implant the device. All central catheters require radiographic confirmation of catheter placement before infusing PN.

Composition of Parenteral Nutrition. The PN formula is tailored to meet the critically ill child's nutritional and fluid requirements (Table 12-16). Children with special nutritional needs resulting from renal disease, hepatic disease, and other conditions may require modified formulations.[194] Initiating PN is a step-by-step process.

◆ TABLE 12-16   Formulating a Total Parenteral Nutrition Solution

Nutrient	Full-term Infant			Child		
	Begin	Advance	Maximum	Begin	Advance	Maximum
Carbohydrate (g/kg/day)	4-6	2-3	10-12	4-6	2-4	10-12
	5-9	3-4	14-17	5-9	3-6	14-17
Fat 20% concentration (g/kg/day)	1-2	1	3-3.5	1-2	1	3
Protein (g/kg/day)	2-2.5		3	1.0-2		2

Adapted from Huddleston K, Ferraro-McDuffie A, Wolff-Small T: Nutritional support of the critically ill child, *Crit Care Clin North Am* 5:72, 1993.
NOTE: Monitor nutritional parameters and tolerance and advance as indicated.

Parenteral protein is supplied in the form of synthetic crystalline amino acids combining essential and nonessential amino acids. Protein provides 4 kcal/g. The type of formulation chosen is based on the child's age and disease state. The selection of the type of amino acid solution may affect the protein use, patient tolerance, and ability to avoid deficiencies. Generally 1 g of protein is equivalent to 1 g of amino acid. Standard PN has inadequate amounts of tyrosine, cystine, and glutamine for infants and children. Trophamine has a similar amino acid pattern to breast milk and is designed for children younger than 6 months of age. Trophamine has higher amounts of tyrosine and histidine, which are essential for infants. Novamine provides essential and nonessential amino acids appropriate for children older than 6 months of age. Special amino acid solutions for children with special needs are also available. Aminosyn RF has a higher ratio of essential to nonessential amino acids and is available for patients with renal failure. Hepatasol is a preparation enriched with branched-chain amino acids for children with severe liver disease. Glutamine added to parenteral formulations may decrease the degree of intestinal atrophy when enteral feedings are not administered.[195] The usual recommendation of parenteral amino acids is 2 to 3 g/kg/day of protein for infants, 1 to 2 g/kg daily of protein for older children, and 1 to 1.5 g/kg daily of protein for adolescents.[5] Nitrogen retention is reduced when protein is supplied parenterally. Therefore when administering protein parenterally, amino acids are supplied in a higher concentration. Children who are well hydrated with normal renal function can receive the full amount of protein recommended at the onset of therapy. When advancing amino acid concentration is necessary, daily increases of 0.5 g/kg are recommended for neonates, whereas 1 g/kg daily is recommended for older infants and children.[196] Care is taken not to administer greater amounts of protein than recommended because azotemia, hyperammonemia, and an increase in minute ventilation and oxygen consumption may occur.

Dextrose is the principal form of carbohydrate supplied and the common energy source of most parenteral regimens. Calories from carbohydrates may provide as much as 40% to 60% of the diet. In parenteral solutions, unlike enteral formulas, dextrose provides 3.4 cal/g, with 10% dextrose providing 0.34 kcal/ml and 20% dextrose providing 0.68 cal/ml. Dextrose is often started at a 10% concentration and then gradually increased over 2 days or as tolerated. With gradual increases in the dextrose concentration, the pancreas is given time to increase its insulin response and avoid hyperglycemia and glucosuria with a secondary osmotic diuresis.[197]

Fat is supplied in the form of a lipid solution produced from either soybean oil alone or a mixture of safflower and soybean oils with egg yolk phospholipid and glycerin as the emulsifying agent. Fat emulsions concentrated at 20% have 200 g/L of fat and 2 cal/ml. In general, higher fat emulsions allow a decrease in carbohydrate administration and may reduce the child's carbon dioxide production and RQ. These lipids are stable for a moderate period at room temperature. The use of intravenous fats provides a concentrated source of energy while preventing essential fatty acid deficiency. To achieve this goal, at least 4% to 8% of the child's diet must be from fat. To prevent essential fatty acid deficiency (EFAD), 0.5 to 1 g/kg/day of Intralipids is recommended.[29] The percentage of fat in the diet, however, should not exceed 50% to 65% of the total calories, or 3 to 4 g/kg daily. Fat intolerance, as indicated by elevated serum triglycerides, may interfere with immune function and should be avoided. When administering lipids, it is important to consider the allergies to soy products and eggs.

Implementation and Advancement. A suggested method of introducing and advancing PN is to begin on day 1 with 2 g/kg of lipid emulsion and 10% dextrose and then on day 2 to advance the lipids by 1 g/kg daily along with advancing the dextrose 5% to 10%. The initiation phase can take 3 to 5 days. A filter is placed on the dextrose and amino acid solution to trap precipitate. Fat emulsions traditionally have been administered separately to prevent clogging of the intravenous catheter; however, modern lipids can be mixed into triple-mixed total nutrient admixtures.[198] Total nutrient admixture (TNA) adds the lipid emulsion to the amino acid and dextrose solution. When administering lipids, an in-line filter is never used because the particles are too large. This method of mixing is economical and conserves nursing and pharmacy time. TNA is a less stable emulsion that traditional PN. Discontinuation of PN is recommended when the GI tract is able to absorb 70% of the child's caloric needs.

Electrolytes, vitamins, and minerals must be added to parenteral solutions to provide nutrients essential for metabolism and cellular function. Pediatric and adult multivitamin preparations are available. Not much definitive information is available concerning the parenteral requirements for vitamins or minerals available for critically ill children. Current guidelines reflect the needs of children who are healthy and are fed orally. The pediatric multivitamin solution used for infants and children younger than 11 years includes vitamin K, lower amounts of the B vitamins, and larger amounts of vitamin D. The adult formulation MVI-12 is used for children older than 11 years. Calcium and phosphorus are necessary for proper bone growth and metabolic functions. Sodium, potassium, calcium, phosphorus, and magnesium are added separately to PN preparations. Depending on the underlying disease and condition, sodium and potassium can be provided in salt forms of chloride, acetate, or phosphate. Zinc, copper, chromium, and manganese are added as trace elements. Intravenous iron is administered to children not receiving iron by enteral means. In children with renal failure, calcium amounts are decreased, and magnesium, phosphorus, and potassium are eliminated.

The dextrose–amino acid component of TPN is stable for up to 30 days; however, with the addition of vitamins and minerals, the solution becomes highly unstable. Refrigeration in a dark place is required, and the solution should be used within 24 hours.

Water is also an essential part of PN. Typically, fluid requirements are calculated by body weight and may be adjusted according to the child's fluid needs. For example, a child with high insensible water loss through a drainage tube, diarrhea, respiratory failure, infection, or elevated temperature may require increased fluids, whereas a child under a radiant warmer or with cardiac disease may require fluid restriction.

Medications can also be mixed or added to TPN to decrease cost, restrict fluids, decrease time, and reduce the risk of potential contamination of the PN.[179] Drug compatibility varies (Table 12-17). PN solutions can inactivate or reduce drug potency and cause precipitation of electrolytes and medications. Drug compatibility is assessed for pharmacokinetics and physical stability.

The success of PN is ensured by effective administration; evaluation of the child's response to therapy; and close, frequent monitoring of complications (Table 12-18). All parenteral nutrition is administered by maintaining a constant rate via an infusion. To establish a baseline of comparison, initial monitoring of the patient on parenteral nutrition includes complete laboratory assessment of fluid and electrolytes, acid-base, renal, hepatic, and nutritional status. During the initial stages of administration, parenteral nutrition requires daily monitoring of many laboratory values. As changes in parenteral solutions become unnecessary and as the disease acuity permits, less frequent monitoring is needed. Hourly accurate intake and output and frequent assessment of fluid requirements are also indicated.

Parenteral nutrition is fraught with complications (Table 12-19). The major catheter-related complication is infection, and local and systemic infections can occur. The most common infections result from *Staphylococcus aureus* and *Candida albicans*. Fat emulsions provide an excellent medium for gram-positive, gram-negative, and fungal growth,

TABLE 12-17 Compatibility of Selected Drugs With Parenteral Nutrition

Drugs	Compatibility
Amikacin*	Incompatible
Amphotericin B	Incompatible
Ampicillin	Incompatible
Cefazolin	Incompatible
Ceftriaxone	Compatible
Chloramphenicol	Compatible
Clindamycin	Compatible
Corticosteroids	Compatible
Diazepam	Incompatible
Digoxin	Compatible
Gentamicin*	Compatible
Imipenem-cilastatin	Incompatible
Metoclopramide	Incompatible
Oxacillin	Compatible
Penicillin G*	Compatible
Phenytoin	Incompatible
Ticarcillin	Compatible
Tobramycin*	Compatible
Vancomycin*	Compatible
Vecuronium	Compatible

Reprinted with permission of Miyagawa C: Drug-nutrient interactions in critically ill patients, *Crit Care Nurse* 13:69-90, 1993.
*Incompatible with parenteral nutrition containing heparin.

whereas crystalline amino acid and dextrose solutions primarily support fungal infections.[186,199] More susceptibility to catheter infection has been observed with central versus peripheral lines, lower limb catheterization versus upper limb, and catheters exiting the neck (internal jugular) versus those exiting the upper chest (subclavian), and multilumen catheters.[200] Sepsis related to PN may result from contamination at the insertion site and migration of bacteria along the catheter.[201] Patients who receive mechanical ventilation via artificial airways seem to be at increased risk for infection. The bacterial colonization associated with mechanical ventilation may contribute to this increased risk.[202]

Preventing catheter-related infection is one of the major challenges in caring for the child receiving PN.[203-205] Adherence to regular and meticulous care of the catheter and site is essential. Strict aseptic technique, including use of an antiseptic agent, is used to clean and maintain the site.[206] A transparent, moisture vapor permeable dressing is then placed over the insertion site and changed at least once a week or when soiled. Daily monitoring of local and systemic signs of infection is important, including observing for redness, pain, swelling, and exudate at the site; fever; and chills.[197,207] Tunneling of the catheter through the subcutaneous tissue before entering the vein may reduce the risk of infection.[20] Unnecessary use of the catheter for blood transfusions or blood sampling is discouraged. To ensure sterility during infusion of PN, a 24-hour expiration period is recommended from time of hanging the fluid. Tubing is changed daily or with every new bottle or bag, using aseptic technique.

TABLE 12-18   Monitoring Parameters for Parenteral Nutrition Support

Variable	Admission	qh	q8h	Daily	Weekly	As Indicated
Growth						
Weight	X			X		X (1-3×/wk for chronically ill, stable patients)
Height	X					X (monthly)
Head circumference (<3 yr)	X					X (monthly)
Skinfold thickness	X					X
Midarm circumference	X					X
Fluid balance (I & O)	X	X				
Temperature	X			X		
Vital signs	X					X
Urine glucose/acetone	X		X			
Catheter site/function		X				
Biochemical Indices						
Sodium	X			X (×1 wk)	X	
Potassium	X			X (×1 wk)	X	
Chloride	X			X (×1 wk)	X	
CO_2	X			X (×1 wk)	X	
Glucose	X			X (×1 wk)	X	
Blood urea nitrogen	X			X (×1 wk)	X	
Creatinine	X			X (×1 wk)	X	
Triglycerides	X				X	
Cholesterol	X				X	
Calcium	X			X (×1 wk)	X	
Magnesium	X			X (×1 wk)	X	
Phosphorus	X			X (×1 wk)	X	
Vitamin B_{12}	X					X (monthly)
Folate	X					X (monthly)
Albumin	X				X	
Alanine aminotransferase (ALT)	X				X	
Aspartate aminotransferase (AST)	X				X	
Alkaline phosphatase	X				X	
Total and direct bilirubin	X				X	
Lactate dehydrogenase	X				X	
Gamma-glutamyltransferase (GGT)	X				X	
Iron	X					X (monthly)
Copper	X					X (monthly)
Zinc	X					X
Selenium	X					X
Ammonia	X					X
Complete blood (cell) count	X					X
Platelet count	X					

Data from Heird W: Parenteral support of the hospitalized patient. In Suskind R, Lewinter-Suskind L, eds: *Textbook of pediatric nutrition,* New York, 1993, Raven Press, pp 225-238; adapted from *The TPN handbook,* ed 5, Boston, 1993, Boston Nutrition Support Service, Children's Hospital.

Whenever catheter-related septicemia is suspected, obtaining blood culture samples is a reasonable recommendation. If the child develops a fever, blood cultures are drawn from the central line and peripheral vein, and antibiotics are started. Cultures are repeated if the initial blood culture result is positive and continued until culture results are negative.

The metabolic complications of PN usually are related to the nutrient components of the parenteral solution.[208] Hyperglycemia is the most common metabolic complica-tion.[209,210] Avoiding hyperglycemia is a prime consideration when increasing the amount of dextrose. Frequent monitoring of glucose metabolism by serum and urine glucose levels is helpful in evaluating hyperglycemia. Hypoglycemia may be seen when dextrose is abruptly stopped. Administering 10% dextrose solution is recommended if the catheter becomes plugged or must be discontinued. Hypercholesterolemia, phospholipidemia, and hypertriglycemia may occur, especially when increasing the amount of lipids administered. Monitoring lipid clearance by routinely

TABLE 12-19 Complications of Parenteral Nutrition

Complication	Cause	Intervention
Infection	Contamination at insertion site	Regular and meticulous site care
	Contamination of infusate	Use an in-line filter
	Equipment contamination	24-Hour hang time for parenteral nutrition solutions
		Refrigerate solutions until used
		Change tubing every 24 hours or with each bottle
		Treat with appropriate antibiotic
Metabolic		
Hyperglycemia	Excessive intake because of hyperosmolarity or high infusion rate	Monitor infusion hourly
		Monitor serum and urine glucose
		Decrease infusion rates
Hypoglycemia	Abrupt cessation of infusion	If parenteral nutrition stopped suddenly, infuse 10% dextrose solution
Azotemia	Excessive amino acid intake	Decrease amino acid content of parenteral solution
Electrolyte, vitamin disorders	Excessive or inadequate intake	Correct composition of parenteral solution
Hypercholesterolemia/ phospholipidemia	Character of or excessive use of lipid emulsion	Reduce lipid rate and monitor
Hypertriglyceremia		Extend length of infusion
Fatty acid deficiency	Limited fat intake	Provide 4%-8% linoleic acid
Hepatic disorders		Avoid excessive calories as protein
Technical		
Peripheral-infiltrations, phlebitis, extravasation	High osmolarity of infusate	Check site every 30 min to 1 h and move peripheral IV as necessary
	Prolonged use of single vein	Clamp catheter
	Break in system	Rotate IV site
		Check site every 30 min to 1 h
Central thrombosis	Frequent blood drawing	Change catheter sites routinely
	Prolonged use of single vein	Monitor sites hourly
Air embolism	Break in system	Immediately clamp catheter
		Place patient in Trendelenburg position with right side up
Pneumothorax/hemothorax	Technique complication	Sedate during insertion
		Radiologically confirm placement
Catheter breakage	Prolonged catheter use, defective, inadvertent puncture	Clamp catheter and repair

checking triglyceride levels becomes important. Appropriate adjustments of nutrients in the infusion may prevent or correct complications.

Other catheter-related complications include the technical complications associated with catheter insertion and use of a venous access system. Catheter malposition, dislodgment, and thrombosis may also occur during use of a venous access system. Clotting within the catheter may be related to the frequency of blood drawing. Facial swelling, edema of the neck and chest, difficulty with the infusion of fluid, and neck pain are all signs of potential catheter thrombosis.[211,212] The signs and symptoms of thrombosis may be subtle and delayed until complete occlusion of the vein occurs.[213] Thrombolytic agents can be used to prolong catheter life and reestablish catheter patency. Urokinase dissolves clots by triggering the body's own fibrinolytic system and was widely used for catheter clearance until a recent citing by the manufacturer. Agencies are now using streptokinase to lyse systemic clots and tissue plasminogen activator for catheter clearance.

SUMMARY

Children in ICUs have demonstrated both an acquired and preexisting tendency toward protein-energy malnutrition. The changes in metabolic demands generated from injury and sepsis make these children's nutritional needs very complex. Nutritional support can positively affect the recovery and survival of hospitalized patients. The nutrition received in childhood may have significant consequences as the child grows, making further work in the area imperative. When caring for a critically ill child, understanding and advocating for the child's metabolic needs are essential.

REFERENCES

1. American Society of Parenteral and Enteral Nutrition (ASPEN). Board of Directors: Guidelines for the use of parenteral and enteral nutrition in adult and pediatric patients, *JPEN J Parenter Enteral Nutr* 17(suppl 4), 1993.
2. Pollack M, Wiley J, Holbrook P: Early nutritional depletion in critically ill children, *Crit Care Med* 9:580-583, 1981.
3. Pollack M, Wiley J, Kanter R et al: Malnutrition in critically ill infants and children, *JPEN J Parenter Enteral Nutr* 6:20-24, 1982.
4. Pollack M, Ruttimann U, Wiley J: Nutritional depletion in critically ill children: association with physiologic instability and increased quality of care, *JPEN J Parenter Enteral Nutr* 9:309-313, 1985.
5. Huddleston K, Ferraro-McDuffie A, Wolff-Small T: Nutritional support of the critically ill child, *Crit Care Nurs Clin North Am* 5:65-78, 1993.
6. Beal Al, Cerra FB: Multisystem organ failure syndrome in the 1990s: systemic inflammatory response and organ dysfunction, *JAMA* 271:226-233, 1994.
7. Lehmann S: Nutrition support in the hypermetabolic patient, *Crit Care Nurs Clin North Am* 5:97-103, 1993.
8. Konstantinides N, Lehmann S: The impact of nutrition on wound healing, *Crit Care Nurs* 13:25-33, 1993.
9. Trujillo EB: Effects of nutritional status on wound healing, *J Vasc Nurs* 11:12-18, 1993.
10. Wilkes G: Nutrition: the forgotten ingredient in cancer care, *Am J Nurs* 100:46-52, 2000.
11. Holmes S: The incidence of malnutrition in hospitalised patients, *Nursing Times* 92:43-45, 1996.
12. Murphy L, Conforti C: Nutritional support of the cardiopulmonary patient, *Crit Care Nurs Clin North Am* 5:57-64, 1993.
13. Schlichtig R, Sargent S: Nutritional support of the mechanically ventilated patient, *Crit Care Clin* 6:767-784, 1990.
14. Agusti A, Torres A, Estopa R et al: Hypophosphatemia as a cause of failed weaning: the importance of metabolic factors, *Crit Care Med* 12:142-143, 1984.
15. Dhingra S, Solven F, Wilson A et al: Hypomagnesemia and respiratory muscle power, *Am Rev Respir Dis* 129:497-498, 1984.
16. Viart P: Hemodynamic findings in severe protein calorie malnutrition, *Am J Clin Nutr* 30:334-348, 1977.
17. Alexander J: Nutrition and translocation, *JPEN J Parenter Enteral Nutr* 14:170s-174s, 1990.
18. Pollack M: Nutritional support of children in the intensive care unit. In Suskind R, Lewinter-Suskind L, eds: *Textbook of pediatric nutrition,* ed 2, New York, 1993, Raven Press.
19. Kinney JM: Metabolic responses of the critically ill patient, *Crit Care Med* 11:569-586, 1995.
20. Lennie T: The metabolic response to injury: current perspectives and nursing implications, *Dimens Crit Care Nurs* 16:79-87, 1997.

21. Monk DQ, Plank LD, Franch-Arcas G et al: Sequential changes in the metabolic response in critically ill patients in the first 25 days after blunt trauma, *Ann Surg* 223:395-405, 1996.
22. Biffl WL, Moore EE, Moore FA et al: Interleukin-6 in the injured patient: marker of injury or mediator of inflamation? *Ann Surg* 224:647-664, 1996.
23. Barton R: Nutrition support in critical illness, *Nutr Clin Pract* 9:127-134, 1994.
24. Frankenfield D, Smith JS, Cooney R: Accelerated nitrogen loss after traumatic injury is attenuated by achievement of energy balance, *JPEN J Parenter Enteral Nutr* 21:324-329, 1997.
25. Steinhorn DM, Green TP: Severity of illness correlates with alteration in metabolism in the pediatric intensive care unit, *Crit Care Med* 19:1503-1509, 1991.
26. Jeejeebhoy K: How should we monitor nutritional support: structure and function? *New Horiz* 2:131-138, 1994.
27. Hamill P, Drizd T, Johnson C et al: Physical growth: National Center for Health Statistics percentiles, *Am J Clin Nutr* 23:607-629, 1979.
28. Jeejeebhoy K: Nutritional assessment, *Gastroenterol Clin North Am* 27:347-369, 1998.
29. Jew R, ed: *Children's Hospital of Philadelphia pharmacy handbook and formulary,* Ohio, 1998, Lexi-Comp.
30. Frisancho A: New norms of upper limb fat and muscle areas for assessment of nutritional status, *Am J Clin Nutr* 34:2540-2545, 1981.
31. Lowrie EG, Lew N: Death risk in hemodialysis patients: the predictive value of commonly measured variables and the evaluation of death rate difference between facilities, *Am Kidney Dis* 15:458-482, 1990.
32. Figueroa-Colon R: Clinical and laboratory assessment of the malnourished child. In Suskind R, Lewinter-Suskind L, eds: *Textbook of pediatric nutrition,* Philadelphia, 1993, WB Saunders.
33. Prealbumin in Nutritional Care Consensus Group: Measurement of visceral protein status in assessing protein and energy malnutriton: standard of care, *Nutrition* 11:169-171, 1995.
34. Petersen SR, Holaday NJ, Jeevanandam M: Enhancement of protein synthesis efficiency in parenterally feed trauma victims by adjuvant recombinant HGH, *J Trauma* 36:726-733, 1994.
35. Trujillo E, Robinson M, Jacobs D: Nutritional assessment in the critically ill, *Crit Care Nurse* 19:67-78, 1999.
36. Doweiko JP, Nompleggi DJ: The role of albumin in human physiology and pathophysiology. III. Albumin and disease states, *JPEN J Parenter Enteral Nutr* 15:476-483, 1991.
37. McClave SA, Snider H; Use of indirect calorimetry in clinical nutrition, *Nutr Clin Pract* 7:207-221, 1992.
38. Gebara B, Gelmini M, Sarnaik A; Oxygen consumption, energy expenditure and substrate utilization after cardiac surgery in

children, *Crit Care Med* 20:1550-1554, 1992.
39. Jones MO, Hammond PP, Lloyd DA: The metabolic response to operative stress in infants, *J Pediatr Surg* 28:1258-1263, 1993.
40. Thomson MA, Bucolo S, Quirk P et al: Measured versus predicted resting energy expenditure in infants: a need reappraisal, *J Pediatr* 126:21-27, 1995.
41. Branson R: The measurement of energy expenditure: instrumentation, practical considerations and clinical application, *Respir Care* 35:640-659, 1990.
42. Fung E: Estimating energy expenditure in critically ill adults and children, *AACN Clin Issues Crit Care Nurs* 11:4, 2000.
43. Zemel BS, Kawchaak DA, Cnaan A et al: Prospectice evaluation of resting energy expenditure, nutritional status, pulmonary function, and genotype in children with cystic fibrosis, *Pediatr Res* 8:578-586, 1996.
44. Edes T, Walk B, Austin J: Diarrhea in tube-fed patients: feeding formulas not necessarily the cause, *Am J Med* 88:91-93, 1990.
45. Weissman C, Kemper M: Metabolic measurements in the critically ill, *Crit Care Clin* 11:169-197, 1995
46. Schears GJ, Deutschman CS: Common nutritional issues in pediatric and adult critical care medicine, *Crit Care Clin* 13:669-690, 1997.
47. Uehara M, Plank L, Hill G: Components of energy expenditure in patients with severe sepsis and major trauma: a basis for clinical care, *Crit Care Med* 27:1295-1302, 1999.
48. Frankenfield D, Wiles III CE, Bagley S et al: Relationships between resting and total energy expenditure in injured and septic patients, *Crit Care Med* 22:1796-1804, 1994.
49. Letton RW, Chwals WJ, Jamie A et al: Early postoperative alterations in infant energy use increase the risk of overfeeding, *J Pediatr Surg* 30:988-993, 1995.
50. Powis MR, Smith K, Rennie M et al: Effect of major abdominal operations on energy and protein metabolism in infants and children, *J Pediatr Surg* 33:49-53, 1998.
51. National Research Council, Food and Nutrition Board: *Recommended dietary allowance,* ed 10, Washington, DC, 1989, National Academy Press.
52. World Health Organization: *Energy and protein requirements* FAO/WHO/UUN, Expert Consultation, Geneva, 1985, World Health Organization.
53. Choban PS, Burge JC, Scales D et al: Hypoenergetic nutrition support in hospitalized obese patients: a simplified method for clinical application, *Am J Clin Nutr* 66:546-550, 1997.
54. Schofield WN, Schofield C, Jamer WPT: Basal metabolic rate-review and prediction, together with annotated bibliography of source material, *Hum Nutr Clin Nutr* 39C(suppl 1):5-41, 1985.
55. Sentongo T, Tershakovec AM, Mascarenhas MR et al: Resting energy expenditure and predictive equations in young children with

failure to thrive, *J Pediatr* 136:345-350, 2000.

56. Cerra F: The role of nutrition in the management of metabolic stress, *Crit Care Clin* 2:807-819, 1986.

57. Cerra F: Hypermetabolism, organ failure and metabolic support, *Surgery* 101:1-14, 1987.

58. Cerra F: How nutrition intervention changes what getting sick means, *JPEN J Parenter Enteral Nutr* 14:164S-169S, 1990.

59. Weissman C, Kemper M, Damask M et al: The effect of routine intensive care interaction of metabolic rate, *Chest* 86:815-818, 1984.

60. Clifton G, Robertson C, Choi S: Assessment of nutrition status of head injured patients, *J Neurosurg* 64:895-901, 1986.

61. Swinamer D, Prang P, Jones R et al: Effect of routine administration of analgesia on energy expediture in critically ill patients, *Chest* 92:4-10, 1988.

62. Shanbhogue R, Lloyd D: Absence of hypermetabolism after operation in the newborn infant, *JPEN J Parenter Enteral Nutr* 16: 333-336, 1992.

63. Chwals W, Lally K, Woolley M et al: Measured energy expenditure in critically ill infants and young children, *J Surg Res* 44:467-472, 1988.

64. Leibel RL, Rosenbaum M, Hissrch J: Changes in energy expenditure resulting from altered body weight, *N Engl J Med* 332:621-628, 1995.

65. Chwals W: Overfeeding the critically ill child: fact or fiction, *New Horiz* 2:147-155, 1994.

66. Pinard B, Geller E: Nutritional support during pulmonary failure, *Crit Care Clin* 11:705-715, 1995.

67. Pomposelli JJ, Bristrian BR: Is total parenteral nutrition immunosuppressive? *New Horiz* 2:224-229, 1994.

68. Lipsky J, Nelson LD: Ventilatory response to high caloric loads in critically ill patients, *Crit Care Med* 22:796-802, 1994.

69. Heymsfield SB, Hill JO, Evert M et al: Energy expenditure during continuous intragastric infusion of fuel, *Am J Clin Nutr* 45:526-533, 1987.

70. Patino JF, de Pimiento SE, Vergara A et al: Hypocaloric support in the critically ill, *World J Surg* 23:553-559, 1999.

71. Zaloga GP, Robert P: Permissive underfeeding, *New Horiz* 2:257-263, 1994.

72. Holland KA, Gillespie RW, Lewis NM et al: Estimating energy needs of pediatric patients with burns, *J Burn Care Rehabil* 16:458-460, 1995.

73. Kaplan AS, Zemel BS, Neiswender KM et al: Resting energy expenditure in clinical pediatrics: measured versus prediction equations, *J Pediatr* 127:200-205, 1995.

74. Klein S, Alpers D, Grand G et al: Advances in nutrition and gastroenterology: summary of the 1997 ASPEN research workshop, *JPEN J Parenter Enteral Nutr* 22:3-13, 1998.

75. Imura K, Okada A: Amino acid metabolism in pediatric patients, *Nutrition* 14:143-148, 1998.

76. Ishibashi N, Plank L, Sando K et al: Optimal protein requirements during the first 2 weeks after the onset of critical illness, *Crit Care Med* 26:1529-1535, 1998.

77. Twyman D: Nutritional management of the critically ill neurologic patient: update on neurologic critical care, *Crit Care Clin* 13:39-49, 1997.

78. Meredith JW, Ditesheim JA, Zaloga GP: Visceral protein levels in trauma patients are greater with peptide diet than with intact protein diet, *J Trauma* 30:825-829, 1990.

79. Diboune M, Ferard G, Ingenbleek Y et al: Composition of phospholipid fatty acids in red blood cell membranes of patients in intensive care units: effects of different intakes of soy oil, medium chain triglycerides and black currant seed oil, *JPEN J Parenter Enteral Nutr* 16:136-141, 1992.

80. Bower R, Cerra F, Bershadsky B et al: Early enteral administration of formula (Impact) supplemented with arginine, nucleotides and fish oil in intensive care unit patients: results of a multicenter prospective randomized clinical trial, *Crit Care Med* 23:436-449, 1995.

81. Daly J, Lieberman M, Goldfine J et al: Enteral nutrition with supplemental arginine, RNS and omega 3 fatty acids in patients after operation: ourimmunologic, metabolic and clinical outsome, *Surgery* 112:56-67, 1992.

82. Jeevandam M, Shahbazian LM, Persen S: Proinflammatory cytokine production by mitogen stimulated peripheral blood mononucleus cells (PBMCs) in trauma patients fed immune enhancing enteral diets, *Nutrition* 15:842-847, 1999.

83. Lacey J, Wilmore D: Is glutamine a conditionally essential amino acid? *Nutr Rev* 48:297-309, 1990.

84. Daly J, Reynolds J, Sigal R et al: Effect of dietary protein and amino acids on immune function, *Crit Care Med* 18:S86-S92, 1990.

85. Wilmore DW, Shabert K: Role of glutamine in immunologic responses, *Nutrition* 14: 618-626, 1998.

86. Barbul A: Arginine and immune function, *Nutrition* 6:53-58, 1990.

87. Evoy D, Lieberman MD, Fahey TY III et al: Immunonutrition: the role of arginine, *Nutrition* 14:611-617, 1998.

88. Skeie B, Kvetan V, Gil K et al: Branched chain amino acids: their metabolism and clinical utility, *Crit Care Med* 18:549-571, 1990.

89. Grimm H, Tibell A, Norrlind B et al: Immunoregulation by parenteral lipids: impact of the ω-3 to ω-6 fatty acid ratio, *JPEN J Parenter Enteral Nutr* 18:417-421, 1994.

90. Charnock JS: Omega 3 polyunsatured fatty acids and ventricular fibrillation: the possible involvement of eicosanoids, *Prostaglandins Leukot Essent Fatty Acids* 61:243-247, 1999.

91. Connor J: Importance of ω-3 fatty acids in health and disease, *American J Clin Nutr* 71(suppl 1):1715-1755, 2000.

92. Simopoulous AP: Essential fatty acids in health and disease, *Am J Clin Nutr* 70(suppl):560S-569S, 1999.

93. Carli F, Webster JD, Halliday D: Growth hormones modulates amino acid oxidation in the surgical patients: leucin kinetics during fasting and fed state using moderate nitrogenous and caloric diet and recombinant human growth hormone, *Metabolism* 46:23-28, 1997.

94. Hammarquist MD, Stromberg C, Vonder Decken A et al: Biosynthetic human growth hormone preserves both muscle protein synthesis and the decrease in muscle free glutamine and improves whole body nitrogen economy after operation, *Ann Surg* 216:184-191, 1992.

95. Petersen SR, Jeevanandam M, Shahbazian, Holaday NJ: Reprioritization of live protein synthesis from recombinant human growth hormone supplementation in parenterally fed trauma patients: the effect of growth hormone in the acute phase response, *J Trauma* 42:987-995, 1997.

96. Gottardis M, Benzer A, Koller W et al: Improvement of septic syndrome after administration of recombinant human growth hormone (rhGH). *J Trauma* 31:81-86, 1991.

97. Voerman H, Van Schijndel SJM, Groenveld AB et al: Effects of recumbinant human growth hormone in patients with severe sepsis, *Ann Surg* 216:648-655, 1992.

98. Kemen M, Senkal M, Homann H et al: Early post-operative enteral nutrition with arginin, ω-3 fatty acids and ribonucleic acid-supplemented diet versus placebo in cancer patients: an immunologic evaluation of Impact, *Crit Care Med* 23:652-659, 1995.

99. Mendez C, Jurkovich G, Garcia I et al: Effects of an immune-enhancing diet in critically injured patients, *J Trauma* 42:933-940, 1997.

100. Saffle JR, Wiebke G, Jennings K et al: Randomized trial of immune-enhancing enteral nutrition in burn patients, *J Trauma* 42:793-800, 1997.

101. Bagley S: Nutritional needs of the acutely ill with wounds, *Crit Care Nurs Clin North Am* 8:159-167, 1996.

102. Cerra RB, Benitez MR, Blackburn GL et al: ACCP Consensus statement: applied nutrition in intensive care unit patients: a consensus statement of the American College of Chest Physicians, *Chest* 111:769-778, 1997.

103. Lipman TD: Grains or veins: is enteral nutrition really better than parenteral nutrition? A look at the evidence, *JPEN J Parenter Enteral Nutr* 22:167-182, 1998.

104. Klein S, Kinney J, Jeejeebhoy K et al: Nutrition support in clinical practice: review of published data and recommendations for future research directions, *Am J Clin Nutr* 66:683-706, 1997.

105. Heyman DR: Nutritional support in the critically ill patient, *Crit Care Clin* 14:423-440, 1998.

106. Lowry S: The route of feeding influences injury responses, *J Trauma* 30:S10-S15, 1990.

107. Moore F, Feliciano D, Andrassy R: Early enteral feedings compared with parenteral reduces postoperative septic complications: the results of a meta analysis, *Ann Surg* 216:172-183, 1991.

108. Schroeder D, Gillanders L, Mahr K et al: Effects of immediate postoperative enteral nutrition on body composition, muscle function and wound healing, *JPEN J Parenter Enteral Nutr* 15:376-383, 1991.

109. Toto K: Endocrine physiology: a comprehensive review, *Crit Care Nurs Clin North Am* 6:637-659, 1994.

110. Chellis M, Sanders S, Webster H et al: Early enteral feeding in the pediatric intensive care unit, *JPEN J Parenter Enteral Nutr* 20:71-73, 1996.

111. Kudsk K, Croce M, Fabian T et al: Enteral versus parenteral feeding effects on septic morbidity after blunt and penetrating head trauma, *Ann Surg* 215:503-511, 1992.

112. Langkamp-Henken B, Donovan TB, Pate L et al: Increased intestinal permeability following blunt and penetrating trauma, *Crit Care Med* 23:660-664, 1995.

113. Minard G, Kudsk K: Is early feeding beneficial? How early is early? *New Horiz* 2:156-163, 1994.

114. Moore FA, Moore EE, Jones T: Benefits of immediate jejunostomy feeding after major abdominal trauma: a prospective randomized study, *J Trauma* 26:874-881, 1996.

115. Nyswonger GD, Helmchen R: Early enteral nutrition and length of stay in stroke patients, *J Neurosci Nurs* 24:220-223, 1992.

116. Trocki O, Michelini A, Robbins ST et al: Evaluation of early enteral feeding in children less than 3 years old with smaller burns (8-25% TBSA), *Burns* 21:17-23, 1995.

117. Alexander J, Gottschleck M: Nutrition immunomodulation in burn patients, *Crit Care Med* 18:149-153, 1990.

118. Braga M, Gianotti L, Vignali A et al: Artificial nutrition after major abdominal surgery: impact of route of administration and composition of the diet, *Crit Care Med* 26:24-30, 1998.

119. Rossi TM, Lee PC, Young C et al: Small intestinal mucous changes, including epithelia cell proliferation activity in children receiving total parenteral nutrition, *Dig Dis Sci* 38,1608-1613, 1993.

120. American Society for Parenteral and Enteral Nutrition (ASPEN): Standards for nutrition support: hospitalized pediatric patients, *Nutr Clin Pract* 4:33-37, 1989.

121. American Academy of Pediatrics, Committee on Nutrition: *Pediatric nutrition handbook,* ed 3, Chicago, 1993, American Academy of Pediatrics.

122. Beaudry M, Dufour R, Marcoux S: Relation between infant feeding and infectious during the first 6 months of life, *J Pediatr* 126:191-197, 1995.

123. Dewey KG, Heinig MJ, Nommsen-Rivers LA: Differences in morbidity between breast fed and formula fed infants, *J Pediatr* 126, 696-702, 1995.

124. Hawkes JS, Bryan D-L, James MJ et al: Cytokines (Il-1B, Il-6, TNF, TGF-B1 and TGF-B2) and prostaglandin E2 in human milk during the first 3 months postpartum, *Pediatr Res* 46:194-199, 1999.

125. Report of the Dietary Guidelines, Advisory Committee on the Dietary Guidelines for Americans: Hyattsville, Md, 1990, US Department of Agriculture.

126. Garza C, Butt N, Goldman A: Human milk and infant formula. In Suskind R, Lewinter-Suskind L, eds: *Textbook of pediatric nutrition,* ed 2, New York, 1993, Raven Press.

127. Jones R: Strategies to promote preterm breast feeding, *Mod Midwife* March 8-11, 1995.

128. Turnbull F: Promoting health: breastfeeding in PICU, *Paediatr Nurs* 11:39-41, 1999.

129. Walker M: Breastfeeding in the preterm infant, *NAACOGS Clin Issu Perinat Womens Health Nurs* 3:620-633, 1992.

130. Fraser R: Breast-feeding support in neonatal surgical unit, *Nursing Times* 19:54-56, 1997.

131. The Human Milk Banking Association of North America: *Recommendations for collection, storage, and handling of a mother's milk for her own infant in the hospital setting,* West Hartford, Conn, 1993, The Human Milk Banking Association of North America.

132. Moore F, Moore E, Kudok K et al: Clinical benefits of an immune enhancing diet for postinjury feeding, *J Trauma* 37:607-615, 1997.

133. DeSouza DA, Green LJ: Pharmacologic nutrition after burn injury, *J Nutr* 128:797-803, 1998.

134. Grant MJ, Martin S: Delivery of enteral nutrition, *AACN Clin Issues Crit Care Nurs* 11:507-516, 2000.

135. Lord L: Enteral access devices, *Nurs Clin North Am* 32:685-703, 1997.

136. Sax JM, Ledgerwood AM, Lucas CE et al: Lower esophageal sphincter dysfunction precludes safe gastric feedings after head injury, *J Trauma* 37:581-585, 1994.

137. Montecalvo MA, Steger KA, Farber HN et al: Nutritional outcome and pneumonia in critical care patients randomized to gastric versus jejunal tube feedings, *Crit Care Med* 20:1377-1387, 1992.

138. Chellis M, Sanders S, Dean M et al: Bedside transpyloric feeding tube placement in the pediatric intensive care unit, *JPEN J Parenter Enteral Nutr* 20:80-90, 1996.

139. Dimand RJ, Veereman-Wauters G, Braner DA: Bedside placement of pH guided transpyloric small bowel feeding tubes in critically ill infants and small children, *JPEN J Parenter Enteral Nutr* 21:112-114, 1997.

140. Salasidis R, Fleiszer T, Johnston R: Air insufflation technique of enteral tube insertion: a randomized, controlled trial, *Crit Care Med* 26, 1036-1039, 1998.

141. Ugo P, Mohler P, Wilson G: Bedside postpyloric placement of weighted feeding tubes, *Nutr Clin Pract* 7:284-287, 1992.

142. Walsh S, Banks L: How to insert a small-bore feeding tube safely, *Nursing 90* 20:55-59, 1990.

143. Zaloga G: Bedside method of placing small bowel feeding tube in critically ill patients: a prospective study, *Chest* 100:1643-1646, 1991.

144. Harrison A, Clay B, Grant MJ et al: Nonradiologic assessment of enteral feeding tube position, *Crit Care Med* 25:2055-2059, 1997.

145. Kraft-Jacobs B, Persinger M, Carver J et al: Rapid placement of transpyloric feeding tubes: a comparison of pH assisted and standard insertion techniques in children, *Pediatrics* 98:242-248, 1996.

146. Cirgin-Ellet ML, Beckstrand J: Examination of gavage tube placement in children, *J Soc Pediatr Nurs* 4:51-60, 1999.

147. Ellett ML: What is the prevalence of feeding tube placement errors and what are the associated risk factors? *Online Journal of Knowledge Synthesis* 4(doc 5)[35 paragraphs]28 ref, 1997, at www.stti.iupui.edu/library/.

148. Ellett ML, Maahs J, Forsee S: Prevalence of feeding tube placement errors and associated risk factors in a pediatric sample, *MCN Am J Matern Child Nurs* 23:234-239, 1988.

149. Metheny N, Hampton K, Williams P: Detection of inadvertent respiratory placement of small-bore feeding tubes: a report of 10 cases, *Heart Lung* 19:631-638, 1990.

150. Metheny N, McSweeney M, Wehrle M et al: Effectiveness of the auscultatory method in predicting feeding tube placement, *Nurs Res* 39:262-267, 1990.

151. Metheny N, Smith L, Wehrle MA, et al: pH, color and feeding tubes, *RN* 61:25-27, 1998.

152. Metheny N Reed L, Berglund B et al: Visual characteristics of aspirates from feeding tubes as a method for predicting tube location, *Nurs Res* 43:282-287, 1994.

153. Metheny N, Ciouse R, Clark J et al: PH testing of feeding aspirates to determine placement, *Nutr Clin Pract* 9:195-190, 1994.

154. Metheny N, Aud MA, Ignatavicius DD: Detection of improperly positioned feeding tubes, *J Healthc Risk Manag* 18:37-48, 1998.

155. Metheny N, Reed L, Wiersema L et al: Effectiveness of pH measurements in predicting feeding tube placement: an update, *Nurs Res* 42:324-331, 1993.

156. DeChicco R, Matarese L: Selection of nutrition support regimens, *Nutr Clin Pract* 7:239-245, 1992.

157. Ho HS, Ngo H: Gastrostomy for enteral access: a comparison among placement by laparotomy, laparoscopy, and endoscopy, *Surg Endosc* 13:991-994, 1999.

158. Naureckas SM, Chistoffel K: Nasogastric or gastrostomy feedings in children with neurologic disabilities, *Clin Pediatr* 30:353-359, 1994.

159. Brant CQ, Stanich P, Ferrari AP: Improvement of children's nutritional status after enteral feeding by PEG: an interim report, *Gastrointest Endosc* 50:183-188, 1999.

160. Neal J, Slayton D: Neonatal and pediatric PEG tubes, *MCN Am J Matern Child Nurs* 17:184-191, 1992.

161. Payne KM, King TM, Eisenach JB: The technique of percutaneous endoscopic gastrostomy: a safe and cost effective alternative to operative gastrostomy, *J Crit Illn* 6:617-619, 1991.

162. DiLorenzo J, Dalton B, Miskovitz P: Percutaneous endoscopic gastrostomy, *Postgrad Med* 91:277-296, 1992.

163. Hall IC: Low profile gastrostomy, *Nursing 97* 27:62-67, 1997.

164. Kaufman MV, Faller NA, Lawerence L: Low profile gastrostomy devices, *Gastroenterol Nurs* 18:171-176, 1995.

165. Steele N: The Button: replacement of gastrostomy device, *J Pediatr Nurs* 6:421-424, 1991.

166. Borkowski S: The Mic-Key experience with the pediatric patient, *J Wound Ostomy Continence Nurs* 21:195-198, 1994.

167. Lazarus BA, Murphy JB, Culpepper L: Aspiration associated with long term gastric versus jejunal feeding: a critical analysis of literature, *Arch Phys Med Rehabil* 71:46-50, 1990.

168. Grant J, Denne SC: Effect of intermittent versus continuous enteral feeding on energy expenditure in premature infants, *J Pediatr* 118:928-932, 1991.

169. Irving S, Simone S, Hicks F, Verger J: Nutrition for the critically ill child: enteral and parenteral support, *AACN's Clinical Issues* 11:541-558, 2000.

170. Smith C, Manrie L, Brogdon C et al: Diarrhea associated with tube feeding in mechanically ventilated critically ill patients, *Nurs Res* 39:148-152, 1990.

171. Maka D, Murphy L: Drug-nutrient interaction: a review, *AACN Clin Issues Crit Care Nurs* 11:580-589, 2000.

172. Ibanez J, Panafiel A, Raurich JM et al: Gastrointestinal reflux in intubated patients receiving enteral nutrition: effect of supine and semirecumbant positions. *JPEN J Parenter Enteral Nutr* 16:419-422, 1992.

173. Parrish CR, McCray SF: Protocols for practice applying research at the bedside, *Crit Care Nurse* 19:91-94, 1999.

174. Taylor T: Comparison of two methods of nasogastric tube feeding, *Neurol Nurs* 14:49-55, 1992.

175. Dive A, Miesse C, Galanti Jamart J et al: Effect of erthromycin in gastric motility in mechanically ventilated critically ill patients: a double blind, randomized placebo controlled study, *Crit Care Med* 23:1356-1362, 1995.

176. Jooste CA, Mustoe J, Collee G: Metoclopamide improves gastric motility in critically ill patients, *Intensive Care Med* 25:464-468, 1999.

177. Powell KS, Marcuard SP, Farrior ES et al: Aspirating gastric residuals causes occlusion of small bowel feeding tubes, *JPEN J Parenter Enteral Nutr* 243-245, 1993.

178. Marian AM, Allen P: Nutrition support for patients in long term acute care and subacute care facilities, *AACN Clin Issues Crit Care Med* 9:427-440, 1998.

179. Miyagawa C: Drug-nutrient interactions in critically ill patients, *Crit Care Nurs* 13:69-90, 1993.

180. Doak KK, Haas CE, Dunnigan KJ et al: Bioavailability of phenytoin acid and phenytoin sodium with enteral feedings, *Pharmacology* 18:637-645, 1998.

181. Marvel ME, Bertino JS: Comparative effects of an elemental and a complex enteral feeding formulation on the absorption of phenytoin suspension, *JPEN J Parenter Enteral Nutr* 15:316-318, 1991.

182. Belknap DC, Seifert CF, Petermann M: Administration of medications through enteral feeding catheters, *Am J Crit Care* 6:382-392, 1997.

183. Gill N, Behnke M, Conlon M et al: Nonnutritive sucking modulates behavioral state for preterm infants before feeding, *Scand J Caring Sci* 6:3-7, 1992.

184. Miller H, Anderson G: Nonnutritive sucking: effects on crying and heart rate in intubated infants requiring assisted mechanical ventilation, *Nurs Res* 42:305-307, 1993.

185. Bazyk S: Factors associated with the transition to oral feeding in infants fed by nasogastric tubes. *Am J Occup Ther* 44:1070-1078, 1990.

186. Worthington P, Gilbert K, Wagner B: Parenteral nutrition for the acutely ill adult, *AACN Clin Issues Crit Care Nurs* 11:4, 2000.

187. Camp-Sorrell D: Advanced central venous access devices selection, catheters, devices, nursing management, *J Intraven Nurs* 13:361-370, 1990.

188. Acra SA, Rolin SC: Principles and guidelines for parenteral nutrition in children, *Pediatr Ann* 28:113-120, 1999.

189. Andris DA, Krzda EA: Central venous access: clinical practice issues, *Nurs Clin North Am* 32:719-739, 1997.

190. Crowley JJ, Pereira JK, Harris L et al: Peripherally inserted central catheters: experience in 483 children, *Radiology* 204:577-521, 1997.

191. Dubois J, Garel L, Tapiero B et al: Peripherally inserted central catheters in infants and children, *Radiology* 204:582-586, 1997.

192. Frey AM: Pediatric perhipherally inserted central catheter program report: a summary of 4,536 catheter days, *J Intraven Nurs* 18:280-291, 1995.

193. Marcoux C, Fisher S, Wong D: Central venous access devices in children, *Pediatr Nurs* 16:123-133, 1990.

194. Lipsky C: Recent advances in parenteral nutrition neonatal/perinatal, *Nutrition* 22:141-155, 1995.

195. Fishm J: A prospective randomized study of glutamine-enriched parenteral compared with enteral feeding in postoperative patients, *Am J Clin Nutr* 65:977-983, 1997.

196. Fisher AA, Poole RL, Machie R et al: Clinical pathway for pediatric parenteral nutrition, *Nutr Clin Pract* 12:76-80, 1997.

197. Kuhn M: Nutritional support for the shock patient, *Crit Care Nurs Clin North Am* 2:201-220, 1990.

198. Driscoll DF: Total nutrient admixtures: therapy and practice, *Nutr Clin Pract* 10:114-119, 1995.

199. Thompson B, Robinson L: Infection control of parenteral nutrition solutions, *Nutr Clin Pract* 6:49-54, 1991.

200. Early T, Gregory R, Wheeler J et al: Increased infection rate in double lumen versus single lumen Hickman catheters in cancer patients, *South Med J* 83:34-36, 1990.

201. Salzman MB, Isenberg HD, Shapiro JF et al: A prospective study of catheter hub as the portal of entry for organisms causing catheter related sepsis, *J Infect Dis* 167:487-490, 1993.

202. Holtzman G, Warner S, Melnik G et al: Nutritional support of pulmonary patients: a multidisciplinary approach, *AACN Clin Issues Crit Care Nurs* 1:300-312, 1990.

203. Garland J, Dunne M, Havens P et al: Peripheral intravenous catheter complications in critically ill children: a prospective study, *Pediatrics* 89:1145-1150, 1992.

204. Jones GR: A practical guide to evaluation and treatment of infections in patients with central venous catheters, *J Intraven Nurs* 21:134-142, 1998.

205. Sitges-Serra A, Hernandez R, Maistro S et al: Prevention of catheter sepsis: the hub, *Nutrition* 13:30S-35S, 1997.

206. U.S. Department of Health and Human Service, Public Health Service, Center for Disease Control: Guidelines for prevention of intravascular device related infections. Part I. Intravascular device-related infections: an overview. Part 2. Recommendations for prevention of intravascular device related infections, *Infect Control Hosp Epidemiol* 17:438-473, 1996.

207. Wickham R, Purl S, Welker D: Long term central venous catheters: issues for care, *Semin Oncol Nurs* 8:133-147, 1992.

208. Rosmarin DK, Wardlow GM, Mirtallo J: Hperglycemia associated with high continuous infusion rates of total parenteral nutrition dextrose, *Nutr Clin Pract* 11:151-156, 1996.

209. Orr M: Hyperglycemia during nutrition support, *Crit Care Nurs* 12:64-70, 1992.

210. Pomposelli JJ, Baxter JK, Babineau TJ et al: Early postoperative glucose control predicts nosocomial infection rate in diabetic patients, *JPEN J Parenter Enteral Nutr* 22:77-81, 1998.

211. Beers T, Burnes J, Fleming C: Superior vena caval obstruction in patients with gut failure receiving home parenteral nutrition, *JPEN J Parenter Enteral Nutr* 14:474-479, 1990.

212. Timsit JF, Furkas JC, Boyer JM et al: Central venous catheter-related thrombosis in intensive care patients: incidence, risk factors and relationship with catheter related sepsis, *Chest* 114:207-213, 1998.

213. Brown-Smith J, Stoner M, Barley Z: Tunneled catheter thrombosis: factors related to incidence, *Oncol Nurs Forum* 17:543-549, 1990.

Clinical Pharmacology

Donna M. Kraus

The safe and rational use of medications in critically ill children requires a thorough understanding of pediatric pharmacology and proper medication administration. Age-related differences in drug disposition, metabolism, excretion, and pharmacodynamic effects, coupled with the special pharmacologic considerations of the critically ill, can make the pediatric intensive care patient a pharmacotherapeutic challenge for the clinician. Critically ill children usually receive multiple medications; many of which are extremely potent and require careful titration. Oftentimes the use of medications in critically ill children falls outside of the product labeling approved by the Food and Drug Administration (FDA). In addition, the proper dosage form and concentration of many medications may not be readily available for these patients. Thus the PICU patient is at a great risk for many drug misadventures including miscalculation of doses, use of non-optimal or untested doses, improper dilution and administration of medications, and

multiple drug interactions. This chapter will review pediatric pharmacokinetics, pharmacodynamics, drug dosing, therapeutic drug monitoring, medication administration, and drug interactions in the PICU patient.

PEDIATRIC AGE GROUP TERMINOLOGY

The normal developmental maturation of body composition, physiologic parameters, weight, and size that occur throughout infancy and childhood dramatically influence pharmacokinetic parameters, pharmacodynamics, and dosing recommendations of medications in children. In fact, pediatric dosing recommendations are usually specified according to specific age group terms. For many drugs, the mg/kg recommended dose is different for children of different ages.[1] Categorizing an individual by the wrong age group term could result in significant overdosing or underdosing of the patient. Therefore it is important for PICU clinicians to know the definitions of the various age group terminology. These terms are listed in Table 13-1.

MONITORING PARAMETERS

Many clinical monitoring parameters used in adults for assessing medication efficacy or toxicity are also used in the critically ill child. However, normal values for infants and children may differ. One must be aware of these differences in laboratory parameters and normal vital signs in order to adequately monitor pharmacotherapy in PICU patients. For example, children, especially neonates and young infants, have lower blood pressures and higher respiratory and heart rates, compared to adults. Proper references should be consulted for the normal values for age when providing clinical care to critically ill children.

PEDIATRIC PHARMACOKINETICS

Pharmacokinetics mathematically describes the concentration of a drug or its metabolites in the body (i.e., in the blood, body fluids and tissues) over a period of time.[2]

TABLE 13-1 **Definition of Age Group Terminology**

Gestational age (GA)	The time from conception until birth. More specifically, gestational age is defined as the number of weeks from the first day of the mother's last menstrual period (LMP) until the birth of the baby. Gestational age at birth is assessed by the date of the LMP and by physical exam (Dubowitz score).
Postnatal age (PNA)	Chronologic age since birth
Postconceptional age (PCA)	Age since conception. Postconceptional age is calculated as gestational age plus postnatal age (PCA = GA + PNA).
Neonate	A full-term newborn 0-4 weeks postnatal age. This term may also be applied to a premature neonate whose postconceptional age (PCA) is 42-46 weeks
Premature neonate	Neonate born at <38 weeks gestational age
Full-term neonate	Neonate born at 38-42 weeks (average ~40 weeks) gestational age
Infant	1 month to 1 year of age
Child/Children	1-12 years of age
Adolescent	13-18 years of age
Adult	>18 years of age

Reproduced with permission from Taketomo CK, Hodding JH, Kraus DM: *Pediatric dosage handbook,* ed 6, Hudson, OH, 1999, Lexi-Comp, 13.

Clinically, pharmacokinetics is used to describe the time-dependent changes of the drug plasma concentration following administration of a medication. The concentration of a drug in the plasma is dependent upon numerous factors including: the absorption of the drug from the site of administration into the systemic circulation, distribution of the drug into tissues and fluids of the body, metabolism or biotransformation of the drug, and elimination or excretion of the drug from the body. Mathematic pharmacokinetic models can be used to characterize absorption, distribution, metabolism and elimination of a drug and can predict the drug concentration in the plasma at a given time. This is clinically important. For many drugs, the plasma drug concentration is proportional to the concentration of the drug at the receptor site. Therefore the plasma concentration can be related to the pharmacodynamic and clinical effects of the drug.[3] This section will define pharmacokinetic terminology and discuss important age-related differences in drug absorption, distribution, metabolism, and excretion as they clinically relate to the PICU patient.

Absorption

Administration of medication by any route, except intravenous, requires the drug to be absorbed from the site of administration into the systemic circulation. Once a drug reaches the systemic circulation, it can then be distributed throughout the body and to the drug receptor site (i.e., site of drug action). "Bioavailability" is a pharmacokinetic term that estimates the *extent* of absorption of a drug. Bioavailability is defined as the percent of an administered dose that reaches the systemic circulation.[4] Several factors can affect drug bioavailability, including the dissolution characteristics of the dosage form (e.g., capsule, tablet, sustained-release product), physicochemical characteristics of the drug (e.g., solubility, degree of ionization, salt from), route of administration, and extent of metabolism by the liver or gut before the drug reaches the systemic circulation. Drugs that are

administered orally must first pass through the gastrointestinal mucosa and into the portal circulation of the liver before reaching the systemic circulation. Therefore orally administered drugs can be metabolized by enzymes located in the gastrointestinal mucosa or the liver before reaching the systemic circulation. This phenomena is called the "first-pass effect." A large first-pass effect will result in a lower bioavailability for a drug and a larger difference between the recommended oral and intravenous doses. Drugs that are administered IV do not have to pass through the liver to reach the systemic circulation. Therefore IV drugs do not have a first-pass effect and have a bioavailability of 100%. Propranolol is an example of a drug with an extensive first-pass effect; its oral bioavailability is only 30% to 40%.[1] The usual oral dose of propranolol to treat arrhythmias in children is 0.5 to 1 mg/kg given every 6 to 8 hours, whereas the recommended IV dose is only 0.01 to 0.1 mg/kg. As one can see by this example, the bioavailability of a drug must be taken into consideration when changing the route of administration of a medication. If it is not, serious and potentially fatal overdoses or underdoses may occur. Other examples of drugs with low bioavailability and significant differences between the IV and oral dose include: hydralazine, labetalol, midazolam, morphine, and verapamil.[1]

Bioavailability may also be different for different dosage forms of the same drug. For example, the oral bioavailability of digoxin elixir can be as low as 70%, whereas the bioavailability of digoxin capsules can be 100%.[1] This 30% difference in bioavailability dictates that a dosage adjustment must be made when one dosage form is changed to the other. Thus bioavailability needs to be considered not only when changing the route of administration, but also when changing dosage forms.

Many factors can affect the absorption of enterally administered medications in the pediatric intensive care patient. Significant age-related maturational changes of gastric emptying time, gastric acidity, intestinal motility and integrity, enzymatic activity, biliary function, and bacterial colonization occur during the first 2 years of life and can influence drug absorption. For example, gastric emptying time can be delayed in neonates for as long as 6 to 8 hours and adult values may not be reached until 6 to 8 months of age.[5] Disease states, drugs, and diet may also influence gastric emptying time and gastrointestinal motility. A longer gastric emptying time may delay drug absorption in the small intestine. This can result in a decreased peak serum drug concentration and a longer time to reach the peak concentration of an enterally administered medication.

Gastric acidity and duodenal pH also affect drug ionization and absorption.[5,6] Drugs are absorbed across membranes in the un-ionized form. In general, acidic drugs are better absorbed in an acidic environment because these drugs would be in the un-ionized form. However, a basic drug in an acidic environment will be mostly ionized and therefore less well absorbed. Similarly, in an alkaline or more basic environment, acidic drugs will be ionized and less well absorbed, whereas basic drugs will be un-ionized and better absorbed. Therefore age-related changes in gastric pH can affect drug absorption. Gastric acidity is decreased in neonates, especially in preterm newborns.[7] This decrease in gastric acid output is often termed "relative achlorhydria" and results in a higher (more alkaline) gastric pH. This may result in a decrease in the bioavailability of acidic drugs (e.g., phenobarbital, phenytoin) and an increase in the bioavailability of acid-labile drugs (e.g., ampicillin, erythromycin, penicillin).[5,8] Although gastric acidity is generally lower in the neonatal period, maximal gastric acid output does not reach adult values until 2 years of age.[5,7] Thus infants and young children may have age-related differences in drug absorption related to gastric pH.

Differences in the formulation of an enterally administered medication can also affect drug absorption. Sustained-release products are made to release a drug over an extended period of time (e.g., 12 hours). However, in young infants, the gastrointestinal transit time may be less than 8 hours. Thus the use of a sustained release preparation (such as theophylline) in a young infant, may result in incomplete and highly variable absorption (i.e., the sustained release product may be excreted in the stool before the drug is completely absorbed). This is why fast (or prompt) release oral products (i.e., non–sustained-release products) are usually used in neonates and infants.[1]

The absorption of enterally administered medications may also be delayed or decreased in patients who have decreased perfusion to the gastrointestinal tract (e.g., critically ill patients, patients in shock, patients with congestive heart failure) or decreased gastrointestinal function (e.g., postoperative patients recovering from anesthesia). Therefore medications are not usually administered enterally to these patients. In addition, medications commonly used in PICU patients may influence gastrointestinal drug absorption. Anticholinergics may prolong gastric emptying time and delay drug absorption, while metoclopramide may shorten gastric emptying time and hasten the time to drug absorption.[9] Medications that are used to increase gastrointestinal pH, such as antacids, histamine-2 receptor blockers

(e.g., cimetidine, ranitidine) and proton pump inhibitors (e.g., omeprazole) may also affect the absorption of medications. For example, the oral absorption of ketoconazole (which requires an acidic pH for proper absorption) is decreased by these agents.[1] Medications, such as ß-blockers, may decrease liver blood flow and increase the oral bioavailability of certain drugs that normally rely on liver blood flow for a large first-pass effect.[9]

Even food can interfere with the absorption of drugs and some medications are better absorbed on an empty stomach. Continuous NG feedings can decrease the enteral absorption of phenytoin, carbamazepine, hydralazine, levothyroxine, and warfarin.[10] These drug-nutrient interactions require holding enteral feedings for a period of time (to allow the drug to be absorbed), close monitoring of the patient, and measurement of serum drug concentrations.

For some of these agents (e.g., phenytoin, carbamazepine) holding the feedings for 2 hours before and 2 hours after a dose is recommended, if possible.[1,10] If the continuous feedings cannot be interrupted for that period of time, the IV route of administration or alternative drugs may need to be considered. Sucralfate will interact with continuous enteral feedings by binding to the protein in the food. It is not recommended in these patients because of the prolonged period of time that feedings would need to be held.[10]

The rectum has been used as an alternative route of pediatric drug administration, especially when the oral route is not feasible and IV access is not readily available. However, routine use of the rectal route is discouraged, especially for certain drugs (e.g., aminophylline) because of unpredictable drug absorption and potential toxicities.[8] In general, the slow and unpredictable absorption by this route of administration makes rectal administration of medications in the intensive care setting undesirable.[11] However, if one utilizes the proper drug and dosage formulation, rapid and efficient rectal absorption can occur. For example, rectally administered diazepam and valproic acid have been used to treat status epilepticus. In fact, rectally administered diazepam solution for injection produced comparable serum concentrations to IV use and rectal use of valproic acid syrup produced concentrations similar to those from oral administration.[12,13] A recently marketed diazepam rectal gel formulation (Diastat) is approved for use in children ≥2 years and adults for intermittent episodes of increased seizure activity.[1] Rectal administration of diazepam, midazolam, and morphine has also been successfully used for analgesia or pre-anesthetic sedation in children.[11]

Drug absorption following intramuscular (IM) administration is dependent upon several factors including: blood flow, muscular contractions, muscle mass, and physico-chemical characteristics of the drug.[5,6,8] In critically ill patients with low cardiac output or hypotension, the rate and extent of IM drug absorption may be decreased as a result of compromised perfusion of the injection site. In addition, the low degree of muscular activity and muscle contractions in immobile, severely ill, or paralyzed PICU patients can also decrease the rate of IM drug absorption. Because IM absorption is also affected by the surface area of the muscle over which the medication has spread, patients with a low muscle mass to total body mass ratio (e.g., neonates) may also display a decrease in IM absorption of drugs. The physicochemical properties of a drug also play an important role in IM absorption. Phenytoin, for example, will precipitate at the site of IM injection, due to its physicochemical properties and the relative pH of the muscle.[8] This precipitation or crystallization of the drug acts as a depot of medication in the muscle. Absorption of the drug is decreased initially, but the medication continues to be absorbed over a prolonged period of time (even after the IM injections are discontinued). The erratic absorption of IM phenytoin, and the pain associated with precipitation of the drug in the muscle, make the IM route of administration unacceptable for this medication.[14] Fosphenytoin, a prodrug of phenytoin, is water soluble and is FDA approved for IM administration in adults; however, limited studies in children have been conducted.[1] Although certain drugs, such as the aminoglycosides, penicillins, and phenobarbital, can be administered IM, in general, because of variable absorption, the IM route of administration should be avoided in critically ill pediatric patients.[1,11]

The potential absorption of medications through the skin should not be overlooked in the PICU patient. Percutaneous absorption of drugs can be increased in neonates, especially preterm newborns, as a result of the increased hydration of the skin, decreased thickness of the stratum corneum (outer layer of the epidermis), and the higher ratio of surface area per kilogram body weight.[5,6] Toxicities have been reported following topical application of boric acid, corticosteroids, epinephrine, hexachlorophene, iodine, and salicylic acid in neonatal patients.[15] Although skin barrier development may be fully developed by 2 to 3 weeks after birth,[15] it is important to remember that the ratio of body surface area to kilogram body weight is still increased in infants and young children, compared to adults. Because of this higher surface area/weight ratio, infants and young children will absorb more drug per kilogram for an equal application of topical medication. In addition, disruptions in the integrity of the skin, such as abrasions, open lesions, or burns, and occlusive dressings can also increase the percutaneous absorption of medications in any aged patient. Therefore the young PICU patient may potentially be at risk for toxicities from the topical application of medications.

Distribution

Once a drug is absorbed or enters the bloodstream (i.e., the central compartment), it then can be delivered to other sites in the body, including the site of action and the site of elimination. Drug "distribution" is the process of drug movement to the various body tissues, organs, and fluids. The "distribution phase" refers to the time during which the drug is distributing throughout the body. Clinically, for many drugs, the serum drug concentration *after* distribution more closely correlates with the concentration of drug at the receptor site. Thus serum concentration determinations for most drugs must be obtained after the distribution phase. Some drugs (like digoxin) have a very long distribution phase (6 to 8 hours).[1] If a digoxin serum concentration is

obtained too soon after the dose, it will reflect drug in the central compartment and will be extremely elevated. This example illustrates the importance of understanding the concept of distribution phase as it clinically applies to the PICU patient.

The "volume of distribution" (Vd) represents the hypothetical volume that would "account for the total amount of drug in the body if it were present throughout the body at the same concentration found in the plasma."[4] Clinically, a small volume of distribution indicates that the drug has minimal distribution and is largely retained in the central compartment (e.g., in adults, the Vd of gentamicin is 0.25 L/kg). A large volume of distribution indicates that the drug distributes well into peripheral compartments (tissues, organs and body fluids) and may even concentrate in certain tissues or organs (e.g., in adults, the Vd of digoxin is 7 L/kg).[1] For a given drug, provided other factors remain constant, patients with larger volumes of distribution will require larger doses to obtain the same serum concentration as patients with smaller volumes of distribution. Understanding the variables that affect drug distribution will help explain some of the special dosing requirements of critically ill pediatric patients.

Drug distribution is dependent upon the physicochemical properties of the drug (molecular weight, degree of ionization, solubility in water and lipids) and various patient-specific physiologic factors. These factors include: the composition and size of body compartments (e.g., total body water, intracellular and extracellular water, and adipose tissue), membrane permeability, pH, protein binding, and hemodynamic variables such as cardiac output, tissue perfusion and regional blood flow.[16] Many of these factors, especially body composition and protein binding, are age related and can be influenced by various disease states observed in PICU patients.

Total body water and extracellular water, when expressed as a percentage of weight, are increased in the newborn and decrease throughout childhood with increasing age. The total body water of a full-term newborn is 75%, but it is 60% in a three-month old and 55% in an adult.[17] Extracellular water is approximately 50% of body weight in premature infants, 35% in infants 4 to 6 months old, 25% in a 1-year-old child, and 19% in adults.[18] The higher total body water and extracellular water observed in newborns and infants generally results in a larger Vd for water-soluble drugs, compared with older children and adults. Additionally, the Vd for aminoglycosides (e.g., gentamicin) and other drugs that distribute into the extracellular water compartment roughly correlates to the volume of the extracellular water compartment. The Vd for these drugs is larger in neonates and infants; therefore a larger mg/kg loading dose is needed to achieve similar initial concentrations compared to older children and adults.

The Vd for gentamicin can also be increased in patients with increased extracellular water, such as those patients with ascites, third spacing, or congestive heart failure. In fact, the mean Vd for gentamicin in PICU patients (0.42 L/kg) was found to be greater than the mean Vd reported in children in the literature (~0.31 L/kg).[19]

This larger Vd and other alterations in pharmacokinetic parameters suggest that critically ill children may need initial gentamicin doses closer to 9 mg/kg/day to produce therapeutic serum concentrations (using traditional q8h dosing) rather than the standard recommended doses of 7.5 mg/kg/day.

In contrast, smaller milligrams per kilogram loading doses of fat-soluble drugs (e.g., diazepam) are recommended in neonates and young infants. Neonates and young infants have much less adipose tissue compared with adults. The adipose tissue content of a preterm newborn is only 1% to 2%, but it is 15% in a term newborn.[17] This lower amount of adipose tissue (and the higher water content of adipose tissue in newborns) may result in a decreased Vd for fat-soluble drugs, and thus smaller mg/kg loading doses for fat-soluble drugs.

The plasma protein binding of many medications is lower in neonates and infants for several reasons. Neonates have (1) a decreased affinity for drugs by fetal albumin; (2) lower concentrations of binding proteins (e.g., albumin, alpha$_1$-acid glycoprotein); (3) a lower plasma pH (which can decrease binding of acidic drugs to protein); and (4) higher concentrations of endogenous substances (such as bilirubin and free fatty acids) or other substances acquired transplacentally (e.g., medications, hormones) that may compete with medications for protein-binding sites.[5,20] The affinity of albumin for acidic drugs and total plasma protein concentrations increase with age and may approach adult values at 10 to 12 months of age.[6] Thus PICU patients less than 1 year of age may have an age-related decrease in protein binding compared to older patients. In addition, PICU patients with disease states that result in low concentrations of albumin or total protein, acidosis, hyperbilirubinemia, or uremia may have decreased protein binding for certain drugs. Clinically, these changes are important for drugs that are highly protein bound, such as phenytoin, valproic acid, and warfarin.

Decreased protein binding results in an increase in the percent of drug that is free or unbound in the plasma. This higher proportion of free drug or "free fraction" can result in an increase in the Vd for a medication, as only the free or unbound drug can cross membranes and distribute into tissues. One would think that an increase in the free fraction of a drug would also lead to an increase of free drug at the receptor site and thus an increased drug effect. However, the free or unbound drug is also available to distribute into tissues where the drug has no receptors and is available to organs for metabolism (inactivation) or elimination from the body.[9] The overall result of decreased protein binding is that the free *fraction* of the drug in plasma is increased, the free *concentration* of the drug is not significantly altered, but a *decrease* in the *total* concentration of the drug occurs. Therefore changes in protein binding will alter the clinical interpretation of serum drug concentrations. An example will help to illustrate this point. The therapeutic range of phenytoin in a patient with normal protein binding is 10 to 20 µg/ml. If normal protein binding of phenytoin is considered to be 90%, then the normal free concentration would be 1 to 2 µg/ml (10% of 10 to 20). Therefore if a patient with

normal protein binding had a serum phenytoin concentration of 10 µg/ml, and their free fraction was 10%, then their free concentration would be 1 µg/ml. Remember it is the free *concentration* that best correlates with drug effect. If a patient had low protein binding (such that their free fraction was 20%), but their serum phenytoin concentration was only 5 µg/ml, their free concentration would still be 1 µg/ml (20% of 5). If a clinician only looked at the measured serum phenytoin concentration, they may misinterpret it to be subtherapeutic, when in reality it is comparable to a concentration of 10 µg/ml in a person with normal protein binding. This example illustrates the importance of identifying clinical situations that alter protein binding. In this case, a measurement of the free or unbound concentration of phenytoin can be determined to better assess therapy.

Metabolism

In general, most drugs are relatively lipid soluble and need to be converted into more polar (water-soluble) compounds in order to become inactivated and excreted from the body. However, there are a few exceptions to this statement. Some medications (e.g., enalapril) are inactive "prodrugs" that need to be metabolized into an active form (enalaprilat) before they can have a pharmacologic effect. Other drugs may have active metabolites that contribute to the pharmacologic effect of the drug or that may accumulate with decreased renal function and cause toxicities. For example, meperidine is metabolized to normeperidine, an active metabolite that can accumulate in patients with renal dysfunction and cause tremors or seizures.[1] These examples illustrate the importance of understanding the metabolism of medications used in PICU patients.

Drug metabolism can take place in a variety of sites (e.g., GI tract, skin, plasma, kidney, lungs), but most drugs are metabolized in the liver via hepatic enzymes and most drug metabolites are eliminated by the kidneys or biliary tract. Drugs may undergo hepatic metabolism via Phase I and Phase II reactions. During Phase I reactions the molecular structure of the drug may be altered via oxidation, reduction, demethylation, and hydrolysis. Phase II reactions are synthetic in nature and include conjugation with glucuronide, sulfate, glycine, hippurate, and glutathione; methylation; and acetylation.[21]

Both Phase I and Phase II biotransformation reactions are significantly decreased in the newborn, but increase (mature) with age. However, the degree of enzyme maturation at birth varies for the different hepatic enzyme reactions and the different enzyme pathways mature at different rates and for different substrates (drugs). For example, for Phase I reactions, the level of activity of cytochrome P-450 hepatic enzymes in full-term newborns is only ~ 50% of the adult value.[22] This results in decreased oxidation of certain medications (e.g., phenobarbital, phenytoin, theophylline, diazepam).[5,21] However, cytochrome P-450 oxidative reactions can mature relatively early in relation to other enzymes. The hydroxylation of phenobarbital and phenytoin increases to adult levels as early as 2 to 4 weeks after birth in full-term newborns, but can be delayed in infants who are born premature. Although oxidative metabolism is reduced in the newborn, it increases to 2 to 5 times that of an adult by 1 year of age. This has important clinical relevance. For drugs that are primarily excreted by the liver, metabolism helps determine the drug's clearance from the body (i.e., the amount of blood or plasma completely cleared of the drug per unit time). Clearance of the drug helps determine the recommended maintenance dose. Drug that have a high clearance will require a higher mg/kg maintenance dose, whereas drugs with a low clearance will require lower mg/kg maintenance doses. Thus for drugs that are primarily oxidized by the P-450 enzyme system (e.g., phenobarbital), the recommended maintenance doses will be lower on a mg/kg basis during the neonatal period (3 to 4 mg/kg/day), but will significantly increase during the first year of life and throughout early childhood (1 to 5 years: 6 to 8 mg/kg/day). Interestingly, this high P-450 enzyme activity in early childhood decreases during adolescence to a lower level in adulthood (see Figure 13-1). The age-related changes in P-450 enzyme activity will, in part, dictate the

mg/kg maintenance doses for drugs metabolized by this system. Therefore after early childhood, the mg/kg maintenance dose of phenobarbital decrease to 4 to 6 mg/kg/day for 5 to 12 year old patients and 1 to 3 mg/kg/day for adolescents and adults.[1] Prediction of doses based on maturation of hepatic enzymes can be complex because different enzymes mature at different rates, and more than one enzyme may be involved in the metabolism of a drug. For example, the hydroxylation of theophylline matures to adult levels by 40 weeks postconceptional age, but clearance of theophylline does not significantly increase until 55 weeks postconceptional age, when the N-demethylation pathway matures.[23] Like phenobarbital and other drugs that are metabolized via the P-450 enzyme system, the clearance of theophylline (and therefore the dose of theophylline on a mg/kg/day basis), increases dramatically during the first year of life and exceeds adult values on a per kilogram basis in early childhood.

Phase II reactions, such as acetylation, glucuronide conjugation, and glycine conjugation are also decreased in the newborn; however, methylation and sulfonation are functionally more mature at birth.[21,24] Most infants younger than 2 months are phenotypically slow acetylators. This results in decreased acetylation of drugs such as sulfonamides and hydralazine. In general, glucuronide conjugation does not fully mature until 6 to 18 months of age, but maturation of glucuronide conjugation differs for different substrates. Because of the decreased rate of conjugation, metabolism of drugs such as chloramphenicol, corticosteroids, lorazepam, morphine and trichloroethanol (active metabolite of chloral hydrate) can be significantly decreased in neonates and young infants. In fact, the "gray baby syndrome" (manifested by shock and cardiovascular collapse) was caused by the accumulation of chloramphenicol in neonates who were not given reduced doses to accommodate the reduced metabolism of the drug. Glycine conjugation is an important pathway for the metabolism of the preservatives benzyl alcohol and benzoic acid. This pathway is decreased in neonates, but matures by approximately 8 weeks of age. Because of this decreased metabolism, neonates (especially preterm neonates) who are given excess benzyl alcohol and benzoic acid may develop the "gasping syndrome." This potentially fatal syndrome consists of severe metabolic acidosis, gasping respirations and multiple organ system failure.[25] As a result of these problems, the FDA advises the use of preservative-free IV medications, diluents, and solutions in neonatal patients.[26]

In addition to age-related differences in drug metabolism, certain disease states and drugs utilized in the PICU may increase (induce) or decrease (inhibit) hepatic enzyme activity. Decreased cardiac output, decreased liver perfusion, liver dysfunction, or hypoxia may decrease the activity of hepatic enzymes and decrease drug clearance. This decrease in drug clearance may result in an increase in drug levels and toxicities, unless proper dosage adjustments are made (see dosing of drugs in hepatic failure below). Drugs that inhibit specific hepatic enzymes can decrease the metabolism of other drugs that are normally metabolized by those specific hepatic enzymes. Inhibition of an enzyme that normally metabolizes a drug can cause significant eleva-

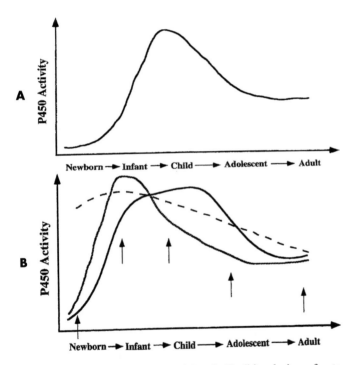

Fig. 13-1 P-450 Enzyme activity. **A,** Traditional view of cytochrome P-450 development. The development of functional P-450 activity is traditionally viewed as being limited in newborn infants but increasing in the first year of life to levels in toddlers and older children that generally exceed adult capacity. Near the onset of puberty, oxidative drug biotransformation begins the decline to adult levels. **B,** Developmental profiles of hypothetic cytochromes P-450. Not all P-450s share the "traditional" developmental profile. Overall drug biotransformation capacity represents a composite of the individual drug metabolism pathways and is dependent on the isoforms and amounts of P-450s (and other drug metabolizing enzymes) expressed. Therefore for a given pediatric patient, the apparent drug metabolism "phenotype" is a function of that individual's unique complement of drug metabolizing enzymes and stage of development (*vertical arrows*). (From Leeder JS, Kearns GL: Pharmacogenetics in pediatrics: implications for practice. *Pediatr Clin North Am,* 44:67, 1997).

tions of drug concentrations and toxicities. For example, erythromycin inhibits certain P-450 enzymes, and can increase the serum concentrations of drugs metabolized by those enzymes (e.g., midazolam, carbamazepine, phenytoin, cisapride, cyclosporine, theophylline).[1] The elevation in serum drug concentrations can cause serious toxicities. In contrast, drugs that induce hepatic enzymes, such as phenobarbital, phenytoin, and rifampin, may increase the metabolism of medications that are normally metabolized by these enzymes. This can result in subtherapeutic serum concentrations of the concurrently administered agent. For example, rifampin induces certain P-450 hepatic enzymes and may decrease the serum concentrations of drugs such as barbiturates, methadone, digoxin, verapamil, quinidine, cyclosporine, corticosteroids, warfarin, theophylline, chloramphenicol, ketoconazole, and oral contraceptives.[1] The decrease in serum concentration may be very significant. For instance, an alternative form of contraception should be strongly considered in women taking both oral contraceptive agents and rifampin (even short courses of rifampin). Before starting any medication, each potential drug interaction should be carefully evaluated. For many drug interactions involving hepatic metabolism, avoidance of an agent, dosage modification, or close monitoring may be advised. To better evaluate specific drug-drug interactions, a more detailed text should be consulted.[1,27]

Elimination

Several pharmacokinetic terms need to be defined to better understand drug elimination. *Total body clearance* is the intrinsic ability of the body to remove drug from the plasma or blood.[4] It does not indicate the amount of drug being removed from the plasma or blood, but indicates how much plasma or blood would be totally cleared of the drug if it were present. Therefore clearance is usually expressed as milliliters per minute (i.e., volume per time). In pediatrics, clearance is standardized per kilogram (ml/min/kg) or per body surface area (ml/min/meter^2) to better compare individuals of different ages and body size. Total body clearance is actually the sum of drug clearance of each organ of elimination. For many drugs, total body clearance is equal to hepatic clearance plus renal clearance. Renal clearance is determined by the clearance of unchanged drug in the urine. In the liver, drug clearance can occur via biotransformation to a metabolite and/or excretion of unchanged drug into the biliary tract. *Half-life* is an indirect measurement of clearance that is used to quantify elimination. Half-life is the time it takes for the drug concentration to be decreased by one-half (Figure 13-2). Clearance and volume of distribution determine half-life. Although half-life is not a very good indicator of drug elimination, it does help to determine an appropriate dosing interval for medication regimens. It also can be used to determine the time it takes to achieve steady-state and the time for a drug to be completely removed from the body. *Steady-state* (Figure 13-3) occurs when the rate of drug administration is equal to the rate of drug elimination; the drug concentration remains constant at steady-state.[4] When a patient begins a new medication regimen, it will take 3 to 5 times the half-life of the drug to

reach steady-state. Thus it will take a longer period of time to reach steady-state for a drug with longer half-life. For example, if the half-life of a drug is 1 hour, it will take 3 to 5 hours to reach steady-state. If the half-life of a drug is 24 hours, it will take 3 to 5 days to reach steady-state. Similarly, it takes the body 3 to 5 times the half-life to remove a drug from the body, once a medication is discontinued.

For many drugs and metabolites, the kidney is the most important route of excretion. The kidney has three physiologic functions: glomerular filtration, tubular secretion, and tubular reabsorption. Renal elimination of medications is dependent on the balance of these three functions. Some drugs are primarily eliminated by glomerular filtration (e.g., aminoglycosides, vancomycin). Clearance of these agents (and therefore dosing) is well correlated with glomerular filtration rate. Other drugs are also eliminated by proximal tubular secretion (e.g., penicillins, thiazides, furosemide). Tubular reabsorption of drugs also affects total body clearance. Therefore age or disease-related changes in any of these renal functions can affect the renal clearance and dosing of medications used in the PICU.

At birth, all three physiologic functions of the kidney (glomerular filtration, tubular secretion and tubular reabsorption) are decreased in the newborn compared to adults. This results in a decreased clearance for drugs that are eliminated via the kidneys. Therefore the maintenance doses of these drugs must also be reduced. Renal function matures with age. However, the rates of maturation for the individual physiologic functions are different, making it difficult to predict the renal clearance of drugs that are eliminated by more than one of these mechanisms. At birth, glomerular filtration is only 10 to 20 ml/min/1.73 m^2; it doubles by 2 weeks of age, but does not reach adult values until 3 to 5 months of age.[28,29] Tubular secretion is only 20% to 30% of adult values at birth; it reaches adult values at approximately 8 to 10 months of age, and values 10 times higher

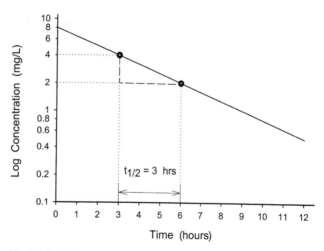

Fig. 13-2 The half-life of a drug can be calculated by plotting the logarithm of the serum drug concentration (following a dose given at time 0) versus time. The half-life of a drug is the time it takes for the serum drug concentration to fall by one-half. In this example, the serum drug concentration is 4 mg/L at 3 hours and falls to 2 mg/L at 6 hours. Thus the half-life ($t_{1/2}$) of the drug is 3 hours.

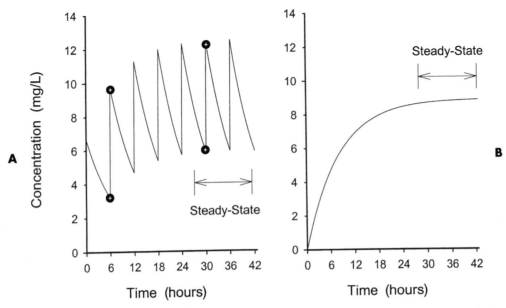

Fig. 13-3 Steady-state occurs when the rate of drug administration is equal to the rate of drug elimination. This produces drug concentrations that are constant. Steady-state occurs at 5 times the drug's half-life. (Clinically, 3 to 5 times the drug's half-life is used to estimate steady-state). In A, an intermittent dose of a drug with a half-life of 5.5 hours is administered every 6 hours. Serum drug concentrations increase after each dose to a peak amount and then decline to a trough concentration (right before the next dose is given). With repeated dosing the peak and trough concentrations increase (as a result of drug accumulation) until steady-state is achieved. At steady-state, all the peak concentrations are equal and all the trough concentrations are equal. In this example, steady state occurs at 27.5 hours (5 times the half-life of 5.5 hours). In B, the same drug is administered via a continuous infusion at the same dose per day. Steady-state occurs at the same time (27.5 hours or 5 times the half-life of 5.5 hours). Because the same amount of drug was given per day, the steady-state concentration in B is equal to the average steady-state concentration in A.

than birth by 1 year of age.[5,6] Tubular reabsorption is decreased in the neonate and the normal diurnal variation in urinary pH is not evident until 2 years of age. Thus the kidney's capacity for clearance via all three physiologic functions may not be fully developed until 2 years of age. Clinically then, PICU patients less than 2 years of age may have age-related alterations in renal clearance of medications that are normally eliminated by the kidney. This is probably more significant for patients who are 1 year of age or less. Medical conditions, such as decreased cardiac output, decreased renal perfusion, renal disease, and asphyxia may also decrease glomerular filtration and drug clearance. Whenever renal function is decreased, proper dosage adjustment of drugs that are normally eliminated by the kidney, must be made so that accumulation of drug and toxicity does not occur (see dosing of drugs in renal failure below).

PHARMACODYNAMICS

Pharmacodynamics is the study of the time-dependent actions or biologic effects of a drug in the human body that result from the interaction of the drug and its receptor.[2] Pharmacodynamics uses mathematic models to describe the relationship between the drug dose or the plasma concentration and the pharmacologic effect of the drug. One such

model is the sigmoidal model (Figure 13-4), which approximates an S-shaped curve.[30] In this model, the pharmacologic effect of the drug only slightly increases as one begins to increase the dose or concentration. As the dose or concentration continues to increase, the pharmacologic effect of the drug then increases greatly, almost in a linear fashion. As one continues to increase the dose even higher, a leveling off of the effects occur. This leveling off of the curve indicates that there is a maximum amount of drug, above which no further increase in effect is seen. In conjunction with the pharmacologic effects, adverse effects or toxicities that are dose or concentration related may also occur. Pharmacodynamic modeling tries to identify a dose that will produce an optimal level of pharmacologic effect, with a minimal amount of dose-related side effects.

Pharmacodynamic modeling may also help identify the range of therapeutic serum drug concentrations. Concentrations below the therapeutic range are usually subtherapeutic and concentrations above the therapeutic range are usually toxic. Serum drug concentrations are only useful when they closely relate to the concentration of drug at the receptor.[31] The "therapeutic index" of a drug uses the serum concentrations of the therapeutic range and is the ratio of the maximum serum concentration in the therapeutic range to the minimum serum concentration in the therapeutic range. If a drug has a "narrow therapeutic index," it

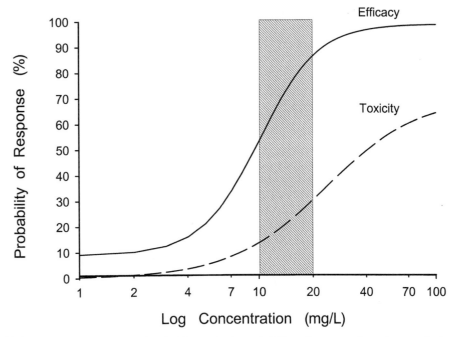

Fig. 13-4   Pharmacodynamic model. In this graph, the probability of response for a pharmacologic effect (efficacy) and toxicity are plotted versus the logarithm of the serum drug concentration. The efficacy line displays the traditional sigmoidal shaped curve. In this example, as the serum drug concentration increases from 0 to 4 mg/L, the probability of a pharmacologic effect is low and barely increases. At concentrations from 6 to 30 mg/L the probability of effect increases greatly, almost in a linear fashion. Note that as concentrations increase to greater than 30 mg/L the probability of an effective response does not significantly increase. However, the probability of toxicity continues to increase with increasing serum drug concentrations. The shaded area represents an identified therapeutic range of 10 to 20 mg/L. At these concentrations, the probability for efficacy would be about 50% to 85%, although the probability for toxicity would be only 10% to 30%.

means that the serum concentration (or dose) that produces a subtherapeutic effect is very close to the serum concentration (or dose) that produces a toxic effect. Proper monitoring of serum drug concentrations for drugs with a narrow therapeutic index can optimize dosing and pharmacologic effect, while minimizing toxic effect (see therapeutic drug monitoring below).

Dosing of Medication in Critically Ill Children

The pharmacodynamics and pharmacokinetics of a drug must be taken into consideration when dosing guidelines are designed. Pediatric dosing guidelines must take into account all of the developmental pharmacokinetic issues discussed above, plus any age-related differences in pharmacodynamic response. Medications are dosed in PICU patients according to their age and body size (either weight or body surface area). Pediatric doses are usually expressed as mg/kg/day or mg/kg/dose with the dosing interval specified. Potent medications that are given as continuous infusions (such as catecholamines), are dosed as μg/kg/min.[1] For many drugs, the mg/kg dose is different for different age groups. Although there is a good correlation of body surface area with body functions (i.e., cardiac output, glomerular filtration rate) and growth and development, measurement of body surface area can be difficult (espe-

cially in small infants). Therefore surface area is usually used to dose certain medications that require very accurate dosing (e.g., chemotherapeutic agents).

Normally, for most PICU patients, the individual's actual body weight (total body weight) is used to calculate mg/kg doses. However, special dosing considerations must be made for certain medications in patients who are extremely obese. Unfortunately, very few studies have examined the pharmacokinetics and dosing of drugs in obese pediatric patients. Therefore much has to be extrapolated from studies performed in obese adults. Several pharmacokinetic differences exist between obese and non-obese adults.[32,33] In obese patients, the Vd per kilogram of actual body weight will be decreased for water-soluble drugs (e.g., gentamicin). This is expected, because the excess weight in obese patients is adipose tissue, and water soluble drugs will not penetrate well into adipose tissue. However, the Vd per kilogram of actual body weight for lipid-soluble drugs is less predictable, with an increase in Vd for some lipid-soluble drugs (benzodiazepines, carbamazepine, verapamil) and a decrease in Vd for others (cyclosporine, propranolol). This suggests that other factors besides lipid-solubility play an important role in tissue distribution.[32] Generally, total body clearance of drugs that are hepatically metabolized by oxidation, reduction, or conjugation is not decreased in obese patients. However, clearance may be increased for prednisolone, halothane, and some benzodiazepines. Renal clearance of aminogylcosides in L/hr is significantly higher in obese adults compared with the non-obese.[33] These pharmacokinetic differences require that different dosage adjustments be made for different drugs. For example, in obese patients, the dose of lorazepam and vancomycin should be based on total body weight.[32,33] Vecuronium, however, should be dosed on ideal body weight. The initial dose of an aminoglycoside should be based on an adjusted body weight, which is calculated by adding the ideal body weight to 40% of the difference between the total body weight and the ideal body weight.[33] Subsequent doses of aminoglycosides should be based upon serum drug concentrations. Practical guidelines for dosing other drugs in obese adults have been proposed.[32,33] Clinical use of these guidelines, especially in obese children, requires close monitoring of the patient and serum drug concentration determinations to best optimize the dose.

Loading Doses. As stated before, when a dosing regimen is started, it will take 3 to 5 times the half-life of the drug to achieve steady-state. If the dosing regimen has been properly designed, it should achieve a steady-state serum drug concentration that is therapeutic. However, for drugs that have a long half-life, it will take a longer time to reach steady-state and therefore a longer time to reach a therapeutic serum drug concentration. If the time it will take to achieve the steady-state therapeutic drug concentration is too long for the clinical condition being treated, then a loading dose may be given. In other words, a loading dose is given to rapidly achieve a therapeutic serum drug concentration; it will NOT affect the time it takes to get to a steady-state condition.[4]

An example may better illustrate this point. Let's say we have a 4-year-old patient who requires phenobarbital to control his active seizure activity. The half-life of phenobarbital in this child may range from 37 to 73 hours.[1] Therefore if just a maintenance dose of phenobarbital was started, we could expect steady-state to occur in approximately 5 to 15 days (3 to 5×37 to 73 hours). If the maintenance dose was correct, then the patient would also achieve therapeutic serum concentrations at around the same time (5 to 15 days). Obviously, 5 to 15 days is too long to wait for a therapeutic effect, so a loading dose of phenobarbital should be given. The loading dose will rapidly achieve a therapeutic serum concentration, so that the patient's seizure activity can be controlled. After the loading dose, the patient should be started on a phenobarbital maintenance dose. It will still take 5 to 15 days of phenobarbital maintenance therapy to achieve steady-state. However, this patient's serum concentration should remain in the therapeutic range during this time. As the phenobarbital concentration from the loading dose begins to decline over time, the phenobarbital concentrations from the maintenance doses should accumulate over time. The overall result will maintain the concentrations within the therapeutic range.

Dosing of Drugs in Renal Failure. When PICU patients develop significant renal dysfunction, the dose of medications that are renally eliminated must be reduced or

the dosing interval for these drugs must be lengthened. With either method, the amount of drug that the patient receives per day is reduced. If the dose of a renally eliminated drug is not adjusted in a patient with renal dysfunction, the drug will accumulate in the patient and clinical toxicities may occur. Box 13-1 lists some common PICU medications that may require dosage reduction in patients with clinically significant renal dysfunction. Dose reduction may be required at different levels of renal dysfunction based on creatinine clearance. Dose reduction also depends on the amount of drug that is eliminated unchanged in the urine. Thus for a given creatinine clearance, the degree of dosage reduction will be different for different drugs. Several methods of adjusting the dose of medications in renal failure have been described.[1,11,34] Serum drug concentrations of certain medications (e.g., amikacin, digoxin, gentamicin, tobramycin, vancomycin) should be monitored in patients with renal dysfunction to optimize the dose.

Patients with renal failure and other conditions may also undergo dialysis, which can remove medications from the body. The amount of drug removed by dialysis de-

---

Box 13-1

Common PICU Medications That May Require Dosage Reduction in Patients With Significant Renal Dysfunction

Acyclovir	Fluconazole
Amikacin	Ganciclovir
Amoxicillin	Gentamicin
Ampicillin	Hydralazine
Atenolol	Imipenem-Cilastatin
Aztreonam	Lisinopril
Bretylium	Meperidine
Captopril	Meropenem
Cefazolin	Methadone
Cefepime	Methicillin
Cefotaxime	Mezlocillin
Cefotetan	Milrinone
Cefoxitin	Morphine
Ceftazidime	Nizatidine
Ceftizoxime	Oxacillin
Cefuroxime	Pancuronium
Cephalothin	Penicillin
Cimetidine	Pentamidine
Codeine	Piperacillin
Digoxin	Procainamide
Disopyramide	Quinidine
Enalapril	Ranitidine
Enalaprilat	Sulfamethoxazole
Enoxaparin	Ticarcillin
Famciclovir	Tobramycin
Famotidine	Trimethoprim
Fentanyl	Vancomycin
Flecainide	Verapamil

Specific dosing guidelines to reduce the dose of these drugs when used in patients with renal dysfunction can be found in Taketomo CK, Hodding JH, Kraus DM: *Pediatric dosage handbook,* ed 6, Hudson, Ohio, 1999, Lexi-Comp.

pends upon several properties of the drug (i.e., molecular size/weight, water solubility, protein binding and volume of distribution), as well as the type of dialysis used.[34] Significant differences in drug removal occur between hemodialysis, peritoneal dialysis, and the three main types of continuous renal replacement therapy (CRRT) (i.e., continuous arteriovenous or venovenous hemofiltration [CAVH/CVVH], continuous arteriovenous or venovenous hemodialysis [CAVHD/CVVHD], and continuous arteriovenous or venovenous hemodiafiltration [CAVHDF/CVVHDF]).[35] (See Chapter 21.) Doses of medications for PICU patients undergoing dialysis must be individualized and serum drug concentrations should be monitored to help optimize doses.

Dosing of Drugs in Hepatic Failure.   Many drugs are eliminated by the liver, either by metabolism to inactive forms or by excretion via the biliary tract. Therefore these drugs must be used with caution and doses may need to be decreased in patients who have hepatic dysfunction or biliary tract obstruction. If doses of hepatically eliminated drugs are not decreased in patients with hepatic dysfunction, the drug may accumulate and clinical toxicities may occur. Certain drugs, such as valproic acid and felbamate, are contraindicated in patients with hepatic dysfunction because they are hepatotoxic.[1] Common PICU drugs that are significantly metabolized by the liver include carbamazepine, cyclosporine, diazepam, ketamine, midazolam, labetalol, lidocaine, phenytoin, procainamide, propranolol, and vecuronium. Dosage reduction may be required at different levels of hepatic dysfunction (e.g., moderate or severe) and will depend upon the percent of drug that is eliminated by the liver. Specific guidelines for dosing of many drugs in hepatic dysfunction are not well developed. Unlike how serum creatinine can easily assess renal function, there is not one simple clinical marker that can reliably assess the degree of hepatic dysfunction in a patient. Thus for certain medications, dosage adjustment may be made based on clinical assessment of hepatic function, liver enzymes, and/or bilirubin serum concentrations. Oftentimes, the dose may be adjusted based on the patient's clinical response and signs of drug toxicity or adverse effects. Serum concentrations for specific hepatically metabolized drugs (e.g., carbamazepine, cyclosporine, lidocaine, phenobarbital, phenytoin, procainamide) should be monitored to best optimize therapy.

Therapeutic Drug Monitoring

Many medications that have a narrow therapeutic range are utilized in the PICU and require therapeutic drug monitoring (e.g., aminoglycoside antibiotics, phenobarbital, phenytoin, theophylline, and vancomycin). Proper obtainment of serum drug concentrations in relation to the dose and duration of therapy is essential in order to best interpret the concentrations and make correct dosage adjustments. Table 13-2 lists the therapeutic range and time to obtain serum concentrations for these agents. The peak serum drug concentration (i.e., the maximum concentration achieved) occurs shortly after administration of an IV dose, or after absorption into

the blood stream when the drug is administered via other routes. The trough serum drug concentration (i.e., the minimum concentration achieved with a dosing regimen) occurs right before the next dose. The optimal time to measure the peak and trough serum drug concentration has been determined with clinical studies for each drug. These studies have related the drug concentrations obtained at certain times to the optimal clinical effect. Therefore drug concentrations must be drawn at the appropriate times in order to best utilize their results.

It is also important for PICU clinicians to document the time that the dose was administered (i.e., start and stop time of the infusion) and the time that the serum drug concentration was obtained. Using this information, the dose, other patient information, and the results of the serum drug concentrations, the clinical pharmacist can calculate the patient's individual pharmacokinetic parameters and optimize the dose. One should remember that drawing blood samples from central catheters where the drug was just infused may falsely elevate the drug concentration, even if extra blood is taken from the catheter. The measured serum drug concentrations and calculated pharmacokinetic parameters should always be utilized in conjunction with the patient's clinical condition.

MEDICATION ADMINISTRATION IN THE PICU

IV Administration

Pediatric total daily fluid requirements (in ml/day) are much smaller than adults. In addition, pediatric patients cannot tolerate large volumes of fluid. Therefore the *volume* of fluids that an IV medication can be delivered into a pediatric patient is limited. Additionally, the *rate* of drug infusion is also limited. This is not only because of the limitations of volume, but also because of the limitations of the physico-chemical properties of the drug and the adverse effects it may cause in high concentration to the smaller diameter veins. This problem is compounded in the PICU patient who may be fluid restricted because of renal, respiratory or cardiac disease.[11] Table 13-3 lists the maximum concentration, method of infusion and rate of infusion for select PICU medications.

The method of IV drug administration in pediatric patients can affect drug delivery. The slow IV infusion rates for maintenance fluids used in infants and young pediatric patients (e.g., <25 ml/hr) can cause a delay in drug delivery, especially if medications are administered via volumetric chamber devices (Metriset or Buretrol). Even when factors such as tubing diameter, drug volume, and infusion rates have been taken into consideration, the actual delivery of drug to the patient may be delayed up to 2 hours if these devices are used.[36] In addition, administration of drugs at a Y-site, instead of using a syringe pump at the site closest to the patient, can also affect drug delivery. A delay in peak aminoglycoside concentrations of 1.5 hours and a mean decrease in peak concentrations of 2.5 μg/ml was seen in neonates, when tobramycin was administered via Y-site

TABLE 13-2 Blood Level Sampling Time Guidelines			
Drug	**Infusion Time**	**Therapeutic Range**	**When to Draw Levels**
Amikacin sulfate			
IV	30 min	Peak: 20-30 µg/ml	Peak: 30 min after end of 30-min infusion
		Trough: <10 µg/ml	Trough: Within 30 min before next dose
IM			Peak: 1 hr after IM injection
			Trough: Within 30 min before next dose
Carbamazepine		4-12 µg/ml	Just before next dose
Chloramphenicol			
IV	30 min	Peak: 15-25 µg/ml	Peak: 90 min after end of 30-min infusion
			Trough: Just before next dose
PO			Peak: 2 hr post-PO dose
Cyclosporine		BMT 100-200 ng/ml	Just before next dose
IV/PO		Liver transplant 200-300 ng/ml	
		Renal transplant 100-200 ng/ml	
Digoxin IV/PO		Age and disease related: 0.8-2 ng/ml	6 hr postdose to just before next dose
Ethosuximide PO		40-100 µg/ml	Just before next dose
Flucytosine PO		25-100 µg/ml	Peak: 2 hr after at least 4 days of therapy
Fosphenytoin (measure phenytoin levels)		Phenytoin: 10-20 µg/ml	
IV			Peak: 2 hr after end of an infusion
IM			Peak: 4 hr after IM injection
Gentamicin			
IV	30 min	Peak: 4-10 µg/ml	Peak 30 min after end of 30-min infusion
		Trough: 0.5-2 µg/ml	Trough: Within 30 min before next dose
IM			Peak: 1 hr after IM injection
			Trough: Within 30 min before next dose

Drug	Infusion time	Therapeutic level	Sampling time
Phenobarbital		15-40 µg/ml	Trough: just before next dose
Phenytoin PO, IV		10-20 µg/ml	Trough: just before next dose Post-load/peak: 1 hr after end of infusion
Theophylline IV bolus	30 min	10-20 µg/ml	Peak: 30 min after end of 30-min infusion
Continuous infusion			16-24 hr after the start or change in a constant IV infusion
PO liquid, fast-release tablet (Somo-phyllin, Slo-Phyllin liquid and tablet)			Peak: 1 hr postdose Trough: Just before next dose
PO slow-release (Theo-Dur, Slo-Phyllin GC, Slo-bid)			Peak: 4 hr postdose Trough: Just before next dose
Tobramycin IV	30 min	Peak: 4-10 µg/ml Trough: 0.5-2 µg/ml	Peak: 30 min after end of 30-min infusion Trough: Within 30 min before next dose
IM			Peak: 1 hr post-IM injection Trough: Within 30 min before next dose
Trimethoprim IV, dose 20 mg/kg	60 min	Peak: 5-10 µg/ml	Peak: 30 min after end of 60-min infusion
IV, dose 8-10 mg/kg		Peak: 1-3 µg/ml	Peak: 1 hr postdose
PO			Trough: Just before next dose
Valproic acid PO		50-100 µg/ml	Trough: Just before next dose
Vancomycin	60 min	Peak: 25-40 µg/ml Trough: 5-15 µg/ml	Peak: 20-30 min after end of 60-min infusion* Trough: Within 30 min before next dose

*Some institutions may draw vancomycin peak 1 hour after 1-hour infusion and accept the lower range of therapeutic.
From Taketomo CK, Hodding JH, Kraus DM: *Pediatric dosage handbook*, ed 6, Hudson, OH, 1999, Lexi-Comp.

TABLE 13-3   Maximum Concentrations of Select Medications for IV Infusion in Pediatric Patients

Drug	Method of Infusion/Rate	Maximum Concentration
Amikacin	Intermittent infusion over 30 min	5 mg/ml
Aminophylline	Usual: infuse over 20-30 min	1 mg/ml
	Maximum: 0.36 mg/kg/min, no faster than 25 mg/min	25 mg/ml
Amphotericin B (conventional)	Peripheral infusion over 2-6 hr	0.1 mg/ml
	CVP over 2-6 hr	0.5 mg/ml
Ampicillin	IVP over 3-5 min; max: 100 mg/min	100 mg/ml
	Intermittent infusion over 15-30 min	30 mg/ml
Bretylium	Life-threatening situation:	
	IVP over <30 sec	50 mg/ml
	Non–life-threatening situation:	
	Slow IVP over at least 8 min	10 mg/ml
Ceftriaxone	Intermittent infusion over 10-30 min	40 mg/ml
Cimetidine	Intermittent infusion over 15-30 min	6 mg/ml
	Slow IVP over at least 15 min	15 mg/ml
Dobutamine	Continuous infusion	5 mg/ml
Dopamine	Continuous infusion	3.2 mg/ml
		6 mg/ml has been used in large veins in extreme fluid restriction
Epinephrine	Continuous infusion	64 µg/ml
Gentamicin	Intermittent infusion over 30-60 min	2 mg/ml
	Slow IV over 15 min	10 mg/ml
Isoproterenol	Continuous infusion	20 µg/ml
		64 µg/ml has been used in extreme fluid restriction
Norepinephrine	Continuous infusion	4 µg/ml
		16 µg/ml has been used in extreme fluid restriction
Ranitidine	Intermittent infusion over 15-30 min	0.5 mg/ml
	Slow IVP over at least 5 min	2.5 mg/ml
Tobramycin	Intermittent infusion over 30-60 min	2 mg/ml
	Slow IV over 15 min	10 mg/ml
Vancomycin	Intermittent infusion over 60 min	5 mg/ml

Adapted from Taketomo CK, Hodding JH, Kraus DM: *Pediatric dosage handbook,* ed 6, Hudson, OH, 1999, Lexi-Comp.

compared to the syringe pump.[37] Therefore inappropriate IV drug administration can result in lower measured peak concentrations, and calculations of inappropriately large volumes of distribution and prolonged half-life for a drug. Whenever calculated pharmacokinetic parameters seem suspiciously high or low, the method of drug administration should be closely evaluated.

Certain methods of drug delivery may also cause medical problems. In adults patients, many drugs are administered via IV "piggyback" or in IV "riders." With this method of administration, the dose of medication is added to 50 or 100 ml of D_5W or NS. This method of drug delivery should not be used in small patients (e.g., those <10 kg), because of the excess amount of fluid, free water (from D_5W), and sodium (from NS) that will be delivered. Other potential problems or errors in pediatric drug administration techniques are listed in Box 13-2.

Pediatric Dosage Forms

Pediatric patients, especially those who are critically ill, are not able to swallow solid dosage forms. However, not all oral drugs are commercially available in a liquid formulation. Oftentimes, an extemporaneous liquid preparation must be compounded by the pharmacist using either an oral solid dosage form or an injectable product.[1,38] Information regarding the preparation and stability of pediatric extemporaneous formulations is limited.[39] In addition, extemporaneous products take much time to prepare and may not be readily available at all institutions.

The lack of liquid medications results in alternative methods to administer solid dosage forms to pediatric critically ill children. In general, regular-release tablets may be crushed, and administered either orally or through a nasogastric (NG) tube after being mixed with a small amount of water. This can be done, unless the medication

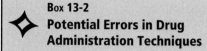

Box 13-2
Potential Errors in Drug Administration Techniques

Factors Involving Drug (Dose) Preparation

- Inappropriate dilutions
- Similarity in appearance of dose units
- Loss of potentially large amounts of drug dose in the dead space of a syringe; infusion Y-site, etc.
- Unsuitable drug formulations for administration
- Unlabeled or undesirable ingredients in dosage forms
- Undesirable drug concentrations and/or osmolalities
- Errors in interpreting drug orders and/or dose calculations

Factors Involving IV Drug Administration

- Loss of drug consequent to routine changing of IV sets
- Reduction in serum concentrations for drugs with rapid plasma clearance that are infused slowly
- Extreme increase in plasma drug concentrations consequent to rapid infusion of drugs with small central compartment volume of distribution
- Delayed infusion of total dose when IV line is not flushed Inadvertent mixture of drugs by the manual IV retrograde method
- Large distance between the site of drug infusion into an IV line and the insertion of the line into the patient
- Potential loss of large volume doses in the overflow syringe with the IV retrograde technique
- Possible loss of drug because of binding to IV tubing
- Use of large intraluminal diameter tubing for small patients
- Infiltrations not detected by pump alarms
- Infusion of multiple medications/fluids at different rates by means of a common "hub"
- Oscillations in fluid/dose rate of potent medications infused with piston-type pumps

Factors Involving Other Routes of Drug Administration

- Loss in delivery (nasogastric tube dead space) or from oral cavity
- Leakage of drug from IM or SC injection site
- Expulsion of drug from the rectum
- Misapplication to external sites (i.e., ophthalmic ointment in young infants)

From Blumer JL, Reed MD: Principles of neonatal pharmacology. In Yaffe S, Aranda JV, eds: *Pediatric pharmacology: therapeutic principles in practice*, ed 2, Philadelphia, 1992, WB Saunders, p. 168.

will produce irritation to the oral mucosa, is extremely bitter in taste (does not apply to NG use), contains dyes or could directly stain mucosal tissue or teeth, or is potentially carcinogenic.[40] Enteric-coated, sublingual, and extended-release dosage forms should not be crushed. Enteric-coated tablets are designed to stay intact in the acid environment of the stomach and to release the drug in the intestines. If enteric-coated tablets are crushed and administered gastrically, the drugs (1) may cause stomach irritation when they come into contact with the stomach mucosa; (2) may be destroyed by the acids in the stomach; or (3) may have an earlier onset of action. Sublingual tablets are meant to be

rapidly absorbed via the blood vessels under the tongue and in the mouth. This rapid absorption and fast onset of action will be lost if sublingual tablets are crushed and administered into the stomach or intestines. Extended-release dosage forms commonly have one of the following abbreviations after their trade name: CR (controlled release), CRT (controlled-release tablet), LA (long acting), SR (sustained release), TR (time release), TD (time delay), SA (sustained action), XL (extended release), or XR (extended release). These products are designed to release the drug slowly over a prolonged period of time. Thus the amount of drug contained in extended-release dosage forms is typically greater than regular-release dosage forms. If extended-release dosage forms are crushed and administered, all of the drug contained in the tablet or capsule will be released and absorbed at one time, resulting in very high serum concentrations and toxicities in the patient.

A comprehensive listing of oral dosage forms that should not be crushed has been published recently.[40] A summary of some common PICU medications that should not be crushed is listed in Table 13-4. Oftentimes the mg strength of a commercially available tablet may be too large for a child. In general, regular-release tablets can be cut in half to administer partial doses, but enteric-coated and extended-release products should not be cut.

Transdermal patches are occasionally used in older children and adolescents to deliver certain medications. These products can be used intact, provided that the milligram strength of the transdermal delivery system and dose delivered is appropriate for the patient's age and body size (i.e., weight). Different types of transdermal patches exist and some types should not be cut to deliver partial doses. For example, transdermal patches for clonidine (Catapress-TTS) and fentanyl (Duragesic) are membrane-controlled systems. If these types of patches are cut, the semipermeable membrane can be damaged and the rate of drug delivery may be affected. Contents of the patch reservoir may also leak. In addition, by cutting the patch, the patch may not adhere to the skin as well and the drug's stability or potency may be affected by exposure to air or sunlight. Therefore these patches should not be cut.[41]

Partial doses of patches may be delivered by covering a portion of skin with an impermeable adhesive bandage (i.e., blocking the patch). The area of the skin covered with the adhesive bandage should be proportional to the amount of dose reduction. An adhesive bandage may then be placed over the whole system to secure it in place.[41]

Pediatric Medication Administration Decision Making

Critically ill pediatric patients are often given highly potent medications that are dosed by body weight and administered by continuous IV infusion. In emergency situations, drugs such as dopamine, dobutamine, epinephrine, norepinephrine, and isoproterenol, need to be mixed appropriately and prepared for immediate administration. Proper calculation of the patient's dose, concentration for infusion, and milliliter-per-hour infusion rate are essential. Errors in

TABLE 13-4   Common PICU Medications That Should Not be Crushed

Type of Formulation	Example Drugs	Comments
Enteric coated	Biscodyl	Use suppository or powder form
	Erythromycin	Use suspension form
	Ferrous sulfate	Use liquid form
	Pancrelipase	Use powder form
	Sulfasalazine	Use suspension or regular tablets*
Extended-release	Acetazolamide	Use regular tablets or extemporaneous liquid preparation
	Carbamazepine	Use suspension or regular tablets
	Chlorpromazine	Use liquid preparation or regular tablets
	Diltiazem	Open capsule (do not crush beads); mix with applesauce and swallow immediately (do not chew) or flush beads down gastric tube with sterile water
	Disopyramide	Open capsule (do not crush beads); flush beads down gastric tube with sterile water; or use extemporaneous liquid preparation
	Lansoprazole	Open capsule (do not crush beads); mix with apple juice and flush through gastric tube
	Metoprolol	Use regular tablets
	Morphine	Use liquid form
	Omeprazole	Gastric tube: Mix capsule with apple juice or cranberry juice; stable 30 min after mixing
		Jejunostomy tube: Dissolve capsule in 8.4% sodium bicarbonate to make final concentration of 2 mg/ml
	Procainamide	Use regular tablets or extemporaneous liquid preparation
	Propranolol	Use liquid preparation
	Quinidine	Use regular tablets or extemporaneous liquid preparation
	Theophylline	Use liquid preparation
	Valproic Acid	Use liquid preparation
	Verapamil	Use regular tablets or extemporaneous liquid preparation

Adapted from Mitchell JF: Oral dosage forms that should not be crushed: 2000 update, *Hosp Pharm* 35:553-557, 2000; Engle KK, Hannawa TE: Techniques for administering oral medications to critical care patients receiving continuous enteral nutrition, *Am J Health Syst Pharm* 56:1441-1444, 1999; and Taketomo CK, Hodding JH, Kraus DM: *Pediatric dosage handbook,* ed 6, Hudson, OH, 1999, Lexi-Comp.
*"Regular tablets" means regular-release tablets (i.e., not extended release, not enteric coated, not sublingual)

calculations can result in significant overdose (and toxicities) or underdose (and lack of response). To complicate matters, many different combinations of concentration and rates can be used to deliver the same μg/min dose. Basically, there are three ways to calculate doses for proper administration of these agents: (1) the standard concentration method; (2) the "rule of 6s"; and (3) individualization of concentrations based on rates of infusion and dose. Each of these methods requires knowing the patient's weight and the intended μg/kg/min dose. Then, if the concentration is known, the rate of administration can be calculated; if an intended rate of administration is known, the concentration of the infusion can be calculated.

Standard concentrations for continuous infusions can be developed by weight, so that the rates of infusion are acceptable when the medication is dosed within the usual dosage range.[42] For example, standard concentrations for dopamine can be 200 μg/ml for infants 2 to 3 kg; 400 μg/ml for infants 4 to 8 kg; 800 μg/ml for children 9 to 15 kg and 1600 μg/ml for patients >15 kg. To calculate the ml/hr rate of infusion, first multiply the μg/kg/min dose times the kg weight, then times 60 (min/hr) and divide by the standard concentration. For example, let's say we wanted to deliver a dose of dopamine at 5 μg/kg/min to a 10-kg infant. Multiply

5 μg/kg/min times 10 kg to get 50 μg/min; multiply this by 60 min/hr to get 3000 μg/hr; then divide by the standard concentration of 800 μg/ml to get 3.75 ml/hr and round to 3.8 ml/hr. So, for this patient, 3.8 ml/hr of an 800 μg/ml solution will provide 5 μg/kg/min. The advantage of standard concentrations is that no patient calculations are needed to prepare the IV bag. Thus the IV bag can be quickly prepared or hung while the dose and rate are being calculated.

The rule of 6s is based on the fact that there are 60 minutes in an hour. With this method, a calculation based on the patient's body weight is made to determine the amount of medication to add to 100 ml of solution. Because the calculation uses the rule of 6's, the ml/hr infusion rate very easily relates to the dose in μg/kg/min. For dopamine and dobutamine, 6 times the patient's body weight is added to 100 ml; then 1 ml/hr will equal 1 μg/kg/min. For epinephrine, norepinephrine, and isoproterenol, 0.6 times the patient's body weight is added to 100 ml; then 1 ml/hr will equal 0.1 μg/kg/min.[1] Let's use this method to deliver a dose of dopamine at 5 μg/kg/min to a 10-kg infant. Multiply 10 kg × 6 to get 60; this is the amount of drug (60 mg) that should be added to 100 ml of IV solution. Then 1 ml/hr will equal 1 μg/kg/min and 5 ml/hr will equal

5 µg/kg/min. This method has the advantage of utilizing a milliliter-per-hour rate that very simply relates to the µg/kg/min dose. However, the disadvantage of this method is that patient-based calculations must be performed in order to make the IV solution.

With either of these methods, the ml/hr rate may be too large for some patients (e.g., if the patient requires fluid restriction). To individualize the concentration of the infusion, first multiply the µg/kg/min dose times the kilogram weight, then multiply times 60 (min/hr) and divide by the intended rate of infusion. For example, let's say we wanted to deliver a dose of dopamine at 5 µg/kg/min to a 10-kg fluid-restricted infant at 2 ml/hr. First multiply 5 µg/kg/min times 10 kg to get 50 µg/min; multiply this by 60 min/hr to get 3000 µg/hr; then divide by the intended rate of infusion of 2 ml/hr to get a concentration of 1500 µg/ml. For this patient, 2 ml/hr of a 1500 µg/ml solution will provide 5 µg/kg/min. This method has the advantage of being able to select the amount of fluid that the patient receives. However, it requires patient-specific calculations in order to make the IV solution.

Each PICU team should decide which of these methods to use to calculate continuous infusions of emergency medications. Some institutions elect to use a combination of methods. For example, standard concentrations can easily be prepared by the PICU staff during emergency situations. If the patient then requires fluid restrictions, the pharmacy can perform the necessary calculations to concentrate the infusion.

Changing patients from the IV route of administration to the oral or enteral route can result in significant cost savings. However, clinicians should keep in mind that patients should not be switched to the enteral route until the GI tract is well perfused and functioning. Otherwise, GI absorption may be compromised and the pharmacologic effects of the drug may be decreased. In addition, the oral versus IV bioavailability of the specific medication needs to be addressed when changing routes of administration (see Absorption above). If a drug with low oral bioavailability is given orally in the same dose as IV, an underdose will occur and minimal systemic effects may be seen. However, if a drug with low oral bioavailability is given IV in the same dose that is recommended orally, an overdose will occur and toxicities will result. Thus the recommend dose of a medication should be verified when changing routes of administration.

PRINCIPLES OF DRUG INTERACTIONS

Interactions can occur between two drugs (drug-drug interaction) or between a drug and a nutrient (drug-nutrient interaction). Drug-drug interactions can be pharmacokinetic or pharmacodynamic in nature. Pharmacokinetic drug-drug interactions result from alterations in absorption, distribution, metabolism or elimination. Absorption may be altered if a drug changes gastric pH, GI motility, GI mucosa or flora, alters the first-pass effect, or complexes with another drug in the GI tract. Drugs may affect distribution by altering protein binding. Metabolism may be altered when drugs inhibit or induce hepatic enzymes, or if two drugs compete for metabolism by the same enzyme. Drugs may affect excretion by altering renal elimination of unchanged drug or hepatic elimination via the biliary tract.[27] Examples of pharmacokinetic drug-drug interactions and drug-nutrient interactions have been given throughout this chapter.

Pharmacodynamic drug interactions occur when one drug modifies the pharmacologic effect of another. This type of interaction may take place at the receptor level, may include different cellular mechanisms of action, may involve alterations of the cellular environment, or may occur from the neutralization of one drug by another in the body.[27] At the receptor level, drugs may act as agonists (by stimulating the receptor), or antagonists (by blocking the receptor). (Some drugs may act as partial agonists by both stimulating and blocking the receptor.) An example of a drug-drug pharmacodynamic interaction that occurs at the receptor level would be albuterol and propranolol. Albuterol is a ß-adrenergic receptor agonist, and propranolol is a ß-adrenergic receptor antagonist (ß-blocker). If these two drugs are administered in the same patient, the bronchodilation effects of albuterol would be blocked by propranolol. Clinically, bronchoconstriction may be observed.

Two drugs may interact because of different cellular mechanisms of action that may either increase or decrease the pharmacologic response. For example, diuretics may enhance the antihypertensive effects of captopril, and indomethacin may decrease the antihypertensive effects of propranolol. Each of these drugs has a different mechanism of action. Drugs may interact by altering the cellular environment. For example, diuretics such as furosemide may cause hypokalemia which may increase the risk of digoxin toxicities. Drugs may also interact by neutralization. For example, protamine will neutralize heparin and reverse its pharmacologic effects.

Clearly the PICU patient is at risk for drug-drug and drug-nutrient interactions because of the many medications that they receive. The clinician should be aware of these problems and evaluate all drugs and nutrients for potential adverse interactions. In addition, clinicians must be aware of physical and chemical incompatibilities of IV medications. Certain medications will precipitate with or inactivate other medications. For example, when furosemide is injected into IV lines containing amrinone or milrinone, a precipitate will form. Aminoglycosides can be inactivated by penicillins. Sodium bicarbonate is incompatible with calcium salts, catecholamines and atropine and should not be mixed with or administered with other medications. Other incompatibilities of common PICU medications are listed in the Appendixes.

In summary, PICU patients require many special pharmacologic considerations. The age-related and disease state differences of pharmacokinetics and pharmacodynamics in these patients, along with the lack of appropriate dosage forms and use of multiple medications, can pose a pharmacotherapeutic challenge for the clinician. By having a better understanding of clinical pharmacology, including pharmacokinetics, pharmacodynamics, drug dosing, therapeutic drug monitoring, medication administration, and drug interactions, the PICU clinician will be better equipped to optimize the care of critically ill children.

REFERENCES

1. Taketomo CK, Hodding JH, Kraus DM: *Pediatric dosage handbook,* ed 6, Hudson, OH, 1999, Lexi-Comp.
2. Kearns GL: Pharmacokinetics in infants and children, *Inflamm Bowel Dis* 4 (2):104-107, 1998.
3. Danish M: Clinical pharmacokinetics. In Yaffe SJ, Aranda JV, eds: *Pediatric pharmacology: therapeutic principles in practice,* Philadelphia, 1992, WB Saunders.
4. Winters ME: *Basic clinical pharmacokinetics,* ed 3, Vancouver, Wash, 1994, Applied Therapeutics.
5. Morselli PL: Clinical pharmacology of the perinatal period and early infancy, *Clin Pharmacokinet* 17(suppl 1):13-28, 1989.
6. Besunder JB et al: Principles of drug disposition in the neonate: a critical evaluation of the pharmacokinetic-pharmacodynamic interface, Part I, *Clin Pharmacokinet* 14:189-216, 1988.
7. Yahav J: Development of parietal cells, acid secretion, and response to secretagogues. In Lebenthal E, ed: *Human gastrointestinal development,* New York, 1989, Raven Press.
8. Radde IC: Mechanisms of drug absorption and their development. In Radde IC, MacLeod SM, eds: *Pediatric pharmacology and therapeutics,* St Louis, 1993, Mosby Year Book.
9. Rudy AC, Brater DC: Pharmacokinetics. In Chernow B, ed: *The pharmacologic approach to the critically ill patient,* ed 3, Baltimore, 1994, Williams & Wilkins.
10. Engle KK, Hannawa TE: Techniques for administering oral medications to critical care patients receiving continuous enteral nutrition, *Am J Health Syst Pharm* 56:1441-1444, 1999.
11. Notterman DA: Pediatric pharmacotherapy. In Chernow B, ed: *The pharmacologic approach to the critically ill patient,* ed 3, Baltimore, 1994, Williams & Wilkins.
12. Seigler RS: The administration of rectal diazepam for acute management of seizures, *J Emerg Med* 8:155-159, 1990.
13. Cloyd JC, Kriel RL: Bioavailability of rectally administered valproic acid syrup, *Neurology* 31:1348-1352, 1981.
14. Tozer TN, Winter ME: Phenytoin. In Evans WE, Schentag JJ, Jusko WJ, eds: *Applied pharmacokinetics: principles of therapeutic drug monitoring,* ed 3, Vancouver, WA, 1992, Applied Therapeutics.
15. Barrett DA, Rutter N: Transdermal delivery and the premature neonate, *Crit Rev Ther Drug Carrier Syst* 11(1):1-30, 1994.
16. Radde IC: Growth and drug distribution. In Radde IC, Macleod SM, eds: *Pediatric pharmacology and therapeutics,* St Louis, 1993, Mosby.
17. Friis-Hansen B: Water distribution in the foetus and newborn infant, *Acta Paediatr Scand* 305(suppl):7-11, 1983.
18. Friis-Hansen B: Body water compartments in children: changes during growth and related changes in body composition, *Pediatrics* 28:169-181, 1961.
19. Kraus DM, Dusik CM, Rodvold KA et al.: Bayesian forecasting of gentamicin pharmacokinetics in pediatric intensive care unit patients, *Pediatr Infect Dis J* 12:713-718, 1993.
20. Radde IC: Drugs and protein binding. In Radde IC, Macleod SM, eds: *Pediatric pharmacology and therapeutics,* St Louis, 1993, Mosby.
21. Radde IC, Kalow W: Drug biotransformation and its development. In Radde IC, Macleod SM, eds: *Pediatric pharmacology and therapeutics,* St Louis, 1993, Mosby Year Book.
22. Aranda JV, MacLeod SM, Renton KW et al: Hepatic microsomal drug oxidation and electron transport in newborn infants, *J Pediatr* 85:534-542, 1974.
23. Kraus DM, Fischer JH, Reitz SJ et al: Alterations in theophylline metabolism during the first year of life. *Clin Pharmacol Ther* 54:351-359, 1993.
24. Leeder JS, Kearns GL: Pharmacogenetics in pediatrics: implications for practice, *Pediatr Clin North Am* 44:55-77, 1997.
25. Gershanik J, Boecler B, Ensley H et al: The gasping syndrome and benzyl alcohol poisoning, *N Engl J Med* 307:1384-1388, 1982.
26. Food and Drug Administration: Benzyl alcohol may be toxic to newborns. *FDA Drug Bulletin* 12:10-11, 1982.
27. Rudy AC, Brater DC: Drug interactions. In Chernow B, ed: *The pharmacologic approach to the critically ill patient,* ed 3, Baltimore, 1994, Williams & Wilkins.
28. Radde IC: Renal function and elimination of drugs during development. In: Radde IC, Macleod SM, eds: *Pediatric pharmacology and therapeutics,* St Louis, 1993, Mosby.
29. Vanpee M, Blennow M, Linne T et al: Renal function in very low birth weight infants: normal maturity reached during early childhood. *J Pediatr* 121:784-788, 1992.
30. Lalonde RL: Pharmacodynamics. In Evans WE, Schentag JJ, Jusko WJ, eds: *Applied pharmacokinetics: principles of therapeutic drug monitoring,* ed 3, Vancouver, Wash, 1992, Applied Therapeutics.
31. Schumacher GE: Introduction to therapeutic drug monitoring. In Schumacher GE, ed: *Therapeutic drug monitoring,* Norwalk, Conn, 1995, Appleton & Lange.
32. Cheymol G: Clinical pharmacokinetics of drugs in obesity, *Clin Pharmacokinet* 25:103-114, 1993.
33. Bearden DT, Rodvold KA: Dosage adjustments for antibacterials in obese patients: applying clinical pharmacokinetics, *Clin Pharmacokinet* 38:415-426, 2000.
34. Matzke GR, Millikin SP: Influence of renal function and dialysis on drug disposition. In Evans WE, Schentag JJ, Jusko WJ, eds: *Applied pharmacokinetics: principles of therapeutic drug monitoring,* ed 3, Vancouver, Wash, 1992, Applied Therapeutics.
35. Frye RF, Matzke GR: Drug therapy individualization for patients with renal insufficiency. In Dipiro JT et al, eds: *Pharmacotherapy: a pathophysiologic approach,* ed 4, Stamford, Conn, 1999, Appleton & Lange.
36. Nahata MC: Intravenous infusion conditions: implications for pharmacokinetic monitoring, *Clin Pharmacokinet* 24:221-229, 1993.
37. Nahata MC, Powell DA, Durrell DE et al: Effect of infusion methods on tobramycin serum concentrations in newborn infants, *J Pediatr* 104:136-138, 1984.
38. Nahata MC, Hipple TF: *Pediatric drug formulations,* ed 3, Cincinnati, 1997, Harvey Whitney Books.
39. Nahata MC: Lack of pediatric drug formulations, *Pediatrics* 104:607-609, 1999.
40. Mitchell JF: Oral dosage forms that should not be crushed: 2000 update, *Hosp Pharm* 35:553-557, 2000.
41. Lee HA, Anderson PO: Giving partial doses of transdermal patches, *Am J Health Syst Pharm* 54:1759-1760, 1997.
42. Campbell MM, Taeubel MA, Kraus DM: Updated bedside charts for calculating pediatric doses of emergency medications, *Am J Hosp Pharm* 51:2147-2152, 1994.

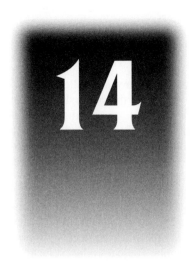

14

Thermal Regulation

Mary Frances D. Pate

ESSENTIAL PHYSIOLOGY OF TEMPERATURE REGULATION
    Physiologic Control of Body Temperature
    Behavioral Control of Body Temperature
    Mechanisms of Thermoregulation

NURSING INTERVENTIONS TO MAINTAIN NORMOTHERMIA
    Assessment and Maintenance of Normal
        Body Temperature
    Assessment of Temperature Imbalance
    Thermoregulation Devices

ABNORMALITIES OF BODY TEMPERATURE REGULATION
    Hyperthermia
    Drug Fever
    Malignant Hyperthermia
    Nursing Care of Patients With Elevated
        Body Temperature
    Hypothermia
    Nursing Care of Patients With Decreased
        Body Temperature

SUMMARY

Heat is a natural byproduct of metabolism. It is constantly produced and continuously lost to the environment. When the quantity of heat produced is equal to the amount lost, homeostasis exists. If heat production and heat loss are not in balance, body temperature will rise or fall.

Normal thermoregulatory function serves to maintain body temperature within a narrow range. Both environmental and maturational factors can cause or contribute to *ineffective thermoregulation*—the inability to maintain normal body temperature in the presence of adverse or changing environmental factors.[1] Critically ill infants and children are at high risk for ineffective thermoregulation

resulting from both environmental and maturational factors (Table 14-1). Critical care nurses play an essential role in protecting patients from adverse environmental factors and in identifying patients at risk from maturational factors that may impair effective thermoregulation.

Many patients in the pediatric intensive care unit (PICU) may experience a *risk for altered body temperature*—the state in which the individual is at risk for failing to maintain body temperature within a normal range.[1] Abnormal body temperature may be the result of illness (such as infection, surgery, or shock) or its therapy.

Internal factors that contribute to or are risk factors for altered body temperature include pathophysiologic and treatment-related factors. For example, traumatic brain injury or congenital central nervous system (CNS) malformations may produce recurrent, transient elevations in body temperature. In contrast, certain hypothalamic lesions produced by cerebrovascular hemorrhage, neurosurgical procedures, or tumors may result in low body temperature, resulting from decreased ability to produce heat. Furthermore, a depressed or injured CNS results in a diminished response to cold and minimizes shivering as a means of generating heat.

Shock states limit peripheral perfusion in response to hypotension and endogenous catecholamine-mediated subcutaneous vasoconstriction. These responses reduce peripheral blood flow, thereby diminishing heat dissipation and resulting in increased core temperature.

Treatment-related factors leading to alterations in body temperature include medications (e.g., vasopressors or sedatives), parenteral fluids or blood transfusions, renal dialysis, anesthesia, and surgery. For instance, anesthesia inhibits most of the body's heat-producing and heat-conserving mechanisms. When infants or children are unconscious or paralyzed (either pharmacologically or nonpharmacologically), postural changes are no longer possible because muscular activity is obliterated. Anesthetic agents may also depress the hypothalamic thermoregulatory center, causing vasodilation and depression of the metabolic rate, thereby reducing heat production and increasing heat loss.[2] Induced hypothermia for extracorporeal circulation, exposure to cold ambient temperature, and exposure of the thoracic cavity during open heart surgery are specific treatment-related risk factors for infants and children. The consequences of intraoperative hypothermia are often not manifested until the postoperative phase. Small incremental drops in temperature markedly increase oxygen consumption at a time when oxygen supply to tissues is marginal, resulting in hypoxemia.[3]

Pediatric critical care nurses are in a position to appreciate a variety of environmental, situational, and individual factors that can result in either altered body temperature or ineffective thermal regulation. Care of infants and children based on an understanding of the dynamic interface between the patient and the environment can maximize the nurse's ability to assist patients in maintaining a normal body temperature despite the stress of illness. Regardless of the thermoregulatory issue with which the nurse is confronted, interventions that are evidence based are critical to the well-being of the patient.

TABLE 14-1   Factors Related to Ineffective Thermoregulation

Environmental	Maturational
Changing environmental temperature	Extremes of age
Insufficient heating or humidification	Large ratio of body surface area to body mass
Physical contact with or proximity to cold or warm objects	Metabolic immaturity and decreased heat production
Wet or exposed body surfaces	Rapid metabolic rate
Excessive or insufficient clothing or coverings	Thin layer of subcutaneous fat

ESSENTIAL PHYSIOLOGY OF TEMPERATURE REGULATION

Physiologic Control of Body Temperature

Heat production and heat loss are controlled in two states. First, the transfer of heat to the body skin surface from the central core establishes an internal thermal gradient. Second, heat is dissipated from the skin surface to the surrounding environment. This balance is critical to normal thermoregulatory function and is summarized in Fig. 14-1.

Body temperature regulation is controlled almost exclusively by intricate nervous system feedback mechanisms located in the hypothalamus. Heat-sensitive neurons located in the preoptic area of the hypothalamus are the body's most influential temperature receptors. These receptors respond to rising temperature by increasing their impulse output and to falling temperature by decreasing their output.

Additional temperature receptors found in the skin consist of both warmth and cold receptors. There are 4 to 10 times as many cold as warmth receptors. These receptors convey nerve impulses to the hypothalamus, where the information is used to regulate body temperature. Receptors in the spinal cord itself, the abdomen, and other internal body structures also transmit signals, primarily cold signals, to the CNS to help in temperature control. Peripheral thermoreceptors dispatch signals to the posterior hypothalamus, where they are integrated to control heat loss and heat production.[4] This "hypothalamic thermostat" is the primary temperature control mechanism in the body.

The Body's Response to Heat. Overheating of the hypothalamic thermostatic area increases the pace of heat loss by two essential processes. The first prompts the sweat glands to boost evaporative heat loss from the body. The second inhibits sympathetic centers in the posterior hypothalamus. This reaction allows vasodilation and, consequently, increased heat loss from the skin.[4]

The Body's Response to Cold. When the body cools down to a normal temperature (37° C), several mechanisms reduce heat loss and escalate heat production. Vasoconstriction of the epidermal vessels is one of the body's earliest

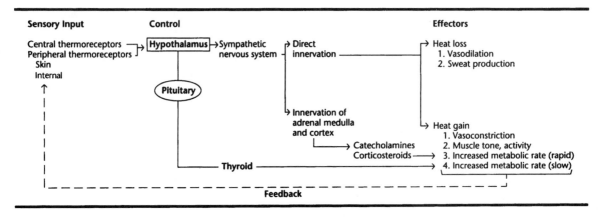

Fig. 14-1 Thermoregulation. (Reprinted by permission of *Neonatal Netw* 13:15, 1994, Fig. 1.)

efforts to enhance heat conservation. The posterior hypothalamus mobilizes the sympathetic nervous system and initiates powerful vasoconstriction throughout the body. This effect decreases conduction of heat from the internal core to the skin. When vasoconstriction develops, the only heat loss that persists is that via the fat insulators of the skin. Vasoconstriction can diminish heat loss eightfold and can very forcefully conserve heat. When the temperature of the hypothalamic thermostat falls below normal body temperature, the elimination of sweating is absolute. This response arrests evaporative cooling except for insensible evaporation (e.g., from the respiratory tract).[4]

The body also increases heat production in the event of cold stress. This occurs in three distinct ways when body temperature drops below 37° C. First, hypothalamic stimulation of shivering occurs. The primary motor center for shivering is located in the posterior hypothalamus. Cold stress stimulates and heat inhibits this nerve center. When muscle tone is increased to a critical level in response to cold stress, shivering begins. As a result, heat production can increase 4 to 5 times the normal amount.

Second, chemical thermogenesis commences. The rate of cellular metabolism increases as a result of sympathetic stimulation or circulating epinephrine. In the adult, this generally accounts for an increase in heat production of no more than 10% to 15%. In infants, however, chemical thermogenesis can increase the rate of heat production as much as 100% and is a crucial mechanism.[4]

Thermogenesis in infants is different than in older children or adults. In infants, brown fat is the biochemical substance used in chemical thermogenesis. Brown fat cells are approximately one-half the size of white fat cells. Brown fat is found in the subcutaneous tissue, adjacent to the major blood vessels of the neck, abdomen, and thorax, between the scapulae, and in large quantities in the suprarenal areas. At birth, 2% to 6% of the infant's body weight consists of brown fat.[2] Brown fat cells contain finely scattered lipid droplets and are rich in cytoplasm in mitochondria, which facilitates energy transformation and heat production.

Cold stress produces a release of norepinephrine and thyroid hormones. This response in turn triggers a lipolytic process in the brown fat stores. Triglycerides in the fat are broken down into fatty acids and glycerol. These fatty acids then enter the thermogenic pathways that produce the common pool of metabolic acids. Besides thermogenesis, glycolysis may be stimulated, resulting in a transient increase in serum glucose levels. Because infants are unable to shiver or actively alter their environment, they depend on nonshivering (chemical) thermogenesis, that is, use of brown fat, to increase heat production.[5]

If cold stress is sustained, increased thyroxine production results in an elevated rate of cellular metabolism throughout the body. This mechanism requires several weeks to become operative, and thus it cannot be considered a primary response to cold stress.[4] (See Fig. 14-2 for a summary of physiologic consequences of cold stress.)

Behavioral Control of Body Temperature

The most obvious thermoregulatory responses are behavioral.[6] When the temperature of the preoptic area of the hypothalamus rises, this produces the sense of being warm; cooling of the skin and possibly other receptors produces the awareness of being cold. Older children and adolescents who experience either of these sensations usually take steps to reestablish a feeling of comfort.

Effective behavioral control of temperature depends on both an intact sensory-motor system and an ability to communicate perceptions. For example, regulation of body temperature is inadequate below the level at which the sympathetic nerves leave the cord in spinal cord transection. This occurs because the hypothalamus can no longer control skin blood flow or the degree to which sweating is possible. To maintain thermal homeostasis, the affected person needs to rely on responses to cold and hot sensations in the region of the head to make suitable behavioral and environmental adaptations.[4]

Critically ill infants and children have a limited ability to alter their environment in response to their perception of temperature variations. Moreover, their ability to communicate their perceptions is often limited by their developmental stage and the severity of their illness.

Mechanisms of Thermoregulation

The normal body temperature measured rectally is 37° C. Practitioners have assumed that rectal temperatures are 1° C higher and that axillary temperatures are 1° C lower than

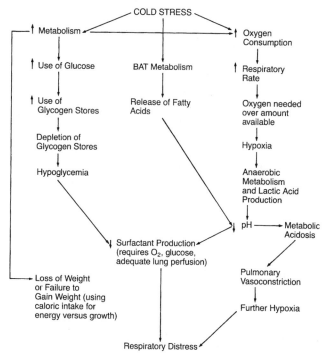

Fig. 14-2 Physiologic consequences of cold stress in infants. *BAT,* Brown adipose tissue. (From Blackburn ST, Loper DL: *Maternal, fetal, and neonatal physiology,* Philadelphia, 1992, WB Saunders, p 692.)

Box 14-1

Comparable Clinical Temperatures in a Resting Afebrile Subject With Rectal Temperature as a Reference

Rectal approximately 37° C
Oral 0.3°-0.5° C lower than rectal
Esophageal 0.2° C lower than rectal
Pulmonary artery 0.2°-0.3° C lower than rectal
Tympanic membrane 0.05°-0.25° C lower than rectal
Bladder temperature 0.1°-0.2° C lower than rectal
Axillary temperature 0.6°-0.8° C lower than rectal

From Holtzclaw BJ: Monitoring body temperature, *AACN Clin Issues Crit Care Nurs* 4:49, 1993; Holtzclaw BJ: New trends in thermometry for the patient in the ICU, *Crit Care Nurs Q* 21:18, 1998.

oral temperatures. However, studies have demonstrated that the difference is considerably less[7] (Box 14-1). The core body temperature varies by 1.1° C during the day, with the highest temperature occurring in late afternoon or evening and the lowest occurring around 4 AM. Presumably, this holds true in critically ill infants and children. Once thought to be the result of exogenous factors, such as muscular exercise or feeding activity, it is now clear that these periodic fluctuations in temperature are the result of the operation of an endogenous system.[8] Despite the influence of certain conditions that alter the regulation of body temperature, among them fever, the human organism is capable of immense thermoregulatory adaptations and changes.

Circadian cycles influence childhood temperature. Temperature variation is one of the earliest rhythms to develop in infants and begins to appear after the first week of life. These rhythm changes develop progressively until the age of 5 years, when the adult pattern is present.[8]

The stability of body temperature varies inversely with the size of the body. This means that in infants with a rapid metabolic rate and somewhat large body surface area, the oral and rectal temperatures may vary through a range perhaps twice that of adults.[9] Because of the infant's small size, increased ratio of body surface area to mass, and elevated thermal conduction rate, the thermoregulatory ability of infants is restricted and easily overwhelmed by the environment.[2] Conversely, adults exhibit very stable body temperature mechanisms.

Heat Loss. The amount of heat loss that occurs varies according to atmospheric conditions, such as the speed of air currents passing over the body and the relative humidity of the air. The common modes of heat loss are via (1) radiation, conduction, and convection from the skin; (2) evaporation of sweat and insensible perspiration; (3) warming and humidifying of inspired air; and (4) urine and stool. Only the first two are under direct physiologic control. Of the sources under direct control, radiation accounts for approximately 50% of the total heat loss and convection, about 15%. Most of the remainder (about 30%) occurs through evaporation of water.[9]

Radiation is the loss of heat that radiates from the body to surroundings that are cooler than the body itself. It involves

the transfer of heat between two objects, independent of the environmental temperature. The difference in temperature between the body and objects in the environment directly affects the rate at which a body cools via radiation.[9] For example, radiative heat losses can occur even when nude infants are in warm but transparent, single-walled incubators, particularly when near a cold wall or window. The total radiating surface of infants or children also influences heat loss. In fact, radiative heat loss is proportionately greater in smaller infants and children and represents the most serious source of heat loss for this group.[2]

Conductive heat loss involves the transfer of heat between two surfaces that are in direct contact with each other. The intensity of conductive heat loss depends on the temperature gradient between the body and the surface it contacts, the total body surface area, and the conductivity of the material contacting the body. In addition, physiologic factors influencing conductive heat loss are the velocity of cutaneous blood flow and the thickness of the body's subcutaneous insulating tissue.[2]

Convection is simply the movement of air. Heat loss by convection refers to heat conducted to the air and then carried away by convection currents. Insignificant amounts of convection always occur because heated air naturally rises away from the body. The degree of convective heat loss depends on several conditions, including the temperature of the air, volume of airflow, and the specific heat of the flowing air. Exposure of infants or children to drafts or increased airflow causes convective heat loss and is a stimulus for increased oxygen consumption.

Evaporative losses, primarily through the skin and lungs, account for a significant portion of heat loss. Infants are particularly vulnerable because their skin is thinner than that of older children, which increases evaporative losses. When water evaporates from the skin, 0.58 calories of heat are lost for every gram of water that evaporates. Under normal conditions, nearly 20% of the total body heat loss occurs from evaporation. Little can be done about this in terms of body temperature regulation because evaporative heat loss results from continuous diffusion of water molecules at any body temperature. However, excessive evaporative loss can be controlled by regulation of sweating, primarily by environmental manipulation.

Besides transepidermal evaporation, the respiratory system also serves as a route of evaporative heat loss. Evaporative losses via the respiratory tract are higher in infants as a result of their higher minute ventilation (the product of respiratory rate and tidal volume) in relation to body weight. Adequate environmental humidity minimizes evaporative losses from the lungs and skin surfaces. Physical factors affecting the rate of evaporation include relative humidity, velocity of airflow, and minute ventilation. Physiologic factors include infants' ability to sweat and their rate of minute ventilation.[2]

The neutral thermal zone of infants is the range of ambient temperatures at which the metabolic rate is minimal and temperature regulation is achieved by nonevaporative physical processes.[2] The neutral thermal environment (NTE) is further described as the ambient temperature and humidity in which the control of body temperature is achieved by vasomotor adjustments, with minimal oxygen consumption and heat production. This narrow range of temperatures in infants varies with gestational age, postnatal age, weight, and clothing. With increasing age and weight, the NTE widens, and lower environmental temperatures are tolerated.[10]

Sweating. Sweating is an important means of controlling heat balance. Full-term infants, for example, begin to sweat with rectal temperatures of 37.5° to 37.9° C and an ambient temperature higher than 35° C. As body temperature rises, the anterior part of the hypothalamus is stimulated. The impulses from this area are transmitted through the anatomic pathways to the spinal cord and through the sympathetic outflow to the sweat glands in the skin throughout the body.[4] When the body temperature increases as little as 1° C, the sweat glands secrete large amounts of sweat to the skin surface.[11] This reaction produces evaporative cooling of the body. The rate of sweating varies according to environmental factors.

Excessive sweating can deplete extracellular fluid levels of electrolytes, particularly sodium and chloride. Cholinergic sympathetic nerve fibers ending on or near the glandular sweat cells elicit the secretions, which contain large amounts of sodium chloride. Similar to its effect on the renal tubules, aldosterone works in the sweat glands by augmenting the rate of active reabsorption of sodium by the ducts. This process also carries chloride with it because of the electrical gradient that develops across the epithelium with the reabsorption of sodium. Aldosterone can minimize the loss of sodium chloride in sweat when the plasma concentration is already low. Becoming acclimated to the heat can diminish this loss because of increased aldosterone production resulting from decreased salt reserves in the body.[4]

NURSING INTERVENTIONS TO MAINTAIN NORMOTHERMIA

Nurses can help to maintain the body temperature of critically ill infants and children within normal limits primarily by managing external factors. The environment may be manipulated based on the principles of conduction, convection, radiation, evaporation, and the impact of each on body temperature. Factors such as ambient air temperature, humidity, airflow velocity, and the temperature of objects in direct contact with children's skin are all considered part of the environment. Each of these factors should be considered when making alterations to support an NTE.

Keeping infants and children (especially their heads), clothing, and bed linens dry can minimize evaporative losses. Humidifying and warming inspired gases can minimize evaporative and conductive losses from respiratory mucosa. In contrast, gases may be humidified and cooled when infants or children are hyperthermic. High humidity tends to reduce insensible water losses and evaporative losses; however, it also encourages the growth of gram-negative bacilli on the skin, including *Escherichia coli* and *Pseudomonas aeruginosa*. Hence, a relative level of humid-

ity, approximately 50%, provides optimal environmental conditions.[12]

Conductive heat losses can be reduced by ensuring that cold surfaces are not in direct contact with children's skin and by using various types of thermal insulation, such as blankets and head coverings. Nurses can position children to avoid drafts and maintain the environmental temperature within the neutral thermal zone to avoid convective losses. Increasing the room temperature, using external heating devices, and applying thermal insulators, such as plastic or aluminized plastic sheeting, can minimize radiant heat loss.

Assessment and Maintenance of Normal Body Temperature

The medical and surgical treatment of critically ill or injured infants and children often aggravates heat loss through skin and body cavity exposure, administration of cold intravenous fluids and blood products, and anesthetic administration. Hypothermia may contribute to inaccuracies in patient assessment and may complicate resuscitation of injured infants or children. Because the risk for alterations in body temperature are greater for critically ill infants and children, assessment of temperature and the body's thermoregulatory capabilities must be accurate and ongoing.

Frequent monitoring of critically ill infants' or children's body temperatures is necessary to establish baseline parameters and to guide nursing interventions. Temperature should be measured at recommended intervals for age and condition. Various techniques are used to measure core, regional, and skin temperatures in critically ill infants and children. Each is evaluated based on its relative advantages and disadvantages. The method selected is based on individual patient needs and the net balance of advantages and disadvantages of the system accurately monitoring body temperature. The site selected for estimating infants' or children's temperatures is recorded and used consistently in serial measurements. Because of the inaccuracy of many thermometers in clinical use, the same thermometer is used consistently for an individual patient. To decrease the possibility of inaccuracy, electronic and infrared devices are regularly scheduled for calibration.[13]

Internationally, the Celsius scale is the standard of temperature measurement. However, in the United States, the Fahrenheit scale is still widely used. Nurses may not be comfortable with converting temperatures from one scale to another and also may not be aware of the severity of temperature changes when measured on the Celsius scale.[13]

Core Temperature Monitoring. The core or central temperature is the temperature of the blood flowing through the branches of the carotid arteries to the hypothalamus. Pulmonary artery catheters and esophageal, tympanic, or nasopharyngeal probes monitor the temperature of blood, which approximates the temperature of the carotid artery and may be used for continuous assessment of core temperature.[14] Although useful, esophageal and nasopharyngeal temperature probes are not routinely used in PICU settings. Urinary bladder temperature (UBT), using a urinary catheter with an indwelling temperature-sensing element, may also be measured. Tympanic thermometers have been found to be less accurate than esophageal readings but more accurate than rectal, axillary, or bladder readings for core temperature over a wide range of temperatures in pediatric surgery patients.[15]

The accepted standard for measurement of core body temperature is a thermistor in the pulmonary artery.[16] Pulmonary artery temperatures are approximately 0.2° lower than blood returning from the brain.[15] Because of the invasive nature, pulmonary artery temperature is only assessed in critically ill infants and children who also require advanced hemodynamic monitoring.

Peripheral Temperature Monitoring. Noncentral temperature measurement does not reflect core temperature but, rather, regional temperature. Regional temperature is affected by a variety of factors that may affect regional blood flow, such as intravascular volume, vascular tone, or environmental conditions. These methods are convenient and useful in monitoring changes and trends in temperature but lack the accuracy of most core temperature techniques. In contrast to core temperature reading techniques, regional temperature monitoring can detect physiologic decompensation in response to persistent hypothermia or hyperthermia. When hypothermia persists, for example, children's increased metabolism fails to compensate for the body cooling and results in regional blood flow shifts, causing metabolic acidosis and, eventually, apnea.[14]

Generally, regional temperatures are measured using electronic thermometers. Temperature measuring sites include the oral, rectal, and axillary locations. In the critical care setting, the oral route is infrequently used, whereas rectal or axillary routes predominate. Measuring rectal temperature is generally unnecessary. The risk of rectal perforation, cross-contamination, and the repeated invasiveness of the procedure are probably not warranted, particularly in young infants.[7,10] Rectal temperature probes can be influenced by the presence of stool in the rectum, which can act as an insulator and produce markedly delayed responses to core temperature changes.[2] In addition, relying solely on rectal temperature measurements that may not reflect rapid changes in core temperature may lead to delayed recognition of temperature extremes. Rectal probes and temperatures are always avoided in infants and children with inflammatory bowel disease, absolute neutropenia, or evidence of coagulation disorders or thrombocytopenia. Axillary temperatures are less hazardous to patients but have been shown to underestimate core temperature and be affected by ambient temperature.[7]

Skin temperature may be measured either by electronic thermometers or by electronic skin temperature thermistor probes that provide continuous assessment. They are a useful adjunct to other standard temperature-measuring devices but can be affected by poor perfusion, equipment dysfunction, or improper application. Critically ill patients who require the use of overbed warmers or warming blankets are continuously monitored for skin temperature with appropriate alarms for underheating or overheating. When skin temperature is continuously monitored, temperature is also measured periodically with an electronic thermometer.

For critically ill infants or children, a combination of temperature-measuring techniques is often indicated. This approach is necessary to detect variations in temperature that occur in response to physiologic dysfunction associated with critical illness or injury. Because significant differences may occur between peripheral and core temperatures, critical care nurses require skill in interpreting the implications of these differences considering the patient's physiologic status.

Assessment of Temperature Imbalance

Wide variations in temperature produce alterations in cardiac output, oxygen consumption, and insensible water losses. With hyperthermia, heart rate increases, whereas with hypothermia, heart rate commonly decreases. Blood pressure can also be affected. For instance, blood pressure and cardiac output drop precipitously as hypothermia becomes more severe. Cardiac dysrhythmias, such as conduction delays and abnormal atrial and ventricular rhythms, may be evident. Respiratory rates may also vary. For example, hypothermic infants may experience periods of apnea or shallow breathing; in contrast, infants or children with fever or hyperthermia may become tachypneic.

Neurologic function may be impaired when infants or children experience temperature imbalance. For example, severe hypothermia (a core temperature lower than 35° C) may complicate neurologic assessment as pupils dilate, level of consciousness declines, reflexes and respirations diminish, and varying degrees of amnesia occur. Cerebral blood flow has been estimated to decrease 6% to 7% for every 1° C decrease in body temperature.[17] This is of particular concern for infants or children who have experienced multiple trauma or multiorgan dysfunction syndrome. All patients with hypothermia are monitored for changes in level of consciousness, signs of irritability or lethargy, diminished ability to arouse, and changes in muscle tone. Hence, measures to promote thermal neutrality are instituted as early as possible to ensure accurate neurologic assessment. Seizures may occur after periods of hypothermia as a result of ischemic brain injury and cerebral edema.

Oxygen consumption and tissue perfusion are important assessment parameters. Oxygen saturation using arterial or mixed venous blood can provide an important indicator of oxygen consumption. Often oxygen saturation of mixed venous blood indicates changes in physiologic status before changes in heart rate, pulmonary capillary wedge pressure (PCWP), or blood pressure are evident.[18] Supplemental oxygen may be necessary to combat hypoxemia, particularly in hypothermic infants and children.

Tissue perfusion assessed from skin color, temperature, and capillary refill must be routinely monitored. Pale, cool skin is an early manifestation of the vasoconstrictive response to cold stress or a decrease in core temperature. With hyperthermia, the skin may appear flushed as vasodilation occurs. Flushing may also come about because oxygen is not liberated from hemoglobin as readily when either low temperatures or overheating occurs.[19] Evidence of sweating is monitored in hyperthermic children.

Increased muscle activity is associated with heat production, whereas diminished muscle activity is often indicative of reduced heat production. Infants and children who are experiencing either elevated or reduced temperature may manifest changes in motor activity and therefore are monitored for such changes.

Routine assessment for the presence of shivering permits early detection and intervention. Shivering develops in a predictable fashion, beginning with masseter contractions and then proceeding to contractions of the trunk and long muscle groups. It culminates with generalized body shaking and teeth chattering.[20] Assessment for the presence of shivering includes palpation of the mandible for vibration and close inspection of facial, neck, and chest muscles for fasciculation. Core and peripheral temperatures are routinely assessed and compared. Assessment for shivering is continued until central and peripheral temperatures are normal.[18]

Fluid balance and renal function are carefully monitored when body temperature becomes deranged. Because the rate of fluid loss increases as a result of hyperthermia, adequate hydration is maintained. Adequate hydration prevents the complications of dehydration and promotes heat dissipation. When infants and children are hypothermic and peripherally vasoconstricted, fluids are carefully regulated during rewarming. When patients have vasoconstriction, fluid requirements are diminished; as warming occurs, the intravascular space expands, thereby increasing fluid requirements to maintain cardiac output. Infants' and children's ability to concentrate urine is impaired as hypothermia worsens. Acute tubular necrosis may occur as a result of diminished cardiac output and renal perfusion and myoglobinuria. Measurement of fluid balance enables nurses to prevent fluid overload or deficit. Fluid deficit following a period of hypothermia is often the result of increased insensible water loss during rewarming.

Laboratory data are routinely monitored to detect metabolic, biochemical, and hematologic derangements often associated with thermal instability. For example, excessive sweating can deplete extracellular fluid levels of electrolytes, particularly sodium and chloride. Serum electrolytes, blood urea nitrogen, creatinine, measures of acid-base balance, serum and urine osmolarity, hemoglobin, hematocrit, platelets, and other specific biochemical determinations are assessed regularly.

Hypothermia may cause metabolic acidosis. Acidosis coupled with hypothermia results in a left shift in the oxyhemoglobin dissociation curve, thereby impairing oxygen release at the tissue level. Arterial blood gases are monitored closely, and measures are instituted to prevent episodes of hypoxemia and acidosis. Hyperthermia can cause biochemical changes, depending on the underlying cause.

Hypoglycemia is another common finding in infants who experience alterations in temperature. This condition results from depletion of glycogen stores in the attempt to maintain core temperature in the normal range. In contrast, a transient hyperglycemic response is a common finding in older infants and children with alterations in temperature. This condition occurs as part of the body's response to stress, which liberates glucose to fuel the response.

Laboratory studies used in determining the source of fever or hyperthermia may include indirect and direct studies. Indirect studies, such as the white blood cell count and the erythrocyte sedimentation rate, reflect the body's response to infection. Indirect tests may serve as screening devices for identifying subgroups of infants and children at high risk of occult bacteremia (Table 14-2). Direct studies include blood and urine culture and sensitivity and rapid tests for detection of bacterial antigen. Direct tests allow detection of the specific causative organism.[21]

Other diagnostic tests may include cerebrospinal fluid examination or urinalysis. In addition, examinations such as radiographs; ultrasounds and computed tomographic (CT) scans; magnetic resonance imaging (MRI); or other nuclear medicine studies of the lungs, abdomen, and other organs may be indicated to determine the underlying cause of the temperature derangement.

Thermoregulation Devices

Maintaining a neutral thermal environment and a normothermic body temperature are common nursing goals when caring for critically ill infants and children. Various thermoregulation devices are used regularly in the critical care setting. This is particularly crucial when transferring infants or children to other units within the hospital or to another facility.

Warming Devices. In addition to manipulating environmental conditions to alter the ambient temperature,

---

◆ **TABLE 14-2 Risk of Occult Bacteremia**

	Low Risk	High Risk
Age	>3 yr	<2 yr
Temperature	<39.4° C	>40° C
WBC count (per microliter)	>5000 and <15,000	<5000 or >15,000
Observational variables	Normal	Abnormal
		History of contact with *Haemophilus influenzae* or *Neisseria meningitidis*
		History of bacteremia
		Immunologic impairment

From Kline MW, Lorin MI: Fever without source. In Oski FA, DeAngelis CD, Feigin RD et al, eds: *Oski's principles and practice of pediatrics,* Philadelphia, 1999, Lippincott Williams & Wilkins, p 844.
WBC, White blood cell.

specialized equipment is often necessary to maintain an NTE. Various types of devices are used for this purpose. For infants, some type of closed warming device is commonly used, such as single- or double-walled incubators. These convection-warmed devices are used for thermal regulation of the infant's ambient air. Standard closed incubators control infant temperature by recirculation of warmed and humidified air. Infant size and postnatal age determine the temperature of the air in the incubator.[10] Plastic blankets or heat shields inside the incubator also reduce convective and evaporative losses. Disadvantages of this type of device include heat losses when the incubator is entered, potential variations in both incubator and infant temperatures during heating cycles, and diminished accessibility of infants for assessment and treatment.[22]

Open radiant warmers are useful to regulate temperature, particularly when infants and children require frequent monitoring and interventions. A radiant warmer consists of an electrically heated element that emits radiation within the infrared region of the electromagnetic spectrum. Radiation within this range allows optimal absorption of the energy by the skin. Heating of the skin causes vasodilation and increased blood flow to the skin. Moreover, it provides an avenue for heat transfer from the skin surface to the blood and eventually to deeper structures.

The advantages of radiant warmers include a superior servocontrol mechanism, greater consistency in surface temperature, improved patient access, and easier cleaning. The disadvantages associated with infrared radiation used in radiant warmers include risk of cataracts, flash burns of the skin, and heat stress.[22] In addition, radiant warmers promote insensible water loss, increase oxygen consumption, and slightly increase metabolic rate in infants, depending on weight and gestational age. Fluid requirements may be increased by 10% to 20%, particularly when radiant warmers are used in conjunction with phototherapy. Hence fluid requirements are adjusted depending on clinical and biochemical data. Radiant warmers are generally servocontrolled with the temperature probe attached to the abdomen.[19]

Servocontrolled devices automatically adjust heat output to maintain the temperature at a predetermined level in response to changes in patients' skin temperature. Some use an anterior abdominal wall temperature servocontrol mechanism to regulate skin temperature within a thermal-neutral range (36° to 36.5° C) by automatic air temperature control.[19] Core temperature is measured frequently when servocontrol is used to avoid overheating if the skin sensor loosens. In addition, accurate assessment of the infant's temperature may be compromised when a servocontrol device is used because the temperature is regulated to maintain the temperature at the predetermined level.

For older children, external heat sources, such as radiant warmers or heating blankets, are often used. Circulating water mattresses may be used to raise a patient's temperature and reduce conductive heat losses. Water-filled heating blankets are used judiciously in infants and children because when children are cold and peripherally vasoconstricted, the ability of surface capillaries to dissipate heat is diminished, increasing the risk for burns. Hence continuous monitoring of temperature and assessment of responses to interventions

for rewarming are crucial to avoid tissue injury. The fluid temperature in the heating blanket should never exceed 39° C, and several layers of material are placed between the patient and the heating blanket to avoid burns.[23]

Forced air heating blankets have been shown to be the most clinically effective warming device intraoperatively.[24] This modality transfers the greatest amount of heat to the patient, when compared with other warming modalities.

When rapid rewarming is necessary, cardiopulmonary bypass may be used. This technique allows direct perfusion of the central circulation with warmed blood, reducing cardiac irritability and the risk of ventricular fibrillation and cardiac arrest. Alternatively, body cavities such as the chest, peritoneum, or gastrointestinal tract may be irrigated with warmed fluids.

Cooling Devices. When infants or children become hyperthermic, surface cooling techniques, such as removing heat-conserving clothing or blankets or packing in ice, may be used. Most commonly, external cooling blankets are applied, and in the majority of cases, the decision to use this modality is made by the critical care nurse.[25] A comparison of the effectiveness of posterior versus anterior positioning of the blanket and cooling effectiveness after placement is needed. If the blanket is placed posteriorly, care is taken to avoid decubitus ulcers. A recent development in cooling is the use of cold air blankets. These blankets are thought to be more comfortable for patients and may be more effective than circulating water blankets; however, this assumption has not been substantiated by research studies.[25] Whatever method is used for surface cooling, the patient's vital signs, perfusion, and skin integrity are assessed frequently. If additional temperature reduction is needed, body temperature can be reduced by core cooling. Lavage of gastric or peritoneal cavities and the administration of iced intravenous fluids can achieve this goal.

Extreme variation in temperature, hypothermia or hyperthermia, can result in death or serious injury, and thus alarm systems and range controls of all equipment used to regulate temperature require regular testing.

ABNORMALITIES OF BODY TEMPERATURE REGULATION

Hyperthermia

Hyperthermia is a state in which a person has a sustained elevation in body temperature (more than 37.8° C orally or 38.8° C rectally) because of internal or external factors.[1] Internal factors, such as fever, malignant hyperthermia, or heat-related illnesses, and external factors, such as extreme environmental conditions or accidental overheating, contribute to the development of hyperthermia. The most common cause of hyperthermia is fever. Although relatively uncommon, malignant hyperthermia may also necessitate a patient's admission to a critical care unit.

Fever is distinguished from other types of elevations in body temperature. First, the "set-point" is that temperature around which body temperature is regulated by the thermostat-like mechanism in the hypothalamus. "Hyperthermia" is that situation in which body temperature exceeds the set-point. This usually results from conditions producing more heat than the body can dissipate (e.g., in heatstroke, aspirin toxicity, or hyperthyroidism). "Fever" is an elevation in the set-point such that body temperature is regulated at a higher level.[26] In any discussion of fever, it is important to remember that fever is a *symptom,* not a disease, and should be viewed as reflecting an underlying disorder.

Fever may result from abnormalities in the brain itself, the presence of toxins that affect the brain's temperature control areas, infection, dehydration, or other causes.[4] Generally, fever results from a pyrogen-mediated elevation in the hypothalamic set-point. The major problems resulting in fever include an increase in the hypothalamic thermoregulatory set-point, excess heat production, and defective heat loss.[27]

Instrumental in resetting the hypothalamic thermostat are pyrogens, substances that cause the set-point to be increased. These pyrogens may be proteins, breakdown products of proteins, or certain other substances (e.g., lipopolysaccharide toxins secreted by bacteria). Pyrogens may be present during disease states. When the set-point is elevated, all the body's efforts turn to decreasing heat loss and increasing heat production. Heat production is increased via increased muscle tone, activity, and metabolic rate, whereas heat loss is decreased through peripheral vasoconstriction.[28] These changes help the body to reach its new temperature within hours.[4]

The pathophysiologic mechanism of fever includes the production of hormonelike mediators by macrophages and cells of the reticuloendothelial system. This results in (1) an increase in CNS production of prostaglandin E_2, which increases the hypothalamic set-point and temperature; (2) an increase in neutrophil release from the bone marrow; (3) a decrease in serum iron and zinc; (4) a change in hepatic protein production; and (5) an increased T-lymphocyte proliferation. Interleukin-1 (IL-1) is a substance common to these pathways.[29] Undesirable effects of fever are listed in Box 14-2.

For healthy infants and children, these demands pose no particular threat. For those with underlying disease, especially that involving the heart or lungs, the increased demands are potentially harmful or even fatal. In susceptible infants and children 6 months to 5 years old, fever can precipitate seizures. Generally, these seizures are benign, but they are very upsetting to both parents and children and

may result in invasive, expensive, and probably unnecessary procedures.[28]

Febrile conditions share several characteristics. Chills occur when the hypothalamic set-point abruptly rises to a higher-than-normal level because of tissue destruction, presence of pyrogenic substances, or dehydration. As the body attempts to attain its new temperature setting, the blood temperature is lower than the set-point temperature for several hours. Autonomic responses to increased body temperature occur, such as chills, vasoconstriction, and shivering. When the blood temperature reaches the set-point temperature, the person feels neither hot nor cold. As long as the factor producing the fever continues, the body temperature is regulated normally but at a higher level. If the factor producing the fever is suddenly removed, the set-point abruptly decreases to its normal lower level. The body then feels "overheated" and reacts with intense sweating and hot skin, resulting from a general vasodilation caused to dissipate heat more quickly. This reaction is known as the "crisis" or "flush."[4]

Fever has several other causes. Traumatic brain injury or congenital CNS malformations can produce recurrent, transient elevations in body temperature. Other noninfectious causes of fever are (1) iatrogenic (e.g., heavy blankets, overdressing, mechanical); (2) thrombophlebitis, resulting from intravenous catheterization; (3) infusions of irritating fluids; and (4) endocrine disorders. Certain hypothalamic lesions produced by cerebrovascular hemorrhage, neurosurgical procedures, or tumors may produce decreased thermoregulatory ability. Drugs that produce fever include lysergic acid diethylamide (LSD), cocaine, amphetamines, phencyclidine (PCP), salicylates, anticholinergics, prostaglandin E_1, and tricyclic antidepressants.[30,31]

Treatment of Fever.   The decision to treat fever can be difficult. An important principle is that not all fevers *need* to be treated; body temperature does not always need to be completely normal. The importance of fever as an indicator of disease, not as inherently harmful, should be expressed to the patient's significant others, who may be experiencing "fever paranoia."[32] Recommendations for treatment include (1) high fever (40° C or above), (2) fever in infants and children at risk for febrile seizures, (3) fever in infants and children with underlying neurologic or cardiopulmonary disease, or (4) fever in any situation in which heat illness (e.g., heatstroke) is suspected. Treating fever for patient comfort should not be condemned.[28] Once the decision to treat a fever has been made, the choice of a specific modality is based on a number of considerations. Because fever is the result of an elevated hypothalamic set-point, the most logical means of treating the fever is by restoring the set-point to a normal level. Aspirin, acetaminophen, and ibuprofen all work in this way. Aspirin and acetaminophen are equally effective at similar doses. Ibuprofen is effective at a slightly lower dose and has a longer duration of action. Given the minimal difference in the effectiveness of aspirin and acetaminophen, selection should be based on potential toxicities and cost rather than efficacy.[28]

In therapeutic doses, aspirin is the most toxic of the choices. Potentially serious side effects are gastritis, gastro-

---

**Box 14-2
Undesirable Effects of Fever**

Patient discomfort
Increased metabolic rate
Elevated oxygen consumption
Increased carbon dioxide production
Increased cardiovascular and pulmonary system demands

From Lorin MI: Pathogenesis of fever and its treatment. In Oski FA, DeAngelis CD, Feigin RD et al, eds: *Oski's principles and practice of pediatrics,* Philadelphia, 1999, Lippincott Williams & Wilkins, pp 848-850.

TABLE 14-3	Use of External Cooling Methods for Treating Elevated Temperature
Cooling Method	**Indications**
Tepid sponging **instead of** antipyretic drugs	Very young infants Severe liver disease History of hypersensitivity to antipyretic drugs
Tepid sponging **plus** antipyretic drugs	High fever (>40° C) History of febrile seizures, neurologic disorders, or brain damage Infection plus suspicion of overheating Septic shock*
Cold sponging **alone**	Heat illness

From Lorin MI: Pathogenesis of fever and its treatment. In Oski FA, DeAngelis CD, Feigin RD et al, eds: *Oski's principles and practice of pediatrics,* Philadelphia, 1999, Lippincott Williams & Wilkins, p 850.
*May require cold sponging.

intestinal bleeding, diminished platelet functioning, decreased urinary sodium excretion, and lowered immune response. These effects are seen often with aspirin, less often with ibuprofen, and not at all with acetaminophen. In fact, acetaminophen has no side effects at therapeutic levels. However, one study found that when administered rectally, the absorption of acetaminophen was found to be erratic.[25] Aspirin, and possibly ibuprofen and naproxen, because of their pharmacologic similarity, has been implicated in the development of Reye's syndrome.[28]

Another method of fever reduction is external cooling, generally by sponging with tepid water. This may be used with or without the administration of antipyretic medications. Henker[25] provided evidence that the combination of acetaminophen with sponging was significantly more effective in decreasing temperature than acetaminophen alone. External cooling is the treatment of choice for heat-related illnesses. Its use in fever is generally recommended only if a heat-related illness may be the partial or total cause of the elevated body temperature[28] (Table 14-3).

Sponging as a method of fever reduction usually adds nothing other than discomfort when used with previously well infants or children with non–life-threatening fever. When ice water is used, cooling is more rapid and more uncomfortable; therefore it is used only in the case of heat illness. Sponging is useful in infants or children with neurologic disorders because many have abnormal temperature control mechanisms and respond poorly to antipyretics. Sponging is preferable in infants and children with demonstrated hypersensitivity to antipyretics or in those who have liver disease. Sponging is normally done with tepid water (approximately 30° C). Alcohol is not used because the fumes may be absorbed through the lungs and possibly skin, and it may produce alcohol intoxication.[28]

External cooling devices may also be effective in reducing body temperature.

Treatment of fever associated with suspected bacteremia generally includes antibiotics. Ideally, with the emergence of antibiotic-resistant organisms, blood cultures are obtained before instituting antibiotic therapy.[33] Specific antibiotic recommendations are directed at the most common bacterial pathogens. In any case, the patient is followed carefully to monitor the effectiveness of the treatment regimen. When infants and children are critically ill and febrile, parenteral antibiotic therapy may be initiated in tandem with the diagnostic workup. Infants younger than 30 days, children with underlying disorders that predispose them to serious bacterial infections, and children who appear toxic are generally treated with antibiotics before culture results are returned, to decrease the possibility of an overwhelming sepsis.[21] Moreover, if the source of the fever is determined to be infectious, proper infection control and therapeutic measures are initiated.

Drug Fever

Fever may be a complication of drug therapy. This response to medications can increase the duration of hospital stay and the number of diagnostic tests performed.[34] Particular drugs associated with drug fever include phenytoin, histamine blockers, procainamide, and antibiotics, most notably sulfonamides.[35] Drug fever is considered if a clinically improved patient develops an unexplained fever after receiving drugs known to produce febrile reactions 7 to 10 days after their institution. Drugs that raise the basal metabolic rate, produce increased skeletal muscle activity, or lower cutaneous blood flow may produce an increase in body temperature that will normalize after the drug is stopped.[30] Drug-associated fever can be extremely elevated in some patients and can take up to 5 days to resolve after discontinuation of the drug.[35]

Malignant Hyperthermia

Malignant hyperthermia (MH) is a hypermetabolic crisis triggered by the administration of a certain quantity of potent volatile anesthetic agents or a depolarizing muscle relaxant, usually succinylcholine (SCH). The mean age of a patient experiencing a MH episode is 22 years of age.[36] MH is a familial disease, but the mode of genetic transmission remains unclear. The syndrome was originally thought to be transmitted as an autosomal dominant trait. Further investigation suggests that the inheritance in most families is multigenetic with variable expression.[37] Reports of MH vary between countries. In the United States, the incidence is highest in the Midwest.[36]

The incidence of MH ranges from 1 in 14,000 pediatric patients to 1 in 40,000 adult patients. The difference in occurrence may occur because adults are often induced with sodium thiopental and a nondepolarizing muscle relaxant, both of which inhibit triggering of MH. Children, on the other hand, are often induced with halothane followed by SCH, a combination that constitutes an effective trigger for MH.[37]

The site of the primary lesion implicated in the pathogenesis of MH is skeletal muscle and is related to disturbed calcium metabolism. Traditional theory is that a defect in the muscle cell membrane causes loss of control of intracellular ionized calcium levels, leading to an increase in calcium in skeletal muscle and abnormal muscle activity. As hyperthermia continues, the myoplasmic calcium concentration remains elevated, producing continued muscle contraction and heat production. A new developing theory is that MH is a disorder of the ion channels that control skeletal muscle, that is, a channelopathy.[38,39]

Initially, an anesthetic-induced increase in aerobic and anaerobic metabolism occurs, manifested by massive production of heat, carbon dioxide, and lactic acid. This results in respiratory and metabolic acidosis, along with a rapid increase in temperature. Tachycardia is accompanied by other signs of circulatory and metabolic stress. Abnormal muscle activity develops, which may progress to whole-body rigidity. An increase in muscle permeability produces increased serum levels of potassium, phosphorus, calcium, sodium, and creatine phosphokinase (CPK). Muscle edema develops, and an excessive release of myoglobin from muscle results in gross myoglobinemia. Disseminated intravascular coagulopathy and cardiac or renal failure may develop. Death may result from a combination of gross electrolyte disturbances, especially hyperkalemia, leading to cardiac failure.[37,38]

The clinical course of MH is extremely variable. It can be fulminant, rapidly progressing to metabolic acidosis and death if not diagnosed and treated promptly. Rarely, the onset can be delayed for some hours. The sequence and severity of clinical events depend on (1) the types and concentrations of anesthetics involved, (2) the nature and extent of underlying myopathy, and (3) the promptness of diagnosis and initiation of appropriate treatment.[43]

The first systemic effect of MH is increased metabolism (increased oxygen consumption and carbon dioxide production). The cardiovascular and respiratory systems respond to this increased demand by increasing their output. Therefore the first clinically evident signs and symptoms of MH are tachycardia and tachypnea. However, an increased end-tidal carbon dioxide value precedes these signs and symptoms[40] (Table 14-4).

Tachycardia occurs in 96% of all patients with MH within 30 minutes of anesthesia induction.[41] Rapid ventricular arrhythmias (e.g., bigeminy and ventricular tachycardia) may occur. Tachycardia and/or dysrhythmias usually occur before fever, and thus MH is suspected when these signs occur, unless there are other obvious causes for them. Cardiac arrhythmias result from the stress of MH on the myocardium, probably caused by the hypermetabolic state. The electrocardiographic tracing shows tall, peaked T waves, and/or ST-segment depression.[42]

Muscle rigidity may or may not occur. If seen, it usually occurs first in the muscles of the jaw, extremities, or chest usually after the administration of SCH. Instead of relaxing, the jaw tightens, making intubation and ventilation difficult or impossible.[42] Facial muscle fasciculation may be present. Rigidity then travels through other skeletal muscles.

Fever is the clinical hallmark of MH and results from many biochemical derangements. It is a somewhat late sign and may not occur at all if dantrolene is promptly administered.[43] Without treatment, the body temperature can rise 1° C every 5 minutes and exceed 43° C.[38]

Patients undergoing anesthesia are observed for evidence of fever. Signs of fever during surgery include hot, flushed skin; a hot anesthetic rebreathing bag; and hot tissue around the operative site. A change in skin color may accompany the development of MH. Flushed, rosy skin (similar to the familiar "atropine flush") may occur from the increased production of body heat. To dissipate the heat, vasodilation occurs. The flushed skin subsequently becomes mottled and then cyanotic. Simultaneously, the surgeon notes dark blood at the operative site.[43]

Treatment of MH includes early recognition, discontinuation of the anesthetic agent, cooling, hyperventilation with 100% oxygen, restoration of acid-base balance, administration of medications to treat dysrhythmias, and relax skeletal muscle contractions.[38,44] All interventions are carried out simultaneously. In addition, dantrolene sodium is administered without delay because MH is potentially fatal if not treated immediately with this medication. The mortality rate from MH reached 70% before the use of dantrolene. Earlier diagnosis of MH and advent of dantrolene have decreased the mortality rate to less than 5%.[38]

Dantrolene is a lipid-soluble hydantoin derivative with direct effects on skeletal muscle. It is given intravenously, initially 2 mg/kg, increasing to a total of 10 mg/kg. Dosing in this manner provides therapeutic blood levels with a half-life of at least 10 hours in children and adults.[38]

TABLE 14-4   Clinical Presentation of Malignant Hyperthermia

Clinical Findings	Laboratory Findings
Tachycardia	Marked elevation of end-tidal carbon dioxide
Tachypnea—spontaneous ventilation	Hypercarbia—central venous and arterial
Unstable blood pressure	Acidosis—respiratory and metabolic
Fever—rapid rise (1° C every 15 min)	Central venous and arterial desaturation
Sustained rise (to 43° C)	Hyperkalemia
Rigidity—especially trismus	Elevated creatine phosphokinase (CPK), myoglobinemia
Cyanosis—dark blood in surgical field, mottling of skin	
Profuse sweating	

From Ryan JF: Malignant hyperthermia. In Ryan JF, Todres ID, Cote CJ, et al, eds: *A practice of anesthesia for infants and children,* ed 2, Philadelphia, 1993, WB Saunders, pp 417-428; Gronert GA, Antognini JF, Pessah IN: Malignant hyperthermia. In Miller RD, ed: *Anesthesia,* 2 vols, ed 5, New York, 2000, Churchill Livingstone, pp 1033-1052.

Nursing Care of Patients With Elevated Body Temperature

Hyperthermia may be treatable by nursing intervention alone (e.g., by correcting external causes such as inappropriate clothing for environmental conditions, exposure to the elements, or dehydration). In other cases, such as MH, nursing intervention alone is insufficient, and medical and other interventions may be necessary.

The impact of core hyperthermia on an already compromised patient can be deleterious. Oxygen consumption rises 10% to 12% for every 1° C temperature elevation.[45] The increased metabolic demand in response to hyperthermia may produce progressive metabolic acidosis, as oxygen delivery to the tissues is compromised.[46] Arterial blood gases and biochemical balance are monitored closely to detect acid-base imbalances and hypoxemia. Proper treatment of acidosis is promptly instituted to prevent untoward effects.

Sustained tachycardia in hyperthermic infants and children may compromise myocardial perfusion and diastolic filling and may lead to greater stress on an already compromised heart. Moreover, infants or children experiencing hyperthermia are observed for sweating and peripheral vasodilation, both of which greatly increase loss of heat from the skin.

Regardless of the measures instituted to reduce temperature, shivering is not stimulated. Shivering is a normal compensatory response to heat loss, but in the hemodynamically compromised patient, the effects can be deleterious. Shivering increases metabolic rate, carbon dioxide production, and myocardial oxygen consumption, all of which eventually increase the myocardial workload. Arterial oxygen saturation decreases and systemic vascular resistance and heart rate increase with shivering. In addition, oxygen consumption increases 500%,[47] and the production and accumulation of lactic acid accelerate, which may culminate in lactic acidosis.

Nurses focus on determining the proper combination of interventions to reduce temperature and avoid shivering. If shivering develops, measures are instituted to avoid the metabolic and hemodynamic consequences. Appropriate nursing interventions for shivering modify the rate of heat loss from the skin and interfere with the body's determination of heat loss.[48] Various techniques have been suggested. Intravenous narcotics have been used to suppress shivering but may also produce side effects such as nausea or hypotension.[49] An alternative is wrapping the extremities with towels during surface cooling with a hypothermia blanket.[48]

Psychologic support is particularly important when dealing with critically ill infants and children who are further distressed by both the discomfort of fever and its treatment. Interventions are based on the developmental stage and cognitive ability of the patient.

Hypothermia

Hypothermia is defined as any core body temperature less than 35° C. Degrees of hypothermia are detailed in Table

14-5. At low body temperatures (below 34° C), the hypothalamus functions minimally, and below 29° C, it cannot regulate temperature at all. Loss of temperature-regulating capability produces a rapid decrease in body temperature and eventually results in death.[4] When temperature drops low enough to trigger thermoregulatory control mechanisms, shivering thermogenesis and a generalized catecholamine release occur. Responses of the sympathetic nervous system prompt many other physiologic responses to produce the diagnostic characteristics of hypothermia (Box 14-3).

Infants and children are among high-risk groups for hypothermia, especially if unconscious, immobile, sedated, or malnourished. Mild hypothermia often can be observed in infants and children admitted to critical care units because of cold ambient temperatures. Box 14-4 outlines predisposing factors. Moderate to severe hypothermia is often present in patients who have suffered trauma, exposure, drowning, ingestion of poisons, or shock. Infants or children with unexplained altered responsiveness are evaluated for hypothermia by measuring core temperature.[50]

Many pharmacologic agents may contribute to hypothermia. Phenothiazines and barbiturates exert a direct effect on the anterior hypothalamus, decreasing its responsive-

TABLE 14-5 Levels of Clinical Hypothermia

Level	Temperature (° C)
Normothermia	37
Mild hypothermia	32-35
Moderate hypothermia	28-32
Severe hypothermia	<28

Heimbach D, Jurkovich GJ, Gentilello LM: Accidental hypothermia. In Grenvik A, Ayres SM, Holbrook PR et al, eds: *Textbook of critical care,* ed 4, Philadelphia, 1999, WB Saunders, pp 377-383.

Box 14-3
Diagnostic Characteristics of Hypothermia

Major (80%-100% of Cases)

Rectal temperature of <35.5° C
Cool skin
Pallor (moderate)
Shivering (mild)

Minor (50%-79% of Cases)

Mental confusion, drowsiness, restlessness
Decreased pulse and respirations
Cachexia, malnutrition

Data from Carpenito LJ: *Nursing diagnosis: application to clinical practice,* ed 8, Philadelphia, 2000, JB Lippincott, p 147.

ness to cold. Neuromuscular blocking agents and phenothiazines decrease the body's ability to engage in shivering thermogenesis. Vasodilators inhibit the peripheral vascular vasoconstrictor response and increase heat loss, thus decreasing temperature stability. Long-term use of vasopressors depletes catecholamine reserves and alters receptor function, thus impairing the peripheral vascular response to cold stress.[50]

One clinical phenomenon that may produce severe hypothermia is cold water drowning (i.e., drowning in freezing water). Even in warm climates, however, the temperature of pool water can be significantly lower than air temperature. Moderate water temperatures are lower than body temperature. The relatively large body surface area of infants and children predisposes them to rapid heat loss in water. As a consequence, small infants or children can become hypothermic even in relatively warm pool water in a moderate climate.

Therapeutic, induced, or controlled hypothermia is used to reduce metabolic demands during cardiac surgery. Induced hypothermia for cardiac surgery involves both systemic and cardiac cooling. Systemic hypothermia is achieved by cooling the blood as it circulates through the heat exchanger of the cardiopulmonary bypass pump. Cardiac hypothermia is achieved directly by a cooled perfusate. Initially, a regional temperature gradient occurs because the core (heart and brain) is cooled first and the peripheral tissues remain warm. Gradually, the skin temperature drops and eventually approximates the core temperature as heat is dissipated. During this time, the body's inherent thermoregulatory mechanisms cease, resulting in profound hypothermia.[51] Rewarming is initiated by warming the blood circulated through the body and discontinuing extracorporeal circulation. During this phase, the core is warmed first, and the regional and peripheral areas (rectum, bladder, and skin) remain cooler, creating another temperature gradient. As the patient's thermoregulatory function returns, the patient is vulnerable to shivering.

Box 14-4

✦ **Factors Predisposing Infants and Children to Thermal Instability**

Relatively large body surface area
Relatively limited nutritional reserve
Impaired cardiac, renal, hepatic, or endocrine function
Impaired behavioral, neural, and endocrine responses (from underlying physical and physiologic states)
Impaired neuroendocrine response (from pharmacologic agents)
Cardiopulmonary resuscitation, anesthesia, or extended radiographic procedures

Data from Brink LW: Abnormalities in temperature regulation. In Levin DL, Morris FC, eds: *Essentials of pediatric intensive care,* New York, 1999, Churchill Livingstone, pp 548-559, and St Louis, Quality Medical Publishing; and Heimbach D, Jurkovich GJ, Gentilello LM: Accidental hypothermia. In Grenvik A, Ayres SM, Holbrook PR et al, eds: *Textbook of critical care,* ed 4, Philadelphia, 1999, WB Saunders, pp 377-383.

Nursing Care of Patients With Decreased Body Temperature

Once the diagnosis of hypothermia is made, continuous core body temperature measurement is initiated while evaluating thoroughly for risk factors (Table 14-6) and potential complications. Important assessments following the diagnosis of hypothermia include (1) electrocardiographic monitoring (significant arrhythmias may occur because of myocardial irritability); (2) arterial blood pressure monitoring; and (3) frequent evaluation of acid-base status, serum electrolytes, and blood glucose levels. External and/or core rewarming is instituted promptly.

Interpretation of arterial blood gas results in the hypothermic patient may necessitate the use of correction curves or values on rewarmed specimens. This is recommended because low temperatures cause carbon dioxide solubility to change, forcing the oxygen dissociation curve to shift to the left. When a specimen is drawn from a hypothermic patient and warmed to 37° C, the solubility of carbon dioxide decreases, resulting in a higher $Paco_2$ and lower pH than exists in the patient. Pao_2 values are corrected for temperature because warming the blood increases the solubility of oxygen and results in Pao_2 values significantly higher than in the patient.[50] According to Shapiro and Cane,[52] however, if the patient's temperature is 35° to 39° C, little is to be gained in correcting blood gas values. If the patient's temperature falls outside this range, it may be clinically useful to correct blood gas values with an uncorrected Pao_2 less than 60 torr or an uncorrected $Paco_2$ less than 30 torr because these values may be higher than actual measurements.

Shivering thermogenesis begins at temperatures of 30° to 35° C. This condition results in a small increase in heat production, whereas oxygen consumption and metabolic rate increase significantly. Transient hyperglycemia may result from glycogenolysis in the liver and muscles. The catabolism of fat can produce ketosis. Lactate production ends in metabolic acidosis, and compensatory respiratory alkalosis follows. These changes peak at 34° to 35° C.[50]

As hypothermia deepens, shivering thermogenesis ceases. Nonshivering thermogenesis occurs as the core temperature falls below 30° C. Heat production and metabolic rate both fall below baseline requirements at this point.[50,53] Total oxygen consumption is proportionately decreased. There is a 6% fall in oxygen consumption for every degree Celsius that the core temperature decreases. However, the extent of reduction of metabolism varies in each organ system.[50] When the temperature is normal, oxygen consumption is highest in the kidney, which is the organ most rapidly affected by hypothermia.

Cold diuresis is a term used to describe the renal response to cold. This response denotes adequate urine output despite a significant impairment in renal blood flow and glomerular filtration rate. Diuresis may continue despite systemic hypotension, dehydration, and hyperosmolarity, presumably because of a defect in renal tubular reabsorption of water.[50]

Changes in the cardiovascular system occur with hypothermia. The initial catecholamine-induced tachycardia is transient. During the phase of shivering thermogenesis,

TABLE 14-6 Risk Factors for Hypothermia

Cause	Mechanism
Exposure Trauma Drowning	Increased heat loss, especially conductive heat loss (wet clothes or immersion) or convective losses (wind)
CNS depression Head injury Cerebral hemorrhage, tumor, or infection	Direct central effect on thalamic temperature center
Drug-induced Narcotics Barbiturates Phenothiazines Alcohol General anesthesia	CNS depression and vasodilation CNS depression α-Adrenergic block, impaired shivering thermogenesis, lowered set-point CNS depression (and associated trauma, exposure, and impaired behavioral responses) CNS depression with vasodilation
Endocrine Abnormalities Hypoglycemia Hypothyroidism Hypopituitarism	Impaired thermogenesis, limited metabolic response to cold Impaired hypothalamic response to cold
Spinal Cord Transection	Interrupted sensory afferent Inability to sense cold Impaired central reflex and behavioral responses
Skin Disorders Erythrodermas Burns Stevens-Johnson syndrome	Increased transdermal water and heat losses
Therapeutic Treatment of Reye's syndrome Cardiopulmonary bypass	CNS depression

Data from Brink LW: Abnormalities in temperature regulation. In Levin DL, Morris FC, eds: *Essentials of pediatric intensive care,* New York, 1999, Churchill Livingstone, p 553, and St Louis, Quality Medical Publishing.
CNS, Central nervous system.

TABLE 14-7 Cardiac Dysrhythmias in Hypothermia

Core Temperature	Arrhythmia
<34° C	Atrial fibrillation (more severe bradydysrhythmias noted with cooling)
<30° C	First-degree atrioventricular block
<20° C	Third-degree atrioventricular block

Data from Brink LW: Abnormalities in temperature regulation. In Levin DL, Morris FC, eds: *Essentials of pediatric intensive care,* New York, 1999, Churchill Livingstone, p 553, and St Louis, Quality Medical Publishing.

there is a decrease in cardiac conductivity and automaticity and an increase in the refractory period.[50] Table 14-7 outlines the characteristic cardiac effects of various levels of hypothermia. These arrhythmias may not be treatable until core rewarming occurs. However, electrocardiographic monitoring may be useful in identifying the severity of hypothermia. The J-point elevation, for example, is potentially useful in diagnosing the severity of hypothermia.[50]

Another significant effect of hypothermia is hemodynamic. Both myocardial contractility and vasomotor tone are impaired by hypothermia. This effect may produce profound hemodynamic collapse. During rewarming, significant hypotension may occur in response to peripheral vasodilation. Severe hypothermia may make cardiac resuscitation impossible, and thus rewarming should continue during resuscitation.[54] Resuscitation is continued until a core temperature of *at least* 30° C has been obtained, particularly if the primary cause of the cardiac arrest is hypothermia. Resuscitation efforts are applied thoughtfully in the severely hypothermic child. Core temperature below 28° C places the child at high risk for ventricular fibrillation, which may be induced by cardiac compression. If the child presents with a nonarrest cardiac rhythm, chest compression is not implemented, even in the face of severe bradycardia. However, chest compression is necessitated in patients with asystole or ventricular fibrillation.[49] Hypothermic patients are not declared legally dead until a core temperature of 32° C or greater is achieved.[55]

The respiratory system shows less uniform effects. Initially, cold stimulates tachypnea. Shivering thermogenesis may produce compensatory alkalosis; however, below 30° C, hypoventilation is often seen. Central apnea occurs as hypothermia progresses.[50] In addition, oxygen consumption rises and may produce hypoxia.

The CNS response varies with the degree of hypothermia. Mild to moderate hypothermia can produce confusion and behavioral changes. As the core temperature continues to drop, stupor worsens, and coma results. Below 26° C, unresponsiveness; flaccidity; and fixed, dilated pupils follow. The CNS can benefit from the reduced metabolic and oxygen demands that result from hypothermia. Factors that determine the degree of benefit include (1) degree and duration of hypothermia, (2) underlying disease processes, (3) cardiorespiratory status, and (4) prior or concomitant medication usage. Because the effects of hypothermia on the CNS may be profound, rewarming to a temperature higher than 35° C is recommended before evaluation of brain death is undertaken.[50]

Pharmacologic effects of hypothermia are varied. Moderate to severe hypothermia produces such a serious decrease in metabolic rate that oxygen consumption and the rate of biochemical reactions slow considerably. As a result, drug levels and effects are difficult to evaluate in hypothermic patients. Decreased cardiac output, dehydration, slowed hepatic metabolism, impaired glomerular filtration, and abnormal renal tubular filtration and reabsorption can all result in reduced drug clearance.[50] Hypothermia, for example, elevates the toxic dose of digitalis, whereas it decreases the inotropic dose. Potassium- and calcium-induced cardiac arrhythmias are possible because of increased myocardial sensitivity during hypothermia. Finally, temperatures below 26° C depress the cardiotonic effects of catecholamines; mild to moderate hypothermia, however, enhances their effects.[50] Other pharmacologic effects include heightened sensitivity to anesthetic agents and barbiturates. Both barbiturates (because of their depressant effect) and phenothiazines (because of their α-adrenergic blocking effects) potentiate hypothermia.

With body temperature below 30° C, hyperviscosity and hypercoagulability of the blood may occur. This results from a rising hematocrit level resulting from the cold diuresis that accompanies hypothermia. Infection is also a danger as a result of neutropenia, and coagulopathies can be accentuated because of thrombocytopenia.[50]

Generally, external warming devices are used to return the patient's temperature to the normal range in the case of mild to moderate hypothermia (i.e., core temperature of 30° to 35° C). Radiant warmers, heating blankets or pads, warmed blankets, and head coverings are commonly used. Reflective blankets (lightweight metallic blankets that reflect up to 80% of radiant heat to the body)[56] and buntings insulated with Thinsulate[57] have been recommended. A combination of modalities may be superior to a single rewarming technique.[58]

When instituting such measures, nurses are vigilant in their assessment of the patient's responses to the treatments. Radiant warmers are used only with the servocontrol option to avoid thermal injury to the skin. Heating pads and blankets and other warming devices are used with caution. Critically ill infants or children are not likely to be able to perceive a thermal injury or communicate it to nurses.

Severe hypothermia (core temperature lower than 30° C), for example, as a result of cold-water submersion, often requires active internal warming methods in addition to external warming measures. In such circumstances, measures such as heated humidified air, warmed intravenous fluids, and gastric or colonic lavage with warmed solutions or peritoneal dialysis may be implemented.[53] Extracorporeal rewarming (ECR) may be required in the most severe circumstances.[49] ECR has been advocated as a rewarming technique in hypothermic patients to reduce the problems of rewarming shock, dysrhythmias, and thermal injury associated with external warming devices.[17,59]

ECR diverts a significant portion of the patient's cardiac output through the extracorporeal membrane oxygenator and blood warmer. Gradual rewarming is facilitated by maintaining a warming gradient of approximately 10° C between the perfusate in the extracorporeal circuit and the patient's core temperature until body temperature reaches a normal range.[60] Slow rewarming avoids the sudden recirculation of cold, acidotic blood from the vasoconstricted peripheral vascular beds to the central circulation. This phenomenon, called "rewarming shock" or "afterdrop," is manifested by a continued decline in core temperature and serum pH after removal from the cold.[53] Because rapid rewarming increases the risk of ventricular fibrillation, gradual rewarming is the goal in any severely hypothermic patient, regardless of the intervention selected. Throughout the rewarming phase, the patient is closely monitored for cardiac dysrhythmias and coagulopathies resulting from systemic heparinization if ECR is used. Another option is the use of continuous arteriovenous rewarming. Femoral arterial and venous catheters and the patient's own blood pressure create a circulatory system that drives blood through a heat exchanger.[53]

SUMMARY

The incidence of altered body temperature and ineffective thermoregulation is significant among patients in the PICU. The risks to physiologic stability in critically ill infants and children are high. Critical care nursing practice can correct environmental factors leading to altered body temperature, support thermoregulatory processes, provide physical comfort during interventions to normalize body temperature, and ensure physiologic stability in patients with altered body temperature or ineffective thermoregulation.

REFERENCES

1. Carpenito LJ: *Nursing diagnosis: application to clinical practice,* ed 8, Philadelphia, 2000, JB Lippincott.

2. Bissonnette B, Davis PJ: Temperature regulation: physiology and perioperative management in infants and children. In Motoyama EK, Davis PJ, eds: *Smith's anesthesia for infants and children,* ed 6, St Louis, 1996, Mosby.

3. Gauntlett I, Barnes J, Brown T et al: Temperature maintenance in infants undergoing anaesthesia and surgery, *Anaesth Intensive Care* 13:300-304, 1985.

4. Guyton AC, Hall JE: *Human physiology and mechanisms of disease,* ed 6, Philadelphia, 1997, WB Saunders.

5. Perlstein P: Physical environment. In Fanaroff AA, Martin RJ, eds: *Neonatal-perinatal medicine: diseases of the fetus and infant,* ed 6, 2 vols, St Louis, 1997, Mosby.

6. Bolton DPG: Energy metabolism and temperature regulation. In Bray JJ, Cragg PA, Macknight ADC et al, eds: *Lecture notes on human physiology,* ed 4, Oxford, 1999, Blackwell Science.

7. Schwartz P: *Whaley & Wong's nursing care of infants and children,* ed 6, St Louis, 1999, Mosby.

8. Matusik MC: Chronobiology. In Colon AR, Ziai M, eds: *Pediatric pathophysiology,* Boston, 1985, Little, Brown.

9. Livingston RB: Neurophysiology. In West JB, ed: *Best and Taylor's physiological basis of medical practice,* Baltimore, 1991, Williams & Wilkins.

10. Blake WW, Murray JA: Heat balance. In Merenstein GB, Gardner SL, eds: *Handbook of neonatal intensive care,* ed 4, St Louis, 1998, Mosby.

11. Quinton PM: Sweating and its disorders. *Annual Review of Physiology,* 34, 429-452, 1983.

12. Amlung SR: Neonatal thermoregulation. In Kenner C, Lott JW, Flandermeyer AA, eds: *Comprehensive neonatal nursing: a physiologic perspective,* ed 2, Philadelphia, 1998, WB Saunders.

13. Holtzclaw BJ: New trends in thermometry for the patient in the ICU, *Crit Care Nurs Q* 21:12-25, 1998.

14. Vacanti FX, Ryan JF: Temperature regulation. In Ryan JF, Todres ID, Cote CJ et al, eds: *A practice of anesthesia for infants and children,* ed 2, Philadelphia, 1993, WB Saunders.

15. Robinson JL, Seal RF, Spady DW et al: Comparison of esophageal, rectal, axillary, bladder, tympanic, and pulmonary artery temperatures in children, *J Pediatr* 133:553-556, 1998.

16. Henker R, Coyne C: Comparison of peripheral temperature measurements with core temperatures, *AACN Clin Issues Crit Care Nurs* 6:21-30, 1995.

17. Reuler JB: Pathophysiology, clinical settings and management, *Ann Intern Med* 89:519-527, 1978.

18. Earp JK: Thermal gradients and shivering following open heart surgery, *Dimens Crit Care Nurs* 8:266-273, 1989.

19. Anderson S: Thermoregulation. In Deacon J, O'Neill P, eds: *Core curriculum for neonatal intensive care nursing,* ed 2, Philadelphia, 1999, WB Saunders.

20. Holtzclaw BJ: Postoperative shivering after cardiac surgery: a review, *Heart Lung* 15:292-299, 1985.

21. Kline MW, Lorin MI: Fever without source. In Oski FA, DeAngelis CD, Feigin RE et al, eds: *Principles and practice of pediatrics,* ed 3, Philadelphia, 1999, Lippincott Williams & Wilkins.

22. Kirsch EA, Thompson-Bush L: Temperature-sensing and temperature-regulating devices. In Levin DL, Morriss FC, eds: *Essentials of pediatric intensive care,* ed 2, New York, 1997, Churchill Livingstone and St Louis, Quality Medical Publishing.

23. Cote CJ: Pediatric equipment. In Ryan JF, Todres ID, Cote CJ et al, eds: *A practice of anesthesia for infants and children,* ed 2, Philadelphia, 1993, WB Saunders.

24. Sessler DI: Consequences and treatment of perioperative hypothermia, *Anesth Clin North Am* 12:425-456, 1994.

25. Henker R: Evidence-based practice: fever related interventions, *AACN Clin Issues Crit Care Nurs* 8:481-487, 1999.

26. Wong D: *Whaley & Wong's nursing care of infants and children,* ed 6, St Louis, 1999, Mosby.

27. Lovejoy Jr FH: The etiology and treatment of fever: current concepts, *Pediatric update: new developments in fever management,* 1989. (Available from Department of Medical Affairs, MacNeil Consumer Products, Camp Hill Rd, Fort Washington, Pa 19034.)

28. Lorin MI: Pathogenesis of fever and its treatment. In Oski FA, DeAngelis CD, Feigin RD et al, eds: *Principles and practice of pediatrics,* Philadelphia, 1999, Lippincott Williams & Wilkins.

29. Zeisberger E: Fever and antipyresis. In Gluckman PD, Heymann MA, eds: *Pediatrics and perinatology: the scientific basis,* ed 2, New York, 1997, Oxford University Press.

30. Littlefield LC: Management of fever. In Hoekelman RA, Blatman S, Friedman SB et al, eds: *Primary pediatric care,* St Louis, 1987, Mosby.

31. Curley FJ, Irwin RS: Disorders of temperature control: hypothermia. In Rippe JM, Irwin RS, Fink MP et al, eds: *Intensive care medicine,* ed 3, Boston, 1996, Little, Brown.

32. Alpern ER, Henretig FM: Fever. In Fleisher GR, Ludwig S, Henretig FM et al, eds: *Textbook of pediatric emergency medicine,* ed 4, Philadelphia, 2000, Lippincott Williams & Wilkins

33. Isaacman DJ, Bhisitkul DM: Fever. In Burg FD, Ingelfinger JR, Wald ER et al, eds: *Gellis & Kargan's current pediatric therapy,* ed 16, Philadelphia, 1999, WB Saunders.

34. Henker R, Kramer D, Rogers S: Fever, *AACN Clin Issues Crit Care Nurs* 8:351-367, 1997.

35. Zaleznik DF: Hospital-acquired and intravascular device-related infections. In Fauci AS, Martin JB, Braunwald E et al, eds: *Harrison's principles of internal medicine,* ed 14, New York, 1999, McGraw-Hill.

36. Mikhail, MS, Thangathurai D: Hyperthermia. In Grenvik A, Ayres SM, Holbrook PR et al, eds: *Textbook of critical care,* ed 4, Philadelphia, 1999, WB Saunders.

37. Sessler DI: Temperature regulation. In Gregory GA, ed: *Pediatric anesthesia,* ed 3, New York, 1994, Churchill Livingstone.

38. Gronert GA, Antognini JF, Pessah IN: Malignant hyperthermia. In Miller RD, ed: *Anesthesia,* 2 vol, ed 5, New York, 2000, Churchill Livingstone.

39. Bond EF: Channelopathies: potassium-related periodic paralyses and similar disorders, *AACN Clin Issues Crit Care Nurs* 11:261-270, 2000

40. Ryan JF: Malignant hyperthermia. In Ryan JF, Todres ID, Cote CJ et al, eds: *A practice of anesthesia for infants and children,* ed 2, Philadelphia, 1993, WB Saunders.

41. Henschel EO, ed: *Malignant hyperthermia: current concepts,* New York, 1987, Appleton-Century-Crofts.

42. Harris MF, Landers DF: Malignant hyperthermia. In Levin DF, Morriss FC, eds: *Essentials of pediatric intensive care,* 2 vol, ed 2, New York, 1997, Churchill Livingstone and St Louis, Quality Medical Publishing.

43. Wlody GS: Malignant hyperthermia: potential crisis in patient care, *AORN J* 50:286-298, 1989.

44. Hopkins PM, Ellis FR: Neuromuscular pathology and malignant hyperthermia. In Prys-Roberts C, Brown BR, eds: *International practice of anaesthesia,* 2 vols, Woburn, Mass, 1996, Butterworth-Heinemann.

45. Buran NJ: Oxygen consumption. In Pinsky MR, Snider JV, eds: *Oxygen transport in the critically ill,* St Louis, 1987, Mosby.

46. Buck SH, Zaritsky AL: Occult core hyperthermia complicating cardiogenic shock, *Pediatrics* 83:782-784, 1989.

47. Pflug AE, Aasheim GM, Foster C: Prevention of post-anesthesia shivering, *Can Anesth Soc J* 25:43-49, 1978.

48. Holtzclaw BJ: Control of febrile shivering during amphotericin B therapy, *Oncol Nurs Forum* 17:521-522, 1990.

49. Kiley JA, Robinson MD: Environmental heat and cold injuries. In Fuhrman BP, Zimmerman JJ, eds: *Pediatric critical care,* ed 2, St Louis, 1998, Mosby.

50. Brink LW: Abnormalities in temperature regulation. In Levin DL, Morriss FC, eds: *Essentials of pediatric intensive care,* 2 vols, ed 2, New York, 1997, Churchill Livingstone and St Louis, Quality Medical Publishing.

51. Lerman J: Special techniques: acute normovolemic hemodilution, controlled hypotension and hypothermia, and extracorporeal membrane oxygenation. In Gregory GA, ed: *Pediatric anesthesia,* ed 3, New York, 1994, Churchill Livingstone.

52. Shapiro BA, Cane RD: Interpretation of blood gases. In Shoemaker WC, Ayres S, Grenvik A et al, eds: *Textbook of critical care,* 2 vol, ed 2, Philadelphia, 1989, WB Saunders.

53. Heimbach D, Jurkovich GJ, Gentilello LM: Accidental hypothermia. In Grenvik A, Ayres SM, Holbrook PR et al, eds: *Textbook of critical care,* ed 4, Philadelphia, 1999, WB Saunders.

54. Rogers MC: *Textbook of pediatric intensive care,* ed 3, Baltimore, 1996, Williams & Wilkins.

55. Rowin ME, Christensen D, Allen EM: Pediatric drowning and near-drowning. In Roger MC, ed: *Textbook of pediatric intensive care,* ed 3, Baltimore, 1996, Williams & Wilkins.

56. Crayne HL, Miner DG: Thermo-resuscitation for postoperative hypothermia using reflective blankets, *AORN J* 47:222-227, 1988.

57. Holtzman IR: A method to maintain infant temperature, *Am J Dis Child* 139:390-392, 1985.

58. Topper WH, Stewart TP: Thermal support of the very-low-birth-weight infant: role of supplemental conductive heat, *J Pediatr* 105:810-814, 1984.

59. Feldman KW, Morray JP, Schallar RT: Thermal injury caused by hot pack application in hypothermic children, *Am J Emerg Med* 3:38-41, 1985.

60. Bolte RG, Black PG, Bowers RS et al: The use of extracorporeal rewarming in a child submerged for 66 minutes, *JAMA* 260:377-379, 1988.

15

Host Defenses

Mary Jo C. Grant

Host defenses are of considerable importance to the pediatric critical care nurse because of the age and vulnerability of the patient population and the complexities of critical care illness and the critical care environment. Host defenses may be altered because of developmental, situational, or congenital stressors. Whatever the process or mechanism of alteration, the outcome of altered host defenses ranges from hyperactivity of the immune system, manifested clinically as hypersensitivity (allergies or autoimmune disease), to hypoactivity of the immune system, manifested as an increased susceptibility to infection. This chapter focuses on the most common alterations in host defenses experienced by the pediatric critically ill patient.

ESSENTIAL EMBRYOLOGY

The fetus and neonate occupy a special niche in terms of immunity and the external environment. The developing immune system must learn to tolerate host constituents while preparing to battle with external pathogens. The fetal immune system is capable of significant immune reactivity fairly early in life. Protective immune responses are present in the human fetus as early as the seventh week of gestation, shortly after recognizable T cells can be detected. Before 7 to 12 weeks of gestation, protection against infection must be provided exclusively by the mother. Further protection of the developing fetus is provided by transplacentally acquired maternal immunoglobulin G (IgG). Beginning at 8 to 10 weeks and accelerating during the last trimester, this placental transfer is active and specific for IgG. The newborn is more susceptible to infection than the adult. The development of normal immunity is a gradual process, probably reflecting the effect of progressive and continuous exposure to antigenic stimulation. The human immune system matures rapidly; in normal children, most immune functions assume adult values at 2 to 3 years of age.[1]

MATURATIONAL ANATOMY AND PHYSIOLOGY OF THE IMMUNE SYSTEM

The most notable function of the immune system is host defense, or the active protection of the host from invading microorganisms. The other functions of the immune system are related to host defense but serve in the role of proactive maintenance. Homeostasis, the second function of the immune system, is the process by which the immune system maintains a balance between the old and new immune cells as a part of normal physiologic functioning. Homeostasis is the removal of old cells and debris resulting from normal catabolism, growth, and injury. Homeostasis keeps the body's internal environment clean and easy to survey. The third function of the immune system, surveillance, is the process in which the immune cells differentiate self from mutated self cells (nonself).

Nonspecific Versus Specific Immunity

Every person, whether healthy or immunocompromised, is in contact with millions of actual and potential microorganisms on a daily basis. The well-orchestrated, complex, and efficient cadre of defenses provided through the immune system is a barrier to these invaders. Host defenses can be classified as nonspecific or specific. Nonspecific defenses are generic host responses to a foreign agent. These responses are not tailored to an individual agent but are the same responses to any agent at any time. Nonspecific host defenses include first and second lines of defense, the natural barriers and the inflammatory responses, respectively. In contrast, specific defenses depend on the exposure to a foreign agent, recognition of the agent as foreign, and the host's individual reaction to that agent. The specific immune responses of the host are the third line of defense and include humoral immunity (immunoglobulin) and cell-mediated immunity.

Concept of Human Defense

Normal immune defense is maintained through the protection of self and the destruction of nonself. To perform host defense, yet maintain the integrity of self, a genetic blueprint (deoxyribonucleic acid [DNA] code) at the molecular level assists the immune system in discriminating self from nonself or altered self. Nonself is composed of foreign or alien molecular structure and is referred to as antigenic, or as an antigen.

The specific immune system discriminates between self and nonself through the major histocompatibility complex (MHC) molecules for each species. The MHC molecules specific to the human species are human leukocyte antigens (HLAs). HLAs are inherited according to mendelian laws, with a genotype determined by one paternal and one maternal haplotype. Close relatives share some of these

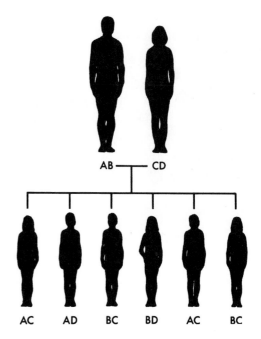

Fig. 15-1 Human lymphocyte antigens (HLAs) are inherited from parents: one set of HLAs is inherited from the mother, and the second set is inherited from the father. Each set of inherited antigens is co-dominant (i.e., each set is co-expressed on the surfaces of the pertinent body cells).

antigens, whereas identical twins share all of these antigens. Fig. 15-1 reflects the diagrammatic representation of inheritance of the HLAs in a family.

Although first discovered on white blood cells and coined "human leukocyte antigens," HLAs are actually located on the surfaces of most nucleated cells in the body, as well as platelets. HLAs of the MHC are divided into two classes (class I and II) based on function, types of cell antigens expressed on the cell membrane surfaces, and structure. Class I includes HLAs A, B, and C antigens and is found on all nucleated cell surfaces and platelets. Class II includes HLAs D and DR antigens and is located nearly exclusively on the surfaces of certain immune cells (macrophages and B lymphocytes).

Once thought to be important only in the transplantation process, HLAs are now known to play a comprehensive role in determining self versus nonself and in autoimmune disease processes. Class I antigens serve as identification markers of self and assist in the elimination of cells infected with intracellular microorganisms, mutated or malignant cells, or rejection of tissue grafts. Class II antigens serve as identification markers of exogenous antigens and assist in the elimination of extracellular microorganisms.

The Lymphoid System

The lymphoid system is composed of tissues, organs, and interconnecting vessels and is responsible for the production, maturation, storage, and activation of host defense cells, particularly the lymphocytes. The lymphoid system is divided into primary or secondary lymphoid tissues. Primary (central) lymphoid tissue or organs are sites for lymphopoiesis (development and maturation of B cells and T cells), whereas secondary (peripheral) lymphoid tissues and organs are the environment in which immune cells are activated to conduct host defense.

Although traditionally primary and secondary lymphoid tissue is categorized as two discrete groups, there are exceptions to this approach. For instance, the bone marrow, although thought of as a primary lymphoid organ, is also considered a secondary lymphoid organ because it stores lymphocytes. Conversely, the spleen and liver, usually categorized as secondary organs, can serve as primary organs. In the face of bone marrow failure, the spleen and liver can become the centers of hematopoiesis.[2]

Primary Lymphoid Tissue and Organs. The primary (central) lymphoid tissues include the thymus and the bone marrow. The thymus gland is an encapsulated structure located in the anterior mediastinum directly behind the sternum. The thymus is very large relative to fetal body size at birth (10 to 15 g), reaches peak mass at puberty (30 to 40 g), and then begins and continues to involute throughout adult life. The primary function of the thymus is the maturation and differentiation of T cells. In addition, the production and secretion of thymosin and other thymic hormones influence lymphopoiesis and the maturation and differentiation of the various subsets of T cells.

The human bone marrow is the location for hematopoiesis, a series of events that begin with the pluripotent stem cell and progress to the development of a full line of functional blood cells. Through hematopoiesis, the pluripotent stem cell is capable of creating all lines of differentiated cells, including erythrocytes, granulocytes, monocytes and macrophages, lymphocytes, and platelets. In adults, hematopoiesis occurs in red bone marrow contained primarily in the flat bones, such as the sternum, ribs, skull, iliac crest, and proximal ends of long bones. However, in infancy, hematopoiesis occurs in nearly all bones. The bone marrow is also the location for B cell maturation and differentiation.

The bone marrow and associated hematopoietic function may be altered by many diseases and treatments. Malignancies can have a direct impact through bone marrow infiltration by malignant cells or an indirect impact through the side effects of cytotoxic agents. Other diseases affect hematopoiesis through destruction of an individual cell line, such as that occurring in acquired immunodeficiency syndrome (AIDS) (helper T cell) or all cell lines, such as those in aplastic anemia (pluripotent stem cell). Bone marrow aspiration and biopsy provide quantitative and qualitative information regarding bone marrow function.

Secondary Lymphoid Tissue and Organs. The secondary organs include the lymph system, spleen, liver, and the mucosa-associated lymphoid tissues (MALTs), including the tonsils and Peyer's patches of the gut. The secondary tissues and organs serve as the environment in which the white blood cells (WBCs), specifically the lymphocytes, travel to and enter any part of the body to perform their host defense functions. Lymphocyte storage and activation occur in the secondary lymphoid tissues.

Bone marrow, in addition to being a primary lymphoid organ, is also a secondary lymphoid organ.

Lymphatic System. The lymphatic system is composed of nodes, lymphatic fluid (lymph), and lymphatic vessels and is an accessory route by which fluids can flow from the interstitial spaces into the blood. The lymphatic vessels parallel the venous system and drain into either the thoracic duct or the right lymphatic duct and eventually into the central venous circulation.

The amount of fluid or lymph collected and transported through the lymphatic system is approximately 120 ml/hr.[3] As the lymph is transported through this network, it also travels through lymph nodes. Lymph nodes are strategically located at junctions of lymphatic vessels and are usually kidney-shaped, bean-size organs. The lymph node serves as a filtering station for the WBCs to identify, process, and remove particulate matter or antigens. The lymph node also adds lymphocytes to the lymph fluid to increase the numbers of circulating lymphocytes. A lymph node biopsy and lymphangiography reveal information on the function of the lymphatic system.

Spleen. The spleen is the largest lymphoid organ and lies in the upper left quadrant of the child's abdomen. It comprises two types of tissue: red pulp and white pulp. The red pulp, containing venous sinusoid areas, is primarily involved with the destruction and removal of old or damaged erythrocytes, whereas the white pulp contains lymphoid tissue. The function of the spleen is to filter the blood as it travels through the splenic tissue. Antigens are trapped in the filtering mechanisms, where resident B cells and T cells are activated and destroy the antigen.

After loss of the spleen (surgical splenectomy or autosplenectomy resulting from sickle cell anemia), patients experience an increased risk of overwhelming postsplenectomy infection (OPSI), predominantly from encapsulated bacteria. In the asplenic pediatric patient, this risk is exacerbated because of other immunologic deficits, such as diminished phagocytic and complement function and reduced immunoglobulin levels. In the asplenic patient, the liver assumes the spleen's role in clearing mature and damaged red blood cells (RBCs).[2]

Liver. Located in the upper right quadrant of the abdomen, the liver serves as a filtering organ for the blood returning from the gastrointestinal (GI) tract. Venous sinusoids within the liver are lined with large, fixed macrophages, referred to as Kupffer cells, which are highly phagocytic. Because venous portal blood has drained from the intestines, it usually contains considerable quantities of particulate matter and bacteria. Kupffer cells are capable of removing more than 99% of all particulate matter in the portal venous blood before the blood completes its course through the entire sinusoidal passages.[4]

Laboratory tests, such as for hepatic enzymes and bilirubin, can indicate the quality of liver function. A liver biopsy or noninvasive procedures, such as computed tomography (CT) or magnetic resonance imaging (MRI), provide information on the structure and function of the liver.

Mucosa-Associated Lymphoid Tissues. Throughout the body there are dispersed aggregates of nonencapsu-

TABLE 15-1 Normal White Blood Cell (WBC) Values

Cell Type	Differential (%)	Absolute Number (mm³)
Total WBC count	100	
Birth		9000-30,000
24 hours		9400-34,000
1 month		5000-19,500
1-3 years		6000-17,500
4-7 years		5500-15,500
8-13 years		4500-11,000
>13 years		5000-10,000
Granulocytes		
Neutrophils	60-70	3000-7000
Segmented	56	2800-5600
Bands	3-6	150-600
Eosinophils	2-5	50-400
Basophils	<1	25-100
Monocytes	2-8	100-800
Lymphocytes	20-40	1000-4000
T cells	60-88*	600-2200
B cells	3-21*	100-400
Natural killer cells	5-10*	50-400

Modified from Tribett D: Immune system function: implications for critical care nursing practice. *Crit Care Nurs Clin North Am* 1:727, 1989; Behrman RE, Vaughn VC III, eds: *Nelson textbook of pediatrics,* ed 13, Philadelphia, 1989, WB Saunders.
*Percentage of total lymphocyte count rather than percentage of total WBC count.

lated lymphoid tissues. These tissues, MALTs, are found in a variety of places, especially in the submucosal areas of the GI (Peyer's patches, tonsils), respiratory, and urogenital tracts.[5] These tissues function like other secondary lymphoid tissues but are strategically placed close to potential sites of invasion. Both macrophages and lymphocytes are present to allow nonspecific and specific activity, respectively, to occur as needed.

Cells of Host Defense

White Blood Cells. WBCs, or leukocytes, are the mobile units of the immune system and are colorless blood cells that defend the body against infection. These cells are categorized as granulocytes, monocytes and macrophages, and lymphocytes. Granulocytes are critical in engulfing and phagocytizing microorganisms and are nonspecific in nature. They are further categorized as neutrophils, eosinophils, and basophils. Monocytes and macrophages also engulf microorganisms but more importantly are a link between the nonspecific and specific immune responses. Lymphocytes (B and T cells) are the key players in specific, acquired response. Table 15-1 reviews the normal values for each of the WBCs, and each is discussed separately.

Neutrophils develop and mature in the bone marrow for approximately 10 days. They spend approximately 12 hours in the circulation before migrating to the tissues, where they

live for only a few days. The primary function of neutrophils is to move to the site of invasion and destroy microorganisms through the process of phagocytosis. Neutrophils are the first WBCs to respond and the most numerous WBCs found at the site of tissue injury.

A mature neutrophil is described as a polymorphonuclear leukocyte (PMNL) or segmented neutrophil because of the appearance of the nucleus. Normally, segmented neutrophils or "segs" constitute the majority of circulating neutrophils. Neutrophilia, an increased number of circulating neutrophils, is often accompanied by an increase in the number of bands because the bone marrow releases a supply of neutrophils in response to the body's demands without regard to the cell's maturity or readiness for release. Neutrophilia is also observed in situations that stimulate secretion of epinephrine, adrenocorticotropic hormone (ACTH), or adrenal corticosteroids and cause increases in cardiac output. Therefore neutrophilia is observed in patients experiencing infection; stress response from surgery, hemorrhage, or emotional distress; and metabolic disorders, such as diabetes. The presence of greater than normal numbers of immature neutrophils in the circulation (*neutrophilia*) is clinically significant because the immature neutrophil's ability to phagocytize is less effective than that of a mature neutrophil and, more importantly, may signify that a problem exists.

Neutropenia, a decreased number of circulating neutrophils, is often associated with a pathologic or malignant condition. Conditions such as aplastic anemia or treatment with cytotoxic agents result in neutropenia. Neutropenia is technically defined as less than 3000 cells/mm³ of absolute neutrophils.

Eosinophils. Eosinophils account for approximately 2% to 5% of the circulating WBCs in healthy, nonallergic individuals but up to 50% in patients with parasitic infections or (less often) allergic conditions.[6] Following maturation in the bone marrow, the eosinophil is released into the circulation and remains there for a brief time before migrating to the tissues. Unlike other cells, eosinophils can recirculate back and forth from the circulation to the tissues. Their time in the tissues is approximately 12 days. Although eosinophils have the ability to phagocytize, the process is less efficient than that of the neutrophil. The eosinophil's role in host defense is not exactly known but is believed to be involved in the "turning off" of the immune response because it arrives last to the site of infection.

Eosinophils, like neutrophils, basophils, and mast cells, can be triggered to degranulate. Degranulation is the process in which intracellular granules fuse with the target cell's plasma membrane and cellular contents are released to the outside of the cell. If the target is too large to phagocytize, the eosinophils can shower the target with toxins located in their granules.

As previously mentioned, eosinophilia, an increased number of circulating eosinophils, is observed in patients with parasitic infection and allergic conditions. It is also observed in patients with chronic skin infections, GI conditions, such as ulcerative colitis and Crohn's disease, and rare conditions such as hypereosinophilia. Eosinopenia, a decreased number of circulating eosinophils, is observed in pl atients with acute mononucleosis and other acute infections, as well as conditions or therapies stimulating adrenal steroid production.

Basophils and Mast Cells.   Basophils represent the smallest proportion of granulocytes in the circulation, usually less than 1% of circulating WBCs. The basophil's production, distribution, and lifespan are not thoroughly understood. Basophils possess granules containing heparin, histamine, and other mediators, which can degranulate with the proper stimulus. Basophilia, an increased number of circulating basophils, is seen in leukemia and is seen less often with allergies and infectious diseases such as tuberculosis, influenza, and chickenpox. A decreased basophil count is observed in patients with allergic reactions or in those who are receiving prolonged steroid therapy.

The mast cell is often indistinguishable from the basophil, but the two cells do differ. Mast cells do not circulate in the bloodstream but instead are found throughout the body's tissues, particularly the skin and mucosal linings of the respiratory and GI tracts. Like the basophil, mast cells store granules with histamine and other potent mediators that are important in the inflammatory response and tissue repair. When the mast cell or basophil is inappropriately activated, these granules may lead to an allergic response. Because mast cells do not circulate, the suffixes "philia" and "penia" are not usually used to refer to abnormal numbers of mast cells. An abnormal accumulation of mast cells is termed *mastocytosis* and can range from benign skin lesions to organ infiltration resulting in organ dysfunction and death.

Monocytes and Macrophages.   Monocytes are large, nongranular leukocytes with kidney-shaped nuclei that make up 2% to 8% of total circulating WBCs. After their release from the bone marrow, monocytes spend only a brief time in the circulatory system (12 days) before they migrate to their primary site of action, the tissues. Following migration into the tissue, monocytes undergo differentiation into macrophages. Like neutrophils, monocytes (in the circulatory system) and macrophages (free and fixed, but usually in various tissues) have the ability to phagocytize.

Because monocytes are circulating WBCs, they can be quantified in the differential WBC count. Monocytosis, an increase in the number of circulating monocytes, is observed in patients with viral, parasitic, or rickettsial infections, although this finding may indicate a recovery phase and may be a favorable sign. A decrease in the circulating monocyte count, monocytopenia, is not clinically significant but may be observed in patients with human immunodeficiency virus (HIV) infection or in patients receiving prednisone therapy.

The macrophage is capable of phagocytizing larger and greater numbers of particles than the neutrophil. It has a primary role in nonspecific defense through its phagocytic activities but also in specific defense by its processing and presentation of the antigen to the helper T cell. Thus the macrophage serves as a link between the nonspecific and specific host defenses. The macrophage is also involved in the production and release of cytokines. It produces interleukin-1 (IL-1), a known pyrogen and mediator of the inflammatory response. The macrophage also produces interferon in the presence of viral invasion.

Lymphocytes.   The lymphocyte is a small, mononuclear cell that makes up 20% to 40% of the circulating WBCs. The lymphocyte is produced in the bone marrow and migrates to other parts of the body for differentiation and maturation into several distinct subsets of lymphocytes. Lymphocyte subsets include B cells, T cells, and natural killer (NK) cells based on differences in their immune function and surface molecules (phenotypic markers).

Although these cells are normally measured in the periphery, lymphocytes circulate through a network of interconnected passages referred to as the recirculating pathway. In the recirculating pathway, lymphocytes survey the body for invading organisms or antigens by traveling among the blood, lymphatic vessels, lymphoid tissue, and bone marrow and back to the blood. Lymphocytes can also be found in specialized tissue collections, spleen, thymus, mucosa of the GI tract, and many other body tissues.

Lymphocytosis, an increase in the number of circulating lymphocytes, is seen in patients with viral infections, such as infectious mononucleosis and infectious hepatitis, lymphocytic leukemia, and lymphoma. Lymphopenia, a decrease in the number of lymphocytes, is commonly seen in patients with congenital immunodeficiencies, AIDS, uremia, or Cushing's disease or after the administration of cortisol or ACTH.

B Cells.   B cells make up approximately 10% to 15% of the total lymphocyte count, with alterations in the number of B cells considered clinically significant (Table 15-2). The B cell is primarily responsible for humoral immunity through its transformation into a plasma cell that secretes immunoglobulin. Humoral immunity primarily protects the host from bacterial infection and viral invasion.

The term *immunoglobulin* refers to a group of serum proteins that are composed of antibody molecules. Immunoglobulins are specialized molecules synthesized by plasma cells serving as flexible adapters connecting immune cells and antigens. *Antibody* is the term reserved for an individual immunoglobulin molecule, one for which the "destiny" antigen is known. The primary purpose of the antibody is to bind to its destiny or predetermined antigen and either neutralize it or enable the cells of the immune system to destroy it.

Immunoglobulins are composed of polypeptides (chains of amino acids) formed into a basic Y-shaped structure. The basic immunoglobulin molecule consists of two identical long (heavy) chains and two identical short (light) chains held together by chemical bonds (Fig. 15-2). Both the heavy and the light chains have a variable segment at one end of the molecule and a constant segment at the other end of the molecule. The variable segment binds to the antigen for which it was made, and is referred to as the antigen-binding fragment (Fab).[7] Although the variable segment is unique, the sequence of amino acids that creates the constant segment of the immunoglobulin molecule remains identical within each class of immunoglobulin and is thus referred to as the constant fragment (Fc).

Human immunoglobulin molecules are divided into five classes based on the structure of their constant segments: IgG, IgA, IgM, IgE, and IgD. Phagocytes and other immune cells have receptors on their surfaces into which the constant Fc portion of the Ig molecule fits. This receptor is called an Fc receptor. Table 15-3 is a review of the major classes of

◆ TABLE 15-2   Lymphocytes: Laboratory Analysis and Clinical Significance of Alterations

Cell Type	Total Lymphocyte Count (%)	Absolute Count (per mm³)*	Clinical Significance of Alterations

T cells	60-88	600-2200	Decreased:
			    Malignant disease
			    AIDS
			    Postviral infection (temporary)
			    Severe combined immunodeficiency
			    DiGeorge syndrome
			    Nezelof syndrome
			Increased:
			    Graves' disease

Helper T	34-67	493-1191	Decreased: AIDS
Cytotoxic-suppressor T	10-49	182-785	Decreased: Overall lymphopenia

B cells	3-21	100-400	Decreased:
			    X-linked hypogammaglobulinemia
			    Selective deficiency of IgG/IgA/IgM
			    Lymphoma
			    Multiple myeloma
			    Nephrotic syndrome

Natural killer cells	5-10	50-400	Increased:
			    Lymphocytic leukemia
			    Lupus erythematosus

Data from Fischbach FT: *A manual of laboratory and diagnosis tests,* ed 4, Philadelphia, 1992, JB Lippincott; Tribett D; Immune system function: implications for critical care nursing practice, *Crit Care Nurs North Am* 1:727, 1989.
*These values most accurately reflect the older child or adolescent. Recent evidence reveals that absolute lymphocyte counts may be higher in the infant and young child.

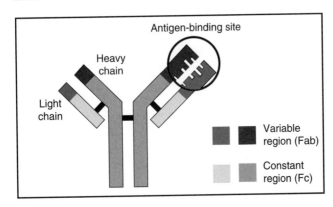

Fig. 15-2 Structure of immunoglobulin molecule. Fab segment is variable and attaches to its destiny or predetermined antigen. Fc segment can attach to any cell that has an Fc receptor. (From Schindler LW: *The immune system—how it works.* United States Department of Health and Human Services, Bethesda, Md. NIH publication number 92-3229, p. 6, 1992.)

human immunoglobulins with their respective serum levels, mechanisms of action, and location.

T Cells. After production in the bone marrow, T cells differentiate in the thymus and are rereleased into the circulation, where they make up 80% of all lymphocytes. In general, T cells are responsible for cell-mediated immunity, which protects the host from infections with intracellular organisms, such as viruses, fungi, protozoa, and helminth parasites. T cells are also involved in the elimination of mutant or tumor cells and are involved in the immune response triggered during tissue graft or organ transplant rejection.

During differentiation in the thymus, T cells develop into one of four distinct subclasses: helper T cell, suppressor T cell, cytotoxic T cell, or memory T cell. Helper T cells have many functions, such as producing lymphokines, which then stimulate the cloning and differentiation of B cells. Helper T cells are also active in several nonspecific host responses, such as attracting macrophages and neutrophils. Following helper T cell activation and the production of lymphokines, suppressor T cells are activated. Suppressor T cells curb the immune response. Cytotoxic T cells (effector cells) are responsible for direct destruction of target cells in the specific immune response. Memory cells are formed with the initial antigen contact and are involved in subsequent contacts with the antigen.

Because helper T cells orchestrate the entire immune response, it is essential to have adequate numbers of these cells. Normally, there are twice as many helper T cells as there are cytotoxic and suppressor T cells. Although some clinicians measure the ratio of helper T cells to cytotoxic and suppressor T cells, this comparison is less clinically useful than absolute numbers or percentages of the T cell subclasses. Alterations in the numbers of T cells and their subclasses are considered clinically significant (see Table 15-2).

Natural Killer Cells. NK cells make up approximately 5% to 10% of the total lymphocyte count. Many

◆ **TABLE 15-3 Human Immunoglobulins**

Ig	% in Serum	Location	Activity and Function

IgG	75	Intravascular, extravascular	Opsonization
			    Neutralization
			    Complement fixation

IgA	15	Found in mucous membrane secretions, intravascular	Neutralization Prevention of surface attachment
IgM	10	Intravascular	Agglutination Complement fixation
IgE	0.1	Bound to mast cells and basophils	Release of histamine and other mediators from mast cells and basophils
IgD	<1	Located on surface of B cells	Function not yet defined May be important to B cell differentiation

Adapted from Grady C: Host defense mechanisms: an overview, *Semin Oncol Nurs* 4:92, 1988.

terms are used to describe the NK cell; it is often referred to as "null," "blank," or "non-T non-B cell" because of the lack of T or B cell identification markers. The NK cell is a member of a group of large, granular lymphocytes (LGLs) with nonspecific cytotoxic abilities that act through a mechanism similar to that of cytotoxic T cells. The target cell for the NK cell is the tumor cell or virally infected cell. The NK cell's cytotoxic abilities are nonspecific in nature because the cell can destroy its target without prior sensitization.

LGLs may be stimulated in the laboratory with interleukin-2 to become lymphokine-activated killer (LAK) cells. Although these cells remain nonspecific, they respond to a greater diversity of targets than the NK cell. Protocols employing LAK cells are undergoing clinical trials in the treatment of many malignancies.

ASSESSMENT OF IMMUNE FUNCTION

In comprehensive assessments of the critically ill child, the inclusion of an immunologic component is imperative. Assessing the patient's host defenses begins with the identification of risk factors. The critically ill child displays many factors that are known to impair host defense or immune function. These risk factors include young age; presenting illness and associated interventions; poor nutritional status; and past medical history, including immunization, childhood diseases, and stress. Although these factors and their associated effects are reviewed in other sections of this chapter, they must be assessed as part of the patient history and addressed in the patient's plan of care.

Assessment of childhood immunizations, in addition to immunizations received for foreign travel, is included in the patient's history. With the discovery and use of vaccinations, the incidence of several childhood infectious diseases has been greatly reduced and, in some cases, eradicated.[8] Compliance with immunization schedules is credited to many school systems, which mandate up-to-date immunization records for matriculated children. However, many young children not yet enrolled in school may lack immunizations.

The results of recent tuberculosis screening, either through skin testing or chest radiographs, are included in the patient's history. Blood component transfusion history includes the patient's experience with and total number of past transfusions, as well as the year in which these transfusions occurred. These data help identify patients who may have developed antibodies to cells or substances in blood components and patients who are at risk for blood-borne infections, such as hepatitis B or C, cytomegalovirus (CMV), and HIV.

Adolescents and young adults should also have a sexual history completed because sexual activity is a risk factor for impaired immune function. Unprotected sexual intercourse increases the likelihood of exposure to and acquisition of HIV infection and other sexually transmitted diseases. This risk is increased with intercourse involving multiple, homosexual, or intravenous drug–abusing partners.

The child's past medical history should include details of chronic or recurrent infections. A careful, detailed history assists in separating the immunologically competent child from the child with "too many infections." A healthy young child may experience six to eight respiratory infections per year and more than eight if the child is exposed to siblings or other children in day-care settings.[9] Cues, such as repeated infections without a symptom-free interval, increased dependency on antibiotics, unexpected or severe complications to infection, or infection with an unusual or opportunistic organism, are often a significant part of the history of a child with primary immunodeficiency.

Although a primary immunodeficiency may be suspected in the young child who presents with a life-threatening infection in the first year of life or with a history of chronic or recurrent infections, it is also important to consider nonimmunologic causes of "too many infections."[10] In addition to exploring the medical history of the patient, a comprehensive family history is helpful. Primary immunodeficiencies, in particular, may have a clear pattern of inheritance.[9]

First Line of Defense

The most primitive defense mechanisms of any host, healthy or compromised, are the natural barriers that provide protection from the environment. The major components of the first line of defense include the unique functions of each of the following tissues and organ systems: integumentary, respiratory, GI, genitourinary, and ophthalmologic. These barriers include epithelial surfaces with their unique physical, chemical, and mechanical capacities that impede the entrance of microorganisms. The structure and function of each of these barriers vary; therefore each is discussed separately, followed by the developmental alterations noted in the infant and young child. Barriers and their unique characteristics are summarized in Table 15-4. Any sign of a disruption in host defense or an infectious process is noted, documented, and addressed in the patient's plan of care. Table 15-5 reflects physical assessment findings from the immunologic perspective. Pediatric critical care nurses can easily incorporate an immunologic assessment into a routine nursing assessment.

Laboratory assessment of the first line of defense includes cultures of sputum, wound, stool, urine, and other body fluids. Bedside analysis of gastric and urinary pH assists in determining the status of the child's chemical barriers.

Colonization and Bacterial Interference. All body tissue and organ systems exposed to the external environment are composed of epithelial cell surfaces. These epithelial surfaces are normally colonized by indigenous bacterial flora that aid in the process of host defense and the prevention of infection. Colonization, the residence of microorganisms, is influenced by a variety of environmental factors, including dietary intake, sanitary conditions, air pollution, and hygienic habits.[11] Generally, two types of flora are harbored by a host: normal resident (indigenous) flora that, if disturbed, reestablishes residency easily, and transient flora that may colonize the host for varying periods, from hours to weeks, without taking up permanent residence.

The presence of indigenous bacterial flora is thought to prevent or retard colonization by other potentially harmful organisms through a variety of mechanisms, but the exact phenomenon of bacterial interference is not completely understood. Known mechanisms of indigenous flora that prevent or retard colonization by other organisms include

---

TABLE 15-4 Barriers: The First Line of Defense

Integumentary	Intact skin
	Intact mucous membranes
	Acidic pH
	Bacterial interference
	Sweat glands—lysozyme
	Sebaceous glands—sebum/fatty acids
Respiratory	Intact mucous membranes
	Aerodynamic filtration
	Humidification
	Mucociliary transport system
	Bacterial interference
	Alveolar macrophages
	Lysozyme
	Secretory IgA
	Sneeze, cough, gag reflexes
Gastrointestinal	Intact mucous membranes
	Gastric acidity
	Pancreatic and intestinal secretions
	Intestinal motility
	Bacterial interference
	Secretory IgA
	Phagocytic cells
	Breast milk (lactating females)
Genitourinary	Flushing action of urination
	Acidic pH of urine
	Length of urethra (male)
	Prostatic secretions (male)
	Acidic pH of vagina (female)
	Secretory IgA
	Bacterial interference
Eye	Flushing action of tearing
	Lysozyme
	Secretory IgA
	Blink reflex

Adapted from Adams A: External barriers to infection, *Nurs Clin North Am* 20:146, 1985.

TABLE 15-5 Immunologic Physical Assessment Findings

Category/System	Assessment Findings
Skin/hygiene	Altered temperature, diminished turgor, dehydration, signs of infection, oral lesions, breaks in integrity, purpura, palpable lymph nodes, rhinitis dermatitis, urticaria, eczema
Mobility/comfort	Decrease in level of activity, muscle weakness, fever, chills, joint swelling or tenderness
Respiratory	Altered rate/depth of respirations, wheezing, crackles, bronchospasm, cough, hypoxemia
Cardiovascular	Vasculitis, pale skin and mucous membranes
Gastrointestinal	Altered bowel sounds, vomiting, chronic diarrhea, hepatosplenomegaly, protuberant abdomen (not age appropriate)
Neurologic	Altered level of consciousness, deficits in sensory and/or motor function, diminished cranial nerve function (blink, tear, cough, swallow, and gag)

Modified from Rosenthal CH: Immunosuppression in the pediatric critical care patient, *Crit Care Nurs Clin North Am* 1:781, 1989.

competition for the same nutrients, competition for the same receptors on host cells, and production of products that are toxic to other organisms. In addition, indigenous flora provides continuous stimulation and keeps the immune system alert to respond.

Although the newborn's skin is essentially sterile at birth,[12] the acquisition and maintenance of normal epithelial flora contribute to the newborn's development of the first line defense. Within 48 hours, the newborn begins to colonize organisms that are easily obtained from the environment, nursery personnel, and family. Within approximately 6 weeks of age, the newborn's skin flora is quantitatively comparable to that of older children and adults.[13]

Integumentary: Skin and Mucous Membranes.
The intact skin is an effective physical barrier to the penetration of microorganisms. Few organisms can directly and effectively penetrate the skin; instead they must rely on a vector (an organism that will transmit infection), a primary lesion, or a (synthetic) device for entrance.[11] Few organisms find the skin conducive for growth because the skin is a generally dry, mildly acidic (pH 5 to 6) environment. Besides containing secretory IgA, sweat also posses sufficient salt to create a high osmotic pressure.[14] In addition, desquamation, or the natural sloughing process, hampers residence on epithelial surfaces.

The skin serves as a chemical and physical barrier for the body's internal environment through the secretion of lysozyme and sebum. Secreted by the sweat gland, lysozyme can attack and lyse the cell membranes of gram-positive and gram-negative bacteria. Sebum, secreted by the sebaceous glands, is an oily substance that has been postulated to have antifungal and antibacterial properties, although none of these claims have been substantiated.

The external epithelial surfaces are not the only ones with these physical and chemical properties. Mucous membranes and the internal epithelial surfaces are colonized with numerous organisms that assist with the phenomenon of bacterial interference. Virtually all secretions of mucous membranes contain lysozyme, as well as IgA and IgG, and significant amounts of iron-binding proteins, such as lactoferrin. Lactoferrin, among other iron-binding proteins, maintains the level of free iron below the level in which bacteria flourish.

The newborn's skin is about 1 mm thick at birth and increases to approximately twice that thickness at maturity. The newborn has scant amounts of stratum corneum, the barrier component of the skin, resulting in increased skin permeability.[4] The stratum corneum develops quickly and is considered an adequate barrier at 2 weeks of age. It is similar to that of the adult by about 4 months of age.

The sebaceous glands at birth are well developed and are active during the neonatal period under the influence of maternal androgens acquired transplacentally.[4] Following the neonatal period, the sebaceous glands involute and produce only small amounts of sebum until puberty.

The sweat glands are formed with associated patent ducts by the end of the second trimester of gestation,[15] although sweating has a delayed onset of several days in the newborn. Sweating is noted first on the face, then on the palms of the hands and feet, and later on the remainder of the body. The differences noted in sweating may be related to the immaturity of autonomic (sympathetic) control of sweating rather than the structural immaturity of the glands. Complete neural control of sweat glands is noted between 2 and 3 years of age. Diminished sweat production may result in lower quantities of bactericidal and fungicidal substances and, in some, alteration in the physical barrier of the infant or young child's skin.

Respiratory System.
The respiratory tract has numerous nonspecific and specific defense mechanisms. The nonspecific mechanisms are composed of the aerodynamic filtration; the mucociliary transport system; sneeze, cough, and gag mechanisms; and alveolar macrophages. Many foreign particles come into contact with the mucous membranes of the respiratory tract because of the turbulent airflow that is characteristic of the upper airway and tracheobronchial tree. Most particles escaping this filtration system are eliminated by the mucociliary transport system, by being entrapped in mucus and swept upward by the cilia and then expectorated or swallowed. These mechanisms are normally efficient and eliminate approximately 90% of inhaled particles.

Another major function of the upper respiratory tract, humidification, aids the filtration capacities of the lung. Small hydroscopic organisms or particles absorb water from the moist respiratory tract, enlarge in size, and are more easily phagocytized.[11] The respiratory tract has detoxification defenses that include diluting substances with bronchial secretions and alveolar fluids and phagocytizing substances by the alveolar macrophages.

The small airways of the infant and young child make a significantly greater contribution to airway resistance compared with those in the adult.[4] This increase in resistance to flow places the child at greater risk for airway occlusion resulting from edema or inflammatory exudate. Normal defense mechanisms of the respiratory tract may be disrupted by such narrowing or obstruction.

Gastrointestinal System.
Defense mechanisms of the GI tract include saliva; antibacterial effect of gastric acid, digestive enzymes, pancreatic secretions, intestinal secretions, and bile; intestinal motility; and indigenous flora.[11,16,17] Most organisms enter the GI tract through the mouth and are readily destroyed either in the mouth by saliva containing antimicrobial factors, such as lysozyme and IgA, or in the stomach by the highly acidic (normal gastric pH <4) environment. Organisms in partially digested food particles encounter both a thick intestinal mucous layer and an intact mucosal epithelium as deterrents to their viability. Pathogen attachment to mucosal epithelium is also discouraged through peristalsis.

Secretory IgA, a component of the third line of defense (specific immune response), is the predominant immunoglobulin on all mucosal surfaces. It assists in the prevention of attachment and invasion of microorganisms and in the limitation of the amount of food antigen that enters the systemic circulation from the GI mucosa.[7]

Secretory IgA is a form of antibody that is particularly adapted to the unique needs of the GI tract. Its three unique features are that it is a double molecule, resists digestion, and does not activate complement. The epithelial cells of the GI tract provide secretory IgA with a molecule called the "secretory piece." This secretory characteristic prevents secretory IgA from being easily destroyed by the various digestive secretions and enzymes. At birth, newborn saliva contains no secretory IgA, although half of infants have detectable secretory IgA levels by 28 days of age.[18] Mellander and co-workers[19] have found that levels of secretory IgA can increase toward adult levels within a few weeks of life if the host is subjected to intense exposure to microbes. Secretory IgA concentrations rise more quickly than serum IgA concentrations. Some evidence indicates that there are only a few secretory IgA–producing cells in the submucosa of the GI tract at birth and that breast-feeding may be required to obtain optimal levels of secretory IgA in that area.[20]

Young children's serum level of IgA remains low for months, and they are dependent on an exogenous source of IgA. Breast milk provides this exogenous source of IgA, as well as lactoferrin, lysozyme, and lymphocytes.[17] Breast milk can offer as much as 0.5 to 1 g of secretory IgA antibodies to the fully breast-fed infant daily.[21] This amount of secretory IgA is equivalent to approximately one-third that normally produced by an average adult for defense.

Breast milk, with its many components, may aid the infant's mucosal defenses, but the exact role that each of these components plays is still undefined. It is generally accepted that breast milk provides the GI tract some protection from food allergies and microorganisms until the infant's mucosal immune system matures. Colostral antibodies do not cross the newborn's gut after the first 24 hours of life and do not have a role in the newborn's systemic immunity.[22]

An additional chemical property of the GI tract is the acidity of the stomach. At birth, the gastric pH is approximately 6, but normally reaches a pH of 2 to 3 within the first 24 hours of life. Acidity of the stomach gradually increases through childhood, and then it plateaus to adult levels at 10 years of age. Peristalsis propels the antigen through the GI tract, decreasing the opportunity for the antigen to settle and attach. The continual shedding of epithelial cells in the intestinal tract also limits the efficacy of an infectious process.

Peristaltic motion is intact at birth, with evidence that even the newborn's peristaltic contractions occur at the same frequency as the adult's.[23] However, unlike the adult's, the newborn's intestinal epithelium allows certain molecules to pass into the systemic circulation. The maturation of the intestinal epithelium is thought to occur in response to hormones and a variety of growth factors.

Genitourinary Tract. Organisms in the lower urinary tract are normally eliminated during urinary evacuation. In addition, normally acidic urine maintains the sterility of urine. In the male, the length of the urethra provides a physical protective barrier to pathogens. Antimicrobial substances, such as prostatic fluid secretions and secretory IgA, also assist in urinary tract defenses.

The female's vagina supports a large amount of indigenous microorganisms, primarily lactobacilli. The epithelial surfaces of the vagina contain increased amounts of glycogen, which is then metabolized into lactic acid by the bacterial flora. This creates an acidic and unfavorable environment for most potential pathogens.

Urine levels of secretory IgA may be an indication of the degree of risk for urinary tract infection (UTI). Fliedner and co-workers[24] found that girls with a history of a UTI have lower levels of secretory IgA in the urine during noninfected periods than girls without previous UTIs.

Ophthalmologic Defenses. The eye is equipped with eyelashes and the blink reflex to mechanically augment defenses. Tearing is the major external defense for the eye. Tears drain through the lacrimal duct and deposit organisms into the nasopharynx for the mucociliary transport system to eliminate. Tears contain high concentrations of lysozyme. Tearing is present by approximately 6 weeks of age, and lysozyme levels in the normal infant and the adult are comparable.

Second Line of Defense

Penetration of microorganisms into the internal environment signifies a breach of the first line of defense. Once the internal environment is threatened through an extrinsic insult (vascular access, Foley catheter, burn, trauma, etc.) or an intrinsic insult (thrombosis, malignancy, etc.), the second line of defense is triggered. These secondary defenses, like first-line defenses, are nonspecific and occur immediately and independently of the body, recognizing the specific antigen. Preexisting cell types and chemical mediators form the second line of defense, which consists of inflammation, phagocytosis, and complement activation.

Inflammation. The goals of the inflammatory response are distinct and are consistently well described in the literature; these goals are to localize, dilute, and destroy the offending antigen (if present), to maintain vascular integrity and minimize tissue damage, and to transport cells and substances to the area requiring tissue repair. The inflammatory process is triggered by any cell or tissue injury. The hallmark of the inflammatory response is the release of chemical mediators, such as histamine, bradykinin (and other kinins), serotonin, and prostaglandins. The process generally begins as a localized response accompanied by classic symptoms that include erythema, edema, warmth, and pain. The systemic response marks the inability of the local response to fulfill the goals of containment and is manifested by leukocytosis, neutrophilia, fever, and others. The mechanisms of the localized inflammatory response are described first.

The immediate response to injury is vasoconstriction so that the formation of the fibrin plug and margination of leukocytes, erythrocytes, and platelets can begin. The brief period of vasoconstriction is followed by a longer period of vasodilation, manifested by redness, heat, and increased capillary permeability. Increased capillary permeability allows plasma and cells to leak out of the vascular space and attend to the tissue injury. The result of this plasma and cell movement into the tissue is interstitial swelling (edema) and the formation of an inflammatory exudate. Although the development of swelling may be physically restricting in the inflamed area, the inflammatory exudate ultimately assists in accomplishing the previously stated goals of inflammation. Pain of the inflammatory site is the result of various events, but predominant it is the release of kinins and swelling or restriction of the site.

In response to the inflammation, leukocytes are released from the bone marrow and marginating pool into the circulation. Leukocytosis is indicated by an increase in WBC count from a normal count up to 30,000 cells/mm^3. The cells and bacteria at the site of cellular or tissue injury release substances that attract neutrophils to the site within minutes of the initial insult. The neutrophil response in inflammation predominates for the initial 24 to 48 hours. Monocytes are subsequently attracted to the site to augment the neutrophil's phagocytic activity.

Once in the general area of the inflamed tissue, the neutrophil will line up against the blood vessel wall (pavement) and migrate through the epithelial gaps of the vessel into the interstitial space by a process called diapedesis. Once in the injured tissue, the neutrophil and other phagocytes continue their purposeful movement, referred to as chemotaxis, to the site of inflammation. Chemotactic substances are chemical substances that attract or move phagocytes to necessary sites.

Following the initial neutrophil response to inflammation, the monocyte and macrophage response predominates. This phase of the inflammatory process varies, depending on several factors. If a virus is present, the monocyte arrives and produces α-interferon, which has antiviral properties. The monocyte may also migrate into the tissue to further differentiate into a macrophage and efficiently phagocytize bacteria, cellular debris, and dead neutrophils. The activated macrophage may then release the cytokine IL-1 to act as an endogenous pyrogen that causes fever and inhibits further microorganism growth. The monocyte and macrophage response is a vital link between the nonspecific and specific immune responses. The response signifies the need for specific cells to enter the inflammatory response.

If the amount or virulence of a microorganism is overwhelming or the injury is extensive, signs of a systemic inflammatory process can be seen (leukocytosis, neutrophilia, malaise, inability to gain weight or weight loss, and fever). The American College of Chest Physicians (ACCP) and the Society of Critical Care Medicine (SCCM) held a consensus conference to provide a conceptual and practical framework of various clinical syndromes (bacteremia, sepsis, trauma, etc.) involving a systemic inflammatory response.[25] The proposed terminology recognizes that the host is an active participant in the immune response to both infectious and noninfectious insults. Although the details of the proposed terminology can be found elsewhere,[25] the term *systemic inflammatory response syndrome* (SIRS) is the most applicable to this chapter. SIRS is defined as a systemic or nonlocalized response to a variety of infectious but also noninfectious insults.[25] As previously mentioned, the ACCP-SCCM consensus conference has proposed

objective criteria characterizing the SIRS (see Chapter 27 for further information about SIRS).

The presence or absence of the inflammatory response is directly assessed by the nurse, with phagocytosis and complement activation indirectly demonstrated by pus formation and fever. All disruptions in epithelial surfaces are assessed for the cardinal signs and symptoms of the inflammatory response. It is important to note those situations in which the cardinal signs of the local inflammatory response (redness, inflammation, induration, and drainage) may be diminished or absent in newborn infants, neutropenic patients, or patients receiving medications suppressing the inflammatory response. In addition, the newborn may have a delayed or limited ability to localize infection. In these patients, the most reliable sign of local inflammatory response is often pain at the site of infection.

In critical care patients, fever is the most reliable sign of systemic inflammation. Fever is caused by pyrogens, exogenous or endogenous substances that cause the hypothalamus to adjust the temperature set-point upward. Exogenous pyrogens are derived outside of the host and are commonly microbial products, toxins, or the microbes themselves. The lipopolysaccharide produced by gram-negative bacteria is an example of an exogenous pyrogen and is commonly called an endotoxin. Endogenous pyrogens are polypeptides that are produced by host immune cells, most commonly IL-1 produced by the monocyte and macrophage. Numerous other cytokines, including tumor necrosis factor (TNF), α-interferon, and IL-6, are also pyrogenic.

Temperatures above 39° C can contribute to host defense by augmenting T cell and B cell activity and leading to cytotoxic T cell generation and immunoglobulin synthesis. In addition, in vitro microbial growth is suppressed at elevated temperatures. Despite these advantages in host defense, fever is often treated with antipyretics and other fever-reducing measures. This is especially true in the critically ill child because fever increases the child's already high metabolic rate. Whether reducing an elevated temperature adversely affects the outcome of patients with fever is debated.[26]

Phagocytosis. The primary role of phagocytic cells is to destroy foreign substances or microorganisms. Once phagocytes are mobilized, the process of phagocytosis may begin. Phagocytosis is multiphasic. Neutrophils (and other white cells) recognize the target to be ingested, attach, ingest, and finally digest the target through a variety of intracellular antimicrobial mechanisms. Phagocytes ingest organisms by nonspecific mechanisms; that is, they are not specifically sensitized to the antigens of the particle they ingest. Fig. 15-3 presents a schematic representation of phagocytosis.

To function effectively, the neutrophil and other phagocytes must be able to migrate to the site of inflammation and then ingest and kill the target cell through bactericidal activity. An important note is that the contact between the phagocyte and the target cell is mediated by opsonins, and phagocytosis of these target cells may be diminished because of the reduced quantities of circulating opsonins, such as complement proteins or immunoglobulins. Although

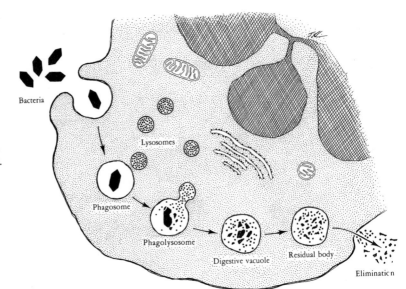

Fig. 15-3 Schematic representation of phagocytosis showing ingestion process and intracellular digestion.

bactericidal activity of the newborn phagocyte has been reported as normal or equal to adult bactericidal activity, strong evidence has shown that bactericidal activity is diminished in the presence of stress or secondary illness, such as respiratory distress syndrome or sepsis.[27,28]

Although the quantity of peripherally circulating neutrophils is similar in the infant and the adult, the infant has considerably smaller numbers of stored neutrophils per kilogram of body weight than the adult. The infant's smaller neutrophil storage pool results in less ability to repeatedly replace the number of circulating neutrophils; therefore the infant's neutrophils can easily be depleted in the face of an infection, leading to neutropenia.

The storage pool of neutrophils also contains various stages of developing neutrophils that are released at a time of need.[29] The result may be the release of neutrophils that are too immature to effectively function during times of increased demand or diminished supply. Release of immature neutrophils can be observed in all patients, but animal data suggest that it may be exaggerated in the infant and young child.

Another developmental difference noted in the inflammatory response is the movement and mobility of phagocytic cells, particularly the neutrophil. Data suggest that the newborn's neutrophil chemotaxis is altered.[30] This neutrophil chemotactic hypoactivity remains unchanged for the first 24 months of life and may not reach adult activity until approximately 16 years of age.[31] Monocyte chemotactic activity in infants and children is less well understood. Klein and co-workers[31] found that monocyte chemotaxis in the infant and young child under the age of 6 years may be extremely poor and significantly less than that of older children and adults.

The available data suggest that the ability of the human neonate to increase neutrophil production in response to infection may be limited.[30] The infant's neutrophils have less ability to aggregate and are less deformable than the adult's.[32] The phagocyte's capacity for deformability is

essential for chemotaxis and for movement through small intercellular spaces. The infant's neutrophil surface is more rigid, which may impair the neutrophil's movements though capillary walls and bone marrow sinusoids. This effect may partially explain impaired chemotaxis and thus the inability to localize infection.

Impaired phagocyte function increases the infant and young child's risk of infection and impairs their ability to localize infection. The clinical consequence is a higher incidence of severe recurrent bacterial infections.

Complement System. The complement system is a complex group of more than 20 interacting proteolytic enzymes and regulating proteins that are found in plasma and extracellular fluids. The complement system, like the coagulation system, reacts sequentially in a series of enzymatic reactions in a cascading manner (Fig. 15-4).

Complement may be activated by several factors, such as the release of plasmin or protease from damaged cells or microorganisms, the formation of antigen-antibody complexes, the presence of viruses or bacteria in the circulation, the release of endotoxin by gram-negative bacteria, or the aggregation of immunoglobulins or platelets. The complement system consists of two separate but interrelated enzyme cascades: the classical pathway and the alternative pathway. Both pathways lead to the generation of C3 and C3b and a final common pathway. Activation of the classical pathway is only initiated by antibody-antigen complexes, whereas the alternative pathway does not have an absolute requirement for antibody for activation.[33] The importance of the alternative pathway is that by not requiring specific antibody, it provides an early protective mechanism that is effective before the development of specific immunity.

Activation of either pathway of the complement cascade leads to enhancement of inflammation, mediation in the opsonization process, mediation of lytic destruction of cells, and assistance in chemotaxis.[34]

Complement proteins gradually increase to 60% to 80% of normal adult levels at birth for the classical pathway and

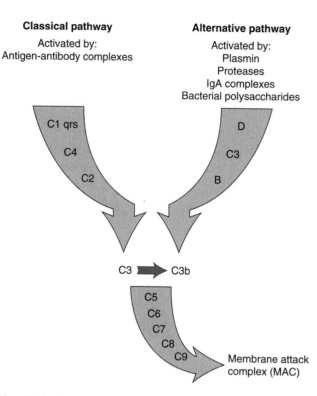

Classical pathway
Activated by:
Antigen-antibody complexes

C1 qrs
C4
C2

Alternative pathway
Activated by:
Plasmin
Proteases
IgA complexes
Bacterial polysaccharides

D
C3
B

C3 → C3b

C5
C6
C7
C8
C9

Membrane attack complex (MAC)

Fig. 15-4 Complement system consists of two separate but interrelated enzyme cascades: classical and alternative pathways. Each is activated by different stimuli, but the result is a final common pathway leading to enhancement of inflammation, assistance in chemotaxis, mediation of opsonization, and target membrane rupture. (Adapted from Frank MM: Complement and kinin. In Stites DP, Terr AI, Parslow TG, eds: *Basic and clinical immunology,* ed 8, Norwalk, Conn, 1994, Appleton & Lange, p. 125.)

lower percentages for the alternative pathway,[30] but serum complement levels are not within normal adult range until about 3 to 6 months of age. Low complement levels at birth may contribute to the newborn's afebrile and absent leukocytic response to infection.

Third Line of Defense

If nonspecific defenses fail, a specific acquired response is triggered. The specific immune response is complex and still not fully understood. Specific immunity is composed of two different mechanisms: humoral immunity (HI), primarily involving the B cell, and cell-mediated immunity (CMI), primarily involving the T cell. Each of these two forms of immunity involves different cells, mediators, and means of function, but significant interaction and interdependence occurs between the two immunities.

The distinguishing features of an acquired immune response are specificity, heterogeneity, and memory. Specificity refers to the characteristic by which an individual lymphocyte responds to its destiny or predetermined antigen. Specific immunity is also characterized by heterogeneity. Heterogeneity is the involvement of a variety of different cells and cell products that work together in diverse ways to protect the host. Memory, an attribute acquired by lymphocytes while participating in a first immune response with an

antigen, enables lymphocytes to recall subsequent exposures to their destiny antigen. This first encounter with an antigen triggers a primary immune response. A second or subsequent exposure to an antigen, occurring months to years later, will stimulate an accelerated and augmented response because of the immunologic memory of lymphocytes.

The third line of defense, specific immunity, is assessed through a comprehensive examination of the patient's history, clinical course, and data from laboratory testing. Laboratory testing is used to reveal the immune system's ability to recognize and process foreign antigens, recall previous exposure to antigens, and produce normal amounts of effector cells to the antigens. The laboratory tests also evaluate the competence of these effector cells to antigens. Testing is often categorized into those tests that measure individual elements of the immune system (quantitative) and those tests that measure the immune response to an antigen (qualitative).

Acquisition of Specific Immunity. Specific immunity may be "acquired" either actively or passively. Specific immunity is acquired actively when the body is exposed to a particular antigen, mounts an immune response to that antigen, and results in the formation of immunologic effector and memory cells. Contracting mumps or receiving a vaccine is an example of actively acquiring specific immunity. Specific immunity also may be acquired passively through the transfer of sensitized cells or their products (i.e., immunoglobulin) from one person to another. Maternal transfer of antibody across the placenta to the fetus is an example of passively acquiring specific immunity. The characteristics of passive and active specific immunity are contrasted in Table 15-6.

Components of Acquired Immunity. The specific immune response (Fig. 15-5) is often divided into three phases or limbs: afferent, central, and efferent. The afferent limb involves the recognition and presentation of an antigen to the B cell or T cell. The central limb involves the cloning and differentiation of activated cells, as well as the production and release of cytokines. The efferent limb involves the actual elimination of the target cell or antigen. Memory cells are developed during the central and efferent limbs of the specific immune response.

Recognition Phase (Afferent Limb). The first phase of the specific immune response involves the recognition and processing of the antigen. Each lymphocyte (B cell, helper T cell, and cytotoxic T cell) requires the formation of a complex with the antigen-presenting cell and antigen to recognize the antigen as foreign and begin the activation process. The manner in which a B cell and a T cell recognize an antigen is different.

The B cell recognizes its destiny antigen when the antigen contacts the immunoglobulin projecting from the B cell's surface. Although most B cell recognition of antigens occurs with great assistance from the T cells, certain antigens can trigger B cells with little T cell assistance. This response is sometimes called "T cell independent" activation and occurs most often with exposure to encapsulated bacteria, such as *Haemophilus influenzae* and *Streptococcus pneumoniae.* B cells activated in this

TABLE 15-6   Comparison of Passive and Active Immunity

	Passive	Active
Genesis	No participation of the host; a transfer of preformed substances or sensitized cells from an immunized host to a nonimmune host	Active participation of host following exposure to antigen either naturally (subclinical or clinical disease) or by immunization (vaccination)
Components of humoral and cell-mediated immunity	Cells and their products (immunoglobulin and cytokines)	Effector cells (helper T cells, cytotoxic T cells, B cells) and memory cells and their respective products
Onset of action	Immediate	Delayed, following recognition and preparation phase of acquired immunity
Duration	Temporary	Long lived
Clinical application	IVIg in immune deficiency states Prophylaxis, such as hepatitis B immunoglobulin, VZV immunoglobulin	Vaccination

Modified from Herscowitz HB: Immunophysiology: cell function and cellular interactions in antibody formation. In Bellanti J, ed: *Immunology III,* Philadelphia, 1985, WB Saunders, p 117.
IVIg, Intravenous immunoglobulin; *VZV,* varicella zoster virus.

manner do not form memory cells to protect against future exposure to the microbe; in addition, these B cells can only produce the IgM class of antibody.

In contrast to the B cell, T cells recognize antigen only when the antigen is combined with HLAs. Class II HLAs are required for helper T cell activation, whereas class I HLAs are required for cytotoxic T cell activation.

Helper T cell antigen recognition begins with a macrophage ingesting an antigen and converting (processing) the antigen into a form that is easily recognized by the helper T cell. The macrophage reexpresses the antigen on its cell membrane along with the class II HLA DR antigen. The antigen-HLA complex is then presented to the unprimed helper T cell and combines with the T cell destiny antigen receptor. Helper T cell antigen recognition is also facilitated by numerous cytokines, such as IL 1, which is produced by the macrophage during its processing of the antigen. Other signals may be required for helper T cell activation and are the focus of intense research.

Cytotoxic T cells require antigen to be combined with class I HLAs. For example, a cell infected with a virus projects viral antigens on its surface in combination with the cell's class I HLAs. The antigen-HLA complex is then presented to the appropriate, unprimed cytotoxic T cell and combines with the T cell destiny antigen receptor. IL 2, produced by the helper T cell, serves as a second signal for the cytotoxic T cell.

In utero, maternal host defense mechanisms shield the fetus from exposure to environmental antigens, and the placenta provides a shield from maternal host defenses. Although the infant is born with the capacity to perform nonspecific host defenses, the product of immunologic experience (specific host defense) is acquired. Before 7 to 12 weeks of gestation, exclusively the mother must provide protection against infection. Further protection of the developing fetus is provided by transplacentally acquired maternal IgG. Beginning at 8 to 10 weeks and accelerating

during the last trimester, this placental transfer is active and specific for IgG. By 14 weeks of gestation, the thymic cortex and medulla are demarcated and B lymphocytes in blood reach normal adult levels.

Preparation Phase (Central Limb). Once an antigen is presented to the unprimed lymphocyte, the second phase of the specific immune response, the preparation phase, begins. During this phase, lymphocytes undergo activation, cloning, and differentiation to form effector cells and memory cells. (The cloning of lymphocytes during the preparation phase accounts for the lymphadenopathy that accompanies infection. The lymph nodes are swollen because of the extensive cloning of the activated B and T cells.) Fig. 15-6 is a review of the primary and secondary clonal expansion of lymphocytes in response to an antigen.

Produced by activated lymphocytes, cytokines function as regulators of the immune response. They serve as intercellular signals to support the growth and differentiation of various immune cells, the cytotoxic mechanisms of killer cells, and other effector cell functions.

In the past, certain cytokines were believed to be produced only by the lymphocytes; these were referred to as lymphokines. Others were believed to be produced only by monocytes or macrophages and were referred to as monokines. Lymphokines and monokines are now known to be produced by many classes of cells; hence, the term *cytokines* is the most accurate. However, the terms *lymphokine* and *monokine* continue to be commonly used.

Effector cells are immune cells that produce the expected result of antigen destruction. Effector cells include helper T cells, which augment the entire immune response; B cells, which indirectly attack the invader through the secretion of antibody from plasma cells; and cytotoxic T cells, which directly attack the invader. The preparation phase culminates with the creation of effector cells for effective and efficient elimination of the target. Memory cells produced

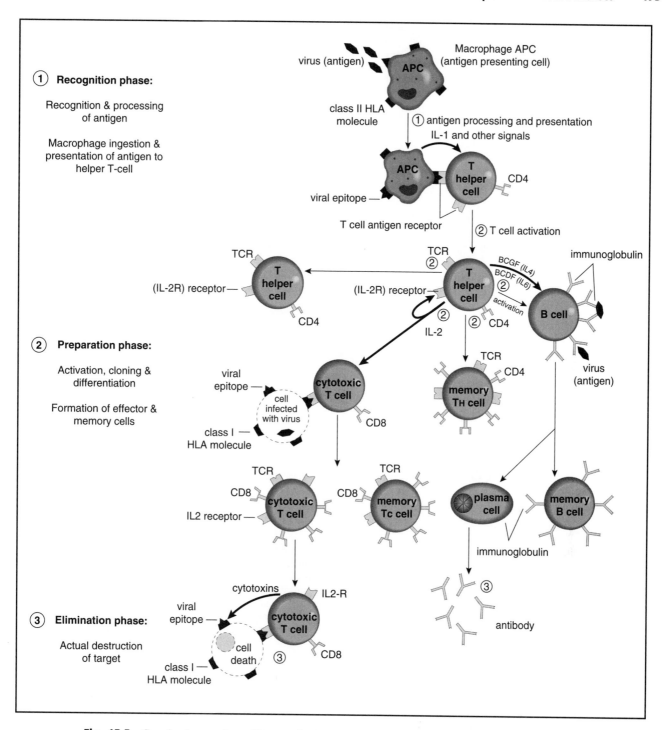

Fig. 15-5   Grand scheme of specific, acquired immunity is made up of humoral (immunoglobulin) immunity (HI), orchestrated by the B cell, and cell-mediated immunity (CMI), orchestrated by the T cell. Note the interdependence between the B and T cells. The three phases of specific immune response are indicated by the numbers in the figure: (1) recognition phase, (2) preparation phase, and (3) elimination phase. Activated helper T cell expresses IL-2 receptors and produces B cell growth factor *(BCGF)* (IL-4) and B cell differentiation factor *(BCDF)* (IL-6). B cell activation usually requires three signals: following the binding of the B cell with its destiny antigen (first signal), BCGF (second signal) stimulates proliferation of the B cell. BCDF (third signal) induces differentiation. Two signals are needed for cytotoxic T cell activation, binding of the cytotoxic T cell receptor with the class I HLA–antigen complex and IL-2 production. The activated helper T cell expresses IL-2 receptors and produces IL-2, which triggers cloning of helper T cells and production of cytokines, such as BCDF (IL-4) and BCGF (IL-6). (Adapted from Goodman JW: The immune response. In Stites DP, Terr AI, Parslow TG, eds: *Basic and clinical immunology,* ed 8, Norwalk, Conn, 1994, Appleton & Lange, p. 43.)

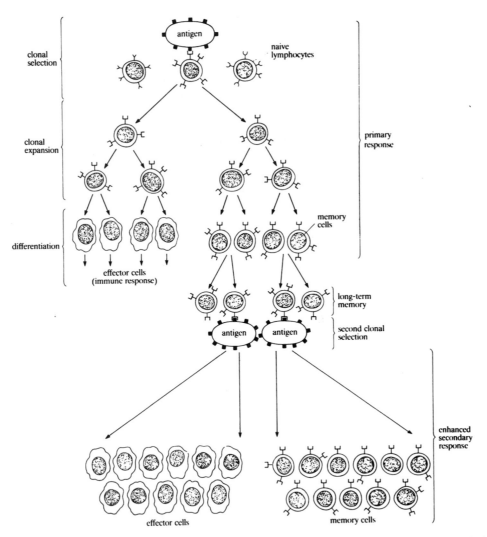

Fig. 15-6   T cells and B cells carrying specific antigen receptors are produced in the primary lymphoid organs and from the unprimed lymphocyte pool. After activation by their destiny antigens, lymphocytes clone and differentiate into either effector cells (e.g., cytotoxic T cells, helper T cells, or antibody-secreting plasma cells) or memory cells. This cellular proliferation constitutes the primary response. When memory cells are again stimulated by their destiny antigens, they will clone also (secondary response). Some of these memory cells mature into effector cells, whereas other memory cells remain as memory cells, thus increasing the size of both effector and memory cell pools. (From Davey B: *Immunology: a foundation text,* Englewood Cliffs, NJ, 1990, Prentice Hall, p. 23.)

after activation circulate throughout the body to survey for subsequent encounters with that antigen.

Activation of helper T cells occurs early in the immune response because of their pivotal role in the orchestration of many other immunologic events. For instance, activated helper T cells secrete IL-2, which assists in the cloning and differentiation of themselves, other helper T cells, and cytotoxic T cells. Activated helper T cells also play a key role in B cell activation through the secretion of B cell growth factor (BCGF) and B cell differentiation factor (BCDF) and other cytokines.

Two communication signals are required for activation of the helper T cell. One signal is completed through the binding of the helper T cell with the macrophage. The second signal is obtained through the secretion of IL-1, which is produced during macrophage processing of the

antigen. These two signals result in helper T cell expression of IL-2 receptors on its surface membrane and the production of IL-2. The primary function of IL-2 is to amplify the response initiated by the binding of the helper T cell and macrophage and to amplify the growth of additional helper T cells expressing IL-2 receptors.

Most often, activation of the B cell requires three signals: one signal from the antigen and two (or more) signals from the activated helper T cell. After the binding of the B cell with its destiny antigen, BCGF (IL-4) stimulates proliferation of the B cell. BCDF (IL-6) induces the activated B cell to differentiate into antibody-secreting plasma cells. A number of B cells do not differentiate into plasma cells but form a pool of memory cells. The speculation is that these memory cells receive insufficient amounts of BCDF to become antibody-secreting plasma cells.[35]

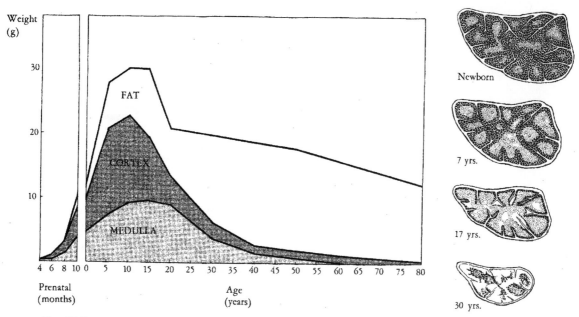

Fig. 15-7 Schematic representation of changes in weight and composition of the thymus gland with maturation, showing involution of gland with age. (From Bellanti JA, Kadlec JV: General immunobiology. In Bellanti J, ed: *Immunology III,* Philadelphia, 1985, WB Saunders, p. 44.)

Activation of the cytotoxic T cell, like that of the helper T cell, requires two signals. The first signal is the binding of the cytotoxic T cell receptor with the class I antigen complex; the second signal results from the IL-2 produced after helper T cell activation.

Developmental alterations of the central limb are primarily noted in the development of lymphoid cell lines and their respective function. Cytokine production and release (IL-1, IL-2, BCGF, and BCDF) necessary for activation, differentiation, and cloning of lymphocytes are intact and effective.

By the ninth gestational week, the thymus has begun to develop and becomes populated with precursor T cells, called thymocytes. Direct contact with the various regions of the thymus epithelium is thought to be required for development of mature T cells. The thymocytes mature as they progress from the outer to inner regions of the thymus. Within the thymus, there are three distinct stages of thymocyte differentiation, described according to their surface markers.[36,37] The most immature thymocytes are found in the periphery of the cortex. Mature thymocytes are found in the thymic medulla and express either the CD4 or the CD8 surface marker. These cells also express class I HLAs.[36-38] Fig. 15-7 shows a pictorial representation of thymus gland changes with age.

The numbers of mature T cells gradually increase in the fetal circulation with gestational age. However, the numbers of T cells present at birth vary and may depend on the method used for measurement. Sources reporting slightly elevated levels, compared with that of an adult, state that this finding is related to the increased numbers of suppressor T cells found in the newborn.[20,39] Other sources report significantly lower percentages than those found in the adult.[40]

Alterations in T cell response can be illustrated by delayed hypersensitivity skin testing in which the infant and young child may not react to certain intradermal antigens. Altered helper T cell response may also be illustrated clinically by altered B cell production of immunoglobulin. Because helper T cells play a key role in influencing the class of immunoglobulin that is made, a deficiency in helper T cells (number or function) can result in an alteration in the type of immunoglobulin produced by B cells. A normal mature response is the elicitation of an IgM antibody response followed by an IgG antibody response within 6 to 7 days. In the newborn, the IgM response can last for 20 to 30 days with no subsequent IgG response. This diminished reaction was previously thought to be solely the result of lack of previous antigen exposure; however, the reduced number and function of helper T cells also contribute.

B cell differentiation is a discontinuous process that occurs in two distinct stages: antigen-independent and antigen-dependent phases. The first stage, which is genetically predetermined, involves the differentiation of stem cells into pre–B cells. Although the first stage of B cell differentiation begins in the fetal liver, further B cell differentiation occurs in the bone marrow when that location becomes the primary site of hematopoiesis (at 20 weeks' gestation).[38] The earliest cells committed to antibody production are termed pre–B cells, and they lack surface immunoglobulins.[41] B cells with surface immunoglobulin are found in the fetal peripheral blood, bone marrow, and spleen by the eleventh week of gestation but are generally restricted to the IgM class. As development continues, the remaining classes and subclasses of immunoglobulin appear on the surface of the mature B cell clones.

The second stage of B cell differentiation is initiated by the binding of an antigen to the unprimed, resting B cell. After contact with antigen, activated B cells clone and differentiate into plasma cells to secrete antibody from a

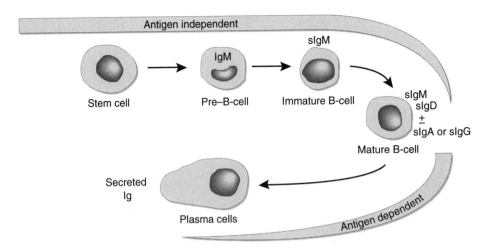

Fig. 15-8 Developmental stages of B cells. Diagram depicts discontinuous stages of development: antigen independent and antigen dependent. Earliest cells are termed pre–B cells and contain immunoglobulin M *(IgM)* in their cytoplasm. Immature B cells contain IgM on their surface *(sIgM)*. As development continues, remaining classes of immunoglobulin appear on the surface of mature B cell clones (also depicted with an *s* before *Ig*). The antigen-dependent phase begins antigen binding to the unprimed mature B cell, which then differentiates into plasma cells and memory cells (not depicted in figure). (Redrawn from Lawton AR. In Twomey JJ, ed: *The pathophysiology of human immunologic disorders.* Baltimore, 1982, Urban & Schwarzenberg.)

TABLE 15-7   Serum Immunoglobulins in the Fetus, at Birth, and Age With Mature Levels

Ig	Synthesis by Fetus (Gestation—Weeks)	% of Adult Levels at Birth	Age at Which Adult Levels Are Achieved
IgM	10.5 weeks	10%	1-2 years
IgD	14 weeks	Small amount	1 year
IgG*	12 weeks	110%†	4-10 years
IgA	30 weeks	Small amount or none	6-15 years
IgE	10.5 weeks	Small amount	6-15 years

From Rosenthal CH: Immunosuppression in the pediatric critical care patient, *Crit Care Nurs Clin North Am* 1:775, 1989.
*Crosses placenta.
†Greater than or equal to maternal level.

single immunoglobulin class or into memory B cells. Fig. 15-8 presents B cell differentiation.

Despite early differentiation of the B cell population, the infant's B cells are deficient in producing comparable adult levels and subclasses of immunoglobulins. Serum Ig levels and degree of synthesis at birth and the age in which the levels are comparable to the adult are reflected in Table 15-7. Although the IgG level seems comparable in the newborn and adult, the level reflects the transplacental acquisition of maternal antibody during, primarily, the third trimester of gestation. The infant is lowest in immunoglobulin concentrations at about 4 to 5 months of age when maternal IgG begins to decrease through natural catabolism and when infant synthesis of immunoglobulin is low.[30] This period is referred to as one of physiologic hypogammaglobulinemia, and during this time, the infant is most susceptible to infections caused by viruses, *Candida,* and acute inflammatory bacteria *(Staphylococcus aureus, S. haemolyticus, Streptococcus pneumoniae, H. influenzae* type B, and *Neisseria*

meningitidis). This state can range in duration from patient to patient and can be prolonged to such an extent that the young child suffers from recurrent and severe infections.

Numerous explanations are given for minimal synthesis of fetal and newborn immunoglobulin. The rare numbers of plasma cells and small amount of immunoglobulin synthesized by the fetus are thought to reflect the normally sterile intrauterine environment and lack of antigenic exposure in utero.[40] Maternal antibodies in the newborn's circulation may exert a strong immunosuppressive effect on the infant's ability to mount an independent immune response and to subsequently produce antibodies. In addition, the dominance of newborn suppressor T cells[20] and bilirubin levels higher than 15 mg/dl[42] have also been implicated in the increased numbers of newborn immature B cells and decreased Ig production.

As the infant's exposure to antigen increases, a repertoire of antibodies to antigens is developed, and the memory component to humoral immunity is heightened through the development of the various IgG subclasses. Intrauterine infection may also accelerate the fetus's immunoglobulin production dramatically. Following intrauterine infection and the experience with such intense antigenic stimulation, the infant may be born with adult levels of IgM and increased levels of IgG and IgA.[38]

Elimination Phase (Efferent Limb). The actual elimination of the target cell or antigen occurs in the efferent limb of the specific immune response. To ensure effective destruction of the antigen, the efferent limb usually consists of a dual response by circulating antibody (HI) and effector T cells (CMI). Specific immunity elimination of the antigen occurs through the mechanisms of immunoregulation, cytotoxicity, and memory.

Immunoregulation. Immunoregulation is not well understood but appears to be the fine balance and feedback that occur between the helper T cells and suppressor T cells. When properly balanced, there is just enough of an immune response to eliminate the invading organism but not enough to cause host injury.

Data on the immunoregulatory function of pediatric T cells are complex. Investigators note that adult T cells are better equipped than newborn T cells at helping B cells synthesize immunoglobulin.[43] Newborn T cells exhibit more suppressor activity compared with adults. Controversy exists regarding the basis of these findings. These findings may be partly related to newborn helper T cells being less functional (see Cytotoxicity), whereas other investigators suspect an intrinsically more functional suppressor T cell or enhanced suppressor T cell function as a remnant of fetal life. Altman, Handzel, and Levin[44] suggest that the fetus has increased suppressor T cell activity to prevent maternal rejection, but this increased suppressor activity remains apparent after birth. In summary, this question remains: Is increased newborn suppressor T cell activity (1) the result of the immaturity of newborn helper T cells; (2) related to newborn suppressor T cells being intrinsically more active than those of adults; or (3) a remnant of fetal life to prevent maternal rejection?

Cytotoxicity. The actual killing of antigen is accomplished through cytotoxic T cell activity and is sometimes called cell-mediated cytotoxicity. Cell-mediated cytotoxicity includes three basic yet distinct phases: (1) the effector cell binds to the target or antigen; (2) it degranulates, showering the target cell membrane with toxins that destroy the antigen; and (3) certain cytokines are released by activated cytotoxic T cells (i.e., TNF and γ-interferon), which can, by themselves, cause direct cytotoxic effects and death of the targeted cell.[45]

Cytotoxicity is diminished in the newborn period,[40] whether the elimination of the target is through the activity of the cytotoxic T cell, NK cell, or antibody-dependent cellular cytotoxicity (ADCC) (see Antibody-Antigen Interaction). The reason for this finding is unknown but may be related to the newborn T cell's diminished ability to produce cytokines, such as γ-interferon and IL-4.[38,46] Reduced γ-interferon appears to be related to the reduced numbers of memory T cells. As previously reviewed, once the macrophage presents the antigen to the helper T cell, the activated

T cell secretes γ-interferon and IL-2. γ-Interferon subsequently activates the macrophages to ingest and kill the invading intracellular pathogen. Macrophages that are not γ-interferon activated do not kill as efficiently. The clinical consequence of this phenomenon is a diminution of macrophage antiviral properties[39,47] and may contribute to the severity of viral illness seen in many newborns.

Although NK cell activity is diminished, cytotoxic activity from LAK cells is not diminished. The addition of IL-2 in vitro to nonspecific lymphocytes results in the recruitment of cells that display strong nonspecific cytotoxic activity. Newborns have been found to have an equivalent, if not a heightened, degree of LAK cell cytotoxic activity.[48]

Antibody-Antigen Interaction. The six major antibody antigen interactions are neutralization, agglutination, precipitation, opsonization, complement fixation, and lysis. When antibody neutralizes a microorganism, it renders the microorganism ineffective or incapable of action. Thus when enough antibody molecules bind to a microorganism, it may no longer pose a risk to a host cell. Antibody may also bind to toxins, thus preventing the toxin from attaching to and poisoning a host cell. Antibody can also agglutinate or precipitate an antigen, rendering it inactive by causing it to form clumps or solidify, respectively.

Antibody greatly enhances nonspecific immune responses. For instance, opsonization, the process in which antibody coats the antigen, greatly enhances the ability of phagocytes to engulf the foreign particle. The binding of antibody to antigen may also lead to activation of the complement cascade. Certain complement components produced in this process are tremendously important in enhancing phagocytosis through opsonization, attracting phagocytes through chemotaxis, and lysing bacteria.

Antibody molecules can be instrumental in destroying an antigen through ADCC. During this process, the variable segment (Fab) of the antibody molecule attaches to an antigen while the constant segment (Fc) fits into the Fc receptor on a monocyte, neutrophil, eosinophil, NK cell, or cytotoxic T cell. This antibody Fc receptor connection stimulates the involved immune cell (monocyte, neutrophil, eosinophil, NK cell, or cytotoxic T cell) to release poisonous chemicals to destroy the antigen by lysis.

As previously mentioned, ADCC depends on antibody (immunoglobulin). The diminished ability of newborns to destroy target cells via ADCC is related to reduced levels of antibody or reduced B cell production of immunoglobulin. Clinical ramifications of this finding include the increased number of bacterial infections noted in infants.

Memory. Memory cells reside in the host to await subsequent exposures to their destiny antigen. The memory cell reacts in subsequent exposures to that antigen by producing an augmented response, as compared with the primary exposure.

The secondary response to an antigen characteristically differs from the primary response in that there is a shorter latent period, a more rapid rate of antibody synthesis, and a higher peak titer of antibody that persists for a longer period. In addition, the dose of the antigen required to elicit a secondary response is normally much less than that required to initiate a primary response. These differences are directly related to the number of antigen-sensitive cells, called memory cells.

The infant and young child have fewer memory cells. The reduced secondary immune response in these patients may be the result of either the reduced numbers of memory cells or a reduced effectiveness of these cells during secondary immune response.

DIAGNOSING DYSFUNCTION

Laboratory Tests

White Blood Cell Count

Total WBC Count.   The normal total WBC count is 5000 to 10,000 cells/mm^3 and may vary, depending on the time of day. However, total WBC count varies with the age of the infant and young child. The WBC count only reflects the circulating WBCs, not those WBCs marginated to vessel walls, circulating in the lymphatic system, or sequestered in body tissues. As a general screening test for immune function, the total WBC count serves as an indicator of the inflammatory response or disease states, presence of an infection, and response to therapy.

Increases and decreases in the total WBC count from normal levels are called leukocytosis and leukopenia, respectively. Leukocytosis is usually the result of an increase in one type of WBC rather than a proportional increase in all types of WBCs and commonly indicates the presence of infection. Leukocytosis can result from release of additional WBCs from the bone marrow in response to infection, trauma, and physical or emotional stress, but it also can be the result of increased production of abnormal WBCs, as in leukemia. Any condition that increases blood flow or cardiac output will result in the recruitment of WBCs into the circulation from the marginating pool. Leukopenia, on the other hand, is associated with conditions that either depress the bone marrow's hematopoietic function or stress the bone marrow by exceeding bone marrow supplies or ability to replenish supplies.

Differential WBC Count.   The differential WBC count is a report of the five different types of WBCs (neutrophils, basophils, eosinophils, monocytes, and lymphocytes) as a percentage of the total WBC count. The reported percentage for each cell type determines the number of mature circulating WBCs and the absolute number of the various types of WBCs. The differential count evaluates the bone marrow's ability to produce those particular cells. The differential WBC count also reflects the morphology of cells, such as the presence of abnormal WBCs or atypical lymphocytes. Lymphocyte subclasses are not a component of the differential WBC count and are not routinely quantified because the process requires specialized equipment. However, the AIDS epidemic has increased the availability of lymphocyte subclass measurements because these measurements are integral to treatment decisions in these patients. Neutropenia, rather than neutrophilia, is a common observation noted in septic newborns and young infants. This finding is most likely the result of several mechanisms, including depletion of a relatively small neutrophil storage pool, a disturbed regulation of bone marrow release, and an inability of the stem cells to proliferate at a faster rate.[49]

Under certain clinical conditions, the WBC differential may reveal an excess of immature WBCs or an excess of aged WBCs. These alterations are often referred to as "shifts." The presence of an excess number of immature cells (bands) is called a "shift to the left." It is usually an indication of severe infection in which an increased quantity of immature neutrophils is released from the bone marrow. The more severe the infection, the greater the shift to the left noted in the differential count. A "right shift" usually refers to an increased number of circulating mature neutrophils, which can be observed in patients experiencing pernicious anemia, morphine addiction, or vitamin deficiency (folate or B$_{12}$).

On the other hand, some clinicians use the term *right shift* in a different context. Instead of viewing a shift as a reflection of the developmental stage of neutrophils (immature versus mature), a shift is viewed as the type of cell excessively prominent. In this context, a "right shift" indicates lymphocytosis seen in viral infections. Considering the different meanings, it is important and accurate to describe the laboratory observation rather than merely stating "shift to the right" or "shift to the left."

Absolute Neutrophil Count.   The absolute neutrophil count (ANC) quantifies the total number of circulating neutrophils per cubic millimeter. The ANC includes mature neutrophils ("polys" and "segs") and immature neutrophils ("bands"). The ANC serves as a reliable barometer of the patient's degree of risk of infection in that the lower the cell count and the longer the time the patient experiences the neutropenic state, the higher the patient's risk of infection. In general, the risk of infection significantly increases if the ANC falls to certain levels (slightly increased with an ANC of 1500/mm^3, moderately increased with an ANC of 1000/mm^3, and greatly increased with an ANC of 500/mm^3). However, the patient's primary disease process also influences the risk of infection. Patients with a low ANC are at high risk of infection from their own GI flora in addition to exogenous gram-negative bacteria; gram-positive bacteria, such as *S. aureus* and *S. epidermitis;* and fungal infections, such as from *Candida* and *Aspergillus*. To calculate an ANC, see Table 15-8. The absolute cell count may be determined for any cell type using the same process shown in Table 15-8.

Absolute Lymphocyte Count and Lymphocyte Subsets.   Although lymphocyte counts were once thought to be comparable in patients of all ages, recent evidence refutes this belief. This is exemplified in the change in prophylaxis of *Pneumocystis carinii* pneumonia in infants and children with HIV infection. Prophylaxis in young children is no longer started at lymphocyte counts below 200 cells/mm^3 but rather at higher and more age-appropriate levels. Apparently, although the total lymphocyte count and lymphocyte subsets are an equivalent percentage of the total WBC count in all ages of patients, the infant and young child's higher WBC count yields greater absolute numbers

TABLE 15-8   Calculation of Absolute Neutrophil Count (ANC)

1. Obtain patient's total WBC count.	WBC = 5 k/mm³
2. Translate the total WBC count into an absolute number ("k" means 1000 cells).	5 × 1000 = 5000 Absolute WBC count = 5000/mm³
3. Obtain WBC differential* and add the percentages of "polys" plus "bands."†	Polys = 60% Bands = 10% 60% + 10% = 70%
4. Translate the percentage of "polys" plus "bands" into an absolute number by dividing by 100.	70% ÷ 100 = 0.7
5. Multiply the absolute WBC count by the absolute "poly" plus "band" count.	5000 × 0.7 = 3500 ANC = 3500/mm³

*Generally, the WBC differential count is based on a sample of 100 cells. In persons with severe leukopenia, the differential count may be based on a sample of 50 cells. Conversely, in persons with leukocytosis, the differential count may be based on a sample of 200 cells. Regardless of the number of cells used for the count, the individual cells will represent an overall percentage of the total, and the same procedure outlined above is used to determine an ANC.
†Although bands are immature neutrophils, they are included in the ANC because they are relatively functional.

of lymphocytes and subsets of lymphocytes. Therefore age is an important consideration in the interpretation of the total lymphocyte count and subsets of lymphocytes, especially in children with HIV infection.[50,51]

Other Laboratory Tests

Erythrocyte Sedimentation Rate. The erythrocyte sedimentation rate (ESR) is a laboratory test that is a nonspecific indicator of systemic inflammation. In many cases, the ESR is so nonspecific that it has little clinical use. However, in the immunocompromised child, it may be one of the few objective measurements of response to therapy or relapse. The ESR is useful as a prognostic marker for evaluating the resolution of certain infectious diseases during therapy (e.g., osteomyelitis).

C-Reactive Protein. C-reactive protein (CRP) is normally present in low levels in serum; levels increase several hundred times within 6 to 8 hours after onset of infection or injury. With successful antimicrobial treatment, CRP levels fall rapidly. A normal CRP or ESR level does not exclude a pathologic condition.

Complement System. The complement system is sometimes evaluated because of the pivotal role these proteins play in the inflammatory response and in humoral immunity. The most common test of the function of the entire complement cascade is the CH_{50}, which measures the function of the classical and terminal complement pathways. When defects in the alternative pathway are being considered, an analogous test evaluating alternative-pathway function is requested.[34] Individual complement proteins,

such as C3 and C4, can be quantified and the function of certain complement components evaluated. C4 levels are critical to the function of the classical pathway, with normal serum levels ranging from 10 to 30 mg/dl. A reduction of levels of individual complement proteins or CH_{50} can be the result of either underproduction of complement or excess complement activation or both. Therefore additional complement function testing may be necessary to identify the exact nature of the presenting patient problem. Serum complement activity is reduced in preterm infants in proportion to the magnitude of their immaturity.[52] In contrast, complement levels in healthy full-term infants range from 60% to 100% of those in healthy adults.

Total Immunoglobulin Levels. The total Ig level and levels for the various classes and subclasses can be determined. Normal Ig levels vary with age; therefore use of age-adjusted values is imperative for all comparisons. Ig levels can be diagnostic for congenital primary immunodeficiencies. However, if Ig levels are normal despite suspected immunodeficiency, an examination of the function and effectiveness of the immunoglobulin to an antigen may be indicated (qualitative testing).

Serologic Testing. Serologic testing for either antibodies or antigens can also be performed to detect current or past infection (bacterial, viral, fungal, or parasitic). A well-known example of serologic testing is the enzyme-linked immunosorbent assay (ELISA) that is used to screen blood products for and identify persons infected with HIV. The presence of antigens of a particular organism is an indication that the patient is currently infected with that organism. For example, the presence of *Clostridium difficile* toxin in the stool indicates the child is infected with *C. difficile.*

The presence of antibodies to a microorganism indicates an infection; the particular class of antibody can indicate if the infection occurred in the past, is occurring acutely, or is chronic. During an acute infection the initial manufactured Ig is IgM. If the infection is particularly severe, the microorganism's antigens may overwhelm and exceed the neutralizing capacity of antibody, resulting in the presence of measurable antigen in the serum. Later, the main Ig manufactured is IgG, and the antigen will no longer be measurable because the immune response successfully eradicated the infection. A child with an acute CMV infection will have anti-CMV IgM, whereas anti-CMV IgG would indicate past CMV infection. During chronic infections, the serum may contain both IgG and IgM antibodies to the microorganism, as well as antigens of the microorganism.

Delayed Hypersensitivity Testing. Cell-mediated immune function (T cell responsiveness) is evaluated by using delayed hypersensitivity (DH) skin testing. Testing involves the intradermal administration of antigens and is reliable in children who are over 1 year of age. The premise of DH skin testing is that if sensitized T cells to that antigen are present, the injection will cause the body to mount an inflammatory response. DH skin testing is performed by using one or more of the following widely accepted antigens injected intradermally: intermediate-strength *Candida,* *Trichophyton,* tetanus, streptococcal antigens, or mumps antigen. Because DH response depends on the T cell's prior exposure to the specific antigen, as well as normal cellular chemotaxis, remembering developmental differences in the infant and young child is imperative. The demonstration of intact DH skin testing confirms the presence of functional CD4+ T cells and excludes most of the congenital defects in cell-mediated immunity.[53]

In contrast to DH skin testing, immediate hypersensitivity testing determines a patient's sensitivity to allergens such as dust, and animal hair. DH and immediate hypersensitivity skin testing differ in purpose, immune cells involved, antigens used, technique of administration, and the time that the tests are read.

Chest Radiograph.   The chest radiograph is a valuable tool for assessing the second line of defense. However, just as other signs and symptoms of infection are masked during neutropenia, the chest radiograph may be unreliable in revealing pneumonia in the immunocompromised child, particularly the child with neutropenia. The immune response in the neutropenic child may be so diminished that even in a child with fulminant pneumonia, the chest film may appear normal. In this patient population, once the neutrophil count begins to increase to a near-normal level, the chest x-ray film result may often worsen, revealing the existing pneumonia.

SUPPORT OF IMMUNE FUNCTION

Support of the immune system includes maintaining external barriers, infection control procedures, and manipulation or augmentation of the immune system. Maintenance of these practices help to limit the incidence of nosocomial infections that can result from impaired host defenses.

Maintain External Barriers

The incidence of nosocomial infection reflects the numerous invasions of the child's natural barriers (first line of defense). Intact skin and mucous membranes can be preserved by maintaining adequate perfusion and oxygenation and accurate fluid intake (including modification for fever and daily insensible water losses). The pediatric intensive care unit (PICU) nurse most often performs a complete assessment of the child's skin integrity during the daily bath and associated activities. Any sign of redness or disruption in the skin are monitored. Adding small measures to routine nursing care can contribute significantly to host defense. For example, using a nonacetone adhesive remover when loosening tape or electrodes (ensuring that this solution is removed) and skin preparation solutions before applying dressings can preserve the outer layers of the child's epidermis. Routine and careful mouth, eye, and perineal care may protect the child's mucous membranes and body orifices.

Endotracheal tube (ETT) intubation affects the first and second lines of defense by directly bypassing the respiratory tract's local host defenses, increasing the incidence of bacterial colonization, and acting as a foreign object in the airway. In bypassing the upper respiratory tract, the ETT facilitates direct access of microorganisms to the lower respiratory tract. The presence of the ETT decreases the effectiveness of the cough reflex by interfering with glottic closure. Local mucosal irritation and trauma and repeated introduction of suction catheters impede the function of the mucociliary transport.[54]

Respiratory secretions and the ETT itself can act as reservoirs for bacteria, specifically *Pseudomonas aeruginosa.*[55-57] Proliferation of bacteria occurs because the ETT serves as a haven for bacteria growth and is sequestered from host defenses and antibiotics.[58] Colonization of the child's airway occurs within 72 hours of intubation.[59]

Aspiration of bacteria from a previously colonized oropharynx or tracheobronchial tree constitutes the cause of the majority of nosocomial pneumonias. Despite inflation of the cuff, aspiration around an ETT cuff can occur.[60] With the use of uncuffed ETTs in the pediatric population, the incidence of aspiration can be assumed to occur often. One survey reports aspiration in up to 70% in intubated infants and children.[61]

The mere presence of the ETT can lead to increased mucous secretion, stagnation of mucus, airway inflammation, and tracheal mucosal injury.[60] As a reflex to any foreign object in the airway, secretion of mucus is increased and results in stagnation and pooling. The tracheal mucosa may be traumatized by the pistonlike motion of the ETT tip along the tract of tube insertion during breathing, as well as by cuff injury (in the older child) to the tracheal wall. This mechanical trauma evokes an inflammatory response and bacterial colonization.[60,62] Pistonlike motion may be increased in the younger critically ill child because of the presence of an uncuffed ETT.

Promoting the evacuation and cleansing of organ systems such as the respiratory, GI, and genitourinary tracts is vital. Each of these epithelial-lined tracts is protected with a combination of secretory IgA, lactoferrin, lysozyme, and acidic lipid secretions that decrease pathogen takeover. Recognizing the importance of pulmonary, gut, bowel, and urinary evacuation in limiting the growth of enteric flora can diminish the child's risk of infection.[63-65] Nursing interventions may include implementing pulmonary toilet, maintaining adequate hydration, monitoring bowel activity, establishing a bowel routine, and facilitating the patency and functioning of the GI or urinary drainage systems.

Narcotics, often used to facilitate artificial ventilation, affect the function of cilia and pulmonary macrophages. Lack of movement increases the risk for atelectasis and subsequent superinfections. Antacids and H_2 blockers alter gastric acidity and thus alter the gastric fibra. Chest tubes also contribute to poor clearance of respiratory secretions by creating resistance to chest wall movement because of pain and immobility.[66] The result is poor clearance of respiratory secretions, decreased compliance with pulmonary toilet exercises, and thus increased incidence of pneumonias.

The presence and duration of use of intravascular lines significantly increase the child's risk for bacteremia and, subsequently, nosocomial infection. Infection rates are highest when catheters are placed under emergency conditions. All catheters must pass through the first line of defense, the epithelial surface, either through direct percutaneous or surgical cutdown insertion. With the passage of the catheter through the skin surface, the catheter has the potential to become colonized with indigenous or hospital-acquired flora. In addition, a fibrin sheath soon forms around the inserted catheter and provides an environment for bacterial growth and migration down the catheter and toward the bloodstream. These catheters may also become contaminated through the infusing solution or entry sites, such as stopcocks and injection ports, and by microorganisms from other infected sites in the body.[67,67a]

The 1996 Centers for Disease Control and Prevention (CDC) Guidelines for Prevention of Intravascular-Device-Related Infection suggest that intravenous tubing and transducers of regular intravenous fluids be changed only every 72 hours; lipids, blood, and blood products be changed every 24 hours; and dressings be replaced only when the dressings becomes damp, loosened, or soiled. The guidelines make no recommendations for frequency of catheter replacement except for pulmonary artery catheters, which is 5 days.[68]

Many critically ill children require nasogastric (NG) tube placement, and the result is essentially the same in all patients, regardless of age. Tubes placed through the nose place a patient at risk for obstruction of the ostia of the sinuses and eustachian tubes. The presence of the tube is thought to hinder the closure of the esophageal sphincter and to promote the reflux of gastric contents, leading to a risk of aspiration pneumonia.[59] Because 25% to 35% of children younger than 6 months of age are thought to experience some degree of reflux without the placement of a gastric tube,[61] the placement of a gastric tube significantly increases this risk.

A urinary catheter attached to a closed urinary drainage system facilitates bacteremia in the host in a variety of ways. During placement, the catheter will "push" or "drag" urethral organisms into the bladder, and the indwelling catheter enhances bladder colonization by serving as a conduit for organism growth and movement.[69] Urine can no longer flow through the urethra and flush microorganisms from the body.

Diagnosis of a UTI may be challenging because the infant or young child is often unable to communicate the presence of symptoms. In addition, the child in the PICU may often have multiple reasons for a fever or abdominal pain.[70] Children often have age-specific signs and symptoms of UTIs[71] and experience more asymptomatic bacteriuria than adults.[72] These findings pose an increased risk of delayed recognition and treatment of UTI in children. The diagnosis is established by urinalysis and urine culture. Infection is defined as more than 100,000 organisms per milliliter of voided urine, 1000 or more organisms per milliliter from urine obtained by catheterization, or any organisms from urine obtained by bladder aspiration.

The importance of handwashing cannot be overemphasized. Unfortunately, handwashing is often forgotten. Studies of intensive care units and outpatient facilities have shown that physicians wash their hands less than 50% of the time before and after they examine a child.[73] Hands should be washed before and after each patient contact.

Provide Nutritional Support

The link between nutritional status and immunocompetence has been established.[39] The PICU nurse has an active role in determining the timing, route, and tolerance of nutritional support. In the critically ill child, the GI tract is used to provide nutritional support, if appropriate. The use of the GI tract for enteral feeding, rather than parenteral nutrition, is well documented as being advantageous because it decreases the incidence of bacterial translocation across the gut lining.[74] In addition, infants with lactating mothers are given breast milk as a component of their nutritional support because of the many advantages of breast milk in mucosal immunity.

If the child is able to take nutrition by mouth, encouragement of the child's food and fluid intake includes consideration of the child's likes and dislikes, the manner in which the child prefers food (fried versus boiled), and the time at which the child is accustomed to eating. The PICU nurse ensures that the child has a "safe time" to eat without actual or perceived interruption, threat, or invasion. The child's developmental needs are especially important to consider in the promotion of nutritional intake.

Reduce Stress

Investigators of psychoneuroimmunology, the exploration of the interactions between the brain and the immune system and the influence on health, suggest that stress adversely affects immune function.[75,76] A growing body of evidence has demonstrated an inverse relationship between stress and immune function; the end result is an increased susceptibility to infection.[77] The immune system and nervous system are interconnected by a complex system of chemical signals in the form of cytokines and hormones. Through these signals, each system communicates with and influences the functioning of the other system. The immune system communicates with the nervous system through cytokines released by activated immune cells. The nervous system influences immune system functioning through the action of hormones such as ACTH released from the pituitary (under the influence of the hypothalamus), norepinephrine released from the sympathetic nerves, epinephrine released by the adrenal medulla, and glucocorticoids released by the adrenal cortex.[76] Data from animal studies suggest that stress, unaccompanied by injury, depresses CMI.[78] The individual's cognitive, behavioral, and physical response to stress may also modulate or amplify the effect of stress on the immune system. In other words, stress alone may not be as immunosuppressive as maladaptive coping to stress.[75] The young child is particularly vulnerable to psychologic stress because of limited or immature cognitive and developmental levels and lack of understanding of the critical care environment and interventions.[79]

Reducing stress in the critically ill child can be a challenge. Recognizing the child's cognitive and physical age and the associated developmental tasks and fears is the first step in planning stress reduction for the child. A basic stress-reducing intervention includes respecting the child as an individual and respecting the right to privacy and personal body space. Recognizing and accepting the child's need for regression while providing as calm, caring, and reassuring an environment as possible are vital to the coping of the critically ill child and family. Reducing the stress of parents and siblings has an indirect but beneficial effect on the child and should be incorporated into the child's plan of care.

Optimize Patient Comfort

Striving for and establishing comfort in the pediatric critical care patient are important not only because of the body-mind link of psychoneuroimmunology but also in assisting the child's relative degree of cooperation with the environment, staff, and nursing and medical regimens. Nurses often play a pivotal role in determining the need for and the adequacy of analgesics and sedative medication. Administration of analgesics, sedatives, and narcotics (opiates) aids in comforting the child during physically and psychologically painful experiences. However, long-term use of these medications may also alter immune function and host defenses. The PICU nurse maintains the balance between enhanced child comfort and overmedicating, which may reduce immune function.

Prevent Infection

The Hospital Infections Program (HIP), a part of the CDC's National Center for Infectious Diseases, has a major role in providing information and guidance to hospital infection control programs. Coordinated by the HIP, the National Nosocomial Infection Surveillance (NNIS) system collects data on the incidence of nosocomial infections in more than 150 U.S. hospitals. The Hospital Infection Control Practices Advisory Committee (HICPAC) was established in 1991 to provide advice and guidance to the HIP and the CDC regarding the practice of hospital infection control and strategies for surveillance, prevention, and control.[80]

Limit Exposure to Reservoirs. Prevention of infection can be facilitated by limiting the child's exposure to reservoirs, which are environments in which organisms replicate and persist. The child's room and bedside area are damp dusted[64] and the floor mopped[12] every 24 hours and monitored for standing collections of water or other liquids.[64] All containers of normal saline or sterile water for irrigation purposes are labeled with date and time opened and replaced every 24 hours. It is also important to avoid contamination of these solutions during use. Humidity is provided in the PICU environment for the benefit of the infant and child's small airways and for reduction of organisms that thrive in dry environments.[64] Medical equipment and supplies that must be kept sterile or aseptic include medications, total parenteral and enteral nutrition, humidifiers, face masks, manual resuscitation bags, large-bore suction catheters, suction tubing, and canisters.[64,65] Other po-

tential reservoirs include hand lotions,[65] baby oil and bath supplies, nonprescription ointments, and children's toys.

Proper handwashing decreases the transmission or reduces carriage of potential nosocomial pathogens by the contaminated hands of healthcare workers. In general, hands should be washed before and after patient contact; after contact with body fluids and substances, mucous membranes, nonintact skin, and objects that are likely to be contaminated; before performing invasive procedures; and after removing gloves.[80]

In addition to the environment, supplies, and equipment, healthcare workers, parents, siblings, and other visitors within the critical care environment are potential exogenous reservoirs. Some 15% to 20% of healthy individuals are carriers of *S. aureus* in the nasal antrum and could potentially shed these organisms into the environment.[65] Healthcare workers and visitors may also be infectious with other bacterial or viral organisms.

Visiting policies and traffic control measures must limit unnecessary visitors and limit the PICU environment to essential staff, patient family members, and significant others. All persons entering the PICU (including pediatric visitors) require compliance with strict handwashing procedures before and after patient visitation.[80a] Thorough, frequent handwashing remains the most important method of preventing the transmission of pathogens between the patient and healthcare team member or visitor.[12,64,65]

Healthcare workers require protection from the significant infectious risks inherent in patient care; conversely, patients and other healthcare workers need to be protected from exposure to healthcare workers with communicable diseases. Integrating management and prevention strategies to accomplish these two goals requires close collaboration between hospital infection prevention and control programs and occupational health departments.

A comprehensive employee health program does not replace sound judgment in determining exposure of infectious persons to critically ill infants and children. The nurse has an active and vital role in patient advocacy and carefully monitors self, team members, and visitors for evidence of an infectious process. Patients with altered host defenses should not be cared for or visited by infectious persons without appropriate safety precautions. Guiding infectious persons in delaying their visit or in handwashing and using disposable masks in the child's room may lower the risk of transmission. Unlike exogenous reservoirs, which are often identified, disinfected, or eliminated, little can be done to eradicate pathogens from the endogenous reservoir, the patient.[65] Many opportunistic organisms are present in a patient's system and may cause infection in a patient in a compromised state.[65,81]

Prevent Antigen Exposure. In addition to identifying the known allergies of the infant or young child, recognition of the numerous substances that the child is exposed to on a daily basis in the PICU and identification of potential or actual antigens are critical. Most critical care units minimize the presence of flowers, plants, and pets in the unit and encourage other age-appropriate sources of pleasure, such as mobiles, radios, and tape players. Flexibility and exceptions are common in the PICU environment and are evident by the use of closed terrariums rather than potted plants, changing water in flower vases every 8 hours, or showing videotapes or photographs of pets in between the planned visits by pets. Recognizing the presence of potential antigens and vectors of infection is important. Awareness of their impact on the child and other patients in the unit and planning interventions accordingly are vital.

Consider the Cost/Benefit Ratio of Invasive Techniques. Exposure to invasive medical devices or procedures represents a significant risk for nosocomial infection. Despite the risks, these devices and procedures are an integral part of the pediatric critical care environment and will continue to be in the future. Assisting in the careful comparison of the benefits versus the risks of these invasive techniques is important because most preventable infections are related to the use of invasive devices or procedures. Once the decision is made that the benefit outweighs the risk, care is taken to follow institution-specific standards for invasive techniques and procedures, as well as the care and maintenance of the invasive devices.

Survey for and Identify Infection. Monitoring fever patterns is essential to assist in the identification of the cause of infection. With the exception of the newborn and young infant, the body's ability to mount a febrile response usually remains intact and therefore is the best indicator of infection.[82] Gram-negative sepsis is often accompanied by a pattern of intermittent fevers, whereas a slowly rising but steady fever may indicate the presence of a fungal infection.[82] Fever may also be a manifestation of a reaction to certain medications, such as antibiotics. In this situation, fever closely follows the medication administration, and the medication may temporarily be discontinued to evaluate whether the fever resolves. Close attention to the proper use, method, and care of the temperature-taking device is prudent because treatment decisions are made with the data obtained from temperature taking.

Identification of the source of infection becomes a primary concern in the presence of the febrile patient. Particular attention is targeted toward the lungs and the skin (especially sites of intravenous insertion access, and perioral and perirectal areas). All indwelling catheters, whether suspected or not, are sampled for culture. In addition, two peripheral blood samples are obtained from separate venipuncture sites. Other cultures the nurse may anticipate include routine urinalysis and urine culture, a stool examination and culture (if diarrhea is present), and a chest radiograph. In the febrile neutropenic patient, these cultures and diagnostic tests are anticipated, despite the absence of other clinical symptoms.[83]

Treat Infection

Antibiotic therapy is anticipated in a critically ill child with signs and symptoms of infection. Recognition of the goal of antibiotic therapy by all members of the healthcare team is important. This includes knowledge of whether the drug is empiric or definitive therapy for a suspected or an established infection.[84] The properties of an ideal antibiotic are demonstrated efficacy through controlled clinical trials, nontoxic effects, no alteration in normal patient or environmental flora, facilitation of rapid discharge of the patient from the hospital, and inexpensive cost.

Antimicrobial Therapeutics. Antibiotics are among the most widely prescribed drugs in the acute care setting, often accounting for 15% to 25% of inpatient pharmacy budgets. The rational use of antibiotics in the ICU continues to present a challenge to the healthcare provider. Antibiotics are typically used in three basic ways: (1) for treatment of primary infections; (2) for treatment of secondary or iatrogenic infections; and (3) for prophylaxis of potential or anticipated infections.[85] Treatment rationales include prophylactic treatment, direct or therapeutic treatment, presumptive treatment, and empiric treatment.

Antibiotic selection is an ongoing process with continual evaluation of the indications for antibiotic therapy, the patient's response, and laboratory data.[84] During the course of therapy, additional information is used to adjust the antibiotic regimen to ensure coverage against all suspected or identified microorganisms. The patient's response or lack of response and side effects may lead to the adjustment of the antibiotic regimen. This may result in an antibiotic that has more or all the properties of an optimal antibiotic.

Broad-spectrum antibiotics are usually begun immediately after careful initial examination and collection of specimens for culture and sensitivity testing. Selection of broad-spectrum antibiotics is often based on organisms typically found in a particular institution, whether the patient is neutropenic and the duration of the neutropenia, organisms associated with unique patient populations, and the underlying pathophysiologic condition (e.g., renal failure). Broad-spectrum antibiotic therapy is never a substitute for the careful evaluation of the suspected infection. Pretreatment specimens are always desirable to determine the infectious organism; therefore all desired cultures are accurately obtained in a timely fashion.[82] Once the appropriate antibiotic regimen is chosen, the medication must be administered as soon as possible. Regardless of the method of antibiotic delivery (slow intravenous push, metered chamber, or syringe pump), close attention to the rate of the administration, location of administration, and the dead space of the intravenous tubing ensures that the child receives the drug completely and consistently.

Antibiotic serum drug concentrations (SDCs) are obtained, when appropriate. These are often ordered by the practitioner as peak and trough drug levels. Results are used to adjust drug doses to maximize therapeutic efficacy (to ablate microorganism growth) while minimizing or avoiding toxicity. The determination of when a SDC is obtained is based on the underlying condition of the patient and the point at which the drug reaches a steady-state condition. In the clinical setting, this is often defined according to a specific drug regimen (e.g., following the third administered dose of gentamicin). However, in the critically ill child or the child with organ dysfunction resulting in altered elimination of that drug, SDC may be obtained after the first administered dose. To reach and maintain a therapeutic SDC, it is imperative that all antibiotic doses be given on schedule, regardless of other scheduled diagnostic procedures or regimens.

SDC specimens are accurately collected and labeled to ensure that the derived data are accurate. The actual time the specimen was drawn, as well as the antibiotic infusion start and completion times, should be noted directly on the laboratory specimens. Administration techniques can produce misleading SDC results if the delivery time is miscalculated.[86] The administration time, administration method, infusion duration, specimen collection container, collection time, and concomitant administered medications influence the SDC obtained.

Trough levels are always obtained before administration of an antibiotic dose. Peak levels vary depending on the class of antibiotic; for example, aminoglycoside peak concentrations are obtained from 30 to 60 minutes after a 30-minute infusion, whereas vancomycin peak concentrations are obtained 60 minutes after a 60-minute infusion. If toxicity is suspected, SDCs may be obtained at any time in the dosing schedule.

Many procedures are available for testing the susceptibility of various microorganisms to antiinfective drugs. The greatest dilution of antibiotic associated with the inhibition of bacterial growth is called the minimum inhibitory concentration (MIC). If the sample can be diluted further without a recurrence of bacterial growth, then this dilution is also the minimum bactericidal concentration (MBC) for the drug. MIC and MBC values provide some indication of the potency of the antibiotic with regard to the infecting pathogen.

Simultaneous use of two or more antimicrobials is applied to achieve a broad spectrum of antimicrobial activity when empirical therapy is initiated to minimize the possibility that drug resistance might emerge to a single antimicrobial agent and to exploit synergistic antimicrobial properties.

Antimicrobial-Resistant Microorganisms. The rapid emergence of pathogens resistant to multiple antimicrobial agents (e.g., vancomycin-resistant enterococci, gram-negative bacteria producing extended-spectrum β-lactamases) and the widespread dissemination of these resistant microorganisms constitute an unprecedented crisis for hospitals worldwide. The mechanisms involved in the emergence and spread of antimicrobial resistance are complex but are facilitated undoubtedly by intense selection pressure caused by overuse and misuse of antimicrobial agents in hospitals, particularly newer broad-spectrum agents.[86a] Dissemination of resistant strains is facilitated by poor compliance with handwashing and isolation precaution procedures.

At least eight distinct mechanisms of antibiotic resistance have been described in bacteria. Resistant enterococci to vancomycin has been classified as A, B, or C based on levels of resistance to vancomycin. One method of resistance is enzymatic inhibition, which is due mainly to the production of enzymes that inactivate antibiotics, cause alterations of bacterial membranes (both outer and inner membranes), and alter binding capacity of the antibiotic. Further resistance has been demonstrated by enteric gram-negative organisms,

which have the capacity to actively efflux tetracycline back across the cell membrane. Resistance to a wide variety of antimicrobial agents, including tetracyclines, macrolides, and aminoglycosides, may result from alteration of ribosomal binding sites. Failure of the antibiotics to bind to its target site or sites on the ribosome disrupts its ability to inhibit protein synthesis and cell growth. Large glycopeptide molecules prevent the incorporation of precursor antibiotic targets, such as vancomycin in the cell wall. β-Lactam antibiotics inhibit bacteria by binding covalently to penicillin-binding protein in the cytoplasmic membrane. In gram-positive bacteria; resistance to β-lactam antibiotics may be associated either with a change in the affinity of penicillin-binding protein for the antibiotic or with a change in the amount of penicillin-binding protein produced by the bacterium.[87]

New drug discoveries have remained one step ahead of the bacterial pathogens. Nonetheless, the rapid evolution of resistance has limited the duration of the effectiveness of specific agents against certain pathogens. The best hope for the future is the development of a greater understanding of how antimicrobial resistance spreads and the implementation of effective infection control strategies. New antimicrobial agents have had a substantial impact in decreasing human morbidity and mortality rates over the past half-century. Expanding surveillance of antibiotic resistance determinants and exercising caution in dispensing antibiotics to maximize their continued efficacy are critical to the continued effectiveness of these agents.[87]

Antifungal Drugs. Amphotericin B is considered by most to be the gold standard for systemic antifungal drugs. It is the agent to which all new antifungal drugs must be compared before clinical acceptance. Fluconazole is the first in a series of new triazole antifungal agents providing an effective and less toxic therapy than amphotericin B. Many other antifungal agents are available, including flucytosine, itraconazole, griseofulvin, synthetic imidazoles, and topical nystatin.

Antiviral Drugs. Antiviral drugs such as acyclovir and ganciclovir are effective in the treatment of localized and disseminated herpes simplex virus infections. Amantadine and rimantadine have been used against influenza A viruses. Considerable controversy surrounds the use and true clinical effectiveness of ribavirin. Ribavirin may be of clinical value in the treatment of severe lower respiratory tract viral infections caused by influenza A and B viruses and respiratory syncytial virus. Currently the American Academy of Pediatrics suggests use in selected patient population only (see Chapter 19).

Antiprotozoal Drugs. Pentamidine isethionate is considered a second-line drug for the treatment of *P. carinii* pneumonia in patients who fail to respond to co-trimoxazole (trimethoprim-sulfamethoxazole) and used increasingly in patients with AIDS.

Antimalarial Drugs. Chloroquine is used primarily for the treatment of malaria; however, today many chloroquine-resistant and multidrug-resistant strains of malaria exist. Quinine is also indicated for malaria prophylaxis or in the treatment of the acute disease; however, the drug is much less effective and more toxic than chloroquine.[88]

Immunotherapy and Immunomodulation

Immunotherapy involves the use of immune factors, alone or in combination, to enhance immunity or prevent unwanted physiologic responses and tissue destruction. These factors include immunoglobulin (e.g., antitoxins, monoclonal antibodies), WBC transfusions, and cytokines. *Biotherapy* is a broad term used to refer to various biologic treatment modalities employed to augment, restore, or modify the immune response or hematopoiesis. Through advanced biotechnologic methods, such as recombinant engineering techniques, many naturally occurring immunologic substances in the body are produced in sufficiently large quantities for clinical trials and therapeutic application.[89,90] Biotherapy may be used to augment or restore the immune system in the treatment of cancer, immunodeficiencies, HIV disease, and septic shock. Biotherapy is also used to suppress or restrict the immune response, such as in the prevention, diagnosis, or treatment of graft rejection and graft versus host disease (GVHD) or in the treatment of autoimmune disease. Biotherapy has also become a new tool to reverse drug toxicity. Certain forms of biotherapy have nonclinical applications; they are used in the laboratory to diagnose diseases or infections, determine blood and tissue types, and differentiate between B cells and T cells.

An important nursing consideration for the use of biotherapy, because it is often investigational, is to ensure that the informed consent process is complete. In addition to the parents' or guardians' consent, it is important to obtain the child's assent, when appropriate, to participate in the research process and protocol.

Another significant nursing implication in caring for the child receiving biotherapy is knowledge about the contraindications, complications, and side effects. In general, the long-term effects of biotherapy are unknown; hence, this therapy is used only when clearly indicated, part of a research protocol, or for compassionate use. Complications of therapy are variable and may be acute or chronic, nearly universal, or rare. Each biotherapy agent has unique side effects, but most agents are associated with a flulike syndrome of fever, chills, myalgia, headache, and fatigue.

Biotherapy generally involves the administration of one form or a combination of the following: (1) immunoglobulins; (2) cytokines, such as colony-stimulating factors (CSFs), interferons, or interleukins; (3) monoclonal antibodies (MoAbs); (4) genetically engineered enzymes; (5) autologous activated immune cells (tumor-infiltrating lymphocytes [TILs] and LAK cells); and (6) gene transfer therapy. Each category of biotherapy is discussed individually, but as with all other immunologic events, these substances do not act independently or in isolation.

Immunoglobulin. Intravenous immunoglobulin (IVIg) is a solution of immunoglobulin containing many antibodies normally present in adult human blood. It is obtained from plasma-pooled whole blood of thousands of diverse adult donors, ensuring a broad spectrum of antibodies. Immune globulin therapy is rapidly shifting from standard pooled preparations to specific immune globulin preparations. High-titer specific immune globulin preparations are prepared by screening or immunizing donors. Examples include cytomegalovirus immune globulin (CMV-Ig), respiratory syncytial virus immune globulin (RSV-Ig), and varicella-zoster immune globulin (VZIg). Hepatitis B immune globulin (HBIg) is used to prevent hepatitis B infection, and VZIg can prevent or modify the course of chickenpox in immunocompromised patients.

Intravenous immunoglobulin. More than 90% of IVIg solution consists of IgG. The manufacturing process ensures that the levels of IgA and IgM are low to reduce the rare incidence of anaphylaxis (predominantly resulting from anti-IgA antibodies) and hemolytic transfusion reaction (predominantly resulting from IgM antibodies of the ABO and Rh blood system).

IVIg has many clinical applications, but the mechanism of action may vary related to the disease state for which the IVIg is given. Table 15-9 illustrates the various disease states and clinical conditions for which IVIg has been administered; however, the efficacy in many of these states remains unclear.[91] It was initially developed to provide passive immunity and prevent infections in persons with primary immunodeficiencies who were unable to produce or maintain adequate levels of IgG.

IVIg is used in many other clinical conditions because it has immunomodulatory effects that are not well characterized but are the focus of intense research. Evidence of these immunomodulatory effects has led to the use of IVIg in the treatment of inflammatory or autoimmune conditions such as Kawasaki syndrome or, rarely, idiopathic thrombocytopenic purpura (ITP).

TABLE 15-9 Conditions in Which IVIg Has Been Used

Primary Immunodeficiency
Hypogammaglobulinemia
Common variable immunodeficiency
Severe combined immunodeficiency
Wiskott-Aldrich syndrome

Secondary Immunodeficiency
Pediatric acquired immunodeficiency syndrome (AIDS)
Bone marrow transplantation

Inflammatory or Autoimmune Disorders (Immunomodulatory)
Kawasaki syndrome
Guillain-Barré syndrome
Immune hemolytic anemia
Immune neutropenia
Idiopathic thrombocytopenic purpura (ITP)

Condition With Increased Risk of Infection
Low birth weight

Adapted from NIH Consensus Conference: Intravenous immunoglobulin: prevention and treatment of disease, *JAMA* 26:3189-3193, 1990.

Several brands of IVIg are available in the United States; all are purified and processed to remove or inactivate HIV, hepatitis B virus, and other microorganisms. Dosages for IVIg may vary tenfold depending on the disorder for which it is being administered. IVIg is given by slow infusion usually over several hours, with an initial infusion rate of 0.5 ml/kg/hr for 30 minutes, gradually increased at subsequent 15- to 30-minute intervals to a maximum of 2 to 4 ml/kg/hr. The patient should be observed for acute reactions; slowing or stopping the infusion for 15 to 30 minutes usually alleviates the reaction.

As the result of a significant number of adverse-event reports of renal dysfunction and acute renal failure associated with the administration of IVIg, the U.S. Food and Drug Administration recently published recommendations for IVIg use. Preliminary evidence suggests that IVIg products containing sucrose may pose a greater risk for this complication.[92]

Respiratory syncytial virus immune globulin. RSV-Ig contains high titers of RSV immune globulin. Concerns about the requirement of monthly administration requiring intravenous cannulation and infusion over several hours and the fluid volume and protein load have restricted the use of RSV-Ig.[92a] Efforts have been directed to the development of a monoclonal IgG antibody and prophylaxis against RSV. A randomized, multicenter, double-placebo-controlled trial involving 1502 premature infants with or without chronic lung disease receiving palivizumab prophylaxis reduced the incidence of RSV hospitalizations by 55% compared with placebo recipients (p <0.001).[93] Current recommendations include considering palivizumab in neonates who meet predefined criteria. Palivizumab is not indicated for infants with congenital heart disease and for the treatment of RSV disease.

CMV-Ig. CMV-Ig ensures high titers of CMV-specific antibody and is highly efficacious in the prevention and treatment of CMV infections in kidney and bone marrow transplant patients.[94] Several products with a high antibody titer to a specific pathogen have been available for many years to prevent, modify, or treat a variety of infections.[73]

Cytokines. Cytokines are soluble substances produced primarily by cells of the immune system that act as powerful communication signals between cells. In this sense, cytokines function much like hormones or neurotransmitters. Cytokines regulate or influence the immune response by affecting a variety of cellular activities, especially in regard to HI and CMI. Like antibodies, cytokines are generally released in response to the presence of antigen[95]; however, unlike antibodies, cytokines are not specific to a particular antigen.

Cytokines can be categorized as CSFs, interferons, and interleukins. Other cytokines, such as TNF-α, lymphotoxin (TNF-β), and IL-1, have unique effects that defy categorization.

Colony Stimulating Factors. CSFs are involved principally in the production of neutrophils and monocytes. They were discovered because of their ability to stimulate the formation of colonies of granulocytes, monocytes, and macrophages in cultured bone marrow cells and were named according to the primary cell colony type that they elicited.

CSFs are a group of glycoproteins that are extensively involved in hematopoiesis, the process by which blood cells proliferate, differentiate, and mature.[96,96a] Each CSF binds to and activates the corresponding receptors found on the surface of its target cell (each CSF may have a variety of target cells).[96,96a] Upon binding to its receptor membrane, the CSF signals the target cell to initiate particular intracellular processes, such as protein synthesis and replication of genetic material, which leads to differentiation, cloning, maturation, and, in some cases, functional activation of that target hematopoietic cell.[96,96a]

Recombinant CSFs, produced by genetic engineering, have three major therapeutic applications. Two applications are to restore hematopoietic function by raising cell counts from suppressed levels and to augment host defense against infection by enhancing the sensitivity and function of immune cells. The third application is an indirect role in containing or eliminating malignant cells. By far the most common applications of CSFs are to reverse anemia, thrombocytopenia, and neutropenia following cytotoxic and radiation therapy during the treatment of cancer. Bone marrow suppression, with its consequent risks of life-threatening infection or bleeding, is the primary dose-limiting factor of cytotoxic drugs for the treatment of cancer. CSFs accelerate bone marrow recovery, which reduces the period of severe neutropenia and thrombocytopenia, thereby permitting higher doses of chemotherapy and possibly higher rates of remission or cure. Research is ongoing in using various CSFs for these multiple purposes.

Five major endogenous human CSFs are granulocyte CSF (G-CSF), granulocyte macrophage CSF (GM-CSF), macrophage CSF (M-CSF), interleukin-3 (IL-3), and erythropoietin. Table 15-10 reviews individual CSFs according to their cellular source, action, and therapeutic application.

Interferons. Interferons are substances produced by the immune cells primarily in response to viral infection. All of the interferons are antiviral, antiproliferative (cloning), and immune modulating, but the different types of interferons may vary in efficacy when exerting these effects. Like other biologic response modifiers (BRMs), interferons cause a flulike syndrome.[97,98] Table 15-11 lists the various interferons with their respective cellular sources, actions, and therapeutic applications in pediatric critical care.

Interleukins are a form of BRMs that have received much attention. More than 17 interleukins have been identified, and their unique function and contribution to the immune response are not completely understood. IL-2, the most commonly administered interleukin, increases lymphocyte proliferation (cloning) and NK cell activity.[99-101]

Lymphokines and Monokines. During infection, genes for nearly all the cytokines are expressed. The cytokine family, through a complex web of interactions, functions to initiate and then regulate both proinflammatory and antiinflammatory responses.[102] Considerable experimental and clinical interest has focused on the proinflammatory cytokines TNF-α and IL-1 as important early mediators in the pathogenesis of sepsis and meningococcal

TABLE 15-10   Selected Colony-Stimulating Factors (CSFs)

CSF	Cellular Source	Action	Therapeutic Application
Erythropoietin (EPO)	Renal cells	Stimulates production and speeds maturation of erythrocytes	Reverse anemia related to: • Chronic renal failure • HIV disease • Zidovidine therapy for HIV
IL-3 (Multi-CSF)	T cells	Stimulates growth of precursors to granulocytes, macrophages, RBCs, platelets, and mast cells	Reverse thrombocytopenia related to: • Cancer therapy
Granulocyte (G)-CSF*	Monocytes Macrophages Endothelial cells Fibroblasts	Stimulates growth and activation of neutrophils	Reverse neutropenia related to: • Cytotoxic therapy • Radiation therapy • HIV disease • Congenital neutropenia • Cyclic neutropenia
Macrophage (M)-CSF	Monocytes Macrophages Endothelial cells Fibroblasts	Stimulates growth and activation of monocytes	Expedite bone marrow recovery following autologous bone marrow transplant
GM-CSF	T cells Endothelial cells Fibroblasts	Stimulates the growth and activation of neutrophils, eosinophils, and macrophages Enhances ability of macrophages and neutrophils to ingest bacteria and kill antibody-coated tumor cells	Expedite bone marrow recovery following autologous bone marrow transplant

Data from Herberman RB, ed: *Cetus immunoprimer series.* Part 3. Cytokines, Emoryville, Calif, 1989, Cetus Corporation.
*It is relatively easy to transfuse RBCs to reverse anemia or platelets to reverse thrombocytopenia. In contrast, granulocyte transfusions to reverse neutropenia are logistically difficult to perform. In addition, their therapeutic efficacy has not been reliably established.

TABLE 15-11   Selected Interferons

Agent	Cellular Source	Action	Pediatric Critical Care Therapeutic Application
α-Interferon	T, B, NK cells Macrophages Fibroblasts Epithelial cells	Enhance NK activity Antiviral Induces HLA-I antigen expression Induces fever Generates cytotoxic T-cells Induces macrophage killing of tumor cells	Non-Hodgkin's lymphoma Hepatitis B HIV disease Under investigation in: Hepatitis B or C
β-Interferon	Fibroblasts Macrophages Epithelial cells	See α-interferon actions	Multiple sclerosis

γ-Interferon	T and NK cells	Antiviral
		Induces HLA-I antigen expression
		Induces microorganism and tumor cell killing of macrophages
		Regulates action of certain cytokines
		Increases NK cell activity
		Induces production of T cell suppressor factor
		Increases expression of Fc receptor
			Chronic granulomatous disease
			Under investigation in:
			    HIV disease
			    Rheumatoid arthritis
			    Chronic mycobacterial infections
			    (*Mycobacterium avium*)

Data from Herberman RB, ed: *Cetus immunoprimer series.* Part 3. *Cytokines,* Emoryville, Calif, 1989, Cetus Corporation.

disease, as demonstrated by a correlation between morbidity and mortality and high serum levels of TNF-α and IL-1.[103] The basis for the potential therapeutic use of these two cytokines in human disease states involves two clinically distinct hypotheses: (1) excessive cytokine production results in host immune injury leading to severe shock, and (2) deficient cytokine production renders a host susceptible to infection by invasive pathogens. Research and future clinical trials will attempt to inhibit endotoxin release or limit TNF-α and IL-1 production and function. Current clinical trials are also focusing on the TNF-α and IL-1 synthesis with the administration of corticosteroids either before or during antibiotic administration and the use of pentoxifylline a methylxanthine derivative to block TNF-α transcription and production.[103]

Monoclonal Antibodies. MoAbs are laboratory-produced antibodies for a single destiny antigen. The process in which MoAbs are produced in the laboratory is reflected in Fig. 15-9. MoAbs are used to prevent, diagnose, and treat graft rejection and GVHD; perform diagnostic testing; treat disease (e.g., cancer, autoimmune disease); and

monitor response to treatment to eliminate toxins and reverse drug toxicity. Each therapeutic application of MoAbs is discussed separately.

The use of monoclonal antiendotoxin antibodies to inhibit the binding of endotoxin to its target cell is promising although more effective if given earlier during sepsis syndrome.[104] Anti–T cell MoAbs, such as OKT3, are effective agents widely used in heart, liver, pancreas, and bone marrow transplants to prevent, diagnose, or treat graft rejection or GVHD. To prevent graft rejection, OKT3 is administered to prevent the child's mature T cells from rejecting the grafted or transplanted organ. To prevent GVHD in bone marrow transplant patients, the donor marrow is incubated with anti–T cell MoAbs before the marrow is infused into the recipient to purge the donor marrow of immunocompetent T cells. MoAbs can also be used to monitor subsets of T cells at the site of organ graft to assist in the diagnosis or monitoring of graft rejection.[105,106]

MoAbs may also be used on serum, urine, and stool samples to diagnose infections with microorganisms such as

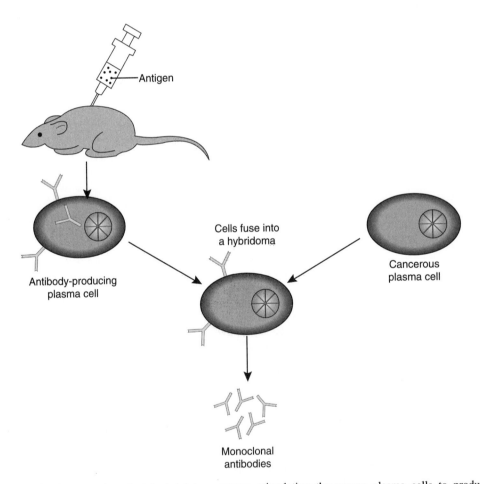

Fig. 15-9 Target antigen is injected into a mouse, stimulating the mouse plasma cells to produce antibodies to that destiny antigen. Mouse plasma cells are then harvested and fused with immortal laboratory-grown plasma cell. These cells are then cloned and referred to as hybridomas. This hybridoma will secrete the "made-to-order" antibody for an indefinite period. Through this process, research has mimicked the immune system's humoral immunity. (Adapted from Schindler LW: *The immune system—how it works.* United States Department of Health and Human Services, Bethesda, Md, 1992, NIH publication number 92-3229, p. 22.)

herpes simplex virus, streptococci, and *Chlamydia*. In addition, MoAbs assist in the identification of cells and tissues (e.g., B cell and T cell differentiation or HLA or blood typing).

MoAbs to various tumor antigens or tumor products can be used to confirm the diagnosis of certain types of cancers (glioma, cancer of the pancreas, lung, kidney, and others). A radioactive tracer can be attached to MoAbs so that after the MoAbs are administered, a body scan may reveal where the cancer is located within the body.

Antitumor MoAbs can also be used therapeutically. They attach to tumor cells, opsonizing these cells, and enhancing the tumor cells' destruction. Antitumor antigen MoAbs that are attached to toxins are called conjugated MoAbs. Often these conjugated MoAbs are combined with radioactive or other agents to assist in the treatment of various cancers, such as acute lymphocytic leukemia. In theory, these will attach solely to the tumor cells rather than harming healthy cells.[107]

More commonly in the PICU, MoAbs are used to reverse drug toxicity or minimize toxic effects. For example, in a child experiencing digoxin toxicity, the MoAb Digibind "binds" to the excess digoxin, preventing it from exerting its toxic effects. MoAbs to microbe toxins have been developed against *Escherichia coli* and *P. aeruginosa* to name a few. Murine MoAbs against TNF may improve survival in certain patients; however, at this time, clinical usefulness is limited.[108]

Integrins and Selectins. Neutrophil adherence to and migration through the capillary endothelium is a critical early event in the acute inflammatory response. The adhesive interactions between leukocytes and endothelial cell surfaces are regulated by two families of glycoproteins: the integrins and the selectins. Monoclonal antibodies to integrins and selectins are being tested in animal models.[103]

Genetically Engineered Enzymes. Some diseases affecting children occur as a consequence of genetic defects that result in the lack of one or more key enzymes for cell growth and metabolism. For such diseases, genetically engineered enzyme replacement therapy may halt the disease process. This involves administering the deficient enzyme in adequate amounts. Because such endogenously administered enzymes may last only a short time within the body, molecules such as *polyethylene glycol* (PEG) can be attached to the enzyme to prolong its half-life.[109]

Autologous Activated Immune Cells. LAK cells and TILs are forms of biotherapy that are undergoing investigation as a treatment of cancer. In some clinical trials, the cells have effectively produced tumor regression in cancers that were unresponsive to conventional therapy. Both forms of therapy involve removing lymphocytes from a person with cancer, activating these cells with IL-2, and then returning the activated cells to the patient. Theoretically, either type of activated cell would be expected to lyse tumor cells while sparing normal cells.

In LAK cell therapy, the patient is first given IL-2 and then undergoes pheresis in which lymphocytes are removed. These lymphocytes are incubated with IL-2 and then returned to the patient in the hope that these cells will attack the tumor. TILs are normal lymphocytes that are harvested directly from the patient's malignant tumor. Thus in contrast to LAK cells, TILs are theoretically "programmed" against the tumor cells from which they are found. TILs are also incubated with IL-2, stimulated to clone, harvested, and reinfused into the patient.[110,111]

ALTERATION IN IMMUNE FUNCTION

Transient Immune Dysfunction

Etiology. The critically ill child often experiences iatrogenic interference to host defenses. Common PICU diagnostic and therapeutic interventions interfering with host defense and immunologic function include anesthesia procedures[112,113]; pharmacologic interventions such as neuromuscular blockers, narcotics, sedatives, and barbiturates; immunosuppressive therapies such as chemotherapy, radiation, and corticosteroids; and extensive blood component administration.[114] The child is also subjected to numerous invasive procedures in the PICU, such as tracheal intubation, and catheterization or cannulation of body orifices and cavities. Each of these stressors disrupts the child's physical, mechanical, and chemical barriers and increases the risk of nosocomial infection.

Transient immune dysfunction may result indirectly from the cause for the child's admission to the PICU. Severe musculoskeletal trauma, thermal injury, or major surgery are examples of overwhelming tissue injuries that can produce transient immunocompromise. Regardless of the type of tissue injury (trauma vs. thermal injury), the resultant immunocompromise is similar and involves all components of the immune system. Infection is the most frequent fatal complication after major tissue injury[78,115]; the more severe the injury, the greater the immune system dysfunction and the higher the risk of sepsis and death.[78] Every investigated component of the immune system has revealed an alteration in function after major tissue injury.

Incidence. In addition to penetration of the natural barriers as described earlier, the younger the child in the PICU, the higher the risk for infection. Infants 1 month old or younger have a 2 to 3 times higher risk for infection than patients who were at least 2 years old.[116]

Several studies of nosocomial infections in hospitalized patients suggest that infection rates are actually lower in the pediatric patient population compared with adults.[117-120] The cumulative incidence of nosocomial infections (number of nosocomial infections per 100 discharges) for pediatric services and normal newborn nurseries is lower than for most other services. Length of hospitalization is an important factor in assessing rates of nosocomial infection because the cumulative probability that an individual will experience at least one nosocomial infection increases with increasing exposure to the hospital. To minimize the effect of differences in length of hospitalization, rates of nosocomial infection are expressed as an incidence density (the number of nosocomial infections per 1000 patient days).[121]

The majority of nosocomial pneumonias are caused by bacteria and are associated with mechanical ventilation.[121a] The rate of ventilator-associated pneumonia has been reported at 6 per 1000 ventilator days,[122] which includes viral causes of pneumonia. Mechanical ventilation is a major risk factor not only for nosocomial pneumonia but also for sinusitis and otitis media because the nasotracheal tube interferes with normal drainage of the ostia of the sinuses and the eustachian tube.[121] The majority of nosocomial pneumonias are polymicrobial and often include both gram-positive and gram-negative bacteria. The pathogenesis of ventilator-associated pneumonia is complex but can be reduced to two general mechanisms: aspiration of microorganisms colonizing the stomach and oropharynx and inhalation of contaminated aerosols.

Rates of bloodstream infection associated with central venous catheters in PICUs are reported to be 8 per 1000 central line days. This is higher than rates reported in adult ICUs.[122] These data do not distinguish rates of infection associated with specific catheter types, nor do these distinguish which catheter is the source of the infection in patients with multiple catheters. A recent review suggests that rates of bloodstream infection are lower in totally implanted (0.1 to 0.7 infections per 1000 catheter days) than tunneled (0.4 to 7.8 per 1000) catheters.[123] Arterial line–related septicemia ranges from 0% to 4%[124,125] depending on populations, definitions of infection, practices related to insertion, and duration of use.[126] Current information is not sufficient to state whether the site of insertion of central venous catheter affects the risk of infection. Nearly a third of infections are caused by coagulase-negative staphylococci. Other gram-positive bacteria, including *S. aureus* and *Enterococcus* species, account for another third.

Patients undergoing surgical procedures are at risk for a variety of nosocomial infections. A 1-year study of more than 600 pediatric patients undergoing surgical procedures found that surgical-site infection was the most common nosocomial infection after surgery, occurring in 3.5% of patients.[127] A study of more than 300 children undergoing cardiovascular surgery found an infection rate of 7.1%.[128] Infection rates were higher among patients in whom the sternum was left open after surgery (27.6% in patients with open sternums vs. 5% in patients with closed sternums), although this occurrence may be related to severity of illness.

UTIs are *not* the most common nosocomial infection in the pediatric population, as they are in the adult population,[66,69] but are second to upper respiratory tract infections. UTIs represent only 10% or less of all hospital-acquired infections in children in the National Nosocomial Infections Surveillance System report,[122] although the incidence is higher in the critically ill child.

Pathophysiology. The interference of the lines of defense create an environment that facilitates the development of nosocomial infection. Malnutrition leads to a mosaic of changes affecting both nonspecific and specific host defenses.[129,130] Factors that interfere with adequate tissue perfusion and oxygen delivery, such as hypoxemia, shock, and hypothermia, affect inflammatory response, phagocytosis, and wound healing. The efficiency of neutrophils in killing bacteria is related to a level of oxygen in the tissues not just in the circulation. For example, because an activated phagocyte's oxygen consumption increases 10 to 20 times over its resting metabolism,[131] it must have access to adequate oxygen to perform its phagocytic functions.

All patients with chronic renal failure, regardless of age, experience a high incidence of infection, with approximately 40% of patients dying of an infectious complication.[132] Although data are inconclusive and often contradictory, many factors in the patient with renal failure are thought to contribute to altered host defenses and increased susceptibility to infection.

The primary immune abnormality seen in patients with both acute and chronic renal failure is lymphocytopenia and a sequestration of lymphocytes to the bone marrow.[132] Apparently the uremic state and its effect on the blood sera are responsible for the defects seen in cellular immunity. Washed uremic lymphocytes incubated in normal blood sera respond normally, as opposed to lymphocytes in uremic blood sera.[132]

Hypothermia and cardiopulmonary bypass are often used during cardiac surgery. Induced hypothermia has also been associated with an increased risk for bacterial infection.[78,133] Laboratory studies reveal that the increased risk of infection may be a result of depressed neutrophil migration in low-temperature states.[134]

Gram-positive cocci account for approximately one half of the isolates of surgical-site infections.[134a] *S. aureus* is the most common isolate, but coagulase-negative staphylococci and *Enterococcus* species are also common. Cardiopulmonary bypass can be viewed as an iatrogenic cause of immune dysfunction. The movement of the immune cells and proteins through the heart-lung bypass machine causes cellular destruction, complement activation, and other changes that result in impaired immune function.[78] It has been reported in animals and adults that the rapid flow through the bypass machine results in decreased complement levels, decreased immunoglobulin levels, increased leukocyte adherence, depressed phagocytosis, and a transient neutropenia.[135] Similar findings are reported in children after cardiac surgery.[136] Depressed complement levels have been noted postoperatively in children and were still observed 24 hours after surgery.[136] This finding is in contrast to the observation in adults of a return to preoperative complement levels within 4 hours postoperatively.[137] Other immunologic findings following pediatric cardiac surgery include lymphopenia, decreased helper T cells, and decreased levels of IgG and IgM.[136] Minimal information is available on the effect of extracorporeal membrane oxygenation (ECMO) or cardiac assist devices on host defenses.[137a,137b]

Critical Care Management. Malone and Larson[138] demonstrated the introduction of the Occupational Safety and Health Administration (OSHA) Blood-borne Pathogen Exposure Control Plan, and Body Substance Isolation and a barrier hand foam were associated with a significant reduction in nosocomial infection rates. The CDC has developed a comprehensive guideline for the prevention of nosocomial pneumonia.[139] Empiric antimicrobial therapy of nosocomial pneumonia in the patient supported on mechanical ventilation should be guided by Gram stain of the endotracheal aspirate. Treatment duration has not been studied, and, generally, 10 days of therapy are given.[121]

Potential bloodstream infections are evaluated with at least two blood cultures, including at least one blood culture drawn by venipuncture before the institution of antibiotic therapy. Empiric antimicrobial therapy for suspected bloodstream infection while awaiting culture results is based on local knowledge of the relative frequency and susceptibility patterns of nosocomial pathogens. Empiric treatment should include an antibiotic effective against gram-positive bacteria and most gram-negative bacteria.

The majority of critical care management focuses on maintaining external barriers. Review the previous section for specific interventions that protect and enhance the first and second lines of defense.

Primary Alterations in Immune Function

Etiology and Incidence. More than 40 primary immune deficiency disorders are currently recognized by the World Health Organization. Most are clinically heterogeneous and probably represent similar manifestations of separate defects in a particular cellular or molecular pathway. The overall incidence of primary immune deficiency has been estimated at approximately 1 case in 10,000 individuals in the population. Antibody deficits constitute approximately 50% of immune deficiencies; T cell defects are next at 30% to 40%.[140] The relative distribution of immunodeficiencies is shown in Fig. 15-10. Primary immunodeficiencies are conventionally divided into disorders involving B cells, T cells, phagocytes, complement, or a combination.

B Cell Disorders. B cell deficiency states are associated with quantitative or qualitative antibody deficit caused by (1) lack of all immunoglobulin classes (e.g., agammaglobulinemia), (2) lack of one immunoglobulin class (e.g., IgA deficiency), (3) lack of immunoglobulin subclass(es) (e.g., IgG2 deficiency), or (4) lack of functional antibody. B cell deficiencies are often intertwined with T cell

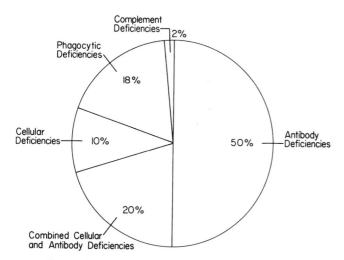

Fig. 15-10 Relative distribution of primary immunodeficiencies. (From Stiehm ER: Immunodeficiency disorders: general considerations. In Stiehm ER, ed: *Immunological disorders in infants and children,* ed 3, Philadelphia, 1989, WB Saunders, p. 158.)

dysfunction. Patients typically present with recurrent bacterial infections.[141] Antibody deficiencies are the most common B cell disorders and are present in approximately one half of the patients with primary immunodeficiency.[9,142] Because patients with B cell disorders have a diminished ability to form immunoglobulins, they are unable to generate effective antibody-antigen interactions.[143]

The pattern of infection associated with B cell disorders is characteristically recurrent sinopulmonary tract infections with encapsulated bacteria and, less frequently, gram-negative organisms.[143] Pyogenic bacteria, such as pneumococci, meningococci, streptococci, *H. influenzae,* and enteroviruses are common etiologic organisms. Patients with antibody deficiency should not receive live virus vaccines.

T Cell Disorders. T cell disorders are present in approximately 40% of patients with primary immunodeficiencies[142]; however, 75% of these cases are associated concomitantly with antibody deficiencies. Patients with T cell disorders have a limited ability to produce mature T cells and therefore are unable to assist with the activation of the immune response.

T cell defect may be due to a stem cell defect, a thymus defect, an enzyme deficiency, or a postthymic defect. The DiGeorge syndrome is an example of a T cell deficiency secondary to a thymus defect. Patients with T cell deficiency present primarily with opportunistic infections or autoimmune disease.

Phagocytic Disorders. Patients with phagocytic disorders have either an insufficient number or inadequate function of neutrophils and monocytes or macrophages. Impaired phagocytic function may be further classified as chemotactic, opsonic, ingestion, or killing defects. Children with neutrophil dysfunction experience recurrent infections of the skin and soft tissue, abscesses, lung infections, and periodontal disease. Patients with phagocytic disorders involving inadequate functioning are considered at risk for infection despite a "normal" WBC count. Infections should be treated aggressively with prolonged use of systemic antibiotics and surgical drainage of abscesses.

Complement Deficiencies. Deficiencies have been described for each of the key components of complement; however, an increase in the susceptibility to infection is commonly noted for deficiencies in C2, C3, C5, C6, C7, and C8.[39] Infection patterns vary depending on which component of complement is deficient. For instance, infections in a child with deficiencies of C2 and C3 are similar to those in a child with a B cell disorder. The child with a complement deficiency in terminal complement components (C5 through C8) has infections from meningococcal or gonococcal organisms.[39]

Combined Immunodeficiencies. Several rare disorders are based on a combined immunodeficiency of both HI and CMI. These disorders are the most severe of all the immunodeficiencies because the child is unable to form antibody and lacks T cells to orchestrate the immune response and to destroy cells infected with intracellular microorganisms. Persons with combined B and T cell disorders suffer from multiple severe infections (bacterial, fungal, viral, and protozoal), diarrhea, and muscle wasting.

A well-known example of a combined B and T cell disorder is severe combined immunodeficiency disease (SCID). SCID is a rare inherited disorder occurring in only 1 in 1 million live births in the United States. SCID may be caused by several immunologic abnormalities, but all result in the lack of development or function in B cells and T cells.

Acquired Immunodeficiency

Human Immunodeficiency Virus

Etiology and Incidence. HIV disease is defined as the spectrum from exposure to the virus until death. AIDS is that part of the HIV disease spectrum during which opportunistic illnesses have begun to develop until death. Pediatric AIDS refers to those cases that have been reported in children under 13 years of age. In 1981, 16 cases of AIDS were first reported among children below the age of 13.[144] By June 1999, 8596 cases of pediatric AIDS had been reported.[145]

From 1982, when the first cases of AIDS in children were reported, through June 1997, 7902 cases of AIDS had been reported in the United States.[146] Of these cases, the majority were infected through mother-infant transmission, with a smaller number infected through receipt of infected blood, blood products, or tissue or through receipt of contaminated blood products used for hemophilia treatment. The number of children with perinatally acquired HIV disease has steadily declined since 1993 from over 900 per year to 225 in 1998. From 1996 to 1997, the number of children who were diagnosed with HIV declined 40%, principally reflecting several factors: the continued success of efforts to reduce perinatal transmission through promoting voluntary HIV testing and zidovudine therapy for pregnant HIV-infected women and their infants[145] and increased use of antiretroviral drugs to treat HIV infection in pregnant women.

Worldwide, the HIV epidemic has left an estimated 8.2 million children orphaned and 1.1 million children living with HIV.[147] Through December 1997, 641,086 persons with AIDS had been reported to the CDC by state and local health departments. Of these, 1.2% were children younger than 13 years old.

By midyear 1999, 1803 children were reported to be living with HIV and 3669 to be living with AIDS. A total of 4975 children with AIDS have died, the majority of whom were African American, followed by Hispanics, making up the second largest ethnic group.[145] Of the 678 children reported with AIDS in 1999, 91% had a mother with or at risk for HIV infection, 4% were infected through blood or blood products, 3% were hemophiliacs or had a clotting disorder, and 2% had other or no reported risks.[145] Adolescents tend to become infected by routes of transmission associated with risky behaviors. These include unprotected sexual intercourse with infected partners, intravenous drug use, and contamination with infected blood.[148]

Despite a decreased number of children diagnosed with HIV, more children affected by this disease are being admitted to PICUs for intense medical and nursing management because of multisystem organ involvement and subsequent organ failure, The average length of hospital stay in 1997 was 8.1 days.[145]

Extraordinary progress has been made in developing highly active antiretroviral therapies (HAARTs), as well as continuing progress in preventing and treating opportunistic infections (OIs). HAART has reduced the incidence of OIs and extended lives substantially. In addition, prophylaxis against specific OIs continues to provide survival benefits even among persons who are receiving HAART.[149] However, in comparison with Caucasians, African Americans received inferior care on six selected measures of service and pharmaceutical use.[150] Compared with children who died in 1990, HIV-infected children who died in 1996 were significantly older, more symptomatic, and more likely to have a greater number of organ system involvement and to have received antiviral therapy and OI prophylaxis.[151]

Pathophysiology and Transmission. A great deal of information has been learned about the transmission of HIV since it was first isolated in 1983. HIV is a very fragile virus and cannot survive for long periods once it is outside the body. The length of time it does survive depends on the size of the droplet that the virus is in and the concentration of HIV within that droplet.[152] The larger the droplet, the longer the survival time of the virus. HIV is killed as the droplet dries.

HIV has been isolated from all body fluids, including blood, semen, vaginal fluid, tears, saliva, sweat, sputum, urine, breast milk, and cerebrospinal fluid. It has also been isolated from some body tissues, including bone marrow, lymph nodes, and brain tissue.[153-155] Blood, semen, vaginal fluid, and breast milk are the only fluids that have been implicated in the transmission of HIV.[156]

Body fluid exposure is dependent on two variables: the amount of viral particles present within the fluid and the ability of that fluid to reach the target T4 lymphocytes. For HIV to produce an infection, it must be able to enter the recipient's bloodstream and attach itself to the T4 lymphocyte.

There are three modes of transmission for HIV.[155,157-160] The first is unsafe vaginal or anal sexual contact with an infected individual. Direct inoculation with infected blood or blood products is the second mode of transmission. Mechanisms that allow this transmission to occur include inoculation through transfusions, needles not cleansed properly after intravenous drug use, inoculation with infected blood through small cuts, and inoculation through needlesticks or percutaneous exposure. The risk of transmission through blood transfusions has significantly decreased since 1985, when the ELISA was implemented into the process of blood screening. Since 1985, all donated blood has been screened for the presence of HIV.[161]

The third mode is vertical transmission from mother to fetus or during birth. Vertically infected children exhibit a bimodal pattern disease of progression.[162] About 10% to 25% of infected children develop profound immunosuppression, *Pneumocystis carinii* pneumonia, severe encephalopathy, organomegaly, and multiple opportunistic infections in the first few months of life; without treatment, few of these children survive more than 2 years.[163] Most children have a slower progression to AIDS with mean times to AIDS of 6 to 9 years.[162] Factors contributing to the variable rates of disease progression include the route and timing of infection, the amount and phenotype of the virus, and host immunogenetic factors.[164]

Being an HIV-positive mother does not guarantee that her baby will develop HIV disease. However, babies born to infected women will test positive because of maternal antibody transmission to the fetus during development.[165,166] Maternal antibodies remain in the baby's system for up to 15 months[161]; therefore it is not currently possible to determine the true HIV status of a baby until the effects of maternal antibodies have resolved. The widespread use of zidovudine has led to a decline in the number of children becoming perinatally infected with HIV. The rate of mother-infant transmission has declined by 50% or more in many areas of the United States.[167] Because the number of children born to HIV-infected women each year has remained about the same in recent years, the declining transmission rate has already contributed to fewer children being reported with AIDS nationwide. Several maternal, delivery, and newborn factors appear to be associated with higher risk for mother-infant transmission. One of the maternal risk factors most consistently found across studies is the stage of the mother's HIV infection, as measured by clinical, immunologic, or virologic markers.[167] Also, if a woman has given birth to an HIV-positive baby in the past, there is a 65% chance that the woman will give birth to another HIV-positive baby.[168]

Zidovudine (AZT) has proved to be effective in the prevention of perinatal transmission of HIV.[169] In a study of 364 HIV-positive women, AZT therapy was associated with a 67.5% decrease in perinatal transmission. As a result of this study, the Public Health Service recommends that HIV-positive women be informed that AZT substantially reduces the risk of HIV transmission to their unborn baby but does not eliminate it. Also, because this study did not examine teratogenicity, the recommendation is that AZT not be started before the fourteenth week of gestation if it is being given for the sole purpose of reducing perinatal transmission.[169]

Incubation Period. When HIV was first identified, the belief was that individuals were diagnosed as being HIV positive, developed AIDS, and then died within a very short time. The pace of HIV disease progression in children is accelerated compared with adults. This difference is presumably a consequence of the acquisition of infection at a time of immunologic immaturity and the availability of increased numbers of susceptible target cells. Children infected through nonvertical routes may have a course more similar to that of adults, with longer median time to AIDS diagnosis and death.[164] The mean age of AIDS diagnosis is 12 months for children with disease acquired through perinatal transmission and 24.4 months for children with transfusion-acquired disease.[170]

Viral Replication. HIV is classified as a retrovirus. A retrovirus must first translate, or convert, its RNA into DNA to replicate. Once translation has taken place, the virus can

then insert itself into host DNA, which allows the host cell to produce more retroviral particles.[171] The translation from RNA to DNA requires the presence of reverse transcriptase, an enzyme that is present in retroviruses but not present in normal host cells.[153] Some of the current therapies to slow the progression of HIV disease are reverse transcriptase inhibitors that prevent this translation from taking place.

Initially, HIV enters the bloodstream of the host and attaches itself to the CD4 receptor, on the T4 helper lymphocyte. Once this attachment has taken place, the virus uncoats or sheds its outer envelope. The HIV RNA is transcribed into DNA via reverse transcriptase after the virus is uncoated and inside the host cell. Once translation is complete, the HIV replication process continues. Next, the viral DNA is incorporated into the host DNA. At this point, the virus can remain dormant for up to several years or begin replication immediately.

At the end of a latent stage, the cell in which the virus is located becomes activated by an antigen. It is uncertain what antigen causes the cell to become activated. New virions are formed and released into the bloodstream through a process called budding. These new viral cells then attach to other uninfected cells. The host cell ruptures, releasing many viral particles at once and causing death to that cell. All the particles released into the bloodstream can now continue the cycle. This mechanism causes the immune system to be gradually depleted of T4 cells, leaving the host open to massive infections and malignancies, which eventually lead to the individual's death.[153,159,171,172]

Fig. 15-11 illustrates the process of viral replication. There are two subsets of T cells: the T4 and T8 cells.

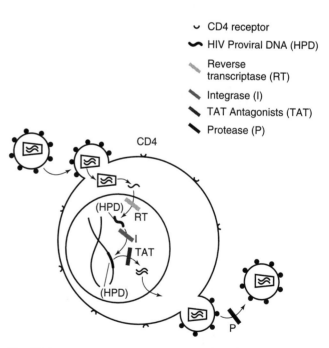

∨ CD4 receptor

∽ HIV Proviral DNA (HPD)

╲ Reverse transcriptase (RT)

╲ Integrase (I)

╲ TAT Antagonists (TAT)

╲ Protease (P)

Fig. 15-11 Replication cycle of human immunodeficiency virus. The life cycle of HIV is shown with the points at which research is ongoing for pharmacologic agents that may block viral maturation, including points for inhibition of reverse transcriptase, integrase, TAT transportation, and protease.

T4 cells are also called inducer, or helper, cells and are sometimes referred to as the conductor of the immune system because of their immunomodulatory function. The T4 cells release lymphokines, which activate the other cells of the immune system and signal warning that nonhost cells are present.[172] The T4 cell is responsible directly or indirectly for the induction of a wide array of functions of multiple limbs of the immune response, as well as for certain nonlymphoid cell functions. Decreased CD4 helper-inducer cells with an expanded CD8 cell population result in an inverted CD4/CD8 ratio, usually with a number much less than 1.

Classification. The CDC has developed a classification system to assist the healthcare provider in staging the progression of HIV disease because of the huge spectrum that exists. The system classifies infected children into mutually exclusive categories according to infection status, clinical status, and immunologic status.[173] This system is outlined in Box 15-1.

Laboratory Diagnosis of HIV Infection. Polymerase chain reaction (PCR) is a procedure that examines an individual's genes within the DNA strand to detect the presence of HIV. HIV DNA PCR is the preferred virologic method for diagnosing HIV infection during infancy. A meta-analysis of published data from 271 infected children indicated that HIV DNA PCR was sensitive for the diagnosis of HIV infection during the neonatal period.[174] HIV culture has sensitivity similar to that of DNA PCR for the diagnosis of infection and is considered the gold standard.[175] However, HIV culture is more complex and expensive to perform than is DNA PCR, and a definitive result may not be available for 2 to 4 weeks.

The ELISA detects the presence of antibodies to the whole virus.[176] Though the ELISA is sensitive and specific, other antibodies within the patient's body can react with the material used in the ELISA to produce a false-positive result.[152] The Western blot test is designed to detect the presence of anti–HIV-1 antibodies and antigens. The precise criteria for what constitutes a positive Western blot test remain controversial; however, it is used as a confirmatory test for a positive ELISA.

Although use of standard and immune-complex dissociated p24 antigen tests are highly specific for HIV infection and have been used to diagnose infection in children, the sensitivity is less than that for the other HIV virologic tests. This assay measures the amount of free viral protein (p24) present in the plasma or tissue culture supernatant. p24 antigen testing alone is not currently recommended to exclude infection or for the diagnosis of infection for infants younger than 1 month because of a high frequency of false-positive assays during this time.[177] Initial testing is recommended by 48 hours of age because nearly 40% of infected infants can be identified at this time. Infants with positive virologic test results before age 48 hours are considered to have early (i.e., intrauterine) infection, whereas infants with negative virologic test results during the first week of life and subsequent positive tests are considered to have late (i.e., intrapartum) infection.

Because the routine tests are limited in infants, an alternative approach is the repeated (longitudinal) collection of serum samples and batch assay to establish a rising anti-HIV antibody titer. The increasing titer is evidence of HIV infection. Johnson and colleagues[178] demonstrated that up to 85% to 90% of infected infants will be detected by 6 months of age.

It is not uncommon for HIV antibody tests to be ordered and performed in the PICU. Anxiety can develop in the patient or parent because of a lack of understanding concerning the meaning of the test or the possibility that the test will be positive. Therefore pretest and posttest counseling is very important and required by law in many states. PICU nurses must understand these tests, be able to explain their meaning and purpose, and clarify the misconception that a positive HIV test result equals AIDS. It is also essential for nurses to be aware of local and national resources of written literature to provide to the parents.

Evaluation of Immunologic Status. Human lymphocytes possess specific glycoproteins on their surface that play an important role in cell activity and function. CD4+ lymphocytes are the primary targets of HIV infection, and the CD4 receptor is the primary binding site of HIV-1. The loss of these cells is associated with development of the characteristic OIs and malignancies of AIDS and an important determinant of clinical staging. The numbers of CD4 and CD8 cells are measured through the use of specific monoclonal antibodies and flow cytometry.[179]

Clinicians interpreting CD4+ T lymphocyte number in children must consider age as a variable. A pediatric clinical and immunologic staging system for HIV infection has been developed that includes age-related definitions of immune suppression. Values should be obtained as soon as possible after a child has a positive virologic test result for HIV and every 3 months thereafter.[180]

Viral burden in peripheral blood can be determined using quantitative HIV RNA assays. Coincident with the body's humoral and cell-mediated immune response, viral RNA levels decline 6 to 12 months after acute infection, reflecting the balance between ongoing viral production and immune elimination. The HIV RNA pattern in perinatally infected infants includes persistently high copy numbers for prolonged periods.[177] HIV RNA patterns may be correlated with disease progression and mortality. However, the predictive value of specific HIV RNA levels for disease progression and death for an individual child is only moderate. In addition, specimen storage, delay in specimen processing, and different HIV RNA assays make direct extrapolation of the predictive value of the HIV RNA levels difficult.

AIDS-Defining Illnesses. A wide range of manifestations of HIV infection are present in children. There are generally two patterns of disease presentation: one that is associated with a rapidly progressive disease with a poorer prognosis and the other associated with a slower process. However, regardless of the manifestation, once a child develops an AIDS-defining illness, the prognosis is poor.

AIDS-defining illness can be caused by viruses, fungi, parasites, bacteria, or cancers.[181] One of these opportunistic infections must be present for the diagnosis of AIDS to be used. All of the organisms that cause these illnesses are ubiquitous in nature.

Box 15-1

◆ Clinical Categories for Children With Human Immunodeficiency Virus (HIV) Infection

Category N: Not Symptomatic

Children who have no signs or symptoms considered to be the result of HIV infection or who have only one of the conditions listed in Category A.

Category: Mildly Symptomatic

Children with two or more of the conditions listed below but none of the conditions listed in Categories B and C.
- Lymphadenopathy (≥0.5 cm at more than two sites; bilateral = one site)
- Hepatomegaly
- Splenomegaly
- Dermatitis
- Parotitis
- Recurrent or persistent upper respiratory infection, sinusitis, or otitis media

Category B: Moderately Symptomatic

Children who have symptomatic conditions other than those listed for Category A or C that are attributed to HIV infection. Examples of conditions in clinical Category B include but are not limited to:
- Anemia (<8 g/dl), neutropenia (<1000/mm^3), or thrombocytopenia (<100,000/mm^3) persisting ≥30 days
- Bacterial meningitis, pneumonia, or sepsis (single episode)
- Candidiasis, oropharyngeal (thrush), persisting (>2 months) in children >6 months of age
- Cardiomyopathy
- Cytomegalovirus infection, with onset before 1 month of age
- Diarrhea, recurrent or chronic
- Hepatitis
- Herpes simplex virus (HSV) stomatitis, recurrent (more than two episodes within 1 year)
- HSV bronchitis, pneumonitis, or esophagitis with onset before 1 month of age
- Herpes zoster (shingles) involving at least two distinct episodes or more than one dermatome
- Leiomyosarcoma
- Lymphoid interstitial pneumonia (LIP) or pulmonary lymphoid hyperplasia complex
- Nephropathy
- Nocardiosis
- Persistent fever (lasting >1 month)
- Toxoplasmosis, onset before 1 month of age
- Varicella, disseminated (complicated chickenpox)

Category C: Severely Symptomatic*

Children who have any condition listed in the 1987 surveillance case definition for acquired immunodeficiency syndrome, with the exception of LIP.
- Serious bacterial infections, multiple or recurrent (i.e., any combination of at least two culture-confirmed infections within a 2-year period), of the following types: septicemia, pneumonia, meningitis, bone or joint infection, or abscess of an internal organ or body cavity (excluding otitis media, superficial skin or mucosal abscesses, and indwelling catheter–related infections)
- Candidiasis, esophageal or pulmonary (bronchi, trachea, lungs)
- Coccidioidomycosis, disseminated (at site other than or in addition to lungs or cervical or hilar lymph nodes)
- Cryptococcosis, extrapulmonary
- Cryptosporidiosis or isosporiasis with diarrhea persisting >1 month
- Cytomegalovirus disease with onset of symptoms at age >1 month (at a site other than liver, spleen, or lymph nodes)
- Encephalopathy (at least one of the following progressive findings present for at least 2 months in the absence of a concurrent illness other than HIV infection that could explain the findings): (a) failure to attain or loss of developmental milestones or loss of intellectual ability, verified by standard developmental scale or neuropsychologic tests; (b) impaired brain growth or acquired microcephaly demonstrated by head circumference measurements or brain atrophy demonstrated by computed tomography or magnetic resonance imaging (serial imaging is required for children <2 years of age); (c) acquired symmetric motor deficit manifested by two or more of the following: paresis, pathologic reflexes, ataxia or gait disturbance
- HSV infection causing a mucocutaneous ulcer that persists for >1 month; or bronchitis, pneumonitis, or esophagitis for any duration affecting a child >1 month of age
- Histoplasmosis, disseminated (at a site other than or in addition to lungs or cervical or hilar lymph nodes)
- Kaposi's sarcoma
- Lymphoma, primary, in brain
- Lymphoma, small, noncleaved cell (Burkitt's), or immunoblastic or large cell lymphoma of B cell or unknown immunologic phenotype
- *Mycobacterium tuberculosis,* disseminated or extrapulmonary
- *Mycobacterium,* other species or unidentified species, disseminated (at a site other than or in addition to lungs, skin, or cervical or hilar lymph nodes)
- *Myobacterium avium* complex or *Mycobacterium kansasii,* disseminated (at site other than or in addition to lungs, skin, or cervical or hilar lymph nodes)
- *Pneumocystis carinii* pneumonia
- Progressive multifocal leukoencephalopathy
- Salmonella (nontyphoid) septicemia, recurrent
- Toxoplasmosis of the brain with onset at >1 month of age
- Wasting syndrome in the absence of concurrent illness other than HIV infection that could explain the following findings: (a) persistent weight loss >10% of baseline OR (b) downward crossing of at least two of the following percentile lines on the weight-for-age percentile chart (e.g., 95th, 75th, 50th, 25th, 5th) in a child ≥1 year of age OR (c) <5th percentile on weight-for-height chart on two consecutive measurements, ≥30 days apart PLUS (a) chronic diarrhea (i.e., at least two loose stools per day for ≥30 days) OR (b) documented fever (for ≥30 days, intermittent or constant)

*See the 1987 AIDS surveillance case definition for diagnosis criteria.

From Centers for Disease Control and Prevention: 1994 Revised classification system for human immunodeficiency virus infection in children less than 13 years of age; Official authorized addenda: human immunodeficiency virus infection codes and official guidelines for coding and reporting ICD-9-CM, *MMWR* 43:RR-12, 1994.

TABLE 15-12 Clinical Manifestations of Pediatric HIV Infection

Nonspecific	Infectious Complications
Recurrent fever	Pyogenic infections
Failure to thrive*	Mycobacterial
Parotiditis	Tuberculosis
Diffuse lymphadenopathy	Atypical*
Hepatosplenomegaly	Candidal infections
Anorexia*	Tineal infections
Hyperviscosity	Viral infections
	Measles*
Organ System–Related	Cytomegalovirus*
Diseases	Hepatitis A, B, C
Progressive encephalopathy*	Herpes zoster virus
Peripheral neuropathy	Herpes simplex virus
Lymphoid interstitial	Epstein-Barr virus
pneumonia	*Pneumocystis carinii**
Cardiomyopathy*	*Toxoplasma gondii**
Arteriopathy*	Cryptosporidiosis
Hepatitis	Cryptococcal infections*
Chronic diarrhea/	Malignancies*
malabsorption	Lymphomas, particularly
Neuropathy/nephritis	non-Hodgkin's type
Hypertension	
Anemia/leukopenia/	
thrombocytopenia	
Endocrinopathies	
Dermatitis	

From Hoyt LG, Oleske JM: The clinical spectrum of HIV infection in infants and children: an overview. In Yogev R, Connor E, eds: *Management of HIV infection in infants and children*, St Louis, 1992, Mosby, pp 227-246.
*Associated with a graver prognosis.

Common clinical manifestations of HIV infection in infants and children are listed in Table 15-12. The presenting signs and symptoms are often nonspecific and may include recurrent fevers, failure to thrive, diffuse lymphadenopathy, hepatosplenomegaly, and anorexia. These may be caused by chronic viral infection, malnutrition, and immunodeficiency.

The most common clinical manifestation early in the disease process is lymphadenopathy. This condition is often associated with hypergammaglobulinemia and splenomegaly. In addition, skin disorders, such as candidal dermatitis, in particular, are common clinical manifestations.

Acute Respiratory Failure. Pulmonary complications leading to acute respiratory failure (ARF) are the most common reason for admission of pediatric AIDS patients to the PICU. Pulmonary diseases cause significant morbidity and mortality in pediatric HIV patients. Table 15-13 outlines the infectious and noninfectious pulmonary diseases that can occur in HIV-infected children.

Pneumonias caused by *Pneumocystis carinii* pneumonia (PC), RSV, CMV, *Mycobacterium avium-intracellulare, P. aeruginosa, Candida albicans, H. influenzae, S. aureus,* Klebsiella, and lymphoid interstitial pneumonitis (LIP) have all been reported as reasons for ARF. Of these, PCP and LIP are by far the most common.

Pneumocystis carinii Pneumonia. PCP remains the most common opportunistic infection in children with HIV infection. PCP was reported in 34% of U.S. children with perinatally acquired AIDs through 1997.[146] PCP has been shown to be an important cause of mortality among children infected with HIV. In 1992 the estimated median survival of children after a diagnosis of PCP was 19 months.[182]

PCP is considered either a protozoan parasite or a fungus and exists as a cyst containing eight intracystic

TABLE 15-13 Pulmonary Diseases in Children With AIDS

Infectious	
1. Parasitic	*Pneumocystis carinii, Toxoplasma gondii, Strongyloides stercoralis*
2. Viral	Respiratory viruses: respiratory syncytial virus, influenza virus, parainfluenza virus, adenovirus
	Measles
	Opportunists: cytomegalovirus, herpes simplex, varicella zoster virus
3. Bacterial	*Streptococcus pneumoniae, Haemophilus influenzae, Staphylococcus aureus*
	Nosocomial: enteric bacilli, *Pseudomonas aeruginosa*
	Actinomycetes: *Nocardia* sp.
	Mycobacterial: *M. tuberculosis, M. avium-intracellulare*
4. Fungal	*Cryptococcus neoformans, Histoplasma capsulatum, Coccidioides immitis, Candida* sp., *Aspergillus* sp.
Noninfectious	
1. Lymphoid diseases	Pulmonary lymphoid hyperplasia
	Lymphocytic interstitial pneumonia
	Polyclonal polymorphic B cell lymphoproliferative disorder
2. Bronchiectasis	
3. Kaposi's sarcoma	

From Berkowitz ID, Berkowitz FE, Johnson JP: The critically ill child and human immunodeficiency virus. In Rogers MC, ed: *Textbook of pediatric intensive care*, Baltimore, 1992, Williams & Wilkins.

bodies.[183] These bodies are released from the cysts and form new cysts, which then attach to type I alveolar cells. As a result, alveolitis and interstitial edema develop, leading to ventilation perfusion mismatch, decreased pulmonary compliance, hypoxia, and an increased alveolar-arterial (A-a) gradient.[183]

The clinical course of PCP is highly variable, ranging from the acute onset of fever and marked respiratory distress to a more insidious onset with a subacute course. The presenting signs are often nonspecific and include fever, cough, tachypnea, and hypoxemia. Chest auscultation may be normal even with the presence of tachypnea and clinical evidence of respiratory distress. Early in the course, the chest radiograph may also be normal. As roentgenographic findings develop, a diffuse bilateral interstitial pattern is most often seen. Patients may rapidly progress to respiratory failure and death if the diagnosis of PCP is not made early.

Guidelines exist for prophylaxis against PCP for children infected with or perinatally exposed to HIV.[184] Prophylaxis is determined by the child's CD4+ count, CD4+ percent, and age. Trimethoprim-sulfamethoxazole (TMP-SMX) remains the drug of choice for prophylaxis. Alternative regimens include the use of dapsone or aerosolized pentamidine.[184] Because PCP is relatively safe, effective, and inexpensive chemoprophylaxis is available, preventing PCP has been a major priority in the care of children infected with HIV.

PCP may be diagnosed with noninvasive or invasive techniques. Analysis of sputum, endotracheal secretions, and gastric washings may show evidence of the organism and is attempted first. Other methods may include bronchoalveolar lavage, transbronchial biopsy, or open lung biopsy.[175] Open lung biopsy is reserved for children in whom other methods have not provided a diagnosis. The latter three are the most reliable methods for diagnosis.[185]

Management of the child with PCP includes oxygen therapy, antibiotic therapy, steroids, positive end-expiratory pressure (PEEP) or continuous positive airway pressure (CPAP), and mechanical ventilation. The standard antibiotic therapy for PCP is the administration of TMP-SMX or pentamidine isethionate. TMP-SMX is given orally or intravenously at 20 mg/kg/day, with the initial administration being intravenous. Oral administration can begin once improvement has taken place. Because many patients become neutropenic when treated daily with TMP-SMX, administration 3 times a week may be used; this approach appears equally effective and causes less neutropenia.[186] Therapy is recommended to continue for 21 days.

Intravenous pentamidine is instituted when no response to TMP-SMX is seen. Aerosolized pentamidine, although effective in adults with less severe cases of PCP, is of limited use in children because of uneven delivery of the drug to the smaller airways.[187] The recommended dose is 4 mg/kg/day given in a single dose for 14 to 21 days. The drug is administered by slow intravenous infusion because hypotension may result if administered rapidly. Side effects that may result with use of pentamidine are hypoglycemia, hyperglycemia, neutropenia, thrombocytopenia, and azotemia. Table 15-14 lists the dosage and side effects of these drugs.

Lymphoid Interstitial Pneumonitis. LIP is a common symptom of pulmonary involvement in children with HIV infection.[188] LIP is very common in pediatric HIV infection and has been found in up to 30% to 40% of HIV-infected infants and children with pulmonary disease.[188]

LIP involves the diffuse lymphoid infiltration of the lung parenchyma; a related disorder, pulmonary lymphoid hyper-

TABLE 15-14 Treatment Options for Moderate to Severe *Pneumocystis Carinii* Pneumonia

Treatment Regimen	Dose(s), Route, Frequency	Side Effect(s)
Trimethoprim (TMP)-sulfamethoxazole (SMX)	15 mg/kg (TMP), IV, divided every 6-8 hr*	Rash,† fever, N/V, ↑ liver function tests, ↑ K+, neutropenia
Pentamidine isethionate	3-4 mg/kg, IV, once daily	Nephrotoxicity, ↑ K+, ↓ Ca2+/Mg2+, ↑ amylase, ↓↑ glucose‡
Trimetrexate plus leucovorin ± dapsones§	45 mg/m², IV, once daily, plus 20 mg/m², PO, every 6 h ± 100 mg, PO, once daily	Neutropenia, thrombocytopenia, rash, fever, ↑ liver function tests, hemolytic anemia (check G6PD level), methemoglobinemia; limited experience with children
Clindamycin plus primaquine	1800 mg, IV, divided every 6-8 hr plus 30 mg (base), PO, once daily	Rash, N/V, diarrhea, hemolytic anemia (check G6PD level), methemoglobinemia; limited experience with children

Adapted from Stansell JD, Huang L: *Pneumocystis carinii* pneumonia. In Sande MA, Volberding PA, eds: *The medical management of AIDS*, ed 5, Philadelphia, 1997, WB Saunders, p 287.
*TMP-SMX is dispensed as a fixed combination.
†Mild rash that does not cause bullous skin lesions and does not involve mucous membranes can often be treated with antihistamines first and should not necessarily result in discontinuation of drug.
‡Avoid other nephrotoxic agents (nonsteroidal antiinflammatory agents, aminoglycosides, foscarnet, amphotericin B). Risk of hypotension can be minimized if infusion is given over a 2- to 3-hour period.
§A study is in progress comparing TMP-SMX with trimetrexate-dapsone (plus leucovorin).
IV, Intravenous; *PO*, orally; *N/V*, nausea and vomiting; *G6PD*, glucose-6-phosphate dehydrogenase; ↑ = increased; ↓ = decreased.

plasia (PLH), involves hyperplasia of bronchus-associated lymphoid tissue. In the 1994 CDC Revised Classification System for Human Immunodeficiency Virus Infection in Children, LIP is classified as a category B symptom, one attributed to and indicative of an HIV-related immunologic deficit.[149]

Clinical manifestations of LIP can range from asymptomatic disease with isolated radiographic abnormalities to severe bullous lung disease with pulmonary insufficiency. Children with symptomatic LIP often present during the second or third year of life with the insidious onset of dyspnea, fatigability, tachypnea, cough, and occasionally fever associated with salivary gland enlargement and lymphadenopathy.[189]

Clinical and radiographic findings may lead to a presumptive diagnosis. However, the definitive diagnosis is made by lung biopsy. The specimen will show the typical lymphocytic infiltrates. LIP responds to systemic corticosteroids, but no controlled studies have been performed to assess the efficacy of steroids for LIP.[189] Treatment with steroids is usually reserved for patients with significant hypoxemia and symptoms of pulmonary insufficiency, including tachypnea, dyspnea on exertion, and exercise intolerance.

Tuberculosis. Tuberculosis is less common in children than adult patients with AIDS. The increase in cases of tuberculosis reported to the CDC between 1986 and 1992 not only represented a 20% increase in total cases but also a 33% increase in the number of cases reported in children.[190] Children with tuberculosis are almost always infected by an adult in their environment, usually a close household contact. It is less common in the child with AIDS, with little information available on the incidence and clinical characteristics.

Tuberculosis may be caused by either *Mycobacterium tuberculosis* or *M. bovis,* although disease with *M. bovis* is seen only in the rare circumstances of vaccine-associated infection. *M. tuberculosis* is a small, weak gram-positive rod, which is a slow-growing, obligate aerobe.

Nonimmunocompromised children who develop primary tuberculosis demonstrate lymph node enlargement in the hilar, mediastinal, and cervical areas. Pulmonary infiltrates with consolidation, atelectasis, pleural effusion, and tuberculous meningitis can also be seen.[191] The clinical manifestations in HIV-infected children are usually nonspecific and include fever, weight loss, and cough. On chest radiograph, localized patchy infiltrates and hilar lymphadenopathy are seen. Because of the immunosuppression that accompanies the disease, skin testing alone is not conclusive for diagnosis of tuberculosis. Cerebrospinal fluid and blood cultures, in addition to gastric and bronchial washings, are necessary. Children tend to swallow their sputum, so acid-fast stains of gastric washings are more helpful than sputum stains in establishing the diagnosis. Gastric washings are obtained very early in the morning before the patient has any oral intake.

Isoniazid, rifampin, pyrazinamide, and ethambutol or streptomycin are recommended for initial treatment while awaiting susceptibility results. In the case of disseminated disease, a bactericidal agent may be used. The duration of therapy ranges from 6 to 9 months, determined by infection site, response to therapy, and the sensitivity of the organism. A 12-month duration of therapy is recommended for those children with miliary tuberculosis, bone and joint tuberculosis, or tuberculous meningitis.[192]

Infection control is a critical nursing concern in caring for children with HIV infection and tuberculosis. Children with cavitary lesions, endobronchial tuberculosis, or positive gastric washing or sputum cultures are placed on respiratory isolation.[193] Family members should wear a tuberculosis mask during visits, and careful monitoring of the infection status of these children is necessary.

Cardiovascular Dysfunction. Cardiac disease in children with HIV infection may be common, extensive, and clinically significant. Some suggest that approximately 20% of HIV-infected children will have some type of cardiac complication, the two most common being cardiovascular failure secondary to septic shock and cardiomyopathy.[194]

Cardiomyopathy is the second most common cardiac PICU presentation of children with AIDS, with 33% of the deaths occurring in the setting of significant cardiovascular disease.[195] Although the degree of cardiac dysfunction may be difficult to determine because of multiorgan involvement, autopsy findings of these children have shown biventricular dilation, myocardial hypertrophy, interstitial fibrosis, myocardial necrosis, and endocardial thickening.[196] Conduction disturbances secondary to vasculitis, myocarditis, or fibrosis have also been described.[197]

Left ventricular dysfunction, often a precursor to dilated cardiomyopathy and congestive heart failure; is the most common cardiac manifestation of HIV infection among children. Left ventricular dysfunction is often asymptomatic and is diagnosed echocardiographically.[195]

Cardiac dysrhythmias have been reported in HIV-infected children, although the occurrence is uncommon and nonspecific. Isolated incidences of ventricular and atrial ectopy have been reported.[198]

The cause of HIV-associated cardiomyopathy is unknown. Many factors may be involved, including HIV infection, infection with other agents, an abnormal host response, and drug toxicity.[199] Despite the autopsy findings, the pathogenesis of this dilated cardiomyopathy has yet to be fully explained. The virus itself may cause myocardial damage by releasing mediator-infected monocytes, or the host immune system may play a role by producing an autoimmune response.[200]

Congestive heart failure is the predominant clinical manifestation of later-stage cardiac involvement, although it may be difficult to diagnose in the HIV-infected child. Tachypnea and rales may be secondary to pulmonary disease or insufficiency, tachycardia may be due to fever or anemia, and hepatosplenomegaly is typically present in many children with HIV infection. Therefore these symptoms cannot be relied on as specific to congestive heart failure. From the experience gained at several institutions, the most reliable clinical indicators of congestive heart failure in these children are the presence of a gallop rhythm associated with tachypnea and tachycardia and cardiomegaly on chest x-ray film.[194,201]

Septic shock may be the primary cardiovascular cause for PICU admission of HIV-infected children. Serious bacterial infections often occur in children with AIDS. *Streptococcus pneumoniae; Salmonella, Pseudomonas,* and *Enterobacter* species; *H. influenzae; Enterococci; S. aureus* and *S. epidermidis;* and *E. coli* have all been identified as causative pathogens.

Nursing care for the HIV-infected child is the same as for any child exhibiting low cardiac output secondary to septic shock or cardiomyopathy and includes inotropic support, afterload reduction, and appropriate antimicrobial therapy. Treatment of congestive heart failure secondary to cardiomyopathy includes preload reduction and the administration of digoxin for diminished pump function.

Central Nervous System Dysfunction.   HIV-related central nervous system (CNS) abnormalities are a common and important complication of HIV disease in children, causing significant morbidity and mortality. Encephalopathy has been reported to be the presenting manifestation of AIDs in as many as 18% of children.[202] CNS dysfunction in the HIV-positive child may be caused by secondary infection by usual or opportunistic pathogens, as well as by primary HIV infection of the brain.

Children may develop bacterial meningitis associated with usual pathogens such as *H. influenzae, S. pneumoniae,* and *N. meningitidis,* as well as various gram-negative bacilli. Meningitis and encephalitis may also result from infection by numerous viral pathogens. Other CNS infections include mycobacterial and fungal meningitis.[203]

Primary CNS lymphomas are the most common intracranial mass lesions that develop in children with HIV, although they are relatively rare. The symptoms usually seen are seizure activity, mental status changes, and neurologic deficits.

The primary neurologic manifestation of HIV infection of the brain is HIV encephalopathy, and it is present in more than 50% of HIV-infected children.[183] This manifestation can present as a rapid course of deterioration or may be static.

Children can exhibit signs of static encephalopathy, demonstrated by an inability to achieve developmental milestones in some or all areas.[204] Also, progressive encephalopathy has been reported in children. This condition has been described as either a loss of developmental milestones or intellectual deficits, associated with impaired brain growth; weakness with bilateral pyramidal tract signs, ataxia, and, less commonly, seizures; and coma.[204,205] In a study performed by Epstein and co-workers,[206] the most common CT scan finding was cerebral atrophy, with secondary enlargement of the subarachnoid spaces and ventricles. The damage to the CNS may be caused by the direct effect of the virus in the brain tissue. Progressive encephalopathy develops and worsens proportionally to the increasing immunodeficiency.[207] The most common neurologic diagnoses that necessitate admission of the HIV-infected child to the PICU are CNS infection, lymphoma, and strokes.

Strokes are an infrequent but potentially devastating complication of AIDS. They may result from the inflammation of the cerebral blood vessels, causing an ischemic infarction, or they may result from cerebral hemorrhage. HIV-associated progressive encephalopathy is the clinical corollary of the direct and indirect effects of CNS or systemic HIV infection. The predominant clinical neurologic findings include impaired brain growth, progressive motor dysfunction, and loss or plateauing of neurodevelopmental milestones. Treatment includes antiretroviral drugs, rehabilitation, immunomodulatory therapy, and psychoactive medications.

Hematologic Dysfunction.   Hematologic dysfunction related to HIV infection includes autoimmune thrombocytopenia, anemia, leukopenia, granulocytopenia, and lymphomas.[186] Primary bone marrow failure also occurs in some children.[203]

Thrombocytopenia may be an early manifestation of HIV infection. B cell dysfunction is postulated to lead to the production of autoantibodies and immune complexes, resulting in peripheral platelet destruction.[208] Therapies to treat thrombocytopenia in the HIV-infected child include corticosteroids, splenectomy, danazol, vincristine, and intravenous IgG.[208]

Anemia is a prominent diagnosis of HIV disease. Although the anemia is generally mild and nonprogressive, in a child with multiple opportunistic infections, this may be significant. Many factors may cause anemia, one being that the virus may infect erythroid precursors in the bone marrow, inhibit the production of red cells, and cause sequestration of the red cells in the spleen and liver.[208] Zidovudine (AZT) may also cause anemia.

Leukopenia commonly occurs in children with HIV infection, often in combination with anemia. Granulocytopenia can also occur and is usually accompanied by a left shift in the differential portion of the complete blood count. The cause is probably multifactorial, including immune dysfunction resulting in hypogammaglobulinemia and production of autoantibodies and immune complexes. Antibodies against granulocytes have also been observed.

Malignancies, such as non-Hodgkin's lymphoma, have been reported in HIV-infected children. These tumors are almost always of B cell origin. Also, primary CNS lymphoma has been reported in children with perinatally acquired infection.

HIV-infected patients with anemia who are symptomatic are recommended to receive transfusion of irradiated packed RBCs. Also, G-CSF with erythropoietin for children with zidovudine toxicity has been found to be effective in correcting anemia.[208] Further information regarding RBC and platelet disorders is found in Chapter 24.

The primary method of treatment of HIV-associated leukopenia and granulocytopenia is the use of granulocyte growth factors. Both recombinant GM-CSF and G-CSF have been found to be effective. Short-term chemotherapy is usually the treatment of choice in children with malignancies because most of these children will not tolerate the immunosuppressive effects of long-term chemotherapy.[208]

Other Organ Dysfunction.   Abnormalities of all organ systems can be seen in HIV-infected children, whether induced by the HIV infection itself or by opportunistic infections. Hepatitis is commonly seen without an easily documented infectious cause. Pancreatitis with elevated serum amylase and lipase levels has also been seen in HIV-infected children. HIV-associated renal disease with azotemia and proteinuria has been described in children.[209] As many as 30% of HIV-infected children may develop one of several forms of renal disease.[183]

Critical Care Management of the Patient With HIV.   In 1999 the U.S. Public Health Service and Infectious Diseases Society of America developed disease-specific recommendations for prevention of OIs and an immunization schedule for HIV-infected children.[210] Prophylaxis to prevent the first episode of OI in infants and children infected with HIV include TMP-SMX against PCP, isoniazid against isoniazid-sensitive *M. tuberculosis,* clarithromycin against *M. avium,* VZIg, and influenza vaccine.[210] PCP occurs most often between 3 and 6 months of age in perinatally infected children, so PCP prophylaxis is recommended to be initiated at 4 to 6 weeks of life for all HIV-exposed infants and continued until 12 months of age.

Antiretroviral Therapy.   Ongoing viral replication is the driving force behind immunologic destruction. The goal of antiretroviral therapy in children is to suppress viral replication to extremely low levels; if replication continues, ongoing mutation will lead to drug resistance.[175]

As of January 1998, 11 antiretroviral agents were approved for use in HIV-infected adults and adolescents in the United States; 6 of these have approved pediatric indications. The agents available fall into three major classes: (1) nucleoside analogue reverse transcriptase inhibitor (NRTI) agents, (2) nonnucleoside analogue reverse transcriptase inhibitor (NNRTI) agents, and (3) protease inhibitor (PI) agents. NRTI agents are potent inhibitors of the HIV reverse transcriptase enzyme, which is responsible for the reverse transcription of viral RNA into DNA; this process occurs before integration of viral DNA into the chromosomes of the host cell. This is the first class of antiretroviral drugs available for the treatment of HIV infection. NRTI agents require intracellular phosphorylation to their active form by cellular kinases. The phosphorylated drug acts to competitively inhibit viral reverse transcriptase and to terminate additional elongation of viral DNA after its incorporation into the DNA chain. Because these drugs act as a preintegration step in the viral life cycle, they have little or no effect on chronically infected cells in which proviral DNA has already been integrated into cellular chromosomes. Although resistance eventually develops to these agents during the course of long-term, single-drug therapy, combination therapy with these drugs may prevent, delay, or reverse the development of resistance.[177]

NNRTI agents specifically inhibit reverse transcriptase activity by binding directly to the active site of the enzyme without previous activation. At this time, no NNRTI agents are approved for pediatric use; however, phase I trials are underway. PI agents inhibit the HIV protease enzyme that is required to cleave viral polyprotein precursors and to generate functional viral proteins. The protease enzyme is crucial for the assembly stage of viral replication that occurs after transcription of proviral DNA to viral RNA and subsequent translation into viral proteins. Because PI agents act at a postintegration step of the viral life cycle, they are effective in inhibiting replication in both newly infected and chronically infected cells.[177] By 1998, 85% of patients with CD4+ T cell counts below 500/mm^3 were being treated with PI or NNRTIs.

In addition to the drugs listed previously, new classes of drugs are being developed that will work at different points in the viral life cycle. Among these are drugs that block binding of HIV to cells and integrate inhibitors and zinc finger inhibitors (zinc fingers are parts of proteins that bind to nucleic acids and are essential for the assembly of new virus particles).

Combination antiretroviral therapy is recommended for HIV-infected children with clinical symptoms of HIV infection (i.e., clinical category A, B, or C) or evidence of immune suppression. Ideally, antiretroviral therapy should be initiated in all suspected HIV-infected infants. Issues associated with adherence to treatment are especially important in considering whether and when to initiate therapy. Antiretroviral therapy is most effective in patients who have never received therapy and who therefore are less likely to have antiretroviral-resistant viral strains. Lack of adherence to prescribed regimens and subtherapeutic levels of antiretroviral medications, particularly PI agents, may enhance the development of drug resistance. Participation by caregivers and child in the decision-making process is crucial, especially in situations for which definitive data concerning efficacy are not available.[177]

Nutrition.   Appropriate nutrition is a fundamental and necessary part of a child's medical therapy. Nutrition affects the management of children with HIV infection by affecting GI tract function, CNS development, immune function, recovery from infection, bioavailability of therapeutic agents, growth, and quality of life. Growth delay affecting both height and weight is one of the earliest effects of HIV disease in infants and children. Management includes longitudinal assessment of growth-estimating energy requirements, and dietary assessment. The approach to maximizing nutritional support and avoiding malnutrition in children with HIV infection is accomplished by attention to the following goals of nutritional management: (1) treat underlying GI or infectious diseases that interfere with nutrient intake and absorption or increase nutrient loss and (2) provide sufficient nutrition for catch-up growth. Tube or parenteral feedings may be required.[175]

Psychosocial Issues.   As previously stated, developmental delays are a common occurrence in the child with HIV infection. Nursing care involves assessment of the child's developmental level and gearing communication at that level. In addition, some children may display depressive symptoms, such as apathy, social withdrawal, or anorexia.[211] These symptoms are often an indication of other issues, and a psychotherapist should be consulted. Nurses caring for the child may also need to consider that the child may have lost a parent to the same disease. Excellent communication skills and support are necessary.

A diagnosis of HIV infection also has a major impact on the family. Often, the child may be diagnosed before the parent. The psychosocial stress that the diagnosis of HIV places on the family is unique in that in most cases, the child and parent are both ill.[211] Problems that are faced include (1) coping with the diagnosis of a potentially fatal illness; (2) dealing with the healthcare of the child; (3) approaching the emotional, financial, and time demanding aspects of a sick child; and (4) facing potential ostracism from family members and the community.[209]

Working with these families often poses a major challenge for the PICU nurse. The sight of the ICU to a parent who is also infected may be overwhelming because it may represent to the parent his or her future.[212] Parents may blame themselves and have difficulty even visiting their child.

Many parents are also dealing with the problem of substance abuse. Working with these families may be especially difficult for the nursing staff. Open communication, establishment of a relationship, and referral to appropriate resources are critical to family-centered care of the child.

Infectious Diseases Unique to Pediatrics

Toxic Shock Syndrome. Toxic shock syndrome (TSS) was first described in 1978 as a disease characterized by high temperature, hypotension, and diffuse macular erythroderma with desquamation 1 to 2 weeks after onset of illness. In 1980, a profound increase in disease incidence was recognized to be associated almost exclusively with the use of superabsorbent tampons in menstruating women. The mean mortality rate is 3%,[212a] primarily related to adult respiratory distress syndrome, heart block, and dysrhythmias.

TSS is a clinical diagnosis supported by the isolation of *S. aureus* from a focal or enclosed infection, and in some cases, TSS toxin-1 (TSST-1). TSST-1 is a very potent stimulus in vitro for the release of IL-1B, TNF-α, and IL-2.- TSS will become a fulminate disease without proper early intervention. Untreated TSS may evolve to include shock, cardiomyopathy, pericarditis, hepatitis, acute respiratory distress syndrome, renal failure, disseminated intravascular coagulation, and encephalopathy.

After the initial evaluation, if the patient is demonstrating signs of poor perfusion, intravenous (IV) fluids are initiated immediately. While IV fluids are being administered, possible foci of infection are identified, foreign bodies including sutures are removed, and Gram stains and cultures are obtained. The mainstay of therapy consists of supportive care aimed at preservation of vital organ function. Rapid reversal of hypotension is imperative; infusion of large volumes of fluid may be necessary to maintain an adequate cardiac output, venous return, and blood pressure.[213]

Antistaphylococcal β-lactamase–resistant antibiotics are given IV in maximally recommended doses. Commercial preparations of IVIgs contain high levels of antibody to TSST-1 and potentially to the staphylococcal enterotoxins.[213] Administration of IVIg has been shown to be beneficial in a rabbit model of TSS, although it has not yet been systematically studied in humans. Ongoing research includes investigations into the use of MoAbs to IL-1, TNF, and TSST-1.[214]

Infant Botulism. Infant botulism was first recognized as a distinct clinical entity in 1976. Of all forms of human botulism (food borne, wound, and infant), infant botulism is now the most common in the United States. More than 90% of reported cases come from the United States, and within the United States, more than half of the cases come from California, Utah, and southeast Pennsylvania. This finding is likely a consequence of high concentrations of *Clostridium botulinum* spores in the soil of these regions.[215]

C. botulinum is a ubiquitous gram-positive, spore-forming, obligate anaerobe with soil and dust as its natural habitat. Infant botulism typically affects previously well infants within the first 4 to 6 months of life (median 10 weeks) and is caused by ingestion of spores of *C. botulinu*m that germinate and produce toxin in the GI tract. The toxin irreversibly blocks the peripheral cholinergic synapses throughout the body, most importantly at the neuromuscular junction. The toxin does not cross the blood-brain barrier.[216]

Constipation is characteristically an early sign, followed by signs of listlessness and becoming progressively more weak. Symmetric descending paralysis is the rule; the cranial nerves are the first so be affected. The diagnosis is confirmed by detection of the organism or its toxin in the infant's stool.

Aggressive respiratory and nutritional care are the mainstays of treatment. Many infants require intubation and prolonged mechanical ventilation. Physical and occupational therapies are crucial in maintaining range of motion and functional positioning of patients. Prognosis for complete recovery is excellent with meticulous, supportive care. Infant botulism is a self-limited illness lasting a total of 2 to 6 weeks with progressive symptoms. It is universally recommended that honey and corn syrup not be fed to infants younger than 1 year of age to prevent the occurrence of infant botulism.[217]

Rocky Mountain Spotted Fever. Rocky Mountain spotted fever (RMSF) caused by *Rickettsia rickettsii* is the most prevalent rickettsial disease in the United States, and more than two thirds of patients are under 15 years of age.

After the bite of an infected tick, *R. rickettsii* multiply within the endothelial cells of the small blood vessels and then become widely disseminated, resulting in the pathologic lesion of widespread vasculitis and a resulting petechial rash. Clinical manifestations include fever, rash, headache, meningoencephalitis, inflammation of the heart, pulmonary edema, and myalgias. Rash is present in 78% of patients and may be very atypical.

The typical rash involves the palms and soles and begins on the wrists and ankles to spread rapidly in hours up the extremities.[213,218]

Diagnosis of RMSF is made on clinical and epidemiologic grounds. Nonspecific laboratory abnormalities include anemia (30%), thrombocytopenia, and hyponatremia (50%). Treatment consists of supportive care and either chloramphenicol, doxycycline, or tetracycline. Doxycycline is thought to be most favorable in children younger than 9 years of age because of its documented effectiveness, broader margin of safety, and reduced risk of drug-related adverse effects.[219]

Reye's Syndrome.   As acute postinfectious encephalopathy with hepatic dysfunction, Reye's syndrome (RS) was first described by Dr. Reye in 1963. The case fatality rate was 41% during the 1973 to 1974 outbreak and 12% in 1980, probably reflecting an improvement in the level of sophistication of pediatric critical care. In 1980 a statistically significant association was noted between RS and the use of aspirin for the preceding viral illness.[220] Over the past decade, the use of aspirin in young children for minor viral illnesses has decreased significantly, as has the incidence of RS from a peak of 555 cases in 1980 to no more than 36 cases per year since 1987.[213,221] This may be a reflection of better diagnostic techniques and criteria for inborn errors of metabolism that mimicked RS, as most patients originally diagnosed with RS are now known to have metabolic disorders.[222]

Criteria for diagnosis of RS include acute onset of disturbance in consciousness, elevation of serum glutamic-oxaloacetic transaminase (SGOT) and serum glutamic-pyruvate transaminase (SGPT) to twice-normal concentrations, and histologic changes consistent with the syndrome seen in biopsy specimens of liver or postmortem material. Persistent vomiting is usually the first symptom; as the vomiting begins to decrease, confusion appears. The complete neurologic sequence progresses from stage I, in which the child is frightened and confused, to stage V, with a loss of brainstem reflexes.

No specific therapy is available; intensive supportive care is critical with respect to airway maintenance, tissue oxygenation, and control of cerebral edema. Because Reye's syndrome is now very rare, any infant or child suspected of having this disorder should undergo extensive investigation to rule out the treatable inborn metabolic disorders that can mimic Reye's syndrome.[221]

EXPERIMENTAL THERAPIES

Gene transfer therapy is a revolutionary means of actually replacing defective genes within the body.[210] This highly experimental procedure was first used in children with SCID related to ADA deficiency[223] and in familial hyperlipoproteinemia, a lipid disorder. Like the administration of LAK cells and TILs, one method of gene transfer therapy is a multistep treatment that requires the removal of specific cells from the patient, modification of these cells in the laboratory, and return of the modified cells to the patient.[224,225] Gene transfer therapy shows tremendous potential in the cure of other diseases that are the result of a defective gene, such as cystic fibrosis.[226]

Nitric oxide is a membrane-permeable gas that functions in the regulation of vascular tone, the inhibition of platelet aggregation, and leukocyte adhesion and has antitumor and antimicrobial activity. Increased production of nitric oxide observed during septic shock may be largely responsible for sepsis-induced hypotension and myocardial depressions. The use of nitric oxide synthase inhibitors may improve survival in severe septic shock by increasing mean arterial pressure and restoring vascular responsiveness to catecholamines. At this time, beneficial effects on clinical outcomes, including survival, only are suggested in human clinical trials.[227]

SUMMARY

Knowledge of immunology is increasingly important for the pediatric critical care nurse for two reasons. All PICU patients experience altered host defenses; most commonly, these are changes in the structure and function of the first line of defense. In addition, the pediatric critical care nurse's knowledge of the immune system is often limited. With increasing technology and expanding knowledge of the intricacies of immunologic events, expertise in the field of immunology is imperative.

Caring for the child with altered host defenses is a challenge. Children in the PICU are at risk developmentally and situationally for altered host defense. Recognition of this fact provides the basis for a thorough immunologic assessment, which will further identify the child at risk. Many of the interventions, including medical efforts, involve expert nursing care to promote the best possible outcome for the child.

REFERENCES

1. Infante AJ: Evaluation of immune function. In Jenson HB, Baltimore RS, eds: *Pediatric infectious diseases: principles and practice,* Norwalk, Conn, 1995, Appleton & Lange.
2. Rhoades R, Pflanzer R: *Human physiology,* ed 2, Philadelphia, 1992, Saunders College Publishing.
3. Guyton A, Hall JE: The microcirculation and the lymphatic system: capillary fluid exchange, interstitial fluid, and lymph flow. In *Textbook of medical physiology,* ed 9, Philadelphia, 1996, WB Saunders.
4. Guyton AC, Hall JE: *Textbook of medical physiology,* ed 9, Philadelphia, 1996, WB Saunders.
5. Lydyard P, Grossi C: The lymphoid system. In Roitt IM, Brostoff J, Male DK, eds: *Immunology,* ed 2, Philadelphia, 1989, JB Lippincott.
6. Jett MR, Lancaster LE: The inflammatory-immune response: the body's defense against invasion, *Crit Care Nurse* 3:64-86, 1983.

7. Heinzel FP: Antibodies. In Mandell G, Demett JE, Dolin R, eds: *Principles and practice of infectious disease,* ed 5, New York, 2000, Churchill Livingstone.

8. Slota MC: The cutting edge of pediatric critical care, *Crit Care Nurs* 13(suppl 3):22-23, 1993.

9. Wood RA, Sampson HA: The child with frequent infections, *Curr Probl Pediatr* 19: 234-281, 1989.

10. Stiehm ER: Immunodeficiency disorders: general considerations. In Stiehm ER, ed: *Immunological disorders in infants and children,* ed 3 Philadelphia, 1989, WB Saunders.

11. Tramont EC: General or nonspecific host defense mechanisms. In Mandell GL, Douglas RG, Bennett JE, eds: *Principles and practice of infectious disease,* ed 3, New York, 1990, Churchill Livingstone.

12. Donowitz LG: The critical care patient. In Donowitz LG, ed: *Hospital acquired infection in the pediatric patient,* Baltimore, 1988, Williams & Wilkins.

13. Leyden JJ: Bacteriology of newborn skin. In Maibach HI, Boisits EK, eds: *Neonatal skin: structure and function,* New York, 1982, Marcel Dekker.

14. Pauw BE, Donnelly JP: Infections in the immunocompromised host: general principles. In Mandell G, Demett JE, Dolin R, eds: *Principles and practice of infectious disease,* ed 5, New York, 2000, Churchill Livingstone.

15. Hashimoto K, Gross BG, Lever WF: The ultrastructure of the skin of human embryos: the intraepidermal eccrine sweat duct, *J Investig Dermatol* 45:139-151, 1965.

16. Adams A: External barriers to infection, *Nurs Clin North Am* 20:145-149, 1985.

17. Bousvaros A, Walker WA: Development and function of the intestinal mucosal barrier. In MacDonald T, ed: *Ontogeny of the immune system of the gut,* Boca Raton, Fla., 1990, CRC Press.

18. Selner JC, Merrill DA, Claman HN: Salivary immunoglobulin and albumin: development during the newborn period, *J Pediatr* 72:685-689, 1968.

19. Mellander L Carlsson B, Jalil F et al: Secretary IgA antibody response against *Escherichia coli* antigen in infants in relation to exposure, *J Pediatr* 107:430-433, 1985.

20. Goldman AS, Ham-Pong AJ, Goldblum RM: Host defenses: development and maternal contributions, *Adv Pediatr* 32:71-100, 1985.

21. Hanson LA, Adlerberth I, Carlsson B et al: Antibody-mediated immunity in the neonate, *Padiatr Padol* 25:371-376, 1990.

22. Rote NS: Immunity. In McCance K, Huether SE, eds: *Pathophysiology: the biologic basis for dosage in adults and children,* ed 5, St Louis, 1990, Mosby.

23. Morriss FH, Moore M, Weisbrodt NW et al: Ontogenic development of gastrointestinal motility: duodenal contractions in preterm infants, *Pediatrics* 78:1106-1113, 1986.

24. Fliedner M, Mehls O, Rauterberg E et al: Urinary sIgA in children with urinary tract infection, *J Pediatr* 109:416-421, 1986.

25. ACCP-SCCM Consensus conference: Definitions for sepsis and organ failure and guidelines for the use of innovative therapies in sepsis, *Crit Care Med* 20:864-874, 1992.

26. Henker R: Evidence-based practice: fever-related interventions, *Am J Crit Care* 8:481-487, 1999.

27. Anderson DC, Hughes BJ, Edwards MS et al: Impaired chemotaxigenesis by type III group B streptococci in neonatal sera: relationship to specific anticapsular antibody and abnormalities of serum complement, *Pediatr Res* 17:496-502, 1983.

28. Wright WC, Ank BJ, Herbert J et al: Decreased bactericidal activity of leukocytes of stressed newborn infants, *Pediatrics* 56:579-584, 1975.

29. Nauseef WM, Clark RA: Granulocytic phagocytes. In Mandell G, Demett JE, Dolin R, eds: *Principles and practice of infectious disease,* ed 5, New York, 2000, Churchill Livingstone.

30. Lewis DB, Wilson CB: Developmental immunology and role of host defenses in neonatal susceptibility to infection. In Remington JS, Kelin JO, eds: *Infectious disease of the fetus and newborn infant,* Philadelphia, 1995, WB Saunders.

31. Klein RB, Fischer TJ, Gard SE et al: Decreased mononuclear and polymorphonuclear chemotaxis in human newborns, infants, and young children, *Pediatrics* 60: 467-472, 1977.

32. Miller ME: Immunocompetence of the newborn. In Chandra RK, ed: *Primary and secondary immunodeficiency disorders,* New York, 1983, Churchill Livingstone.

33. Frank MM: Complement and kinin. In Stites DP, Terr AI, Parslow TG, eds: *Basic and clinical immunology,* ed 8, Norwalk, Conn, 1994, Appleton & Lange.

34. Densen P: Complement system. In Mandell G, Demett JE, Dolin R, eds: *Principles and practice of infectious disease,* ed 5, New York, 2000, Churchill Livingstone.

35. Goodman JW: The immune response. In Stites DP, Terr AI, Parslow TG, eds: *Basic and clinical immunology,* ed 8, Norwalk, Conn, 1994, Appleton & Lange.

36. Bellanti JA, Kadlee JV: General immunobiology. In Bellanti JA, ed: *Immunulogy III,* Philadelphia, 1985, WB Saunders.

37. Wilson M: Immunology of the fetus and newborn: lymphocyte phenotype and function, *Clin Immunol Allergy* 5:271-286, 1985.

38. Lawton AR, Cooper MD: Ontogeny of immunity. In Stiehm ER, ed: *Immunologic disorders in infants and children,* ed 3, Philadelphia, 1989, WB Saunders.

39. Cooper MD, Buckley RH: Developmental immunology and the immunodeficiency diseases, *JAMA* 248:2658-2669, 1982.

40. Miller ME: Immunodeficiencies of immaturity. In Stiehm ER, ed: *Immunologic disorders in infants and children,* ed 3, Philadelphia, 1989, WB Saunders.

41. Vogler LB, Lawton AR: Ontogeny of B cells and humoral immune functions, *Clin Immunol Allergy* 5:235-252, 1985.

42. Nejedla Z: The development of immunological factors in infants with hyperbilirubinemia, *Pediatrics* 45:102-104, 1970.

43. Hayward AR, Lawton AR: Induction of plasma cell differentiation of human fetal lymphocytes: evidence for functional immaturity of T and B cells, *J Immunol* 119:1213-1217, 1977.

44. Altman Y, Handzel ZT, Levin S: Suppressor T-cell activity in newborns and mothers, *Pediatr Res* 19:123-126, 1984.

45. Rook G: Cell-mediated immune responses. In Roitt IM, Brostoff J, Male D, eds: *Immunology,* ed 2, Philadelphia, 1991, JB Lippincott.

46. Parkman R: Cytokines and T-lymphocytes in pediatrics, *J Pediatr* 118:s21-s23, 1991.

47. Bryson YJ, Winter HS, Gard SE et al: Deficiency of immune interferon production by leukocytes of normal newborns, *Cell Immunol* 55:191-200, 1980.

48. Sancho L, Martinez-A C, Nogales A et al: Reconstitution of natural-killer-cell activity in the newborn by interleukin-2, *N Engl J Med* 314:57-58, 1986.

49. Polin RA, St Geme JW: Neonatal sepsis, *Adv Pediatr Infect Dis* 7:25-61, 1992.

50. Denny T, Yogev R, Gelman R et al: Lymphocyte subsets in healthy children during the first 5 years of life, *JAMA* 267:1484-1488, 1992.

51. Kotylo PK, Fineberg NS, Freeman KS et al: Reference ranges for lymphocyte subsets in pediatric patients, *Am J Clin Pathol* 100: 111-115, 1993.

52. Notarangelo LD, Chirico G, Chaira A: Activity of classical and alternative pathway of complement in preterm and small for gestational age infants, *Pediatr Res* 18:281-285, 1984.

53. Holland SM, Gallin UI: Evaluation of the patient with suspected immunodeficiency. In Mandell G, Demett JE, Dolin R, eds: *Principles and practice of infectious disease,* ed 5, New York, 2000, Churchill Livingstone.

54. Gal TJ: How does tracheal intubation alter respiratory mechanics? *Probl Anesthes* 2: 191-200, 1988.

55. Ramphal R, Guay P, Pier G: *Pseudomonas aeruginosa* adhesions for tracheobronchial mucin, *Infect Immun* 55:600-603, 1987.

56. Sheth NK, Franson TR, Rose HD et al: Colonization of bacteria on polyvinyl chloride and Teflon intravascular catheters in hospitalized patients, *J Clin Microbiol* 18: 1061-1063, 1983.

57. Sottile FD, Marrie TJ, Prough DS et al: Nosocomial pulmonary infection: possible etiologic significance of bacterial adhesion to endotracheal tubes, *Crit Care Med* 14: 265-270, 1986.

58. Stamm WE: Infections related to medical devices, *Ann Intern Med* 89:764-769, 1978.

59. Riggs CD, Lister G: Adverse occurrences in the pediatric intensive care unit, *Pediatr Clin North Am* 34:93-117, 1987.

60. Levine SA, Niederman MS: The impact of tracheal intubation on host defenses and

risks for nosocomial pneumonia, *Clin Chest Med* 12:523-543, 1991.

61. Browning DH, Graves SA: Incidence of aspiration with endotracheal tubes in children, *J Pediatr* 102:582-584, 1983.

62. Steen JA: Impact of tube design and material on complications of tracheal intubation, *Probl Anesthes* 2:211-224, 1988.

63. Espersen S: Nursing support of host defenses, *Crit Care Q* 9:51-56, 1986.

64. Griffin JP: Nursing care of the critically ill immunocompromised patient, *Crit Care Q* 9:25-34, 1986.

65. Massanari RM: Nosocomial infections in critical care units: causation and prevention, *Crit Care Nurs Q* 11:45-57, 1989.

66. Hoyt NJ: Host defense mechanisms and compromises in the trauma patient, *Crit Care Nurs Clin North Am* 1:753-765, 1989.

67. Merritt WT: Noscomial infections in the pediatric intensive care unit. In Rogers MC, ed: *Textbook of pediatric intensive care,* ed 2, Baltimore, 1992, Williams & Wilkins.

67a. Wynsma LA: Negative outcomes of intravascular therapy in infants and children, *AACN Clin Issues Crit Care Nurs* 9:49-63, 1998.

68. Pearson ML: Guidelines for prevention of intravascular device-related infections Hospital Infection Control Practice Advisory Committee, *Infect Control Hosp Epidemiol* 17:438-473, 1996.

69. Warren JW: The catheter and urinary tract infection, *Med Clin North Am* 75:481-493, 1991.

70. Cobb JP, Danner RL: Nosocomial infections in the practice of pediatric critical care. In Holbrook PR, ed: *Textbook of pediatric critical care,* Philadelphia, 1993, WB Saunders.

71. Sherbotie JR, Cornfeld D: Management of urinary tract infections in children, *Med Clin North Am* 75:327-338, 1991.

72. Stull TL, LiPuma JJ: Epidemiology and natural history of UTI in children, *Med Clin North Am* 75:287-297, 1991.

73. Fischer GW: Immunotherapy and immunomodulation. In Jenson HB, Baltimore RS, eds: *Pediatric infectious diseases: principles and practice,* Norwalk, Conn, 1995, Appleton & Lange.

74. Mainous MR, Block EF, Deitch EA: Nutritional support of the gut: how and why, *New Horiz* 2:193-201, 1994.

75. Locke SE: Stress, adaption and immunity: studies in humans, *Gen Hosp Psychiatry* 4:49-58, 1982.

76. Sternberg EM, Chrousos GP, Wilder RL et al: The stress response and the regulation of inflammatory disease, *Ann Intern Med* 117:854-866, 1992.

77. Peterson PK, Chao CC, Molitor T: Stress and pathogenesis of infectious disease, *Rev Infect Dis* 13:710-720, 1991.

78. Hauser GJ, Holbrook PR: Immune dysfunction in the critically ill infant and child, *Crit Care Clin* 4:711-732, 1988.

79. Rosenthal CH: Immunosuppression in the pediatric critical care patient, *Crit Care Nurs Clin North Am* 1:775-785, 1989.

80. Huskins WC, Goldman DA: Prevention and control of nosocomial infections in hospitalized children. In Feigin RD, Cherry JD, eds: *Textbook of pediatric infectious diseases,* ed 4, Philadelphia, 1998, WB Saunders.

80a. Donowitz LG: Handwashing techniques in a pediatric intensive care unit, *Am J Dis Child* 141:683-685, 1987.

81. Halliburton P: Impaired immunocompetence. In Carrieri VK, Lindsey AM, West CM, eds: *Pathophysiological phenomena in nursing: human responses to illness,* Philadelphia, 1986, WB Saunders.

82. Rostad ME: Current strategies for managing myelosuppression in patients with cancer, *Oncol Nurs Forum* 18(suppl 2):7-15, 1991.

83. Pizzo PA: Combating infections in neutropenic patients, *Hosp Pract* 24:93-110, 1989.

84. Crawford GE: Empiric selection of antibiotics, *Probl Crit Care* 6:1-20, 1992.

85. Mackersie RC: Toward the rational use of antibiotics in the intensive care unit, *Formulary* 34:836-850, 1999.

86. Gilman JT: Therapeutic drug monitoring in the neonate and paediatric age group: problems and clinical pharmacokinetic implications, *Clin Pharmacokinet* 19:1-10, 1990.

86a. Tenover FC, Hughes JM: The challenges of emerging infectious diseases: development and spread of multiply-resistant bacterial pathogens, *JAMA* 275:300-310, 1996.

87. Opal SM, Mayer KH, Medeiros AA: Mechanisms of bacterial antibiotic resistance. In Mandell G, Demett JE, Dolin R, eds: *Principles and practice of infectious disease,* ed 5, New York, 2000, Churchill Livingstone.

88. Reed MD, Goldfarb J, Blumer JL: Anti-infective therapy. In Jenson HB, Baltimore RS, eds: *Pediatric infectious diseases principles and practice,* Norwalk, Conn, 1995, Appleton & Lange.

89. Haeuber D: Future strategies in the control of myelosuppression: the use of colony-stimulating factors, *Oncol Nurs Forum* 18:16-21, 1991.

90. Johnson J: Introduction, *Oncol Nurs Forum* 18(suppl 2):2, 1991.

91. NIH Consensus Conference: Intravenous immunoglobulin: prevention and treatment of disease, *JAMA* 264:3189-3193, 1990.

92. Epstein JS, Zoon KC: Department of Health and Human Services, Food and Drug Administration, Drug warning letter, September 29, 1999.

92a. Groothuis JR, Simoes EA, Levin MJ et al: Prophylactic administration of respiratory syncytial virus immune globulin to high-risk infants and young children: The Respiratory Syncytial Virus Immune Globulin Study Group, *N Engl J Med* 329:1524-1530, 1993.

93. Meissner CH, Welliver RC, Chartrand SA et al: Immunoprophylaxis with palivizumab, a humanized respiratory syncytial virus monoclonal antibody, for prevention of respiratory syncytial virus infection in high risk infants: a consensus opinion, *Pediatr Infect Dis J* 18:223-229, 1999.

94. Snydman DR, Werner BG, Heinze-Lacey B et al: Use of cytomegalovirus immune glob-ulin to prevent cytomegalovirus disease in renal-transplant recipients, *N Engl J Med* 317:1049-1054, 1987.

95. Herberman RB, ed: Cetus immunoprimer series. Part 3. Cytokines, Emoryville, Calif, 1989, Cetus Corporation.

96. Haeuber D, DiJulio JE: Hemopoietic colony stimulating factors: an overview, *Oncol Nurs Forum* 16:247-255, 1989.

96a. Clay TM, Custer MC, Spiess PJ et al: Potential use of T cell receptor genes to modify hematopoietic stem cells for the gene therapy of cancer, *Pathol Oncol Res* 5:3-15, 1999.

97. Figlin RA: Biotherapy with interferon in solid tumors, *Oncol Nurs Forum* 14(suppl): 23-26, 1987.

98. Roth MS, Foon KA: Biotherapy with interferon in hematologic malignancies, *Oncol Nurs Forum* 14(suppl 6):16-22, 1987.

99. Byram DA: The immunocompromised patient: future experiences for critical care nurses: competence in immunotherapy, *Crit Care Nurs Clin North Am* 1:707-806, 1989.

100. Jassak PF, Sticklin LA: Interleukin-2: an overview, *Oncol Nurs Forum* 13:17-22, 1986.

101. Padavic-Shaller K: IL-2: nursing applications in a developing science, *Oncol Nurs Forum* 4:142-150, 1988.

102. Borish L, Rosenwasser LJ: Update on cytokines, *J Allergy Clin Immunol* 97:719-730, 1996.

103. LaPine TR, Cates KL, Hill HR: Immunomodulating agents. In Feigin RD, Cherry JD eds: *Textbook of pediatric infectious diseases,* ed 4, Philadelphia, 1998, WB Saunders.

104. Ziegler EJ, Fischer CJ Jr, Sprung CL et al: Treatment of gram-negative bacteremia in septic shock with HA-1A human monoclonal antibody against endotoxin: a randomized, double-blind placebo-controlled trial. The HA-1A Sepsis Study Group, *N Engl J Med* 324:429-436, 1991.

105. Mahon PM: Orthoclone OKT3 and cardiac transplantation: an overview, *Crit Care Nurs* 11:42-50, 1991.

106. Shaefer M, Willis L: Nursing implications of immunosuppression in transplantation: update on drug intervention, *Nurs Clin North Am* 26:291-314, 1991.

107. DiJulio JE: Treatment of B-cell and T-cell lymphomas with monoclonal antibodies, *Oncol Nurs Forum* 4:102-106, 1988.

108. Baumgartner JD, Calandra T: Treatment of sepsis: past and future avenues, *Drugs* 57:127-132, 1999.

109. Hershfield MS: Enzyme therapy for an inherited immunodeficiency disease, *Immune Deficiency Foundation Newsletter,* Columbia, Md, September 1989, Immune Deficiency Foundation.

110. Brogley JL, Sharp EJ: Nursing care of patients receiving activated lymphocytes, *Oncol Nurs Forum* 17:187-193, 1990.

111. Corey BS, Collins JL: Implementation of an RIL-2/LAK cell clinical trial: a nursing perspective, *Oncol Nurs Forum* 13:31-36, 1986.

112. Blackburn GL, Menkes E: Surgical immunology. In Chandra RK, ed: *Primary and secondary immunodeficiency disorders,* New York, 1983, Churchill Livingstone.

113. Tsuda T, Kahan BD: The effects of anesthesia on the immune response. In Chandra RK, ed: *Primary and secondary immunodeficiency disorders,* New York, 1983, Churchill Livingstone.

114. Schot JDL, Schuurman RKB: Blood transfusion suppresses cutaneous cell-mediated immunity, *Clin Exp Immunol* 65:336-344, 1986.

115. Howard RJ: Effect of burn injury, mechanical trauma, and operation on immune defenses, *Surg Clin North Am* 59:199-211, 1979.

116. Milliken J, Tait GA, Ford-Jones EL et al: Nosocomial infections in a pediatric intensive care unit, *Crit Care Med* 16:233-237, 1988.

117. Horan TC, White JW, Jarvis WR et al: Nosocomial infection surveillance, 1984, *Morb Mortal Wkly Rep CDC Survell Summ* 35:17ss-29ss, 1986.

118. Donowitz LG, Wenzel RP, Hoyt JW: High risk of hospital-acquired infection in the ICU patient, *Crit Care Med* 10:355-357, 1982.

119. Wenzel RP, Thompson RL, Landry SM et al: Hospital-acquired infections in intensive care unit patients: an overview with emphasis on epidemics, *Infect Control* 4:371-375, 1983.

120. Brown RB, Hosmer D, Chen HC et al: A comparison of infections in different ICUs within the same hospital, *Crit Care Med* 13:472-476, 1985.

121. Huskins WC, Goldman DA: Nosocomial infections. In Feigin RD, Cherry JD, eds: *Textbook of pediatric infectious diseases,* ed 4, Philadelphia, 1998, WB Saunders.

121a. Richards MJ, Edwards JR, Culver DH et al: Nosocomial infections in medical intensive care units in the United States: National Nosocomial Infections Surveillance System, *Crit Care Med* 27:887-892, 1999.

122. National Nosocomial Infections Surveillance System: National Nosocomial Infection Surveillance (NNIS) semi-annual report, *Am J Infect Control* 23:277-385, 1995.

123. Weiner ES: Catheter sepsis: the central venous line Achilles' heel, *Semin Pediatr Surg* 4:207- 214, 1995.

124. Ducharme FM, Gauthier M, Lacriox J: Incidence of infection related to arterial catheterization in children: a prospective study, *Crit Care Med* 16:272-276, 1988.

125. Norwood SH, Cormier B, McMahon NG et al: Prospective study of catheter related infection during prolonged arterial catheterization, *Crit Care Med* 16:836-842, 1988.

126. Mantese VA, German DS, Kaminski DL et al: Colonization and sepsis from triple-lumen catheters in criticaly ill patients, *Am J Surg* 154:597-601, 1987.

127. Bhattacharyya N, Kosloske AM, Macauthus C: Nosocomial infection in pediatric surgical patients: a study of 608 infants and children, *J Pediatr Surg* 28:338-343, 1993.

128. Pollock EM, Ford-Jones EL, Rebeyka I et al: Early nosocomial infections in pediatric cardiovascular surgery patients, *Crit Care Med* 18:378-384, 1990.

129. Gershwin ME, Beach RS, Hurley LS: *Nutrition and immunity,* Orlando, 1985, Academic Press.

130. Chandra RK: Malnutrition. In Chandra RK, ed: *Primary and secondary immunodeficiency disorders,* New York, 1983, Churchill Livingstone.

131. Hotter AN: Wound healing and immunocompromise, *Nur Clin North Am* 25:193-203, 1990.

132. Slavin RG: Immunologic effects of uremia. In Stites DP, Terr AI, eds: *Basic and clinical immunology,* ed 7, Norwalk, Conn, 1990, Appleton & Lange.

133. Bohn DJ, Biggar WD, Smith CR et al: Influence of hypothermia, barbiturate therapy, and intracranial pressure monitoring on morbidity and mortality after near-drowning, *Crit Care Med* 14:529-534, 1986.

134. Lewin S, Brettman LR, Holzman RS: Infections in hypothermic patients, *Arch Intern Med* 141:920-925, 1981.

134a. Mangram AJ, Horan TC, Pearson ML et al: Guideline for prevention of surgical site infection: Centers for Disease Control and Prevention (CDC) Hospital Infection Control Practices Advisory Committee (1999), *Am J Infect Control* 27:97-132, 1999.

135. Utley JR: The immune response to cardiopulmonary bypass. In Utley JR, ed: *Pathophysiology and techniques of cardiopulmonary bypass,* vol 1, Baltimore, Md, 1982, Williams & Wilkins.

136. Hauser GJ, Chan MM, Casey WF et al: Immune dysfunction in children after corrective surgery for congenital heart disease, *Crit Care Med* 19:874-880, 1991.

137. Chiu RCJ, Samson R: Complement (C3, C4) consumption in cardiopulmonary bypass, cardioplegia, and protamine administration, *Ann Thorac Surg* 37:229-232, 1984.

137a. Coffin SE, Bell LM, Manning M et al: Nolocomial infections in neonates receiving extracorporeal membrane oxygenation, *Infect Control Hosp Epidemiol* 18:93-96, 1997.

137b. Douglass BH, Keenan AL, Purohit DM: Bacterial and fungal infection in neonates undergoing venoarterial extracorporeal membrane oxygenation: an analysis of the registry data of the extracorporeal life support organization, *Artif Organs* 20:202-208, 1996.

138. Malone N, Larson E: Factors associated with a significant reduction in hospital-wide infection rates, *Am J Infect Control* 24:180-185, 1996.

139. Tablan OC, Anderson LJ, Arden et al: Guideline for prevention of nosocomial pneumonia, *Infect Control Hosp Epidemiol* 15:587-627, 1994.

140. Infante AJ: Primary immune deficiency disorders. In Jenson HB, Baltimore RS, eds: *Pediatric infectious diseases: principles and practice,* Norwalk, Conn, 1995, Appleton & Lange.

141. Horowitz SD: In Fuhrman BP, Zimmerman JJ, eds: *Pediatric critical care,* ed 2, Baltimore, 1998, Mosby.

142. Rotrosen D, Gallin JI: Evaluation of the patient with suspected immunodeficiency. In Mandell GL, Douglas RG, Bennett JE, eds: *Principles and practice of infectious disease,* ed 3, New York, 1990, Churchill Livingstone.

143. Heinzel FP: Infections in patients with humoral immunodeficiency, *Hosp Pract* 24: 99-130, 1989.

144. Centers for Disease Control and Prevention: HIV/AIDS surveillance report: first quarter edition, 5:1-19, 1993.

145. Centers for Disease Control and Prevention: HIV/AIDS surveillance report: mid-year 1999 edition, 11, 1999.

146. Centers for Disease Control and Prevention: US HIV and AIDS cases reported through December 1997, HIV/AIDS surveillance report, 9:1, 1997.

147. Joint United Nations Programme on HIV/ AIDS and World Health Organization: Report on the Global HIV/AIDS Epidemic, Geneva, 1997, World Health Organization.

148. Gayle HB, D'Angelo J: The epidemiology of AIDS and HIV infection in adolescents. In Pizzo PA, Wilfert CM, eds: *Pediatric AIDS: the challenge of HIV infection in infants, children and adolescents,* Baltimore, 1990, Williams & Wilkins.

149. Centers for Disease Control and Prevention: 1994 Revised classification system for human immunodeficiency virus infection in children less than 13 years of age; Official authorized addenda: human immunodeficiency virus infection codes and official guidelines for coding and reporting, ICD-9-CM, *MMWR* 43:1-10, 1994.

150. Shapiro MF, Morton SC, McCaffrey DF et al: Variations in the care of HIV-infected adults in the United States: results from the HIV Cost and Services Utilization Study, *JAMA* 281:2305-2315, 1999.

151. Johann-Lang R, Cervia JS, Noel GJ: Characteristics of human immunodeficiency virus-infected children at the time of death: an experience in the 1990s, *Pediatr Infect Dis J* 16:1145-1150, 1997.

152. Centers for Disease Control and Prevention: Recommendations for prevention of HIV transmission in health-care settings, *MMWR* 36:3S-18S, 1987.

153. Levy JA: Features of HIV and the host response that influence progression of disease. InSande MA, Volberding PA, eds: *The medical management of AIDS,* ed 2, Philadelphia, 1990, WB Saunders.

154. McMahon KM: The integration of HIV testing and counseling into nursing practice, *Nurs Clin North Am* 23:803-821, 1988.

155. Newman CL, Quinn TC: Acquired immunodeficiency syndrome. In Harvey AM, Johns RJ, McKusick VA et al, eds: *The principles and practice of medicine,* ed 22, Norwalk, Conn, 1988, Appleton & Lange.

156. Wofsy CB: Prevention of HIV transmission. In Sande MA, Volberding PA, eds: *The management of AIDS,* ed 2, Philadelphia, 1990, WB Saunders.

157. Barrick B: Light at the end of a decade, *Am J Nurs* 90:37-40, 1990.

158. Bartlett J: *Medical management of HIV infection,* Coleview, Ill, 1994, Physicians & Scientists.

159. Michael NL, Burke DS: Natural history of human immunodeficiency virus infection, *Dermatol Clin North Am* 9:429-441, 1991.

160. Flaskerud JH: Health promotion and disease prevention. In Flaskerud JH, Unguarski PJ, eds: *HIV/AIDS: a guide to nursing care,* ed 3, Philadelphia, 1995, WB Saunders.

161. Boland M, Czarniecki L: Nursing care of the child. In Flaskerud JL, Unguarski PJ, eds: *HIV/AIDS: a guide to nursing care,* ed 3, Philadelphia, 1995, WB Saunders.

162. Barnhart HX, Caldwell MB, Thomal P et al: Natural history of human immunodeficiency virus disease in perinatally infected children: an analysis from the Pediatric Spectrum of Disease Project, *Pediatrics* 97:710-716, 1996.

163. Mayaux MJ, Burgard M, Teglas JP et al: Neonatal characteristics in rapidly progressive perinatally acquired HIV-1 disease: The French Pediatric HIV Infection Study Group, *JAMA* 275:606-610, 1996.

164. Aldrovandi GM: Natural history of pediatric HIV disease. In Zeichner SL, Read JS, eds: *Handbook of pediatric HIV care,* Philadelphia, 2000, Lippincott Williams & Wilkins.

165. Bastin N, Tamayo OW, Tinkle MB et al: HIV disease and pregnancy. Part 3. Postpartum care of the HIV-positive woman and her newborn, *J Obstet Gynecol Neonatal Nurs* 21:105-111, 1992.

166. Tinkle MB, Amaya MA, Tamayo OW: HIV disease and pregnancy. Part 1. Epidemiology, pathogenesis, and natural history, *J Obstet Gynecol Neonatal Nurs* 21:86-93, 1992.

167. Simonds RJ, Steketee R, Nesheim S et al: Impact of zidovudine use on risk and risk factors for perinatal transmission of HIV, *AIDS* 12:301-308, 1998.

168. Smeltzer SC, Whipple B: Women and HIV infection, *Image J Nurs Sch* 23:249-256, 1991.

169. Centers for Disease Control and Prevention: Zidovudine for the prevention of HIV transmission from mother to infant, *MMWR* 43:285-287, 1994.

170. Mendez H: Natural history and prognostic factors. In Yogev R, Connor E, eds: *Management of HIV infection in infants, children and adolescents,* St Louis, 1992, Mosby.

171. Tramont EC: The human immunodeficiency virus, *Dermatol Clin North Am* 9:397-401, 1991.

172. Grady C: The immune system and AIDS/HIV infection. In Flaskerud JH, ed: *AIDS/HIV infection: a reference guide for nursing professionals,* Philadelphia, 1989, WB Saunders.

173. Centers for Disease Control and Prevention: 1994 revised classification system for human immunodeficiency virus infection in children less than 13 years of age, *MMWR* 43(RR-12):1-10, 1994.

174. Dunn DT, Brandt CD, Krivine A: The sensitivity of HIV-1 DNA polymerase chain reaction in the neonatal period and the relative contributions of intrauterine and intra-partum transmission, *AIDS* 9:F7: 1995.

175. Pavia AT, Christenson JC: Pediatric AIDS. In Sande MA, Volberding PA, eds: *The medical management of AIDS,* ed 6, Philadelphia, 1999, WB Saunders.

176. Grady C, Vogel S: Laboratory methods for diagnosing and monitoring HIV infection, *J Assoc Nurses AIDS Care* 4:11-21, 1993.

177. Oleske J: Working group on Antiretroviral Therapy and Medical Management of Infants, Children and Adolescents with HIV Infection: Antiretroviral therapy and medical management of pediatric HIV infection, *Pediatrics* 102:1005-1062, 1998.

178. Johnson JP, Nair P, O'Neil KM et al: HIV infection in infants: natural history and serologic diagnosis of children, *Am J Dis Child* 143:1147-1153, 1989.

179. Grant RM, Saag MS: Laboratory testing for HIV-1. In Sande MA, Volberding PA, eds: *The medical management of AIDS,* ed 6, Philadelphia, 1999, WB Saunders.

180. El-Sader W., Olske, J.M., Agins B.D. et al (1994). Evaluation and management of early HIV infection. Clinical Practice Guideline No. 7. AHCPR Publication No. 94-0572. Rockville, MD: Agency for Health Care Policy and Research, Public Health Service, US Dept of Health and Human Services.

181. Centers for Disease Control and Prevention: 1993 revised classification system for HIV infection and expanded surveillance case definition for AIDS among adolescents and adults, *MMWR* 41(RR-17):1-10, 1992.

182. Simonds RJ, Oxtoby MJ, Caldwell MB et al: *Pneumocystis carinii* pneumonia among United States children with perinatally acquired HIV infection, *JAMA* 270:470-473, 1993.

183. Farley JJ, Englander R, Tressler RL et al: The critically ill child with human immunodeficiency virus infection. In Rogers MC, ed: *Textbook of pediatric intensive care,* Baltimore, 1996, Williams & Wilkins.

184. Centers for Disease Control and Prevention: 1995 revised guidelines for prophylaxis against *Pneumocystis carinii* pneumonia for children infected with or perinatally exposed to human immunodeficiency virus, *MMWR* 44(RR-4):1-11, 1995.

185. Tribett D: Immune system function: implications for critical care nursing practice, *Crit Care Nurs Clin North Am* 1:725-740, 1989.

186. Wasserman R: AIDS. In Levin DL, Morriss FC, eds: *Essentials of pediatric intensive care,* St Louis, 1990, Quality Medical Publishing.

187. Hauger SB Powell KR: Infectious complications in children with HIV infection, *Pediatr Ann* 19:422-433, 1990.

188. Centers for Disease Control and Prevention: AIDS indicator conditions reported in 1996 by age group, United States, *HIV/AIDS Surv Rep* 8:18, 1996.

189. Wood L: Pulmonary problems. In Zeichner SL, Read JS, eds: *Handbook of pediatric HIV care,* Philadelphia, 1999, Lippincott Williams & Wilkins.

190. Ussery XT, Valway SE, McKenna M et al: Epidemiology of tuberculosis among children in the United States: 1985-1994, *Pediatr Infect Dis J* 15:697-704, 1996.

191. Stamos JK, Rowley AH: Pediatric tuberculosis: an update, *Curr Probl Pediatr* 25:131-136, 1995.

192. Centers for Disease Control and Prevention: *Core curriculum on tuberculosis: what the clinician should know,* ed 3, Atlanta, 1994, CDC.

193. Burroughs MH, Edelson PJ: Medical care of the HIV-infected child, *Pediatr Clin North Am* 38:45-67, 1991.

194. Stewart JM, Kaul A, Gromisch DS et al: Symptomatic cardiac dysfunction in children with human immunodeficiency virus infection, *Am Heart J* 117:140-144, 1989.

195. Luginbuhl LM, Orav EJ, McIntosh K et al: Cardiac morbidity and related mortality in children with HIV infection, *JAMA* 269:1869-1875, 1993.

196. Joshi VV, Gadol C, Connor E et al: Dilated cardiomyopathy in children with acquired immunodeficiency syndrome, *Hum Pathol* 19:69-73, 1988.

197. Bharati S, Joshi V, Connor V et al: Conduction system in children with acquired immunodeficiency syndrome, *Chest* 96:406-413, 1989.

198. Lipschultz SE, Chanock S, Sanders SP et al: Cardiovascular manifestations of human immunodeficiency virus infection in infants and children, *Am J Cardiol* 63:1489-1497, 1989.

199. Kavanaugh-McHugh A, Ruff AJ, Rowes A et al: The challenge of HIV infection in infants, children, and adolescents. In Pizzo PA, Wilfert CM, eds: *Pediatric AIDS,* Baltimore, 1991, Williams & Wilkins.

200. Vogel RL: Cardiac manifestations of pediatric acquired immunodeficiency syndrome. In Yogev R, Connor E, eds: *Management of HIV infection in infants and children,* St Louis, 1992, Mosby.

201. Castello FV, Pena RM: Adult respiratory distress syndrome (ARDS) in children with AIDS, *Crit Care Med* 18:s232, 1990.

202. Scott GB, Hutto C, Makuch RW et al: Survival in children with perinatally acquired HIV-1 infection, *N Engl J Med* 321:1791-1796, 1989.

203. Wilkinson JD, Greenwald BM: The acquired immunodeficiency syndrome: impact on the pediatric intensive care unit, *Crit Care Clin* 4:831-843, 1988.

204. Belman AL: Acquired immunodeficiency syndrome and the child's central nervous system, *Pediatr Neurol* 39:691-714, 1992.

205. Caldwell MB, Rogers MF: Epidemiology of pediatric HIV infection, *Pediatr Clin North Am* 138:1-16, 1991.

206. Epstein LG, Sharer LR, Oleske JM et al: Neurologic manifestations of human immunodeficiency virus in children, *Pediatrics* 78:678-687, 1986.

207. Mintz M, Rapaport R, Oleske JM et al: Elevated serum levels of tumor necrosis factor are associated with progressive encephalopathy in children with acquired im-

munodeficiency syndrome, *Am J Dis Child* 143:771, 1989.

208. Warrier I, Lusher JM: Hematologic manifestations of HIV infection. In Yogev R, Connor E, eds: *Management of HIV infection in infants and children,* St Louis, 1992, Mosby.

209. Falloon J, Eddy J, Wiener L et al: Human immunodeficiency virus infection in children, *J Pediatr* 114:1-30, 1989.

210. Centers for Disease Control and Prevention: 1999 USPHS/IDSA guidelines for the prevention of opportunistic infections in persons infected with human immunodeficiency virus: US Public Health Service (USPHS) and Infectious Diseases Society of America (IDSA), *MMWR* 48:1-63, 1999.

211. Spiegel L, Mayers A: Psychosocial aspects of AIDS in children and adolescents, *Pediatr Clin North Am* 38:153-167, 1991.

212. Czarniecki L, Dillman P: Pediatric HIV/AIDS, *Crit Care Nurs Clin North Am* 4:447-456, 1992.

212a. Broome CV: Epidemiology of toxic shock syndrome in the United States: overview, *Rev Infect Dis* 11:14-21, 1989.

213. Chesney PJ: Pediatric infectious disease-associated syndromes. In Fuhrman BP, Zimmerman JJ, eds: *Pediatric critical care,* ed 2, St Louis, 1998, Mosby.

214. Parsonnet J: Mediators in the pathogenesis of TSS: overview, *Rev Infect Dis* 11(S1): 263-269, 1989.

215. Ferrari N, WeisseM: Botulism, *Adv Pediatr Infect Dis* 10:81-88, 1995.

216. Tardo C, Steele RW: Infant botulism, *Clin Pediatr* 36:591-594, 1997.

217. Glatman-Freedman A: Infant botulism, *Pediatr Rev* 17:185-186, 1996.

218. Abramson JS, Givner LB: Rocky Mountain spotted fever, *Pediatr Infect Dis J* 18:539-540, 1999.

219. Cale DF, McCarthy MW: Treatment of Rocky Mountain spotted fever in children, *Ann Pharmacother* 31:492-494, 1997.

220. Centers for Disease Control and Prevention: Reye syndrome: United States, *MMWR* 34: 13, 1984.

221. Belay ED, Bresee JS, Holman RC et al: Reye's syndrome in the United States form 1981 through 1997, *N Engl J Med* 340:1377-1382, 1999.

222. Orlowski JP: Whatever happened to Reye's syndrome? Did it ever really exist? *Crit Care Med* 27:1582-1587, 1999.

223. Blaese RM: Development of gene therapy for immunodeficiency: adenosine deaminase deficiency, *Pediatr Res* 33(suppl 1):s49-s53, 1992.

224. Antoine FS: Landmark gene therapy trial progresses, *NIH Record,* XLII (18), Bethesda, Md, 1990, The National Institutes of Health.

225. Garnett C: First human gene therapy trial debuts at NIH, *NIH Record,* XLII (20), Bethesda, Md, 1990, The National Institutes of Health.

226. Wallace CS, Hall M, Kuhn RJ: Pharmacologic management of cystic fibrosis, *Clin Pharm* 12:657-674, 1993.

227. Natanson C, Hoffman WD, Suffredini AF et al: Selected treatment strategies for septic shock based on proposed mechanisms of pathogenesis, *Ann Intern Med* 120:771-783, 1994.

16

Skin Integrity

Sandy M. Quigley
Darlene E. Whitney

The skin is one of the largest, most accessible, and easily examined organs of the human body. It provides a variety of protective functions essential to life, facilitates sensory input, and can be a source of great comfort or discomfort. Easily seen and touched, the skin allows ready access to information about its integrity. Illness and internal organ dysfunction are also often evident through integumentary manifestations. In childhood, the routine discomforts caused by rashes, dry skin, and sunburn are usually quickly diagnosed and relieved with gentle cleansing and over-the-counter products.

Integumentary resilience and wound healing are influenced by maturation. Healthy children enjoy the benefits of strong, supple skin that resists injury and heals quickly. The bruises, scrapes, and cuts that are inevitable byproducts of normal childhood development are usually healed with the comfort of a loving caregiver and the application of a cartoon bandage. Critically ill or injured children, however, are influenced by powerful internal and external factors that place them at significant risk of developing wounds that will not heal without nursing expertise.

Impairment in skin integrity places an already compromised child at risk for serious complications and significant discomfort. Skin breakdown can negatively impact a child's ability to eat, sleep, or move. Disruptions in the body's outer layer of defense leaves a child vulnerable to infection. Increased loss of fluids and a decreased ability to retain body heat can add further stress to an already taxed child. Routine skin care practices that promote skin integrity, that allow for the early identification of children at high risk for breakdown, and that incorporate individualized preventive strategies can minimize complications.

Optimizing wound healing through skillful, scientifically based care can improve patient outcomes, maximize resource allocation, and decrease cost. Pediatric critical care nurses often provide an array of expert wound care. Managing surgical wounds efficiently and effectively are essential aspects of everyday nursing practice. Minimizing the impact of iatrogenic wounds (including pressure ulcers, irritant contact diaper dermatitis, and intravenous infiltrate injuries) through aggressive prevention, early identification, and prompt treatment is predominately a nursing responsibility. As direct bedside caregivers, nurses play an integral role in promoting skin integrity and enhancing the potential for positive patient outcomes.

INTEGUMENTARY STRUCTURE AND FUNCTION

The skin consists of two distinct anatomic layers, the epidermis and dermis, supported by underlying subcutaneous tissue. These layers, together with epidermal derivatives including hair, nails, mucous membranes, and glands, make up the functioning units of the integumentary system.

Epidermis

The avascular epidermis is the outermost layer of the skin. It consists of five distinct cell layers and functions as a protective barrier between the environment and the body, as well as a membrane that holds in body fluids. The inner, basal cell layer of the epidermis is nourished by the blood supply of the dermis and is responsible for epithelial cell division. As basal cells multiply, they are pushed up by the remaining layers of the epidermis and are gradually filled with keratin, a waterproofing protein.[1] The result of keratinization is 25 to 30 rows of dead, flat, dry, tightly adhered cells making up the outermost layer of the epidermis. These keratinocytes provide an effective barrier against microorganisms and irritating chemicals and impede the exchange of fluids and electrolytes between the body and the environment. The continual replacement and shedding of keratinocytes help to prevent excessive microbial colonization of the skin surface. Melanocytes, which produce the granules of melanin, are also found in the basal layer of the epidermis. The amount and distribution of the cells that manufacture melanin, the brown pigment, determine whether we are black or white.[2] In black skin, the granules are larger and more evenly distributed throughout the cell, whereas in white skin, they are smaller and tend to be clumped together.[3] They are responsible for pigmentation and provide some but not complete protection from ultraviolet rays. Langerhans' cells are found throughout the epidermis and serve the protective function of phagocytosis.[1]

The epidermal layer of newborns and infants is thinner and functionally immature as compared to adults.[4] Infants experience higher levels of water loss and have a greater permeability to chemicals than older children.[5] This, coupled with a larger ratio of skin surface area to body weight, increases the risk of dehydration and the systemic toxicity from transcutaneously absorbed chemicals. The thin epidermis is also more likely to blister and become damaged from mechanical trauma and the use of adhesives.

Dermis

The dermis is a highly vascular layer of the skin secured beneath the epidermis. It is comprised of collagenous and elastic fiber connective tissue embedded with blood vessels, lymphatics, nerve endings, hair follicles, and sebaceous glands. Collagen, produced by fibroblasts and macrophages, gives the skin substance, mechanical strength, and elasticity. It allows the skin to withstand frictional stress and remain pliable over joints. The dermal vasculature nourishes both the dermal and epidermal cells, as well as facilitates thermal regulation. Sebaceous glands secrete a mixture of fat,

cholesterol, protein, and salt called sebum.[1] Sebum helps to keep skin soft and hydrated by limiting evaporation. Black skin has more sweat glands to help with temperature control, as it absorbs heat.[2]

The dermal layer in infants and children is thinner and produces less sebum. Dermal thickness increases slowly after 1 year of age and doubles between the ages of 3 and 7. Sebaceous glands are functional at birth, but sebum production remains low until 8 to 10 years of age, providing less protection against evaporation and drying.[6]

Subcutaneous Tissue

Subcutaneous tissue, located below the dermis, is an important supporting layer of the skin. It is composed of adipose tissue embedded with the same structures found in the dermis plus the secretory portion of sudoriferous, or sweat, glands. Subcutaneous tissue serves as a cushion to trauma, a heat insulator, and an important source of energy metabolism. Sweat, which is a mixture of water, salt, urea, acids, ammonia, and sugar, functions as a body temperature regulator and waste eliminator.[1] Lysozyme is also secreted by sweat glands and provides chemical protection against harmful bacteria.[7] Newborn infants have less subcutaneous tissue than older infants and children and are therefore more at risk for thermal instability.

PHASES OF WOUND HEALING

A wound is defined as tissue trauma associated with an interruption in tissue continuity. Virtually all critically ill children experience wounds from trauma, surgery, or invasive procedures, including intravascular access. Wounds are a potential source of significant morbidity and mortality. Wound healing is the process in which injured tissue is replaced through regeneration or repair. Regeneration is the replacement of tissue with like tissue. Superficial and partial thickness wounds of the epidermis and upper dermis heal by regeneration. Some tissues, including subcutaneous and muscle tissue, cannot regenerate and must heal by formation of new connective tissue (scar) to fill the defect. Wound healing affects and is affected by critical care management decisions and has a profound impact on patient outcomes.

The cellular process of wound healing can be divided into three phases: the inflammatory phase, the proliferative phase, and the maturation phase (Table 16-1). Although these phases overlap and intertwine, each has a predictable sequence of events that distinguishes it.[8-12] When this orderly cascade of events is allowed to proceed, most wounds can be expected to heal in 3 to 4 weeks. If the sequence is interrupted, healing will be delayed, and the wound may become chronic in nature.

Inflammatory Phase

The first of the three phases of wound healing, the defensive or inflammatory phase, is the body's immediate response to injury and can last up to 6 days. The function of this phase is to clear away dead cells and bacteria and to stimulate the

TABLE 16-1   Phases of Wound Healing

Phase	Clinical Observation	Cellular Activities
Inflammatory Phase Typically begins at time of injury and lasts approximately 3 days	Erythema, warmth, edema, and pain	*Vasoconstriction:* platelets form along injured blood vessels; platelets release vasoconstrictive substances and promote fibrin clot to prevent hemorrhage *Vasodilation:* vasodilatory substances allow leakage of plasma into wound Leukocytes migrate through vessel walls to phagocytose bacteria and foreign materials Monocytes differentiate into macrophages, which give rise to tissue repair process
Proliferative Phase Overlaps with inflammatory phase and continues until wound is healed	Beefy, red granulation tissue	*Macrophages* secrete growth-promoting substances that mediate granulation tissue and epithelialization *Collagen synthesis:* performed by fibroblasts; provides tensile strength to wound *Angiogenesis:* regeneration of a vascular network to restore capillary system to dermis
	Thin, silvery, epithelial layer surrounding granulation tissue	*Epithelialization:* cell migration across a wound
	Wound shrinkage	*Contraction:* myofibroblasts migrate through tissue to facilitate closing the wound
Maturation Phase Begins 3 weeks after wounding and may continue for several years	Shrinking, thinning, paling of scar	Remodeling of tissue matrix as fibroblasts migrate away from the wound while fibrous bundles of collagen increase the tensile strength of the scar

healing process by initiating a cascade of interdependent reactions. The major events during this phase are hemostasis and inflammation.

The vascular response in the inflammatory phase is responsible for the clinical observations of the wound. Immediately after the injury, a short period of vasoconstriction lasting 5 to 10 minutes occurs. Vasoconstriction slows blood flow through the area and aids in hemostasis.[13] This activates coagulation factors and causes platelet aggregation, resulting in fibrin clot formation. The clot provides initial wound closure and helps prevent excessive blood loss. Vasoconstriction is followed by active vasodilation induced by the release of bradykinin and histamine.[12] Vascular permeability increases, allowing serum to gain entry into the wound. Fluid, protein, and enzymes normally found in the intravascular compartment leak through the vessel walls into the extracellular space, causing edema and erythema.[14]

The cellular response during the inflammatory phase triggers the healing cascade and begins the debriding process. During this period, vessel walls become lined with platelets, leukocytes, and erythrocytes. Platelets release cytokines or growth factors, which are thought to trigger the healing cascade and to stimulate the growth of local venular endothelial cells that give rise to new blood vessels.[15] Neutrophils migrate to the wound area to ingest bacteria and debris. They are short lived (2 to 3 days) and become part of the wound exudate. Macrophages orchestrate the healing process through ingestion of debris, angiogenesis, and the release of a protein that stimulates the formation of fibroblasts necessary for the next phase of wound healing. The overall result of the inflammatory phase of wound healing is control of bleeding and establishment of a clean wound bed.

Antiinflammatory agents, particularly corticosteroids, given before the injury or during the inflammatory phase can markedly reduce the necessary inflammatory response needed to stimulate healing.[12] Vitamin A has been found to counteract the antiinflammatory response of corticosteroids, but when given systemically, it can also attenuate the anticipated systemic steroid effect. A persistent decrease in wound blood flow, as seen in dehydration or impaired cardiac output, can also delay the onset of inflammation.

Proliferative Phase

The proliferative phase is the primary phase of cell regeneration and repair that occurs approximately 4 to

20 days after the injury. The major processes occurring during this phase include macrophage replication, fibroblast production, collagen synthesis, angiogenesis, epithelialization, and wound contraction. The clinical observations are a moist, beefy red, granulation tissue surrounded by a thin, silvery epithelial layer. As the phase progresses, epithelialization is completed, and wound contracture occurs, serving to reduce the size of the wound defect.

The macrophages and platelets seen in the inflammatory phase trigger many of the events that occur in the proliferative phase.[15a,16] Granulation tissue is beefy red, moist, and friable and has a shiny, cobblestone appearance as a result of newly formed collagen and blood vessels (Fig. 16-1). Fibroblasts are responsible for collagen synthesis. Platelet growth factor, macrophage activity, lactic acid, and ascorbic acid are necessary for fibroblast proliferation.[12,16] Fibroblast migration into the wound occurs along local fibrin strands from the initial wound coagulation, as well as any remaining collagen strands. Peak collagen synthesis occurs from 5 to 7 days in primary healing wounds and may continue for more than a year in chronic wounds.[10] Fibroblast activity and continued proliferation are dependent on the adequacy of local oxygen supply and neovascularization.

Angiogenesis, or the development of new blood vessels, takes place just behind the advancing edges of fibroblasts. The immature collagen produced by fibroblasts provides vital structural support for new friable capillaries. Without the collagen support, these new blood vessels would not be able to withstand the pressure of arterial blood flow. Impaired perfusion, tissue hypoxia, and the lack of nutrients, such as vitamin C, zinc, magnesium, and amino acids, will retard the angiogenesis process.[9,10,12,16]

Epithelialization is the migration of epithelial cells from the wound borders to resurface the defect. Normally, new cells form from the basal layer and migrate vertically. However, when there is loss of epidermal tissue, adjacent basal cells become reprogrammed. They appear to detach from their basement membrane, divide, and migrate toward

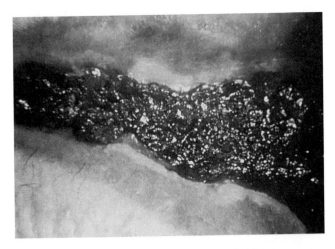

Fig. 16-1 Granulation tissue—red, beefy, and shiny appearance without evidence of infection.

and across the wound forming a sheet of epithelium.[12] Once a single layer of epithelium develops, additional layers are created from mitotic division of these epidermal cells. If any hair follicles are present in the center of the wound, the epithelial tissue around them will reproduce and form islands of pink epithelial tissue that migrate toward other islands.[17]

The reepithelialization process can be rapid (i.e., 3 to 5 days in a partial thickness wound) or may require several months depending on the size of the wound, nutrient supply, and the wound environment. Optimal environmental conditions for epithelial migration are a moist, protected wound bed free of necrotic tissue. A surface barrier that is permeable to water vapor and oxygen and able to absorb wound exudate while allowing for cell migration has been demonstrated to improve wound healing.[18] This is the premise for many of the wound dressings that are discussed later in the chapter.

Wound contraction is the final process that occurs during the proliferative phase. Contraction is the process by which a large wound with tissue loss is reduced in area by the inward migration of normal tissue.[16] The mechanism of contraction, which shrinks the wound, is the generation of cellular forces in the contractile elements of myofibroblasts. Wound contraction decreases the amount of surface area that needs to be filled by granulation and epithelialization. Effective contracture can only occur if the surrounding tissue is pliable enough to allow movement.[19] Wound contraction is exemplified by the closure of a tracheostomy, gastrostomy, or enterocutaneous fistula. If the loss of tissue is too great and the defect is not closed by contraction, surgical intervention may be required.

Maturation Phase

The last phase of healing begins approximately 20 days after the injury and continues or up to a year or longer. Its primary purpose is to remodel the wound and provide a scar that has maximum tensile strength. The clinical observations of this phase include shrinking, thinning, and paling of the wound scar. Black skin seems to be more prone to overgrowth of scar tissue after wounding (keloid scars), and when injured, it turns blacker.[3] A keloid is a benign dense growth of connective tissue that forms in the dermis after trauma. The lesions are often firm, raised, pink, and rubbery. They may be tender or pruritic. Increasing wound strength is accomplished through the maturation of collagen, the protein that provides structural strength and integrity to body tissue. Collagen establishes the wound's tensile strength, the maximum amount of pressure that can be applied to a wound without causing rupture.[16] Collagen synthesis becomes mature, increasingly organized, and consequently stronger during the maturation phase. In the first 2 weeks of healing, a wound can regain 30% to 50% of its original strength. By 3 months, the tensile strength of the wound nears 80%. However, a wound will never regain more than 80% of its original strength.[19]

PROMOTING SKIN INTEGRITY

Routine practices that protect healthy skin surfaces are essential standards of care in the pediatric intensive care unit (PICU). All critically ill children share an increased risk of skin compromise because of factors such as suboptimal nutrition, impaired sensation, immobility, decreased tissue perfusion and oxygenation, immunosuppression, and the use of medical devices, restraints, and invasive procedures. Furthermore, they are particularly vulnerable to the adverse effects of compromised skin integrity, including infection, discomfort, interference with needed treatments, delayed wound healing, and prolonged hospitalization. Healthcare providers need to be knowledgeable regarding skin integrity characteristics of various ethnic groups. Promoting skin integrity through nursing practice guidelines can maximize the potential for achieving desired patient outcomes (Box 16-1).

Assess and Individualize Skin Care Practices. Vigilant assessment of all skin surfaces (including oral mucosa and eye integrity) supports the critical evaluation and necessary individualization of skin care practice guidelines. Identifying the adequacy of existing practice before significant alteration in skin integrity occurs is central to effective care. Comprehensive documentation facilitates continuity, assists in identifying trends, and is helpful with tracking evolving issues.

Bathe Daily With pH-Balanced Cleanser. Daily baths with a liquid, alcohol-free, and pH-balanced cleanser supports the skin's protective barrier function and minimizes the risk for infection. The tightly adhered epidermal cells of intact skin provide an effective physical barrier against microbial invasion.[20] The epidermal surface is dry, mildly acidic, continually shedding, and possesses the antimicrobial properties of sebum and lysozyme.[7,16] Healthy skin is also colonized with indigenous bacteria that inhibit the growth of potentially harmful microorganisms. The mechanical forces exerted with gentle cleansing facilitate the protective shedding of epidermal cells. The shed layers are darker if the nuclei have more melanin. Thus when the skin

of an African-American child is cleansed with an alcohol wipe, for instance, the wipe will look darker than it does when white skin is wiped, not because of dirt but because of shed cells with rich melanin deposits.[21] Avoiding antimicrobial products for routine cleaning helps maintain the skin's natural bacterial flora. Soap is alkaline and can increase skin pH, creating a more hospitable environment for bacterial growth. It removes protective sebum and lysosome. Jackson[22] reports that black skin tends to be dry and to use soap sparingly. Bar soap carries the additional risk of supporting bacterial growth and acting as an infectious reservoir. Infants are at greater risk for epidermal drying and cracking because they produce less lubricating sebum and may therefore benefit from less frequent washing with minimal use of cleansers. Shampooing need only be done once a week or after electroencephalogram (EEG) lead removal. Smith and Burns[21] discuss the anatomic and physiologic features of African-American hair and skin. They report that the process of hair lubrication takes longer to occur in African-American hair than in the hair of Caucasians or Asians; therefore it is drier. Because it takes longer to get a natural sheen between shampoos, African Americans tend to wash their hair less often than do other racial groups.[23] Often oil-based shampoos, not water based, are used. Discussing hair care regimens with patients or their families is important.

Keep Skin Surfaces Dry. Moisture is universally noted as a major risk factor contributing to bacterial growth, skin breakdown, and pressure ulcer development. Jiricka and colleagues[24] concluded that skin breakdown was 4 times more likely in patients exposed to moisture. Skin exposure to moisture from perspiration, secretions, wound drainage, gastric output, urine, and stool leads to bacterial growth, maceration, rashes, and, in extreme cases, cellulitis that weakens the natural barrier of the epidermis.[25] Measures to keep skin dry include maintaining a slightly cool ambient temperature, careful attention to skin folds during bathing, frequent linen and diaper changes, efficient removal or containment of excess exudates, and the consistent application of topical products that provide a moisture barrier to areas of the skin considered at risk.

Use Moisture Barrier Products on Incontinent Infants and Children. Although all incontinent patients can benefit from vigilant care and the routine application of protective ointments, identifying children at increased risk for developing perineal breakdown and implementing consistent prevention strategies can greatly reduce the incidence of irritant contact diaper dermatitis.[26] Some common causes that place children at risk for perineal breakdown include increased moisture from urinary incontinence, coupled with friction forces; short gut syndrome; changes in bowel flora resulting in loose, watery stools; and intestinal adaption to adjustments in enteral feedings. The initial impact of stool on the perineum after closure of an ileostomy or colostomy can also produce significant skin breakdown. Diapers should be changed as soon as they are wet or soiled. Cleansing can be done with a pH-balanced cleanser and water, mineral oil, or disposable diaper wipes that are free of perfumes and alcohol. Products containing alcohol are drying and irritat-

---

Box 16-1
Skin Care Practice Guidelines

Assess and individualize skin care practices
Bathe daily with pH-balanced cleanser
Keep skin surfaces dry
Use moisture barrier products on incontinent infants and children
Maintain skin hydration
Avoid products that contain perfumes, alcohol, or latex
Minimize the use of adhesives
Minimize the impact of medical devices
Keep mucous membranes clean and moist
Keep eyes moist and protected
Maximize nutritional status
Support tissue perfusion and oxygenation
Promote immunocompetence
Minimize hazards of immobility

ing to sensitive skin; therefore these products should be avoided.

Avoid the frequent use of plain water and excessive friction motion during cleansing.[27] Apply a protective moisture barrier product with each diaper change. Choose barrier products that are free of alcohol and perfumes, easy to apply and remove, and cost efficient. Products such as petroleum jelly, A&D ointment, or zinc oxide preparations are often sufficient to protect at-risk skin.

Maintain Skin Hydration. Skin hydration is maintained through adequate systemic hydration and the judicious use of topical moisturizers. Children exhibit the adverse effects of dehydration more readily than adults and are particularly sensitive to fluid losses because they have a proportionally higher body composition of water. Dehydration adversely affects tissue perfusion and is a factor in pressure ulcer development. Even mild fluid volume deficits can result in poor skin turgor and a dry, cracked epithelial surface. This condition leaves the body vulnerable to chemical absorption and bacterial invasion. Dry skin can add to patient discomfort, and scratching can lead to further breakdown. Identify and compensate for additional fluid losses from stool and gastric output, fever, tachypnea, diaphoresis, open wounds, radiant warmers, phototherapy, and extracorporeal membrane oxygenation support to the extent that each child's condition allows. Topical moisturizers applied to extremely dry skin will lessen fluid losses to the environment and enhance patient comfort, but these should be used cautiously on the thin and more permeable epidermal layer of infants. Moisturizers are particularly beneficial when adequate systemic hydration is contraindicated or when the underlying cause of integumentary dehydration is the result of non–fluid-related factors, such as liver dysfunction, radiation therapy, or autoimmune mediators (i.e., eczema).

Avoid Products That Contain Perfumes, Alcohol, or Latex. Contact dermatitis is a hyperimmune-mediated response to an antigenic product that results in a sequence of inflammatory changes in the dermis and epidermis. Cutaneous manifestations can include erythema, swelling, vesicle formation, pruritus, and ulceration. Use of multiple skin care products containing chemicals increases the risk of ingredient interactions and skin sensitivity. Exposure to latex may cause an allergic response, either locally at the site of contact (Type IV), or an IgE-mediated systemic reaction (Type I, anaphylaxis). Latex is found in a wide array of medical devices and skin care products. Children at increased risk for developing a latex allergy are those with myelomeningocele and/or a history of chronic or recurrent instrumentation of the genitourinary tract. At-risk children should be placed on "latex precautions," and the use of all latex-containing products should be carefully avoided to minimize the risk of an allergic reaction (see www.latexfree.com for an up-to-date list of latex-containing and alternative, latex-free products).

Minimize the Use of Adhesives. Adhesive-based products are widely used in the pediatric critical care setting. Although often necessary, adhesives are a potential skin irritant and can cause significant skin trauma if applied or removed improperly. Use alternative products, including gel electrodes, Velcro ties, Montgomery straps, and cloth wraps whenever possible (Figs. 16-2 and 16-3). Moisture vapor permeable, transparent film dressings allow better visualization of underlying skin and may be less irritating. Applying a thin pectin- or hydrocolloid-based product as an "anchor" under adhesives will protect the skin from irritation and trauma caused by prolonged or repeated tape removal. When tape is required, consider the use of skin barrier films to provide a protective interface between the skin and adhesive product. Avoid the use of benzoin as a skin barrier under adhesives because it can irritate the skin and has the potential to be absorbed systemically. To prevent epidermal separation from the dermis, epidermal stripping, adhesives should be secured around a tube or line before being attached to the skin to limit tension on the epidermal layer. Careful attention to the location of devices before taping, such as securing endotracheal tubes midline, and the use of padding under pressure points will

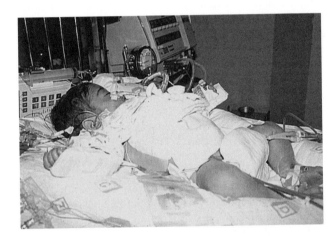

Fig. 16-2 Montgomery straps on a liver transplant patient.

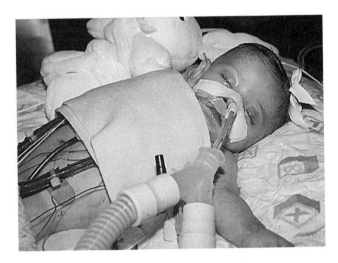

Fig. 16-3 Chest wound with Stockinette.

lessen the risk of localized pressure injury. When removing adhesive-based products, the underlying skin should be supported while applying gentle traction to the product using water or an adhesive remover. Adhesive remover is highly irritating and should be washed off the skin immediately after applying to avoid the development of contact dermatitis.

Minimize the Impact of Medical Devices. A myriad of medical devices are used in the assessment and treatment of critically ill children. Each line, tube, probe, electrode, catheter, and dressing carries with it the potential to disrupt the skin's protective barrier and to cause iatrogenic tissue injury. Limiting the adverse impact of medical devices on the integumentary system requires careful adherence to manufacturers' guidelines on usage and care. General guidelines include using the fewest devices possible, alternating pressure points regularly (moving oxygen saturation probes, blood pressure cuffs), padding areas of persistent pressure (nasal bridge from oxygen delivery mask), minimizing the use of high-risk devices (heating lamps and cooling blankets), and frequently assessing affected areas.

Keep the Mucous Membranes Clean and Moist. Oral cavity assessment and care provided every 4 hours for intubated patients and every 8 hours for patients who are not intubated, combined with suctioning of oral secretions every 2 hours, can decrease the incidence of nosocomial pulmonary infection.[28] Studies have also shown that there are benefits to providing oral care at least every 2 hours in critically ill adults, the elderly, and adult oncology patients.[29-32] Products that provide atraumatic cleaning include soft bristle toothbrushes, toothettes, tap water, normal saline, sodium bicarbonate, hydrogen peroxide, and mouth rinses containing clorhexidine.[31-34] Use of lemon-glycerine swabs and mouth rinses that contain alcohol should be avoided to prevent chemical irritation and drying of the oral mucosa.[35] The hyperpigmented oral mucosa of many dark-skinned patients is a normal finding. Nasal mucosa and lips should be kept moisturized with the frequent application of petrolatum or water-soluble lubricants. If the tongue becomes swollen and exposed, it should be kept covered with petroleum gauze to prevent drying. Significant tongue edema may require a dental consult to evaluate the benefit of using a mouth guard or prop to prevent pressure injury. Dental appliances should be removed and cleaned regularly with mouth care.

Keep Eyes Moist and Protected. Prevent corneal epithelial breakdown by keeping eyes moist and protected from chemical and foreign body irritants. Many critically ill children are at risk for iatrogenic corneal injury because of a diminished or absent blink response. Eye moisture can be maintained with artificial tears or lubricant in nonparalyzed children with insufficient tear production, incomplete lid closure, or diminished blink response. Chemically paralyzed children and those with absent blink response should have their eyes protected with a moisture chamber created by instilling normal saline drops every 2 hours and covering the eyes with plastic wrap to seal in the moisture[36] (Fig. 16-4). The plastic wrap should be changed daily or more frequently as needed to prevent infection.

Maximize Nutritional Status. Maximize each child's nutritional status through careful assessment and the early initiation of enteral and/or parenteral feedings. Most critically ill children experience some degree of suboptimal nutrition as a result of increased metabolic demands, altered tolerance of enteral feedings, impaired intake, or preexisting malnutrition. The assessment of nutritional status, the calculation of protein-energy need, and the implementation of nutritional support are multifactorial and require multidisciplinary collaboration. Nutritional deficits that contribute to pressure ulcer development include hypoproteinemia, anemia, ascorbic acid deficiency, and trace mineral deficiency. These deficits alter the quality and integrity of the components of soft tissue, particularly collagen.[37] The release of stress hormones triggered by critical illness result in the accelerated breakdown of protein for energy. Depletion of amino acids interferes with cell membrane integrity. Capillary leak and hypoalbuminemia contribute to interstitial edema, which impedes the cellular exchange of metabolites and increases the skin's fragility by stretching collagen fibers.[38] Insufficient intake of protein, calories, vitamins, and minerals also has a profound effect on wound healing. Consultation with the nutritional support team is helpful in determining whether specialized enteral feedings or vitamin and mineral supplementation would be beneficial. The early initiation of enteral feedings and a proactive evaluation of the need for central parenteral nutrition based on each child's history and expected trajectory are essential in maintaining skin integrity.

Support Tissue Perfusion and Oxygenation. Decreased cardiac output with inadequate tissue perfusion is a final common pathway for a wide range of pediatric critical care phenomena. Decreased perfusion of the skin and subcutaneous tissue is mediated by the compensatory mechanism of the sympathetic nervous system, which

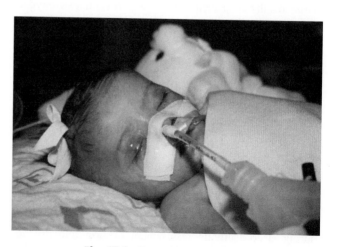

Fig. 16-4   Eye moisture chamber.

shunts blood flow to vital organs during low-output states. Inadequate tissue oxygenation is usually the result of hypoxemia in children, although hypovolemia alone can have the same effect.[39] The impact of hypoxemia on the skin is similar to that of inadequate tissue perfusion. Peripheral vasoconstriction and hypoperfusion can contribute to delayed wound healing.

Promote Immunocompetence. Critically ill infants and children are particularly vulnerable to acquiring nosocomial infections resulting from immature immune responses, multiple stressors, invasive procedures, and the use of immunosuppressive therapies.[40] Disruptions in the epidermis from numerous catheters, surgical wounds and drains, external fixation devices, and traumatic injury leave the body susceptible to invasion from indigenous and opportunistic microorganisms. Localized and systemic infection can place a child with immune dysfunction from serious illness or injury at significant risk for increased morbidity and mortality. Promoting immunocompetence requires a multidisciplinary effort to address a broad spectrum of care, including nutrition, iatrogenic stressors, comfort or sedation, and medical alterations of immunologic function. Systemic infection increases the risk of opportunistic skin infections, skin breakdown, and pressure ulcer development.[16,41] Preventing infection requires strict adherence to the Centers for Disease Control and Prevention Guidelines (see www.cdc.gov), including good handwashing, the appropriate use of barrier precautions, patient cohorting, the early identification and treatment of infections, and the proper maintenance of lines, dressings, and medical devices. Children receiving immunosuppressive therapy are at additional risk for skin integrity impairment as a result of increased skin fragility, decreased elasticity, gingival hypertrophy, increased risk of avascular necrosis, and interference with the normal phases of wound healing.[16,42]

Minimize the Hazards of Immobility. Impaired physical mobility and sensation often accompany serious illness and can predispose skin over bony prominences to prolonged or excessive pressures. Pressure that compromises capillary blood flow to the skin and underlying soft tissue results in inadequate tissue perfusion and oxygenation, metabolic acidosis, ischemia, and necrosis seen clinically as a pressure ulcer. Routine assessment for pressure ulcer risk and the early tracking of at-risk patients into preventive protocols are essential in reducing the morbidity and mortality associated with pressure injury. However, virtually all patients can benefit from frequent position changes, encouraging the highest level of mobility possible, range-of-motion exercises, and the judicious use of physical and chemical restraints. Children confined to bed rest, those developmentally unable to roll, and those with neuromuscular or sensation impairment should be repositioned with small moves at least every 2 hours.[43,44] Removal of physical restraints at least every 2 hours when a child is awake and every 4 hours during sleep facilitates assessment of skin integrity and perfusion.

PROBLEMS ENCOUNTERED IN CRITICAL CARE

Pressure Ulcers

Pressure ulcers are localized areas of tissue destruction that develop when soft tissue is compressed between a bony prominence and an external surface for a prolonged period[45] (Fig. 16-5). Continued pressure on tissues compresses capillary blood flow, resulting in tissue ischemia with eventual necrosis if pressure is not relieved. The general belief is that the amount of pressure required to collapse capillaries must exceed capillary pressure. Capillary pressures of 12 to 32 mmHg are commonly used as the numerical "standard" for capillary closing pressure.[16] Whenever external pressure is exerted that exceeds capillary closing pressure, tissue hypoxia and cellular death can occur. Pressure ulcers usually occur over bony prominences, although pressure from external medical equipment devices, such as face masks, endotracheal tubes, abdominal binders, limb restraints, enteral feeding tube flanges, and plaster or fiberglass casts, can result in pressure ulcers.

Pressure ulcers can be debilitating to patients for weeks or even months after development. The large expense to prevent and the much greater expense to treat pressure ulcers are of increasing concern in acute, rehabilitative, and home care patients. Healthcare providers need to appropriately allocate finite resources while maintaining quality care for patients with potential or actual alterations in skin integrity. A plethora of nursing research is available on the incidence, prevalence, and expense of pressure ulcer prevention and management in adults (most of which is noted in the clinical practice guideline, Pressure Ulcers in Adults: Prediction and Prevention, Agency for Health Care Policy and Research[46]). However, little empirical data exist to guide pediatric nursing practices. Care of infants and children is extrapolated from practices developed primarily for adults. Adding to this complexity are numerous wound care products and specialty support surfaces of varying costs thought to help prevent or manage pressure ulcers in

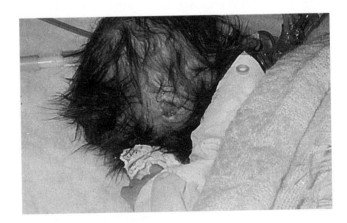

Fig. 16-5 Occiput pressure ulcer.

children but that are derived from clinical trials conducted with adults.

Risk Assessment. The most important nursing intervention in preventing skin breakdown in critically ill infants and children is the early identification of risk factors.[47] In 1996, Quigley and Curley adapted the adult-based Braden scale for Predicting Pressure Sore Risk,[48] Modified Braden Q scale (Table 16-2), for use in the pediatric population. The Braden scale was selected because it has been extensively tested in diverse adult clinical areas, including intensive care, and contains vivid categorical descriptors.[25,49]

The Braden Q scale is composed of seven subscales: mobility, activity, sensory perception, skin moisture, friction and shear, nutrition, and tissue perfusion and oxygenation. All seven subscales are rated from 1 (least favorable) to 4 (most favorable). Each level is mutually exclusive, with only one choice for each category. The range of possible scores for the Braden Q is 7 (highest risk for skin breakdown) to 28 (no risk for breakdown). The Braden Q scale was originally tested on 178 children on bed rest by a group of expert pediatric nurses who scored the patients and who concurrently rated each child's level of risk for skin breakdown as high, moderate, or low. Comparing the Braden Q score with the subjective rating for each child showed that children considered at low risk for skin breakdown scored an average of 25 points on the Braden Q scale. Children at moderate risk averaged 21 points, and children at high risk for skin breakdown averaged 16 points. Confidence intervals indicated that children scoring less than 23 points were at moderate or high risk for skin breakdown. Thus patients with a Braden Q score of less than 23 points are considered at risk for alterations in skin integrity.

The necessary frequency of reassessment of pressure ulcer risk is unknown. Braden and Bergstrom[50] explored the impact of assessment intervals on the ability to optimally predict pressure ulcers in a nursing home population. They recommended that the interval for risk assessment should be determined according to the stability of the patient population.[50] Carlson, Kemp, and Shott[51] found that among 82% of the patients who had pressure ulcers, the ulcers developed by the third day after admission to an ICU, indicating the need to routinely monitor risk for pressure ulcers during the initial days in the ICU. Quigley and Curley[52] recommend that all pediatric patients with skin breakdown, as well as all immobile patients, undergo a risk assessment evaluation by a registered nurse on admission and every 24 hours thereafter. Risk assessment, as the first step in the nursing process, cannot be delegated to assistive personnel.[53] All patients at risk for pressure ulcer development should have a systematic skin inspection at least once every 24 hours, particularly over all bony prominences.

Prevention and Risk Modification. Once a child at risk for pressure ulcer development has been identified, a management plan should be developed to modify or eliminate known risk. Quigley and Curley[52] developed a skin care algorithm (Fig. 16-6) to establish practice guidelines for the prevention of alterations in skin integrity. After a patient has been identified as being at risk for skin

breakdown based on a Braden Q score of less than 23, a prevention protocol is instituted. The protocol was extrapolated from the recommendations in the Agency for Health Care Policy and Research (AHCPR) Clinical Practice Guideline No. 3, Pressure Ulcers in Adults: Prediction and Prevention.[54]

Patient positioning and mobility are systematically assessed because it is generally accepted that unrelieved pressure of sufficient duration leads to the development of pressure ulcers over bony prominences. Both intensity and duration of pressure are equally important. For example, high pressures for short durations equal the same risk as low pressures for long duration. Among experts, no general agreement exists regarding the exact level of intensity or duration needed for pressure ulcer formation.

Regular repositioning has been shown to significantly decrease the incidence of pressure ulcer development. The recommendation that at-risk individuals be repositioned every 2 hours is derived from two classic studies. Kosiak[55] used animal control studies to demonstrate that pressure-induced ischemic injury occurs within 1 to 2 hours of exposure. In his study, he applied 70 mmHg for 1 hour to rat muscle fibers, and this caused no damage. However, an application of the same pressure for 2 hours caused "moderate" muscle damage. Norton, McLaren, and Exton-Smith[56] divided a sample of 100 hospitalized adult patients into three groups based on the number of times they were repositioned in 24 hours. The incidence of pressure ulcers in the group turned every 2 to 3 hours was lower than the group turned every 4 hours and the group turned 2 to 4 times a day. They concluded that if pressure is not relieved by regular 2-hour changes in positioning, pressure ulcers would eventually develop.

The AHCPR recommendations are that any individual in bed who is assessed to be at risk for pressure ulcer development should be repositioned at least every 2 hours if this is consistent with the patient's overall goals. Evidence shows that small shifts in body weight can be used as an adjunct to the standard repositioning schedule to further decrease the exposure of at-risk individuals to high pressure.[57] Neidig, Kleiber, and Oppliger[58] significantly decreased the incidence of occipital pressure ulcers from 16.9% to 4.8% in a sample of postoperative cardiac surgery children by instituting a prevention protocol in which the primary intervention was repositioning the head at least every 2 hours. The routine use of gel pillows under the occiput of critically ill immobile infants is also warranted to reduce pressure.

The way patients are repositioned is critically important as well. Seiler and Stahelin[59] recommend repositioning at-risk patients from supine to right and left 30-degree oblique positions. The 30-degree oblique position more evenly distributes pressure over the five major bony prominences. Alvarez[60] identified the classic ulcer sites as being over the sacrum, greater trochanter, ischial tuberosities, lateral malleoli, and heels. When the patient is lying on his or her side, all of the weight is distributed over one or two bony prominences. The lateral decubitus position (surface at

◆ **TABLE 16-2   Modified Braden Q Pressure Ulcer Risk Assessment Tool**

	1	2	3	4	Score
Intensity and Duration of Pressure					
Mobility (ability to change and control body position)	**1. Completely immobile:** Does not make even slight changes in body or extremity position without assistance.	**2. Very limited:** Makes occasional slight changes in body or extremity position but unable to completely turn self independently.	**3. Slightly limited:** Makes frequent though slight changes in body or extremity position independently.	**4. No limitations:** Makes major and frequent changes in position without assistance.	
Activity (degree of *current* physical activity)	**1. Bedfast:** Confined to bed.	**2. Chairfast:** Ability to walk severely limited or nonexistent. Cannot bear own weight or must be assisted into chair or wheelchair.	**3. Walks occasionally:** Walks occasionally during day but for very short distances, with or without assistance. Spends majority of each shift in bed or chair.	**4. If ambulatory, all patients too young to ambulate *or* walk frequently:** Walks outside the room at least twice a day and inside room at least once every 2 hours during waking hours.	
Sensory perception (ability to respond in a *developmentally* appropriate way to pressure-related discomfort)	**1. Completely limited:** Unresponsive (does not moan, flinch, or grasp) to painful stimuli as result of diminished level of consciousness or sedation **or** limited ability to feel pain over most of body surface.	**2. Very limited:** Responds only to painful stimuli. Cannot communicate discomfort except by moaning or restlessness **or** has sensory impairment that limits the ability to feel pain or discomfort over one half of body.	**3. Slightly limited:** Responds to verbal commands but cannot always communicate discomfort or need to be turned **or** has some sensory impairment which limits ability to feel pain or discomfort in one or two extremities.	**4. No impairment:** Responds to verbal commands. Has no sensory deficit, which would limit ability to feel or communicate pain or discomfort.	
Tolerance of the Skin and Supporting Structure					
Moisture (degree to which skin is exposed to moisture)	**1. Constantly moist:** Skin is kept moist almost constantly by perspiration, urine, drainage, etc. Dampness is detected every time patient is moved or turned.	**2. Very moist:** Skin is often but not always moist. Linen must be changed at least every 8 hours.	**3. Occasionally moist:** Skin is occasionally moist, requiring linen change every 12 hours.	**4. Rarely moist:** Skin is usually dry; routine diaper changes; linen only requires changing every 24 hours.	

Friction and shear
(*friction*: occurs when skin moves against support surfaces; *shear*: occurs when skin and adjacent bony surface slide across one another)

1. Significant problem:
Spasticity, contracture, itching, or agitation leads to almost constant thrashing and friction.

2. Problem:
Requires moderate to maximum assistance in moving. Complete lifting without sliding against sheets is impossible. Frequently slides down in bed or chair, requiring frequent repositioning with maximum assistance.

3. Potential problem:
Moves feebly or requires minimum assistance. During a move, skin probably slides to some extent against sheets, chair, restraints, or other devices. Maintains relative good position in chair or bed most of the time but occasionally slides down.

4. No apparent problem:
Able to completely lift patient during a position change; moves in bed and in chair independently and has sufficient muscle strength to lift up completely during move. Maintains good position in bed or chair at all times.

Nutrition
(*usual* food intake pattern)

1. Very poor:
NPO and/or maintained on clear liquids or IVs for more than 5 days **or** albumin <2.5 mg/dl **or** never eats a complete meal. Rarely eats more than half of any food offered. Protein intake includes only 2 servings of meat or dairy products per day. Takes fluids poorly. Does not take a liquid dietary supplement.

2. Inadequate:
Is on liquid diet or tube feeding/TPN, which provides inadequate calories and minerals for age **or** albumin <3 mg/dl **or** rarely eats a complete meal and generally eats only about half of any food offered. Protein intake includes only 3 servings of meat or dairy products per day. Occasionally will take a dietary supplement.

3. Adequate:
Is on tube feedings or TPN, which provide adequate calories and minerals for age **or** eats over half of most meals. Eats a total of 4 servings of protein (meat, dairy products) each day. Occasionally will refuse a meal, but will usually take a supplement if offered.

4. Excellent:
Is on a normal diet providing adequate calories for age. For example: eats most of every meal. Never refuses a meal. Usually eats a total of 4 or more servings of meat and diary products. Occasionally eats between meals. Does not require supplementation.

Tissue perfusion and oxygenation

1. Extremely compromised:
Hypotensive (MAP <50 mmHg; <40 in a newborn) or the patient does not physiologically tolerate position changes.

2. Compromised:
Normotensive; serum pH is <7.40; oxygen saturation may be <95%; hemoglobin maybe <10 mg/dl; capillary refill may be >2 seconds.

3. Adequate:
Normotensive; serum pH is normal; oxygen saturation may be <95%; hemoglobin may be <10 mg/dl; capillary refill may be >2 seconds.

4. Excellent:
Normotensive; serum pH is normal; oxygen saturation >95%; normal Hgb; capillary refill <2 seconds.

TOTAL: If <23, refer to Skin Care Algorithm

From Quigley S, Curley MAQ: Skin integrity in the pediatric population: preventing and managing pressure ulcers, *J Soc Pediatr Nurs* 1:7-18, 1996. *IV*, Intravenous; *TPN*, total parenteral nutrition; *NPO*, nothing by mouth; *MAP*, mean arterial pressure.

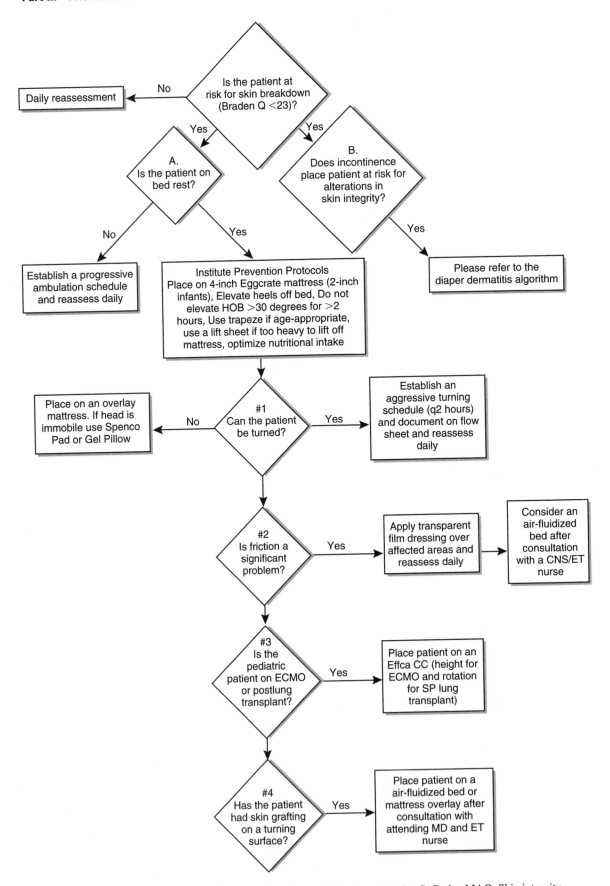

Fig. 16-6   Skin care algorithm. (Reproduced with permission from Quigley S, Curley MAQ: Skin integrity in the pediatric population: preventing and managing pressure ulcers, *J Soc Pediatr Nurs* 1:7-18, 1996.)

90 degrees to the patient's back) should be avoided because it places the skin over the greater trochanter and lateral malleolus at greatest risk for pressure necrosis.[5] Murdoch and Storman[61] found that turning to a variety of positions, including the prone position, was possible even in the most critical patients. Colin and colleagues[44] compared the effect of 30-degree with 90-degree turns on trochanteric and retrotrochanteric oxygen supply in 20 healthy adults on a foam mattress. After 20 minutes, a 90-degree turn position caused significant trochanteric hypoxia, although retrotrochanteric hypoxia did not occur in the 30-degree position. Therefore Colin and colleagues concluded that 30-degree turns may be better in helping to prevent the development of pressure ulcers.

Because of the small surface area of the heels, it is particularly difficult to redistribute the pressure. Sheepskin heel protectors have long been thought to offer some pressure-reducing benefit. Norton and Young[62] monitored the incidence of intraoperative acquired heel pressure ulcers in a pediatric surgical population receiving epidural anesthesia after converting from sheepskin protectors to heel elevation. They reported no incidents of heel pressure ulcers with intraoperative foot elevation, as compared with the reported occurrence of heel pressure ulcers when positioned with sheepskin protectors. To totally relieve the pressure, the heels should be elevated slightly off the bed surface. Suspending the heels can be accomplished by distributing the weight of the leg across a larger surface area based on the patients' size, using positioning devices underneath the lower leg, and leaving the popliteal space free of pressure while supporting the ankle. For example, some devices used include cotton gauze padding on premature infants and neonates and infant blankets, pillows, or commercial positioning devices marketed to lift heels off the bed for infants to young adults.

Shear and friction are forces that can lead to localized skin breakdown and pressure ulcer development. A shear injury occurs when the epidermal layer of the skin is pulled in a direction away from its underlying dermis, causing trauma to the basement membrane. Clinically, shear is exerted when the head of the bed is elevated greater than 30 degrees or when a patient sitting in a chair slides down in the chair. In these positions, the skin and superficial fascia remain fixed against the bed linens or chair while the deep fascia and skeleton slide downward.[54] As a result of shear, blood vessels in the sacral area are likely to become twisted and distorted, and tissue may become ischemic and necrotic.[63] Shear forces may be a factor in the development of undermining and deep tissue injury seen in some sacral pressure ulcers. The head of the bed should not be elevated more than 30 degrees for periods greater than 2 hours unless medically contraindicated. A draw sheet should be used when repositioning to avoid dragging and pulling the epidermis away from underlying tissue.

Friction, which is associated with blister and abrasion development, occurs when the skin slides against linens or the bed surface. Casts and orthopedic devices are other

TABLE 16-3	Staging of Pressure Ulcers
Stage I	Nonblanchable erythema of intact skin; the heralding lesion of skin ulceration. Discoloration of skin, warmth, or hardness also may be indicators. *Note:* Reactive hyperemia can normally be expected to be present for one-half to three-fourths as long as the pressure-occluded blood flow to the area; it should not be confused with a stage I pressure ulcer.
Stage II	Partial-thickness skin loss involving epidermis and/or dermis. The ulcer is superficial and presents clinically as an abrasion, blister, or shallow crater.
Stage III	Full-thickness skin loss involving damage or necrosis of subcutaneous tissue that may extend down to but not through underlying fascia. The ulcer presents clinically as a deep crater with or without undermining of adjacent tissue.
Stage IV	Full-thickness skin loss with extensive destruction, tissue necrosis, or damage to muscle, bone, or supporting structures (e.g., tendon or joint capsule). *Note:* Undermining and sinus tracts may also be associated with stage IV pressure ulcers.

sources of friction.[37] Placing a trapeze on a patient's bed, if developmentally appropriate, to allow the patient to assist with lifting during repositioning decreases friction. Using a lift sheet to facilitate moving a patient and not dragging his or her skin across the linens or bed surface also eliminates friction. Trauma to the epidermal layer over bony prominences can be seen from the friction forces generated by patients with frequent restless movements. Friction injury can be reduced by the use of lubricants (such as cornstarch and creams), protective dressings (such as film dressings), and protective padding (such as genuine sheepskin).[46,64]

The impact of nutritional status, fluid and electrolyte balance, moisture, and tissue oxygenation and perfusion on the development of pressure ulcer development has been previously discussed.

Management. Despite the implementation of preventative skin care practices within the critical care environment, pressure ulcers may be difficult to prevent and heal.

Staging. Assessment of injury is the first step in the treatment of a patient with a pressure ulcer. The pressure ulcer is staged according to the recommendations of the International Association for Enterostomal Therapy (IAET) and the National Pressure Ulcer Advisory Panel (NPUAP) (Table 16-3). This classification serves as a guideline for both assessment and intervention. However, a wound cannot be staged if there is eschar or necrotic tissue present in the wound bed because the depth of tissue damage cannot be determined.

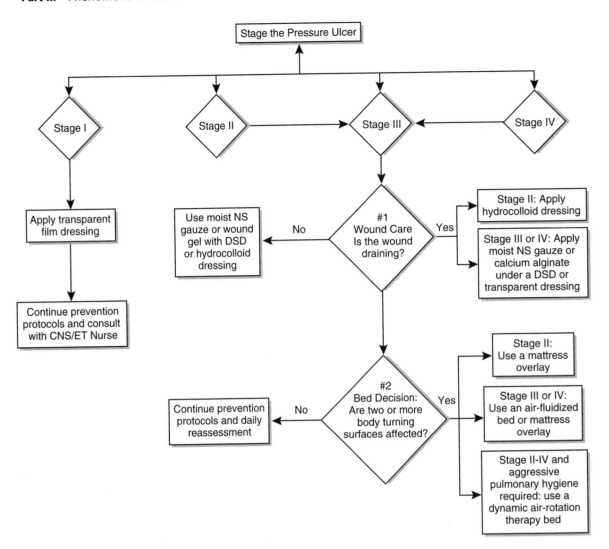

Fig. 16-7 Pressure ulcer algorithm. *CNS,* Clinical nurse specialist; *DSD,* dry sterile dressing; *ET,* enterostomal therapist; *NS,* normal saline. (Reproduced with permission from Quigley S, Curley MAQ: Skin integrity in the pediatric population: preventing and managing pressure ulcers, *J Soc Pediatr Nurs* 1:7-18, 1996.)

Pressure Ulcer Algorithm. Quigley and Curley developed a pressure ulcer algorithm (Fig. 16-7), which is consistent with the AHCPR clinical practice guideline, Treatment of Pressure Ulcers.[54] The purpose of the algorithm was to standardize pressure ulcer interventions and decrease variation in treatment practices. There has been an explosion of wound care products and support surfaces, making product selection difficult and complex. Pressure ulcer dressing selection is based on wound location, the presence or absence of infection, the presence of undermining or tunneling, the condition of the periwound skin integrity, ease or difficulty of dressing application, and cost. No single dressing provides the optimal environment for all pressure ulcers throughout the entire wound healing continuum. If a dressing is nonadherent and needs to be stabilized, whenever possible, Montgomery strap dressings (Johnson & Johnson Medical, Inc., Arlington, Tex.) are used to minimize epidermal stripping to the periwound skin from

frequent adhesive removal. A pectin-based wafer can also be applied on either side of the wound to serve as a tape anchor. A protective barrier is recommended under tape to protect the skin from further injury and irritation. Pressure ulcers change over time and require ongoing reassessment of the efficacy of the dressing in optimizing wound healing.

Dressing Principles. When choosing a dressing, there are seven basic principles that facilitate healing by creating an optimal microenvironment. These principles are to (1) remove necrotic tissue, which can be accomplished by mechanical, chemical, or autolytic methods; (2) eradicate infection—all wounds are contaminated, but not all wounds are infected (indications for culture and sensitivity sampling include signs of local or systemic infection or evidence of bone involvement); (3) absorb excess exudate; (4) obliterate dead space; (5) maintain a moist wound surface, which facilitates cellular migration; (6) insulate the wound; and (7) protect the wound from further trauma and bacteria.

Tables 16-4 and 16-5 provide information on products that meet these principles.

Therapeutic Support Surfaces. A variety of therapeutic support surfaces are available, categorized according to their ability to counteract forces contributing to pressure ulcer development (Tables 16-6 and 16-7). The capillary closing pressure of 12 to 32 mmHg is used as a measure of efficacy of support surfaces to minimize the occlusion of capillary blood flow and pressure ulcer formation. Although significant improvements had been made to bed frames, not until the late 1980s were pressure reduction mattresses introduced to replace foam overlays and reduce the need for costly specialty rental beds. These mattress replacement systems (MRSs) have multiple layers of high-resiliency, antimicrobial solid foam, which more readily conforms and distributes weight as compared with standard vinyl-covered mattresses. The inner foam core quality is defined by density (weight of one cubic foot of foam), with the higher density foams ensuring that the original resiliency will endure after repeated compressions, and indentation force load deflection (IFD), which is a measure of load-bearing capacity. Most of the MRSs have water-repellent, antibacterial, nylon top covers that offer benefits of low shear and low friction. When MRSs are introduced, most institutions can safety eliminate the use of 4-inch convoluted foam overlays.

Advances in medical technology have produced a multitude of products to prevent and treat pressure ulcers, including those that reduce pressure and those that relieve pressure. Currently a universal set of evaluation criteria related to the selection and use of different types of pressure-reducing and pressure-relieving surfaces indicated for a given patient situation is not available.

Pressure-reducing surfaces can lower the external pressure exerted over bony prominences, as compared with standard hospital mattresses. Of importance to note is that they do not consistently reduce pressure to *less than* capillary closing pressure and therefore may not prevent pressure ulcer development.

Pressure-relieving devices differ from pressure-reduction devices in that they consistently maintain pressures less than capillary closing pressures, allowing blood to flow unimpeded through the skin's microcirculation. Specialized therapeutic beds are the largest and most sophisticated group of pressure-relieving devices available. They are also designed to reduce or eliminate damage from shear, friction, and maceration on a short-term basis. Unfortunately, specialty beds are an expensive care option, and most institutions have limited resources available for bed rentals. The use of therapeutic mattress overlays or beds is reserved for those patients at high risk for skin breakdown despite optimal nursing care. Children that often warrant and can benefit most from this level of intervention include those with skin grafts on a turning surface or extensive skin integrity compromise, including burns, purpura fulminans, and pressure ulcers on more than one turning surface.

Several types of specialty beds are currently available. When deciding which bed is most appropriate for children, a clear understanding of their present risk factors, treatment goals, and projected illness trajectory is necessary.

Static low-air-loss beds consist of independently inflated air-filled cushions that provide pressure relief. They can adjust manually to a variety of positions, and they are available in small and crib sizes. Most are covered with nonabsorbent nonstick sheets, and some have special features, such as built-in scales. Disadvantages of these beds include cost and bulky size, the fact that the bed does not actively change the patient's position, and that the bed does not absorb fluids, which may lead to maceration, infection, and delayed wound healing. Children most likely to benefit from this type of bed are those at high risk for developing skin breakdown, those who tolerate some movement, and those who do not have extensive wounds and in whom the primary treatment goal is to prevent pressure breakdown until their underlying condition has improved.

Kinetic therapy beds are a group of beds that can be programmed to rotate a patient's position at set intervals. Rotation beds are a type of kinetic bed in which the entire bed frame moves to rotate the patient. They are often made of flat, firm foam surfaces with foam support cushions and straps. These beds are optimal for treating patients with unstable traumatic injury in whom the treatment goals are to prevent pressure breakdown, mobilize pulmonary secretions, and stimulate gastrointestinal mobility. Disadvantages of these beds include cost, size, waterproof cushions that may promote sweating and fluid contact with skin, and the risk of shearing injury with movement. These beds are used only until patients' initial traumatic injuries have been stabilized and they can be safely moved to a bed with less risk of shearing or maceration.

Another subgroup of kinetic therapy beds is the active *low-air-loss bed.* These beds consist of independently inflated air-filled cushions that either pulsate or rotate the patient from side to side. The advantages that these beds offer include selected pressure relief, a variety of bed positions, cushions that dry quickly, and bed movement that may stimulate capillary blood flow and loosen pulmonary secretions.[65] Disadvantages include cost, size, and bed movement that is relatively limited when compared with manual turning. Children who benefit most from active low-air-loss beds include those who do not tolerate manual turning but require repositioning as an essential aspect in the care of their underlying illness.

Air fluidized or *static high-air-loss beds* have absorptive ceramic beads that are blown by warm air to create a fluidlike motion. The beads are contained within a thin filter sheet. The beads absorb fluid and keep both the sheet and patient continually dry. The filter sheet and chemical makeup of the beads also help to reduce the risk of infection. The fluid movement of these beds is superior to air cushions in placing minimal pressure on tissues. Temperature regulation of the bed's airflow can be manipulated to meet patient care needs. Disadvantages include cost, size, weight, the inability to adjust bed height, limited bed positions, and the bed's drying effect, which may overly dry open wounds and thicken pulmonary secretions. These beds are used when the primary objective is optimal wound healing in infants and children with severe skin disorders, movement disorders,

TABLE 16-4 Properties of Commonly Used Dressing Materials

Dressing Categories	Examples	Indications	Advantages	Disadvantages	Considerations
Dry gauze/fine mesh gauze		Stage III, IV	Absorb wound exudate, protect wound, effective delivery of topical solutions if kept moist.	When left to dry in the wound, it may remove viable tissue; labor intensive.	Helps to physically debride necrotic tissue; excellent for packing and undermining; use rolled gauze for packing large wounds; pack loosely; use wide mesh gauze for debriding; do not use cotton-filled materials on wound surface.
Moisture vapor permeable membranes (MVP films)	Acuderm, Bio-clusive, Blister Film, Clear Skin, Ensure It, Op Site, Tegaderm, Omiderm, Polyskin	Intravenous sites; superficial abrasions; blisters; minor burns; donor sites; stage I, II, or III pressure ulcers	Maintains physiologic environment; provides bacterial barrier; transparent; conforms to wound; waterproof; reduces pain; can be used with gauze to absorb leakage.	Adhesive can damage new wound surface epithelium upon dressing removal; nonabsorbent; some products difficult to apply; can promote wound infection.	Protect friable wound margins; avoid in wounds with infection, copious drainage, or tracts; change only if dressing leaks. Stretch and "lift off" wound bed.
Hydrocolloids	Cutinova Hydro, Comfeel, DuoDerm, Restore, Hydra Pad, Intact, IntraSite, Sween-a-Peel, Tegasorb, Ultec, RepliCare	Stage I, II, or III pressure ulcers; dermal ulcers; donor sites; second degree burns; abrasions	Creates a moist environment by interacting with wound fluid; provides barrier to external bacteria; protects from reinjury; fosters autolytic debridement; waterproof; reduces pain; absorbent; nonadhesive to healing tissue; easy to apply; flexible to mold over difficult areas.	May soften and lose shape with heat and friction; the interaction between wound exudate and barrier material produces a yellow to brown drainage, which can be confused with purulent drainage.	Frequency of changes depends on amount of exudate (change as needed for leakage); avoid in wounds with infection or in sinus tracts; may cause periwound trauma when removed.

Type	Examples	Indications	Function	Comments	Application
Foam dressings Polymeric and composite polymeric dressing	Allevyn, Biobrane, Epi-Lock; Kontour, LYOfoam, Primaderm, Synthaderm; Viasorb; Mitraflex	Stage I, II, or III pressure ulcers; dermal ulcers; donor sites; burns; abrasions; lacerations; partial-thickness wounds; graft sites; highly exudative chronic wounds; dressing for tracheostomy drain sites.	Insulates wound; provides some padding; maintains physiologic environment; reduces pain; permits some autolytic debridement; nonadherent to wound.	Poor barrier; nontransparent; requires taping of edges.	One layer usually absorbs or wicks exudate while another layer maintains moist environment while adhering to skin; change every 24 hours or when leaking occurs.
Wound exudate absorbers, powders, pastes	Bard Absorption Dressing, Comfeel Ulcer Powder, DuoDerm Granules, Comfeel Paste, DuoDerm paste granules, Hollister wound exudate absorber, Pharmaseal, HydraGram, Envisan	Hydrophilic compounds that attract bacteria, exudate debris through osmotic forces in wound. Heavily draining chronic wounds; autolytic debridement.	Absorbs in varying degrees; maintains moist environment; facilitates debridement. Decreases number of dressing changes required.	Can cause pain with application; requires cover dressing; materials leak from dressing edges if not well taped; difficult to remove from tracts and deep pockets.	Partially fill wound to allow for expansion of materials; not for wounds with fistulas/tracts that prevent or hinder removal; monitor electrolytes if copious drainage; may increase wound pH. Avoid in infected wounds; change every 8 hours.
Wound gels	Carrington Gel, Geliperm, IntraSite, Spand-Gel, Dermal wound gel, Biolex	Stage I, II, or III ulcers.	Good "filler" for small, deep wounds; easy to apply; maintains moist environment; helps to soften or slough eschar in necrotic wound.	Requires a cover dressing; variable absorbency.	
Calcium alginates	Kaltostat, Sorbsan, Curasorb, Algosteril, AlgiDerm	Highly exudating wounds.	Nonadherent to wound; absorbent dressing made from seaweed; may be used with infected wounds; nonwoven fiber dressings that convert to a firm gel/fiber mat when mixed with wound exudate.	Requires less frequent dressing changes; highly absorbent; excellent for packing and undermining; requires cover dressing; characteristic odor to dressing when removed.	

Reprinted from Hagelgans NA: Pediatric skin care issues for the home care nurse, *Pediatr Nurs* 19:504, 1993.

TABLE 16-5 Topical Agents Used for Wound Care

Category	Examples	Considerations	Nursing Intervention
Isotonic solutions	Normal saline	Nontoxic to healing tissue; readily available	Used for rinsing, irrigating, and packing; used to cleanse wound before obtaining a culture.
Antiseptic solutions	Acetic acid 0.25%	Cytotoxic to fibroblasts; effective against *Pseudomonas*	Use as 0.25% solution for irrigating or continuous moist packing; discontinue use as soon as granulation tissue is noted.
	Hydrogen peroxide 3%	Cytotoxic to fibroblasts; potential for air emboli when used as an irrigant under pressure	Avoid using as irrigant in deep wounds or wounds with tunneling; limit use to removing dried blood; dilute to ½ strength.
	Povidone-iodine 1%	Cytotoxic especially in detergent form; when used at 0.001% concentration, it has a bactericidal and noncytotoxic effect; absorbed by RBCs, therefore potentially causes metabolic acidosis, renal problems, cardiac instability if used in large wounds over a period of time	Use in concentration of 10% or less if used for packing; change dressing frequently to maintain activity; discontinue when wound is clean and granulating.
	Sodium hypochloride 0.2% (Dakin's solution)	Cytotoxic to fibroblasts at full strength; used at 0.005% concentration, it has a bactericidal with no cytotoxic effect	If used as packing, moisten frequently to maintain activity; discontinue use when wound is clean and granulating; reduce concentration if patient complains of stinging.

Reprinted from Hagelgans NA: Pediatric skin care issues for the home care nurse, *Pediatr Nurs* 19:504, 1993.

TABLE 16-6 Pressure Reduction/Relief Devices

Description	Advantages	Disadvantages	Examples
Overlay: A Device That Is Made to Fit Over a Regular Hospital Mattress			
1. Foam: varying density; 2-4 inch convoluted and nonconvoluted.	Primarily pressure reduction, although in children may have pressure relief advantages; can be cut to fit cribs.	Can soil with incontinent patient; inability to reduce skin moisture resulting from lack of airflow.	Aerofoam, BioGard, DuraPedic, GeoMatt, Ultra Form Pediatric
2. Gel/water filled: pressure reduction; water or gel conforms to patient's contours.	One time charge; low cost for water; gels are expensive.	Gravity displacement can lead to inadequate flotation; potential for leaks; heavy; question safety indications for CPR.	Aqua-Pedics (water and gel), Tender Gel and Water, Theracare (water and gel)
3. Alternating pressure mattress: an overlay with rows of air cells and pump. Pump cycles air to provide inflation and deflation over pressure points.	Constant low-volume air flow; manages excess skin moisture.	Cost of pump rental; ongoing monitor and maintenance of equipment; some complain pumps are noisy.	AeroPulse, AlphaBed, AlphaCare, BetaBed, Bio Flote, Dyna-CARE, Lapidus, PCA Systems, Pillo-Pump, Tenderair
4. Static air: designed with interlocking air cells that provide dry flotation. Inflated with a blower.	May be more effective than foam; easy to clean; has been documented in adult studies to reduce pressure.	Inflation level must be checked frequently by caregiver to maintain therapeutic levels; may cause increased perspiration because of plastic surface.	DermaGard, K-Soft, KoalaKair, Roho, Sof-Care, Tenderair
5. Specialty mattress overlay: fitted air-filled cushions placed over entire bed; pressures can be set and controlled by a pump.	Surface materials are constructed to reduce friction and shear and to eliminate moisture; pressure relief; can be used for prevention and/or treatment of ulcers.	Surface mattress and pump are a rental item; not available for cribs. Side rails on some beds may not adequately contain large patients.	ACUCAIR, BioTherapy, Clini-Care, CRS 4000, RibCor Therapeutic Mattress Pad

Reprinted from Hagelgans NA: Pediatric skin care issues for the home care nurse, *Pediatr Nurs* 19:504, 1993.

TABLE 16-7 Specialty Beds

Description	Advantages	Disadvantages	Examples
*Specialty beds are "high-tech" beds used in place of the standard hospital bed, are usually used on a rental basis, and are intended for short-term use. They provide pressure relief and eliminate shear, friction, and maceration and in some cases provide lateral rotation and chest physiotherapy.			
1. Low-air-loss beds: surface consists of inflated air cushions; each zone is adjusted for optimal pressure relief for patient's body size; some models have built-in scales.	Provides pressure relief in any position; treatment for Stages II-IV pressure ulcers; available in pediatric crib sizes. Ideal for treatment of heel and occipital pressure sores.	Difficult for the patient to move around in bed.	FlexiCair, Air Plus, KinAir, Mediscus; Cribs: Pedcare, PediKair, PNEU-CARE/ Pedi
2. Air-fluidized beds: air is blown through silicone beads to "float" patient.	Treatment for deep-pressure sores, burns, posterior flaps; draws fluid away from patient.	Airflow may dry out wound if latex sheet is not used. Bed weighs 1500 lb; difficult to transfer patient.	CLINITRON, FluidAir Plus, Skytron
3. Continuous lateral rotation beds; cushion beds: microprocessor-controlled low-air-loss bed inflates and deflates cushions to achieve lateral rotation. Some models include percussion, vibration, pulsation. Some raise patient high enough for ECMO support. *Table based:* Without low-air-loss cushions, achieves lateral rotation by turning complete bed frame.	Indicated for patients with a high degree of immobility, severe respiratory distress, and who are hemodynamically unstable when moved. Must have stable spine. *Table based:* same as above and suitable for some patients without a stable spine.	Cost	*Cushion based:* Efica (RESCUE), BioDyne, *Table based:* RotoRest, Keane Mobility

Data from Doughty D: The process of wound healing: a nursing prospective, *Progressions* 2:3-12, 1990; Glavis C, Barbour S: Pressure ulcer prevention in critical care: state of the art, *AACN* 1:602-613, 1990; Krasner D: Patient support surfaces, *Ostomy Wound Manage* 38:57-60, 1991.
Reprinted from Hagelgans NA: Pediatric skin care issues for the home care nurse, *Pediatr Nurs* 19:504, 1993.
*This list is a representative sampling of products, which is not intended to be all inclusive. No endorsement of any product is intended. Within each category, products must be individually evaluated on their efficacy as comfort, pressure-reducing, or pressure-relieving devices. All products within a category do not necessarily perform equally.
ECMO, Extracorporeal membrane oxygenation.

extensive skin breakdown, heavily draining or large open wounds, or large grafted areas.

Alternating *low-air-loss overlay mattresses* are applied over the existing hospital mattress. They are dynamic, using electricity to alternately inflate and deflate and thus decreasing tissue interface pressures lower than capillary closing pressure. Many overlays are pressure-reducing not pressure-relieving products. The advantages of these overlays are a low daily rental fee (compared with entire specialty bed units), placement while patient is on bed, no storage of existing hospital bed, quick deflation for emergencies, and easy movement and cleaning of bed. Disadvantages are that assembly is required, motor may be noisy, sensation of inflation and deflation may bother the patient, and electricity is required.

A variety of therapeutic support surfaces are available to provide an environment to prevent or assist in the management of a pressure ulcer. Therapeutic support surfaces are only one component of a comprehensive management plan.

Irritant Contact Diaper Dermatitis

Irritant contact diaper dermatitis is an inflammation of the skin resulting from contact with urine and stool. The resultant diaper dermatitis is often characterized by any of the following: erythema, maceration, erosions, or a candidal (monilial) rash throughout the perianal, perineal, and genital area. The epidermal layer may or may not be intact. The more severe forms include ulcerations scattered throughout the perineal area, sometimes including the genital area and groin. At this phase, nerve endings are exposed, and pain is experienced. The clinical features of a candidal rash are erythema with "satellite" papules and pustules often associated with pruritus.

Diaper Dermatitis Algorithm. A diaper dermatitis algorithm (Fig. 16-8) was developed to standardize the care of patients with perianal, perineal, or buttock skin impairment. The guidelines use pH-balanced skin cleansers, oatmeal or astringent soaks to promote healing, moisture barrier creams or ointments to protect the skin, and antifungal

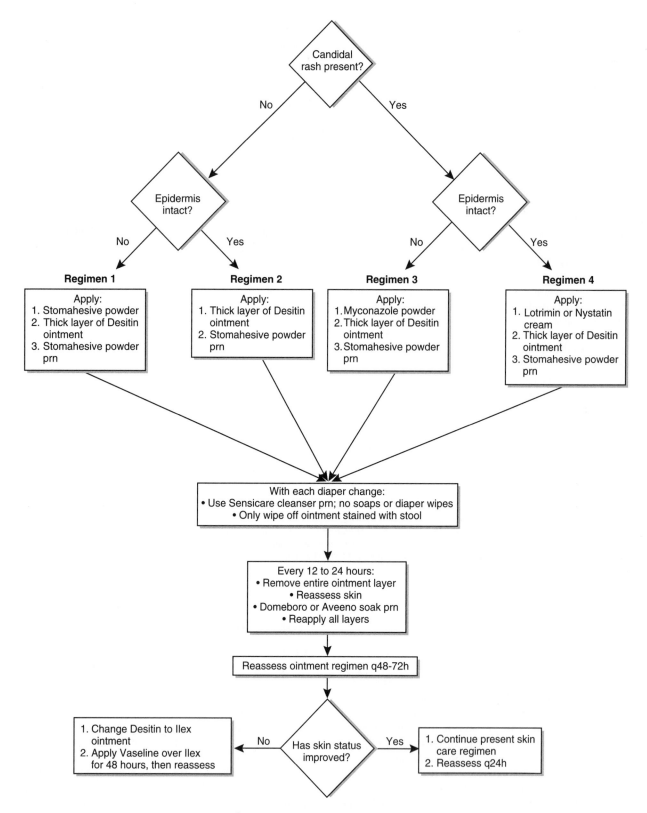

Fig. 16-8 Diaper dermatitis algorithm.

topical products to treat candidal yeast infections that may be associated with irritant contact diaper dermatitis.

Frequent diaper changes and proper cleansing of the skin, with the application of topically applied barrier powders, creams, or ointments, promote healing of compromised skin. The practice of leaving the diaper area open to air or blowing oxygen onto the skin is not supported in research. However, researchers do know that the systemic circulation of oxygen is critical to wound healing. Furthermore, wounds heal more readily in a moist environment rather than a dry one. Leaving the diaper area open to air only facilitates the recognition of when a patient defecates.

The use of pectin-based wafers, such as Stomahesive or Duoderm (Convatec, Chicago, Ill.) over the buttocks is not advised. Stool tends to accumulate around the edges of the wafer, and the "meltdown" it produces within the moist environment of a diaper can cause further trauma to the skin on removal. Often the area with the most skin integrity compromise is in the gluteal crease, and the barrier wafers do not conform and adhere well. The use of heat lamps is also strongly discouraged because they can burn the perineal area.

The diaper dermatitis algorithm guides interventions based on accurate assessment of skin integrity status. It is not necessary to remove the entire protective barrier with each diaper change. Each time the skin is cleansed, by taking the barrier layer completely off, there is an increased likelihood that new epithelial growth can be disrupted. Therefore removing only that portion of the protective barrier that is soiled is advised, along with reapplication of the barrier layer. Every 12 to 24 hours it is recommended to soak or bathe off the entire protective barrier layer to reassess and document efficacy of treatment and skin condition.

Therapeutic soaks or baths, such as oatmeal colloidal soaks (Aveeno, S.C. Johnson & Son, Racine, Wis.), for 5 to 10 minutes every 12 to 24 hours may be indicated for relief of irritated, pruritic skin, which is often associated with candidal yeast rashes. Astringent agents, such as Domeboro (Bayer Corp., Elkhart, Ind.), may be indicated for relief of inflammatory skin conditions requiring "drying out" of denuded, weepy skin.

Regimen 1. If the epidermal layer is not intact and no candidal rash is present, then, as first layer, apply Stomahesive powder to absorb moisture and provide a dry base, which will enhance the adherence of a moisture barrier ointment or cream. Next, apply a thick layer of moisture barrier, cover with powder for first 48 to 72 hours, and then reevaluate and document skin integrity status. If no improvement occurs, refer to regimen 1 for the sequence of moisture barrier layers to apply.

Regimen 2. If the epidermal layer appears intact with the presence of erythema and no coexisting candidal rash, the regimen is as follows: Apply, as first layer, a thick layer of zinc oxide–based ointment or cream (i.e., Desitin, Pfizer, Inc., New York, N.Y.) as a moisture barrier layer to protect skin from contact with urine and stool. Cover the barrier with Stomahesive powder (Convatec, Princeton, N.J.) to decrease the adherence of the ointment into the absorbent gel layer in disposable diapers for the first 48 to 72 hours, then reevaluate and document skin integrity status. If no improvement is seen, change the barrier layer to Ilex paste (Medcom Industries, Grafton, Mass.) covered with petroleum jelly for the next 48 to 72 hours, then reevaluate and document skin integrity status. If no improvement is noted or skin integrity worsens, change the barrier layer to Criticaid paste (Coloplast/Sween Corp., N. Mankato, Minn.) covered with Stomahesive powder for 48 to 72 hours and then reevaluate and document.

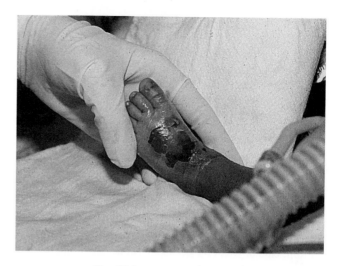

Fig. 16-9 Extravasation injury.

Regimen 3. If epidermis is not intact and a coexisting candidal rash is present, then, as first layer, apply an antifungal powder to open, denuded areas and antifungal ointment or cream to surrounding intact skin and refer to regimen 1 for the sequence of moisture barrier layers to apply.

Regimen 4. If the epidermis is intact and a coexisting candidal rash is present, then, as first layer, apply an antifungal cream or ointment and refer to regimen 1 for the sequence of moisture barrier layers to apply.

Evaluation. Daily evaluation and documentation of the skin integrity are critical to assess the outcome of interventions. Consistency is the key to a successful skin care regimen. Changing the regimen with every nursing shift only diminishes the ability to know effectiveness of any one particular intervention. Moderate to severe perineal skin breakdown often does not show signs of healing for several days, particularly if stool frequency persists. Therefore changes to a skin care program are not initiated until after 48 to 72 hours after implementation.

Intravenous Infiltrate Injury

Virtually all critically ill pediatric patients have an intravascular access device in place for blood sampling, pressure monitoring, or delivery of a wide variety of fluids and medication. Intravenous therapy is an essential aspect of care that carries significant risks, including extravasation injury. Extravasation or infiltration is the leakage of intravenous fluid or medication into interstitial tissues. It is a potentially serious complication that can cause morbidity through direct skin and tissue damage (Fig. 16-9).

Infiltration occurs through cannula dislodgment, punctures in the venous wall, seepage around insertion sites, or increased permeability of the infiltrate through damaged endothelium. The extent of tissue damage sustained from extravasation depends on the physical and chemical nature of the infiltrate, the volume infiltrated, and the patient's clinical condition at the time of the injury.[66,67] Effects can range from mild erythema, edema, and discomfort, which resolve spontaneously to extensive necrosis and loss of epidermal, dermal, and subcutaneous tissue that require extensive wound care over an extended period. Severe extravasation injuries can impact limb function, sensation, and cosmetic appearance.

Infiltrates that have the potential to cause the most significant injury if extravasation occurs include those that are hyperosmolar, vasoconstrictive, alkaline, poorly water soluble, or directly cytotoxic.[68] Hyperosmolar fluids have a higher osmolality than serum and are irritating to venous endothelium, resulting in inflammation and capillary leak. Once in the interstitial space, hyperosmolar agents cause edema, vasoconstriction, ischemia, and necrosis. Hyperosmolar solutions include dextrose concentrations greater than 10% and those containing high amino acid or electrolyte additives. Undiluted electrolytes including potassium, calcium, and bicarbonate also have extremely high osmolalities.

Vasoconstrictive drugs cause tissue damage when infiltrated by reducing blood flow to the affected area, causing localized tissue ischemia. Vasopressor medications such as dopamine, dobutamine, epinephrine, and norepinephrine all have the potential to cause vasoconstrictive tissue damage. Alkaline agents, including sodium bicarbonate and sodium thiopental, cause direct cellular injury once infiltrated. Drugs with low water solubility, such as lorazepam, diazepam, phenytoin, digoxin, and nitroglycerin, can form cytotoxic precipitates if infiltrated undiluted.[68] Most antineoplastic agents are directly cytotoxic. Vesicants, such as doxorubicin, daunorubicin, dactinomycin, nitrogen mustard, vincristine, and vinblastine, carry the highest risk for extensive tissue damage if infiltrated.[67]

Prevention.   Prevention of extravasation injury begins with careful selection of catheter type, size, and location. Ideally, collaborative decision making that accurately reflects a child's current condition and anticipated trajectory guides vascular access placement. Often this goal is unrealistic, given emergent patient conditions, difficult or limited access sites, and evolving care issues. Central venous access should be secured as soon as possible if high-risk intravenous agents are required. Peripheral catheters made of soft plastic are better choices than rigid steel needles, which have been shown to increase the risk of infiltration.[69] When possible, a peripheral cannulation site should be chosen that minimizes the risk of dislodgment from movement. Joint spaces should be avoided because even when arm board restraint is used to limit flexion, catheter displacement from rotation can result. Manufacturers' guidelines on the proper dilution and infusion rates of medications should be followed, whether given centrally or peripherally. When an infusion pump is used to deliver solutions peripherally, a volumetric cassette pump with a maximum delivery pressure of less than 20 pounds per square inch is safest.[68] Syringe pumps often have higher flow pressures and should be used with caution.

Management.   Vigilant assessment of the intravenous site once an infusion is in place is essential to detect early signs of infiltration, prevent large volume infiltrates, and minimize tissue injury. Signs to watch for include swelling, blanching, coolness, firmness, leakage around the insertion

site, decreased flow rate, or increased resistance with flushing. It is not appropriate to rely on patient-reported discomfort to detect intravenous extravasation. Children have relatively loose subcutaneous tissue that can hold a significant amount of infiltrated fluid before becoming painful, and many critically ill children are too young, too sick, or too sedated to reliably alert anyone that an infiltrate is occurring. Frequent observation is aided by not obscuring the intravenous site with excessive tape, gauze wrap, "welcome" sleeves, or protective covers. The use of a transparent adhesive dressing facilitates visualization.

The goal of treatment after the identification of an extravasation is to limit the extent of skin and tissue damage incurred. For all infiltrates, the first intervention is to stop the infusion and attempt to aspirate fluid through the cannula. The catheter is left in place until a collaborative decision is made on the administration of an antidote. Further treatment is based on staging the infiltrate (Table 16-8). When staging an infiltrate, it is important to realize that the extent of injury may not be apparent during the initial assessment. Some infiltrates, including dopamine, norepinephrine, calcium, potassium, sodium bicarbonate, vancomycin, amphotericin B, dextrose concentrations of 20% or more, and most chemotherapeutic agents, can cause progressive damage to tissues over hours to days.[67]

Treatment of stage I and II infiltrates usually includes site elevation to decrease edema and the application of warm or cold compresses. Warm compresses are applied to extrava-

TABLE 16-8 Staging of Intravenous (IV) Infiltrates

Stage	Characteristics
I	Painful IV site
	No erythema
	No swelling
II	Painful IV site
	Slight swelling (0%-20%)
	No blanching
	Good pulse below infiltration site
	Brisk capillary refill below infiltration site
III	Painful IV site
	Marked swelling (30%-50%)
	Blanching
	Skin cool to the touch
	Good pulse below infiltration site
	Brisk capillary refill below infiltration site
IV	Painful IV site
	Extensive swelling (>50%)
	Blanching
	Skin cool to the touch
	Decreased or absent pulse*
	Capillary refill >4 seconds*
	Skin breakdown or necrosis*

From Flemmer L, Chan JJ: A pediatric protocol for management of extravasation injuries, *Pediatr Nurs* 19:424, 1993.
*The presence of any one of these characteristics constitutes a stage IV infiltrate (see Millam DA: Managing complications of IV therapy, *Nurs 88* 18:34-42, 1988).

sations of noncaustic solutions regardless of osmolarity.[70] Warmth improves circulation to the affected area and increases the rate of fluid absorption. Cold compresses help to reduce ulceration when applied to infiltrate sites of caustic or highly irritating agents.[70] In addition to these measures, stage III or IV infiltrates require immediate and aggressive interdisciplinary intervention because they carry a high risk for extensive deep tissue damage.[66] Despite aggressive treatment, some extravasation injuries result in tissue damage that requires surgical intervention and extensive wound care. A plastic surgery consult done soon after discovery is helpful in addressing physical, functional, and cosmetic issues.

Antidotes. Several substances have been found to be useful in limiting the extent of tissue injury associated with extravasations.[71-73] These antidotes are administered through the infiltrated catheter, multiple subcutaneous injections, or topical application (Table 16-9). Hyaluroni-

◆ TABLE 16-9   Antidotes

Medication	Antidote	Dose
Acyclovir	Hyaluronidase 15 U/mL	0.2 ml × 5 doses SQ
Aminophylline	Hyaluronidase 15 U/mL	0.2 ml × 5 doses SQ
Amphotericin	Hyaluronidase 15 U/mL	0.2 ml × 5 doses SQ
Amsacrine (AMSA)	Cold compresses	qid × 72 hr
Calcium salts	Hyaluronidase 15 U/ml	0.2 ml × 5 doses SQ
Carmustine	Sodium bicarbonate 2.1% dilution	Infiltrate area with 1-3 ml, leave for 2 min and aspirate off again
Chloramphenicol	Hyaluronidase 15 U/ml	0.2 ml × 5 doses SQ
Cisplatin	Cold compresses	
	Sodium thiosulfate—1/6 M solution (4 ml of 10% sodium thiosulfate 100 mg/ml mixed with 6 ml of sterile water)	Infiltrate 2 ml of this 1/6 M solution for each 100 mg of cisplatin
Dacarbazine (DTIC)	Cold compresses	qid × 72 hr
	Sodium thiosulfate 1/6 M solution (dilute as with cisplatin)	Multiple SQ injections for a total of 4-5 ml
Dactinomycin (actinomycin D)	Cold compresses	
	Sodium thiosulfate 1/6 M solution (dilute as with cisplatin)	Multiple SQ injections for a total of 4-5 ml
	Ascorbic acid	50 mg SQ
	Hydrocortisone	50-100 mg SQ
Daunorubicin	Initial (first 24 hours): Dimethyl sulfoxide (DMSO) Hydrocortisone cream Cold compresses	Apply DMSO topically q2 hr, followed by hydrocortisone cream and 30 min of cold compresses
	Subsequent 14 days: Dimethyl sulfoxide (DMSO) Hydrocortisone cream *or*	Apply DMSO topically q6 hr alternating with hydrocortisone cream q6h
	Sodium bicarbonate 2.1% dilution	Infiltrate area with 1-3 ml, leave for 2 min and aspirate off again
Dextrose 10%	Cold compresses	q8h until perfusion restored
	Hyaluronidase 15 U/ml *or* nitroglycerin ointment 2%	0.2 ml × 5 doses SQ 4 mm/kg
Diazepam	Hyaluronidase 15 U/ml	0.2 ml × 5 doses SQ
Dobutamine	Phentolamine Neonates: dilute 2.5-5 mg in 10 ml normal saline All others: dilute 5-10 mg in 10 ml normal saline	Neonates: multiple SQ injections not to exceed 0.1 mg/kg or 2.5 mg All others: multiple 0.5 mg SQ injections not to exceed 10 mg
	Nitroglycerine ointment 2%	4 mm/kg q8h
Dopamine	Phentolamine Neonates: dilute 2.5-5 mg in 10 ml normal saline All others: dilute 5-10 mg in 10 ml normal saline	Neonates: multiple SQ injections not to exceed 0.1 mg/kg or 2.5 mg All others: multiple 0.5 mg SQ injections not to exceed 10 mg
	Nitroglycerine ointment 2%	4 mm/kg q8h

Courtesy Kathleen Gura, BS, RPh, Clinical Pharmacist; Patricia A. Berry, RN; Staff Nurse III, MICU, Children's Hospital, Boston.   *Continued*

TABLE 16-9 **Antidotes—cont'd**

Medication	Antidote	Dose
Doxorubicin (Adriamycin)	Initial (first 24 hours): Dimethyl sulfoxide (DMSO) Hydrocortisone cream Cold compresses	Apply DMSO topically q2h, followed by hydrocortisone cream and 30 min of cold compresses
	Subsequent 14 days: Dimethyl sulfoxide (DMSO) Hydrocortisone cream	Apply DMSO topically q6h alternating with hydrocortisone cream q6h
Epinephrine	Phentolamine Neonates: dilute 2.5-5 mg in 10 ml normal saline All others: dilute 5-10 mg in 10 ml normal saline	Neonates: multiple SQ injections not to exceed 0.1 mg/kg or 2.5 mg All others: multiple 0.5 mg SQ injections not to exceed 0.1-0.2 mg/kg or 5 mg
	Nitroglycerine ointment 2%	4 mm per kg q8h
Erythromycin	Hyaluronidase 15 U/ml	0.2 ml × 5 doses SQ
Etoposide (VP-16)	Warm compresses Hyaluronidase 150 U/ml	1-6 ml SQ via multiple injections; repeat over several hours
Gentamicin	Hyaluronidase 15 U/ml	0.2 ml × 5 doses SQ
Mannitol	Hyaluronidase 15 U/ml	0.2 ml × 5 doses SQ
Mechlorethamine (nitrogen mustard)	Cold compresses Sodium thiosulfate 1/6 M solution (dilute as with cisplatin)	Inject 2 ml of solution for each mg of mechlorethamine
Methicillin	Hyaluronidase 15 U/ml	0.2 ml × 5 doses SQ
Mitomycin	Sodium thiosulfate 1/6 M solution (dilute as with cisplatin)	Multiple SQ injections for a total of 4-5 ml
Nafcillin	Hyaluronidase 15 U/ml	0.2 ml × 5 doses SQ
Norepinephrine	Phentolamine Neonates: dilute 2.5-5 mg in 10 ml normal saline All others: dilute 5-10 mg in 10 ml normal saline	Neonates : multiple SQ injections not to exceed 0.1 mg/kg or 2.5 mg All others: multiple 0.5 mg SQ injections not to exceed 0.1-0.2 mg/kg or 5 mg
	Nitroglycerine ointment 2%	4 mm/kg q8h
Oxacillin	Hyaluronidase 15 U/ml	0.2 ml × 5 doses SQ
Parenteral nutrition	Hyaluronidase 15 U/ml	0.2 ml × 5 doses SQ
	Nitroglycerin ointment 2%	4 mm/kg q8h
Penicillin G	Hyaluronidase 15 U/ml	0.2 ml × 5 doses SQ
Phenytoin	Hyaluronidase 15 U/ml	0.2 mL × 5 doses SQ
Piperacillin	Hyaluronidase 15 U/ml	0.2 mL × 5 doses SQ
Potassium salts	Cold compresses Hyaluronidase 15 U/ml	0.2 ml × 5 doses SQ
Radiocontrast dye	Hyaluronidase 15 U/ml	0.2 ml × 5 doses SQ
Rifampin	Hyaluronidase 15 U/ml	0.2 ml × 5 doses SQ
Sodium bicarbonate	Hyaluronidase 15 U/ml	0.2 ml × 5 doses SQ
Teniposide (VM-26)	Warm compresses Hyaluronidase 150 U/ml	qid × 72 hr 1-6 ml SQ via multiple injections; repeat over several hours
Tobramycin	Hyaluronidase 15 U/ml	0.2 ml × 5 doses SQ
Tromethamine	Hyaluronidase 15 U/ml	0.2 ml × 5 doses SQ
Vancomycin	Hyaluronidase 15 U/ml	0.2 ml × 5 doses SQ
Vinblastine	Warm compresses Hyaluronidase 150 U/ml	qid × 72 hr 1-6 ml SQ via multiple injections; repeat over several hours
Vincristine	Warm compresses Hyaluronidase 150 U/ml	qid × 72 hr 1-6 mL SQ via multiple injections; repeat over several hours

Courtesy Kathleen Gura, BS, RPh, Clinical Pharmacist; Patricia A. Berry, RN; Staff Nurse III, MICU, Children's Hospital, Boston.

dase is useful in treating most irritating but nonvasopressor infiltrates. Hyaluronidase works by temporarily dissolving normal interstitial barriers, allowing the infiltrated solution to diffuse over a greater area, become dilute, and absorb faster. The usual dosage is a concentration of 15 U/ml administered by five subcutaneous injections of 0.2 ml each into the affected area.[74] Hyaluronidase is most effective if administered within 2 hours of the infiltrate, but benefits can be seen up to 12 hours after extravasation.[75] Hyaluronidase has few known side effects but may rarely cause urticaria.

Phentolamine is an α-adrenergic blocker that directly reverses the vasoconstrictive effects of infiltrated vasopressor agents. The dosage range is 5 to 10 mg diluted in 10 ml of normal saline administered by multiple subcutaneous injections of 0.5 mg each into the affected area. Phentolamine is most effective if given within 12 hours of the extravasation. Careful assessment must be made before treating a child with phentolamine because it has the potential to cause significant hypotension caused by vascular smooth muscle relaxation. Phentolamine can also cause tachycardia and dysrhythmias.

Glyceryl trinitrate in the form of transdermal nitroglycerin patches or ointment may be a safer and less invasive treatment option than injections of hyaluronidase or phentolamine in the treatment of extravasations that result in ischemia. The beneficial effects of topical nitroglycerin have been demonstrated in the treatment of children with vasopressor extravasations,[76,77] parenteral nutrition extravasations,[78] and purpura fulminans.[79] Nitroglycerin is a nonspecific vascular smooth muscle relaxant that can improve collateral circulation to localized areas of peripheral ischemia. The recommended dosage is 4 mm of 2% nitroglycerin ointment per kilogram of body weight applied topically over the affected area every 8 hours until perfusion is restored.[77] Local vasodilation effects occur within 15 to 30 minutes of application. To minimize the potential for systemic hypotension, caution is taken in using topical nitroglycerin on infants younger than 21 days old and in children with existing skin breakdown because absorption may be increased.

Hydrocortisone and dexamethasone may mitigate inflammation associated with infiltrate injury. Case reports suggest that sodium thiosulfate, sodium bicarbonate, ascorbic acid, and sodium edetate may also be beneficial in treating some extravasation injuries.[68] It is thought that these drugs help to inactivate some infiltrated drugs or decrease their binding to cellular deoxyribonucleic acid (DNA).

Follow-up care for all intravenous infiltrate injuries includes the ongoing assessment and documentation of circulation, sensation, motor function, and wound appearance until healing is complete.

WOUND CARE

General Principles

Critical care nurses make assessments and plan interventions related to skin integrity and wound management on a daily basis. These interventions can either enhance or delay the wound healing process. Effective wound management involves proper identification of the cause of the wound, wound assessment, proper dressing selection, and systematic documentation. The wound location should be clearly documented in relation to anatomic landmarks such as the right scapula, left trochanter, or the right upper quadrant of the abdomen. The wound size should be measured with the length, width, and depth calculated in centimeters (not compared with an object such as a dime). If it is a full-thickness wound, determine if tunnels or undermining are present by gently "probing" with a sterile cotton-tipped applicator. Document presence of tunnels in relation to the hands of a clock (i.e., 3-cm tunnel at 6 o'clock) for objective reassessment to determine wound progression. The presence or absence of wound drainage should be assessed. Describe the amount, color, and odor of exudate if present. The character of the wound tissue should be assessed, including the presence of granulation tissue, slough (nonviable tissue), or eschar. The presence of infection, which will damage tissue or impair healing, should be assessed. The condition of periwound skin integrity should be noted. Protecting the healthy skin around the wound is essential. This can be achieved by using skin sealants (3M No-Sting Protective Wipes, 3M Healthcare, St. Paul, Minn.) or moisture barrier creams (Aquaphor, Beiersdorf, Wilton, Conn.).

Successful wound healing depends on proper cleansing, treatment of infection, wound debridement if clinically indicated, a moist wound base, and proper selection of a dressing. In 1962, George Winter[80] revolutionized the approach to wound care. His research demonstrated that wound healing is optimized in a moist wound environment. With a moist wound environment, collagen synthesis and granulation tissue formation are improved; cell migration and epithelial resurfacing occur faster; and scabs, crusts, and eschars do not form.[81] If serous exudate dries in a wound bed, epithelialization is delayed because epithelial cells are forced to migrate below the eschar instead of migrating across a moist wound bed. Routine general cleansing to remove exudate and debris from the wound is indicated to assess the wound bed and determine the appropriate dressing. The general consensus among wound care experts is that normal saline is the best wound cleanser and irrigant, and it is cost effective as well. Following wound cleansing, the wound margins should be carefully patted dry.

Dressings should be considered in categories, and their actions, indications, and contraindications should be known so that the healthcare team can appropriately match the right dressing to the right wound (see Table 16-4). The principal function of a wound dressing is to provide an optimal healing milieu. Wound healing is a dynamic process, with changes occurring in the wound environment at different stages of the healing process. Appropriate dressing selection requires knowledge of dressing design classifications and their ability to perform in specific scenarios. Before a new dressing is applied, the old dressing should be carefully removed and analyzed. Has the previous dressing adequately absorbed the exudate, has it protected the wound bed, has it adhered to new granulation tissue, and has it provided a moist wound

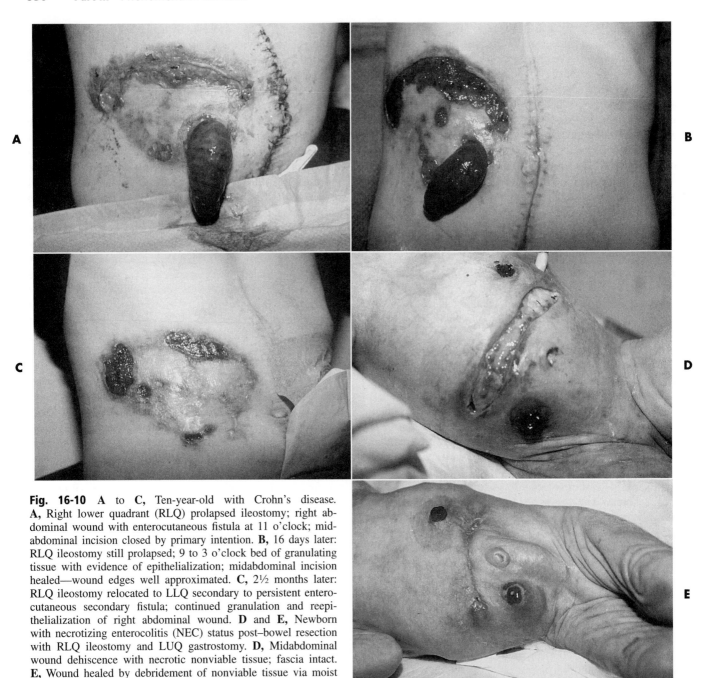

Fig. 16-10 A to **C,** Ten-year-old with Crohn's disease. **A,** Right lower quadrant (RLQ) prolapsed ileostomy; right abdominal wound with enterocutaneous fistula at 11 o'clock; midabdominal incision closed by primary intention. **B,** 16 days later: RLQ ileostomy still prolapsed; 9 to 3 o'clock bed of granulating tissue with evidence of epithelialization; midabdominal incision healed—wound edges well approximated. **C,** 2½ months later: RLQ ileostomy relocated to LLQ secondary to persistent enterocutaneous secondary fistula; continued granulation and reepithelialization of right abdominal wound. **D** and **E,** Newborn with necrotizing enterocolitis (NEC) status post–bowel resection with RLQ ileostomy and LUQ gastrostomy. **D,** Midabdominal wound dehiscence with necrotic nonviable tissue; fascia intact. **E,** Wound healed by debridement of nonviable tissue via moist wound healing over 14 days, then surgically closed by tertiary intention.

environment? Correct selection of a dressing is essential for optimal wound healing.

All dressings are classified as either primary or secondary types. A primary dressing is placed in direct contact with the wound bed and may provide absorptive capacity and adhesion of the secondary dressing to the wound. A secondary dressing is applied over a primary dressing to provide further protection, absorption, compression, and occlusion. Dressing changes should be made as frequently as demanded by the accumulation of fluid and debris, overload of absorbent material, and degree of infection.

Surgical Wounds

Wound closure occurs by primary, secondary, and delayed primary or tertiary intention.[10,17] Fig. 16-10 demonstrates characteristics of this classification system. Primary intention refers to a wound that is surgically closed with the edges approximated by sutures, staples, or tape. There is minimal tissue loss and potential for infection. A wound healing by secondary intention is left open and allowed to heal by formation of new blood vessels and the production of connective (scar) tissue. Examples of secondary-intention healing are pressure ulcers and open abdominal wounds.

Skin sealant: liquid copolymer that provides protective layer to skin surface by protecting skin from shearing force of removing tapes and adhesives	Used under adhesive tape and adhesive portion of ostomy face plate; is not necessary under solid wafer barrier; alcohol-based produces should not be used on premature infant or fragile skin	Most contain alcohol and will "sting" irritated skin; compound tincture of benzoin contains allergens that can cause irritation; the bond formed between benzoin and tape is stronger than underlying epidermal-dermal bond; therefore when tape is removed from skin of premature infant where benzoin is used, it can cause epidermal stripping; available in wipes and liquid form	*Alcohol-based products:* ConvaTec: AllKare Smith & Nephew: Skin-Prep Mentor: Skin Shield Bard: Protective Film Barrier Non Alcohol Based products: Smith & Nephew: No-Sting; Stoma Laboratories: Stoma Care *Benzoin preparations*
Ostomy pouch: used to collect effluent	One piece: precut and cut to fit; urinary and fecal drainage	Usually has flexible barrier, which is excellent for pouching stomas in a crease or fold; most are odorproof	ConvaTec: Little Ones* Active Life Dansac* Hollister: Pouchkins Incutech: Premie Pouch Bard: Fistula Pouch (Fecal Only)
	Two piece: precut and cut to fit; urinary and fecal drainage; snap-on pouch to flange wafer	Good for flat pouching surface; pouch can be removed or replaced while face plate remains intact; wafer flange and pouch flange must match; snap-on system may be painful in immediate postoperative period; however, pouch and wafer can be applied as one unit; odorproof	ConvaTec: Little Ones* SurFit Hollister: Pouchkins Coloplast United

Adapted from Hagelgans NA, Janusz BH: Pediatric skin care: issues for the home care nurse, part 2, *Pediatr Nurs* 20:72-73, 1994.
*Made specifically for infants and young children.

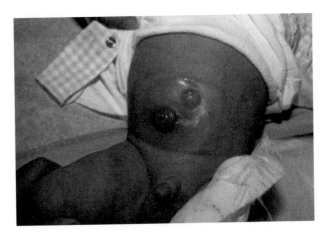

Fig. 16-11 Candidal yeast rash surrounding colostomy.

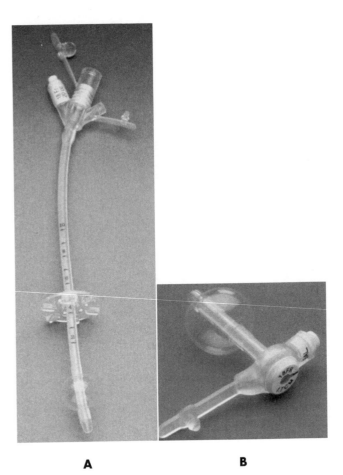

A   **B**

Fig. 16-12 A, MIC® tube. B, MIC-KEY® tubes. (Courtesy Kimberly-Clark/Ballard Medical Products, Draper, Utah.)

No-Sting barrier (3M Healthcare, St. Paul, Minn.), before applying the new ostomy appliance. Changing the pouch every 24 to 48 hours may be indicated to reapply the antifungal powder and reevaluate the skin integrity based on the severity of the infection.

Preterm Infant Considerations. Special considerations are necessary when caring for an infant with a stoma, particularly if the patient is a preterm infant weighing less than 2 kg. Maintaining pouch adherence may be quite challenging because there are few pouch options and often a limited pouching surface.

Preterm infant skin is more permeable, and therefore ingredients contained in products must be fastidiously examined before application. Diminished cohesion exists between the epidermal and dermal layer, and the epidermis can easily be traumatized. Minimize use of all tapes, adhesives, sealants, and solvents on the skin. Use pectin-backed wafers and nonalcohol-based sealants to protect peristomal skin. Gently peel ostomy wafers and adhesive tape slowly, supporting the abdominal skin surface with the fingertips to decrease the tension and pulling the epidermis from the dermal layer. Monitor pouch adherence closely and remove the appliance if effluent leaking under the barrier adhered to the skin to avoid irritant contact dermatitis. Cleansing agents that have a neutral pH or warm, sterile water alone are the safest choices. Rubbing skin surfaces should be avoided to prevent chafing and irritation.

Enteral Feeding Tubes

Enteral feedings are indicated for children with a functional gastrointestinal tract who are unable to consume adequate nutrients to meet their nutritional requirements. Data suggest that there are advantages to using enteral over parenteral nutrition to meet the nutritional requirements of the critically ill patient (see Chapter 12). If it is clinically determined that enteral feedings are anticipated to be necessary for a prolonged period, then a gastrostomy or jejunostomy is created. A gastrostomy may be created by surgical, endoscopic, or radiologic approaches. Enteral feedings into the jejunum may be accessed via radiographic guidance through

an existing gastrostomy site or surgically. The care and management of various feeding tubes and interventions for commonly encountered problems are discussed here.

Some of the most common ICU problems of enteral feeding tubes are inadvertent dislodgment, migration, tract enlargement, peristomal skin compromise caused by leakage, and clogging of the tube lumen.

Preventing Dislodgment. Tube stabilization is critical, particularly the first 6 weeks postoperatively, as the tract heals. Before stabilization, tube placement should be determined if the tube is not sutured in place. If it is a balloon-inflated device, such as a Foley or Mic Tube (Medical Innovations Corporation, division of Ballard Medical Products, Draper, Utah) (Fig. 16-12), securely hold tube at abdominal surface, withdraw fluid from balloon, and then gently reinflate. Check placement by gently pulling up on tube until resistance is felt. If there is no skin compromise, then apply split gauze around tube entry site. If it is a Foley catheter, use the slit-tape method to secure tube. Slit the tape in half, halfway down the length of the tape, and position the tape to the halfway slit up to the base of the tube on the abdominal surface. Apply the tape to the skin, wrapping half of the slit end up and around the shaft of the tube. There are several commercially available anchoring devices, including the Hollister Drain Tube Attachment Device

(Hollister, Libertyville, Ill.) and Flexi-Trak Anchoring Device (ConvaTec, Princeton, N.J.). To further secure the tube, a tabbed piece of tape is placed onto tube and pinned to the patients' diaper. Routine daily cleansing of the tube insertion site with normal saline or mild soap and water to assess site is indicated. If tube is a balloon-inflated low-profile skin level device, such as a MIC-KEY (see Fig. 16-12) or Hide-A-Port (Ross Products Div., Abbott Lab, Columbus, Ohio), then checking balloon inflation and taping across the external flange to avoid inadvertent displacement if the balloon breaks constitute sound practice.

Migration and Tract Enlargement. A variety of french sizes, as well as shaft lengths, are available in balloon-inflated, low-profile, skin-level devices. Ideally, the intragastric end of the tube is gently placed against the stomach wall, and the external flange is anchored on the abdominal surface. If excess shaft length remains, the tube can migrate in and out of the track. This scenario usually results in granulation tissue protruding from the stoma site and gastric juices leaking onto the peristomal skin surface. Granulation tissue is treated with silver nitrate cauterization until no longer protruding from the stoma or with the application of steroid creams (i.e., triamcinolone 0.1% bid for 5 to 7 days). The excess space between the abdominal surface and the external flange is managed by placing gauze or foam dressings to minimize the movement in and out of the tract.

Peristomal Skin Compromise. Skin compromise is treated with topical powders, such as Stomahesive powder (ConvaTec, Princeton, N.J.), to absorb moisture, antifungal creams or ointments to treat candidal yeast infections, therapeutic soaks with Aveeno (S.C. Johnson & Son, Racine, Wis.) or Domeboro (Bayer Corp., Elkhart, Ind.) to promote healing and comfort, and gauze or foam dressings changed daily and as needed.

If peristomal erythema or maceration is present from excess gastric leakage onto the skin, then using a high-absorbency foam dressing may be indicated, such as Allevyn (Smith & Nephew, Largo, Fla.) or Sof-Foam (Johnson & Johnson, Arlington, Tex.), changed daily and as needed. Concomitant superficial candidal yeast infections often are present, evidenced by erythema, macular or papular rash, and characteristic "satellite" lesions (Fig. 16-13). Treatment consists of a topical antifungal agent, such as nystatin (Mycostatin) powder, and an absorbent dressing. If left untreated in a moist environment, the organisms may proliferate and increase in the surface area affected. Often, when a peristomal candidal infection is present, the patient may have a coexisting oral candidiasis (thrush). Thrush appears as white, slightly raised patches resembling milk curds, which, when removed, expose a hyperemic area that may bleed slightly on the buccal mucosa. Treatment usually is with topical nystatin oral suspension 100,000 U/ml 0.5 to 1 ml placed inside of each cheek tid for 7 to 10 days.

A referral is indicated to a qualified enterostomal therapy nurse or clinical nurse specialist familiar with enteral tubes if an increase in severity of peristomal skin compromise or

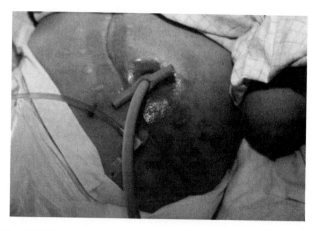

Fig. 16-13 Candidal yeast rash surrounding gastrostomy tube.

no improvement with aforementioned interventions is seen within 48 to 72 hours.

LEECH THERAPY

The medicinal use of leeches dates back to 1500 BC Egypt.[87] Present-day leech therapy is used to relieve venous congestion at surgical sites with inadequate venous drainage and to relieve damaging pressure on tissues adjacent caused by large hematomas. The surgical disruption of small blood vessels can lead to venous insufficiency, placing tissues at risk for edema, thrombosis, and necrosis. Digit transplantation and free-flap tissue grafts, which are prone to venous congestion, have increased survival rates when leech therapy is used postoperatively until adequate collateral circulation can be established.[87] Venous regeneration during wound healing can take up to 22 days.

Leeches attach to skin with both ends of their body: a sharp three-jawed feeding mouth and a rear anchor. Leeches are efficient blood removers, sucking 5 to 15 ml of blood, up to 10 times their body weight, within 15 to 60 minutes.[88] Leech saliva contains a potent anticoagulant called hirudin that inhibits the conversion of prothrombin to thrombin and prevents localized blood clotting. The major therapeutic effect of leech application occurs during the postbite period when the wound continues to ooze for up to 10 hours.[89] While feeding, a vasodilator in the leech saliva improves blood flow to the area of attachment.[90] Leech saliva also contains an anesthetic that facilitates painless feeding.[91] Once a leech is satiated, it will fall off of the skin.

Medicinal leeches, *Hirudo medicinalis,* require specialized care to ensure their health and containment. Unfed leeches are thin, slippery, efficient climbers and move relatively quickly.[89] They are generally stored in large, specially designed containers filled with sterile water that allow airflow and movement but prevent escape. Water in the container should be changed every 3 to 5 days or sooner if cloudy.[92] The container should be kept covered to block out light and in a room temperature of 60° to 68° Fahrenheit.[92] Estimating and ordering enough leeches for a 3-day period will help to ensure adequate availability for treatment while limiting the need to care for an excess number of leeches.

Initiation of Therapy

Patients undergoing leech therapy are treated with prophylactic antibiotics to reduce the risk of infection from the bacteria *Aeromonas hydrophila* found in the leech's digestive tract.[93] Antibiotics are often continued for 1 week after completion of leech therapy to protect the open, slow-to-heal bites from other infectious pathogens. Systemic anticoagulation may also be initiated before beginning leech therapy and requires frequent monitoring of coagulation parameters and hematocrit. The area to be leeched should be elevated to reduce swelling and congestion. A transparent, semipermeable dressing; gauze; or layer of bacitracin is applied to the healthy skin surrounding the area to be leeched.[89,92] This discourages the leeches from attaching to healthy skin. Orifices near the leech sites are packed to prevent migration. An absorbent pad is placed under the area to be leeched to help contain the expected continuous ooze. Patient and family teaching before the initiation of therapy is essential to allay the fear and anxiety that may accompany this unfamiliar and unusual treatment. Therapeutic play, role-playing, diversion, and shielding can be helpful.

Application. The frequency of leech application varies according to the degree of venous congestion present. Intervals of 1 to 6 hours are often needed at the initiation of therapy.[92] As venous drainage improves, the therapy is weaned slowly by gradually spacing applications and carefully assessing for the return of venous insufficiency, which is seen as edema and blue-purple discoloration. The area to be leeched is cleaned with water and patted dry to encourage attachment. Leeches are contaminated with blood and require universal precautions when handled. After preparing the site to be leeched, to prevent migration, the leech is removed from its container using a nontoothed forceps with a gauze pad underneath to prevent accidental dropping.[89] The leech is placed on the skin and watched for successful attachment, as evidenced by a rhythmic sucking motion. If the leech does not attach, a drop of glucose water is applied to the site.[92] If attachment is still not achieved, the leech is removed and another tried. Refusal of multiple leeches to attach could indicate inadequate tissue perfusion and arterial insufficiency, which require immediate physician evaluation.

Monitoring. Once applied, the leech must be under continuous observation to ensure that it has not migrated or fallen off. Leeches should remain attached to the site for 15 minutes to 1 hour before they drop off or are removed. Encouraging the wound to continue bleeding after the leech is gone is an important aspect of leech therapy. The bite is left uncovered and any locally formed clots are removed gently with sterile gauze. The leeched area should be actively oozing blood for up to 10 hours and should not appear dusky or engorged. Evidence of venous congestion should be evaluated and may necessitate more frequent leech application. Patients undergoing prolonged leech therapy must have frequent monitoring of their hematocrit level. Leech therapy over a 3 days or more may necessitate blood transfusions.

Removal and Disposal. Leeches generally detach from the skin after becoming satiated. If the leech has not dropped off after 1 hour, it should be removed by stroking it gently with an alcohol swab until it falls off.[92] Stroking the leech with an alcohol swab allows it to release its teeth. Pulling the leech off can cause the teeth to remain in the skin and cause the leech to regurgitate into the wound, increasing the risk of infection.[92] A used leech should be picked up with forceps and placed in a covered container of 70% alcohol. The container should be discarded in a biohazard waste receptacle in accordance with universal precautions. Leeches are disposed of after a single use because they are contaminated with the patient's blood and they may not be ready to feed again for up to 1 month.

SUMMARY

This chapter has presented information about the pediatric integumentary system and wound healing as they relate to the critically ill child. The concepts are an essential part of every critical care nurse's knowledge base in providing quality patient care. Although nurses may not have control over many of the factors that place critically ill infants and children at risk for skin breakdown and delayed wound healing, nurses have the ability to positively influence patient care outcomes through knowledgeable assessment, prevention, treatment, and evaluation.

REFERENCES

1. Tortora GJ: The integumentary system. In Tortora GJ, ed: *Principles of human anatomy*, ed 4, New York, 1986, Harper & Row.
2. Special report: skin care for special groups, *Nursing Times* 92:48-50, 1996.
3. Murray D: *Scientific skin care*, London, 1983, Arlington Books.
4. Harpin VA, Rutter N: Barrier properties of the newborn infant's skin, *J Pediatr* 102:419-425, 1983
5. Malloy MB, Perez-Woods RC: Neonatal skin care: prevention of skin breakdown, *Pediatr Nurs* 17:41-48, 1991.
6. Nicol NH, Hill MJ: Altered skin integrity. In Betz CL, Hunzberger M, Wright S, eds: *Family centered nursing care of children*, ed 2, Philadelphia, 1994, WB Saunders.
7. Holbrook KA, Sybert V: Basic science. In Schachner LA, Hansen RC, eds: *Pediatric dermatology*, New York, 1988, Churchill Livingstone.
8. Hudson-Goodman P, Girard N, Brewer-Jones M: Wound repair and the potential use of growth factors, *Heart Lung* 19:379-384, 1990.
9. Sieggreen MY: Healing of physical wounds, *Nurs Clin North Am* 22:439-447, 1987.
10. Wysocki A: Surgical wound healing, *AORN J* 49:502-518, 1989.
11. Carrico TJ, Mehrhof A, Cohen IK: Biology of wound healing, *Surg Clin North Am* 64:721-733, 1984.

12. Orgill D, Demling RH: Current concepts and approaches to wound healing, *Crit Care Med* 16:899-908, 1988.

13. Alvarez OM, Goslen JB, Eaglstein WH et al: Wound healing. In Fitzpatrick TB, Eisen AZ, Wolff K et al, eds: *Dermatology in general medicine,* ed 3, New York, 1987, McGraw-Hill.

14. Hotter A: Physiologic aspects and clinical implications of wound healing, *Heart Lung* 11:522-530, 1982.

15. Hunt TK, Halliday B: Inflammation in wounds: from "laudable pus" to primary repair and beyond. In Hunt TK, ed: *Wound healing and wound infection: theory and surgical practice,* New York, 1980, Appleton-Century-Crofts.

15a. Hunt A, Eriksson E: Management of burn wound, *Clin Plast Surg* 13:57-67, 1986.

16. Bryant R: Wound repair: a review, *J Enterostomal Ther* 14:262-266, 1987.

17. Pollock SV: Wound healing: a review of the biology of wound healing, *J Dermatol Surg Oncol* 5:389-392, 1979.

18. Winter GD: A note on wound healing under dressings with special reference to perforated film dressing, *J Invest Dermatol* 45:299, 1965.

19. Hunt TK, VanWinkle W: Normal repair. In Hunt TK, Dunphy JE, eds: *Fundamentals of wound management,* New York, 1979, Appleton-Century-Crofts.

20. Tramont EC: General or nonspecific host defense mechanisms. In Mandell GL, Douglas RG, Bennett JE, eds: *Principles and practice of infectious disease,* ed 3, New York, 1990, Churchill Livingstone.

21. Smith W, Burns C: Managing the hair and skin of African American pediatric patients, *J Pediatr Health Care* 13:72-78, 1999.

22. Jackson F: The ABC's of black hair and skin care, *ABNF J* 9:100-104, 1998.

23. Laude T: Approach to dermatologic disorders in black children, *Semin Dermatol* 14:15-20, 1995.

24. Jiricka MK, Ryan P, Carvalho MA et al: Pressure ulcer risk factors in an ICU population, *Am J Crit Care* 4:361-367, 1995.

25. Bergstrom N, Braden BJ, Laguzza A et al: The Braden scale for predicting pressure sore risk, *Nurs Res* 36:205-210, 1987.

26. Kramer D, Honig PJ: Diaper dermatitis in the hospitalized child, *J Enterostomal Ther* 15:167-170, 1988.

27. Zimmerman R, Lawson K, Calvert C: The effects of wearing diapers on skin, *J Pediatr* 101:721-723, 1986.

28. Anonymous: Infection control feedback to SICU staff lowers rates, *Hosp Infect Control* 18:132-133, 1991.

29. Ginsberg MK: A study of oral hygiene nursing care, *Am J Nurs* 61:67-69, 1961.

30. DeWalt EM: Effect of timed hygienic measures on oral mucosa in a group of elderly subjects, *Nurs Res* 24:104-108, 1975.

31. Beck S: Impact of a systematic oral care protocol on stomatitis after chemotherapy, *Cancer Nurs* 2:185-199, 1979.

32. Beck SL, Yasko JM: *Guidelines for oral care,* Crystal Lake, Ill, 1993, Sage Products.

33. Ezzone S, Jolly D, Replogle K et al: Survey of oral hygiene regimens among bone marrow transplant centers, *Oncol Nurs Forum* 20:1375-1380, 1993.

34. Kenny SA: Effect of two oral care protocols on the incidence of stomatitis in hematology patients, *Cancer Nurs* 13:345-353, 1990.

35. Warner LA: Lemon-glycerine swabs should not be used for routine oral care, *Crit Care Nurs* 6:82-83, 1986.

36. Cortese D, Capp L, McKinley S: Moisture chamber versus lubrication for the prevention of corneal epithelial breakdown, *Am J Crit Care* 4:425-428, 1995.

37. Braden B, Bergstrom N: A conceptual schema for the study of the etiology of pressure sores, *Rehabil Nurs* 36:205-229, 1987.

38. Mechanic HF, Perkins BA: Preventing tissue trauma, *Dimens Crit Care Nurs* 7:210-218, 1988.

39. Chang N, Goodson WH, Grottup F et al: Direct measurement of wound and tissue oxygen tension in postoperative patients, *Ann Surg* 197:470-478, 1983.

40. Milliken J, Tait GA, Ford-Jones EL et al: Nosocomial infections in a pediatric intensive care unit, *Crit Care Med* 16:233-237, 1988.

41. Piloian BB: Defining characteristics of the nursing diagnosis "high risk for impaired skin integrity, *Decubitus* 5:32-47, 1992.

42. Doughty D: The process of wound healing: a nursing perspective, *Progressions* 2:3-12, 1990.

43. Norton D, McLaren R, Exton-Smith AN: *An investigation of geriatric nursing problems in hospital,* London, 1975, Churchill Livingstone.

44. Colin D, Abraham P, Preault L et al: Comparison of 90 degree and 30 degree laterally inclined positions in the prevention of pressure ulcers using transcutaneous oxygen and carbon dioxide pressures, *Adv Wound Care* 9:35-38, 1996.

45. National Pressure Ulcer Advisory Panel: Pressure ulcers: incidence, economics, risk assessment. Consensus Development Conference statement, *Decubitus* 2:24-28, 1989.

46. Agency for Health Care Policy and Research: *Pressure ulcers in adults: prediction and prevention* (AHCPR publication 92-0047), Rockville, Md, 1992, The Agency.

47. Goodrich C, March K: From ED to ICU: a focus on prevention of skin breakdown, *Crit Care Nurs Q* 15:1-13, 1992.

48. Braden BJ, Bergstrom N: Clinical utility of the Braden scale for predicting pressure sore risk, *Decubitus* 2:44-51, 1989.

49. Bergstrom N, Demuth PJ, Braden BJ: A clinical trial of the Braden scale for predicting pressure sore risk, *Nurs Clin North Am* 22:417-428, 1987.

50. Braden B, Bergstrom N: Predictive validity of the Braden Scale for pressure sore risk in a nursing home population, *Res Nurs Health,* 17:459-470, 1994.

51. Carlson EV, Kemp MK, Shott S: Predicting the risk of pressure ulcers in critically ill patients, *Am J Crit Care* 8:262-269, 1999.

52. Quigley SM, Curley MA: Skin integrity in the pediatric population: preventing and managing pressure ulcers, *J Soc Pediatr Nurs* 1:7-18, 1996.

53. American Association of Critical Care Nurses: *Delegating of nursing and nonnursing activities in critical care: a framework for decision making,* Aliso Viejo, Calif, 1990, Author.

54. Agency for Health Care Policy and Research: *Treatment of pressure ulcers* (AHCPR publication 95-0652), Rockville, Md, 1994, Author.

55. Kosiak M: Etiology and pathology of ischemic ulcers, *Arch Phys Med Rehabil* 40:62-69, 1959.

56. Norton D, McLaren R, Exton-Smith AN: *An investigation of geriatric problems in hospital,* Edinburgh, 1975, Churchill Livingstone.

57. Oertwich PA, Kindschuh AM, Bergstrom N: The effects of small shifts in body weight on blood flow and interface pressure, *Res Nurs Health* 18:481-488, 1995.

58. Neidig J, Kleiber C, Oppliger R: Risk factors associated with pressure ulcers in the pediatric patient following open-heart surgery, *Prog Cardiovasc Nurs* 4:99-106, 1989.

59. Seiler WO, Stahelin HB: Decubitus ulcers: treatment through five therapeutic principles, *Geriatrics* 40:30-44, 1985.

60. Alvarez OM: Pressure ulcers: critical considerations in prevention and management, *Clin Mater* 8:209-222, 1991.

61. Murdoch I, Storman M: Improved arterial oxygenation in children with the adult respiratory distress syndrome: the prone position, *Acta Paediatr* 83:1043-1046, 1994.

62. Norton E, Young MA: Perioperative patient positioning: a focus on quality improvement for pediatric patients, *Surg Serv Manag* 5:14-20, 1999.

63. Reichel SM: Shearing force as a factor in decubitus ulcers in paraplegics, *JAMA* 166:762-763, 1958.

64. Marchand AC, Lidowski H: Reassessment of the use of genuine sheepskin for pressure ulcer prevention and treatment, *Decubitus* 6:44-47, 1993.

65. Lovell HW, Anderson CL: Put your patient on the right bed, *RN* 53:66-72, 1990.

66. Flemmer L, Chan JS: A pediatric protocol for management of extravasation injuries, *Pediatr Nurs* 19:355-358, 424, 1993.

67. Millam DA: Managing complications of IV therapy, *Nurs 88* 18:34-42, 1988.

68. MacCara ME: Extravasation: A hazard of intravenous therapy, *Drug Intell Clin Pharm* 17:713-717, 1983.

69. Tully JL, Friedland GH, Baldini LM, Goldman DA: Complications of intravenous therapy with steel needles and Teflon catheters: a comparative study. *Am J Med,* 70:702-706, 1981.

70. Hastings-Tolsma MT, Yucha CB, Tompkins J et al: Effect of warm and cold applications on the resolution of IV infiltrations, *Res Nurs Health* 16:171-178, 1993.

71. Brusko C: Treatment of extravasation caused by intravenous drugs, *Clin Trends Hosp Pharm* 4:39-43, 1990.

72. Dorr RT: Antidotes to vesicant chemotherapy extravasation, *Blood Rev* 4:41-60, 1990.

73. Larsen DL: Treatment of tissue extravasation by antitumor agents, *Cancer* 49:1796-1799, 1982.

74. Zenk K: Management of intravenous extravasations, *Infusion* 5:77-79, 1981.

75. Young TE, Mangum OB: *Neofax, a manual of drugs used in neonatal care,* ed 4, Columbus, Ohio, 1991, Ross Laboratories.

76. Denkler KA, Cohen BE: Reversal of dopamine extravasation injury with topical nitroglycerin ointment, *Plastic Reconstr Surg* 84:811-813, 1989.

77. Wong AF, McCulloch LM, Sola A: Treatment of peripheral tissue ischemia with topical nitroglycerin ointment in neonates, *J Pediatr* 121:980-983, 1992.

78. O'Reilly C, McKay FM, Duffty P et al: Glyceryl trinitrate in skin necrosis caused by extravasation of parenteral nutrition, *Lancet* 2:565-566, 1988 (letter).

79. Irazuzta J, McManus ML: Use of topically applied nitroglycerin in the treatment of purpura fulminans, *J Pediatr* 117:993-995, 1990.

80. Winter GD: Formation of scab and rate of epithelialization on superficial wounds in skin of domestic pig, *Nature* 193:293-294, 1962.

81. Krasner D: Resolving the dressing dilemma: selecting wound dressings by category, *Ostomy Wound Manage* 35:62-69, 1991.

82. Meehan PA: Open abdominal wounds: a creative approach to a challenging problem, *Progressions* 4:3-11, 1992.

83. Brown CD, Zitelli JA: Choice of wound dressing and ointments, *Otolaryngol Clin North Am* 28:1081-1090, 1995.

84. Boarini JH: Principles of stoma care for infants. *J Enterostomal Ther* 16:21-25.

85. Adams DA, Selekof JL: Children with ostomies: comprehensive care planning, *Pediatr Nurs* 12:429-433.

86. Embon C: Ostomy care for the infant with necrotizing enterocolitis: nursing considerations, *J Perinat Neonatal Nurs* 4:56-63, 1990.

87. Golden MA, Quinn JJ, Partington MT: Leech therapy in digital replantation, *AORN* 62:364-375, 1995.

88. Kocent LC, Spinner SS: Leech therapy: new procedures for an old treatment, *Pediatr Nurs* 18:481-483, 1992.

89. White RL, Fries CM: Leech therapy: new applications for an old treatment, *Nurs Spectrum* 3:10-12, 1999.

90. Rivera ML, Gross JE: Scalp replantation after traumatic injury, *AORN J* 62:175-184, 1995.

91. Graham CE: Leeches, *BMJ* 310:603, 1995.

92. LoRe H, White J: Leech therapy. In *Nursing policy and procedure manual,* Boston, 1999, Children's Hospital.

93. Biopharm Ltd: *Biopharm leeches,* United Kingdom, 1996, Walters Printers.

17 Caring Practices: Providing Comfort

Linda L. Oakes

New technology and drug regimens for the treatment of children with critical illnesses and injuries have led to increasingly successful outcomes. However, with this success comes the clinical challenge of providing optimal management of children's distress associated with intensive care therapy. Nonpharmacologic and pharmacologic approaches to the relief of pain, anxiety, and agitation and for the promotion of rest are well-recognized goals in the nursing care of critically ill infants and children.

Discomfort is an almost universal consequence of critical illness. Chest, endotracheal, and nasogastric tubes are unpleasant interventions associated with some degree of pain. Exposure to an environment characterized by excessive stimulation: bright overhead lights; strange noises associated with monitors, ventilators, suctioning; and medical emergencies, even those involving other patients; and lack of diurnal variation contribute to children's distress and anxiety often exhibited as agitation. Although young children cannot always explicitly describe what stresses they are feeling, older patients in the pediatric intensive care unit (PICU) can do so and report their experiences while being supported on mechanical ventilation. These patients indicate that they experienced distress caused by pain, inability to speak or reposition themselves when uncomfortable, the tugging of ventilator tubing, the discomfort of being suctioned, and the hectic pace of the unit interfering with rest.[1,2]

Pain is defined by the International Association of Pain[3] as "an unpleasant sensory and emotional experience associated with actual or potential tissue damage, or described in terms of such damage." The implication of this definition is that pain is both a sensory and emotional experience. *Anxiety* is a sustained state of apprehension in response to a real or perceived threat associated with motor tension, autonomic activity, and vigilance scanning. *Agitation* is excessive, often nonpurposeful motor activity associated with internal tension and accompanied by anxiety, panic, depression, delusions, hallucinations, and delirium. *Delirium* is the state of reduced ability to appropriately respond to external stimuli, usually manifested as disorganized thinking (rambling, incoherent speech), decreased level of consciousness, altered sensory perception, disorientation, or altered level of psychomotor activity, including agitation.[4] A key problem with agitation is the potential for physical injury. Agitation can be the result of children experiencing intolerable levels of pain and anxiety. However, agitation can also result from hypoxia, bronchospasm, or inadequate ventilatory support. Nurses are challenged to sort out what the causes may be in agitated infants and children to provide the appropriate interventions.

Pain and anxiety often coexist and magnify each other. Minimizing pain and anxiety is an essential treatment goal in the PICU, leading experts to develop treatment protocols using psychosocial interventions, pharmacologic agents, and the provision of the least stressful environment for children. The goals of analgesics and sedatives are to (1) alleviate anxiety or distress, (2) improve comfort, (3) facilitate medical procedures, (4) promote sleep, (5) prevent later memory of particularly distressing interventions, (6) tolerate having an endotracheal tube, (7) enable safe and effective ventilation, (8) reduce oxygen consumption, (9) control intracranial pressure, and (10) optimize cerebral perfusion pressure.

Conventionally, pain management was initiated after noxious stimuli, such as surgery. Recent advances in our understanding of the responses to pain have generated interest in active intervention to prevent it from occurring.[5] Preemptive analgesia is a strategy in which analgesia administered before the painful stimulus is given to prevent or reduce subsequent pain and analgesic requirements. The hypothesis is that this strategy prevents or reduces the "memory" of pain in the nervous system. The benefit of preemptive analgesia has been well established in animal studies, although results from clinical studies are at best mixed.[6] Despite these mixed results, preemptive analgesia appears to be an appropriate and humane goal of clinical practice.

During the last decade, interest and research regarding pain in infants and children has mushroomed. A heightened awareness of pain in such patients has led to improved measures in the prevention, assessment, and treatment of pain in all age groups.[7-10] This shift in practice has been the result of recent basic and clinical research, as well as more attention to appropriate pain management by accrediting healthcare organizations and national commissions.[11] However, even today, the general consensus is that pain and anxiety are often underrecognized and undertreated. There continues to be inadequate amounts of analgesics and sedatives ordered by physicians and insufficient administration of these prescribed medications by nurses.[2,7,10,12,13]

Despite advances in healthcare, unrelieved pain remains a problem, and adults who can describe their hospitalization continue to relate pain as a major stressor and their worst memory of critical care.[14,14a] Examination of barriers to effective pain management in children may help to explain this suboptimal treatment.

BARRIERS TO EFFECTIVE PAIN MANAGEMENT IN CHILDREN

Patients, families, and even healthcare professionals continue to have a lack of knowledge and many misconceptions about treatment options, especially regarding the use of opioids (narcotics) leading to addiction. These misunderstandings continue to prevent the timely and appropriate treatment of patients of all ages. Confusion exists regarding three terms associated with use of opioids: addiction, physical dependency, and tolerance. These terms are often used inappropriately and interchangeably, perpetuating misconceptions.

Drug addiction is defined as a pattern of compulsive drug use characterized by a continued craving for a drug and the need to use it for effects other than relief of symptoms such as pain.[15] Persons who are addicted obtain drugs for their mind-altering properties, not for medicinal purposes. A behavioral pattern is established, characterized by spending time acquiring or using drugs, abandoning normal social or occupational activities because of the need for the drug, and using the drugs despite adverse psychologic or physical effects.[16] Public attention has been needed regarding the very real concern of young people becoming abusers of unprescribed substances, including narcotics. However, the media campaign of constantly warning citizens to "just say no to drugs" has not made it clear that this does not extend to the use of narcotics under the supervision of healthcare providers. (In light of the negative perception induced by the using the word *narcotic*, the term *opioid* is used throughout the remainder of the chapter when pertaining to medically prescribed analgesics.) Parents continue to have fears that their children will get "hooked" and become addicts. Yet less than 1% of children and adults treated with opioids for medical reasons develop addiction, unless they have had prior history of substance abuse.[2,16,17] Therefore withholding adequate pain relief from a suffering patient on the theoretical grounds of addiction is inappropriate.

Physical dependence means that the patient has developed a physical need for the drug, such that rapid withdrawal will manifest as a specific set of symptoms. It is a well-recognized phenomenon that occurs after prolonged opioid, benzodiazepine, barbiturate, and steroid administration or other nonprescribed substances, such as nicotine. *Tolerance* is the development of a need to increase the dose to achieve the same effect previously attained with a lower dose. Patients appropriately treated with opioids, benzodiazepines, and barbiturates can become tolerant and physically dependent, and these terms are clinically important only because they influence the choice of the appropriate dosage and schedule for weaning patients from these medicines.

In addition, concerns exist regarding the safety of the administration of opioids to infants and children. Opioids are no more dangerous for children than they are for adults when appropriately administered. Some differences are found in opioid pharmacodynamics and pharmacokinetics used in infants younger than 6 months of age, but adequate analgesia can still be provided safely with appropriate dosages, intervals of drug administration, and rate of administration of parenteral preparations. Even today an excessive and unfounded concern over young children's immature metabolic capacity causing drug accumulation and subsequent adverse effects has been a major deterrent to administering opioids to pediatric patients. Acknowledgement that respiratory depression is a serious and well-known side effect of opioids is appropriate. However, this effect rarely occurs in children. Of important note is that pain acts as a natural antagonist to the analgesic, and opioid side effects making respiratory depression less likely in children who are experiencing acute pain.

This apparent deafness to patients' complaints does not reflect a lack of compassion. Instead, it is a product of a pattern of a lack of knowledge about pain management interventions and the need for easier methods of recognizing untreated pain. Physicians and nurses mistakenly continue to believe that neuromuscular blocking agents (NMBAs), such as pancuronium, have anxiolytic or analgesic effects, as well as being unaware of the harmful physiologic effects of unrelieved pain. Continued undertreatment reflecting limitations in training about pain assessment, analgesic pharmacology, and behavioral interventions is still prevalent in healthcare. Also, a misunderstanding remains regarding neurodevelopment, such as believing that young children do not have the neurologic system maturity to feel pain, which may promote an underestimation of children's pain experiences. Some healthcare professionals hold onto the now refuted theory that infants and young children have no memory of painful or anxiety-provoking experiences, leading to the erroneous conclusion that optimal pain management is not necessary.

Healthcare professionals may cite the "resiliency" of children or their ability to "bounce back" as indicators that children do not feel pain as much as adults do. In fact, children's ability to cope with distress through playing or watching television is useful as a positive coping mechanism. However, caregivers may interpret these observations as children are not suffering, resulting in the withholding of appropriate analgesics.

The reasons that pain has been ineffectively managed in pediatric patients lie in the subjective nature of pain and the need to verbally communicate its presence and intensity. Developmental stages of young children may preclude effective communication of their pain. Pain is a complex and individualized sensation that is difficult to quantify, particularly for children. As early as 1968, McCaffery[7] recommended to those in clinical practice to consider that "pain is whatever the experiencing person says it is, existing whenever he say it does." However, assessment tools in which children can use self-report are limited to those who are at the very least older than 3 years of age. Children who are critically ill may have less ability to demonstrate behavioral signs of pain because of neurologic deficits associated with their illness or suppression by NMBAs. Therefore clinicians in the ICU rely on their own informal observations to determine whether children are hurting.

Even when children can self-report, it has been shown that pediatric nurses do not routinely use self-report and pediatric pain tools in their practice, despite their ease of use and proven validity and reliability.[8,17a] Some nurses continue to use self-report only to confirm other indicators of pain.[18] This discrepancy in practice may lead to large variability in pain assessments and thus inconsistency in pain management interventions for a child.

Inadequate documentation of pain management continues to lead to overall ineffective pain management. Pain experts and organizations continue to stress the need to make pain more visible. Unlike other vital signs, pain is not displayed in a prominent place on the chart or at the bedside. Strategies offered by pain organizations, such as the American Pain Society, have recommended including the measurement of pain intensity as a fifth vital sign, making this data more available to those making treatment decisions. However, institutions have been slow to comply with this recommendation.[7] Even when pain is assessed by clinicians, failure to accept children's report of pain is still a problem, especially if pain is reported in the absence of objective signs of tissue damage. Few things dismay all patients more than sensing that their doctors and nurses are questioning whether their pain is "real."

Further complicating pain assessment strategies is the premise supported by society that pain is to be expected and endured, as evidenced with the phrases "no pain, no gain," or "pain builds character," or that by asking for analgesics, a person is being "weak." For children with medical problems, this premise needs to be replaced with "pain can kill." Children may deny pain if they believe they are supposed to be brave or if they anticipate receiving an injection for pain. For example, a child may suffer in silence for fear of being given a "shot," particularly if he or she does not understand the concept that asking for pain medication will result in pain relief. Therefore children often cannot or will not report pain to their care providers; thus nurses must anticipate pain, recognize subtle indications of pain, and intervene to relieve pain.

ANATOMY AND PHYSIOLOGY

Pain involves a response of the peripheral nervous system, the autonomic and skeletal motor systems, and the central nervous system. A simple stimulus-response model is often used to describe pain transmission and pain perception. Although this model is useful, it must be remembered that individual response to pain often defies straightforward anatomic and physiologic explanation. A one-to-one relationship does not exist between a noxious stimulus and an individual's response to the pain.

Peripheral Nervous System

Nociception is the term used to describe normal pain transmission. This process begins in the periphery (skin, subcutaneous tissue, visceral or somatic structures), where primary afferent neurons, called nociceptors, are distributed. Nociceptors are free nerve endings with the capacity to distinguish between noxious and harmless stimuli. When tissue is exposed in sufficient quantity to noxious stimuli, tissue damage occurs, followed by the release of chemical substances, called mediators, from damaged cells, initiating and facilitating the movement of the pain impulse from the periphery to the spinal cord. Substance P is one of these mediators that transmits pain by the ascending spinal tracts. Prostaglandin E sensitizes tissues to bradykinin. Histamine, potassium, and bradykinin are released from mast cells and are actively involved in the inflammatory response to painful injuries. Peripherally acting agents such as aspirin, acetaminophen, and nonsteroidal antiinflammatory agents (NSAIDs) inhibit prostaglandin synthesis and activation of the nociceptors.

A stimulus is activated in response to thermal, chemical, or mechanical trauma, causing an impulse to be transmitted by nociceptor fibers. Two types of nociceptor fibers, C fibers and A-delta fibers, are responsible for the transmission of pain from the periphery to the spinal cord.[6] The A-delta fibers are thinly myelinated neurons that conduct impulses at rapid velocity and have a low threshold for firing. Once activated, these fibers are associated with what is described as "first pain": a sharp, intense, and well-localized sensation. The C fibers are unmyelinated; they conduct impulses at a slower speed and have a relatively high firing threshold. They are associated with a later onset or "second pain," which is described as a poorly localized, dull, burning, prolonged sensation.

Both A-delta and C fibers share the property of sensitization, which has clinical implications. Both nociceptors become more sensitive and more reactive with repeated episodes of noxious stimulation. Injuries such as burns, bruises, and abrasions are often accompanied by hyperesthesia (increased sensitivity to mild stimuli) or hyperalgesia (increased sensitivity to painful stimuli). The threshold to sensory stimulation is decreased, and even commonly innocuous stimulation is experienced as painful.

Peripheral nociceptors remain unmyelinated or thinly myelinated throughout the life cycle from infancy to adulthood. Lack of myelination does not imply lack of conduction and perception but, rather, slower conduction. Therefore the lack of myelination of peripheral nerves in the infant does not support the assertion that infants cannot appreciate pain. Moreover, the slower conduction velocity characteristic of unmyelinated nerves may well be offset by the shorter distances that the nerve impulse travels in a small infant.

Spinal Cord

Pain stimuli are delivered by sensory neurons from the peripheral site of trauma to the spinal cord. Nociceptors and other sensory fibers travel to and converge on cells within the dorsal horn of the spinal cord. The dorsal horn cells activate several central mechanisms involved in the appreciation and response to painful stimuli. Some dorsal root neurons initiate a protective, spinal reflex in response to pain; for example, pulling one's hand away from a hot stove even before the heat and burning are consciously realized. Some dorsal horn cells are involved with inhibition of further incoming nociceptive input. When these cells become damaged from nerve injury and inhibition is removed, pain sensation increases. Most importantly, dorsal horn cells activate central transmission tracts that relay peripheral input to higher brain centers. These messages travel to the thalamus and, finally, to the brain.

Central Nervous System

The spinothalamic and the spinoreticular tracts are the main central pathways of pain impulse transmission. These tracts synapse in different areas of the thalamus and then continue and ultimately terminate in various areas of the cortex. The spinothalamic tract travels to and synapses in the lateral thalamus. From here, the tract continues to and terminates in the somatosensory cortex. The spinothalamic tracts "map" information onto the somatosensory cortex so that individuals are able to identify and localize pain.

The spinoreticular pathway ascends to the brainstem reticular formation. Some of these communications continue to the lateral thalamus and onward to the somatosensory cortex. Others travel to the medial thalamus, which continues to the association cortex or, more specifically, to the limbic system and the frontal cortex. These higher cortical areas recruit a sophisticated response to pain, which involves the appreciation of pain intensity, the desire to escape from pain, and the anxiety that accompanies the need to be rid of painful stimuli. This sophisticated response determines the impact that emotions, personality, culture, gender, past experience with pain, and the meaning of the pain have on an individual's perception and response to pain. The spinothalamic and the spinoreticular tracts are completely myelinated by 30 weeks of gestation.

The cerebrum and thalamus are known as the control centers that process and register the experience of pain. Once the impulse enters the higher centers of the brain, information about the pain, such as location and intensity, is processed, as well as other factors that include fear of the situation, past and present experiences, and the child's current emotional status. In addition to receiving and interpreting information from peripheral input, the central nervous system acts as a sensory modulation system. The brain may respond by blocking further pain impulses from reaching the higher centers or by producing endogenous opioids (i.e., endorphins), which saturate receptor sites along the spinal cord and in the brain, providing an analgesic effect. These endogenous compounds are identical pharmacologically to morphine in their action on opioid receptors. Opioid receptors are present throughout the body, with higher concentrations in the dorsal horn of the central nervous system. The action of endogenous opioids and opioid analgesics on these central receptors is thought to provide analgesia. Opioid receptors are also present in many tissues that are not involved in analgesia. The action of opioids on these receptors is responsible for many of the side effects and complications seen with opioid administration.

Physiologic Effects of Untreated Pain and Anxiety

The importance of providing effective comfort measures cannot be overemphasized as more clinicians recognize the benefits of effective therapies beyond the obvious humanitarian reasons. Inadequate management leads to significant deleterious consequences of a superacute and unnecessary arousal of the stress response. All infants and children, even the critically ill, respond to noxious stimuli with biochemical and physiologic responses that if untreated can lead to increased patient morbidity and mortality.[2] These responses are well documented, including increases in respiratory rate, heart rate, blood pressure, cardiac contractility, afterload, dysrhythmias, and myocardial oxygen consumption.[2]

The effects of unrelieved pain lead to inefficient ventilation, resulting in hypoxia. Respiratory dysfunction is the most common result of pain associated with abdominal or thoracic surgery because the child reduces the muscle movement of his chest and abdominal muscles in an attempt to splint the area and to prevent painful movements, resulting in atelectasis. Also, splinting interferes with the ability to cough and clear secretions, contributing to lobar collapse and infection. The hormonal and endocrine responses to pain include the release of corticosteroids, growth hormone, and catecholamines, as well as a decrease in insulin secretion. This response leads to hyperglycemia and a breakdown of carbohydrate and fat stores. Use of fat for energy may cause metabolic acidosis, resulting from an increase in blood lactate, pyruvate, ketone bodies, and fatty acids. If allowed to continue, this catabolic process results in a poor environment for healing.

Ongoing research efforts by clinicians emphasize the importance of analgesia. Anand and co-workers[19] demonstrated that preterm infants undergoing frequent distressing procedures (i.e., heel sticks, insertion of feeding tubes) had marked changes in cerebral blood flow and oxygen delivery. These changes were seen to be temporally associated with an increased risk for intraventricular hemorrhage and periventricular leukomalacia, thus leading to significant neurodevelopmental sequelae. Pain impairs the immune system and even enhances growth of cancerous tumors.[2,20,21]

CHILDREN'S RESPONSES TO PAIN AND ANXIETY

Historically, children have been undertreated for pain and anxiety because of the belief that children neither respond to nor remember painful experiences to the same degree as adults. This is simply untrue. Now it is known that even neonates experience pain. Studies of long-term effects of early and prolonged exposure to pain during infancy suggests a process whereby peripheral injury leads to

changes in the structure and function of the pain system.[22] Longitudinal studies in preterm infants have shown that repeated painful experiences have demonstrable and prolonged effects on the infant nervous system and behavior long after the exposure to pain. Relationships between neonatal pain and emotional temperament in infancy or childhood further suggest the widespread distribution of these neurobiologic changes. Studies indicate that repeated painful procedures are associated with an increase in depression, a pattern of "learned helplessness" insomnia, feeding patterns, and impaired coping responses.[9,22] Infants circumcised at birth demonstrated an increased pain response to routine immunizations months later and that minimizing the pain of circumcision with lidocaine-prilocaine (EMLA) attenuated the pain response.[23]

Preschool children are very egocentric in their thinking and believe that all events and sensations originate from their internal world. They have little understanding of cause-and-effect relationships, often misconstruing the meaning and cause of pain. They may view pain as a punishment for past misdeeds or bad thoughts. Young children are to be repeatedly reassured that procedures or painful experiences are not punishments. Breakdowns in skin integrity from cuts, abrasions, or incisions are extremely threatening to children because of their fears of bodily injury and mutilation. They believe that all of their body and blood will leak out. Band-Aids and dressings hold a special power for children as they fix the "leak" and hold the body in.

School-age children become more logical and reasonable in their thinking. They are in the process of gaining greater command over their world and tend to be achievement oriented. Because these children are often organized by "rules," they respond well to rituals to cope with painful events. Once these rituals and routines are established, they must be followed consistently to be effective.

Adolescents are capable of abstract thinking and have an understanding of "if-then" relationships. Although capable of adult-level problem solving, adolescents lack the life experiences that facilitate consistent mature responses. During stressful situations, adolescents may vacillate between adult responses and regression to immature behaviors.

TYPES OF PAIN

Clinicians must identify the type of pain to determine appropriate interventions to relieve it. Pain is often categorized by duration, such as (1) acute (relatively brief pain that subsides as healing takes place) or (2) chronic (pain existing for as long as 3 to 6 months after the healing has presumed to have occurred). Chronic pain treatment plans are complex, with the need for a multidisciplinary team to offer multimodal approaches, usually with strong behavioral and rehabilitation components.

Another method of classifying pain is by the inferred pathophysiologic condition, specifically, either nociceptive or neuropathic in origin. *Nociceptive pain* arises from stimuli from somatic (bone, joint, muscle, skin, or connective tissue) and visceral (arising from organs such as the gastrointestinal system) structures, as described in the previ-

TABLE 17-1   Useful Mnemonic to Obtain a Pain History

P	Palliative and provocative factors	What makes the pain better? (e.g., hot or cold packs, immobilizing painful body part, repositioning, sleeping)
		What makes the pain worse? (e.g., eating, fatigue, movement)
Q	Quality	What does the pain feel like? (e.g., shooting, throbbing, stabbing, pulsing, burning, tingling)
R	Region and radiation	Where is the pain?
		Does it spread anywhere else?
S	Severity	How bad is the pain?
		Use pain-rating scales to aid communication of pain intensity
T	Timing	When did the pain start?
		How long have you had the pain?
		Is the pain constant or intermittent?

ous section on anatomy and physiology of pain. Somatic pain is described as aching or throbbing and is generally well localized. Visceral pain, which is characterized as deep and aching, is often not well localized and referred to other areas of the body. For example, visceral pain related to hepatomegaly may radiate to the right shoulder. Nociceptive pain usually can be blocked by opioids, NSAIDs, and steroids.

Neuropathic pain is associated with injury, dysfunction, or altered excitability of portions of the peripheral or central nervous system, with the pain commonly described as a burning, stabbing, "pins and needles," or shooting sensations along the damaged nerve tract. The level of intensity and the duration of the pain often greatly exceed the time in which the injury would be expected to resolve. Though many mechanisms have been proposed, the general consensus is that the injury leads to repetitive spontaneous depolarization and transmission of pain. Patients at risk for this type of pain are those who are recovering from surgery involving nerves; illnesses associated with nerve damage, such as Guillain-Barré syndrome; or those receiving medications associated with neuropathies as side effects, such as chemotherapy (i.e., vincristine). A specific type of neuropathic pain that is particularly disturbing is that following an amputation of a limb, producing "phantom limb sensations."

PAIN ASSESSMENT

Successful assessment and control of pain depends, in part, on a positive relationship between healthcare professionals, children, and their families. For children who are able to communicate their discomforts directly, pain assessment is easier to obtain. However, fear, confusion, developmental immaturity, and the severity of illness hinder children's ability to communicate with caregivers. Children are quite capable of describing many aspects of their pain. Through a brief but comprehensive interview, the caregiver may learn much about a child's pain. Fundamentally, caregivers are to ask the child or parent what word they use for pain, such as "owie" or "boo-boo." A basic assessment must include at least the intensity (severity) and location of the pain. Further assessment in a systematic manner can be done, if possible, encompassing the description of the pain (sharp, pulsing,

dull), as well as its duration, any influencing factors (aggravating or relieving), or any radiation to other areas. Information regarding aspects of the pain such as using the format of "PQRST" will help to delineate the problem so that management can be more effective (Table 17-1). In many instances, such as postoperative care, nurses need to be alert to a child's pain within the situational context. For example, after bowel surgery, a child may experience incisional pain, as well as gas pain. It is important to differentiate between the two because incisional pain responds best to opioids, whereas gas pain worsens with opioids and responds to increased activity and movement by the child.

Self-report is the most critical component of pain assessment. Children are to be encouraged to describe their pain because their statements reflect the most reliable indicator of pain. When self-report is available, it represents the "gold standard" for assessing children's pain.[24]

Self-Report Scales

The easiest and most accessible method commonly used in assessing the presence of pain in adolescents and adults is to ask them verbally to rate pain intensity with a 0 to 10 scale, with 0 meaning no pain and 10 being the worst pain one could ever imagine. To use the numeric scale, the patient must be able to count to 10 and understand the principles of rank and order. Therefore, for children between 3 and 13 years of age, scales better suited to their cognitive ability are more useful.

Many pediatric self-report pain tools have been tested in clinical settings with diverse populations to determine their reliability and validity. Several scales use pictures of faces in various levels of pain for younger children to rate pain intensity (Figs. 17-1 and 17-2). They present faces ranging from happy and not hurting to sad and hurting arranged linearly along a vertical or horizontal line. Younger children tend to respond at the extreme points on pain-rating scales, perhaps signifying their limited cognitive capacity to make the discriminations of which older children are capable. The Eland color scale is unique in that it addresses both pain location and intensity (Fig. 17-3). The child is presented with back and front views of a body outline and is asked to

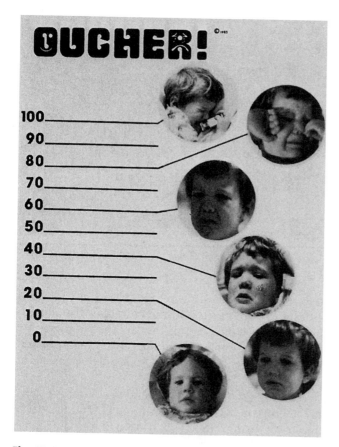

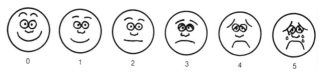

Fig. 17-2 Faces rating scale. Explain to the child that each face is for a person who feels happy because he or she has no pain (hurt) or sad because he or she has some or a lot of pain. Face 0 is very happy because the person doesn't hurt at all. Face 1 hurts just a little bit. Face 2 hurts a little more. Face 3 hurts even more. Face 4 hurts a whole lot, but face 5 hurts as much as you can imagine, although you don't have to be crying to feel this bad. Ask the child to choose the face that best describes how he or she is feeling. This rating scale is recommended for persons of age 3 years and older. (From Whaley L, Wong D: *Nursing care of infants and children,* ed 6, 1999. Copyrighted by Mosby, Inc. Reprinted by permission. The Wong-Baker Faces Pain Scale may be reproduced for clinical and research use, provided the copyright information is retained with the scale.)

choose four color crayons to represent different levels of pain. The location of the pain may be marked directly on the body parts affected. Pain intensity is indicated by the color that the child chooses to color or mark the painful part. The Eland tool has been shown numerous times to be a very sensitive tool for identifying painful locations.[25] Pain intensity scales provide a means for communication between child and caregiver, as well as between caregivers. Understanding how a child is rating pain intensity over a continuum of time and activities gives more information about the child's experience. Changes in therapy can be geared to meeting the deficiencies in pain coverage.

Believing the child is important. If the child perceives that he or she is not believed, he or she will not report accurately, making assessment more difficult. If the child fears that admitting pain will result in an intramuscular injection or a painful examination, he or she will often deny pain. Healthcare professionals must assure the child that he or she will be included in deciding how to best treat the pain.

Observational Scales

Self-report tools are not feasible in children who are preverbal (generally younger than 3 years of age) or unable

to communicate because of the severity of their illness. Yet critically ill children who are unconscious, sedated, mechanically ventilated, or paralyzed may be experiencing severe pain but unable to communicate to others. Clinicians are to realize that pain will be expressed differently depending on the age and development level. Learning each individual's response to pain requires awareness and time to get to know the child. The nurse is then able to make pain assessments that incorporate the individual patient's behavioral responses to discomfort. Inferring pain from behavior is fraught with difficulties, however, because there are frequent discordances between pain behavior and self-report. The concordance between behavior and self-report of pain is often best for brief, sharp pain, such as pain from a needle. Behaviors seen with nonprocedural pain may differ dramatically from those seen in a child suffering from acute pain episodes for invasive procedures. Overt signs of pain may be suppressed. Instead, the child may sleep more, have a decrease in appetite, and appear depressed and withdrawn. On the other hand, a child who is experiencing pain may be active and playing "normally" as a way to distract attention from the pain and attempting to enjoy a favorite activity. Behaviors such as watching television, playing, or sleeping can be distraction strategies used for coping with acute pain. Therefore clinicians are to be wary of depending on general observation because it will often lead to underassessment and therefore undertreatment of pain in children. The absence of behaviors associated with pain does not indicate the absence of pain.

Interpretation of behaviors of infants and children to determine the presence of pain without a reliable and valid assessment tool presents several problems. Pain estimates may vary, depending on the behavioral criteria used by each observer to infer pain. Although one health professional may believe that a patient's behavior indicates pain, another may interpret the behaviors as signs of anxiety or emotional distress. Several behavioral observation pain scales have been developed to help caregivers be more objective, systematic, and consistent in their assessment of pain behaviors. These scales use behavioral criteria, with some scales

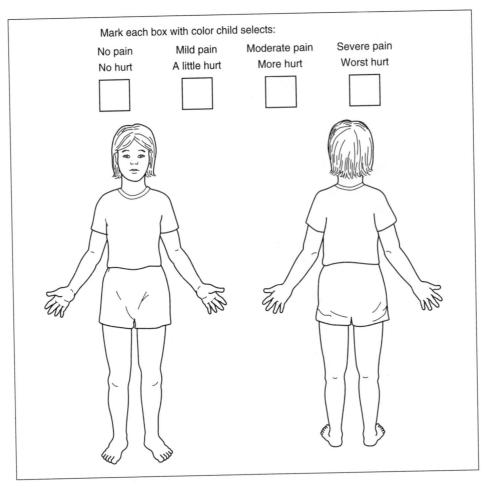

Mark each box with color child selects:

No pain | Mild pain | Moderate pain | Severe pain
No hurt | A little hurt | More hurt | Worst hurt

Fig. 17-3   Eland color scale. Redrawn with permission of the author, who also gives permission for this to be duplicated for use in clinical practice. (Permission from Joann M. Eland.)

also including physiologic criteria, therefore not depending on the child's verbal ability or cooperation. Healthcare professionals need to recognize that these scales cannot, for the most part, discriminate well between the physical response of pain and other forms of stress or discomfort.

Researchers have defined specific distress behaviors as indicators of pain: the character of any crying or other vocalizations, facial expression, motor responses (ranging from restlessness to not wanting to move at all), body posture such as guarding a body part, and general activity or appearance of the child. These symptoms provide a basis for the development of observational tools reported in the literature, including the CRIES and, more recently, the FLACC. However, these nonverbal behaviors are not to be used instead of or to refute a patient's verbal complaints of pain.

The *CRIES,* an acronym of the indicators of the scale to assist raters' memory of the assessment parameters, was developed for determining postoperative pain in infants[26] (Table 17-2). Consisting of five physiologic and behavioral indicators, each indicator is rated on a 3-point scale (0, 1, 2) that results in a total score ranging from 0 to 10. The psychometric properties of the measure were established with infants (32 to 60 weeks' gestational age) cared for in NICUs and PICUs. Although tested thoroughly for reliabil-

ity and validity, the feasibility and clinical usefulness of the measures have not been formally assessed. However, to date the CRIES is the most promising measure available for assessment of postoperative pain in infants.[27]

The *FLACC,* an acronym for the assessment criteria as well, has been found to have interrater reliability and preliminary validity for scoring postoperative pain in young children of ages 2 months to 7 years, thus providing a simple consistent method for clinicians to identify, document, and evaluate pain[28] (Table 17-3). A pain score ranging from 0 to 10 is derived from each category with a subscore of 0 to 2. Further testing in other populations needs to be done.

These scales have limitations in reliably selecting all patients in pain and therefore must be used in combination with knowledge of the clinical and environmental context of the pain assessment. Because these observations may indicate other sources of distress, it is important to examine the context or situation in which changes in the behaviors are seen. Healthcare professionals may ask themselves: Given the infant's or child's diagnosis and treatments, is it reasonable to infer that this child is experiencing pain? Do these behavioral changes respond to analgesics? What other factors may be contributing to the child's distress?

TABLE 17-2   CRIES Neonatal Postoperative Pain Measurement Score

Criteria	0	1	2
Crying	No	High pitched	Inconsolable
Requires O_2 for saturations >95%	No	<30%	>30%
Increased vital signs	HR and BP less than or equal to preop	Increase in HR or BP <20% of preop	Increase in HR or BP >20% of preop
Expression	None	Grimace	Grimace/grunt
Sleepless	No	Wakes at frequent intervals	Constantly awake

Coding Tips for Using CRIES

Crying	The characteristic cry of pain is *high pitched*. If no cry or cry that is not high pitched, score 0. If cry high pitched but baby is easily consoled, score 1. If cry is high pitched and baby is inconsolable, score 2.
Requires O_2 for sats >95%	Looks for *changes* in oxygenation. Babies experiencing pain manifest decreases in oxygenation as measured by transcutaneous monitoring or pulse oximetry. If no O_2 is required, score 0. If <30% O_2 is required, score 1. If >30% O_2 is required, score 2. (Consider other causes of changes in oxygenation such as atelectasis, pneumothorax, oversedation.)
Increased vital signs	Note: measure BP last because this may wake child, causing difficulty with other assessments. Use baseline preoperative parameters from a nonstressed period. Multiply baseline HR × 0.2; then add this to baseline HR to determine the HR, which is 20% over baseline. Do likewise for BP. Use mean BP. If HR and BP are both unchanged or less than baseline, score 0. If HR or BP is increased but increase is <20% of baseline, score 1. If either one is increased >20% over baseline, score 2.
Expression	The facial expression most often associated with pain is a grimace. This may be characterized by brow lowering, eyes squeezed shut, deepening of the nasolabial furrow, open lips and mouth. If no grimace present, score 0. If grimace alone present, score 1. If grimace and noncry vocalization grunt present, score 2.
Sleepless	This parameter is scored based on the infant's state during the hour preceding this recorded score. If he or she is continuously asleep, score 0. If awakened at frequent intervals, score 1. If awake constantly, score 2.

From Krechel SW, Bildner J: CRIES: a new neonatal postoperative pain measurement score: initial testing of validity and reliability, *Pediatr Anesth* 5:53-61, 1995. Neonatal pain assessment tool developed at the University of Missouri-Columbia.

TABLE 17-3   FLACC Scale

Categories	Scoring		
	0	1	2
Face	No particular expression or smile	Occasional grimace or frown, withdrawn, disinterested	Frequent to constant quivering chin, clenched jaw
Legs	Normal position or relaxed	Uneasy, restless, tense	Kicking or legs drawn up
Activity	Lying quietly, normal position, moves easily	Squirming, shifting back and forth, tense	Arched, rigid or jerking
Cry	No cry (awake or asleep)	Moans or whimpers, occasional complaint	Crying steadily, screams or sobs, frequent complaints
Consolability	Content, relaxed	Reassured by occasional touching, hugging, or being talked to; distractible	Difficult to console or comfort

Each of the five categories—face (F), legs (L), activity (A), cry (C), and consolability (C)—is scored from 0-2, resulting in a total score range of 0 to 10.

From Merkel SI, Voepel-Lewis T, Shayevitz JR et al: The FLACC: a behavioral scale for scoring postoperative pain in young children, *Pediatr Nurs* 23:293-297, 1997.

A major limitation for observational scales that depend on motor activity is that they cannot be used in children with neurologic deficits or receiving NMBAs. Researchers[29,30] recommend a continued effort to develop a reliable and valid observational scale for such infants and children.

Physiologic Indicators

Children in acute pain most often have an elevated heart rate, respiratory rate, and blood pressure. The cardiovascular and respiratory responses are a result of the release of catecholamines from the adrenal medulla in the body's preparation for "fight or flight." Preterm and newborn infants may respond somewhat differently with an increase or decrease in heart rate.[30a] The magnitude and intensity of the change in heart rate are related to the duration and intensity of the stimulus and the temperament of the individual infant.

The body cannot sustain the stress response for extended periods. Physiologic adaptation will occur, sometimes within minutes of the painful stimulus. Vital signs will return to normal, and other physical parameters associated with acute pain, such as sweating and pupillary dilation, will cease. A nurse assessing a child for pain may be misled by the presence of "normal" physiologic parameters. Although appealing as concrete markers, physiologic indicators often are not sensitive for distress of a prolonged nature. Other more complex modalities, such as serum cortisol or endorphin levels, are relatively invasive and not practical for real-time usage, and techniques such as palmar sweat measurement require complex apparatus for evaluation, which is well beyond most routine clinical settings.

Other Considerations in Assessment

Culture plays a role in children's reports and responses to pain. As racial and cultural diversity increases in the United States, clinicians should be familiar with beliefs and practices common to the cultural groups they serve and have their pain assessment tools translated into languages of their patients. A clear standard of care has emerged requiring that routine measurement of pain be done at regular intervals using consistent and valid criteria.[11] For critically ill infants and children, this practice includes assessment intervals of every 4 to 8 hours at a minimum,[31] as well follow-up for any pharmacologic and nonpharmacologic interventions administered to them.

In children who cannot report on their own pain, parent ratings may be the best proxy measure available. Most parents provide information on how to ask the children about pain and which cues to look for. Parents appear to be highly aware of particular behaviors exhibited by their children when experiencing pain in the postoperative setting. Parents' perceptions of their children's pain are also important, and nurses can encourage them to participate in pain assessment.[32] More needs to be known about parents' rating of their own children's pain.

ASSESSMENT OF AGITATION

Agitation is a form of behavioral communication for patients who are unable to communicate their discomfort verbally because of age, illness, neurologic status, or intubation. Agitation is not a diagnosis; it is simply a sign that something is wrong and may be caused by life-threatening events, such as hypoxia; emotional distress, such as anxiety; physical distresses from pain or nausea; drug reactions or withdrawal when physiologically dependent; or environmental factors. Environmental reasons for agitation may be related to a cold or hot room temperature, noises associated with anticipated unpleasant procedures, or lack of parental presence.

Assessing and managing severe agitation in an infant present a challenge to pediatric nurses. Nurses must constantly review a mental "checklist" of possible causes for agitation in their patients using a calm, systematic approach to determine the cause of the behavior, such as the rapid decisions outlined in the algorithm in Fig. 17-4. If a patient is supported on a ventilator, a quick check for technologic causes by hand ventilation with a bag-mask device may determine if this is the cause of the agitation. In general, pain is to be considered and ruled out as a contributing factor in a patient with repeated episodes of agitation. A trial of analgesics, even in the absence of a clear pain source, is appropriate and is to be included in the systematic approach to managing agitation in a critically ill child.

Treatment of agitation becomes critical to reduce a child's own harmful activities, such as self-extubation, removal of arterial and venous catheters, increased systemic and myocardial oxygen consumption, and a lack of cooperation with medical treatments. Opioids and sedatives are administered to reach the desired clinical outcome to reduce pain and anxiety. Undersedation is more easily detectable because agitation behaviors include overt symptoms of hypertension, tachycardia, respiratory distress, and physical movements to displace catheters. However, oversedation is often more difficult to assess because it has a more insidious onset caused by drug accumulation and difficulty in differentiating it from the severity of the underlying illness. Noting oversedation is especially important because its side effects include respiratory depression and problems in weaning from the ventilator, hemodynamic instability, gastrointestinal stasis, muscle wasting, and decreased ability to communicate.[1,33] Additional risks for prolonged effects and toxicity from accumulated metabolites of sedatives occur in some patients, such as those with renal or hepatic failure, because of impaired excretion of these medications.

The goal of sedation is to provide a level of medication to promote sleep and reduce anxiety for the child yet allow caregivers to arouse him or her for assessment and provide ongoing medical interventions. Specifically, sedation allows compliance with mechanical ventilation but also prevents awareness of the potentially very frightening environment of the PICU. Nurses often rely on subjective methods to determine the effectiveness of the sedative regimen rather than standardized tools such as sedation scales, which hampers consistent documentation of levels of sedation and thus communication within the team of caregivers. A wide

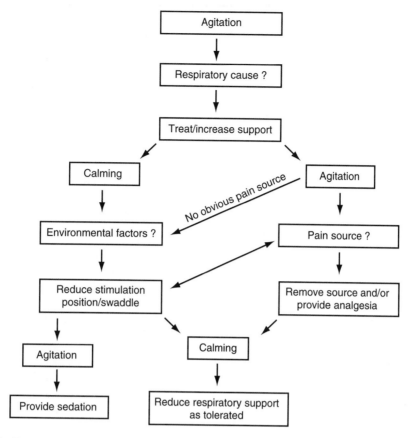

Fig. 17-4   Decision flowchart for assessment and management of agitated infants. (Adapted from Gordin PC: Assessing and managing agitation in a critically ill infant, *MCN Am J Matern Child Nurs* 15:26-32, 1990.)

range of adjectives with ambiguous definitions are commonly applied to describe an appropriately sedated patient, such as "snowed," "chilled," or "fidgety."

Clearly, a means of reliably measuring the level of sedation in ICU patients on a continuous basis, including both physiologic parameters and behavioral responses to the therapy, would be advantageous. Currently, limited clinical research is available on the use of assessment tools for measuring the depth of sedation in the critically ill that could be used to titrate sedatives. Plasma concentration monitoring is generally not useful, and drug therapy monitoring is better accomplished using observational and objective criteria.

Observational Tools

One of the earliest scales to be developed was the Ramsey scale, which is considered the criterion reference method for assessing sedation. This tool is often used in adult and pediatric ICU settings as the principal method for numerically ranking a patient's level of consciousness because of its availability and ease of use. However, it has not been tested for its reliability and validity. Other limitations are that it is not designed to be a continuous method of assessment, with overlapping categories not clearly defined.[1,33,34] For example, it is not clear if the Ramsey score is defined as a level 1 or level 4 for a patient who is asleep but responds to a light stimulus by becoming anxious or

agitated. Also, it is not clear how to rate a patient's sedation if he or she is unresponsive to a voice but yet is biting the endotracheal tube (ETT). Responsiveness scales such as the Ramsey scale have a major limitation regarding the need to measure the arousability of the patient, which is counterproductive to the goal of sedation in a critically ill child because he or she is repeatedly disturbed from rest.

Recently, other scales have been developed to overcome these shortcomings. The Comfort Scale is an eight-dimensional observational scale used to measure general distress in PICU patients without requiring arousability as a criteria[35] (Table 17-4). This tool encompasses the physiologic and behavioral responses associated with pain, anxiety, and fear. Following staff training of 2 hours, it is reported to be clinically useful, valid, and reliable, with an administration time of 3 minutes. Other critical care professionals have demonstrated adequacy of sedation within a target score ranging from 17 to 26 out of a total score of 40.[36] Although not validated for preterm infants, it has been used to assess levels of sedation and an increase in agitation at the time of withdrawal of morphine infusion.[19]

Two similar scales in the literature for adult ICU patients are the Motor Activity Assessment Scale (MAAS) and the Sedation-Agitation Scale (SAS). The MAAS categorizes patients across a wide cognitive spectrum, from those unresponsive to usual stimuli to those who are dangerously agitated[33] (Table 17-5). Clear and concise descriptions are

TABLE 17-4 Comfort Scale

Criteria/Descriptor	Score	Criteria/Descriptor	Score
Alertness		**Heart Rate Baseline** _____	
Deeply asleep	1	Heart rate below baseline	1
Lightly asleep	2	Heart rate consistently at baseline	2
Drowsy	3	Infrequent elevations ≥15% above	3
Fully awake and alert	4	baseline (1-3) during observation period	
Hyperalert	5	Frequent elevations of ≥15% above baseline	4
Calmness/Agitation		(more than 3)	
Calm	1	Sustained elevation of ≥15%	5
Slightly anxious	2	**Muscle Tone**	
Anxious	3	Muscles totally relaxed; no muscle tone	1
Very anxious	4	Reduced muscle tone	2
Panicky	5	Normal muscle tone	3
Respiratory Response		Increased muscle tone and flexion of fingers	4
No coughing and no spontaneous respiration	1	and toes	
Spontaneous respiration with little or no response to ventilation	2	Extreme muscle rigidity and flexion of fingers and toes	5
Occasional cough or resistance to ventilator	3	**Facial Tension**	
Actively breathes against ventilator or coughs regularly	4	Facial muscles totally relaxed	1
Fights ventilator, coughing or choking	5	Facial muscle tone normal; no facial muscle tension evident	2
Physical Movement		Tension evident in some facial muscles	3
No movement	1	Tension evident throughout facial muscles	4
Occasional, slight movement	2	Facial muscles contorted and grimacing	5
Frequent, slight movement	3		
Vigorous movement limited to extremities	4		
Vigorous movement including torso and head	5		
Blood Pressure (MAP) Baseline _____			
Blood pressure below baseline	1		
Blood pressure consistently at baseline	2		
Infrequent elevations of 15% or more (1-3)	3		
Frequent elevations of 15% or more (more than 3)	4		
Sustained elevation ≥15%	5	Total Score = _____	

From Marx CM, Smith P, Lowrie LH et al: Optimal sedation of mechanically ventilated pediatric critical care patients, *Crit Care Med* 22:163-170, 1994.

TABLE 17-5 Modified Motor Activity Assessment Scale

Score	Description	Definition
−3	Unresponsive	Minimal or no response to noxious* stimulus; does not communicate or follow commands.
−2	Responsive only to noxious stimuli	Opens eyes or raises eyebrows or turns head toward stimulus or moves limbs with noxious stimulus.
−1	Responsive to touch or name	Opens eyes or raises eyebrows or turns head toward stimulus or moves limbs with touch or when name is spoken; drifts off after stimulation; follows simple commands.
0	Calm and cooperative	No external stimulus is required to elicit movement; calm, awakens easily, and follows commands.
+1	Restless and cooperative	No external stimulus is required to elicit movement; picking at tubes but consolable.
+2	Agitated	No external stimulus is required to elicit movement; attempting to sit or move limbs to get up and inconsolable despite frequent attempts; requires physical restraint, biting ETT.
+3	Dangerously agitated, uncooperative	No external stimulus is required to elicit movement; patient unsafe—attempting to pull at ETT/catheters; desaturating; thrashing side-to-side; climbing over the rail; striking at staff.

Modified by Boston Children's Hospital from Devlin JW, Boleski G, Mlynarek M et al: Motor activity assessment scale: a valid and reliable sedation scale for use with mechanically ventilated patients in an adult surgical intensive care unit, *Crit Care Med* 27:1271-1275, 1999, via personal communication from Curley MAQ, 1999.
*Noxious stimulus, suctioning or 5 seconds of nail bed pressure.
ETT, Endotracheal tube.

used for each of the six categories, with higher scores indicating increasing levels of agitation. Beginning efforts to establish validity and reliability of the MAAS are being done in a surgical ICU setting with patients over 18 years of age receiving mechanical ventilation,[33] as well as in a PICU.[37] Nurses have found the MAAS to be easy to use in assessing and documenting the level of sedation following administration of sedative agents, as well as accurately reflecting the patient's true level of sedation. One problem is that only motor ability is assessed, not physiologic indicators, such as heart rate, which might be useful in neurologically impaired patients.

The SAS involves rating agitated behavior that is already occurring, such as thrashing movements, or actually stimulating the calmer adult to determine his or her arousability.[34] Each patient assessment took 2 to 5 minutes, and studies to indicate its use as a reliable and valid tool for describing sedation and agitation in adult ICU patients have begun.[38]

These scales are limited to those children with otherwise normal neurologic responses because many criteria within them require some form of motor movement. Researchers have not defined the optimal level of sedation using either the MAAS or SAS. For all three scales, clinicians must know that the satisfactory or appropriate level of sedation will vary from patient to patient and at different times for the same patient. A clear end point as the optimal level of sedation needs to be defined yet targeted for individual patients.

Bispectral Index

Anesthesiologists have long sought to catalog specific electroencephalogram (EEG) changes induced by various anesthetic and sedative agents. Despite predictions that the EEG could be a clinically useful monitor of "anesthetic depth," multiple technical problems and clinical complexities precluded its routine use as a monitor of anesthetic effect. A recently developed EEG machine (Aspect, A-1000, Natick, Mass.) converts the continuous output of the raw EEG pattern into continuous trends for a number of derived variables, such as the bispectral index (BIS).[39] The BIS has proven to be a valid and reliable measure of hypnotic drug effect in the operating room, but it has only recently been considered for use in ICU. Simmons and colleagues[38] explored use of this technique in assessing sedation as propofol was titrated in adult patients supported on mechanical ventilation who were recovering from surgery or trauma and comparing it with the SAS. The depth of sedation could be better estimated by using the BIS than by using clinical signs alone.[39]

The BIS measures a state of the brain, not a concentration of a particular drug. Interpretation of the BIS is predicated on the assumption that sedation is intended to produce a state of sleep that includes a lack of awareness and a lack of recall, whereas analgesia is intended to produce a state of reduced pain perception manifested by decreased autonomic responses to noxious stimuli. In general, a BIS score is a discrete value between 0 and 100, with awake patients scoring in the mid to upper 90s, conscious sedation dropping the BIS to 70s to 80s, and general anesthesia having scores in the 40 to 60 range.[38] No identification of a "best" level of sedation has been determined. This new monitoring technique is promising; however, more investigation is necessary to determine the reliability of the BIS and how it can be used to provide optimal sedation and analgesia, including its economic impact, before it can be incorporated into routine clinical practice in the future.

NONPHARMACOLOGIC MANAGEMENT OF PAIN AND AGITATION

Although the research is not as well established, nonpharmacologic interventions for the reduction of pain and agitation have long been recognized as enhancing or complementary to other medical interventions. Key recommendations are that these interventions work best when introduced early in the course of illness as a part of a multimodal treatment approach and that they should not be considered as a substitute for analgesics.[7,11] The best management involves an integrated approach that considers both pharmacologic and nonpharmacologic strategies with the overall goal to provide comfort. A wide array of interventions is available and effective in making pain more tolerable for some children, especially during medical procedures.[40] Still, nonpharmacologic interventions are often neglected. However, many of these methods fall within the independent scope of nursing practice and contribute to a holistic approach to pain management building trusting relationships with children and their families.

Patients and parents are increasingly willing to try complementary and alternative therapies that involve mind-body interactions, including meditation, prayer, massage therapy, and healing or therapeutic touch, as part of their treatment.[41,42] Proponents of these interventions explain that by receiving caring and purposeful touching of the skin or in the form of pleasant distractions, the stress response is reduced, including a release of endogenous opioids, and pain is relieved. More controversy lies in the insistence that human energy fields can be manipulated to promote comfort and healing, such as that espoused by those who advocate therapeutic touch.[43,44]

Patients can learn to use music for both distraction and relaxation, as found effective in many settings such as PICUs or cancer units, particularly if patients are allowed to choose the type of music they want to hear.[45] Having available small, portable tape players with headsets to block out environmental noises and building a library of audiotapes with a variety of musical styles and artists have been found useful.

In addition, nurses are to take time to provide basic comfort measures. Attention to mouth care, eye care, preventing the pulling of tubes, itching, muscle cramps, and thirst may calm an agitated patient. A child can be positioned in neutral alignment, with all parts of the body supported and the joints slightly flexed. Frequent position changes are important and may be necessary more often than every 2 hours, depending on the medical status of the child. Positioning a patient so that self-calming behaviors (e.g., sucking a thumb or fingers) are supported is a simple way to assist patients to cope with the stressors inherent in PICU care.

Environmental Control

The PICU is a brightly lit and noisy place that is often overwhelming even to healthy adults who visit and work there. Thus the impact on sick infants and children as they are surrounded by unfamiliar equipment that looks and sounds threatening may be very disturbing. With the combination of the critical illness affecting many vital organs and the discomfort of many medical procedures, it is not surprising that some children become confused, agitated, or even combative. Behavioral conditioning may actually occur when a seemingly nonnoxious stimulus is paired with an unpleasant experience on a regular basis. Some common examples of this are the pairing of ventilator alarms with suctioning and handling of extremities before needlesticks for blood sampling or intravenous (IV) insertion. Some patients begin to expect that whenever they hear a ventilator alarm or feel someone touch their foot that something unpleasant will happen. This association can result in agitated behavior that seems to occur without any consistent pattern. Careful structuring of the patient's experiences to "unlearn" these associations is necessary to treat this cause of distress. However, preventing this type of learning is much easier than unlearning it after a problem develops. Using pleasant interventions, such as massage or music, to provide a signal to the child that a particular period is safe for them to relax is useful as well.

Promoting sleep both enhances psychologic health and provides physical benefits by promoting growth and healing, and it has become a focus of critical care study. Researchers have acknowledged that it is not safe or realistic to provide complete darkness or lack of assessment of a child in the PICU at night; however, they do point out that noise could be reduced by minimal alarm sounds and a concerted effort by staff to communicate in lowered tones and to refrain from past rituals of bathing children during the night shift.[46] Nurses can organize care by clustering assessments, medications, and interventions to allow maximum periods of undisturbed rest and sleep. A lack of sleep results in increasing anxiety and sensitivity to pain and discomfort, hyperactivity, and aggression, all leading to delirium. ICU psychosis, a pattern of agitation and delirium associated with being in the ICU 3 to 5 days, is most often caused by a combination of such factors as the patient's premorbid coping mechanisms and the environment, including a frightening atmosphere, lack of sleep, unusual and disturbing sounds, lack of windows, and deprivation of day-night cycles.[47] Simple strategies such as reducing unpleasant noises, such as applying rubber stoppers to the ends of suction tubing when not in use, are useful. Decreasing environmental stimulation has been particularly recommended for the treatment of mild opioid or benzodiazepine withdrawal.[31] Because many interactions are potentially threatening to children in the PICU, they may begin to generalize their distress toward all approaches by care-givers. When treatments and procedures are unexpected, children are kept in a constant state of tension and readiness. They may become distressed and hypersensitive to seemingly benign, routine procedures of care. Advocating for protected periods in which children are allowed freedom from the intrusive examinations and treatments, unless an unstable condition arises, may provide a sense of control for children. Whenever possible, nurses can provide a "routine" to children to introduce predictability into this chaotic environment, which may then help them cope with the many distressing experiences.

Infants and children with neurologic damage may be unable to regulate their own motor responses to the excessive sensory input of ICU. They may react positively to swaddling because it provides boundaries to the incoming stimuli and their ability to respond to it with disorganized motor responses.

Toddlers and older children need to understand what is happening to them. Not telling children that a procedure will be painful reduces their trust in the PICU staff. Toddlers and young children respond to brief honest explanations as to what is happening to them, as well as having whatever control is possible within the situation. The approach may be as simple as saying, "I know that this will hurt; however, if you take a deep breath and blow out slowly, it may hurt less." It is important to follow a procedure with praise for any cooperative behaviors. Even young children may be assigned a small "job" such as holding the tape, pouring saline on the dressing, or pulling off the old dressing. By being active participants in their care, children feel more in control rather than feeling controlled by their pain. Choices can be offered to the child whenever possible. For example, "Should we start with the burn dressing or the central line dressing change?"

Children say that parents are their greatest source of strength when facing pain.[24] Excluding a parent from observing an invasive procedure has been the traditional approach in PICUs, based on fears of parental interference or because of the view that it is better for the parent "not to see." This tradition is perceived by many parents as a major source of anxiety at a time that parents may perceive that it is crucial to the child's course of recovery to be there. A study by Powers and Rubenstein[48] challenges these assumptions as they surveyed parents of children undergoing intubation, central venous catheter placement, and chest tube placement, as well as the nurses involved in the procedure. Parental presence significantly reduced the parental anxiety related to the procedure. The reasons for this finding centered on the fact that the parents found that the actual procedure was far less noxious than what they had imagined and that they believed their presence was a comfort to their child until the sedation was given. Also, 94% of the nurses found a parent's presence helpful to the child and to the parents. None of the physicians in the study thought that the parents interfered or were in the way of them successfully performing all procedures.

Positive evidence has shown that parents are fairly accurate in predicting how distressed their children will be about an upcoming procedure. This finding seems to be due to the parents' knowledge of their children's usual pattern of reactions. Nurses should advocate for parent involvement in their children's care and praise them for providing soothing, nurturing behaviors in this high-tech environment. Because children may react to their parents' fears, parents should be provided with adequate support so that they can be effective with their critically ill child. They can learn how to use many of the cognitive/behavioral and physical comfort strategies described in the next sections.[49]

Cognitive Behavioral Techniques

Children have incredible inner resources that give them the ability to cope with distress: their imaginations, their ability to focus to the extent of being unaware of their surroundings, their ability to distract themselves through play, and their motivation to try new things. Nurses may tap into these resources and teach children, as well as their parents as their children's coaches, systematic strategies to cope with painful events.

This process can begin by assessing the degree the child can follow directions. Distraction is a highly effective method of relieving mild anxiety and pain because the child pays attention to the activity, not the painful stimulus.[50] For toddlers and preschool children, diversion activities such as counting and reciting nursery rhymes are easy to do, work well, and involve parental coaching of the children. Use of soothing, familiar music in the form of lullabies or tapes featuring the parents' voices may serve to divert children's attention and permit relaxation.

Play therapy and medical play are important for any child who is undergoing medical treatment. Through play, children gain more command and control over their hospital experience. Most patients in the PICU may not be able to actively participate in a program of medical play, but they can benefit from hearing stories or tapes about the hospital. As patients improve, more active play alternatives can be offered. By allowing children to play with and manipulate devices such as stethoscopes and needleless syringes, they gain a sense of mastery over the objects and become less sensitized to the presence of these objects at their bedside. After a distressing procedure, nurses should encourage children to express their feelings about pain. Medical play with dolls is a way of "working through" what has happened to them, whereas older children may want to draw pictures. If developmentally appropriate, the child can be encouraged to explore medical instruments, role-play procedures using dolls, and reenact procedures in a nonthreatening environment.

For children older than 6 years of age, focusing on a pleasant mental picture or mentally traveling to a place of contentment provides another means of coping with a painful activity. Such guided imagery is most effective if all of the senses are evoked (vision, hearing, smell, taste, movement). Another approach would be to have the child think of a favorite television show and becoming one of the characters. This strategy can also be used to rehearse mentally or prepare for a stressful situation, such as being a soldier fighting a battle; to decrease feelings of powerlessness.[50] A similar mind process is used when a child is coached to use positive self-talk: "I will be okay; this procedure will help make me well."

Controlled breathing to promote relaxation is another easy technique to use with children as they focus their attention on the movement of air in and out of their bodies during the procedure or "blowing away the pain." This can be followed with techniques promoting muscle relaxation of voluntary skeletal muscles for older children. Use of props such as blowing bubbles or party blowers have been found to be helpful.

The specific interventions used with a specific patient depend on the developmental stage, type of pain the child is experiencing, and personal preference and, for optimal learning, can be introduced and practiced when the child is not agitated or distressed. Additional interventions such as biofeedback and hypnosis are not as useful because they require specialized training, and children in the PICU are too tired or ill to participate.

Physical Comfort Measures

Massage techniques include simple rhythmic rubbing, stroking, and kneading of muscle and soft tissues and are effective in reducing edema, stiffness, and pain, especially in myofascial trigger points. Trigger points are small, circumscribed hypersensitive areas located within a tight band of muscle that develop as a result of acute or chronic muscle strain. Any area of the body can be massaged; favorite sites are the back, hands, and feet. Clinicians are to avoid massaging areas of thrombophlebitis, infection, or tissue necrosis and malignancies. This technique can easily be taught to parents.

For infants, rhythmic movement in the form of rocking helps with relaxation and decreases pain. Nonnutritive sucking with a pacifier is also comforting. Pretreatment of newborns up to 6 weeks of age with oral sucrose has shown a rapid and significant calming effect lasting for at least 4 minutes following a heel lance.[9] The theory is that sucking of sucrose reduces the stress response through endogenous opioids because subsequent administration of naloxone reverses the process.

Superficial heating or cooling techniques decrease sensitivity to pain. Because of the variable uses and contraindications to these techniques in relation to a specific injury, nurses must collaborate with physical therapists for specific uses. Warm compresses or a heating pad applied to the to painful site promotes relaxation and healing by improving circulation and availability of nutrients at the injured site, as well as reducing inflammatory edema. Heat is not to be used over areas of circulatory compromise or irradiated tissues. Cold compresses or ice packs reduce muscle spasms, skin sensitivity, inflammation, and joint stiffness. Precautions should be taken to ensure that the hot or cold packs are wrapped, allowing comfortable sensation of cold or heat without damaging the skin. Nurses should rotate ice packs to a new site at intervals no longer than 10 minutes.

Another form of cutaneous stimulation is transcutaneous electrical nerve stimulation (TENS), a battery-operated device that delivers a low-voltage electrical current through electrodes placed on skin. This method is most often used for musculoskeletal discomfort, phantom limb pain, or postoperative pain and is usually monitored by a physical therapist.

PHARMACOLOGIC MANAGEMENT OF PAIN AND AGITATION

A variety of medications are currently available to manage pain, including opioid and nonopioid analgesics, given systemically by different types of delivery systems, as well as regional and local anesthetic techniques. The goals of therapy must be to optimize pain control while minimizing side effects and adverse outcomes. For patients who are anxious or agitated, sedatives or anxiolytics are used to promote comfort by promoting relaxation and sleep, reducing anxiety, and increasing tolerance of common ICU interventions. The intricacy of treating relatively brief periods of acute, intense pain requires clinicians to follow principles of thinking preemptively. Nurses must be familiar with the time interval to onset of action, as well as expected duration of action of any analgesic or sedative given to their patients (Table 17-6).

The pharmacokinetics and pharmacodynamics of analgesics, anxiolytics, anesthetics, and sedatives are significantly altered in critically ill patients, requiring careful attention to individualizing the regimen for a specific patient. Drug toxicity may be a problem in critically ill patients, especially those with renal or hepatic compromise who are more likely to exhibit decreases in clearance, which results in longer durations of action from accumulation of the opioids, as well as any active metabolites, leading to prolonged sedation.

Opioids

Opioids remain the single most important group of medications for the relief of moderate to severe pain in PICU patients. Analgesia is achieved primarily by binding to μ-receptors in the peripheral, spinal, and supraspinal opioid receptors and, subsequently, inhibiting the release of several neurotransmitters, including substance P from the primary afferent terminals. In addition, inhibition of the conduction of pain up the spinothalamic tract by the opioid prevents the fibers from signaling to the brain that a painful situation exists.

Key Concepts Related to Opioids

Equianalgesia. Opioids bind to receptors with varying strengths, which contributes to different analgesic potency between different opioids.[10] The term *equianalgesia* refers to the fact that different opioids require different doses to provide approximately the same pain relief, usually comparing all available opioids to a specific dose of parenteral morphine. A common misconception is that the more potent a drug is, the more therapeutically superior it is. Potency is the ratio of the dose of two analgesics required to

produce the same analgesic effect. Fentanyl is more potent than morphine because the dose of morphine required to achieve the same analgesia as fentanyl is 100 times the fentanyl dose. However, fentanyl is not a more effective or superior opioid. Lack of knowledge regarding this concept often leads to undertreatment of pain.

Recommended Dosages. Most clinicians find it helpful to refer to a chart, such as Table 17-6, to provide a list of doses, both oral and parenteral, that are approximately equal to each other in their ability to provide pain relief. Such tables provide an initial dose as they convert from one opioid to another or when changing the route of administration; however, these guidelines are only to be considered as dosing estimates. Traditionally, the child's weight has been used to determine the starting opioid dose. Numerous variables can influence the appropriate dose for the individual patient. The optimal dose is to be determined always by titration.[51]

Ceiling Dose. Most drugs have a ceiling dose in which the recommended maximum dose is not to be exceeded because no further benefit will be gained yet side effects will be increased. However, opioids have no ceiling dose for analgesia, meaning that as doses are increased, further increases in analgesia continue to be achieved. Doses of opioids are escalated until pain relief occurs or side effects intervene. There is no predetermined maximum dose of an opioid.

Considerable variation, as much as a tenfold difference, is found among patients in their opioid requirements during the postoperative period.[52] All opioid analgesics have recommended initial doses (see Table 17-6). For children who remain alert and are still experiencing pain, it is safe to titrate further doses, using doses equivalent to half the initial dose. Opioid response increases linearly with the log of the dose. Thus a dose increment of less than 30% to 50% is not likely to improve analgesia significantly for those in moderate to severe pain.[52] Very high doses of opioids may be required in patients with terminal cancer or extensive burns (because of hypermetabolism).[53] This wide variability reinforces the need for prompt and individualized attention to unrelieved pain.

Tolerance. Continued exposure to opioids results in tolerance, which is a pharmacologic property of opioids and benzodiazepines in which higher doses are required to gain the same effect. It is usually managed by increasing the dose, although the addition of other analgesics, sedatives, or both may be clinically beneficial. The rate at which tolerance develops depends on the pattern of use. If treatment is intermittent, adequate sedative and analgesic effects are possible with standard doses of opioids and benzodiazepines for a longer period. However, if the drug is given continuously, significant tolerance can develop more quickly. Tolerance is not related to an increase in the rate of metabolism but rather to alterations in receptor numbers and sensitivities. When tolerance to a specific opioid develops, incomplete cross-tolerance to other opioids develops. By changing from one opioid to another, the analgesia achieved is often improved with lower doses of the newer opioid, even using appropriate calculations to account for differences in potency. Therefore when patients are switched to another opioid, the starting dose of the new drug can be reduced to 50% to 75% of the equianalgesic dose to account for this incomplete cross-tolerance.[52]

Physical dependence is also a pharmacologic property of opioids that is defined by a withdrawal syndrome following sudden discontinuation of the opioid or administration of an opioid antagonist. Generally, physical dependence is assumed to develop after 2 to 7 days of opioid therapy.[2,31,49] Further details on how to wean a patient from opioids are offered in a later section of this chapter.

Management of Side Effects

Central nervous system effects include drowsiness, confusion, and dizziness, which can occur initially but usually disappear within a few days. Nurses should ensure that a sedated patient can be easily aroused during this time; otherwise, this is a warning that further opioid doses could lead to respiratory depression. A patient who has been in severe pain may be sleep deprived; once the pain is controlled, he or she may be "catching up" on sleep. This is not a sign of overdosage as long as the patient is arousable. Other effects from opioids include myoclonus, which is the involuntary jerking of the muscles. Although the mechanism for its cause is unclear, a benzodiazepine or barbiturate may be useful in its management.

Clinically significant respiratory depression is the most feared of the opioid-induced side effects. Like sedation, tolerance to respiratory depression develops over days. The longer the patient receives opioids, the wider the margin of safety. Patients most at risk are infants younger than 6 months of age. A decreased metabolic rate and a less restrictive blood-brain barrier predispose the neonate to a greater risk of opioid-induced respiratory depression. Therefore correct dosing and careful monitoring are crucial when newborns and young infants are treated with opioids.

Pain is a potent respiratory stimulant and counteracts opioid-induced respiratory depression. Patients do not succumb to opioid-induced respiratory depression while awake and in pain.[15] No additional doses of opioids are to be given to children who are somewhat sedated but have no signs of respiratory compromise. They are to be assessed frequently for break-through pain and further need for analgesia. Mild respiratory depression can be managed by reducing the opioid dose, whereas with moderate to severe depression, stimulation, airway support, and bag-mask ventilation are to be considered. If administration of opioid antagonists such as naloxone (Narcan) becomes necessary, it is to be given in frequent low-dose boluses because it is not a benign medication. Giving too much naloxone or giving it too rapidly can increase sympathetic activity, leading to hypertension, tachycardia, ventricular dysrhythmias, vomiting, pulmonary edema, and cardiac arrest, in addition to precipitating severe pain that is extremely difficult to control. One method is to mix an ampule (0.4 mg) with 10 ml of normal saline and slowly

administer a dose of 0.5 ml IV every 2 minutes until respirations improve.[15] Nurses should discontinue administering the naloxone as soon as patients are responsive to physical stimulation and are able to take deep breaths. Patients who have been receiving opioids for more than 1 week may be exquisitely sensitive to antagonists.[53,54] Sometimes administering more than one dose of naloxone is necessary because the half-life for naloxone is significantly shorter than that of opioids, thus requiring continuous monitoring for the first few hours. The goal is to reverse the respiratory depression without compromising analgesia. Obviously, the potential for respiratory depression is of less concern in infants and children receiving mechanical ventilation.

Cardiovascular effects theorized as the result of histamine release can cause vasodilation, resulting in hypotension, especially when patients are hypovolemic or have poor cardiovascular reserves. Pruritus, usually confined to the face and hairline and not associated with a rash, is presumed to result from the histamine release. Treatment consists of giving antihistamines, such as diphenhydramine (Benadryl), or changing to another opioid in which pruritus may not occur. Infusions of low-dose opioid antagonists, such as naloxone, sometimes prescribed for prevention and treatment of pruritus, have been proposed but require close monitoring to ensure avoidance of reversing the analgesic effects as well.[54] Genitourinary effects from increased smooth muscle tone within the bladder can lead to sphincter spasm and urinary retention. Tolerance develops quickly, but urinary catheterization may be necessary for short-term management.

Nausea and vomiting usually subside after a few days of use of opioids. Slow and steady opioid titration helps to reduce nausea. Historically, clinicians have added an antiemetic with the additional idea that it will potentiate the analgesic effect of the opioid. However, there is no scientific basis for the belief that phenothiazines such as promethazine enhance the analgesic effects of opioids.[54] In fact, some studies indicate that promethazine increases sensitivity to pain and increase the amount of opioids required to produce satisfactory pain relief.[54]

Constipation is of concern for those patients receiving around-the-clock (ATC) opioid regimens of more than a few days. Stool softeners often are not enough to prevent constipation with chronic opioid use. Clinicians must be vigilant to signs of constipation and consider administering a laxative. Other therapies such as oral naloxone have received some attention because it is poorly absorbed following oral administration, and its effects may be limited to the gastrointestinal system[52] without reversing the needed analgesic effects.

Simply decreasing the opioid dose often is sufficient to eliminate or make a side effect more tolerable, or if this strategy is ineffective, children may benefit from a change in opioid. Some patients may not tolerate a particular opioid but will do well with another. The exact reasons for this are not fully explained. Vigilant pain assessment and evaluation of the patient's response to the new opioid guide further titration of the new opioid.

TABLE 17-6 Pharmacologic Management of Pain and Agitation

Drug	Initial Dose	Approximate Equianalgesic Dose	Onset of Action	Duration of Action	Half-life With Active Metabolites
Opioid Analgesics					
Morphine	Intermittent IV bolus: 0.05-0.3 mg/kg q2-4h Continuous IV infusion: 0.03-0.06 mg/kg/hr with initial bolus of 0.05 mg/kg Oral: 0.15-0.3 mg/kg q4h	IV: 10 mg	IV: 2-10 min	IV: 2-5 hr	Infants and toddlers: 1-12 hr Older children: 1-3 hr
Fentanyl	Intermittent IV bolus: 1-2 μg/kg Continuous IV infusion: 1-3 μg/kg/hr Epidural: continuous infusion: 0.4-1 μg/kg/hr	IV: 0.1 mg	3-5 min	0.5-1 hr	IV:3 hr (may be up to 36 hr after long-term infusions)
Hydromorphone (Dilaudid)	Intermittent IV bolus: 0.015 mg/kg/dose q4-6h	IV: 1.5 mg	2-10 min	3-4 hr	1-3 hr
Methadone	Intermittent IV bolus or oral: 0.1 mg/kg (maximum: 10 mg/dose); for either route, give q4h for 2-3 doses, then every 12 hr as needed	IV or oral: 10 mg	IV: 10-20 min Oral: 30-60 min	IV: 4-6 hr Oral: 6-8 hr; increases to 22-48 hr with repeated doses	4-62 hr
Oxycodone	Oral: 0.1 mg/kg q4h	Oral: 10 mg	10-15 min	3-6 hr	1.2-3 hr
Nonopioids					
Choline magnesium trisalicylate (Trilisate)	Oral: 10-15 mg/kg q8-12h (maximum: 1 g/dose or 3 g/day)	NA	30-60 min	4-6 hr	NA
Ketoralac (Toradol)	IV bolus: 0.5 mg/kg q6h (maximum: 30 mg/dose with no more than 5 days of use)	NA	30-60 min	4-6 hr	NA

Drug	Dose		Onset	Duration	Half-life
Acetaminophen (Tylenol)	Oral: 10-15 mg/kg q4h (maximum: 75 mg/kg/dose)	NA	30-60 min	3-4 hr	NA
Gabapentin (Neurontin)	Oral: 5 mg/kg or 100 mg bid; increase gradually to 300-400 mg PO tid	NA	NA	NA	NA
Sedatives/Anxiolytics/Anesthetics					
Lorazepam	Oral and IV: 0.03-0.1 mg/kg q6h (maximum: 2 mg/dose)	NA	IV: 1-5 min PO: 30-60 min	3-4 hr	10-20 hr
Midazolam	IV bolus: 0.05-0.15 mg/kg Continuous IV infusion: IV loading dose of 0.05-0.2 mg/kg followed by infusion of 1-2 µg/kg/min	NA	IV: 1-3 min PO: 10-30 min	1-3 hr	2-20 hr
Pentobarbital	Oral: 0.5-0.75 mg/kg (maximum dose: 20 mg) IV bolus: 0.5-1 mg/kg followed by repeated doses of 1 mg/kg q3-5min (maximum total dose of 6 mg/kg)	NA	1-10 min	1-4 hr	NA
Haloperidol	PO/IV: 0.1-0.5 mg/kg/day given in 2-3 divided doses; maximum: 0.15 mg/kg/day IM: 1-3 mg/dose q4-8h to a maximum of 0.15 mg/kg/day	NA	PO: Peak concentration 2-6 hr IM: 1-3 hr IV: 1-2 hr	PO: 8 hr IM/IV: 4-8 hr	NA
Chloral hydrate	PO/PR: 25-50 mg/kg; may repeat × 1	NA	10-60 min	2-8 hr	8-30 hr
Ketamine	IV bolus: 0.25-2 mg/kg/dose IV continuous infusion: 5-100 µg/kg/min	NA	0.5-1 min	3-10 min	NA
Propofol	IV bolus: 0.5-3 mg/kg Continuous IV infusion: 50-200 µg/kg/min	NA	0.5-3 min	5-20 min	8-12 min

From Yaster M, Krane EJ, Kaplan RF et al, eds: *Pediatric pain management and sedation handbook*; 1997, St Louis, 1997, Mosby; St. Jude Children's Research Hospital Pharmaceutical Department: *Formulary handbook*, Hudson, Ohio, 2000, Lexi-Comp; Harvey MA: Managing agitation in critically ill patients, *Am J Crit Care* 5:12, 1996; Yaster M, Berde C, Billet C: The management of opioid and benzodiazepine dependence in infants, children, and adolescents, *Pediatrics* 98:135-139, 1996; Gordin PC: Assessing and managing agitation in a critically ill infant. *MCN Am J Matern Child Nurs* 15:26-32, 1990; Chambliss CR, Anand KJS: Pain management in the pediatric intensive care unit, *Curr Opin Pediatr* 9:248-253, 1997.

NA, Not applicable or no available information.

Specific Opioids

Morphine is considered the "gold standard" of opioids. The clearance of morphine is increased in patients with extensive burns or sickle cell disease, thus requiring higher doses titrated to clinical effect.[2,53] Septic shock and renal disease decrease the clearance of morphine and its active glucuronide metabolites, respectively.

Hydromorphone (Dilaudid) is similar to morphine with anecdotal reports of less risk of pruritus. However, a metabolite may accumulate in renal failure, resulting in neurotoxicity and cognitive impairment.

Fentanyl has several advantages in the critical care setting: a rapid onset of action; relative short duration, which makes it useful for short-term procedural-related pain; and because fentanyl administration is not associated with histamine release, it has become a popular analgesic for critically ill patients at risk for hypotension and bronchospasm. It is suitable for continuous infusions or transdermal delivery. A new preparation, oral transmucosal fentanyl citrate (OTFC), has good oral bioavailability by sublingual absorption and can be used as an effective preoperative analgesic and sedative, especially when IV access is not available. However, several disadvantages with fentanyl by any route are seen clinically. Tolerance and dependence predictably develop much more quickly than with other opioids, as soon as after only 5 to 10 days of continuous fentanyl infusions, leading to frequent dose escalation.[2] The clearance is dependent on hepatic blood flow and thus may be decreased in cardiac failure. Chest wall rigidity may follow rapid IV administration of doses greater than which would best be managed by administering a neuromuscular blocking agent, naloxone, or both. More potent opioids similar to fentanyl are sufentanil and alfentanil. However, they are less useful in PICUs because of cost and familiarity in dosing and do not offer any significant pharmacokinetic advantage over fentanyl.[53]

Methadone is a synthetic opioid with a long half-life following IV or oral administration[2] and produces less sedation and gastrointestinal effects than other opioids. Thus it is useful in providing a smooth transition from IV to oral opioids as an effective analgesic, while suppressing withdrawal symptoms even at low doses.

Oxycodone, often compounded with other agents such as acetaminophen (Percocet), is also useful in mild to moderate pain. However, this opioid is not available in a parenteral form. Clinicians are to be mindful of the fact that although there is no ceiling dose of oxycodone, there is one for acetaminophen (75 mg/kg/day or 15 mg/kg/dose) to avoid the risk of hepatic toxicity. Therefore clinicians can use the noncompounded form, oxycodone, with its long-acting form, called OxyContin, for those patients in which hepatic toxicity is to be avoided. *Hydrocodone* (Lortab, Vicodin) is also useful in treating mild to moderate pain. However, it is available in the United States only as a compounded product with acetaminophen.

No advantages of using meperidine over morphine have been proven. Yet the use of meperidine has a distinct disadvantage over other opioids; its metabolite (normeperidine) may accumulate in patients with impaired renal function, leading to central nervous system irritability and seizures. Therefore it is no longer recommended for critically ill patients.[2] Clinicians should not give naloxone for meperidine-associated seizures because doing so will only add to the neurotoxicity. By an unclear mechanism, meperidine does provide effective reversal of shivering secondary to anesthesia and amphotericin-associated rigors, making an occasional bolus the only justified use of this opioid.

Mixed agonists-antagonists opioids *(nalbuphine, butorphanol)* have the theoretical advantage of causing less respiratory depression than pure opioids. Their use in severe pain is limited by their ceiling effects and their potential to reverse pure opioid agents previously given and precipitate withdrawal[2] and therefore are not recommended for use for continuing painful states, such as those that children experience during critical illness.

Special considerations are necessary when giving opioids to young infants. Generally, morphine given to infants younger than 6 months of age tends to have a longer elimination half-life and a lower clearance rate.[55] The duration of action of morphine is highly variable among infants in this age group. Because of the unpredictability in response, opioid titration in young infants must be conservative, with a recommended morphine starting dose of 0.01 to 0.03 mg/kg. The infant's response to an opioid dose is to be assessed carefully. Once the infant's response is known, it becomes easier to titrate further doses of opioid.

Drug Delivery Systems

Medical conditions in PICU patients such as an ileus or recent gastrointestinal surgery, along with concerns for poor drug absorption, may preclude the use of oral agents. The availability of IV access eliminates the necessity for intramuscular injections to provide analgesia for children.

Traditional approaches to pain management have been through as-needed (prn) doses of analgesics, which, by design, dictate that patients experience reemergence of pain before each new request, as well as requiring the child to notify the caregiver that he or she is experiencing pain. Younger children may not understand the concept between requesting pain medication and obtaining pain relief, whereas older children will often deny or endure pain to avoid an intramuscular injection. Many as-needed dosing regimens result in patients receiving no or little analgesics. Analgesics are always more effective, actually with less dosage, in preventing pain rather than overcoming established pain by "chasing it." An as-needed schedule is appropriate for children who have intermittent (pain separated by pain-free intervals), unpredictable pain, or pain related to specific activities.

PICU patients often experience pain continuously. Therefore effective pain management strategies include techniques that permit continuous delivery of analgesics, such as ATC scheduled dosing or continuous infusions, and provision of additional analgesic doses for break-through pain.[13,15] For continuous pain, effective analgesia requires the maintenance of constant serum and cerebrospinal fluid concentrations of the opioids, achieved by continuous IV infusions. For patients receiving continuous infusions of opioids, titrating or adjusting the dose according to anticipated responses of the patients to problems or procedures provides critical care nurses a prevention-based focus for care. Continuous infusions avoid the peaks and troughs of blood concentrations associated with side effects and inadequate analgesia. On the other hand, bolus dosing offers rapid onset of analgesia when the patient is either about to experience pain or the level of pain intensity has suddenly increased. "Rescue doses" are supplemental doses offered to patients on ATC schedules to treat pain that "breaks through" the baseline analgesic level. The size and frequency of rescue dosing vary with the route of administration. As baseline doses are escalated, rescue doses need to be adjusted. Adjustment of the opioid dose is essential throughout the patient's course of illness.

A common way of offering patients an interactive method of treating their own pain by way of self-administration of the rescue doses is with the use of patient-controlled analgesia (PCA) devices. These devices allow parenteral delivery of opioids on demand, according to parameters set by the healthcare team. The pump can be programmed to provide a background, continuous infusion yet allow the child to push a button to deliver a rescue dose at programmed intervals. Although the child may push the PCA button frequently, the PCA device will only successfully deliver a opioid dose when the preset lockout time has passed. For safety, a total hourly maximum setting limits the overall availability of opioid to the patient.

Patients must be alert, oriented, and physically able to push a button. Although usage of the PCA requires adequate understanding of instructions by the child, pumps are routinely effective in children 7 years of age and older and have been used successfully in children as young as 5 years of age.[10,24] For young children or those who are developmentally delayed and not cognitively able to understand how to self-administer analgesics, some experts advocate for family-controlled analgesia and nurse-activated dosing. Potential candidates for parent-controlled analgesia are to be considered carefully. Because the child's safety is paramount, caregivers are to carefully evaluate parents in terms of their ability to provide parent-controlled analgesia. Parents who successfully manage the care of a chronically ill child at home may be very capable of assuming the responsibilities for parent-controlled analgesia. They may wish to retain some control over their child's care during a hospital stay and are often familiar with hospital routines. On the other hand, parents of children who are undergoing a single elective procedure may not be the best candidates to provide parent-controlled analgesia. These families are unfamiliar with the hospital routine and the care of their child after surgery.

PCA addresses the variations in analgesic requirements between individuals. With a PCA, the patient is able to finely titrate the amount of opioid delivered to simultaneously maximize analgesia and minimize side effects. Patients gain an element of self-control when using PCA. They are no longer as dependent on healthcare providers to

ensure pain relief. Most patients report greater satisfaction with pain relief when using PCA in comparison with more traditional methods of pain management.[6] Extensive experience has been reported with various opioids. A common regimen for morphine includes a loading dose, if needed, of 0.05 mg/kg, followed by a moderate basal rate (0.03-0.06 mg/kg/hr), with rescue doses 30% to 50% of the hourly continuous dose every 10 to 15 minutes.

Nonopioids

Nonopioids, including acetaminophen and acetylsalicylic acid, or other NSAIDs, such as ibuprofen, are employed for mild to moderate pain. Unfortunately, these medications do have a ceiling effect that makes them inappropriate for treating severe pain. However, they can be used in combination with opioids to lower the opioid dose requirements and incidence of opioid-related side effects.

NSAIDs act peripherally to provide their analgesic effect by interfering with the synthesis of prostaglandin, through the inhibition of cyclooxygenase (COX). There are two isoenzymes of COX: COX-1 and COX-2. The COX-1 isoform is expressed primarily in the kidney, gastrointestinal tract, and platelets. In contrast, the COX-2 isoform is found in low levels in tissues but is induced during inflammation. By selectively inhibiting the COX-2 isoform, prostaglandin pathways are influenced, decreasing pain and inflammation and avoiding the toxicities of the inhibition of COX-1. Most NSAIDs are nonselective inhibitors of COX. At present, two selective COX-2 inhibitors are available (celecoxib and rofecoxib) for which platelet aggregation does not appear to be effected at indicated dosages.[56] However, limited pediatric data is available for dosing, as well as side effects for these selective COX-2 inhibitors. Also, the COX-2 inhibitors are not recommended for use in patients with advanced renal disease.

Serious side effects of nonselective NSAIDs include (1) gastrointestinal irritation and bleeding, (2) coagulopathies from decreased platelet aggregation, and (3) nephrotoxicity. Prolonged administration (greater than 5 to 7 days) or concurrent use with other nephrotoxic drugs are to be avoided, especially for children with preexisting renal dysfunction.[52] The nonselective NSAID, choline magnesium trisalicylate (Trilisate) is preferred in patients who have a risk of bleeding because it has less effect on platelet aggregation and no effect on bleeding time at the usual clinical doses.[52]

Ketorolac (Toradol) is the only parenteral NSAID with a potency similar to opioids and has been shown to be effective in postoperative pain in children, especially if given preemptively and continued on an ATC schedule. However, all NSAIDs are to be used with extreme caution in patients with extensive surgical dissection, such as posttonsillectomy, because clinical trials of NSAID therapy have demonstrated increased postoperative blood loss.[2] Also, ketorolac is useful in treating vasoocclusive crises in sickle cell disease.

Acetaminophen is an effective oral analgesic and antipyretic with a low side-effect profile (no reduction in platelet activity and minimal gastric irritation). However, it is a weak antiinflammatory agent, and hepatotoxicity is of concern with doses of more than 75 mg/kg/day.

Medicines for Neuropathic Pain

Early recognition and aggressive therapy improve the prognosis for the resolution of neuropathic pain. Although some patients report relief using NSAIDs and other nonopioid analgesics, neuropathic pain is less responsive to opioids than nociceptive pain[52,57] without dosages leading to unacceptable side effects. Several classes of drugs that are not traditional analgesics are more often useful, including (1) tricyclic antidepressants such as amitriptyline (Elavil) and (2) anticonvulsants such as gabapentin (Neurontin), phenytoin (Dilantin), or carbamazepine (Tegretol).

The analgesic effects of tricyclic antidepressants (TCAs) result from their pharmacologic activity of "calming" damaged nerves, not through their antidepressant activity. Because these drugs can cause cardiac rhythm disturbances, baseline electrocardiograms (ECGs) may be indicated for patients with heart disease or other risk factors for dysrhythmias. The anticonvulsant gabapentin has been used with moderate success and avoids the concern with side effects of TCAs, such as dysrhythmias. Both the TCAs and anticonvulsants require a period of at least 3 to 5 days to achieve analgesic effects. Each is to be given an adequate period of time at full dosage before adding the next because additional drugs produce additional side effects. It is important that the dose ordered is given each day, usually at night to avoid daytime drowsiness, so that a steady state is achieved.

Local Analgesics

Injections, chest tube insertions, bone marrow aspirates, lumbar punctures, and insertion of peripheral intravenous needles (PIVs) are major sources of discomfort and distress to children in the PICU. Children develop conditioned anxiety responses to painful procedures and associated objects. In addition, most children do not adapt to the discomfort of repeated procedures over time but instead experience greater levels of anxiety with repeated painful procedures. Anesthetics delivered preemptively are given to block the generation and propagation of the pain impulses by peripheral nerves, yet children fear the pain associated with subcutaneous drug delivery by needles. Increasing interest in administering local anesthetics by other methods has led clinicians to the use needleless approaches to providing local anesthesia.

A combination of lidocaine-prilocaine *(EMLA)* was the first available and effective percutaneously applied anesthetic cream for use on intact skin, and it has been used to provide local anesthesia for venipuncture and minor superficial procedures, with effective analgesia to a depth of 5 mm. However, effective analgesia requires this cream be left in place for 60 to 90 minutes,[58] precluding its use for emergency procedures. Systemic absorption of EMLA is extremely low, resulting in a wide margin of safety. However, caution must be exercised when using this cream

on diseased skin and in young infants because of the possibility of methemoglobinemia included by the metabolites of prilocaine. Amethocaine gel (Ametop), composed of 4% tetracaine, is a new topical anesthetic that requires a shorter application time (30 to 45 minutes) for skin anesthesia as a result of its greater lipophilicity than EMLA.[59,60] Other advantages of Ametop include a lower risk of methemoglobinemia and a longer duration of action (4 to 6 hours) compared with EMLA. However, as of 2000, it is available in the United Kingdom and Canada but not in the United States.

A novel method for subcutaneous drug delivery of local anesthetics is called Numby Stuff, which is a battery-operated unit using iontophoresis as the method for administering ionizable drugs such as lidocaine through the skin with the electrical current of a small battery. This method shortens the administration time to 10 to 15 minutes,[61] an advantage in emergency procedures performed in the PICU. However, the invasive procedure must be done immediately after using Numby Stuff because the lidocaine rapidly dissipates from the prepared site. Found to provide local analgesia to a depth of 8 mm, it is useful in patients who have chronic painful procedures, such as dialysis needle insertion in pediatric patients.[61] Adverse side effects associated with the iontophoresis of lidocaine appear to be limited to transient blanching and erythema at the site of the drug delivery and dispersal electrodes. Some children do not tolerate iontophoresis secondary to the electrical sensation (tingling) associated with its use.[61] PICU clinicians often have to administer lidocaine to deeper tissues, which are not penetrable by the creams or Numby Stuff. Because the pH of lidocaine is acidic, especially if epinephrine is added to prolong the analgesia by vasoconstriction, mixing the lidocaine with sodium bicarbonate in a 10:1 ratio, respectively, will hasten the effect and minimize the burning sensation associated with nonbuffered solutions.[62]

Epidural Analgesia

Delivery of drugs by the epidural route is accomplished by threading a catheter through a needle into the epidural space (Fig. 17-5). Diffusion of morphine or fentanyl through the dura into the cerebral spinal fluid (CSF) and then into the spinal cord directly to the analgesic action site (receptors in the dorsal horn of the spinal cord) leads to direct analgesia, eliminating many of the systemic side effects of opioids without having any effect on motor or sympathetic function. Potential side effects of the epidural opioid infusions include the previously discussed effects associated with opioid administration. The risk of respiratory depression after intraspinal opioids occurs with concomitant therapy of intravenous opioids as well; therefore using both routes must be done with caution, most often provided by having the anesthesiology service write orders for pain and sedation. It is critical to monitor the patient's sedation level and respiratory status and to decrease the epidural opioid dose if excessive sedation is detected. Because infants under 6 months of age are the highest risk for clinically significant, opioid-induced respiratory depression, many clinicians recom-

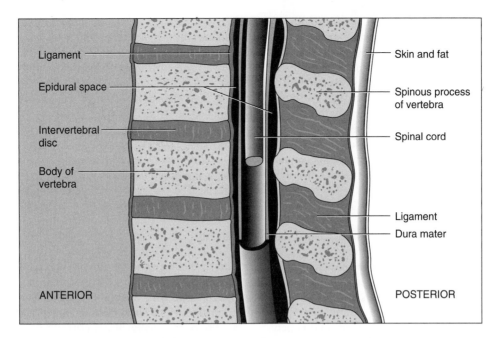

Fig. 17-5   Epidural space depicted with surrounding anatomy. (Modified from Sinatra R: Spinal opioid analgesia: an overview. In Sinatra RS, Hord AH, Ginsberg B, Preble LM, eds: *Acute pain: mechanisms and management,* St Louis, 1992, Mosby, p 107.)

mend that these patients be monitored by pulse oximetry or cardiac/apnea monitors during administration.

Infusions of dilute concentrations of local anesthetics are administered epidurally to provide synergistic effects with the opioids, resulting in better analgesia and fewer side effects at lower doses than would be possible if opioids were administered alone. Evidence shows that a combination of opioids and local anesthetics is more effective than using either agent alone.[6] Children are subject to the adverse effects of local anesthetics (sensory and motor deficits, hypotension, and neurotoxicity, such as seizures). The occasional occurrence of minor temporary numbness of lower extremities usually is resolved easily by decreasing the dose or removing the local anesthetic from the epidural analgesia solution. To reduce adverse effects, doses are carefully titrated to a maximum dose to avoid these complications. The rate of a bupivacaine infusion is to be maintained less than 0.4 to 0.5 mg/kg/hr. Lower doses in infants younger than 6 months may be necessary because of lower clearance rates in this age group.

Only preservative-free solutions that have been approved for intraspinal use are to be used to prevent local damage to the spinal cord. Catheters and IV tubing (without rubber injection ports) that is distinctive for epidural infusions, such as being color coded and boldly labeled, are recommended to prevent accidental introduction of unintended medications into the epidural space. Infection of the epidural space is a very rare (less than 0.0015%) but a serious complication,[54] especially if it leads to formation of an epidural abscess resulting in spinal cord compression and, in extreme cases, paralysis. This complication is thought to be more common when epidural catheters are left in place for a prolonged time, such as to treat chronic pain,[54] and are more often associated with poor aseptic technique or

migration of localized skin infection at the epidural catheter entry site. Early signs and symptoms of an epidural infection can be difficult to detect because skin site infection and fever may not be present.

Puncture of epidural blood vessels during the placement of the epidural catheterization leading to the formation of an epidural hematoma that results in paraplegia is a potential risk, although rare. This complication is best prevented by careful screening of candidates for epidural catheter use, such as establishing a minimal platelet count of $70,000/mm^3$ and ensuring that coagulation test results are in the normal range before placement.

Clinical signs of an abscess or hematoma of the epidural space are similar: increasing diffuse back pain or tenderness, pain or paresthesia on epidural injection, and bowel or bladder dysfunction. As an epidural abscess or hematoma grows within the epidural space, sensory and motor deficits increase. Patient recovery without neurologic injury depends, in large part, on early recognition, followed by confirmation of the compression by computed tomography (CT) or magnetic resonance imaging (MRI). Treatment ranges from antibiotics to surgical removal of the abscess or hematoma.

Children can ambulate and perform all of the routine recovery activities expected of them to the extent of their medical or surgical condition. Research suggests that epidural anesthesia in the postoperative setting may facilitate earlier recovery and improved outcome by reducing the incidence of thromboembolisms and pulmonary and gastrointestinal complications after major surgery.[63]

Most state boards of nursing in the United States have approved the administration of epidural boluses by nurses who possess the necessary knowledge and skills and where institutional policy and procedure support this function.[54]

Vascular uptake or injection of the local anesthetic directly into the systemic circulation can result in adverse reactions related to high blood levels of local anesthetic. Before injecting a bolus, the nurse is to gently aspirate the catheter. If other than a scant (less than 1 ml) of clear liquid is aspirated, the nurse must collaborate with the anesthesia staff before administering the bolus or continuing the infusion. Free-flowing clear fluid (CSF) return indicates that the catheter may be in the subarachnoid space. Free-flowing blood aspirate return indicates that the catheter may be in a blood vessel.

Sedatives

For both infants and children, adequate pain control may preclude the need for other sedatives. However, if agitation persists, agents such as benzodiazepines and barbiturates are commonly used as first-line sedative agents. Proper selection and administration of drugs require knowledge of their comparative effects, characteristics, and limitations. The goal is to have the child be free from pain and anxiety, able to tolerate medical procedures such as suctioning, but able to be aroused easily from light sleep, enabling effective neurologic assessment. For some patients, reaching the desired clinical outcome may require larger-than-recommended drug doses. Dose response varies greatly not only among patients but also over time within an individual patient because of tolerance over time to the beneficial effects leading to receptor down-regulation and competitive drug interactions, as well as changes in pH, serum albumin, autonomic activity, or renal and liver function. When a continuous infusion rate proves to be subtherapeutic, increasing the rate alone is not effective. An additional small dose must also be given, or it will take 4 to 5 half-lives to reach a new steady state.

Benzodiazepines most commonly used in the PICU include midazolam (Versed) and lorazepam (Ativan). These agents possess sedative, anxiolytic, hypnotic, muscle relaxant, and anticonvulsant effects but no analgesic effects. Although they have minimal negative cardiovascular effects, dose-related effects include respiratory depression, most commonly related to patient-specific factors, such as age; concurrent disease; and drug cotherapy. The presence of active metabolites with all of them except lorazepam complicates their use during periods of prolonged use. Combinations of benzodiazepines and opioids are synergistic in producing sedation. Tolerance to the sedating effects has been reported in pediatric patients.[49]

Diazepam (Valium) has become less popular with the arrival of newer, more water-soluble, less irritating, and shorter-acting benzodiazepines. However, it is the least expensive. When used over several days, diazepam is stored in body fat, and active metabolites can accumulate, leading to long half-lives (greater than 100 hours), especially in those patients with renal failure.[64] *Lorazepam* (Ativan) does not accumulate in lipid stores. Well absorbed from oral and parenteral sites, it undergoes primarily hepatic glucuronidation, a process relatively resistant to

hepatic dysfunction. In contrast to other injectable benzodiazepines, the pharmacokinetics of lorazepam do not change significantly with critical illness.[53] Because of the slower onset of action, alterations in continuous infusion rates are to be preceded by a small bolus dose to avoid excessive dose administration and oversedation. Many recommend it as the agent of choice for long-term sedation in the ICU because of its lower cost and favorable properties.[53]

Midazolam (Versed) produces effective sedation, antegrade amnesia, and anxiolysis, with relatively few adverse effects. The major risk is hypoventilation and subsequent hypoxemia. Onset of action is very short (less than 3 minutes). A low-dose infusion of midazolam provides smooth sedation without the peaks and troughs seen with intermittent doses. In addition to an infusion, "rescue doses" or intermittent doses ordered for break-through agitation provide appropriate titration in response to a patient's changing needs for sedation. Although promoted as a sedative with a short duration, many studies challenge this assertion, especially in the critically ill.[53] It has an active metabolite that can accumulate over days of use and extend the half-life to 12 to 20 hours in many patients,[64] especially in patients with renal failure. However, in ICU patients without significant end-organ disease, clearance does not appear to be decreased. The clearance may be reduced by concurrent use of calcium-channel blocking agents, erythromycin, and triazole antifungal agents.[53]

For further details on these agents, see Table 17-6. Administration of high doses of benzodiazepines increases the risk of developing moderate to severe withdrawal reactions. All benzodiazepines appear to have an equal likelihood of producing such physical dependence. Benzodiazepine-induced sedative and respiratory effects can be reversed with incremental doses of flumazenil (Romazicon) 0.01 mg/kg every 1 to 2 minutes until a total dose of 1 mg is given.[65] However, it is not effective in reversing barbiturates. Clinicians are warned to use this agent with caution because administration may precipitate seizures, particularly in children taking benzodiazepines for seizure control, as well as an increase in intracranial pressure from the spontaneous awakening in a distressed state. Therefore flumazenil is rarely used in the ICU.

Barbiturates are used in the ICU primarily for anesthetic induction, cerebral protection, and treatment of seizures. These agents possess long half-lives and are not as well suited for routine sedation of critically ill patients because they are difficult to titrate to achieve a desired sedative effect without significant general depression of the central nervous system, resulting in respiratory depression and hypotension. However, they are useful for sedating patients with acute head injury because they decrease cerebral metabolic oxygen consumption by as much as 50%. Barbiturates may actually increase a patient's sensitivity to pain and are never substituted for analgesics.[53] *Pentobarbital* is the most commonly used barbiturate in the ICU to induce barbiturate coma for improving control of increased ICP for patients with severe head injury. Because it does not have any active metabolites, its pharmacokinetics are not altered in renal failure. Hyperdynamic states, such as sepsis, have correlated with increased barbiturate clearance.

To promote sleep and control agitation, *choral hydrate* and *haloperidol* (Haldol) are recommended in specific situations (see Table 17-6 for details regarding dosing). Although choral hydrate is available for only oral or rectal routes, it is rapidly absorbed and has the advantage of only limited effects on cardiopulmonary function. However, clinicians must be aware that it has no analgesic properties, and excitement and delirium may result if given to patients in pain.[47] Because of the accumulation of active metabolites, its use is not recommended for infants younger than 3 months of age or patients with liver dysfunction.[66] Haloperidol has been found useful when less potent sedatives are ineffective and has been found especially beneficial for the treatment of delirium in critically ill patients.[4,66] This sedative-hypnotic has a rapid onset of action, leading to minimal respiratory depression, and has no active metabolites. However, adverse effects include hypotension, dystonia, and extrapyramidal effects. Haloperidol may cause QT prolongation on the ECG, leading to torsade de pointes (a specific form of ventricular tachycardia), and should be used with caution in conjunction with other drugs that may also lead to this abnormality.

Deep Sedation

Other agents may be used to offer a deeper level of sedation associated with painful procedures or to increase tolerance to the stresses of having mechanical ventilation. *Ketamine* is a nonbarbiturate derivative of phencyclidine (PCP) that produces "dissociative anesthesia," a cataleptic state in which the eyes remain open with a slow nystagmic gaze. Commonly classified as an anesthetic, when administered in lower doses, it produces intense analgesia and amnesia[67] (see Table 17-6 for specific dosages). Although the child appears to be awake, he or she is not able to feel pain or communicate. For those children with a risk of hypotension from other sedatives, ketamine actually leads to the reverse, an elevation in blood pressure. Clinicians should be aware that it is a potent cerebral vasodilator, thus to be avoided in children who are at risk for increased intracranial pressure. A set of symptoms reported by older patients as visual, auditory, proprioceptive, and strange illusions, called the emergence phenomena, can occur when the drug is discontinued, especially in patients older than 16 years.

Propofol is an ultrashort-acting sedative-hypnotic agent useful as a bolus for deep sedation for a stressful procedure in nonintubated patients, as well as a bolus followed by a continuous infusion for patients requiring mechanical ventilatory support in the ICU. Its advantages are its rapid onset of action and rapid dissipation of effects.[68] The patient's level of sedation can be regulated by titrating the propofol, much like blood pressure regulation by a dopamine infusion. Although the half-life is 1 to 3 days, the sedative effects typically dissipate within 5 to 10 minutes after the infusion is discontinued, which makes it so useful. If the time to extubate a patient is approaching and the patient has been receiving other sedative agents, it may be appropriate to discontinue those agents and begin a propofol infusion. This will allow minute-to-minute balancing between oversedation and respiratory depression on one hand, yet prevent anxiety related to the ventilatory weaning process on the other. Propofol may also be an appropriate choice in ICU patients with neurologic problems because it decreases cerebral metabolic rate and intracranial pressure while maintaining cerebral perfusion pressure. Propofol has no analgesic effects; other analgesics must be added for ongoing or procedurally related pain. One unusual effect is discoloration of the urine to a green tint. Infusions for critically ill adults have been found to be satisfactory and safe. The cardiovascular and respiratory effects of propofol are similar to those of barbiturates. Decreases in blood pressure and heart rate are common after treatment with propofol is started. Data on its use in children are limited, and adverse events in this population have been reported, centering on unexplained metabolic acidosis and hyperkalemia leading to cardiac arrest in pediatric patients who were receiving an infusion of propofol.[69,70] Why propofol might produce metabolic acidosis is unknown. Some advocate its use with caution in pediatric patients.[69] It is administered in a lipid solution, which increases cost and can increase the risk of infection. Transient elevation of triglycerides has been reported.

Inhalational Agents

The use of inhalational anesthetic agents such as isoflurane (Forane) is another alternative useful in providing comfort to complex patients who are unresponsive to maximal conventional therapy.[71] Advocates for their use convey their benefits: rapid onset, rapid awakening on discontinuation, and ease of control of the depth of sedation. Additional benefit from its effect of bronchodilation makes it an attractive agent for patients who have severe reactive airway diseases. However, several logistical problems may limit their usefulness outside of the operating room. Rules and regulations regarding who should regulate the inspired concentration of the agent is complex and may be not sanctioned to be done by nursing staff. Effective scavenging devices are necessary to prevent environmental pollution.

Discontinuation of Analgesics and Sedatives

Strategies to appropriately discontinue opioids and benzodiazepines in infants and children recovering from critical illness are one of the most challenging aspects of critical care nursing. Comprehensive management is based on accurate and repetitive clinical assessment and a compassionate interplay of pharmacologic and nonpharmacologic measures used in a complementary manner. The nurse should assure the child and family that this does not mean the child is addicted to the medicines. It means the child is temporarily physically dependent on them in the same fashion as steroids.

The ICU nurse must monitor for subtle clues indicative of withdrawal while continuing to serve as an advocate for patient comfort. Early recognition and management of withdrawal symptoms are imperative. Many of the signs and symptoms associated with withdrawal are similar to those associated with pain or the agitation itself. Use of an objective assessment tool such as the Neonatal Abstinence Scoring Tool (NAST) may assist the caregiver in identifying the presence of withdrawal symptoms because it is easy to overlook these individual symptoms or attribute them to other causes when scoring.[72] As shown in Table 17-7, the NAST was developed to assess and mange the opioid-addicted newborn; it identifies behaviors consistent with withdrawal and assigns a score to each behavior. A score of 8 or greater indicates neonatal abstinence syndrome. Although the tool has not been validated for use in older children, it may provide an objective means of assessment for caregivers in the PICU setting.[49]

Clinical features of *opioid withdrawal* include gastrointestinal dysfunction (poor feeding, uncoordinated sucking, vomiting, diarrhea), autonomic signs (dilated pupils, piloerection, increased sweating, nasal congestion, fever, mottling), neurologic excitability (high-pitched crying, insomnia, hallucinations, increased motor tone, tremors, seizures).[31] Signs of withdrawal are more severe in older children than in younger children and infants. Clinical features of *benzodiazepine withdrawal* differ marginally from those of opioid withdrawal. In addition to those found in opioid withdrawal, severe anxiety, confusion, perceptual disorders, depression, facial grimacing, choreoathetoid movements, dyskinetic movements of the mouth, myoclonus, ataxia, poor visual tacking, and opisthotonos have also been reported following abrupt discontinuance of benzodiazepines.[73] Experts have found that some signs of withdrawal (movement disorders) persist for up to 6 to 8 weeks after the discontinuation of midazolam and are only partially responsive to treatment with other benzodiazepines.[31]

Symptoms are not only extremely uncomfortable for the patient and anxiety provoking for the family, it may further

TABLE 17-7 Neonatal Abstinence Score Sheet

System	Signs and Symptoms	Score
Central nervous system disturbances	Excessive high-pitched (or other) cry	2
	Continuous high-pitched (or other) cry	3
	Sleeps <1 hour after feeding	3
	Sleeps <2 hours after feeding	2
	Sleeps <3 hours after feeding	1
	Hyperactive Moro reflex	2
	Markedly hyperactive Moro reflex	3
	Mild tremors when disturbed	1
	Moderate to severe tremors when disturbed	2
	Mild tremors when undisturbed	3
	Moderate to severe tremors when undisturbed	4
	Increased muscle tone	2
	Excoriation	1
	Myoclonic jerks	3
	Generalized convulsions	5
Metabolic and vasomotor or respiratory disturbances	Sweating	1
	Fever of 37.2° C to 38.2° C (99° F to 100.8° F)	1
	Fever >38.4° C (101° F)	2
	Frequent yawning (more than 3 to 4 times/interval)	1
	Mottling	1
	Nasal stuffiness	1
	Sneezing (more than 3 to 4 times/interval)	1
	Nasal flaring	2
	Respiratory rate >60/min	1
	Respiratory rate >50/min with retractions	2
Gastrointestinal disturbances	Excessive sucking	1
	Poor feeding	2
	Regurgitation	2
	Projectile vomiting	3
	Loose stools	2
	Watery stools	3

Adapted from Finnigan LP, Kron RE, Cannaughton JF et al: A scoring system for evaluation and treatment of neonatal abstinence syndrome: a new clinical and research tool. In Morselli PL, Garattini S, Sereni F, eds: *Basic and therapeutic aspects of perinatal pharmacology*, New York, 1975, Raven Press; reprinted from the *J Perinat Neonatal Nurs* July 1990, p 70.

complicate a patient's PICU course. The agitation accompanying withdrawal triggers the release of endogenous catecholamines and other stress hormones such as glucagon and corticosteroids that can lead to cardiovascular compromise. Attempts to wean from ventilatory support may be disrupted by increasing oxygen consumption and carbon dioxide production. Withdrawal symptoms expend energy and calories needed for healing and may at times mimic the onset of sepsis.

Previous use of other agents to control withdrawal, such as phenobarbital, has been done to minimize withdrawal symptoms. However, these have side effects of their own. Therefore experts recommend the slow weaning of their respective doses and converting to other agents, such as methadone and clonidine, as useful in preventing withdrawal symptoms. Because of methadone's prolonged half-life, plasma levels of the drug will decline slowly, allowing gradual weaning.[31] Some use methadone in the weaning process at doses of 0.1 mg/kg given enterally every 12 hours while gradually decreasing and eventually discontinuing infusions of fentanyl and morphine.[49]

It is now known that α_2-aderenergic receptors and μ-opioid receptors activate the same potassium channel, albeit via different proteins. Therefore administration of clonidine, an α_2-aderenergic receptor agonist, is another method of preventing opioid withdrawal symptoms; it may "mimic" opioids at the subreceptor level, thus allowing a decrease in the opioid dose without the occurrence of signs or symptoms of withdrawal using oral doses of 3 to 5 μg/kg every 4 to 8 hours.[31,49] In addition, clonidine's central nervous system effects produce mild sedation and a sense of well-being and calmness that also help ameliorate the symptoms of withdrawal. Patients can be weaned off the drug in 1 to 2 weeks as it is reduced by 0.1 to 0.2 mg each day.

Patients can benefit from institutions developing standardized approaches for such discontinuance of opioids and benzodiazepines (Fig. 17-6). The general recommendation is to avoid simultaneous decrease in both drugs at the same time at intervals providing time for reassessment of the child and attainment of a new steady state before the next decrease in dose. Patients who have been treated with continuous infusions of high doses of opioids require up to 2 to 3 weeks to be weaned.[31]

NURSING'S ROLE IN PAIN MANAGEMENT

Nurses have primary responsibility for assessing children's distress and coordinating pharmacologic, environmental, and social interventions to optimize comfort. Their role in providing patients and families with factual information about pain and analgesics is an extremely important nursing intervention directed toward breaking down the many barriers to its effective management. Nurses need to make pain management a priority, starting with establishing the standard in PICU that pain assessment be done with the same frequency and attention as measurement of vital signs and checking the crash cart. Nurses are in a crucial position to advocate for their patients with the fundamental obligation to manage pain and relieve patient suffering as a crucial element of their professional commitment to patient care. These are not merely lofty ideals; effective pain and anxiety management produces myriad patient benefits, including reduced morbidity and mortality.[11]

Nurses' participation is necessary in developing and establishing the institutional systems that promote quality care in the area of pain management. Research has shown that clinical protocols can be implemented by critical care nurses to guide sedation strategies in such a way that the duration of mechanical ventilation can be reduced at the same time comfort can be provided.[74] Nurses should actively decide which pain assessment tools will be used and ensure that they are readily available for staff and patients to use. For example, a selection of pain assessment tools may be compiled on a single sheet of paper, copied, and placed on every bedside clipboard. Nurses can also influence patient documentation systems to include a specific section for pain assessments. Pain flow sheets[22] have demonstrated that patients who are assessed more frequently experience less pain and receive more opioid analgesics. Overall, there is still a lack of accountability of healthcare systems, specifically critical care units, to make pain as a recognized priority. Many experts advocate that the first step is establishing a trigger point in the pain intensity assessment scale, such as that pain needs to be less than 50% of the total scale (i.e., less than 3 on a 0- to 5-point scale), or a trigger point requiring an intervention aimed at providing pain relief.[54]

In recent years, extensive work in pain management guideline development has been done, with accompanying recommendations for quality improvement monitoring. Nurses may be actively involved with the implementation of well-recognized guidelines such as that of the Agency for Health Care Policy and Research (AHCPR).[11] Increasing efforts have been made by the Joint Commission on Accreditation of Health Care Organizations to hold healthcare professionals responsible for assessing and relieving pain.[7,75]

SUMMARY

Caregivers must believe in the authenticity of a child's pain and that the benefits of adequate analgesia far outweigh the potential side effects. Adequate and early pharmacologic interventions for pain relief minimize patient suffering, maintain normal homeostasis, and improve a patient's tolerance of ICU therapies and nursing interventions. The appropriate selection and method of delivery of the pharmacologic strategy is determined by the intensity of the pain experienced, the expected treatment goals, and the child's overall condition. Even for the sickest child, adequate analgesia can be provided using the interventions, both pharmacologic and nonpharmacologic, as outlined in this chapter.

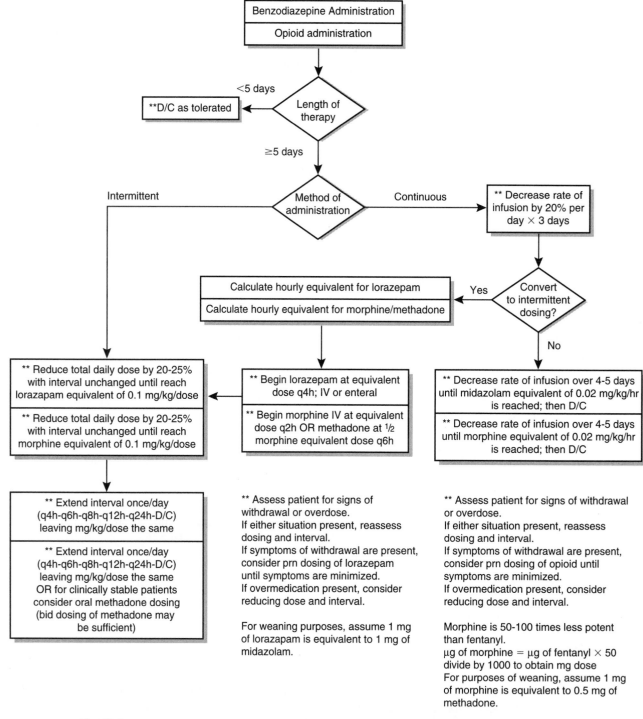

Fig. 17-6 Algorithm for weaning benzodiazepines and opioids. (Data from Cincinnati Children's Hospital Medical Center: *Therapeutic concepts: narcotic/benzodiazepine withdrawal,* 1996, pp 1-4.)

REFERENCES

1. Creasey J: Sedation scoring: assessment tools, *Nurs Crit Care* 1:171-177, 1996.
2. Chambliss CR, Anand KJS: Pain management in the pediatric intensive care unit, *Curr Opin Pediatr* 9:248-253, 1997.
3. International Association for the Study of Pain, Subcommittee on Taxonomy: Pain terms: a list with definitions and notes on usage, *Pain* 6:249-252, 1979.
4. Shapiro BA, Warren J, Egol AB et al: Practice parameters for intravenous analgesia and sedation for adult patients in the intensive care unit: an executive summary, *Crit Care Med* 23:1596-1600, 1995.
5. McCaffery M, Portenoy RR: Overview of three groups of analgesics. In McCaffery M, Pasero C, eds: *Pain: clinical manual,* ed 2, St Louis, 1999, Mosby.
6. Scull T, Motamed C, Carli F: The stress response and pre-emptive analgesia. In Portenoy RK, Kanner RM, eds: *Pain management theory and practice,* Philadelphia, 1996, FA Davis.
7. McCaffery M: Pain management: problems and progress. In McCaffery M, Pasero C, eds: *Pain: clinical manual,* ed 2, St Louis, 1999, Mosby.

8. Higgins SS, Turley KM, Harr J et al: Prescription and administration of around the clock analgesics in postoperative pediatric cardiovascular surgery patient, *Prog Cardiovasc Nurs* 14:19-24, 1999.

9. Anand KS, Grunau RE, Oberlander TF: Developmental character and long-term consequences of pain in infants and children, *Child Adolesc Psychiatr Clin N Am* 6:703-725, 1997.

10. Macfadyen AJ, Buckmaster MA: Pain management in the pediatric intensive care unit, *Crit Care Clin* 15:185-200, 1999.

11. Agency for Health Care Policy & Research: *Clinical practice guideline: acute pain management—operative or medical procedures and trauma* (AHCPR Pub No 92-0032), Rockville, Md, 1992, US Department of Health and Human Services, Public Health Service.

12. McRae ME, Rourke DA, Imperial-Perez MA et al: Development of a research-based standard for assessment, intervention, and evaluation of pain after neonatal and pediatric cardiac surgery, *Pediatr Nurs* 23:263-271, 1997.

13. Hamers JP, Abu-Saad HH, van den Hout MA et al: Are children given insufficient pain-relieving medication postoperatively? *J Adv Nurs* 27, 30-36, 1998.

14. Stanik-Hutt JA: Pain management in the critically ill, *Crit Care Nurs* 18:85-88, 1998.

14a. Meehan DA, McRae ME, Bourke DA et al: Analgesic administration, pain intensity, and patient satisfaction in cardiac surgical patients, *Am J Crit Care* 4:435-442, 1995.

15. American Pain Society: *Principles of analgesic use in the treatment of acute pain and cancer pain,* Pensacola, Fla, 1999, The Society.

16. Krane E, Yaster M: Transition to less invasive therapy. In Yaster M, Krane EJ, Kaplan RF et al, eds: *Pediatric pain management and sedation handbook,* St Louis, 1997, Mosby.

17. Porter J, Jick H: Addiction rare in patients treated with opioids, *N Engl J Med* 302:123, 1980.

17a. Colwell C, Clark L, Perkins R: Postoperative use of pediatric pain scales: children's self-report versus nurse assessment of pain intensity and affect, *J Pediatr Nurs* 11:375-382, 1996.

18. Pederson C, Matthies D, McDonald S: A survey of pediatric critical care nurses' knowledge of pain management, *Am J Crit Care* 6:289-295, 1997.

19. Anand KJS, McIntosh N, Lagercrantz H et al: Analgesia and sedation in preterm neonates who require ventilatory support: results from the NOPAIN trial, *Arch Pediatr Adolesc Med* 153:331-338, 1999.

20. Page GG, Ben-Eliyahu S, Yirmiya R et al: Morphine attenuates surgery-induced enhancement of metastatic colonization in rats, *Pain* 54:21-28, 1993.

21. Fitzgerald M, Anand KJS: Developmental neuroanatomy and neurophysiology of pain. In Schechter NL, Berde CB, Yaster M, eds: *Pain in infants, children, and adolescents,* Baltimore, Md, 1993, Williams & Wilkins.

22. Stevens B: Pain assessment in children: birth through adolescence, *Child Adolesc Psychiatr Clin North Am* 6:725-743, 1997.

23. Taddio A, Katz J, Ilersich AL et al: Effect of neonatal circumcision on pain response during subsequent routine vaccination, *Lancet* 349:599, 1997.

24. Agency for Health Care Policy & Research: *Quick reference guide for clinicians. Acute pain management in infants, children, and adolescents: operative and medical procedures* (AHCPR Pub No 92-0020), Rockville, Md, 1992, US Department of Health and Human Services, Public Health Service.

25. Eland JM: Pain in children. In Hockenberry M, Coody D, eds: *Pediatric hematology-oncology: perspectives in care,* St Louis,1986, CV Mosby.

26. Krechel SW, Bildner J: CRIES: a new neonatal postoperative pain measurement score: initial testing of validity and reliability, *Pediatr Anesth* 5:53-61, 1995.

27. Stevens B: Pain in infants. In McCaffery M, Pasero C, eds: *Pain: clinical manual,* ed 2, St Louis, 1999, Mosby.

28. Merkel SI, Voepel-Lewis T, Shayevitz JR et al: The FLACC: a behavioral scale for scoring postoperative pain in young children, *Pediatr Nurs* 23:293-297, 1997.

29. West N, Oakes L, Hinds PS et al: Measuring pain in pediatric oncology ICU patients, *J Pediatr Oncol Nurs* 11:64-68, 1994.

30. Porter F: Pain assessment in children: infants. In Schechter NL, Berde CB, Yaster M, eds: *Pain in infants, children, and adolescents,* Baltimore, Md, 1993, Williams & Wilkins.

30a. Schade JG, Joyce BA, Gerkensmeyer J et al: Comparison of three preverbal scales for postoperative pain assessment in a diverse pediatric sample, *J Pain Symptom Manage* 12:348-359, 1996.

31. Anand KS, Ingraham J: Tolerance, dependence, and strategies for compassionate withdrawal of analgesics and anxiolytics in the pediatric ICU, *Crit Care Nurs* 16:87-93, 1996.

32. Miller D: Comparisons of pain ratings from postoperative children, their mothers and their nurses, *Pediatr Nurs* 22:145-149, 1996.

33. Devlin JW, Boleski G, Mlynarek M et al: Motor activity assessment scale: a valid and reliable sedation scale for use with mechanically ventilated patients in an adult surgical intensive care unit, *Crit Care Med* 27:1271-1275, 1999.

34. Riker RR, Picard JT, Fraser GL: Prospective evaluation of the sedation-agitation scale for adult critically ill patients, *Crit Care Med* 27:1325-1329, 1999.

35. Ambuel B, Hamlett KW, Marx CM et al: Assessing distress in pediatric intensive care environments: the Comfort Scale, *J Pediatr Psychol* 17:95-109, 1992.

36. Marx CM, Smith PG, Lowrie LH et al: Optimal sedation of mechanically ventilated pediatric critical care patients, *Crit Care Med* 22:163-170, 1994.

37. Curley MAQ: Modified motor activity assessment scale, personal communication, 1999.

38. Simmons LE, Riker RR, Prato BS et al: Assessing sedation during intensive care unit mechanical ventilation with the Bispectral Index and the Sedation-Agitation Scale, *Crit Care Med* 27:1499-1504, 1999.

39. Struys M, Bersichelen L, Byttebier G et al: Clinical usefulness of the bispectral index for titrating propofol target effect-site concentration, *Anaesthesia* 53:4-12, 1998.

40. McCaffery M, Pasero C: Practical nondrug approaches to pain. In McCaffery M, Pasero C, eds: *Pain: clinical manual,* ed 2, St Louis, 1999, Mosby.

41. Dossey B: Holistic modalities and healing moments, *Am J Nurs* 98:44-47, 1998.

42. Weiss SM: The emerging acceptance and importance of alternative medical therapies, *Cancer Control* 5(suppl 1):50-52, 1998.

43. Wetzel WS: Healing touch as a nursing intervention, *J Holistic Nurs* 11:277-285, 1993.

44. Rosa L: A close look at therapeutic touch, *JAMA* 279, 1005-1010, 1998.

45. Smith NK, Pasero C, McCaffery M: Using nondrug methods during procedures, *Am J Nurs* 97:18-20, 1997.

46. Cureton-Lane RA, Fontaine DK: Sleep in the pediatric ICU: an empirical investigation, *Am J Crit Care* 6:56-63, 1997.

47. Yaster M, Bean JD, Schulman SR et al: Pain, sedation, and postoperative anesthetic managment in the pediatric intensive care unit. In Rogers MC, Helfaer MA, eds: *Handbook of pediatric intensive care,* ed 3, Baltimore, 1999, Williams & Wilkins.

48. Powers KS, Rubenstein JS: Family presence during invasive procedures in the pediatric intensive care unit: a prospective study, *Arch Pediatr Adolesc Med* September, 153:955-958, 1999.

49. Banks LJ, Lindsay CA: Opioid and benzodiazepine dependence. In Levin DL, Morriss FC, eds: *Essentials of pediatric intensive care,* ed 2, New York, 1997, Churchill Livingstone.

50. Vessey JA, Carlson KL, McGill J: Use of distraction with children during an acute pain experience, *Nurs Res* 43:369-372, 1994.

51. Pasero C, Portenoy RK, McCaffery M: Opioid analgesics. In McCaffery M, Pasero C, eds: *Pain: clinical manual,* ed 2, St Louis, 1999, Mosby.

52. Zuckerman LA, Ferrante FM: Nonopioid and opioid analgesics. In Portenoy RK, Kanner RM, eds: *Pain management theory and practice,* Philadelphia, 1996, FA Davis.

53. Wagner BKJ, O'Hara DA: Pharmacokinetics and pharmacodynamics of sedatives an analgesics in the treatment of agitated critically ill patients, *Clin Pharmacokinet* 33:426-453, 1997.

54. Pasero C: *Epidural analgesia for acute pain management,* Pensacola, Fla, 1999, American Society of Pain Management Nurses.

55. Lin Y, Krane E, Yaster M: Challenging pain problems. In Yaster M, Krane EJ, Kaplan RF et al, eds: *Pediatric pain management and sedation handbook,* St Louis, 1997, Mosby.

56. Searle: *Brief summary—Celebrex,* Chicago, Ill, 1999, GD Searle.

57. Dellemijn D: Are opioids effective in relieving neuropathic pain? *Pain* 80:453-462, 1998.

58. Lander J, Hodgins M, Nazarali S et al: Determinants of success and failure of EMLA, *Pain* 64:89-97, 1996.

59. Bishai R, Taddio A, Bar-Oz B et al: Relative efficacy of amethocaine gel and lidocaine-prilocaine cream for Port-a-Cath puncture in children, *Pediatrics* 104:31, 1999.

60. Lawson RA, Smart NG, Gudgeon AC et al: Evaluation of an amethocaine gel preparation for percutaneous analgesia before venous cannulation in children, *Br J Anaesth* 75:282-285, 1995.

61. Zempsky WT, Ashburn MA: Iontophoresis: noninvasive drug delivery, *Am J Anesthesiol* 25:158-162, 1998.

62. Anderson A: Sedation and analgesia in the emergency department. In Yaster M, Krane EJ, Kaplan RF et al, eds: *Pediatric pain management and sedation handbook,* St Louis, 1997, Mosby.

63. Ballantyne JC, Carr DB, deFerranti S et al: The comparative effects of postoperative analgesic therapies on pulmonary outcome: cumulative meta-analyses of randomized, controlled trials, *Anesth Analg* 86:598-612, 1998.

64. Harvey MA: Managing agitation in critically ill patients, *Am J Crit Care* 5:7-16, 1996.

65. Yaster M, Coté C: Sedatives, hypnotics, anxiolytics, and amnestics. In Yaster M, Krane EJ, Kaplan RF, eds: *Pediatric pain management and sedation handbook,* St Louis, 1997, Mosby.

66. Deshpandé JK, Anand KJS: Basic aspects of acute pediatric pain and sedation. In Deshpandé JK, Tobias JD, eds: *The pediatric pain handbook,* St Louis, 1996, Mosby.

67. Yaster M: General anesthetics. In Yaster M, Krane EJ, Kaplan RF et al, eds: *Pediatric pain management and sedation handbook,* St Louis, 1997, Mosby.

68. Covington H: Use of propofol for sedation in the ICU, *Crit Care Nurs* 18:34-39, 1998.

69. Strickland RA, Murray MJ: Fatal metabolic acidosis in a pediatric patient receiving an infusion of propofol in the intensive care unit: is there a relationship? *Crit Care Med* 23:405-409, 1995.

70. Cray SH, Robinson BH, Cox P: Lactic acidemia and bradyarrhythmia in a child sedated with propofol, *Crit Care Med* 26:2087-2092, 1998.

71. Curley MAQ, Molengraft JA: Providing comfort to critically ill pediatric patients: isoflurane, *Crit Care Nurs Clin North Am* 7:267-274, 1995.

72. Finnegan LP, Kron RE, Cannaughton JF et al: A scoring system for evaluation and treatment of neonatal abstinence syndrome: a new clinical and research tool. In Morselli PL, Garattini S, Sereni F, eds: *Basic and therapeutic aspects of perinatal pharmacology,* New York, 1975, Raven Press.

73. Fonsmark L, Rasmussen YH, Peder C: Occurrence of withdrawal in critically ill sedated children, *Crit Care Med* 27:196-199, 1999.

74. Brook A, Ahrens TS, Schaiff R et al: Effect of a nursing-implemented sedation protocol on the duration of mechanical ventilation, *Crit Care Med* 27:2609-2823, 1999.

75. Joint Commission on Accreditation of Health Care Organization: CAMH Update 3. Standard for pain: PE 1.4, August 1999.

Final Common Pathways

This section presents state-of-the-art nursing care for patient problems within each body system. A focus on the final common pathways of many disease states is presented so that system dysfunction is viewed broadly and addressed within a nursing framework. The etiology, incidence, and pathogenesis of specific disorders that lead to development of a final common pathway are also presented when appropriate. Critical care management is focused broadly on the final common pathways of system dysfunction and specifically on patient care unique to a particular disorder.

18 Cardiovascular Critical Care Problems

Janet Craig
Lori D. Fineman
Paula Moynihan
Annette L. Baker

Cardiovascular dysfunction necessitates admission to a critical care setting across the lifespan. The percentage of pediatric intensive care unit (PICU) patients with cardiovascular dysfunction was 13% to 38% in one multi-center study[1] and 19% in the American Association of Critical Care Nurses 1999 role delineation study.[2] Cardiovascular dysfunction may be the consequence of hypovolemia, myocardial dysfunction, cardiac rhythm disturbances, increased afterload, or pericardial tamponade. It is important to note that myocardial dysfunction may be either the result of a primary cardiac problem or the final pathophysiologic consequence of a variety of other problems. Cardiovascular dysfunction can result in a low-flow shock state and inadequate tissue perfusion.

ASSESSMENT OF PATIENTS WITH CARDIOVASCULAR DYSFUNCTION

The clinical picture of the patient with inadequate tissue perfusion can be clearly identified because low cardiac output results in physiologic compensation that is readily apparent on physical examination.

A common first sign of physiologic distress in infants and children is tachycardia. Tachycardia occurs with fever, anemia, hypovolemia, dyspnea, activity, and excitement or anxiety. In fact, it is an ominous sign of cardiac dysfunction if heart rate does not increase in the face of physiologic distress. Persistent tachycardia during sleep is generally nonphysiologic and warrants further evaluation. In addition, following trends in heart rate over time is useful.

Tachycardia related to physiologic distress is the result of sympathetic nervous system (SNS) stimulation. SNS stimulation also results in increased minute ventilation, whereby respiratory rate and depth can increase.

SNS stimulation also results in peripheral vasoconstriction. As a consequence, arterial blood pressure is maintained, even in situations when cardiac output is low. Vasoconstriction elevates the diastolic blood pressure and narrows the pulse pressure, maintaining mean and systolic pressure at normal levels. Peripheral vasoconstriction is clinically apparent by weak peripheral pulses, cool extremities, pallor, mottling, and prolonged capillary refill. These are classic early signs of low cardiac output and decreased tissue perfusion, even in the presence of "normal" blood pressure.

If increased heart rate and peripheral vasoconstriction are not sufficient to support decreased cardiac output, continued SNS stimulation results in regional redistribution of blood flow to ensure perfusion of vital organs. Blood is shunted away from the skin, gastrointestinal tract, kidneys, and liver to maintain circulation to the heart, lungs, and brain. Decreased perfusion of the skin and subcutaneous tissue is evident in mottling and cooling of the extremities (Fig. 18-1). Inadequate perfusion of the gastrointestinal tract is apparent when infants or children develop feeding intolerance that may progress to the development of paralytic ileus and/or gastrointestinal necrosis. Decreased urine output is the consequence of inadequate renal blood flow because the glomerular filtration rate is decreased. Acute tubular necrosis (ATN) can be the eventual outcome. Impaired hepatic function is evidenced by abnormalities in coagulation, the development of jaundice, and increases in liver function tests.

Determination of electrolyte, acid-base, and substrate abnormalities is important in the care of pediatric patients

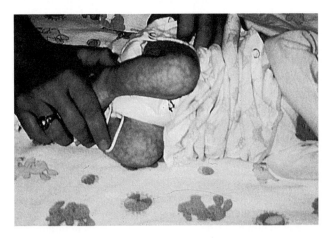

Fig. 18-1 Marked mottling of the skin in infant with regional redistribution of blood flow caused by congestive heart failure.

with impaired tissue perfusion because of their effect on cardiac performance. These abnormalities occur as the consequence of decreased tissue perfusion and can compound cardiac dysfunction. Serum electrolytes, calcium, glucose, urea nitrogen, and creatinine are measured to establish their baseline values in patients with low cardiac output, with measurements repeated at intervals determined by the individual patient's physiologic status.

Arterial blood gases, pH, and base excess or deficit provide specific information about the adequacy of tissue perfusion and oxygenation. Metabolic acidosis develops when tissues are inadequately perfused, with the subsequent development of anaerobic metabolism. Lactic and other organic acids accumulate and require buffering by the buffer bases. This results in rapid use of the base buffers and a resultant base deficit. Metabolic acidosis causes decreased myocardial contractility and decreased adrenergic receptor sensitivity and predisposes to myocardial irritability and lethal cardiac rhythm disturbances.

FINAL COMMON PATHWAYS

Regardless of the cause of inadequate tissue perfusion, if cardiovascular performance cannot be restored, the outcome is similar in all. The possible consequences include impaired cardiac performance, cardiac arrhythmias, cardiac arrest, pulmonary edema, acute respiratory distress syndrome, and irreversible central nervous system ischemia. Clearly the goal is to intervene successfully in a timely manner before these devastating sequelae occur.

PROVIDING BASELINE SUPPORT

Baseline care of patients with cardiovascular dysfunction is predicated on minimizing metabolic demands, support of respiratory function, and provision of nutritional needs. Therapy is escalated as indicated according to patient needs and expected outcomes.

Conserving energy and minimizing stress lower oxygen demand and reduce myocardial work. Promoting rest is of primary importance. Close monitoring of physiologic status allows the timely identification of adverse effects, and clustering of care allows periods of undisturbed rest. If extreme restlessness or irritability is present, the underlying cause must be identified and corrected. If necessary, sedation is provided to minimize anxiety and agitation.

Work of breathing is supported to conserve energy and decrease metabolic demands. In children with left-to-right shunt lesions or in congestive heart failure, concurrent pulmonary edema, decreased lung compliance, low lung volumes, and airway obstruction can be present. All of these pathologic phenomena contribute to increased work of breathing, tachypnea, retractions, rales, and orthopnea. Often the supine position is not well tolerated because of increased pulmonary congestion and decreased lung volumes. The best position for these children is in semi-Fowler's to facilitate displacement of blood in the systemic venous bed and augment lung volumes. In addition, a head-up position displaces the liver and abdominal organs downward, permitting greater chest excursion. Administration of diuretics helps to control pulmonary venous congestion and edema.

Administration of humidified oxygen may be necessary to promote alveolar oxygen diffusion or to treat pulmonary hypertension. However, because of its pulmonary vasodilatory effects, oxygen should be used judiciously in patients with increased pulmonary blood flow or when trying to balance pulmonary-systemic blood flow (as in hypoplastic left heart syndrome) because this intervention can worsen heart failure in these patients. Mechanical ventilation is implemented to take over the work of breathing and to minimize the metabolic demands of the respiratory muscles.

Metabolic rate is increased in children with cardiovascular dysfunction. Unfortunately, many infants and small children cannot consume enough calories to meet metabolic needs. Nutritional support is critically important in these patients. Caloric needs are continually assessed, and growth is monitored over time on an age-appropriate growth chart (see Appendix II). High-calorie formulas are often recommended for infants to maintain weight gain. Nasogastric or nasojejunal feedings are implemented if the infant does not demonstrate normal weight gain despite increasing caloric density. The critically ill child will require monitoring of serum protein, albumin, glucose, electrolytes, and lipids to maximize nutritional support.

Maintenance of normal body temperature conserves energy because both hypothermia and fever result in thermal stress. Wide variations in body temperature produce alterations in oxygen consumption, affecting cardiac output. Hyperthermia increases heart rate, whereas severe hypothermia can result in precipitous drops in cardiac output and blood pressure.

CONGESTIVE HEART FAILURE

Congestive heart failure (CHF), regardless of the age of the patient, is the inability of the cardiovascular system to meet the metabolic demands of the body. Specific causes and clinical presentations vary with age (Box 18-1 and Table 18-1). Manifestations of CHF primarily are due to the physiologic compensatory mechanisms that are results of low cardiac output reflecting the body's attempt to compensate. To understand the pathophysiologic and clinical manifestations of heart failure, the nurse must have a thorough understanding of the normal determinants of cardiac output (see Chapter 7 for review).

Etiology

Congenital heart defects are the most common causes of heart failure in infants. Structural heart disease can impose either a pressure or volume load on the heart. Defects with a left-to-right shunt (ventricular septal defect, patent ductus arteriosus) impose a volume load. Clinical manifestations are dependent on the size of the shunt and pulmonary vascular resistance. Generally, these infants become symptomatic within the first 6 weeks of life. Obstructive lesions (particularly left-sided lesions: aortic stenosis, hypoplastic

left heart syndrome, coarctation) impose a pressure load on the heart. Symptoms become apparent during the first few days of life once the ductus arteriosus closes.[3,4] Anomalies of the coronary arteries can result in myocardial ischemia with subsequent ventricular pump dysfunction and heart failure. Corrective or palliative surgery can result in resolution of CHF or slow its progression.

Acquired heart disease is the most common cause of CHF in children over 1 year of age. Acquired disease includes cardiomyopathy, endocarditis, myocarditis, Kawasaki disease, and rheumatic heart disease. These diseases (with the exception of rheumatic heart disease) result in impaired myocardial contractility. Diminished contractility can ultimately result in volume overload, with subsequent pulmonary and venous congestion. Rheumatic heart disease can result in significant mitral or aortic valve regurgitation, cardiac dilation, and pulmonary congestion.

Tachyarrhythmias or bradyarrhythmias can result in heart failure. Acute-onset tachycardia (supraventricular tachycardia, junctional ectopic tachycardia) can result in heart failure if not identified and treated in a timely manner. Incessant, chronic tachyarrhythmias (atrial ectopic tachycardia, premature junctional reciprocating tachycardia) can result in CHF if the tachycardia occurs throughout the day. In some

---

Box 18-1
Causes of Heart Failure

Alterations in Workload

Volume Overloading of the Ventricles

Large left-to-right shunt
    Ventricular septal defect
    Atrioventricular septal defect
    Patent ductus arteriosus
Valvular insufficiency
    Aortic, mitral, pulmonary
Systemic arteriovenous fistulas

Pressure Overloading of the Ventricles

Obstruction to outflow
    Aortic stenosis
    Pulmonary stenosis
    Coarctation of the aorta
Obstruction to inflow
    Mitral stenosis
    Cortriatriatum
    Tricuspid stenosis

Alterations in Inotropic Function

Inflammatory disease
Electrolyte disturbances
Metabolic disease
Coronary artery lesions

Alterations in Chronotropic Function

Tachyarrhythmias
Profound bradycardia
    Complete heart block

TABLE 18-1 Likely Causes of Heart Failure Related to Timing of Its Development

CHF at Birth or Shortly After

Myocardial dysfunction
  Asphyxia
  Sepsis
  Hypoglycemia
  Hypocalcemia
  Myocarditis
  Transient myocardial ischemia
  Hematologic abnormalities
  Anemia
Hyperviscosity syndrome (hematocrit >65%)

Structural abnormalities
  Tricuspid regurgitation
  Pulmonary regurgitation
  Total anomalous pulmonary venous return with
    obstruction
Heart rate abnormalities
  Supraventricular tachycardia
  Congenital complete heart block

CHF in the First Week of Life

Myocardial or heart rate abnormalities
Same as above, except asphyxia less likely as a cause
Structural abnormalities
  Patent ductus arteriosus
  Hypoplastic left heart syndrome
  Aortic stenosis
  Total anomalous pulmonary venous return
  Coarctation of the aorta
Renal disorders
  Renal failure
  Systemic hypertension

Pulmonary abnormalities
  Upper airway obstruction
  Bronchopulmonary dysplasia
  Central nervous system hypoventilation
  Persistent pulmonary artery hypertension

Endocrine disorders
  Neonatal hyperthyroidism
  Adrenal insufficiency

CHF in Early Infancy (1-6 Weeks)

Myocardial abnormalities
  Endocardial fibroelastosis
  Anomalous origin left coronary artery
  Myocarditis
Dilated cardiomyopathy
Renal disorders
  Same as above

Structural abnormalities
  Coarctation
  Ventricular shunt (VSD, AVSD, SV)
  Aortic shunt (PDA, truncus, AP window)

Endocrine disorders
  Hypothyroidism
  Adrenal insufficiency

CHF After Infancy

Acquired heart disease
  Cardiomyopathy
  Myocarditis
  Vasculitis (Kawasaki disease)
Other
  End-stage pulmonary disease
  Cystic fibrosis
  Primary pulmonary artery hypertension
  Tachyarrhythmia

Congenital heart disease
  Preoperative patients
    Eisenmenger's syndrome
    Pulmonary stenosis (rare)
    Ebstein's anomaly with increasing TR
    Aortic regurgitation
    Mitral regurgitation
    With onset of tachycardia
  Postoperative patients
    Ventriculotomy
    Large residual left to right shunt
    Valvular regurgitation, especially MR, AR
    Obstructed conduit or mechanical valve
    Prosthetic valve malfunction
  Coronary artery injury
  Ventricular dysfunction

AP, Aortopulmonary; *AR,* aortic regurgitation; *AVSD,* atrioventricular septal defect; *CHF,* congestive heart failure; *MR,* mitral regurgitation; *PDA,* patent ductus arteriosus; *SV,* single ventricle; *TR,* tricuspid regurgitation; *VSD,* ventricular septal defect.

patients, cardiomyopathy may be the result of incessant abnormal tachycardias. Once the rhythm is controlled, the cardiomyopathy resolves. Complete heart block with a slow ventricular rate can be responsible for CHF; once the heart block is treated, the CHF resolves as well.

Heart failure may develop as a consequence of acidemia, hypoxia, lung disease, or drug ingestion. Low Pao_2, low pH, and elevated $Paco_2$ depress myocardial function and elevate pulmonary resistance. Chronic lung disease results in pulmonary hypertension and right heart failure. Inborn errors of metabolism can result in cardiomyopathy and CHF. Although rare, heart failure can be iatrogenically induced by excessively rapid infusion of fluid, calcium channel blocker overdose, and β-blocker overdose.

Pathogenesis

The pathogenesis of heart failure is the result of interplay between hemodynamic, neurohormonal, and cellular factors and abnormal autonomic responses. The normal compensatory responses to heart failure initially serve to support cardiovascular function for a limited period. However, if protracted, these compensatory responses may actually be detrimental to the failing heart (Fig. 18-2).

Determinants of Cardiac Performance. The factors that control cardiac output are preload or diastolic volume; afterload or the ventricular wall tension developed during ventricular ejection; contractility or the inotropic state of the myocardium; and heart rate. In addition, significant myocardial structural and maturational issues affect cardiac output in neonates and young infants.

When compared with those in the adult, immature myocytes are thinner, less compliant, and less well organized. The developing heart is also thought to have a relative decrease in contractile mass, with a predominance of noncontractile elements. At birth there is right ventricular dominance that progresses to left ventricular dominance over the first few months of life.[5,6] The newborn heart, at baseline, functions at the peak of the Frank-Starling curve, exhibiting a greater resting tension for any degree of stretch indicating limited ventricular compliance. Therefore volume loading and increased stretch can actually decrease cardiac output. Because of a high intrinsic heart rate, the infant has limited ability to increase cardiac output through an increase in heart rate. Increases in afterload are not well tolerated in neonates and infants because of limited compliance and diminished contractile function.

In newborns the sarcoplasmic reticulum (SR) is poorly organized and less well developed compared with adults. Normally in mature cells the SR is the primary source of intracellular calcium for modulation of contraction. However, because of relative immaturity, the newborn myocyte is dependent on serum calcium for contraction. The contractile proteins (actin and myosin) increase their sensitivity to calcium with maturation, increasing inotropic response with age.[6] In addition, maturational changes in the autonomic nervous system lead to developmental differences in response to autonomic stimulation by endogenous and exogenous adrenergic agonists.

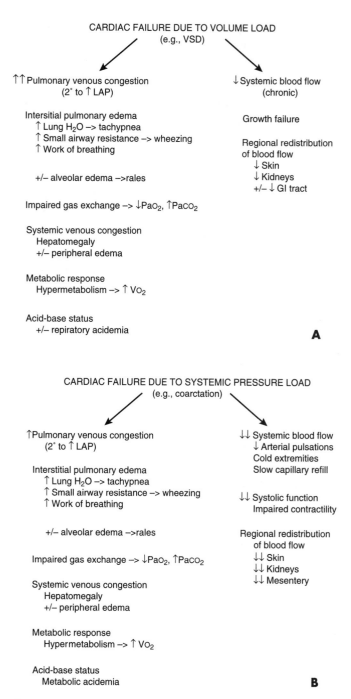

Fig. 18-2 Diagrammatic representations of cardiac failure caused by volume load (**A**) and pressure load (**B**). *VSD,* Ventricular septal defect; *LAP,* left atrial pressure; *GI,* gastrointestinal.

Hemodynamic Characteristics. The hemodynamic abnormalities of heart failure are due to reduced ejection (systolic dysfunction) or diminished ability to receive venous return (diastolic dysfunction). In systolic dysfunction, there is impaired ventricular contraction with a subsequent decrease in the ability to increase stroke volume with volume loading. In this scenario, small increases in afterload are not well tolerated, leading to a decline in cardiac output. Conversely, small decreases in afterload may contribute to a significant improvement in cardiac output. Causes for systolic dysfunction include lesions with left-to-right shunts, dilated cardiomyopathy, and myocardial ischemia. Depending on the underlying cause, systolic dysfunction can lead to volume or pressure overload or both.[7]

Diastolic dysfunction is due to decreased ventricular compliance requiring high venous pressures to support ventricular filling. Causes of diastolic dysfunction include lesions that limit ventricular filling (atrioventricular [AV] valve stenosis, pulmonary venous obstruction), lesions that contribute to reduced intrinsic compliance (hypertrophic cardiomyopathy), and pericardial effusion or tamponade.

Neurohormonal Factors. A decrease in cardiac output triggers a neurohormonal response that is vital to survival in acute low-output states. This is accomplished through enhanced activity of the SNS and the renin-angiotensin-aldosterone system (RAAS). Initially, this results in improved contractility, fluid and sodium retention, and vasoconstriction to support blood pressure. However, when sustained, these compensatory mechanisms may exacerbate hemodynamic abnormalities and accelerate myocardial cell death. Fig. 18-3 depicts the neurohormonal response to low cardiac output and the consequences. SNS stimulation initially improves cardiac output by increasing heart rate, blood pressure, and ejection fraction. With sympathetic stimulation, there is a subsequent increase in ventricular afterload resulting from vasoconstriction. This mechanism supports blood pressure acutely, but eventually it contributes to increased ventricular work. Unfortunately, the long-term sequelae of SNS stimulation lead to increased myocardial oxygen consumption, increased ventricular wall stress, and diminished myocardial oxygen supply.

RAAS stimulation causes salt and water retention, which initially augments preload. Chronic sodium and water retention results in long-term pulmonary congestion and peripheral edema. Vasoconstriction is also augmented by angiotensin II (following conversion of angiotensin I to angiotensin II in the lung). In the short term, it serves to maintain blood pressure for vital organ perfusion. Long-term effects are those of increased afterload: exacerbation of systolic dysfunction and increased energy requirements. Besides promoting salt and water retention, aldosterone is also responsible for the development of ventricular fibrosis and promotion of collagen synthesis in heart failure. These mechanisms are responsible for decreased myocardial capillary density, increased ventricular stiffness, and diastolic dysfunction.[6,8]

Increased SNS and RAAS activity contributes to cardiac toxicity through cell necrosis and apoptosis. Necrosis is a passive process characterized by inflammation that occurs as a result of a number of cytotoxic mechanisms. Apoptosis is an active process that is secondary to activation of genes encoded for programmed cell death. Apoptosis is activated in clinical conditions in which vascular remodeling, hypertension, and ischemia occur.[6]

Cellular Factors. Ventricular dilation occurs in response to the increased stress imposed by volume or pressure overload. An increase in ventricular end-diastolic volume, even in the face of diminished fiber shortening, supports stroke volume. However, chamber dilation requires an increase in wall tension to maintain systolic pressure, increasing myocardial oxygen requirements. This physiologic mechanism is limited in that excessive wall stretch will exceed the heart's ability to contract forcefully. Conse-

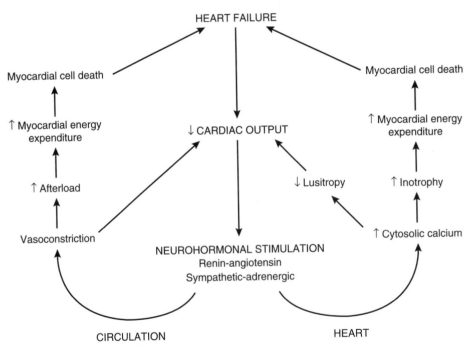

Fig. 18-3 Diagrammatic representation of consequences of neurohormonal response in heart failure. (Adapted from Katz AM: Cardiomyopathy of overload, *N Engl J Med* 322:100-110, 1990.)

quently, a fall in systolic function and stroke volume will occur. As mentioned previously, fibrosis and collagen formation occur in heart failure with a subsequent loss of myocytes. These phenomena contribute to progressive cardiac dilation, decrease in capillary density, and a relative deficit of energy-producing mitochondria. Because of changes in calcium intrusion into the cytosol with energy deficit, ventricular relaxation (lusitropy) diminishes (relaxation is more sensitive to energy deficit than contraction).

Hypertrophy of the overloaded ventricle is a complex process brought about by changes in actin, myosin, and collagen contributing to cardiac remodeling. Adding new sarcomeres aids the heart in adapting to chronic ventricular overload. However, chronic hypertrophy is associated with abnormal gene expression leading to progressive myocardial damage, fibrosis, and cell death. Chronic hypertrophy prolongs the action potential, leading to electrophysiologic abnormalities and cardiac rhythm disturbances. Hypertrophy also impairs relaxation of the heart, leading to diastolic dysfunction. In infants and children, relief of increased ventricular afterload allows regression of hypertrophy.

Abnormal Autonomic Responses. Acutely, SNS compensatory activation improves cardiovascular function through an increase in chronotropic, inotropic, and lusitropic responses. Over time, with sustained sympathetic overstimulation, a subsequent down-regulation of β-receptors occurs. Ultimately the myocytes fail to respond normally to endogenous and exogenous adrenergic agonists, with a substantial decrease in responsiveness to adrenergic stimulation.

Clinical Manifestations

The signs of heart failure in infants and children can be subtle and are dependent on the underlying etiology and age of the child. They can be organized into three general categories: signs related to impaired myocardial performance and those resulting from pulmonary and systemic venous congestion.

Impaired Myocardial Performance. The cardiac manifestations of heart failure primarily are due to the neurohormonal compensatory mechanisms that are activated because of low cardiac output. In addition, cardiac failure presents additional specific symptoms related directly to poor myocardial function.

Cardiac enlargement on chest radiograph is a consistent sign of impaired function, representing ventricular dilation or hypertrophy. Only in the earliest stages of heart failure is cardiac size normal. Tachycardia is commonly seen with cardiac failure and represents an adaptive mechanism to support cardiac output and oxygen delivery to tissues. An S_3 gallop rhythm noted at the apex is often appreciated because of rapid filling of a stiff, noncompliant ventricle.[3] Vasoconstriction decreases peripheral perfusion, signaled by cool extremities, weak peripheral pulses, slow capillary refill, and mottling. In high output failure, pulse pressure may be increased and arterial pulsation bounding. Severe anemia (hemoglobin level lower than 5 g/dl) causes a similar phenomenon. Vasoconstriction most often maintains blood pressure in the normal range, even when tissue perfusion is inadequate. Hypotension is a late and ominous sign.

Many infants and small children in heart failure cannot ingest enough calories to support growth, particularly with the concurrent increase in metabolic demands. This phenomenon is usually secondary to fatigue and poor feeding. As a result of sympathetic activation, diaphoresis with feeding can be noted.[9] Severely ill infants may fatigue so quickly with feeding that it is physically impossible for them to take in an adequate volume of formula. Therefore growth failure results, necessitating increasing caloric density of formula or the institution of tube feedings.

Pulmonary Congestion. Pulmonary congestion occurs secondary to increased pulmonary blood flow, left ventricular failure, or pulmonary venous obstruction. Normally the pulmonary lymphatics remove accumulated lung fluid to prevent alveolar edema. If capacity of the lymphatics is exceeded because of pulmonary overcirculation or pulmonary venous congestion, then pulmonary edema ensues.[3] Tachypnea is a common sign of heart failure indicating pulmonary interstitial edema and decreased lung compliance. Intercostal retractions, grunting, wheezing, and cough may also be present. Older children will complain of dyspnea on exertion or orthopnea. Rales are generally a late sign and may not be appreciated in infants. Wheezing may be due to bronchial edema or compression of the airways by distension of the pulmonary arteries or left atrium.

Systemic Venous Congestion. Hepatomegaly is the most consistent sign of systemic venous congestion. Enlargement of the liver reflects an increase in systemic venous volume or right atrial pressure. Tenderness of the liver and the absence of a firm, discrete liver edge can be elicited even in older children with heart failure. Jaundice may occur with hepatic congestion but is generally a late sign.

Systemic venous congestion can be evaluated in older children by observing the jugular venous vein (this cannot be assessed in infants). Normally when the child is supine and lying at a 45-degree angle, the jugular vein should not rise above the imaginary line drawn across the manubrium of the sternum. If the vein is visible above this line, then jugular venous distension is present, indicating CHF. Peripheral edema is a rare finding in infants, although periorbital edema can sometimes be detected. In older children, peripheral edema and, occasionally, ascites and generalized anasarca may be present.[9] These clinical signs are more often appreciated in the child with severely compromised myocardial function.

Diagnosis. In addition to history and physical examination findings, the diagnosis of heart failure is aided by a number of noninvasive and invasive laboratory studies. Chest radiography is necessary to assess cardiac size; it also permits assessment of pulmonary congestion. The electrocardiogram (ECG) is not particularly useful, unless an arrhythmia is the cause for cardiac failure. Echocardiography permits assessment of myocardial function from ventricular dimensions, fiber-shortening rate, and ejection fraction. Diastolic function is evaluated from estimates of isovolumetric relaxation time, diastolic dimensions, filling time, and other parameters.

Critical Care Management

Treatment of cardiac failure is determined by the underlying cause. Structural heart disease in infants or children who are in CHF should be repaired or palliated in a timely manner. Early surgical repair can lead to reversal of neurohormonal and cellular abnormalities that lead to ventricular dilation and hypertrophy. Preoperative use of prostaglandin E_1 (PGE_1) to maintain ductal patency in ductal-dependent lesions permits stabilization and an elective approach to surgery.

Medical management in acute heart failure is directed at support of cardiac output through manipulation of preload, afterload, and contractility. (See Chapter 7 for a complete discussion on volume replacement and medications.) Volume status is normalized through diuresis and judicious fluid management. Inotropes, either intravenous or oral, are instituted to improve contractility. Afterload-reducing agents are instituted if appropriate and are being used increasingly to decrease ventricular work. If the cause of heart failure is incessant, tachyarrhythmia antiarrhythmics are used for conversion to sinus rhythm or for rate control.

Mechanical assist (ventricular assist device, intraaortic balloon pump, or extracorporeal membrane oxygenation) is used in the severely decompensated patient for temporary support or as a bridge to heart transplantation (see Chapter 7, section on mechanical assist.)

Maneuvers to manipulate the pulmonary vascular bed are implemented in select patients to maximize pulmonary: systemic flow. Oxygen, alkalosis, hyperventilation, nitric oxide, prostacyclin, and afterload reduction decrease pulmonary vascular resistance, therefore augmenting pulmonary blood flow. These interventions are to be used in patients with pulmonary hypertension and should be avoided in children with large left-to-right shunts. In the latter, increased pulmonary blood flow will be at the expense of systemic flow, contributing to systemic underperfusion. Inhaled carbon dioxide or nitrogen will increase pulmonary vascular resistance, decreasing pulmonary blood flow. These two maneuvers are generally reserved for infants with hypoplastic left heart syndrome or single-ventricle physiology who require careful balancing of systemic-to-pulmonary blood flow.

Diuretic Therapy. In treating chronic failure, diuretic therapy is aimed at correcting the clinical problems of pulmonary and systemic venous congestion. Diuretic agents are useful to maximize sodium excretion and thereby increase the volume of urine excreted. Table 18-2 lists the various types of diuretic agents useful as adjuncts in treating patients with heart failure.

Because all diuretic agents increase sodium excretion, hypovolemia and hyponatremia are potential complications of their use. Acid-base imbalances can occur. Metabolic alkalosis is common with administration of the potent loop diuretics, owing to chloride depletion and volume contraction. Metabolic acidosis is a potential complication of carbonic anhydrase inhibitors, but this usually is mild. Hypokalemia is the consequence of potassium wasting. Hypokalemia can be avoided by diuretics given every other day, potassium supplementation, or the concurrent use of a potassium-sparing diuretic.

Neurohormonal Modulation. As the understanding of the pathophysiologic mechanisms underlying heart failure increases, so have novel therapeutic interventions. Newer treatment modalities are aimed at blocking or resetting neurohormonal overstimulation. Presently used agents include angiotensin-converting enzyme inhibitors (ACEIs), digoxin, β-blockers, aldosterone antagonists, and angiotensin-receptor blockers.

Angiotensin II is responsible for vasoconstriction, aldosterone secretion, myocardial fibrosis, and cellular remodeling in heart failure. ACEIs inhibit the enzyme responsible for the conversion of angiotensin I to angiotensin II. They also inhibit degradation of bradykinin and inhibit norepinephrine release, thus augmenting vasodilation. These

◆ TABLE 18-2 Diuretic Agents for Heart Failure

Drug	Action
Loop Diuretics	
Furosemide	Block Na and Cl reabsorption widely at multiple medullary and cortical sites
Bumetanide	Cautions: volume contraction (free water reabsorption is blocked); hypokalemia
Ethacrynic acid	
Cortical Diluting Segment Agents	
Thiazide diuretics	Block Na and Cl reabsorption at the ascending limb; less loss of K
Metolazone	Caution: volume contraction (especially with metolazone)
Potassium-Sparing Agents	
Spironolactone	Aldosterone antagonist; impairs Na reabsorption and increases K and H ion secretion
	No effect on water production or reabsorption
Carbonic Anhydrase Inhibitors	
Acetazolamide	Inhibits carbonic anhydrase to decrease Na and Cl reabsorption at distal sites
	Less effect on free water production and reabsorption, but K excretion is increased
	Diuretic effects are mild only

Cl, Chloride ions; *H,* hydrogen ions; *K,* potassium ions; *Na,* sodium ions.

agents have long been used for afterload reduction to decrease ventricular wall stress and work. Angiotensin II and norepinephrine (along with increased ventricular wall stress) are also known to contribute to ventricular remodeling and fibrosis. ACEIs have been shown to prevent fibrosis and limit myocyte necrosis and apoptosis.[10] Clinically, these agents have been shown to produce symptomatic improvement and reduce mortality.[6]

Digoxin is extensively used to treat heart failure, improving hemodynamics through the enhancement of systolic function. Digoxin also enhances parasympathetic stimulation, therefore opposing sympathetic overstimulation. The mechanism by which digoxin potentiates parasympathetic stimulation is not well understood.

β-Blockers, albeit counterintuitive, have been shown to improve ventricular function and decrease mortality in both children and adults. These agents are usually employed once diuretic, afterload-reducing, and inotropic medications have been maximized.[11-13] Mechanism of action is thought to be the prevention and reversal of SNS-mediated myocardial remodeling and dysfunction. Initially, β-blockers can worsen failure, so starting doses are low with slow incremental increases in dose up to maximum therapeutic dose or clinical effect. Dosage adjustment is tailored to the patient and may take weeks. Cardio-selective third-generation agents (carvedilol) are generally well tolerated with few side effects.[14] Carvedilol is believed to have antioxidant effects, theoretically providing protection against cytotoxic biologic modifiers.[6,11] Further studies are necessary to evaluate β-blockers in children because of the variable causes and natural history of heart failure in pediatrics.

Aldosterone, as part of the RAAS, plays a significant role in the pathophysiology of heart failure. It promotes sodium and water retention, myocardial fibrosis, and collagen formation. Spironolactone is an aldosterone-receptor antagonist, potassium-sparing diuretic long used in pediatrics to avoid potassium replacement but is avoided in adults because of potential hyperkalemia. The Randomized Aldactone Evaluation Study (RALES)[8] demonstrated significant clinical improvement and reduction in mortality in adults with CHF who were prescribed spironolactone. This randomized, double-blinded study was halted prematurely because the observed improvement in outcome in the spironolactone group exceeded prespecified end points. Mechanism of action is thought to be prevention of sodium and water retention, prevention of myocardial fibrosis, and blocking of collagen formation.

Angiotensin II antagonists (losartan, candesartan) are new agents currently under investigation in adults to selectively block angiotensin II receptors, mitigating the effects of the RAAS. Currently they are used for patients who are refractory to ACE inhibition, and are generally prescribed concurrently.[10] To date, no pediatric clinical trials have been published.

Nutrition. Nutrition is one of the most important aspects of the management of children in heart failure. Small children and infants in heart failure often cannot consume enough calories to support growth. Tachypnea and fatigue can interfere with normal nursing or nippling. Many infants in heart failure require up to 150 calories/kg/day. A number of biologic markers can be used to assess nutritional status. In the PICU, serum albumin or prealbumin can be measured. Prealbumin is a better marker of nutritional state because it has a shorter half-life than albumin and correlates with positive nitrogen balance. In an effort to maximize caloric intake, formula or breast milk can be fortified to increase caloric density. In general, formula should not be increased to greater than 30 calories/ounce to prevent an excessive osmotic and protein load. Tube feedings are implemented if the infant continues to fail to thrive. These feedings can be nasogastric or nasojejunal, given throughout the day or at night only. Any infant with structural heart disease who does not gain weight appropriately on maximum calories and medical management constitutes a medical failure and should undergo surgical intervention.

CYANOSIS AND HYPOXEMIA

Cyanosis and hypoxemia are commonly encountered clinical problems in pediatric patients. Cyanotic infants often present a confusing diagnostic picture. The first task is differentiating cardiac disease from pulmonary disease in these infants. A general rule of thumb is that children who improve with oxygen have lung disease and those who do not have cyanotic heart disease. In some cases, this does not always hold true, prompting further diagnostic investigation. Echocardiography is an important diagnostic tool used in concert with clinical presentation and other ancillary tests (chest x-ray film, ECG).

Etiology and Clinical Presentation in Cyanotic Infants

Structural heart diseases that produce cyanosis can have decreased pulmonary blood flow (PBF) or variable PBF. Defects that result in decreased PBF are characterized by right heart atresia or right ventricular outflow obstruction (severe pulmonary stenosis, pulmonary atresia, and tetralogy of Fallot). These defects are manifested by cyanosis that is often severe following closure of the ductus arteriosus, is intensified by crying, and may be episodic. It is not relieved by the administration of oxygen, even at high concentrations. Tachypnea not accompanied by dyspnea, retractions, grunting, or nasal flaring (which are also characteristic of pulmonary disease or edema) is indicative of a cyanotic congenital heart defect with decreased PBF.

Cardiac defects with left-to-right shunts and increased PBF may or may not develop cyanosis. Pulmonary vascular resistance (PVR) determines the presence of cyanosis in this population. If PVR is elevated, there can be right-to-left or bidirectional shunting. This generally occurs in the neonate. Once PVR falls to normal levels, cyanosis will not be evident unless the infant develops a concurrent respiratory illness. Mixing lesions, such as transposition of the great arteries, develop severe cyanosis once the ductus arteriosus closes. Infants and children with pulmonary venous obstruction with associated pulmonary hypertension will be cyanotic until obstruction is relieved.

With recent surgical advances, many infants' defects are repaired early, so long-standing cyanotic heart disease is becoming less of an issue. However, a large number of adolescents and young adults who received palliative treatment in infancy never underwent surgical correction. Eisenmenger's syndrome develops in the presence of long-standing increased PBF (left-to-right shunt). At some point, depending on the size of the shunt and characteristics of the patient, pulmonary vascular disease develops secondary to pulmonary pressure and volume load. When pulmonary artery pressure exceeds systemic pressure, then shunt reversal (right to left) and chronic cyanosis result. If PVR is not reactive to pulmonary vasodilators (oxygen, nitric oxide), then the patient is considered inoperable for repair of the primary cardiac defect, and referral for heart-lung transplant may be considered.

A number of other clinical clues help to differentiate cardiac and pulmonary disease. Chest radiographs, although not always conclusive, are often helpful in detecting pulmonary disease in infants. Arterial blood gas analysis may reveal helpful differential findings. In lung disease, the $Paco_2$ may be elevated, whereas it is normal or even decreased because of tachypnea in patients with cardiac disease. Acid-base balance is initially maintained, but inadequate tissue perfusion, which may be the consequence of ductal closure, results in lactic acidosis.

Pathogenesis of hypoxemia and cyanosis with respect to specific cardiac lesions are discussed in the section on congenital heart disease. Acute hypoxemia associated with respiratory disease is discussed in Chapter 19.

Acute Hypoxia.   Acute hypoxic episodes have the potential to occur in critically ill infants and children for various reasons, most of them pulmonary in nature. Acute hypoxia produces pulmonary hypertension, which is usually transient and reversible in healthy individuals. However, in patients with preexisting heart disease, pulmonary hypertension (particularly in the postoperative cardiac surgery patient) is not well tolerated. In these patients, hypoxia can result in acute pulmonary hypertensive crisis. This serious problem is characterized by an acute rise in pulmonary artery pressure and central venous pressure (CVP) with a subsequent fall in left atrial pressure (LAP), cardiac output, and systemic oxygen saturation. Without timely intervention, metabolic and respiratory acidosis ensues, further exacerbating pulmonary hypertension. Interrupting the vicious cycle of right ventricular dysfunction, inadequate PBF, severe hypoxemia, and low cardiac output can be extremely difficult. These crises may be fatal despite aggressive attempts to reverse the condition. Interventions include analgesia or sedation, hyperventilation with 100% oxygen, maintenance of normothermia, and skeletal muscle relaxation.

Chronic Hypoxia.   Chronic cyanosis and hypoxemia have deleterious effects on many body systems and have been recognized for decades. These effects include changes in the following tissues and organs:

1. *Blood:* Chronic hypoxia stimulates overproduction of red blood cells in the bone marrow, resulting in polycythemia. When polycythemia is severe (hematocrit of 70% to 75%), blood viscosity increases dramatically. Despite elevated red cell counts, red cell indices are frequently abnormal, with iron deficiency anemia requiring iron replacement therapy. In the face of hypoxemia, the body attempts to increase oxygen delivery by increasing cardiac output. Therefore these patients can have a "relative" anemia if hemoglobin concentration is "normal" (e.g., following blood loss or trauma). In this scenario, these patients will act like they are anemic (hyperdynamic, with signs of increased cardiac output). Keeping hemoglobin level between 16 to 18 g/dl is beneficial in this population. Thrombocytopenia, impaired platelet aggregation, and reduction in clotting factors are additional complications of polycythemia. Bleeding disorders can result, primarily in older children.

2. *Central nervous system:* As a result of polycythemia and hyperviscosity, acute or transient cerebral insults may occur from cerebral infarcts. Strokes can also occur as a result of decreased deformability of the microcytic red blood cells. In addition to the risk of stroke, an increased incidence of brain abscesses is seen among those who are older. These can occur because venous bacteria are shunted into the systemic circulation without undergoing the normal filtering process afforded by the pulmonary macrophages.

3. *Heart:* Hypoxia evokes compensatory cardiac changes, including coronary vasodilation and the development of myocardial collateral circulation. Hyperviscosity increases systemic and pulmonary afterload and decreases coronary artery perfusion. Consequently, myocardial function is depressed, leaving older cyanotic children with limited exercise capacity.

4. *Lungs:* Increased viscosity contributes to increased PVR. Increased PVR increases right-to-left shunting, exacerbating cyanosis and hypoxia.

Treatment of Polycythemia.   Generally, patients do not exhibit symptoms until hematocrit reaches 70%. Clinically, manifestations include headache, joint and chest pain, anorexia, and visual disturbances. Historically, these patients would receive a phlebotomy before the development of symptoms. However, clinical effects are short lived because hematocrit again increases as a normal physiologic response to hypoxemia. Currently the recommendation is to phlebotomize symptomatic patients only. This procedure is performed as a partial exchange transfusion, removing small aliquots of blood and replacing them with normal saline or albumin, down to a hematocrit of 60% to 65%. Patients experience immediate symptomatic relief, but unfortunately, some become quite dependent on this intervention and frequently request it.

CONGENITAL HEART DISEASE

The incidence of congenital heart disease is approximately 1% of all live births. Worldwide, 1.5 million children are born with a congenital heart defect yearly, and in the United States, approximately 40,000 newborns are affected each year. Of these children, 5% to 8% have associated chromosomal anomalies or syndromes. At least one third of the infants born in the United States with a congenital heart defect will be critically ill or require surgical therapy during their first year of life.[15] Despite major advances in the management of these children, congenital heart disease accounts for a large proportion of infant mortality and is a major reason for admission to the PICU.

The etiology of congenital heart disease is a rapidly growing field of interest and research. Known risk factors include environmental exposures, drug exposures, maternal diabetes, maternal reproductive history, and a family history.[16] Despite these risk factors, the exact cause of congenital heart disease is poorly understood. Cardiac formation begins on day 18 of gestation when the cardiac mesoderm begins to form and ends on day 45 of gestation when the ventricular septum has closed.[17] Each cardiac malformation can be determined to have occurred during a specific time during gestation. Like many congenital defects, cardiac malformation has often occurred before pregnancy is detected. Although formation is complete early in gestation, the heart continues to mature until well after birth.

In the past, there has been a reluctance to do primary surgical repairs on neonates and young infants because of the potential increased risk of cardiac surgery in these patients. As a result, palliative and staged procedures had been preferred. Refinements in surgical techniques, cardiopulmonary bypass, myocardial preservation, and postoperative management has led to the recent trend toward primary repairs of congenital heart defects in neonates and young infants. This current philosophy has resulted in a change in the patient population and the patient care management in PICUs today. Although the majority of patients are neonates and young infants, many older children, adolescents, and adults, who had previously received palliative treatment, are reentering PICUs for additional surgery or for treatment of sequelae.

Several classification systems exist to categorize congenital heart defects. One system that is clinically useful is based on the presence or absence of cyanosis and an estimate of the volume of PBF. These characteristics are determined by physical examination and radiographic examinations and are diagnosed by echocardiography (Box 18-2).

Acyanotic Heart Defects With Increased PBF

Congenital heart defects that produce a left-to-right shunt at varying points in the circulation lead to an increase in PBF. The most common lesions associated with increased PBF include patent ductus arteriosus, atrial septal defect, ventricular septal defect, and AV septal defect. (Table 18-3 summarizes the findings on cardiac examination, ECG, and chest radiograph of children with these defects.)

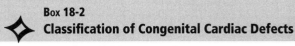

Box 18-2

◆ Classification of Congenital Cardiac Defects

Acyanotic Defects With Increased PBF

Patent ductus arteriosus
Atrial septal defect
Ventricular septal defect
Atrioventricular septal defect

Acyanotic Defects That Obstruct Flow

Coarctation of the aorta
Aortic stenosis
Pulmonary stenosis

Cyanotic Defects With Decreased PBF

Tricuspid atresia
Tetralogy of Fallot
Pulmonary atresia with intact ventricular septum

Cyanotic Defects With Increased PBF

Total anomalous pulmonary venous connection
Truncus arteriosus
Hypoplastic left heart syndrome

Cyanotic Defects With Variable PBF

Transposition of the great arteries
Double-outlet right ventricle
Double-inlet left ventricle
Single ventricle

PBF, Pulmonary blood flow.

Patent Ductus Arteriosus. The ductus arteriosus is formed during the fifth to seventh week of gestation. It is a vascular communication between the junction of the main and left pulmonary arteries and the lesser curvature of the descending aorta just distal to the left subclavian artery. The ductus is approximately 1 cm in length, slightly less than 1 cm in diameter, and has a sphincterlike muscle in its wall. The ductus begins to close within 10 to 15 hours of birth, and closure is usually completed by 3 weeks of age. Although a ductus can close spontaneously at any time other than the newborn period, this is very unlikely to occur after the age of 1 year because of the absence of normal physiologic mediators that contribute to closure.

At birth, with the removal of the placenta (major source of prostaglandin in utero) and with the concurrent onset of respiration, PVR decreases with a subsequent rise in Pao_2. The combination of an increased Pao_2 and a fall in prostaglandins results in ductal constriction. Eventually anatomic closure occurs, and the ductus becomes fibrous, forming the ligamentum arteriosus. If these processes do not occur or are interrupted, a patent ductus arteriosus (PDA) is the result (Fig. 18-4). Prematurity, hypoxia, and scarring of the ductus from rubella during fetal life are all factors that can prevent ductal closure.

The size of the shunt through the PDA is determined by the relative pressure differences between the systemic and

TABLE 18-3 Acyanotic Congenital Heart Defects With Increased Pulmonary Blood Flow

Defect	Cardiac Examination	Electrocardiogram	Chest Radiograph
PDA	"Machinery" murmur heard throughout systole and diastole; best heard at left upper sternal border and under left clavicle; palpable cardiac thrill (with large PDA) at left sternal border	May be normal or demonstrate left ventricular hypertrophy	Increased pulmonary vascularity, prominent pulmonary arteries, enlargement of the left ventricle and aorta
ASD			
Ostium secundum and sinus venosus	Normal S_1; Soft systolic ejection murmur best heard at second left ICS; fixed and widely split S_2	May be normal, but right axis deviation, right ventricular hypertrophy, RSR' in V_1	Increased pulmonary vasculature, enlargement of right atrium, right ventricle, and pulmonary artery; aorta smaller than normal
Ostium primum	Same as above	Left axis deviation, RSR' in V_1	
VSD			
Small, muscular	Loud, harsh systolic murmur localized to left sternal border; associated cardiac thrill	Normal	Normal heart size and PBF
Moderate to large	Rumbling murmur heard best at lower left sternal border; radiates across the left chest sometimes as far as the midaxillary line; pulmonary component of S_2 loud and widely split	Left ventricular dominance and left ventricular hypertrophy	Cardiomegaly, enlarged left atrium, enlarged left ventricle, prominent pulmonary vascular markings
Eisenmenger's complex	Quieter heart murmur; loud single P_2	Right ventricular hypertrophy	Normal or enlarged right atrium, right ventricle, and pulmonary artery; small distal pulmonary vessels; variability in size of left atrium and left ventricle
AVSD			
Incomplete; competent mitral valve	Same as for ASD	Same as for ostium secundum ASD	Same as for ASD
Mitral insufficiency	Systolic murmur best heard apically; radiates to the axilla	Left ventricular hypertrophy	Enlargement of left ventricle and left atrium
Complete	Combination of ASD, VSD, and atrioventricular valve insufficiency murmurs; no murmur may be present; with pulmonary artery hypertension, P_2 is loud and widely split	Left axis deviation and biventricular hypertrophy	Cardiomegaly and increased pulmonary vascular markings

ASD, Atrial septal defect; *AVSD,* atrioventricular septal defect; *ICS,* intercostal space; *P_2,* pulmonary component of second heart sound; *PBF,* pulmonary blood flow; *PDA,* patent ductus arteriosus; *S_1,* first heart sound; *S_2,* second heart sound; *VSD,* ventricular septal defect.

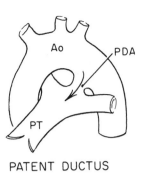

Fig. 18-4 Patent ductus arteriosus. *Ao,* Aorta; *PDA,* patent ductus arteriosus; *PT,* pulmonary trunk. (From Perloff JK: *The clinical recognition of congenital heart disease,* ed 4, Philadelphia, 1994, WB Saunders, p 510.)

pulmonary vascular beds and the size of the PDA. After birth, with the normal fall in PVR and rise in systemic vascular resistance, the shunt is left to right. If the PDA is large or moderate in size, this will lead to pulmonary overcirculation and left heart enlargement. However, if there is some degree of lung disease or elevation of PVR, the shunt can be bidirectional or right to left.

Clinical Presentation and Course. When occurring in isolation, clinical symptoms vary with the size of the PDA and the degree of shunt. Small PDAs may not be appreciated on auscultation and can be hemodynamically insignificant. Large PDAs can contribute to CHF once PVR has fallen. These infants and children can have signs and symptoms of CHF, including tachypnea, poor feeding, and diaphoresis.

On auscultation the classic finding is one of a continuous murmur audible in the left upper chest. However, if PVR is elevated (with subsequent decreased shunt) or the PDA is small, the murmur may be soft or inaudible. Generally, the pulses are bounding, and in the older child the pulse pressure will be wide (low diastolic pressure). Echocardiogram is adequate to make the diagnosis and in determining the size and configuration of the PDA for possible coil occlusion.

Management. Asymptomatic children with hemodynamically insignificant PDAs require no medical treatment before elective closure between 2 to 5 years of age. Endocarditis prophylaxis is necessary for dental work or contaminated surgical procedures.[18] Controversy exists regarding whether small "silent" PDAs should be closed because the risks of intervention may exceed the lifetime risk of endocarditis.

The premature infant or any child in CHF requires anticongestive therapy with fluid restriction, diuretics, and digoxin. If, however, CHF cannot be controlled by these measures, then closure is recommended. Indomethacin, a prostaglandin inhibitor, is advocated in the preterm population in an attempt to close the PDA without surgery. Indomethacin is usually given at a dose of 0.2 mg/kg orally or intravenously as a single dose and, if necessary, repeated after 8 and 16 hours. Because indomethacin is an acetylsalicylic acid, it cannot be given to the infant with poor renal function, necrotizing enterocolitis, bleeding dyscrasias, hyperbilirubinemia, internal bleeding, and shock or myocardial ischemia. When this drug is administered, close assessment for signs and symptoms of abnormal bleeding is crucial. Larger infants and older children may undergo coil occlusion or surgical division of the PDA.

Coil Occlusion. PDAs can be coil occluded in the catheterization laboratory if the PDA is of the right size and configuration. Small to moderate, conically shaped PDAs are most amenable to this intervention; however, a snare-assisted technique has been used successfully to occlude large PDAs.[19,20] The usual technique for coil occlusion involves a retrograde approach via the femoral artery to the PDA. One or more coil can then be deployed until a shunt is no longer seen on angiography. Complications include embolization of the coil into the pulmonary artery or aorta, improper placement, or residual shunt.[21] Benefits include short hospital stay and no surgical incisions. In many institutions, catheter occlusion is the treatment of choice for PDA (with the exception of the preterm neonate).

Surgical Correction. Surgical repair of a large PDA is performed off cardiopulmonary bypass and is recommended for those patients with a large, unusually shaped, or short PDA. Some centers will not coil occlude PDAs in small patients because of the risk of embolization and pulmonary artery occlusion with the device, so surgery is recommended. The defect may be ligated, divided, or occluded with a hemoclip. The surgery is performed through a posterolateral incision in the fourth left intercostal space (ICS). In the neonate a hemoclip is used. In the older infant or child, the ductus is usually ligated with heavy suture to prevent recanalization or hemorrhage, which may occur with incomplete ligation, or the ductus can be divided between clamps and the severed ends closed by sutures. Postoperative complications are rare except in the premature infant, for whom other factors, such as respiratory distress, complicate recovery. The incidence of laryngeal nerve palsy of the vocal cords is about 4%, with smaller neonates at the greatest risk.[22] Recently video-assisted thorascopic surgery (VATS) has been successfully applied for closure of a PDA.

These patients are usually extubated in the operating room and generally do not go to the PICU. Postoperative issues include pain control and wound care. Assessment of peripheral pulses, heart sounds, pulse oximetry, and breath sounds is important. Rarely, ligation of nonductal vascular structures (usually the left pulmonary artery) has occurred.

Atrial Septal Defect. An atrial septal defect (ASD) exists when a nonphysiologic communication between the left and right atrium persists beyond the perinatal period. The atrial septum is formed between the fourth to sixth week of gestation. The septum is composed of septum primum and septum secundum. An opening, called the foramen ovale, persists in the atrial septum throughout intrauterine existence. This opening permits blood to bypass the lungs. After birth, with an increase in left atrial pressure, the foramen ovale closes. It should be noted that up to 30% of normal adolescents and adults have a probe-patent, valve-competent foramen ovale that is not considered an ASD and is capable of producing an atrial shunt.[23] ASDs develop

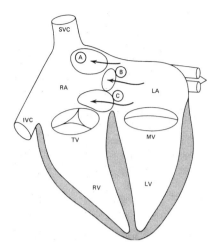

Fig. 18-5 Three locations of atrial septal defect (ASD). *A*, Sinus venosus ASD; *B*, ostium secundum ASD; *C*, ostium primum ASD. *IVC*, Inferior vena cava; *LA*, left atrium; *LV*, left ventricle; *MV*, mitral valve; *RA*, right atrium; *RV*, right ventricle; *SVC*, superior vena cava; *TV*, tricuspid valve. (From Smith JB: *Pediatric critical care*, Albany, NY, 1985, Delmar.)

from the defective development of the septum secundum or the septum primum.

ASDs are classified according to their location in the atrial septum. The most common site is at the center of the atrial septum at the level of the foramen ovale; this is called an ostium secundum ASD. If the defect occurs high in the atrial septum, it is called a sinus venosus ASD. This defect, located near the junction of the superior vena cava and the right atrium, can also be associated with partial anomalous pulmonary venous connection. When the defect occurs low in the septum, it is identified as an ostium primum ASD (Fig. 18-5). Primum ASDs are often associated with AV valvar abnormalities or AV septal defects. A rare defect, the coronary sinus type (unroofed coronary sinus), is located at the roof of the coronary sinus.

The hemodynamic significance of ASDs depends on the size of the defect, the location, associated cardiac anomalies, and right heart compliance. During the postnatal transition period, PVR is generally elevated, and right heart compliance is decreased; therefore shunting may be minimal at first (even with large defects). In older infants and children, the right heart is more compliant than the left; therefore the atrial shunt is left to right. Left-to-right atrial shunt imposes a volume load on the right heart, resulting in right heart enlargement.

Clinical Presentation and Course. Children with small shunts will be asymptomatic, and it is not unusual for this defect to be missed until school age or adolescence. Those with large shunts will have a systolic murmur and a fixed, widely split second heart sound. With secundum ASDs, clinically significant CHF and growth failure are unusual, although this can occur with primum defects. Echocardiogram is sufficient to make the diagnosis and to determine the location and size of the defect, and cardiac catheterization is almost never needed.

Management. Isolated secundum ASDs do not usually require medical management before elective surgical closure. Children with an ostium primum ASD and associated AV valve abnormalities that present with CHF are treated with anticongestive therapy. Small and some moderately sized ASDs will close spontaneously during the first few years of life. Closure of small, hemodynamically insignificant (no right heart enlargement) ASDs remains controversial because the risks of cardiopulmonary bypass may outweigh the benefits. Endocarditis prophylaxis is not recommended for secundum ASDs. It is generally agreed that moderate to large defects should be closed in childhood to prevent the future development of pulmonary vascular disease with subsequent pulmonary hypertension.

Device Closure. For some centrally located secundum defects that are not excessive in size (less than 22 mm), closure with an occluding device can be done in the cardiac catheterization laboratory.[21] A number of devices are currently under Food and Drug Administration (FDA) investigation. Risks include embolization of the device, thrombus, malposition, and residual shunt. Long-term risks and outcomes have yet to be defined.

Surgical Correction. Repair is traditionally recommended between 3 and 5 years of age.[24] Surgical correction is performed by means of a median sternotomy incision. Today many surgeons use a ministernotomy technique. The child is placed on cardiopulmonary bypass, and either suture or a patch of pericardium or synthetic material is used to close the ASD. With sinus venosus defects the patch is placed so as to close the ASD and to direct any anomalous pulmonary venous drainage into the left atrium. Because of the proximity of the sinus node to the sinus venosus baffle, damage to the sinoatrial (SA) node can occur. Repair of ostium primum defects can result in damage to the AV node or bundle of His.

Intravenous vasoactive agents are rarely needed following surgery, and most patients can be extubated in the operating room or shortly thereafter. Postoperative concerns include pain control, bleeding, and wound care. Complications include heart block, residual shunt, AV valve regurgitation (particularly following primum repairs), and atrial arrhythmias. The potential development of atrial arrhythmias remains a complication for a lifetime.[25]

Pericardial effusions are quite common following ASD repair and may not manifest until after the child is discharged from the hospital. A friction rub, increased heart size on chest radiograph, and echocardiographic evidence of pericardial fluid are diagnostic. Most effusions respond to ibuprofen or steroids; rarely is pericardiocentesis indicated.

Ventricular Septal Defect. A ventricular septal defect (VSD) is a communication between the ventricles. The ventricular septum is established in fetal life during the fourth to eighth week of gestation. The ventricular septum is formed from muscular and membranous tissues that fuse with the endocardial cushions and bulbus cordis. If development of these tissues is interrupted in fetal life, a VSD results. The size of a VSD varies from that of a pinpoint to the absence of the entire septum. Types of VSDs include perimembranous, subpulmonary, muscular, and malaligned canal type.

Generally, a VSD shunt is left to right; however, a number of variables determine the direction and degree of shunting. These include the size of the defects and the relative pressure differences between the right and left ventricle. Small VSDs can be hemodynamically insignificant with very little shunt; many of these close spontaneously during the first few years of life.

At birth, when PVR is elevated, there may be no or very little shunt. However, during normal postnatal transition, as PVR and right heart pressures fall below systemic pressures, a left-to-right shunt will develop. Because this occurs over time, many VSDs are not detected until 4 to 6 weeks of age. Exceptions to this are very large VSDs that can produce CHF early or lung disease that can contribute to prolonged elevation of PVR, therefore protecting the pulmonary vascular bed from overcirculation.

Once PVR normalizes, a left-to-right shunt with pulmonary overcirculation develops. The size of the shunt directly influences the child's initial clinical presentation and the effect of excessive blood flow on the pulmonary vasculature. Increased PBF will impose a volume load on the left heart, with subsequent left heart enlargement. Over time, pulmonary overcirculation contributes to progressive structural and functional abnormalities in the pulmonary vascular bed, with the subsequent development of pulmonary hypertension.[26]

If the defect is not closed in a timely manner, then irreversible pulmonary vascular disease can occur with fixed (does not respond to pulmonary vasodilators) pulmonary hypertension. In the presence of suprasystemic pulmonary artery pressure, the ventricular shunt is reversed (right to left) and the patient becomes chronically cyanotic. Fixed pulmonary hypertension in the presence of left-to-right shunt lesions is known as Eisenmenger's complex. These patients are no longer candidates for primary cardiac repair and require heart/lung transplantation. Fig. 18-6 illustrates possible hemodynamic variations of VSD.

Clinical Presentation and Course. Children with small VSDs will be asymptomatic and generally do not develop CHF. Moderate to large VSDs will result in CHF in the absence of pulmonary hypertension. Infants will display tachypnea, poor feeding, and poor weight gain. Echocardiogram is sufficient to determine the size, location, and hemodynamic significance of the VSD; cardiac catheterization is not indicated unless pulmonary vascular disease is a concern.

Management. Spontaneous closure of small perimembranous or muscular VSDs occurs in up to 50% of patients. Although controversial, many clinicians do not recommend closing small VSDs that do not result in left heart enlargement or cardiomegaly because the risks of open heart surgery may outweigh the benefits of closure. However, data have shown that small VSDs are not necessarily benign defects during adulthood because of the risk of endocarditis, arrhythmias, and progressive aortic regurgitation.[27] Endocarditis prophylaxis is recommended for all patients with a VSD, regardless of the size.

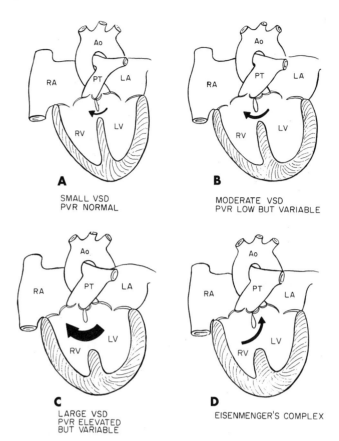

Fig. 18-6   **A** to **D,** Illustrations of small, moderately restrictive, and nonrestrictive (large) perimembranous ventricular septal defect *(VSD).* PVR, Pulmonary vascular resistance; *Ao,* Aorta; *LA,* left atrium; *LV,* left ventricle; *PT,* pulmonary trunk; *RA,* right atrium; *RV,* right ventricle. (From Perloff JK: *The clinical recognition of congenital heart disease,* ed 4, Philadelphia, 1994, WB Saunders, p 402.)

Children in CHF require anticongestive therapy consisting of diuretics, digoxin, and afterload reduction (ACE inhibitors). Many of these infants also require nutritional supplementation to increase the caloric density of their formula or tube feedings. If the infant does not gain weight appropriately despite medical management, then surgical closure or pulmonary artery band is recommended.

Transcatheter Closure. Various umbrella devices are currently under investigation for nonoperative, transcatheter closure of VSDs. These devices are currently under FDA investigation and are generally used in apical muscular VSDs and in children who are considered poor surgical candidates.[21] Complications include embolization of the umbrella arms and residual shunt.

Surgical Management. Pulmonary artery banding is used in some patients who are deemed too small for definitive correction, have multiple VSDs, or have medical disorders that preclude definitive surgery.[28] The band is then removed in the operating room just before definitive correction. Corrective repair of VSD is achieved via a median sternotomy incision. Cardiopulmonary bypass and deep hypothermia are required. Sutures or a patch are used to close the defect. Most defects are closed through a transatrial approach; rarely is a ventriculotomy required. Because of the proximity of the AV node and His bundle to many septal defects, care is taken to avoid damage to the conduction system because this can result in acquired heart block.

Postoperative complications may include residual VSD, heart block, low cardiac output, and junctional ectopic tachycardia. In patients with elevated pulmonary pressures preoperatively, right heart failure can occur. Aortic insufficiency can develop after repair of subarterial defects and is identified by the presence of a widened pulse pressure and a diastolic murmur.[29]

In the absence of pulmonary vascular disease, most patients can be extubated and weaned from oxygen quickly. Those with pulmonary hypertension may require longer ventilatory and oxygen therapy. If there is preoperative pulmonary hypertension, then a pulmonary artery (PA) catheter is usually inserted intraoperatively before closure of the chest. Maneuvers to decrease PVR (oxygen, nitric oxide, alkalosis) are implemented until PA pressures decrease or normalize.

If concern remains about a residual VSD and a PA and right atrial (RA) line are in place, then simultaneous PA and RA oxygen saturations can be obtained to help evaluate for a residual septal defect. A step up (increase) in the PA saturation from the value obtained from the RA, especially if the PA saturation is greater than 80%, strongly suggests the presence of a residual VSD. In this scenario a high-frequency systolic murmur will also be appreciated. The exception to this would be the presence of equal ventricular pressures without significant left-to-right shunt; therefore a step up or murmur may not be appreciated.

Atrioventricular Septal Defect.   An atrioventricular septal defect (AVSD) generally involves a primum ASD, AV valve abnormalities, and a VSD. However, this defect is quite variable and is classified as balanced, unbalanced, incomplete, and complete. When the ventricles are of equal size, the defect is balanced. An unbalanced defect is when one ventricle is larger than the other (i.e., right ventricle [RV] dominant). An incomplete defect primarily consists of a primum ASD and two AV valve orifices with a cleft mitral valve. A complete defect consists of a primum ASD, VSD, and a common AV valve with five leaflets. This defect is prevalent in children with trisomy 21 (Down syndrome).

During fetal life, the endocardial cushions are responsible for the development of the mitral and tricuspid valves, the upper ventricular septum, and the lower atrial septum. The endocardial cushions also play a role in the placement of the AV conduction system. These developments occur between the fourth and eighth week of gestation. Inadequate development of these fetal structures may result in a variant of AVSD. The sections that follow contrast the incomplete and the complete types of AVSD.

Incomplete AVSD.   The infant or child with an incomplete AVSD presents with an ostium primum ASD, as well as variable degrees of AV valve abnormalities. A cleft mitral valve (Fig. 18-7) is the classic associated anomaly. Hemodynamic alterations are determined by the size of the septal defect, degree of mitral valve incompetence, and

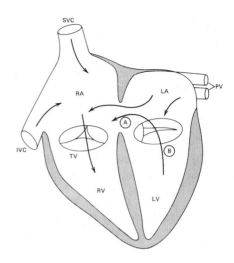

Fig. 18-7 Incomplete atrioventricular septal defect (AVSD). *A,* Ostium primum atrial septal defect; *B,* cleft mitral valve. *IVC,* Inferior vena cava; *LA,* left atrium; *LV,* left ventricle; *RA,* right atrium; *RV,* right ventricle; *SVC,* superior vena cava; *TV,* tricuspid valve. (From Smith JB: *Pediatric critical care,* Albany, NY, 1985, Delmar.)

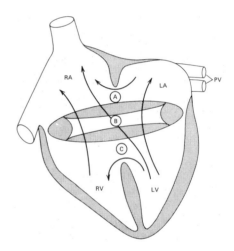

Fig. 18-8 Complete atrioventricular septal defect (AVSD). *A,* Ostium primum atrial septal defect; *B,* Common atrioventricular valve; *C,* Ventricular septal defect. *LA,* left atrium; *LV,* left ventricle; *PV,* pulmonary vein; *RA,* right atrium; *RV,* right ventricle. (From Smith JB: *Pediatric critical care,* Albany, NY, 1985, Delmar.)

PVR. Once PVR falls to normal, the shunt is left to right. If the mitral valve is competent, despite an anatomic abnormality, hemodynamics will be the same as an ostium primum ASD. A cleft mitral valve that is insufficient will produce a left ventricular to right atrial shunt (through the ASD) increasing the volume load on the right heart. If the ASD is small, mitral insufficiency will increase LAP and volume.

Complete AVSD.   In the complete form of AVSD, an ostium primum ASD, a VSD in the upper ventricular septum, and a common AV valve are present (Fig. 18-8). These defects generally allow significant left-to-right shunt (in the absence of pulmonary vascular disease) with pulmonary overcirculation. The right atrium can receive blood from two intracardiac sources. During systole, a left ventricle to right atrial shunt can occur via the insufficient mitral valve and the ASD. Blood can also enter the right atrium from the right ventricle via the incompetent tricuspid valve. This increase in right heart volume and pulmonary overcirculation can contribute to the development of pulmonary hypertension if the defect is not closed in a timely manner. Factors that play an important role in determining the degree of shunting are pulmonary resistance, systemic resistance, ventricular pressures, and myocardial compliance.

Clinical Presentation and Course. Infants and children with incomplete AVSD may be asymptomatic, or they may have the same clinical symptoms as those with a primum ASD. If mitral regurgitation is significant, then signs and symptoms of CHF may develop. Those infants with complete AVSD generally develop CHF early, unless they have pulmonary hypertension.

Echocardiogram is sufficient to diagnose the defect, size of the septal defects, and hemodynamic significance (heart size and function). Cardiac catheterization is indicated if pulmonary vascular disease is a concern or if questions remain regarding anatomy and intracardiac pressures.

Management

Incomplete AVSD. The infant or child with an incomplete AVSD is treated in the same way as children with a primum ASD. Endocarditis prophylaxis is indicated because of mitral valve abnormalities. If CHF occurs secondary to significant mitral insufficiency, then anticongestive therapy is indicated with digoxin and diuretics.

Complete AVSD. An infant with complete AVSD generally requires anticongestive therapy once PVR falls and the left-to-right shunt becomes significant (commonly by 2 months of age).[30] These children are also at high risk for the development of respiratory infections (particularly respiratory syncytial virus) and pneumonia, which may preclude surgical repair at the time of active respiratory illness. Therefore respiratory infections should be treated aggressively. Auscultatory or echocardiographic evidence of developing pulmonary hypertension may also be an indication for surgical intervention.

Surgical Management. Surgery is recommended for those who fail medical management or who fail to thrive. Surgery is generally recommended before the child reaches 1 year of age because the development of severe pulmonary vascular obstructive disease is likely thereafter. Early repair is indicated in patients with Down syndrome because of the proclivity to develop early pulmonary vascular disease in this population. Complete intracardiac repair of complete AVSD is achieved between 6 and 12 months of age when heart failure is present and generally not later than 2 years of age in those without severe symptoms.

Corrective surgery is performed via a midline sternotomy incision with deep hypothermia and cardiopulmonary bypass. An incomplete AVSD is repaired with autologous (pericardium) or synthetic patch closure of the ASD and by suturing the cleft in the mitral valve.[30] Relative to synthetic patches, autologous patches have been associated with a decreased incidence of hemolysis. Corrective repair of a complete AVSD involves either a single- or two-patch repair of the ASD and VSD and repair of the mitral or tricuspid valves or both. The AV valves are reconstructed using available tissue from the common AV valve leaflets with the objective of achieving valve competence. Mitral valve replacement may be necessary on rare occasions. Close care is taken during suturing to prevent heart block. Postoperative complications may include heart block, arrhythmias, residual shunt, and AV valve insufficiency. A small percentage of these patients will require mitral valve replacement in the future for persistent mitral regurgitation.[28]

Many of these patients will have transthoracic atrial (right and left) and PA catheters in place for pressure monitoring. The timely diagnosis of the cause of left atrial (LA) and PA pressure elevation will dictate therapy. Treatment of pulmonary hypertension includes oxygen, sedation, alkalosis, normothermia, and possibly nitric oxide (see Chapter 7). Elevation of LA pressure can indicate left heart failure. Aggressive volume resuscitation should be avoided because it can initiate a vicious cycle of annular dilation, increased left AV valve regurgitation, low cardiac output, and hypotension. Inotropes and afterload reduction are the initial intervention. Mechanical support (intraaortic balloon pump [IABP], ventricular assist device [VAD], extracorporeal membrane oxygenation [ECMO]) or reoperation may be necessary.[30]

Acyanotic Defects That Obstruct Flow

Coarctation of the aorta and aortic stenosis are two common cardiac lesions that result in increased left ventricular work. When occurring in isolation because no abnormal intracardiac connections are present, shunting of blood does not occur, PBF is normal, and cyanosis is absent.

Pulmonary stenosis, unless very severe, is a third common defect that does not produce cyanosis. If severe, pulmonary stenosis will result in increased right ventricular work and hypertrophy. (Table 18-4 summarizes the findings on cardiac examination, ECG, and chest radiograph of children with these defects.)

Isolated mitral stenosis, an uncommon defect, obstructs pulmonary venous return and does not cause an alteration in oxygen saturation. Mitral atresia or marked hypoplasia is representative of the spectrum of infants with hypoplastic left heart syndrome. Isolated mitral stenosis is not discussed here.

Coarctation of the Aorta. Coarctation of the aorta is a narrowing of the aorta distal to the left subclavian artery at the insertion of the ductus arteriosus (juxtaductal). Like other congenital heart defects, aortic coarctation exists along a spectrum; however, it is usually described as neonatal or adult coarctation and typically presents in neonates, infants, or older children. This lesion possibly exists as a result of decreased antegrade blood flow across the isthmus during fetal development. In addition, ectopic ductal tissue that exists in the aorta at the insertion of the ductus arteriosus may constrict at birth, resulting in aortic coarctation.[31]

◆ **Table 18-4** **Acyanotic Congenital Heart Defects That Obstruct Flow**

Defect	Cardiac Examination	Electrocardiogram	Chest Radiograph
Coarctation of the aorta	Systolic murmur left upper chest and midscapula; decreased or absent femoral pulses; arm/leg BP gradient; upper extremity hypertension	Varying degrees of left ventricular hypertrophy	Normal or cardiomegaly; enlarged left atrium and left ventricle; dilated ascending aorta; rib notching in children over 8 years of age with extensive collateral circulation
Aortic stenosis			
Valvular (mild to moderate)	Ejection click best heard at the fourth ICS to the left of the sternum; rough, harsh murmur best heard at base of the heart to the right of the sternal border	Left ventricular hypertrophy, or may be normal	May appear normal; possible left ventricular enlargement and dilated ascending aorta
Moderate to severe	Palpable thrill best felt at the suprasternal notch and at the second right ICS; diminished S_2	Left ventricular hypertrophy; possible ST and T wave changes, or may be normal	Same as for mild to moderate AS; pulmonary congestion may be seen
Subvalvular	Similar to valvular AS, with absence of ejection click	Same as for valvular AS	Similar to valvular AS, but dilation of aorta absent
Supravalvular	Normal S_1; absent ejection click; ejection systolic murmur; palpable thrill may be present	Same as for valvular AS	Ascending aorta smaller than normal; descending aorta normal in size
Pulmonary stenosis			
Valvular (mild to moderate)	Systolic ejection click after, followed by systolic ejection murmur best heard at upper left sternal border and radiating widely; possible palpable thrill at second left ICS; right ventricular lift	Normal or right ventricular hypertrophy	Normal or right ventricular and main pulmonary artery enlargement; normal left heart and pulmonary vascular markings
Severe	Murmur increased in duration and intensity, obscuring S_2; no ejection click audible	Right ventricular and right atrial hypertrophy	Same as above, with right atrial enlargement
Infundibular (fibrous ring)	Similar to valvular PS, but no ejection click	Same as for valvular PS	Right ventricular enlargement; normal pulmonary artery, left heart, and pulmonary vascular markings
Subvalvular	No ejection click; short systolic murmur ending before S_2, best heard at third or fourth left ICS; palpable thrill with severe stenosis; bulging of lower precordium; right ventricular heave	Same as for valvular PS	Same as for fibrous ring infundibular PS
Supravalvular	Systolic ejection murmur heard over sites of obstruction, radiating through pulmonary vasculature; occasional continuous murmur; normal S_1 and S_2; no ejection click	Normal or RVH	Normal or variable enlargement of right heart chambers and main pulmonary artery

AS, Aortic stenosis; BP, blood pressure; ICS, intercostal space; PS, pulmonary stenosis; RVH, right ventricular hypertrophy; S_1, first heart sound; S_2, second heart sound.

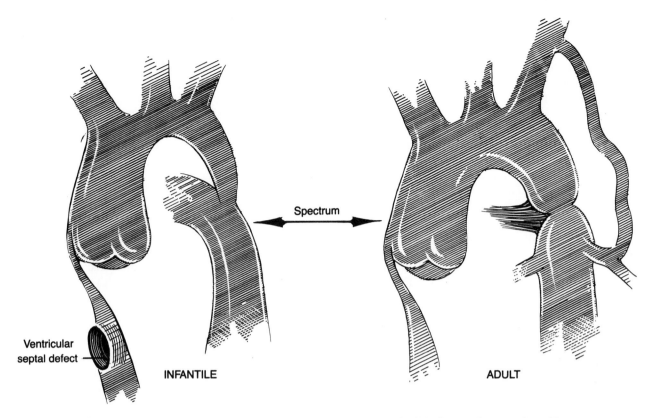

Fig. 18-9 Schematic showing difference between infantile and adult forms of coarctation. (From Castenada AR, Jonas RA, Mayer JE et al: *Cardiac surgery of the neonate and infant,* Philadelphia, 1994, WB Saunders.)

Associated lesions include PDA, tubular hypoplasia of the aortic arch, bicuspid aortic valve, patent foramen ovale, ASD, and VSD. Aortic coarctation in neonates often presents with a PDA and varying degrees of hypoplasia of the distal aortic arch. Lower body perfusion is often dependent on ductal patency. Associated cardiac lesions are common, yet major collateral arteries are typically absent in neonates.

Older children who present with the adult type of aortic coarctation usually have an isolated discrete coarctation at the location of the ligamentum arteriosum. This condition is often associated with a bicuspid aortic valve; however, other associated cardiac defects are unusual, and the proximal aortic arch is typically well developed. Coarctation in these children appears as an hourglass narrowing with associated arterial collateral vessels between the upper and lower body. Fig. 18-9 depicts both infantile and adult coarctation.

Coarctation of the aorta may be part of a spectrum of left-sided obstructive defects referred to as Shone's complex. This spectrum includes varying forms of mitral stenosis, hypoplastic left ventricle, subaortic stenosis, aortic stenosis, and coarctation of the aorta. In addition, aortic coarctation can appear in combination with other more severe forms of congenital heart disease, including hypoplastic left heart syndrome, Taussig-Bing anomaly, and transposition of the great arteries with tricuspid atresia.

Neonatal Coarctation. The pathophysiology of coarctation in newborns is dependent on the degree of aortic obstruction, the patency of the ductus arteriosus, and the presence of associated intracardiac lesions. Constriction of the aorta in a neonate will result in left ventricular failure and cardiovascular collapse. Although the PDA will supply the lower body with blood flow, sudden closure will also result in cardiovascular collapse. Left ventricular failure will eventually lead to elevated LAP and pulmonary edema. The presence of a VSD will result in a left-to-right shunt and possible delay of left ventricular dysfunction.

Adult Coarctation. Constriction of the aorta leads to increased afterload for the left ventricle with the development of left ventricular hypertrophy. Collateral arterial vessels from the upper body to the lower body provide adequate perfusion distal to the coarctation.

Clinical Presentation and Course

Neonatal Coarctation. Presentation of neonatal coarctation is dependent on the pathophysiologic condition, specifically, the amount of constriction and the timing of ductal closure. With severe coarctation and acute ductal closure, neonates can have acute cardiovascular collapse, metabolic acidosis, and end-organ ischemia. This can result in intracranial hemorrhage, renal failure, and necrotizing enterocolitis. When the development of the coarctation is slow and ductal closure is delayed, these patients can present in early infancy with CHF and differential blood pressure between their upper and lower extremities.

Adult Coarctation. Adult aortic coarctation typically presents in older children and adolescents on routine physical examination. Clinical signs include systemic hypertension, arm/leg pressure gradient, and diminished pulses in the lower extremities. If undiagnosed, these patients can develop complications such as myocardial infarction, cerebral vascular accidents, endocarditis, aortic aneurysms and dissection, CHF, headaches, lower body symptoms, and epistaxis.[32]

Management

Neonatal Coarctation. Neonates who present with cardiovascular collapse are aggressively resuscitated and treated with a continuous infusion of PGE_1 to maintain ductal patency and adequate lower body perfusion. In addition to opening the ductus arteriosus, PGE_1 may relax the area of aortic coarctation where ductal tissue exists. If left ventricular dysfunction is present, the administration of inotropic agents may be necessary. Administration of sodium bicarbonate to correct the metabolic acidosis is important to improve cardiac performance. Endotracheal intubation and mechanical ventilation may be necessary for the unstable neonate. In those infants with a VSD overoxygenation and hyperventilation should be prevented to avoid lowering PVR and subsequent pulmonary overcirculation. The overall goal should be the prevention of end-organ ischemia. If this exists, reversal of the process with recovery should be accomplished before surgery.

Adult Coarctation. The older child whose coarctation is detected on routine physical examination requires close assessment of blood pressure. Significant hypertension may require the use of antihypertensive agents preoperatively. If significant hypertension is present at rest, exercise restriction may be recommended. Antibiotic prophylaxis for bacterial endocarditis prevention is recommended preoperatively and postoperatively in children with associated bicuspid aortic valve.

Transcatheter Dilation. Balloon angioplasty performed in the catheterization laboratory has been shown to be successful in dilating both native and recurrent coarctation of the aorta. In general, balloon dilation of recurrent coarctation is thought to be safer than native coarctation due to supporting scar tissue that can reduce the risk of aortic rupture.[33] However, with improved technique and skill level, this intervention has been successfully used in some centers to treat native coarctation.[34] Risks of aortic rupture are slightly increased in neonates.

In addition, stents have been successfully placed in the aorta to relieve mild native and recurrent coarctation. Because of the size of the introducer, this technology is primarily reserved for school-aged, adolescent, and adult patients.

Surgical Management. Neonates and infants with ductal-dependent systemic blood flow are surgically repaired on presentation following adequate resuscitation and recovery of end-organ ischemia. Children with systemic hypertension who are otherwise asymptomatic have traditionally undergone surgery between the age of 3 to 5 years. The current trend, however, is to repair on presentation to avoid the postoperative complications of residual hypertension and postcoarctectomy syndrome.

The surgical technique used for repair depends on the type of coarctation and institutional preference. Current techniques include the resection-and-anastomosis technique, subclavian flap aortoplasty, and the synthetic patch aortoplasty. These techniques are performed without the use of cardiopulmonary bypass. When associated intracardiac lesions are involved, the coarctation may be repaired initially, followed by a later procedure for intracardiac repair. When patent, the ductus arteriosus is ligated.

The coarctation repair is preformed via a posterolateral thoracotomy incision. The aorta is temporarily clamped proximal and distal to the coarctation. The resection-and-anastomosis techniques most commonly include a resection of the ductal tissue, coarctation, and narrowed segment of the aorta, followed by an end-to-end or end-to-side anastomosis. The end-to-side anastomosis involves bringing the distal end of the aorta more proximal and performing the anastomosis underneath the aortic arch. The advantage of the resection-and-anastomosis technique is the removal of the ductal tissue along with the coarctation. The disadvantages include the potential for tension on the suture line, a greater degree of technical difficulty, more extensive dissection, and the presence of a circumferential scar.[31]

With the subclavian-flap angioplasty technique, the subclavian artery is ligated, and an incision is made from the proximal subclavian artery along the area of aortic coarctation. Hypoplastic tissue is removed, and the flap of subclavian artery is folded down and used to patch the aorta. Advantages of this approach include use of native tissue, avoidance of tension on the suture lines, and no circumferential scar. Disadvantages include interruption of blood flow to the left arm with potential growth alteration, retention of abnormal ductal tissue in the aorta, and potential for development of an aneurysm.[31]

With the patch aortoplasty technique, the area of coarctation is incised, and a patch of pericardial tissue or a synthetic patch is placed to widen the area of hypoplasia. The advantages and disadvantages of this procedure are similar to the subclavian-flap technique; however, left arm perfusion is not interrupted with the patch aortoplasty.

Systemic hypertension is the most common postoperative problem after surgical repair for coarctation of the aorta. Although seen in neonates and infants, this is more common in children and adolescents who have sustained longer periods of altered lower body perfusion. The cause of hypertension is thought to be multifactorial, including the presence of increased catecholamines, derangement of the RAAS, and disrupted baroreceptor response.[32] Systemic hypertension can lead to bleeding along the aortic suture lines or from collateral arteries if present. A continuous infusion of sodium nitroprusside or esmolol is often recommended to control hypertension. The short half-life of sodium nitroprusside provides rapid initial treatment and allows quick adjustments in titration. The presence of postoperative hypertension may be transient or may last for days or months. Long-term administration of afterloading agents, such as captopril or β-blockers, may be indicated. Maintenance of appropriate blood pressure also requires control of postoperative pain and agitation. These interventions can be crucial in avoiding postoperative bleeding.

Postcoarctectomy syndrome may be caused by mesenteric arteritis secondary to the introduction of pulsatile blood flow to the lower body and subsequent vessel injury or reflex vasoconstriction after surgery.[32] This syndrome is rarely seen in neonates and infants and is more common in older children who have severe coarctation and preoperative systemic hypertension. Symptoms include abdominal pain, abdominal distension, nausea, ascites, fever, and leucocytosis. It is often associated with postoperative systemic hypertension. Treatment includes nasogastric decompression and the administration of intravenous fluids. Oral feedings are withheld until symptoms resolve.

Spinal cord ischemia is a potential complication that is rarely seen in neonates and infants. The cause, although not completely understood, may be secondary to abnormal spinal artery anatomy or inadequate collateral circulation during the aortic clamp time. A complete neurologic assessment, specifically, evaluation of lower body movement, is critical to assess for this complication.

Additional potential complications that require nursing assessment in the postoperative period include injury to thoracic structures obtained secondary to the surgical thoracotomy. Damage to the thoracic duct leading to the development of a chylothorax, damage to the laryngeal nerve leading to vocal cord paralysis and stridor, or damage to the phrenic nerve leading to diaphragm paralysis are possible complications that must be evaluated.

Residual coarctation may develop after neonatal and infant repair during the first year after surgery. Management may include reoperation or balloon dilation. Four-extremity blood pressure assessment in the early postoperative period is important to evaluate for a residual gradient between upper and lower body measurements.

In addition to the observation and management of potential complications, it is important for the nurse to question the presence of associated intracardiac lesions, especially in neonates and infants. This may alter the postoperative management plan or present additional complications. For example, the presence of a large VSD may alter the postoperative mechanical ventilation plan to avoid excessive left-to-right intracardiac shunting and pulmonary overcirculation.

Aortic Stenosis. Aortic stenosis can be defined as a lesion that results in obstruction of blood flow from the left ventricle to the aorta. Aortic stenosis is categorized into three subgroups depending on the location of the obstruction. These include valvar aortic stenosis, subvalvar aortic stenosis, and supravalvar aortic stenosis (Fig. 18-10).

Valvar Aortic Stenosis. Valvar aortic stenosis exists along a spectrum of disease with variable obstruction. Most patients have an isolated bicuspid aortic valve and remain asymptomatic until they are adults. Valvar aortic stenosis in neonates and young infants is commonly called critical aortic stenosis and often presents in the neonatal period with cardiogenic shock. In this case, the valve commissures may

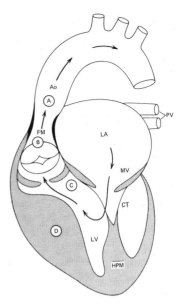

Fig. 18-10 Four locations of aortic stenosis (AS). *A,* Supravalvular AS; *B,* valvular AS; *C,* discrete subvalvular AS; *D,* idiopathic hypertrophic subaortic stenosis. *Ao,* Aorta; *CT,* chordae tendineae; *FM,* fibrous membrane; *HPM,* hypertrophic papillary muscle; *LA,* left atrium; *LV,* left ventricle; *MV,* mitral valve; *PV,* pulmonary vein. (From Smith JB: *Pediatric critical care,* Albany, NY, 1985, Delmar.)

be fused, the valve annulus may be small, and the valve leaflets may be thick and deformed. Neonates may also have a hypoplastic ascending aorta and left ventricle. Older infants may have valvar stenosis and left ventricular hypertrophy. Older children usually have a bicuspid aortic valve with thickened valve leaflets. Associated lesions include supravalvar aortic stenosis, mitral valve abnormalities, and coarctation of the aorta. Aortic insufficiency and endocardial fibroelastosis may be present as a result of the valvar aortic stenosis.

Neonates with critical aortic stenosis will receive systemic blood flow after birth through a PDA. The left ventricle, however, will be dilated and poorly contractile, and coronary perfusion may depend on retrograde flow and be compromised. Left ventricular dysfunction will lead to elevated LAP and the development of pulmonary edema and pulmonary hypertension. When the ductus arteriosus closes, circulatory shock can result with the development of renal failure, necrotizing enterocolitis, and intracranial hemorrhage. Older children with valvar aortic stenosis typically have left ventricular hypertrophy secondary to the chronic pressure overload.

Clinical Presentation and Course. Neonates with critical aortic stenosis present with dyspnea and tachypnea, irritability, pallor, narrowed pulse pressure, oliguria, and metabolic acidosis when the ductus arteriosus closes. Older children are often asymptomatic, presenting with a murmur. When moderate to severe obstruction exists, they can present with syncope, exercise intolerance, angina, and possibly sudden death.

Management.   Neonates with cardiogenic shock are aggressively treated with a continuous infusion of PGE_1 to maintain ductal patency and ensure systemic blood flow. Mechanical ventilation, inotropic support, and administration of sodium bicarbonate are often necessary to treat the shock. When the shock state has been reversed, invasive intervention is performed.

The management of older children depends on their symptoms and the severity of the obstruction. The presence of a gradient greater than 50 mmHg across the obstruction along with symptoms of angina or ST-T segment changes in the ECG usually warrants surgical intervention.[32] Asymptomatic children with mild to moderate obstruction may be medically managed and followed for signs of worsening obstruction. Vigorous physical activity may be limited in these patients to prevent the risk of sudden death. These patients are particularly prone to bacterial endocarditis and require prophylaxis with antibiotic therapy for invasive procedures. Treatment for valvar aortic stenosis in neonates and young infants includes percutaneous balloon dilation or surgical valvotomy or both.

Transcatheter Dilation.   In balloon dilation, a balloon catheter is placed retrograde across the aortic valve, the balloon is inflated, and the valve is dilated. This approach has reduced the need for surgical valvotomy in some patients. In others, it serves to palliate the infant or small child until definitive repair with a Ross procedure. When aortic valve regurgitation is present or the balloon dilation is not successful, a surgical valvotomy may be indicated.

Surgical Management.   With the use of cardiopulmonary bypass, an aortic incision is made, and valve commissures are incised in a way that avoids worsening aortic insufficiency.

In older children, the goal of management is to preserve left ventricular function; therefore the obstruction must be removed before permanent damage occurs. When surgery is indicated, options include surgical valvotomy, valvuloplasty, or aortic valve replacement. Aortic valve replacement options include the Ross procedure or prosthetic valve replacement. With the Ross procedure, the aortic valve is replaced with a pulmonary autograft, and a pulmonary homograft is placed in the right ventricular outflow tract to the pulmonary artery. Coronary artery reimplantation into the neoaorta is necessary with this procedure. Criteria for the Ross procedure may include the presence of a normal pulmonary valve, absence of pulmonary insufficiency, and absence of rheumatic and connective tissue disease. Although with advances in surgical skill, these criteria are being broadened.[35] Anticoagulation is not needed after the Ross procedure, and the new aortic valve will grow with the patient. Valve replacement may also include the use of a mechanical valve. In this case, anticoagulation is required, and the valve will need replacement when the patient grows.

The Konno operation is another surgical option for aortic stenosis. In this procedure, the aortic valve is approached through a right ventriculotomy and an incision in the ventricular septum. A patch is used to augment the left ventricular outflow tract, and the valve is replaced with a mechanical valve or a pulmonary autograft.[32]

Postoperative management depends on the age of presentation, the degree of obstruction, the condition of the left ventricle before surgery, and the specific procedure performed. Neonates are typically very ill after surgery and suffer from left ventricular dysfunction. Older children usually have an uneventful postoperative course, unless significant preoperative left ventricular dysfunction exists. Left ventricular dysfunction may result in low cardiac output and ventricular arrhythmias in the postoperative period, requiring inotropic support, afterloading reduction, and antiarrhythmics.

Specific surgical procedures have potential complications. For example, complete heart block can occur after the Konno operation. Myocardial ischemia can occur after the Ross procedure if problems arise with the coronary artery translocation.

Postoperative echocardiography provides information regarding the presence of aortic insufficiency. When present, additional afterload reduction may be necessary. Anticoagulation is necessary with mechanical valve placement. This is initially provided with continuous infusions of heparin, followed by the initiation of warfarin therapy later in the postoperative course. Anticoagulation can be difficult in neonates and infants secondary to immature liver function and unreliable metabolism of anticoagulation agents.

Subaortic Stenosis.   Subaortic stenosis is described as an obstruction to outflow from the left ventricle to the aorta that is beneath the aortic valve. This defect is most commonly an isolated lesion in older children. In neonates and infants, it can exist in combination with a VSD or coarctation of the aorta. Additional associated defects include double-chamber right ventricle, AV canal defects, and the presence of aortic insufficiency.[32] Types of subaortic stenosis include membranous, fibromuscular, and hypertrophic. Membranous stenosis consists of a discrete ring of tissue beneath the aortic valve and is usually seen in older children. Fibromuscular obstruction involves a segment of muscle tissue that can extend from below the aortic valve to the mitral valve. Hypertrophic cardiomyopathy includes a variety of obstructive lesions; however, it usually involves hypertrophy of the ventricular septum (see section on hypertrophic cardiomyopathy).

Pressure overload of the left ventricle results in progressive left ventricular hypertrophy and possible failure. Turbulent blood flow below the aortic valve can cause abnormalities of the valve and lead to the development of aortic valve insufficiency and regurgitation.

Clinical Presentation and Course.   Although present at birth, subaortic stenosis is rarely severe enough to cause symptoms in neonates and young infants. Older children can present with aortic insufficiency, left ventricular failure, syncope, and angina. Bacterial endocarditis and sudden death are potential complications.

Management.   Surgical intervention will depend on the type of subaortic stenosis and the presenting symptoms. When a significant gradient develops, surgery is performed to prevent left ventricular failure. The development of aortic insufficiency and the presence of associated intracardiac lesions may also warrant surgery. When surgery is performed, a median sternotomy is used with the institution of cardiopulmonary bypass. For discrete membrane formation beneath the aortic valve, the membrane and muscle are surgically removed through an aortic incision. When extensive muscle excision is required for a tunnel type of stenosis, muscle is removed via an aortic incision or the Konno procedure. A combined Ross-Konno operation may be necessary for complex aortic stenosis with left ventricular outflow tract obstruction.[32]

Postoperative management after the removal of a discrete subaortic membrane is usually uneventful. When extensive muscle removal is warranted, left ventricular dysfunction and the development of left bundle branch block or complete heart block are possible. Inotropic support, afterload reduction, and temporary or permanent pacemaker therapy may be indicated. Aortic insufficiency can develop or worsen if present preoperatively. Mitral valve damage can also occur with extensive muscle resection, resulting in mitral valve regurgitation.

Supravalvar Aortic Stenosis.   Supravalvar aortic stenosis is defined as an obstruction to blood flow occurring in the ascending aorta above the aortic valve. This can include the presence of a fibrous membrane, hypoplasia of the ascending aorta, or the presence of an "hourglass" deformity of the aorta. Supravalvar aortic stenosis is often found in children with Williams' syndrome, who have characteristic faces (elfin), developmental delay, and personality changes. Hypercalcemia, peripheral pulmonary stenosis, aortic coarctation, and renal artery stenosis may also be present in these children. Supravalvular aortic stenosis occurs less often than all other forms of aortic stenosis.

As with other forms of aortic stenosis, this type of obstruction can result in left ventricular hypertrophy and dysfunction from the pressure overload. When the coronary arteries are filled under pressure from the obstruction, coronary artery abnormalities and ischemia can result.

Clinical Presentation and Course.   This disease is progressive and often reoccurs despite surgical intervention. Patients with Williams' syndrome should always be evaluated for the presence of supravalvar aortic stenosis. Symptoms include poor growth, exercise intolerance, angina, and syncope. Bacterial endocarditis and sudden death are possible complications. Indications for surgical intervention include the development of a significant gradient, myocardial ischemia, clinical symptoms, and the development of coronary artery abnormalities.

Management.   Supravalvular aortic stenosis is amenable to operative treatment if the narrowing is discrete and can be widened with insertion of a patch. Surgery is performed via a median sternotomy and the use of cardiopulmonary bypass. A vertical incision of the stenosed area is made, and a patch is inserted to enlarge the aortic diameter. Secondary aortic valve damage may occur as a result of this surgery.

Postoperative care is usually more complicated after surgical intervention compared with other types of aortic stenosis. Extensive suture lines along the aorta can result in systemic hypertension and bleeding. Treatment with afterload-reducing agents may be required. When coronary abnormalities are present, myocardial ischemia may occur. Aortic insufficiency may be present if aortic valve damage is present preoperatively or is a complication of the surgery.

Pulmonary Stenosis.   Pulmonary stenosis is the result of an obstructive lesion that interferes with blood flow from the right ventricle to the pulmonary artery. This lesion can occur at a number of locations in the right ventricular outflow tract and pulmonary artery. Subcategories include valvar pulmonary stenosis, subvalvular pulmonary stenosis, and supravalvular pulmonary stenosis (Fig. 18-11). Valvar pulmonary stenosis typically presents with a bicuspid valve that is fused at the commissures. This is the most common form of pulmonary stenosis. Subvalvular pulmonary stenosis includes double-chamber right ventricle and infundibular pulmonary stenosis. Double-chamber right ventricle typically consists of a fibrous or muscle ring of tissue below the pulmonary valve within the right ventricle. Infundibular stenosis involves muscle extension in the right ventricular outflow tract. Supravalvular pulmonary stenosis can occur within the main pulmonary artery or within any of its branches. Often, multiple areas of stenosis exist throughout the pulmonary vasculature. This is a rare defect and may be associated with other arterial abnormalities.

Regardless of the specific location of the pulmonary stenosis, the hemodynamic result is obstruction of blood ejected from the right ventricle in systole. This obstruction places a pressure burden on the right ventricle.

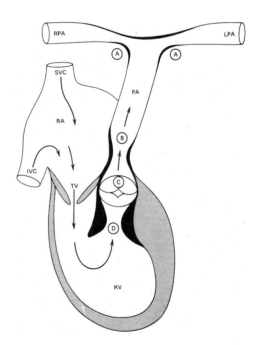

Fig. 18-11   Four locations of pulmonary stenosis (PS). *A,* Branch pulmonary artery stenosis; *B,* discrete supravalvular PS; *C,* valvular PS; *D,* subvalvular PS. *IVC,* Inferior vena cava; *LPA,* left pulmonary artery; *RA,* right atrium; *RPA,* right pulmonary artery; *RV,* right ventricle; *PA,* pulmonary artery; *SVC,* superior vena cava; *TV,* tricuspid valve. (From Smith JB: *Pediatric critical care,* Albany, NY, 1985, Delmar.)

Valvular Pulmonary Stenosis. Obstruction to ventricular emptying and the resultant increase in right ventricular pressure cause right ventricular and main pulmonary artery enlargement. The right ventricle enlarges as its muscular wall hypertrophies in response to the increased afterload it must overcome. The main pulmonary artery enlargement is characteristic of poststenotic dilation. However, pressure in the pulmonary trunk is normal or lower than normal, and therefore the peripheral pulmonary vasculature and the left heart are unaffected. When severe valvar pulmonary stenosis is present, right atrial pressure may also increase, with resultant enlargement of the right atrial chamber.

Subvalvular Pulmonary Stenosis. Double-chamber right ventricle and infundibular pulmonary stenosis are characterized by right ventricular hypertrophy that develops in response to the increased pressure in the ventricle as it pumps against an obstruction. However, the increased force is dissipated over an area of obstruction that is larger than that of valvular pulmonary stenosis, and, as a result, the main pulmonary artery remains normal in size. Pressure in the main pulmonary artery is normal or reduced.

Supravalvular Pulmonary Stenosis. Unlike the other forms of pulmonary stenosis, supravalvular lesions produce hypertension in the main pulmonary artery as well as in the right ventricle. However, ventricular and pulmonary artery enlargement vary with the severity and location of the lesions.

Clinical Presentation and Course. Children with pulmonary stenosis are followed closely to detect, as early as possible, progression of their stenosis with growth. Although progression is less likely in children with pulmonary stenosis than in those with aortic stenosis, it is detected by changes in the murmur (increased intensity, loss of ejection click, the development of a palpable thrill), increased right ventricular hypertrophy on ECG, or increased clinical symptoms. Children with pulmonary stenosis have a low risk of developing bacterial endocarditis, but antibiotic prophylaxis with dental work or other surgical procedures is generally provided.

Management. Treatment of pulmonary stenosis is recommended when the pressure gradient across the right ventricular outflow tract is 50 to 60 mmHg.

Transcatheter Dilation. Discrete valvular pulmonary stenosis can be treated successfully by balloon valvoplasty in the cardiac catheterization laboratory. In general, this approach is quite successful, resulting in a gradient of less than 50 mmHg, RV pressure of less than half systemic, and mild pulmonary insufficiency. In many patients, this is the treatment of choice without any required subsequent surgical intervention. Exceptions are those patients with dysplastic pulmonary valves.

Surgical Management. In patients who are not candidates for balloon dilation, surgical valvotomy is performed. Cardiopulmonary bypass is used, and an incision is made in the pulmonary artery. Incising the fused commissures as widely as possible relieves valvular stenosis. The right ventricular infundibulum is palpated through the newly enlarged pulmonary valve to detect localized muscular or fibrotic obstruction. Subvalvular stenosis is excised widely by means of a right ventriculotomy or through an incision in the pulmonary artery.

Postoperatively, children who have had repair of valvular pulmonary stenosis may have some degree of pulmonary valve regurgitation, but this is generally not significant and is well tolerated. Patients who, before surgery, have significant right ventricular hypertension and hypertrophy may develop some degree of right-sided CHF postoperatively and require digoxin or diuretic therapy for variable periods. Most children recover uneventfully and continue to grow and develop normally.

Cyanotic Congenital Heart Defects With Decreased PBF

Cyanotic structural defects with decreased PBF generally have obstruction within the right heart in combination with an intracardiac shunt. These lesions result in intracardiac mixing and systemic desaturation. Tetralogy of Fallot and its variants are the most common lesion in this subgroup. Other lesions include pulmonary and tricuspid atresia. Table 18-5 summarizes the clinical, ECG, and radiographic findings of this population.

Tetralogy of Fallot. Tetralogy of Fallot (TOF) accounts for approximately 10% of all congenital heart defects (CHDs). It consists of four primary cardiac defects resulting from hypoplasia of the right ventricular infundibulum. These include a malaligned VSD, infundibular pulmonary stenosis, right ventricular hypertrophy, and aortic override of the ventricular septum (Fig. 18-12). These four defects result in a spectrum of disease dependent on the variations and degree of right ventricular outflow tract obstruction (RVOTO). TOF can be further categorized as TOF with pulmonary stenosis (TOF-PS) and TOF with pulmonary atresia (TOF-PA).

Tetralogy of Fallot With Pulmonary Stenosis. Although variations exist, typically the RVOTO seen in TOF-PS includes hypoplasia of the infundibulum, pulmonary valve stenosis, hypoplasia of the pulmonary annulus, and hypoplasia of the pulmonary trunk. The branch pulmonary arteries are usually continuous and not hypoplastic. The right ventricular hypertrophy is secondary to the pressure load induced by outflow tract obstruction. The VSD is always malaligned. In approximately 3% of patients with TOF-PS, a second VSD exists that is usually muscular. Additional anatomic abnormalities can include coronary artery abnormalities, a right aortic arch, and a persistent left superior vena cava.

The degree of RVOTO, which determines the amount of obstruction to PBF, determines the pathophysiology of this defect. With a large VSD, the two ventricles essentially function as a single ventricle; therefore systemic vascular resistance may also contribute to the amount of PBF. A decrease in systemic vascular resistance can decrease PBF, whereas an increase in systemic vascular resistance can increase PBF. When RVOTO is minimal, there may actually be a left-to-right shunt across the VSD, resulting in pulmonary overcirculation and signs of CHF. These patients often have systemic arterial oxygen saturations of greater than 90% and are called "pink tets." When RVOTO is

TABLE 18-5 Cyanotic Congenital Heart Defects With Decreased Pulmonary Blood Flow

Defect	Cardiac Examination	Electrocardiogram	Chest Radiograph
Tetralogy of Fallot	Loud systolic murmur with palpable thrill along the entire left sternal border; single S_2; prominent inferior sternum and right ventricular impulse	Right axis deviation and right ventricular hypertrophy; occasional right atrial hypertrophy	Normal cardiac size with concavity in main pulmonary artery area; decreased pulmonary vascular markings; boot-shaped heart silhouette; right aortic arch common
Pulmonary atresia with intact ventricular septum	Heart murmur may be absent; when detected, usually holosystolic blowing murmur of tricuspid regurgitation and continuous, "machinery" murmur of PDA; single S_2	Absence of or decrease in right ventricular forces; left ventricular dominance	Cardiomegaly with significant right atrial enlargement; decreased pulmonary vascular markings
Tricuspid atresia	No tricuspid S_1; S_2 also often a single sound: no pulmonary S_2; variable systolic (VSD and PS) murmurs or diastolic (mitral flow) murmur; often, no murmur is audible	Left axis deviation; left ventricular, left atrial, and right atrial hypertrophy; no right ventricular forces	Normal overall heart size with concavity in main pulmonary artery area; right atrial, left atrial, left ventricular, and aortic enlargement; decreased pulmonary vascular markings

PDA, Patent ductus arteriosus; *PS*, pulmonary stenosis; *S₁*, first heart sound; *S₂*, second heart sound; *VSD*, ventricular septal defect.

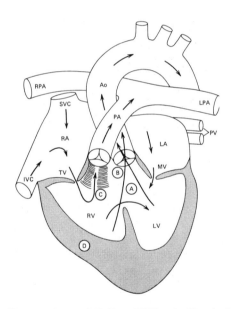

Fig. 18-12 Tetralogy of Fallot (TOF). *A*, Ventricular septal defect; *B*, aorta overriding ventricular septum; *C*, pulmonary stenosis; *D*, right ventricular hypertrophy. *Ao*, Aorta; *IVC*, inferior vena cava; *LA*, left atrium; *LPA*, left pulmonary artery; *LV*, left ventricle; *MV*, mitral valve; *PA*, pulmonary artery; *PV*, pulmonary vein; *RA*, right atrium; *RPA*, right pulmonary artery; *RV*, right ventricle; *SVC*, superior vena cava; *TV*, tricuspid valve. (From Smith JB: *Pediatric critical care*, Albany, NY, 1985, Delmar.)

moderate, there is protection from pulmonary overcirculation and a small right-to-left shunt across the VSD with mild cyanosis and oxygen saturations of about 90%. These patients are commonly asymptomatic. When RVOTO is severe, there is a significant right-to-left shunt across the VSD with oxygen saturations of 70% to 80%. In these patients, decreased oxygen saturations can lead to severe

hypoxemia and acidosis. The effect on the heart of these changes in hemodynamics includes an increase in the size and work of the right ventricle. The right atrium is usually unaffected. An increased volume load on the left ventricle results; however, it remains normally compliant.

Tetralogy of Fallot With Pulmonary Atresia. With TOF-PA, no outflow exists from the right ventricle to the pulmonary artery. The source of PBF is variable and further describes the subcategories of this defect. In newborns with valvar pulmonary atresia, the PBF is dependent on a PDA. At the other end of the spectrum, complete absence of a main pulmonary artery is evident, and the presence of branch pulmonary arteries is variable. PBF, in this case, is dependent on multiple aortopulmonary collateral arteries (MAPCAs) (Fig. 18-13). The number, size, and origin of the MAPCAs is variable and further describes the pathophysiology and prognosis of TOF-PA.

Without forward flow from the right ventricle to the pulmonary artery, a complete right-to-left shunt occurs across the VSD. The amount of cyanosis and severity of disease depend on the source of PBF, which is provided either by the PDA or by MAPCAs. The presence of what would be true branch pulmonary arteries is variable. Neonates with TOF-PA and ductal-dependent PBF have a normal pulmonary trunk and branch pulmonary arteries. These neonates will be severely cyanotic and in extreme distress when the ductus begins to close. Newborns with TOF-PA and MAPCAs usually have an adequate source of PBF in the early infant period; however, they will be cyanotic. The amount of PBF and cyanosis depends on the size, number, and condition of the MAPCAs.

Clinical Presentation and Course

Tetralogy of Fallot With Pulmonary Stenosis. Symptoms vary depending on the degree of RVOTO and shunt. Patients can be asymptomatic and acyanotic or severely

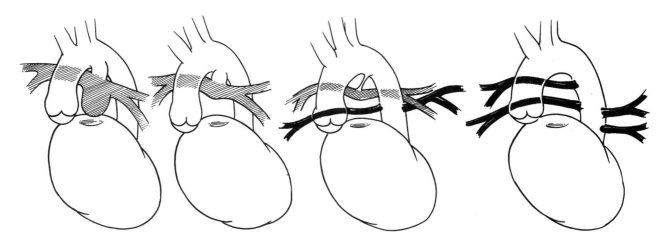

Fig. 18-13 Tetralogy of Fallot with pulmonary atresia. In groups I and II, the pulmonary arteries are well developed, and blood flow is supplied by a large patent ductus arteriosus. The main pulmonary artery is absent in group II. In group III, the ductus is either absent or very small. Both left and right pulmonary arteries are diminutive, connecting to variable numbers of bronchopulmonary segments; the more important sources of pulmonary blood flow are APCAs. In group IV, there are no mediastinal pulmonary arteries, and all bronchopulmonary segments are supplied entirely by APCAs. (From Castenada AR, Jonas RA, Mayer JE et al: *Cardiac surgery of the neonate and infant,* Philadelphia, 1994, WB Saunders.)

cyanotic and distressed. Persistent hypoxemia in infants stimulates bone marrow production of red blood cells, however, microcytic and hypochromic anemia can result from deficient iron stores. Cyanosis eventually leads to increased hemoglobin levels and hyperviscosity. RVOTO and the degree of cyanosis worsens over time and hypercyanotic spells may occur more frequently with age. Patients are at risk for cerebral abscess, cerebral vascular accidents, or death resulting from hypercyanotic spells. Late complications include bacterial endocarditis, hemorrhagic disorders, and complications of prolonged cyanosis. This disease is progressive and there is no chance for spontaneous recovery, therefore a definitive surgical repair is always indicated. Early corrective surgery is preferred to normalize the physiology and avoid these complications. Echocardiography is usually adequate to make the appropriate preoperative diagnosis for patients with TOF-PS. Even with multiple VSDs and abnormal coronary artery anatomy, echocardiography has proven to be sufficient. Cardiac catheterization may be indicated in patients with previous palliation, symptoms suggestive of aortopulmonary collaterals, concerns about coronary artery anatomy, or pulmonary vascular disease.

Hypercyanotic Spells. Hypercyanotic or "tet" spells can occur in infants and children with TOF-PS and are probably caused by intermittent worsening of RVOTO. Usually preceded by periods of agitation, these spells include symptoms of increased distress followed by hyperpnea, worsening cyanosis, and syncope. If severe or untreated, severe hypoxemia can result in brain injury or death. Anything that distresses the infant can precipitate a hypercyanotic spell. Careful attention must be paid to patients who are admitted preoperatively to avoid procedures that may stimulate a hypercyanotic spell.

Initial treatment includes oxygen administration, sedation, and volume expansion. If severe, a phenylephrine infusion may be initiated to increase systemic vascular resistance and therefore decrease the right-to-left shunt and improve PBF. Positioning the infant or child in a knee-chest position has been advocated to increase systemic venous return and systemic vascular resistance; however, some children may not be comfortable in this position, and their distress may actually be worsened. Emergency surgery for either a Blalock-Taussig shunt or a complete repair may be indicated. The primary goal of early complete repair, however, is to avoid these spells as the disease progresses, thereby avoiding their complications.

Tetralogy of Fallot With Pulmonary Atresia. These patients are cyanotic at birth because of the obligatory right-to-left intracardiac shunt. The degree of oxygen desaturation depends on the source of PBF. Newborns with ductal-dependent PBF have severe distress, hypoxemia, and rapid deterioration when the ductus begins to close. Patients with MAPCAs have variable oxygen saturations depending on the number and level of obstruction to flow within the MAPCAs. Unobstructed MAPCAs could possibly result in pulmonary overcirculation and signs of CHF.

Management
Tetralogy of Fallot With Pulmonary Stenosis. Although controversy exists regarding the timing and approach to the surgical management of TOF-PS, the increasing trend is to avoid palliation and to provide a complete surgical repair in the neonatal or early infant period. However, some centers prefer early surgical palliation followed by a complete surgical repair in late infancy or early childhood. The goals of early complete repair are to avoid complications of surgical palliation, correct the cyanosis, avoid a second surgery, and to normalize the cardiopulmonary physiology.

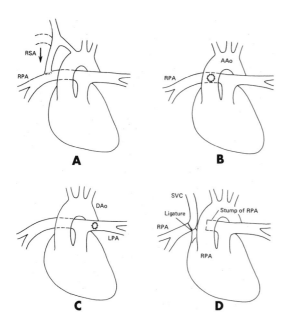

Fig. 18-14 Palliative shunts to increase pulmonary blood flow. **A,** Blalock-Taussig anastomosis; **B,** Waterston anastomosis; **C,** Potts-Smith-Gibson anastomosis; **D,** Classic Glenn anastomosis. (From Smith JB: *Pediatric critical care,* Albany, NY, 1985, Delmar.)

The timing of a primary surgical repair in these patients depends on the patient's symptoms and the institutional philosophy. Patient subtypes of TOF-PS can be categorized into three groups that can assist in the timing decision of when to perform surgery. Patients with TOF-PS who have ductal-dependent PBF and have cyanotic spells in the newborn period when the ductus closes require surgery in the neonatal period. Patients who are asymptomatic with arterial oxygen saturations of 75% to 90% can be electively repaired between 1 and 3 months of age or when they become symptomatic. Patients with arterial oxygen saturations greater than 90% (pink tets) can electively undergo repair between the age of 2 of 4 months. However, any patient who becomes symptomatic, presenting with cyanosis or any history of hypercyanotic spells, should be immediately considered for surgical repair or palliation to avoid complications and possible death.

Palliative Surgical Management. Palliative surgical intervention involves the placement of a systemic-to-pulmonary artery shunt to improve PBF. The modified Blalock-Taussig shunt is generally performed. In this procedure, a Gore-Tex shunt is anastomosed from the subclavian artery to the branch pulmonary artery (Fig. 18-14). Although this is a low-risk procedure, potential complications including branch pulmonary artery stenosis with partial or complete occlusion, thrombosis of the shunt resulting in acute worsening of cyanosis and possible death, or the development of pulmonary vascular obstructive disease, exist. In addition, with surgical palliation, the patient's cardiopulmonary physiologic condition remains abnormal and cyanosis persists, which may have long-term effects on the developing organs.

Complete Surgical Repair. Through a median sternotomy, this surgery is performed with the use of cardiopulmonary bypass, aortic cross clamping, and the administration of cardioplegia solution. Any previously placed aortopulmonary shunts are taken down, and the pulmonary artery is reconstructed if necessarily. The surgical approach for repair depends on the location and degree of RVOTO. Without pulmonary valve annulus hypoplasia, the VSD, subpulmonary artery stenosis, or pulmonary valve stenosis can be repaired through a combined transatrial and transpulmonary approach, thereby avoiding a right ventricular incision. When pulmonary valve annulus hypoplasia exists, a right ventriculotomy is made. The VSD and RVOTO are repaired through this incision, and a transannular patch or infundibular patch is used to correct the RVOTO. Typically these patches are made with the use of the patient's preserved pericardial tissue. A patent foramen ovale (PFO) is often maintained or incised to allow a right-to-left atrial shunt in the presence of right ventricular dysfunction in the postoperative period. This shunt allows the maintenance of systemic cardiac output regardless of right ventricular dysfunction. Cyanosis, which is usually well tolerated, results. The PFO closes spontaneously when right ventricular dysfunction resolves.

Tetralogy of Fallot With Pulmonary Atresia. In neonates with TOF-PA and ductal-dependent PBF, a PGE_1 infusion is maintained until a palliative shunt or complete repair can be performed in the early neonatal period. Diagnosis is made by echocardiography, and cardiac catheterization is rarely required. Many centers prefer an early complete repair to avoid the complications of palliation and provide early normal cardiopulmonary physiology. After the initiation of cardiopulmonary bypass and aortic cross clamp, a right ventricular incision is made in all cases. Through this incision, the VSD is closed, right infundibular obstruction is repaired, and a right ventricular to pulmonary artery valved homograft is placed. These neonates often have left branch pulmonary artery stenosis at the site of the ductus arteriosus, requiring surgical repair. A PFO is often maintained to allow right-to-left atrial shunting and the maintenance of systemic cardiac output.

For patients with TOF-PA with MAPCAs, the surgical approach is based on institutional preference, symptoms, and the patient's individual anatomy and physiology. Cardiac catheterization is always required to determine the location, size, and flow patterns of the MAPCAs. The goal of surgery is to unifocalize all aortopulmonary collateral vessels to the true branch pulmonary arteries, to place a right ventricular to pulmonary artery homograft conduit, and to close the VSD. This can be accomplished with a one-stage complete repair with VSD closure, a complete unifocalization of the MAPCAs leaving the VSD open, or through a staged unifocalization. In a staged approach, the right and left collateral arteries are unifocalized through separate thoracotomy procedures. At a later date, a midline sternotomy is performed to place a right ventricle to pulmonary artery homograft conduit and to close the VSD.

Postoperative Management

Tetralogy of Fallot With Pulmonary Stenosis. The primary postoperative issues after complete surgical repair for TOF-PS include the management of right ventricular dysfunction and arrhythmias. The development of right bundle branch block is common secondary to the VSD closure. Sinus tachycardia and junctional ectopic tachycardia (JET) are also common and may be difficult to differentiate. Careful evaluation of the atrial waveform for the presence of cannon *a* waves and an atrial ECG assist in the diagnosis. Sinus tachycardia is a compensatory response to improve cardiac output in the face of right ventricular dysfunction. JET occurs frequently in postoperative neonates and infants, with heart rates as high as 180 to 230 beats/min. It usually presents during the first 24 hours following cardiopulmonary bypass and is often associated with hemodynamic instability, warranting treatment. Maintaining normothermia, core cooling to temperatures of 35° C, or the use of antiarrhythmic agents may be indicated.

The right ventricle is hypertrophied and noncompliant. This, in association with cardiopulmonary bypass and the surgical procedure, results in postoperative right ventricular dysfunction. The degree of right ventricular dysfunction depends on the amount of right ventricular hypertrophy, the preoperative anatomy and pathophysiologic condition, the amount of right ventricular infundibular muscle removal, the requirement of a right ventriculotomy or transannular patch, and the length of the cardiopulmonary bypass and aortic cross clamp times. In general, pink tets require very little RVOT muscle resection and do not require a right ventricular incision or transannular patch. Their postoperative course is usually uneventful, resulting in endotracheal extubation by postoperative day 1 or 2. Patients with more complex anatomy and preoperative cyanosis require more extensive surgery often prolonging their postoperative recovery. The presence of a transannular patch results in some degree of pulmonary insufficiency, which can contribute to the right ventricular dysfunction and prolong the postoperative recovery. The presence of residual lesions, including any residual VSD or RVOTO, also contributes to the degree of right ventricular dysfunction. A transesophageal echocardiogram (TEE) is performed at the end of the surgical procedure to evaluate for the presence of residual lesions. If present, a return to cardiopulmonary bypass with further surgery may be required.

Manifestations of right ventricular dysfunction include tachycardia and elevated right atrial pressures. The high right atrial pressure is usually necessary to maintain adequate preload for the right ventricle. If the foramen ovale is patent, right-to-left shunting may occur when right atrial pressure exceeds left atrial pressure. This will maintain left ventricular output, yet result in cyanosis. If a PFO is not present, right ventricular dysfunction and failure can result in inadequate systemic cardiac output and inadequate tissue oxygen delivery. The management of right ventricular dysfunction includes inotropic support, right atrial pressure monitoring, evaluation of systemic cardiac output, observing for signs of atrial shunting, and the treatment of situations that increase oxygen demands, such as fever,

agitation, and pain. Endotracheal intubation is usually required until right ventricular dysfunction improves, as indicated by diuresis and decreased requirement for inotropic support.

Tetralogy of Fallot With Pulmonary Atresia. Neonates who undergo a complete repair for TOF-PA have a similar postoperative course as do neonates following repair for TOF-PS. The complications requiring treatment include cardiac arrhythmias and right ventricular dysfunction. The degree of right ventricular dysfunction, however, may be less than that seen in patients with TOF-PS. This is secondary to the absence of both extensive RVOT muscle resection and a transannular patch. The presence of a right ventricular to pulmonary artery homograft may result in some degree of pulmonary insufficiency possibly contributing to right ventricular dysfunction.

The postoperative course for patients after surgical procedures for TOF-PA with MAPCAs depends on the specific procedure performed and the postoperative physiology. Potential complications following unifocalization procedures include lung injury, right ventricular hypertension and dysfunction, problems with oxygenation and ventilation, organ system dysfunction, and bleeding. Lung injury can result from reperfusion injury, pulmonary contusions, or pulmonary hemorrhage and is manifested by hypoxemia, pulmonary edema, and pleural effusions. The need for endotracheal intubation and mechanical ventilation is often prolonged until recovery occurs. Right ventricular hypertension occurs secondary to the resistance created by the small and abnormal pulmonary arteries and the resistance created by extensive suture lines. Right ventricular dysfunction results from these factors in addition to the reasons outlined for patients with TOF-PS. Oxygenation and ventilation can be impaired because of abnormal lung and pulmonary artery development, atelectasis, and the presence of reactive airway disease, requiring bronchodilator therapy and prolonged periods of mechanical ventilation. Bleeding is secondary to the extensive suture lines required for the unifocalization, the length of cardiopulmonary bypass, and the presence of a coagulopathy. These patients are highly complex to care for, especially when their physiology remains abnormal in the postoperative period.

Pulmonary Atresia With Intact Ventricular Septum.

Pulmonary atresia with intact ventricular septum (PA-IVS) (Fig. 18-15) is a rare congenital heart defect. In this defect, atresia of the pulmonary valve results in complete obstruction to blood flow from the right ventricle to the pulmonary artery. In addition, the ventricular septum is intact, and the right ventricle is hypertrophied. The right ventricular size is variable, ranging from extremely hypoplastic to larger than normal. The tricuspid valve size and structure are also variable, although it is often hypoplastic and stenotic. The main pulmonary artery is generally of normal size, and a large ASD is always present.

A significant finding in patients with PA-IVS is the presence of abnormal coronary circulation. Approximately 10% of these patients have coronary artery stenosis or atresia of the major coronary arteries. When this occurs, the coronary arteries distal to the stenosis or atresia are perfused

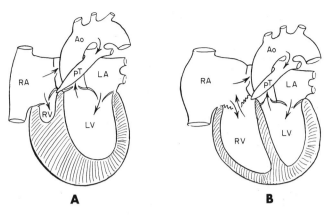

Fig. 18-15 Pulmonary atresia with intact ventricular septum. **A,** Type 1; **B,** type 2. *Ao,* Aorta; *LA,* left atrium; *LV,* left ventricle; *pT,* pulmonary trunk; *RA,* right atrium; *RV,* right ventricle. (From Perloff JK: *The clinical recognition of congenital heart disease,* ed 4, Philadelphia, 1994, WB Saunders, p 599.)

via fistulas between the right ventricle and the coronary artery bed. Coronary artery abnormalities are usually associated with severe right ventricular and tricuspid valve hypoplasia and occur when right ventricular pressure is greater than systemic pressure.

With PA-IVS, no forward flow of blood occurs across the pulmonary valve, and the right ventricle is hypertrophied and noncompliant. Right ventricular pressure is often supersystemic, and usually some degree of tricuspid valve regurgitation exists. Pressure in the right atrium is greater than that in the left, resulting in a right-to-left shunt across the ASD and cyanosis.

When coronary artery stenosis or atresia exist, the distal coronary artery beds are supplied with right ventricular blood from fistulous communications. These intramyocardial sinusoids result in retrograde coronary blood flow from the desaturated blood in the right ventricle to the coronary arteries. As long as right ventricular hypertension persists, this may not have an immediate impact in the neonate. However, if the right ventricle is decompressed, distal coronary artery perfusion will decrease, resulting in myocardial ischemia. Long-term perfusion of coronary arteries from venous blood can result in both right and left ventricular ischemia and subsequent fibrosis.

Clinical Presentation and Course. Neonates born with PA-IVS are cyanotic secondary to the obligatory right-to-left shunt across the atrial septum. Their PBF is dependent on PDA; therefore when ductal closure occurs, these infants will become severely distressed, hypoxemic, and acidotic. Death can occur rapidly if emergency treated is not initiated. The long-term course of these patients depends on the individual anatomy, ranging from single-ventricle palliation to complete two-ventricle repair. In the presence of coronary artery fistula with evolving myocardial ischemia, cardiac transplant may be indicated.

Management. Management of the newborn with PA-IVS includes the correction of hypoxemia and acidosis and the administration of PGE_1 to maintain patency of the ductus and ensure PBF. Endotracheal intubation and me-

chanical ventilation are often required. Arterial oxygen saturations should be maintained between 75% and 85%. Administration of sodium bicarbonate and infusions of inotropic agents may be necessary to treat hypoxemia and acidosis. Echocardiography is performed to establish the diagnosis of pulmonary atresia, right ventricular size, and tricuspid valve morphology. In most instances, cardiac catheterization is also necessary to determine the abnormalities in coronary artery anatomy and the presence of right ventricular fistula. Cardiac catheterization can also provide information regarding right ventricular pressure and tricuspid valve regurgitation.

A surgical procedure is necessary in the early neonatal period to provide a reliable source of PBF. Given the spectrum of this defect, the exact surgical procedure depends on the individual anatomy and ranges from a two-ventricular repair to a single-ventricle palliation. The goal of neonatal surgery is to provide adequate oxygenation with a balance of systemic and pulmonary circulations and to provide forward flow across the pulmonary valve into the pulmonary artery whenever possible. This approach allows growth of the right ventricle, with the goal of achieving a two-ventricle repair in the future. When the right ventricle is extremely hypoplastic, however, a systemic-to-pulmonary artery shunt is placed, the ductus is ligated, and the patient's management is like that of other single-ventricle defects.

The presence of coronary artery fistula also determines the surgical management. When present, the elevated right ventricular pressure provides the coronary artery perfusion to the distal bed. If forward flow is surgically provided across the pulmonary valve, right ventricular pressure will decrease, coronary artery perfusion will diminish, and myocardial ischemia will result. In these patients, a systemic-to-pulmonary artery shunt is placed, and the patient's condition is managed like other single-ventricle defects. A cardiac transplant may be indicated in the future.

In a small number of patients with PA-IVS, the right ventricle is of normal size with mild tricuspid valve disease and the absence of coronary artery fistula. In these cases, reconstruction of the right ventricular outflow tract without the placement of a systemic-to-pulmonary shunt can be performed. However, in most cases a combination of systemic-to-pulmonary artery shunt with right ventricular outflow tract reconstruction is provided. Even when the pulmonary valve and outflow tract are repaired, the small size of the right ventricle, along with its limited compliance, results in a decreased cardiac output ejected to the pulmonary artery. The systemic-to-pulmonary artery shunt is necessary to provide adequate PBF. Additional future surgery will most likely be necessary in these patients.

The overall goals for postoperative management depend on the individual anatomy and the type of surgical procedure performed. When severe right ventricular hypoplasia exists and an isolated systemic-to-pulmonary artery shunt is placed in the neonate, management is similar to that of other neonates with single-ventricle palliation, with the goal of balancing the systemic and pulmonary circulations (see section on hypoplastic left heart syndrome). In addition, if right ventricular sinusoids and abnormal coronary artery circulation exist, the patient should be carefully monitored for signs of myocardial ischemia, including ECG changes, ventricular arrhythmias, and signs of low cardiac output.

When a combination of right ventricular outflow tract reconstruction and placement of a systemic-to-pulmonary artery shunt is performed, the patient must be monitored for signs of balanced circulations and right ventricular function. Signs of pulmonary overcirculation, including wide systemic arterial pulse pressure, oliguria, poor peripheral perfusion, metabolic acidosis, and elevated arterial oxygen saturations, may indicate excessive PBF. In this case the right ventricle may be adequate to provide an entire cardiac output to the pulmonary bed, and the systemic-to-pulmonary artery shunt may be too large or is not needed.

In older patients who receive a two-ventricle repair with closure of the ASD and takedown of the systemic-to-pulmonary artery shunt, signs of right ventricular failure should be monitored. Elevated right atrial pressure, signs of low cardiac output, and the development of ascites or pleural effusions may indicate right ventricular failure. This situation may indicate the need for a communication between the right and left atria to allow right-to-left shunting and the maintenance of adequate systemic cardiac output.

Tricuspid Atresia. Tricuspid atresia consists of an absent tricuspid valve and no opening from the right atria to either ventricle. In most cases, tricuspid valve tissue is not evident, but rather the floor of the atria is muscular. There are varying degrees of right ventricular hypoplasia. A communication between the left ventricle and the hypoplastic right ventricle exists via a VSD (bulboventricular foramen) and can often be a site of obstruction to blood flow. The great vessels may be normally related or transposed. Type I tricuspid atresia refers to absence of the tricuspid valve with normally related great vessels, whereas type II

refers to absence of the tricuspid valve with transposition of the great vessels. Further classification depends on the degree of obstruction to PBF, which can be (1) pulmonary valve atresia, (2) pulmonary valve stenosis, or (3) unrestricted PBF. An atrial communication is always present, although it is often restrictive. A PDA is usually present at birth, but closes spontaneously within a few days. Most commonly, tricuspid atresia exists with hypoplasia of the right ventricle, normally related great vessels, and some obstruction to PBF (type Ib) (Fig. 18-16).

Regardless of the various defects associated with tricuspid atresia, blood flow through the heart is essentially the same. With no outlet from the right atria to the right ventricle, the entire systemic venous return shunts across the atrial septum from the right to the left atrium via a PFO or an ASD. Here systemic venous blood mixes with pulmonary venous blood and passes into the left ventricle. From the left ventricle, some blood is ejected to the aorta, and some is shunted across the VSD (bulboventricular foramen) out the right ventricular infundibulum to the pulmonary artery. The amount of PBF is determined by how restrictive the VSD is or the obstruction to flow at the pulmonary valve. This lesion is usually not ductal dependent unless coexisting pulmonary atresia is present.

Clinical Presentation and Course. Infants with tricuspid atresia present in the neonatal period with cyanosis from the right-to-left atrial shunt and a murmur. If PBF is inadequate once the ductus arteriosus closes, neonates may become distressed, hypoxemic, and acidotic. Rarely is unrestricted PBF present, in which case signs of CHF would be evident.

Management. If PBF is ductal dependent, a continuous infusion of PGE$_1$ is necessary to maintain ductal patency. Although PBF may be decreased, it is usually not

TRICUSPID ATRESIA WITHOUT TRANSPOSITION

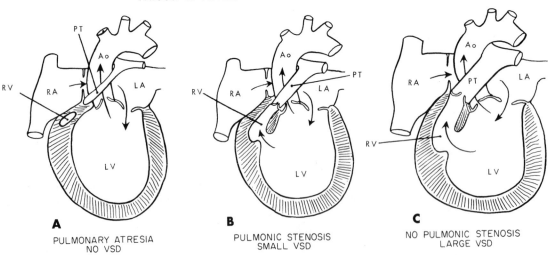

A	B	C
PULMONARY ATRESIA NO VSD	PULMONIC STENOSIS SMALL VSD	NO PULMONIC STENOSIS LARGE VSD

Fig. 18-16 Illustrations of tricuspid atresia with normally related great arteries. In all, the only outlet for right atrial *(RA)* blood is interatrial communication. Variations in ventricular septum and pulmonary valve are depicted. *Ao,* Aorta; *LA,* left atrium; *LV,* left ventricle; *PT,* pulmonary trunk; *RV,* right ventricle. (From Perloff JK: *The clinical recognition of congenital heart disease,* ed 4, Philadelphia, 1994, WB Saunders, p 616.)

ductal dependent; therefore most neonates can tolerate spontaneous ductal closure. A balloon atrial septostomy may be necessary if the atrial septum is restrictive.

A palliative surgical procedure is usually required in the neonatal period. Typically, a systemic-to-pulmonary artery shunt is placed to improve PBF. If the atrial septum is restrictive, an atrial septectomy can be performed at this time to provide adequate mixing of blood at the atrial level. In rare situations when PBF is excessive, a pulmonary artery band is placed to limit pulmonary overcirculation and optimize systemic blood flow. In either case, the presence of right ventricular hypoplasia does not allow a two-ventricle repair; therefore these patients require additional palliative procedures for single-ventricle physiology, typically including the bidirectional Glenn anastomosis at 4 to 6 months, followed by the Fontan procedure later in childhood. For a complete description of these procedures, see the section on hypoplastic left heart syndrome.

Some newborns with tricuspid atresia have relatively balanced systemic and pulmonary blood flow and may not require a surgical procedure in the newborn period. These infants receive a primary bidirectional Glenn anastomosis in infancy (4 to 6 months of age), followed by a Fontan procedure later in childhood.

The postoperative management issues depend on the preoperative pathophysiologic condition, specifically, the presence of too much to too little PBF, and the surgical procedure performed. Typically, a systemic-to-pulmonary shunt is placed to provide a reliable source of PBF, and the goal of postoperative care includes the balancing of systemic and pulmonary circulations (see section on hypoplastic left heart syndrome). Usually a regimen of oral aspirin (5 to 10 mg/kg/day) is started in these patients to maintain shunt patency.

Cyanotic Congenital Heart Defects With Increased PBF

Cyanotic CHDs with increased PBF include total anomalous pulmonary venous connection (TAPVC), truncus arteriosus, and hypoplastic left heart syndrome (HLHS). These conditions can occur in isolation or in combination with other structural defects. Table 18-6 summarizes the findings on cardiac examination, ECG, and chest radiograph of children with these defects.

Total Anomalous Pulmonary Venous Connection. TAPVC results in anomalous pulmonary venous drainage into a systemic venous structure rather than the left atrium. Of note is that partial anomalous pulmonary venous return can occur as well. In this defect some of the pulmonary veins drain to the left atrium, and some drain abnormally to systemic veins in the thorax or directly to the right atrium. This can occur in isolation or in association with other cardiac structural defects. In isolation, partial anomalous pulmonary venous connection is uncommon, and patients are often asymptomatic; therefore it is not discussed here.

The pulmonary venous system develops at about the third week of gestation. The splanchnic plexus, which is con-

---

TABLE 18-6 Cyanotic Congenital Heart Defects With Increased Pulmonary Blood Flow

Defect	Cardiac Examination	Electrocardiogram	Chest Radiograph
TAPVC With obstruction	Cardiac murmurs minimal or absent	Right ventricular hypertrophy	Increased pulmonary vascular markings; normal-sized heart
Without obstruction	Systolic ejection murmur best heard high in left chest; middiastolic murmur best heard low in left chest; widely split S_2	Right axis deviation, right atrial hypertrophy, right ventricular hypertrophy	Supracardiac: "figure eight" or "snowman" configuration; all defects: enlarged right atrium, right ventricle, and main pulmonary artery; increased pulmonary vascular markings
Truncus arteriosus	Normal S_1, single S_2, ejection click; loud, continuous (PDA type) murmur with unrestricted PBF; murmur shortened and softened by decreasing PBF	Left ventricular hypertrophy; biventricular hypertrophy seen occasionally	Nonspecific except for alteration in pulmonary vascular markings; may detect right-sided aortic arch, and pulmonary vessels may arise abnormally high in the chest
HLHS	Dominant RV impulse, decreased impulse at apex; single S_2 with increased intensity; diminished peripheral pulse; gallop rhythm in some, soft systolic murmur at LSB, middiastolic rumble at apex	Right ventricular hypertrophy; in some, right atrial enlargement	Cardiomegaly, increased pulmonary vascular markings

HLHS, Hypoplastic left heart syndrome; *LSB,* left sternal border; *PBF,* pulmonary blood flow; *PDA,* patent ductus arteriosus; S_1, first heart sound; S_2, second heart sound; *TAPVC,* total anomalous pulmonary venous connection.

nected to the umbilical vitelline veins and the cardinal veins, is in direct communication with the lung buds. The common pulmonary vein, which arises in the common atrium, grows to join the splanchnic plexus. Once the common pulmonary vein and the splanchnic plexus are joined, the cardinal veins and vitelline veins are no longer connected to the splanchnic plexus. The pulmonary veins then drain into the left atrium via the common pulmonary vein. Gradually, the common pulmonary vein is absorbed into the body of the left atrium,

and four distinct pulmonary veins draining into the left atrium persist. Failure in any of these embryologic processes can lead to the malformation of the four pulmonary veins, resulting in partial or total anomalous pulmonary venous connection.

TAPVC may occur in four forms: (1) supracardiac, whereby the pulmonary veins course via a vertical vein to the innominate vein that drains into the superior vena cava (Fig. 18-17, *A*); (2) cardiac, whereby the pulmonary veins

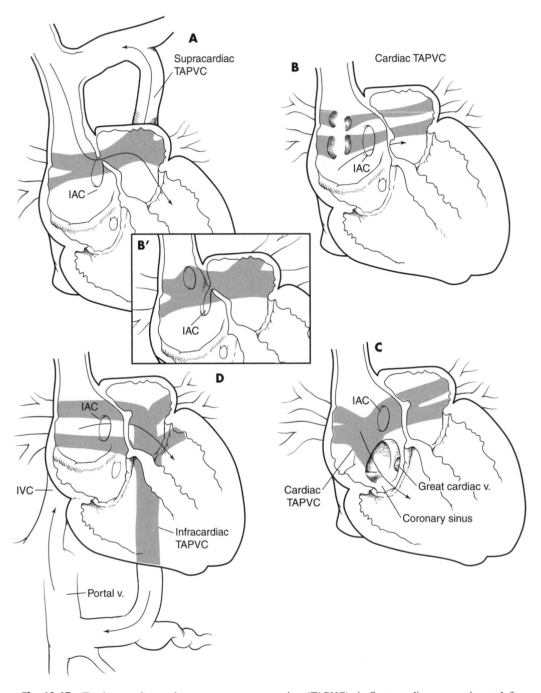

Fig. 18-17 Total anomalous pulmonary venous connection *(TAPVC)*. **A,** Supracardiac connection to left innominate vein. **B,** Cardiac connection to four separate veins. **B′,** Cardiac connection by single common orifice. **C,** Cardiac connection to coronary sinus. **D,** Infradiaphragmatic TAPVC via the portal venous system. *IAC,* Interatrial communications; *IVC,* inferior vena cava. (Reproduced with permission. Garson A, Bricker JT, Fisher DJ et al: *The science and practice of pediatric cardiology,* Baltimore, 1998, Williams & Wilkins.)

drain into the coronary sinus or directly into the right atrium (Fig. 18-17, *B* and *C*); (3) infracardiac, whereby the pulmonary veins drain into a descending vein and join the portal venous system (Fig 18-17, *D*); and (4) mixed, which includes variants of the previous three forms. Supracardiac TAPVC accounts for most of the cases. Essentially the anatomic malformation is such that pulmonary venous return is to the right atrium. Because of this defect, an ASD is necessary for oxygenated blood to reach the left atrium.

TAPVC may occur with or without obstruction in the pulmonary venous pathway. TAPVC with obstruction occurs predominantly in the infradiaphragmatic type. Obstruction with infradiaphragmatic TAPVC can occur at a number of sights along the anomalous venous pathway. Discrete obstruction can occur from constriction of the vein as it passes through the diaphragm. Diffuse obstruction occurs when the anomalous attachment enters the portal system. A restrictive atrial communication will obstruct flow from the right to left atrium, therefore obstructing pulmonary venous return to the systemic circulation.

TAPVC With Obstruction. Blood from both the pulmonary and the systemic venous systems returns to the right atrium. However, because of the presence of an obstruction in the pulmonary venous connection, pulmonary venous flow to the right atrium is restricted. This results in elevated pulmonary venous pressure with the subsequent development of progressive pulmonary hypertension and pulmonary edema. As PVR increases, so does right heart pressure. Decreased right ventricular compliance and right atrial hypertension result in a right-to-left shunt at the atrial level producing systemic hypoxemia. This right-to-left shunt decompresses the right heart, so cardiomegaly does not typically develop. Progressive hypoxemia contributes to metabolic acidosis and end-organ failure. Without surgical correction, death will ensue. Because of common clinical features, TAPVC with obstruction is often mistaken for persistent pulmonary hypertension of the newborn (PPHN). Specific diagnosis with echocardiogram is critical because therapeutic interventions for each are quite different.

TAPVC With Restrictive Intraatrial Connection. An atrial connection (ASD or PFO) is critical to the immediate survival of these infants. The size of the atrial shunt determines the degree of mixing and subsequent systemic oxygen saturations. A restrictive atrial communication results in right atrial volume overload, pressure elevation, and enlargement. As PVR falls, pulmonary overcirculation ensues that results in CHF and cardiac dysfunction. Generally, this occurs over the first few weeks of life, although clinical presentation can be variable. Elevated right atrial pressure results in systemic venous congestion.

TAPVC Without Obstruction. In the unobstructed forms, free communication occurs between the two atria. The relative pulmonary and systemic vascular resistances and cardiac compliance determine atrial shunt. As PVR falls, PBF increases, with subsequent volume load to the right heart. If not surgically addressed in a timely manner, pulmonary hypertension can develop secondary to pulmonary overcirculation.

Clinical Manifestations and Course. Neonates without obstruction may have mild to moderate cyanosis dependent on the degree of atrial mixing and pulmonary resistance. As PVR falls and PBF increases, the signs and symptoms of CHF can develop. The physical examination is often similar to that of a large ASD, although hepatomegaly or cyanosis may also be noted (atypical for isolated ASD).

Neonates with obstruction have quite different symptoms. These infants are typically critically ill, poorly perfused, acidotic, and cyanotic. Institution of supportive therapies is necessary shortly after birth with intubation, mechanical ventilation, and inotropes. Some require extracorporeal membrane oxygenation (ECMO) or high-frequency ventilation before surgery. Every effort should be made to make the diagnosis before cannulation for ECMO because emergent corrective surgery is the preferred treatment.

Management. As mentioned earlier, neonates with obstruction require early and aggressive intervention with mechanical ventilation, inotropes, volume, correction of acid-base disorders, maneuvers to decrease pulmonary resistance (nitric oxide), and possibly ECMO. In some, balloon atrial septostomy may stabilize the neonate's condition.[36] If stabilization does not occur, a true surgical emergency exists.

Management of TAPVC without obstruction is directed toward controlling CHF with anticongestive therapy and treating failure to thrive. If the patient is relatively asymptomatic, surgery can be performed at any age; however, many centers believe that the optimal time is at presentation or during the first year of life. Untreated infants who survive to older childhood or early adulthood may develop fixed pulmonary artery hypertension; therefore surgery should not be delayed.

Definitive Surgical Correction. Surgical correction is performed via a midline sternotomy incision using cardiopulmonary bypass and hypothermia. Some centers also employ circulatory arrest during a portion of the perioperative period. Surgical repair involves anastomosing the pulmonary venous confluence to the left atrium, resulting in proper drainage. The connecting vein to the systemic venous circulation is ligated, and the ASD is closed. Potential postoperative problems include low cardiac output, respiratory insufficiency, pulmonary hypertension, and arrhythmias. TAPVC with obstruction has a high postoperative mortality rate from pulmonary hypertension and respiratory failure.

Monitoring PA and LA pressures in the postoperative period can aid in the identification of residual or progressive pulmonary venous obstruction that constitutes a surgical emergency. Volume resuscitation is judicious because of decreased left heart compliance. Maneuvers to decrease PVR are employed in those patients with preoperative and postoperative pulmonary hypertension.

Truncus Arteriosus. Truncus arteriosus is the result of failure of the primitive arterial trunk (the truncus arteriosus) to septate and divide into a distinct aorta and pulmonary artery. The aorta and the pulmonary artery normally develop from the common truncus arteriosus at the

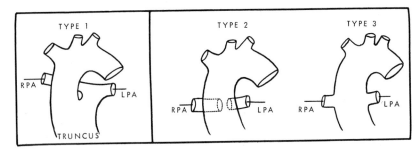

Fig. 18-18   Illustrations of various types of truncus arteriosus. In type 1 a short main pulmonary artery arises from the truncus. In types 2 and 3 the branch pulmonary arteries arise directly from walls of the truncus. *LPA,* Left pulmonary artery; *RPA,* right pulmonary artery. (From Perloff JK: *The clinical recognition of congenital heart disease,* ed 4, Philadelphia, 1994, WB Saunders, p 688.)

end of the third week and during the fourth week of gestation. This occurs by virtue of the unique development of conotruncal ridges that spiral and separate to form the great arteries. Failure of septation of the common trunk results in the persistence of a single vessel that gives rise to the systemic and pulmonary arteries and contains only one valve (truncal valve), which is often dysmorphic. The truncus arteriosus overlies a VSD that is always seen in conjunction with this defect and is an integral part of its pathophysiology.

Truncus arteriosus exists in three anatomically distinct variations. These occur with respect to the size and site of origin of the pulmonary arteries. In type 1, a short pulmonary trunk arises from the truncus and divides into the branch pulmonary arteries. In type 2, both branch pulmonary arteries arise in close proximity directly from the truncus without a main pulmonary artery. In type 3, the separate origins of the branch pulmonary arteries arise some distance apart from the lateral sides of the aorta (Fig. 18-18). Type 4 is characterized by no main or branch pulmonary arteries with multiple small collateral arteries arising from the descending aorta. This defect is really a misnomer and is more appropriately described as a variant of pulmonary atresia. Truncus arteriosus is a conotruncal anomaly and is associated with the genetic syndrome commonly referred to as 22q deletion.[37]

Because of the large VSD, right and left ventricular pressures are equal. Mixing of oxygenated and deoxygenated blood occurs at the level of the ventricles. The single great artery (truncus) arising from the right and left ventricles receives the entire cardiac output of both ventricles. Flow to the pulmonary and systemic vascular beds is secondary to the relative resistances. As PVR falls, PBF increases, with subsequent pulmonary overcirculation and the development of CHF. Because both great arteries arise from the truncus, they will both have the same systolic pressure, which is markedly elevated (relative to normal) for the pulmonary artery, resulting in pulmonary hypertension.

The competence of the truncal valve can be quite variable, ranging from normal to severe regurgitation to stenotic. Truncal regurgitation results in ventricular volume load, cardiac dysfunction, and worsening heart failure. Truncal stenosis imposes a pressure load on both ventricles.

Clinical Presentation and Course.   As PVR falls and PBF increases, the neonate develops signs and symptoms of CHF. Cyanosis may become less pronounced over the first few days to weeks of life because of a decrease in right-to-left shunt and an increase in PBF. A systolic murmur is usually heard in the first few days of life, and the second heart sound is single.

Management.   Truncus arteriosus is usually diagnosed in the neonatal period. If left untreated, this lesion carries a mortality rate of 87% by 6 months of age and 91% by 1 year of age.[37] Initial management consists of anticongestive therapy, and early surgical intervention is now generally recommended in the neonatal period. The only absolute contraindication for surgery is Eisenmenger's syndrome.

Definitive Surgical Correction.   Surgery is performed via a median sternotomy. Deep hypothermia with low-flow technique or circulatory arrest is employed. The pulmonary arteries are excised from the aortic root and anastomosed to a valved conduit (homograft). The homograft is interposed between the right ventricle and pulmonary arteries, resulting in right ventricular to pulmonary artery continuity. The VSD is patched in a manner that isolates the truncus arteriosus and truncal valve to the left of the septum, where it functions as the aorta. Surgery is repeated if the conduit becomes stenotic or insufficient or as it becomes inadequate in size as the child grows, requiring replacement with a larger one.

Caring for these infants can be challenging because of the potential for the development of postoperative pulmonary hypertension, right ventricular dysfunction, and arrhythmias (particularly JET). The use of usual ventilatory and nursing maneuvers to treat pulmonary hypertension helps to decrease PVR and pulmonary hypertensive crises. If pulmonary hypertension is unresponsive to these measures, nitric oxide or mechanical assist (ECMO, VAD) should be considered. Information obtained from a transthoracic PA line helps to evaluate for pulmonary hypertension, residual VSD, or RVOTO. Arrhythmias require immediate treatment because they are poorly tolerated, particularly JET.

Hypoplastic Left Heart Syndrome.   HLHS includes a spectrum of disease involving varying degrees of underdevelopment of the mitral valve, left ventricle, aortic valve, and aorta (Fig. 18-19). Typical variations include aortic and

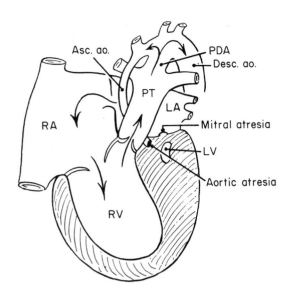

Fig. 18-19 Hypoplastic left heart syndrome (HLHS). *Asc ao,* Ascending aorta; *Desc ao,* descending aorta; *LA,* left atrium; *LV,* left ventricle; *PDA,* patent ductus arteriosus; *PT,* pulmonary trunk; *RA,* right atrium; *RV,* right ventricle. (From Perloff JK: *The clinical recognition of congenital heart disease,* ed 4, Philadelphia, 1994, WB Saunders, p 727.)

mitral atresia, aortic and mitral stenosis, aortic atresia and mitral stenosis, or aortic stenosis and mitral atresia. Hypoplasia of the left ventricle is always present, making it incapable of supporting systemic circulation. The aorta is always hypoplastic but provides adequate coronary blood flow in both the preoperative and postoperative period. The left atria may be small, and an ASD or a PFO exists. Occasionally the atrial communication can be restrictive. HLHS is rarely associated with other cardiac anomalies. Associated extracardiac and chromosomal anomalies may be present, including central nervous system abnormalities.[31]

Survival in the newborn period is dependent on a PDA to maintain systemic circulation. When ductal closure occurs, and without aggressive medical management, circulatory shock develops rapidly, and death will result. With HLHS, systemic venous blood returns to the right atrium normally, and pulmonary venous blood returns to the left atrium normally. With no outflow from the left atrium to the left ventricle, there is a complete left-to-right shunt across an ASD or a PFO. Mixing of blood occurs in the right atrium, flows across the tricuspid valve into the right ventricle, and out the pulmonary artery. Some blood will flow to the lungs, and some will shunt right-to-left across the PDA to the aorta. In the aorta, blood flow will be antegrade to the descending aorta and retrograde around the aortic arch, head vessels, ascending aorta, and coronary arteries. The amount of systemic and pulmonary blood flow will depend on the relative resistance of the two vascular beds.

Clinical Presentation and Course. Typically newborns with HLHS present with cyanosis, respiratory distress, and variable degrees of circulatory collapse during the first 24 to 48 hours of life. When cyanotic congenital heart disease is suspected, an infusion of PGE₁ should be administered immediately to maintain ductal patency and sustain systemic circulation. Diagnosis of HLHS is made by echocardiography. Cardiac catheterization is not necessary to make the diagnosis. Because of short postpartum hospital stays, a newborn with HLHS will occasionally be discharged home before diagnosis. Failure to make the diagnosis can occur when the ductus arteriosus has remained patent and the systemic and pulmonary circulations are adequately balanced. When the ductus arteriosus eventually closes, the patient will rapidly deteriorate, presenting "late" with profound shock and signs of multiple organ system failure. If resuscitation is successful, recovery of end-organ ischemia may be necessary before surgical palliation. The presence of a restrictive foramen ovale or ASD will severely limit the left-to-right atrial shunt and result in inadequate PBF. In this case, the neonate would present early with severe cyanosis and metabolic acidosis.

In the current era, HLHS is often diagnosed on prenatal ultrasound or fetal echocardiography. The advantage to prenatal diagnosis is that the delivery and newborn resuscitation can be arranged before the birth. In fact, prenatal diagnosis of HLHS is associated with improved preoperative hemodynamics and improved survival following neonatal palliation, compared with neonates diagnosed after birth.[38]

Preoperative Management. A PGE₁ infusion is initiated immediately on suspicion of HLHS to maintain ductal patency and ensure adequate systemic circulation. If end-organ ischemia is present, support and adequate recovery of organ function are critical to provide optimal conditions for the stage 1 palliative surgical procedure. Often these patients require endotracheal intubation, mechanical ventilation, and inotropic support to optimize hemodynamics. Metabolic acidosis should be aggressively treated and may require the administration of sodium bicarbonate or tromethamine.

The overall goal of medical management of any preoperative neonate with single-ventricle physiology is to provide a balance of the systemic and pulmonary circulations. Newborns with single-ventricle physiology are often dependent on a large systemic-to-pulmonary communication (the ductus arteriosus) for the delivery of blood to their lungs or to their systemic circulation. When the ductus arteriosus is widely patent (PGE₁ administration), the distal PVR is often the major determinant of the balance of flow between the lungs and body. Preoperatively, two major clinical problems can be seen: pulmonary overcirculation or pulmonary undercirculation. Pulmonary overcirculation occurs when PBF is so generous that it is at the expense of systemic output. It is manifested as high systemic saturations (90%), poor peripheral perfusion, and low diastolic blood pressure. Because it is the result of a very low distal PVR, management strategies are directed at increasing PVR, which can be achieved by supporting the infant by ventilation with a hypoxic gas mixture (17% to 20% oxygen) or by inducing respiratory acidosis (pH 7.25 to 7.35).

A hypoxic gas mixture is achieved by adding nitrogen to the gas mix. The resultant decrease in alveolar Po₂ will augment pulmonary vasoconstriction and decrease PBF. Supplemental nitrogen therapy has been shown to be efficacious in maintaining systemic saturations of about 75% in infants with single-ventricle physiology without long-term sequelae.[39]

Respiratory acidosis may be achieved by decreasing the minute ventilation or adding CO_2 to the ventilator gas mixture. Available data suggest that the beneficial effects of inhaled CO_2 are mediated through resulting respiratory acidosis. Pulmonary vasoconstriction should result in an improvement in systemic perfusion, an increase in diastolic blood pressure, and a decrease in systemic oxygen saturation.[40] Clearly a potential advantage of using inhaled CO_2 is that the respiratory acidosis can be induced without the use of severe hypoventilation, which may induce atelectasis.

Clearly these therapies have potential morbidity, and extreme hypoxia and acidosis should be avoided. Pulmonary undercirculation occurs when the PVR is too high, resulting in severe hypoxemia despite a PDA. This is often the result of failure of the PVR to normally decrease at birth, and management strategies are directed at decreasing PVR. This can be achieved by providing the infant ventilation with 100% oxygen and inducing an alkalosis (pH 7.50 to 7.55) by a combination of hyperventilation and sodium bicarbonate administration. Inhaled nitric oxide may also be beneficial in this setting.

Typically, pulmonary overcirculation occurs in preoperative patients with HLHS because lowering of PVR in the newborn period. Oxygen administration is generally avoided to prevent pulmonary vasodilation and overcirculation. A systemic arterial oxygen saturation of 75% to 80% usually indicates appropriate PBF.

Surgical Management. Current options for treatment include palliative reconstructive surgery, cardiac transplantation, and withholding of treatment. With the more recent improvements in reconstructive surgery and associated outcomes in some centers, withholding of treatment has becomes much less common. Cardiac transplantation has had success; however, the lack of available neonatal donors has made this option less appealing. Reconstructive surgery along the Fontan pathway has been the most common approach to the overall management of neonates with HLHS.

Stage 1 Palliative Reconstruction. The goal of neonatal reconstructive surgery for HLHS is to provide a dependable source of systemic and pulmonary blood flow. In addition, efforts are made to provide the best conditions for future bidirectional cavopulmonary shunt and Fontan operation. Preventing problems such as ventricular hypertrophy, arrhythmias, pulmonary artery hypertension, tricuspid valve regurgitation, and pulmonary artery distortion will provide optimal conditions for later reconstructive procedures.

Success with the staged surgical approach to HLHS was first described in 1983.[41] The first-stage palliation, often referred to as the Norwood procedure, accomplished two primary objectives: the establishment of permanent unobstructed flow from the right ventricle to the aorta and regulation of PBF. Through a median sternotomy and the use of cardiopulmonary bypass, the ductus arteriosus is

ligated, and the main pulmonary artery is ligated from the branch pulmonary arteries. An incision is made in the descending aorta retrograde to the aortic valve, avoiding injury to the coronary arteries. The pulmonary artery root is then anastomosed to the aorta, and a homograft patch is used to augment the wall of the neoaorta (Fig. 18-20). An aortopulmonary shunt, most commonly a modified Blalock-Taussig shunt, is placed to provide the single source of PBF. An atrial septectomy is performed to allow adequate mixing of systemic and pulmonary venous blood. Often, hypothermic circulatory arrest is used to perform the aortic reconstruction. However, recent attempts have been made to use low-flow cardiopulmonary bypass via cannulation in the head and neck vessels, thereby avoiding the potential neurologic complications associated with circulatory arrest.

With this reconstruction, systemic and pulmonary venous blood enter and mix in the common atria, enter the single right ventricle via the tricuspid valve, cross the native pulmonary valve, and enter the neoaorta. Blood will flow antegrade to the systemic circulation, and the coronary arteries will be perfused during diastole. When blood enters the aorta, some will flow across the aortopulmonary shunt into the pulmonary circulation.

Bidirectional Cavopulmonary Shunt. The goal of the second-stage palliative procedure is to decrease the volume load of the single ventricle, thereby decreasing work and preserving myocardial function, tricuspid valve function, and myocardial perfusion. Typically, the procedure performed is the bidirectional cavopulmonary shunt, commonly called the bidirectional Glenn shunt. Through a median sternotomy, the superior vena cava is divided from the right atria and anastomosed to the right branch pulmonary artery. The modified Blalock-Taussig shunt is removed, and the cardiac end of the superior vena cava is oversewn (Fig. 18-21). The azygous vein is usually ligated

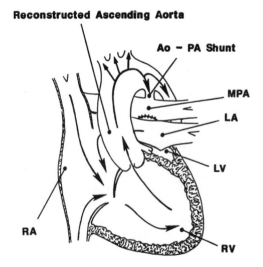

Fig. 18-20 Circulatory pathway after Stage I reconstructive surgery for HLHS. *RA,* Right atrium; *Ao-PA shunt,* aorta pulmonary shunt; *MPA,* main pulmonary artery; *LA,* left atrium; *LV,* left ventricle; *RV,* right ventricle. (From Smith JB, Vernon-Levett P: Care of infants with HLHS, *AACN Clin Issues Crit Care Nurs* 4:33, 1993.)

to decrease a source of decompression of the upper systemic veins to the atria. Additional surgical procedures that may be performed at this time to optimize conditions for the Fontan procedure may include a pulmonary arterioplasty and a tricuspid valvuloplasty.

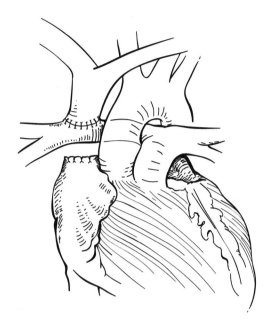

Fig. 18-21 Bidirectional superior cavopulmonary anastomosis (bidirectional Glenn). (From Chang A, Hanley F, Wernovsky G et al: *Pediatric cardiac intensive care,* Baltimore, 1998, Williams & Wilkins.)

With this anatomy, systemic venous blood from the head and neck directly enters the pulmonary circulation. The systemic venous blood from the inferior vena cava enters the common atria, where it mixes with the coronary sinus and pulmonary venous blood. This blood exits the heart through the aorta, resulting in a systemic arterial oxygen saturation of 75% to 85%. Although this decreases the volume load and subsequent work of the single ventricle, problems with this procedure include the late development of arterial desaturation, pulmonary arteriovenous malformations, and aortopulmonary collaterals.[42]

Fontan Operation. The goal of the third and final palliative procedure is to provide a separation of the systemic and pulmonary circulations and correct arterial desaturation. Many revisions of the Fontan operation have evolved over the years in an attempt to improve the outcome of patients with single-ventricle physiology. Currently, the two procedures most commonly performed include the intraatrial lateral tunnel Fontan and the extracardiac conduit Fontan.

With the lateral tunnel Fontan operation, a right atrial incision is made, and a Gore-Tex patch is sewn around the orifice of the inferior vena cava along the lateral wall of the right atria toward the superior vena cava.[42] The upper end of the superior vena cava is then anastomosed to the right branch pulmonary artery, creating a tunnel from the inferior vena cava, through the right atria, to the pulmonary artery (Fig. 18-22). The superior vena cava has been previously anastomosed to the pulmonary artery when the bidirectional cavopulmonary shunt was performed.

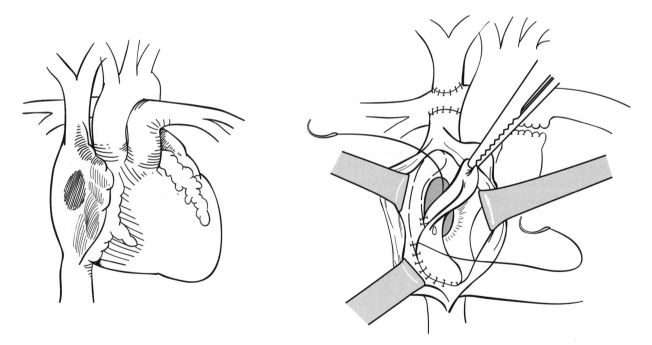

Fig. 18-22   Lateral tunnel cavopulmonary Fontan procedure. (From Chang A, Hanley F, Wernovski G et al: 1998) *Pediatric cardiac intensive care,* Baltimore, 1998,Williams & Wilkins.)

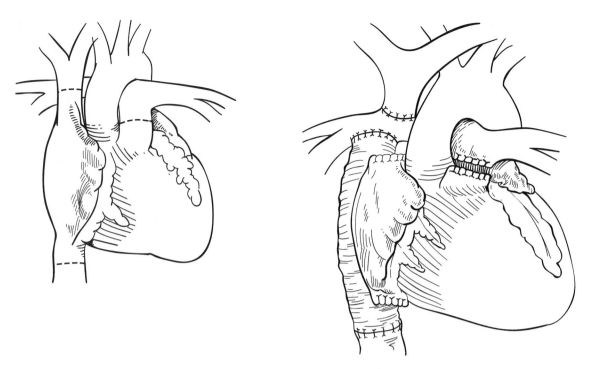

Fig. 18-23   Extracardiac Fontan procedure. (From Chang A, Hanley F, Wernovski G et al: *Pediatric cardiac intensive care,* Baltimore, 1998, Williams & Wilkins.)

With the extracardiac conduit Fontan operation, the inferior vena cava is transected from the right atria. A Gore-Tex conduit is sewn to the inferior vena cava and connected to the right pulmonary artery (Fig. 18-23). Possible advantages of this technique include the avoidance of right atrial suture lines and the elimination of elevated right atrial pressure, resulting in potentially fewer atrial arrhythmias and effusions.

With either Fontan operation, all the systemic venous blood is directly diverted to the pulmonary circulation. The coronary sinus blood enters the atria, mixes with the pulmonary venous blood, and is ejected into the systemic circulation, resulting in a systemic arterial oxygen saturation of approximately 95%. In some cases an atrial fenestration (connection from the systemic venous connection to the left atrium) may be inserted, which allows shunting of systemic venous blood to the atria in the event of elevated pulmonary artery pressure, thereby preventing complications of low cardiac output and effusions.

Postoperative Management

Stage 1 Palliative Procedures.   The primary goals in the postoperative management of complex reconstructive procedures, such as the Norwood procedure, include the management of low cardiac output and balancing of the systemic and pulmonary circulations. Low cardiac output is managed with continuous infusions of inotropic and afterload-reducing agents. Volume administration is given judiciously to avoid distension of the single ventricle. Hemodynamics are monitored closely, and signs of low cardiac output, including poor peripheral perfusion, oliguria, tachycardia, hypotension, and metabolic acidosis, should prompt aggressive intervention. Delayed sternal

closure is often performed to prevent mechanical cardiac tamponade in the early postoperative period. The hematocrit is maintained greater than 45% to improve oxygen delivery in the face of chronic arterial desaturation. Oxygen demand is minimized with the aggressive management of pain and agitation and the careful performance of nursing procedures. Procedures, such as suctioning and dressing changes, must be performed carefully to avoid a stimulus response that may result in acute hemodynamic deterioration. Acid-base abnormalities should be aggressively treated to avoid further depression of myocardial function.

Similar to the preoperative setting, infants with single-ventricle physiology who have a systemic-to-pulmonary communication as their source of PBF (i.e., Norwood procedure) may suffer from postoperative pulmonary over-circulation or undercirculation. In this setting, altering the PVR, as previously described, may be lifesaving. In the postoperative period, however, it must be remembered that the surgically placed systemic-to-pulmonary communication (vascular shunt) may need to be modified if these other measures fail.

Bidirectional Cavopulmonary Anastomosis.   Postoperative management of these patients is fairly straightforward. Typically, these patients can be extubated within 12 to 24 hours of surgery. Inotropic infusions are common after the use of cardiopulmonary bypass. Two important postoperative management issues following the bidirectional Glenn procedure include the assessment of elevated superior vena cava (SVC) pressure (SVC syndrome), and hypoxemia. SVC syndrome can be the result of an obstruction at the anastomosis site, pulmonary artery distortion, or elevations in PVR.[42] Clinical signs include upper body plethora and edema, with demarcation across the chest. Significant elevations in SVC pressure can limit cerebral blood flow and result in cerebral ischemia. Prevention and management strategies include elevating the head of the bed and keeping the head and neck midline. This positioning optimizes passive flow of blood from the head and neck to the pulmonary circulation. If PVR is elevated, vasodilation with oxygen and afterload-reducing agents may be necessary. Frequent nursing evaluation for the development of SVC syndrome, along with examination of the neurologic status, is critical in the postoperative period because an increase in SVC pressure can be detrimental to cerebral perfusion. Atrial pressure is maintained at 6 to 8 mmHg to avoid interference with pulmonary venous return to the heart.

Hypoxemia with Glenn physiology may be caused by pulmonary venous desaturation (pneumothorax, pleural effusion, pulmonary edema), systemic venous desaturation (anemia, low cardiac output), or decreased PBF (elevated PVR, pulmonary venous hypertension).[42] When the systemic arterial oxygen saturation is less than 70%, careful evaluation for these problems must be performed to identify the cause and provide the appropriate treatment. Careful respiratory assessment along with radiographic examination will provide critical information regarding the cause of hypoxemia. The patient's hematocrit should be maintained at greater than 45% to optimize oxygen delivery compensating for the cyanosis.

Fontan Operation.   The postoperative management of patients after the Fontan operation may be dependent on the type of procedure performed and the preoperative hemodynamics. Postoperative complications include low cardiac output, hypoxemia, and effusions. Low cardiac output after this operation is commonly caused by myocardial dysfunction or inadequate preload. Preload is completely dependent on adequate PBF and pulmonary venous return to the single ventricle. Therefore an elevation in PVR becomes a major contributing factor in the development of low cardiac output. Elevations in PVR may be demonstrated by a low atrial pressure and an elevated systemic venous pressure. If a fenestration is present, right-to-left shunting can occur, providing adequate cardiac output in the face of elevated PVR. Any obstruction in the systemic veins could also result in inadequate PBF and low cardiac output. Myocardial dysfunction is supported with the use of continuous infusions of inotropic and afterload-reducing agents. Volume administration is frequently needed, particularly when effusions result in excessive loss of fluid.

The cause of cyanosis in these patients is similar to that seen with bidirectional Glenn physiology. In particular, patients with Fontan physiology are at risk for the development of pleural effusions, which can result in hypoxemia. Vigilant pulmonary assessment along with radiographic examination is critical to determine the cause of hypoxemia in these patients. When a fenestration is present, cyanosis may be the result of right-to-left shunting of blood. Typically, systemic arterial oxygen saturation in unfenestrated patients is 95% to 97%. When a fenestration is present, the saturation depends on the amount of shunting.

PBF in these patients is completely dependent on passive flow from the systemic circulation to the pulmonary circulation. This results in a natural elevation of systemic venous pressure, and any rise in PVR will further elevate systemic venous pressure. These mechanisms result in the leaking of serous fluid from the systemic veins to the extravascular spaces. Pleural effusions, pericardial effusions, and ascites can develop. Chest tube output must be carefully monitored to provide an adequate assessment of fluid intake and output. Fluid replacement may be necessary if losses become excessive. Diuretic therapy is frequently administered to decrease the systemic venous pressure and volume, potentially preventing the development of effusions. Typically, effusions resolve within 1 to 2 weeks following surgery once the systemic veins have adapted to higher pressures.

Infants and children who undergo procedures in which caval-to-pulmonary communications are used (Glenn or Fontan procedures) are dependent on a low PVR to maintain adequate PBF and systemic output. Because PBF is passively driven, minor increases in PVR may have profound physiologic effects in the postoperative period. Sedation, ventilator, and vasodilator strategies should be implemented as described for patients with pulmonary hypertension. However, despite these measures, these children have a very high morbidity and mortality rate. Problems with increased PVR in this patient population often indicate unfavorable physiology. Surgical options (fenestration of the Fontan, takedown of the Glenn or Fontan) must be considered before significant multisystem organ dysfunction results.

Cyanotic Congenital Heart Defects With Variable PBF

Some complex cyanotic CHDs present with a number of anatomic variations that result in alterations in the volume of PBF. Complete transposition of the great arteries is a common defect in this group, whereas all others (double-outlet right ventricle, double-inlet left ventricle, and single ventricle) are rare. These last defects are not discussed in this text.

Transposition of the Great Arteries.   In transposition of the great arteries (TGA), the aorta arises from the morphologic right ventricle and the pulmonary artery from the morphologic left ventricle. The most common form of TGA occurs when the ventricles are normally positioned and the aorta is anterior and to the right of the pulmonary artery (D-TGA). Coexisting cardiac lesions occur in about one half of infants with TGA. The most common is VSD (with or without subpulmonary stenosis), coarctation or interrupted aortic arch, and coronary artery abnormalities.

Between the third and fourth week of gestation, the truncus arteriosus is divided into the pulmonary artery and the aorta. This results from spiral growth of the conotruncal ridges. Failure of the conotruncal ridges to spiral or rotate completely results in transposing of the aorta and the pulmonary artery relative to the ventricles. Therefore the aorta arises from the right ventricle, and the pulmonary artery arises from the left ventricle. Without a PDA, PFO, ASD, or VSD, the result will be two parallel circulations.

D-TGA, as initially described here, is contrasted to *corrected transposition of the great arteries* (L-TGA). Corrected transposition exists when the morphologic right and left ventricles and AV valves are transposed. This results in the pulmonary artery arising from the systemic venous ventricle (right-sided, morphologic LV), and the aorta arising from the pulmonary venous ventricle (left-sided, morphologic RV). Therefore systemic venous blood (desaturated) flows to the pulmonary artery and pulmonary venous blood (saturated) to the aorta, and cyanosis is not present. L-TGA can occur in isolation or in combination with other structural defects and is often associated with progressive heart block. Heart failure can occur in young adulthood because the morphologic RV serves as the systemic pump, a function that it is not structurally intended to perform for a prolonged period. The rest of this section focuses on the identification and treatment of D-TGA.

The child with D-TGA essentially has two independent parallel circuits of circulation. Venous blood from the body flows to the right atrium, to the RV, and out the aorta to the body and returns again to the right atrium. Thus systemic perfusion is with persistently desaturated blood. Oxygenated blood from the lungs flows to the left atrium, LV, and out the pulmonary artery to the lungs and returns again to the left atrium. Thus the lungs are perfused with completely saturated blood. The systemic arterial oxygen saturations are dependent on adequate mixing with oxygenated blood. Immediately after birth, the PDA and PFO are present. These two structures allow mixing at the level of the great arteries (bidirectional between aorta and pulmonary artery through PDA) and the atrium (left to right through the PFO) until the normal postnatal changes occur that induce ductal and PFO closure (Fig. 18-24). Survival in these patients is predicated on maintaining mixing until surgical correction.[43]

The infant with D-TGA and VSD generally has adequate mixing across the VSD (bidirectional) and the PFO (left to right).[44] Desaturated blood will go from the RV to the LV, and saturated blood will go from the left atrium to the right; therefore these patients are only mildly cyanotic but can develop pulmonary overcirculation when PVR falls (Fig. 18-25).

D-TGA, VSD, and pulmonary stenosis (PS) may have an appropriate amount of mixing with protection of the pulmonary vascular bed (by PS) without pulmonary overcirculation. The degree of PBF is determined by the degree of PS, which can be quite variable. Frequently the PS will

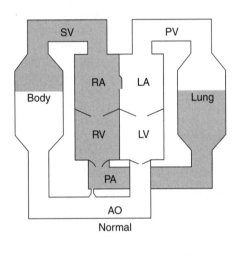

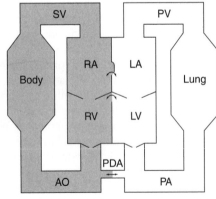

Fig. 18-24 Diagram of circulatory pathways in transposition of the great arteries. *AO,* Aorta; *PV,* pulmonary vein; *LA,* left atrium; *RA,* right atrium; *LV,* left ventricle; *RV,* right ventricle; *PA,* pulmonary artery; *SV,* systemic vein; *PDA,* patent ductus arteriosus. (From Garson A, Bricker JT, Fisher DJ et al: *The science and practice of pediatric cardiology,* Baltimore, 1998, Williams & Wilkins.)

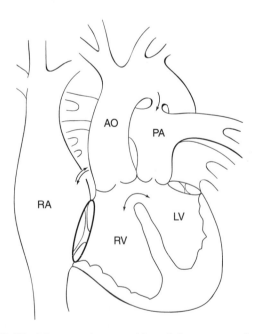

Fig. 18-25 Diagram of transposition of the great arteries indicating the possible sites of mixing of blood between systemic and pulmonary circulations *(arrows). AO,* Aorta; *PA,* pulmonary artery; *LV,* left ventricle; *RV,* right ventricle; *RA,* right atrium. (From Garson A, Bricker JT, Fisher DJ et al: *The science and practice of pediatric cardiology,* Baltimore, 1998, Williams & Wilkins.)

progress; therefore PBF will decrease, and the infant will become progressively cyanotic.[45]

Clinical Presentation and Course. Table 18-7 summarizes the clinical findings in infants with TGA. In infants with simple D-TGA (without VSD), once the PDA closes, the infant will develop significant metabolic acidosis, cyanosis, and ultimately death if not treated. Those with associated defects may be acyanotic or only mildly cyanotic.

Echocardiogram is sufficient to make the diagnosis; cardiac catheterization is only required if concerns remain about coronary artery anatomy or associated structural defects.

Management. Management in the newborn is aimed at ensuring adequate mixing and supporting systemic oxygen delivery. Maintaining patency of the PDA with prostaglandins will increase PBF and mixing. In addition, balloon atrial septostomy is performed to augment mixing and to decompress the volume load of the left heart. Septostomy can be performed at the bedside under echocardiographic guidance or in the catheterization laboratory.[43] Rarely will an infant not respond to PGE_1 or balloon septostomy. These children will have persistent cyanosis, poor perfusion, and metabolic acidosis. Intravenous inotropes are instituted to support contractility. If pulmonary hypertension is the cause of poor mixing, then maneuvers to decrease PVR are implemented (oxygen, alkalosis, nitric oxide). Some will require emergent surgery; however, these unstable infants can have a difficult postoperative course. Digoxin and diuretic therapy are indicated in the infant with large VSDs and CHF.

Surgical Management. Surgical repair of TGA is an example of progress and "change" in pediatric cardiac surgery that has occurred over the last 30 to 40 years. Some of the progress is the result of interest in "old" ideas. The first repairs of TGA were attempts at anatomic correction, that is, placing the pulmonary artery and aorta in their normal anatomic positions. These operations, performed by Bailey and colleagues in 1954[46] and by Kay and Cross in 1955,[47] did not include transfer of the coronary arteries and resulted in universal mortality. Mustard and co-workers also performed an anatomic correction in 1954, with transfer of the left coronary artery, but also without success.

The focus of attempts to repair TGA then shifted from anatomic correction to "physiologic repair" by rerouting pulmonary and systemic venous return through a baffle of Dacron or pericardium, such that each atrium emptied into the opposite ventricle (atrial switch procedure; Fig. 18-26). First successfully applied by Senning,[48] the procedure was modified by Mustard.[49] Although risk of mortality was low, long-term complications became apparent. Complications include systemic (right) ventricular dysfunction, heart failure, exercise intolerance, and symptomatic atrial arrhythmias.[50,51] In general, the Mustard and Senning procedures are no longer performed for straightforward TGA. However

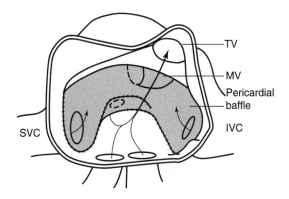

Fig. 18-26 Atrial switch procedure, whereby atrial septum is excised and atrial baffle is placed. Short, curved arrows designate systemic venous flow through the baffle toward the mitral valve *(MV)*, left ventricle, and pulmonary artery. Bold arrow indicates pulmonary venous flow behind and around the baffle to the tricuspid valve *(TV)*, right ventricle, and aorta. *IVC,* Inferior vena cava; *SVC,* superior vena cava. (From Emmanouilides GC, Riemenschneider TA, Allen HD et al: *Heart disease in infants, children, and adolescents,* Baltimore, 1995, Williams & Wilkins.)

◆ TABLE 18-7	Cyanotic Congenital Heart Defects With Variable Pulmonary Blood Flow (TGA)		
Defect	**Cardiac Examination**	**Electrocardiogram**	**Radiograph**
Uncomplicated TGA	Murmur may not be present, single S_2	Right ventricular hypertrophy, possible right atrial hypertrophy, right axis deviation; may be normal in newborn	Cardiomegaly, narrow mediastinum, increased pulmonary vascular markings; may be normal in newborn
TGA with VSD	Single S_2; holosystolic murmur best heard at fourth ICS to left of sternum; thrill may be present	Right ventricular hypertrophy or biventricular hypertrophy	Cardiomegaly, narrow mediastinum, increased pulmonary vascular markings
TGA with VSD and sub-PS	Single S_2; holosystolic murmur; ejection systolic murmur best heard along left sternal border	Right ventricular hypertrophy	Cardiomegaly, narrow mediastinum, decreased pulmonary vascular markings

ICS, Intercostal space; S_2, second heart sound; *sub-PS,* subvalvular pulmonary stenosis; *TGA,* transposition of the great arteries; *VSD,* ventricular septal defect.

surgical innovations have resurrected this procedure for select patients with complex AV and ventriculoarterial discordance. The so-called double-switch procedure uses the atrial (Mustard or Senning) and arterial switch procedures in an attempt to provide functionally normal hemodynamics.[52]

Even before recognition of the long-term problems associated with atrial correction of TGA, attempts at developing a successful method of anatomic correction continued. Interest heightened as complications of older procedures became apparent. Jatene and associates[53] performed the first successful arterial switch operation (ASO) in 1975. Initially, the ASO was used only in infants diagnosed with TGA and a VSD. Use of the ASO was later expanded to include those patients with TGA and intact ventricular septum (IVS). Currently, the ASO is performed with the same low mortality expected with either atrial correction and is the operation of choice for infants with TGA. ASO consists of transecting the aorta and pulmonary artery and reanastomosing the great arteries to the correct ventricle (i.e., PA to RV and aorta to LV). Transection of the great artery is performed above the semilunar valve; therefore the native pulmonary valve becomes the new aortic valve, and visa versa. The coronary arteries must also be moved to the new aortic connection. Significant PS may preclude the ASO because PS will become aortic stenosis after the arterial switch. These patients may require an atrial switch repair or an RV-to-PA conduit.

After the arterial switch, the left ventricle must be able to eject against systemic resistance. Timing for surgical repair is critically important because the LV will not be able to function against systemic resistance if surgery is delayed. This is due to the fact that the LV has become "deconditioned" because it has only been required to support the low-resistance pulmonary vascular circuit. The exact time when the LV becomes deconditioned is unknown, but clinical experience would suggest that the LV remains adequately prepared for at least 2 to 4 weeks after birth.[43] The exception would be a large unrestricted VSD in which the LV and RV pressures are equal or the presence of PS. In some infants who present late or in older patients with failed atrial baffle procedures, concerns may arise about LV function and ability to support systemic circulation. Under these conditions a two-stage procedure may be undertaken in select patients.[54] The stages include banding of the pulmonary artery to increase LV pressure (and work), followed in a few days by the arterial switch and takedown of the PA band.

After the ASO, myocardial ischemia or arrhythmias resulting from the operative transfer of the coronary arteries may occur. Ultimately this will produce left ventricular dysfunction and possibly failure. This effect is manifested as an increase in LA pressure, worsening mitral regurgitation, poor peripheral perfusion, low blood pressure, and metabolic acidosis. Inotropic support is initially instituted, and mechanical support can be implemented for those infants who fail medical management.

Described and possible late complications include supravalvar PS, failure of the native pulmonary valve to function in the aortic position, RVOTO, and possible coronary artery abnormalities.[55]

PERIOPERATIVE MANAGEMENT OF PEDIATRIC CARDIAC SURGICAL PATIENTS

Advances in the surgical management of infants and children with CHDs have significantly affected postoperative management and outcomes. Improved understanding of the anatomy and pathophysiology of structural defects and neonatal physiology, along with technologic advances in hypothermia, cardiopulmonary bypass, circulatory arrest, critical care management, and pharmacologic intervention, have combined to improve postoperative outcomes.[56] Currently, many complex lesions are amenable to partial or complete repair during infancy.

Repair of CHD early in life can prevent or diminish the pathologic sequelae that result from prolonged abnormal hemodynamics and cyanosis. However, unique features of the physiologic responses of young cardiac surgery patients continue to provide challenges to nurses and physicians involved in their care.

Following birth, parents of critically ill infants are often faced with the immediate transport of their infant to a tertiary care center that is specifically equipped to treat infants with congenital heart disease. Transport to a center many miles away is coupled with the stress of unexpected surgical intervention necessary to treat their newborn. Prenatal diagnosis permits planning to expedite the management of the infant known to have a heart defect,[57] as well as affording time for parental preparation and education. In addition, parents of older infants and children may not have their usual support system immediately available and are therefore not immune to the stress of cardiac surgery.

Preoperative Preparation

An uncomplicated operative and postoperative course for cardiac surgery patients begins with preoperative assessment and preparation. All infants and children must have a careful history and physical examination conducted before surgery. It is important to evaluate for the presence of acute illnesses (upper respiratory infection, pneumonia, otitis media) that would necessitate rescheduling elective surgery. Chronic medical problems, such as diabetes, asthma, arrhythmias, and seizure disorders, that would require special management are identified.

Routine laboratory and radiology assessments are performed. A chest radiograph is obtained on all patients. For those children having closed heart operations of an elective nature, generally only a complete blood count and urinalysis are required. Seriously ill patients and those scheduled for open heart operations generally have coagulation studies, platelet count, and serum electrolytes obtained in addition. These tests may identify problems that would require correction before or special attention during surgery.

Newborn infants with severe obstructive CHDs may present with severe heart failure, poor perfusion, oliguria, and acidosis, or severe cyanosis as the ductus arteriosus closes. Stabilization can be achieved for some with PGE_1. Infants with ductal-dependent heart lesions can be stabilized when ductal patency is maintained, thereby increasing systemic oxygenation. Preoperative measures to stabilize the infant's physiologic status may prevent emergency surgery in a very ill baby and possible subsequent end-organ complications.

Another necessary prelude to corrective cardiac surgery in some patients is the demonstration that PVR is either low enough to allow safe surgery or can be lowered sufficiently to allow recovery from surgery. Therefore cardiac catheterization, which allows the calculation of baseline PVR and response to vasodilator therapy, has been the standard method of preoperative evaluation of the pulmonary circulation. Unfortunately, this approach is not a very sensitive indicator of perioperative morbidity and mortality. For example, the fact that baseline PVR is high and cannot be lowered does not prove that surgery cannot be performed safely, and the fact that PVR can be lowered at cardiac catheterization does not ensure a safe postoperative course. In addition, exactly how high the PVR must be to preclude surgical repair is uncertain. PVR more than 15 Wood units is associated with very poor short- and long-term results, although notable exceptions exist. For example, if the patient has coexisting pulmonary disease, recatheterization after intensive pulmonary therapy may show a decrease in PVR. Similarly, if the patient lives at altitude, recatheterization after 4 or more weeks of oxygen therapy may show a decrease in PVR. More studies are necessary to identify better predictors of postoperative morbidity secondary to pulmonary hypertension.[58]

Perioperative Techniques

Since the introduction of the heart-lung machine nearly 40 years ago, efforts have continued toward the development of safe and reliable methods to control circulation during cardiac surgery. Refinement of these methods has improved outcomes over the past years; nonetheless, cardiopulmonary bypass, hypothermia, circulatory arrest, and aortic cross clamping can precipitate physiologic derangements in major organs during surgery that continue into the postoperative period.[59]

Cardiopulmonary Bypass. Cardiopulmonary bypass (CPB) provides tissue perfusion and oxygenation through the use of a mechanical pump and oxygenator, thereby bypassing the patient's own heart and lungs. To reroute blood, cannulas are placed in the right atrium and in the ascending aorta. Blood is removed from the right atrium, circulated through the oxygenator, and returned to the ascending aorta. Balanced crystalloid priming solution or citrated whole blood are used to prime the pump and dilute the hematocrit to 20% to 25%.[59] Heparin is used to prevent clot formation within the circuit and oxygenator.

Myocardial Protection. Bypass of the heart and lungs necessitates attention to protection of the myocardium during cardiac surgery. Both hypothermia and chemical preservation of the myocardium are currently employed.

Hypothermia and Circulatory Arrest. Moderate (20° to 25° C) and deep (15° to 18° C) hypothermia decreases the body's oxygen consumption, thereby protecting the brain and other vital organs during low circulatory flow with CPB. The protective effect of hypothermia is generally attributed to decreased cellular metabolic activity, reflected by both decreased oxygen consumption and glucose use. Core or surface cooling may be used singly or in combination. Surface cooling begins before the incision is made and is facilitated by decreasing the environmental temperature and through the use of hypothermia blankets or ice packs. Core cooling is accomplished using the heat exchanger in the bypass circuit. Heart rate and blood pressure decrease as body temperature falls, with asystole generally occurring between 22° to 24° C. In deep hypothermia, cooling is continued to a body temperature of less than 20° C. With deep hypothermia, circulatory arrest (the cessation of CPB) can be used. This method allows removal of intracardiac cannulas, thereby providing the surgeon an unobstructed surgical field, which enables repair of complex defects on very small patients.

Most data regarding the physiologic changes of organ systems associated with hypothermic circulatory arrest are based on animal research. Overall, these studies indicate that relatively short periods of hypothermic arrest are not associated with significant end-organ injury or dysfunction. Nevertheless, potential complications include renal insufficiency, necrotizing enterocolitis, liver necrosis, and atelectasis secondary to a low-flow state.

Impairment of the functional integrity of the brain after hypothermia and circulatory arrest has been the focus of intensive investigation since the 1960s. Experimental animal studies indicate that cerebral hypothermia protects against the development of, although it cannot prevent, metabolic and structural changes that lead to functional neurologic impairment.[59] Prolonged periods of cerebral hypothermia, without circulatory arrest, produce irreversible brain injury in animal models. Adverse neurologic sequelae after periods of hypothermia and circulatory arrest include seizures, choreoathetosis, paresis, rigidity, muscular hypotonia, intellectual impairment, coma, and death.[59] A period of 45 to 60 minutes of hypothermia and circulatory arrest is judged to be "safe."[59] A nomogram can be used to estimate the probability of a "safe" circulatory arrest time (Fig. 18-27).

Aortic Cross Clamping and Chemical Myocardial Protection. With initiation of CPB and cooling, the aorta can be cross clamped to prevent backflow into the left ventricle, thereby creating a bloodless surgical field. Decreasing metabolic and oxygen requirements with hypothermia achieves some myocardial protection from ischemia. During CPB, electromechanical arrest is also achieved via an injection of hypothermic (4° C) cardioplegic solution into the aortic root. This results in immediate cessation of cardiac activity. Although it is protective in the older infant and child, efficacy of cold cardioplegia for myocardial protection in the immature myocardium remains to be defined.

The ideal cardioplegia solution would provide rapid and complete cardiac arrest, maintain the myocardial electrolyte environment, deliver substrates, wash out metabolites, and

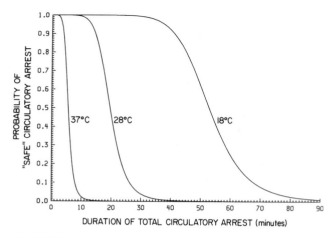

Fig. 18-27 Nomogram of probably safe circulatory arrest times in patients at various degrees of hypothermia. (From Kirklin JW, Barratt-Boyes BG, eds: *Cardiac surgery,* ed 2, New York, 1993, John Wiley & Sons, p 74.)

maintain cellular pH at a protective level.[60] Although many different solutions are used in cardiac surgery today, the search for a "perfect" solution continues. Most cardioplegic solutions are similar to extracellular fluid, with the exception of large amounts of added potassium to induce diastolic cardiac arrest. Increased concentrations of potassium and magnesium (another component of cardioplegia) are thought to prevent calcium influx, inhibit calcium release from the sarcoplasmic reticulum, and reduce mitochondrial uptake of calcium. This approach is believed to be protective because calcium release and uptake may be related to ischemic cell membrane damage and to subsequent myocardial cellular swelling and death. Cardioplegic solutions provides myocardial protection because the heart is ideally maintained in diastole with minimal metabolic requirements and rebeating is prevented.

Rewarming. When the intracardiac repair is completed, surface and core warming are begun. If circulatory arrest is used, then CPB is resumed and the aortic cross clamp removed. Spontaneous ventricular contractions usually occur at a temperature of 30° to 32° C. If the heart does not begin to beat spontaneously, electrical defibrillation may be needed. When the body temperature is nearly normal, bypass is discontinued.

Potential Postoperative Complications

The potential for complications is high following cardiac surgery in infants and children. Timely assessment, identification, and intervention improve outcomes.

Inadequate Tissue Perfusion. Tissue perfusion is dependent on the adequacy of cardiac output, which in the immediate postoperative period may change rapidly. Continuous assessment of the patient's hemodynamic status by evaluating peripheral pulses and temperature of the extremities, capillary refill, core temperature, arterial blood pressure, and filling pressures are key to the early identification of problems. Tissue perfusion is dependent on myocardial contractility, intravascular volume (preload), resistance to

ventricular ejection (afterload), and heart rate. Low cardiac output and impaired perfusion can be the consequence of (1) decreased intravascular volume from excessive losses, inadequate replacement, cardiac tamponade, or excessive diuresis; (2) increased systemic or pulmonary vascular resistance from vasoconstriction or hypertension; (3) decreased ventricular contractility from myocardial injury secondary to inadequate intraoperative protection, hypoxia, acidosis, or electrolyte imbalance; (4) alteration in heart rate or rhythm; or (5) inadequate intracardiac repair with residual shunts or valve lesions. These causes are summarized in Table 18-8.

Inadequate Intravascular Volume. Adequate preload is essential to maintain cardiac output. Postoperatively, volume replacement may be necessary because of postoperative bleeding, expansion of the vascular space during rewarming, third spacing of fluid, or diuresis. Postoperative bleeding may be surgical or due to inadequate heparin reversal at the end of CPB. Coagulation disorders are assessed and corrected. Surgical bleeding is suspected when chest tube drainage is greater than 3 ml/kg/hr for over 3 hours or 5 to 10 ml/kg in any 1 hour. Volume loss of this nature is significant in light of total blood volume in infants and children (i.e., neonates, 85 to 90 ml/kg; infants, 75 to 80 ml/kg; children, 70 to 75 ml/kg) and may require reoperation.

The type and amount of fluid administered when preload is inadequate are based on the patient's hematocrit and the nature of the fluid lost. Packed red blood cells are administered to patients who are bleeding or have a significantly decreased hematocrit. Optimal hematocrit is dependent on patient condition, operative procedure, hemodynamics, and residual defects. Fresh frozen plasma or cryoprecipitate are administered to replace clotting factors. To treat hypovolemia unrelated to bleeding, colloid or crystalloid may be infused. Boluses of fluid or blood are administered in volumes of 10 ml/kg over several minutes while filling pressures are carefully assessed. In general, increasing LAP to greater than 14 to 16 mmHg rarely provides any additional improvement in cardiac performance and may contribute to left ventricular dysfunction.

Tamponade. Cardiac tamponade causes compression of the atria, restricts venous return to the heart, and results in decreased ventricular preload. Because early cardiac tamponade results from persistent surgical bleeding not being sufficiently evacuated by the chest drains, mediastinal or chest drainage tubes must be kept patent. Signs of potential or real tamponade include abrupt cessation of chest tube output, elevated venous pressures, equalization of atrial pressures, neck vein distension, systemic arterial hypotension, and narrow pulse pressure. Associated hypotension may not be responsive to volume administration. Cardiac tamponade necessitates prompt intervention, such as Fogarty striping of chest tubes or surgical reexploration to evacuate the pericardial hematoma and control bleeding.

Occasionally, in infants following complex surgery myocardial swelling, chamber dilation, respiratory compromise, persistent bleeding, or the need for ECMO will prevent chest closure at the conclusion of surgery. Leaving

TABLE 18-8 Differential Diagnosis of Inadequate Tissue Perfusion

Cause	Critical Signs*
Inadequate Preload	
Fluid volume deficit	Low ventricular filling pressures
Increased losses	LAP, RAP <3-5
Inadequate replacement	CVP <5-8
Cardiac tamponade	Acute increase in filling pressures
Pericardial hematoma	LAP, RAP, CVP rise
Myocardial swelling	Acute decrease in chest drainage
Excessive Afterload	
Increased SVR	Normal to increased systemic arterial pressure
Decreased tissue perfusion	Cool, mottled extremities
SNS stimulation	Decreased peripheral pulses
Increased PVR	Acute rise in PA pressures
Hypoxia, hypercarbia	Cyanosis
Suctioning	Bradycardia
Agitation, pain	Death (a potential consequence)
Myocardial Dysfunction	
Chemical	High ventricular filling pressures
Hypothermia	LAP, RAP >12
Acidosis	CVP >15-18
Electrolyte imbalance	
Hypoxia	
Functional	
Preoperative dysfunction	
Prolonged ischemic time	
Residual hemodynamic problems	
Cardiac rhythm disturbances	ECG abnormalities

*Seen in addition to the typical clinical signs of inadequate tissue perfusion.
CVP, Central venous pressure; *ECG*, electrocardiogram; *LAP*, left atrial pressure; *RAP*, right atrial pressure; *SNS*, sympathetic nervous system.

the sternum open with the mediastinum covered with an impermeable dressing is an option in this scenario. Once myocardial swelling or bleeding has subsided and both cardiac and pulmonary function have stabilized, the sternum can be closed electively in the PICU usually 2 to 3 days after surgery. Adjustment of ventilatory settings and inotropic support may be indicated after chest closure because significant changes in hemodynamics and respiratory physiology can occur.[61]

Increased Systemic Afterload. Increased systemic vascular resistance (SVR) is most often the consequence of SNS stimulation in an attempt to compensate for low cardiac output. Increased SVR may be poorly tolerated in the postoperative period if myocardial performance is already near maximal levels or if ventricular function is depressed. Elevated SVR is signaled by normal to increased systemic arterial pressure accompanied by cool, mottled extremities; delayed capillary refill; poor peripheral pulses; and metabolic acidosis. Treatment is aimed at reduction of afterload with vasodilator therapy.

Pulmonary Hypertension. The status of the pulmonary circulation is crucial in the perioperative management of many children with congenital heart disease. This is most pronounced is two subgroups of patients: those with increased PBF or increased pulmonary venous pressure, in

which the development of pulmonary hypertension could increase perioperative morbidity or mortality, as well as exclude surgical options, and those with single ventricle physiology, in which the status of the pulmonary circulation will not only determine the level of oxygenation but also determine systemic output.

Chronic and acute elevations in PVR remain a major source of morbidity and mortality following surgical correction of congenital heart disease. Chronic elevation in PVR results from structural changes of the pulmonary vascular bed that decrease cross-sectional area. After successful surgery, if these structural changes are reversible, PVR will begin to decrease in the postoperative period. However, complete normalization of the structural changes may take months[26]; therefore postoperatively the right ventricle may work against an elevated PVR for a prolonged period. Acute elevation in PVR results from the active contraction of structurally abnormal pulmonary arteries during a period of extreme vasoreactivity in the immediate postoperative period. This decreases cardiac output, produces acidosis and hypoxemia, and may result in significant morbidity and mortality. This period of extreme vasoreactivity is caused by the degranulation of platelets and leukocytes following CPB and hypothermia, with the subsequent release of potent vasoconstrictors. The postoperative management of patients with preoperative increases in pulmonary arterial pressure and PVR is directed at preventing acute pulmonary hypertensive crises during this period of extreme vasoreactivity and subacute support of the right ventricle.[62] Care of these children can be quite challenging and requires a thorough understanding of the pulmonary circulation.

Immediately after surgery with CPB, a period of enhanced pulmonary vascular reactivity is seen in children with preoperative pulmonary hypertension.[63] This period of enhanced reactivity, which may last up to approximately 5 to 7 days after CPB, is most likely a manifestation of altered endothelial/smooth muscle cell interactions in a previously altered pulmonary circulation. During CPB, several factors, including the disruption of normal PBF, complement activation, and neutrophil activation, induce pulmonary vascular endothelial dysfunction. For example, impaired endothelium-dependent pulmonary vasodilation, altered eicosanoid metabolism, abnormal von Willebrand factor (a marker of endothelial injury), and ultrastructural changes of the pulmonary vascular endothelium have all been noted in patients after undergoing CPB. This results in increased vasoconstricting factors produced by the endothelium, such as endothelin 1 and thromboxane A_2, and decreased vasodilating factors, such as nitric oxide.

Acute increases in PVR initiate a cascade of cardiopulmonary interactions that may lead to cardiovascular collapse. During pulmonary hypertensive crises, there is an acute increase in right ventricular afterload, producing right ventricular ischemia and failure. The resulting increase in right ventricular end-diastolic volume shifts the intraventricular septum to the left, decreasing left ventricular volume and cardiac output. Decreased cardiac output results in decreased systemic perfusion and metabolic acidosis. Increased PVR and right ventricular failure also decrease PBF, leading to increased dead space ventilation. Distension of the pulmonary arteries and perivascular cuffing with edematous fluid produce large and small airway obstruction, respectively, worsening ventilation/perfusion mismatch and lung compliance. Clinically, this may be manifested as inability to move the chest wall with mechanical ventilation; accidental extubation or pneumothoraces should also be considered. These ventilatory derangements produce hypoxemia and hypercapnia. The resulting acidosis (either metabolic or respiratory) and hypoxia further increase PVR, perpetuating this cascade.[64]

Prevention of pulmonary hypertensive crises is accomplished by avoiding those stimuli known to increase PVR, including hypoxia, acidosis, agitation, overdistension of the lung, and polycythemia. Alveolar hypoxia with systemic arterial hypoxemia and acidosis (metabolic or respiratory) increases PVR; their combination is synergistic. Agitation and pain acutely increase PVR secondary to catecholamine release and receptor activation.[62,64] Positive pressure ventilation with high peak inspiratory and end-expiratory pressures overdistend the lung and increase PVR. However, the appropriate use of positive pressure ventilation improves ventilation and oxygenation, which decreases PVR. Polycythemia (hematocrits >55%) increases blood viscosity and PVR.

Myocardial Dysfunction. Low cardiac output may be due to myocardial dysfunction when signs of inadequate tissue perfusion are accompanied by increased filling pressures. Drugs, anesthesia, ischemia, hypoxia, acidosis, extensive ventriculotomy, myocardial resection, or residual hemodynamic abnormalities may depress myocardial performance. Both inotropic and afterload-reducing agents are useful in improving cardiac performance. If pharmacologic therapy is ineffective, a mechanical assist device or ECMO may be useful.

Cardiac Rhythm Disturbances. Cardiac arrhythmias are not uncommon after cardiac operations. Temporary epicardial pacing wires are often placed before leaving the operating room. Although many arrhythmias do not require treatment because hemodynamics are not compromised, treatment may be necessitated if the ventricular rate is either too slow or too rapid to maintain adequate cardiac output. In addition to specific treatment, it is important to correct electrolyte and acid-base disturbances, if present. For treatment of specific rhythm disorders, see the section on cardiac rhythm disturbances.

Critical Care Management

The management of pediatric patients recovering from cardiac surgery is best provided by a coordinated multidisciplinary team with expertise in cardiac surgery, cardiology, anesthesia, intensive care, cardiac nursing, and respiratory therapy. The primary objective in the care of these patients is the ongoing assessment and monitoring of hemodynamic parameters to detect postoperative problems as early as possible, to intervene effectively, and to ensure adequate oxygen delivery. Both invasive and noninvasive methods are useful to monitor hemodynamic stability and tissue perfusion. Heart rate and rhythm, preload, afterload, and contractility are continuously assessed. Decisions to provide pharmacologic or mechanical support are based on careful attention to hemodynamic status.

Hemodynamic Assessment. Invasive hemodynamic monitoring and clinical assessment are the cornerstone of postoperative assessment. The critical care nurse must possess not only astute clinical assessment skills but also understand the use and limitations of technologic assessment tools. For an in-depth review of invasive hemodynamic monitoring, see Chapter 7.

Heart Rate and Rhythm. Arrhythmias have the potential to compromise cardiac output if they interrupt diastolic filling or AV synchrony. Continuous ECG monitors heart rate and rhythm. The postoperative period represents a period of physiologic stress; therefore heart rate is anticipated to be elevated.

Cardiac rhythm disturbances are not uncommon after cardiac operations. Potential causes during the operation include the surgical sequelae, effects of anesthesia, effects of CPB or hypothermia, damage to the conduction system, or high levels of endogenous or exogenous catecholamines. Additional causes include metabolic and electrolyte imbalances, volume changes, hypoxemia, and temperature instability. Exogenous catecholamines can contribute to arrhythmogenesis, as can digoxin toxicity (particularly in the setting of hypokalemia). If arrhythmias are noted, potassium, magnesium, calcium, and phosphorus levels must be checked and corrected to normal.

Ventricular arrhythmias and atrial fibrillation are uncommon outside the older adolescent or adult age group. Automatic tachycardias such as atrial ectopic tachycardia or JET are more common in infants than in the older child. Conduction delay or heart block is associated with repairs of septal defects, septal myectomy, and AV valve abnormalities. For more complete review of arrhythmia management, see the section on cardiac rhythm disturbances.

Systemic Arterial Blood Pressure. Continuous monitoring of arterial pressure is achieved via an indwelling arterial catheter and allows beat-to-beat assessment of blood pressure. Noninvasive blood pressure measurements may not be accurate in the early postoperative period because of rapid changes in vascular tone and hemodynamics. The potential for low cardiac output and inadequate tissue perfusion is high in the early hours following cardiac surgery and is related to a number of physiologic phenomena. These include fluid shifts, bleeding, rhythm abnormalities, and abnormalities of contractility and vascular tone. It is important to remember that hypotension is generally a late sign of low cardiac output. Data from direct measurement of arterial pressure allows the timely identification of potential postoperative blood pressure problems.

Monitoring Atrial Pressures. CVP or right atrial pressure (RAP) provides information about the systemic venous return and right heart preload and function. In the absence of tricuspid valve disease, the CVP and RAP reflect right ventricular end-diastolic pressure (RVEDP). Low CVPs indicate hypovolemia. Right ventricular failure is more common in infants than in adult patients. Elevated RAP (often as high as 15 to 18 mmHg) may indicate right ventricular failure or pulmonary hypertension.

LAP provides information about pulmonary venous pressure and left heart preload and function. In the absence of mitral valve disease, LAP reflects left ventricular end-diastolic pressure (LVEDP). Low LAP indicates hypovolemia. Elevated LAP indicates left ventricular failure or increased left ventricular afterload.

In addition to monitoring the mean atrial pressures to determine preload and ventricular function, assessment of the waveform yields important information about cardiac structure and function. Cannon *a* waves result from increased resistance to ventricular filling (mitral or tricuspid stenosis, aortic or pulmonary stenosis, pulmonary hypertension) or when the atria contract against a closed AV valve, as occurs with nodal rhythm or AV dissociation. The *a* waves are absent in atrial fibrillation. Tall *v* waves are seen in mitral or tricuspid regurgitation, VSD, ASD, or CHF.

Monitoring Pulmonary Artery Pressure. Pulmonary artery pressure (PAP) monitoring provides information about right ventricular function, right ventricular outflow tract patency, PVR, pulmonary venous pressure, and pulmonary wedge pressure (if balloon-tipped catheter is used). PAP is monitored as systolic, diastolic, and mean pressures. PA diastolic pressure corresponds to the LAP in the absence of pulmonary hypertension and mitral valve disease. Under normal circumstances, systolic PAP is the same as the right ventricular systolic pressure.

Systemic or suprasytemic PAP in postoperative patients can be life threatening, contributing to significant hemodynamic compromise. Measures to decrease PVR, such as oxygenation, sedation, alkalosis, and possibly nitric oxide, may be necessary.

Monitoring Oxygenation.   Systemic arterial oxygen saturation is routinely monitored by continuous pulse oximetry. An understanding of the patient's unique postoperative physiology will assist in the interpretation of pulse oximetry data. Invasive monitoring of mixed venous oxygen saturation also provides important data regarding the adequacy of oxygen delivery. This information is most accurately obtained from a pulmonary artery catheter, whereby a true mixed venous sample of blood can be obtained. Continuous or intermittent monitoring of mixed venous blood provides valuable information regarding oxygen supply and demand. An elevation in mixed venous oxygen saturation may occur in patients with high cardiac output states or left-to-right intracardiac shunts. Decreased mixed venous oxygen saturation may be seen in patients with decreased cardiac output, anemia, decreased systemic arterial oxygen saturation, and increased oxygen consumption states, such as fever.

Oxygen saturation measurements obtained from the right atrium are dependent on the location of the catheter, anatomy, and streaming (or blood flow) within the right atrium or vena cava. Samples of blood from the SVC, inferior vena cava (IVC), and coronary sinus will have different oxygen saturations and may not accurately reflect the mixed venous oxygen saturation. Blood samples from the SVC may reflect a slight decrease in saturation relative to IVC blood in the awake patient who is breathing room air. However, the reverse is true in the deeply sedated or anesthetized patient.[65] Blood samples obtained from the coronary sinus or hepatic veins will be desaturated relative to a true mixed venous sample (obtained from the PA).[66] Right atrial oxygen saturations are monitored for trends; interventions are determined based on these data along with clinical correlation of patient condition.

Caring for Patients With Transthoracic Intracardiac Catheters.   Transthoracic intracardiac catheters are placed at the conclusion of surgery for hemodynamic monitoring and management of postoperative patients. These consist of directly placed RA, LA, or PA catheters. On arrival to the PICU, chest radiographs demonstrate catheter placement (Fig. 18-28). Most intracardiac catheters are reserved for hemodynamic monitoring and the continuous infusion of vasoactive medications.

Morbidity associated with the use of transthoracic intracardiac catheters includes nonfunction, thrombus, and infection.[67] In addition, air or clot embolus from the LA line can have devastating consequences if it embolizes to the coronary or cerebral circulations. Careful attention must be made to avoid any air entry into LA lines; therefore these lines are typically used for monitoring of LA pressure only.

Once intracardiac lines are no longer indicated, specially trained nurses or physicians accomplish removal in the PICU. All possible data that may be needed from these lines

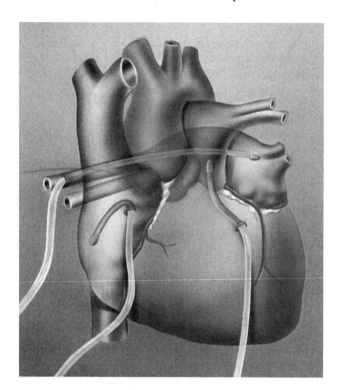

Fig. 18-28 Transthoracic, intracardiac line locations. (From Barker S: *CV Nurse,* Second Issue, 1993.)

are obtained before their removal. Examples include RA and PA oxygen saturations, an LA tracing to demonstrate elevated *v* waves, and a PA pullback pressure to assess for RVOTO.

Morbidity associated with the removal of intracardiac catheters include bleeding, need for intervention (chest tube placement for hemothorax or pneumothorax, catheter wiring for retained catheter, chest tube suctioning), and hemodynamic compromise. Bleeding is the most common complication and occurs more often with LA catheter removal and in patients with genetic abnormalities and thrombocytopenia. Excessive bleeding can result in cardiac tamponade, anemia, hypovolemia, hemothorax, and hemodynamic compromise. Careful assessment after the removal of intracardiac catheters must be performed to evaluate the development of these complications. Hemodynamic compromise occurs more often after the removal of catheters in the LA or PA position and in patients with thrombocytopenia.[67]

Respiratory Care. After undergoing cardiac surgery, most patients arrive in the PICU intubated and mechanically ventilated. Initial assessment of the patient includes auscultation of the lungs to determine appropriate endotracheal tube position and adequacy of ventilation. Chest radiographs and arterial blood gas analysis help to support clinical assessment. The size and position of the endotracheal tube are documented, and the tube is secured in place.

Initially patients are ventilated with an F_{IO_2} of 1.0, unless the patient has undergone palliation of single-ventricle physiology with an aortopulmonary shunt. In these infants, hyperoxia may decrease PVR and increase PBF at the expense of systemic perfusion. These patients typically receive an F_{IO_2} of 0.25 to 0.30. F_{IO_2} is weaned rapidly in most patients based on continuous pulse oximeter measurements of oxygen saturation or arterial blood gas. Although this can be institution specific, generally volume-cycled ventilation is used for postoperative support. Tidal volume and rate are selected based on individual patient need to best ensure ventilation and oxygenation. Titration of ventilator settings is based on arterial blood gas analysis and clinical condition. Occasionally, pressure-cycled ventilation is used to support very small infants.

Suctioning of the endotracheal tube is reserved for episodes of increased pulmonary secretions or episodes of high airway pressure (caused by possible endotracheal tube occlusion) and is executed with extreme caution. Ventilation and oxygenation are ensured by manual ventilation before and after each passage of the suction catheter, or an in-line suction device can be used. In some patients, hand ventilation with 100% oxygen and mild hyperinflation and hyperventilation may protect them from hypoxemia and hypercarbia during suctioning, although this technique remains controversial. Patients with single-ventricle physiology or aortopulmonary connection can develop pulmonary overcirculation in response to hyperoxia or hypocarbia. These infants should receive manual ventilation that simulates the mechanical ventilation while monitoring pulse oximetry to ensure that PBF does not increase or decrease dramatically. An in-line suction device can be quite helpful in this patient population. Conversely, pulmonary vasospasm can be induced when ventilation with suctioning is inadequate, particularly in newborns and in infants and children with pulmonary artery hypertension. Acute pulmonary hypertensive episodes can result in sudden decreases of systemic cardiac output and cardiac arrest.

The length of time required for mechanical ventilation depends on the complexity of the cardiac repair and the postoperative course. It may be longer in patients with pulmonary vascular congestion from large left-to-right shunts or heart failure and in those with complex heart defects. Mechanical ventilation is continued until the patient is hemodynamically stable and able to sustain adequate respiratory function independent of the ventilator. As the patient awakens and begins to initiate respiration, the ventilator can be weaned. Readiness for extubation is based on physical assessment and arterial blood gas analysis. Extubation can be accomplished when the patient is hemodynamically stable with little or no inotropic support on minimal ventilator settings, awake, able to clear pulmonary secretions spontaneously, and breathing spontaneously.

Patients who are unable to be extubated and do not have pulmonary disease require investigation of potential cardiac problems that could be contributory. Poor myocardial contractility or residual defects may be responsible. Paralysis of the diaphragm from intraoperative injury to the phrenic nerve may result in inability to extubate. Ultrasound or fluoroscopic examination of the diaphragm assists in the identification of this problem.

Vigorous diuresis in postoperative patients may result in the development of metabolic alkalosis and can contribute to delayed extubation. Careful monitoring of fluid and electrolytes and appropriate electrolyte replacement may be helpful. Acetazolamide (Diamox) therapy or chloride replacement with arginine chloride may be helpful in the ventilator-dependent patient whose total bicarbonate level approaches or exceeds 40 mEq/L. These maneuvers may help treat contraction alkalosis, thereby normalizing serum bicarbonate, minimizing alkalosis, and resulting in improved respiratory effort.

Fluid and Electrolyte Replacement.   Institutional preference prevails in recommendations regarding postoperative intravenous fluids. Some institutions restrict sodium intake for the first 24 hours, given the mild tendency for sodium retention following CPB, administering 5% dextrose in water solutions to infants and children and 10% dextrose to newborns. Solutions are changed to 5% or 10% dextrose with 0.2% normal saline after the first postoperative day. Others recommend routine use of dextrose-containing solutions with 0.2% saline on the first postoperative day to avoid hypovolemia. The volume of fluid administered is generally restricted to 50% of maintenance for patients who have required CPB for the first 24 hours. Fluids are increased to full maintenance as determined by patient physiology, clinical condition, fluid balance, chest radiograph, and need for diuretics. In those patients not requiring CPB, full maintenance fluids may be started immediately after surgery. All sources of fluid intake, including flushes of intravascular and intracardiac catheters, are measured with care and included in the calculated fluid requirement.

Fluid balance is assessed from heart rate, intracardiac filling pressures, systemic arterial blood pressure, urine output, and acid-base status. Volume is administered to support filling pressures and cardiac output while preventing fluid overload. In the immediate postoperative period, rewarming can result in peripheral vasodilation and expansion of the vascular space, necessitating administration of blood or colloid to maintain adequate intravascular volume.

Edema is present postoperatively to some extent in all patients who undergo cardiac surgery with CPB and hypothermia. Other contributing factors include length of the surgery, type of procedure, and amount of fluid administered intraoperatively. Total body water accumulation during cardiac surgery may be as much as 600 to 1000 ml.[56] After the first postoperative night, diuretics are administered to augment diuresis and treat third spacing. Low-dose dopamine (3 µg/kg/min) may also be advantageous. The use of diuretics mandates attention to fluid, electrolyte, and acid-base balance.

CPB, diuretic administration, and acid-base balance affect serum potassium levels. Hypokalemia is known to contribute to ventricular irritability, especially in patients receiving digoxin, and can cause rhythm disturbances. Parameters for electrolyte replacement are specific to patient condition and institutional preference. Hypokalemia is treated with potassium chloride supplements of 0.25 to 1 mEq/kg administered as a continuous infusion over 1 to 2 hours if urine output is adequate or added to the maintenance fluids. Care is taken to ensure that potassium supplements are not administered rapidly or in an excessively concentrated infusion because of the potential for hyperkalemic cardiac arrest. Hyperkalemia is rare, unless postoperative renal dysfunction is present. Treatment consists of removing all potassium from intravenous fluids and the administration of polystyrene sulfonate (1 g/kg every 4 hours) by mouth or rectum until renal function improves. Occasionally, hemodialysis is required.

Mild hyponatremia is common but does not often require treatment beyond administration of diuretics and restriction of free water intake. Patients with serum sodium less than 125 mEq/L are at risk for seizures and other neurologic symptoms and require diuresis, water restriction, and cautious administration of normal saline.

Hypocalcemia is most often seen in newborns, those with DiGeorge syndrome, and in patients receiving large amounts of blood products. Transfused blood is preserved with citrate phosphate dextrose that produces precipitation of serum calcium with subsequent hypocalcemia. Administration of serum albumin also binds ionized calcium, resulting in hypocalcemia. Documented hypocalcemia requires replacement therapy to support contractility.

Infants are at risk for the development of hypoglycemia because of high metabolic rate and limited glycogen stores. Hypoglycemia can depress myocardial function and may cause seizures.

Acid-base balance is monitored with care because myocardial performance is adversely affected by acidosis. Metabolic acidosis indicates impaired tissue perfusion, usually the result of inadequate cardiac output. Treatment necessitates correction of the underlying hemodynamic problem or administration of intravenous sodium bicarbonate (1 mEq/kg/dose). Adequate ventilation must be ensured because the buffering action of bicarbonate results in the formation of carbon dioxide. Tromethamine (THAM) is an alternative buffering agent for patients with severe metabolic acidosis and impaired renal function or hypernatremia.

Renal Function.   Urine output is a sensitive indicator of cardiac output and tissue perfusion after cardiac surgery. Urine output of 1 ml/kg/hr is anticipated in infants and young children; 0.5 ml/kg/hr (or 20 to 40 ml/hr) is expected urine production in older children and adults. If urine flow decreases, but physical examination and laboratory results suggest adequate cardiac output, the diminished urine flow is most likely caused by stimulation of hormones designed to retain fluid and maximize cardiac output. These hormonal modulators can be caused by CPB, low atrial pressures, decreased renal blood flow, and decreased cardiac output. The RAAS is stimulated by a decrease in renal blood flow, restoring cardiac output by sodium and water retention, which increase intravascular volume. Urine output can also be diminished by the secretion of antidiuretic hormone (ADH) stimulated by CPB.

Diminished urinary output should not be the sole indicator for the administration of diuretics. Other clinical parameters should be used such as filling pressures, hepatomegaly, fluid balance, and chest radiograph. Administration of tubular diuretics is not likely to alter the outcome of vasomotor nephropathy, which may have resulted from diminished perfusion during CPB or subsequent hemodynamic instability. Acute renal failure can occur in infants and children after open heart surgery. Serum potassium, blood urea nitrogen (BUN), and creatinine are key to assessing renal function. If, despite adequate cardiac output, urine output remains inadequate with an upward trend in BUN and creatinine or the development of hyperkalemia, renal replacement therapy may be indicated with continuous veno-veno hemofiltration or dialysis.

Thermal Regulation.   Although induced hypothermia for cardiac surgery is reversed at the conclusion of the procedure, core temperature may be low, and peripheral vasoconstriction persists when the patient arrives in the PICU. Hypothermia prolongs postoperative bleeding and may delay hemodynamic stabilization; may lead to acidosis, hypoglycemia, hypoxemia, increased PVR; and may induce shivering. Active rewarming is achieved with warming devices. Infants have a higher loss of heat via conduction, convection, radiation, and evaporation and may be slow to rewarm despite efforts to reestablish normothermia while weaning off CPB.

Establishment of a neutral thermal environment (NTE) is key to postoperative thermal regulation. Newborns and small infants are cared for in an infant warmer bed using a servocontrol mechanism. Postoperative assessment includes measurement of core temperature and the differential between core and peripheral temperatures, as well as assessment of the extremities for coolness and capillary refill. When cool extremities are noted with an elevated core temperature, low cardiac output is suspected (this results from redistribution of the cardiac output away from the extremities). Conversely, loss of temperature regulation can result in heat retention and a high core temperature. Capillary refill is expected to be brisk when the cardiac surgery patient has been rewarmed and hemodynamic stability is achieved. In the newborn, normal refill may take 3 to 5 seconds owing to peripheral vascular adaptation. Refill time longer than 5 seconds is abnormal and reflects diminished peripheral perfusion.

Feeding and Nutrition.   Generally, oral feedings are begun as soon as possible. Some patients (mechanically ventilated, infants who are poor feeders) may require nasogastric or nasojejunal feedings. In patients who have had straightforward cardiac repairs and are recovering well, feedings can be rapidly advanced. Exceptions may include newborns with umbilical artery catheters or those who had limited gut perfusion preoperatively because of the association between necrotizing enterocolitis (NEC) and feeding. Patients having repair of coarctation of the aorta are not fed until hypertension is controlled and bowel sounds are active to prevent reactive mesenteric enteritis and its complications. Nasogastric or transpyloric feedings are considered early for patients unable to resume oral intake within 48 to 72 hours of surgery. Because of its expense, parenteral nutrition is considered only if the gastrointestinal tract cannot be used for an extended period postoperatively. Newborns may require as much as 120 to 150 calories/kg/day for weight gain. Older infants and children are likely to have a similar increase in nutritional requirements.

Wound Care.   Following cardiac operations, the surgical incision is generally covered with a dry sterile dressing, separated from the chest tube and intracardiac lines. After lines and chest tubes are removed, at approximately 24 to 48 hours, the dressing is usually removed, and the incision is left uncovered.

A standard technique for wound care has not been established for patients in whom sternal closure is delayed. Maintenance of sterility and protecting the patient from infection are priorities. A nonpermeable patch (Silastic, Gore-Tex, bovine pericardium) is generally sutured to the wound edges and then covered with a dressing. The site is assessed continuously for fluid accumulation that can lead to tamponade. The most common signs are fullness and bulging of the membrane. Immediate evacuation of the incision is indicated if this occurs. When the sternum is left open, the water seal chamber of the chest tube collection chamber should bubble, and the patient is kept sedated and possibly chemically paralyzed.

Infection Prophylaxis.   Most patients receive prophylactic antibiotics before surgery and in the immediate perioperative period. When to terminate these antibiotics is dependent on the individual center and is often open to debate. Antibiotics given during the perioperative period can decrease the risk of infectious complications, including catheter sepsis, pneumonitis, urinary tract infection, and mediastinitis. Unfortunately the increased use of broad-spectrum antibiotics has encouraged the development of multiple resistant organisms and fungi. Therefore the use of empiric antibiotics should be carefully evaluated. Once all invasive catheters and tubes have been removed, antibiotics should be discontinued unless they are being given for a documented or suspected infection.

Central Nervous System Assessment.   Neurologic complications after cardiac operations may be the consequence of cerebral ischemia, hypoxia, electrolyte imbalances, metabolic acidosis, hypoglycemia, or cerebral emboli. Seizures are the most common neurologic complication. Hypoglycemia, hypocalcemia, and hypomagnesemia are causes for seizures in infants, and therefore levels should be monitored and replacement given as indicated. Anticonvulsants are administered as indicated for seizure control, and these may need to be continued for some months after surgery.

Pain Management.   An essential component of patient management after congenital heart surgery is the maintenance of adequate analgesia and sedation to provide comfort. Often a combination of drugs, such as opioids and benzodiazepines, are used, thereby keeping total drug dose to a minimum. Analgesia requirements for young children can be difficult to assess, particularly when they are paralyzed and supported on a ventilator. Increases in blood pressure and heart rate and decrease in arterial oxygen saturation are measures of inadequate anxiety and pain control in critically ill infants and children, although these physiologic changes may also be caused by a number of other clinical conditions, including seizures.

Other approaches to postoperative analgesia are common, although intravenous narcotic analgesics are employed in most settings for at least 24 to 48 hours postoperatively. Other interventions include local nerve blockade with pleural catheters and epidural administration of narcotics. The additional around-the-clock administration of acetaminophen (Tylenol) or nonsteroidal antiinflammatory drugs (NSAIDs) is useful in augmenting pain control when given concurrently with narcotics.[68]

ACQUIRED HEART DISEASE IN INFANTS AND CHILDREN

Acquired heart disease in pediatric patients includes a group of diseases, sometimes of unknown cause, in which the central feature is involvement of the heart muscle itself. An exception is Kawasaki disease, in which the coronary arteries are primarily involved. *Idiopathic cardiomyopathy* is the term used to describe diseases involving the heart muscle that are of unknown cause. These myocardial diseases in infants and children are not the consequence of ischemic, hypertensive, congenital, valvular, or pericardial disease.[60] Specific heart muscle diseases (also called *secondary cardiomyopathy*) have a known cause and include myocarditis, hypertension, and tachyarrhythmias. Although less common than CHDs, acquired heart disease in infants and children can lead to significant cardiac dysfunction, morbidity, and mortality.

Acute Myocarditis

Myocarditis is a generalized myocardial inflammation characterized histologically by lymphocytic infiltration and myocardial necrosis. Myocarditis may result in impaired cardiac function that may be subclinical or asymptomatic. If the inflammation is severe, it can result in critical sequelae, including CHF, arrhythmias, and possibly death.

Etiology.   Virtually any infectious agent can produce cardiac inflammation. Myocarditis has been described during and following a wide variety of viral, bacterial, rickettsial, fungal, and protozoan infections. The most common etiologic agents in North America are viruses, specifically Coxsackie and other enteroviruses. In addition to infectious agents, drugs (doxorubicin [Adriamycin], cocaine), chemicals (carbon monoxide), hypersensitivity reactions, autoimmune diseases and vasculitis, or Kawasaki disease may cause myocardial inflammation.

Incidence.   Myocarditis has been documented in 25% of pediatric autopsies.[69,70] However, only 0.3% of patients seen by pediatric cardiologists have clinically significant evidence of myocarditis.[71] A large percentage of asymptomatic or subclinical cases accounts for the discrepancy between the autopsy findings and clinical incidence.

The incidence of myocarditis is highest in children younger than 1 year of age. Between 5% and 12% of children infected with either influenza viruses or Coxsackie virus develop clinical myocarditis. Forty percent of older children with infectious mononucleosis have myocardial involvement that is most often subclinical.[71] With the advent of polymerase chain reaction (PCR), compared with enteroviruses, adenovirus has been identified more often as a causative agent.[72]

Pathogenesis.   Infectious agents produce myocardial damage by direct invasion of the myocardium, production of a myocardial toxin, or immune-mediated inflammation of the myocardium. Viruses injure myocardial tissue by direct destruction of the myofibrils and by cytotoxic T cell destruction of myocytes. Strong evidence shows that in viral myocarditis, a cell-mediated immunologic reaction is a principal mechanism of cardiac involvement. Adjacent cells may be destroyed by complement-mediated antibody action.

The time between the onset of inflammation and the initial clinical manifestations of disease varies. Generally within a week of infection, myocardial necrosis develops. However, the subsequent inflammatory and autoimmune response to viral infection becomes the primary mediator of clinical disease. Cellular immunity (T lymphocytes, macrophages), humoral immunity (antibodies), and cytokines (tumor necrosis factor, interleukins) are responsible for myocardial and coronary vascular injury. Vascular endothelial injury leads to vascular permeability with subsequent myocardial edema, increased ventricular wall thickness, and decreased ventricular function.[73]

Clinical Manifestations.   The clinical presentation of patients with myocarditis ranges from those who are asymptomatic to those with severe cardiac dysfunction progressing rapidly to fulminant CHF and death. Typically, newborns and young infants manifest a sudden onset of symptoms with rapid progression to critical illness.

Young patients with myocarditis present with lethargy, fever, and tachycardia. Respiratory distress, cyanosis, and vomiting may also occur. Older children present with fever, malaise, myalgia, gastroenteritis, pharyngitis, and meningitis but generally do not appear as ill as infants. In addition to tachycardia out of proportion to the fever, the cardiovascular examination reveals poor peripheral perfusion, thready pulses, cool extremities, and pallor. The heart sounds may be muffled if a pericardial effusion is present. With severe cardiac dysfunction, a gallop rhythm and a high-frequency, holosystolic (loudest at the apex) murmur of mitral regurgitation may be auscultated.

Diagnosis.   Many laboratory studies are indicated when myocarditis is suspected. Typically, patients with myocarditis have an elevated white blood cell count without a left shift, elevated erythrocyte sedimentation rate (ESR), abnormal liver function tests, and elevation of lactate dehydrogenase (LDH) isoenzyme 1, creatine phosphokinase (CPK) MB fraction, and troponin I. Of note is that myocarditis can still be present with a normal ESR. Bacterial infection is ruled out by blood culture. The nasopharynx and stool are cultured for viral isolation. Because viral cultures and convalescent viral titers may be nonspecific for determining the cause, PCR is used to amplify specific viral genomes through quantitation of specific viral RNA (if it is present in the tissue). PCR is more specific than culture for the amplification and identification of the specific causative virus.[74]

Chest radiographs may demonstrate cardiomegaly. Pulmonary venous markings are increased when heart failure is present. The ECG can reveal life-threatening cardiac rhythm disturbances that often accompany myocarditis. The classic electrocardiographic changes for myocarditis are low-voltage QRS, low or inverted T waves, and decreased or absent Q waves in V_5 and V_6. Echocardiography is used to evaluate cardiac function and detect the presence of a pericardial effusion. Most often the left ventricle is dilated, with increased left ventricular dimensions at end systole and end diastole. Global myocardial depression or wall motion abnormalities of the left ventricular free wall may be noted.

Historically the definitive diagnosis of myocarditis was made by myocardial biopsy, the gold standard, which demonstrates myocyte necrosis or degeneration associated with inflammatory infiltration,[72,75] the so-called *Dallas criteria*. The Dallas criteria define the characteristics of myocarditis from histologic examination of endomyocardial biopsy tissue obtained by cardiac catheterization (Fig. 18-29) and permit accurate diagnosis and systematic investigation of myocarditis. In addition, myocardial tissue can be can be sent for PCR analysis to determine viral etiology.

Unfortunately, the focal and patchy nature of myocarditis, as well as the small size of tissue samples obtained at biopsy, makes it difficult to obtain a definitive diagnosis in many cases, and false-negative results can occur. Therefore the absence of a positive biopsy result does not rule out myocarditis, and treatment is based on clinical symptoms and other diagnostic findings.

Critical Care Management.   Management of infants and children with myocarditis remains supportive rather than specifically aimed at a causative organism. Ensuring bed rest during the acute phase (7 to 14 days) is often recommended to decrease demands on the heart. In addition, animal studies also suggest that bed rest during the acute phase of myocarditis decreases viral replication and improve outcomes.[76] Administration of supplemental oxygen or mechanical ventilation may be often necessary to maintain adequate oxygen delivery in the face of CHF. Because the potential for complete recovery of myocardial function exists even in critically ill patients with myocarditis, treatment of cardiac dysfunction is aggressive.

Anticongestive Therapy.   The overall goal of treatment in patients with myocarditis is to increase cardiac output. In the critically ill patient, early and aggressive therapy is instituted, usually combining inotropic and afterload-reducing agents. Treatment includes single or combination drug therapy with dobutamine, dopamine, milrinone, amrinone, nitrovasodilators, or ACEIs. Dobutamine serves as an inotrope and is especially effective in patients with refractory CHF. Milrinone and amrinone have both inotropic and vasodilating properties that serve to decrease ventricular work. Diuretic therapy is prescribed to reduce volume load. (See Chapter 7 for an in-depth discussion on vasoactive and diuretic medications.) The goal of fluid balance is to provide adequate hydration to preserve preload and provide adequate ventricular filling pressures without fluid overload.

ACEIs provide afterload reduction by interfering with the formation of angiotensin II (a strong vasoconstrictor). In controlled studies, the use of ACEIs, such as captopril and enalapril, has been effective in slowing the course of heart failure, decreasing symptoms, and potentially prolonging survival in patients with mild to severe left ventricular dysfunction.[77,78]

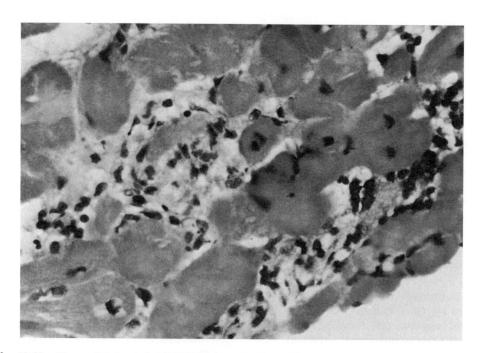

Fig. 18-29   Myocardial tissue showing focal, interstitial, lymphocytic infiltrate, and myocyte degeneration. Degenerating myocytes show closely apposed lymphocytes around it and attached to the membrane. (From Baker A: Acquired heart disease in infants and children, *Crit Care Nurs Clin North Am* 6:183, 1994.)

Some patients who recover from severe cardiac dysfunction require long-term oral anticongestive therapy. Digoxin, furosemide, and an ACEI are commonly employed. Some clinicians avoid administering digoxin during the acute phase of illness because of suggested increased digoxin toxicity in the inflamed myocardium.[73]

Arrhythmia Management. With myocardial dysfunction, cardiac rhythm disturbances can be life threatening, and aggressive therapy is warranted. Supraventricular tachycardia (SVT), ventricular ectopy, and heart block can develop in a subset of patients with myocarditis. Tachyarrhythmias are controlled to help prevent further deterioration of ventricular function. Antiarrhythmic agents are used to control symptomatic SVT, ventricular tachycardia, and premature ventricular contractions. The possibility of any negative inotropic or proarrhythmic effects should be considered when choosing an antiarrhythmic agent. If second- or third-degree AV block develops, a temporary transvenous or epicardial AV sequential pacemaker may be used. Persistence of complete heart block beyond 2 weeks is an indication for elective placement of a permanent pacemaker.[71,79]

Anticoagulation. Although controversial, anticoagulation therapy is used by some clinicians in patients with the potential for thrombus formation as a result of severely compromised ventricular function and stasis of blood flow. Systemic mural thrombi can potentially embolize to the cerebrovascular system, causing neurologic sequelae.

Coagulation parameters are followed closely, and therapy is adjusted to maintain an adequate anticoagulatory state. Because of the possibility of cerebral emboli, neurologic status is monitored closely, and changes in the patient's mentation or responsiveness are evaluated immediately. Signs and symptoms of pulmonary emboli, which include acute onset of shortness of breath, tachycardia, hypoxemia, and chest pain, are assessed. The risk of systemic emboli is also present and may manifest as a change in color, temperature, or perfusion of an extremity.

Antiinflammatory Treatment. Suppression of inflammatory mediators may help limit the severity of illness and shorten the clinical course. Unfortunately, no clinical regimen consistently ameliorates the acute phase of illness. Use of antiinflammatory agents, such as prednisone, azathioprine, and cyclosporin, is controversial.[73,80] Initial animal studies suggested a poorer outcome when steroids are administered early in the course of illness (during viral replication), suggesting that immunosuppression may enhance myocardial damage during this period. Subsequent human studies have suggested a benefit, but the studies were nonrandomized and are difficult to interpret because 45% to 50% of patients with myocarditis improve spontaneously.[81] The timing of this intervention accounts for the difference in outcome, so consideration should be given to delaying antiinflammatory treatment until the phase of lymphocytic infiltration and myocardial necrosis is decreased.[82,83] NSAIDs have been associated with worsening of myocardial damage and increased mortality.[73]

Intravenous immune globulin (IVIG) has been reported to have beneficial effect in patients with myocarditis. Left ventricular function improved and mortality decreased at 1 year following presentation in patients treated with high dose (2 g/kg) IVIG.[84,85] Although the specific mechanism of active is unknown, IVIG may interfere with the humoral immunity and autoantibodies responsible for myocardial cell damage. Associated side effects of IVIG are headaches, chills, and malaise.

Other Therapies. Antiviral agents, immunomodulatory agents, and antilymphocytic monoclonal antibodies are all currently under investigation for treatment of myocarditis. Unfortunately, many of these agents work best immediately following viral inoculation, making clinical application difficult. Interferon and monoclonal antibody to the infectious agent would provide specific effect and are under investigation in animal models.

Mechanical Assist Devices and Extracorporeal Support. If conventional therapy is unsuccessful, other means of support may be attempted. Chang and co-workers[86] reported the successful use of a left ventricular assist device in a patient with acute myocarditis. The use of intraaortic balloon pump and ECMO has been reported in patients who do not respond to conventional therapy; however, experience is limited. If cardiac function fails to improve, cardiac transplantation may be considered.

Preventing Complications. As is the case with any critically ill patient, the high potential for nosocomial infection is an important consideration. Multiple venous and arterial lines are required for the infusion of cardioactive drugs and continuous hemodynamic monitoring. Protecting patients from infection and vigilant assessment for early signs of localized or systemic infection are both important.

Decreased tissue perfusion in the acutely ill patient in combination with immobility increases the potential for ischemia and skin breakdown. Skin integrity is an important concern. Attention is directed toward alleviating pressure, repositioning to whatever extent is possible on a regular basis, and employing methods to prevent skin breakdown.

Attention to the patient's nutritional requirements is crucial to promote healing and to provide a positive nitrogen balance. Because the acutely ill patient is usually not able to take food orally, adequate nutrition must be provided intravenously or enterally (nasogastric or nasojejunal). Nutrition should be instituted early in the course of illness to fulfill caloric requirements.

Kawasaki Disease

Kawasaki disease is an acute systemic vasculitis that was first described in Japan in 1967. The acute illness itself is self-limiting, but 15% to 25% of untreated children with Kawasaki disease suffer damage to the coronary arteries, resulting in dilation or aneurysm formation.[87] Although damage can occur in any medium-sized muscular artery, the vessels most often affected are the coronary arteries, making Kawasaki disease the leading cause of acquired heart disease in children in the United States.

Etiology. The cause of Kawasaki disease is unknown. An infectious agent is suggested for a number of reasons. First, it is almost exclusively a pediatric disorder, suggesting the development of passive immunity by adulthood. Geographic outbreaks occur with an increase in the number of cases in the late winter and early spring. Lastly, many clinical similarities to other infectious diseases (i.e., scarlet fever, adenovirus) are seen. However, there is no evidence of spread from person to person. In the absence of a known agent, several researchers have begun to explore the possibility that the inflammation in Kawasaki disease may represent a "final common pathway" and that one agent may not be responsible. Epidemiologic studies have found associations between the occurrence of Kawasaki disease and recent exposure to carpet cleaning and residence near a body of stagnant water; however, these data are weak, and definitive cause and effect have not been established. Kawasaki disease is reported more often among children from higher socioeconomic groups and in those of Asian descent.

Incidence. The first cases of Kawasaki disease in the United States were described in the early 1970s. Although Japanese children have the highest incidence of this illness, Kawasaki disease occurs in all races. African Americans have the second highest rate of occurrence; Caucasian children follow. Eighty percent of cases occur in children under age 5, with the greatest incidence in the toddler age group (1- to 2-year-olds).[88] Infants often present in an atypical fashion, without fulfilling diagnostic criteria; however, this age group (especially infant males) has the highest risk for the development of severe coronary artery disease. Recent research has also documented a higher incidence of coronary artery aneurysms in children older than 6 years of age.[89] Males are affected more often than females (1.5:1). The actual incidence of Kawasaki disease in this country is not known because reporting to the Centers for Disease Control and Prevention (CDC) is accomplished via a voluntary, passive surveillance system.

Pathogenesis. The overall mortality in Kawasaki disease is 0.3%, with almost all deaths related to the cardiac sequelae.[90] Kawasaki disease causes diffuse acute vasculitis of medium-sized arteries and small arterioles and venules throughout the body, with a predilection for the coronary arteries. The involvement of small peripheral blood vessels is evidenced in the inflammatory signs and symptoms that characterize this illness. During the initial acute phase, inflammation of the small arteries and venules is evident. Inflammation then progresses to involve the medium-sized muscular arteries, including the coronary arteries, with the potential development of coronary artery aneurysm. The inflammatory process is an immune-mediated response in which the T cells and macrophages produce inflammatory cytokines that infiltrate the coronary arteries and myocardium. During the acute phase, there is often evidence of pericarditis, myocarditis, and valvulitis. Enlargement (ectasia) of the coronary arteries can be seen by echocardiogram as early as day 7 after the onset of fever. Affected vessels may continue to enlarge for some time, reaching their maximum dimension at approximately 28 days from the onset of fever. In dilated vessels, the potential for thrombus exists. Over time, affected vessels heal by the process of myointimal proliferation, which can result in stenosis,

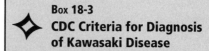

Box 18-3
CDC Criteria for Diagnosis of Kawasaki Disease

Fever >5 days unresponsive to antibiotics and at least four of the five following physical findings with no other more reasonable explanation for the observed clinical findings:
1. Bilateral conjunctival injection
2. Oral mucosal changes (erythema of lips or oropharynx, strawberry tongue, or drying or fissuring of the lips)
3. Peripheral extremity changes (edema, erythema, or generalized or periungual desquamation)
4. Rash
5. Cervical lymphadenopathy >1.5 cm in diameter

From Centers for Disease Control: Kawasaki disease—New York, *MMWR* 29:61-63, 1980.

especially at the distal ends of aneurysms. The myocardium is involved directly in almost all cases, with myocellular hypertrophy, degeneration of myocytes, and endocardial changes that lead to myocarditis and decreased ventricular function. Myocardial dysfunction is subclinical in most patients.

Clinical Manifestations. A definitive diagnostic test for Kawasaki disease does not exist. Rather, the diagnosis is based on the presence of certain clinical criteria developed by Dr. Kawasaki and outlined by the CDC (Box 18-3). The presence of prolonged fever plus four of the five diagnostic criteria, without evidence of another known disease, is required to meet diagnostic criteria. The conjunctivitis in Kawasaki disease is bilateral nonexudative with limbal sparing. The lips and oropharynx are red. The filiform papillae of the tongue slough off, creating the classic "strawberry tongue." The hands may be edematous and red in this phase. The rash of Kawasaki disease is never vesicular or bullous. It is accentuated in the groin in 50% of cases and often is accompanied by local desquamation of this area.[91] The lymphadenopathy is nonsuppurative, with one node at least 1.5 cm or larger in the anterior cervical chain. In addition to these symptoms, a number of associated clinical and laboratory findings are often present and support the diagnosis (Box 18-4). Irritability is often extreme and may persist over the entire course of the illness. Analysis of cerebrospinal fluid may demonstrate mild aseptic meningitis. Arthritis occurs in one third of patients, usually affecting the small joints initially with progression to the large weight-bearing joints. Diarrhea, nausea, and vomiting are not uncommon. Hydrops of the gallbladder and abdominal pain may also be present. The diagnostic criteria should be viewed only as a guideline because some children develop aneurysms without meeting diagnostic criteria (atypical Kawasaki disease). Atypical disease is especially common in infants who often present symptoms with subtle or incomplete findings.

Kawasaki disease is an acute, self-limiting illness. Complete resolution of clinical symptoms and return of laboratory results to normal often require 6 to 8 weeks. The

---

Box 18-4

Associated Clinical and Laboratory Findings in Kawasaki Disease

Elevated sedimentation rate (resolves 6-8 weeks after the onset of fever)

Leukocytosis with a left shift

Aseptic meningitis

Urethritis with sterile pyuria: microscopic examination reveals mononuclear cells

Elevated liver transaminases: commonly 2-3 times normal

Thrombocytosis: peaking 3-4 weeks after onset

Hydrops of the gallbladder, right upper quadrant abdominal pain

Anemia that persists until the resolution of inflammation

Irritability (can last for 6-8 weeks)

Diarrhea and vomiting

---

course of the illness can be divided into three stages: acute, subacute, and convalescent phases.

The **acute phase** begins with the abrupt onset of fever, which lasts for at least 5 days (average of 11 days without treatment). Over the first week, the diagnostic findings become evident. All of the clinical features may not be present at the same time, making the diagnosis challenging. Small joint arthritis is seen in approximately one third of patients. Echocardiography is performed at the time of diagnosis to evaluate cardiac function and establish a baseline for evaluation of coronary artery size and shape. Mild to moderate CHF from myocarditis, left ventricular dysfunction, and pericardial effusion may be detected. Although unusual, cardiac rhythm disturbances may occur, including first- or second-degree AV block, prolonged QT interval, abnormal ST segment and T wave, and low R wave amplitude.

The **subacute phase** begins with resolution of fever, although multisystem involvement is still evident. During this stage the characteristic periungual desquamation occurs (peeling of the skin of the palms and soles beginning under the fingertips and toes). Arthritis, if present, generally affects the larger weight-bearing joints in this phase. Laboratory studies reveal a hypercoagulable state with significant thrombocytosis. The sedimentation rate continues to be elevated, and a normocytic, normochromic anemia is common. In those patients who develop coronary artery abnormalities, dilation or aneurysms become evident by echocardiogram in this phase.

The third stage is a **convalescent phase,** during which the child continues to recover and laboratory values return to normal. Unfortunately (if untreated), although the child seems clinically improved, coronary aneurysms may continue to enlarge during this stage, reaching their maximum dimension approximately 28 days from the onset of illness.

Cardiac Findings.   During the acute phase of illness, at least some degree of myocarditis is present in all children with Kawasaki disease, as demonstrated by both biopsy and autopsy findings.[92] The majority of cases are subclinical;

however, severe cases can result in CHF and cardiogenic shock. Physical examination often reveals tachycardia and a gallop rhythm during the acute phase (often out of proportion to the degree of fever). Echocardiography can reveal decreased left ventricular contractility in the acute phase. This condition may persist for several months and is improved by treatment with IVIG.[93]

In the acute phase, the most common ECG changes include a prolonged PR interval and nonspecific ST and T wave changes. The arrhythmias seen in the acute phase of Kawasaki disease are not usually life threatening and are consistent with myocarditis. Later, abnormal ECGs may reflect myocardial infarction or ischemia in the most severely affected patients.

Valvulitis can occur in the acute phase. Mitral regurgitation is sometimes present and is thought to be the result of myocarditis in the acute stage or myocardial ischemia later. Late-onset aortic regurgitation sometimes requiring valve replacement is a late, rare finding.[94]

The most important sequelae from Kawasaki disease are coronary artery aneurysms. Of untreated children, 15% to 25% develop damage to the coronary arteries, resulting in ectasia (dilation) or aneurysm formation of one or more vessels. Duration of fever is the strongest predictor of aneurysm formation: the longer the fever persists, the greater the risk of the development of coronary aneurysms.[69,95,96] Aneurysm formation and healing (regression) is a dynamic process. In the acute phase of the illness, inflammation of the coronary arteries causes weakness in the vessel wall. Over the course of subsequent weeks, the damaged vessel increases in diameter, resulting in ectasia or aneurysm formation. The Japanese Ministry of Health defines an aneurysm as an internal lumen diameter greater than 3 mm in a child younger than 5 years of age or greater than 4 mm in a child of age 5 years or older. In addition, any segment that is 1.5 times larger than an adjacent segment is considered abnormal, as is a vessel with an obviously irregular lumen. These criteria are based on age and do not take into account the differences in body size of individual patients. Recent data show that body surface area (BSA)-adjusted z-scores (standard deviations from the average) in patients with Kawasaki disease were actually larger than expected, even in patients with coronary arteries that would be classified as normal by the Japanese criteria.[97]

Coronary artery abnormalities are not often evident until the second week after the onset of fever; however, they have been detected as early as day 7 of illness. The affected vessels can continue to enlarge through the fourth week of illness, at which time their maximum dimension is generally reached. Echocardiography is highly sensitive for detection of enlargement of aneurysms in the proximal coronary arteries.

Thrombocytosis occurs during the subacute phase of illness, with platelet counts that can approach 1 million. Sluggish blood flow through enlarged coronary vessels, in combination with an elevated platelet count, increases the risk of thrombosis in patients with aneurysms and places these children at risk for the development of thrombus with subsequent myocardial ischemia or infarction. At greatest

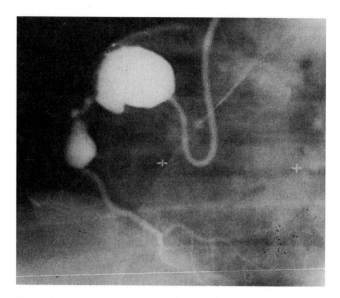

Fig. 18-30 Right coronary arteriogram demonstrating giant proximal aneurysm and smaller distal one.

risk for clot development are those with "giant aneurysms," which measure more than 8 mm in diameter (Fig. 18-30).

Over time, regression of aneurysms can occur. The majority of healing occurs during the first year or two after the onset of illness. In 50% to 66% of cases, the internal lumen diameter of aneurysmal vessels actually returns to its normal size by a process of myointimal proliferation. The amount of healing or regression in an individual patient is most closely related to the extent of damage. The larger the aneurysm, the less likely it is to return to its normal size. Regardless of the internal diameter of the coronary artery, affected vessel walls are not truly "normal" in terms of either histology or reactivity to coronary vasodilators because of thickening and calcification that occurs in the process of healing.[91,98] These vessels may be at greater risk of developing premature atherosclerotic disease. Although less common, aneurysms may occur in other arteries, most commonly the axillary (often palpable), subclavian, brachial, iliac, or femoral vessels and sometimes in the abdominal aorta and renal arteries.[99] These areas are generally affected only in patients who also have significant coronary aneurysms.

Over years, stenotic areas may develop in affected coronary arteries, occurring most commonly at either the proximal or distal end of aneurysms as the vessel walls heal inward. The incidence of stenosis increases over the lifespan, especially in patients with giant aneurysms. As a consequence of progressive stenosis, blood flow to the myocardium may be impeded or occluded. If adequate collateral circulation has not developed, myocardial ischemia or infarction may result. Stenoses are not easily detectable by echocardiogram, so patients must be carefully monitored over time to detect myocardial ischemia by stress testing, myocardial perfusion scans, and ECG. Cardiac catheterization accurately detects stenotic areas and is generally performed a year after the onset of illness or at

any time that noninvasive testing suggests signs of myocardial ischemia.

Management. The majority of patients with Kawasaki disease do not require critical care. Typically, a 1- or 2-day admission is necessary during the acute phase for monitoring and providing IVIG. Those with acute ventricular dysfunction and symptoms of myocardial ischemia or infarction and those who require systemic heparinization or thrombolytic therapy also require close monitoring.

γ-Globulin Therapy. The use of IVIG shortens the acute phase of Kawasaki disease and decreases the risk of coronary damage.[100] This treatment is currently the standard of care in Kawasaki disease. The recommended dose of IVIG is 2 g/kg given intravenously in a single infusion over 8 to 12 hours.[101] In an National Institutes of Health funded, multicenter study, γ-globulin was shown to decrease the incidence of aneurysms threefold to fivefold when given within the first 10 days of illness.[100] For best outcomes, IVIG should ideally be given within the first 10 days of illness. However, it should be administered after this time to any child diagnosed late with persistent fever, aneurysms, or signs or symptoms of ongoing inflammation. Retreatment with IVIG is given to patients who have persistent or recrudescent fever 48 to 72 hours after the administration of IVIG.[102]

Careful cardiac monitoring is necessary during the administration of γ-globulin. Approximately 40 ml/kg of fluid is administered with the γ-globulin over an 8- to 12-hour period. Patients with myocardial dysfunction can experience acute CHF. Many centers administer diphenhydramine (Benadryl) before the infusion of IVIG to decrease the risk of a reaction to this product.

Aspirin Therapy. Historically, aspirin has been given as part of the treatment for Kawasaki disease in both antiinflammatory and antiplatelet doses. In prospective studies, the administration of aspirin has never been shown to have an effect on whether a patient develops aneurysms. High doses of aspirin (20 to 25 mg/kg/dose every 6 hours) are used initially for their antiinflammatory effect. When the patient has been afebrile for 2 to 3 days, the dose is decreased to an "antiplatelet" dose (3 to 5 mg/kg/day). Low-dose aspirin is continued through the convalescent phase and then discontinued in patients without coronary involvement.

Antithrombotic Therapy in Patients With Aneurysms. Children with coronary aneurysms require long-term antithrombotic therapy. The potential for thrombosis of the coronary arteries is actually greatest after the acute phase when thrombocytosis occurs along with ongoing vasculitis, creating a hypercoagulable state. This is especially true in patients with rapidly increasing coronary artery dimensions or with giant aneurysms. Aspirin therapy remains the most common therapy for the majority of these patients. Dipyridamole (Persantine) is sometimes added at a dose of 3 to 6 mg/kg/day in three doses in patients, although its efficacy in these situations has never been documented.

If "giant" aneurysms are diagnosed, systemic heparin therapy is often instituted, especially in patients in whom the aneurysms are rapidly increasing in size. When an adequate anticoagulation state is reached, oral warfarin (Coumadin) is substituted and administered in addition to aspirin, maintaining an international normalized ratio (INR) in the 2.0 to 2.5 range. This is the most common regimen for patients with giant aneurysms. Low-molecular-weight heparin is occasionally used instead of warfarin; however, this treatment requires twice daily injections. Experience with newer inhibitors of platelet aggregation, such as clopidogrel and ticlopidine, is very limited in pediatrics. The risks and potential benefits of various anticoagulation regimens are considered on an individual basis.[103]

Patients taking chronic aspirin therapy should receive yearly influenza vaccines. Other therapies should be substituted if the child develops influenza or varicella infection because of the risk of Reye's syndrome. In addition, because the varicella vaccine is a live vaccine, aspirin should be substituted with another regimen for 6 weeks after receiving this vaccine.

Thrombolytic Therapy. Clots may occur even with antithrombotic therapy, especially in patients with giant aneurysms causing blood flow in the area of the aneurysm to be very sluggish. Thrombolytic therapy is considered if clot formation is detected, through either signs or symptoms of myocardial ischemia or infarction or by echocardiography. Because no large clinical trials have been conducted in children, the use of thrombolytic agents is based on studies in adults with coronary thrombosis. Urokinase and streptokinase have both been used to restore vessel patency.[104-106] The earlier thrombolytic therapy is instituted after clot formation or the onset of ischemic symptoms, the greater is its efficacy. The adjunct use of other therapies such an antagonists to glycoprotein IIb-IIIa receptor (i.e. Abciximab) have been encouraging in adults and small pediatric studies; however, further data are required to determine safety and efficacy in the pediatric population.[107] If reperfusion is achieved, systemic heparin therapy and aspirin are administered to maintain vessel patency, followed by oral antithrombotic regimens. Close assessment of laboratory measures of coagulation and cardiac function is a priority in these patients.

Anticongestive Therapy. CHF in patients with Kawasaki disease is most often a consequence of ischemic cardiomyopathy, although it may occur acutely in patients with marked myocarditis. In those rare patients, intravenous inotropes and afterload reduction may be necessary. More often, patients with CHF from ischemic disease and coronary insufficiency require therapy with oral digoxin, diuretics, β-blockers, or ACEIs.

Surgical Intervention. Coronary bypass surgery, although technically difficult with small vessels, has been performed in children with severe coronary artery disease. The indications for bypass surgery in children are not well established; however, surgery may be indicated if (1) coronary stenosis or occlusion is progressive, (2) collateral blood supply is not adequate, (3) the portion of myocardium to be perfused via the graft is still viable, and (4) the vessel proximal to the planned graft site is healthy.[99] In addition to the technical difficulty of coronary artery bypass surgery in pediatric patients, children often develop collateral circula-

tion around a coronary occlusion over time. Because grafts need to remain patent for many decades, surgery is usually recommended only for those with life-threatening vascular disease.

Coronary bypass surgery is contraindicated in patients with acutely inflamed or excessively small coronary vessels. Coronary artery anatomy in some also precludes bypass operation. In addition, the disease may damage the internal mammary arteries (most often used as graft vessels in children).

Interventional Cardiac Catheterization Techniques. Over the past decade, significant advances have been made in catheterization interventions in patients with Kawasaki disease. Percutaneous transluminal coronary angioplasty (PTCA) has been performed in children with coronary artery stenosis with varying success. PTCA is a more difficult technique in patients with Kawasaki disease than in adults with coronary artery disease mainly because the areas of stenosis are often very stiff and calcified. The balloon pressures necessary to dilate these areas can predispose the patient to late aneurysm formation. Rotational ablation techniques and stent placement have also been used in this population.[108]

Cardiac Transplantation. Cardiac transplantation has been performed in a small number of patients with Kawasaki disease.[109] This operation is obviously a last resort for patients with severe ischemia and is only used in situations in which surgery or catheter intervention is not possible.

Cardiomyopathy

Cardiomyopathy is a disease of the heart muscle itself. Cardiomyopathy may be idiopathic, primary (i.e., of unknown cause), or secondary to a known cause or systemic disease that affects the heart muscle. Cardiomyopathy is further classified into the following three types:

1. Dilated, characterized by ventricular dilation, systolic (contractile) dysfunction, and signs and symptoms of CHF
2. Hypertrophic, usually with preserved or enhanced contractile performance and diastolic dysfunction (compliance)
3. Restrictive, marked by impaired diastolic filling (Fig. 18-31)

Because of overlap, the distinction between one category and the next is not absolute. The basic characteristics of each type are outlined in Table 18-9. Restrictive cardiomyopathy is rare in children and is not considered in the sections that follow.

Dilated Cardiomyopathy. Dilated cardiomyopathy (DCM) is the most common cardiomyopathy in pediatric patients (characterized by increased ventricular volume with ventricular dilation). DCM results from a group of diverse disorders that affect myocardial contractile proteins, leading to decreased contractility. DCM is characterized by systolic dysfunction. Typically, the left ventricle (and sometimes the right) is enlarged, thin walled, and poorly contractile.

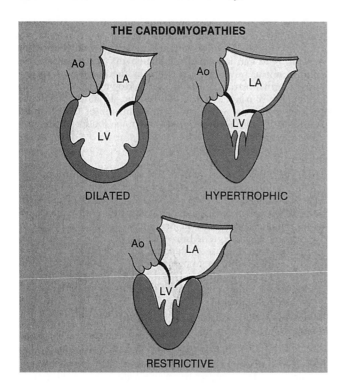

Fig. 18-31 Comparison of three morphologic types of cardiomyopathy. *Ao,* Aorta; *LA,* left atrium; *LV,* left ventricle. (Modified from Roberts WC, Ferrans VJ: Pathologic anatomy of the cardiomyopathies, *Hum Pathol* 6:287, 1975. In Wyngaarden JB, Smith LH, Bennett JC: *Cecil textbook of medicine,* ed 19, Philadelphia, WB Saunders, 1991, p 332.)

Etiology. The etiology can be heterogeneous and multifaceted. In the majority of patients, the cause of DCM is unknown, although a link to myocarditis is often presumed. Myocarditis that leads to the development of DCM is an important factor. In some patients with "primary" cardiomyopathy, retrospective evidence of a postviral disorder includes inflammatory changes on endocardial biopsy, high antibody viral titers, and others.[60] In addition, research evidence shows that patients with idiopathic cardiomyopathy have abnormalities of both cellular and humoral immunity. Antimyocardial antibodies, cytotoxic T cells, suppressor T cells, and natural killer cells have been identified in some studies.[110] Possibly a prior myocarditis incorporates viral components in cardiac cells, which then serve as an antigenic source that directs the immune system to attack the myocardium.

Up to 25% of patients with idiopathic DCM have a familial form of the disease.[111] This condition can be caused by autosomal dominant inheritance, with first-degree relatives having the highest risk for development of DCM.[112]

Familial disorders such as neuromuscular disorders and inborn errors of metabolism are associated with the development of DCM. Duchenne and Becker muscular dystrophy are the most commonly encountered neuromuscular disorders that develop cardiomyopathy.[113] The inborn errors of metabolism include but are not limited to, glycogen storage disease, fatty acid oxidative disorders, and mucopolysaccharidosis. Endocardial fibroelastosis can also cause DCM.

Cardiovascular structural disease, arrhythmias (incessant tachycardia), coronary artery disease, Kawasaki disease, and hypertension may lead to DCM. Secondary myocardial disease results from systemic causes in which the primary illness is extracardiac. DCM may result from nutritional deficiencies, carnitine deficiency, obesity, radiation, malignancy, drug toxicity (alcohol, chemotherapy), and other systemic infections and illnesses.[113]

Incidence. DCM is the most common form of cardiomyopathy. Reported annual incidence in the United States is 2 to 8 cases per 100,000.[114]

Pathogenesis. The ventricles become dilated and thin walled and the atria become enlarged. Ventricular hypertrophy is sometimes seen, but the thickness of the ventricular wall is inadequate for the degree of dilation present. Poor contractility permits stasis of blood, particularly in the ventricular apex, thereby setting the stage for thrombus formation.

Histologic features include fibrosis, myocyte hypertrophy, possible necrosis, and occasionally lymphocytes. Structural changes in the mitochondria have been found on electron microscopy. Genetic analysis has discovered mutations in beta-myosin, troponin, and dystrophin—all important cardiac contractile proteins.

Many of these patients develop arrhythmias, particularly ventricular arrhythmias. These can be a significant cause of sudden death in this population.[115]

Clinical Manifestations. Pediatric patients with DCM may be asymptomatic for months, despite systolic dysfunction and ventricular dilation. Many present with signs and symptoms of CHF. A few children are not identified as having DCM until severe ventricular dysfunction occurs and cardiogenic shock with low output is present. Occasionally, ventricular ectopy or syncope may be the presenting sign.

Physical examination may reveal pulmonary congestion, a quiet precordium, a prominent S_3 gallop, and hepatomegaly. If left ventricular dilation and dysfunction are severe, the murmur of mitral regurgitation may be heard at the apex.

Diagnosis. Chest radiographs reveal marked cardiomegaly and pulmonary edema (Fig. 18-32). The ECG may be normal or can show nonspecific ST-T wave abnormalities, atrial enlargement, left bundle branch block, ventricular strain, QRS prolongation, or sinus tachycardia. An important aspect is that the presence of left bundle branch block is an ominous sign.[116] Echocardiography shows enlargement of one or both ventricles and provides quantitative analysis of ventricular function. Shortening and ejection fractions are both decreased, and in some, regional wall motion abnormalities are detected. Mural thrombi may be evident by echocardiogram, especially in the left ventricular apex and left atrial appendage.

Histologic examination and PCR of myocardial tissue obtained via cardiac catheterization[117] aid further in elucidation of the cause. Cardiac catheterization also aids in determining hemodynamic measurements and cardiac output.

Urine tests for organic and amino acids may be useful in diagnosing metabolic or inborn errors of metabolism as the

TABLE 18-9   Classification of Cardiomyopathies

	Dilated	Restrictive	Hypertrophic
Symptoms	Congestive heart failure, particularly left sided Fatigue and weakness Systemic or pulmonary emboli	Dyspnea, fatigue Right-sided congestive heart failure Signs and symptoms of systemic disease: amyloidosis, iron storage disease, etc.	Dyspnea, angina pectoris Fatigue, syncope, palpitations
Physical examination	Moderate to severe cardiomegaly; S_3 and S_4 Atrioventricular (AV) valve regurgitation, especially mitral	Mild to moderate cardiomegaly; S_3 or S_4 AV valve regurgitation; inspiratory increase in venous pressure (Kussmaul's sign)	Mild cardiomegaly Apical systolic thrill and heave; brisk carotid upstroke S_4 common Systolic murmur that increases with Valsalva maneuver
Chest roentgenogram	Moderate to marked cardiac enlargement, especially left ventricular Pulmonary venous hypertension	Mild cardiac enlargement Pulmonary venous hypertension	Mild to moderate cardiac enlargement Left atrial enlargement
Electrocardiogram	Sinus tachycardia Atrial and ventricular arrhythmias ST segment and T wave abnormalities Intraventricular conduction defects	Low voltage Intraventricular conduction defects AV conduction defects	Left ventricular hypertrophy ST segment and T wave abnormalities Abnormal Q waves Atrial and ventricular arrhythmias
Echocardiogram	Left ventricular dilation and dysfunction Abnormal diastolic mitral valve motion secondary to abnormal compliance and filling pressures	Increased left ventricular wall thickness and mass Small or normal-sized left ventricular cavity Normal systolic function Pericardial effusion	Asymmetric septal hypertrophy (ASH) Narrow left ventricular outflow tract Systolic anterior motion (SAM) of the mitral valve Small or normal-sized left ventricle
Cardiac catheterization	Left ventricular enlargement and dysfunction Mitral or tricuspid regurgitation, or both Elevated left and often right-sided filling pressures Diminished cardiac output	Diminished left ventricular compliance "Square root sign" in ventricular pressure recordings Preserved systolic function Elevated left- and right-sided filling pressures	Diminished left ventricular compliance Mitral regurgitation Vigorous systolic function Dynamic left ventricular outflow gradient

From Wynne J, Braunwald E: The cardiomyopathies and myocarditides. In Braunwald E, ed: *Heart disease,* ed 4, Philadelphia, 1992, WB Saunders, p. 1396.

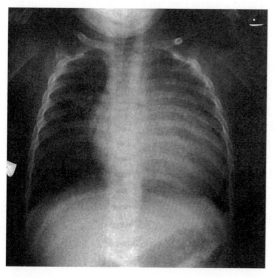

Fig. 18-32   Chest x-ray film of infant with cardiomegaly and pulmonary edema/congestive heart failure. (From Baker A: Acquired heart disease in infants and children, *Crit Care Nurs Clin North Am* 6:182, 1994.)

etiology. Molecular analysis, if available, may aid in the diagnosis of genetic causes.

Critical Care Management. If an underlying cause is identified, such as carnitine deficiency or a metabolic disorder, this finding can direct specific replacement or dietary interventions.

Anticongestive therapy is initiated to support cardiac function. Diuretics are implemented for volume reduction. The critically ill child may require intravenous inotropic support and afterload reduction. Dobutamine and phosphodiesterase inhibitors will augment stroke volume. Dopamine is usually kept at renal doses. The nitrovasodilators and phosphodiesterase inhibitors augment vascular relaxation, decrease resistance, reduce ventricular work, and may improve LV relaxation. Frequently intubation and mechanical ventilation is necessary during acute illness for respiratory support and to decrease the metabolic work of the respiratory muscles. Bed rest and or sedation are implemented as needed to decrease metabolic demands.

If the patient is well enough for oral agents, then digoxin and ACEIs are frequently employed. Third-generation β-blockers (carvedilol) have been found to decrease symptoms and improve survival in patients with DCM.[14,118] It has been postulated that β-blockers lower adrenergic activity and prevent β-receptor up-regulation, therefore attenuating one of the neurohumoral responses associated with heart failure (see section on CHF).

Although controversial, some clinicians institute anticoagulation therapy in patients with intracavity stasis to prevent thrombus formation in the dilated and poorly contractile heart. Management of ventricular rhythm disturbances may be necessary for some patients. Selection of antiarrhythmics is based on negative inotropic and proarrhythmic side effects. Amiodarone has been shown to be efficacious in suppression of ventricular ectopy without significant negative inotropic effects.[119,120] Occasionally a patient with intractable, refractory ventricular tachycardia or ventricular fibrillation will require implantation of an internal automatic defibrillator.

Serial monitoring of cardiac function with echocardiography is performed to evaluate improvement or deterioration after the institution of medical management. If the patient is unresponsive to medical management or if symptoms are rapidly progressive, cardiac transplantation may be considered. Ventricular assist devices have been used as a bridge to transplantation in this population.

Hypertrophic Cardiomyopathy. Hypertrophic cardiomyopathy (HCM) is a heterogeneous disorder that is characterized by a hypertrophied, nondilated left ventricle in the absence of hypertension, coronary artery disease, aortic stenosis, and coarctation of the aorta. Infants often have biventricular hypertrophy.

The pathophysiologic consequence of histologic changes and hypertrophy of the left ventricle is abnormal relaxation or diastolic dysfunction. Diastolic dysfunction can lead to exercise intolerance, cardiac rhythm disturbances, and sudden death.

The age of onset can be quite variable, and sudden death can be the first manifestation of HCM. Most patients present in adolescence or early adulthood. Sudden death occurs most often between 15 to 35 years of age, and many of these patients are asymptomatic or only mildly symptomatic before death.[114,121]

Etiology. HCM is a familial, genetically linked autosomal dominant disease in at least 50% of cases.[122] Significant advances in molecular genetics have found a large number of heterogeneous mutations in genes that encode for myocardial contractile proteins. In HCM the causative mutations are generally in the sarcomeric proteins known as: beta-myosin heavy chain, troponin I, troponin T, troponin C, light chains of myosin, and cardiac binding protein.[123] Although a single family may share the same genetic protein defect, clinical presentation and manifestations can be quite varied.

HCM has also been reported to be associated with tacrolimus[124,125] and long-term high-dose steroid therapy.[126] Transient HCM has been reported in infants of diabetic mothers and secondary to fetal distress.[127] Noonan's syndrome, Pompe's disease, Beckwith-Wiedemann syndrome, and infiltrative diseases are also associated with HCM.

Incidence. Because the onset of HCM is so variable, the absolute incidence is unknown. In addition, many patients can have subclinical disease, making patient identification difficult. Although reports vary, HCM may have an incidence of up to 2.5% per 100,000 and accounts for up to 30% of pediatric primary myocardial disease.[114]

Pathogenesis. Histologic features consistent with HCM include fibrosis, myocardial cellular disorganization, myocyte hypertrophy, scarring, and abnormal intramural coronary arteries. Cellular disarray is interspersed throughout the left ventricle and can occur in areas of normal or mildly increased thickness. The intramural arteries are thickened with a narrow lumen and are found around areas of fibrosis and scarring, implying a casual relationship between small vessel disease and ischemia.[128] Myocardial bridging (from hypertrophied muscle) has been reported in 10% of children with HCM and may cause compression of the coronaries with subsequent ischemia.[129] All of these factors may contribute to hypertrophy, impaired diastolic function, arrhythmias, and sudden death.

Structural anomalies include left ventricular hypertrophy and mitral valve abnormalities. Left ventricular hypertrophy (LVH) is usually asymmetric. The anterior ventricular septum and anterolateral free wall typically demonstrate the greatest degree of wall thickening. The pattern and extent of LVH exhibit marked heterogeneity among patients. Infants less than 1 year old can have concentric LVH and right ventricular hypertrophy.[114] In infants and children, significant increases in hypertrophy can occur with age, particularly during the accelerated growth phase of adolescence. Structural abnormalities of the mitral valve (MV) include increased MV area, elongated leaflets, thickened leaflets, and anomalous attachment of the papillary muscle directly into the anterior leaflet without the interposition of the chordae tendineae. MV abnormalities may be secondary to asymmetric hypertrophy and altered flow dynamics.

Many of these patients have left ventricular outflow tract obstruction (LVOTO). This condition can be quite variable and often is dynamic in that it worsens with exercise, tachycardia, dehydration, or anemia. Obstruction can occur in early, mid, or at the end of systole (which is the classic finding). LVOTO can be secondary to septal hypertrophy, anterior displacement of the papillary muscles, or malposition of the MV during systole. Systolic anterior motion (SAM) of the MV causes coaptation of the anterior MV leaflet with the septum producing LVOTO. SAM is felt to be secondary to a high-velocity jet of flow through the LV outflow tract (Venturi effect) or flow drag on the leaflet. The duration and onset of SAM is directly related to the magnitude of the LV outflow tract gradient.[128]

Unlike the older child or adult, infants and young children often develop RVOTO as well from septal hypertrophy.[114] The subpulmonary obstruction tends to be fixed and not dynamic, contributing to overall right ventricular hypertrophy.

Diastolic dysfunction is characteristic of HCM, resulting from decreased chamber distensibility and increased chamber stiffness (poor compliance). Myocyte hypertrophy, fibrosis, myocardial ischemia, and cellular disorganization are all factors in diastolic dysfunction. Although diastolic dysfunction is unrelated to the severity of outflow tract obstruction or distribution of hypertrophy, it can be present when symptoms and LVOTO are absent.[128]

Myocardial ischemia occurs in many patients with HCM and is believed to be responsible for myocardial fibrosis and scarring. Potential causes of myocardial ischemia include abnormal coronaries, increased oxygen demand that exceeds delivery, or elevated ventricular wall tension from prolonged diastolic relaxation interfering with perfusion.

Other pathologic sequelae of HCM include mitral regurgitation, arrhythmias, and, rarely, systolic dysfunction. Mitral regurgitation is secondary to SAM and other MV abnormalities. Arrhythmias are often seen in children with HCM and can be both supraventricular and ventricular. Sustained ventricular tachycardia is thought to be an important cause of sudden death in adults,[130] but this factor has not been shown in children.[115] Systolic function is usually supranormal; however, a patient can progress to a DCM and subsequently develop systolic dysfunction.

Clinical Manifestations. The majority of people with HCM are either asymptomatic or only mildly affected. Often these patients are identified during screening after detection of an affected family member. Early recognition of HCM in children is important because of the increased risk of sudden death in young patients. Death commonly occurs during competitive sports or severe exertion in often asymptomatic or mildly symptomatic children. Sometimes the only previous symptom is syncope. Clinical symptoms are not often appreciated in children over 1 year of age; however, when they do occur, they consist of dyspnea, exercise intolerance, chest pain, presyncope, and syncope. Infants, on the other hand, are often quite symptomatic with tachypnea, tachycardia, poor feeding, and CHF. Children over the age of 1 year rarely present in CHF.[114]

The physical examination may be completely normal in asymptomatic patients. Most children however, have a left ventricular lift, and the apical impulse is often displaced laterally and is unusually forceful. If LVOTO is significant, a thrill may be palpable along the left sternal border. Often a systolic murmur prompts the referral for evaluation by a cardiologist; however, this sign is only found in 40% of patients.[114] The second heart sound may be paradoxically split, and third and fourth heart sounds are frequently audible.

Diagnosis. Chest radiograph often demonstrates cardiomegaly with normal PBF. Most patients will have abnormal ECGs, making this a useful screening tool for HCM. ECG abnormalities include LVH, ST segment changes, ventricular strain, deep Q waves, and QTc and QRS prolongation.[131] Ventricular preexcitation and Wolff-Parkinson-White (WPW) syndrome have also been associated with HCM.[132,133]

Echocardiography is the most useful tool in diagnosing HCM. The degree of LVH, outflow tract obstruction, systolic and diastolic function, MV abnormalities, and SAM can be determined. Serial echoes can help monitor progression of disease and response to therapeutic intervention.

Invasive studies include cardiac catheterization and radionuclide studies. Although echocardiography has all but replaced cardiac catheterization as a diagnostic tool, occasionally biopsy is performed to diagnose mitochondrial disorders as a cause. Thallium perfusion scans are used to detect regional perfusion abnormalities.

If the patient has symptoms in infancy, metabolic studies should be performed to identify causative factors such as glycogen storage disease or mitochondrial disorders. Blood and urine tests for amino and organic acids should be obtained.

Critical Care Management. Overall management of patients with HCM is directed toward alleviating symptoms and reducing the risk of sudden death. Data regarding the natural history of the disorder in pediatric patients are limited. Some patients are stable without symptoms, whereas others have symptoms that rapidly progress. The prognosis for infants who present before 1 year of life is poor, particularly if the initial presentation is CHF.[114]

Alleviating Symptoms. Responses to therapeutic intervention can be highly variable, so therapy must be individually tailored for symptom control. Treatment of asymptomatic children is controversial. Many clinicians treat asymptomatic patients (particularly if there is a malignant family history of sudden death) to try to improve the clinical course of the disease. Note that none of these therapies to date have shown to improve survival, but rather the goal is symptom control. Medical therapy includes the use of negative inotropes, calcium channel blockers, and antiarrhythmics (if warranted).

Negative inotropes such as β-blockers and disopyramide improve symptoms of angina, dyspnea, exercise intolerance, and presyncope. These agents are thought to decrease left ventricular ejection acceleration with subsequent reduction of SAM and LVOTO.[134]

Calcium channel blockers are believed to improve LV relaxation and filling and may reduce myocardial ischemia.[135] These agents are often used in patients who continue to have symptoms while receiving β-blockers.

Verapamil has been used most often; nifedipine and diltiazem have also shown beneficial effects. Care must be used in patients with severe outflow tract obstruction because the vasodilating properties of calcium channel blockers in this scenario can be detrimental.

Arrhythmias are a frequent complication of HCM. QTc prolongation, ventricular tachycardia, WPW syndrome, and atrial fibrillation are associated with sudden death in adults with HCM.[129,136,137] Although whether this phenomena holds true for children is uncertain, many clinicians treat arrhythmias in symptomatic patients, particularly in those with syncope. Amiodarone has been shown to be effective in treating both atrial fibrillation and ventricular tachycardia.[135] Clinical effect, side effects, and concurrent drug interactions determine the choice of a specific antiarrhythmic.

Diuretics are used cautiously as high filling pressure are required to augment cardiac output. Generally diuretics are reserved for infants presenting in CHF. Positive inotropes are contraindicated because they can worsen dynamic LVOTO.

Surgical Intervention. Patients who fail medical management and who remain symptomatic may undergo surgical septal myectomy-myotomy for relief of LVOTO. Myectomy-myotomy can relieve both the obstruction and the mitral regurgitation. Reducing left ventricular systolic pressure decreases myocardial oxygen demand and can improve symptoms in many patients.[138] Perioperative mortality is low, and postoperative management is similar to that of other open heart procedures.[139] Surgical myectomy has not been shown to improve survival in patients with HCM. The rare patient who remains symptomatic after medical and surgical management or who progresses to the dilated form of cardiomyopathy may be considered for cardiac transplantation.

Dual-Chamber Pacing. In select patients who are refractory to medical management, dual-chamber pacing has been implemented. In some patients this approach can decrease LVOTO and improve symptoms.[140,141] The mechanism for improvement remains unclear. It has been postulated that RV apex pacing, along with a short AV interval, changes the septal activation sequence, resulting in dyssynchronous septal contraction, improved diastolic filling, and ventricular remodeling.[142] Occasionally, pharmacologic prolongation of AV conduction time or AV node ablation is required to maintain AV sequential pacing. This treatment modality remains controversial and is not universally embraced by all clinicians.[143]

Reducing the Risk of Sudden Death. HCM is a significant cause of sudden death in adolescents and young adults. Risk factors include malignant family history of sudden death from HCM, syncope, young age, and, in adults, ventricular tachycardia on Holter monitoring.[144] The cause of sudden death is presumed to be either a ventricular arrhythmia or myocardial ischemia. Because sudden death often occurs during exercise, the patient should be restricted from engaging in strenuous exertion or competitive sports.

To date, predicting the clinical course of HCM is impossible because it is so heterogeneous in presentation and progression. Medical and surgical management help control symptoms, but unfortunately, no intervention has been shown to improve survival.

CARDIAC RHYTHM DISTURBANCES

Technologic advances and a better understanding of cardiac electrophysiology have improved accurate diagnosis and management of cardiac rhythm disturbances. In addition, an expanding array of innovative treatment modalities, including new antiarrhythmics, pacing algorithms, and radiofrequency catheter ablation, have improved outcomes.

Arrhythmia diagnosis can be a relatively simple and concise or challenging and complex. The management of abnormal heart rhythms can range from simple vagal maneuvers to antiarrhythmic medication, pacemaker placement, or radiofrequency catheter ablation. The sections that follow detail the diagnosis and management of cardiac rhythm disturbances in infants and children.

Etiology and Pathogenesis

A wide variety of structural and functional cardiac diseases, along with systemic diseases, can be the underlying cause of rhythm disturbances. Most arrhythmias are due to abnormal impulse conduction (reentrant circuits), abnormal impulse generation (increased automaticity or an ectopic focus), or a combination of both.

Generally the sinus node determines heart rate and rhythm. In the presence of sinus node dysfunction or suppression, the distal portions (AV node, His bundle) of the conduction system will take over. The rate of sinus node discharge is primarily determined by autonomic tone. In addition, changes in the cellular milieu can affect sinus node activity (i.e., temperature, pH, Po_2, and extracellular potassium and calcium concentrations).

The presence of an accessory connection, suture lines, or scarring can form the substrate for reentrant arrhythmias. These arrhythmias are triggered by an extrasystole and are propagated over the substrate until they are terminated by block (adenosine, pacing, and cardioversion) in one of the limbs of the reentrant circuit. See the section on ECG interpretation in Chapter 7.

All cardiac cells are excitable and can spontaneously depolarize; this is called *automaticity.* Abnormal automaticity can occur anywhere in the conduction system or in isolated myocytes (ectopic focus). Autonomic tone or conditions that contribute to local changes in cell membrane potential, such as excessive cardiac stretch, ischemia, hypokalemia, and digoxin toxicity, affect these rhythm abnormalities. Ectopic impulse initiation competes with and can suppress normal sinus node activity. Automatic rhythms are generally not responsive to adenosine or pacing for termination.

Diagnosis

Many factors are considered when evaluating a child with a rhythm disturbance. An accurate history is critically important, particularly because many arrhythmias do not happen in a predictable manner. The ability to determine symptoms depends on the age of the child; infants or small children will not be able to adequately describe symptoms associated with palpitations or tachycardia. Older children will be able to identify triggering events, onset, and termination of rhythm abnormalities. In evaluations, the onset and termination of arrhythmias should be identified. Older children can easily describe the sudden onset and termination of supraventricular tachycardia. Automatic tachyarrhythmias are less easily identifiable because of their typical "warm up" (slow increase in heart rate) and "cool down" (slow deceleration). Associated symptoms and should be identified; these include chest pain, fatigue, light-headedness, and syncope. Precipitating events should be investigated as well. Past medical history of congenital or acquired cardiac disease, infectious diseases, or genetic syndromes is investigated. Any family history of cardiac rhythm disturbance or sudden unexplained death in young adults or teenagers should also be investigated. The physical examination concentrates on the cardiovascular system. Cardiac auscultation reveals abnormal murmurs, clicks, and other sounds that are clues to the identification of structural heart disease. The rate and regularity of the cardiac rhythm are assessed. Physical signs that the rhythm disturbance compromises cardiac function or tissue perfusion are noted.

Electrocardiogram. The surface 12- or 15-lead ECG and the cardiac rhythm strip are important tools for ECG interpretation and arrhythmia detection. However, such recordings illustrate cardiac rhythm at a single point in time and may not reveal abnormalities. The mechanism of the arrhythmia also may remain unclear because P waves may be difficult to visualize. Recording the ECG with an esophageal electrode or from epicardial pacing wires provides additional information when the heart rate is rapid or when atrial activity is difficult to distinguish.

Current telemetry and arrhythmia monitoring units are helpful in caring for patients with arrhythmias in the critical care unit. These systems store electrocardiographic strips for analysis and can recognize some types of specific rhythm abnormalities.

Echocardiography. The echocardiogram is performed to evaluate cardiac structure and function. CHDs often associated with cardiac rhythm disturbances are listed in Box 18-5. Decreased ventricular contractility in the face of a rhythm disturbance presents a dilemma. Has the arrhythmia led to a poorly contractile ventricle or is a poorly functioning heart the cause of the rhythm disturbance? Baseline evaluation of ventricular function also is important because antiarrhythmics may depress function further.

Electrophysiology Study. Invasive evaluation of the conduction system is undertaken with an electrophysiologic study (EPS). At cardiac catheterization, multiple catheters in the right heart are used to record the ECG from various sites (the SA node, AV node, and His bundle). With the aid of pacing protocols and manipulation of automaticity (isoproterenol, atropine, β-blockers), automatic foci or accessory pathways can be located. In addition to definitive diagnosis of a rhythm disturbance, EPS permits evaluation of medi-

cation efficacy and therapeutic ablation of an arrhythmogenic substrate.

Sinus Node Abnormalities

Sinus bradycardia, sinus tachycardia, and sinus node disease (SND) (also called sick sinus syndrome) may be seen in pediatric patients in the PICU. Both sinus bradycardia and tachycardia are fairly common and generally are not cardiac in etiology; they result from other underlying causes. SND is more common in children who have extensive atrial incision lines or scarring (Fontan, Mustard, Senning) or who have atrial pressure elevation or dilation (Fontan, mitral stenosis, cardiomyopathy).[145]

Sinus bradycardia is a heart rate less than the lower limits for age. Sinus tachycardia is heart rate greater than age-related normal values (see Table 7-7).

SND manifests as sinus bradycardia or sinus arrest or as a combination of bradycardia and atrial tachyarrhythmias (brady-tachy syndrome). SND can also contribute to the development of junctional rhythm as a result of abnormal sinus node suppression.

Etiology and Clinical Presentation. Sinus bradycardia may be caused by hypoxia, hyperkalemia, vagal stimulation, increased intracranial pressure, hypothyroidism, sedation, anesthesia, hypothermia, or sleep. Cardiac causes include sinus node dysfunction and medications (e.g., digoxin or β-blockers). Sinus tachycardia is a physiologic response to fever, sepsis, pain, anxiety, anemia, hypovolemia, thyrotoxicosis or CHF, or it may be caused by medications (e.g., catecholamines).

SND is most often seen in pediatric patients who have had atrial surgery for CHD, most notably atrial baffling procedures (Senning, Mustard) for transposition of the great vessels or the Fontan procedure. Inadvertent trauma to the SA node or its blood supply has been implicated in the development of SND. Follow-up of patients who had a Mustard, Senning, or Fontan procedure revealed SND in 50%.[146,147] Also at risk for SND, although less commonly affected, are those who have operations for ASD, AVSD, Ebstein's anomaly, and anomalous pulmonary venous return. Infrequently, SND is seen in patients with unrepaired mitral stenosis, ASD, or single-ventricle physiology.

Other nonsurgical causes of SND include myocarditis, cardiomyopathy, and myocardial ischemia. Increased vagal tone can induce SND. Antiarrhythmics (e.g., digoxin, β-blockers, calcium channel blockers, and type I medications) may cause sinus node dysfunction as a side effect.

Many pediatric patients with SND are asymptomatic except when the heart rate is excessively slow. Children with SND may not demonstrate a normal chronotropic response (increase in heart rate) with exercise or stress. Therefore these patients will complain of fatigue, exercise intolerance, presyncope, or syncope. Infants may exhibit poor feeding, lethargy, and CHF.

Critical Care Management. Treatment of sinus bradycardia requires the identification of the underlying cause and assessment of hemodynamic significance. The majority of children with sinus bradycardia respond to stimulation,

Box 18-5
Congenital Heart Defects and Cardiac Rhythm Disturbances

Unoperated Congenital Heart Defects

Eisenmenger's Syndrome (Pulmonary Vascular Obstructive Disease)

Ventricular arrhythmias (ventricular volume and pressure
  overload)
Sudden death
Atrial fibrillation or flutter

Pulmonary Stenosis or Atresia and Cyanosis

SVT
Atrial fibrillation or flutter
Ventricular arrhythmias (especially with marked polycythemia)

Ebstein's Anomaly

SVT
WPW with SVT
Atrial flutter or fibrillation
AV block
Junctional rhythm
Ventricular tachycardia and fibrillation

Corrected Transposition of the Great Arteries

AV block (second or third degree)
WPW with SVT

Tricuspid Atresia

Atrial ectopy, flutter, fibrillation
Ventricular ectopy

Aortic Stenosis and Coarctation of the Aorta

Ventricular arrhythmias (with marked elevation of left
  ventricular pressure)

Tetralogy of Fallot (in Older Patients)

Ventricular arrhythmias
SVT

Atrial Septal Defects (in Older Patients)

Atrial flutter and fibrillation
SVT
Junctional and ectopic atrial rhythms
Sinus node dysfunction (sinus venosus ASD)
AV block (primum ASD)

Postoperative Arrhythmias in Congenital Heart Disease

*Extensive Atrial Surgery/Repairs With Elevated Atrial
Pressure (Fontan Procedure, Mustard or Senning Repair, Total
Anomalous Pulmonary Venous Return, Atrial Septal Defect
[Rare])*

Supraventricular arrhythmias
SVT*
Incisional intraatrial reentrant tachycardia
Sinus node dysfunction
Sinus bradycardia
Ventricular arrhythmias (as patients age)

*Ventricular Septal Surgery (Ventricular Septal Defect,
Tetralogy of Fallot, AV Canal Defects, Subaortic Stenosis)*

AV conduction block
Ventricular tachycardia†

*An unusual form of SVT, junctional ectopic tachycardia, or accelerated junctional rhythm is seen most commonly after repair of tetralogy of Fallot or the Fontan repair.

†Ventricular tachycardia is also noted after repair of the Ebstein's anomaly, coronary artery anomalies, single-ventricle defects with the Fontan procedure, and
  D-transposition of the great arteries.

SVT, Supraventricular tachycardia; *WPW,* Wolff-Parkinson-White syndrome; *ASD,* atrioseptal defect; *AV,* atrioventricular.

oxygen, or hand ventilation. Acute management, if the bradycardia is refractory to the aforementioned interventions, is intravenous administration of atropine or epinephrine. Protracted, hemodynamically significant bradycardia can be treated with temporary atrial pacing (in the absence of AV node block) or isoproterenol.

Treatment of sinus tachycardia lies in remedying the underlying cause of the physiologic response of the heart to demands for increased cardiac output.

Treatment of SND is dependent on symptoms and associated atrial arrhythmias. Permanent pacemaker implantation is indicated for excessively slow heart rates and symptom control. SND and bradycardia increase the risk for atrial fibrillation or flutter.[148,149] Therefore antibradycardia pacing is advocated in this population to suppress the development of atrial tachyarrhythmias.[145]

Atrial Arrhythmias

Atrial arrhythmias can be the consequence of an automatic or reentrant rhythm abnormality. Atrial arrhythmias include premature atrial contractions, supraventricular tachycardia (AV reentrant tachycardia, AV nodal reentrant tachycardia, atrial ectopic tachycardia), atrial fibrillation, atrial flutter, and intraatrial reentrant tachycardia.

Premature atrial contractions (PACs) are common, particularly in infants and children. Isolated PACs are a benign condition (even if they occur frequently) and are not treated, so they are not discussed here.

Supraventricular Tachycardia. SVT is the most common rhythm abnormality in infants and children. SVT is a broad term that encompasses a number of tachycardia mechanisms. It can be caused by either a reentrant or automatic mechanism (Box 18-6).

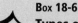

Box 18-6
Types of Supraventricular Tachycardia

Reentry With an Accessory Connection

Wolff-Parkinson-White syndrome (manifest accessory
   connection)
Atrioventricular nodal reentry tachycardia (AVNRT)
Atrioventricular reentry tachycardia (AVRT)
Incisional intraatrial reentry tachycardia (IART)
Permanent junctional reciprocating tachycardia

Ectopic Focus With Increased Automaticity

Atrial ectopic tachycardia (AET)
Junctional ectopic tachycardia (JET)

Etiology and Clinical Presentation

Reentrant SVT. The substrate for reentrant tachycardias is an accessory connection that allows propagation of the tachycardia via retrograde conduction from the ventricles to the atria and antegrade conduction down the AV node.[150] Reentrant mechanisms are responsible for the majority of SVTs and by definition can be initiated and terminated by pacing. Termination can also be achieved by blocking one arm of the circuit (AV node) with adenosine. Atrioventricular reentrant tachycardia (AVRT) and atrioventricular nodal reentrant tachycardia (AVNRT) are specific terms identifying the electrophysiologic cause of the most commonly encountered forms of clinical SVT. AVRT is most often encountered in infants and small children. Substrate for the arrhythmia is an accessory connection (AC) as previously described. Sometimes the AC is not apparent on surface ECG in sinus rhythms. In a subset of patients, the AC is apparent on ECG in sinus rhythm (ventricular preexcitation); this suggests WPW syndrome and is diagnosed by the presence of a delta wave and short PR interval on ECG (see Chapter 7). To truly diagnose WPW syndrome, the patient must have ventricular preexcitation and SVT. Some individuals may have ventricular preexcitation on ECG and no SVT, and therefore they are asymptomatic. There is an increased risk for sudden death in patients with WPW. Sudden death in WPW is due to atrial fibrillation and the rapid anterograde conduction of atrial fibrillation over the AC, resulting in a rapid ventricular rhythm. Cardiac arrest has been reported as the first rhythm abnormality in otherwise asymptomatic patients with WPW.[151]

AVNRT is a reentrant rhythm occurring within the AV node with two distinct AV node pathways (dual AV node physiology). This form of SVT usually manifests in childhood or adolescence. Premature junctional reciprocation tachycardia (PJRT) is another reentrant tachyarrhythmia, but it is rare and is not discussed.

Both AVRT and AVNRT are clinically similar and respond in like manner to therapeutic intervention. The most common ages for occurrence of SVT are the first year of life and puberty. Infants usually present with poor feeding, pallor, and irritability. Up to 50% can present in CHF.[150,152]

Older children complain of palpitations or heart racing that is sudden in onset and termination. They may have associated chest pain, light-headedness and, rarely, syncope. Any child with WPW syndrome and syncope warrants EPS for risk stratification and documentation of life-threatening arrhythmia and consideration of radiofrequency ablation.

Automatic SVT. Automatic SVTs are due to enhanced automaticity or a discrete focus in the atrium. These rhythms cannot be terminated or initiated by pacing, although the rhythm can be suppressed by rapid overdrive pacing. Atrial ectopic tachycardia (AET) and JET are the two forms encountered most often in children. AET commonly presents in infancy, and it can be incessant or intermittent.[153,154] This rhythm abnormality can be an important cause of cardiomyopathy if not identified in a timely manner.[155] (See discussion of JET under section on junctional arrhythmias.)

Clinically this rhythm can be difficult to identify because it can mimic sinus tachycardia, as the rates may not be excessively high. Palpitations are uncommon; more typically the patient presents in heart failure or with decreased ventricular function.

ECG Characteristics.

AVRT and AVNRT are manifested as a narrow complex, regular tachyarrhythmia that is sudden in onset and termination. Retrograde P waves follow the QRS but may be hard to identify in AVNRT. Rates in infants are 250 to 300 beats/min; in children, up to 250 beats/min; and in adolescents, 150 to 220 beats/min (Table 18-10).

The ECG in AET can be variable, depending on the site of origin in the atria. It exhibits a warm-up and cooldown on initiation and termination, atrial rates vary from 130 to 300 beats/min. P waves before the QRS are visible, but morphology is different from the P wave in sinus rhythm. The PR interval is prolonged, particularly at faster rates. This rhythm does not terminate with AV block.

Critical Care Management.

Management of SVT is determined by the underlying substrate and clinical symptoms. Many patients with reentrant SVT will have infrequent, short episodes of tachycardia that require no intervention. The natural history of most reentrant SVT is benign with an excellent outcome. Approximately 25% to 30% of infants with reentrant tachycardia will have no clinical or inducible SVT by 1 year of age. In addition, infants with WPW syndrome can have loss of ventricular preexcitation (delta wave) on surface ECG at 1 year.[152]

In hemodynamically stable SVT that does not convert spontaneously, vagal maneuvers may be successful. Note that this approach will only terminate reentrant SVT, not AET. The diving reflex can be elicited by applying ice to the face or by submerging the face in ice water. Cold fat necrosis can occur with prolonged applications of ice to the face. It is recommended that ice be applied to the less fatty areas of the infant's face and a cloth barrier be used.[156] Elicitation of the diving reflex works best with infants and young children. Older children can be instructed to bear down, blow against a thumb placed in the lips without exhaling, or stand on their heads.

TABLE 18-10 Characteristics of Sinus and Supraventricular Tachycardia

	Sinus Tachycardia	Supraventricular Tachycardia
History	Febrile illness, dehydration, or volume loss	Lethargy or irritability, poor feeding, pallor, diaphoresis without specific causation
Examination	Consistent with fever, dehydration, or bleeding	Signs of CHF: tachypnea, rales, dyspnea, hepatomegaly, decreased tissue perfusion
Chest x-ray film	Normal heart size, clear lung fields	Cardiomegaly, pulmonary edema
ECG*	Heart rate usually >200 beats/min, slight variation in R-R intervals, P waves visible, narrow QRS	Heart rate >220 beats/min, regular R-R intervals, P waves may be retrograde or nondetectable (50%), narrow QRS (>90%)
Echocardiogram	Usually normal	Ventricular dilation, dysfunction

Data from Hanisch DG, Perron L: Complex dysrhythmias in infants and children, *AACN Clin Issues Crit Care Nurs* 3:255-267, 1992.
*An additional ECG finding, if the onset of the arrhythmia is captured: ST will manifest a gradual acceleration in heart rate as compared with the abrupt onset of SVT.
CHF, Congestive heart failure; *ECG,* electrocardiogram.

Patients with frequent sustained episodes require antiarrhythmic therapy for control. Acute termination of reentrant SVT through AV nodal blockade is accomplished by adenosine. This must be given rapid intravenous push at a port proximal to the patient, followed by a large-volume rapid flush. Occasionally, reonset of SVT will occur despite temporary termination with adenosine. If the tachycardia is incessant and hemodynamically significant, intravenous procainamide or amiodarone is used to convert to sinus rhythm. These patients require close monitoring in the PICU, frequent ECGs to evaluate for associated QTc prolongation, and support of hemodynamics. Once the rhythm is controlled, they can switch to oral antiarrhythmics.

Less critically ill patients with frequent SVT can be managed with oral agents such as β-blockers, digoxin, amiodarone, flecainide, and verapamil, noting that intravenous verapamil is contraindicated in infants under 1 year of age because of related cardiovascular collapse. (See the section on antiarrhythmic therapy in Chapter 7 for detailed review of the listed medications.)

AET can be quite resistant to pharmacologic therapy. Although some children outgrow this rhythm, many develop cardiomyopathy in the interim. Rate control is important, particularly in the face of ventricular dysfunction. Many antiarrhythmics are ineffective, with class IC and III being the most effective.[153,154] Intravenous amiodarone is very effective in the critically ill child with AET.[157] Oral amiodarone, sotalol, and flecainide are effective for chronic therapy.

Overdrive atrial pacing is sometimes used to terminate reentrant SVT that is incessant and refractory to pharmacologic intervention. The atrium is paced (esophageal electrode or epicardial electrodes) at a rate faster than the SVT rate for up to 30 seconds. Initially, if pacing is not successful, the rate can be increased incrementally, but it should not be so rapid as to induce atrial fibrillation. Pacing will not terminate AET.

Radiofrequency catheter ablation is recommended for any children with SVT, WPW syndrome, or AET who have frequent episodes of tachycardia, are refractory to medications, have ventricular dysfunction, or syncope. Complications are rare (approximately 3%), and freedom from arrhythmia recurrence is 70% to 90% (dependent on the arrhythmogenic substrate).[155,158]

Atrial Fibrillation. Atrial fibrillation is rare in children with structurally normal hearts. However, in children with atrial enlargement (Fontan, mitral regurgitation [MR], Ebstein's anomaly, cardiomyopathy) or ventricular dysfunction, it can be hemodynamically significant.[149] Atrial fibrillation can be life threatening in patients with WPW syndrome who have rapid antegrade conduction across their AC.

Etiology and Clinical Presentation. Mechanism of atrial fibrillation involves multiple reentry circuits within the atria. These give rise to small, disorganized electrical waves of activity. AV node conduction is variable, with an irregular ventricular rate. In children, atrial fibrillation generally occurs in the setting of congenital heart disease, thyrotoxicosis, WPW syndrome, or cardiomyopathy, or it can be familial.[150]

Clinically these patients may be asymptomatic, with an irregular heart rate often being a serendipitous finding on routine examination. If the ventricular rate is rapid, the child may complain of palpitations or heart racing. Patients with WPW syndrome may present symptoms of tachycardia, syncope, and cardiac arrest.

ECG Characteristics. No visible P wave with disorganized atrial activity is evident that results in either coarse or fine fibrillatory waves. There is no discrete atrial activity, and the ventricular rate is variable and irregular because of variable AV conduction.

Critical Care Management. Atrial fibrillation is unresponsive to pacing. Synchronized cardioversion is necessary for conversion if the episode does not terminate spontaneously (Box 18-7). Before cardioversion, it must be determined how long the patient has been in atrial fibrillation. Intracardiac thrombus can form if atrial fibrillation has been present for longer than 48 hours, despite anticoagulation. Therefore transesophageal echocardiogram must be performed to evaluate for thrombus, given that the risk for embolization is significant during cardioversion.

Intravenous procainamide may be helpful in converting the rhythm or in making refractory atrial fibrillation responsive to cardioversion. Digoxin is effective in ventricular rate

Box 18-7
Cardioversion and Defibrillation in Pediatric Patients

Indications

Synchronized Cardioversion (R Wave Sensing Ensured)

Intraatrial reentry tachycardia (IART), atrial flutter or fibrillation

Supraventricular tachycardia

Ventricular tachycardia

Not indicated for junctional ectopic tachycardia or chaotic atrial rhythm

Defibrillation (Asynchronous)

Pulseless ventricular tachycardia

Ventricular fibrillation

Sedation

If awake: choice of agent will vary with institutional and clinician preference and is based on the patient's clinical status.

Fentanyl, propofol, midazolam (Versed), lorazepam (Ativan), morphine sulfate, or ketamine can be used as single agents or in combination.

Paddle Size

Infant: 4.5 cm

Child: 8 or 13 cm (ensure good contact with skin)

Multifunction Pad Size

Less than 15 kg: pediatric

Greater than 15 kg: adult

Electrode Placement

Standard

Base at upper right chest

Apex at left anterior axillary line

Anterior-Posterior

Base on anterior chest over the heart

Apex on the back

Energy Dose

Synchronized Cardioversion

0.5-1 watt-second (joule) per kg

Repeat with 2 watt-second/kg if needed

Defibrillation

2 watt-second/kg

Repeat with 4 watt-second/kg if needed

Adapted from Perry JC, Garson A: Diagnosis and treatment of arrhythmias, *Adv Pediatr* 36:177-200, 1989.

---

control by slowing AV node conduction, and it may be helpful in improving hemodynamics to prevent recurrences.

Atrial Flutter/Intraartial Reentrant Tachycardia. Classic atrial flutter (AF) is a regular reentrant atrial rhythm, is usually found in infants with structurally normal hearts, and is rare.[149] Intraatrial reentrant tachycardia (IART) accounts for most of the "atrial flutter" in children and often occurs in patients who have undergone surgical correction of congenital heart disease.

Etiology and Clinical Presentation. AF is rare but can be seen in neonates with structurally normal hearts. Often the diagnosis is made on fetal echocardiogram. The atrial rates are usually 250 to 450 beats/min, with variable AV conduction and ventricular rate. CHF can develop if there is delay in making the diagnosis.

IART is a reentrant rhythm and has slow atrial rates (up to 250 beats/min), which distinguishes IART from classic AF. Atrial surgery (Fontan, Mustard, Senning, ASD, and TAPVR repair) is the usual cause of arrhythmia substrate.[25,159] In addition, conditions that contribute to AV valve regurgitation or stenosis with subsequent atrial dilation (MR, mitral stenosis [MS], tricuspid regurgitation, Ebstein's anomaly) are associated with IART.[51,148] Atrial suture lines, atrial scarring, or abnormal atrial tissue caused by chronic atrial volume and pressure overload form the arrhythmia substrate. An atrial circuit, usually around the suture lines, characterizes the reentrant course of IART, with sufficient recovery time in one limb of the circuit to allow tachycardia propagation.[159]

Clinically, children with AF and IART usually present with a **fixed,** (this can be the key to diagnosis) rapid heart

rate that does not vary with activity or physiologic state (sleep). If the rate is slow, the patient may be asymptomatic. If the ventricular rates are high, the child may complain of palpitations, heart racing, fatigue, and exercise intolerance. If not identified in a timely manner, CHF may ensue. The development of IART often indicates poor hemodynamics and is often seen in children with SND and bradycardia.[51]

ECG Characteristics. AF is characterized by rapid, regular sawtooth flutter waves that are morphologically different from the P waves in sinus rhythm. Variable AV conduction is often present (usually 2:1), so the subsequent ventricular rate is half the atrial rate.

IART is sometimes difficult to identify on ECG. The atrial rate is usually 250 beats/min or less, without the classic sawtooth flutter waves found in AF. The P waves are distinct from the sinus P wave and are frequently of low amplitude. If 2:1 conduction is present, the ventricular rate will be slower than classic AF, making diagnosis difficult. Although adenosine will not usually terminate the arrhythmia, it is helpful in making the diagnosis with ECG because AV block will slow the ventricular rate, making the flutter waves more apparent (Fig. 18-33). This arrhythmia should always be suspected in any patient who has undergone a Fontan, Senning, or Mustard procedure with a fixed, nonvariable heart rate or with a heart rate that is more rapid than expected.

Critical Care Management. In the neonate with a structurally normal heart, AF is easily terminated with synchronized cardioversion or atrial overdrive pacing. Late recurrences are uncommon, and chronic antiarrhythmic therapy is unnecessary.

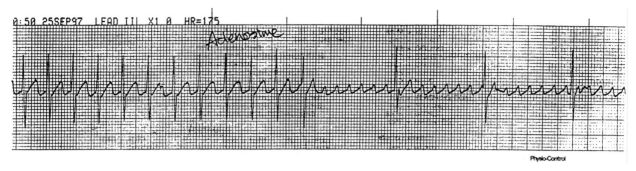

Fig. 18-33 ECG of infant in intraatrial reentrant tachycardia. To confirm diagnosis, a dose of adenosine was given to produce AV block, making flutter waves more apparent.

IART requires conversion to sinus rhythm, along with evaluation of hemodynamics. Medical or surgical interventions to maximize hemodynamics can help control recurrences. Some patients can present in asymptomatic IART and in hindsight may have been in this rhythm for weeks or months. These patients are at risk for the development of intracardiac thrombi resulting from atrial stasis, even if currently on anticoagulation therapy. The risk of embolic phenomena is not insignificant in patients with atrial flutter and can occur with cardioversion.[160] Therefore thrombi must be ruled out with transesophageal echocardiogram (TEE) before cardioversion.[161] Hemodynamically stable patients with intracardiac thrombi present a therapeutic dilemma. If clot is present in the left atrium, then many clinicians advocate anticoagulation with repeat TEE before cardioversion. The ideal period for anticoagulation has yet to be determined. However if ventricular function is decreased, the patient is hemodynamically unstable, or if the clot is on the systemic venous side of the heart, then cardioversion is performed.

Synchronized cardioversion (0.5 to 1 watt/kg) is usually effective in restoring sinus rhythm. Some patients are refractory or may develop recurrence of IART. In this scenario, intravenous procainamide or amiodarone may be effective in either converting the rhythm or improving the ability to electrically cardiovert. Chronic antiarrhythmic therapy is individualized and can consist of amiodarone, procainamide, β-blockers, or sotalol.

Rapid overdrive atrial pacing may also terminate IART. This must be performed in a controlled environment because the atrium is paced at a rate just faster than the atrial tachycardia rate. Rapid atrial burst pacing or the introduction of PACs after rapid atrial pacing will make one limb of the circuit refractory, thereby terminating the arrhythmia. This technique is most effective if the child has not been in IART for a protracted period of time. Coexisting SND and bradycardia are risk factors for the development of IART. Therefore the recommendation is that these patients be permanently paced (modes AAI or DDD at rates of about 80 beats/min) to prevent the development or recurrence of IART.

Radiofrequency catheter ablation, cryoablation, and the Maze procedure have all been advocated as treatment for incessant refractory IART. To date, the success of radiofre-

quency catheter ablation is less than satisfactory, with recurrence as high as 50%.[162,163] Intraoperative cryoablation is currently advocated in some Fontan patients during surgical revision from intracardiac to an extracardiac Fontan, particularly because the atrium cannot be accessed for catheter ablation after this procedure.[164,165] Antitachycardia pacemakers have been implanted during surgery in select patients to terminate postoperative IART.[165] The Maze procedure is infrequently performed in children; however, in adults it is advocated for control of AF or atrial fibrillation. In this operative procedure, a number of surgical incisions are made in the atrium (taking care to prevent injury to the sinus node) to interrupt the reentrant circuit. This surgery can be curative in up to 98% of adult patients.[166]

Atrioventricular Nodal and Junctional Arrhythmias

Junctional arrhythmias are the consequence of abnormal automaticity in the AV node or HIS bundle, which produces JET. They can also be due to sinus node slowing or disease with subsequent junctional escape rhythm. Premature junctional beats or accelerated junctional rhythms are not life threatening so are not discussed in detail. Treatment of SND will generally abolish the junctional rhythm.

Junctional Ectopic Tachycardia. JET is an automatic tachycardia that can be difficult to diagnose and treat.

Etiology and Pathogenesis. JET is an automatic tachycardia caused by enhanced automaticity of the AV node or proximal His bundle. Most often, JET is a transient phenomenon occurring acutely in infants or young children after cardiac surgery (TOF, VSD, TGA). Rarely, JET is seen as a congenital rhythm disturbance in infants with structurally normal hearts.

The pathophysiologic consequences of JET are the result of both the sustained rapid heart rate and associated decrease in ventricular filling caused by loss of "atrial kick" from AV dissociation. In postoperative cardiac surgery patients, profound hypotension and cardiovascular collapse may develop. Infants with congenital JET develop left ventricular dysfunction over several months.[154]

ECG Characteristics. The ECG of JET is characterized by a narrow QRS, the morphology of which is similar to the postoperative sinus rhythm. (This can make it difficult

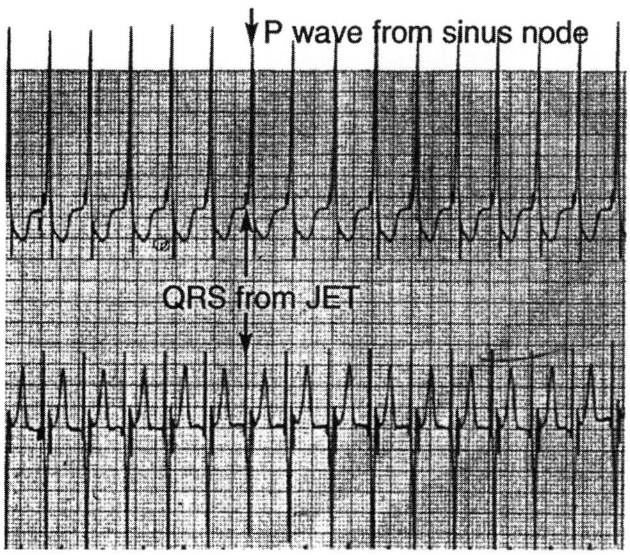

Fig. 18-34 Atrial ECG of infant in junctional ectopic tachycardia *(JET)*. Top recording is from atrial epicardial wires; note that junctional rate is slightly faster than atrial rate.

to distinguish it from an atrial tachycardia.) There is AV dissociation with the ventricular rate faster than the atrial rate. An atrial epicardial or transesophageal ECG is most often necessary to differentiate JET from other types of SVT (Fig. 18-34)

Critical Care Management. Postoperative JET is a transient, self-limiting arrhythmia that resolves spontaneously in hours to days after onset. Mildly increased junctional rates can be well tolerated, but rapid JET results in hemodynamic instability or death. The goal of management is twofold: first, to restore AV synchrony and, second, to slow the junctional tachycardia. AV synchrony is restored, provided the heart rate is less than 200 beats/min, by overdrive atrial or AV sequential pacing at a rate slightly above the junctional rate.

In addition, this rhythm is catecholamine sensitive, so every attempt should be made to decrease or discontinue the infusion of exogenous catecholamines. Unfortunately, poor hemodynamics exacerbate JET, so the risks and benefits of intravenous inotropes must be individually balanced for each patient. Hyperthermia and electrolyte imbalances are treated vigorously.

Early intervention to slow the junctional rate is best achieved by hypothermia to a core temperature of 34° C to 35° C, using a cooling blanket. Occasionally temperatures as low as 33° C are necessary.[167] To prevent shivering, hypothermia necessitates sedation and chemical paralysis with intubation and mechanical ventilation.

Pharmacologic therapy of JET is difficult. Digoxin is generally ineffective in controlling JET, although it may improve hemodynamics. Procainamide alone or in combination with hypothermia has been shown to be effective.[167] Intravenous amiodarone can be used if the JET is refractory to cooling, pacing, or procainamide.[157]

ECMO has been used for emergency support of infants with life-threatening JET. The aim of this therapy is cardiovascular support until the arrhythmia spontaneously resolves.[168] Rarely, catheter ablation has been implemented as a lifesaving maneuver.

Most postoperative patients who develop JET do quite well, as long as ventricular rate is controlled and hemodynamics are supported. If these two goals are not accomplished, death may ensue. Effective therapy usually results in a ventricular rate less than 170 beats/min.

Atrioventricular Conduction Block. Three forms of AV block are discussed here. For further review, see Chapter 7.

Etiology and Clinical Presentation. First-degree heart block is the consequence of slowed impulse conduction through the AV node. It is characterized by a prolonged PR interval on the ECG with a P wave preceding each QRS complex. These patients are asymptomatic because there is no significant hemodynamic impact. This conduction disturbance does not necessitate intervention beyond the identification of its cause. In pediatric patients, digoxin administration is the most common cause of first-degree heart block.

Second-degree heart block occurs when an occasional or patterned block of AV conduction occurs. The ECG characteristics of Mobitz type I and Mobitz type II second-degree heart block have been described in Chapter 7. Mobitz type I second-degree heart block may reflect AV node dysfunction in patients following intracardiac surgical procedures near the AV node or in those with digoxin, β-blocker, calcium channel blocker, or quinidine toxicity. It may be seen in patients without cardiovascular disease, especially during sleep. Most often, treatment is not required because this conduction delay does not compromise cardiac output and it is unlikely to progress to complete heart block.

Mobitz type II second-degree heart block is usually related to His bundle or bundle branch block, most often resulting from surgical injury. Progression to complete heart block can occur.

Complete heart block (CHB) is also called third-degree heart block. It can be related to structural heart disease (L-TGA), it may be congenital in infants with normal cardiac structure, or it may be acquired (myocarditis, surgery). Regardless of the cause, the SA node paces the atria, whereas an independent junctional or ventricular pacemaker establishes the ventricular rhythm. Cardiac output may be compromised if the ventricular rate is excessively slow.

Congenital heart block appears infrequently and most infants have a structurally normal heart. Structural defects associated with congenital heart block are L-TGA, AV septal defects, endocardial fibrosis, and left atrial isomerism. In infants without CHD, a strong association is found between the incidence of congenital CHB and maternal connective tissue disease, typically systemic lupus erythematosus.

Low fetal heart rate usually leads to the prenatal diagnosis of congenital CHB. Fetal echocardiography detects asynchronous and independent contraction of the atria and ventricles. Fetal mortality is high.[169]

After birth, infants with congenital CHB may be asymptomatic, or they may be in severe CHF as manifested by hydrops fetalis, tachypnea, and lethargy. Postnatal mortality is increased if there is associated structural heart disease. After infancy, children with congenital CHB and a structurally normal heart may have exercise intolerance, fatigue, sleep disturbances, or syncope. In these patients, the ventricular rate and the ability to increase heart rate with activity determine their symptoms.

Acquired CHB is most often seen as a complication of intracardiac surgery near the AV junction, although it can also occur secondary to endocarditis, myocarditis, or Lyme disease. Surgical procedures with increased risk for CHB include repair of VSDs or AVSDs, L-TGA, TOF, aortic valve replacement, and mitral or tricuspid valve replacement.[145] Postoperative or acquired CHB may be transient or permanent. In the postoperative period, resumption of sinus rhythm may take up to 2 weeks.

ECG Characteristics.   The P wave in patients with CHB originates in the SA node and is of normal morphology. However, transmission through the AV node is blocked, and an escape rhythm, usually generated by a site high in the His bundle, ensues. The QRS complex may be wide or narrow. The P-P interval is usually regular, as is the R-R interval. The atrial rate is faster than the ventricular rate.

Critical Care Management.   Postoperative heart block is managed acutely by temporary AV sequential pacing, ideally in the DDD mode. If the temporary pacemaker cannot sense the intrinsic atrial rate appropriately, then a DVI or VVI mode can be used (see Chapter 7). Implantation of a permanent pacemaker is recommended in patients with postoperative heart block that persists for 14 days.[79]

The ventricular rate and symptoms determine acute management of CHB. In severe symptomatic, hemodynamically significant bradycardia, a continuous infusion of epinephrine or isoproterenol will increase the heart rate until temporary pacing can be instituted. If the cause of CHB is acquired (other than postoperative CHB), temporary pacing may only be necessary until recovery of the AV node is achieved. If the AV node apparently will not recover, then a permanent pacemaker is needed.

Asymptomatic newborns with congenital CHB are monitored continuously for a number of days before discharge. In newborns, permanent pacing is indicated for CHF, ventricular rate less than 55 beats/min, prolonged QTc, wide QRS escape rhythm, or frequent ventricular ectopy.[169]

Children with congenital CHB are followed closely because symptoms can occur at any age. Exercise testing and Holter monitoring are used to determine heart rate with exercise and to detect ventricular arrhythmias. Frequent ventricular ectopy, exercise intolerance, syncope, low heart rate (6 to 10 years, less than 50 beats/min; 16 to 20 years, less than 45 beats/min), QTc prolongation, or inadequate

heart rate response to exercise are criteria for pacemaker placement.[170,171]

Ventricular Arrhythmias

Infants and children have far fewer ventricular arrhythmias than adults. Premature ventricular contractions and ventricular tachycardia are the ventricular rhythm abnormalities most commonly encountered in pediatric patients.

Premature Ventricular Contractions.   Premature ventricular contractions (PVCs) are recognized on ECG as an early QRS complex with morphology different than that of the sinus QRS. Typically the duration of the QRS complex is prolonged, and the complex is bizarre in appearance. However, a nearly normal appearance and duration of the QRS are not uncommon, particularly in infants.

PVCs can either be single, clustered in groups of two

Box 18-8
Drugs Known to Prolong QTc

Note: These drugs should be avoided if QTc is prolonged or if long QT syndrome is present.

Adrenergic Agents
Adrenaline

Antihistamines
Terfenadine (Seldane)
Astemizole (Hismanal)
Diphenhydramine (Benadryl)

Antibiotics
Erythromycin
Sulfamethoxazole (Septra)
Pentamidine

Antifungals
Ketoconazole
Fluconazole
Itraconazole

GI Medications
Cisapride

Cardiac Medications
Quinidine
Procainamide
Disopyramide
Sotalol
Probucol

Psychotropic Medications
Amitriptyline
Phenothiazines
Haloperidol
Risperidone

(couplets), or occurring in runs (three, four, five, etc., beats in a row). Bigeminy occurs when every other beat is a PVC. The morphology of the PVC should also be evaluated because multiform PVCs may be more ominous. PVCs that are single, uniform, and suppressed with exercise and increased heart rate are benign and do not require treatment in children with structurally normal hearts. These are quite common, noted in as many as 18% of newborns, 6% of infants, 14% of children, and 27% of adolescents.[147] Conversely, children with structural heart defects, multiform PVCs, or couplets are at increased risk for hemodynamic compromise or progression to a lethal ventricular rhythm. Careful surveillance is necessary with periodic Holter monitoring, however, most children with PVCs require only observation and no intervention.

Electrolytes and pH should be monitored in hospitalized children with PVCs, particularly after open heart surgery. Potassium, calcium, and magnesium levels should be kept normal with replacement therapy if necessary. Persistent acidosis should be corrected.

Ventricular Tachycardia. Ventricular tachycardia (VT) is a wide-complex tachycardia with AV dissociation, the origin of which is the ventricle. The ventricular rate will be faster than the atrial rate on ECG. This rhythm can be due to abnormal impulse generation or conduction. Hemodynamic significance of VT depends on the rate, the presence of heart disease, and whether it occurs with exercise. Occasionally a child in SVT will present with wide-complex tachycardia. Clinically significant wide-complex tachycardia should be considered a VT until proven otherwise.

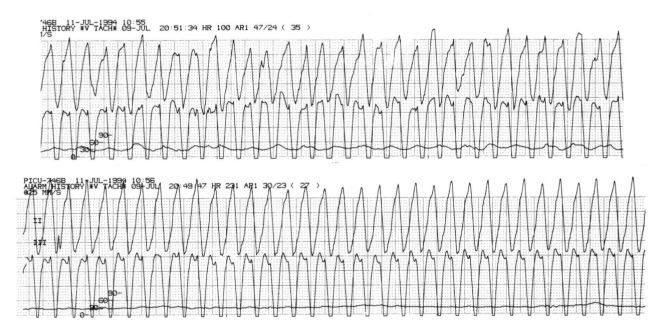

Fig. 18-35   Ventricular tachycardia in 6-month-old with severe left ventricular outflow tract obstruction.

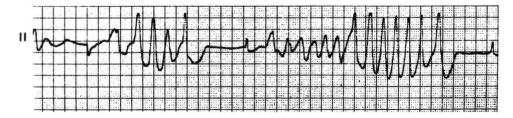

Fig. 18-36   Ventricular tachycardia with torsade de pointes configuration. (From Holbrook PR: *Textbook of pediatric critical care*, Philadelphia, 1993, WB Saunders, p 406.)

Etiology and Clinical Presentation. Causes of VT in infants and children include electrolyte or metabolic disturbances, including acidosis, hypoglycemia, hyperkalemia, hypokalemia, hypercalcemia, hypomagnesemia, and hypothermia. Other potential causes are drug toxicity (digoxin, quinidine, procainamide, sympathomimetics, anesthetic agents, cocaine, caffeine, nicotine) and cardiac pathologic conditions (cardiomyopathy, aortic stenosis, myocarditis, cardiac tumors). VT has been implicated as a cause for sudden death in patients after repair of TOF.[172] Idiopathic or congenital long QT syndrome is characterized by ventricular repolarization abnormalities that can result in polymorphic ventricular tachycardia (torsades de pointes) and sudden death. Idiopathic long QT can be caused by drugs (Box 18-8) or electrolyte imbalances, most notably hypokalemia, hypocalcemia, and hypomagnesemia.[173,174]

Symptoms are dependent on the rate and hemodynamic effects of the VT. If the rate is slow, the tachycardia can be well tolerated, and the patient may be asymptomatic. Rapid rates can result in the sensation of palpitations, light-headedness, syncope, or cardiovascular collapse.

ECG Characteristics. VT occurs at a rate generally between 120 and 300 beats/min. The complexes are wide and can be bizarre in appearance (Fig. 18-35). However, if the VT focus is near the AV node, the QRS may only be slightly prolonged. Torsade de pointes occurs in the presence of QTc prolongation and is characterized as a rapid, spiraling, polymorphic VT, as illustrated in Fig. 18-36.

Critical Care Management. The hemodynamic significance of the rhythm disturbance, age, type of tachycardia, and associated symptoms determine management of VT.

Acute short-term management of hemodynamically significant VT is cardioversion. If the patient is stable, an intravenous bolus of lidocaine followed by a continuous infusion may convert the rhythm to sinus. Intravenous amiodarone can be used in patients who are refractory to lidocaine. Once the rhythm is controlled, attention is directed toward identifying and correcting the underlying cause. Synchronized cardioversion is necessary if the patient is unstable.

Asymptomatic patients with slow ventricular rates and no associated heart disease require no treatment. Various antiarrhythmics can be used for chronic therapy, including amiodarone, β-blockers, flecainide, and propafenone (see Chapter 7).[175]

Radiofrequency catheter ablation can be used to treat some forms of VT, depending on the cause (right or left ventricular outflow tract VT). Surgery to remove intracardiac tumors or to localize and cryoablate hamartomas is advocated if the patient is symptomatic. Automatic internal cardiac defibrillators (AICDs) are implanted in patients with life-threatening ventricular tachycardia and fibrillation.

Patients with long QT syndrome should be treated with chronic β-blocker therapy and occasionally with antibradycardia pacing. The development of torsade de pointes in some of these patients has been shown to be adrenergic dependent—hence the importance of β-blockers. Pacing can help prevent bradycardia and "pause-dependent" torsade de pointes.[176] Treatment of hemodynamically significant torsade de pointes is intravenous magnesium. Defibrillation is used in the patient with cardiovascular collapse.

Ventricular Fibrillation. Ventricular fibrillation (VF) results from erratic firing of multiple ectopic foci in the ventricles, resulting in disorganized electrical activity, ineffective ventricular contraction, and death.

Etiology and Clinical Presentation. VF is uncommon in infants and children. It may occur in patients with structural or functional heart disease or after prolonged resuscitation attempts. VF results in pulselessness and obvious cardiovascular collapse.

ECG Characteristics. An ECG without measurable heart rate in which no P, QRS, or T waves can be identified documents VF. An erratic, wavy baseline is present (Fig. 18-37).

Critical Care Management. Cardiopulmonary resuscitation (CPR) is initiated to maintain circulation and oxygenation while the defibrillator is readied. Rapid asynchronous defibrillation is performed up to three times (2 watt-second/kg the first time and 4 watt-second/kg for

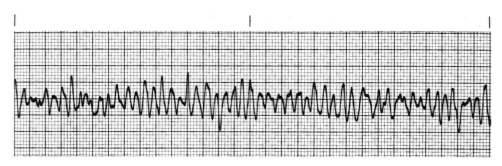

Fig. 18-37 Ventricular fibrillation. (From Curley MAQ: *Pediatric cardiac dysrhythmias,* Bowie, Md, 1985, Brady Communications, p 125. With permission of Appleton & Lange.)

subsequent attempts). If VF persists, intravenous epinephrine (0.01 mg/kg) and lidocaine (1 mg/kg) are administered while CPR continues. Defibrillation (4 watt-second/kg) is attempted 30 to 60 seconds after the medications are administered. Persistent VF is treated with second doses of epinephrine (0.1 to 0.2 mg/kg) and lidocaine (1 mg/kg). Epinephrine may be repeated every 3 to 5 minutes. Bretylium (5 to 10 mg/kg) is considered. Defibrillation (4 watt-second/kg) is repeated 30 to 60 seconds after medication is administered[177] until VF is converted to sinus rhythm or the situation is deemed hopeless and resuscitation attempts are stopped.

SUMMARY

Cardiovascular dysfunction may be the consequence of cardiac rhythm disturbances or of structural, functional, acquired heart diseases. Heart failure, shock, or hypoxemia are the potential final pathways. These phenomena are multifaceted and can occur in any child in the PICU, not only those with the primary diagnosis of heart disease. Care of the critically ill child is optimized by attentive, accurate cardiovascular assessment so that intervention is timely. A sound knowledge base of cardiovascular pathophysiology is important for any nurse caring for critically ill infants and children.

REFERENCES

1. Pollack MM, Getson PR, Rurriman UE et al: Efficiency of intensive care, *JAMA* 258:1481-1486, 1987.
2. Biel M, Eastwood JA, Muenzen P et al: Evolving trends in critical care nursing practice: results of a certification role delineation study, *Am J Crit Care* 8:285-290, 1999.
3. Kohr LM, O'Brien P: Current management of congestive heart failure in infants and children, *Nurs Clin North Am* 30:261-290, 1995.
4. Guidelines for the evaluation and management of heart failure. Report of the American College of Cardiology/American Heart Association Task Force on Practice Guidelines (Committee on Evaluation and Management of Heart Failure), *J Am Coll Cardiol* 26:1376-1398, 1995.
5. Furdon SA: Recognizing congestive heart failure in the neonatal period, *Neonatal Netw* 16:5-13, 1997.
6. Balaguru D, Artman M, Auslender M: Management of heart failure in children, *Curr Probl Pediatr* 30:5-30, 2000.
7. Stewart JM, Hintze TH, Woolf PK et al: Nature of heart failure in patients with ventricular septal defect, *Am J Physiol* 269:H1473-H1480, 1995.
8. Pitt B, Zannad F, Remme WJ et al: The effect of spironolactone on morbidity and mortality in patients with severe heart failure, *N Engl J Med* 341:709-717, 1999.
9. O'Laughlin MP: Congestive heart failure in children, *Pediatr Clin North Am* 46:263-273, 1999.
10. Brunner-La Rocca HP, Vaddadi G, Esler MD: Recent insight into therapy of congestive heart failure: focus on ACE inhibition and angiotension II antagonism, *J Am Coll Cardiol* 33:1163-1173, 1999.
11. Kuklin ML, Kalman J, Charney RH et al: Prospective, randomized comparison of effect of long-term treatment with metoprolol or carvedilol on symptoms, exercise, ejection fraction, and oxidative stress in heart failure, *Circulation* 99:2645-2651, 1999.
12. Shaddy RE: β-blocker therapy in young children with congestive heart failure under consideration for heart transplantation, *Am Heart J* 136:19-21, 1998

13. Shaddy RE, Tani LY, Gidding SS et al: Beta-blocker treatment of dilated cardiomyopathy with congestive heart failure in children: a multi-institutional experience, *J Heart Lung Transplant* 18:269-274, 1999.
14. Gilbert EM, Abraham WT, Olsen S et al: Comparative hemodynamic, left ventricular functional, and antiadrenergic effects of chronic treatment with metoprolol versus carvedilol in the failing heart, *Circulation* 94:2817-2825, 1996.
15. Castaneda AR, Mayer JE, Jonas RA et al: The neonate with critical congenital heart disease: repair: a surgical challenge, *J Thorac Cardiovasc Surg* 98:869-875, 1989.
16. Clark EB: Morphogenesis, growth, and biomechanics: mechanisms of cardiovascular development. In Emmanouilides GC, Riemenschneider TA, Allen HG et al, eds: *Heart disease in infants, children, and adolescents,* Baltimore, 1995, Williams & Wilkins.
17. Van Praagh R: Developmental anatomy: embryology. In Flyer DC, ed: *Nadas' pediatric cardiology,* Philadelphia, 1992, Hanley & Belfus.
18. Dajani AS, Taubert KA, Wilson W et al: Prevention of bacterial endocarditis, *JAMA* 277:1794-1801, 1997.
19. Ing FF, Sommer RJ: The snare assisted technique for transcatheter coil occlusion of moderate to large patent ductus arteriosus: immediate and intermediate results, *J Am Coll Cardiol* 33:1710-1718, 1999.
20. Gatzoulis MA, Rigby ML, Redington AN: Interventional catheterization in paediatric cardiology, *Eur Heart J* 16:1767-1772, 1995.
21. Mandell VS: Interventional procedures for congenital heart disease, *Radiol Clin North Am* 37:439-461, 1999.
22. Chang AD, Wells W: Patent ductus arteriosus. In Chang A, Hanley F, Wernovsky G et al, eds: *Pediatric cardiac critical care,* Philadelphia, 1998, Williams & Wilkins.
23. Vick GW: Defects of the atrial septum including atrioventricular septal defects. In Garson A, Bricker JT, Fisher DJ et al, eds: *The science and practice of cardiology,* Baltimore, 1998, Williams & Wilkins.

24. Chang AD, Jacobs J: Atrial septal defect. In Chang A, Hanley F, Wernovsky G et al, eds: *Pediatric cardiac critical care,* Philadelphia, 1998, Williams & Wilkins.
25. Gatzoulis MA, Freeman MA, Siu SC et al: Atrial arrhythmia after surgical closure of atrial septal defects in adults, *N Engl J Med* 340:839-846, 1999.
26. Rabinovitch M: Structure and function of the pulmonary vascular bed: an update, *Cardiol Clin* 7:227-238, 1989.
27. Neumayer U, Stone S, Somerville J: Small ventricular septal defects in adults, *Eur Heart J* 19:1573-1582, 1998.
28. LeBlanc JG, Russell JL: Pediatric cardiac surgery in the 1990s, *Surg Clin North Am* 78:729-747, 1998.
29. Chang AD, Jacobs J: Ventricular septal defect. In Chang A, Hanley F, Wernovsky G et al, eds: *Pediatric cardiac critical care,* Philadelphia, 1998, Williams & Wilkins.
30. Chang AD, Burke R: Common atrioventricular canal. In Chang A, Hanley F, Wernovsky G et al, eds: *Pediatric cardiac critical care,* Philadelphia, 1998, Williams & Wilkins.
31. Castaneda AR, Jonas RA, Mayer JE et al: *Cardiac surgery of the neonate and infant,* Philadelphia, 1994, WB Saunders.
32. Chang AD, Starnes VA: In Chang A, Hanley F, Wernovsky G et al, eds: *Pediatric cardiac critical care,* Philadelphia, 1998, William & Wilkins.
33. McCrindle B, Jones TK, Morrow WR et al: Acute results of balloon angioplasty of native coarctation versus recurrent aortic obstruction are equivalent, *J Am Coll Cardiol* 28:1810-1817, 1996.
34. Ovaert C, McCrindle BW, Nykanen D et al: Balloon angioplasty of native coarctation: clinical outcomes and predictors of success, *J Am Coll Cardiol* 35:988-996, 2000.
35. Elkins RC, Knott-Craig CJ, Ward KE et al: The Ross operation in children: 10 year follow up, *Ann Thorac Surg* 65:496-502, 1998.
36. Ward KE, Mullins CE: Anomalous pulmonary venous connections, pulmonary vein stenosis, and atresia of the common pulmonary vein. In Garson A, Bricker JT, Fisher DF et al: *The science and practice of*

cardiology, Baltimore, 1998, Williams & Wilkins.

37. Chang AD, Reddy M: Truncus arteriosus. In Chang A, Hanley F, Wernovsky G et al: *Pediatric cardiac critical care,* Philadelphia, 1998, Williams & Wilkins.

38. Tworetzky W, McElhinney DB, Reddy VM et al: Does prenatal diagnosis of hypoplastic left heart syndrome lead to improved surgical outcome? *J Am Coll Cardiol* (suppl A) 31:71A, 1998.

39. Day RW, Barton AJ, Pysher TJ et al: Pulmonary vascular resistance of children treated with nitrogen during early infancy, *Ann Thorac Surg* 65:1400-1404, 1998.

40. Jobes DR, Nicholson SC, Steven JM et al: Carbon dioxide prevents pulmonary overcirculation in hypoplastic left heart syndrome, *Ann Thorac Surg* 54:150-151, 1992.

41. Norwood WI, Lang P, Hansen DD: Physiologic repair of hypoplastic left heart syndrome, *N Engl J Med* 308:23-26, 1983.

42. Wernovsky G, Bove EL: Single ventricle lesions. In Chang A, Hanley F, Wernovsky G et al, eds: *Pediatric cardiac critical care,* Philadelphia, 1998, Williams & Wilkins.

43. Wernovsky G, Jonas R: Transposition of the great arteries. In Chang A, Hanley F, Wernovsky G et al, eds: *Pediatric cardiac critical care,* Philadelphia, 1998, Williams & Wilkins.

44. Neches WH, Park SG, Ettedgui JA: Transposition of the great arteries. In Garson A, Bricker JT, Fisher DJ et al, eds: *Science and practice of cardiology,* Baltimore, 1998, Williams & Wilkins.

45. Grifka RG: Cyanotic congenital heart disease with increased pulmonary blood flow, *Pediatr Clin North Am* 46:405-425, 1999.

46. Bailey CP, Cookson BA, Downing DF et al: Cardiac surgery under hypothermia, *J Thorac Cardiovasc Surg* 27:73-77, 1975.

47. Kay EB, Cross FS: Surgical treatment of transposition of the great vessels, *Surgery* 39:712, 1955.

48. Senning A: Surgical correction of transposition of the great vessels, *Surgery* 45:966-972, 1959.

49. Mustard WT: Successful two-stage correction of transposition of the great arteries, *Surgery* 55:469-474, 1964

50. Turina M, Siehenmann R, Nussbaumer P, et al: Long-term outlook after atrial correction of transposition of the great arteries, *J Thorac Cardiovasc Surg* 95:828-835, 1988.

51. Puley G, Siu S, Connelly M et al: Arrhythmia and survival in patients >18 years of age after the Mustard procedure for complete transposition of the great arteries, *Am J Cardiol* 83:1080-1084, 1999.

52. Yeh T, Connelly MS, Coles JG et al: Atrioventricular discordance: results of repair in 127 patients, *J Thorac Cardiovasc Surg* 117:1190-1203, 1999.

53. Jatene AP, Fontas VF, Saoza LC et al: Anatomic correction of transposition of the great arteries, *J Thorac Cardiovasc Surg* 72:364-371, 1976.

54. Mavroudis C, Backer CL: Arterial switch after failed atrial baffle procedures for trans-position of the great arteries, *Ann Thorac Surg* 69:851-857, 2000.

55. Wernovsky G, Mayer JE, Jonas RA et al: Factors influencing early and late outcome of the arterial switch operation for transposition of the great arteries, *J Thorac Cardiovasc Surg* 109:289-302, 1995.

56. Roth S: Postoperative care. In Chang A, Hanley F, Wernovsky G et al, eds: *Pediatric cardiac critical care,* Philadelphia, 1998, Williams & Wilkins.

57. Marino B, Wernovsky G. Preoperative care. In Chang A, Hanley F, Wernovsky G et al, eds: *Pediatric cardiac critical care,* Philadelphia, 1998, Williams & Wilkins.

58. Fineman JR, Soifer SJ: Pulmonary vascular regulation in newborns, infants and children after surgery for congenital heart disease, *Prog Pediatr Cardiol* 4:125-133, 1995.

59. Mayer J: Cardiopulmonary bypass. In Chang A, Hanley F, Wernovsky G et al, eds: *Pediatric cardiac critical care,* Philadelphia, 1998, Williams & Wilkins.

60. Wynne J, Braunwald E: The cardiomyopathies and myocarditides: toxic, chemical, and physical damage to the heart. In Bruanwald E, ed: *Heart disease,* Philadelphia, 1992, WB Saunders.

61. McElhinney DB, Reddy MV, Parry AJ et al: Management and outcomes of delayed sternal closure after cardiac surgery in neonates and infants, *Crit Care Med* 28:1180-1184, 2000.

62. Burrows FA, Klinck JR, Rabinovitch M et al: Pulmonary hypertension in children: perioperative management, *Can Anaesth Soc J* 33:606-28, 1986.

63. Komai H, Haworth SG: The effect of cardiopulmonary bypass on the lung. In Jonas RA, Elliott MJ, eds: *Cardiopulmonary bypass in neonates, infants, and young children,* Oxford, 1994, Butterworth Heinemann.

64. Wheller J, George BL, Mulder DG et al: Diagnosis and management of postoperative pulmonary hypertensive crisis, *Circulation* 60:1640-1644, 1979.

65. Vargo TA: Cardiac catheterization: Hemodynamic measurements. In Garson A, Bricker JT, Fisher DJ et al, eds: *The science and practice of cardiology,* Baltimore, 1998, Williams & Wilkins.

66. Lock JE, Keane JF, Perry SB: *Diagnostic and interventional catheterization in congenital heart disease,* ed 2, Boston, 2000, Kluwer Academic Publishers.

67. Flori HR, Johnson LD, Hanley FL et al: Transthoracic intracardiac catheters in post-operative congenital heart surgery patients: associated complications and outcomes, *Crit Care Med* 28:2997-3001, 2000.

68. Higgins SS, Turley KM, Harr J et al: Prescription and administration of around the clock analgesics in postoperative pediatric cardiovascular surgery patients, *Prog Cardiovasc Nurs* 14:19-24, 1999.

69. Koren G, Lavi S, Rose V et al: Kawasaki disease: review of risk factors for coronary aneurysms, *J Pediatr* 108:388-392, 1986.

70. Burch GE, Sun S, Chu K et al: Interstitial and coxsackie B myocarditis in infants and children: study of 50 autopsied hearts, *JAMA* 203:1-9, 1968.

71. Moore P, Soifer SJ: Acquired heart disease. In Holbrook PR, ed: *Textbook of pediatric critical care,* Philadelphia, 1993, WB Saunders.

72. Garjarski RJ, Towbin JA: Recent advances in the etiology, diagnosis, and treatment of myocarditis and cardiomyopathies in children, *Curr Opin Pediatr* 7:587-594, 1995.

73. Druker NA, Newburger JW: Viral myocarditis: diagnosis and management, *Adv Pediatr* 44:141-171, 1997.

74. Micevski V: The use of molecular technologies for the detection of enterovirus ribonucleic acid in myocarditis, *J Cardiovasc Nurs* 13:78-90, 1999.

75. Artez HT: Myocarditis: the Dallas criteria, *Hum Pathol* 18:619-624, 1987.

76. Cabinian AE, Kiel RJ, Smith F et al: Modification of exercise-aggravated coxsackie B myocarditis by T lymphocyte suppression, *J Lab Clin Med* 115:454-459, 1990.

77. Abramowitz: Drugs for chronic heart failure, *Med Lett Drugs Ther* 35:40-42, 1993.

78. Pfeffer MA, Braunwald E, Moye LA et al: Effect of captopril on mortality and morbidity in patients with left ventricular dysfunction after myocardial infarction, *N Engl J Med* 327:669-677, 1992.

79. Gregoratos G, Cheitlin MD, Conill A et al: ACC/AHA guidelines for implantation of cardiac pacemakers and antiarrhythmia devices: executive summary, *Circulation* 97: 1325-1335, 1998.

80. Liu P, McLaughlin PR, Sole MJ: Treatment of myocarditis: current recommendations and future approaches, *Heart Failure* 8:33-40, 1992.

81. Tomioka N, Kishimoto C, Matsumori A et al: Effects of prednisone on acute viral myocarditis in mice, *J Am Coll Cardiol* 73:1058, 1986.

82. Monrad ES, Matsumori A, Murphy JC et al: Therapy with cyclosporin in murine myocarditis with encephalomyocarditis virus, *Circulation* 73:1058-1062, 1986.

83. O'Connell JB, Reap EA, Robinson JA: The effects of cyclosporine on acute coxsackie B3 myocarditis, *Circulation* 73:1058-1062, 1986.

84. McNamara DM, Rosenblum WD, Janosko KM et al: Intravenous immune gobulin in the therapy of myocarditis and acute cardiomyopathy, *Circulation* 95:2476-2478, 1997.

85. Drucker NA, Colan SD, Lewis AB et al: Gamma globulin treatment of acute myocarditis in the pediatric population, *Circulation* 89:252-257, 1994.

86. Chang AD, Hanley FL, Weinding SN et al: Left heart support with a ventricular assist device in an infant with acute myocarditis, *Crit Care Med* 20:712-715, 1992.

87. Dajani AS, Taubert KA, Gerber MA et al: Diagnosis and therapy of Kawasaki disease in children, *Circulation* 87:1776-1780, 1993.

88. Melish ME: Kawasaki syndrome, *Pediatr Rev* 17:153-162, 1996.

89. Momenah T, Sanatani S, Potts J et al: Kawasaki disease in the older child, *Pediatrics* 102:e7, 1998.
90. Nakamura Y, Yanagawa H, Kato H et al: Mortality rates for patients with a history of Kawasaki disease in Japan, *J Pediatr* 128: 75-81, 1996.
91. Burns JC, Shike H, Gordon JB et al: Sequelae of Kawasaki disease in adolescents and young adults, *J Am Coll Cardiol* 28:253-257, 1996.
92. Fujiwara H, Hamashima Y: Pathology of the heart in Kawasaki disease, *Pediatrics* 61: 100-107, 1978.
93. Newburger JW, Sanders SP, Burns JC et al: Left ventricular contractility and function in Kawasaki syndrome, *Circulation* 79:1237-1249, 1989.
94. Gidding SS: Late onset valvular dysfunction in Kawasaki disease, *Prog Clin Biol Res* 250:305-309, 1987.
95. Daniels SR, Specker B, Capannari TE et al: Correlates of coronary artery aneurysm formation in patients with Kawasaki disease, *Am J Dis Child* 141:205-207, 1987.
96. Ichida F, Fatica NS, Engle MA et al: Coronary artery involvement in Kawasaki syndrome in Manhattan, New York: risk factors and the role of aspirin, *Pediatrics* 80:828-835, 1997.
97. De Zorzi A, Colan SD, Gauvreau K et al: Coronary artery dimensions may be misclassified as normal in Kawasaki disease, *J Pediatr* 133:254-58, 1998.
98. Dhillon R, Clarkson P, Donald AE et al: Endothelial dysfunction late after Kawasaki disease, *Circulation* 94:2103-2106, 1996.
99. Suzuki A, Kamiya T, Ono Y et al: Aortocoronary bypass surgery for coronary arterial lesions resulting from Kawasaki disease, *J Pediatr* 116:567-573, 1990.
100. Newburger JW, Takahashi M, Beiser AS et al: A single intravenous infusion of gamma globulin as compared with four infusions in the treatment of acute Kawasaki syndrome, *N Engl J Med* 324:1633-1639, 1991.
101. American Academy of Pediatrics: Kawasaki disease. In AAP: *1997 Red Book: report of the Committee of Infectious Disease,* Elk Grove Ill, 1997, AAP.
102. Burns JC, Caparelli EV, Brown JA et al: Intravenous gamma globulin treatment and retreatment in Kawasaki disease" US/Canadian Kawasaki Syndrome Study Group, *Pediatr Infect Dis J* 17:1144-1148, 1998.
103. Newburger JW, Burns JC: Kawasaki disease, *Vasc Med* 4:189-202, 1999.
104. Burtt DM, Pollack P, Bianco JA: Intravenous streptokinase in an infant with Kawasaki disease complicated by myocardial infarction, *Pediatr Cardiol* 6:307-311, 1986.
105. Kato H, Ichinose E, Inoue D et al: Intracoronary thrombolytic therapy in Kawasaki disease: treatment and prevention of acute myocardial infarction, *Prog Clin Biol Res* 250:445-454, 1987.
106. Terai M, Ogata M, Sugimoto K et al: Coronary artery thrombi in Kawasaki disease, *J Pediatr* 106:76-78, 1985.
107. McCrindle B, Shulman S, Burns J et al: Summary and Abstracts of the Sixth International Kawasaki Disease Symposium, *Pediatr Res* 47:544-570, 2000.
108. Sugimara T, Yokoi H, Sato N et al: Interventional treatment for children with severe coronary artery stenosis with calcification after long-term Kawasaki disease, *Circulation* 96:3928-3933, 1997.
109. Checchia PA, Pahl E, Shaddy RE et al: Cardiac transplantation for Kawasaki disease, *Pediatrics* 100:695-699, 1997.
110. Abelman WH, Lorell BH: The challenge of cardiomyopathy, *J Am Coll Cardiol* 13: 1219-1224, 1989.
111. Grunig E, Tasman JA, Kucherer H et al: Frequency and phenotypes of familial dilated cardiomyopathy, *J Am Coll Cardiol* 31:186-194, 1998.
112. Baig MK, Goldman JH, Caforio ALP et al: Familial dilated cardiomyopathy: cardiac abnormalities are common in asymptomatic relatives and may represent early disease, *J Am Coll Cardiol* 31:195-201, 1998.
113. Schwartz ML, Cox GF, Lin AE et al: Clinical approach to genetic cardiomyopathy in children, *Circulation* 94:2021-2038, 1996.
114. Towbin JA: Pediatric myocardial disease, *Pediatr Clin North Am* 46:289-312, 1999.
115. Muller G, Ulmer HE, Hagel KJ: Cardiac dysrhythmias in children with idiopathic dilated or hypertrophic cardiomyopathy, *Pediatr Cardiol* 16:56-60, 1995.
116. Cnota JF, Samson RA: Left bundle branch block in infants with dilated cardiomyopathy conveys a poor prognosis, *Cardiol Young* 9:55-57, 1999.
117. Baker A: Acquired heart disease in infants and children, *Crit Care Nurs Clin North Am* 6:175-196, 1994.
118. Bristow MR, Gilbert EM, Abraham WT et al: Carvedilol produces dose related improvements in left ventricular function and survival in subjects with chronic heart failure, *Circulation* 94:2807-2816, 1996.
119. Brachmann J, Hilbel T, Grunig E et al: Ventricular arrhythmias in dilated cardiomyopathy, *Pacing Clin Electrophysiol* 20(10 Pt 2):2714-2718, 1997.
120. Kowey PR, Levine JH, Herre JM et al: Randomized, double blind comparison of intravenous amiodarone and bretylium in the treatment of patients with recurrent, hemodynamically destabilizing ventricular tachycardia and fibrillation, *Circulation* 92: 3255-3263, 1995.
121. Yetman AT, Hamilton RM, Benson LN et al: Long term outcome and prognostic determinants in children with hypertrophic cardiomyopathy, *J Am Coll Cardiol* 32:1943-1950, 1998.
122. Burch M, Blair E: The inheritance of hypertrophic cardiomyopathy, *Pediatr Cardiol* 20:313-316, 1999.
123. Piano MR: Familial hypertrophic cardiomyopathy, *J Cardiovasc Nurs* 13:46-58, 1999.
124. Atkinson P, Joubert G, Barron A et al: Hypertrophic cardiomyopathy associated with tacrolimus in paediatric transplant patients, *Lancet* 345:894-896, 1995.
125. Baruch Y, Weitzman E, Markiewicz W et al: Anasarca and hypertrophic cardiomyopathy in a liver transplant patient on FK506: relieved after a switch to neoral, *Transplant Proc* 28:2250-2251, 1996.
126. Haney I, Lachance C, van Doesburg NH et al: Reversible steroid-induced hypertrophic cardiomyopathy with left ventricular outflow tract obstruction in two neonates, *Am J Perinatol* 12:271-274, 1995.
127. Vaillant MC, Chantepie A, Casasoprana C et al: Transient hypertrophic cardiomyopathy in neonates after acute fetal distress, *Pediatr Cardiol* 18:52-56, 1997.
128. Wigle ED, Rakowski H, Kimball BP et al: Hypertrophic cardiomyopathy: clinical spectrum and treatment, *Circulation* 92: 1680-1692, 1995.
129. Yetman AT, McCrindle BW, MacDonald C et al: Myocardial bridging in children with hypertrophic cardiomyopathy: a risk factor for sudden death, *N Engl J Med* 339:1201-1209, 1998.
130. Kuck K: Arrhythmias in hypertrophic cardiomyopathy, *Pacing Clin Electrophysiol* 20(10 Pt 2):2706-2713, 1997.
131. Dipchard AI, McCrindle BW, Gow RM et al: Accuracy of surface electrocardiograms for differentiating children with hypertrophic cardiomyopathy from normal children, *Am J Cardiol* 83:628-630, 1999.
132. MacRae CA, Ghaisas N, Kass S et al: Familial hypertrophic cardiomyopathy with Wolff-Parkinson-White syndrome maps to a locus on chromosome 7q3, *J Clin Invest* 96:1216-1220, 1995.
133. Stellbrink C, Kunze K, Hanrath P: Preexcitation in hypertrophic cardiomyopathy: a case of a fasciculoventricular Mahaim fiber, *Pacing Clin Electrophysiol* 18(9 Pt 1):1717-1720, 1995.
134. Sherrid MV, Pearle G, Gunsburg DZ: Mechanism of benefit of negative inotropes in obstructive hypertrophic cardiomyopathy, *Circulation* 97:41-47, 1998.
135. Spirito P, Seidman CE, McKenna WJ et al: The management of hypertrophic cardiomyopathy, *N Engl J Med* 336:775-785, 1997.
136. Cecchi F, Montereggi A, Olivotto I et al: Risk for atrial fibrillation in patients with hypertrophic cardiomyopathy assessed by signal average P wave duration, *Heart* 78: 44-49, 1997.
137. Buja G, Miorelli M, Turrini P et al: Comparison of QT dispersion in hypertrophic cardiomyopathy between patients with and without ventricular arrhythmias and sudden death, *Am J Cardiol* 72:973-976, 1993.
138. Schonbeck MH, Brunner-LaRocca HP, Vogt PR et al: Long term follow up in hypertrophic obstructive cardiomyopathy after septal myectomy, *Ann Thorac Surg* 65:1207-1214, 1998.
139. Theodoro DA, Danielson GK, Feldt RH et al: Hypertrophic obstructive cardiomyopathy in pediatric patients: results of surgical treatment, *J Thorac Cardiovasc Surg* 112: 1589-1599, 1996.
140. Rishi F, Hulse JE, Auld DO et al: Effects of dual chamber pacing for pediatric patients

with hypertrophic obstructive cardiomyopathy, *J Am Coll Cardiol* 29:734-740, 1997.

141. Betocchi S, Losi M, Piscione F et al: Effects of dual chamber pacing in hypertrophic cardiomyopathy on left ventricular outflow tract obstruction and on diastolic function, *Am J Cardiol* 77:498-502, 1996.

142. Nishimura RA, Trusty JM, Hayes DL et al: Dual chamber pacing for hypertrophic cardiomyopathy: a randomized, double blind, crossover trial, *J Am Coll Cardiol* 29:435-441, 1997.

143. Nishimura RA, Symanski JD, Hurrell DG, et al: Dual chamber pacing for cardiomyopathies: a 1996 clinical perspective, *Mayo Clin Proc* 71:1077-1087, 1996.

144. Maki S, Ikeda H, Muro A et al: Predictors of sudden cardiac death in hypertrophic cardiomyopathy, *Am J Cardiol* 82:774-778, 1998.

145. Friedman RA: Sinus and atrioventricular conduction disorders. In Deal BJ, Wolff GS, Gelband H, eds: *Current concepts in diagnosis and management of arrhythmias in infants and children*, Armonk, NY, 1998, Futura Publishing.

146. Garson A, Chronic postoperative arrhythmias. In Gillete DC, Garson A, eds: *Pediatric arrhythmias: electrohysiology and pacing*, Philadelphia, 1990, WB Saunders.

147. Kugler JD: Benign arrhythmias: neonate throughout childhood. In Deal BJ, Wolff GH, Gelband H, eds: *Current concepts in diagnosis and management of arrhythmias in infants and children*, Armonk, NY, 1998, Futura Publishing.

148. Fishberger SB, Wernovsky G, Gentles TL et al: Factors that influence the development of atrial flutter after the Fontan operation, *J Thorac Cardiovasc Surg* 113:80-86, 1997.

149. Gow RM: Atrial fibrillation and flutter in children and in young adults with congenital heart disease, *Can J Cardiol* 12:45A-48A, 1996.

150. Deal BJ: Supraventricular tachycardia, mechanisms and natural history. In Deal BJ, Wolff GH, Gelband H, eds: *Current concepts in diagnosis and management of arrhythmias in infants and children*, Armonk, NY, 1998, Futura Publishing.

151. Wellens HJ, Rodriquez LM, Timmermans C et al: The asymptomatic patient with the Wolff-Parkinson-White electrogram, *Pacing Clin Electrophysiol* 20(Pt II):2082-2086, 1997.

152. Etheridge SP, Judd VE: Supraventricular tachycardia in infancy: evaluation, management and follow-up, *Arch Pediatr Adolesc Med* 153:267-271, 1999.

153. Wren C: Incessant tachycardias, *Eur Heart J* 19:E32-E36, 1998.

154. Case CL, Gillette PC: Automatic atrial and junctional tachycardias in the pediatric patient: strategies for diagnosis and management, *Pacing Clin Electrophysiol* 16:1323-1335, 1993.

155. Lashus AG, Case CL, Gillette PC: Catheter ablation treatment of supraventricular tachycardia-induced cardiomyopathy, *Arch Pediatr Adolesc Med* 151:264-266, 1997.

156. Craig J, Scholz TA, Vanderhooft SL et al: Fat necrosis after ice application for supraventricular tachycardia termination, *J Pediatr* 133:727, 1998.

157. Perry JC, Fenrich A, Hulse JE et al: Pediatric use of intravenous amiodarone: efficacy and safety in critically ill patients from a multi-center protocol, *J Am Coll Cardiol* 27:1246-1250, 1996.

158. Kugler JD, Danford DA, Houston K et al: Radiofrequency catheter ablation for paroxysmal supraventricular tachycardia in children and adolescents without structural heart disease, *Am J Cardiol* 80:1438-1443, 1997.

159. Lesh MD, Kalman JM, Saxon LA et al: Electrophysiology of incisional reentrant atrial tachycardia complicating surgery for congenital heart disease, *Pacing Clin Electrophysiol* 20(Pt II):2107-2111, 1997.

160. Lanzarotti CJ, Olshansky B: Thromboembolism in chronic atrial flutter: is the risk underestimated? *J Am Coll Cardiol* 30:1506-1511, 1997.

161. Feltes TF, Friedman RA: Transesophageal echocardiographic detection of atrial thrombi in patients with nonfibrillatory atrial tachyarrhythmias and congenital heart disease, *J Am Coll Cardiol* 24:1365-1370, 1994.

162. Triedman JK, Bergau DM, Saul P: Efficacy of radiofrequency ablation for control of intraatrial reentrant tachycardia in patients with congenital heart disease, *J Am Coll Cardiol* 30:1032-1038, 1997.

163. Kalman JM, VanHare GF, Olgin JE et al: Ablation of incisional reentrant atrial tachycardia complicating surgery for congenital heart disease, *Circulation* 93:502-512, 1996.

164. Deal BJ, Mavroudis C, Backer CL: Impact of arrhythmia circuit cryoablation during fontan conversion for refractory atrial tachycardia, *Am J Cardiol* 83:563-568, 1999.

165. Marvoudis C, Backer CL, Deal BJ et al: Fontan conversion to cavopulmonary connection and arrhythmia circuit cryoablation, *J Thorac Cardiovasc Surg* 115:547-556, 1998.

166. Ferguson, TB, Cox JL: Surgery for atrial fibrillation. In Zipes DP, Jalife J, eds: *Cardiac electrophysiology: from cell to bedside*, Philadelphia, 1995, WB Saunders.

167. Walsh EP, Saul JP, Sholler GF et al: Evaluation of a staged treatment protocol for rapid automatic junctional tachycardia after operation for congenital heart disease, *J Am Coll Cardiol* 29:1046-1053, 1997.

168. Azzam FJ, Fiore AC: Postoperative junctional ectopic tachycardia, *Can J Anaesth* 45(9):898-902, 1998.

169. Michaelsson M, Riesenfeld T, Jonzon A: Natural history of congenital complete atrioventricular block, *Pacing Clin Electrophysiol* 20(Pt II):2098-2101, 1997.

170. Michaelsson M: Congenital complete atrioventricular block, *Prog Pediatr Cardiol* 4:1-10, 1995.

171. Odemuyiwa O, Camm AJ: Prophylactic pacing for prevention of sudden death in congenital complete heart block, *Pacing Clin Electrophysiol* 15:1526-1530, 1992.

172. Balaji S, Lau YR, Case CL et al: QRS prolongation is associated with inducible ventricular tachycardia after repair of tetralogy of Fallot, *Am J Cardiol* 80:160-163, 1997.

173. Roden DM, Lazzara R, Rosen M et al: Multiple mechanisms in the Long QT syndrome: current knowledge, gaps and future directions, *Circulation* 94:1996-2012, 1996.

174. Vizgirda VM: The genetic basis for cardiac dysrhythmias and the long QT syndrome, *J Cardiovasc Nurs* 13:34-45, 1999.

175. Perry JC: Pharmacologic therapy of arrhythmias. In Deal BJ, Wolff GH, Gelband H, eds: *Current concepts in diagnosis and management of arrhythmias in infants and children*, Armonk, NY, 1998, Futura Publishing.

176. Viskin S, Alla S, Barron HV et al: Mode of onset of torsade de pointes in congenital long QT syndrome, *J Am Coll Cardiol* 28:1262-1268, 1996.

177. Chameides L, Hazinski MF: *Textbook of pediatric advanced life support*, Dallas, 1994, American Heart Association.

19

Pulmonary Critical Care Problems

Mary Jo C. Grant
Martha A.Q. Curley

RESPIRATORY FAILURE

MECHANISMS OF ABNORMAL GAS EXCHANGE

FINAL COMMON PATHWAYS

MECHANICAL ALTERATIONS: DISORDERS THAT INCREASE
   THE WORK OF BREATHING
   Upper Airways Disease
   Lower Airways Obstructive Disease
   Restrictive Disease
   Mixed Obstructive and Restrictive Disease
   Impairment of Respiratory Muscle Function

CIRCULATORY ALTERATIONS

ALTERATIONS IN CONTROL OF BREATHING

SUMMARY

Approximately 24% of pediatric critical care practice involves caring for patients with pulmonary problems.[1] Therefore knowledge of respiratory anatomy and physiology as well as familiarity with the common pathologies leading to respiratory failure are essential. This chapter examines the physiology of the respiratory system and the means by which physiology is altered by disease. Respiratory failure is defined and the mechanisms of abnormal gas exchange are reviewed. A short review of the basic physiology of the developing respiratory system establishes the final common pathways of respiratory failure: mechanical, circulatory, and regulatory alterations. The remaining sections are devoted to specific disorders associated with these final common pathways in infants and children, exploring incidence, etiology, treatment, and nursing management. Whether resulting from chronic or acute processes, impending respiratory failure can be extremely frightening for infants, children, and their families. Consequently, sensitivity and attention to the impact of critical illness on children and their families is as important

as knowledge of the causes and treatment of respiratory failure.

RESPIRATORY FAILURE

Respiratory failure is frequently defined simply in terms of blood gas abnormalities—for example, a Pao_2 of less than 50 mmHg and a $Paco_2$ greater than 50 mmHg in a patient who is spontaneously breathing room air. Quantifying respiratory failure in this fashion, however, lacks specificity and is ultimately inadequate. A child with a congenital heart defect, for example, may have a Pao_2 less than 50 mmHg without respiratory failure. Similarly, a patient with a diuretic-induced metabolic alkalosis may have an increase in $Paco_2$ to greater than 50 mmHg; however, this does not indicate respiratory failure. In addition, in clinical practice, blood gas tensions are often maintained with supplemental oxygen. It follows that respiratory failure is more appropriately understood as an inability of the respiratory system to fulfill its role in transferring oxygen (O_2) and carbon dioxide (CO_2) to and from the venous blood in an amount commensurate with the needs of the patient.

The advantage of this definition is that it emphasizes the important link that exists between the function of the respiratory system and the metabolic requirements of the tissues. For example, the infant with chronic lung disease may be able to meet everyday metabolic demands, but when an infectious process increases those demands, the child's respiratory reserve may be inadequate and respiratory failure will ensue. In fact, fatigue from increased work of breathing, rather than hypoxia, usually precipitates respiratory failure in infants and children. Respiratory failure is also differentiated from respiratory distress, which is manifested by retractions, tachypnea, nasal flaring, and so on. The latter is a judgment made by the clinician regarding the patient's work of breathing or the patient's own perception of dyspnea and does not necessarily imply respiratory failure. The child in status asthmaticus, for instance, may have respiratory distress yet be able to meet metabolic needs. Compensatory mechanisms, involving increased effort and use of addi-

Box 19-1
Pediatric ICU Admission Criteria

1. Endotracheal intubation or potential need for emergency endotracheal intubation and mechanical ventilation, regardless of etiology.
2. Rapidly progressive pulmonary, lower or upper airway, disease of high severity with risk of progression to respiratory failure and/or total obstruction.
3. High supplemental oxygen requirement (FIO_2 0.5) regardless of etiology.
4. Newly placed tracheostomy with or without the need for mechanical ventilation.
5. Acute barotrauma compromising the upper or lower airway.
6. Requirement for more frequent or continuous inhaled or nebulized medications that cannot be administered safely on the general pediatric care unit.

Adapted from American Academy of Pediatrics Committee on Hospital Care and Section on Critical Care Pediatric Section and Admission Criteria Task Force: Guidelines for developing admission and discharge policies for the pediatric intensive care unit *Pediatrics* 103:840-842, 1999.

tional respiratory muscles, can retard the development of respiratory failure, even if it is at an increased energy cost.

In 1999, the American Academy of Pediatrics Committee on Hospital Care and Section on Critical Care Pediatric Section Admission Criteria Task Force developed guidelines for admission and discharge criteria for pediatric intensive care.[2] For patients with severe or potentially life-threatening pulmonary or airway disease, the admission criteria include, but are not limited to, those listed in Box 19-1.

MECHANISMS OF ABNORMAL GAS EXCHANGE

Mechanisms of impaired gas exchange in the lungs may include diffusion, hypoventilation, shunt, and ventilation-perfusion ($\dot{V}/\dot{Q}$) mismatch disorders. Impediments in O_2 diffusion do not represent a significant problem in children; therefore we will concentrate on the remaining three.

Hypoventilation may be defined on the basis of reduced minute alveolar ventilation [(tidal volume – dead space) × (respiratory rate)] and inevitably results in an inability to eliminate CO_2. Because the increased alveolar CO_2 occupies space, O_2 is displaced out of the alveolus and both alveolar and arterial PO_2 are decreased. Supplemental O_2, however, can overcome this displacement, and restore PaO_2 to normal (Fig. 19-1, *B*).

Normally, a small percentage of right ventricular output is returned to the left atrium without passing through ventilated areas of the lung. This represents a physiologic right-to-left shunt. Additional shunting of blood occurs when collapsed alveoli continue to be perfused. Because these alveoli are no longer ventilated, the blood circulating through them is not oxygenated. This blood is mixed with oxygenated blood from other ventilated areas, thereby increasing pulmonary venous admixture, or causing an abnormal *right-to-left* shunt. PaO_2 decreases, but in this case, supplemental O_2 will not entirely abolish hypoxemia because the shunted blood is not exposed to inspired O_2 (Fig. 19-1, *C*). Intrapulmonary shunting does not usually result in an increase in $PaCO_2$ because the respiratory center responds to hypoxemia by increasing ventilation.

$\dot{V}/\dot{Q}$ mismatching is the most common cause of abnormal gas exchange. If ventilation and blood flow are unequal in various regions of the lung, impairment of both O_2 and CO_2 transfer results. Supplemental O_2 will, however, increase the PaO_2 to normal (Fig. 19-1, *D*).

FINAL COMMON PATHWAYS

The principal purpose of the respiratory system is to exchange gases, O_2 and CO_2, with the atmosphere. This process requires the combined function of heart, blood vessels, and lungs. It may be helpful to view the respiratory system as a mechanical pump controlled by a complex feedback system (Fig. 19-2). The pump includes the lung, the chest wall, and the respiratory muscles (primarily the diaphragm, but also the intercostal and abdominal muscles), which, when acting on the chest wall (rib cage and abdomen), expand and compress the lungs. Respiration is regulated by the respiratory center in the brainstem. This center is stimulated directly by CO_2 and hydrogen ions and indirectly via central and peripheral chemoreceptors. In addition, mechanoreceptors in the lung and chest wall convey information about the status of the lungs. The central nervous system integrates all of the data and acts on the respiratory center where the respiratory pattern is established and conveyed through peripheral nerves like the phrenic nerve to the muscles of respiration. The pulmonary circulation completes the respiratory system by establishing a close interface between inspired gas and the blood, which permits delivery of O_2 to the blood and removal of CO_2.

This conceptual model of the respiratory system also delineates the three final common pathways of respiratory failure. These involve mechanical, circulatory, and regulatory alterations. Mechanical (or pump) alterations in pulmonary function can be classified into two major categories: illnesses that increase the work of breathing, and diseases in which the respiratory muscles are unable to perform even the normal amount of work. The former include disorders that increase airway or pulmonary resistance (obstructive disease), those that decrease thoracic compliance (restrictive disease), and mixed disorders resulting in alterations in both resistance and compliance (e.g., bronchopulmonary dysplasia [BPD]). The diseases that affect the respiratory muscles, rendering them incapable of normal work, include disorders of the peripheral nerves (Guillain-Barré syndrome [GBS]), the neuromuscular junction (infant botulism or myasthenia gravis), and the muscle itself (muscular dystrophy). Circulatory alterations involve disturbances in the normal contact between blood and gas within the lungs; pulmonary embolism (PE) and persistent pulmonary hypertension of the newborn are characteristic examples. In these conditions, pulmonary circulation is reduced, physiologic dead space increases, and gas exchange may be impaired. Finally,

Room Air   100% O₂

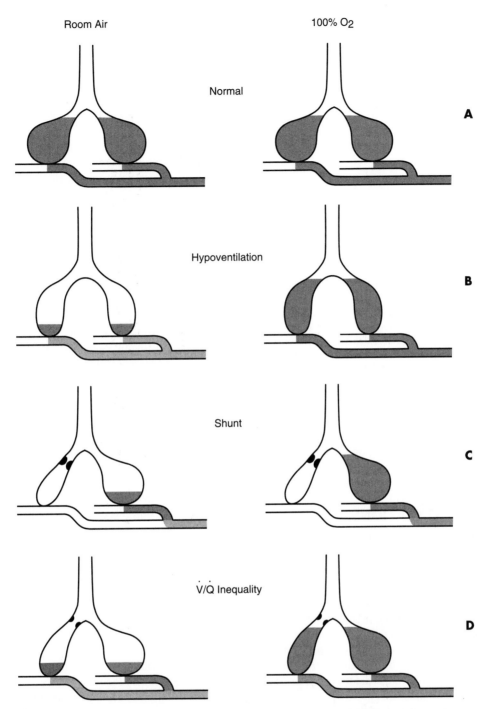

Fig. 19-1 Mechanisms of hypoxemia and effect of increased F_{IO_2} in patients with lung disease. In this schematic representation, the normal lung is composed of two alveolar units with their respective capillaries. **A,** While breathing room air, on the left, the F_{IO_2} in the alveoli (shown by the level of filling of the alveolar units in the figure) is only 0.21. The alveolar P_{O_2} (P_{AO_2}, indicated by the shading inside the alveoli), however, is sufficiently high to produce a normal O_2 hemoglobin saturation in the pulmonary capillaries (shown by the degree of shading inside the capillaries in the figure). Administration of an F_{IO_2} of 1.0 barely increased the O_2 content of the arterial blood. **B,** In the presence of hypoventilation, P_{AO_2} is reduced in room air, and the capillary blood is poorly saturated. Administration of an F_{IO_2} of 1.0 increases both the P_{AO_2} and O_2 content of the capillary blood. **C,** An intrapulmonary shunt allows mixed venous blood to pass through the lungs without being exposed to alveolar O_2. As a result, the arterial O_2 content is decreased. Supplemental O_2 raises only the O_2 content of the capillary blood that is not shunted; therefore arterial O_2 content increased only to a limited extent. **D,** In $\dot{V}/\dot{Q}$ inequality, alveolar units that have a decreased P_{O_2} exist in combination with others that have a normal P_{O_2}. Blood from these two types of units mixes, resulting in a lower than normal arterial O_2 content. Administration of O_2 increases the P_{AO_2} in both hypoventilated and normal units, and the O_2 content of the arterial blood increases as well. (Courtesy J. Julio Perez Fontan, MD, and George Lister, MD, New Haven, Connecticut.)

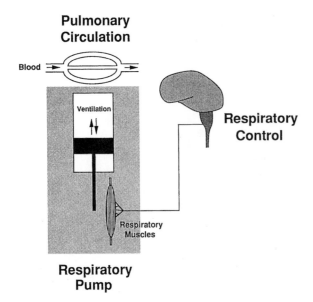

Fig. 19-2 Schematic drawing of the respiratory system. In this schematic representation, the respiratory system consists of a mechanical pump controlled by a complex feedback system. The respiratory pump includes the lung, chest wall, and respiratory muscles. Respiratory control is established by the respiratory center in the brainstem and conveyed (via peripheral nerves) to the muscles of respiration. Finally, the pulmonary circulation establishes an alveolar-capillary interface that permits gas exchange.

alterations in the control of breathing include primary or secondary derangements in the breathing pattern such as apnea and alveolar hypoventilation syndromes.

MECHANICAL ALTERATIONS: DISORDERS THAT INCREASE THE WORK OF BREATHING

Mechanical alterations in pulmonary function in infants and children are often the result of illnesses that cause airway obstruction. Because the signs and symptoms of obstruction depend (in large part) on location, it is helpful to delineate two categories of airway obstruction: extrathoracic or upper airways disease (laryngotracheobronchitis, epiglottitis, foreign body aspiration, and pharyngeal obstruction) and intrathoracic or lower airways disease (asthma, bronchiolitis, and tracheobronchomalacia).

The diameter of an airway is determined by the compliance of the airway wall, coupled with the deforming force exerted upon it. The latter is the pressure difference between the gas inside the airway and the tissues surrounding the airway. This pressure difference, known as the transmural pressure, varies during inspiration and expiration and differs for extrathoracic and intrathoracic airways.

The signs and symptoms of obstruction depend on location (extrathoracic or intrathoracic) and the direction of airflow (inspiration or expiration). During inspiration, airway pressure becomes progressively more negative as the alveoli are approached; a pressure gradient is necessary for airflow to occur inside the airways. On expiration, the pressure within the alveoli becomes positive and the gradient is reversed with pressures inside the airways being always positive but diminishing toward the mouth. In contrast, the influence of inspiration and expiration on the pressure outside the airway depends on whether the airways are extrathoracic or intrathoracic.

Extrathoracic airways (the pharynx, larynx, and a portion of the trachea) are included in the tissues of the neck, where the pressure can be considered to be zero or atmospheric. Because intrathoracic airways are embedded in the chest, however, the pressure affecting their airway caliber is the pleural pressure. During inspiration, extrathoracic airways have a transmural pressure that favors narrowing because intraluminal pressure decreases, whereas the pressure exerted by tissues outside the airway remains constant. Intrathoracic airways dilate during inspiration as pleural pressure becomes more negative than intraluminal pressure (i.e., transmural pressure decreases). During expiration, the situation is reversed; extrathoracic airways dilate as intraluminal pressure becomes positive with respect to atmospheric pressure, and intrathoracic airways narrow as the pressure within those airways decreases with respect to pleural pressure. Airway obstruction causes an exaggeration of these normal changes in airway diameter (Fig. 19-3).

Typical clinical manifestations accompany airway obstruction. First, and perhaps foremost, a relatively slow respiratory rate helps to conserve energy. This can be readily appreciated by breathing through a straw—it is much more difficult to breathe rapidly than to breathe slowly. Additional signs of obstruction include intercostal and/or substernal retractions, which may be pronounced, and nasal flaring or the use of accessory muscles of respiration. Based on the previous discussion of airway dynamics, however, there are substantial differences between extrathoracic (upper airways) and intrathoracic (lower airways) obstruction—differences that can be detected by a careful clinical examination (Table 19-1). Inspiration is prolonged in extrathoracic obstruction, whereas the duration of expiration remains unchanged. The opposite is true in intrathoracic obstruction, in which expiration is prolonged and inspiratory time unchanged. The adventitious sounds heard on auscultation also differ in extrathoracic and intrathoracic obstruction. Inspiratory stridor occurs in extrathoracic obstruction; expiratory wheezing occurs in intrathoracic obstruction. Gas trapping is not a predominant characteristic of extrathoracic obstruction, but occurs often in intrathoracic obstruction.

Upper Airways Disease

The etiology of extrathoracic airway disease with obstruction may vary considerably, but the dynamic consequences of the obstruction are the same: to overcome increased resistance during inspiration, the child must create greater negative pressure inside the airway segment downstream from the obstruction. This segment of the airway tends to collapse, worsening the obstruction and producing a characteristic inspiratory stridor. With extrathoracic obstruction the child's respiratory rate is relatively low, mainly because inspiration is prolonged. Suprasternal and subclavicular retractions occur. In addition, nasal flaring and head bobbing

Inspiration

Expiration

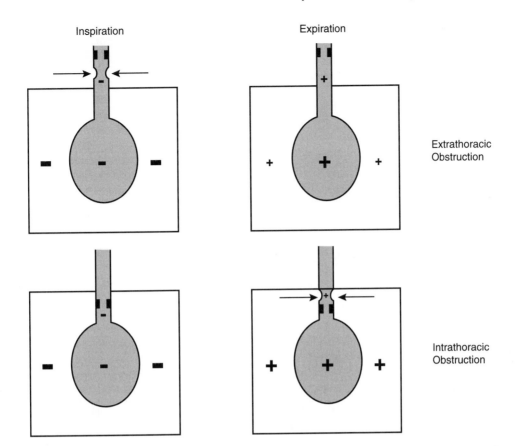

Extrathoracic
Obstruction

Intrathoracic
Obstruction

Fig. 19-3 Effect of the respiratory cycle on upper and lower airway obstruction. Upper airway obstruction worsens during inspiration as intraluminal pressure decreases and the pressure outside the airways remains constant (atmospheric pressure). Lower airway obstruction worsens during expiration when positive pressures outside the airways (pleural pressure) exceed the pressure within the airways downstream from the obstruction. (Adapted from Fontan JJP, Lister G: Respiratory Failure. In Touloukian RJ, ed: *Pediatric trauma,* St Louis, 1990, Mosby.)

◆ TABLE 19-1   Differences Between Upper and Lower Airway Obstruction on Physical Examination

Sign	Upper Airway	Lower Airway
Respiratory rate	Slow	Slow
Duration of inspiration	↑	↔
Duration of expiration	↔	↑
Stridor	+	−
Wheezing	−	+
Gas trapping	−	+

↑, Increased; ↔, unchanged; +, present; −, absent.

(neck extension during inspiration and flexion during expiration) may serve to keep the airway open during inspiration. In the pediatric intensive care unit (PICU), frequent causes of upper airways obstruction are laryngotracheobronchitis, epiglottitis, bacterial tracheitis, foreign body aspiration, pharyngeal obstruction, and tracheobronchomalacia.

Laryngotracheobronchitis (Croup)

Etiology. Laryngotracheobronchitis (croup), a viral illness, is the most commonly occurring upper airway obstruction in pediatrics. It is characterized by airway obstruction that is primarily subglottic. The etiologic organisms are most commonly viral, and they include the parainfluenza viruses (types 1, 2, and 3) and influenza virus A. Bacterial agents may cause laryngotracheobronchitis, including *Mycoplasma pneumoniae* and *Corynebacterium diphtheriae;* however, a bacterial basis is rarely seen.

Incidence. Laryngotracheobronchitis usually occurs in late autumn and winter. More prevalent in males (ratio 1.5:1), infants and toddlers 3 months to 3 years old are primarily affected, with incidence peaking at 9 to 18 months.

Pathogenesis. Children with laryngotracheobronchitis typically present following several days of symptoms consistent with a viral upper respiratory infection: coryza (dry inflammation of the nasal mucus membranes), sore throat, cough, hoarseness, and low-grade temperature. The child commonly has a low-grade fever, may complain of a sore throat, but does not appear very ill. A typical "croupy" cough and stridor develop as a result of swelling of the airway (glottic and subglottic edema). Laryngotracheobronchitis also affects other areas of the airway, but the subglottic area is the most narrow air passage in young children; therefore the clinical manifestations are primarily related to this region. Older children, however, often have tracheitis and even bronchitis.

Typically, laryngotracheobronchitis is a mild disease, and most children can be treated as outpatients. Very young infants appear more acutely ill and are often in more respiratory distress than older infants and children because their airways have a smaller diameter; as a result, a modest amount of edema produces a grater degree of airway obstruction. Stridor and retractions even at rest, tachycardia, restlessness, and cyanosis indicate progressive airway obstruction necessitating close monitoring in a PICU and possibly airway intervention.

Critical Care Management. A child who presents with a croupy cough, stridor, and respiratory distress is carefully evaluated. An anteroposterior neck radiograph usually depicts subglottic narrowing (referred to as the "steeple sign"). Treatment for coup is usually symptomatic. In most instances, treatment with cool-mist O_2 is sufficient to ameliorate symptoms. The efficacy of cool-mist therapy has not been demonstrated; however, many physicians still recommend its use.

In more severe cases, nebulized racemic epinephrine delivered using a small-volume nebulizer 1:1000 (0.5 ml/kg; maximum 4 ml) can provide transient reductions in stridor. A recent meta-analysis of randomized controlled trials examined the effectiveness of glucocorticoid treatment in children with laryngotracheobronchitis.[3,4] The review demonstrated that dexamethasone 0.6 mg/kg as an initial dose followed by 0.15 mg/kg every 6 hours and inhaled budesonide (2 mg) were effective in relieving the symptoms of laryngotracheobronchitis as early as 6 hours after treatment. In addition, fewer cointerventions are used and the length of time spent in the hospital is decreased in patients treated with glucocorticoids.

Heliox (30% O_2 and 70% helium) may be used in patients without a large O_2 requirement. Because the density of helium is lower than the density of air or O_2, helium will rapidly flow through the narrowed upper airway, decreasing the work of breathing and fatigue. Stridor scores have been demonstrated to be lower with helium-O_2 than with O_2-supplemented room air in patients with postextubation stridor.[5] In the unlikely event that endotracheal intubation is required, endotracheal tubes 0.5 to 1.5 mm smaller in diameter than usual for the child's age are used and are prone to obstruction with thick secretions.

Nursing management of the child with laryngotracheobronchitis includes limiting activity that may increase respiratory effort and exacerbate symptoms. The tachypnea that accompanies agitation, for example, may cause an increase in transmural pressure and airway turbulence, both of which lead to further narrowing of the airway. Therefore it is essential to minimize the child's anxiety. Encouraging parental presence and participation in care may go a long way in reducing fears associated with hospitalization. Sedation should be used judiciously. Decreasing the number of times the fearful patient is approached by hospital staff

TABLE 19-2 A Croup Scoring System Based on Four Clinical Signs

Level of consciousness	0	=	Normal
	5	=	Disoriented
Desaturation	0	=	None
	4	=	With agitation
	5	=	At rest
Stridor	0	=	Normal
	1	=	With agitation
	2	=	At rest
Air entry	0	=	Normal
	1	=	Decreased
	2	=	Markedly decreased
Retractions	0	=	None
	1	=	Mild
	2	=	Moderate
	3	=	Severe

Zero represents the normal state or absence of the sign; the highest number represents the most severe distress. The range for each sign is weighted to reflect the clinical implications of the most severe form of that sign.

Adapted with permission from Westly CR, Cotton EK, Brooks JG: Nebulized racemic epinephrine by IPPB for the treatment of croup, *Am J Dis Child* 132:486. Copyright 1978, American Medical Association.

can minimize anxiety and its associated increase in the work of breathing.

Close observation and monitoring of the child's respiratory status includes respiratory rate and effort, heart rate, and Spo_2. Use of a croup scoring system (Table 19-2) may facilitate documentation of the progression or regression of symptoms, and provide a more objective evaluation of the efficacy of various interventions.[6] Intubated children are at high risk for inadvertent extubation because of their young age, mobility, and the difficulty of taping tubes to the face in the presence of copious nasal secretions. Nursing vigilance can minimize the risk by splinting the arms to prevent elbow flexion and extreme care with tube position and fixation. Low dose sedation may be useful, but muscle relaxants or high-dose sedation are generally unnecessary.

Epiglottitis

Etiology and Incidence. Epiglottitis is a bacterial infection of the laryngeal inlet usually caused by *Haemophilus influenzae* type b (Hib). The diagnosis is often confused with laryngotracheobronchitis because both problems present with inspiratory stridor and respiratory distress. The patient with epiglottitis is most likely to be between 2 and 4 years of age. Causes of epiglottitis include *Pneumococcus* group A, *Streptococcus* and *Staphylococcus aureus*, and Hib. In 1988, Hib conjugate vaccines were introduced for use in children aged 18 months to 5 years; the Advisory Committee on Immunization Practices (ACIP) subsequently recommended them for routine use in infants in 1990. Since the introduction of the Hib vaccine in 1988, the incidence of epiglottitis has fallen dramatically, but the vaccine does not offer complete protection and the disease can occur in immunized children. In the prevaccine era (i.e., before 1988), *Haemophilus influenzae* caused approximately 95% of the *Haemophilus influenzae* invasive disease among children aged younger than 5 years. During 1989 through 1995, Hib invasive disease among children aged younger than 5 years declined 95% nationally.[7]

Pathogenesis.   There is an acute onset (usually less than a day) of sore throat, high fever, muffled voice, dysphagia, and lethargy. Dysphagia rapidly progresses to an inability to clear oropharyngeal secretions and signs of obstruction develop, including inspiratory stridor, tachypnea, cyanosis, and retractions. Lying down often increases the degree of obstruction, so children with epiglottitis adopt a characteristic posture: sitting forward, drooling, with minimal head and neck movement. At this point, the child often appears pale and restless. Because ventilation can be maintained only in an upright position, the child should not be forced into a recumbent position.

Critical Care Management.   The maintenance of a patent airway is the primary goal of therapy. Agitation may precipitate laryngospasm and complete laryngeal obstruction, so no detailed physical examination, blood drawing, or other invasive procedures are performed immediately on a child presenting with signs and symptoms suggestive of epiglottitis. It is especially important to avoid any attempt to examine the pharynx before the child can be taken to the operating room for direct visualization of the glottis under anesthesia. O_2 is given as unobtrusively as possible. Before laryngoscopy, a lateral neck radiograph showing a very swollen epiglottic shadow is typical and may be helpful in cases if there is doubt about the diagnosis (Fig. 19-4). However, radiographic examination should not delay therapy in a child in severe distress. In those instances, the child is transported directly to the operating room in the parent's arms. Although respiratory arrest can occur from total airway obstruction, it is usually the result of a combination of partial obstruction and fatigue.

The anatomy may be so distorted from inflammation and edema that the glottic structures will be unidentifiable. As a result of this extensive edema of the glottis, a wide selection of endotracheal tubes with a smaller diameter than predicted, but sufficient length, are made available. Once an appropriate level of inhalation anesthesia is reached, an intravenous line is placed, and visualization of the glottis and intubation are accomplished. The most experienced individual skilled in intubation performs the intubation. In the event that the examination induces laryngospasm and an acute airway obstruction, a tracheostomy will be necessary. Laryngeal and blood cultures are obtained before initiating antibiotic therapy; third-generation cephalosporins (e.g., cefotaxime) are the antibiotics of choice. There is no evidence to suggest that corticosteroids are helpful in the treatment of epiglottitis.

Acute pulmonary edema has been described in children with the relief of airway obstruction. This postobstructive

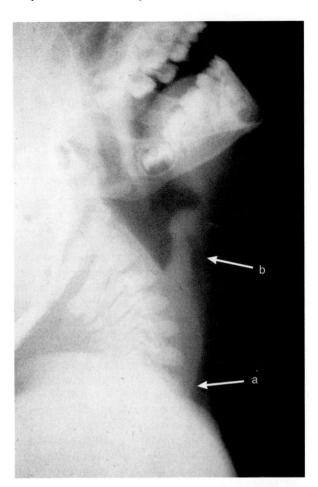

Fig. 19-4 Lateral neck radiograph in epiglottitis. To define the epiglottis, follow the posterior border of the trachea (**A**) to the epiglottis (**B**). Instead of its usual sharp appearance, the epiglottis is swollen. The supraglottic portion of the airway is dilated, while the air column below the laryngeal level is well preserved (i.e., there is no subglottic edema). Please note that a radiograph should not be obtained in any patient with clear signs and symptoms of epiglottitis.

pulmonary edema manifests itself immediately or within a few hours of the relief of obstruction. Several mechanisms have been proposed, including an increased left ventricular transmural pressure gradient from the negative pleural pressure generated against the airway obstruction.[8]

Once the child has been intubated, a primary goal is to maintain the position and patency of the artificial airway. Accidental extubation, particularly early in the course of epiglottitis, is potentially disastrous. The majority of patients with laryngotracheobronchitis or epiglottitis are toddlers or preschoolers in whom egocentricity is prominent, freedom of movement is essential, and separation from parents is a major source of fear and stress. Elbow restraints are necessary to prevent the child from removing the endotracheal tube but are not used in isolation. Additional measures to keep the child calm and quiet should also be taken, including the administration of sedatives, decreasing noxious or threatening stimuli, and encouraging continued family presence and participation in care. If accidental extubation occurs, positioning the child in an upright forward sitting position may facilitate air entry. Bag and mask ventilation may be required if the child is unable to maintain spontaneous ventilation. The child with epiglottitis secondary to *H. influenzae* will also require droplet precautions until 24 hours after the start of effective antibiotic therapy.

Planned extubation of the child is based on revisualization of the supraglottic structures, presence of a leak around the endotracheal tube, and clinical status of the patient. Extubation can usually be accomplished within 48 to 72 hours after antibiotic therapy is started.

Bacterial Tracheitis

Etiology and Incidence. Bacterial tracheitis is thought to be a complication of laryngotracheobronchitis and closely resembles laryngotracheobronchitis. Bacterial tracheitis can produce a complete airway obstruction as a result of copious, mucopurulent secretions. A recent review of 46 children admitted with bacterial tracheitis found the mean age to be 69 months, 57% of whom required tracheal intubation.[9]

Pathogenesis. The child may actually appear to be improving after an episode of viral laryngotracheobronchitis when suddenly there is a new onset of stridor. It may be distinguished from laryngotracheobronchitis because the patient usually has a high fever and may appear very ill. A lateral neck film shows subglottic swelling. In children, predominant organisms include *S. aureus* and *H. influenzae*.[10] *Moraxella catarrhalis* has been identified in 12 (27%) of 45 bacterial respiratory cultures, whereas influenza A virus was recovered from 18 (72%) of 25 viral respiratory cultures in children with bacterial tracheitis.[9]

Critical Care Management. The child who presents with bacterial tracheitis may have significant respiratory distress and a septic appearance. Management is focused on maintenance of a patent airway and treatment of blood pressure instability with fluids and catecholamines as necessary. A superimposed bacterial pneumonia may coexist, and this is likely to cause the child to require mechanical ventilation.

Foreign Body Aspiration

Etiology. A relatively common cause of airway obstruction in children is a foreign body lodged in the tracheobronchial tree, commonly in the bronchi. Infants usually inhale radiolucent food items (peanuts, seeds, pieces of carrot), whereas toddlers inhale radiopaque items (coins, teeth, metal or plastic toy parts). The foreign bodies most commonly found in a review of 639 patients were sunflower seeds (21.1%), beans (10.4%), watermelon seeds (10%), and hazelnuts (9.8%).[11]

Incidence. Foreign body aspiration may affect any age, but occurs most frequently in young children ranging in age from 6 months to 3 years. In a retrospective review of 84 children and 28 adults, the peak incidence of foreign body aspiration was found to occur during the second year of life in children and during the sixth decade of life in adults.[12]

Pathogenesis. Signs and symptoms of foreign body aspiration vary, depending on the location of the object in the airway. A foreign body will usually lodge at or above the larynx, in the trachea or a bronchus. Although a foreign body preferentially lodges in the right bronchial tree in adults, a central location (but not at all exclusive) with air trapping is more common in children.[12] Children may also present with acute asphyxia from tracheal obstruction, wheezing when a mainstem bronchus is occluded, or they may complain solely of a chronic cough or bloody sputum if a smaller or more peripheral airway is involved. Foreign bodies do not usually cause stridor unless the obstruction is at or near the larynx. When a foreign body is lodged in a lobar or segmental bronchus, unilateral physical findings become prominent. Asymmetric breath sounds, absent air entry, and unilateral prolongation of expiration may occur.

Critical Care Management. When foreign body aspiration is suspected, a careful history may reveal a choking episode several days, weeks, or months before symptoms began. In a series of 87 children with foreign-body aspiration, neither clinical signs or symptoms nor radiology had sufficient diagnostic sensitivity, and especially specificity, on which to rely for the diagnosis. Only the choking crisis, when present in the history, had good sensitivity and specificity (respectively, 96% and 76%).[13] Although most aspirated objects are radiolucent, diagnosis may be aided by chest radiographs demonstrating unilateral hyperinflation, atelectasis, or infiltrate (Fig. 19-5). Unilateral hyperaeration, atelectasis, and unilateral parenchymal infiltration are the most common radiologic findings.[11] A forced expiration radiographic technique often reveals persistent air trapping in one location, a finding missed on a conventional chest film because there is increased and uniform expansion of the lung during inspiration. Fluoroscopy may also demonstrate persistent inflation during both phases of respiration, indicating airway obstruction and identifying the location of the foreign body. Even in the absence of a definitive diagnosis, bronchoscopy under general anesthesia is the diagnostic test and the treatment of choice when aspiration of a foreign body below the carina is suspected. The most frequent procedure in children is rigid bronchoscopy.[12]

The use of less direct methods, such as postural drainage, may lead to total airway obstruction by freeing an object that is too large to pass through the larynx. However, when an exact diagnosis cannot be made and a lobar or segmental obstruction is suspected, postural drainage and inhaled bronchodilators may be employed for several days. If there is no improvement, bronchoscopy is performed. For imminent complete obstruction follow Pediatric Advance Life Support recommendations for foreign body aspiration.[14]

Residual irritation after removal of a foreign body by bronchoscopy or postural drainage may necessitate continued administration of supplemental O_2, vigorous pulmonary toilet, and careful monitoring of the child's respiratory status in the PICU. Parent education is also important to help prevent future aspirations. This includes instructing parents that children under 3 years of age are prime candidates for aspiration accidents and aiding them in recognizing the

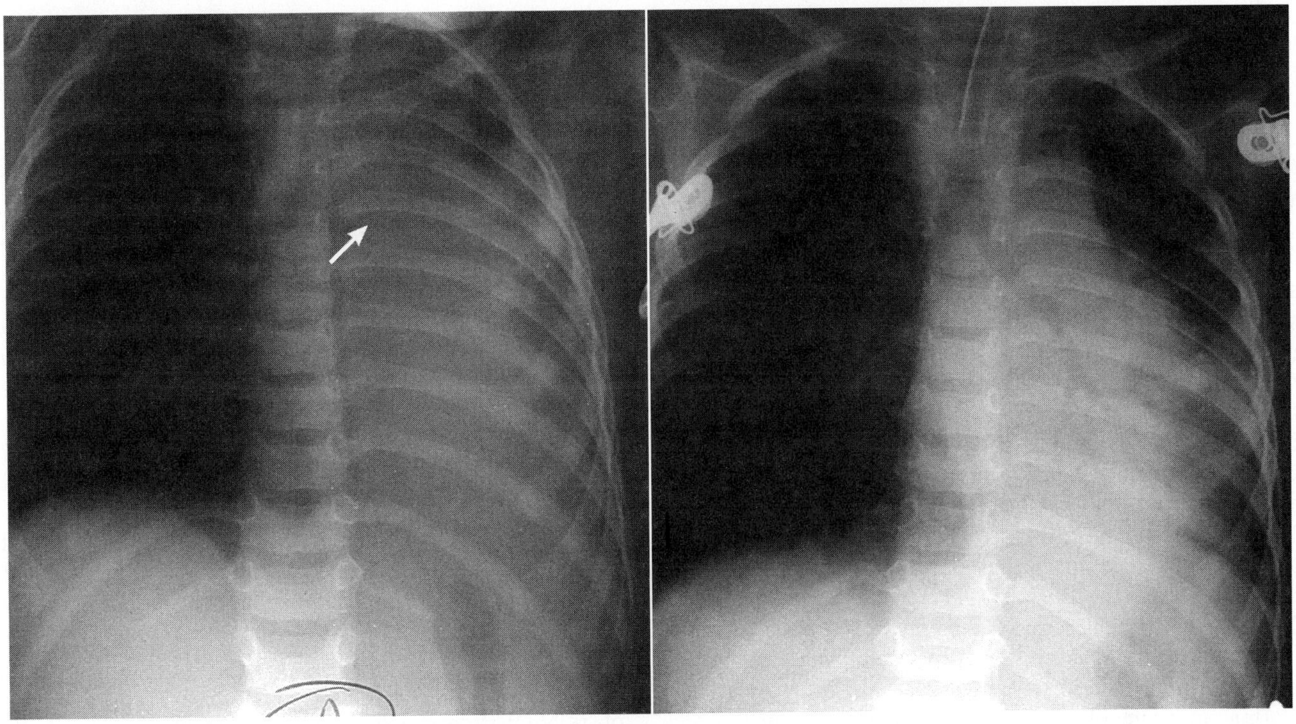

Fig. 19-5 Foreign body chest radiograph. **A,** This AP chest radiograph reveals complete collapse of the left lower lobe with partial aeration of the left upper lobe and lingula. The left main bronchus is well demonstrated containing air through its proximal course where there is an abrupt obstruction to the bronchial lumen. **B,** The AP view of the chest was obtained after the removal of bubble gum from the left mainstem bronchus. Air is now demonstrated throughout the central aspects of the left bronchus including into the periphery of the left lower lobe, which has undergone partial reexpansion compared with the view in **A.** There is partial reexpansion compared with of the upper lobe as well. (Courtesy of Robert Cleveland, MD, Radiology Department, Children's Hospital, Boston.)

importance of safeguarding their children from objects that are commonly aspirated.

Pharyngeal Obstruction

Etiology and Incidence. Pharyngeal collapse or obstruction is a commonly encountered short-term problem in PICU patients. The largest group of patients at risk for pharyngeal obstruction in the PICU are patients who are comatose or are otherwise neurologically impaired. Other high-risk groups are patients who have been extubated after general anesthesia but are not yet fully awake, and those who are heavily sedated. These patients may have little difficulty maintaining a patent airway when awake, but develop sonorous respirations and intermittent airway obstruction when permitted to sleep/rest in the supine position.

Pathogenesis. The pharynx, the most collapsible portion of the extrathoracic airway, is formed by constrictor muscles posteriorly and laterally and pharyngeal dilators located predominantly on the anterior and lateral walls of the pharynx. The constrictor muscles participate primarily in swallowing, whereas the pharyngeal dilators are believed to be important in airway maintenance.[15] During states of decreased consciousness caused by sedatives, anesthesia, or primary central nervous system disease, the activity of these airway muscles and their responses to various stimuli may be depressed, leading to airway collapse during inspiration.

In addition, muscle relaxation may cause airway obstruction by passive posterior displacement of the tongue.

Critical Care Management. Pharyngeal obstruction can usually be overcome simply by side-lying or prone positioning. Placement of a nasopharyngeal airway may also be helpful if the child has an extremely flaccid pharynx or excessive oral secretions. If airway collapse is complete, endotracheal intubation is required.

Because level of consciousness may vary considerably, patients recovering from general anesthesia require close monitoring of both neurologic function and respiratory status. Monitoring Spo_2 ensures adequate oxygenation; physical examination and arterial blood gases (ABGs) provide information about the adequacy of ventilation.

Tracheobronchomalacia

Etiology and Incidence. This rare disease of infancy and childhood is characterized by abnormally high compliance of the tracheal or bronchial wall. Marked delays in the development of the supportive structures of large airways precipitates severe airway obstruction during respiratory maneuvers. The classification of infants with collapsing airways is based on the anatomic area involved, for example, tracheomalacia, tracheobronchomalacia, or bronchomalacia. Tracheomalacia without associated abnormalities is rare. Most cases of abnormally compliant airways are secondary to tracheoesophageal fistula or external compression of the airways by abnormal vascular structures. Prematurity, low birth weight, BPD, and prolonged ventilation predispose patients to the most severe symptoms.[16] Whatever its origin, expiratory collapse of the airway occurs because of inadequate cartilaginous and elastic supporting structures of the trachea and bronchi.

Pathogenesis. Clinical signs and symptoms depend on the location and length of the malacic airway and the severity of the structural abnormality. If the affected segment encompasses both intrathoracic and extrathoracic portions of the trachea (as often occurs), the clinical presentation includes both stridor and wheezing. If the malacic area is only extrathoracic (larynx and trachea), there is only stridor. Airway obstruction may be episodic and is especially pronounced when intrathoracic pressure exceeds airway pressure, for example during forced expiration with Valsalva maneuvers, crying, or agitation. Increased respiratory rate (although slower than one would expect with the degree of respiratory distress), intercostal retractions, and grunting have been described in infants with severe tracheobronchomalacia. Wheezing and marked cyanotic spells requiring immediate intervention have also been reported. During an acute obstructive episode, breath sounds are markedly diminished and hypoxemia and hypercarbia develop.[17]

Critical Care Management. The diagnosis of tracheobronchomalacia is confirmed by examining the airways with bronchoscopy and/or fluoroscopy. Many infants with minor degrees of tracheobronchomalacia and mild or moderate symptoms require no intervention and improve with growth. For infants with severe malacia, however, a tracheostomy is often required. The tracheostomy tube may stint open a semiflaccid trachea, as long as the cannula bypasses the affected area. However, a malacic segment very low in the trachea, or involving the bronchi, will not be supported by a tracheostomy tube alone. In this instance, positive airway pressure during expiration (positive end expiratory pressure [PEEP] or continuous positive airway pressure [CPAP]) may produce the same effect by increasing airway transmural pressure during the critical expiratory phase. Infants with acquired tracheobronchomalacia often benefit from CPAP.[18] Some patients may require a positive airway pressure as high as 25 cm H_2O to maintain airway patency.[19]

A tracheotomy with CPAP may be required by 75% of premature infants and 25% of full-term infants with tracheobronchomalacia. Seventy-one percent of all patients will undergo decannulation without any other surgical intervention.[16] In extreme cases of bronchomalacia, a pneumonectomy or lobectomy may be required because a segmental bronchial resection with end-to-end anastomosis is not feasible. An alternative treatment for patients is a surgically implanted splint that serves to support the collapsing bronchus.

Because tracheobronchomalacia is often a difficult problem to diagnose, it is important to carefully monitor and document episodes that may represent airway collapse. Agitation and attempts by the infant to forcefully exhale

cause airway collapse and complicate management; sedation and even muscle relaxation may be indicated in some patients undergoing mechanical ventilation. Unexplained periods of increased respiratory distress and arterial desaturation (with or without cyanosis) are noteworthy, especially in an infant on long-term ventilation. Documenting events immediately preceding hypoxic episodes is also important, because maneuvers that decrease transmural pressure, for example, crying or straining, may cause a malacic airway to collapse. When an infant with tracheobronchomalacia has acute respiratory decompensation, slow hand ventilation with somewhat higher peak inspiratory pressures than the infant's baseline often relieve the obstruction.[17]

Lower Airways Disease

As with upper airways disease, the respiratory rate of a child with lower airways disease is relatively low. Other signs of respiratory distress may also be prominent including retractions, the use of accessory muscles of respiration (sternocleidomastoids and abdominals), and nasal flaring. However, additional clinical findings distinguish intrathoracic obstruction from its extrathoracic counterpart.

Normally, intrathoracic airways dilate during inspiration (as transmural pressure decreases), and narrow during expiration. These changes are exacerbated when there is obstruction, particularly during expiration, resulting in a prolonged expiratory phase and expiratory wheezes audible on auscultation. Variable regional air entry may also be present. The larger airways tend to collapse during forced expiration, and the combination of large and small airway obstruction leads to air trapping and hyperinflation of the lungs. This may be evidenced by downward displacement of the diaphragm on chest radiographs and a tympanic chest on percussion. Two causes of intrathoracic airway obstruction that commonly lead to PICU admission are bronchiolitis and asthma.

Bronchiolitis

Etiology. Bronchiolitis is an acute inflammatory disease of the lower respiratory tract, resulting in obstruction of small airways. A number of different viral pathogens cause bronchiolitis. Respiratory syncytial virus (RSV) accounts for most cases of bronchiolitis in which a specific agent can be identified. Other viruses that cause bronchiolitis are rhinovirus, parainfluenza virus type 3, adenovirus, and influenza virus. *Mycoplasma pneumoniae* is usually associated with lower respiratory tract disease in older children.

Incidence. RSV is the most common cause of lower respiratory tract disease in infants and young children worldwide.[20] In temperate climates, RSV infections occur primarily during annual outbreaks, which peak during winter months. With inpatient charges of $300 to $400 million per year in the United States, the disease burden of RSV pneumonia is very high in terms of both morbidity and economic costs.[20]

From July 1998 through June 1999, 45 states reported 18,418 positive tests for RSV. In the United States, widespread RSV activity began in early November 1998 and continued for 27 weeks, until late April. Timing of RSV community outbreaks varied from onset (range: September 11 to April 2) to conclusion (range: January 8 to June 18). Overall, RSV outbreaks were observed earlier in laboratories in the South, later in Northeast laboratories, and latest in the West. Although most positive tests (91%) were reported from the week ending November 27 through the week ending April 30, RSV was detected throughout the year.[21] There is no significant difference between using nasal wash and nasopharyngeal wash methods for collecting specimen for RSV testing.[22]

Severe manifestations of RSV infection (e.g., pneumonia and bronchiolitis) most commonly occur in infants aged 2 to 6 months, and hospitalization rates for these diagnoses have been used as an indicator for severe RSV disease among young children. Secretory immunoglobulin A (IgA) antibody secreted in colostrum may provide a protective factor in breast-fed babies. In the United States, bronchiolitis hospitalization rates among children aged less than 1 year increased substantially from 12.9 per 1000 in 1980 to 31.2 per 1000 in 1996; the reasons for this increase are unclear.[23] RSV infection among recipients of bone marrow transplants has resulted in high mortality rates (83%).[24]

Pathogenesis. Bronchiolitis, an acute inflammatory disease in the lower respiratory tract, is also a disease of the lung parenchyma. Whether it is due to alveolar collapse from obstruction, or to primary involvement of the terminal airways and alveoli, many infants have a substantial restrictive component, which may predominate, usually causing a more severe form of the disease. The principal abnormality in gas exchange is hypoxemia. $\dot{V}/\dot{Q}$ mismatching accounts for arterial desaturation because hypoxemia is typically relieved with a modest amount of supplemental O_2.

Most infants, in spite of an increased physiologic dead space–to–tidal volume ratio, are able to maintain normocarbia by increasing minute ventilation ($\dot{V}_E$). Hypercarbia and respiratory failure develop when the infant becomes fatigued and $\dot{V}_E$ falls to predicted basal levels. The high $\dot{V}_E$ is due mainly to the increased respiratory rate, whereas tidal volume is unchanged or somewhat lower than normal. Respiratory muscle fatigue is not surprising considering that most infants increase their work of breathing up to sixfold during acute bronchiolitis. Tachypnea may represent the presence of a restrictive component (alveolitis, edema, or alveolar distension from hyperinflation), an overriding of the mechanism by the infant's cerebral cortex (because of agitation), and/or the work of a feedback mechanism initiated by stretch receptors of the lung and chest wall.

Respiratory distress in bronchiolitis is caused primarily by obstruction of small airways. This results from peribronchiolar cellular infiltration, interstitial edema, and the effects of plugging of small airways by sloughed epithelium and inflammatory exudates. The small size of the developing airways makes infants particularly vulnerable to obstruction owing to these mechanisms. Hypoxemia represents the major abnormality in gas exchange and is the result of underventilation of regions with relatively normal perfusion, that is, low ventilation to perfusion ratio.

Respiratory insufficiency results when the infant, exhausted by the increased work of breathing, can no longer maintain adequate minute $\dot{V}_E$. At this point, air entry is greatly diminished, respiratory pauses and/or apnea may occur, and the infant may develop a respiratory or metabolic acidosis. Crying, feeding, and agitation may exacerbate signs of respiratory distress, which include prolonged expiratory time, crackles and/or wheezing, and substernal and intercostal retractions. Rapidly progressing respiratory distress, increasing O_2 requirements, or an altered mental status are indications for PICU admission and, possibly, assisted ventilation. Smaller infants may also require PICU monitoring because exudates or edema in their small airways produces a comparatively greater degree of obstruction. Apnea in RSV bronchiolitis is not due to upper airway obstruction but rather to a complete absence of respiratory effort.[25]

Critical Care Management. The management of infants with bronchiolitis has changed very little in the past 20 years. Therapy is still largely supportive, consisting of O_2, mechanical ventilation, bronchodilators, and hydration. Supplemental O_2 is generally required by all infants with bronchiolitis and generally reverses the hypoxemia caused by $\dot{V}/\dot{Q}$ abnormalities.

Inhaled bronchodilators may be beneficial; their use is determined by the individual infant's response. Two meta-analyses of bronchodilators in bronchiolitis concluded bronchodilators may produce modest short-term improvement in clinical features of mild or moderately severe bronchiolitis.[26,27] Nebulized epinephrine is also commonly a first-line therapy. Nebulized epinephrine results in significant improvement in clinical scores and airways resistance in children hospitalized with bronchiolitis, causes acute improvement in oxygenation, and decreases length of time in the emergency department and admission rate to the hospital.[28]

Endotracheal intubation is indicated for signs of respiratory failure including worsening respiratory distress, severe tachycardia, listlessness or lethargy, and poor peripheral perfusion. It may also be required for increasing hypoxemia (Pao_2 less than 60 mmHg or O_2 saturation less than 92% in an Fio_2 of 0.4), hypercarbia with respiratory acidosis, metabolic acidosis, apnea, or bradycardia. The routine use of PEEP in infants with bronchiolitis does not consistently improve passive expiratory pulmonary mechanics and may increase the risk of barotrauma from gas trapping.[29]

Nasal CPAP is a reliable alternative to support arterial oxygenation in patients with respiratory failure who are alert and vigorous enough to avoid hypercapnia and respiratory acidosis while breathing spontaneously. In addition, because the patients are able to speak and thus are capable of expressing their feelings, the anxiety observed during respiratory support can be reduced.[30]

In a small randomized, double-blind, controlled, cross-over study and nonrandomized, prospective study Hollman and colleagues demonstrated that inhaled heliox improved the overall respiratory status of children with acute RSV lower respiratory tract infection.[31] The beneficial effects of heliox were most pronounced in children with the greatest degree of respiratory compromise.

A randomized placebo-controlled trial of nebulized corticosteroids in acute RSV bronchiolitis demonstrated no short- or long-term clinical benefits from the administration of nebulized corticosteroids.[32] A second randomized prospective study in infants hospitalized with acute RSV infection showed no effect of systemic prednisolone treatment either in the acute state of RSV infection, nor in the follow-up 1 month and 1 year after admission to hospital. The authors concluded corticosteroid, whether by the systemic route or by inhalation, should not be prescribed to infants with RSV infection.[33]

Ribavirin is generally indicated only to limit the duration of viral shedding.[34] A recent prospective, double-blind, placebo-controlled trial of 41 previously well infants who required ventilation for respiratory distress secondary to RSV bronchiolitis demonstrated the lack of effectiveness of aerosolized ribavirin in reducing the length of ventilation and course of illness in infants with no underlying illness.[35]

Because respiratory failure resulting from bronchiolitis may occur precipitously, it is important to identify high-risk patients upon hospital admission. Continuous monitoring includes heart rate, respiratory rate, and O_2 saturation. Frequent assessment of respiratory effort, breath sounds, and level of consciousness helps detect subtle changes in clinical status. The infant's response to interventions, for example, bronchodilators or chest physiotherapy directs future therapy and is closely evaluated and carefully documented. Any activity that increases the infant's work of breathing is avoided.

Initially, fluid replacement may be necessary to correct fluid deficits resulting from increased insensible loss and poor intake. After replacing losses, fluids are restricted to maintenance requirements or somewhat less to reduce the risk of developing pulmonary edema and further deterioration in respiratory function. The severely tachypneic infant may need to be fed by transpyloric feeding tube.[36] Before endotracheal intubation, placing an oroenteric feeding tube is preferred because a nasoenteric tube will occlude the infant's naris and may worsen respiratory distress by increasing airways resistance.

Attempts are made to maximize ventilation, including elevating the head of the bed and positioning the infant prone to permit freer diaphragmatic movement. When mechanical ventilation is required, sedation may also be necessary to facilitate coordination of the infant's respiratory efforts with the ventilator and minimize coughing paroxysms.

Prevention. No RSV vaccines are available, although both live attenuated and subunit vaccines have entered clinical trials. RSV immune globulin intravenous (RSV-IVIG) and a humanized murine anti-RSV monoclonal antibody (palivizumab) are recommended as prophylaxis for some high-risk infants and young children (e.g., those born prematurely or with chronic lung disease) to prevent serious RSV disease.[37]

Intravenous immunoglobulin is a solution of immunoglobulin containing many antibodies normally present in adult human blood. It is obtained from plasma-pooled whole blood of thousands of diverse adult donors, ensuring a broad spectrum of antibodies. Immune globulin therapy is rapidly shifting from standard pooled preparations to specific immune globulin preparations. High-titer specific immune globulin preparations are prepared by screening or immunizing donors. RSV-IVIG contains high titers of RSV immune globulin. Concerns about the requirement of monthly administration, requiring intravenous cannulation and infusion over several hours and the fluid volume and protein load have restricted the use of RSV-IVIG.

An examination of the effectiveness of RSV-IVIG in reducing hospitalization for treatment of RSV in children with congenital heart disease (CHD) demonstrated a significantly higher frequency of unanticipated cyanotic episodes and of poor outcomes after surgery among children with cyanotic CHD in the RSV-IVIG group (22 of 78, 28%) than in the control group (4 of 47, 8.5%; $P<.001$). At this time RSV-IVIG should not be used for prophylaxis of RSV disease in children with cyanotic CHD.[38]

Efforts have been directed to the development of a monoclonal IgG antibody and prophylaxis against RSV. The Food and Drug Administration recently approved the use of palivizumab, an intramuscularly administered monoclonal antibody preparation. Recommendations for its use are based on a 1502-patient, randomized study demonstrating palivizumab prophylaxis resulted in a 55% reduction in hospitalization as a result of RSV (10.6% placebo versus 4.8% palivizumab).[39] Infants and children with chronic lung disease, formerly designated bronchopulmonary dysplasia, as well as prematurely born infants without chronic lung disease experienced a reduced number of hospitalizations while receiving palivizumab compared with a placebo ($P<.001$).

Both palivizumab and RSV-IVIG are available for protecting high-risk children against serious complications from RSV infections. Palivizumab is preferred for most high-risk children because of ease of administration (intramuscular), lack of interference with measles-mumps-rubella vaccine and varicella vaccine, and lack of complications associated with intravenous administration of human immune globulin products. RSV-IVIG, however, provides additional protection against other respiratory viral illnesses and may be preferred for selected high-risk children, including those receiving replacement intravenous immune globulin because of underlying immune deficiency or HIV infection. For premature infants about to be discharged from hospitals during the RSV season, the American Academy of Pediatrics recommends considering administering RSV-IVIG for the first month of prophylaxis.[37]

RSV infection usually occurs after viral inoculation of the conjunctivae or nasal mucosa by contaminated hands. Guidelines developed by the Centers for Disease Control and Prevention (CDC) addresses common problems encountered by infection-control practitioners regarding the prevention and control of nosocomial pneumonia in U.S. hospitals. Sections on the prevention of bacterial pneumonia in mechanically ventilated and/or critically ill patients, care of respiratory-therapy devices, prevention of cross-contamination, and prevention of viral lower respiratory tract infections (e.g., RSV and influenza infections) have recently been expanded and updated. Traditional preventive measures for nosocomial pneumonia include decreasing aspiration by the patient (transpyloric feedings, elevating the head of the bed at least 15 degrees), preventing cross-contamination or colonization via hands of personnel, appropriate disinfection or sterilization of respiratory-therapy devices, use of available vaccines to protect against particular infections, and education of hospital staff and patients.[40] The CDC specifically recommends contact precautions for all patients with RSV.

Asthma (Reactive Airways Disease)

Etiology.   Asthma (reactive airways disease) is defined as recurrent, reversible episodes of wheezing, or dyspnea caused by airway obstruction. It is classified as extrinsic (an immunologic, allergic response), intrinsic (nonallergic, often triggered by infection), exercise-induced, and/or aspirin induced (the last two types being rare during infancy or childhood).

Asthma is a multifactorial disease that has been associated with familial, infectious, allergenic, socioeconomic, psychosocial, and environmental factors. Atopy, the genetic predisposition for the development of an IgE-mediated response to common aeroallergens, is the strongest identifiable predisposing factor for developing asthma.[41] Decreases in pulmonary functions and exacerbations of asthma have been associated with ambient air pollutants (e.g., ozone, sulfur dioxide, nitrogen dioxide, acid aerosols, and particulate matter), indoor pollutants (e.g., tobacco smoke), and allergens (e.g., dust mites). Approximately 25% of children in the United States reside in areas that exceed the federal standard for ozone.[42]

Incidence.   Asthma is the most common chronic illness in childhood and is characterized by variable airflow obstruction with airway hyperresponsiveness. In the United States, asthma affects an estimated 14 million to 15 million persons, including 4.8 million (6.9%) aged younger than 18 years. During 1980 through 1993, asthma accounted for 3850 deaths among persons aged 0 to 24 years. In 1994, the annual age-specific asthma death rate increased 118% (from 1.7 million to 3.7 per million population) and from 1980 to 1993, the annual hospitalization rate for asthma among persons aged 0 to 24 years increased 28%.[43] Although asthma-associated mortality has increased among persons aged less than 25 years, hospitalizations for asthma have increased primarily among children younger than 5 years of age. The increase among young children may be related to changes in diagnostic practices, changes in coding and reimbursement, or increases in morbidity.[44]

Pathogenesis.   Asthma is a chronic inflammatory disorder of the airways in which many cells and cellular elements play a role, in particular, mast cells, eosinophils, T lymphocytes, macrophages, neutrophils, and epithelial cells. In susceptible individuals, this inflammation causes recurrent episodes of wheezing, breathlessness, chest tightness, and coughing, particularly at night or in the early morning. These episodes are usually associated with widespread but variable airflow obstruction that is often reversible, either spontaneously or with treatment. The inflammation also causes an associated increase in the existing bronchial hyperresponsiveness to a variety of stimuli.[45]

It is hypothesized that airway inflammation can be acute, subacute, and chronic. The acute inflammatory response is represented by the early recruitment of cells to the airway. In the subacute phase, recruited and resident cells are activated to cause a more persistent pattern of inflammation. Chronic inflammation is characterized by a persistent level of cell damage and an ongoing repair process, changes that may cause permanent abnormalities in the airway.[41]

Lung cells recovered from symptomatic patients with asthma generate increased amounts of reactive oxygen species (ROS). Animal and in vitro studies indicate that ROS can reproduce many of the features of asthma. The ability of ROS to produce the clinical features of asthma may depend on an individual's lung antioxidant defenses. Patients with asthma are reported to have reduced antioxidant defenses in peripheral blood, but little is known about the antioxidant defenses of their lung cells.[46]

The differences in the anatomy and physiology of the lungs of infants place them at greater risk for respiratory failure. These differences include greater peripheral airways resistance, fewer collateral channels of ventilation, further extension of airway smooth muscle into the peripheral airways, less elastic recoil, and mechanical disadvantage of the diaphragm.[41]

Severe acute asthma, so-called status asthmaticus, does not respond to routine therapy and necessitates hospitalization. Children whose asthma has caused even one episode of respiratory failure may be more likely to have repeated episodes of respiratory failure and its catastrophic complications, including hypoxic brain injury and death.

The child in status asthmaticus is usually pale and restless, has severe wheezing, and is sometimes cyanotic. Respiratory rate and heart rate are elevated, and a pulsus paradoxus of more than 15 mmHg may be detected. Vomiting and abdominal pain and distension are common, as is dehydration. As airway obstruction increases during an acute attack, ABGs change through a characteristic series of stages. Arterial oxygen tension (Pao_2) is decreased because of a reduced $\dot{V}/\dot{Q}$ ratio caused by the simultaneous occurrence of air trapping and atelectasis. Initially, hypoxemia stimulates the respiratory drive, and the $Paco_2$ decreases, with a normal or slightly elevated pH. Eventually, as muscle fatigue develops and compensatory mechanisms fail, the $Paco_2$ begins to rise, producing respiratory acidosis. Respiratory rate and breath sounds decrease, and extreme restlessness is followed by stupor and unconsciousness. With progression, the $Paco_2$ increases even more, pH falls with a superimposed metabolic acidosis, and Pao_2 becomes markedly reduced.

Critical Care Management.   Treatment is directed at ensuring oxygenation and adequate alveolar ventilation while reversing the primary airway abnormalities: bronchospasm, mucosal edema, and overproduction of tenacious secretions. Because patients in status asthmaticus are often hypoxic, it is essential to provide supplemental O_2 by oxyhood, mask, or nasal cannula. Preexisting $\dot{V}/\dot{Q}$ imbalances may be worsened by treatment with sympathomimetics (agents that ablate hypoxic vasoconstriction in the lungs, thereby increasing venous admixture [see later]); therefore F_{IO_2} is adjusted during treatment to maintain a normal Sp_{O_2}.

To review, sympathomimetics are differentiated by the type of receptor they stimulate: alpha, beta$_1$, or beta$_2$. α-Adrenergic receptors are located in the smooth muscles of all vascular tissue. Stimulation of these receptors results in constriction of arterial and venous vasculature. β_2-Receptors are found in the heart. Stimulating these receptors increases myocardial contractility, automaticity, and heart rate. β_2-Receptors are primarily found in the smooth muscle of the lungs and skeletal muscle arterioles. Stimulation of these receptors results in smooth muscle relaxation, causing bronchodilation in the lungs and increased blood flow in skeletal muscle. Generally, initial management begins with administration of continuous nebulized β_2-agonists.

Short-acting inhaled β_2-agonists, such as albuterol and terbutaline, are indicated for quick relief of acute symptoms. Mechanism of action is bronchodilation through smooth muscle relaxation following adenylate cyclase activation and increase in cyclic adenosine monophosphate (cyclic AMP) producing functional antagonism of bronchoconstriction. Combining a nebulized β_2-agonist with an anticholinergic (ipratropium bromide) may produce better bronchodilation.[47] Anticholinergics, such as ipratropium bromide, cause bronchodilation through competitive inhibition of muscarinic cholinergic receptors, reduce intrinsic vagal tone to the airways, and may decrease mucous gland secretion. Ipratropium bromide may provide some additive benefit to inhaled β_2-agonists in severe exacerbations.

Parenteral corticosteroids are also started immediately. Steroids act not only as antiinflammatory agents, but increase the number of β-adrenergic receptors, enhancing the response of bronchial smooth muscle to both endogenous catecholamines and exogenous β_2-agonists. Therefore early steroid therapy combined with an adrenergic agent is significantly more effective than the adrenergic agent alone, even in infants and toddlers.[48] Clinically, production of the thick tenacious sputum peculiar to asthma is also controlled, and mucosal edema appears to be decreased. Methylprednisolone (preferred over hydrocortisone because it has less effect on sodium and potassium metabolism at high doses) is given intravenously in a dose of 1 mg/kg per dose every 6 hours (maximum single dose 60 mg/day IV). Serious toxicity or adrenal suppression with short-term therapy (less than 2 weeks) is unlikely. Patients in respiratory failure, especially those receiving steroids, routinely receive prophylactic treatment against stress-ulcer bleeding.

Intravenous magnesium sulfate is also administered early in the course. Magnesium sulfate, 25 to 50 mg/kg (up to a maximum dose of 2 g) is administered in a 2-hour infusion; specifically, in severe circumstances, the first half of the dose may be given over the first 15 to 20 minutes, and the remainder of the dose should be administered over 2 hours. The maximum rate of infusion is 125 mg/kg per hour. Serum magnesium levels are obtained 12 hours after the infusion (normal serum magnesium levels = 1.9 to 2.5 mg/dl). The efficacy of intravenous magnesium therapy for moder-

ate to severe asthma exacerbations in 31 pediatric patients was evaluated in a randomized, double-blind, placebo-controlled, clinical trial. Children treated with intravenous magnesium sulfate infusions for moderate to severe asthma had significantly greater improvement in short-term pulmonary function.[49]

When continuous inhaled bronchodilators, steroids, anticholinergics, and magnesium fail to correct hypoxemia and hypercarbia, intravenous terbutaline may provide a reversal of bronchoconstriction and avert the need for endotracheal intubation and assisted ventilation. Terbutaline, a more selective β_2-agonist, has few toxic effects. A loading dose of 10 μg/kg of intravenous terbutaline is administered over 5 minutes followed by a continuous infusion of 1 to 3 μg/kg/min. This maintenance dose may be increased by 0.5 μg/kg per minute as necessary, keeping the heart rate under 200 beats per minute (bpm).

Leukotrienes are potent biochemical mediators released from mast cells, eosinophils, and basophils that contract airway smooth muscle, increase vascular permeability, increase mucous secretions, and attract and activate inflammatory cells in the airways of patients with asthma. Leukotriene modifiers, zafirlukast and zileuton, have been demonstrated to improve lung function and diminish symptoms and the need for short-acting inhaled β_2-agonists in mild to moderate asthma. Zafirlukast, a leukotriene receptor antagonist, or zileuton, a 5-lipoxygenase inhibitor, may be considered an alternative therapy to low doses of inhaled corticosteroids or cromolyn or nedocromil for patients older than 12 years of age with mild persistent asthma.

Heliox has demonstrated mixed results when used during acute asthma. During status asthmaticus in 18 patients, inhaled heliox significantly lowered pulsus paradoxus, increased peak flow, and lessened the dyspnea index.[50] In contrast, in a separate prospective, randomized, double-blind, cross-over study of 11 children with status asthmaticus heliox did not show benefit.[51]

Theophylline and aminophylline are not recommended because they appear to provide no additional benefit to optimal inhaled β_2-agonist therapy and may increase adverse effects.[41] Intravenous isoproterenol is not recommended in the treatment of asthma because of the danger of myocardial toxicity.[52] Antibiotics are also not recommended for asthma treatment and are generally reserved for patients with fever and purulent sputum or evidence of pneumonia.[41]

Most patients respond well to therapy. However, a small minority will show signs of worsening ventilation, whether from worsening airflow obstruction, worsening respiratory muscle fatigue, or a combination of the two. Signs of impending respiratory failure include a declining mental clarity, worsening fatigue, and progressive hypercapnia. Exactly when to intubate is based on clinical judgment. Because respiratory failure can progress rapidly and can be difficult to reverse, early recognition and treatment are critically important.[41] Clinicians should be aware that hypotension commonly accompanies the initiation of positive pressure ventilation, close attention should be given to maintaining or replacing intravascular volume.

Permissive hypercapnia or controlled hypoventilation is the recommended ventilator strategy to provide adequate oxygenation and ventilation while minimizing high airway pressures and barotrauma.[41] It involves administration of as high a FIO_2 as necessary to maintain adequate arterial oxygenation, acceptance of hypercapnia, and treatment of respiratory acidosis with intravenous sodium bicarbonate. Adjustments are made to the tidal volume, ventilator rate, and I:E ratio to minimize airway pressures. Bronchodilators are continued, and even in ventilated patients, aerosol delivery is the route of choice.[53]

Mechanical ventilation with heliox may improve the (A-a) gradient in some patients with status asthmaticus. Although this improvement adds little to routine therapy with supplemental O_2, it does permit reduction in concentration of inspired O_2 to levels that maximize helium concentration and thus permit full benefits of heliox on lung mechanics to be realized in even the most severely ill asthmatics.[54]

Until conventional therapy can be optimized, an intubated mechanically ventilated patient in status asthmaticus may benefit from the use of an inhaled anesthetic that produces a secondary effect of bronchodilation.[55] Isoflurane (Forane), a fluorinated ether, is one such agent. Isoflurane has a low blood-gas solubility coefficient so that changes in the concentration administered will result in an almost immediate alteration of effect—a desirable feature in the ICU setting. The dose of inhaled isoflurane dose is 0.5% (increased in increments of 0.2%). At an inspired concentration of 2%, the hemodynamic side effects (hypotension, tachycardia) may become pronounced and precipitate the need for concomitant inotropic support. Potential adverse reactions are dose dependent and include respiratory depression, hypotension, and junctional dysrhythmias. Management of significant adverse effects includes disconnecting the patient from the isoflurane and ventilating the patient with an FIO_2 of 1.0. Isoflurane is contraindicated in patients with a known or suspected genetic susceptibility to malignant hyperthermia.

Before the introduction of this novel therapy in the ICU, multidisciplinary standards of care and practice guidelines are created and additional nursing competencies are validated. Patients receiving an inhalation agent are continuously observed. In addition to standard ICU monitoring, inspiratory and end-tidal isoflurane concentrations and core temperatures are continuously monitored and recorded hourly. End-tidal concentration should, in general, measure within 0.1% of the inspired concentration. Before suctioning a patient receiving isoflurane, a suctioning plan that takes into consideration the almost immediate reversal of anesthesia and bronchodilation is created, for example, premedication consisting of lidocaine (1 mg/kg) and ketamine (1 to 2 mg/kg). Note that peak lidocaine effect is less than 1 minute.

The importance of continuously monitoring the patient in status asthmaticus cannot be overemphasized. Frequent evaluations are necessary to assess the efficacy of sympathomimetics, and will direct the choice, and frequency of administration, of inhaled bronchodilators. Respiratory as-sessments include respiratory rate and effort, as well as the quality of air movement on auscultation. A fall in SpO_2 below 90% is considered a sign of serious hypoxemia. ABGs also document progression in respiratory failure with an increase in $PaCO_2$ and acidosis. The child's level of consciousness is frequently noted because a decrease in mental status may signal impending respiratory failure.

Assessment of infants is dependent upon physical examination rather than objective measurements. Use of accessory muscles, paradoxical breathing, cyanosis, a respiratory rate greater than 60, and SpO_2 less than 91% are key signs of serious distress.[41] Skilled nursing assessment is necessary not only to monitor the effectiveness of interventions but also to detect negative effects of therapy (Table 19-3).

Caring for the child with asthma after endotracheal intubation presents additional nursing challenges. Routine maneuvers to maintain airway patency may irritate airway receptors and trigger bronchospasm and hypoxia. Heavy sedation and, in some patients, neuromuscular blockade may be required to achieve adequate ventilation and reduce the risks of barotrauma caused by positive pressure ventilation. In particular, the risk of developing a pneumothorax, already increased because of gas trapping, is great in mechanically ventilated patients with asthma. Pneumothorax should be suspected if there is sudden clinical deterioration with hypoxemia, acidosis, hypotension, or the unilateral absence of breath sounds. Equipment to needle aspirate extra-alveolar air (a large-bore intravenous catheter, stopcock, and large syringe) should be kept at the bedside, and equipment necessary for chest tube insertion readily available. Chest physiotherapy is contraindicated during acute exacerbations because it may aggravate the child and his or her airways.

Laboratory studies may help detect actual or impending respiratory failure, however these studies should not delay initiation of treatment. An ABG is helpful in evaluating $PaCO_2$ in patients with suspected hypoventilation. A complete blood count (CBC) may be appropriate in patients with fever or purulent sputum; keeping in mind that modest leukocytosis is common in asthma exacerbations and that corticosteroid treatment causes a further outpouring of polymorphonuclear leukocytes within 1 to 2 hours of administration. It may be prudent to measure serum electrolytes in patients who have been taking diuretics regularly and in patients with coexistent cardiovascular disease, because frequent β_2-agonist administration can cause transient decreased in serum potassium, magnesium, and phosphate. Chest radiography is not recommended for routine assessment but should be obtained in patients suspected of a complicating cardiopulmonary process, such as pneumothorax, pneumomediastinum, pneumonia, lobar atelectasis, or congestive heart failure.[41]

Once an acute episode is controlled, parent and/or patient education becomes a nursing priority. This begins with a careful assessment of the family's understanding of the disease process and the measures necessary to help prevent future attacks.

Monitoring reactive disease in children is difficult because of their inability to cooperate with lung function

TABLE 19-3 **Actions and Clinically Significant Side Effects of Medications Used in the Treatment of Asthma**

Drug	Actions	Side Effects
Inhaled β_2-Agonist		
Albuterol (Ventolin) Terbutaline (Brethine) Metaproterenol (Alupent)	Bronchodilation (largely resulting from local drug effects in the lungs) Improve mucociliary clearance Metaproterenol is somewhat shorter acting and less selective for β-adrenergic receptors	Tachycardia (less than with systemic drugs) Tremor and hyperactivity occur infrequently
Anticholingeric Agent		
Ipratropium bromide	Blocks the action of acetylcholine at parasympathetic sites in bronchial smooth muscle causing bronchodilation.	Tachycardia, flushing, nervousness, headache, drowsiness
Corticosteroids		
Methylprednisolone	Reduce inflammation $\uparrow$ β-adrenergic receptors (enhancing the response of bronchial smooth muscle to catecholamines)	Gastric ulcerations Adrenal insufficiency (with long-term therapy)
Systemic β_2 Agonist		
Terbutaline	Bronchodilation via: — Smooth muscle relaxation — Inhibition of antigen-induced release of histamine and other mediators of inflammation $\uparrow$ heart rate, contractility $\downarrow$ peripheral vascular resistance $\leftrightarrow$ or $\uparrow$ systolic blood pressure $\uparrow$ cardiac output	Tachycardia, hypertension, dysrhythmias, headache, seizures, nausea, and vomiting

tests. In the noncritical patient, the 88%-SAT may be more effective than spirometry for identifying reactive airways disease in young, uncooperative, or developmentally delayed children. The 88%-SAT consists of continuous measurement of Spo_2 while the subject breathes a nonhumidified 12% O_2 and nitrogen mixture for 10 minutes or until Spo_2 decreases to 88%, whichever occurs first.[56]

Prevention. One of the national health objectives for the year 2000 is to decrease asthma morbidity, as measured by a reduction in hospitalizations for asthma, among children younger than or equal to 14 years to no more than 18.3 per 10,000 population. Hospitalizations and mortality related to asthma can be prevented, in part, by improving surveillance, diagnostic measures, and patient management; providing patient education; targeting high-risk populations; and evaluating interventions in the home environment (e.g., reducing levels of house dust mites and exposure to environmental tobacco smoke).[57]

Prolonged breast-feeding and avoidance of early introduction of allergenic foods have been reported to reduce eczema and food sensitization but not to reduce the prevalence of asthma.[41] However, a report of 2187 6-year-old children indicated that the presence of the diagnosis of asthma and wheezing occurring 3 times or more since 1 year of age were associated with exposure to milk that was not breast milk before age 4 months.[58]

The literature is unclear as to when immunotherapy should be initiated for childhood asthma. Although there are suggestions that immunotherapy should be considered for the child with mild or moderate asthma and dust mite sensitivity when pharmacotherapy is not efficacious, the immunomodulatory properties of immunotherapy may actually be more tailored for early intervention in asthma rather than for use once symptoms have occurred.[41,59]

Restrictive Disease

Reduced pulmonary compliance is another mechanical alteration that can produce alterations in pulmonary function and respiratory pump failure. When pulmonary compliance is decreased, a greater airway pressure is needed to distend alveolar units to the same final lung volume; that is, it takes more pressure (and more work) to deliver normal lung volumes to a stiff lung. To reduce the work of breathing yet sustain minute alveolar ventilation, children with decreased thoracic compliance breathe rapidly and shallowly. Diminished compliance also results in intercostal and subcostal retractions, especially in the supple chest wall of the young infant.

In addition to increasing the work of breathing, decreased pulmonary compliance ultimately reduces functional residual capacity (FRC, the amount of air that remains in the lungs at the end of normal expiration). This reduction in FRC may lead to alveolar collapse and result in increased intrapulmonary shunting and hypoxemia.

Frequent causes of decreased lung compliance in PICU patients include pneumothorax, pneumonia, adult respiratory distress syndrome (ARDS), and congenital diaphragmatic hernia.

Pneumothorax

Etiology. A pneumothorax is a collection of air or gas in the pleural space that may occur spontaneously but more frequently results from trauma to the lung parenchyma. A tension pneumothorax exists when air enters the pleural space at such a rate that pressure in the pleural space increases enough to produce circulatory and ventilatory impairment. As extra-alveolar air accumulates, it compresses and shifts the mediastinum toward the unaffected side. If a significant tension pneumothorax is not treated promptly, venous return to the heart falls, cardiac output decreases, and cardiopulmonary arrest ensues. Early detection and timely intervention, however, may prevent this catastrophic chain of events.

Incidence. Although a spontaneous pneumothorax during unassisted breathing is rare, alveolar overdistension then rupture may be seen with the use of use high peak inspiratory or end-expiratory pressures to achieve adequate oxygenation and ventilation.

Pathogenesis. Patients who have regional differences in lung compliance or airways resistance are at risk for the development of extra-alveolar air. A pneumothorax may occur, for example, in a child with ARDS when less affected alveoli are overdistended by the pressure required to inflate noncompliant areas of the lung. In the child in status asthmaticus, a pneumothorax may result if airway obstruction during expiration leads to gas trapping and alveolar hyperinflation.

A pneumothorax may also result from chest trauma. An open pneumothorax (or sucking chest wound) occurs when there is a penetrating injury that creates a communication between the pleural space and the environment. Pleural pressure and atmospheric pressure immediately equilibrate, the lung collapses, and the mediastinum shifts toward the unaffected lung. A small opening in the chest wall that permits air entry but blocks its exit (or a closed lung injury, caused by a broken rib, for example) may cause air to accumulate in the pleural space and result in a tension pneumothorax.

Once the alveolus ruptures, the gas it contains moves into the interstitial space where it dissects into other fascial planes or compartments. This results in air-leak syndrome, for example, interstitial emphysema, pneumopericardium, pneumothorax, pneumomediastinum, subcutaneous emphysema, pneumoretroperitoneum, and/or pneumoperitoneum.

Critical Care Management. The primary therapeutic goals are to identify patients at risk, closely monitor for the signs and symptoms of a pneumothorax, and reduce or eliminate factors that may contribute to the development of extra-alveolar air.

A small, stable pneumothorax may go completely undetected until a chest radiograph reveals its presence (Fig. 19-6). If the pneumothorax increases in size, the child may develop dyspnea, pleuritic chest pain, and tachypnea.

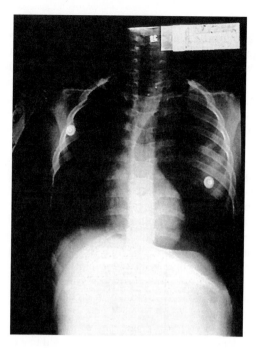

Fig. 19-6 Chest radiograph illustrating pneumothorax with mediastinal shift.

However, a more dramatic presentation frequently occurs in the PICU setting. Commonly, the child undergoing positive pressure ventilation has a sudden deterioration in oxygenation and ventilation as reflected in noninvasive monitors and ABGs. The child becomes tachycardic and hypotensive because of decreased venous return to the heart. A significant pulsus paradoxus (a decrease in blood pressure during inspiration) may also develop as left ventricular output is further compromised by increasing intrathoracic pressures. An infant who develops a large tension pneumothorax may rapidly become hypotensive and develops bradycardia from severe hypoxemia. On physical examination, there may be decreased breath sounds and hyperresonance to percussion on the affected side. However, in infants and small children, breath sounds may be readily transmitted from the unaffected to the affected side, and a decrease in air entry may not be as apparent. Transillumination with a high-intensity light may be helpful in these patients; the side of the chest containing the free air will transmit light well. In older patients, there may also be a contralateral shift of the mediastinum with tracheal deviation toward the unaffected side and lateral displacement of the cardiac apical impulse. Occasionally, subcutaneous emphysema and crepitus may also occur.

To detect the development of a tension pneumothorax, it is necessary to identify and closely monitor those patients at higher risk for developing extra-alveolar air. Patients receiving positive pressure ventilation are assessed frequently to determine the adequacy of their ventilation and detect untoward events, such as right mainstem intubation or asynchronous breathing, which may lead to a pneumothorax. Nursing vigilance in these patients can prevent what is sometimes an iatrogenic complication of treatment.

A tension pneumothorax is a medical emergency that requires immediate intervention. Evacuation of pleural air is attempted whenever a patient has an acute deterioration that is likely to be the result of tension pneumothorax. Although a chest radiograph provides the definitive diagnosis, it should not delay treatment of a suspected pneumothorax in a patient with rapidly deteriorating circulatory function. In the absence of a chest radiograph, transillumination or physical examination can localize a pneumothorax. Initially, a large-bore needle or catheter, attached by a stopcock to a large syringe, may be used to rapidly evacuate the pneumothorax. Once the patient's condition has stabilized, a tube thoracostomy can be performed to permit full reexpansion of the lung and prevent reaccumulation of pleural air.

When a chest tube is required, assessment of the patient's respiratory status is followed by a thorough assessment of the chest tube and drainage system. The chest tube insertion site is covered with an occlusive dressing and kept dry to prevent maceration of the skin. Although usually sutured in at the time of insertion, the chest tube or drainage tubing is also taped to the child's chest wall to minimize the risk of dislodgment. The chest tube is then connected to a drainage system (see Chapter 8).

Pneumonia

Etiology. Most pneumonias in infants and children are viral in origin. However, bacterial pneumonias are still an important cause of severe illness in childhood. In the immunocompetent pediatric patient, the major organisms causing bacterial pneumonia are pneumococcus, streptococcus, and staphylococcus. Certain infectious agents are more prevalent in certain age groups: Group B streptococci predominate in the newborn; pneumococcus in the young child 1 month to 6 years of age; and pneumococcus in the older child. In the immunocompromised patient, *Pneumocystis carinii,* fungi, and opportunistic bacteria such as enteric and atypical mycobacteria are important causative agents.

Incidence. Pneumonia is the most common life-threatening lung disease in pediatric patients.

Pathogenesis. Pneumonia, an inflammatory process in the lungs that progresses to alveolar consolidation, occurs when pulmonary defense mechanisms are altered and an infective agent invades the lung by aspiration or hematogenous spread. Pneumonia can occur anywhere in the lung. As lobes or segments become filled with fluid and cellular debris, lung compliance and vital capacity decrease and the work of breathing increases. Intrapulmonary shunting and $\dot{V}/\dot{Q}$ mismatch result from continued perfusion of consolidated, airless lung and lead to significant hypoxemia. Signs and symptoms of respiratory distress may develop, including tachypnea, dyspnea, cough, and intercostal retractions. Usually, there are localized findings over the affected lung segment with diminished breath sounds or adventitious noises.

Patients with endotracheal intubation are particularly vulnerable to nosocomially acquired pneumonia. Bacterial colonization of the upper respiratory tract commonly occurs in these patients and may promote pneumonia through aspiration of these pathogens. In addition, the child with an artificial airway may be at particularly high risk for pneumonia because of impaired mucociliary clearance, the frequency of airway invasion, and exposure to nosocomial pathogens.

Aspiration pneumonia is an important phenomenon in the PICU patient. When normal airway protective mechanisms are impaired, gastric contents may be aspirated into the airways. This may occur because of a decreased level of consciousness or the presence of an endotracheal tube, which inhibits the child's ability to occlude the larynx.

Critical Care Management. When bacterial pneumonia is suspected, appropriate antibiotic therapy is started as soon as possible. Antibiotic coverage may be changed or extended when the causative organism is identified and antibiotic sensitivities established. Supplemental O_2 is administered to maintain normal Spo_2. If respiratory failure ensues, endotracheal intubation and mechanical ventilation are also required.

Nursing care of the patient with pneumonia is largely supportive. Impaired gas exchange is monitored by following ABGs and Spo_2. When unilateral intrapulmonary shunting predominates, patient positioning becomes critically important. Although pulmonary perfusion is predominately located along the dorsal regions, the pattern of lung inflation depends on how the patient is being ventilated. Lungs inflate from bottom to top during spontaneous breaths and from top to bottom during positive pressure breaths. Optimal position to enhance matching of ventilation to perfusion in patients with unilateral pneumonia is best determined at the bedside with the aid of Spo_2 monitoring.

Acute Respiratory Distress Syndrome

Etiology. In 1967, Ashbaugh and others first described a group of patients who, after injuries such as trauma and sepsis, developed acute dyspnea and hypoxemia that failed to respond to conservative therapy.[60] Today we recognize ARDS as a syndrome of inflammation and increased permeability that is associated with a constellation of clinical, radiologic, and physiologic abnormalities that cannot be explained by, but may coexist with, left atrial or pulmonary capillary hypertension.[61] Although 63% of pediatric patients present with more than one ARDS trigger (an illness that has the potential to cause ARDS),[62] precipitating factors include pneumonia (51%), sepsis (33%), airways disease (18%), pulmonary aspiration (12%), status–post bone marrow transplant (10%), trauma with shock and multiple transfusions (8%), and near-drowning (3%). Sepsis is associated with the highest (40%) progression to ARDS.

To facilitate early recognition and systematic study of ARDS, the American-European Consensus Conference on ARDS provided an operational definition for ARDS in 1994.[61] The group acknowledged the wide spectrum of clinical presentation associated with ARDS. As noted in Table 19-4, the term "acute lung injury" (ALI) was used to describe the less severe end of the spectrum while "ARDS" was used to describe the most severe end of the spectrum.

TABLE 19-4 Recommended Criteria for Acute Lung Injury and Acute Respiratory Distress Syndrome

	Timing	Oxygenation	Chest Radiograph	Pulmonary Artery Wedge Pressure
ALI	Acute onset	Pao_2/Fio_2 ratio ≤300 mmHg (regardless of level of PEEP)	Bilateral infiltrates seen on frontal chest radiograph	≤18 mmHg when measured or no evidence of left atrial hypertension
ARDS	Acute onset	Pao_2/Fio_2 ratio ≤200 mmHg (regardless of level of PEEP)	Bilateral infiltrates seen on frontal chest radiograph	≤18 mmHg when measured or no evidence of left atrial hypertension

From: Bernard GR, Artigas A, Brigham KL et al: The American-European Consensus Conference on ARDS: Definitions, mechanisms, relevant outcomes, and clinical trial coordination, *Am J Respir Crit Care Med* 149:818-824, 1994.

Incidence. Although uncertain, ARDS is thought to account for 3% of all PICU admissions and 8% of all PICU days.[63] Almost 12% of PICU admissions are admitted with an ARDS trigger. Although published pediatric ARDS mortality rates vary, the Pediatric Critical Care Study Group describe overall mortality as 43%.[64] With improvements in supportive care and treatment, mortality rates appear to be decreasing.[65] Fackler describes an 18% mortality rate in extracorporeal membrane oxygenation (ECMO)-eligible children and a 58% mortality rate in ECMO-ineligible children.[62] Specifically, patients thought to be ineligible for ECMO include those with ARDS for longer than 7 days, or patients with chronic lung disease, compromised immune systems, left ventricular failure, or profound acute neurologic injury. Of note, most patients who die with ARDS die of multisystem organ failure—not single organ respiratory failure.

Pathogenesis. Ware and Matthay reviewed what is currently known about the biochemical mediators and products of cellular damage contributing to acute lung injury and recovery (Fig. 19-7, *A* and Fig. 19-7, *B*).[65] The predominant physiologic disturbance is an alteration in the alveolar-capillary interface, which leads to increased capillary permeability and pulmonary edema. Under normal circumstances, the permeability of the alveolar epithelium is relatively constant. Fluid leaves the capillary bed via small clefts located at the junction of the endothelial cells lining the capillary walls, and the lymphatic system is capable of removing excesses. However, when the alveolar capillary membrane is disrupted, large amounts of fluid and protein leak first into the interstitial space, overwhelming the lymphatics, eventually entering the alveolus itself. As a result of this process, for any given pulmonary capillary pressure, lung water is greatly increased. Even at normal pulmonary capillary wedge pressures of 5 to 10 mmHg, there is fluid accumulation in ARDS. However, because measures of lung water and gas exchange correlate poorly, increased lung water is only partially responsible for the refractory hypoxemia seen in ARDS. Of greater consequence is the V̇/Q̇ mismatch associated with the multiple disturbances of pulmonary circulation and alveolar aeration seen in this disease.

The noncardiogenic pulmonary edema of ARDS results in decreased lung compliance (C_L); that is, it takes more pressure (and more work) to deliver normal tidal volumes because the lungs are stiffer. If the force required to inflate the lungs cannot be maintained, overall lung volume decreases, leading eventually to alveolar collapse and a net reduction in FRC. As alveoli collapse, intrapulmonary shunting occurs and hypoxemia develops. Ordinarily, the pulmonary vessels constrict in the face of alveolar hypoxia, a phenomenon called reflex hypoxic vasoconstriction. But in ARDS, reflex hypoxic vasoconstriction may not be intact and poorly ventilated areas continue to be perfused. Collapsed alveoli that remain perfused create a right-to-left shunt, increasing pulmonary venous admixture and causing hypoxemia. The opposite also occurs in the lungs with ARDS; some alveoli may remain ventilated but are not perfused. This may be the result of vasoconstriction, emboli, or destruction of the capillary structure by the disease process. Such areas behave as dead space and may increase $Paco_2$.

Although mechanical ventilation provides an indispensable tool for providing adequate gas exchange and resting respiratory muscles in many disease states, in patients with ALI/ARDS the ventilator strategy required to maintain adequate gas exchange may exacerbate lung injury and cause ventilator-induced lung injury (VILI). In patients with ALI/ARDS, computed tomographic scanning has shown marked heterogeneity in the pattern of lung injury along the vertical axis (Fig. 19-8). Intrapleural pressures become less negative along the vertical axis; specifically, nondependent alveoli are exposed to the greatest transalveolar pressure (alveolar pressure-pleural pressure) so are largest in size, whereas dependent alveoli are exposed to the least transalveolar pressure so are smallest in size. Gattinoini identified three lung zones: responsive, nonresponsive, and recruitable zones. The nondependent lung regions are considered responsive in that they usually remain continuously open to ventilation. The dependent lung regions are considered unresponsive zones in that they usually become consolidated and/or atelectatic. The regions in-between the nondependent and dependent zones are considered recruitable depending on the ventilation strategy.

Normal Alveolus

Injured Alveolus during the Acute Phase

A

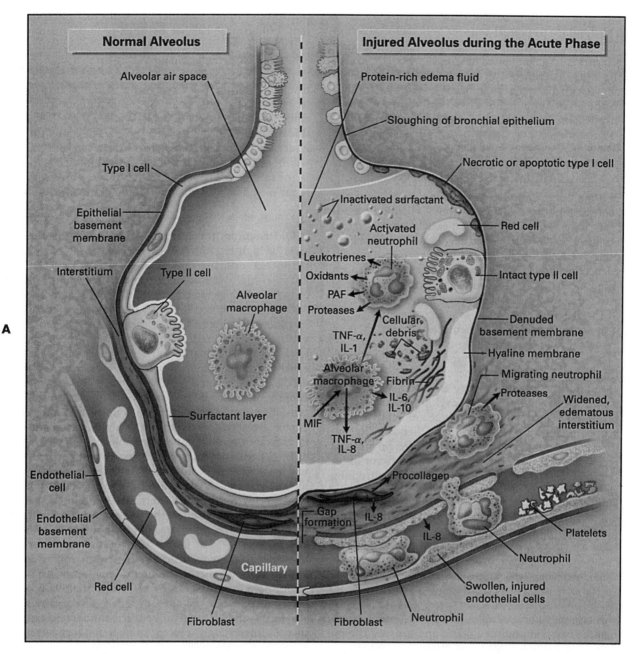

Fig. 19-7 **A,** The normal alveolus (left-hand side) and the injured alveolus in the acute phase of ALI and the ARDS (right-hand side). In the acute phase of the syndrome (right-hand side), there is sloughing of both the bronchial and alveolar epithelial cells, with the formation of protein-rich hyaline membranes on the denuded basement membrane. Neutrophils are shown adhering to the injured capillary endothelium and marginating through the interstitium into the air space, which is filled with protein-rich edema fluid. In the airspace, an alveolar macrophage is secreting cytokines, interleukin-1, -5, -8, and -10 (IL-1, IL-5, IL-8, and IL-10) and tumor necrosis factor–α (TNF-α), which can act locally to stimulate chemotaxis and activate neutrophils. Macrophages also secrete other cytokines, including IL-1, IL-6, and IL-10. IL-1 can also stimulate the production of extracellular matrix by fibroblasts. Neutrophils can release oxidants, proteases, leukotrienes, and other proinflammatory molecules, such as platelet-activating factor (PAF). A number of antiinflammatory mediators are also present in the alveolar milieu, including IL-1–receptor antagonist, soluble tumor necrosis factor receptor, autoantibodies against IL-8, and cytokines such as IL-10 and IL-11 (not shown). The influx of protein-rich edema fluid into the alveolus has led to the inactivation of surfactant. *MIF,* Macrophage inhibitory factor. (From Ware LB, Matthay MA: The acute respiratory distress syndrome, *N Engl J Med* 342:1339, 2000.)

Continued

Fig. 19-7, cont'd   B, Mechanisms important in the resolution of ALI and the acute respiratory distress syndrome ARDS. On the left side of the alveolus, the alveolar epithelium is being repopulated by the proliferation and differentiation of alveolar type II cells. Resorption of alveolar edema fluid is shown at the base of the alveolus, with sodium and chloride being transported through the apical membrane of type II cells. Sodium is taken up by the epithelial sodium channel (EnaC) and through the basolateral membrane of type II cells by the sodium pump (Na^+/K^+-ATPase). The relevant pathways for chloride transport are unclear. Water is shown moving through water channels, the aquaporins, located primarily on type I cells. Some water may also cross by a paracellular route. Soluble protein is probably cleared primarily by paracellular diffusion and secondarily by endocytosis by alveolar epithelial cells. Macrophages remove insoluble protein and apoptotic neutrophils by phagocytosis. On the right side of the alveolus, the gradual remodeling and resolution of intraalveolar and interstitial granulation tissue and fibrosis are shown. (From Ware LB, Matthay MA: The acute respiratory distress syndrome, *N Engl J Med* 342:1339, 2000.)

With marked heterogeneity, providing a noninjurious mode of mechanical ventilation can be difficult. In addition to oxygen toxicity, three types of ventilator-induced lung injury (VILI) have been described: volutrauma, atelectrauma, and biotrauma. Volutrauma, stretch-induced alveolar injury, results from modes of ventilation that allow end-inspiratory alveolar over distension. Atelectrauma, shear-induced alveolar injury, results from modes of ventilation that allow end-expiratory alveolar collapse. Biotrauma, nonpulmonary organ injury, results from end-organ exposure to the pulmonary inflammatory mediators released in response to an injurious mode of mechanical ventila-

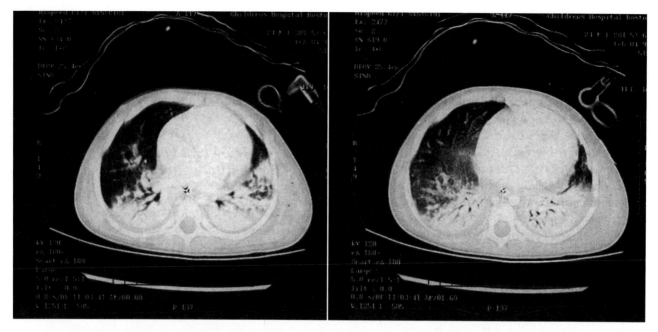

Fig. 19-8 Chest computed tomography images of a 4-year-old girl who developed acute lung injury after laparotomy for gastric perforation. Note the dependent distribution of consolidated lung. (From Doctor A, Arnold J: Mechanical support of acute lung injury: options for strategic ventilation, *New Horizons* 7:361, 1999.)

tion.[66] Evidence for the development of multisystem organ failure secondary to VILI is building. Recently, Ranieri and others were able to document that mechanical ventilation could lead to an increase in cytokine levels in the lung as well as the systemic circulation and that limiting recruitment/derecruitment and overdistention could limit the inflammatory response.[67] They were able to document that the concentration of inflammatory mediators in both blood and bronchial alveolar lavage fluid was significantly lower in the lung-protective strategy group.

Gattinoini and others have also described differences in respiratory mechanics between ARDS originating from pulmonary disease (direct lung injury, for example, pneumonia) and that originating from an extrapulmonary disease (indirect lung injury, for example, sepsis).[68] In patients with direct ARDS they note a prevalence of pulmonary consolidation, stiffer lungs within a highly compliant chest wall, moderate lung recruitment with PEEP, and a tendency to overdistended alveoli placing the patient at risk for barotrauma. In contrast, in patients with indirect ARDS they note a prevalence of pulmonary edema and collapse, compliant lung within a stiffer chest wall, improved compliance and major lung recruitment with PEEP placing the patient at risk for hemodynamic compromise.

After the pulmonary insult, there may be a lag time of several hours to several days before respiratory distress develops. Then, dyspnea develops; the symptom is subjective and can be reported only by an older child. In an infant, increasing respiratory difficulty may be manifested as agitation, sometimes progressing to somnolence. Tachypnea, with intercostal and substernal retractions in smaller children and infants, may persist even after O_2 administration, reflecting the need for increased minute ventilation. Chest auscultation, which can be normal initially, eventually reveals course rales and bronchial breath sounds. The fine,

basilar rales of congestive heart failure are often absent in ARDS. Wheezing may also occur because of narrowing of the terminal airways by peribronchial edema, decreased lung volume, or secretions. The majority of patients require intubation and mechanical ventilation.

Critical Care Management. The treatment for ARDS remains largely supportive.[69] All patients require supplemental oxygen. Although the extent to which the condition is made worse by oxygen is unknown, oxygen toxicity may occur after prolonged exposure to high concentration of F_{IO_2}. In addition, the nitrogen present in an F_{IO_2} less than 0.5 serves as an intra-alveolar splint. With higher concentrations of O_2, decreasing amounts of residual gas remain in the alveoli, and reabsorption atelectasis may occur. Therefore it is prudent to reduce F_{IO_2} as much and as rapidly as possible. The goal is to maintain a Pao_2 of 55 to 80 mmHg, Spo_2 88% to 95%, in an F_{IO_2} less than 0.6.

As illustrated in Fig. 19-9, the pressure-volume curve of the respiratory system in early ALI/ARDS has been described as sigmoid shape with a lower inflection point (P*flex*) representing the pressure required to reopen a collapsed lung and an upper inflection point thought to correspond to overdistention of open units.[70] Restated, the lower inflection point represents a sudden increase in compliance induced by recruiting alveoli that are open while the upper inflection point represents a sudden decrease in compliance induced by alveolar overinflation. The goal of ventilator support in ALI/ARDS is to "open" the lung and keep it open during end-expiration while avoiding overinflation during end-inspiration. Optimal PEEP will obliterate the lower inflection point and the use of tidal volume (Vt)/pressure-limited ventilation will prevent an upper inflection point. Although two conflicting studies exist (Amato and colleagues and Stewart and co-workers), it appears that this ventilation strategy improves oxygenation,

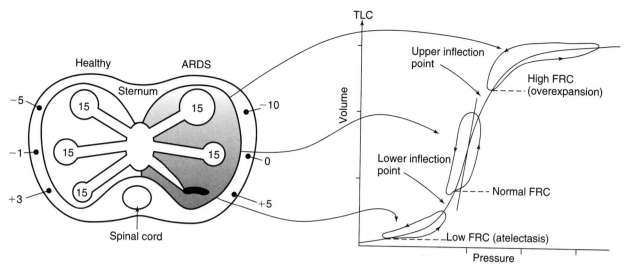

Fig. 19-9 Pressure-volume relationships in ARDS. Intrapleural pressures become less negative along the vertical axis; nondependent alveoli are exposed to the greatest transalveolar pressure so are largest in size, whereas dependent alveoli are exposed to the least transalveolar pressure so are smallest in size. The nondependent lung regions are considered responsive in that they usually remain continuously open to ventilation. The dependent lung regions are considered unresponsive zones in that they usually become consolidated and/or atelectatic. The regions in between the nondependent and dependent zones are considered recruitable depending on the ventilation strategy. The compliance of each region varies as reflected by its location on the pressure-volume curve.

◆ TABLE 19-5	Optimal PEEP-F_{IO_2} Concentration Combinations						
F_{IO_2}	0.3	0.4	0.4	0.5	0.5	0.6	0.7	0.7
PEEP	5	5	8	8	10	10	10	12
F_{IO_2}	0.7	0.8	0.9	0.9	0.9	1.0	1.0	1.0
PEEP	14	14	14	16	18	20	22	24

Levels of PEEP in this scale represent levels set on the ventilator, not levels of total PEEP, auto-PEEP, or intrinsic PEEP.
From The Acute Respiratory Distress Syndrome Network: Ventilation with lower tidal volumes as compared with traditional tidal volumes for acute lung injury and the acute respiratory distress syndrome, *N Engl J Med* 342:1301-1308, 2000.

pulmonary compliance, weaning success, the incidence of barotrauma, and 28-day mortality.[71,72] It should be noted that in day-to-day clinical practice, pressure-volume curves are difficult to construct with the standard super syringe technique and clinicians typically optimize end-expiratory volume by targeting a change in tidal compliance.[73]

PEEP is considered the mainstay of ARDS treatment. When an optimal level of PEEP is added to positive pressure ventilation, alveoli remain open throughout all phases of the respiratory cycle to continually participate in gas exchange. Without PEEP, alveoli collapse on end-exhalation and are forced open during inspiration, causing alveolar atelectrauma. PEEP increases FRC by augmenting the volume of expanded alveoli and by recruiting collapsed units reducing intrapulmonary shunt. PEEP does not remove lung water but improves arterial oxygenation by increasing the number of ventilated alveoli. The implication for nursing is the need to be certain that prescribed levels of PEEP are maintained,

including during endotracheal suctioning, after turning the child, and so on.

As outlined in Table 19-5, the National Institutes of Health (NIH) ARDS Network made recommendations on appropriate PEEP–F_{IO_2} combinations in their low Vt study.[74] When PEEP is increased in an attempt to recruit collapsed alveoli, nondependent alveoli may become overdistended. The proportion of nonoxygenated blood increases as the capillaries surrounding these overdistended areas are compressed, increasing intrapulmonary shunting and hypoxemia. Dead space is increased in the overdistended units and $Paco_2$ may climb. Daily chest radiographs in patients with ARDS are necessary during the acute phase of the disease, not so much to follow the pulmonary edema but to evaluate potential complications of therapy. Complications include pulmonary hyperinflation and air-leak syndrome (barotrauma). Finally, PEEP may cause a decrease in cardiac output primarily in patients with extra-pulmonary ARDS by decreasing systemic venous return to the heart. Myocardial support may be necessary, including both the judicious use of volume to increase preload and the administration of inotropic agents.

As discussed, the traditional approach to mechanical ventilation in the patients with ALI/ARDS was the use of high Vt (10 to 15 ml/kg). This approach is thought to contribute to the development of VILI, specifically, alveolar volutrauma. Recently, the ARDS network compared this traditional approach (Vt 12 ml/kg of predicted body weight, plateau pressure of 50 cm H_2O or less) to a low Vt strategy (Vt 6 ml/kg of predicted body weight, plateau pressure of 30 cm H_2O or less).[74] The primary outcome variables were death and the number of days without ventilator use from day 1 to day 28 (ventilator-free days). The multicenter, randomized trial was stopped after 861 patients were enrolled because mortality was 22% lower in the low Vt group (31% versus 40%). The low Vt group also experienced more ventilator-free days (12 versus 10 days) and, suggesting less lung inflammation, the low Vt group also had a greater reduction in IL-6 concentrations. It was concluded that in patients with ALI/ARDS, mechanical ventilation with a lower Vt than traditionally used results in decreased mortality and an increase in ventilation-free days.

Low Vt strategies will precipitate hypercapnia and a compensated respiratory acidosis. In 1990, Hickling and colleagues first proposed the importance of limiting positive inspiratory pressures (PIP) by reducing Vt even if it resulted in short-term hypercapnia and a deterioration of oxygenation.[75] In a prospective study, Hickling and others demonstrated decreased ARDS mortality using a low-volume, pressure-limited ventilation with permissive hypercapnia strategy.[76] In this study, the mean maximum $Paco_2$ was 66.5 mmHg (range 38 to 158) with a mean arterial pH of 7.23 (range 6.79 to 7.45).

In the low Vt study (described above) the ARDS network study attempted to keep the patient's arterial pH between 7.3 and 7.45 with the use of increased respiratory rates, decreased ventilator dead space, and the use of $NaHCO_3$.[74] Potential side effects associated with the use of permissive hypercapnia include decreased myocardial contractility, cerebral vasodilation, decreased seizure threshold, and hyperkalemia. Although there are no absolute contraindications to permissive hypercapnia, extremes in $Paco_2$ levels should be modified in patients with concomitant cerebral hypertension.

High-frequency oscillatory ventilation (HFOV) is an alternative mode of ventilation that accomplishes the open lung approach desirable in the management of patients with ALI/ARDS (see Chapter 8). Although questionable, HFOV is often reserved for those who fail conventional mechanical ventilation; for example, when a patient requires a PIP greater than 35 cm H_2O, plateau pressures greater than 30 cm H_2O, Paw greater than 18 cm H_2O despite permissive hypercapnia or when chemical paralysis is required. Doctor and Arnold reviewed the advantages for using HFOV, specifically, (1) poorly compliant lungs can be aggressively recruited and maintained, (2) the small Vt and pressure swings may attenuate VILI, and (3) the different flow delivery characteristics may improve V̇/Q̇ matching.[77] When pediatric patients with ALI/ARDS are ventilated using HFOV, an optimal lung volume strategy is used; specifically, Paw are initially set 5 to 8 cm H_2O over what was necessary on conventional therapy then adjusted in an effort to decrease $FiO_2 < 0.6$. Compared with conventional mechanical ventilation, Arnold and colleagues demonstrated significant improvements in oxygenation with an optimal lung volume HFOV strategy and, despite the use of a higher Paw, HFOV was associated with a lower frequency of barotrauma and improved clinical outcomes.[78]

When conventional measures fail and the patient with ARDS still has the potential for a good clinical outcome than ECMO may be considered (see Chapter 8). To date, more than 1700 children have been supported on ECMO for respiratory failure with an overall survival rate of 55%.[79] Although the technical aspects of ECMO are the same, the duration of ECMO support for a pediatric patient with ARDS is usually quite long—up to 2 months.

Considering the volume recruitment priority in ALI/ARDS, endotracheal suctioning (see Chapter 8) should be performed only when clinically indicated. Specifically when there is an increase in airways resistance, a decrease in dynamic compliance, a decrease in delivered Vt, or an increase in PIP with a widening of the PIP-Plateau pressure difference. Recruitment maneuvers, for example the use of higher PIPs or larger Vts breaths with longer inspiratory times are necessary after the suctioning procedure to help rerecruit unstable lung units that collapse with suctioning.

Although controversies abound regarding fluid requirement and restriction in ARDS, it is generally advisable to keep patients relatively fluid restricted. The ultimate goal of fluid therapy is to maintain an adequate cardiac output while keeping microvascular pressures as low as possible. Diuretics may be helpful in shifting extravascular water into the intravascular space if volume overload has occurred. Furosemide is known to be effective in cardiogenic pulmonary edema by virtue of both its diuretic and nondiuretic vascular properties. By lowering central filling pressures through immediate vasodilation (independent of the later diuresis), furosemide can reduce pulmonary shunting and lung water in high permeability pulmonary edema as well.

Other treatment measures include attempts to maximize O_2 delivery. The majority of O_2 is carried by hemoglobin; therefore hemoglobin concentration and O_2 saturation are the important determinants of O_2 content. Maintaining the hemoglobin at normal levels optimizes O_2 carrying capacity without increasing viscosity and limiting tissue perfusion. Continuous Spo_2 monitoring can prove invaluable in monitoring pulmonary perfusion changes that occur during various nursing interventions that may alter V̇/Q̇ matching. Blood pressure is a relatively poor index of cardiac output, which may be measured directly when a pulmonary artery catheter is in place. Noninvasive techniques for measuring cardiac output, such as those based on ultrasound results, provide a valuable alternative. To maximize the availability of O_2 at the cellular level, attempts are made to correct factors that negatively influence oxyhemoglobin dissociation, that is, shift the oxyhemoglobin dissociation curve to the left and impair the release of O_2 to the tissues. Here normothermia is again important, as is the avoidance of metabolic or respiratory alkalosis.

Because hypoxemia is a primary feature of ARDS, measures to reduce O_2 consumption ($\dot{V}o_2$) are critically important. In patients with very large intrapulmonary shunts, fever, anxiety, and physical activity can increase oxygen demand. This in turn decreases the Po_2 of mixed venous blood ($P\bar{v}o_2$), and ultimately lowers Pao_2. Therefore treatment of fever, reduction of anxiety, and sedation are important. Muscle relaxants may be used, not so much to reduce $\dot{V}o_2$ (neuromuscular blockade will not reduce $\dot{V}o_2$ beyond that achieved by adequate sedation[80]) but to overcome desynchrony of the child's respiratory efforts with mechanical breaths and prevent the complications that may bring, for example, barotrauma (pneumothorax or pneumomediastinum).

Hypercarbia is not a predominant feature of ARDS except in severe cases. Here, noninvasive end-tidal CO_2 monitoring may not be as useful except in providing trending information, because the difference between arterial CO_2 and end-tidal values widens with severe $\dot{V}/\dot{Q}$ mismatching. What is ultimately important, however, is not just the Pao_2 but the total amount of oxygen transported to the tissues.

Prone positioning, as first suggested by Bryan in 1974, is a relatively simple maneuver that improves oxygenation and lung mechanics in adults with severe impairments of gas exchange.[81,82] Data suggest that improved oxygenation in the prone position is associated with less variability in end-expiratory lung volume from the dorsal to the ventral regions, resulting in a more even regional inflation/ventilation along the vertical axis, in the absence of a gravity perfusion distribution.[83] A preliminary study did show that pediatric patients improved their oxygenation without serious iatrogenic injury after early, repetitive and prolonged prone positioning.[84] The improved oxygenation resulting from prone positioning allows a reduction in the intensity of ventilator support that may decrease VILI and facilitate patient recovery. However, no randomized, controlled trial has evaluated the safety and effectiveness of early and repeated prone positioning on the clinical outcomes of pediatric patients with ALI/ARDS.

Box 19-2 contains a nursing procedure on prone positioning. Candidates for prone positioning include patients with ALI/ARDS. Patients not considered candidates for prone positioning include those who are experiencing symptomatic hypotension, patients supported on ECMO, or patients with the following clinical problems: cerebral hypertension, spinal instability, unstable long bone fracture, or a nonpulmonary conditions that may be exacerbated by the prone position (e.g., osteogenesis imperfecta or severe skeletal deformities). For maximum lung protection, patients should be positioned prone early in their course of illness for at least 16 to 20 hours/day. Patients are considered "responders" to prone positioning if they experience a 20-mmHg or more supine-to-prone increase in the Pao_2/Fio_2 ratio. Prone positioning is discontinued when the patient is actively weaning from mechanical ventilation.

Patients who require neuromuscular blockade present additional nursing challenges. Although the child may appear calm after neuromuscular blocking agents have been administered, sensory perception and level of consciousness are not altered. Neuromuscular blocking agents have no sedative or analgesic effects; therefore sedatives and/or anxiolytics are *always* administered. Older children and adolescents require reassurance that the paralysis is drug induced and reversible. If painful procedures are to be performed, or if the child's underlying condition or its treatment is inherently painful, analgesics are also administered. Every effort should be made to reduce noxious auditory stimuli around the child, scheduling care to permit quiet time for sleep. The child's response to these interventions can be assessed by monitoring the physiologic consequences of anxiety or pain, that is, tachycardia, hypertension, and pupillary dilatation.

Periodically, the neuromuscular blockade is permitted to wear off to perform at least a summary neurologic evaluation, as well as to determine the need for continued blockade. At times, it may be impossible to allow the patient a honeymoon period from neuromuscular blockade, for example, in the patient who requires high ventilator pressures who immediately has decompensation during dysynchronous breaths. In these cases "train-of-four" monitoring, that is, peripheral nerve stimulation, provides a valuable alternative (see Chapter 8). Several researchers suggest that the consequences of prolonged muscle disuse brought about by neuromuscular blockade in young infants may be more severe than in adults. Reports of microscopic evidence of skeletal muscle growth failure with prolonged use of neuromuscular blockade in preterm infants and residual muscle weakness in newborns after receiving pancuronium for several weeks raise issues relating to the normal growth and development of muscle in the face of prolonged paralysis.[85] It becomes obvious that neuromuscular blockade is used judiciously, especially in infants.

When neuromuscular blockade is necessary, extreme vigilance is required to avoid tissue breakdown from immobility. Chapter 16 provides a review of essential skin and eye care required of the immobilized patient.

Several pharmacologic interventions (inhaled nitric oxide, surfactant, and steroids) have been suggested to help manage ALI/ARDS. Nitric oxide is produced by many cell types in the lung and plays an important physiologic role in the regulation of pulmonary vasomotor tone by several known mechanisms. Nitric oxide stimulates soluble guanylyl cyclase, resulting in increased levels of cyclic guanosine monophosphate (GMP) in lung smooth muscle cells. The gating of K^+ and Ca^{2+} channels by cyclic GMP binding is thought to play a role in nitric oxide–mediated vasodilation. Nitric oxide may also regulate pulmonary vasodilation by direct activation of K^+ channels or by modulating the expression and activity of angiotensin II receptors. Administration of nitric oxide by inhalation (iNO) has been shown to acutely improve hypoxemia associated with pulmonary hypertension in humans and animals.[86] In addition, iNO will

Box 19-2
Prone Positioning Procedure

Preparation for Turning

- Create individually sized head, chest, pelvic, distal femoral, and lower limb cushions using egg crate material (Eggcrate; Span American Medical Systems, Greenville, SC) to allow the patient's abdomen to be unrestrained from the patient's bed and to provide skin protection.
    1. The chest cushion should measure slightly less than the right-to-left greater tubercle of the upper arm; equal to the patient's anterior-posterior width; and wide enough to cover the patient's sternum when compressed.
    2. The pelvic cushion should measure slightly smaller than the right-to-left iliac crest and be slightly smaller than the patient's anterior-posterior width.
    3. The head pillow should allow the patient's head to be slightly higher than his or her chest.
    4. A small cushion should be placed under the distal femur to elevate the patient's knees off the bed.
    5. The lower limb cushion should elevate the patient's toes off the bed.
- Transpyloric enteral feed tube is inserted and checked for placement.
- The security of the endotracheal tube (ETT), vascular lines, and Spo_2 probe is assessed (by applying gentle traction) and reinforced as necessary. The ETT is taped to the upper lip on the side of the mouth that will end in the "up" position. A protective layer of plastic tape is placed over the ETT white adhesive tape to help prevent oral secretions from loosening the white adhesive tape while prone.
- If the patient is receiving a chemical paralytic agent, eye protection is provided. Specifically, both eyes are cleansed, lubricated, and covered with plastic wrap.
- If the patient is supported on high-frequency oscillatory ventilation, a transparent film dressing is placed over the anterior bony prominences to protect the skin from a friction injury.
- EKG electrodes are moved to the lateral aspects of the upper arms and hips.
- The patient's oropharynx is suctioned.
- Nonessential vascular lines and the patient's nasogastric tube are temporarily capped. The start and end point of everything that is left attached to the patient is reviewed.
- The patient is premedicated with comfort medications.

Preplanning the Turn

- Preplanning includes delineation of who is responsible for what patient aspect (e.g., head/ETT: respiratory therapist; chest/arms: Nurse 1; hips/legs: Nurse 2), and technique (smaller patients: levitate up, turn 45 degrees, pause, then gently turn prone, place cushions after patient positioned prone; larger patients: using a draw sheet—gently reposition the patient at the edge of the bed away from the ventilator, turn 45 degrees, pause, position chest and pelvic cushions then position patient prone on cushions). During the turn the patient's head is kept aligned with his or her body by the respiratory therapist—hyperextension is avoided. The patient's arms are contained next to their torso. Legs are supported so that the toes of the upper leg point in the direction of the turn.
- Patients are turned toward the ventilator without disconnecting the patient from the ventilator. The patient is talked through the turn. If the patient requires ETT suctioning, turning is delayed until the patient is suctioned and has returned to presuctioning ventilator settings.

Immediately After the Turn

- The security and patency of all tubes/lines is reassessed. Capped off lines/nasogastric tube are uncapped/reattached.
- Position the patient:
    1. Turn head to side and cushion head and ear with pressure relieving material.
    2. Cushion the upper chest, and pelvis using either a rolled Eggcrate or foam pad—allowing the abdomen to protrude.
    3. Flex arms up.
    4. Position knees and feet off bed using an appropriate sized roll under the distal femur and lower leg.

Maintenance

- Reevaluate oropharyngeal and endotracheal suctioning routine.
- Skin protection:
    1. Use the skin care and pressure ulcer algorithm (see Chapter 16).
    2. Make slight adjustments to the patient's position *at least every 2 hours;* when in the lateral prone position the dependent arm should be down at the patient's side and nondependent arm should be flexed at the elbow up toward the patient's head.
    3. Consult with skin care nurse and physical therapy on all patients as soon as possible after their first turn to assist with skin protection and optimal positioning.
- Elevate head of bed at least 15 degrees.
- Chest films are obtained in the prone position.

---

improve $\dot{V}/\dot{Q}$ matching by vasodilating the pulmonary vascular bed associated with a ventilated alveoli.

Depending on the study, 40% to 60% of patients with ALI/ARDS who receive iNO respond by improving their oxygenation but the effect is rarely sustained over the course of several days. In addition, patients receiving iNO have not demonstrated an improvement in overall survival. Bohn cautions against universal adoption of iNO in ARDS because little is known about its biologic effects; in fact, he notes that it may be time for a moratorium on human studies while more bench research is done.[87]

Potential toxicities to iNO include (1) methemoglobinemia, from the intravascular binding of nitric oxide to hemoglobin and (2) nitric dioxide lung injury, produced from the reaction of iNO with oxygen. Methemoglobin levels are assessed and a level greater than 5% is considered toxic. Both iNO and NO_2 levels are monitored during administration. NO_2 levels greater than 5 parts per million (ppm) are considered toxic. High levels are managed by increasing gas flow and/or blending the iNO and oxygen gases closer to the point to delivery to decrease exposure time.

Considering that one of the hallmarks of ALI/ARDS is endogenous surfactant depletion and inactivation, many have considered the potential impact of surfactant repletion in its acute care management. Willson conducted a multisite, prospective, unblinded, randomized controlled study to describe the use of an exogenous calf lung surfactant (Infasurf) in pediatric respiratory failure.[88] Forty-two patients with acute hypoxemic respiratory failure received intratracheal surfactant (80 ml/m^2 in four equal aliquots in rotating positions, repeated once 12 hours later) within 24 hours of intubation. Patients who received the natural surfactant early in the course of their illness showed rapid improvement in oxygenation, were extubated 4.2 days sooner, and spent 30% fewer days in the PICU than control patients. In addition, there were no difference in mortality or overall hospital stay and no serious adverse effects. A definitive study is currently underway.

Steroids have long stimulated interest for their anti-inflammatory properties. In patients with ARDS, data regarding steroid use are contradictory. Several studies indicate no benefit in the use of pharmacologic doses of steroids even early in the course of the disease except in specific instances—radiation pneumonitis and fat embolism syndrome. As for treatment with high-dose steroids, no improvement in survival rates have been demonstrated and mortality may be higher because of an increase in the number of secondary infections.[89]

Recently Meduri and colleagues hypothesized that, if administered before the development of end-stage fibrosis, methylprednisolone could be effective in improving lung function and outcome in patients with unresolving ARDS.[90] They conducted a randomized, double blind, placebo-controlled trial involving 24 adults with severe ARDS who failed to improve by the seventh day of respiratory failure. In an effort to contain the host defense response, the experimental group (after demonstrating that they were not infected by bronchoalveolar lavage) received methylprednisolone. The initial dose was 2 mg/kg per day and was slowly titrated over 32 days. They were able to document improvement in lung injury, multiorgan dysfunction scores, and mortality in the group receiving prolonged methylprednisolone.

ARDS is not a disorder of the respiratory system alone. Other organs may be adversely affected by the primary disease process (e.g., sepsis), altered oxygen transport, or alteration in organ function directly. Monitoring of various organ function is therefore crucial. The brain may be negatively affected by inadequate O_2 delivery leading to altered levels of consciousness, for example, confusion, combativeness, or coma. Other organs may be involved because, in a more limited way, they undergo the same endothelial injury as the lungs. Therefore disseminated intravascular coagulation (DIC), acute renal failure (ARF), and hepatic dysfunction are common in ARDS.

Mechanical ventilation may be necessary for weeks or months, during which nutritional/caloric needs may greatly exceed maintenance requirement. Nutritional adequacy is established early in the development of ARDS because sustained malnutrition can result in abnormalities in pulmonary defense mechanisms and pulmonary structure and function and may limit the child's ability to wean from mechanical ventilation.[91] See Chapter 12 for transpyloric enteral nutrition.

Because the child's prognosis is frequently uncertain and the intensive care course may be long and fraught with multiple setbacks, parents of the child with ARDS require a tremendous amount of nursing support. It is important to develop a therapeutic relationship with the family early on, to provide consistent and accurate information about their child, and to involve the family in nurturing behaviors.

Congenital Diaphragmatic Hernia

Etiology. Congenital diaphragmatic hernia occurs when the fetal diaphragm fails to develop normally, leaving an opening between the thorax and the abdomen. This permits the abdominal contents to enter the thoracic cavity, interfering with normal development of the lungs.

Incidence. Congenital diaphragmatic hernia occurs in approximately 1 in 2000 births and is the most common cause of pulmonary hypoplasia in the newborn.

Pathogenesis. The diaphragm forms during the eighth to tenth week of fetal life and separates the abdominal and thoracic cavities. Because the left posterior aspect of the diaphragm is usually the last to close, the most common type of diaphragmatic hernia involves this area of the muscle (foramen of Bochdalek). While the diaphragm is forming, the midgut is developing within the umbilical pouch. If the diaphragm has not completely closed when the midgut returns to the abdominal cavity (about the tenth week of gestation), abdominal structures can enter the thoracic cavity—the stomach, large and small intestines in a left-sided defect, or part or all of the liver in the less common right-sided defect. The herniated gut then compresses the developing lung buds, arresting their growth on both the ipsilateral and, to a lesser degree, the contralateral side. As a result, the number of airways and alveoli is markedly reduced. The number of pulmonary arteries is also decreased and their distribution is abnormal. In addition, the amount of smooth muscle in pulmonary arterioles is greater than normal.[92] Therefore infants with congenital diaphragmatic hernia have both lung hypoplasia and increased pulmonary vascular resistance.

At birth, the infant with a significant diaphragmatic hernia is tachypneic and has marked intercostal and substernal retractions. Breath sounds are decreased or absent on the affected side, and the point of maximum impulse (PMI) and heart sounds are shifted to the unaffected side. Typically, the infant's chest diameter is increased and the abdomen is scaphoid. Gas-filled loops of bowel may be evident within the chest on radiograph. Because the hypoplastic pulmonary vascular bed is unable to accommodate the normal increase in postnatal right ventricular output, pulmonary hypertension develops. Blood is shunted right to left across the foramen ovale and patent ductus resulting in refractory hypoxemia and cyanosis.

Critical Care Management. Treatment of infants with congenital diaphragmatic hernia involves the measures used in initial resuscitation of the newborn, ventilatory support, and surgical repair of the lesion. More aggressive support includes the use of ECMO.

Not long ago, it was believed that immediate surgical repair of acutely symptomatic congenital diaphragmatic hernias would permit expansion of the lungs and improve ventilation. However, rather than improving pulmonary mechanics, Sakai and co-workers found that early repair often decreases lung compliance.[93] They attribute this deterioration to postoperative distortion of the diaphragm and chest wall and abdominal distension. Additional clinical data now support a strategy of delaying surgical repair of the defect until the infant's cardiovascular status is more stable.[94-96] Cardiovascular stability is attained by correcting the acidosis, hypoxia, and hypotension that are often present in these critically ill infants. Preoperative stabilization may improve the infant's ability to tolerate surgery.

Often, infants with congenital diaphragmatic hernia are diagnosed prenatally by ultrasound technique, and maternal transport and delivery can be planned at a center equipped to manage the critically ill newborn. Because bag-and-mask ventilation may force air into the gastrointestinal tract and further compromise ventilation, endotracheal intubation is performed immediately after birth.[97] Achieving adequate oxygenation (postductal Pa_{O_2} greater than 100 mmHg) and purposefully producing a metabolic alkalosis may help reduce pulmonary vascular resistance. A metabolic alkalosis can be induced with an infusion of sodium bicarbonate or tromethamine (THAM). This approach may be preferable to aggressive hyperventilation, which poses the risk of barotrauma and pulmonary air leaks.[98] Commonly, sedation and, as a last resort, neuromuscular blockade are necessary to achieve adequate ventilation. For a more thorough discussion of pulmonary hypertension see Persistent Pulmonary Hypertension of the Newborn (PPHN) later in this chapter.

Umbilical arterial and venous access is immediately established to permit monitoring of ABGs and pH and blood pressure and permit the administration of fluids and medications. Hemodynamic support may include crystalloids, transfusions, and/or inotropic agents as needed to maintain adequate peripheral perfusion.

Once the infant's condition has stabilized, the hernia is surgically reduced. A primary repair is attempted, but if this proves impossible, a prosthetic patch is used to close the defect.

If maximal medical measures fail to support ventilation, the infant is placed on ECMO (see Chapter 8). The defect is then repaired after several days of stabilization on ECMO.[99]

In large part, nursing care for the infant with a congenital diaphragmatic hernia focuses on avoiding conditions that increase pulmonary vascular resistance and is discussed within the context of PPHN. Conditions that may increase pulmonary vascular resistance are prevented, including

hypoxemia, acidosis, hypothermia, and hypoglycemia. For the same reason, environmental stressors such as noise, excessive light, and invasive procedures are also minimized.

Weaning mechanical ventilation in the infant with a congenital diaphragmatic hernia presents many of the challenges encountered in infants with BPD and is discussed more thoroughly later. Reductions in ventilatory support occur slowly, but steadily, while the infant's cardiopulmonary status is closely monitored.[97]

The infant's hydration and nutritional status are carefully monitored by evaluating the infant's intake and output, urine specific gravity, liver size, skin turgor, weight, and growth curve. A positive fluid balance may result in worsening respiratory status, which may improve with judicious use of diuretics. Nutritional adequacy promotes healing and growth and decreases the risk of infection, which may prolong the need for ventilatory support.[97]

The infant born with a diaphragmatic hernia typically has a lengthy hospital course that may include extremely intimidating, highly technical interventions. Parents, who may have begun anticipatory grieving at the time of an antenatal diagnosis, require considerable support and are encouraged to verbalize their questions and concerns. The nurse at the bedside can intervene to help parents cope with the sometimes-frightening PICU environment and permit them to connect with their critically ill child.

Mixed Obstructive and Restrictive Disease

For the purpose of more clearly understanding mechanical alterations in pulmonary function, various illnesses are classified by their effect on airways resistance (obstructive disease) or pulmonary compliance (restrictive disease). However, characteristic abnormalities in BPD include both increased airways resistance[100-102] and decreased compliance.[102,103] Therefore BPD is truly a "mixed" disorder, that is, both obstructive and restrictive in nature.

Bronchopulmonary Dysplasia (BPD)

Etiology. BPD, a term originally coined by Northway and colleagues, represents a form of unresolved lung injury of infancy.[104] Clinically defined as oxygen dependency at 1-month postnatal age, BPD most commonly follows severe hyaline membrane disease, but may also occur after meconium aspiration, pulmonary hemorrhage, congestive heart failure, or severe neonatal pneumonia. Although disagreement exists regarding its primary cause, factors contributing to the development of BPD may include O_2 toxicity, positive pressure ventilation and resultant mechanical lung injury, chronic inflammation, and overhydration.

Incidence. Although not limited to the preterm infant, BPD is most commonly associated with prematurity and occurs in up to 40% of mechanically ventilated infants weighing less than 1500 g at birth.[105] Recovery is slow and hospital readmission common, usually because of recurrent respiratory tract infections or the development of significant reactive airway disease.[106]

Pathogenesis. Infants with BPD have both increased airways resistance and decreased compliance. These changes in pulmonary mechanics are most likely the result of inflammation, atelectasis, overdistension, infiltration, increased mucus secretion, and fibrosis, all of which are known to occur in BPD.[107,108] Although minute ventilation can be increased by breathing rapidly, this respiratory pattern has the disadvantage of increasing dead space ventilation.[107] These disturbances in pulmonary function, along with an abnormal distribution of ventilation and perfusion ($\dot{V}/\dot{Q}$ mismatch), lead to characteristic hypoxemia and hypercarbia.

Infants with BPD typically breathe rapidly and shallowly. Increased work of breathing is evidenced by intercostal and substernal retractions. Eventually, respiratory muscle fatigue may lead to episodes of apnea and bradycardia. Crackles and bronchial sounds (sometimes associated with wheezing and decreased air entry when bronchospasm predominates) may be heard on auscultation. Both on physical examination and radiographically, the infant's chest is hyperinflated. Atelectasis also commonly occurs because of inadequate clearing of secretions and airway obstruction.[107] With prolonged respiratory failure, pulmonary hypertension develops, with signs of right-sided heart failure including cardiomegaly, hepatomegaly, and fluid retention.[107] Blood gas abnormalities include marked hypoxemia and hypercarbia.

Critical Care Management. Management of BPD includes ensuring adequate oxygenation, optimizing ventilation, and maximizing the infant's nutritional intake. Oxygen, although perhaps initially contributing to the development of BPD, is the most important medication for the infant with significant disease. Supplemental O_2 to maintain an SpO_2 of 92% to 97% ensures adequate tissue oxygenation and prevents the pulmonary hypertension and cor pulmonale that can result from chronic hypoxemia.[109] Improved growth has also been demonstrated in infants with BPD treated with oxygen during recovery.[110] However, because exposure to high concentrations of oxygen may contribute to lung microvascular and cellular injury, hyperoxia is avoided.

Oxygen therapy, however, is not enough; O_2 delivery to the tissues is also optimized. A hemoglobin of 12 to 15 g/dl maximizes O_2-carrying capacity, and blood transfusions may be necessary to maintain this level. In addition, factors that impair the release of O_2 to the tissues by negatively affecting oxyhemoglobin dissociation, that is, hypothermia and metabolic or respiratory alkalosis, are corrected or avoided. Persistent CO_2 retention results in a compensatory rise in serum bicarbonate concentration that may be further exaggerated by the use of diuretics; this requires close monitoring of serum electrolytes.

The infant with BPD has bronchiolar smooth muscle hypertrophy and hyperreactive airways.[111] Therefore bronchospasm, a condition in which constriction of smooth muscle in the distal airway restricts airflow in and out of the alveoli, commonly occurs in these infants, especially during acute respiratory infections. Bronchodilators may be useful in these circumstances. Theophylline may also increase diaphragmatic strength and diuresis in infants with BPD.[112] Aerosolized beta agonists (e.g., metaproterenol, terbutaline, or albuterol) are also commonly used in the treatment of

bronchospasm in BPD.[100,113-115] (See previous discussion on asthma for more detailed information regarding the treatment of reactive airways.) In addition, diuretics may relieve airway obstruction and improve compliance, probably because of a reduction in interstitial pulmonary edema.[100]

Because the infant with BPD is typically very slow to wean from ventilatory assistance, management of mechanical ventilation becomes a central issue. Attempts to rapidly reduce mechanical ventilation often meet with acute decompensation 24 to 48 hours later when the infant tires and $PaCO_2$ climbs. Therefore it is important to move slowly and allow adequate time for the infant to adjust to decreased ventilator settings. In the infant with BPD, tachypnea with a compensated respiratory acidosis may be "normal." Readiness for weaning from mechanical ventilation may best be demonstrated by a persistent reduction in the infant's baseline spontaneous respiratory rate and $PaCO_2$, accompanied by a sustained weight gain.[116]

When the need for prolonged assisted ventilation is anticipated, a tracheostomy may be considered. A tracheostomy decreases anatomic dead space and permits care to be delivered outside of a critical care setting (at home in some instances), and may prevent the development of subglottic stenosis.[117] However, decannulation may not be accomplished for 12 to 24 months even after assisted ventilation is no longer needed.

In the face of increased work of breathing, caloric intake as high as 170 to 200 Kcal/kg per day may be required for growth in BPD.[117] Nutritional needs are difficult to meet in these infants, not only because of increased calorie demands, but also because of poor feeding tolerance and the need for fluid restriction. Therefore nasogastric, nasojejunum, or gastrostomy tube feeding using concentrated formulas and diuretic therapy to prevent fluid overload are often necessary.

Nursing responsibilities in the care of infants with BPD include ensuring adequate oxygenation and ventilation, monitoring the efficacy of various interventions, and promoting growth and development. To appropriately adjust FIO_2 and treatment regimens, it is especially important to follow SpO_2 during periods of stress (such as feeding), and while administering various treatments. Wheezing or bronchospastic episodes, so-called BPD spells, are treated promptly. Clinicians should document the frequency and precipitating events when spells occur and assess the need for additional O_2, ventilatory support, and/or bronchodilators and the effect of each. Airway obstruction in BPD is, in part, reversible with bronchodilators, provides an opportunity for early intervention during the course of the disease and may possibly reduce its progression.[107]

Minimizing agitation, and the hypoxemia and bronchospasm that often accompany it, is a primary goal. The infant's individual temperament and sensitivities direct nursing measures to reduce stress. These measures may include controlling environmental noise and light, providing therapeutic touch, permitting nonnutritive sucking, and positioning for comfort. At times, sedation may also be required; however, sedation should be administered only after determining that agitation is not the result of inadequate ventilatory support or airway obstruction. Necessary procedures are spaced throughout the day to permit time for recovery, and unnecessary interventions are avoided. For example, clinical assessment and auscultation of breath sounds, not time alone, guide the frequency of chest physiotherapy and suctioning.

The nurse at the bedside may be in the best position to assess the infant's response to reductions in ventilatory support. Once readiness is established, weaning occurs slowly, but on a regular schedule; this is true during the infant's nursery course, and is also frequently necessary when mechanical ventilation is required for respiratory insufficiency later in life. Documenting the infant's respiratory rate and effort, response to activity, $ETco_2$, and Spo_2 after ventilator changes permits objective evaluation of how well weaning is tolerated.

Infants with BPD are at high risk for growth failure into at least their second year and, ironically, growth is the key to recovery.[118] Nutritional assessment includes trending weights, head circumference, and length (and plotting of the infant's growth against a normal curve). Complicating the task of providing sufficient caloric intake is the feeding intolerance frequently experienced in infants with BPD. Nasogastric feedings administered continuously or intermittently may be used, depending in part on the infant's respiratory status. If gastric distension further compromises chest expansion, a continuous infusion is preferred. An intermittent feeding schedule and the use of a pacifier during feedings, however, may help stimulate gastric motility and reduce gastric residuals in some infants. Gastroesophageal reflux and aspiration may also occur and can be minimized by prone positioning with the head elevated to a 30- to 45-degree angle during and immediately after feedings. Infants with BPD are often described as disorganized feeders unable to coordinate sucking, swallowing, and breathing.[119] In the chronically ill hospitalized infant, long-term use of tube feedings or parenteral nutrition can contribute to this behavior and may eventually lead to feeding resistance.[119,120] Helping parents assume the responsibility for feeding their infant and recognizing the social and emotional features of feeding, as well as the technical aspects, is an important part of discharge planning.[120]

Careful monitoring and early intervention are important in detecting and preventing developmental delay in the chronically ill infant. Parental involvement is important in establishing a routine for their infant and providing appropriate stimulation. Resources for ongoing care include child life, occupational, physical, and speech therapy.

Impairment of Respiratory Muscle Function

Impairment of respiratory muscle function is another mechanical alteration affecting the respiratory pump. In this case, diminished respiratory muscle function results in respiratory failure despite normal lung mechanics. Guillain-Barré syndrome (GBS) is one example of the numerous rare illnesses in which the chest wall and lungs are mechanically

sound, but a failure of the respiratory muscles driving the pump leads to respiratory failure.

Guillain-Barré Syndrome

Etiology. GBS is an acute immune-mediated inflammatory disorder of the peripheral nerves and nerve roots characterized by progressive paresis, paralysis, paresthesia, and pain. Paralysis often involves the respiratory muscles. Based on electrophysiologic and pathologic observations, GBS is divided into demyelinating and axonal subtypes. The acute motor axonal neuropathy (AMAN) involves predominantly motor nerve fibers with a physiologic pattern suggesting axonal damage, whereas the acute inflammatory demyelinating polyneuropathy (AIDP) involves both motor and sensory nerve fibers with a physiologic pattern suggesting demyelination.[121]

Incidence. Approximately 1 to 1.5 cases occur annually per 100,000 population with a mortality rate of 4% to 5%.[122] Although GBS affects all ages (the youngest reported case is a 4-month-old infant[123]), children appear to recover more quickly than adults.

Pathogenesis. Criteria necessary to establish the diagnosis of GBS are well established and are summarized in Table 19-6. Typically, symptoms occur within 4 weeks of an infectious process. The antecedent illness is often nonspecific, such as a mild respiratory infection or diarrhea. *Campylobacter jejuni,* a major cause of bacterial gastroenteritis worldwide, is the most common antecedent pathogen. It is likely that immune responses directed toward the infecting organisms are involved in the pathogenesis of GBS by cross-reaction with neural tissues.[124]

Symmetric weakness usually begins in the lower extremities, although it can rapidly ascend to the upper extremities, the trunk, and even the muscles innervated by the cranial nerves. Autonomic dysfunction also occurs frequently in children with GBS, involving the sympathetic and parasympathetic systems. Signs and symptoms of autonomic neu-

TABLE 19-6 Criteria for Diagnosis of Guillain-Barré Syndrome

Features required for diagnosis	Progressive motor weakness of more than one limb
	Areflexia or marked hyporeflexia
Features strongly supportive of the diagnosis	Rapidly developing motor weakness, but no progression by 4 weeks into illness
	Mild sensory signs or symptoms
	Cranial nerve involvement
	Onset of recovery 2-4 weeks after halt of progression
	Autonomic dysfunction
	Initial absence of fever

Data from Asbury AK, Arnason BG, Karp HR et al: Criteria for diagnosis of Guillain-Barré syndrome, *Ann Neurol* 3:565-567, 1978.

ropathy include orthostatic hypotension, hypertension, pupillary disturbances, diaphoresis, cardiac dysrhythmias, constipation, and urinary retention.

Approximately 30% of patients require mechanical ventilation, and these patients are often hospitalized for months before regaining the ability to walk.[122] When respiratory muscle weakness occurs, the child breathes shallowly and is unable to sigh. FRC is reduced, which leads to atelectasis, hypoxemia, and eventually CO_2 retention. Pooling of secretions with an absent or ineffective cough further contributes to alveolar collapse and respiratory compromise. Airway obstruction results from involvement of the pharyngeal muscles, leading to airway collapse during inspiration, passive posterior displacement of the tongue, or an inability to swallow oral secretions. Evaluating cranial nerves IX and X can assess pharyngeal muscle function. When these nerves are involved, there is a decreased ability to swallow or cough, decreased voice volume, and a depressed gag reflex.

Critical Care Management.   Supportive treatment is the mainstay of therapy. In the early stages of the illness, frequent careful assessments are necessary to detect impending respiratory failure, the most serious complication of muscle weakness. Respiratory function can be monitored in older children by measuring forced vital capacity (FVC). When FVC falls to 15 ml/kg, intubation and mechanical ventilation are usually necessary. Although some children are not dyspneic at this level of ventilatory compromise, the risk of aspiration, atelectasis, and pneumonia is minimized by early intervention. Ventilatory support is also indicated whenever there is an increased risk of airway obstruction.

Specific therapy remains a topic of controversy. Because of the inflammatory nature of the disease, corticosteroids were evaluated in a single prospective randomized trail, which failed to show beneficial effects.[125] Immunomodulation is used to improve the recovery rate and shorten hospital stays. Plasma exchange was shown to be effective in improving recovery time in GBS in several controlled trials during the 1980s. Intravenous immunoglobulin (IVIg) therapy has been shown to be equally effective for therapy of GBS and its variants. Although the precise mechanisms of immunomodulation by IVIg are unknown, it probably directly inactivates specific antimyelin antibodies and indirectly inhibits their production. IVIg offers some advantages over plasma exchange by being better tolerated in some patients and being easily administered without special equipment. However, because of the possibility of progression, the treatment of GBS patients requires qualified neurologic and supportive care.[122] Intravenous immunoglobulin (IVIg) therapy in children with very severe GBS was recently evaluated by Singhi and colleagues.[126] In the IVIg group, onset of recovery of muscle power was significantly earlier (day 14.8 of illness versus day 20.9, $P < .05$) and the length of PICU stay significantly shorter (20.5 days versus 50.5 days, $P < .01$).[126]

For older children with rapidly progressive disease, plasmapheresis is now the accepted therapy. Plasmapheresis involves the separation of plasma from cellular components of the blood by centrifugation or filtration. The plasma is replaced with a crystalloid and albumin mixture added to the blood cells and is returned to the body. Three controlled studies of patients over 12 years old have demonstrated that plasmapheresis decreases the severity and improves the outcome of patients with GBS.[127-129] In addition, Epstein and Sladky retrospectively analyzed data from 9 children treated with plasmapheresis, comparing them with 14 similarly affected historical controls.[130] The time to achieve independent ambulation was significantly shorter in the treated patients and there were no significant complications from plasmapheresis. Therefore plasmapheresis is generally recommended for children with severe and worsening disease.[131] The recommended protocol is an exchange of 200 to 250 ml of plasma per kg body weight over 7 to 14 days.[128,132] Why plasmapheresis is helpful is not known. It may be that antibodies such as antiperipheral-nerve antibody or other myelinotoxic or immunopathogenic factors are removed by pheresis.

When there is evidence of progressive disease and significant muscle weakness, the child is moved to the PICU, where frequent monitoring of respiratory status is possible. This is especially true for younger children in whom objective assessment of respiratory function is difficult.[133] Respiratory assessments include respiratory rate, pattern, and effort, as well as the quality of air entry on auscultation. Oxygen saturations are monitored continuously by pulse oximeter. Once the child has been successfully weaned from ventilatory support, swallowing and diaphragmatic function is assessed before removal of the endotracheal tube. In a cooperative child, serial measurements of FVC are obtained at least every 4 hours while muscle weakness is progressing. ABGs also document progression toward respiratory failure with an increase in $Paco_2$ and acidosis. Swallowing ability is also evaluated, as well as the strength of the child's cough and voice. The child's gag reflex is tested periodically. Estimates of peripheral muscle strength are valuable in tracking the course of the illness to determine whether muscle weakness is worsening, has reached a plateau, or strength is returning.

Because autonomic dysfunction is possible, cardiac monitoring is initiated and blood pressure carefully documented. Additional signs of excessive or inadequate activity of the parasympathetic or sympathetic systems are noted and treated as necessary (e.g., placement of a drainage catheter in the case of urinary retention). Hypotension may be especially problematic during plasmapheresis, but it is generally responsive to intravascular volume expansion.

Pain and paresthesias are also commonly present. The most common pain syndrome, present in 83% of 29 children under the age of 6 years, was back and lower limb pain.[134] Lower back pain because of irritation of the nerve roots may be relieved with the careful application of heat, although more severe pain requires the use of analgesics. Successful pain control in adult patients with GBS includes the use of epidural morphine.[135,136]

Because both sensory and motor losses occur, it is important to turn and reposition the child at least every 2 hours. Therapeutic pressure-reducing devices may aid in maintaining skin integrity, but they do not eliminate the need for a routine turning schedule. Passive range of motion is also performed to prevent contractures.

Nutritional adequacy is established early in the course of the illness to avoid excessive muscle wasting. Weakness and dysphagia may necessitate the use of transpyloric feedings and parenteral nutrition.

Especially during the sometimes frightening progression of paralysis, it is important to reassure patients and their families that a near complete, if not full, recovery is expected.

Botulism

Etiology and Incidence. Infant botulism was first recognized as a distinct clinical entity in 1976. Of all forms of human botulism (food borne, wound, and infant), infant botulism is now the most common in the United States. More than 90% of reported cases come from the United States, and within the United States, more than half of the cases come from California, Utah, and southeast Pennsylvania. This is likely a consequence of high concentrations of *Clostridium botulinum* spores in the soil of these regions.[137] Since 1973, a median of 24 cases of food-borne botulism, 3 cases of wound botulism, and 71 cases of infant botulism have been reported annually to the CDC. New vehicles for transmission have emerged in recent decades, and wound botulism associated with black tar heroin has increased dramatically since 1994. Recently, the potential terrorist use of botulinum toxin has become an important concern.[138] It is universally recommended that honey and corn syrup not be fed to infants younger than 1 year of age to prevent the occurrence of infant botulism.

Pathogenesis. *C. botulinum* is a ubiquitous gram-positive, spore-forming, obligate anaerobe with soil and dust as its natural habitat. Infant botulism typically affects previously well infants within the first 4 to 6 months of life (median 10 weeks) and is caused by ingestion of spores of *C. botulinum* that germinate and produce toxin in the gastrointestinal tract. The toxin irreversibly blocks the peripheral cholinergic synapses throughout the body, most importantly at the neuromuscular junction. The toxin does not cross the blood-brain barrier.

Constipation is characteristically an early sign, followed by signs of listlessness and progressive weakness. Symmetric descending paralysis is the rule; the cranial nerves are the first so be affected. Infantile botulism is characterized by poor feeding, difficulty in handling secretions, a weak cry, constipation, and generalized hypotonia. The diagnosis is confirmed by detection of the organism or its toxin in the infant's stool and supportive ancillary testing to rule out other causes of neurologic dysfunction that mimic botulism, such as stroke, the GBS, and myasthenia gravis.

Critical Care Management. Treatment includes supportive care and trivalent equine antitoxin, which reduces mortality if administered early.[138] Aggressive respiratory and nutritional care is the mainstay of treatment. Many infants require intubation and prolonged mechanical ventilation. Physical and occupational therapies are crucial in maintaining range of motion and functional positioning of

patients. Prognosis for complete recovery is excellent with meticulous supportive care. Infant botulism is a self-limited illness lasting a total of 2 to 6 weeks with progressive symptoms.

CIRCULATORY ALTERATIONS

The pulmonary circulation establishes the interface between inspired gas and the blood, thereby permitting delivery of O_2 to the blood and removal of CO_2. The second final common pathway of respiratory failure involves alterations in this circulation. Circulatory alterations disturb the normal contact between blood and gas within the lungs. PE and PPHN are characteristic examples. In these conditions, pulmonary circulation is reduced, physiologic dead space increases, and gas exchange may be impaired.

Pulmonary Embolism

Etiology. PE occurs when materials traveling in the bloodstream become impacted in the pulmonary arterial bed. Although uncommon in childhood, PE may occur after trauma or surgery, and may complicate a number of illnesses and treatments. Thromboembolism is the most commonly occurring form of PE and appears when a blood clot travels from a peripheral vessel through the right side of the heart and lodges in the pulmonary arterial bed. Pulmonary thromboembolism may complicate sickle cell anemia, rheumatic fever, and bacterial endocarditis, or may occur with sepsis or severe dehydration. Risk factors in children include presence of a central venous catheter, immobility, heart disease, ventriculoatrial shunt, and trauma.[139]

Incidence. PE is infrequently diagnosed in children, although clinicians should always have a high index of suspicion, especially when treating a child with the acute onset of respiratory distress or cardiovascular shock. The incidence of PE in children has been estimated to be 3.7% on postmortem examinations.[139]

Pathogenesis. The degree of cardiopulmonary disturbance observed in PE depends on two elements: the previous functional status of the heart and lungs and the severity of the pulmonary vascular occlusion.[140] A major pathophysiologic consequence of acute PE is increased alveolar dead space. This increase occurs because lung units continue to be ventilated despite diminished or absent perfusion. Pulmonary infarction is an uncommon sequela of PE owing to the fact that the lung has three sources of oxygen: pulmonary arteries, the airways, and bronchial arteries.[140]

Hypoxemia is common in acute PE. Regional bronchoconstriction and atelectasis result in $\dot{V}/\dot{Q}$ inequality and intrapulmonary shunting. Because the right ventricle has poor tolerance for an increase in afterload, cardiac output may become inadequate, and mixed venous saturations fall. If pulmonary hypertension develops and there is a patent foramen ovale (or septal defect), right-to-left shunting within the heart also contributes to hypoxemia.

The child's increased respiratory rate usually compensates for the increase in physiologic dead space produced by the arterial occlusion. The $Paco_2$ typically falls below 35 mmHg. However, $Paco_2$ rises in children who cannot adequately increase their minute ventilation (e.g., those with restrictive lung disease, those with neuromuscular disorders, or those receiving chemical paralyzing agents).

The child with a PE is dyspneic, tachypneic, and may complain of acute chest pain. Breath sounds may be clear or there may be scattered crackles. Radiographic findings are nonspecific and may include atelectasis, localized infiltrates, or a pleural effusion. Fever is also often present without other signs of infection. Supportive radiographic tests include a pulmonary angiogram and $\dot{V}/\dot{Q}$ scan. Pulmonary function tests may give abnormal results, but they are again nonspecific.[140]

Critical Care Management. Treatment consists of O_2, hemodynamic support, anticoagulation, and thrombolytic therapy. The treatment of PE goes beyond attempts to lyse the thrombus. In patients with acute respiratory failure, endotracheal intubation and mechanical ventilation is instituted to ensure adequate tissue oxygenation and CO_2 removal. High PEEP may be necessary to achieve oxygenation; however, this may impair venous return to the heart in an already hemodynamically compromised patient.[140]

Once the diagnosis is established, heparin therapy is initiated to prevent further thrombosis. Heparin is given for 7 to 10 days, and is usually initiated by a loading dose of 50 units/kg followed by a continuous infusion of 10 to 25 units/kg/hr, and adjusted according to the child's activated partial thromboplastin time (aPTT). A clotting time of 1.5 to 2.0 times the normal mean aPTT value (usually 50 to 70 seconds) is therapeutic. Approximately 24 to 48 hours after heparin therapy is initiated, warfarin (Coumadin) is begun so that there is an overlap of at least 5 days. Because heparin does not dissolve the clot, a thrombolytic agent such as streptokinase may also be used, although its efficacy in PE is questionable.

Nursing priorities in caring for the child with a PE include maintaining supplemental O_2 (and ventilatory support, if it becomes necessary), evaluating the child's cardiopulmonary status, and assessing the effects of therapy.

Spo_2 monitoring helps ensure adequate oxygenation. The adequacy of ventilation can be determined by evaluating the child's respiratory rate and effort and periodically measuring ABGs. In addition, cardiovascular assessment including heart rate, blood pressure, strength of peripheral pulses, warmth of extremities, and adequacy of urine output helps determine the need for inotropic support or volume expansion.

Because hemorrhage is the major complication of heparin (an untoward effect that may be compounded by thrombolytics), it is especially important to carefully monitor coagulation studies. Initially, aPTT values are measured and the infusion rate adjusted frequently. Daily monitoring is sufficient when a steady dose is achieved. The child is also monitored for signs of bleeding including petechiae, bloody emesis, stools, or gastric aspirates; hemoptysis; and hematuria. Invasive procedures are avoided or minimized.

Persistent Pulmonary Hypertension of the Newborn

Etiology. Persistent pulmonary hypertension of the newborn (PPHN) is a condition in which the high-resistance, low-flow pulmonary circulation of fetal life persists after birth. It is characterized by systemic or suprasystemic pulmonary artery pressures, with significant right-to-left shunting through the ductus arteriosus or foramen ovale. Desaturated venous blood is mixed with saturated arterial blood, resulting in arterial hypoxemia and tissue hypoxia. Right-to-left atrial shunting may be caused by diastolic dysfunction of the less compliant fetal right ventricle or dysfunction of the tricuspid papillary muscle, which causes tricuspid regurgitation.

Delayed relaxation of the pulmonary vascular bed is a feature of many neonatal pulmonary problems, including lung hypoplasia caused by mechanical compression (e.g., congenital diaphragmatic hernia), meconium aspiration pneumonia, perinatal asphyxia, bacterial pneumonia, and sepsis. It may also occur in the absence of obvious triggering diseases, presumably because of abnormal muscularization of pulmonary arterioles or transient defects in endothelial function.[141]

It is possible that PPHN is a process that starts well before birth; therefore birth history may be helpful in identifying those at greatest risk for developing PPHN. Typically, the infant is born at term or postterm, is appropriate in size for gestational age, and had meconium staining or birth asphyxia at the time of delivery.

Incidence. The incidence of PPHN is 1.9 per 1000 live births with a mortality rate of 11%.[142]

Pathogenesis. Manifestations of PPHN often involve dysfunctional pulmonary vasoregulation, with suprasystemic pulmonary vascular resistance causing extrapulmonary shunting, pulmonary parenchymal disease causing intrapulmonary shunting, and systemic hemodynamic deterioration.

Typically, the infant with PPHN develops tachypnea and cyanosis soon after birth. Other signs of respiratory distress also appear including grunting, nasal flaring, and intercostal retractions. The quality of breath sounds depends upon the underlying clinical condition; adventitious sounds are prominent in meconium aspiration, for example, but may be absent in neonatal asphyxia. Neonates with PPHN also demonstrate a wide spectrum of myocardial abnormalities, ranging from mild dysfunction to severe biventricular congestive failure.

The physical examination may be of limited value. A finding of the presence or absence of a murmur is not helpful. Neonates with PPHN may have the murmur of high-velocity tricuspid regurgitation. The chest radiograph may document the parenchymal disease, which is the triggering factor for PPHN. Preductal and postductal blood gas measurements have been used to differentiate PPHN from structural heart disease. Right-to-left shunting through the ductus arteriosus and foramen ovale results in hypoxemia, which often proves refractory to supplemental O_2. Neonates with PPHN may have nearly normal preductal (right arm, head) oxygen tension and oxygen saturation while the postductal (umbilical artery, left arm, lower limbs) right-to-left shunt causes lower oxygen tension and saturation.[141] Echocardiography can usually provide a definitive structural diagnosis. In severe PPHN, hypoxemia is followed rapidly by the development of hypercarbia and acidosis. Hypoxia and acidosis perpetuate the vicious cycle of pulmonary vasoconstriction, pulmonary artery hypertension, and right-to-left intrapulmonary and intracardiac shunting (Fig. 19-10).

Critical Care Management.   Treatment in PPHN is aimed at decreasing the ratio of pulmonary to systemic vascular resistance, thereby reducing or eliminating right-to-left shunting. Historically, this has been accomplished by hyperoxygenation, hyperventilation, and the use of nonspecific vasodilators. However, mortality in infants with PPHN remained high, perhaps in part because of the complications of such aggressive therapy, that is, pneumothorax, pneumomediastinum, barotrauma, and chronic lung disease. Various therapies currently in use include oxygenation, alkalinization, high frequency ventilation, nitric oxide, and ECMO.

Hypoxemia causes reflex pulmonary vasoconstriction in fetal sheep and adult dogs, and may well contribute to the pathophysiology of PPHN. Therefore, in an attempt to reverse pulmonary hypertension, infants with PPHN usually receive high levels of supplemental O_2, the most potent pulmonary vasodilator available.

Through mechanisms that are unclear, an increase in pH also decreases pulmonary vascular resistance. By increasing arterial pH to a "critical level" at which there is a fall in pulmonary artery pressures, a reversal of right-to-left shunting and an increase in Pao_2 appear to be achieved in many cases. The degree of respiratory alkalosis necessary to reverse right-to-left shunting sometimes cannot be achieved with mechanical hyperventilation because of severe lung disease or the development of a metabolic acidosis. There is evidence to suggest, however, that respiratory alkalosis and metabolic alkalosis are equally effective in attenuating hypoxia-induced pulmonary vasoconstriction.[98] However,

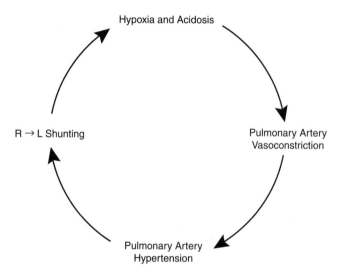

Hypoxia and Acidosis

Pulmonary Artery Vasoconstriction

Pulmonary Artery Hypertension

R → L Shunting

Fig. 19-10   The vicious cycle of persistent pulmonary hypertension of the newborn.

no randomized, controlled trials of hyperventilation versus conservative management are available. An infusion of sodium bicarbonate may produce the desired degree of alkalosis while avoiding the complications of aggressive mechanical hyperventilation; however, serum sodium levels are followed closely. Generally, an infusion of sodium bicarbonate is begun and adjusted to maintain a pH of 7.45 to 7.50. Alternatively, THAM may be used if CO_2 retention or hyponatremia are a problem. A more conservative approach to mechanical ventilation can then be pursued. To prevent the complications of mechanical ventilation, the lowest PIP possible is used to achieve the therapeutic goals.

Because hypoxemia may put the infant with PPHN at risk for cerebral hypoxia, monitoring the infant's neurologic status is important. In a study of 19 infants with PPHN (the majority of whom had birth asphyxia), nine suffered cerebral infarctions.[143] Furthermore, eight of the nine infants with infarction had seizures detected by electroencephalogram (EEG) during periods of neuromuscular blockade. Routine EEGs may be warranted in these patients.

High-frequency ventilation is an alternative approach used in some centers, primarily as a rescue treatment when conventional therapy fails. In high-frequency ventilation, extremely small tidal volumes and high rates are used to provide gas exchange.

The recent discovery of the role of nitric oxide as the endothelium-derived relaxing factor has delivered hope for a selective agent to modulate the neonatal pulmonary vascular resistance.[141] (For a description of iNO, see ARDS on page 679.) Inhaled nitric oxide also reduces the extent to which ECMO is needed in neonates with hypoxemic respiratory failure and pulmonary hypertension.[144] However, again, long-term benefits to these infants have been difficult to demonstrate.

ECMO (see Chapter 8) has been used to support patients with PPHN in whom conventional medical management has failed. The institution of ECMO permits correction of hypoxemia and acidosis. National ECMO experience (through July 2000) derived from ELSO (Extracorporeal Life Support Organization) Registry reported 2227 patients with the primary diagnosis of PPHN have been treated with ECMO with an overall survival rate of 79%.[145] Once the infant is placed on ECMO, ventilator support is reduced to a minimum to avoid any further barotrauma or oxygen toxicity to the lung.[145]

An evaluation of treatment methods used in 12 Level III neonatal intensive care units (before the widespread use of iNO) demonstrated wide variations in practice. Hyperventilation was used in 65% of centers, with a range from 33% to 92%; continuous infusion of alkali was used in 75% of centers, with a range of 27% to 93% of neonates. Other commonly used treatments included sedation (94%; range: 77% to 100%), paralysis (73%; range: 33% to 98%), and inotrope administration (84%; range: 46% to 100%). Vasodilator drugs, primarily tolazoline, were used in 39% (range: 13% to 81%) of neonates.[142]

The nursing care of the infant with PPHN is directed toward avoiding conditions that increase pulmonary vascular resistance, detecting complications of therapy, and whenever possible, minimizing those complications.

As stated earlier, hypoxemia results in increased pulmonary vascular resistance. In an infant in an unstable condition with PPHN, even small reductions in F_{IO_2} can lead to profound hypoxemia. Therefore consistent delivery of O_2 is assured. In the acutely ill infant during the first 24 hours, or in infants exhibiting wide fluctuations in oxygenation, attempts are made to maintain Pa_{O_2} at approximately 100 mmHg. Furthermore, maneuvers that cause hypoxemia, for example, endotracheal suctioning, are avoided unless absolutely necessary. It is not uncommon for these infants to be exquisitely sensitive to any type of tactile stimulation, responding with precipitous drops in Sp_{O_2}.[146] Prohibiting unnecessary handling will help limit episodes of hypoxemia; therefore routine care (e.g., bathing or weighing the infant) is inappropriate. Finally, sedation is used to minimize agitation and its negative effect on pulmonary vascular resistance.

Cold stress, hypoglycemia, and hypoxemia may all result in acidosis that will increase pulmonary vascular resistance. These conditions are avoided by carefully controlling and monitoring the infant's environment and response to therapy. Because ready access to the critically ill infant is necessary, providing a neutral thermal environment is often not possible. Heat loss can be minimized, however, with a radiant warmer. Frequent bedside monitoring of blood glucose is also performed. Preductal and postductal Sp_{O_2} is monitored continuously and blood gases followed to monitor acid-base status, especially when alkalosis is being employed to reduce pulmonary vascular resistance.

Careful assessments of oxygenation and systemic perfusion accompany changes in ventilator settings. In the neonate, a tension pneumothorax may present as sudden hypotension, bradycardia, and hypoxemia and requires immediate needle aspiration and eventual placement of a chest tube. In addition, excessive PEEP may cause an increase in pulmonary vascular resistance. This may increase right-to-left shunting and decrease pulmonary venous return and further reduce systemic flow of oxygenated blood.

Systemic blood pressure must be higher than pulmonary artery pressure to reverse right-to-left shunting; therefore maintenance of adequate systemic blood pressure is essential to correct hypoxemia in PPHN. Intravascular volume is assessed frequently by monitoring heart rate, blood pressure, liver size, capillary refill time, and warmth of extremities. Hydration status can be further evaluated by assessing fluid intake and urine output, urine specific gravity, skin turgor, mucous membranes, and fontanels. As stated earlier, infants with PPHN may have a variable degree of myocardial dysfunction, therefore myocardial depressants such as hypoglycemia, acidosis, and hypocalcemia are avoided. In addition, dopamine may be given to improve cardiac contractility.

The infant undergoing high-frequency ventilation presents additional nursing challenges. These are usually the most critically ill infants in whom conventional mechanical ventilation appears to be failing, or whose course has been complicated by pulmonary interstitial emphysema, pneumothorax, or pneumomediastinum.

The initial PIP used in high-frequency jet ventilation is based on the infant's requirements while on conventional mechanical ventilation. Ordinarily, PIP is set 20% to 33% below the pressure required during conventional treatment.[147] Some infants with severe pulmonary hypertension, however, may have acute deterioration when high-frequency jet ventilation is initiated at lower inflating pressures. Therefore some clinicians suggest that PIP not be lowered initially in infants with PPHN, but should be gradually decreased as determined by the infant's response to therapy (Sp_{O_2} and ABGs).[148] Ventilatory frequency can be adjusted to deliver 300 to 540 cycles per minute (6 to 9 Hz), and is usually started at a rate of 420 cycles per minute (7 Hz).

The infant receiving high-frequency jet ventilation requires continuous monitoring of heart rate, blood pressure, and transcutaneous O_2 and CO_2. Although vibration of the chest and body make monitoring of the infant's respiratory rate impractical, absence of vibration may signal tube obstruction or displacement, or a decrease in C_L, for example, with a tension pneumothorax.[147] Breath sounds are also altered by the ventilator, but subtle changes can be detected with frequent, careful examination.

As with any artificial airway, maintaining airway patency is a primary nursing responsibility. It is possible to suction the endotracheal tube through its main port while maintaining high-frequency jet ventilation. However, some clinicians suggest that this practice may create shearing forces in the trachea (produced by the combination of negative pressure suction and high-frequency positive pressure breaths), which may contribute to the development of necrotizing tracheobronchitis.[148] This particular complication, a severe airway injury that results in sloughing of the tracheal mucosa, is reported with varying frequency and may result from inadequate humidification of inspired gases, shearing forces in the airway, or other factors that have yet to be identified.

ALTERATIONS IN THE CONTROL OF BREATHING

The last final common pathway of respiratory failure includes disorders resulting from abnormalities or deficiencies in the control of breathing, resulting in hypoventilation. This category includes alterations in the neuromuscular control of upper airway patency and abnormalities in respiratory drive that result in alveolar hypoventilation. Apnea, both central and obstructive, and alveolar hypoventilation syndromes are considered.

Apnea

Etiology. Apnea is generally defined as the cessation of breathing for more than 20 seconds or for a shorter period when associated with hypoxemia or bradycardia. Central apnea is characterized by a respiratory pause. In contrast, respiratory efforts continue, sometimes quite vigorously, in obstructive apnea, but there is an absence of airway flow caused by airway obstruction. A mixed picture of central and obstructive apnea may also be observed.

Incidence. The prevalence of apnea of prematurity varies inversely with gestational age. In all births the incidence is 1%.[149] The prevalence of obstructive sleep apnea is 0.7% to 2.9%; peak age of presentation is 2 to 4 years.[150,151]

Pathogenesis. Apnea of prematurity is most commonly central in origin, but obstructive apnea and mixed disorders also occur.[152] Although the cause is unknown, apnea of prematurity is thought to be related not only to an immaturity of the central nervous system, but also to an increase in chest wall compliance. More respiratory work is required to generate a constant tidal volume when the chest wall is highly compliant. Within this context, apnea may represent a strategy to avoid fatigue.

Although central apnea is the classic apnea of prematurity, it occurs in a number of other conditions in which the central nervous system is somehow altered. Sepsis, hypoglycemia, hypothermia, drug intoxication, trauma, and brain tumors may result in apnea. In addition, because their ventilatory response to hypoxia and sensitivity to CO_2 are already depressed, young infants may be especially vulnerable to periods of apnea when they receive narcotics and other respiratory depressants.

In obstructive apnea, upper airway collapse occurs because of poor coordination of the muscles responsible for airway maintenance. Obstructive apnea usually happens during sleep and, in children, it is most often caused by hypertrophy of the tonsils and adenoids. Although sleep is the most common functional condition predisposing to obstructive apnea, other factors that may depress airway-maintaining activity include narcotics, sedatives, alcohol, and some brainstem lesions, particularly those associated with Arnold-Chiari malformation.

Central apnea is evidenced by a cessation of respiratory activity and may be accompanied by a fall in Spo_2 and heart rate. In the preterm infant, respiratory pauses occur more commonly in active sleep and often within the context of periodic breathing. Frequently, these infants also have an obstructive component to their apnea.[152]

Critical Care Management. Physical examination of the sleeping child with obstructive apnea reveals sonorous respirations, retractions, and breathing pauses that may be associated with hypoxemia and bradycardia. Often, vigorous movement occurs during sleep in an attempt to overcome the airway obstruction. Brouillette and co-workers report serious sequelae, including cor pulmonale, failure to thrive, permanent neurologic damage, and behavioral disturbances, hypersomnolence, or developmental delay, in cases in which obstructive sleep apnea had gone untreated.[153]

Although it is unclear what effect apneic periods may have on the preterm infant, frequent episodes accompanied by hypoxemia are usually treated because they may lead to additional neurologic complications. Nasal CPAP may help by preventing lung deflation and chest distortion. Pharmacologic approaches include the use of theophylline or doxapram hydrochloride to increase central respiratory drive and/or improve CO_2 sensitivity.[154] Although caffeine has been used to treat apnea, Henderson-Smart and Steer reported the results of a meta-analysis of two studies examining a total of 104 infants receiving prophylactic caffeine.[155] There were no meaningful differences between the caffeine and placebo groups in the number of infants with apnea, bradycardia, hypoxemic episodes, use of ventilation or side effects in either of the studies. Alternatively, a loading dose of 6 mg/kg of theophylline is followed by a dose of 2 mg/kg given two to three times a day to maintain a serum theophylline level of 8 to 12 mg/L. Doxapram hydrochloride, an analeptic drug, is considered in patients unresponsive to theophylline. To decrease toxic side effects (seizures, hypertension, hyperglycemia, hypothermia) a loading dose of 3 mg/kg is administered over 15 minutes followed by a continuous IV infusion of 1 mg/kg/hr.

Because adenotonsillar hypertrophy is the predominant anatomic cause of obstructive sleep apnea in childhood, tonsillectomy and adenoidectomy often provide the cure.[153,156] Nasal CPAP may effectively relieve obstructive sleep apnea in preterm infants[157] but has rarely been used in children.[158] Tracheostomy is seldom required.

The primary nursing responsibilities in caring for the infant or child with apnea are early detection of the event and monitoring of the effects of treatment. All patients at risk for central or obstructive apnea have continuous cardiac and Spo_2 monitoring. Careful observation and documentation of apneic episodes is essential in establishing the etiology and guiding a treatment plan.

Alveolar Hypoventilation Syndromes

Etiology and Incidence. Alveolar hypoventilation syndromes are rare conditions in which there is no upper airway obstruction, but an insufficient respiratory drive result in hypoventilation. These respiratory control deficits, which originate within the central nervous system, may be congenital (known as Ondine's curse) or acquired, and are characterized by progressive hypoxemia and hypercarbia during sleep, particularly quiet sleep.

Pathogenesis. The severity of hypopnea in congenital hypoventilation syndromes varies widely. The most severe form, central hypoventilation syndrome, is usually diagnosed soon after birth and may be associated with some degree of hypoventilation even during wakefulness.

Alveolar hypoventilation may also be acquired following a brainstem injury. Birth asphyxia can result in central hypoventilation syndrome, as can encephalitis, tumors, and brainstem trauma.[159-161]

The child with alveolar hypoventilation usually has a normal respiratory rate but breathes very shallowly (hypopnea). The respiratory rate is relatively fixed and does not increase in response to progressive hypoxemia or hypocarbia. This phenomenon occurs during quiet sleep when the child is totally dependent on automatic respiratory control systems.

Critical Care Management. Theophylline may be helpful in milder forms of the disorder. A number of other respiratory stimulants have been evaluated in children with hypoventilation, but none has been uniformly effective. In severe cases, ventilatory assistance with positive pressure ventilation or phrenic pacing may be necessary.

SUMMARY

Caring for the patient with pulmonary dysfunction is inherent to the practice of pediatric critical care nursing. This chapter presents the pulmonary illnesses common to pediatric critical care. Within the final common pathway framework of mechanical, circulatory, and regulatory failure, emphasis is placed on nursing and collaborative interventions intended to both support the critically ill patient and prevent iatrogenic injury. Much pediatric specific nursing research is needed to help guide practice related to the care of this vulnerable population and their families. Sensitivity and attention to the impact of critical illness on children and their families is as important as knowledge of the causes and treatment of respiratory failure.

REFERENCES

1. Biel M, Eastwood JA, Muenzen P et al: Evolving trends in critical care nursing practice: results of a certification role delineation study, *Am J Crit Care* 8:285-290, 1999.
2. American Academy of Pediatrics Committee on Hospital Care and Section on Critical Care Pediatric Section and Admission Criteria Task Force: Guidelines for developing admission and discharge policies for the pediatric intensive care unit, *Pediatrics* 103: 840-842, 1999.
3. Ausejo M, Saenz A, Pham B et al: The effectiveness of glucocorticoids in treating croup: meta-analysis. *BMJ* 319:595-600, 1999.
4. Ausejo M, Saenz A, Pham B et al: Glucocorticoids for croup. *Cochrane Database Syst Rev,* 2, 1992.
5. Kemper KJ, Ritz RH, Benson MS et al: Helium-oxygen mixture in the treatment of postextubation stridor in pediatric trauma patients. *Crit Care Med* 19:356-359, 1991.
6. Westley CR, Cotton EK, Brooks JG: Nebulized racemic epinephrine by IPPB treatment of croup: a double blind study. *Am J Dis Child* 132:484-487, 1978.
7. Centers for Disease Control and Prevention: *Haemophilus influenzae* invasive disease among children aged <5 years—California, 1990-1996. *MMWR* 11:737-740, 1998.
8. Travis KW, Todres ID, Shannon DC: Pulmonary edema associated with croup and epiglottitis. *Pediatrics* 59:695-698, 1977.
9. Bernstein T, Brilli R, Jacobs B: Is bacterial tracheitis changing? A 14-month experience in a pediatric intensive care unit. *Clin Infect Dis* 27:458-462, 1998.
10. Brook I: Aerobic and anaerobic microbiology of bacterial tracheitis in children. *Pediatr Emerg Care* 13:16-18, 1997.
11. Pasaoglu I, Dogan R, Demircin M et al: Bronchoscopic removal of foreign bodies in children: retrospective analysis of 822 cases. *Thorac Cardiovasc Surg* 39:95-98, 1991.
12. Baharloo F, Veyckemans F, Francis C et al: Tracheobronchial foreign bodies: presentation and management in children and adults. *Chest* 115:1357-1362, 1999.
13. Metrangelo S, Monetti C, Meneghini L et al: Eight years' experience with foreign-body aspiration in children: what is really important for a timely diagnosis? *J Pediatr Surg* 34:1229-1231, 1999.

14. Chameides L, Hazinski MF, eds: *Pediatric advanced life support,* Dallas, 1997, American Heart Association, American Academy of Pediatrics.
15. Mathew OP, Sant'Ambrogio G: Development of upper airway reflexes. In Chernick V, Mellins RB, eds: *Basic mechanisms of pediatric respiratory disease: cellular and integrative,* Philadelphia, 1991, B.C. Decker.
16. Jacobs IN, Wetmore RF, Tom LW et al: Tracheobronchomalacia in children. *Arch Otolaryngol Head Neck Surg* 120:154-158, 1994.
17. Gordin PC: Assessing and managing agitation in a critically ill infant. *Maternal and Child Nursing* 15:26-32, 1990.
18. Panitch HB, Allen JL, Alpert BE et al: Effects of CPAP on lung mechanics in infants with acquired tracheobronchomalacia. *Am J Respir Crit Care Med* 150:1341-1346, 1994.
19. Kanter RK, Pollack MM, Wright WW et al: Treatment of severe tracheobronchomalacia with continuous positive airway pressure (CPAP). *Anesthesiology* 57:54-56, 1982.
20. Howard TS, Hoffman LH, Stang PE, Simoes EA: Respiratory syncytial virus pneumonia in the hospital setting: length of stay, charges and mortality. *J Pediatr* 137:227-232, 2000.
21. Centers for Disease Control and Prevention: Update: respiratory syncytial virus activity—United States, 1998-1999 season. *MMWR* 10:1104-1106, 1115, 1999.
22. Brenton S: RSV specimen collection methods: nasal vs. nasopharyngeal. *Pediatr Nurs* 23:621-622, 629, 1997.
23. Shay DK, Holman RC, Newman RD et al: Bronchiolitis-associated hospitalizations among US children, 1980-1996. *JAMA* 282:1440-1446, 1999.
24. Wang EEL, Law BJ, Stephens D: Pediatric Investigators' Collaborative Network on Infections in Canada (PICNIC): prospective study of risk factors and outcomes in patients hospitalized with respiratory syncytial viral lower respiratory tract infections. *J Pediatr* 126:212-219, 1995.
25. Helfaer MA, Nichols DG, Rogers MC: Lower airway disease: bronchiolitis and asthma. In MC Rogers, DG Nichols, eds: *Textbook of pediatric intensive care* (ed 3). Baltimore, 1996, Williams & Wilkins.

26. Kellner JD, Ohlsson A, Gadomski AM et al: Efficacy of bronchodilator therapy in bronchiolitis: a meta-analysis. *Arch Pediatr Adolesc Med* 150:1166-1172, 1996.
27. Flores G, Horwitz RI: Efficacy of beta2-agonists in bronchiolitis: a reappraisal and meta-analysis. *Pediatrics* 100:233-239, 1997.
28. Klassen TP: Recent advances in the treatment of bronchiolitis and laryngitis. *Pediatr Clin North Am* 44:249-261, 1997.
29. Smith PG, el-Khatib MF, Carlo WA: PEEP does not improve pulmonary mechanics in infants with bronchiolitis. *Am Rev Respir Dis* 147:1295-1298, 1993.
30. Weksler N, Ovadia LJ: Nasal continuous positive airway pressure: an alternative method for respiratory assistance. *Clin Anesth* 3:442-446, 1991.
31. Hollman G, Shen G, Zeng L et al: Helium-oxygen improves clinical asthma scores in children with acute bronchiolitis. *Crit Care Med* 26:1731-1736, 1998.
32. Cade A, Brownlee KG, Conway SP et al: Randomized placebo controlled trial of nebulized corticosteroids in acute respiratory syncytial viral bronchiolitis. *Arch Dis Child* 82:126-130, 2000.
33. Bulow SM, Nir M, Levin E et al: Prednisolone treatment of respiratory syncytial virus infection: a randomized controlled trial of 147 infants. *Pediatrics* 104:77, 2000.
34. American Academy of Pediatrics Committee on Infectious Diseases: Reassessment of the indications for ribavirin therapy in respiratory syncytial virus infections. *Pediatrics* 97:137-140, 1996.
35. Guerguerian AM, Gauthier M, Lebel MH et al: Ribavirin in ventilated respiratory syncytial virus bronchiolitis: a randomized, placebo-controlled trial. *Am J Respir Crit Care Med* 160:829-834, 1999.
36. Chellis MJ, Sanders SV, Dean JM et al: Bedside transpyloric feeding tube placement in the PICU. *J Parenteral Enteral Nutr* 20:88-90, 1996.
37. American Academy of Pediatrics Committee on Infectious Diseases and Committee of Fetus and Newborn: Prevention of respiratory syncytial virus infections: indications for the use of palivizumab and update on the use of RSV-IGIV. *Pediatrics* 102:1211-1216, 1998.

38. Simoes EA, Sondheimer HM, Top FH Jr. et al: Respiratory syncytial virus immune globulin for prophylaxis against respiratory syncytial virus disease in infants and children with congenital heart disease. The Cardiac Study Group. *J Pediatr* 133:492-499, 1998.

39. The IMpact-RSV Study Group: Palivizumab, a humanized respiratory syncytial virus monoclonal antibody, reduces hospitalization from respiratory syncytial virus infection in high-risk infants. *Pediatrics* 102:531-537, 1998.

40. Centers for Disease Control and Prevention: Guidelines for prevention of nosocomial pneumonia. *MMWR* 3:1-79, 1997.

41. National Heart, Lung, and Blood Institute: *Guidelines for the diagnosis and management of asthma, Expert Panel Report 2.* (National Institutes of Health Publication No. 97-4051). Washington, DC, 1997, U.S. Government Printing Office.

42. Centers for Disease Control and Prevention: Children at risk from ozone air pollution—United States, 1991-1993. *MMWR* 44:309-312, 1995.

43. Centers for Disease Control and Prevention: Asthma Mortality and Hospitalization Among Children and Young Adults—United States, 1980-1993. *MMWR* 45:350-353, 1996.

44. Weiss KB, Gergen PJ, Wagener DK: Breathing better or wheezing worse? The changing epidemiology of asthma morbidity and mortality. *Annu Rev Public Health* 14:491-513, 1993.

45. National Heart, Lung, and Blood Institute: Global initiative for asthma. (National Institutes of Health Publication No. 95-3659), 1995.

46. Smith LJ, Shamsuddin M, Sporn PH, Denenberg M, Anderson J: Reduced superoxide dismutase in lung cells of patients with asthma. *Free Radic Biol Med* 22:1301-1307, 1997.

47. National Heart, Lung, and Blood Institute; National Institutes of Health: *Executive summary: guidelines for the diagnosis and management of asthma* (Publication No. 91-3042A). Washington, DC, 1991, U.S. Government Printing Office.

48. Connett GJ, Warde C, Wooler E et al: Prednisolone and salbutamol in the hospital treatment of acute asthma. *Arch Dis Child* 70:170-173, 1994.

49. Ciarallo L, Sauer AH, Shannon MW: Intravenous magnesium therapy for moderate to severe pediatric asthma: results of a randomized, placebo-controlled trial. *J Pediatr* 129:809-814, 1996.

50. Kudukis TM, Manthous CA, Schmidt GA et al: Inhaled helium-oxygen revisited: effect of inhaled helium-oxygen during the treatment of status asthmaticus in children. *J Pediatr* 130:217-224, 1997.

51. Carter ER, Webb CR, Moffitt DR: Evaluation of heliox in children hospitalized with acute severe asthma: a randomized crossover trial. *Chest* 109:1256-1261, 1996.

52. Maguire JF, O'Rourke PP, Colan SD, Geha RS, Crone R: Cardiotoxicity during treatment of severe childhood asthma. *Pediatrics* 88:1180-1186, 1991.

53. Dhand R, Tobin MJ: Bronchodilator delivery with metered-dose inhalers in mechanically-ventilated patients. *Eur Respir J* 9:585-595, 1996.

54. Schaeffer EM, Pohlman A, Morgan S et al: Oxygenation in status asthmaticus improves during ventilation with helium-oxygen. *Crit Care Med* 27:2666-2670, 1999.

55. Curley MAQ, Molengraft JA: Providing comfort to critically ill pediatric patients: isoflurane. *Crit Care Nurs Clin North Am* 7:267-274, 1995.

56. Wagner CL, Brooks JG, Richter SE et al: The "88% saturation test": a simple lung function test for young children. *Pediatrics* 93:63-67, 1994.

57. Buist AS, Vollmer WM: Preventing deaths from asthma. *N Engl J Med* 331:1584-1585, 1994.

58. Oddy WH, Holt PG, Sly PD et al: Association between breast feeding and asthma in 6 year old children: findings of a prospective birth cohort study. *BMJ* 319:815-819, 1999.

59. Sigman K, Mazer B: Immunotherapy for childhood asthma: is there a rationale for its use? *Ann Allergy Asthma Immunol* 76:299-305, 1996.

60. Ashbaugh DG, Bigelow DB, Petty TL, Levine BE: Acute respiratory distress in adults. *Lancet* 2:319-323, 1967.

61. Bernard GR, Artigas A, Brigham KL et al: The American-European Consensus Conference on ARDS: definitions, mechanisms, relevant outcomes, and clinical trial coordination. *Am J Respir Crit Care Med* 149:818-824, 1994.

62. Fackler JC, Curley MAQ, Green T et al: Improved outcome in the acute respiratory distress syndrome in children using a lung protective ventilation strategy; lessons from an aborted randomized clinical trial of extracorporeal membrane oxygenation. In review.

63. Davis SL, Furman DP, Costarino AT Jr: Adult respiratory distress syndrome in children: associated disease, clinical course, and predictors of death. *J Pediatr* 123:35-45, 1993.

64. Timmons OD, Havens PL, Fackler JC: Predicting death in pediatric patients with acute respiratory failure. *Chest* 108:789-797, 1995.

65. Ware LB, Matthay MA: The acute respiratory distress syndrome. *N Engl J Med* 242:1334-1349, 2000.

66. Slutsky AS, Tremblay LN: Multiple system organ failure: is mechanical ventilation a contributing factor? *Am J Respir Crit Care Med* 157:1721-1725, 1998.

67. Ranieri VM, Suter PM, Tortorella C et al: Effect of mechanical ventilation on inflammatory mediators in patients with acute respiratory distress syndrome: a randomized controlled trial. *JAMA* 282:54-61, 1999.

68. Gattinoni L, Pelosi P, Suter PM et al: Acute respiratory distress syndrome caused by pulmonary and extrapulmonary disease. Different syndromes? *Am J Respir Crit Care Med* 158:3-11, 1998.

69. Moloney-Harmon PA: When the lung fails: acute respiratory distress syndrome in children. *Crit Care Nurs Clin North Am* 11:519-528, 1999.

70. Roupie E, Dambrosio M, Servillo G et al: Titration of tidal volume and induced hypercapnia in acute respiratory distress syndrome. *Am J Respir Crit Care Med* 152:121-128, 1995.

71. Amato MB, Barbas CS, Medeiros DM et al: Effect of a protective-ventilation strategy on mortality in the acute respiratory distress syndrome. *N Engl J Med* 338:347-354, 1998.

72. Stewart TE, Meade MO, Cook DJ et al: Evaluation of a ventilation strategy to prevent barotrauma in patients at high risk for acute respiratory distress syndrome. Pressure- and Volume-Limited Ventilation Strategy Group. *N Engl J Med* 338:355-361, 1998.

73. Suter PM, Fairley HB, Isenberg MD: Effect of tidal volume and positive end-expiratory pressure on compliance during mechanical ventilation. *Chest* 73:158-162, 1978.

74. Acute Respiratory Distress Syndrome Network: Ventilation with lower tidal volumes as compared with traditional tidal volumes for acute lung injury and the acute respiratory distress syndrome. *N Engl J Med* 342:1301-1308, 2000.

75. Hickling KG, Henderson SJ, Jackson R: Low mortality associated with low volume pressure limited ventilation with permissive hypercapnia in severe adult respiratory distress syndrome. *Intensive Care Med* 16:372-377, 1990.

76. Hickling KG, Walsh J, Henderson S et al: Low mortality rate in adult respiratory distress syndrome using low-volume, pressure-limited ventilation with permissive hypercapnia: a prospective study. *Crit Care Med* 22:1568-1578, 1994.

77. Doctor A, Arnold J: Mechanical support for acute lung injury: options for strategic ventilation. *New Horizons* 7:359-373, 1999.

78. Arnold JH, Hanson JH, Toro-Figuero LO et al: Prospective, randomized comparison of high-frequency oscillatory ventilation and conventional mechanical ventilation in pediatric respiratory failure. *Crit Care Med* 22:1530-1539, 1994.

79. Dalton H: Extracorporeal life support in the new millennium: Forging ahead or fading out? *New Horizons* 7:414-432, 1999.

80. Palmisano BW, Fisher DM, Willis M, Gregory GA, Ebert PA: The effect of paralysis on oxygen consumption in normoxic children after cardiac surgery. *Anesthesiology* 61:518-522, 1998.

81. Bryan AC: Comments of a devil's advocate. *Am Rev Respir Dis* 110:143-144, 1974.

82. Curley MA: Prone positioning of patients with acute respiratory distress syndrome: a systematic review. *Am J Crit Care* 8:397-405, 1999.

83. Pelosi P, Tubiolo D, Mascheroni D et al: Effects of the prone position on respiratory mechanics and gas exchange during acute lung injury. *Am J Respir Crit Care Med* 157:387-393, 1998.

84. Curley MA, Thompson JE, Arnold JH: The effects of early and repeated prone positioning in pediatric patients with acute lung injury. *Chest* 118:156-163, 2000.

85. Rutledge ML, Hawkins EP, Langston C: Skeletal muscle growth failure induced in premature newborn infants by prolonged pancuronium treatment. *J Pediatr* 109:883-886, 1986.

86. Weinberger B, Heck DE, Laskin DL et al: Nitric oxide in the lung: therapeutic and cellular mechanisms of action. *Pharmacol Ther* 84:401-411, 1999.

87. Bohn D: Nitric oxide in acute hypoxic respiratory failure: from the bench to the bedside and back again. *J Pediatr* 134:387-389, 1999.

88. Willson DF, Zaritsky A, Bauman LA et al: Instillation of calf lung surfactant extract (calfactant) is beneficial in pediatric acute hypoxemic respiratory failure. Members of the Mid-Atlantic Pediatric Critical Care Network. *Crit Care Med* 27:188-195, 1999.

89. Bernard GR, Bradley RB: Adult respiratory distress syndrome: diagnosis and management. *Heart Lung* 15:250-255, 1986.

90. Meduri GU, Headley AS, Golden E et al: Effect of prolonged methylprednisolone therapy in unresolving acute respiratory distress syndrome: a randomized controlled trial. *JAMA* 280:159-165, 1998.

91. Rochester DF, Esau SA: Malnutrition and the respiratory system. *Chest* 85:411-415, 1984.

92. Bohn D, Tamura M, Perrin D et al: Ventilatory predictors of pulmonary hypoplasia in congenital diaphragmatic hernia, confirmed by morphologic assessment. *J Pediatr* 111:423-431, 1987.

93. Sakai H, Tamura M, Hosokawa Y et al: Effect of surgical repair on respiratory mechanics in congenital diaphragmatic hernia. *J Pediatr* 111:432-438, 1987.

94. Breaux CW, Rouse TM, Cain WS et al: Improvement in survival of patients with congenital diaphragmatic hernia utilizing a strategy of delayed repair after medical and/or extracorporeal membrane oxygenation stabilization. *J Pediatr Surg* 26:333-338, 1991.

95. Langer JC, Filler RM, Bohn KJ et al: Timing of surgery for congenital diaphragmatic hernia: Is emergency operation necessary? *J Pediatr Surg* 23:731-734, 1988.

96. Shanbhogue LKR, Tam PKH, Ninan G et al: Preoperative stabilization in congenital diaphragmatic hernia. *Arch Dis Child* 65:1043-1044, 1990.

97. Kent PA, Curley MAQ: Challenges in nursing: infants with congenital diaphragmatic hernia. *Heart Lung* 21:381-389, 1992.

98. Schreiber MD, Heymann MA, Soifer SJ: Increased arterial pH, not decreased paCO$_2$, attenuates hypoxia-induced pulmonary vasoconstriction in newborn lambs. *Pediatr Res* 20:113-117, 1986.

99. Troug RD, Schena JA, Hershenson MB et al: Repair of congenital diaphragmatic hernia during extracorporeal membrane oxygenation. *Anesthesiology* 72:750-753, 1990.

100. Kao LC, Warburton D, Cheng MH et al: Effect of oral diuretics on pulmonary mechanics in infants with chronic bronchopulmonary dysplasia: Result of a double-blind crossover sequential trial. *Pediatrics* 74:37-44, 1984.

101. Kao LC, Warburton D, Platzker ACG et al: Effects of isoproterenol inhalation on airway resistance in chronic bronchopulmonary dysplasia. *Pediatrics* 74:509-513, 1984.

102. Loeber N, Morray J, Kettrick R et al: Pulmonary function in chronic respiratory failure of infancy. *Crit Care Med* 8:596-601, 1980.

103. Wilkie R, Bryan M: Effect of bronchodilators on airway resistance in ventilator dependent neonates with chronic lung disease. *J Pediatr* 111:278-282, 1987.

104. Northway WH, Rosan RC, Porter DY: Pulmonary disease following respirator therapy of hyaline membrane disease: bronchopulmonary dysplasia. *N Engl J Med* 276, 357-368, 1967.

105. HiFi Study Group: High-frequency oscillatory ventilation with conventional intermittent mechanical ventilation in the treatment of respiratory failure in preterm infants: neurodevelopmental status at 16 to 24 months of postterm age. *J Pediatr* 117:939-946, 1990.

106. Gibson RL, Jackson JC, Twiggs GA et al: Bronchopulmonary dysplasia. Survival after prolonged mechanical ventilation. *Am J Dis Child* 142:721-725, 1988.

107. Bancalari E, Gerhardt R: Bronchopulmonary dysplasia. *Pediatr Clin North Am* 33:1-23, 1986.

108. Lee R, O'Brodovich H: Airway epithelial damage in premature infants with respiratory failure. *Am Rev Respir Dis* 137:450-457, 1988.

109. Goodman G, Perkin RM, Anas NG et al: Pulmonary hypertension in infants with bronchopulmonary dysplasia. *J Pediatr* 112:67-72, 1988.

110. Groothuis JR, Gutierrez KM, Lauer BA: Respiratory syncytial virus infection in children with bronchopulmonary dysplasia. *Pediatrics* 82:199-203, 1988.

111. Smyth JA, Tabachnik E, Duncan WJ et al: Pulmonary function and bronchial hyperreactivity in long-term survivors of bronchopulmonary dysplasia. *Pediatrics* 68:336-340, 1981.

112. Frank M: Theophylline: a closer look. *Neonatal Network* 6:7-13, 1987.

113. Brudno D, Parder D, Slaton G: Response of pulmonary mechanics to terbutaline in patients with bronchopulmonary dysplasia. *Am J Med Sci* 297:166-168, 1989.

114. Gomez-Del-Rio M, Gehardt T, Hehre D et al: Effect of a beta agonist nebulization on lung function in neonates with increased pulmonary resistance. *Pediatr Pulmonol* 2:289-291, 1986.

115. Motoyama E, Fort M, Klesh K et al: Early onset of airway reactivity in premature infants with bronchopulmonary dysplasia. *Am Rev Respir Dis* 136:50-57, 1987.

116. Morray JP, Fox WW, Kettrick RG et al: Clinical correlates of successful weaning from mechanical ventilation in severe bronchopulmonary dysplasia. *Crit Care Med* 9:815-818, 1981.

117. Spitzer AR: Neonatal respiratory care. In Dantzker D, Marini J, Dakow E, eds: *Comprehensive respiratory care.* Philadelphia, 1995, W.B. Saunders.

118. Meisels SJ, Plunkett JW, Roloff DW et al: Growth and development of preterm infants with respiratory distress syndrome and bronchopulmonary dysplasia. *Pediatrics* 77:345-352, 1986.

119. Lund CH, Collier SB: Nutrition and bronchopulmonary dysplasia. In Lund CH, ed: *Bronchopulmonary dysplasia.* Petaluma, Calif, 1990, Neonatal Network.

120. Pridham KF, Martin R, Sondel S et al: Parental issues in feeding young children with bronchopulmonary dysplasia. *J Pediatr Nurs* 4:177-185, 1989.

121. Lu JL, Sheikh KA, Wu HS et al: Physiologic-pathologic correlation in Guillain-Barre syndrome in children. *Neurology* 54:33-39, 2000.

122. Sater RA, Rostami A: Treatment of Guillain-Barre syndrome with intravenous immunoglobulin. *Neurology* 51:S9-15, 1998.

123. Carroll JE, Jedziniak M, Guggenheim AM: Guillain-Barré syndrome: Another cause of the "floppy infant." *Am J Dis Child* 131:699-700, 1977.

124. Hahn AF: Guillain-Barre syndrome. *Lancet* 352:635-641, 1998.

125. Hughes RAC, Newsom-Davis JM, Perkin GD et al: Controlled trial of prednisolone in acute polyneuropathy. *Lancet* 2:750-755, 1978.

126. Singhi SC, Jayshree M, Singhi P et al: Intravenous immunoglobulin in very severe childhood Guillain-Barre syndrome. *Ann Trop Paediatr* 19:167-74, 1999.

127. French Cooperative Group of Plasma Exchange in Guillain-Barré Syndrome: Efficiency of plasm exchange in Guillain-Barré syndrome: role of replacement fluids. *Ann Neurol* 22:753-761, 1987.

128. Guillain-Barré Study Group: Plasmapheresis and acute Guillain-Barré syndrome. *Neurology* 35:1096-1104, 1985.

129. Osterman PO, Lundmo G, Pirskanen R et al: Beneficial effects of plasma exchange in acute inflammatory polyradiculoneuropathy. *Lancet* 2:1296-1299, 1984.

130. Epstein MA, Sladky JT: The role of plasmapheresis in childhood Guillain-Barré syndrome. *Ann Neurol* 26:448, 1989.

131. Shahar E, Murphy G, Roifman CM: Benefit of intravenously administered immune serum globulin in patients with Guillain-Barré syndrome. *J Pediatr* 116:141-144, 1990.

132. McKann GM, Griffin JW, Cornblath DR et al: Plasmapheresis and Guillain-Barré syndrome: analysis of prognostic factors and the effect of plasmapheresis. *Ann Neurol* 23:347-353, 1988.

133. Ouvrier RA, McLeod JD, Pollard J: Acute inflammatory demyelinating polyradiculoneuropathy. In Ouvrier RA, McLeod JD, Pollard J, eds: *Peripheral neuropathy in childhood,* New York, 1990, Raven Press.

134. Nguyen DK, Agenarioti-Belanger S, Vanasse M: Pain and the Guillain-Barre syndrome in children under 6 years old. *J Pediatr* 134:773-776, 1999.

135. Connelly M, Shagrin J, Warfield C: Epidural opioids for the management of pain in a patient with the Guillain-Barré syndrome. *Anesthesiology* 72:381-383, 1990.

136. Rosenfield B, Burel C, Hanley D: Epidural morphine treatment of pain in Guillain-Barré syndrome. *Arch Neurol* 43:1194-1196, 1986.

137. Ferrari ND III, Weisse ME: Botulism. *Adv Pediatr Infect Dis* 10:81-91, 1995.

138. Shapiro RL, Hatheway C, Swerdlow DL: Botulism in the United States: a clinical and epidemiologic review. *Ann Intern Med* 129:221-228, 1998.

139. Buck JR, Connors RH, Coon WW et al: Pulmonary embolism in children. *J Pediatr Surg* 16:385-390, 1981.

140. Evans DA, Wilmott RW: Pulmonary embolism in children. *Pediatr Clin North Am* 41:569-584, 1994.

141. Zahka KG, Patel CR: Cardiovascular problems of the neonate. In AA Fanaroff, RJ Martin, eds: *Neonatal-perinatal medicine: diseases of the fetus and infant* (ed 6). St Louis, 1997, Mosby.

142. Walsh-Sukys MC, Tyson JE, Wright LL et al: Persistent pulmonary hypertension of the newborn in the era before nitric oxide: practice variation and outcomes. *Pediatrics* 105:14-20, 2000.

143. Klesh KW, Murphy TF, Scher MS et al: Cerebral infarction in persistent pulmonary hypertension of the newborn. *Am J Dis Child* 141:852-857, 1987.

144. Clark RH, Kueser TJ, Walker MW et al: Low-dose nitric oxide therapy for persistent pulmonary hypertension of the newborn. Clinical Inhaled Nitric Oxide Research Group. *N Engl J Med* 342:469-474, 2000.

145. Stork EK: Rescue therapies for cardiovascular failure. In Fanaroff AA, Martin RJ, eds: *Neonatal-perinatal medicine: diseases of the fetus and infant* (ed 6). St Louis, 1997, Mosby.

146. Beachy P, Powers LK: Nursing care of the infant with persistent pulmonary hypertension of the newborn. *Clin Perinatol* 11:681-693, 1984.

147. White C, Richardson C, Raibstein L: High-frequency ventilation and extracorporeal membrane oxygenation. *AACN Clinical Issues in Critical Care Nursing* 1:427-444, 1990.

148. Spitzer AR, Davis J, Clarke WT et al: Pulmonary hypertension and persistent fetal circulation in the newborn. *Clin Perinatol* 15:389-413, 1988.

149. Henderson-Smart DJ: The effect of gestational age on the incidence and duration of recurrent apnoea in newborn babies. *Aust Paediat J* 17:273-276, 1981.

150. Ali NJ, Pitson DJ, Stradling JR: Snoring, sleep disturbance, and behaviour in 4-5 year olds. *Arch Dis Child* 68:360-366, 1993.

151. Gislason T, Benediktsdottir B: Snoring, apneic episodes, and nocturnal hypoxemia among children 6 months to 6 years old: an epidemiologic study of lower limit of prevalence. *Chest* 107:963-966, 1995.

152. Roberts JL, Mathew OP, Thach BT: The efficacy of theophylline in premature infants with mixed and obstructive apnea and apnea associated with pulmonary and neurologic disease. *J Pediatr* 100:968-970, 1982.

153. Brouillette RT, Fernback SK, Hunt CE: Obstructive sleep apnea in infants and children. *J Pediatr* 100:31-40, 1982.

154. Bairam A, Boutroy M, Badonnel Y et al: Theophylline versus caffeine: comparative effects in treatment of idiopathic apnea in the preterm infant. *J Pediatr* 110:636-639, 1987.

155. Henderson-Smart DJ, Steer PA: Prophylactic methylxanthine for preventing of apnea in preterm infants. *Cochrane Database Syst Rev* 2, CD000432, 2000.

156. Frank Y, Kravath RE, Pollak CP, Weitzman EK: Obstructive sleep apnea and its therapy: clinical and polysomnographic manifestations. *Pediatrics* 71:737-742, 1983.

157. Miller MJ, Carlo WA, Martin RJ: Continuous positive pressure selectively reduces obstructive apnea in preterm infants. *J Pediatr* 106:91-94, 1985.

158. Guilleminault C: Obstructive sleep apnea syndrome and its treatment in children: areas of agreement and controversy. *Pediatr Pulmonol* 3:429-436, 1987.

159. Brazy JE, Kinney HC, Oakes WJ: Central nervous system structural lesions causing apnea at birth. *J Pediatr* 111:163-175, 1987.

160. Jensen TH, Hansen PB, Brodersen P: Ondines's curse in *Listeria monocytogenes* brain stem encephalitis. *Acta Neurol Scand* 77:505-506, 1988.

161. Quera-Salva MA, Guilleminault C: Post-traumatic central sleep apnea in a child. *J Pediatr* 110:906-909, 1987.

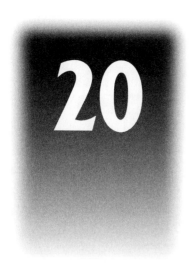

20 Neurologic Critical Care Problems

Paula Vernon-Levett

In pediatric critical care, a large percentage of intensive care admissions result from severe neurologic dysfunction. Numerous congenital and acquired neurologic disorders exist; however, most result in two final common pathways: intracranial hypertension and global hypoxic ischemia. This chapter focuses on these two major patient problems from a critical care nursing perspective.

Intracranial hypertension results from an uncompensated increase in one or more of the three intracranial volumes. Although the pathogenesis and medical management vary among these disorders, nursing care of patients with intracranial hypertension, regardless of the cause, is similar. The mechanisms and consequences of intracranial hypertension are presented, followed by a discussion of critical care management strategies intended to prevent secondary neuronal injury. After the general discussion, specific neurologic disorders that cause intracranial hypertension are presented, including the priorities in management.

The second final common pathway, global hypoxic ischemia, produces primary neuronal injury. Like intracranial hypertension, a number of pathophysiologic events and disorders can result in this final common pathway. A general discussion of the consequences of global hypoxic ischemia is presented, as well as common supportive strategies. Victims of near drowning experience global hypoxic ischemia and are, unfortunately, common in the pediatric population[1]; specific collaborative measures unique to this population are discussed.

Despite state-of-the-art critical care management, some patients develop irreversible brain damage. Specific guidelines and controversies in pediatric brain death are presented.

Because primary neuromuscular dysfunction is seldom the only reason for intensive care hospitalization, disorders of this type are briefly mentioned. Acquired disorders, for example, Guillain-Barré syndrome and spinal cord trauma, are presented in Chapters 19 and 28, respectively. To complement the discussion on care of the patient after a craniotomy, care of the patient after spinal fusion is presented.

INTRACRANIAL HYPERTENSION

Intracranial hypertension is a term used to define a sustained elevation in intracranial pressure (ICP). No single value defines intracranial hypertension for all patients, but it is age related. Normal ICP in adults is between 10 to 15 mmHg, and in children it is less than 10 mmHg. Likewise, the treatment threshold for intracranial hypertension is age related, with children requiring intervention at a lower threshold.[2] Intracranial hypertension is not a disease itself but a final common pathway for a diverse group of neuropathologic conditions that elevate ICP. These diseases can be broadly classified into four groups: conditions that (1) increase blood volume, (2) increase brain volume, (3) increase cerebrospinal fluid (CSF) volume, or (4) increase a combination of the preceding three volumes. Common diseases or conditions among patients seen in the pediatric intensive care unit (PICU) that potentially increase ICP are status epilepticus and arteriovenous malformations (increased cerebral blood volume [CBV]); intracranial tumors, meningitis, and encephalitis (increased brain tissue); and hydrocephalus (increased CSF). In addition, many patients are admitted to the PICU because of traumatic head injuries. Traumatic brain injury can potentially increase CBV, brain tissue, or CSF, resulting in increased intracranial pressure (IICP) on a multidimensional basis.

Uncontrolled intracranial hypertension eventually causes distortion and herniation of brain tissue, as well as a local or generalized reduction in cerebral blood flow (CBF). Initially, an expanding intracranial mass or diffuse edema occludes the subarachnoid spaces, preventing translocation of CSF into the spinal subarachnoid space. Eventually, the CSF cistern collapses, and the arachnoid villi are compressed, preventing reabsorption of CSF. As intraparenchymal pressure increases, vascular collapse may occur with venous outflow obstruction.[3,4] In an effort to maintain CBF with an elevated ICP, compensatory changes in the arterial vascular beds may occur with increased arterial resistance. With an alteration in vascular resistance, capillary pressure may increase, promoting cerebral edema.[3-5] At some critical point, autoregulation of CBF is lost, and CBF becomes passively dependent on arterial pressure and cerebral perfusion pressure (CPP). Local or generalized brain ischemia, anoxia, and neuronal death results, as well as herniation and distortion of brain tissue. Fig. 20-1 shows drawings of normal intracranial contents and intracranial contents with intracranial hypertension.

Brain Herniation Syndromes

A pressure gradient between intracranial compartments may cause a shift in structures from one compartment to another. The cranial cavity is divided into compartments by the dura mater, which is fibrous and relatively rigid. The *falx cerebri* partially separates the supratentorial space as it drops into the longitudinal fissure. The *tentorium cerebelli* is a tentlike structure located in the posterior fossa. It separates the cerebellum and brainstem from the occipital lobe of the cerebral hemispheres. The tentorial notch refers to the central opening of the tentorium. The *foramen magnum* is a bony opening at the base of the skull that anatomically separates the intracranial contents from the spinal cord. Fig. 20-2 illustrates the anatomic compartments of the brain.

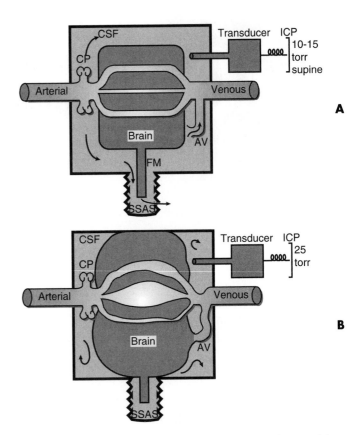

Fig. 20-1 **A,** Schematic representation of normal intracranial contents. Arrows indicate direction of cerebrospinal fluid *(CSF)* flow, and heavy dark lines represent the skull. **B,** Schematic representation of intracranial contents during intracranial hypertension. *SSAS,* Spinal subarachnoid space; *FM,* foramen magnum; *ICP,* intracranial pressure; *AV,* arachnoid villi; *CP,* choroid plexus. (From Shapiro HM: Intracranial hypertension, *Anesthesiology* 43:446, 1975.)

Supratentorial Herniation. Brain herniation syndromes are usually classified into two broad categories: supratentorial and infratentorial. Supratentorial herniation syndromes are further classified into three types. First, *uncal herniation* refers to unilateral displacement of the uncus (medial aspect of the temporal lobe) from the middle fossa to the posterior fossa through the tentorium (Fig. 20-3). Second, *central herniation* refers to a symmetric downward displacement of both cerebral hemispheres through the tentorial notch. This syndrome occurs more often in infants and children, especially those with hydrocephalus.[6] Last, *cingulate herniation* refers to displacement of the cingulate gyrus under the falx cerebri into the opposite hemisphere.[7-9] Compression of the ipsilateral or bilateral anterior cerebral arteries and internal cerebral vein may occur, leading to infarction of the paracentral lobes.

Infratentorial Herniation. Infratentorial herniation occurs less often than supratentorial herniation.[8] Of two types of infratentorial herniation syndromes, the most common is downward displacement of one or both of the cerebellar tonsils through the foramen magnum, which results in

Lateral view

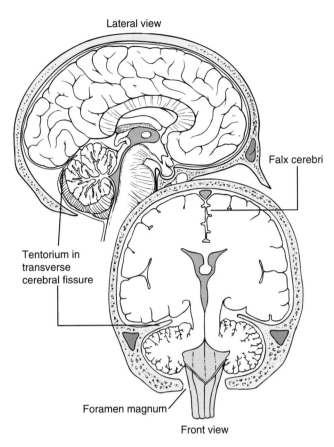

Falx cerebri

Tentorium in transverse cerebral fissure

Foramen magnum

Front view

Fig. 20-2 Falx cerebri and tentorium. (From Snyder M, Jackle M: *Neurologic problems: a critical care nursing focus,* Bowie, Md, 1981, Prentice-Hall, p 21.)

compression of the medulla oblongata and cervical spinal cord (Fig. 20-4). The second type, which is rare, is upward displacement of the cerebellum or lower brainstem through the tentorial notch into the supratentorial compartment.[7-9]

Cerebral Edema

Three types of cerebral edema develop in response to injury.[10] First, *cytotoxic edema* represents intracellular swelling resulting from hypoxia and ischemia. Cell membranes of neurons and glial cells are affected, resulting in a disruption of the internal ionic pump mechanism. It reflects neuronal cell death and is not very amenable to therapy. *Vasogenic edema* is clinically the most common type of edema. It results from an alteration in permeability of brain capillary endothelial cells, allowing extravasation of protein-rich plasma into the brain. Vasogenic edema is commonly seen around abscesses, tumors, and hematomas. In contrast to cytotoxic edema, it is more easily treated. *Interstitial edema* results from increased CSF hydrostatic pressure, commonly seen with obstructive hydrocephalus. There is transependymal movement of CSF from the ventricular system into adjacent tissue, which is easily treated with shunting procedures.

With many acute brain insults or neuropathologic conditions, cerebral edema may result from a combination of the

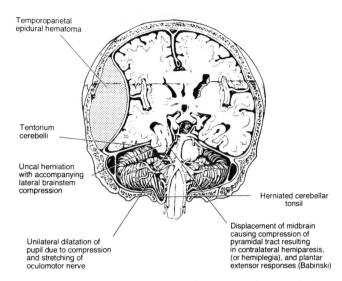

Temporoparietal epidural hematoma

Tentorium cerebelli

Uncal herniation with accompanying lateral brainstem compression

Herniated cerebellar tonsil

Unilateral dilatation of pupil due to compression and stretching of oculomotor nerve

Displacement of midbrain causing compression of pyramidal tract resulting in contralateral hemiparesis, (or hemiplegia), and plantar extensor responses (Babinski)

Fig. 20-3 Cross-section showing herniation of part of the temporal lobe through the tentorium caused by a temporoparietal epidural hematoma. (From Kintzel KC: *Advanced concepts on clinical nursing,* ed 2, Philadelphia, 1977, JB Lippincott.)

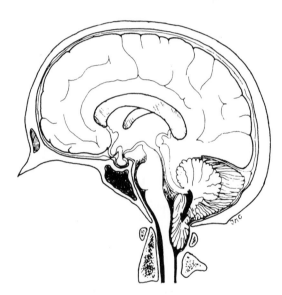

Fig. 20-4 Herniation of cerebellar tonsils into the foramen magnum is the final outcome of increased intracranial pressure. Respiratory centers within medulla oblongata are compressed, and apnea in sleep often leads to cardiac arrest and death. (From Smith RR: *Essentials of neurosurgery,* Philadelphia, 1980, JB Lippincott.)

edema types described earlier. For example, a traumatic brain injury (TBI) may have components of both vasogenic and cytotoxic edema. Vasogenic edema may develop directly from a hematoma, and cytotoxic edema may occur from ischemia and hypoxia. Generalized cerebral swelling in response to severe head injury has been frequently reported and was originally thought to be due to hyperemia.[11] However, recent studies suggest that the cerebral swelling is most likely due to cytotoxic edema from early posttraumatic ischemia.[12,13]

Critical Care Management

Assessment. In the comatose patient, continuous ICP monitoring is the only accurate means of assessing early changes in intracranial pressure and compliance and determining the effectiveness of therapy. (See Chapter 10, Intracranial Dynamics, for a description of nursing care related to ICP monitoring.) In the absence of ICP monitoring, serial assessments of the patient's neurologic status are the best means of identifying intracranial hypertension. Clinical signs and symptoms of IICP are numerous and vary, depending on a number of factors: the specific location or compartment of a mass or swelling, the acuteness of the rise in ICP, and the age of the patient.

With slowly expanding uncal or central herniation syndromes, neurologic signs are usually progressive in a rostral to caudal sequence.[4,8] Within the infratentorial compartment, a clear-cut syndrome does not occur with IICP and herniation. However, late signs of both supratentorial and infratentorial herniation are indistinguishable, that is, cardiovascular collapse and apnea.[3]

Clinical signs and symptoms of IICP also depend on how acutely ICP increases. Early signs and symptoms include an alteration in level of consciousness (restlessness or confusion), motor weakness or paresis, vomiting, headache, and pupillary changes. Late signs and symptoms are more characteristic of brainstem dysfunction: depressed level of consciousness (coma), motor dysfunction (decorticate or decerebrate posturing), respiratory irregularities terminating with apnea, and impaired cranial nerve function (gag, corneal, oculocephalic, oculovestibular reflexes). Cushing's triad, a late sign indicative of brainstem compression, includes the classic signs of increased systolic pressure, which produces a wide pulse pressure, bradycardia, and bradypnea that is often irregular. Table 20-1 summarizes the progressive signs and symptoms of central and uncal herniation.

Neurologic signs of IICP can also be intermittent. Transient signs and symptoms usually last only a few minutes and are most often seen at the peak of plateau waves when CPP is compromised. Common clinical signs and symptoms include headache, blurred vision, change in level of consciousness, pallor, obtundation, paresis, and changes in pupillary reaction.

When chronic IICP exists (e.g., pseudotumor cerebri, slow-growing tumor, slowly increasing hydrocephalus), the patient clinically may be less symptomatic or may display more nonspecific symptoms. The absence of papilledema does not exclude the presence of IICP; however, when present, it is almost always indicative of IICP. It can develop as early as 48 hours after IICP but more often is seen as a chronic sign.[14]

Many signs and symptoms of IICP are also age dependent. In general, the younger the child, the more nonspecific the signs and symptoms. The older child typically complains of headache (especially on awakening in the morning) and blurred vision. Infants and preverbal toddlers cannot report a headache. They usually express a headache by holding

---

◆ **TABLE 20-1   Progressive Signs and Symptoms of Uncal and Central Herniation**

	Early	Late
Uncal Herniation Syndrome		
Level of consciousness	Restlessness, may progress quickly to coma	Coma
Motor function	May have contralateral hemiparesis, hemiplegia, decerebration	Flaccidity
Respirations	Normal	Progresses to Cheyne-Stokes (Diencephalon-midbrain) → Central neurogenic hyperventilation (midbrain-upper pons) → Shallow (lower pons-upper medulla) → Ataxic, apnea (medulla)
Pupil signs	Unilateral, sluggish, nonreactive/dilated ipsilateral pupil	Bilateral, fixed and dilated pupils
Extraocular signs	May have ipsilateral ptosis, slight weakness of oculomotor innervated muscles	Oculomotor paralysis
Central Herniation Syndrome		
Level of consciousness	Agitated, drowsy, then stuporous	Coma
Motor function	Contralateral hemiparesis to hemiplegia, progresses to decorticate posturing	Flaccidity with occasional decerebrate posturing
Respirations	Cheyne-Stokes, progresses as above	Ataxic, then apnea
Pupil signs	Bilateral small and reactive, may progress to unequal and nonreactive	Dilated and fixed
Extraocular signs	Normal or slightly roving, then difficulty with upward gaze	Dysconjugate gaze

Adapted from Hickey JV: *Clinical practice of neurologic and neurosurgical nursing*, ed 2, Philadelphia, 1986, JB Lippincott, pp 259-260.

their head or exhibiting irritability and anorexia.[14] Papilledema is less commonly seen in infants, presumably because of their expansible skull. Progressive signs and symptoms of IICP that are unique to the infant include a large full anterior fontanelle, "setting sun" eyes, "cracked pot" sound on skull percussion, and a progressive increase in head circumference. Separation of cranial sutures (diastasis) or delayed closure of fontanelles may be seen in both infants and young children with IICP because of unfused sutures. Late signs and symptoms of brainstem compression from IICP are more similar than different among the different age groups.

Collaborative Management. Intracranial hypertension results from abnormal increases in intracranial volume components and loss of normal intracranial compensatory mechanisms. Management goals for patients with intracranial hypertension are directed toward improving intracranial compliance and maintaining adequate CBF. In some patients with a localized mass, ICP is normalized after surgical excision. In other cases, the neuropathologic condition is not amenable to surgical correction, and the complexity of the pathologic changes requires a combination of therapies to control intracranial hypertension and prevent cerebral ischemia. In general, specific interventions are introduced in a stepwise approach with the least invasive therapies used first and removed last.

Cerebral Blood Volume Reduction. Mechanisms that increase CBV and increase ICP include cerebrovascular vasodilation, hypercapnia, hypoxia, volatile anesthetics, and venous outflow obstruction.[4,15,16] Fig. 20-5 illustrates the changes in CBF resulting from alterations in Pao_2, $Paco_2$, and blood pressure.

Hyperventilation. Historically, induced, controlled hyperventilation has been widely advocated during the first few days following a severe traumatic brain insult that produces intracranial hypertension.[17,18] The theoretical benefits of hyperventilation are based on the relationship between $Paco_2$ and cerebral vasoreactivity. Cerebral vascular changes are directly affected by the pH of surrounding interstitial fluid and indirectly by changes in $Paco_2$. Low pH results in cerebral vasodilation, whereas high pH results in cerebral vasoconstriction.[19] Induced hypocarbia from hyperventilation may prevent or reverse brain and CSF acidosis, which, in turn, produces vasoconstriction of the precapillary cerebral arterioles and decreases CBF, CBV, and ICP. Because CO_2 readily crosses the blood-brain barrier, an immediate reduction in cerebral interstitial CO_2 occurs, followed by a reduction in hydrogen ion concentration.

Despite the theoretical benefits of hyperventilation, the indiscriminate use of hyperventilation as a prophylactic therapy to control IICP has been questioned.[2,20,21] It is no longer believed that the majority of pediatric patients with a TBI have acute hyperemia. In fact, the opposite is believed to be true; CBF may be critically reduced in the first hours following a closed head injury.[19,22] Consequently, it is thought that hyperventilation may, in some patients, convert borderline cerebral ischemia to frank ischemia. Furthermore, the effects of hyperventilation on CSF, pH, and thus arteriolar diameter are short lived (less than 24 hours).[19] This latter problem is believed to be the result of decreased buffer capacity associated with a low bicarbonate concentration. The cerebral vasculature may be more sensitive to changes in $Paco_2$, and the patient may not tolerate transient increases in $Paco_2$ that occur with nursing care, such as position changes or endotracheal suctioning.

Despite the controversy over the use of hyperventilation, in specific situations its use is generally recommended by most experts: first, in emergent situations when signs of herniation are present or death is imminent; second, in patients with documented hyperemia with abnormally elevated ICP; and last, in patients in which intracranial hypertension is refractory to all other forms of therapy.[20]

When indicated, controlled hyperventilation in the child is achieved with endotracheal intubation, muscle paralysis, and assisted ventilation. To ensure beneficial effects and minimize ischemic risk, arterial oxygen tension (Pao_2) is kept in a normal range, $Paco_2$ is kept in a range of 30 to 35 mmHg, and pH is kept slightly alkalotic.[2] Only rarely is $Paco_2$ lowered significantly below this level. In all situations when hyperventilation is used, monitoring cerebral circulation (e.g., jugular venous oxygen saturation) is desirable and often necessary.[2,23] To summarize, hyperventilation is used with specific indications, for a short time, and withdrawn slowly while monitoring ICP.

Neuromuscular Blockade. Muscular paralysis with neuromuscular blocking agents is often used to facilitate ventilatory control and hyperventilation in the child with intracranial hypertension. Chemical paralyzing agents can also be used to prevent increases in arterial blood pressure associated with isometric muscle contraction (e.g., decerebrate or decorticate posturing).[24] Sedatives and analgesics are administered with neuromuscular agents to minimize anxiety and pain.[25] There are a variety of sedative agents available for use in the pediatric patient.[26,27] However, when managing ICP, agents should be short-acting and

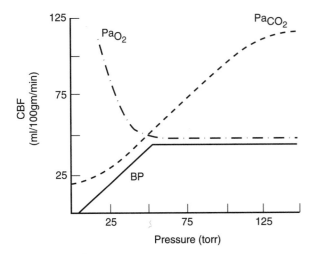

Fig. 20-5 Cerebral blood flow changes caused by alterations in $Paco_2$, Pao_2, and blood pressure *(BP)*. The other two variables remain stable at normal values when the remaining variable is altered. *Pao_2,* Partial pressure of oxygen; *$Paco_2$,* partial pressure of carbon dioxide; *CBF,* cerebral blood flow. (From Shapiro HM: Intracranial hypertension, *Anesthesiology* 43:446, 1975.)

free of cardiovascular side-effects. Furthermore, abrupt reversal of sedatives is avoided to prevent acute increases in CBF and ICP.[28]

Anticonvulsants. In the patient with minimal intracranial buffering capacity, small increases in CBF can cause significant increases in ICP. Seizures increase CBF, CBV, and ICP, and therefore are prevented or controlled on an emergent basis. A variety of anticonvulsants are used depending on whether the therapy is to treat status epilepticus, prevent break-through seizures, or be used prophylactically. Electroencephalogram (EEG) monitoring is necessary to detect seizures in the chemically paralyzed patient.

Barbiturates. Barbiturates have been used to treat intracranial hypertension since the early 1970s.[29] Continuous intravenous infusion of barbiturates to induce coma is reserved for patients in whom conventional therapy has been unsuccessful in controlling intracranial hypertension. Barbiturates decrease ICP by reducing the cerebral metabolic rate, which is followed by a reduction in CBF and CBV.[30,31] The most commonly used barbiturate is pentobarbital. Protocols for initiating a barbiturate coma vary slightly among institutions. The Brain Trauma Foundation[32] recommends a loading dose of 10 mg/kg over 30 minutes, followed with 5 mg/kg every hour for a total of three doses. The maintenance infusion is 1 mg/kg/hr. The actual titration dose of a specific barbiturate also varies among institutions. Some titrate the dose to a desired serum level, others titrate to obtain burst suppression on EEG, and still others titrate to a particular ICP level.[32,33] Barbiturate therapy is associated with significant cardiac effects: decreased cardiac output, decreased cardiac contractility, dysrhythmias, and subsequent hypotension. When continuous barbiturate therapy is administered, bedside EEG monitoring and close monitoring of arterial blood pressure and thermodilution cardiac output measurements are necessary. Vasopressors, specifically epinephrine, are often needed to counteract the hypotensive effects of barbiturate use.

Even when barbiturate therapy is successful in controlling ICP, long-term patient outcome has not been commensurately improved.[33,34] Few controlled studies exist to substantiate the efficacy of this therapy. As a result, barbiturate therapy is not routinely recommended for all cases of refractory intracranial hypertension.

Brain Volume Reduction. Brain tissue itself can also increase the total intracranial volume. The usual causes include tumors, infections, and edema. In the case of a tumor, definitive therapy is straightforward, at least theoretically, with surgical removal. Brain edema is not a disease entity but the consequence of other neuropathologic conditions (e.g., infections, hypoxic-ischemic insult). Therapy is directed at preventing the development of edema or removing the excess fluid.

Hyperosmolar Therapy. Several osmotic agents have been used to treat intracranial hypertension. The theory is that they exert their effect by producing an osmotic gradient between the intravascular compartment and the surrounding brain tissue. A net influx of water enters the bloodstream and is excreted by the kidneys. The end result is a reduction in brain bulk with a decrease in ICP.

Serum osmolality is routinely calculated to monitor hyperosmolar therapy, as well as detect inappropriate antidiuretic hormone (ADH) secretion or diabetes insipidus. Serum osmolality can be calculated by using the following formula:

$$2 \times [Na^+] + [BUN]/2.8 + [glucose]/18$$

where *BUN* is blood urea nitrogen and *Na$^+$* is sodium.

Normal serum osmolality is 270 to 290 mOsm/L. With hyperosmolar therapy, serum osmolality is maintained just above the high normal range (300 to 310 mOsm/L). When serum osmolality is above 320 to 330 mOsm/L, there is an increased risk of cerebral infarction and renal tubular damage. Patients may be at even greater risk for renal failure with preexisting renal disease or when other potentially nephrotoxic medications are being administered concurrently.

Currently, mannitol (Osmitrol) is the most commonly used osmotic agent to treat intracranial hypertension. In addition to its osmotic effects, evidence shows that mannitol reduces CBV and ICP by causing cerebral vasoconstriction.[35] The belief is that in patients with intact autoregulation, low to moderate doses of mannitol (less than 1 g/kg) decrease blood viscosity, which causes autoregulatory vasoconstriction of cerebral arterioles. Because decreased blood viscosity reduces resistance to blood flow, CBF remains unchanged.[35-37]

A wide range of mannitol doses (0.25 to 2 g/kg) have been prescribed for either intermittent administration or as a continuous intravenous infusion. However, reports indicate that beneficial effects and fewer side effects are achieved with more frequently administered lower doses of mannitol.[38-40] Mannitol, administered long term or in high doses, may eventually move into the interstitial space, reducing or reversing the osmotic gradient between the intravascular and interstitial compartments. This theoretical "rebound" effect results in the movement of water into brain tissue.

Osmotic agents are contraindicated in patients with hyperemia associated with acute brain injury. In these patients, CBV is already increased, and osmotic agents would further increase CBV and ICP. Osmotic agents are also contraindicated in patients with a suspected loss of an intact blood-brain barrier. In this situation, the osmotic agent readily crosses into brain interstitial fluid with a net influx of water into the surrounding brain tissue.

Oral glycerol has been used to treat cerebral edema since the 1960s. However, the oral administration route has limited use in the patient with acute elevation in ICP because of delayed onset of action (30 to 60 minutes) and gastrointestinal side effects.[41] However, Takagi and associates[42] recently found improved absorption and lowering of ICP when oral glycerol was administered via an Entero-Duodenal tube. Intravenous glycerol is available, but early studies reported severe side effects, such as hemoglobinuria, hemolysis, and renal failure.[43,44] More recent evidence shows fewer complications when 10% to 20% solutions are administered over several hours.[41,45] The recommended intravenous dose of glycerol is 0.5 to 1 mg/kg every 4 to 6 hours, not to exceed 1 g/kg/hr.[46,47]

Clinical use of urea (Ureaphil) is rare today.[36] Urea is believed to cross the blood-brain barrier more readily than either mannitol and glycerol.[41] Thus there is a higher incidence of a "rebound" effect in ICP.

Diuretics. Furosemide (Lasix) is a potent loop diuretic that has been found to effectively lower ICP in some cases.[48] Several mechanisms are thought to be responsible for the observed lowering of ICP: total reduction in body fluids, inhibition of CSF production, and a direct reduction in sodium transport into the brain.[48,49] Furosemide has been successfully used alone and in combination with osmotic diuretics and oncotic agents.[41,49] The theoretical benefit of using furosemide with mannitol is that furosemide accentuates the osmotic gradient in the renal tubules.[50] It is used most successfully in patients with head injury and pulmonary edema or when used with pulmonary artery hemodynamic data.[36] The usual dose of furosemide in children is 0.5 to 1 mg/kg.[46]

Corticosteroids. The use of steroids in the treatment of intracranial hypertension is unclear. The theoretical basis for the use of steroids stems from their success in treating intracranial hypertension from neuropathologic conditions (e.g., tumors, discrete hematomas) associated with vasogenic edema.[51] The exact mechanism of action is unknown. The use of high-dose steroids in the treatment of severe head injury has been found to have no beneficial effect.[52-54] Furthermore, Dearden and co-workers[53] reported a poorer outcome, assessed at 6 months with the Glasgow Outcome Scale, among head-injured patients with elevated ICP receiving steroids. Thus steroid therapy is usually reserved for conditions associated with vasogenic edema.

Fluid and Electrolyte Monitoring. Fluid and electrolyte status is assessed in the patient with intracranial hypertension. The goal of fluid therapy is maintenance of optimal CBF. However, when brain edema is an issue, optimal fluid administration is unclear. In the past, many experts advocated fluid restriction as a means of limiting total brain edema. Recently, increased awareness of ischemic injury has emphasized the importance of maintaining normal CPP with fluids and electrolytes. Despite this uncertainty, the consensus is that the patient's hemodynamic status should be closely monitored to prevent marked hypovolemia, which could compromise mean arterial pressure (MAP) and, subsequently, CBF.

Although hypotonic intravenous solutions are avoided, evidence supports the use of hypertonic intravenous solutions to reduce ICP.[55,55a,55b] Fisher and co-workers compared the effects of 3% saline boluses and 0.9% saline on IICP in children with traumatic brain injury.[55c] Three percent saline significantly reduced elevated ICP in patients compared with 0.9% solution. Intravascular dehydration, a more common complication with the use of diuretics and hyperosmotic agents, did not occur during the study period. A similar study using a continuous infusion of 3% saline reported similar conclusions.[55d]

Fluid and electrolyte imbalances may also occur in patients with neurologic dysfunction. Common causes include syndrome of inappropriate antidiuretic hormone (SIADH) secretion and diabetes insipidus. Serum and urine electrolytes and osmolalities are monitored. A central venous pressure line is placed to manage fluid balance.

Cerebrospinal Fluid Volume Reduction. Mechanisms that increase CSF volume may also cause elevated ICP. These mechanisms include increased CSF production, decreased CSF absorption, or obstruction of CSF circulation.

Cerebrospinal Fluid Drainage. Ventricular shunting is standard therapy for increased ICP related to hydrocephalus. In other situations, an intraventricular catheter may be placed in one of the lateral ventricles in patients with acute intracranial hypertension. The catheter is used to drain CSF to avoid significant increases in ICP (see Chapter 10). Ventricular drainage may be intermittent or continuous, depending on the size of the ventricles and the type of neuropathologic condition.

Reduced Cerebrospinal Fluid Production. CSF formation can be reduced by a number of drugs. Medications that have been shown to transiently reduce ICP by slowing CSF production include acetazolamide (Diamox) and furosemide (Lasix). However, the efficacy of these agents for long-term control of ICP is unproven.[17,56]

Nursing Care: Decreased Adaptive Capacity

Decreased adaptive capacity, intracranial, is a nursing diagnosis proposed by Mitchell[15] to describe failure of normal intracranial compensatory mechanisms. It occurs in patients with intracranial hypertension but is not synonymous with this pathophysiologic state. Rather, its use identifies patients at risk for disproportionate increases in ICP in response to a variety of nursing care activities. Nursing interventions are designed to reduce intracranial adaptive demands and increase adaptive capacity.

The goals for managing decreased intracranial adaptive capacity are to reduce intracranial volume and improve intracranial compliance. A number of nursing care activities have been shown to alter ICP.[57-59] However, the patient's response to a specific nursing care measure is often variable and depends on the patient's intracranial compliance at a given point in time. Thus all nursing interventions are specific to the patient. In addition to serial neurologic assessments, a number of independent nursing interventions can be used to reduce adaptive demand (i.e., decrease CBV and CSF volume) and increase adaptive capacity (i.e., shift the intracranial volume/pressure [V/P] curve to the left).

Maintain Oxygenation and Ventilation. To avoid cerebral vasodilation, hypercarbia and hypoxemia are avoided or corrected expeditiously when they occur. Nursing measures to prevent hypercarbia and hypoxemia include maintaining a patent airway and judicious, careful airway suctioning. Although considerable variation in patient response to endotracheal tube suctioning (ETTS) does exist, routine suctioning of patients has been shown to increase ICP, presumably resulting from tracheal stimulation, hypercarbia, or hypoxemia.[60,61] Thus suctioning is reserved for documented cases of accumulated airway secretions. The exact suctioning procedure is chosen according to patient response. However, usual steps in the procedure include preoxygenation with an FIO_2 of 1.0, limiting the suction time to less than 10 seconds per catheter insertion, and limiting the number of passes to two per procedure.[8,59,62,63] Crosby and Parsons[64] reported that a stepped rise in ICP, commonly seen with multiple suctioning passes, could be avoided. They recommend a minimum of 60 seconds of manual hyperventilation between each ETTS pass. They also found that the patient should be left undisturbed for at least 2 minutes after ETTS to allow ICP, mean arterial pressure (MAP), and CPP to return to baseline. Similarly, a recent study[65] demonstrated that transient increases in ICP and MAP that occur with ETTS did not impair cerebral oxygenation when preceded by preoxygenation.

Several investigators have found intravenous lidocaine (1.5 mg/kg) given 1 to 2 minutes before suctioning to be effective in blunting increases in ICP related to endotracheal suctioning.[66,67] Both intravenous and endotracheal routes are effective in blunting rises in ICP; however, endotracheal tube (ETT) administration of lidocaine has been shown to be more effective.[67,68] Despite the benefits of ETT administration, Brucia, Owen, and Rudy[68] warn that the ETT route can induce coughing, which may cause an actual rise in ICP. Few data are available comparing the relative effectiveness of other medications in preventing increases in ICP associated with endotracheal suctioning. White and co-workers[69] found thiopental (Pentothal) 3 mg/kg and fentanyl 1 μg/kg to be ineffective in altering an increase in ICP associated with endotracheal suctioning. However, this same study found that succinylcholine (Anectine, Quelicin) 1 mg/kg was effective in blunting ICP associated with suctioning. To summarize, critical care nurses must pay close attention to the details of suctioning protocols, as well as adapting practice to individual patient responses.

Serial monitoring of the patient's respiratory status allows early detection of impaired oxygenation and ventilation. Respiratory rate, depth, and pattern should be regular. Breath sounds should be clear bilaterally without adventitious breath sounds. Further diagnostic monitoring includes the use of pulse oximetry, end-tidal CO_2 ($ETco_2$) monitoring, and serial arterial blood gas (ABG) measurement.

Promote Venous Outflow. Patient position has a dramatic impact on CBV and ICP by altering venous outflow from the cranium. Nursing interventions that promote venous outflow from the cranium include maintaining the head in a midline neutral position, avoiding extreme flexion of the hips and neck, and log rolling the patient while turning. The infant may require elevation of the trunk to allow the head to fall backward into a neutral position. Tape used to secure ETTs should be applied without constricting jugular venous drainage.

The head of bed (HOB) is usually elevated 15 to 30 degrees. However, extreme elevation of the HOB is discouraged because of the possibility of compromising CPP and CBF. This risk particularly applies to patients who are hypovolemic or hypotensive. Rosner and Coley[70] reported that the CPP declines as head elevation increases because of hydrostatic decreases in systemic arterial blood

pressure as the head is positioned above the heart. These authors further state that as CPP reduction occurs, vasodilation follows, which increases CBV and ICP. CBF decreases further, and a vicious cycle results. Although there is agreement that HOB elevation greater than 30 degrees should be avoided, controversy remains over moderate HOB elevation (15 to 30 degrees). In general, most patients with intracranial hypertension benefit from HOB elevation up to 30 degrees, providing that an adequate CPP (70 to 90 mmHg) exists.[71-73] Thus elevation of the HOB is individually determined in each patient while monitoring both ICP and CPP.

An increase in intraabdominal or intrathoracic pressure can also impede cerebral venous outflow. Nursing measures to prevent or minimize increased abdominal and intrathoracic pressure include gastric decompression and prevention of coughing, gagging, vomiting, and a Valsalva maneuver. In addition, isometric muscle activity should be avoided and replaced with passive range of motion. Mechanical or manual ventilation with high tidal volume and positive end-expiratory pressure (PEEP) may also increase ICP and require close monitoring of the patient's response. Any procedure that normally requires the use of the Trendelenburg position (e.g., central line insertion, postural drainage) is avoided. In general, the need for any intervention that has the potential to obstruct venous outflow is assessed. Later, when the patient is able to tolerate enteral feedings, it is important to avoid gastric residuals, administer stool softeners, and maintain good hydration to prevent constipation and straining.

Minimize Noxious Stimuli. Many routine nursing interventions used to care for the child with IICP are unpleasant and painful and may cause elevations (spikes) in ICP.[74,75] Painful procedures are minimized, physiologic pain is controlled, and environmental stressors (e.g., loud noises, jarring of the bed, conversations about the patient) are avoided. When noxious activities cannot be avoided, therapeutic touch may be used.[8,76] Mitchell and co-workers[77] studied the effect of touch on ICP in 13 children. They noted occasional, rather profound decreases in ICP with stabilization following parental stroking.

Data are conflicting when comparing the effects of rest between planned nursing care activities and clustering of care activities at one time.[75,78] Because not all patients respond to noxious stimuli or to clustering of nursing care activities in the same way, specific nursing interventions and how and when they are performed are individually determined for each patient. Risks versus benefits need to be determined when identifying priorities in nursing care for a patient with intracranial hypertension. In patients who cannot tolerate multiple nursing care activities (i.e., respond with sustained elevations in ICP), nursing interventions are restricted to required care, eliminating less critical interventions.

Pain management in the patient with an alteration in consciousness is challenging. Pain assessment is often restricted to physiologic responses (e.g., increased heart rate, blood pressure, and ICP). Pain is especially detrimental in the patient with intracranial hypertension because pain can further increase ICP. Concern is often raised over pharmacologic management of pain because of blunting effects on neurologic assessment and potential decrease in MAP and thus CPP. However, if the patient can perceive pain, appropriate analgesics are required to prevent further increases in ICP.

Control Cerebral Metabolism. Many patients with IICP cannot tolerate an increase in cerebral metabolism. Thus any actual or potential situation that increases cerebral metabolism is monitored and aggressively treated. The injured brain is sensitive to temperature variations: hypothermia is protective, and hyperthermia potentiates ischemic and traumatic brain damage. Core temperature has generally been assumed to equal brain temperature. However, a recent investigation measuring direct brain temperature has shown that in brain-injured patients, brain temperature can be significantly higher than core temperature.[79] Therefore core or brain temperature is monitored frequently, and normothermia or mild hypothermia (~36° C) is maintained. If hyperthermia develops, the cause is investigated and aggressively treated while the hyperthermic condition is reversed. Acetaminophen, fans, and a cooling blanket may be used to treat hyperthermia, and shivering is always prevented. Based on recent clinical and laboratory work, a renewed interest is seen in the use of moderate systemic hypothermia (32° C) to protect the brain from secondary injury.[80,81]

Seizures may occur in patients with neurologic dysfunction. This complication significantly increases cerebral metabolism and may cause an uncoupling or imbalance of cerebral metabolic supply and demand. Further ischemic damage and elevated ICP may develop. Patients, especially if they are chemically paralyzed, are assessed closely for signs of seizure activity. If seizure activity does occur, oxygenation and ventilation requirements are met, and anticonvulsants are promptly administered.

Promote CSF Drainage. Most interventions to control CSF volume are collaboratively managed medical therapies. However, Mitchell[82] demonstrates that patient position can transiently increase CSF obstruction. Body positions that obstruct venous outflow also obstruct CSF flow between the cranial and spinal subarachnoid spaces. A side-lying position with a neutral position of the head is recommended.

Even though the majority of nursing interventions are directed toward reducing adaptive demands, a few nursing interventions may improve intracranial compliance. Farley[58] reviewed the literature and reported the stabilization of ICP with therapeutic touch. Preoxygenation and premedication with lidocaine before suctioning may also transiently improve intracranial compliance so that adaptive capacity is not reduced during a noxious stimulus.[82]

STATUS EPILEPTICUS

A seizure is not a disease itself but is a symptom of a number of diseases and conditions. Seizures represent a sudden abnormal electrical discharge from neurons within the cerebral cortex that produces a disturbance in behavior, sensation, or motor function. Status epilepticus is defined as

"a condition characterized by epileptic seizures that is so frequently repeated or so prolonged as to create a fixed and lasting condition."[83] Minimum actual duration of a seizure necessary for definition as status epilepticus varies; however, most authorities use 30 minutes as the minimum duration.

The exact incidence of status epilepticus is unknown; it is not a reportable disease and is not classified consistently among reported series. However, a recent population-based study reported the incidence of status epilepticus to be 41 patients per year per 100,000 persons.[84] This study further reported the incidence by age and found a bimodal distribution, with the highest values in adults over 60 years of age and in infants. In patients with known epilepsy, a common cause of status epilepticus is abrupt discontinuation of anticonvulsant drugs or a suboptimal drug level.

A number of classification systems have been used to categorize seizures according to clinical manifestations, electrical activity, etiology, or response to therapy. The International Classification of Epileptic Seizures categorizes seizures according to the clinical nature of the onset of the seizure. Two major categories include generalized and partial seizures. Generalized tonic-clonic status epilepticus is the most common form in children. Box 20-1 provides a list of categories of epileptic seizures.

Pathogenesis. In many cases, the precise cause of status epilepticus is unknown. However, it is usually due to an acute event that adversely affects the central nervous system or to an exacerbation of symptomatic epilepsy.[85] Specific etiologies associated with status epilepticus are highly age dependent. For example, the major cause of status epilepticus in children younger than 2 years of age is a febrile illness, whereas stroke and subtherapeutic levels of antiepileptic medications are more common causes in adults.[86] The specific effects of a prolonged seizure or repeated seizures on the developing human brain are unknown. Reports of systemic alterations and neurophysiologic changes associated with status epilepticus are for the most part based on adult studies and animal models. Table 20-2 summarizes the systemic changes associated with seizures and status epilepticus.

If a seizure is allowed to progress beyond a critical point, CBF may become inadequate to meet the increased metabolic demand of the brain. An uncoupling of cerebral oxygen supply and demand occurs with neuronal damage. In the patient with preexisting IICP, the increase in CBF associated with a seizure can cause further increases in ICP with herniation.

Clinical Manifestations. A significant number of patients in the PICU have the potential to develop seizures. Seizure activity associated with status epilepticus in children is most often described as generalized clonic, generalized tonic, or myoclonic. During the tonic phase, signs and symptoms reflect autonomic overactivity: salivation, pupillary dilation, tachycardia, and increased blood pressure. Apneic episodes may occur but are usually short in duration. In the postictal period, the patient is usually drowsy or sleeping, followed by lethargy and confusion.

TABLE 20-2   Physiological Changes Associated With Seizures and Status Epilepticus

Parameter	Seizures	Status Epilepticus	Complications
Blood pressure	↑	↓	Shock
Pao_2	↓	↓	Hypoxia
$Paco_2$	↑	↑ →	↑ ICP
pH	↓	↓ →	Acidosis
Temperature	↑	↑	Fever/hyperpyrexia
Autonomic activity	↑	↑	Arrhythmia
Pulmonary secretions	↑	↑	Atelectasis shunt
K^+	↑	↑	Arrhythmias
CPK and myoglobin	Normal	↑	Renal failure
CBF	↑ (550%)	↑ (200%)	Intracranial hemorrhage
$CMRo_2$	↑ (300%)	↑ (300%)	Neuronal death
Blood glucose	↑	↓	Hypoglycemia, neuronal cell injury or death

CPK, Creatinine phosphokinase; *CBF,* cerebral blood flow; *CMRo₂,* cerebral metabolic rate (O_2 consumption).

 Box 20-1

The International Classification of Epileptic Seizures

I. **Partial (focal, local) seizures**
   A. Simple partial seizures (consciousness not impaired)
      1. With motor symptoms
      2. With somatosensory or special sensory symptoms
      3. With autonomic symptoms
      4. With psychic symptoms
   B. Complex partial seizures (with impairment of consciousness)
      1. Beginning as simple partial seizures and progressing to impairment of consciousness
      2. With impairment of consciousness at onset
   C. Partial seizures evolving to secondarily generalized seizures
      1. Simple partial seizures evolving to generalized seizures
      2. Complex partial seizures evolving into generalized seizures
      3. Simple partial seizures evolving to complex partial seizures to generalized seizures
II. **Generalized seizures (convulsive or nonconvulsive)**
   A. Absence seizures
      1. Absence seizures
      2. Atypical absence seizures
   B. Myoclonic seizures
   C. Clonic seizures
   D. Tonic seizures
   E. Tonic-clonic seizures
   F. Atonic seizures (astatic seizures)
III. **Unclassified epileptic seizures**
   Includes all seizures that cannot be classified because of inadequate or incomplete data and some that defy classification in hitherto described categories. This includes some neonatal seizures, e.g., rhythmic eye movements, chewing, and swimming movements.

Adapted from Dreifuss FE: Classification of epileptic seizures and the epilepsies, *Pediatr Clin North Am* 36:265, 1989.

In the patient with intracranial hypertension, signs and symptoms of cerebral herniation may be present. The chemically paralyzed patient experiencing a seizure may develop a sudden onset of tachycardia, systemic hypertension, elevated ICP, and, occasionally, pupil dilation.

The EEG is useful in evaluating some patients with seizures. The EEG pattern demonstrates bilateral symmetric polyspike discharges that coincide with myoclonic jerks.[85] Because generalized convulsive status epilepticus is easily diagnosed clinically, an ictal EEG is rarely helpful.[87] However, if any question exists regarding the seizure type, an EEG is done immediately. The sooner the EEG is obtained, the greater the likelihood a specific abnormality can be identified.[88] Continuous EEG monitoring is often used in patients considered to be at high risk for seizure activity and is mandatory in heavily sedated or chemically paralyzed patients.

Collaborative Management.   Once the patient's airway is stabilized, oxygenation is maintained, and perfusion is adequate, anticonvulsant therapy is initiated. The three most common classes of anticonvulsants used in children are benzodiazepines, phenytoin, and barbiturates. Table 20-3 lists the most commonly used anticonvulsants for status epilepticus.

When status epilepticus is refractory to conventional anticonvulsant therapy, aggressive therapy is required to terminate seizure activity to avoid further brain injury. High-dose barbiturate therapy is used most often to depress cerebral activity.[86] However, cardiovascular instability is often associated with barbiturate coma and may, in some patients, limit its use. Continuous benzodiazepine infusion and propofol anesthesia have also been reported to be successful in terminating refractory status epilepticus without cardiovascular side effects.[89-91] In all cases, EEG monitoring is mandatory.

The goals in managing care of a child with status epilepticus are to ensure adequate cardiorespiratory function, reverse seizure activity, and assist in the identification and treatment of etiologic and precipitating factors.

TABLE 20-3   Initial Anticonvulsants to Control Status Epilepticus

Drug	Dose	Rate of Administration	Time to Effect	Side Effects
Rapid-Acting Agents				
Diazepam (undiluted)	Begin 0.25 mg/kg IV and titrate to effect	<1 mg/min	1-2 min	Respiratory depression; thrombophlebitis
Lorazepam 2 mg/ml	0.1 mg/kg × 4, 20 min apart, max 4 mg	1 mg/min	2-3 min	Drowsiness, confusion, ataxia
Longer-Acting Agents				
Phenytoin 50 mg/ml; dilute in normal saline 1:10	15 mg/kg, up to 45 mg/kg	20-50 mg/min	~20 min	Heart block; hypotension
Phenobarbital 130 mg/ml	10 mg/kg, up to 30 mg/kg	30 mg/min	10-12 min	Respiratory depression; hypotension

From Blumer JL: *A practical guide to pediatric intensive care,* ed 3, St Louis, 1990, Mosby.

Box 20-2 outlines specific assessments that should be noted when observing a child during a seizure.

Initial management ensures adequate oxygenation and ventilation. The child's body is rolled to the side to facilitate drainage of secretions. If the airway is obstructed with secretions, the mouth is suctioned. Hard objects are not forced into the mouth. Oxygen is administered promptly. Frequently, patients in status epilepticus require intubation. For the patient who has recently eaten, intubation is performed using rapid-sequence induction.

The next step is directed toward protecting the patient from injury. The child is positioned to avoid injury, and the use of restraints is limited. Hard toys and other objects are removed from the child's bed, and the side rails are padded.

Once intravenous access is secured, blood is obtained for study. Capillary blood is tested for glucose, and dextrose 25% in water is administered for hypoglycemia. A number of anticonvulsants may be required to stop the seizure.

Hyperthermia is commonly associated with status epilepticus in children. When present, antipyretics and sponging with tepid water are helpful interventions while the source of infection is determined and treated.

ARTERIOVENOUS MALFORMATION

Arteriovenous malformations (AVMs) of the brain are anomalous connections between arteries and veins without an interposed capillary bed. Fig. 20-6 is a drawing of an AVM over the cerebral cortex. AVMs vary in size from a few millimeters in diameter to more than several centimeters.[92] An AVM is characteristically cone shaped with thin-walled vessels. Although the actual incidence of intracranial AVMs is unknown, approximately 2000 new cases are identified each year.[93]

Pathogenesis. Arteriovenous malformations occur early in fetal development from failure of capillaries to develop. Blood is shunted directly from the artery into the vein. As the child's brain grows, additional arterial contributions are acquired. The size of the vessels increases because they offer less resistance to blood flow than the surrounding vascular beds with capillaries.[94] As the AVM enlarges, blood is diverted from adjacent brain tissue (steal

---

 Box 20-2
Guidelines for Seizure Record Documentation

Onset
1. Activity before seizure: Describe what patient was doing, that is, running, watching TV, sleeping.
2. Aura: Anything noticed at the start of the seizure activity, for example, bizarre behavior, chewing and lip smacking, yelling, sees lights, hears noises.
3. Focal: Only one area of the body involved (record area).
4. Generalized: Entire body involved.
5. Focal to generalized: Begins in one area and progresses to involve the entire body (describe).

Seizure Activity
1. Tonic: Becomes tense or stiff (arms and legs in extension).
2. Clonic: Rapid rhythmic jerking/flexion of extremities.
3. Tonic/clonic: Tonic followed by clonic phase (may be repeated several times).
4. Brief sudden jerk: Myoclonic jerks—may be focal or generalized.
5. Loss of muscle tone: For example, falls to floor or slumps forward, remains limp.
6. Staring: Does not respond to name, no blink response, stares into space, may be seen alone or with eye blinking or other activity (describe).
7. Chewing and lip smacking: Check if present (describe).
8. Unusual behavior: Screaming, biting, pulling at clothing, nonpurposeful behavior, and so on (describe).
9. Level of consciousness: Unresponsive, confused, easily aroused, responds to commands.
10. Eyes: Describe eye movements, for example, roll up, roll to side, nystagmus; status of pupils.
11. Other: Incontinent, vomit, tongue biting.
12. Duration: Time from onset of seizure activity to cessation of seizure activity.

Postictal State
1. Recovery time: In seconds, minutes, and so on.
2. Sleep: Duration.
3. Changes in behavior: Becomes aggressive, fighting, combative, and so on.
4. Paralysis: Location, type (weakness or flaccidity), duration.

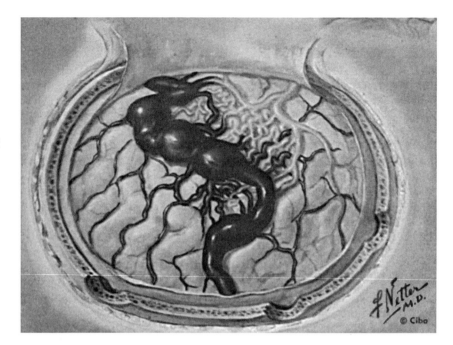

Fig. 20-6 Arteriovenous malformation over the cerebral cortex. (Copyright 1996 by CIBA-GEIGY Corporation. Reprinted with permission from the Ciba Collection of Medical Illustrations, illustrated by Frank Netter, MD. All rights reserved.)

effect), resulting in tissue hypoxia.[95,96] Gliosis (scarring) of the surrounding tissue from focal hemorrhage or ischemia is common. Neurologic symptoms and dysfunction can occur as a result of direct compression of brain tissue. Hydrocephalus can develop from obstruction of CSF pathways or from extension of the AVM into the choroid plexus.[8] Intracranial hemorrhage is the most life-threatening complication.

Clinical Manifestations. Only half of patients with a known AVM are symptomatic, with the majority of manifestations presenting in adulthood.[97] The usual presentation of an AVM is from intracranial hemorrhage, a seizure, or symptoms associated with a space-occupying lesion. In children, spontaneous subarachnoid, intracerebral, or intraventricular hemorrhages are the most common initial manifestation.[97-99] With a hemorrhage, the child may have a history of intermittent headaches or a sudden severe headache. Manifestations of meningeal irritation are common with a subarachnoid hemorrhage. Rapid deterioration in level of consciousness usually occurs with hemorrhage into the ventricular system.[99] Focal neurologic deficits may also develop and are related to the location of the hemorrhage.

A seizure is the next most common initial manifestation of an AVM. The seizure may be simple or complex and focal or general. Seizures occur presumably from ischemic changes in tissue surrounding the AVM.

Less commonly, initial clinical manifestations of an AVM include headache, vomiting, developmental delay, visual disturbances, progressive hemiparesis, behavioral abnormalities, and hydrocephalus. Congestive heart failure is usually the presenting sign in the neonate because of the large runoff in the AVM producing increased blood return to the heart and high-output failure.[100]

Bruits have been auscultated over the head in as many as 50% of children with an intracranial AVM. A cranial bruit in infants younger than 4 months of age almost always represents an AVM.[98] In neonates, the bruit is loud, harsh, and best heard over the fontanelles.[100] However, cardiac manifestations are extremely variable in intensity, and in some infants, the only presenting sign is asymptomatic cardiomegaly.[101] A dural AVM is more likely to be auscultated than an intracranial AVM because of its close proximity to the skull. Bruits are less commonly audible in older children and adults.

Studies commonly used to diagnose an AVM are computed tomography (CT) with contrast enhancement, magnetic resonance imaging (MRI), and angiography. The CT scan can outline the blood clot and, on enhanced study, may detail feeding and draining vessels. MRI can demonstrate flowing blood in AVMs and associated hematomas, but it does not eliminate the need for angiography. Cerebral angiography is required in the planning stages of therapy. It clearly identifies the numbers, size, and location of arterial feeders and draining vascular channels.

Collaborative Management. Many treatment modalities are available to manage the child with an AVM, and these are categorized on two levels. The first level is conservative medical management, and the second level is definitive therapy that consists of surgical resection or an interventional neuroradiologic technique. The specific strategy selected depends on the size and location of the AVM, age of the patient, physician preference, cerebral dominance, technical support, condition of the patient, and characteristics of feeder vessels supplying the AVM.

Conservative management entails close observation without surgical intervention. The AVM is allowed to take its natural course. Investigators in one study reviewed 191 cases with cerebral AVM and found the average yearly risk for first hemorrhage between 2% and 3%. Risk of rebleeding increased with advancing age.[102] The risk of death with each hemorrhage is 20% to 30%.[103] Symptomatic treatment of seizures, headaches, and nausea may also be required.

Total surgical excision of an AVM is ideal but is not always possible because of an inaccessible location. A rare but major complication of surgical excision is a phenomenon known as "normal perfusion pressure breakthrough."[104] It is characterized by massive dilation of vessels around the AVM and loss of autoregulation in these vessels. Without autoregulation, increased blood flow under high pressure occurs, resulting in cerebral edema or hemorrhage. This complication may be reduced with a staged surgical approach (i.e., removal of the AVM by surgical excision or embolization with more than one operation).

In smaller lesions, proton-beam irradiation or focused laser therapy can obliterate the lesion. Proton-beam radiation is done as a stereotactic procedure and is noninvasive. Stereotactic neurosurgery employs a mechanical device to precisely position probes, electrodes, radiation, and other instruments in three-dimensional space. It is usually recommended for surgically inaccessible AVMs. Proton irradiation causes thickening of the vascular elements of the AVM with gradual shrinkage. The risk to the patient is minimal, and hospitalization time is short. The disadvantages are that it may take up to 2 years for optimal effects to occur and the procedure may not completely eliminate the AVM.

Laser therapy is also an alternative therapy for inaccessible lesions. Stereotactic technique is used to locate the target tissue so that the laser can be focused on a particular area. The light beam causes photocoagulation of vessels in the AVM with subsequent shrinkage of vessels.[8,104]

Interventional neuroradiologic techniques using balloon or coil occlusion of the larger feeding vessel may be indicated for inaccessible lesions.[105] One technique uses the femoral artery approach. A catheter is advanced to the cervical area into one of the carotid vessels, depending on the feeder vessel of the AVM. The tip of the catheter is then positioned as close as possible to the area requiring embolization. Embolization material is injected and carried by blood flow until it occludes a vessel. Total occlusion of an AVM may not be possible, but the lesion may be reduced to a more optimal size for surgical excision.[106]

In the patient with a suspected AVM without hemorrhage, nursing assessment and management are directed toward prevention of intracranial bleeding. An initial baseline neurologic assessment is performed, followed by serial assessments. If the child has a large AVM with a high risk for bleeding, special precautions are taken: maintenance of strict bed rest, control of hypertension, and provision of a quiet environment. If hemorrhage has occurred, signs and symptoms of intracranial hypertension are assessed and monitored. Management of intracranial hypertension has been discussed earlier. The principles of postcraniotomy nursing care are discussed in a later section on brain tumors.

If embolization therapy is performed using a femoral artery, postprocedure care is similar to postcardiac catheterization care. The leg is immobilized, and the patient remains on bed rest for 24 hours. The catheter site dressing is assessed for bleeding, and distal pulses and vital signs are monitored closely until stable.

Box 20-3

✦ Classification of Brain Tumors in Children

I. Tumors of neuroepithelial tissue
   A. Glial tumors
   B. Neuronal tumors
   C. "Primitive" neuroepithelial tumors
   D. Pineal cell tumors
II. Tumors of meningeal and related tissue
   A. Meningiomas
   B. Meningeal sarcomatous tumors
   C. Primary melanocytic tumors
III. Tumors of nerve sheath cells
   A. Neurilemmoma
   B. Anaplastic neurilemmoma (schwannoma, neurinoma)
   C. Neurofibroma
   D. Anaplastic neurofibroma
IV. Primary malignant lymphomas
V. Tumors of blood vessel origin
VI. Germ cell tumors
   A. Germinoma
   B. Embryonal carcinoma
   C. Choriocarcinoma
   D. Endodermal sinus tumor
   E. Teratomatous tumors
   F. Mixed
VII. Malformative tumors
VIII. Tumors of neuroendocrine origin
IX. Local extensions from regional tumors
X. Metastatic tumors
XI. Unclassified tumors

Adapted from Rorke LB et al: Revision of the WHO classification of brain tumors for childhood brain tumors, *Cancer* 56:1869, 1985.

BRAIN TUMORS

Primary intracranial tumors are the second most common form of childhood cancer and the most common solid tumor.[107-108] Various types of intracranial tumors have been identified in children, with astrocytomas having the highest incidence, followed by medulloblastomas, brainstem gliomas, and ependymomas.[107,109] The majority of brain tumors in children are located in the posterior fossa.

A universally accepted histologic classification system for brain tumors does not exist. The most extensively used classification system, developed by the World Health Organization (WHO), grades tumors based on site, histologic type, and degree of malignancy. In 1985, this classification system was modified to specifically address central nervous system (CNS) tumors in children.[110] Box 20-3 is an abbreviated list of this revised classification of brain tumors.

Cerebellar astrocytomas represent approximately one third of all posterior fossa tumors and 12% of total brain tumors found in children younger than 15 years of age.[111,112] They are derived from astrocytic neuroglial cells and typically consist of a single large cyst with a solid mural nodule. A smaller percentage involves a solid mass located in the vermis.[109]

Supratentorial astrocytomas are the most common form of supratentorial tumor.[111] Supratentorial astrocytomas are classified according to four grades that reflect their increasing tendency toward malignancy. Grades I and II are considered low-grade astrocytomas with a better outcome than grades III and IV. Approximately 25% of tumors in children are low-grade astrocytomas. Most supratentorial hemispheric tumors occur within the parenchyma without distinct boundaries.[107]

Medulloblastoma is the most common tumor of the posterior fossa and accounts for 15% to 20% of intracranial tumors.[113] Of all childhood tumors, it has shown the greatest improvement in survival. This rapidly growing tumor is a primitive neuroectodermal tumor with nonspecific differentiation. Histologic analysis demonstrates that these tumors may differentiate along several cell lines and may represent a tumor of stem cell origin.[109]

Ependymomas are derived from ependymal cells and may arise from any part of the ventricular system. Typically, one third of tumors are supratentorial, and two thirds are infratentorial. Ependymomas occur more often in young children, with a mean age at diagnosis of 5 to 6 years.[109] In young children, ependymomas are predominantly located in the fourth ventricle, whereas in older children and adolescents, they are more often located in the lateral ventricles.[111,114]

Pathogenesis. The molecular and cellular origins of CNS tumors are not clear in all cases. Evidence shows that genetic factors may play a role in the development of some tumors. Other tumors (e.g., craniopharyngiomas, some medulloblastomas) are congenital and may represent maldevelopment.[115] The immune system may also play a role in the development of CNS tumors. The effect of teratogens and other environmental factors in predisposing the brain to tumors is unclear.

CNS tumors tend to be more compressive than destructive. The pathophysiology of intracranial tumors is based on an expanding mass that increases the intracranial volume. The expanding mass compresses and distorts adjacent tissue, compromises CBF, and obstructs CSF circulation. Left untreated, ischemic and herniation syndromes develop, resulting in death.

Clinical Manifestations. Clinical manifestations of CNS tumors can be classified into general and localized findings. General findings represent all of the potential signs and symptoms associated with increasing ICP. Classic signs and symptoms of increased ICP in a child with a posterior fossa tumor is one in which the child has flulike gastrointestinal symptoms for several mornings. The symptoms resolve and are absent for several weeks, followed by a return of symptoms that are more intense.[111] Localized symptoms vary and depend on the location and degree of involvement of the tumor. Table 20-4 highlights the clinical manifestations of brain tumors based on location.

The diagnostic evaluation of the child with symptoms suggestive of a brain tumor is accomplished with high-resolution CT scanning or MRI. Ancillary studies may be used to further evaluate the tumor. These studies include

TABLE 20-4   Clinical Manifestations of Brain Tumors, According to Location

Frontal lobe	Seizures
	Motor weakness
	Personality and behavioral changes
Parietal lobe	Perceptual problems
	Sensory disturbance
	Dyslexia
Occipital lobe	Visual disturbance
Temporal lobe	Auditory disturbance
	Impaired memory
	Visual field deficits
	Dysarthria
	Personality changes
Midline	Visual loss
	Endocrinopathies
	Nonlocalizing signs of IICP
	Personality changes
Cerebellum	Gait, balance, and coordination disturbance
Brainstem	Cranial neuropathies
	Hydrocephalus
	Hemiparesis/quadriparesis
	Late IICP
	Hyperthermia/hypothermia

IICP, Increased intracranial pressure.

arteriography, EEG, plain skull films, ultrasound (infants), and positron emission tomography (PET).

Collaborative Management. Standard medical management of childhood brain tumors involves one or more of the following therapies: surgery, radiation, and chemotherapy. Even though surgery has many limitations (e.g., accessibility, damage to adjacent tissues), it remains the procedure of choice for most brain tumors. Total removal of the tumor is usually not possible, but debulking surgery improves the effectiveness of radiation therapy and chemotherapy, as well as providing palliation of symptoms from mechanical obstruction or compression. In addition, tumor specimens can be obtained for histologic evaluation and more accurate chemotherapeutic treatment. The effectiveness of surgical removal continues to improve as novel surgical techniques evolve. Currently, ultrasonography during surgery has permitted better localization of tumors. Stereotactic technology together with neuroimaging localizes and maps tumors with better precision.

Radiation therapy has contributed to overall survival in most patients. Ionizing radiation produces its lethal effects by destroying the cell nucleus. It can be delivered to the entire brain, a local area of the brain, or the craniospinal axis. The dosage, timing, and location of radiation are determined by the type of tumor and its potential to spread to other parts of the CNS or seed into the CSF. Some patients with small, inoperable, benign tumors are treated with cobalt radiation using a stereotactic technique. This technique is able to deliver a single high dose of radiation to a precisely defined area, thus preserving surrounding normal tissue.[116]

In general, chemotherapy has been less effective in treating CNS tumors compared with results for neoplasia in other parts of the body because of difficulty reaching the CNS. Several factors account for this outcome. First, the blood-brain barrier provides a physiologic barrier that restricts choices for chemotherapeutic agents. Gliomas also have cellular characteristics that act as physiologic barriers. Astrocytomas have the ability to secrete a hormone that allows the tumor to increase its nutrient supply, thus reducing chemotherapeutic effectiveness. Last, many chemotherapeutic agents that successfully treat systemic tumors cannot be used in concentrations necessary to treat regionally confined tumors, for example, CNS tumors.[117] However, in recent years, there has been an increase in clinical trials of chemotherapeutic agents for treating childhood tumors.[109] Chemotherapy protocols continue to be developed and reexamined.

Postoperative Craniotomy. Many children undergoing craniotomy require intensive care after surgery. Baseline postoperative cardiovascular and neurologic assessments are completed on admission to the PICU and compared with preoperative examination. Surgical dressings are assessed for blood and CSF drainage. Hemorrhage may occur postoperatively, especially in the posterior fossa, producing rapid neurologic deterioration. Signs include alternation in level of consciousness, ataxic respirations, quadriparesis, significant alterations in blood pressure associated with small pupils, and dysconjugate gaze.[118]

Routine care also involves proper positioning of the patient. For supratentorial craniotomy, the HOB is usually elevated 20 to 30 degrees with the patient positioned on either side or on the back. For infratentorial craniotomy, the HOB is usually flat with the patient positioned on either side. In both cases, the neck should not be flexed.[119]

The most common postoperative problems include elevated ICP, ineffective airway clearance, meningitis, hyperthermia, and seizures. Because of extensive manipulation and irritation of brain tissue, edema may develop and elevate ICP. Debulking surgery may also create a pressure gradient between intracranial compartments, causing shift and herniation of brain tissue. ICP peaks at approximately 72 hours. ICP monitoring is not routine, but if a ventriculostomy is in place, monitoring is easily accomplished. Clinical manifestations and treatment of elevated ICP were described earlier.

Respiratory difficulties are a potential problem, especially in the unconscious child who cannot cough effectively and clear secretions. Pulmonary toilet, adequate hydration, and frequent position changes are required. Hypercarbia is avoided because of its adverse effects on CBV and ICP.

Inflammation of the meninges may occur from operative contaminants or from blood remaining in the subarachnoid space. Clinical signs are characteristic of meningeal irritation. Nursing care is similar to that provided to the child with bacterial meningitis. Aseptic technique is used with dressing changes and invasive procedures. Evidence of CSF drainage on the dressing (i.e., the halo sign, in which the center of the drainage is bloody or serosanguinous and the outer periphery is clear or yellow) is promptly reported. A dural tear may be present, placing the patient at risk for an intracranial infection.

Hyperthermia may result from infection or dehydration, as well as from alteration of the temperature-regulating centers in the hypothalamus and brainstem. Antibiotics are administered for infection, and acetaminophen is administered for fever. Fluid and electrolyte status is assessed. Because diabetes insipidus (DI) and SIADH are potential postoperative complications, fluid and electrolyte status is vigilantly assessed. Urine output is closely monitored, as well as levels of serum and urine electrolytes and osmolalities. To prevent cerebral edema, fluids may be restricted or titrated to maintain a predetermined serum osmolality.

Seizures are a potential postoperative problem, especially after the child has recovered from anesthesia. It is at this time that the seizure threshold is lowered.[120] However, seizures may occur at any time before, during, or after surgery. Approximately one third of all patients with a brain tumor have seizures.[116] Many patients receive prophylactic anticonvulsants, and seizure precautions are maintained.

MENINGITIS

Many different types of pathogens (e.g., bacteria, viruses, fungi) can cause infection within the CNS. The most common types of CNS infections seen in children are bacterial and viral meningitis. The Pediatric Task Force on Diagnosis and Management of Meningitis[121] defines meningitis as an "inflammation of the meninges that is identified by an abnormal number of white blood cells (WBCs) in CSF." Aseptic meningitis is defined as meningitis without detectable bacterial pathogens in CSF by usual laboratory techniques.[121] The overwhelming majority of cases of aseptic meningitis are caused by viruses.[122]

The incidence of bacterial meningitis varies over time and by geographic region. Consequently, precise epidemiological data are difficult to report.[123] In general, incidence is age specific; bacterial meningitis peaks between 6 and 12 months of age and declines thereafter. Before widespread immunization, *Haemophilus influenzae* type b was the most common pathogen causing meningitis in children. Currently, *Neisseria meningitides* and *Streptococcus pneumoniae* are responsible for the majority of cases in children.[124] In newborns, the most common etiologic agents are group B streptococcus and *Escherichia coli*.

Viral meningitis is less common than bacterial meningitis and occurs sporadically. It is present in all ages, with the highest incidence found in children. Enteroviruses are the most common cause of viral meningitis.[122]

Pathogenesis. In most cases of bacterial meningitis, pathogens enter the CNS indirectly from a distant site. Less commonly, pathogens enter the CNS directly from penetrating trauma or from a ruptured intracranial abscess. Typically, colonization of a pathogen occurs in the upper respiratory tract and enters the bloodstream through small vessels.[122] The blood-borne organisms then seed in the meninges and colonize the CSF, producing inflammation of the brain and meninges. Throughout the progressive pathogenic stages, the inciting organism overcomes sequential host defenses, resulting in invasion and replication in the CSF.[125] The bacteria and subsequent inflammation produce a cascade of interrelated pathophysiologic events that, if left untreated, may result in cerebral edema, intracranial hypertension, and herniation.

The pathogenesis of viral meningitis remains unclear. Viral meningitis is spread from person to person, with the mouth and nose as the usual ports of entry. Viral pathogens are believed to disseminate through the bloodstream to the CNS. The clinical course is usually self-limiting, with improvement seen in 7 to 14 days.

Clinical Manifestations. Clinical manifestations of meningitis vary and result largely from the host response to pathogen invasion of the CSF. The most common clinical manifestations of bacterial meningitis in children are fever, vomiting, lethargy, headache, and alteration in level of consciousness. In progressive stages, signs and symptoms are characteristic of increased ICP, which, if left untreated, can result in life-threatening cerebral herniation (e.g., oculomotor palsy, irregular respirations, and cardiovascular collapse). No one clinical sign is pathognomic, but signs and symptoms of meningeal irritation include photophobia, back pain, nuchal rigidity, Brudzinski's sign (flexion of the hips and knees with passive flexion of the neck), and Kernig's sign (back pain and resistance after passive extension of the lower legs). Focal neurologic signs (e.g., hemiparesis or quadriparesis, visual deficits), as well as hearing deficits and ataxia, occur in some children. A petechial rash is commonly seen when *N. meningitides* is the etiologic agent and is most pronounced on the extremities. A diffuse maculopapular eruption with or without petechiae is commonly associated with viral illnesses. The clinical manifestations in infants are less specific and include fever, lethargy, poor feeding, vomiting, diarrhea, a bulging anterior fontanelle, hypothermia or hyperthermia, and hypoglycemia or hyperglycemia. Seizures may occur in all age groups. Definitive diagnosis of bacterial meningitis is made by finding a bacterial pathogen in cultures of the CSF. CSF from a lumbar puncture is analyzed for color, glucose, protein, and WBC count. Usual abnormalities seen in the CSF of infants and children with bacterial and viral meningitis are contrasted in Table 20-5. CSF characteristics in the newborn with bacterial meningitis are less definitive and may not vary substantially from normal values.[121]

Clinical manifestations of viral meningitis are those of meningeal irritation, such as fever, photophobia, headache, and nuchal rigidity. Rarely, severe systemic disease occurs in patients with viral meningitis. CSF characteristics of viral meningitis are increased WBCs, normal or slightly increased protein, normal glucose, and no bacteria present on Gram stain or culture.[8,122]

Collaborative Management. Antimicrobial therapy is the mainstay of treatment for bacterial meningitis. Antibiotic therapy is divided into two phases: empiric and definitive. Before CSF results are known, broad-spectrum antibiotics are selected, empirically based on the most likely etiologic agent. In the newborn, empiric therapy usually includes an aminoglycoside with ampicillin and sometimes cefotaxime or, more recently, cefotaxime plus ampicillin. Current recommendations for empiric treatment beyond 3 months of age are a third-generation cephalosporin in high dose with vancomycin 60 mg/kg/day divided into four doses.[123]

Once CSF results are obtained, specific antibiotics are selected based on bacterial sensitivity, patient age, and patient allergies. High doses of multiple antibiotics are often necessary to achieve adequate brain concentrations.[123] With the development of newer cephalosporins, a large selection of antimicrobials are now available. Recommendations for specific antimicrobial therapy and dosages change often. Infectious disease specialists and authoritative sources should be consulted.[125,126] Beyond symptomatic treatment and supportive care, there is no specific therapy for viral meningitis.

Seizures have the potential to adversely effect the child with infectious meningitis. Whether prophylactic anticonvulsants are beneficial in all cases is unclear. However,

---

◆ **TABLE 20-5   Characteristics of Cerebrospinal Fluid (CSF) in Meningitis***

CSF Analysis	Normal Values	Bacterial	Aseptic (Viral)
Pressure (mmHg)	60-100	Increased	Normal or increased
Color	Clear, odorless	Cloudy	Clear to slightly cloudy
WBC (mm³)	≤5	100-60,000	Usually <1000
Predominant WBC type	Mononuclear	Polymorphonuclear	Mononuclear†
Glucose (mg/dl)	>⅔ of blood glucose >60	Decreased, <½ to ⅔ of blood glucose	Normal to slightly decreased or increased
Protein (mg/dl)	15-45	>100	Normal to slightly increased 50-200
Gram stain	Negative	Positive	Negative

*Children beyond the neonatal period.
†An early polymorphonuclear reaction may be present.
WBC, White blood cell.

when seizures do occur, prompt and aggressive treatment is recommended.

Several studies support the use of adjunctive dexamethasone (Decadron) for the treatment of bacterial meningitis in children, particularly in preventing deafness.[127,128] The Committee on Infectious Diseases, American Academy of Pediatrics[129] also stated that dexamethasone probably reduces the likelihood of hearing loss after *H. influenzae* meningitis. The reported benefits of dexamethasone are demonstrated primarily when used to treat *H. influenzae* and include a reduction in cerebral edema, stabilization of the blood-brain barrier, reduction of rapid bacterial lysis, and reduction of biologically active cytokines.[130] Dexamethasone is most effective when 0.15 mg/kg is given intravenously 20 minutes before initiation of antibiotic therapy and, thereafter, every 6 hours for 2 days.[131]

Despite increasing use of dexamethasone, its use is being questioned because of the decline in reported cases of *H. influenzae*. The benefits of dexamethasone use in treating *S. pneumoniae* or *N. meningitidis* are less clear. Consequently, the benefits and possible risks (e.g., gastrointestinal bleeding) are weighed in each patient.

H. influenzae type b polysaccharide vaccine was first licensed in 1985 for administration for children 24 months or older. In October 1990, one of the currently licensed vaccines (HbOC) was approved for administration to infants beginning at 2 months of age.[132] Although the incidence of *H. influenzae* disease is believed to have decreased since the licensure of the vaccine, precise epidemiologic data do not exist.

The use of ICP monitoring for patients with clinical signs of intracranial hypertension is controversial. Controlled studies do not exist, and decisions to monitor ICP are based on individual professional practice.

Along with frequent measurements of vital signs and serial neurologic assessments, the neurologic examination includes assessment of meningeal irritation and IICP. Head circumference is measured daily in infants.

Nursing interventions include promoting patient comfort, preventing patient injury, and controlling elevated ICP. Patient comfort measures include maintaining normothermia, providing a quiet environment, shielding the patient from bright lights, and administering analgesics for headache. The patient is protected from injury by placing crib rails and bed rails up and maintaining seizure precautions. With bacterial meningitis, the infectious process should be halted and reversed as soon as possible. Intravenous antibiotics are administered promptly following blood and CSF culture collections. If intracranial hypertension is presumed, nursing measures to control ICP are instituted, as described earlier. Respiratory isolation is instituted in all patients with suspected meningitis until the specific pathogen is identified. If bacterial meningitis results from *N. meningitidis* or *H. influenzae,* an additional 24 hours of respiratory isolation after the start of antimicrobial therapy is required. Aseptic meningitis requires enteric precautions for 7 days after the onset of disease.[133]

Individuals who were in close contact (e.g., household, day care, nursery school) to patients with known bacterial meningitis from *N. meningitidis* require chemoprophylaxis. The drug of choice is rifampin (Rifadin, Rimactane) 10 mg/kg (maximum dose, 600 mg/day) every 12 hours for a total of four doses during 2 days. Infants may require a lower dose. Household contacts (younger than 48 months of age) of patients with meningitis from *H. influenzae* also require chemoprophylaxis with rifampin. Prophylaxis is not recommended when household contacts are all 48 months or older. Rifampin 20 mg/kg (maximum dose, 600 mg/day) is administered once daily for 4 days. Again, infants younger than 1 month may require a lower dose. Definitive recommendations for chemoprophylaxis for day care and nursery school contacts of *H. influenzae* meningitis have not been established.[132]

VIRAL ENCEPHALITIS

Viral encephalitis is an acute inflammation of the brain and meninges. The exact incidence is unknown. A large epidemiologic study conducted in Olmsted County, Minnesota, between 1950 and 1981 reported an incidence of 8.1 per 100,000 persons per year.[134] This same study reported the highest incidence in children 5 to 9 years of age. Numerous viruses are known to cause encephalitis; however, in the United States the most common are the herpes simplex viruses and arboviruses (California, Eastern equine, Western equine, St. Louis). With the advent of immunizations, encephalitis associated with measles, mumps, and rubella has disappeared almost entirely.

Pathogenesis. Viral growth begins in extraneural tissue and then spreads to the CNS via the bloodstream. It can enter the CSF by passing or growing through the choroid plexus. Passive transfer through the blood-brain barrier may also occur. Less commonly, spread can occur along the peripheral nerves or via the olfactory system.[135] Injury to the CNS occurs from perivascular inflammation with neuronal destruction; demyelination; and subsequent necrosis, hemorrhage, and cavitation. Untreated herpes encephalitis may have associated cerebral edema and intracranial hypertension.

Clinical Manifestations. Many of the clinical features of viral encephalitis are similar to those of aseptic meningitis, as described earlier. However, changes in cortical function from parenchymal involvement differentiate the two. The patient may exhibit abnormal behavior, agitation, seizures, headache, fever, and severe alteration in consciousness. Meningeal signs may be present, depending on the age of the child and degree of meningeal involvement.

The extent of clinical features depends on the severity of the infection, specific focus of infection, and the specific viral pathogen. Patients may develop mild sensory loss or cranial nerve palsies characteristic of a specific area of brain involvement. Herpes simplex viruses are particularly virulent and devastating if untreated. Early manifestations include nausea and vomiting, headache, confusion, seizures, bizarre behavior, hallucinations, and focal neurologic deficits. Late manifestations represent increased ICP and herniation.

Presumptive evidence of encephalitis includes increased ICP, a rise in antibody titer to pathogen, and CSF alterations. CSF changes that are suggestive of encephalitis include elevated WBCs with a predominance of lymphocytes, mildly elevated protein, and mildly reduced glucose. The CSF may also be completely normal. The EEG is abnormal in most cases. CT and MRI may demonstrate signs of cerebral edema, hyperemia, obstructive hydrocephalus, or disseminated lesions. Definitive diagnosis is made by isolating or culturing the viral pathogen from CSF or via a brain biopsy.

Collaborative Management. With few exceptions, treatment of viral encephalitis is primarily supportive and symptomatic. Anticonvulsants are used for seizures, analgesics for pain and headaches, and antipyretics for hyperthermia. SIADH secretion may occur. Thus fluid and electrolyte status and signs of the development of cerebral edema are closely monitored. Antiviral therapy with intravenous acyclovir (Zovirax) (30 mg/kg/day) over 10 days is recommended for herpes encephalitis.[136] Acyclovir has been recommended in severe cases of varicella encephalitis.[137]

Nursing assessment of viral encephalitis is similar to that for meningitis. Management is largely supportive and also similar to that for meningitis. Measures to ensure adequate respiratory and circulatory function, fluid and electrolyte balance, ICP control, and nutritional support are provided.

HYDROCEPHALUS

Hydrocephalus is a condition characterized by a pathologic increase in CSF within the ventricular system that is, or has been, under increased pressure. A discrepancy exists between the amount of CSF produced and absorbed, with a net increase causing dilation of the ventricles. The estimated incidence of hydrocephalus with spina bifida is approximately 7 to 9 cases per 10,000 births.[138] The estimated incidence of congenital hydrocephalus without spina bifida as reported by the Centers of Disease Control is 5.84 cases per 10,000 births.[139]

Terms that more accurately describe the etiology of hydrocephalus are "communicating" and "noncommunicating" hydrocephalus. Communicating hydrocephalus indicates that CSF flows freely from the ventricular spaces into the spinal and cranial subarachnoid spaces. An accumulation of CSF occurs as a result of impaired absorption of CSF by the pacchionian granules or from a blockage within the subarachnoid space. Noncommunicating hydrocephalus indicates that a blockage is somewhere within the ventricular system. Communicating and noncommunicating hydrocephalus are often classified according to both cause and anatomic site of obstruction or abnormality (Box 20-4).

Pathogenesis. Hydrocephalus is caused by obstruction, increased production, or reduced absorption of CSF. The majority of cases of hydrocephalus occur as a result of CSF obstruction. Regardless of the cause, the secondary effects of hydrocephalus on the CNS are potentially the same. The secondary effects result from transependymal

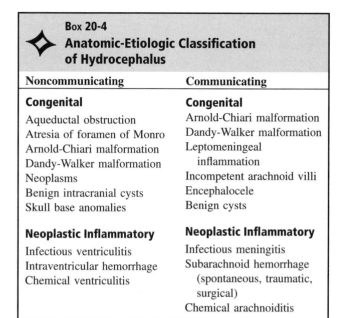

Box 20-4

Anatomic-Etiologic Classification of Hydrocephalus

Noncommunicating	Communicating
Congenital	**Congenital**
Aqueductal obstruction	Arnold-Chiari malformation
Atresia of foramen of Monro	Dandy-Walker malformation
Arnold-Chiari malformation	Leptomeningeal
Dandy-Walker malformation	inflammation
Neoplasms	Incompetent arachnoid villi
Benign intracranial cysts	Encephalocele
Skull base anomalies	Benign cysts
Neoplastic Inflammatory	**Neoplastic Inflammatory**
Infectious ventriculitis	Infectious meningitis
Intraventricular hemorrhage	Subarachnoid hemorrhage
Chemical ventriculitis	(spontaneous, traumatic,
	surgical)
	Chemical arachnoiditis

From Carey CM, Trillous MW, Walker ML: In Cheek WR et al, eds: *Pediatric neurosurgery,* Philadelphia, 1994, WB Saunders, p 189.

flow of CSF and from increased ICP. With acute hydrocephalus, increased CSF pressure causes enlargement of the lateral ventricles, followed by enlargement of the third and fourth ventricles. Spontaneous rupture of the ventricles has been reported.[140] Increased CSF pressure also splits the ependymal lining of the ventricles, enhancing its permeability. The net result is increased transependymal leak of CSF into the surrounding white matter. Interstitial edema is likely the cause of cerebral atrophy and may contribute to thinning of the cerebral mantle (gray matter covering the cerebral hemispheres). Cerebral mantle thinning also occurs from compression of the dilated ventricles and loss of extracellular water.[141] The increased mass effect and increased CSF pressure of hydrocephalus can also reduce CBF to ischemic levels, and herniation of intracranial contents may occur.

Clinical Manifestations. The clinical manifestations of hydrocephalus depend on several factors: age of the patient, degree of obstruction, acuteness of progression, and cause or associated neuropathology. In the infant, the most common clinical sign of hydrocephalus is enlargement of the head. In older children, focal neurologic signs are more common. Box 20-5 lists common clinical manifestations of hydrocephalus in infants and older children. Associated findings that may indicate infantile hydrocephalus include hypotonicity of the lower extremities, decreased active leg motion, and ankle clonus.[138]

Diagnostic studies used to confirm the clinical presentation of hydrocephalus include a number of neuroimaging procedures, as well as a variety of secondary procedures. The primary neuroimaging techniques used to diagnose hydrocephalus are CT scanning (Fig. 20-7), nuclear MRI, and cranial ultrasonography. Secondary studies used to gather prognostic data include CSF analysis, radionuclide studies, ICP monitoring, perfusion and infusion studies, neuropsychologic tests, and CBF studies.

Infant	Child
Increased head circumference	Nausea
"Setting sun" eyes	Vomiting
Spread sutures	Headache
Tense fontanelle(s)	Alteration in consciousness
Increased transillumination	Incontinence
"Cracked pot" sound	Papilledema
Dilated scalp veins	Diplopia
Nonspecific signs	Seizures
Irritability	Cranial nerve palsies
Lethargy	
Poor feeding	
Vomiting	
High-pitched cry	
Seizures	
Alteration in consciousness	

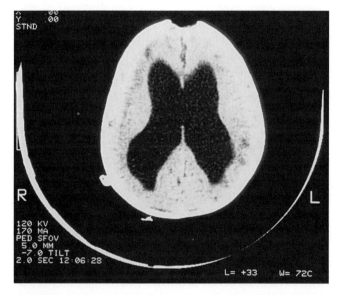

Fig. 20-7 Computed tomographic scan of infant with hydrocephalus, showing selection dilation of occipital horns. (From McLaurin RL, Epstein F, Schut L et al, eds: *Pediatric neurosurgery: surgery of the developing brain,* Philadelphia, 1982, WB Saunders.)

Collaborative Management. Definitive treatment of hydrocephalus is to remove the obstruction. Although removal is the ideal, it is possible in only a small number of patients who have a resectable cyst or tumor. More commonly, the obstruction is bypassed with a shunt, and the majority of children with hydrocephalus are treated with a valve-regulated shunt. Many commercially available systems exist, and all have three major components: proximal catheter, distal catheter, and valve. The proximal catheter is most often placed in the lateral ventricle to drain CSF. The distal catheter can be placed in a number of receptacles; however, the preferred site is the peritoneal cavity, and the

second is the right atrium. The last component of the shunt is a one-way valve that controls the flow of CSF from the proximal catheter into the distal catheter. A description of available shunt systems has been reviewed.[142]

Reservoirs or flush chambers can be added to most shunt systems. Flush devices are either single chambered or double chambered and can be used for withdrawing CSF, instilling medications or contrast material in the ventricles, and assessing shunt patency. Most reservoirs connect directly to the proximal ventricular catheter and provide access to the ventricles for instillation of medications and dye and for withdrawal of CSF. Unlike flush chambers, reservoirs cannot be flushed.[142]

For the most part, medical management of hydrocephalus has not been helpful. Intravenous mannitol (Osmitrol) and urea (Ureaphil) have been used to decrease brain extracellular fluid, but they are not practical agents for long-term management. One study reported a success rate of greater than 50% in avoiding a shunt with the use of acetazolamide (Diamox) and furosemide (Lasix) in infants.[143] This combination therapy decreases CSF production; however, it is reserved for patients with borderline or slowly progressing hydrocephalus.

Nursing management of the infant or child with suspected hydrocephalus begins with obtaining a baseline neurologic assessment. Particular emphasis is placed on head circumference (in children younger than 2 years of age) and on progressive signs and symptoms of increased ICP. The nutritional status of the patient may be compromised because of anorexia and vomiting. Nutritional intake, fluid and electrolytes, and weight are closely monitored. Supportive nursing care includes frequent position changes and head support to prevent neck strain, discomfort, and pressure sores on the scalp.

Nursing care after a shunt insertion is similar to that for all patients following craniotomy. Ventricular shunting is not without complications and requires close nursing surveillance. The most common complication is mechanical malfunction from obstruction or disconnection of the component parts of the shunt.[144] Separation of the ventricular catheter from the rest of the shunt system has become less frequent as one-piece ventricular catheter reservoirs are used. Malfunction of a shunting device can produce signs and symptoms of increased ICP. If the obstruction is intermittent, the clinical manifestations may also be intermittent.

The second most common complication is infection. Infection may occur external to the shunt device, involving the subcutaneous tissue, or it may be internal (i.e., within the system). Signs and symptoms of external infection include the usual systemic signs of acute infection, as well as a detectable reddened streak along the subcutaneous tract of all or a portion of the shunt. Internal infection involves the CSF and is usually less virulent with less acute inflammation.[144] Peritonitis and meningitis may develop. Managing shunt infections is variable and involves a combination of systemic and interventricular antibiotics with or without the removal of the shunt. Often the shunt is externalized, and antibiotics are administered into the shunt for a short period.

Once the infection resolves, a new shunt is surgically placed.

First reported in 1979, latex allergy is a real public health concern. Approximately 65% of patients with spina bifida have a type I latex allergy,[145] and consequently, latex precautions have been instituted for this group. Because patients with spina bifida comprise a significant population with hydrocephalus, maintaining latex precautions has become routine in their nursing care. See Chapter 16 for a detailed discussion of nursing care related to latex allergy.

TRAUMATIC BRAIN INJURY

TBI is defined by the National Head Injury Foundation[146] as an insult to the brain, not of a degenerative or congenital nature, but caused by an external physical force, that may produce a diminished or altered state of consciousness, which results in impairment of cognitive abilities or physical functioning. It can also result in the disturbance of behavioral or emotional functioning. These impairments may be either temporary or permanent and cause partial or total functional disability or psychosocial maladjustment.

Beyond the first year of life, head injury represents the leading cause of death in children.[147,148] Epidemiology, clinical manifestations, and description of specific head injuries are discussed in Chapter 28.

Pathogenesis. CNS development is incomplete at birth and continues to mature over several years. As a consequence, the mechanisms of injury, specific types of injury, and response to injury are age specific. By far, the majority of acute intracranial injuries in children originate from a closed head injury. In contrast to adults, penetrating TBI with direct tissue disruption is less common in children. Although the most common cause of a TBI in adults is from motor vehicle and motorcycle accidents, infants most often sustain a TBI from a fall or domestic abuse. The older child is commonly injured from a motor vehicle accident as a passenger, pedestrian, or cyclist.

The CNS of the infant and young child is not only quantitatively different from that of adolescents and adults, but it is qualitatively different as well. The immature CNS is thought to respond to traumatic injury differently than the mature CNS. In general, closed head injuries that produce a diffuse injury are more common in children. In contrast, brain contusions, focal parenchymal lesions, intracerebral hematomas, and diffuse brain injury (immediate impact type) are more common in adults.[149]

TBIs are most commonly classified according to chronologic events. Primary injuries are those sustained at the time of impact or within milliseconds of the impact; external mechanical forces cause physical or functional disruption of brain tissue. Secondary injuries are physiologic conditions that develop in response to postinjury factors or from extraneous or iatrogenic causes. For example, a severe primary TBI can set into motion complex, interrelated cellular responses, such as alterations in vasoregulation, disruption of the blood-brain barrier, and release of neurotransmitters and neurochemical mediators.[25] Extraneous or iatrogenic causes of secondary injury include hypotension, hypovolemia, and hypoxia.

The cumulative effect of secondary brain injury is cell death and cerebral edema, with or without elevated ICP. Specific clinical conditions producing increased ICP in infants and children are cerebral hyperemia, hypoxia, and hypercarbia (increase CBV); cerebral edema, hematomas, and contusions (increase brain tissue); and subarachnoid hemorrhage obstructing CSF flow and absorption (increase CSF).

Skull radiographs have been used more often in the past to evaluate a child with TBI. However, of more concern than skull disruption is intracranial damage. Thus, for those patients who require CT scanning, skull radiographs usually add very little to the neurodiagnostic evaluation, and vital therapy should not be delayed to obtain them. Skull radiographs can complement the CT scan with some pathologic conditions (e.g., to evaluate those with depressed skull fractures and child abuse or to localize foreign bodies). The CT scan is generally preferred over MRI because of its shorter examination time, ease of monitoring unstable patients, lower cost, and more accurate diagnosis of acute subarachnoid hemorrhage or acute parenchymal hemorrhage if taken within 72 hours after the injury.[150] MRI is useful in the subacute or chronic stages and to assess diffuse axonal injury and brainstem injury.[151]

Collaborative Management. Principles of emergency management of the child with a TBI are similar to those for any resuscitation: respiratory and cardiovascular status are of primary concern. In a patient with an altered level of consciousness or suspected severe injury, intracranial hypertension is assumed, and precautions are taken to avoid further increases in ICP. If the child's airway is patent, spontaneous hyperventilation usually occurs. Intubation may be necessary to control a compromised airway or to provide controlled hyperventilation. Sedation and paralysis are used to avoid increases in ICP induced by the intubation procedure. An ETco$_2$ monitor is helpful to ensure adequate trending of CO$_2$. If intracranial hypertension is suspected, an ICP monitoring device is inserted in the emergency department. Mannitol is commonly administered in the early treatment of head injuries when elevated ICP is present or suspected. A CT scan is obtained as soon as the patient's condition is stabilized.

Beyond the resuscitation phase, management is directed toward correcting the underlying pathologic condition, when possible. When intracranial hypertension results from a hematoma, surgery is usually indicated. More often in children, TBI is diffusely distributed throughout the cerebral hemispheres and brainstem. A variety of therapies are available to treat intracranial hypertension, as discussed earlier. A specific regimen is selected based on the underlying cause.

Early seizures (within 7 days of injury) are a frequent complication in children following TBI. However, they are thought to be an acute reaction to the injury rather than epilepsy (i.e., unprovoked seizures).[152] Anticonvulsants are not usually given for an isolated, self-limited posttraumatic seizure but are indicated for recurrent or late seizures, severe cortical contusions, cerebral lacerations, or a prior history of epilepsy. Phenytoin (Dilantin) is used more often than phenobarbital (Luminal) because it produces less CNS depression. In the patient with preexisting severe CNS depression (e.g., Glasgow coma scale [GCS] score of less than 5), phenobarbital may be used because further CNS depression is irrelevant.

Other systemic complications observed in children after a TBI include neurogenic pulmonary edema, SIADH secretion, and infection. The exact mechanism for the development of neurogenic pulmonary edema is unclear. Treatment involves correcting the underlying neuropathologic state. Respiratory management may require ventilatory support with PEEP, diuretics, pulmonary toilet, and fluid restriction.

Signs and symptoms of SIADH include decreased urine output, hyponatremia, increased ICP, falling Pao_2, and decreased serum osmolality (sometimes difficult to recognize with mannitol administration). Serum and urine electrolytes and osmolality levels are monitored closely. Fluids are often restricted, and intake and output are accurately recorded.

All patients with traumatic stress are at risk for infection. Antibiotics are not routinely administered but are reserved for patients with penetrating injuries or open fractures. Meticulous care of invasive lines, maximizing nutritional support, and close surveillance for signs of a local and systemic infection help prevent or reverse an infectious process.

The key to preventing secondary brain injury in the child is control of hypoxia, hypercarbia, hypotension, and increased ICP. If the patient has inadequate oxygenation, ventilation, or perfusion, the neurologic assessment is delayed until they are restored.

The next step is to obtain a brief but pertinent history. Because the majority of TBIs are closed injuries, they are often anticipated based on history and mechanism of injury. Specific questions inquire how the injury occurred; where the patient was found; what (if any) type of restraint was used; whether the patient was unconscious when found, or if there was a lucid interval; if were drugs ingested; and whether the patient required resuscitation. A brief but thorough neurologic examination is performed, followed by a complete systems review. Repeated assessments are performed during and after the initial management phase.

Beyond the initial stabilization phase, care is focused on correcting the primary TBI and preventing secondary injury from intracranial hypertension, hypoxia, and ischemia. Because operative lesions are less common in children, management is primarily directed toward controlling ICP.

As with all patients with intracranial hypertension, the guiding principles for management are to control the three components of the intracranial space: blood, brain tissue, and CSF. Nursing interventions to decrease CBV include promoting venous outflow from the cranium, maintaining normothermia, and controlling seizures. Nursing interventions to control increased brain bulk include administration and monitoring of hyperosmotic agents and diuretics, routine postoperative craniotomy care for operative lesions,

and close monitoring of respiratory and cardiovascular status (to prevent hypoxia, ischemia, and cerebral edema). Nursing interventions directed toward controlling CSF include management and monitoring of CSF drainage (ventriculostomy) and administration and monitoring of medications to inhibit CSF production.

Complications of a TBI include gastric dysfunction, fluid and electrolyte imbalances, and malnutrition. Stress ulcers and paralytic ileus may occur in the head-injured patient. Gastric pH is monitored closely, and antacids are administered to correct low pH or maintain pH at a level above 4. Paralytic ileus is common in children after trauma and may compromise diaphragmatic movement. Gastric decompression with a orogastric tube may be required, but caution is used to prevent regurgitation and laryngospasm. An orogastric tube is used in place of a nasogastric tube when head and facial trauma is present and cribriform plate fracture may be a possibility.

Fluid and electrolyte imbalances may occur from volume resuscitation, diuretics, hyperosmotic agents, and SIADH. Fluid intake and output are closely monitored, as are serum and urine electrolyte levels, serum and urine osmolality, urine specific gravity, and blood component counts. With fluid overload, ICP is monitored for elevation, and the pulmonary system is assessed for the development of edema.

Patients with a severe TBI often develop a hypermetabolic response, resulting in negative nitrogen balance and loss of lean body mass. Generally, nutritional support is instituted as soon as the patient's condition is stabilized, with the primary goals of maintaining lean body mass and preventing complications. Enteral feedings are desired as the first choice of nutritional support.[153] If the patient is at risk for pulmonary aspiration related to ineffective airway protective reflexes, alternative therapies such as parenteral nutrition are considered.

Because accidental injuries are often thought to be preventable, families of victims with a TBI are at risk for family dysfunction. Whether or not feelings are justified, parents often feel guilty, ashamed, and defensive. The degree to which a family handles this situational crisis depends on many variables, such as age and developmental level of the child, severity of the injury, and preexisting family personalities and relationships. It is important that the family receive multidisciplinary support. Accurate explanations regarding the child's injuries and subsequent care are provided, directed toward dispelling irrational fears and guilt. Chapter 3 presents specific approaches in supporting the family.

HYPOXIC ISCHEMIC ENCEPHALOPATHY

Basic and advanced life support techniques have been increasingly successful in reversing cardiopulmonary arrest. However, irreversible brain damage continues to occur in a significant number of patients following the return of spontaneous circulation. As a result, cardiopulmonary-cerebral resuscitation (CPCR) and its science, reanimatology, have emerged to further elucidate the pathophysiology, reversibility, and treatment of patients suffering cardiopulmonary arrest.

Cardiopulmonary arrest is caused by a number of insults, which include asphyxiation, exsanguination, ventricular fibrillation, and electromechanical dissociation. In adults, primary cardiac arrest usually results from ventricular fibrillation associated with myocardial dysfunction because of coronary artery disease. In children, the usual event is a cardiopulmonary arrest from acute asphyxiation (e.g., airway obstruction or apnea). Asphyxial cardiac arrest is more injurious to the CNS than primary cardiac arrest because of the period of hypoxic tissue acidosis that exists before cardiac standstill.[154]

Terminology

Ischemia and hypoxia are two mechanisms that can cause irreversible damage to the brain. Ischemia refers to a reduction in blood flow. The reduction may be global or focal and complete or incomplete. Global ischemia involves the entire brain, and focal ischemia involves only a portion. With global or focal ischemia, perfusion can be completely absent, as with total circulatory arrest, or incomplete (i.e., on a continuum between perfusion and total absence, such as might occur with hypotension or bradycardia). Pathologic signs of decreased CBF can be detected when flow falls below 25 to 30 ml/min/100 g tissue; however, compensation usually occurs. When CBF falls below this level, a critical infarct threshold is reached, and neuronal function will cease. The exact ischemic threshold varies among patients and depends on many factors (e.g., preexisting injury, age, medications).[155,156]

Hypoxia refers to a reduction in the delivery of oxygen. Oxygen delivery can be reduced from a number of causes, such as anemia (anemic hypoxia), low cardiac output (ischemic hypoxia), severe pulmonary disease (hypoxic hypoxia), and carbon monoxide poisoning (anoxic hypoxia).

Clinically, hypoxia and ischemia are most often seen together. In the adult with primary cardiac arrest, respirations stop shortly after cardiac standstill or electromechanical dissociation. In the child, asphyxia is the usual cause of cardiopulmonary arrest. Typically, a prolonged period of anoxic or hypoxic perfusion of the brain occurs before cardiac standstill. Global cerebral ischemia is the result of cardiopulmonary arrest, regardless of the events that precipitate the arrest.

The terms used to describe hypoxic brain insults and cerebral resuscitation are familiar. Primary and secondary cerebral injury, discussed in relation to traumatic brain injury, are also used when describing brain insults from hypoxia and ischemia. In both situations, the definition of the terms is the same. A primary brain injury describes the immediate damage to brain tissue, and secondary injury refers to the subsequent insults to brain tissue in response to the primary injury.

The mainstay of treatment for hypoxic ischemic brain injury is cerebral resuscitation, that is, application of therapeutic measures to prevent a secondary brain injury. In contrast to cerebral resuscitation, cerebral protection describes prophylactic measures to prevent a primary injury. An example is deep hypothermia used during circulatory arrest for congenital heart surgery.

Pathogenesis

Over the last two decades, numerous studies have examined the pathophysiologic consequences of complete global ischemia.[156-158] However, interpretation and comparison of these studies remain difficult for several reasons. First, the majority of research to date has been performed on animals of various species, limiting application to human subjects. Second, some studies do not clearly differentiate between asphyxial and cardiac arrest. Third, some studies do not differentiate between in-hospital and prehospital arrest. In short, how precisely these experimental studies translate to the clinical situation, especially in patients with a developing CNS, remains unclear.

Laboratory and clinical studies identify numerous pathophysiologic processes following complete global ischemia to the brain.[158-161] These biochemical changes begin with the initial ischemic anoxic period during total circulatory arrest and may continue with resumption of normal perfusion pressure (reperfusion injury). The specific mechanisms of injury include energy failure, calcium-mediated injury, and accumulation of neurotoxic substances (e.g., intracellular proteases, oxygen radicals, free fatty acids).

Ischemic-Anoxic Injury. The biochemical changes that occur in the brain during global cerebral ischemia result from the depletion of vital metabolic substrates and accumulation of toxic byproducts. The brain requirement for oxygen and glucose is very high compared with that for other organs. However, the storage capacity of these substrates is very limited. With the cessation of circulation, oxygen is depleted immediately, but glucose continues to be supplied briefly from the breakdown of brain glycogen stores. However, glycolysis in the brain is inefficient, and neuronal death occurs quickly. Lactic acidosis, which results from anaerobic metabolism, contributes to cellular damage. Hydrogen ion accumulation may cause disruption of adenosine triphosphate (ATP)–dependent ionic pumps and intracellular homeostasis.[162] There is a loss of intracellular potassium with influxes of sodium, chloride, and calcium. Calcium influx causes uncoupling of oxidative phosphorylation and a reduction in ATP production. Lipid peroxidation also occurs with accumulation of free fatty acids. The combination of the aforementioned processes forms necrotizing cascades.[154] If complete circulatory arrest continues without reperfusion, uniform autolysis of the brain results after about 1 hour.[163] Fig. 20-8 is a schematic drawing of proposed mechanisms by which global cerebral ischemia may cause CNS injury.

Reperfusion Injury. In addition to injury that results from the ischemic phase, evidence also shows that additional injury occurs during reperfusion. Postischemic injury is believed to result from a number of interrelated pathophysiologic processes, including CBF alterations, calcium influx, increased oxygen free radical production, and microcirculatory obstruction. These secondary neurotoxic

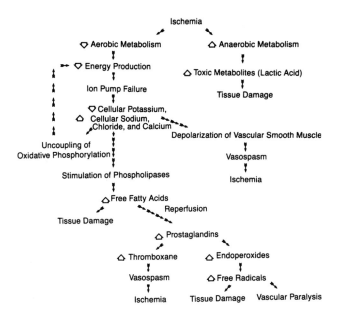

Fig. 20-8   Proposed mechanisms by which global ischemia may cause irreversible vascular and tissue injury. (From Kirsch JR et al: Current concepts in brain resuscitation, *Arch Intern Med* 146:1413-1419, 1986. Copyright 1986 by American Medical Association.)

the outer orbit, making them very reactive. Because of their reactivity, they are also short lived, making direct measurement difficult. During reperfusion following an episode of ischemia, an increase is thought to occur in the production of oxygen free radicals from several pathways. In short, oxygen free radicals undergo a reaction enhanced by superoxide dismutase and form hydrogen peroxide. Hydroxyl radicals eventually form and cause a cascade of biochemical changes that produce widespread cellular injury.[167]

Safar[163] also hypothesizes that blood sludges during the ischemic phase (stasis) and deteriorates. Once circulation is resumed, obstruction of the microcirculation occurs from red blood cell deformity, aggregates of thrombocytes and granulocytes, calcium-induced vasospasm, and mediators of coagulopathy.[154,165] Thus hypoperfusion or no perfusion exists locally or diffusely, producing more cellular damage.

Critical Care Management

Assessment.   Following global cerebral ischemia, historical data are collected from individuals witnessing the events leading to the cardiopulmonary arrest. In addition to routine questions concerning the patient's present and past medical history, details are obtained regarding the cardiopulmonary arrest and resuscitation. Specific questions include duration of apnea and circulatory arrest, precipitating event (e.g., aspiration, trauma, cardiac arrest), duration of basic and advanced life support, body temperature, and metabolic status (if hospitalized). The prehospital and in-hospital resuscitation records should also be reviewed for specific interventions and pharmacologic agents administered.

Clinical assessment of the patient begins with examination of the cardiopulmonary status. A good neurologic outcome depends on adequate oxygenation and cardiac output. Cardiopulmonary status is assessed in the usual fashion.

Once oxygenation, ventilation, and circulation are restored, the child's neurologic status can be assessed. Depending on specific variables of the global cerebral ischemia (e.g., duration of ischemia, type of arrest, metabolic status), the patient's neurologic status may range from complete orientation to coma. The comatose patient should be systematically assessed, starting with level of consciousness and progressing to motor function, respiratory patterns, pupillary signs, and ocular movements. Because a number of resuscitative therapies and conditions can alter the child's neurologic response (e.g., catecholamines, atropine, hypothermia, chemical paralysis), special consideration is required when interpreting results.

Routine ICP monitoring is not recommended after global cerebral ischemia; therefore detection of intracranial hypertension is based on clinical manifestations.[168] Increases in ICP occur transiently during the hyperemic phase of reperfusion but quickly return to normal.[163] Increased ICP may occur more often following asphyxial arrest (e.g., near-drowning); however, the threshold for poor outcome appears to be lower than the threshold for increased ICP

cascades often negate any beneficial effect that occurs with resumption of CBF.

A characteristic pattern of CBF following global cerebral ischemia has been supported by several studies using different animal models and different species.[157-159] Safar[163] describes the resumption of CBF progressing through four stages: (1) immediate multifocal absence of reperfusion ("no-flow phenomenon"); (2) transient increase in CBF (hyperemia) above the preischemic level lasting 15 to 30 minutes; (3) delayed, prolonged global hypoperfusion lasting hours to days; and (4) resolution, continuance, or worsening. The magnitude of postischemic hyperemia followed by hypoperfusion appears to be related to the duration of the ischemic insult. The combination of diffuse hyperemia and loss of vasoreactivity to $Paco_2$ is associated with poor outcome.[164] The ischemic threshold in adults as determined by CBF is reported to be below 10 ml/min/100 g of tissue.[165] At this level, ionic pump failure occurs, which results in cell death. The ischemic threshold in infants and young children is unknown.

Calcium influx associated with cerebral ischemia also occurs in smooth muscle cells of the cerebral vasculature. This influx is believed to contribute, in part, to postischemic hypoperfusion by causing vasospasm in the smooth muscle of cerebral vessels.[165] Other hypothetical detrimental effects of increased intracellular calcium in the brain include neurotransmitter release with neuronal excitability and postischemic hypermetabolism; energy depletion during reperfusion; and free fatty-acid release, which may cause enzymatic dysfunction.[166]

Oxygen-derived free radicals have also been implicated in reperfusion injury. Free radicals are molecules or molecular fragments that have an extra unpaired electron in

development.[169] That is, when increased ICP does develop, it most likely reflects the severity of the primary insult and not an opportunity to prevent secondary injury.

To prevent further uncoupling of supply (CBF) and demand (cerebral metabolic rate of oxygen [$CMRO_2$]), the presence of seizure activity is monitored closely. Body temperature is assessed for hyperthermia, and adequacy of pain control is optimized.

Airway patency and the ability to protect the airway are determined. Serial ABG values quantify the adequacy of oxygenation and ventilation. Pulse oximetry and $ETco_2$ monitoring are also helpful in assessing respiratory status.

Cardiovascular status is monitored closely for hypertension, hypotension, and dysrhythmias. Invasive hemodynamic monitoring is necessary if the cardiovascular system is unstable. Myocardial hypoxic damage is assessed with serial electrocardiograms (ECGs) and cardiac isoenzyme determinations. When induced hemodilution is used, the hematocrit level is monitored frequently.

Urine output is assessed, and specific gravity is monitored. Serum electrolytes are monitored at regular intervals. SIADH secretion is detected by a drop in urine output, decreased serum osmolality, and hyponatremia. Infants may quickly become hypoglycemic following cardiopulmonary arrest; therefore serum or capillary glucose is monitored.

Neurodiagnostic tests are often helpful in further assessing the child's neurologic status after cardiopulmonary arrest. The EEG is extremely sensitive to cerebral cortical hypoxia or ischemia and can provide prognostic information. Slight to moderate insults are demonstrated on the EEG as changes in peak frequency or asymmetric rhythms from homotopic regions in each hemisphere. With a severe hypoxic-ischemic insult, there is progressive flattening of the EEG tracing. Subcortical function can be assessed using evoked potential techniques.[156] CBF can be assessed in the postresuscitation phase using a variety of techniques. Limitations of each of these techniques must be considered when evaluating the patient and the response to therapy. Somatosensory and auditory evoked potentials, as well as CSF biochemical markers (e.g., lactate, creatinine phosphokinase, BB-isoenzyme, lactate dehydrogenase) can provide important adjunctive information.

Collaborative Management. A multitude of interrelated biochemical changes have been identified during and following global cerebral ischemia. Consequently, the efficacy of traditional approaches to patient management during the postischemic phase is questioned, and novel approaches remain to be supported by clinical research.

Traditional. The single best therapy to treat global cerebral ischemia is prevention. Often, nothing can be done to prevent the initial cardiopulmonary arrest, but rapid response and effective intervention can reduce the cerebral ischemic time. Thus, basic and advanced pediatric life support are the first steps in cerebral resuscitation.

The foundation for good neurointensive care following the ischemic phase is to ensure adequate oxygenation, ventilation, perfusion, and fluid and electrolyte homeostasis. In addition to postarrest care, specific interventions to overcome the multifocal no-reflow phenomenon have been

recommended. Safar[163] suggests induced moderate arterial hypertension for 1 to 5 minutes with restoration of circulation. Beyond this period, normotension is maintained with plasma volume expansion and intravenous vasoactive medications. Administering fluids with glucose is controversial in patients with cerebral ischemia. Several studies have shown that hyperglycemia may enhance cerebral ischemic injury.[170-172] Blood glucose is monitored closely; hypoglycemia is avoided in the neonate, and hyperglycemia is avoided in the older child.[168] Ischemia can also worsen with seizures; therefore they are controlled immediately with anticonvulsants.

Hyperventilation. Although intracranial hypertension is not always present after global cerebral ischemia, ICP-directed management continues to be used.[163,166] In the past, induced hyperventilation was one of the most frequently recommended interventions in cerebral resuscitation protocols. However, the benefit of this intervention is unproven. Theoretically, hyperventilation may reduce CBV during the hyperemic phase; on the other hand, it may produce further ischemia during the hypoperfusion phase. To date, no evidence shows that hyperventilation has a sustained beneficial effect, and its use is avoided.

Barbiturates. Barbiturates have been shown to have a beneficial effect in controlling ICP and seizures. However, until recently, the effect of barbiturates in humans after global cerebral ischemia was unknown. In the early 1980s, a multiinstitutional trial was devised to determine the risks and benefits of thiopental loading in 262 comatose cardiac arrest patients.[173] Although barbiturates may be effective for focal cerebral ischemia or for cerebral protection in certain situations (e.g., coronary artery bypass), the results of this study do not support the routine use of thiopental after cardiac arrest.[165,174]

Experimental. A number of novel therapeutic interventions have been proposed to treat global cerebral ischemia; however, the interventions remain in the experimental stage. These interventions stem from current understanding of the pathophysiologic processes described earlier.

Cerebral Blood Flow. A major emphasis in cerebral resuscitative therapies is to improve cerebral microcirculatory flow, especially during hypoperfusion. Therapies studied to enhance blood flow have been directed toward decreasing coagulation and blood viscosity. Although heparin prophylaxis has not been widely supported, some protocols recommend moderate hemodilution.[156,175]

Calcium Antagonists. Intracellular calcium influx has been hypothesized to cause neuronal injury by various mechanisms. As a result, numerous studies have investigated the potential beneficial effects of calcium antagonists. The most common experimental agents include flunarizine, lidoflazine, and nimodipine. Of the three, nimodipine has had the most encouraging results.[176] Use of these drugs remains investigational.[177]

Free Radical Scavengers. Because oxygen-derived free radicals have been hypothesized to be mediators of neuronal injury during reperfusion, the efficacy of free radical scavengers has been studied in animals. Some preliminary reports have been encouraging and have stimulated interest

Chapter 20 Neurologic Critical Care Problems **719**

in the field.[178,179] Limitations of these agents include a short half-life, rapid rate of free radical reactions, and difficulty of some agents in crossing the blood-brain barrier.[180]

Selective Brain Cooling. The beneficial effects of prophylactic hypothermia as a cerebral protective therapy is unquestioned. The same neuroprotective benefits have also been documented in patients with TBI and cerebral ischemia. However, systemic hypothermia is not a benign procedure, and significant deleterious systemic side effects may occur. To avoid these systemic side effects, selective mild brain cooling has been attempted.[181-183] However, the results are conflicting. For example, Park and associates[182] found systemic hypothermia to be more neuroprotective that selective brain cooling. Further study in children is required before widespread use of this therapy is recommended.

Numerous investigational therapies have been proposed to manage global cerebral ischemia (Box 20-6). However, the best therapeutic interventions have not yet been determined.

Nursing Care. Because cerebral resuscitation therapies remain experimental with less than enthusiastic results, the single best approach to preventing neuronal damage is to minimize the ischemic time. The significance of the prompt recognition of impending cardiopulmonary arrest and immediate intervention to restore circulation and breathing cannot be overstated.

Once circulation and breathing are restored, efforts to maintain hemodynamic stability may be required to ensure adequate CBF. Vasopressors and volume expanders are titrated to achieve optimal cardiac output. Dysrhythmias are treated promptly.

Secondary hypoxic hypoxia is prevented. Controlled ventilation with muscle paralysis may be required to ensure adequate oxygenation. Frequent turning and chest physiotherapy are used to avoid atelectasis and promote drainage of pulmonary secretions.

If intracranial hypertension develops, nursing care (as described earlier) to control ICP and improve CBF is instituted. Seizures are treated promptly with anticonvulsants, hyperthermia is reversed with antipyretics, and pain is controlled with analgesics.

Urine output is greater than 5 ml/kg/hr, serum electrolytes levels are in a normal range, and glucose is at a normal level. Stress ulcers are prevented with administration of antacids. Nutrition is supported with enteral and parenteral fluids as appropriate. Infection control is maintained with close surveillance of invasive lines, body temperature, and blood cell counts.

General supportive care is required. Skin integrity is maintained with frequent position changes and skin protective devices (e.g., sheepskin, heel pads). Passive range of motion and other physical therapy help to maintain muscle tone and joint mobility. Artificial tears are used to maintain eye moisture.

NEAR DROWNING

Various terms are used to describe submersion injuries. *Drowning* refers to death by asphyxiation after submersion in water or some other type of liquid. *Near drowning* is the term used to describe survival for at least 24 hours after a submersion episode. The term *secondary drowning* describes delayed death or complications from pulmonary insufficiency after a submersion episode.[184,185] *Dry drowning* describes an entity in which the drowning victim never aspirates water into the lungs or aspirates only a very small amount. It occurs in approximately 10% to 15% of all drowning incidents.

Drowning is the second leading cause of accidental death in children and adolescents 0 to 14 years of age.[186] It is the leading cause of death resulting from injury in children younger than 5 years of age.[187] Within the pediatric population, the two age groups at greatest risk are toddlers and teenagers. As with most accidental injuries, males predominate. By far, the majority of drowning occurs in fresh water, with the backyard swimming pool presenting the greatest risk. Domestic drowning (e.g., bathtub, hot tub, buckets of water, toilet) is greatest in infants and preschoolers. Drowning in lakes and rivers is greatest in teenagers.[1]

Pathogenesis. Karpovich,[188] in his classic study with animals, described the sequence of events during drowning. Following submersion, there is an initial period of struggle and panic with a small amount of water entering the throat causing laryngospasm. Subsequently, large amounts of water are swallowed with vomiting and aspiration of water. In a small percentage of cases (10% to 15%), laryngospasm persists without aspiration of water.[189]

In the past, the type of fluid (fresh versus salt) aspirated was thought to be important in terms of fluid and electrolyte balance. However, clinical information on near-drowning patients does not support this earlier animal research. The discrepancy between the laboratory and the clinical setting

Box 20-6
Investigational Therapies for Cerebral Resuscitation

Hemodilution
Barbiturates
Calcium antagonists
  Flunarizine
  Lidoflazine
  Nimodipine
Glutamate antagonists
  Competitive
  Noncompetitive
Free radical scavengers
  Superoxide dismutase
  21-Aminosteroids
Opiate receptor antagonists
Artificial blood substitutes
Dimethyl sulfoxide (DMSO)
Indomethacin
Cardiopulmonary bypass
Hypertension
Diazepam
Hyperbaric oxygen

is attributed to the fact that humans do not aspirate as large a volume of fluid as was used to simulate drowning in animal studies.

Dramatic circulatory changes have been noted in some animals when submerged. These circulatory changes are commonly called the "diving seal reflex." A redistribution of blood flow occurs with selective shunting away from the cutaneous and splanchnic vascular beds to the coronary and cerebral circulations. Blood pressure is maintained, but heart rate drops significantly.[190] Similar changes, to a lesser degree, were also noted in humans with submersion of the face and were thought to be protective.[191] The diving reflex may be enhanced by cold water submersion and fear.[192]

Hypothermia is commonly defined as a core temperature of less than 35° C. Controlled hypothermia is known to have a protective effect against cerebral hypoxemia. Based on a recent review of prolonged (greater than or equal to 15 minutes) ice-water submersions, several cases of survival with good neurologic outcome were reported.[193] However, many more cases of death from ice-water submersion go unreported. The belief is that the accidental hypothermia that occurs in a few reported miraculous cases may simulate therapeutic hypothermia, which is routinely induced in a controlled setting and thus has a protective effect.

The initial pathologic event during submersion is anoxia. If the patient's airway is not resuscitated promptly, cardiac standstill occurs, causing ischemia. Potentially, every organ in the body can sustain injury from the combination of anoxia and ischemia. However, the CNS is most vulnerable and is primarily associated with outcome. The multiorgan effects of asphyxia are diagrammed in Fig. 20-9.

After submersion, anoxia occurs, but cardiac output usually continues for a brief time. During this period, blood continues to flow to the brain, delivering glucose and other nutrients in the absence of oxygen. Anaerobic metabolism develops, producing lactic acid and other toxic waste products. Once cardiac standstill occurs, all blood flow and substrate delivery cease and cellular metabolism stops. The extent of neurologic injury depends on the duration of anoxia and ischemia. The pathobiologic processes that occur during ischemia and reperfusion are numerous, interrelated, and not well understood. In severe cases, diffuse neuronal death causes cytotoxic cerebral edema, which leads to a vicious cycle of increased ICP, decreased CBF, ischemia, and further CNS damage.

Regardless of the type of fluid aspirated, pulmonary surfactant is altered with submersion injuries. Fresh water causes dilution of surfactant, whereas salt water causes inactivation; both produce alveolar collapse.[194] Aspiration of stomach contents or contaminated water also produces pulmonary injury. Injury to the pulmonary capillaries and alveolar membranes results in abnormally increased permeability. Protein-rich fluid accumulates in the alveoli, causing pulmonary edema. The end result is intrapulmonary shunting and persistent hypoxia.

The heart, like all organs, can sustain injury from hypoxia and ischemia. Metabolic and electrolyte abnormalities may further compromise myocardial function; however, permanent damage is uncommon. Ventricular fibrillation may occur with severe hypothermia.

Other organs may also sustain damage and further complicate recovery. However, most extracerebral injuries and complications are responsive to therapy and rarely determine survival in a patient with intact neurologic function.

Clinical Manifestations.   A large percentage of patients who have a submersion accident are rescued immediately and either do not require resuscitation or need only brief artificial ventilation. This group of patients usually recovers completely. On the other end of the spectrum, if cardiopulmonary resuscitation (CPR) is not begun promptly or the patient was submerged for a long time, significant anoxic-ischemic injury occurs. The primary clinical prob-

Fig. 20-9   Pathophysiology of anoxia and ischemia during submersion injury. *DIC,* Disseminated intravascular coagulation; *ICP,* intracranial pressure. (From Rogers, MC: *Textbook of pediatric intensive care,* ed 2, Baltimore, 1992, Williams & Wilkins, p 887.)

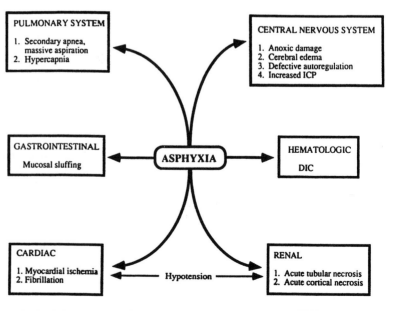
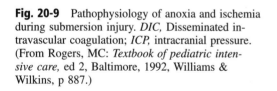

lems for these victims are related to the neurologic and pulmonary systems.

After a mild to moderate submersion injury, neurologic findings most often include restlessness or lethargy and hyporeflexia, all of which are usually transient. Seizures may occur in the acute phase. In contrast, the patient with significant global cerebral ischemia enters the hospital in a coma, is apneic and requires CPR, and has a low serum pH. The depth of coma varies, depending on the extent of neurologic injury. Hypothermia can depress neurologic function. Core temperatures below 30° C result in a clinical picture of brain death (i.e., unconscious, dilated pupils).[192] Signs and symptoms of intracranial hypertension may develop from cytotoxic cerebral edema.

Clinical features of respiratory dysfunction also vary considerably and depend on the degree of anoxic-ischemic injury and the amount and type of fluid aspirated. Common symptoms include cough, shallow rapid breathing, substernal burning, pleuritic chest pain, expectoration of pink frothy sputum, dyspnea, adventitious lung sounds, and shortness of breath.[194a] Apnea may be present with severe submersion injuries but is due primarily to neurologic dysfunction. The chest radiographic findings vary and do not correlate well with other clinical findings. ABG levels are usually abnormal, showing hypoxemia and metabolic acidosis.[195]

Atrial and ventricular fibrillation commonly occurs when the core temperature is lower than 28° C. Acute renal necrosis is the most common renal complication from anoxia and ischemia. Gastric dysfunction is often manifested by abdominal distension, vomiting, and bloody diarrhea.

Collaborative Management.   The primary goal of managing near-drowning victims is prevention of secondary injury. Thus intensive care management has focused efforts in four major areas: cardiopulmonary stabilization, hypothermia correction, ICP maintenance, and cerebral resuscitation.

Once the apneic and pulseless patient is rescued, CPR is begun immediately in hopes of limiting the anoxic-ischemic time. In the PICU, measures are taken to ensure adequate oxygenation, ventilation, and perfusion. Significant hypoxemia is corrected with supplemental oxygen, intubation, and ventilatory support. PEEP is used when pulmonary injury is present because it restores functional residual capacity and improves gas exchange. When high levels of PEEP (10 to 15 cm H_2O) are used, pulmonary artery catheterization is helpful to facilitate hemodynamic support. Diuretics may be required when pulmonary edema is present; however, caution is exercised in the presence of hypovolemia. Serial ABGs, Pao_2/Fio_2 ratio, and $ETco_2$ are often used to assess effectiveness of therapy.[196]

Although fluid restriction is often used to manage cerebral edema, adequate cardiac output and CBF must be ensured. If shock is present, vasopressors and volume expanders may be required. Invasive monitoring is indicated for ongoing assessment, titration of drugs, and determination of therapeutic effectiveness. Cardiac dysrhythmias

usually resolve spontaneously with correction of metabolic abnormalities and hypothermia.

Regardless of the air and water temperature, all patients with a submersion episode are at risk for *postarrest* hypothermia. Children are particularly at risk because of their large body surface area. Hypothermic patients often require rewarming to stabilize their cardiopulmonary status. Hemodynamically stable patients with moderate hypothermia (32° C) can be safely rewarmed with active external rewarming, such as heating blankets, radiant warmer, and warm bath.[192] Active core rewarming with warmed peritoneal or intravenous fluids and inhaled gas is recommended in patients with core temperatures below 32° C to avoid "afterdrop" of core temperature and rewarming shock (see Chapter 14).

In the past, authorities advocated the use of standard intracranial hypertension management (i.e., hyperventilation, mild hypothermia, osmotherapy, diuretics, ICP monitoring, and barbiturates). Despite effective control of ICP, patient outcome did not improve.[197-199] Thus most centers have abandoned routine ICP monitoring and aggressive ICP management. Increases in cerebral metabolism are avoided with aggressive treatment of seizures and maintenance of normothermia.

As described earlier, cerebral resuscitation therapies remain experimental without controlled human clinical trials. Thus protocols for near-drowning victims continue to emphasize excellent cardiopulmonary care.

Obtaining a clear history surrounding the submersion episode is very important in determining injuries and predicting outcome. Specific questions include location of submersion, type of water media, precipitating event (e.g., diving, seizure), duration of submersion, and water temperature. After the rescue, it is important to determine whether a pulse was present, how long apnea persisted, whether spontaneous breathing resumed, when resuscitation began, and what type of resuscitative efforts were performed.

Physical assessment begins with examining airway, breathing, and circulation. This rapid assessment is performed in the usual manner according to American Heart Association guidelines. Core temperature is an important parameter to assess early because of the neurologic depression that occurs with severe hypothermia. Even when the patient clinically appears to have severe irreversible neurologic damage, resuscitation continues until core body temperature is elevated above 32° C.[192] Careful rewarming of the severely hypothermic patient is required to prevent ventricular fibrillation.

Once the patient's cardiopulmonary status is stabilized, a neurologic assessment is performed. Clinical signs and symptoms of intracranial hypertension may develop from cerebral cytotoxic edema. Emphasis is placed on excluding other potential causes of neurologic dysfunction, for example, drug or alcohol intoxication, spinal cord injury, head injury, or hypothermia.

Ongoing respiratory assessment includes monitoring physical assessment findings for significant changes; trending ABGs, $ETco_2$, and pulse oximetry values; and determining effectiveness of ventilatory support. A baseline chest radiograph is obtained early to compare with follow-up radiographs.

Cardiovascular function is determined by assessing heart rate, blood pressure, peripheral pulses, and end-organ perfusion. When the patient is hemodynamically unstable, invasive monitoring of arterial, central, and pulmonary pressures is often required. Continuous infusions of vasopressors require close monitoring of patient response.

Hourly intake and output measurements are necessary to guide fluid therapy and assess renal function. Serum electrolytes, blood urea nitrogen (BUN), creatinine, glucose, and a complete blood count are followed for trends to assess for complications. Abdominal distension, gastric pH, and blood and stool Hematests are used to assess gastrointestinal function.

The goal of nursing management is to maintain or restore adequate oxygenation, ventilation, and perfusion so that secondary injury can be prevented or minimized. Hypoxia is the major threat for secondary injury to organs and is corrected promptly. Supplemental oxygen is the first-line management for respiratory support. If the patient cannot maintain a patent airway or has hypoxemia refractory to supplemental oxygen, manual ventilation followed by intubation is required. The early use of PEEP and generous tidal volumes (15 to 20 ml/kg) are often needed to overcome poor lung compliance.[200] Pulmonary toilet and chest physiotherapy are needed.

Cardiovascular management requires routine assessment of cardiac output. Determination of response to inotropic medications and titration of continuous vasopressor infusions are required in the hemodynamically unstable patient.

Effective management of neurologic damage is yet to be determined. Intracranial hypertension may develop in near-drowning victims. Noninvasive nursing interventions to control ICP are often used to increase adaptive capacity (e.g., HOB elevated 30 degrees, alignment of head and neck). Patient complications that increase cerebral metabolic requirements (e.g., seizures, temperature alterations) are prevented or corrected promptly. A number of other nursing interventions are commonly used in the care of near-drowning victims. They relate to complications that are observed in many pediatric patients with multisystem failure in the intensive care unit. These complications include infection, malnutrition, impaired physical mobility, and renal failure.

BRAIN DEATH

Despite state-of-the art technology and expert collaborative management, some pediatric critical care patients will sustain extensive and irreversible brain damage resulting in death. Before the 1960s, death was defined as the absence of breathing and circulation. However, with the advent of advanced life support techniques and artificial control and maintenance of breathing and circulation, an expanded definition of death was required. Currently in the United States, the diagnosis of death is determined by irreversible cessation of respiration and circulation or irreversible cessation of neurologic functions (brain death). Brain death

is further defined as absence of cerebral and brainstem functions (i.e., whole brain death). Spinal reflexes may persist after death.

A diagnosis of brain death has never been required to withhold or withdraw life support when the patient's condition is terminal and life-sustaining procedures would only serve to prolong the inevitable. However, with the evolution of transplantation and organ procurement, it became critical both legally and ethically to establish criteria by which brain death can be determined. In 1968 the Ad Hoc Committee of the Harvard Medical School published the first set of guidelines for the determination of brain death in adults.[201] Since that time, numerous other reports have set forth specific guidelines for determining brain death, primarily in adults.

The legal and medical definition of death is the same for infants and children as it is for adults. However, concern remains about how brain death is accurately diagnosed in the infant and young child. In the past, caution was recommended when applying adult criteria to children younger than 5 years of age. This arbitrary "age of caution" was used not because of some biologic phenomena but because of the paucity of data describing pediatric brain death. Furthermore, the common belief, though unproven, was that children are more resilient to neurologic damage.[202,203]

In 1987 the Ad Hoc Task Force for the Determination of Brain Death in Children published the first widely accepted guidelines for pediatric brain death.[204] These guidelines apply to children and to term infants beyond the first 7 days of life. Specific issues addressed in these guidelines are critical historical information, physical examination criteria, age-related observation periods, and laboratory testing. Table 20-6 summarizes these guidelines.[204]

The most critical historical piece of information that must be determined is proximate cause of coma. By knowing exactly what caused the brain dysfunction, the possibility of a reversible condition can be more reliably eliminated. Reversible conditions that can invalidate the clinical examination include metabolic disorders, sedatives, paralytic agents, hypothermia, hypotension, and surgically treatable lesions.

To meet the medical and legal definition of brain death, the entire brain must be assessed as irreversibly damaged. The clinical determination of cortical death is difficult.[205,206] In general, the comatose patient with cortical dysfunction presents with flaccid tone, absence of spontaneous movement, and failure to respond to external stimuli. Cortical function is dependent on an intact reticular activating system, diffusely located in the brainstem, for maintenance of arousal.

Brainstem function is examined by eliciting various brainstem reflexes. Absence of a single brainstem reflex does not define brainstem death in all persons. Thus it is the combination of absent brainstem reflexes that determines brainstem demise. The Task Force for the Determination of Brain Death in Children[204] defines absence of brainstem function as fully dilated, midposition pupils that are nonreactive to light; no spontaneous or induced (i.e., oculocephalic or oculovestibular) eye movements; no move-

TABLE 20-6 Guidelines for the Determination of Brain Death in Children

Physical examination*	1. Coma
	2. Absence of brainstem function
	   a. Midposition or fully dilated pupils, nonreactive to light
	   b. Absence of spontaneous eye movements, induced by oculocephalic and oculovestibular testing
	   c. Absence of bulbar musculature
	   d. Apnea
	3. Flaccid tone, absence of spontaneous or induced movements†

Observation period (for patient age)	1. Seven days to 2 months: two examinations separated by at least 48 hours 2. Two months to 1 year: two examinations separated by at least 24 hours 3. Over 1 year: observation period of at least 12 hours when irreversible cause known
Laboratory testing	1. Seven days to 2 months: two EEGs separated by at least 48 hours 2. Two months to 1 year: two EEGs separated by at least 24 hours 3. Over 1 year: laboratory testing not required when irreversible cause is known

Data from Task Force for the Determination of Brain Death in Children: Guidelines for the determination of brain death in children, *Neurology* 37:1007, 1987.
*The physical examination should remain unchanged during the entire observation and laboratory testing periods. Severe hypothermia and hypotension must be excluded.
†Spinal cord reflexes may be present.
EEG, Electroencephalogram.

ment of bulbar musculature, including facial and oropharyngeal muscles; no corneal, gag, cough, sucking, and rooting reflexes; and no spontaneous respirations.

Apnea and coma must coexist for brain death to be diagnosed clinically. After all other physical examination criteria for brain death have been met, apnea testing is performed. Confirmation of apnea is the single most important finding when determining brain death.[207] Standard apnea testing for children has been described in the literature.[208]

For the apnea test to be valid, three conditions must be met while the patient is disconnected from the ventilator. First, the apneic period should be of sufficient duration for $Paco_2$ to rise to a level normally sufficient to stimulate breathing. The exact apneic threshold in children is unknown. It is recommended that an apneic trial of 10 minutes be used initially. If the $Paco_2$ does not reach 60 mmHg (corrected for altitude) after that period of time, a second apneic trial of 15 minutes is used.[207] The second condition that must be met during apnea testing is maintenance of adequate oxygenation. Thus continuous flow of an Fio_2 of 1.0 is delivered by cannula in the airway. Oxygen saturations are monitored via pulse oximetry. The last condition that needs to be ensured during apnea testing is adequate perfusion. Hypotension must be corrected before apnea testing can be initiated. If cardiovascular deterioration occurs during the observation period, the test is discontinued and attempted at a later time.

The recommended observation period for infants and children suspected to be brain dead varies according to age and laboratory test used.[204] In general, the younger the age, the longer the observation period. Laboratory testing (i.e., EEG) is required for infants. However, when an irreversible cause is known in the child older than 1 year, laboratory testing is not required.

Although a number of tests exist to evaluate CBF and brainstem-evoked responses, the EEG remains that single most used laboratory test to confirm brain death. Electrocerebral silence must be demonstrated over a 30-minute period based on guidelines developed by the American Electroencephalographic Society.[209] Cerebral death may be confirmed with a cerebral radionuclide angiogram in infants older than 2 months of age. Fig. 20-10 diagrams the decision-making process in determining brain death in children.

Controversies

Even though the Task Force report[204] on pediatric brain death is widely accepted and endorsed, it is not without controversy.[210-213] Uncertainty regarding the diagnosis of brain death persists in relation to newborns. The irreversibility of a condition is determined by knowing the reason for absent brain functions. In newborns, most hypoxic-ischemic injuries occur in utero. Thus the severity and possible reversibility of the injury are difficult to determine with certainty. Also, concerns exist regarding the accuracy of clinical criteria and EEG or angiographic studies during the neonatal period.[213] However, the Task Force[214] maintains that no reported pediatric survivors fulfilled the combination of criteria used to diagnose brain death. Until better scientific data are available, Freeman and Ferry[211] recommend that brain death determination in children should remain a clinical decision by a qualified physician.

NEUROMUSCULAR DISORDERS

Although relatively rare, numerous diseases affect the motor unit in children, producing neuromuscular dysfunction. The motor unit is divided into four distinct parts: the anterior horn cell, the axon, the neuromuscular junction, and the

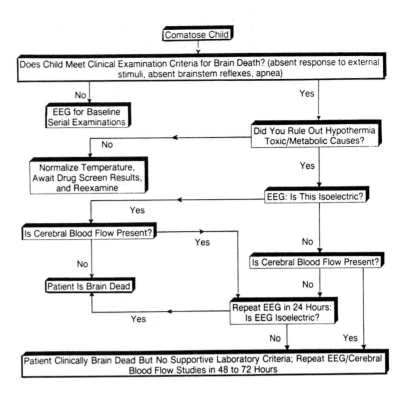

Fig. 20-10 Evaluation for suspected brain death in a child. Flow diagram indicates specific diagnostic studies and decision-making point for determination of brain death. *EEG,* Electroencephalogram. (Reproduced by permission of *Pediatrics* 78:111, Copyright 1986.)

Box 20-7

Classification of Neuromuscular Disease

Anterior Horn Cell

Inherited
  Werdnig-Hoffmann disease
Acquired
  Poliomyelitis

Peripheral Nerves

Axonal
  Lead poisoning
  Some organic compounds
Trauma
  Phrenic nerve paralysis
  Brachial plexus injury
Demyelination
  Guillain-Barré syndrome
  Diphtheria

Neuromuscular Junction

Autoimmune
  Myasthenia gravis
Congenital
  Familial infantile myasthenia gravis
Toxic
  Botulism
  Organophosphate poisoning

---

muscle fibers innervated by the anterior horn cell. Descriptions of disorders are usually grouped together based on the primary level of motor unit involvement. The final common pathway of all disease entities affecting the motor unit is loss of motor output. Box 20-7 outlines the most commonly seen neuromuscular diseases in children based on the level of motor unit involvement.

Specific disease entities causing neuromuscular dysfunction are rarely the primary cause for PICU admission. When admission is required, it is usually from secondary respiratory failure or inability to protect the airway. The presentation of symptoms may be in the form of an acute illness or an exacerbation or progression of a chronic process. Many neuromuscular disorders are progressive and untreatable, and others are self-limiting. In both cases, the mainstay of therapy is supportive care. Chapter 19 presents a more detailed discussion of respiratory management of the pediatric patient with neuromuscular dysfunction.

MUSCULOSKELETAL DISORDERS

The only patients with musculoskeletal disorders that are frequently cared for in the PICU are those who require spinal fusion. Scoliosis is a lateral curvature of the spine greater than 10 degrees.[215,216] It can vary from minor alterations that are visually undetectable to severe curvatures with significant disfigurement. The curve is described according to the directed side of convexity and the location in the spinal column (e.g., right thoracolumbar). With severe cases, females predominate. Scoliosis is most often diagnosed in the preadolescent and adolescent years during routine physical examinations. In approximately 80% of the cases, the cause of scoliosis is idiopathic (unknown). Of the 20% of known causes, they are most often congenital (e.g., congenital rib fusions, hemivertebrae, myelomeningocele), neuromuscular (e.g., cerebral palsy, neurofibromatosis, and muscular dystrophy), and inherited disorders of connective tissue (e.g., Marfan syndrome, Ehlers-Danlos syndrome, and homocystinuria).

| **Box 20-8** |
| **Internal Vertebral Fixation Devices** |

Harrington rod instrumentation	Metal rod attached by hooks placed in vertebra at upper and lower portions of the curve
Dwyer instrumentation	Titanium cable attached to vertebra through cannulated screws
Luque rod instrumentation	Flexible L-shaped metal rod fixed by wires to the bases of the spinous processes

Scoliosis rarely presents as a life-threatening illness, but severe curvatures may compromise pulmonary function. Nonoperative treatment of scoliosis is bracing and is usually recommended in patients with curves between 15 and 40 degrees.[216,217] There are no absolute indications, but surgery is usually recommended when the curvature progresses beyond a 45- to 50-degree range.[218] Surgical technique usually consists of spinal realignment and strengthening with bone grafts and internal fixation with metal rods or wires. The bone graft is taken from the iliac crests or tibia. The surgical approach traditionally has been posterior. However, an anterior approach with or without posterior spinal fusion has become more common in the treatment of spinal disorders. In general, posterior spinal fusion is primarily used for thoracic curves, whereas the anterior approach is used for thoracolumbar and lumbar curves.[217] The anterior approach allows a fewer number of vertebrae to be fused but presents a greater degree of risk to the patient related to the thoracotomy.[219] The Harrington rod is the most commonly used apparatus for internal vertebral fixation. Box 20-8 describes additional surgical techniques for internal fixation.

Spinal fusion is an elective procedure that allows adequate preparation of the acute- and long-term phases of care. Because of potential life-threatening complications and frequent monitoring, patients are usually admitted to the PICU for the first 24 hours following surgery. After 24 hours, the patient is transferred to a general care unit. The patient is usually discharged home with an external fixation device (e.g., splint, cast, jacket). The remaining section focuses on the postoperative nursing care in the intensive care unit.

Care of the Patient After Spinal Fusion

In addition to routine postoperative assessments, a baseline neurovascular assessment is performed on all extremities. Incisional pain and muscle spasms are common and are assessed immediately. The surgical procedure is long, and significant blood loss is common. The wound and graft sites are inspected for bleeding and hematoma formation. Surgical drains may be present. Suction is applied to these drains, and the admission output is recorded. If the chest was opened during surgery (as is the case for an anterior spinal fusion), the chest drainage system is evaluated for proper functioning. The patient is assessed for reexpansion of the lungs, as well as the presence of hemothoraces and pneumothoraces. A paralytic ileus is common postoperatively. The abdomen is assessed for distension and presence of bowel sounds. A nasogastric tube is assessed for patency. Baseline laboratory specimens are obtained, including hemoglobin and hematocrit values, serum electrolytes, and urine specific gravity levels. Continuing assessment focuses on three major objectives: early recognition of complications, promotion of comfort, and promotion of wound healing.

Thoracic excursion and subsequent tidal volume may be impeded from immobility, anesthesia, or pain. Ongoing respiratory assessment emphasizes adequacy of ventilation and oxygenation. The patient is positioned for comfort and optimal respiratory excursion. Careful log rolling is required. Ventilation and tidal volume may need to be supported with incentive spirometry or mechanical ventilation. Airway clearance is maintained with frequent turning, coughing and deep-breathing, chest physiotherapy, and suctioning. Bronchodilators may be required in patients with reactive airway disease.

Because the surgical procedure is long and blood loss is significant, the adequacy of cardiac output and tissue perfusion is determined. A slight oozing of drainage from the wound is normal. The amount, consistency, and color of drainage is recorded. The spinal dressing may need to be reinforced. Clear, odorless drainage from the spinal dressing is reported immediately to rule out CSF leakage. Hemoglobin and hematocrit levels are followed for trends, and intravenous fluids and blood products are administered and adjusted as needed. Autotransfusion of blood is possible in some cases. Heart rate and rhythm, end-organ perfusion, and blood pressure are assessed frequently.

Significant postoperative pain may be present from the surgical incisions, immobility, surgical instrumentation, or muscle spasms. An age-appropriate assessment is performed at frequent intervals. Pain control management is specific to the patient. Often, a continuous morphine infusion is started in the immediate postoperative period and converted to a patient-controlled analgesia (PCA) device when appropriate. The patient is repositioned frequently, and uninterrupted rest periods are provided. Diversional activities and relaxation techniques are also helpful.

Spinal surgery can potentially damage or traumatize spinal nerves intraoperatively. Baseline and continuous neurovascular assessment of the lower extremities includes movement (dorsiflexion, plantar flexion, inversion, eversion, movement of toes), sensation (numbness, tingling, decreased sensation), and circulation (pedal and posterior tibial pulses, color, capillary refill, temperature). Significant alterations in assessment are reported immediately.

Fluid and electrolytes may be altered related to the lengthy anesthesia time and alteration in gastric function. Serum electrolytes, serum osmolarity, and urine specific gravity levels are monitored closely. Intake and output with close attention to nasogastric drainage are recorded at frequent intervals. Once bowel sounds are present, the nasogastric tube is discontinued and oral intake is resumed.

SUMMARY

Pediatric critical care nurses are challenged to care for infants and children with a variety of neurologic insults. This chapter has discussed the most common neurologic disorders seen in the PICU in the context of two final common pathways: intracranial hypertension and global hypoxic ischemia. Discussion of each of these final common pathways included the pathophysiology and common elements of critical care management. Associated pathologic conditions were described in terms of pathogenesis, clinical manifestations, and specific collaborative management approaches. Additional sections presented information on brain death and organ donation, neuromuscular disorders, and care of the child after spinal fusion.

As with all infants and children in the PICU, psychosocial support of the family is an essential component of critical care management. Parents of children with a CNS insult are at particular risk because of the unique threats of the CNS injury or illness and the potential chronicity of illness. In these situations, families benefit from multidisciplinary support. Parent-to-parent support groups and illness-specific organizations (e.g., the National Head Injury Foundation) are particularly helpful.

REFERENCES

1. Quan L, Gore E J, Wentz K et al: Ten year study of pediatric drownings and near-drownings in King County, Washington: lessons in injury prevention, *Pediatrics* 83:1035-104, 1989.
2. Luerssen TG: Intracranial pressure: current status in monitoring and management, *Semin Pediatr Neurol* 4:146-155, 1997.
3. Kotagel S: Increased intracranial pressure. In Swaiman KF, Ashwal S, eds: *Pediatric neurology principles and practice,* St Louis, 1999, Mosby.
4. Shapiro HM: Intracranial hypertension: therapeutic and anesthetic considerations, *Anesthesiology* 43:445-471, 1975.
5. Johnston IH, Rowan JO: Raised intracranial pressure and cerebral blood flow: venous outflow tract pressure and vascular resistances in experimental intracranial hypertension, *J Neurol Neurosurg Psychiatry* 37:392-402, 1974.
6. Milhorat TH: Pediatric neurosurgery, *Contemp Neurol Surg* 16:1-389, 1978.
7. Boss BJ: Concepts of neurologic dysfunction. In McCance KL, Huether SE, eds: *Pathophysiology: the biologic basis for disease in adults and children,* St Louis, 1990, Mosby.
8. Hickey JV: *The clinical practice of neurological and neurosurgical nursing,* ed 2, Philadelphia, 1986, JB Lippincott.
9. Morrison CAM: Brain herniation syndromes, *Crit Care Nurse* 7:34-38, 1987.
10. Fishmann RA: Brain edema, *N Engl J Med* 293:706-711, 1975.
11. Zimmerman RA, Bilaniuk LT, Bruce D et al: Computed tomography of pediatric head trauma: acute general cerebral swelling, *Radiology* 126:403-408, 1978.
12. Barzo P, Marmarou A, Fatouros P et al: Contribution of vasogenic and cellular edema to traumatic brain swelling measured by diffusion-weighted imaging, *J Neurosurg* 87:900-907, 1997.
13. Ito J, Marmarou A, Barzo P et al: Characterization of edema by diffusion-weighted imaging in experimental TBI, *J Neurosurg* 84:97-103, 1996.
14. Bell HE: Increased intracranial pressure-diagnosis and management, *Curr Probl Pediatr* 8:1-62, 1978.

15. Mitchell PH: Decreased adaptive capacity, intracranial: a proposal for a nursing diagnosis, *J Neurosci Nurs* 18:170-175, 1986.
16. Reivich M: Arterial PCO_2 and cerebral hemodynamics, *Am J Physiol* 206:25-35, 1964.
17. Bruce DA: Treatment of intracranial hypertension. In Wonsiewicz M, ed: *Pediatric neurosurgery,* Philadelphia, 1989, WB Saunders.
18. Marshall LF, Marshall SB: Medical management of intracranial pressure. In Cooper PR, ed: *Head injury,* Baltimore, 1987, Williams & Wilkins.
19. Muizelaar JP, van der Poel HG, Li Z et al: Pial arteriolar vessel diameter and CO_2 reactivity during prolonged hyperventilation in the rabbit, *J Neurosurg* 69:923-927, 1988.
20. Marion DW, Firlik A, McLaughlin MR: Hyperventilation therapy for severe traumatic brain injury, *New Horiz* 3:439-447, 1995.
21. Muizelaar JP, Marmarou A, Ward JD et al: Adverse effects of prolonged hyperventilation in patients with severe head injury: a randomized clinical trial, *J Neurosurg* 75:731-739, 1991.
22. Eker C, Asgiersson B, Grande P et al: Improved outcome after severe head injury with a new therapy based on principles for brain volume regulation and preserved microcirculation, *Crit Care Med* 26:1881-1886, 1998.
23. Shapiro K, Giller CA: Increased intracranial pressure. In Levin DL, Morris FC, eds: *Essentials of pediatric intensive care,* St Louis, 1991, Quality Medical Publishing.
24. Gabriel EM, Borel CO: Managing severe head injury in the intensive care unit, *J Crit Illn* 11:171-181, 1996.
25. Zink BJ: Traumatic brain injury, *Emerg Med Clin North Am* 14:115-150, 1996.
26. Albanese J, Viviand X, Potie F et al: Sufentanil, fentanyl, and alfentanil in head trauma patients: a study on cerebral hemodynamics, *Crit Care Med* 27:407-416, 1999.
27. Mirski MA, Muffelman B, Ulatowki JA et al: Sedation for the critically ill neurologic patient, *Crit Care Med* 23:2038-2053, 1995.
28. Chiolero RL, de Tribolet N: Sedative and antagonists in the management of severely

head-injured patients, *Acta Neurochir Suppl* 55:43-46, 1992.
29. Shapiro HM, Galindo A, Wyte SR et al: Rapid intraoperative reduction of intracranial pressure with thiopentone, *Br J Anesthesiol* 45:1057-1062, 1973.
30. Donegan JH, Traystman RJ, Koehler RC et al: Cerebrovascular hypoxic and autoregulatory responses during reduced brain metabolism, *Am J Physiol* 249:H421-429, 1985.
31. Wilberger JE, Cantella D: High-dose barbiturates for intracranial pressure control, *New Horiz* 3:469-473, 1995.
32. Brain Trauma Foundation: The use of barbiturates in the control of intracranial hypertension, *J Neurotrauma* 13:711-714, 1996.
33. Ward JD, Becker DP, Miller JD et al: Failure of prophylactic barbiturate coma in the treatment of severe head injury, *J Neurosurg* 62:383-388, 1985.
34. Trauner D: Barbiturate therapy in acute brain injury, *J Pediatr* 109:742-746, 1986.
35. Muizelaar JP, Wei EP, Kontos HA et al: Mannitol causes compensatory cerebral vasoconstriction and vasodilation in response to blood viscosity changes, *J Neurosurg* 59:822-828, 1983.
36. Bullock R: Mannitol and other diuretics in severe neurotrauma, *New Horiz* 3:448-452, 1995.
37. Muizelaar JP, Lutz HA, Becker DP: Effect of mannitol in ICP and CBF and correlation with pressure autoregulation in severely head-injured patients, *J Neurosurg* 61:700-706, 1984.
38. Brain Trauma Foundation: The use of mannitol in severe head injury, *J Neurotrauma* 13:705-709, 1996
39. McGraw CP, Alexander E, Howard G: Effect of dose and dose schedule on the response of intracranial pressure to mannitol, *Surg Neurol* 10:127-13, 1978.
40. McGraw CP, Howard G: Effect of mannitol on increased intracranial pressure, *Neurosurg* 13:269-271, 1983.
41. Quandt CM, de los Reyes RA: Pharmacologic management of acute intracranial hypertension, *Drug Intell Clin Pharm* 18:105-112, 1984.

42. Takagi H, Tsuyusaki H, Endo M et al: Pharmacokinetics of serum glycerol and changes of ICP: comparison of gastric and duodenal administration, *Acta Neurochir Suppl (Wien)* 71:34-36, 1998.

43. Hagnevik K, Gordon E, Lins LE et al: Glycerol-induced hemolysis with hemoglobinuria and acute renal failure, *Lancet* 1:75-77, 1974.

44. Gilsanz F, Rebollar JL, Buencuerpo J et al: Controlled trial of glycerol vs dexamethasone in the treatment of cerebral edema in acute cerebral infarction, *Lancet* 1:1049-1051, 1975.

45. MacDonald JT, Uden DL: Intravenous glycerol and mannitol therapy in children with intracranial hypertension, *Neurology* 32:437-444, 1982.

46. Dean JM, Rogers MC, Traystman RJ: Pathophysiology and clinical management of the intracranial vault. In Rogers MC, ed: *Textbook of pediatric intensive care*, Baltimore, 1992, Williams & Wilkins.

47. Pitlick WH, Pirikitakuhlr P, Painter MJ et al: Effects of glycerol and hyperosmolality on intracranial pressure, *Clin Pharmacol Ther* 31:466-471, 1982.

48. Cottrell JE, Robustelli A, Post K et al: Furosemide-and mannitol-induced changes in intracranial pressure and serum osmolality and electrolytes, *Anesthesiology* 47:28-33, 1977.

49. Wilkinson HA, Rosenfeld S: Furosemide and mannitol in the treatment of acute experimental intracranial hypertension, *Neurosurgery* 12:405-441, 1983.

50. Roberts PA, Pollay M, Engles C et al: Effect on intracranial pressure of furosemide combined with varying doses and administration rates of mannitol, *J Neurosurg* 66:440-446, 1987.

51. French LA, Galicich JH: The use of steroids for control of cerebral edema, *Clin Neurosurg* 10:212-223, 1964.

52. Braakman R, Schouten HJ, Dishoeck MB et al: Megadose steroids in severe head injury: results of a prospective double-blind clinical trial, *J Neurosurg* 58:326-33, 1983.

53. Dearden NM, Gibson JS, McDowall DG et al: Effect of high-dose dexamethasone on outcome from severe head injury, *J Neurosurg* 64:81-88, 1986.

54. Kelly DF: Steroids in head injury, *New Horiz* 3:453-455, 1995.

55. Suarez JI, Qureshi AI, Bhardwaj A et al: Treatment of refractory intracranial hypertension with 23.4% saline, *Crit Care Med* 26:1118-1122, 1998.

55a. Simma B, Burger R, Falk M et al: A prospective, randomized, and controlled study of fluid management in children with severe head injury: lactated Ringer's solution vs. hypertonic saline, *Crit Care Med* 26:1265-1270, 1998.

55b. Schatzmann C, Heissler HE, Konig K et al: Treatment of elevated ICP by infusions of 10% saline in severely head injured patients, *Acta Neurochir Suppl (Wien)* 71:31-33, 1998.

55c. Fisher B, Thomas D, Peterson B: Hypertonic saline lowers raised intracranial pressure in children after head trauma, *J Neurosurg Anesthesiol* 4:4-10, 1992.

55d. Peterson B, Khanna S, Fisher B et al: Prolonged hypernatremia controls elevated ICP in head-injured pediatric patients, *Crit Care Med* 28:1136-1151, 2000.

56. Bruce DA: Treatment of intracranial hypertension. In McLaurin RL, Schut L, Venes JL et al, eds: *Pediatric neurosurgery: surgery of the developing nervous system*, Philadelphia, 1989, WB Saunders.

57. Chudley S: The effect of nursing activities on intracranial pressure, *Br J Nurs* 3:454-459, 1994.

58. Farley JA: The comatose child: analysis of factors affecting intracranial pressure, *Dimens Crit Care Nurs* 9:216-222, 1990.

59. Hobdell EF, Adamo F, Caruso J et al: The effect of nursing activities on the intracranial pressure of children, *Crit Care Nurs* 9:75-79, 1989.

60. Fisher DM, Swedlow D, Frewan T: Increase in intracranial pressure during suctioning-stimulation vs rise in Paco₂, *Anesthesiology* 57:416-417, 1982.

61. Perlman JM, Volpe JJ: Suctioning in the preterm infant: effect on cerebral blood flow velocity, intracranial pressure, and arterial blood pressure, *Pediatrics* 72:329-334, 1983.

62. Drummond BL: Preventing increased intracranial pressure *Focus Crit Care* 17:116-122, 1990.

63. Rudy EB, Turner BS, Baun M et al: Endotracheal suctioning in adults with head injury, *Heart Lung* 20:667-674, 1991.

64. Crosby L, Parsons LC: Cerebrovascular response of closed head injured patients to suctioning, *J Neurosci Nurs* 24:40-48, 1992.

65. Kerr ME, Weber BB, Seveika SM et al: Effect of endotracheal suctioning on cerebral oxygenation in traumatic brain-injured patients, *Crit Care Med* 27:2776-2781, 1999.

66. Donegan MF, Bedford RF: Intravenously administered lidocaine prevents intracranial hypertension during endotracheal suctioning, *Anesthesiology* 52:516-518, 1980.

67. Yano M, Nishiyama N, Yokota N, et al: Effect of lidocaine on ICP response to endotracheal suctioning, *Anesthesiology* 64:651-653, 1986.

68. Brucia J, Owen D, Rudy E: The effects of lidocaine on ICP, *J Neurosci Nurs* 24:205-213, 1992.

69. White PF, Schlobohn RM, Pitts LH et al: A randomized study of drugs for preventing increases in intracranial pressure during endotracheal suctioning, *Anesthesiology* 57:242-244, 1982.

70. Rosner MJ, Coley IB: Cerebral perfusion pressure, intracranial pressure, and head elevation, *J Neurosurg* 65:636-641, 1986.

71. Beitel J: Positioning and intracranial hypertension implications of the new critical pathway for nursing practice, *Off J Can Assoc Crit Care Nurs* 9:12-18, 1998.

72. Meixensberger J, Baunach S, Amschler J et al: Influence of body position on tissue Po₂, cerebral perfusion pressure, and ICP in patients with acute brain injury, *Neurol Res* 19:249-253, 1997.

73. Simmons BJ: Management of intracranial hemodynamics in the adult: a research analysis of head positioning and recommendations for clinical practice and future research, *J Neurosci Nurs* 29:44-49, 1997.

74. Boortz-Marx R: Factors affecting intracranial pressure: a descriptive study, *J Neurosurg Nurs* 17:89-94, 1985.

75. Parsons LC, Peard AL, Page MC: The effects of hygiene interventions on the cerebrovascular status of severe closed head injured persons, *Res Nurs Health* 8:173-181, 1983.

76. Walleck CA: Controversies in the management of the head-injured patient, *Crit Care Nurs Clin North Am* 1:67-74, 1989.

77. Mitchell PH, Habermann-Little B, Johnson F et al: Critically ill children: the importance of touch in a high-technology environment, *Nurs Adm Q* 9:38-46, 1985.

78. Bruya MA: Planned periods of rest in the intensive care unit: nursing care activities and intracranial pressure, *J Neurosurg Nurs* 13:184-194, 1981.

79. Rumana CS, Gopinath SP, Uzura M et al: Brain temperature exceeds systemic temperature in head-injured patients, *Crit Care Med* 26:562-567, 1998.

80. Clifton GL: Hypothermia and hyperbaric oxygen as treatment modalities for severe head injury, *New Horiz* 3:474-478, 1995.

81. Prendergast V: Current trends in research and treatment of intracranial hypertension, *Crit Care Nurs Q* 17:1-8, 1994.

82. Mitchell PH: Neurologic disorders. In Kinney MG, Packa DR, Dunbar SB, eds: *AACN's clinical reference for critical-care nursing*, New York, 1988, McGraw-Hill.

83. Gastaut H: *Dictionary of epilepsies*. Part 1. *Definitions*, Geneva, 1973, World Health Organization.

84. DeLorenzo RJ, Hauser WA, Towne AR et al: A prospective, population-based study of status epilepticus in Richmond, Virginia, *Neurology* 46:1029-1035, 1996.

85. Pellock JM: Status epilepticus. In Swaiman KF, Ashwal S, eds: *Pediatric neurology principles and practice*, St Louis, 1999, Mosby.

86. Pellock JM, DeLorenzo RJ: Status epilepticus. In Porter RJ, Chadwick D, eds: *The epilepsies 2*, Boston, 1997, Butterworth-Heinemann.

87. Holmes GL: *Diagnosis and management of seizures in children*, Philadelphia, 1987, WB Saunders.

88. Trauner D: Seizure disorders. In Wiederholt WC, ed: *Neurology for the non-neurologist*, Philadelphia, 1988, Grune & Stratton.

89. Harrison AM, Lugo RA, Schunk JE: Treatment of convulsive status epilepticus with propofol: case report, *Pediatr Emerg Care* 13:420-422, 1997.

90. Igartua J, Silver P, Maytal J: Midazolam coma for refractory status epilepticus in children, *Crit Care Med* 27:1982-1985, 1999.

91. Stecker MM, Kramer TH, Raps EC et al: Treatment of refractory status epilepticus

with propofol: clinical and pharmacokinetic findings, *Epilepsia* 39:18-26, 1998.

92. DeVeber G: Cerebrovascular disease in children. In Swaiman KF, Ashwal S, eds: *Pediatric neurology principles and practice,* St Louis, 1999, Mosby.

93. Williams MH: Arteriovenous malformations: complications of surgical intervention and implications for nursing, *J Neurosurg Nurs* 17:14-21, 1985.

94. Dembo M: Arteriovenous malformations of the brain: a review of the literature since 1960, *Arch Phys Med Rehabil* 63:565-568, 1982.

95. Callahan SW: Arteriovenous malformations, *Am J Nurs* 96:30-31, 1996.

96. Vaiden RE, White WR: Arteriovenous malformations of the brain, *AORN J* 46:37-47, 1987.

97. Menkes JH: *Textbook of child neurology,* ed 4, Philadelphia, 1990, Lea & Febiger.

98. Golden GS: Cerebrovascular disease. In Swaiman KF, ed: *Pediatric neurology: principles and practice,* St Louis, 1989, Mosby.

99. Humphreys RP: Arteriovenous malformations of the brain. In Wonsiewicz M, ed: *Pediatric neurosurgery,* Philadelphia, 1989, WB Saunders.

100. Wiggins CW, Loisel D, Budock AM: Intracranial arteriovenous malformation in a neonate: aneurysm of the great vein of Galen, *Neonatal Netw* 9:7-17, 1991.

101. Garcia-Monaco R, DeVictor D, Mann C et al: Congestive cardiac manifestations from cerebrocranial arteriovenous shunts, *Childs Nerv Syst* 7:48-52, 1991.

102. Graf CJ, Perret GE, Torner JC: Bleeding from cerebral arteriovenous malformations as part of their natural history, *J Neurosurg* 58:331-337, 1983.

103. Guertin SR: Neurological intensive care: selected aspects. In Fuhrman BP, Zimmerman JJ, eds: *Pediatric critical care,* St Louis, 1992, Mosby.

104. McNair N: Arteriovenous malformations, *Crit Care Nurse* 8:35-34, 1988.

105. Burrows PE, Lasjaunias PL, Ter Brugge KG, et al: Urgent and emergent embolization of lesions of the head and neck in children: indications and results, *Pediatrics* 80:386-394, 1997.

106. Willis D, Harbit MD: Transcatheter arterial embolization of cerebral arteriovenous malformations, *J Neurosci Nurs* 22:280-284, 1990.

107. Albright L: Pediatric brain tumors, *Cancer* 43:272-288, 1993.

108. Lacayo A, Farmer PM: Brain tumors in children: a review, *Ann Clin Lab Sci* 21:26-35, 1991.

109. Cohen ME, Duffner PK: Tumors of the brain and spinal cord including leukemic involvement. In Swaiman KF, ed: *Pediatric neurology: principles and practice,* St Louis, 1999, Mosby.

110. Rorke LB, Gilles FH, Davis RL et al: Revision of the World Health Organization classification of brain tumors for childhood brain tumors, *Cancer* 56:1869-1886, 1985.

111. Duffner PK, Cohen ME, Freeman AI: Pediatric brain tumors: an overview. *CA Cancer J Clin* 35:287-301, 1985.

112. Sutton LN, Schut L: Cerebellar astrocytomas. In Wonsiewicz M, ed: *Pediatric neurosurgery,* Philadelphia, 1989, WB Saunders.

113. Laurent JP, Cheek WR: Brain tumors in children. In Fishman MA, ed: *Pediatric neurology,* New York, 1986, Grune & Stratton.

114. Hendrick EB, Raffel C: Tumors of the fourth ventricle: ependymomas, choroid plexus papillomas, and dermoid cysts. In Wonsiewicz M, ed: *Pediatric neurosurgery,* Philadelphia, 1989, WB Saunders.

115. Menkes JH, Till K: Tumors of the nervous system. In Menkes JH, ed: *Textbook of child neurology,* Philadelphia, 1990, Lea & Febiger.

116. Barker E: Brain tumor: frightening diagnosis, nursing challenge, *RN* 53:46-55, 1990.

117. Leahy NM: Intraarterial cisplatin infusion: nursing implications, *J Neurosci Nurs* 18:296-301, 1986.

118. Vernon-Levett P, Geller M: Posterior fossa tumors in children: a case study, *AACN Clin Issues Crit Care Nurs* 8:214-226, 1997.

119. Rudy EB: *Advanced neurological and neurosurgical nursing,* St Louis, 1984, Mosby.

120. Stewart-Amidei C: Meningioma: nursing care considerations, *J Post Anesth Nurs* 6:269-278, 1991.

121. Klein JO, Feigin BD, McCracken GH: Report of the task force on diagnosis and management of meningitis, *Pediatrics* 78 (suppl):959-982, 1986.

122. Rubenstein JS: Acute pediatric CNS infections. In Fuhrman BP, Zimmerman JJ, eds: *Pediatric critical care,* St Louis, 1992, Mosby.

123. Snyder RD: Bacterial infections of the nervous system. In Swaiman KF, Ashwal S, eds: *Pediatric neurology principles and practice,* St Louis, 1999, Mosby.

124. Adams WG, Deaver KA, Cochi SL et al: Decline of childhood *Haemophilus influenzae* type-b (Hib) disease in the Hib vaccine era, *JAMA* 269:221-226, 1993.

125. Quagliarello V, Scheld WM: Bacterial meningitis: pathogenesis, pathophysiology, and progress, *N Engl J Med* 327:864-872, 1992.

126. Gilbert DN, Moellering RC, Sande MA: *The Sanford guide to antimicrobial therapy,* ed 28, Hyde Park, Vt, 1998, Antimicrobial Therapy, Inc.

127. Kennedy WA, Hoyt MJ, McCracken GH: The role of corticosteroid therapy in children with pneumococcal meningitis, *Am J Dis Child* 45:1374-1378, 1991.

128. Lebel MH, Freij BJ, Syrogiannopoulos GA et al: Dexamethasone therapy for bacterial meningitis: results of two double-blind, placebo-controlled trials, *N Engl J Med* 3:964-971, 1988.

129. Committee on Infectious Disease, American Academy of Pediatrics: Dexamethasone therapy for bacterial meningitis in infants and children, *Pediatrics* 86:130-133, 1990.

130. Roos KL: The use of adjunctive therapy to alter the pathophysiology of bacterial meningitis, *Clin Neuropharm* 18:138-147, 1995.

131. Perez CO: Dexamethasone effect on the inflammatory response of the central nervous system in bacterial meningitis, *Curr Ther Res* 57(suppl):A:52, 1996.

132. Committee on Infectious Disease, American Academy of Pediatrics: *Report of the committee on infectious disease,* ed 21, Elk Grove, Ill, 1991, American Academy of Pediatrics.

133. Centers for Disease Control: *Guidelines for prevention and control of nosocomial infections,* Atlanta, 1983, CDC.

134. Beghi E, Nicolosi A, Kurland LT et al: Encephalitis and aseptic meningitis, Olmsted County, Minnesota, 1950-1981: I. Epidemiology, *Ann Neurol* 16:283-294, 1984.

135. Weil ML: Infections of the nervous system. In Menkes JH, ed: *Textbook of child neurology,* Philadelphia, 1990, Lea & Febiger.

136. Dyken PR: Viral diseases of the nervous system. In Swaiman KF, ed: *Pediatric neurology: principles and practice,* St Louis, 1989, Mosby.

137. Krywanio ML: Varicella encephalitis, *J Neurosci Nurs* 23:363-368, 1991.

138. McCullough DC: Hydrocephalus: etiology, pathologic effects, diagnosis, and natural history. In Wonsiewicz M, ed: *Pediatric neurosurgery,* Philadelphia, 1989, WB Saunders.

139. Edmonds LD, James LM: Temporal trends in the prevalence of congenital malformations at birth based on the birth defects monitoring program, United States, 1979-1987, *Mor Mortal Wkly Rep CDC Surveill Summ* 39:19-23, 1990.

140. Kapila A, Naidick TP: Spontaneous lateral ventriculocisternostomy documented by metrizamide CT ventriculography: case report, *J Neurosurg* 54:101-104, 1981.

141. Ashwal S: Congenital structural defects. In Swaiman KF, Ashwal S, eds: *Pediatric neurology principles and practice,* St Louis, 1999, Mosby.

142. Post EM: Currently available shunt systems: a review, *Neurosurgery* 16:257-326, 1985.

143. Shinnar S, Gammon K, Bergman EW et al: Management of hydrocephalus in infancy: use of acetazolamide and furosemide to avoid cerebrospinal fluid shunts, *J Pediatr* 107:31-37, 1985.

144. McLaurin RL: Ventricular shunts: complications and results. In Wonsiewicz M, ed: *Pediatric neurosurgery,* Philadelphia, 1989, WB Saunders.

145. Kellett PB: Latex allergy: a review, *J Emerg Nurs* 23:27-36, 1997.

146. National Head Injury Foundation: *Definition of traumatic brain injury,* Southborough, Mass, 1986, National Head Injury Foundation.

147. Conroy C, Kraus JF: Survival after brain injury: cause of death, length of survival, and prognostic variables in a cohort of brain injured people, *Neuroepidemiology* 7:13-22, 1988.

148. Ward JD: Pediatric issues in head trauma, *New Horiz* 3:539-545, 1995.

149. Shapiro K: Head injury in children. In Becker D, Povlishock J, eds: *CNS trauma*

status report, Bethesda, Md, 1985, NINCDS, National Institutes of Health.

150. Snow RB, Zimmerman RD, Gandy SE et al: Comparison of magnetic resonance imaging and computed tomography in the evaluation of head injury, *Neurosurgery* 18:45-52, 1986.

151. Gean AD, Kates RS, Lee S: Neuroimaging in head injury. *New Horizons* 3:549-561, 1995.

152. Temkin NR, Haglund MM, Winn HR, Causes, prevention, and treatment of post-traumatic epilepsy, *New Horiz* 3:518-522, 1995.

153. Roberts P: Nutrition in the head-injured patient, *New Horiz* 3:506-516, 1995.

154. Safar P, Bircher NG: The pathophysiology of dying and reanimation. In Schwartz GR, Cayten CG, Mangelsen MA et al, eds: *Principles and practice of emergency medicine,* Philadelphia, 1992, Lea & Febiger.

155. Bouma GJ, Muizelaar JP: Cerebral blood flow in severe clinical head injury, *New Horiz* 3:384-394, 1995.

156. Wauquier A, Edmonds HL, Clincke GHC: Cerebral resuscitation: pathophysiology and therapy, *Neurosci Biobehav Rev* 11:287-306, 1987.

157. Kirsch JR, Helfaer MA, Blizzard K et al: Age-related cerebrovascular response to global ischemia in pigs, *Am J Physiol* 259:H1551-H1556, 1990.

158. Rosenberg AA: Cerebral blood flow and O_2 metabolism after asphyxia in neonatal lambs, *Pediatr Res* 20:778-782, 1986.

159. Michenfelder JD, Milde JN: Postischemic canine cerebral blood flow appears to be determined by cerebral metabolic needs, *J Cereb Blood Flow Metab* 10:71-76, 1990.

160. Morgenstern LB, Pettigrew LC: Brain protection: human data and potential new therapies, *New Horiz* 5:397-405, 1997.

161. Sweeney MI, Yager JY, Walz W et al: Cellular mechanisms involved in brain ischemia, *Can J Physiol Pharmacol* 73:1525-1535, 1995.

162. Kirsch JR, Dean MJ, Rogers MC: Current concepts in brain resuscitation, *Arch Inter Med* 146:1413-1419, 1986.

163. Safar P: Cerebral resuscitation after cardiac arrest: a review, *Circulation* 74(6 Pt 2): IV138-153, 1986.

164. Prough DS, Johnson JC, Poole GV et al: Effects on intracranial pressure of resuscitation from hemorrhagic shock with hypertonic saline versus lactated Ringer's solution, *Crit Care Med* 13:407-411, 1985.

165. Kirsch JR, Diringer MN, Borel CO et al: Brain resuscitation: medical management and innovations, *Crit Care Nurs Clin North Am* 1:143-154, 1989.

166. Kochanek PM: Novel pharmacologic approaches to brain resuscitation after cardio-respiratory arrest in the pediatric patient, *Crit Care Clin* 4:661-677, 1988.

167. Rogers MC, Kirsch JR: Current concepts in brain resuscitation, *JAMA* 261:3143-3147, 1989.

168. Perkin RM, Ashwal S: Hypoxic-ischemic encephalopathy in infants and older children. In Swaiman KF, Ashwal S, editors:

Pediatric neurology principles and practice, St Louis, 1999, Mosby.

169. Kochanek PM, Uhl MW, Schoettle RJ: Hypoxic-ischemic encephalopathy: pathobiology and therapy of the postresuscitation syndrome in children. In Fuhrman BP, Zimmerman JJ, eds: *Pediatric critical care,* St Louis, 1992, Mosby.

170. Siemkowicz FE, Hansen AJ: Clinical restitution following cerebral ischemia in hypo-, normo-, and hyperglycemic rats, *Acta Neurol Scand* 58:1-8, 1978.

171. Cipolla MJ, Porter JM, Osol G: High glucose concentrations dilate cerebral arteries and diminish myogenic tone through an endothelial mechanism, *Stroke* 28, 405-410, 1997.

172. Sieber FE, Traystman RJ: Special issues: glucose and the brain, *Crit Care Med* 20:104-114, 1992.

173. Brain Resuscitation Clinical Trial I Study Group: Randomized clinical study of thiopental loading in comatose survivors or cardiac arrest, *New Engl J Med* 314:397-403, 1986.

174. Haun SE, Dean JM, Kirsch JR et al: Theories of brain resuscitation. In Rogers MC, ed: *Textbook of pediatric intensive care,* Baltimore, 1992, Williams & Wilkins.

175. Safar P: Resuscitation from clinical death: pathophysiologic limits and therapeutic potentials, *Crit Care Med* 16:923-941, 1988.

176. Steen PA, Gisvold SE, Milde JH, et al: Nimodipine improves outcome when given after complete cerebral ischemia in primates, *Anesthesiology* 62:406-414, 1985.

177. Zornow MH, Prough DS: Neuroprotective properties of calcium-channel blockers, *New Horiz* 4:107-114, 1996.

178. Imaizumi S, Woolworth V, Fishman RA et al: Liposome-entrapped superoxide dismutase reduces cerebral infarction in cerebral ischemia in rats, *Stroke* 21:1312-1317, 1990.

179. Liu TH, Beckman JS, Freeman BA et al: Polyethylene glycolconjugated superoxide dismutase and catalase reduce ischemic brain injury, *Am J Physiol* 256:H589-H593, 1989.

180. Brader E, Jehle D: Cerebral resuscitation, *Top Emerg Med* 11:52-67, 1989.

181. Gilbert DN, Moellering RC, Sande MA: *The standard guide to antimicrobial therapy,* ed 28, Vienna, Va, 1998, Antimicrobial Therapy.

182. Park CK, Jun SS, Kim MC et al: Effects of systemic hypothermia and selective brain cooling on ischemic brain damage and swelling, *Acta Neurochir Suppl* 71:225-228, 1998.

183. Safar P, Klain M, Tisherman S: Selective brain cooling after cardiac arrest, *Crit Care Med* 24:911-914, 1996.

184. Sarnaik AP, Lieh-Lai MW: Near-drowning. In Fuhrman BP, Zimmerman JJ, eds: *Pediatric critical care,* St Louis, 1992, Mosby.

185. Spyker DA: Submersion injury: epidemiology, prevention, and management, *Pediatr Clin North Am* 32:113-125, 1985.

186. Rivara FP: Traumatic deaths of children in the United States: currently available pre-

vention strategies, *Pediatrics* 75:456-462, 1985.

187. Fields AI: Near-drowning in the pediatric population, *Crit Care Clin* 8:113-129, 1992.

188. Karpovich PV: Water in the lungs of drowned animals, *Arch Pathol Lab Med* 15:828-833, 1933.

189. DeNicola LK, Falk JL, Swanson ME et al: Submersion injuries in children and adults, *Crit Care Clin* 13:477-502, 1997.

190. Hochachka P: Brain, lung, and heart function during diving and recovery, *Science* 212:509-514, 1981.

191. Gooden BA: Drowning and the diving reflex in man, *Med J Aust* 2:583-587, 1972.

192. Sarnaik AP, Vohra MP: Near-drowning: fresh, salt, and cold water immersion, *Clin Sports Med* 5:33-46, 1986.

193. Orlowski JP: Drowning, near-drowning, and ice-water submersions, *Pediatr Clin North Am* 34:75-92, 1987.

194. Christensen DW, Dean JM, Setzer NA: Near-drowning. In Rogers MC, ed: *Textbook of pediatric intensive care,* Baltimore, 1992, Williams & Wilkins.

194a. Hanke BK, Fields, AI, Gerace JE et al: Near-drowning. In Schwartz GR, Cayten CG, Mangelsen MA et al, eds: *Principles and practice of emergency medicine,* Philadelphia, 1992, Lea & Febiger.

195. McKinley MG: Near-drowning: a nursing challenge, *Crit Care Nur* 9:52-56, 1989.

196. Glankler DM: Caring for the victim of near drowning, *Crit Care Nur* 13:25-32, 1993.

197. Frewen TC, Sumabat WO, HanVK et al: Cerebral resuscitation therapy in pediatric near-drowning, *J Pediatr* 106:615-617, 1985.

198. Nussbaum E, Maggie JC: Pentobarbital therapy does not improve neurologic outcome in nearly drowned, flaccid-comatose children, *Pediatrics* 81:630-634, 1988.

199. Sarnaik AP, Preston G, Lich-Lai M et al: Intracranial pressure and cerebral perfusion pressure in near-drowning, *Crit Care Med* 13:224-227, 1985.

200. Beyda DH: Pathophysiology for near-drowning and treatment of the child with a submersion incident, *Crit Care Nurs Clin North Am* 3:273-28, 1991.

201. A definition of irreversible coma. Report of the Ad Hoc Committee of the Harvard medical school to examine the definition of brain death, *JAMA* 205:85-88, 1968.

202. Ashwal S, Schneider S: Brain death in children: Part I, *Pediatr Neurol* 3:5-11, 1987.

203. Guidelines for the determination of death. Report of the medical consultants on the diagnosis of death to the President's Commission for the Study of Ethical Problems in Medicine and Biomedical and Behavioral Research, *JAMA* 246:2184-2186, 1981.

204. Task Force for the Determination of Brain Death in Children: Guidelines for the determination of brain death in children, *Neurology* 37:1077-1078, 1987.

205. Moshe SL: Usefulness of EEG in the evaluation of brain death in children: the pros, *Electroencephalogr Clin Neurophysiol* 73:272-275, 1989.

206. Vas CJ: Brain death in children, *Indian J Pediatr* 57:735-742, 1990.

207. Schneider S, Ashwal S: Determination of brain death in infants and children. In Swaiman KF, Ashwal S, eds: *Pediatric neurology principles and practice,* St Louis, 1999, Mosby.

208. Outwater KK, Rockoff MA: Apnea testing to confirm brain death in children, *Crit Care Med* 12:357-358, 1984.

209. American Electroencephalographic Society Guidelines in EEG, 1-7 (revised 1985), *J Clin Neurophysiol* 3:131-68, 1986.

210. Ashwal S: Brain death in the newborn, *Clin Perinatol* 24:859-866, 1997.

211. Freeman JM, Ferry PC: New brain death guidelines in children: further confusion, *Pediatrics* 81:301-303, 1988.

212. Shewmon A: Commentary on guidelines for the determination of brain death in children, *Issues Clin Neurosci* 24:789-791, 1988.

213. Volpe JJ: Brain death determination in the newborn, *Pediatrics* 80:293-297, 1987.

214. Task Force on Brain Death in Children: [Reply], *Issues Clin Neurosci* 24:791, 1988.

215. Kane WJ: Scoliosis prevalence: a call for a statement of terms, *Clin Orthop* 126:43-46, 1977.

216. Skaggs DL, Bassett GS: Adolescent idiopathic scoliosis: an update, *Am Fam Phys* 53:2327-2334, 1996.

217. Roach JW: Adolescent idiopathic scoliosis, *Orthop Clin North Am* 30:353-365, 1999.

218. Behrman RE: *Nelson's textbook of pediatrics,* Philadelphia, 1992, WB Saunders.

219. Ogilvie JW: Anterior spine fusion with Zielke instrumentation for idiopathic scoliosis in adolescents, *Orthop Clin North Am* 19:313-317, 1988.

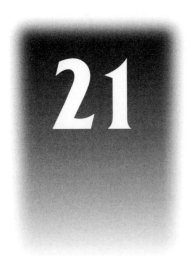

21 Renal Critical Care Problems

Lauren Sorce Grehn
Andrea Kline
Joyce Weishaar

The renal system is an elaborate maze of complex functions that maintains homeostasis in the body. Although the kidney begins as a few tubules, it eventually develops into an intricate organ responsible for homeostatic balance. When the renal system is not functioning appropriately, this balance is in jeopardy. Renal dysfunction that progresses to acute renal failure (ARF) may cause complete cessation of function.

ARF can occur as a primary disease and cause critical illness. In the child, the cause is generally intrinsic to the kidney and urinary tract, compared with multisystem diseases that affect the adult.[1] When ARF is present as a primary disease, the morbidity and mortality are less than when it is associated with additional conditions, such as multiorgan dysfunction syndrome.

The pathogenesis of ARF is multifactorial. Because renal function is dependent on renal blood flow, any diminution in flow potentially alters kidney function. Over time, hypoperfusion results in altered renal function because of changes in the kidney itself. Intrinsic renal failure can occur as a result of ingestion or administration of nephrotoxic agents, which impair renal cell function and cause an alteration in renal tubular reabsorption or secretion.

The clinical presentation and laboratory findings in ARF vary. Following trends in a child's renal status over time best identifies deteriorating renal function. Nursing vigilance, which provides for early identification and management of ARF, can prevent irreversible renal dysfunction.

EMBRYOLOGIC DEVELOPMENT OF THE RENAL SYSTEM

Renal system development goes through three successive bilateral excretory systems in the embryo: the pronephros, the mesonephros, and the metanephros. The pronephros is evident in the embryo in the third week of gestation and degenerates by the fifth week. This structure has no notable excretory function, but it is necessary because it gives rise to the mesonephric duct.[2]

The mesonephric nephrons are noted at approximately the middle of the fourth week of gestation and are caudal to the pronephros. Glomeruli and proximal tubules can be seen in the mesonephros, which is the first functional renal unit of the embryo.[2] The tubules empty into the mesonephric duct, which develops an outgrowth to form the ureteric bud. The ureteric bud in turn leads to the development of the metanephros, the definitive kidney. As the metanephros begins to function, the mesonephric ducts and tubules degenerate in females. In males, they persist and become incorporated into the genital system.[3]

Development of the metanephros begins in the fifth week of gestation.[3] The metanephros is formed from two different embryonic tissues. The excretory portion, including the collecting ducts, calyces, pelvis, and ureter, develops from the ureteric bud. The metanephric blastema gives rise to Bowman's capsule, most of the glomerulus, and the tubules of the nephrons. The collecting ducts and the tubules then

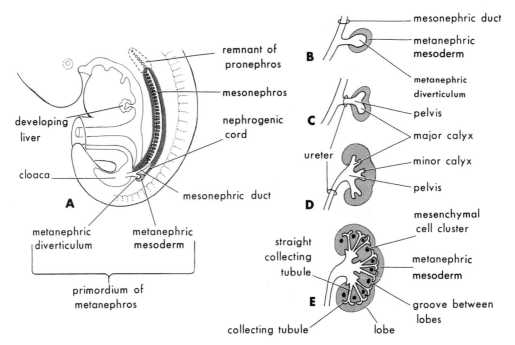

Fig. 21-1 **A,** Sketch of lateral view of 5-week-old embryo showing primordium of the metanephros, or permanent kidney. **B** to **E,** Sketches showing successive stages of development of the metanephric diverticulum (fifth to eighth week) into the ureter, pelvis, calyces, and collecting tubules. Renal lobes illustrated in **E** are visible in the kidneys of newborn infants. External evidence of the lobes normally disappears by the end of the first year. (From Moore KL: *Before we are born: basic embryology and birth defects,* ed 2, Philadelphia, 1985, WB Saunders, p 171.)

make connections, giving rise to an anatomically complete microstructure by 12 to 16 weeks gestation.[4] As the tubules are developing, they are influenced by a variety of growth factors.[3] Fig. 21-1 provides an overview of embryologic development of the kidney.

By full gestation, each human kidney contains approximately 1 million nephrons in different stages of development. The maturest nephrons are found in the renal medulla, and immature nephrons are in the outer cortex. Although maturation of the renal system continues after birth, no additional nephrons are formed.

MATURATIONAL FACTORS

Structure of the Renal System

The kidneys occupy a large portion of the posterior abdominal wall as a result of the ascent and rotation of the kidneys during gestation. They are located in the retroperitoneal space in front and on both sides of the vertebral column. A thin fibrous capsule composed of connective tissue, lymphatics, and blood vessels covers each kidney. The blood vessels, lymphatics, nerves, and ureter enter or exit the kidney in the area known as the hilum. A cross-section of the mature kidney demonstrates an outer area of renal cortex that is approximately 1 cm wide and an inner area of renal medulla that is approximately 5 cm wide. About 85% of the nephrons in each kidney are located within the renal cortex. The remaining 15% are called the

"juxtamedullary nephrons" and are located at the junction of the cortex and medulla. The ureters are proportionately shorter in infancy than in adults. As renal development continues, the ureters grow to adult proportions, and the kidney reaches adult size by adolescence. The kidney's weight is 10 times greater at maturity than at birth.[5] Fig. 21-2 demonstrates the gross structure of the kidney.

At birth, each kidney contains approximately 1 million nephrons. Although these nephrons are in varying maturational stages, each has both a tubular and vascular component. The arcuate artery branches within the kidney to form the afferent arterioles. Afferent arterioles then divide into capillary tufts called glomeruli, which protrude into Bowman's capsule. The tubular component of the nephron is composed of Bowman's capsule, the proximal and distal convoluted tubules, the loop of Henle, and the collecting ducts.

Function of the Renal System

The permanent kidney has a complete microstructure by the fourth month of gestation; nonetheless, renal development continues until adolescence. During this time, the immature kidney can ensure fluid and electrolyte balance, which is essential for growth in the developing infant; however, it is less capable of adjusting to the stress imposed by an acute illness. Table 21-1 summarizes the limitation of immature renal function.

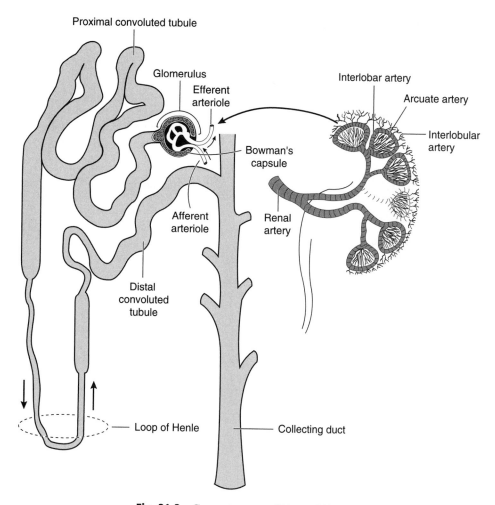

Fig. 21-2 Gross structure of bisected kidney.

TABLE 21-1	**Maturational Limitations of Renal Function**
Characteristics	**Mechanism**
Inability to excrete excessive sodium	Immature tubular function
Lower serum bicarbonate concentrations	Limited capacity to reabsorb bicarbonate and secrete hydrogen ions
Inability to concentrate urine	Cannot generate a sufficient concentration gradient in the inner medulla
Low glomerular filtration rate	Low perfusion pressures, decreased surface area available for filtration, glomerular permeability, and low glomerular plasma flow
Decreased renal blood flow	High renal vascular resistance in afferent and efferent arterioles
	Low cardiac output delivered to kidneys
	Possible incomplete sympathetic innervation

The newborn kidney receives approximately 4% to 6% of the total cardiac output because of a lower mean arterial pressure and high renal vascular resistance. The lower percentage of the cardiac output supplied to the newborn kidney compares with 20% to 25% of cardiac output supplied to the mature kidney.[6] Some data suggest that the higher vascular resistance may be a response to the renin-angiotensin system.[6,7] In addition, a decrease in amount or effectiveness of circulating vasodilators, such as endothelin-derived relaxing factor, may contribute to elevated renal vascular resistance.[6,7] Elevated renal vascular resistance may also be a response to circulating catecholamines and digitalis-like peptides. However, an abrupt decrease in catecholamines or slow decline in digitalis-like peptide does not provide a substantial decrease in renal vascular resistance.[7,8]

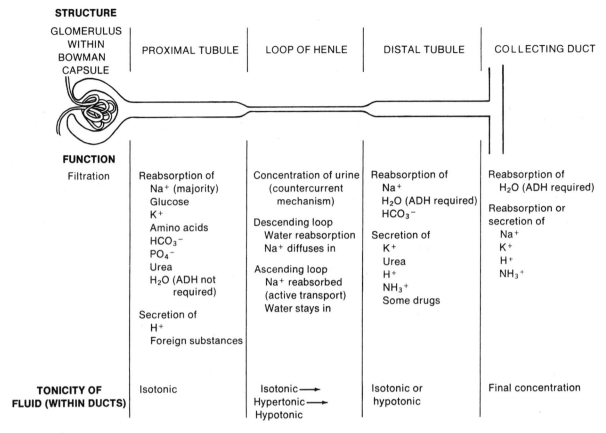

Fig. 21-3 Tubular components of the nephron. (From Whaley LF, Wong DL: *Nursing care of infants and children,* ed 6, St Louis, 1999, Mosby.)

The sympathetic nervous system may also play an important role in renal hemodynamics in infants. Sympathetic innervation may be incomplete, and most of the adrenergic receptor sites may be of alpha type, which produce renal vasoconstriction when stimulated.[8]

Normal urine output averages between 0.5 ml/kg/hr in a well-hydrated adolescent to 1 ml/kg/hr in the child and 2 ml/kg/hr in the infant. Although normal urine specific gravity is between 1.005 and 1.020, infants and children younger than 2 years may not present with high specific gravity because of renal maturational factors.

The urine produced in the newborn's kidneys is dilute. The limited ability to concentrate urine in the newborn is due to short loops of Henle with reduced sodium chloride transport, high protein anabolism, and wide peripapillary fornices.[9,10] The infant cannot excrete very dilute urine in states of overhydration and may be unable to excrete very concentrated urine in response to dehydration.

Renal blood flow (RBF) and glomerular filtration rate (GFR) increase with gestational age. At birth, a variable GFR, which decreases, increases, and decreases all within the first few hours of life, is seen. The newborn's GFR within the first 24 hours averages 25 ml/min/1.73 m². During the first 3 months of life, GFR increases in relation to body size, kidney weight, and surface area of the kidney. Factors affecting the increase in GFR are increased arterial pressure, increased RBF, increased filtration surface area, and increased glomerular permeability.[10] GFR then in-

creases at a slower rate until it reaches adult values between 12 and 24 months of age.[6] GFR may be calculated for children. The calculation for children ages 1 to 6 years is 0.55 × length (in cm)/plasma creatinine (mg %). This yields GFR in millimeters per minute on body surface area corrected to 1.73 m².

Immature tubular function results in less efficient maintenance of sodium and water balance. The decreased urinary excretion of sodium characteristic of the first year of life is directly related to the low GFR and high reabsorption rates at the level of the distal segment of the tubule.[10] Functions in the distal tubules depend on the actions of aldosterone and antidiuretic hormone. In the infant, the distal tubule is relatively insensitive to aldosterone. Hence the infant has limited ability to respond to sodium excess or depletion and may experience impaired secretion of potassium and hydrogen ions. These developmental factors continue to play a role in fluid and electrolyte balance during the first 2 years of life and help to explain the sensitivity of infants and young children to fluid and electrolyte alteration.

Renal function is not limited to the formation of urine but is also responsible for a variety of other activities that maintain the internal stability of other body systems. These activities include the mechanisms of secretion, reabsorption, and active transport that take place in the renal tubules (Fig. 21-3). Secretion clears the serum of unwanted substances. Reabsorption and active transport allow substances to be returned to the serum in appropriate proportions to

TABLE 21-2	**Renal Function**
Function	**Mechanism**
Formation of urine	Secretion, reabsorption, and active transport
Acid-base balance	Hydrogen/bicarbonate ion secretion or absorption
Maintenance of blood pressure	Alteration in circulating blood volume, renin-angiotensin system
Erythrocyte production	Secretion of erythropoietin
Calcium and phosphorus balance	Activation of vitamin D
Vasodilation or vasoconstriction of the renal vasculature	Synthesis of prostaglandins

maintain normal blood levels. The kidneys are also responsible for the excretion of foreign substances and byproducts of metabolism, including urea, toxins, and medications.[11] Table 21-2 summarizes these functions.

Acid-base balance is regulated by the kidneys, lungs, and chemical buffering systems. The kidney selectively secretes or absorbs hydrogen and bicarbonate ions to maintain the serum pH within normal range. Renal regulation of acid-base balance in the immature kidney has certain quantitative differences. Though able to maintain a normal balance, serum pH and bicarbonate levels are generally lower because of low renal threshold for bicarbonate.[10] Under normal conditions the immature kidney is able to maintain acid-base homeostasis, but when challenged with excess acid, the immature kidney is unable to clear it efficiently because of finite availability of urinary buffers.[10]

The kidneys maintain blood pressure by both direct and indirect means. This is accomplished by altering the circulating blood volume and activating the renin-angiotensin system. The outcome of renin-angiotensin system activation is contraction of vascular smooth muscle and aldosterone secretion, which results in renal tubular reabsorption of sodium and water (Fig. 21-4).

The kidney secretes erythropoietin, which stimulates bone marrow to produce erythrocytes. Erythropoietin is released in response to decreased oxygen delivery to the kidneys resulting from low hematocrit or oxygen tension.

Several factors, including vitamin D_3 and parathyroid hormone (PTH), regulate calcium metabolism. Vitamin D_3 is an essential cofactor for PTH in both bone and kidney. After vitamin D_3 is absorbed by the jejunum and ileum, it must be metabolized into its active form first by the liver and then by the kidney. In its active form, vitamin D_3 promotes intestinal absorption of calcium and stimulates bone reabsorption of calcium. In the absence of vitamin D_3, hypocalcemia and disturbances in bone mineralization occur.

Serum calcium and phosphate levels share an inverse relationship (i.e., when serum calcium levels rise, serum phosphate levels decline and vice versa). The interrelationship of calcium phosphate is progressively disrupted during ARF. When the GFR decreases, phosphate is

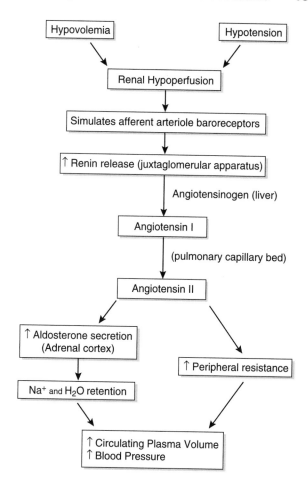

Fig. 21-4 Renin-angiotensin aldosterone cascade to maintain systemic perfusion pressure.

retained by the kidneys. Phosphate retention decreases serum calcium levels. The azotemic state also interferes with vitamin D activation by the kidneys, which is necessary for intestinal absorption of calcium. Both factors contribute to hypocalcemia.

The nephron also synthesizes prostaglandins, which are important in the maintenance of RBF and glomerular perfusion during changes in renal vascular resistance. Vasodilation results in an increase in blood flow and GFR, whereas the opposite occurs during vasoconstriction.

ACUTE RENAL FAILURE

ARF is the abrupt cessation of kidney function with or without oliguria, resulting in fluid and waste product accumulation. Traditionally, ARF has been divided into three categories: prerenal, renal, and postrenal failure. These categories are based on the site of the abnormality thought to be causing the renal insufficiency (Fig. 21-5).

Prerenal Failure

Pathogenesis. Prerenal failure is due to renal hypoperfusion from inadequate preload or heart failure (Table 21-3). There is no structural defect in the kidney itself. Prerenal dysfunction can lead to decreased RBF, GFR, and

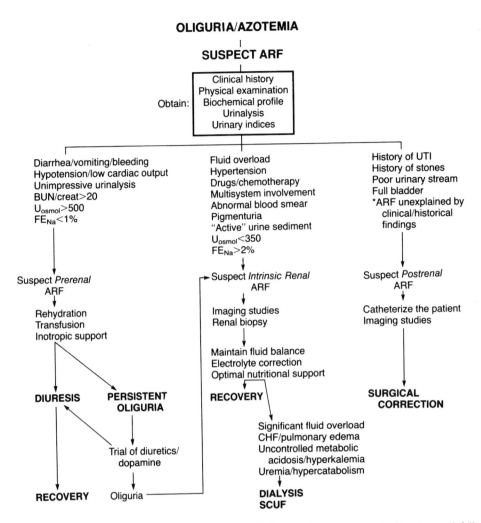

Fig. 21-5 Suggested approach to basic diagnostic and therapeutic management of acute renal failure *(ARF)* in infants and children. *BUN,* Blood urea nitrogen; U_{osmol}, urine osmolality; *UTI,* urinary tract infection; FE_{Na}, fractional excretion of sodium; *SCUF,* slow continuous ultrafiltration. (From Ongkingco JRC, Block GH: Diagnosis and management of acute renal failure in the critical care unit. In Holbrook PR: *Textbook of pediatric critical care,* Philadelphia, 1993, WB Saunders, p 592.)

◆ TABLE 21-3   **Causes of Prerenal Oliguria**

Altered Cardiac Performance	Vasodilation	Altered Vascular Volume	Altered Blood Supply to the Kidney
Cardiogenic shock	Septic shock	Intravascular volume loss	Surgical
Congestive heart failure	Anaphylaxis	Hemorrhage	Cardiac bypass
Congenital heart disease	Allergic	Third space	Aortic cross clamp
Postoperative myocardial	Transfusion	Edema	Umbilical arterial catheter displacement
dysfunction	Vasodilating agents	Peritonitis	Renal artery thrombosis
Dysrhythmias	Drug overdose	Burns	
Cardiomyopathy	Liver failure	Gastrointestinal loss	
Myocarditis		Vomiting	
Cardiac tamponade		Diarrhea	
Positive pressure ventilation		Renal Losses	
Pulmonary embolism		Excessive diuresis	
		Pancreatitis	
		Dermal losses	

urine output. Oliguria is a compensatory mechanism intended to restore intravascular volume when tissue perfusion is inadequate through conservation of sodium and water. Venous return is increased, and tissue perfusion to major organ systems may be improved.

The physiologic responses of the kidney to reduced blood flow depend on the integrity of several intrarenal and extrarenal mechanisms. Autoregulation is an intrarenal mechanism by which the kidney can locally readjust its vascular resistance and regulate blood flow.[12] By varying arteriolar resistance, autoregulation allows organs to regulate blood flow in proportion to metabolic demand and maintain a constant blood flow over a wide range of perfusion pressures.

Autoregulation in the kidney is designed to maintain a relatively constant RBF in the face of changing blood pressure and renal perfusion pressure (RPP). Autoregulation functions independently of humoral and neurogenic factors and keeps RBF in a remarkably narrow range under normal physiologic conditions.[12] To maintain a relatively constant GFR, afferent arteriolar resistance varies in direct proportion to systemic pressure. Systemic hypotension is accompanied by afferent arteriolar vasodilation, which reduces renal vascular resistance and improves RBF. This is an initial short response, followed by vasoconstriction. Blood is then shunted away from the renal cortex to the juxtamedullary nephrons. This results in tubular reabsorption of water, sodium, and urea.[13] With significant vasoconstriction, the kidney will shunt blood to the most vital organs (brain and heart), which can be lifesaving in a patient with shock.[13] If delivery of oxygen to the kidney remains impaired after compensatory mechanisms are applied, the patient is at risk for acute tubular necrosis (ATN) of the kidney. Because arterioles are present at either end of the glomerulus, constriction or dilation of these arterioles alters the perfusion pressure through the glomerular capillaries and regulates glomerular filtration. Changes in GFR ultimately affect the volume and content of the final urine product.

The extrarenal mechanisms that affect renal function include alterations in cardiac output, systemic vascular tone, antidiuretic hormone, corresponding distribution of systemic blood flow, and systemic blood pressure. The importance of the interplay of both intrarenal and extrarenal factors is evident during the physiologic response of the kidney to an acute episode of volume depletion or myocardial dysfunction. For example, a sudden reduction in renal perfusion activates the renin-angiotensin system to normalize renal perfusion and maintain GFR (see Fig. 21-4). The release of renin from the macula densa acts extrarenally to increase systemic vascular resistance and improve systemic blood pressure. In addition, renin stimulates the adrenal cortex to release aldosterone, which acts to increase tubular reabsorption of sodium followed by water. These responses also serve to normalize renal perfusion, thereby maintaining the GFR.

Primary or secondary renal vascular disease may cause a partial or complete obstruction to blood flow, resulting in renal ischemia. In infants, examples of obstruction leading to ischemia include venous and arterial vein thrombosis.

Umbilical venous catheters may lead to renal vein thrombosis, manifested by hematuria, proteinuria, or renal failure. Renal artery thrombosis is more likely to present with hypertension. Renal failure in either case is rare unless the patient has a solitary kidney. Bilateral renal vein occlusion, a more common vascular lesion in infants, has been associated with asphyxia and congenital heart disease.[14]

If compromised renal perfusion persists, the capacity of the intrarenal and extrarenal mechanisms to maintain homeostasis is jeopardized. Urine production decreases, and azotemia may occur. If systemic pressure and volume are not restored after a finite period, true, fixed intrinsic renal failure ensues. Early detection of the subtle signs and symptoms of intrinsic renal failure is crucial to facilitate appropriate management to preserve renal function.

Clinical Presentation. Renal failure can be oliguric or nonoliguric. Nonoliguric ARF describes renal dysfunction associated with a normal or excessive urine volume. The key to early recognition is to be alert for signs of decreased or increased urine volume in relation to overall fluid balance. Acid-base disturbances may be detected early in patients with prerenal failure. An unexplained metabolic acidosis is a sign of decreased tissue perfusion, including renal perfusion.

The diagnosis of renal failure is based on the presence of azotemia. Serum blood urea nitrogen (BUN) and creatinine levels provide an index of glomerular filtration. Both of these substances are nitrogenous end products of protein metabolism normally excreted in urine. As GFR decreases, BUN and creatinine levels increase. In isolation, BUN is not a reliable indicator of renal function because the level may be affected by factors other than nitrogen excretion by the kidney. Extrarenal factors that affect BUN concentration are listed in Table 21-4. Creatinine is an end product of muscle metabolism, which is excreted and eliminated at a constant rate. Serum creatinine is relatively unaffected by extrarenal factors and, therefore, is a more reliable indicator of glomerular function. Because the level of serum creatinine is a function of muscle mass, it is affected by age, muscle mass, and body build.[15] In the face of decreased tubular flow, a greater percentage of urea is reabsorbed into the circulatory system, producing a significant elevation in serum BUN. In the same circumstance, creatinine levels are usually only slightly elevated. The serum BUN/creatinine ratio may also help to differentiate prerenal from intrinsic renal failure (Table 21-5).

Other laboratory values used to differentiate prerenal failure from intrinsic renal failure include measuring tubular reabsorption of sodium and water. Unlike the kidney with parenchymal damage, the underperfused but functionally intact kidney has the capability to actively reabsorb sodium as a compensatory response to hypovolemia. When evaluating a patient with ARF, the single most informative laboratory test is the fractional excretion of sodium (FE_{Na}). The FE_{Na} is calculated as follows:

$$(FE_{Na}) = (Urine\ [Na]/Plasma\ [Na])/(Urine\ [Cr]/Plasma\ [Cr]) \times 100$$

In patients with prerenal azotemia, the FE_{Na} is usually less than 1%, and in patients with ATN, it is generally greater than 1%. These levels may be altered by the administration of diuretics. Loop diuretics inhibit the reabsorption of sodium at the proximal tubule, which improves solute excretion in the urine.

Reabsorption of water also requires a functionally intact renal tubule. Measurement of urine specific gravity is a simple and readily available procedure. A urine specific gravity over 1.020 strongly suggests prerenal failure. The increased concentration of urine indicates decreased RBF and functioning compensatory mechanisms intended to preserve circulating volume.

Chemical testing of the urine has been simplified by the introduction of multiple dipstick tests that detect substances such as glucose, bilirubin, pH, protein, blood, and ketones on a single impregnated paper strip. Dipstick tests can be done quickly and accurately to gather information about the capacity of the kidneys to maintain homeostasis during an acute illness.

Emergent Management.   Assessment and intervention to attenuate renal parenchymal damage are dependent on recognizing high-risk situations that are associated with prerenal failure. Those conditions that alter fluid volume status and cardiac performance place patients at particular risk. Patient outcome depends on early diagnosis and management of inadequate renal perfusion and avoidance or careful monitoring of patient response to nephrotoxic agents listed in Box 21-1. Prompt evaluation and possible discontinuation of both nephrotoxic agents and supplemental potassium may be warranted.

The first step in managing an oliguric patient is to assess and ensure the adequacy of intravascular volume. On physical examination, dry mucous membranes, tachycardia,

 TABLE 21-4   Extrarenal Factors That Affect BUN and Creatinine Levels

Blood Urea Nitrogen

Increased by:	Decreased by:
Hypercatabolic states (e.g., fever, sepsis)	Liver disease
GI hemorrhage	Hypometabolic state
Dehydration/intravenous depletion	Hyperlipidemia
High protein diet	Low protein diet
Starvation	High caloric diet
Medications (i.e., corticosteroids, tetracyclines)	
Low urine flow rate	

Creatinine

Increased by:	Decreased by:
Dehydration	Loss of muscle mass
Rhabdomyolysis	Burns
Cephalosporins	Hyperlipidemia
Large muscle mass	

BUN, Blood urea nitrogen; *GI,* gastrointestinal.

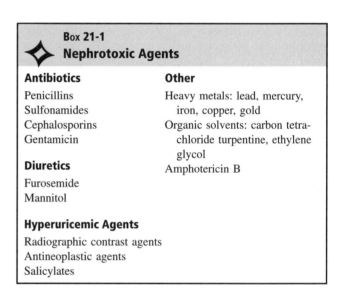

Box 21-1
Nephrotoxic Agents

Antibiotics
Penicillins
Sulfonamides
Cephalosporins
Gentamicin

Diuretics
Furosemide
Mannitol

Hyperuricemic Agents
Radiographic contrast agents
Antineoplastic agents
Salicylates

Other
Heavy metals: lead, mercury, iron, copper, gold
Organic solvents: carbon tetrachloride turpentine, ethylene glycol
Amphotericin B

 TABLE 21-5   Laboratory Values That Differentiate Causes of Oliguria

Laboratory Test	Normal	Prerenal Failure	Renal Failure
Urine specific gravity	1.015-1.022	>1.020	<1.010
Urine osmolality	50-1500 mOsm/L (infant: 50-650)	>500	<400
Urine sodium	40-80 mEq/L	<10 mEq/L	>30 mEq/L (infant >25)
Urine potassium	40-80 mEq/L	30-70 mEq/L	<20-40 mEq/L
Urine creatinine		>100 mg/dl	<70 mg/dl
Urine creatinine/plasma ratio		>30	<20 (infant <10)
Urine urea		>2000	<400
Urine urea:plasma ratio		>14	<6
Serum BUN/creatinine ratio	10:1-15:1	>20:1	<10:1
FE_{NA} (fractional excretion of filtered sodium)	<1%	<1%	>2%

BUN, Blood urea nitrogen.

hypotension, a sunken fontanelle, absence of tears, and decreased urine volume indicate hypovolemia. Ongoing assessment includes direct physical examination, as well as monitoring hemodynamic variables that reflect volume status.

Restoration of intravascular volume is the priority if hypovolemia is detected, to ensure adequate cardiac output regardless of whether renal damage has occurred. Except in the presence of hypervolemia, a 10 to 20 ml/kg fluid challenge, using any volume expander, is administered. Unless the patient is in congestive heart failure, the fluid bolus is repeated, followed by diuretics. After each intervention, the fluid volume status is evaluated.[13] Diuretics can help distinguish prerenal from fixed renal failure and can convert an oliguric to a nonoliguric state. Diuretics may also be useful in restoring and maintaining normal water and electrolyte balance and preventing further renal damage. The desired outcome is to restore circulating blood volume and increase urinary output.

Recovery from prerenal failure depends on astute nursing care focused to attenuate the progression of irreversible renal damage. Outcome is not only related to the underlying cause of renal failure and extent of other organ system damage but also to the ability of healthcare providers to recognize patients at risk and intervene effectively.

Intrinsic Renal Failure

Pathogenesis.   Intrinsic renal failure refers to numerous conditions or primary physiologic events that produce renal parenchymal damage involving the glomerulus or tubular epithelium. Direct injury to the renal parenchyma also can be caused by episodes of acute hypoperfusion or adverse reactions to nephrotoxic agents.

Manifested by proteinuria and/or hematuria, intrinsic renal failure may occur after extensive injury to the glomerular capillary wall. Although the lesion is primarily glomerular, entire nephrons can be destroyed, leading to chronic renal failure. The most common causes of intrinsic oliguria in the pediatric population are listed in Box 21-2. More than 50% of cases of intrinsic renal failure in children are the result of acute glomerulonephritis, hemolytic uremic syndrome, and drug-induced nephritis.

Acute poststreptococcal glomerulonephritis (APSGN) can occur sporadically, which is more common, or in epidemics. It occurs most often in children of preschool and early school-age years. Less than 5% of cases are seen in children under 2 years of age, and 5% to 10% occur in adults older than 40 years.[16] Twenty percent of asymptomatic school children are carriers of streptococci. Though APSGN may be seen without the usual prodromal illness, pharyngitis and pyoderma are common antecedents to APSGN.[16] Treatment of the prodromal illness does not appear to prevent APSGN but may prevent a rise in titers of streptococcal-related antibodies.

The major physiologic disturbance of APSGN is reduced GFR caused by decreased glomerular filtration surface from both infiltration by inflammatory cells and decreased basement membrane permeability. RBF is also decreased, usually in proportion to the decreased GFR. The filtration fraction remains normal, and tubular function is preserved. Decreased filtration, in conjunction with usual oral intake, results in retention of fluid and solute. Edema and hypertension are due to vascular and interstitial volume expansion. If solute filtration is significantly decreased, azotemia with acidemia, hyperkalemia, and hyperphosphatemia become prominent.[16] Most children are not usually critically ill and recover completely following treatment.

Hemolytic uremic syndrome (HUS) is a syndrome of microangiopathic hemolytic anemia with multiorgan involvement. The pathologic state results from endothelial injury and microvascular thrombosis with glomerular injury, ARF, and, at times, cortical necrosis.[17] HUS is discussed in more detail in Chapter 24.

Drug-induced nephritis is a common cause of ARF and often has systemic manifestations of an allergic process. It was first described in association with methicillin and has also been described in relation to use of penicillins, cephalosporins, sulfonamides, allopurinol, cimetidine, ciprofloxacin, and nonsteroidal antiinflammatory medications. The clinical diagnosis can be suspected in the presence of fever, rash, urine sediment revealing red cells and white casts, acute rise in creatinine level temporally related to a medication or infection, eosinophilia, mild proteinuria, and signs of tubular dysfunction. However, cases have been

Box 21-2
Causes of Intrinsic Renal Failure

Immune-Related
Glomerulonephritis
Systemic lupus erythematosus

Vascular
Hemolytic-uremic syndrome
Renal vein artery thrombosis
Disseminated intravascular coagulation
Thrombotic thrombocytopenia purpura

Interstitial Nephritis
Infectious
Drug-related
Malignant

Renal Trauma

Nephrotoxins
Endogenous
  Transfusion reaction
  Cytotoxic therapy
  Tumor lysis
Exogenous
  Anesthetic agents
  Heavy metals
  Organic solvents
  Antibiotics
  Pesticides
  Radiographic contrast agents
  Hyperalimentation

described, especially with nonsteroidal medication use, in which most of these symptoms are absent or variable. Indications for biopsy include uncertainty of diagnosis, advanced renal failure, or lack of spontaneous recovery after cessation of medication administration. Acute interstitial nephritis (AIN) is not medication dose dependent, and its onset may occur from 3 to 5 days to weeks or months after initiation of drug therapy. Major histologic findings on renal biopsy include interstitial edema and interstitial infiltrates of T lymphocytes and monocytes. Sometimes, eosinophils and neutrophils with minimal changes in the glomeruli may be seen. When infection is responsible for AIN, neutrophils are present in large numbers.[18]

The term acute tubular necrosis (ATN) is commonly applied to nephrotoxic and ischemic renal injuries that damage the tubular epithelium. Two types of histologic changes are commonly observed in ATN: necrosis of the tubular epithelium leaving the basement membrane intact, commonly resulting from the ingestion of nephrotoxic agents, and necrosis of the tubular epithelium and basement membrane, commonly associated with renal ischemia. Nephrotoxic injury can also be produced by chemical agents that directly impair renal cell function, participate in immune or inflammatory reactions, or aggravate an underlying renal disorder (see Box 21-2).

Ischemic injuries resulting in ATN occur during an acute period of renal hypoperfusion. If ischemia persists, irreversible renal damage occurs. The amount of renal cell damage depends on the length of the ischemic episode. It has been reported that an ischemic time of 30 minutes or less to the kidney may be well tolerated. In low perfusion states, the autoregulatory properties of the afferent and efferent arterioles of the glomerulus become impaired. The pathologic change produced by renal ischemia is destruction of the tubular epithelium and basement membrane or cortical necrosis. Early responses to ischemia are found in the brush border of the proximal tubule. Even mild ischemia lasting 10 minutes can cause sloughing of the brush border and changes in the proximal tubular histology. In more prolonged periods of ischemia, these changes progress to lethal injury to cells and disruption of the basement membrane.[14] When the basement membrane is destroyed, epithelial regeneration occurs in a random haphazard manner, often leading to obstruction of the nephron at the site of necrosis. Prognosis is therefore dependent on the extent of necrosis.

The mechanisms that lead to a decrease in GFR and associated oliguria in patients with ATN have not been clearly defined. Tubular backleak and obstruction theories have been proposed to explain the oliguria associated with ATN. The tubular backleak hypothesis proposes that glomerular filtration continues normally but tubular fluid "leaks back" from the damaged tubular cells into the renal interstitium rather than being excreted as urine. The tubular obstruction theory proposes that ATN leads to the desquamation of necrotic tubular cells and formation of brush border debris, which occludes the tubule lumina and produce obstruction.[14] Cellular swelling as a result of the initial ischemia may also contribute to obstruction and perpetuate the ischemia. Intratubular pressure increases so that net glomerular filtration pressure is reduced. Tubular obstruction may be an important factor in ATN when prolonged ischemia or ingestion of heavy metals or ethylene glycol occurs.

Clinical Presentation. Infants and children with ATN often present with abrupt-onset oliguria or anuria. It is important to recognize the onset of oliguria and differentiate the cause leading to ATN from prerenal, intrinsic, and postrenal disorders that may cause oliguria. Three phases characterize the clinical course of ATN: oliguria, diuresis, and recovery.

After exposure to a nephrotoxic agent or following an ischemic event, oliguric ATN may develop immediately or several days after renal cell damage occurs. This phase is most often characterized by abrupt reduction in urine production that continues for 24 to 48 hours, though this may vary. During the oliguric phase, serum BUN and creatinine levels rise. Other significant laboratory data resulting from tubular dysfunction and inability to concentrate urine include urine specific gravity less than 1.018, low urine osmolality, and urine sodium greater than 10 mEq/L. Potential complications during the oliguric phase include hypervolemia causing congestive heart failure or pulmonary edema; electrolyte imbalances, particularly hyponatremia and hyperkalemia; and acid-base disturbances.

The diuretic phase of ATN usually lasts 5 to 7 days. Early in the diuretic phase, urea clearance does not keep pace with endogenous urea production despite more than adequate urine output. BUN continues to rise. Later in the diuretic phase, BUN decreases, and azotemia eventually disappears. Because glomerular filtration and subsequent production of urine is the first mechanism to recover, total body fluid and electrolytes may be depleted if replacement is inadequate. To achieve the goal of normovolemia with electrolyte and acid-base balance, astute monitoring is essential. Tubular reabsorption returns next and contributes significantly to the overall improvement in renal function.

The recovery phase from ATN in infants and children is usually longer than in adults; 2 to 4 months may elapse before normal renal function returns. BUN and urine laboratory values gradually return to normal, reflecting a progressive restoration of GFR and tubular function. The level of recovery is variable, especially if preexisting medical problems or renal insufficiency are present. Some patients may be left with some residual renal impairment, such as a permanent decrease in renal function or a urine concentrating defect. The primary cause of death during the recovery phase is infection or complications related to the primary illness that initially compromised renal function.

Nonoliguric ATN, increased urine output with elevated BUN and creatinine levels, is commonly associated with nephrotoxic agents, asphyxia, respiratory distress, and congenital anomalies in the newborn. Compared with patients with oliguric ATN, patients with nonoliguric renal failure have lower overall mortality rate.[14] Nonoliguria facilitates fluid and nutritional management of ARF.

Emergent Management. Currently, no therapy is known to modify the course of intrinsic renal failure. Management strategies for ATN are aimed at improving renal perfusion and removing the cause of the disease by discontinuing the nephrotoxic medications. Some innovative medical therapies have been evaluated for reversal of ATN, but none have proven effective in controlled human studies. Therapy for non-ATN intrarenal failure may involve steroids or other immunomodulating agents. To date, the mainstay of therapy is supportive care and control of complications during renal compromise.[19]

Postrenal Failure

Pathogenesis. Postrenal oliguria results from an anatomic obstruction of the urinary tract and is uncommon in children. Box 21-3 outlines the causes of postrenal oliguria, which may result from obstruction of any portion of the urinary system. Most urinary obstruction in children is the result of a congenital problem. Obstruction increases intratubular pressure and leads to a reduction in RBF and GFR that is manifested by a decrease in urinary output. Oliguria will not occur from unilateral obstruction unless the contralateral kidney is absent or nonfunctional. In children, especially infants, who present with oliguria alone, the first consideration is to determine that the major anatomic components of the renal system (arteries, veins, ureters, and bladder outlet) are intact.

Anomalies in the urinary collecting system may restrict urinary flow from the bladder. Urinary reflux can ultimately increase hydrostatic pressure in the collecting ducts and renal tubules. When hydrostatic pressure in Bowman's capsule increases, GFR decreases, tubular reabsorption is enhanced, and oliguria or anuria develops. Eventually, renal insufficiency results from tissue atrophy.

Bilateral anatomic obstruction occurs more often in male infants than in females because of congenital posterior ureteral valves and/or urethral strictures. Postrenal oliguria may occur in older infants who have an undiagnosed solitary kidney that becomes acutely obstructed. The obstruction may be the result of an anatomic abnormality or an acquired intraluminal lesion, such as renal calculi, blood clot, inflammation, and edema. Extrinsic compression of the

urethral outflow tract by lesions such as periurethral abscess, trauma, Wilms' tumor, or a neuroblastoma are rare but must be suspected in any patient with acute bilateral obstruction.

Clinical Presentation. The infrequent occurrence of obstructive uropathy in the critical care setting does not diminish its importance because early diagnosis and correction can avert permanent parenchymal damage. Diagnostic imaging techniques are used to determine the cause. Children with postrenal oliguria often present with abdominal or flank pain. A palpable mass may suggest an obstructed urinary system, although a mass may be associated with other causes of ARF, such as renal vein thrombosis or polycystic kidney disease. A renal mass associated with a palpable bladder, palpably enlarged kidneys, or abnormal urinary stream in a male may suggest urinary tract obstruction from posterior ureteral valves.[20] Young children may be completely asymptomatic except for failure to thrive. Analysis of urinary sediment associated with obstruction is usually normal unless a coexisting infection exists. Ultrasonography can demonstrate bladder thickening, hydronephrosis, dilation of the posterior urethra, and posterior urethral valves. The diagnosis is made by voiding cystourethrography, which delineates the valves and confirms findings necessary for surgical intervention.

Several invasive radiographic and urodynamic studies can be used to assess the function of the renal system through the detection of disturbances in voiding patterns and structural defects. These include intravenous pyelography (IVP), voiding cystourethrography (VCUG), renal angiography, and renal scan.

Emergent Management. The goal of treatment is decompression of the urinary collecting system by removal of the obstruction or by urinary diversion. Relief of the obstruction may result in a marked increase in urine formation because of increased RBF and improved tubular function. Immediate success of ablative therapy of the obstruction can be demonstrated on VCUG, but resolution of hydroureteronephrosis and reflux generally takes longer. Periodic follow-up is required to detect delayed obstruction caused by stricture or loss of bladder tone.[16]

Critical Care Management

As outlined in Table 21-6, altered renal function affects all body systems. Clinical presentation depends on the length and acuity of the disease process.

Maintenance of Intravascular Volume. During ARF the regulatory factors that control intravascular volume status may be inadequate. The primary goal in fluid management in ARF is to achieve and maintain normal intravascular fluid volume. Because children with ARF have a spectrum of volume disorders, initial and ongoing estimation of fluid status is important. This is monitored by accurate intake and output assessment, weights, vital signs, capillary refill, central venous pressure monitoring, and presence of edema. Laboratory data including serum sodium and FE_{Na} also help determine fluid volume status.

Children with ARF and decreased intravascular volume, despite an oliguric or anuric state, require prompt fluid

---

Box 21-3
Postrenal Causes of Oliguria

Ureteral

Intrinsic

Stones
Blood clot
Ureteropelvic stenosis

Extrinsic

Tumor
Surgical ligation
Radiation injury

Bladder

Blood clots
Neurogenic bladder

Urethral

Posterior urethral valves
Urethral stricture

TABLE 21-6	**Management Priorities During Acute Renal Failure**
Alteration	**Consequence**
Intravascular volume status	Hyper- or hypovolemia manifested
Electrolyte balance	Abnormal K, Na, Ca, Mg, Phos levels
Uremia	Uremic syndrome
Acid-base balance	Metabolic acidosis
Nutritional status	Malnutrition
Immune function	Infection
Anemia, thrombocytopenia	Disruption in oxygen delivery, coagulation
Respiratory	Pulmonary edema
Cardiovascular	Dysrhythmias, hypertension

resuscitation. A delay in therapy jeopardizes renal function recovery, as well as other functions of major organs. Conversely, ARF associated with volume overload requires fluid restriction and diuretics. Hypervolemia is a common manifestation of ARF. Hypertension may result from the increase in circulating volume and interplay of the renin-angiotensin system.

Deteriorating renal function may also result in excessive urinary output. Management strategies such as restricted fluid intake and diuretic therapy contribute to a fluid volume deficit. As a consequence, cardiac output and tissue perfusion may be impaired.

Maintenance fluid requirements are adjusted to the evolving needs of the patient. Daily total output determines intake. Daily intake includes oral and parenteral fluids, blood products, and medications. Often overlooked intake can include fluid for catheter or medication flushes and endotracheal tube lavage with suctioning. This intake can equal as much as 12 ml/kg/day of fluid intake and as much as 2.4 mEq/kg/day of sodium.[14]

Daily output is the sum of urine output and insensible losses, which include gastrointestinal, respiratory, and evaporative losses. Other factors that influence precise calculation of fluid needs include the humidity and temperature of the environment and the use of phototherapy, warming devices, and mechanical ventilation. Sensible fluid output includes urine, stools, emesis, tube drainage, ostomy output, and fistula output. Insensible water output equals approximately 750 ml/m^2/day. Net insensible water loss is approximately equal to one third of calculated maintenance rate. Patients receiving humidified air have less insensible losses; those with burns, tachypnea, or receiving thermal warming therapy have higher losses. Fever increases a patient's insensible water losses by 12.5% per degree Celsius (C) above normal.[14] Although fluid balance can be calculated and is monitored closely, ongoing assessment of tissue perfusion is the best indicator of adequate intravascular volume.

Maintenance of Electrolyte Balance.   Electrolyte disturbances commonly occur during the course of ARF.

Alterations are related to changes in volume status and the inability of the kidneys to regulate electrolyte balance. Because the kidneys are responsible for 90% of potassium excretion, hyperkalemia is a major life-threatening complication of ARF. The catabolic state of the patient further elevates serum potassium. Because of the potentially lethal nature of hyperkalemia, patients at risk require ongoing assessment of laboratory values along with cardiac rhythm assessment (see Chapter 12).

Attention must be given to the administration of potassium-containing intravenous fluid, medications (aqueous penicillin G contains 1.7 mEq potassium per 1 million units) and cold stored blood (blood stored for 10 days can contain up to 30 mEq/L of potassium). Endogenously produced potassium in clinical states of trauma, burns, and tumor lysis syndrome can increase serum potassium.

Sodium imbalance is also prevalent in ARF. Most commonly, hyponatremia is iatrogenic, induced from overestimation of free water needs and inability to diurese excess free water. Important to consider is the variability in the amount of sodium excreted by the kidney. Induced diuresis or the diuretic phase of nonoliguric renal failure can significantly increase urine sodium loss.

Ongoing monitoring of serum sodium levels and urine sodium excretion determines the appropriate type and volume of fluid intake. Hyponatremia may deleteriously affect the clinical status and prognosis of the patient with ARF. Serum sodium levels of 130 mEq/L or less indicate a need for further fluid restriction. In a patient with a serum sodium level of 120 mEq/L or less who is not responding to fluid restriction or experiencing mental status changes, 3% sodium chloride administration (513 mEq/L) is considered. The calculation is for infusing 3% sodium chloride is as follows:

$$\text{mEq of Na} = (125 - \text{observed Na}) \times \text{kg body weight} \times 0.6$$

Three percent sodium chloride is administered slowly over 2 to 4 hours. An estimate of 12 ml/kg of 3% sodium chloride will increase the serum sodium concentration by 10 mEq/L.[14]

Hypocalcemia and hyperphosphatemia are additional electrolyte disturbances that occur rapidly in ARF. Phosphate levels increase because of the limited ability of the kidney to excrete phosphate. This response occurs simultaneously with catabolic increases in phosphate released from tissue. Hypocalcemia in ARF has multiple causes, including hyperphosphatemia, vitamin D_3 deficiency, and hypoalbuminemia. Ionized calcium levels must be monitored to evaluate the unbound form of calcium, which determines physiologic activity.

Parenteral or enteral calcium replacement therapy is more efficient if hyperphosphatemia is managed first. Elevated plasma phosphate concentrations result in the precipitation of calcium phosphate in bone and soft tissues. Reduction of the serum phosphate level is accomplished by diminishing the absorption of phosphorus in the gastrointestinal tract. This usually results in an increase in the serum calcium level. Limiting the intake of parenteral and enteral

TABLE 21-7   Daily Nutrient Intake Recommendations for the Child With Acute Renal Failure Not Requiring Dialysis

Age	0-0.5 yr	0.5-1 yr	1-3 yr	4-6 yr	7-10 yr	11-18 yr
Energy (kcal/kg)	≥108	≥98	102	90	70	40-55
Protein* (g/kg)	2.2	1.6	1.2	1.2	1.0	0.9-1.0

From Mendley SR, Langman CB: Acute renal failure in the pediatric patient, *Adv Renal Replace Ther* 4:96, 1997.
*Once dialysis is initiated, increase the protein intake by ~50%.

sources of phosphate requires a thorough review of phosphorus content in all sources of intake.

Magnesium is another electrolyte that is affected by ARF. Commonly, patients with ARF have mild, asymptomatic hypermagnesemia. Higher levels may be seen with injudicious use of magnesium-containing laxatives or antacids. Hypomagnesemia can occur in patients with renal tubular damage from nephrotoxic agents. Generally, this hypomagnesemia is asymptomatic, but if severe, it will result in neuromuscular effects such as cramps, cardiac arrhythmias, and seizures.[21]

Maintenance of Acid-Base Balance.   Impairment of renal function results in the disturbance of acid-base homeostasis. Metabolic acidosis is the predominant finding. Renal tubular dysfunction results in the inability to reabsorb filtered bicarbonate or regenerate bicarbonate used to buffer the daily acid load.[21] In a healthy person, dietary protein metabolism results in daily generation of approximately 1 mEq of fixed, nonvolatile acids per kilogram of body weight. In ARF, inability to clear acids results in metabolic acidosis. In uncomplicated ARF, the serum bicarbonate falls by about 1 to 2 mEq/L/day. In hypercatabolic states, this level can fall much faster.[21] The mild acidosis that accompanies this isolated disturbance is compensated for by the respiratory system. Disturbances in normal cellular metabolism, caused by hypoxemia or altered tissue perfusion, result in anaerobic metabolism and lactic acid production. Other conditions such as ethylene glycol intoxication, certain inborn errors of metabolism, diabetic ketoacidosis, or the administration of medications may overwhelm renal excretory capacity and worsen metabolic acidosis.

Before initiating treatment for metabolic acidosis, the patient's ability to compensate for the imbalance is considered. Bicarbonate levels of 10 to 13 mEq/L may be managed with administration of intravenous sodium bicarbonate. Before administration, the clinical condition, including current respiratory mechanisms and the potential effect of sodium and volume bolus, must be evaluated. Severe acidosis, particularly in an oliguric patient with fluid overload, may prohibit administration of intravenous bicarbonate and may require emergent dialysis.[21]

Maintenance of Respiratory Status.   Complications of the respiratory system in children with ARF most commonly are due to fluid retention with oliguria. This condition may be demonstrated as pulmonary edema or infection. Acute respiratory distress syndrome (ARDS) is also a complication in critically ill patients with multiorgan

dysfunction syndrome (MODS) and ARF. These children require vigilant monitoring for respiratory distress and may require intubation and mechanical ventilation.

Maintenance of Neurologic Status.   A variety of neurologic complications may occur. These patients may exhibit symptoms ranging from mild myoclonus or muscle twitching to seizures and uremic encephalopathy. Asterixis and lethargy may be early signs of uremia. As ARF progresses, the patient may demonstrate confusion, personality changes, seizures, and eventually a comatose state. Generally, these symptoms respond promptly to dialysis. If symptoms do not improve after initiation of dialysis, other causes of mental status change must be considered, such as a medication effect or a neurologic event. Seizures may be due to uremia, hypertension, hyponatremia, or hypomagnesemia. Electroencephalogram abnormalities are common in patients with uremic encephalopathy. These abnormalities include loss of background alpha activity with the development of slow waves, progressing to diffuse slow wave and spike activity.[21]

Maintenance of Adequate Nutrition.   Many disease processes precipitating or occurring simultaneously with ARF place the child in a hypercatabolic state. Children's nutritional needs are relatively large compared with those of adults (Table 21-7). Normal infants have twice the protein requirement of adults, which must be maintained during critical illness to prevent a negative nitrogen balance.[1] Studies in adults and children have indicated that aggressive nutritional support decreases tissue catabolism, which reduces the accumulation of acids, nitrogenous wastes, and potassium. In addition, hypercatabolic states have been noted as a significant risk factor for ARF.[21]

Meeting a patient's nutritional requirements depends on the function of the gastrointestinal tract, vascular access, and severity of oliguria. Small and frequent enteral feedings are the method of choice. Advantages to the use of the enteral route include oral gratification, decreased risk for septicemia because vascular access is not required, and possible prevention of gut bacterial translocation.

When caloric needs cannot be met through the use of enteral feedings, parenteral nutrition is necessary. With renal replacement therapy, daily protein and caloric intake can be generous (0.5 to 1 to g/kg/day of protein). If the BUN is near 50, the patient may benefit from special "nephro" hyperalimentation solutions, which contain essential amino acids and various nonessential amino acids. Depending on the patient's serum electrolytes, solutions should contain minimal sodium and no potassium.[13] In some cases, especially in patients with oligoanuria, renal replacement therapy may be necessary because of the high volumes of fluid required to meet the child's nutritional needs. Daily monitoring of electrolytes and frequent glucose monitoring are required in the first days of parenteral nutrition.

Prevention of Infection.   The patient with ARF is at high risk for infection because of invasive monitoring and catheters, surgical procedures, and a highly catabolic metabolism. Between 50% to 70% of patients with ARF develop infections, and administration of prophylactic antibiotics does not appear to decrease the high incidence of infection. The most common sites of infection are the chest, urinary tract, and wounds.[21] Difficulty in meeting the patient's nutritional needs compromises immune function. In addition, the patient's ability to fight infection is minimized as a result of defective chemotaxis, absolute or relative granulocytosis, relative lymphopenia, and impaired cell-mediated immunity. The need for indwelling bladder and central venous catheters is reevaluated daily in light of the high risk for infection.

Because manifestations vary, infection during ARF is difficult to identify. Symptoms may include both hypothermia and hyperthermia. White blood cell count may be elevated or diminished. Other subtle signs include tachycardia, tachypnea, lethargy, flushing, and localized inflammatory response. Surveillance cultures may be routinely indicated.

Prophylactic antibiotics are not recommended. Aggressive treatment with appropriate antibiotics is indicated in the case of proven infection. Dosage and frequency of antibiotics are based on renal function.

Maintenance of Hematologic Function.   Hematologic complications in ARF include anemia, platelet dysfunction, bleeding disorders, and leukocytosis. Anemia often results from failure of the kidney to produce erythropoietin and can occur as soon as 10 days after the onset of ARF. Other causes of anemia include blood loss or hemodilution from volume expansion.

Uremic platelets display defective aggregation and adhesion properties. Nitric oxide (NO) and prostacyclin, agents that inhibit platelet aggregation, may be increased in uremia, thus contributing to platelet dysfunction.

Bleeding disorders, in the presence of uremia, are primarily attributed to platelet dysfunction and may be potentiated by increased capillary fragility and anemia. The platelet count is usually normal, but thrombocytopenia may be present in patients with HUS or disseminated intravascular coagulation (DIC). Platelet dysfunction can be detected by a prolonged bleeding time, with the prothrombin time and partial thromboplastin time remaining normal except in the presence of DIC. The bleeding tendencies of uremia can be corrected with red blood cell transfusions, dialysis, or a vasopressin analog such as desmopressin (DDAVP). Leukocytosis generally is due to infection or acute catabolic stress.[21] Monitoring for bleeding, especially from multiple access sites, is imperative in this population.

Laboratory Studies.   Although physical findings are the best guide to adequacy of fluid volume status, several laboratory tests support the presence of ARF.

Urinalysis.   A urinalysis provides invaluable information when evaluating a patient with ARF. Intermediate values may be found in patients with postrenal failure or in those transitioning from prerenal failure to ATN. Use of potent diuretics can invalidate these laboratory findings for up to 24 hours. A urine dipstick with trace to 1+ protein may be consistent with prerenal azotemia or ATN, but larger amounts of protein suggest an interstitial nephritis or glomerulonephritis. However, in an acute episode of congestive heart failure or malignant hyperthermia, significant proteinuria may also be present. Urine dipstick tests do not distinguish between hemoglobin and myoglobin. Therefore a strong presumptive diagnosis of rhabdomyolysis with myoglobinuria can be made by demonstrating a heme-positive urine dip in absence of red cells or on the supernatant of the urine, an elevated serum phosphokinase and aldosterone, and a normal serum color without evidence of hemolysis. The presence of glucosuria when the serum glucose level is normal may suggest a proximal tubular lesion. However, falsely high values may occur in the presence of urine protein, glucose, radiographic dyes, or other high-molecular-weight substances.[22]

Osmolality.   Although a considerable overlap can exist among individuals, prerenal failure is usually associated with a urine osmolality greater than 500 mOsm/L, whereas parenchymal failure is associated with a urine osmolality of less 400 mOsm/L.[21]

Specific Gravity.   With prerenal azotemia, hepatorenal syndrome, and early acute glomerulonephritis, the urine specific gravity is generally elevated at greater than 1.020. Patients with postrenal failure and ATN lose the ability to concentrate urine and generally have a specific gravity similar to that of plasma, which is approximately 1.010.

Urine Sediment.   In prerenal failure, hyaline casts are present in large numbers. Red cells and red cell casts may indicate glomerulonephritis or vasculitis. Heavy oxalate or hippurate may be noted in ethylene glycol ingestion. In drug-induced interstitial nephritis, proteinuria, urinary sediment with hematuria (gross or microscopic), eosinophiluria, and casts may be found. In ATN, the classic urine sediment is brown, containing renal tubular casts, renal tubular cells, and coarsely granular casts.[21] Infectious causes of intrinsic nephritis often have white blood cell casts in the sediment, indicating renal inflammation.

Serum BUN/Creatinine.   The BUN-to-serum creatinine (Cr) ratio is normally 10:1. In prerenal failure, this ratio may reach levels of 60:1.

Antineutrophilic Cytoplasmic Antibody.   The antineutrophilic cytoplasmic antibody (ANCA) is a sensitive marker for detecting ARF caused by Wegener's granulomatosis, polyarteritis nodosa, and approximately 80% of cases previously labeled "idiopathic" crescentic glomerulonephritis. ANCA may have a pathogenic role in activating leukocytes and the resultant inflammatory injury, leading to renal failure.

Without all supporting data available, prerenal azotemia can be suspected if urine specific gravity is greater than

1.016, urine sodium concentration is less than 20 mEq/L, and the BUN/Cr ratio is greater than 20:1. The BUN/Cr ratio can also be elevated in postrenal failure.

Imaging Techniques. The diagnosis of ARF is generally made based on clinical findings and laboratory results. Imaging may determine the correct diagnosis when the cause of ARF is unknown. Table 21-8 provides the various imaging procedures that may be used to diagnose ARF.

Plain Films of the Abdomen. Plain films are the least expensive and most readily accessible imaging technique. This procedure can document the size of the kidneys, thus giving information on the duration of the renal failure. Chronic renal failure is associated with small kidneys, and enlarged kidneys may suggest an acute process.

Gray-scale Ultrasonography. Gray-scale ultrasonography (US) is useful in detecting kidney and bladder size. This imaging technique is generally accepted as a method to exclude renal obstruction as the cause of ARF. It is also very accurate in detecting hydronephrosis. False-negative results may be seen in patients with early renal obstruction and dehydration. Echogenicity of the kidney can also be evaluated with gray-scale US. Most patients with ARF have normal kidney echogenicity and parenchymal thickness. A decrease in parenchymal thickness may be associated with underlying chronic nephropathy.

TABLE 21-8 Imaging Procedures in the Diagnosis of Acute Renal Failure

Procedure	Purpose
Flat plate of the abdomen or nephrotomography	For kidney size, calcification, calculi, abnormal gas collection
Ultrasonography	For kidney size, cysts, calculi, hydronephrosis, mass
Intravenous urography with postvoiding film	For kidney size, function, hydronephrosis, hydroureter, bladder size, bladder outlet obstruction
Computed axial tomography	Better evaluation of retroperitoneal lesions; for renal trauma, renal masses, site of obstruction
Radionuclide scans	For blood flow and function, gallium-67 scan for acute interstitial nephritis
Arteriography and venography	For renal trauma, vascular occlusion, polyarteritis nodosa, renal vein thrombosis

From Cadnapaphornchai P, Alvapati RK, McDonald FD: Differential diagnosis of acute renal failure. In Jacobson HR, Striker GE, Klahr S, eds: *The principles and practice of nephrology,* ed 2, St Louis, 1995, Mosby, p 562.

Duplex Doppler Ultrasonography. Renal dynamics differ in prerenal, renal, and postrenal ARF. Duplex Doppler US is capable of measuring the renal resistive index, which can differentiate between the different categories of renal failure. This technique provides more information than the morphologic view of the kidneys. This device is valuable in distinguishing between prerenal ARF and ATN. Most patients with prerenal failure have normal parenchymal flow, whereas patients with ATN demonstrate markedly abnormal flow profiles and have increased pulsatility with loss of diastolic flow. The course of ATN may be monitored with duplex Doppler US. Improvement on Doppler flow can be seen before clinical signs of function recovery. Duplex Doppler US is also useful in detecting significant urinary tract obstructions.

Both gray-scale and duplex Doppler US provide information useful for diagnosis and management of specific pathologic conditions such as hepatorenal failure, HUS, acute renal thrombosis, and acute renal artery thrombosis.[23]

Unenhanced Computed Tomography. This form of radiologic testing adds clinically important information in patients with indeterminate sonograms. Dilated ureters can generally be located to exact location of obstruction. Computed tomography (CT) can be very useful in detecting renal calculi.[23]

Magnetic Resonance Imaging. In ARF, altered corticomedullary changes can be noted on magnetic resonance imaging (MRI), although these changes are nonspecific. In suspicious postrenal failure, MRI is useful in detecting obstruction and assessing hydronephrosis. Renal perfusion can be assessed using bolus injection of paramagnetic media. MRI may be preferred to contrast-enhanced CT in patients with ARF because no significant nephrotoxicity has been reported related to paramagnetic contrast agents used in common clinical practice.[23]

Excretory Urography. This imaging technique can provide information regarding renal anatomy, chronicity of disease, and presence of urinary tract obstruction with the use of contrast. Dense urographic nephrogram and delayed opacification of the dilated collecting system are indicators of postrenal failure. Similar findings are also noted in prerenal failure, acute glomerulonephritis, renal vein thrombosis, and occasionally ATN. Most patients with ATN and acute bacterial nephritis show an immediate, dense, persistent nephrogram. Striated urographic changes are seen primarily in acute pyelonephritis. In acute occlusion of the main renal artery, the nephrogram is either absent or extremely faint. Similar findings are appreciable in acute cortical necrosis.[23]

Contrast-Enhanced Computed Tomography. Contrast-enhanced CT is much more reliable than excretory urography in detecting structural deformities of the nephrogram and requires considerably less contrast material. Contrast-enhanced CT can generally identify acute renal obstruction, both intrinsic and extrinsic. It is helpful in identifying hydronephrosis, nephritis, and mass lesions such as abscesses.[23]

Angiography. This imaging technique has been valuable in evaluating arterial or venous occlusion as a cause for

ARF. Angiography demonstrates a characteristic pattern of acute cortical necrosis and thromboembolic disease, both arterial and venous. In many clinical situations such as these, Doppler US, CT, and MRI have become the preferred diagnostic tool. However, abnormalities that directly involve the vessels create unique angiographic patterns and are best diagnosed by angiography. There are parenchymal diseases that indirectly alter blood flow, resulting in angiographic findings, which are generally nonspecific. Patchy or diffusely decreased nephrograms occur in many disease states, such as ATN, acute glomerulonephritis, and interstitial nephritis.[23]

Iodinated intravenous contrast agents, which are necessary for excretory urography, contrast-enhanced CT, and angiography, are nephrotoxic and pose a serious clinical problem. Iodinated contrast media account for about 10% of all hospital cases of renal failure, with azotemic patients at greatest risk. Excretory urography, contrast-enhanced CT, and angiography are only performed in the azotemic patient when US, unenhanced CT, and MRI are unavailable.[23]

Renal Biopsy. In cases for which the cause is unknown, renal biopsy can be a useful adjunctive tool for diagnosis, intervention, and prognosis. The diagnoses for which specific treatments are indicated include glomerulonephritis, vasculitis, and AIN.[18]

Renal biopsy in the patient with ARF carries significant risk because of the invasiveness of the procedure. These patients are at increased risk for postbiopsy bleeding as a result of coagulation disorders (including platelet dysfunction and abnormal platelet vessel wall interaction) and anemia. Arterial hypertension and dialysis compound the risk. Before renal biopsy, it is important to check the prothrombin time, partial thromboplastin time, platelet count, and bleeding time.

General postbiopsy patient care includes prone positioning on a rolled sheet or towel to promote hemostasis, strict bed rest for 24 hours, frequent vital sign monitoring, urine monitoring for macroscopic hematuria, and hematocrit check.[18] In renal disease, as with others, the least invasive mode of diagnosis is the preferred diagnostic test.

Renal Pharmacology. Several issues are considered when discussing pharmacology in renal failure. First, various degrees of renal insufficiency may alter the kidney's ability to clear medications, and toxic levels may develop. Second, the initiation of renal replacement therapy may further alter the therapeutic level of medications. Finally, several medications can be considered to enhance renal function to establish homeostasis.

Effect of Renal Insufficiency on Drug Elimination. Renal insufficiency may alter elimination of many drugs in the critically ill patient. With decreased function, the amount of a drug normally eliminated by the kidney is decreased. Drugs that are metabolized in the liver may require renal function to eliminate metabolites. In renal insufficiency, RBF and the ability of the kidney to extract drug are decreased; therefore the total amount of drug excreted per unit of time decreases.[24] Consequently, inefficient drug clearance may lead to metabolite accumulation and production of toxic effects. Adjustments to dosages may be

---

Box 21-4

◆ **Drugs Requiring Dosage Adjustment in Reduced Renal Function**

Acetaminophen	Diphenhydramine
Acyclovir	Gentamycin
Amikacin	Imipenem
Amphotericin B	Penicillin G
Ampicillin	Piperacillin
Ceftazidime	Ranitidine
Cefuroxime	Tobramycin
Digoxin	Vancomycin

---

required to maintain a steady therapeutic state. The goal is to attain an effective drug level while avoiding toxicity. Those drugs that have a wide therapeutic range may need no adjustment because levels can fluctuate without reaching toxicity.

Different methods can be used for adjusting medication dosages in ARF. One method of dosage adjustment is to deliver a loading dose to reach peak serum concentration, followed by delivery of subsequent usual maintenance doses at intervals determined by the elimination half-life of the medication.[25] However, this approach can result in extended intervals between doses, with possible subtherapeutic levels.

Another method of medication adjustment is to decrease the dosage used with normal renal function and deliver the medication at the usual intervals. This approach may provide a more steady state of the drug. In addition, this may be more the accepted method of dosing medications with a narrow therapeutic range.[25] Because of the pharmacokinetics of each drug, it is wise to consult the pharmacology references for the proper dosage. Box 21-4 gives examples of the drugs that require adjustments in renal insufficiency. Many drug formularies determine the adjusted dosages of medications according to the amount of the calculated creatinine clearance.

Effect of Renal Replacement Therapies on Drug Disposition. All renal replacement therapies affect the elimination of drugs. The extent to which the drug is dialyzed determines whether supplemental doses are necessary. The dialyzability of the drug is dependent on several factors. The molecular size of the drug affects its ability to pass through the membrane. Generally, small molecular weight particles pass through the membrane and are dialyzed. Another factor is protein binding of a drug, which is the amount of drug secured to protein in the body. Nonprotein-bound medication is available for dialysis. Distribution affects dialysis in that a drug with a large volume of distribution is less likely to be dialyzed. Solubility is a factor because drugs with high water solubility are more likely to be dialyzed because the dialysate is an aqueous solution. Finally, plasma clearance affects dialyzability of the drug. Plasma clearance is the sum of the renal and the nonrenal clearance. When nonrenal clearance is high, the drug is less likely to be dialyzed.[26] Table 21-9 gives examples of some of the drugs that are

TABLE 21-9   Considerations for Drug Prescription in Renal Failure: Supplement for Hemodialysis, Special Considerations for Peritoneal Dialysis and Continuous Renal Replacement

Drugs	Hemodialysis	Hemofiltration	Peritoneal Dialysis
Amikacin	*	—	+
Cefotaxime	**	0	0
Cefuroxime	**	—	0
Ceftriaxone	0	0	0
Clindamycin	0	0*	0*
Erythromycin	0	0*	0*
Gentamycin	*	—	+
Ticarcillin	**	++	++
Tobramycin	*	—	+
Penicillin G	**	++	++
Piperacillin	**	++	++
Vancomycin	Conventional 0 Permeable membrane—	—	—
Acyclovir	**	3.5 mg/kg/day	++
Amphotericin B	0	0*	0*
Fluconazole	**	++	++
Metronidazole	**	—	0
Trimethoprim-sulfamethoxazole	½ dose**	—	0
Pancuronium (Pavulon)	UK	UK	UK
Morphine	0	0*	0*
Lorazepam	0	0*	0*
Midazolam	0*	0*	0*
Amiodarone	0	0*	0
Digoxin	0	0	0
Dobutamine	UK	UK	UK
Enalapril	**	—	0
Milrinone	UK	UK	UK
Nicardipine	0	0*	0*
Furosemide (Lasix)	0	NA	0
Insulin	0	0*	0*
Ranitidine	½ dose	—	0
Phenytoin (Dilantin)	0	0*	0
Phenobarbital	*	Likely to be removed	75% q12h
Methylprednisolone	Yes	Likely to be removed	UK
Cyclosporine	UK	UK	UK

Adapted from Swan S, Bennett W: Use of drugs in patients with renal failure. In Schrier RW, Gottschalke CW, eds: *Diseases of the kidney,* ed 6, vol III, Boston, 1997, Little, Brown, pp 2963-3017.
+, 30% q24h; ++, dose for GFR <10 (dose for GFR 10-50 ml/min); *, ⅔ normal dose after dialysis; **, dose after dialysis; 0*, unlikely; *UK,* unknown.

affected by the different types of renal replacement therapies.

Drugs That Enhance Renal Output.   Several agents are available to enhance renal output in the presence of renal disease. Table 21-10 outlines the more common agents employed in the pediatric intensive care unit (PICU).

Loop Diuretics.   Loop diuretics are the most common diuretics used in the PICU. They are often prescribed to promote urine output and to facilitate the change of oliguric to nonoliguric ARF.[27] Loop diuretics inhibit the sodium-chloride co-transport mechanism in the thick ascending limb of the loop of Henle, where 20% to 30% of sodium reclamation occurs.[28] Furosemide, a loop diuretic, also is thought to reverse decreased GFRs.[29] Furosemide is mainly

excreted in the kidney, whereas bumetanide undergoes extensive hepatic metabolism and, of the two, is less likely to be excreted. In addition, bumetanide appears to have a more substantially favorable therapeutic index. When a higher dose is required, it offers a substantial improvement in the margin of safety.[28]

Adverse consequences are due to the effects of drug-electrolyte imbalance, fluid depletion, and acid-base balance. Ototoxicity occurs as a result of repeated doses, especially in the presence of renal insufficiency. Newborns do not eliminate loop diuretics efficiently because of decreased renal clearance, which can contribute to the prolonged half-life of the drug seen in early infancy.[30] Rapid fluctuations of fluid and electrolytes may be improved by

TABLE 21-10   **Drugs That Enhance Renal Function**

Therapeutic Class (Drug)	Use	Mechanism of Action	Elimination	Nursing Considerations
Loop Diuretics				
Furosemide	Management of edema associated with congestive heart failure and hepatic or renal disease.	Inhibits reabsorption of sodium and chloride in the ascending loop of Henle and distal renal tubule, thus causing increased excretion of water, sodium chloride, magnesium, and calcium.	80% of IV dose excreted in urine within 24 hours; the remainder is eliminated by other nonrenal pathways, including liver metabolism.	Rate of administration is 0.5 mg/kg/min; maximum infusion rate is 4 mg/min. Adverse reactions include hypokalemia, hyponatremia, dehydration, and potential ototoxicity and hearing loss.
Bumetanide	Management of edema secondary to congestive heart failure or hepatic or renal disease, including nephrotic syndrome.	Inhibits reabsorption of sodium and chloride in the ascending loop of Henle and proximal renal tubule, thus causing increased excretion of water, sodium, chloride, magnesium, calcium, and phosphate.	Partial metabolism occurs in the liver; unchanged drug is excreted in the urine (50%).	Larger doses may be necessary in patients with impaired renal function to obtain the same therapeutic response; light sensitive, may discolor when exposed to light. Adverse reactions include hyperglycemia, hypokalemia, hyponatremia, decreased uric acid excretion, increased serum creatinine.
Osmotic Agents				
Mannitol	Promotion of diuresis in the prevention or treatment of oliguria or anuria caused by acute renal failure.	Increases the osmotic pressure of glomerular filtrate, which inhibits tubular reabsorption of water and electrolytes and increases urinary output.	Primarily unchanged in urine by glomerular filtration.	In-line 5-micron filter set should always be used for mannitol infusion with concentrations of 20% or greater, crystallization may occur at low temperatures; coutraindicated in severe renal disease; adverse effects include circulatory overload, congestive heart failure, hyponatremia, hypokalemia.

From Bell C, Simon D, Sovcik J: *Children's formulary handbook,* Hudson, 1999, Lexi-Comp.
IV, Intravenous.

Continued

using loop diuretic infusions rather than frequent doses to maintain a steady state. This manner of delivery has proven to have a greater cumulative diuretic effect with lower doses, thus avoiding the effects of toxic levels.[28,30,31] Furthermore, potential hypotension with bolus doses is avoided, and hemodynamic stability is maintained. Regardless of the dosing, diuretic tolerance develops with prolonged use. The distal tubule is thought to be the site of action responsible for development of tolerance, although the mechanism is not known. Care is taken in using increased doses in the presence of tolerance to avoid toxicity.

An interesting nonrenal effect of the loop diuretics is an improvement in pulmonary compliance in ventilated patients, which is thought to be a result of a variety of factors, although the exact mechanism is unknown.[30] Occasionally, furosemide is administered as an aerosol to infants with bronchopulmonary dysplasia to increase tidal volumes. This action may provide an additional benefit in children with respiratory distress secondary to fluid retention in ARF.

Osmotic Diuretics. Mannitol is the principal osmotic diuretic used in the clinical setting. Mannitol not only acts as an osmotic agent in the proximal tubule to inhibit the reabsorption of water; it also increases renal filtration pressure and causes a solute diuresis. Because of the large fraction of filtrate normally reabsorbed from the proximal tubule, the distal tubule partially attempts to compensate for this loss. A profound diuresis can be attained by combining mannitol with a more distally acting diuretic. When compared with doses administered for cerebral edema, mannitol doses for ARF are smaller and more frequent to achieve the desired diuretic effect. Because acute mannitol toxicity is directly related to its influence on extracellular osmolality, frequent measurement of serum osmolality during therapy is important.[24] Care is taken in the use of osmotic diuretics in the presence of decreased renal function. Without elimination, accumulation can occur, leading to volume overload, hypernatremia, and hyperkalemic metabolic acidosis.[28]

TABLE 21-10   Drugs That Enhance Renal Function—cont'd

Therapeutic Class (Drug)	Use	Mechanism of Action	Elimination	Nursing Considerations
Thiazides Metolazone	Treatment of edema in congestive heart failure and nephrotic syndrome, especially in patients with impaired renal function.	Inhibits sodium reabsorption in the distal tubule, causing increased excretion of sodium and water, as well as potassium and hydrogen ions.	70%-90% excreted unchanged in the urine; enterohepatic recycling.	When metolazone is used in combination with other diuretics, there is an increased risk of azotemia and electrolyte depletion; metolazone may cause increased digoxin toxicity; adverse reactions include hypokalemia, metabolic alkalosis, hyperglycemia, and tinnitus.
Potassium-Sparing Agents Spironolactone	Management of edema associated with excessive aldosterone excretion; hypertension.	Competes with aldosterone for receptor sites in the distal renal tubule, increasing sodium, chloride, and water excretion while conserving potassium phosphate and hydrogen ions.	Metabolized in the liver, urinary and biliary excretion.	Diuretic effect may be delayed 2-3 days; when combined with angiotensin-converting enzymes inhibitors (e.g., captopril) may additively increase the serum potassium; may decrease digoxin clearance and attenuate its inotropic effects; adverse reactions include arrhythmia, hyperkalemia, dehydration, and hyponatremia.
Adrenergics Dopamine	Both systemic and local renal dopamine actions used to enhance renal output; systemically, dopamine increases cardiac contractility.	Lower doses of 2-5 µg/kg/min are mainly dopaminergic stimulating and produce renal and mesenteric vasodilation.	Metabolized in the plasma, kidneys, and liver (75% to inactive metabolites, 25% to norepinephrine); metabolites are excreted in the urine.	Administer into a large vein to prevent the possibility of extravasation; administration into an umbilical arterial catheter is *not* recommended.

Thiazides.   Thiazides are not commonly used in the PICU because they are exclusively enteral formulations and have a relatively low ceiling of maximal diuretic effect. The site of action overlaps with that of the loop diuretics.[24] Metolazone also has effects in the proximal renal tubule, therefore making it the favored drug in this class. Metolazone may be useful in combination with the loop diuretics to achieve a greater diuretic effect or to overcome diuretic tolerance.

Potassium-Sparing Agents.   Potassium-sparing agents administered independently may have little effect in increasing water excretion, but in combination with more proximally acting diuretics, they may effect a substantial increase in the excretion of sodium and water.[24] Spironolactone has a much longer half-life than other diuretics and is the more common agent used in the PICU.

Dopamine.   Dopamine has been found to be an effective agent to enhance renal function. Renal dose dopamine, 2 to 5 µg/kg/min, is used when the desired effect of drug infusion is to stimulate dopaminergic (DA) receptors without altering blood pressure. The DA receptors are in the renal arteries and the afferent arterioles. When stimulated, the receptors cause renal vasodilation, resulting in improved RBF, GFR, sodium excretion, and creatinine clearance.[32] Dopamine also exerts a synergistic action with furosemide via vasodilation and reversal of ischemia; thus furosemide transport to the loop of Henle improves, subsequently increasing urine output. The combination of low-dose dopamine and furosemide can result in conversion of oliguric to nonoliguric renal failure if adequate intravascular volume and cardiac output are present.

An increase in urine flow does not represent an improvement in renal function, nor effect the natural history of the disease that precipitated the renal failure. However, enhancement of urine output may be valuable in the management of hyperkalemia and fluid overload.[33]

RENAL REPLACEMENT THERAPY

The rationale for initiating renal replacement therapy includes the need to remove excessive intravascular volume and correct significant alterations in electrolyte or acid-base balance. Progressive hypervolemia may result in hypertension and, in the patient whose condition is previously

TABLE 21-11	**Advantages and Disadvantages of Different Forms of Renal Replacement Therapy**	
Method	**Advantages**	**Disadvantages**
Peritoneal dialysis	Gradual process Can be used in hemodynamically unstable patients Vascular access beyond peripheral IV not required No complex equipment needed Inexpensive No heparinization required Greater mobility	Catheter malfunctions Hyperglycemia Slow clearance of fluid and electrolytes—not helpful in hyperkalemic crises Risk for catheter-related sepsis, peritonitis Requires use of abdomen—not optimal status post laparotomy Large protein loss Failure of treatment results in worsened hypervolemia Fluid/electrolyte removal less controllable Diminished ventilation with decreased diaphragm compliance
CVVH or hemofiltration	Very effective with hypervolemia Can be used in hemodynamically unstable patients Continuous treatment allows constant readjustment in therapy Relatively inexpensive Allows parenteral nutrition to be optimized without risk of hypervolemia Can add dialysis	Access complications: infection, clotting, blood leaks, air emboli, bleeding Requires vigilant monitoring Heparinization often required Not quickly effective with hyperkalemia Hemofilter clotting requires immediate intervention
Hemodialysis	Quickly effective in fluid and catabolic overload Intermittent therapy	Access complications: infection, clotting, bleeding Requires special equipment and specially trained personnel Heparinization required Fluid and electrolyte shift during therapy, hypotension Disequilibrium syndrome

CVVH, Continuous venovenous hemofiltration; *IV*, intravenous.

compromised, congestive heart failure and pulmonary edema. Slow, steady increases in serum potassium eventually produce lethal cardiac dysrhythmias. Persistent metabolic acidosis contributes to neurologic deterioration. Other electrolyte imbalances include hyponatremia, hypercalcemia, and an imbalance in the calcium-to-phosphorus ratio. An elevation in BUN, with rapidly rising creatinine, influences the decision-making process to initiate more aggressive therapy. Inadequate nutrition delivery resulting from fluid restriction required in the presence of limited urine output has become a major indication to initiate renal replacement therapy.[34]

Treatment options, intended to mimic renal function, include peritoneal dialysis (PD), continuous venovenous hemofiltration (CVVH), and hemodialysis (HD). The benefits and limitations of each management option are compared in Table 21-11. Determining the type of dialysis to be used includes evaluation of hemodynamic stability, cardiac performance, bleeding tendencies, the presence of sepsis, respiratory issues, nutritional needs, cost, personnel requirements, and local expertise.[35]

All renal replacement therapies function by diffusion or convection. The components of the system include a selectively permeable membrane separating the patient's blood from a second compartment (Fig. 21-6). The membrane may be part of a dialyzer incorporated into an extracorporeal circuit or it may be present in the patient, such as the peritoneal membrane. The second compartment may contain dialysate or form a simple reservoir that collects ultrafiltrate from the plasma. Diffusion is the primary mechanism of solute removal during dialysis. The amount of solute removed depends on permeability of the membrane, molecular weight of the solute, and the concentration gradient on both sides of the membrane. During ultrafiltration, fluid is removed by the hydrostatic or osmotic pressure gradient directed toward the second compartment; solute is pulled with the water particles. This method of solute removal (convection) is not as efficient at removing small solute particles, such as urea.[36]

Peritoneal Dialysis

PD removes fluid and solutes slowly over 2 to 3 days. Because of this time frame, the decision to initiate PD is usually made early, when progressive deterioration in patient status can be reasonably predicted. Earlier intervention is especially beneficial in some patients with multisystem organ failure, for example, in the patient with congenital heart disease who develops ARF after cardiovascular surgery. A study by Sorof and colleagues[37] suggests that placing the PD catheter during cardiovascular surgery in small infants and initiating PD within 24 hours of surgery

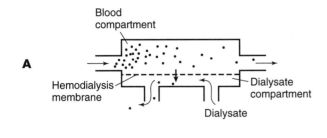

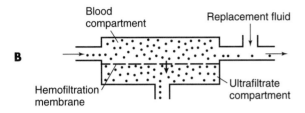

Fig. 21-6   Schematic representation of solute and fluid transport across semipermeable membranes. **A,** Hemodialyzer. Plasma concentration of small solutes *(solid circles)* in the blood inlet is high. Because of the diffusive loss across semipermeable hemodialysis membrane *(dotted line),* plasma concentration in the blood outlet is much lower. Thin arrow across the dialysis membrane represents small amount of fluid loss (which is not necessary for solute removal). High dialysate flow rate is necessary to maintain the concentration gradient across the dialysis membrane. **B,** Hemofilter. Plasma concentration of small solutes in the blood compartment remains unchanged as blood travels the length of the fiber, and is similar to their concentrations in the ultrafiltrate. Hemofiltration membrane *(broken line)* has relatively large pores, which allow necessary removal of large volume of fluid *(heavy arrow).* Replacement of fluid is infused into the blood outlet to lower plasma concentration of solutes and compensate for fluid loss. (From Cheung A: Hemodialysis and hemofiltration. In Greenberg A, ed: *Primer on kidney disease,* ed 2, San Diego, 1998, Academic Press, p 410.

resulted in low complication rates and successful achievement of negative fluid balance.

PD can be successfully initiated in patients with limited vascular access. In addition, because the removal of fluid and solutes is accomplished in a slow manner, patients who are especially sensitive to changes in vascular volume are ideal candidates. PD may be the treatment of choice for ARF in hemodynamically unstable patients or in patients with coagulopathy. PD continues to be a favored modality in the newborn or early infant population.[38-40]

There are no absolute contraindications to PD. However, some experts suggest that the presence of a ventriculoperitoneal shunt and severe respiratory distress are contraindications. Patients better suited to another type of therapy include those with peritonitis, peritoneal adhesions, diaphragmatic defects or those healing from recent abdominal surgery.

Principles of Therapy.   The goal of PD is established before instituting therapy and is reevaluated on a daily basis. For example, the daily goal may include removing a specific amount of fluid over a defined period, decreasing the serum potassium level to within normal limits, or decreasing the BUN to 3 times normal. Achievement of established multidisciplinary goals, ongoing monitoring of the patient's

status, and prevention of complications require vigilant assessment, intervention, and documentation.

With PD, the patient's peritoneum serves as the semipermeable membrane to allow movement of solutes by diffusion and water by osmosis. As a semipermeable membrane, the peritoneum allows some but not all molecules to move across it.

Dialysate fluid, containing a predetermined osmolality and concentration of ions, is infused into the peritoneal cavity. Exchange of solutes and water occurs over the peritoneal membrane. The osmotic gradient that drives the ultrafiltration is created by the glucose in the dialysate. The greater the amount of glucose present, the greater the gradient and the ultrafiltrate removed. Glucose may also move from the peritoneal space to the child's intravenous space, resulting in hyperglycemia. This occurrence is usually temporary until the pancreas is able to increase insulin production. Serum electrolytes diffuse across the peritoneum until equilibrium is reached with the dialysate. Urea and creatinine diffuse against a zero concentration gradient because these two solutes are not present in dialysate. Therefore they are readily cleared from the serum.

The smaller the patient, the larger the ratio of peritoneal space to body mass. Therefore, in general, PD is more efficient in smaller pediatric patients.

Dialysate is commercially available as 1.5%, 2.5%, and 4.25% dextrose concentrations. Except for the addition of glucose and the absence of potassium, dialysate is similar to normal serum. Dialysate generally contains lactate as a buffer. Because of the lactate base, the use of a standard PD solution in a patient with impaired liver function or metabolic acidosis caused by lactic acidosis can be harmful; the substitution of bicarbonate for lactate may be necessary. Table 21-12 shows the components of both standard lactate and bicarbonate-base dialysates. Potassium, heparin, antibiotics, or antifungal medications can be added to the dialysate as needed. Systemic heparinization does not occur in patients with heparin (250 to 500 U/L) added to the dialysate.[41]

Procedure.   PD can be initiated with relative ease in the PICU. Preparation of the patient includes obtaining a baseline weight, abdominal circumference, and placing a urinary catheter. The urinary catheter drains the distended bladder, which decreases the risk of bladder puncture during the procedure.

There are several types of peritoneal catheters. The "acute" catheter is rigid and easy to place percutaneously. The "chronic" catheter (most often the Tenckhoff catheter) is a more flexible catheter that is tunneled through the subcutaneous fat during a surgical procedure. The Tenckhoff catheter may have a cuff that is placed at the level of the peritoneum, which decreases the incidence of leakage.

Before starting the procedure, the PD system used both to deliver dialysate to the peritoneal cavity and collect peritoneal drainage is prepared. Dialysate can be delivered manually or mechanically. Manual instillation requires assembly of equipment, warming of the dialysate (for patient comfort and to enhance solute clearance), and frequent opening of the system to spike the dialysis bags.

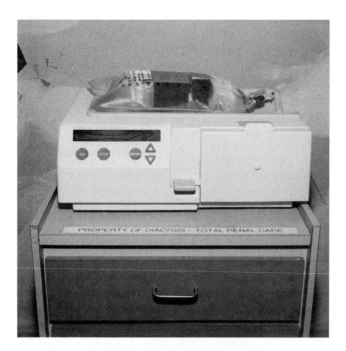

Fig. 21-7 Peritoneal dialysis cycler.

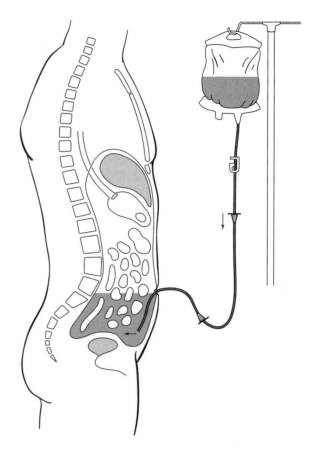

Fig. 21-8 Placement of peritoneal dialysis catheter. (From Hudak C, Gallo B: *Critical care nursing: a holistic approach,* ed 6, Philadelphia, 1994, Lippincott Williams & Wilkins, p 568.)

TABLE 21-12 Peritoneal Dialysis Solutions: Commercially Available Dialysate (Lactate-Based) and Specialized (Bicarbonate-Based) Solution

Constituents	Standard Peritoneal Dialysis Solution	Specialized Bicarbonate Solution
Dextrose (g/L)	15, 25, 42.5	15, 25, 42.5
Sodium (mEq/L)	132	92-100†
Chloride (mEq/L)	92	92-100
Lactate (mEq/L)	40	0
Sodium bicarbonate (mEq/L)	0	40†
Potassium (mEq/L)	0-5*	0-5*
Calcium (mEq/L)	3.5	2-4
Magnesium (mEq/L)	0.5	0.5

From Smoyer W, Maxvold N, Remenapp R et al: Pediatric renal replacement therapy. In Fuhrman B, Zimmerman J, eds: *Pediatric Critical Care,* ed 2, St Louis, 1998, Mosby.
*Standard potassium bath is zero, but up to 5 mEq/L may be added.
†Sodium needs to be supplemented to physiologic levels (130-145 mEq/L).

The PD cycler may have various configurations and controls. An example of a PD cycler is the Baxter Home Choice shown in Fig. 21-7. It provides a relatively easy way to maintain continuous PD, warm the dialysate, and display the cycle status and the amount of spent dialysis per cycle. All PD cyclers have a volume controller that contains an occlusion mechanism to regulate dialysate flow to and from the patient. If the machine has a microprocessor, the PD cycler can store the number of cycles and ultrafiltration parameters in memory, even during electrical power interruptions.[42] Use of a cycler decreases the number of connections and disconnections in a 24-hour period.

PD Catheter Insertion. Paracentesis is usually accomplished in the PICU. Patients younger than 2 years of age, those with poor abdominal tone, those who require chemical paralyzing agents for effective ventilation, or those with a history of abdominal surgery may warrant catheter placement in the operating room. The catheter is usually placed 2 to 3 cm below the umbilicus in the midline, with the tip of the catheter directed toward either the bladder or the lateral pelvic gutters. Initially, 5 ml/kg of ascitic drainage should be removed, followed by initial instillation of 5 to 10 ml/kg of dialysate.[41] To avoid excessive ultrafiltration, 1.5% dextrose solution is used initially. Fig. 21-8 shows placement of the catheter in the body.

During the initial cycle, patient assessment includes evaluation for fluid infiltration around the insertion site, abdominal pain, grossly bloody drainage, fecal-contaminated drainage, and cardiovascular or respiratory compromise. After optimal catheter position is established, a purse-string suture closes the incision around the PD catheter. An occlusive, dry, sterile dressing, which prevents kinking of the PD catheter, is applied.

Catheter Maintenance. Each PD cycle or run consists of three phases: instillation, dwell, and drainage. During the instillation phase, dialysate runs into the peritoneum through the inflow line of the PD system. This occurs rapidly by gravitational flow over 5 to 15 minutes. The volume of dialysate instilled with each run is usually 10 to 20 ml/kg in infants and 35 to 40 ml/kg in children. Depending on patient tolerance, initial volumes can be gradually increased. Increased PD volume increases efficiency of dialysis. However, in patients with tissue edema, increased PD volume may cause dialysate fluid leakage.

During the dwell phase, both the inflow and outflow lines are clamped. The dialysate remains in the peritoneal cavity, allowing water and solute movement across the peritoneum. This phase usually requires 30 to 60 minutes but is dependent on many factors, such as surface area of the peritoneal membrane. Maximal solute transfer occurs at the beginning of the dwell phase. In general, shorter dwell times remove greater amounts of fluid, and longer dwell times are more efficient in solute removal.

The drainage phase begins when the clamp on the outflow line leading to the drainage bag is opened. Although the time required for drainage varies for each patient, the average time is 15 to 20 minutes. Drainage can be enhanced by repositioning the patient.

Modifications in PD therapy are made based on the patient's clinical status, renal function, and laboratory test results. The dialysate concentration is changed with relative simplicity. Variations in concentrations can be obtained by combining different osmolar solutions with each run. Even though initial hyperglycemia may resolve with increased endogenous insulin production, other related side effects usually limit the use of highly osmolar solutions.

The volume of dialysate instilled depends on the patient's tolerance during the dwell phase. Dialysate overfill is a serious complication, as demonstrated by shortness of breath, abdominal discomfort, distension, and pain. Instillation of smaller, more frequent volumes may accomplish the desired goals in the patient who cannot tolerate runs of more than 20 ml/kg every hour.

Initial PD drainage is blood tinged. This bloody drainage should clear after the first few runs. After this, PD drainage takes on a characteristic straw color. Persistently bloody drainage must be investigated. Likewise, development and persistence of cloudy drainage can indicate peritonitis and requires evaluation.

After the first few cycles, a predictable drainage pattern should develop. At times the catheter tip may migrate away from the dialysate in the peritoneal cavity, or the catheter may become occluded by the omentum, impingement of the abdominal organs on the catheter, or fibrin deposits. In these situations, dialysate freely flows into but not out of the peritoneal cavity. Interventions to increase fluid drainage include changing the child's position, elevating the head of the bed, or turning the child gently from side to side.

Catheter-related problems also include leakage at the insertion site. If the volume infused is greater than that drained, the drainage tubing or catheter may be kinked and require straightening. A clotted catheter requires replacement.

Catheter leakage at the insertion site may also indicate catheter displacement. If all PD catheter infusion/drainage sites are contained within the abdomen, an extra external stitch to stop oozing of fluid from around the insertion site may be required. Sometimes catheter leakage results from dialysate overfill, and volumes of dialysate may need to be decreased.

The need for accurate documentation of intake and output cannot be overstated. Twice-daily patient weights may be used to validate fluid assessments if the patient's condition permits. Weights are only useful if a consistent scale is used and the patient is weighed at the same time of day and during a specific phase in a PD cycle.

Laboratory studies are followed at a frequency determined by the acuity of the patient's condition. Following trends of serum electrolytes, calcium, phosphorus, BUN, and creatinine levels is routine. Close monitoring of the patient's neurologic status is important because serum electrolyte and acid-base imbalance may manifest in neurologic changes. Often the parents' observations and concerns about the patient's level of consciousness are early warnings to the nurse and necessitate further evaluation.

The child's level of comfort is continuously monitored. Especially important is the patient's perception of comfort during the different phases of PD. Nonverbal signs of discomfort include tachycardia, tachypnea or shallow breathing, grimacing, splinting, and agitated or unsettled behaviors. In some instances, slowing the rate of dialysate infusion, decreasing the volume used per cycle, further warming of the dialysate, or repositioning the child may alleviate some discomfort. Analgesics and sedatives are used in addition to comfort measures.

Complications. Distending the abdomen with large volumes of dialysate may compromise the patient's respiratory status. Increased abdominal volume and pressure prevent normal downward displacement of the diaphragm and limit functional residual capacity. This effect may predispose the patient to atelectasis with associated intrapulmonary shunting and increased work of breathing. Fatigue, anxiety, and pain further compromise the patient's ability to compensate for existing alterations in oxygenation and ventilation.

Ongoing assessment of the patient's nutritional status includes an appreciation of the protein loss across the membrane during PD. This may potentiate nutritional, immunologic, and infectious problems such as peritonitis.

Instillation of large volumes of dialysate into the peritoneum may also compromise venous return and cardiac output. This effect is especially true when intravascular volume is limited. Close monitoring of cardiovascular status is necessary, especially during the instillation phase. During the drain cycle, hypotension may also be a problem, often related to leaky capillary syndrome in patients with decreased intravascular but increased extravascular volume.[34]

The greatest shift of water and solutes occurs within the first part of the dwell phase. Patient discomfort and respiratory and cardiovascular distress may force a time limit on the dwell phase. These adjustments eventually affect the number of cycles completed within the day, potentially influencing the effectiveness of therapy. As the patient's need for PD lessens, drainage time can be gradually increased, resulting in fewer runs per day.

The use of an acute catheter placed percutaneously leads to the possibility of leakage. Chronic catheters are tunneled and often have cuffs to increase the effectiveness of the seal. In general, the risk of peritonitis increases after day 3 of PD. Guidelines for practice regarding the frequency of system tubing change, catheter insertion site cleansing and dressing, and frequency of catheter change are policies determined within each institution. It is prudent to recommend care that is similar to guidelines for intravascular lines.

Signs of peritonitis include cloudy PD drainage, fever, abdominal pain and tenderness, and a change in the patient's level of consciousness. Daily culture, cell count with differential, and Gram stain of PD drainage are warranted. Peritoneal cell counts exceeding 100 white cells/μl or the presence of greater than 50% neutrophils on differential is suggestive of bacterial peritonitis. Maintaining a closed system, specimens should be aspirated from the PD outflow line and not the drainage bag. To prevent the possibility of contaminated fluid from flowing back into the peritoneum, the drainage bag is never elevated above the level of the abdomen.

Peritonitis does not preclude PD therapy. Treatment includes adding antibiotics to the dialysate. Some commonly used intraperitoneal antibiotics include vancomycin, tobramycin, cefotaxime, and piperacillin. Appropriate systemic antibiotic administration for positive blood cultures is required. Pancreatitis is also a frequent finding in patients undergoing PD. Signs and symptoms include abdominal pain, nausea, vomiting, low-grade fever, and elevated serum lipase and amylase levels.

Documentation. Documentation is crucial to patient management. Fig. 21-9 is an example of a documentation flow sheet for cycler PD (the presence of tidal PD addresses a form of PD not commonly used, wherein a small amount of dialysate is purposely not drained from the patient). If manually performed, documentation also includes the times at which (1) instillation of dialysate begins; (2) instillation ends, and dwell time begins; (3) dwell time ends, and drainage time begins; and (4) drainage time ends, and a new run begins. These times are automatically

---

The Children's Memorial Hospital

CYCLER PERITONEAL DIALYSIS FLOW SHEET

DATE:_____ HEATER BAG:____%D____L LAST BAG(if different):____%D____L EXTRA FLUIDS:____%D____L

ADDITIVES TO BAGS:_____ ____%D____L

_____ ____%D____L

WEIGHT(empty):_____kg

CCPD or TIDAL PD   Total Volume:____ml   Therapy Time:____hr____min   Fill Volume:____ml   Last Fill:____ml   Last Dextrose:_____   # Cycles_____   Avg. Dwell:____min

Tidal Volume:____%   Total (estimated) UF:_____ml   Full Drains:__g__cycles   Tidal Volume:____ml   UF per cycle:____ml

TIME	#CYCLE	*CYCLE ULTRAFILTRATE	*CUMULATIVE ULTRAFILTRATE	PROGRAM CHANGES	ALARMS and COMMENTS	SIGNATURE (initials)
	INITIAL DRAIN	(actual amount)	(day fill - Initial drain)			
	#1					

*When cycler displays (+) UF, record on flow sheet as (−): Patient net fluid loss (removed)
*When cycler displays (−) UF, record on flow sheet as (+): Patient net fluid gain (retained)
*Cycle and Cumulative UF will only be displayed at Full Drains on TIDAL program
*Cumulative UF does not include Initial Drain

Fig. 21-9 Peritoneal dialysis worksheet. (Courtesy The Children's Memorial Hospital, Chicago, Ill.)

programmed in the PD cycler and do not need to be documented.

Ongoing assessment of drainage volume, compared with instilled volume, is important in evaluating the patient's fluid balance. The patient's fluid status is considered to "positive" when the volume instilled is greater than the volume drained. Positive fluid balance can be related to an increase in the patient's serum osmolarity or to an occlusion in the drainage system. If no occlusion is identified in the drainage system and a continued positive fluid balance for two or more runs is obtained, a change in management strategy is required.

The patient is considered to be in "negative" fluid balance when the volume instilled is less than the volume drained. Negative balance, indicating removal of body fluid volume, is generally a goal of PD; however, rapid removal of volume may compromise the child's hemodynamic status. Continuous evaluation of the child's tolerance to fluid removal is necessary to determine the desired goal for hourly fluid balance.

To calculate the 24-hour net body balance, the following equation is used:

$$
\begin{aligned}
&(\text{Total amount of dialysate instilled} + \text{intake}) - \\
&\quad (\text{Total fluid drained from dialysis} + \text{output}) = \\
&\quad\quad\quad\quad\quad\quad\quad\quad \text{Total body balance for 24 hours}
\end{aligned}
$$

To determine the effectiveness of PD, the net gain or loss is calculated by the following equation:

$$
\text{Total dialysate intake} - \text{Total ultrafiltrate output} = \text{Net loss or gain}
$$

Additional documentation specific to PD includes patient and parent education and assessment of their level of understanding and comfort with the information. Documentation also includes a description of the child's tolerance of PD. Appearance of the insertion site, the presence of any fluid leakage, and a description of the fluid drained out of the peritoneal cavity are documented at each shift.

Continuous Arteriovenous/Venovenous Hemofiltration

Continuous arteriovenous hemofiltration (CAVH) and continuous venovenous hemofiltration (CVVH) provide two conceptually similar methods for slow, continuous removal of fluid and solutes from the body, enabling continuous adjustment in the child's fluid status. Slow continuous hemofiltration is especially important in the critically ill child in whom a predictable fluid and solute removal process allows a more liberal approach to intravenous intake of necessary nutrition and medications.

Hemofiltration can usually be successfully initiated in patients in whom PD or hemodialysis is contraindicated. Compared with hemodialysis, special equipment and the need for extra personnel are minimized with CVVH.

Principles of Therapy. Uniquely different from PD and HD, CVVH removes excessive fluid and solutes through ultrafiltration. The process requires continuous extracorporeal circulation of blood through a filter. With CVVH, a hemopump is used to pump blood through the hemofilter using two separate venous cannulas or two separate ports from a single multilumen cannula (Fig. 21-10). Different machinery is available for CVVH, and the simplicity of the therapy is determined by the machine.

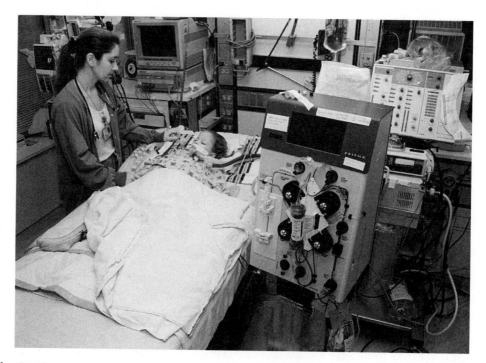

Fig. 21-10 Pump-assisted continuous venovenous hemofiltration (CVVH). (Courtesy The Children's Memorial Hospital, Chicago, Ill.)

As blood moves through the highly permeable hemofilter, water and low-molecular-weight molecules are removed through ultrafiltration. Variations in hemofilter size and shape are commercially available. Cylindric hollow filters or parallel plate filters are two commonly used types. Options in membrane type, surface area, clearance rate, and volume are commercially available.

Similar to that which occurs within the vascular space, ultrafiltration occurs as the net result of the opposing forces of hydrostatic and oncotic pressure. Hydrostatic pressure (determined by the hemopump's blood flow rate) provides the force necessary to filter blood on one side of the membrane, as oncotic pressure (determined by the concentration of plasma proteins) pulls fluid back into the system on the other side of the membrane (see Fig. 21-6). Initially, hydrostatic pressure is greater than oncotic pressure, and thus water and small particles move out of the serum into the ultrafiltration collection fluid. At this point, depending on the concentration of plasma protein that establishes the plasma oncotic pressure, water is pulled back into the venous side of the circuit and ultrafiltrate (UF) is drained into the collection bag.

UF has the same solute load as the patient's serum. Potassium, sodium, chloride, urea, and creatinine are all small molecules that freely move across the hemofilter. Glucose and other moderate-size molecules move slowly across the hemofilter. Plasma proteins, which are large-size molecules, do not cross the hemofilter. Therefore all plasma proteins are returned to the patient and UF is protein free.

As water and small molecules are removed, plasma oncotic pressure increases. The net effect of oncotic and hydrostatic pressures becoming more equal is a decrease in the rate of ultrafiltration over time. At this point the patient's serum osmolarity is maintained as sodium, potassium, and chloride are removed and creatinine, urea, and glucose are filtered in concentrations equal to that of plasma.

The process of fluid and solute removal has distinct features that make hemofiltration the therapy of choice for many children with ARF. The slow process allows relative hemodynamic stability during volume removal. In addition, it is a continuous therapy, allowing constant readjustment in the treatment plan as the patient's needs change. Compared with HD, the extracorporeal circuit volume is small and there is a relatively low risk of bleeding. This aspect is especially important in infants and patients with existing coagulopathy. The major advantage over PD is that ventilation during hemofiltration is not affected by the abdominal distention that occurs during the dwell phase of each PD run.

A disadvantage to simple hemofiltration is that it does not remove solutes such as urea as efficiently as desired for some patients. Large solutes also are poorly cleared. Small ones, although cleared, are removed slowly. Therefore hemofiltration without dialysis may not be the therapy of choice for patients with azotemia.

The clearest indications for simple hemofiltration are fluid overload, which is resistant to diuretic therapy, and electrolyte imbalance. One common use of hemofiltration is to improve nutritional intake for patients who cannot tolerate a positive fluid balance. Increased amounts of parenteral nutrition can be administered because excessive fluid volume can be continuously removed. The controlled fluid management specifically benefits patients with multisystem organ dysfunction syndrome (MODS). In addition, some evidence suggests the effective clearance of cytokines present in children with shock.

CAVH therapy works similarly to that described earlier for CVVH. The main differences include access, adequacy of cardiac output, and interactions with the system. CAVH requires arterial access for blood removal from the body. The driving force is the child's cardiac output. Thus if cardiac output is less than optimal, the hemofiltration will also be less than optimal. Use of a blood pump is not generally required because the child's cardiac output drives the system. Interactions with the system include raising or lowering the ultrafiltration bag to decrease or increase the ultrafiltration amount. Because CAVH is used much less frequently than CVVH, the remainder of this section focuses on CVVH.

Procedure. Venous cannulation sites must accommodate the largest size cannula possible because system performance is directly related to the amount of blood flow through the hemofilter. Infants have adequate filter flow through 7 French (internal lumen) catheters. In the best situation, a double-lumen catheter is used to eliminate the need for two separate sites and catheters. Femoral and jugular access are most common. If two separate cannulas are used, drainage and return cannulas are generally the same size for optimal flow. When the gauge of the drainage cannula is less than optimal, improved circuit flow may be achieved when the return cannula is one to two gauge sizes larger than the drainage cannula. Return cannula size determines resistance of blood flow back to the patient and affects flow throughout the circuit. One venous cannula/line often pulls more effectively than the other. If this is the case, simply reversing the drainage and return lines may improve system performance. The procedure for gaining vascular access is the same as for any central line.

Preparation of the circuit is completed before gaining vascular access. If access is obtained before preparation of the circuit, the cannulas are heparin packed, then capped.

Assembly and priming of the circuit are institution specific. General principles include the maintenance of aseptic technique during flushing of the circuit with 1 to 3 L of heparinized saline, the volume determined by the type of filter used. The concentration of heparin may vary by institution. The system is flushed to remove air and all traces of glycerin, a byproduct of the sterilization process.

Most pediatric patients benefit from priming the hemofilter with packed red blood cells or 5% albumin; again, this is done according to institution policy and patient size. Depending on the size of the hemofilter, the circuit volume varies.

A continuous heparin infusion, attached prefilter, is necessary to keep the system from clotting. It is initially infused at a rate of 10 U/kg/hr and then titrated to maintain an activating clotting time (ACT) within an individual therapeutic range (usually 180 to 200 seconds or 10% over baseline). Patients with thrombocytopenia may not require anticoagulation. Some centers prefer regional heparinization of the hemofilter. This may be accomplished by infusion of sodium citrate, which acts by binding with calcium ions. Side effects of citrate include hypercalcemia, hypercitratemia, and metabolic acidosis.[43]

Once vessel access has been achieved and the circuit has been primed, it is connected to the patient. The drainage side is connected to the patient first. Clamps are used to assist the team in establishing the extracorporeal circuit without air entry or unnecessary blood loss.

Maintenance. Pump-driven CVVH provides the hemofilter with constant blood flow, which results in a consistent ultrafiltration rate (UFR) that can be precisely controlled. Ordered pump speed, adjusted in milliliters per minute, depends on cannula size, intravascular volume, and desired UFR with solute clearance. Pump speeds should be maintained at a certain level depending on the size of the patient to prevent filter clotting.

Fluids need to be infused through the appropriate site on the circuit. Except for albumin, replacement fluids are generally delivered before the filter. Fluid administration before the hemofilter decreases the hematocrit, blood viscosity, and oncotic pressure. In combination, these factors improve blood flow through the hemofilter, decreasing the need for heparin therapy. Also, prefilter replacement fluid administration may prolong the life of the filter and circuit.[43]

Albumin is administered after the filter because it may decrease the patency of the hemofilter. Medications are also administered after the filter to avoid hemofiltration of the medication.

Monitoring. Fluid balance assessment and calculations require vigilant monitoring and documentation, which may be time consuming. Older technology requires manual calculation of fluid balance and use of additional infusion pumps separate from the blood pump. This system requires hourly evaluations of ultrafiltrate removed to determine replacement fluids and hourly balance. The newest technology for CVVH therapy is a system that performs the therapy independent of additional pumps or manipulations of the circuit. The PRISMA pump (Gambro, Lakewood, Colo.) is an example of this type of system (Fig. 21-11). This system infuses and removes fluid based on a computerized weighted system. When programmed, the system achieves a net fluid removal per unit of selected time. This feature saves nurses time by eliminating the need for routine calculations and pump manipulations. It benefits the child by providing immediate fluid replacement from continuously calculated data.

Hemofiltration requires ongoing monitoring of the patient and extracorporeal circuit. Circuit pressures are monitored as a safety alarm to immediately identify inadvertent patient disconnection or changes in pressure in the system. The PRISMA system has the advanced technology of a detailed alarm system that displays alarms in a hierarchy depending on potential risk to the child.

The child's volume status and cardiac output are affected over the time of fluid removal. Trends in laboratory results,

CVVHDF

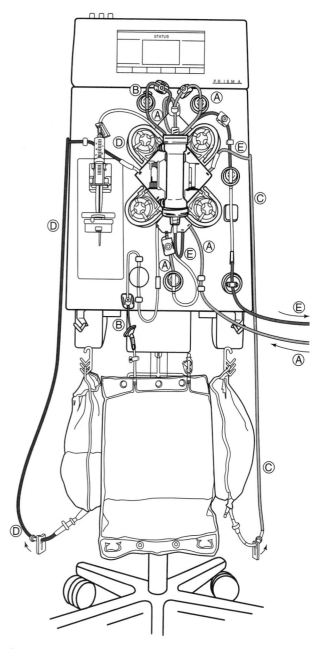

Fig. 21-11 PRISMA machine in use with CVVHDF. Tube *A* represents blood flow from patient to machine and through the filter; *B* represents filtrated fluid, ultrafiltrate; *C* represents replacement fluid; *D* represents dialysate fluid; *E* represents blood flow returning to patient.

intake and output totals, patient weights, and vital signs are critical assessment parameters.

The cardiovascular examination is crucial. Perfusion to the extremities distal to the cannulated vessels may diminish. Ongoing assessment of the presence and quality of pulses and sensation and movement of extremities is necessary. Vigilant monitoring of the patient's hemodynamic status is critical. Inadvertent errors in calculating fluid removal may be discovered by decreases in the blood pressure, central venous pressure or elevated heart rate.

Serum sodium, potassium, and chloride are removed in proportion to the fluid volume filtered, and shifts in these electrolytes occur as a result of the therapy. Changing acid-base status may also affect electrolyte levels. The volume and type of replacement fluid are readjusted, depending on the needs of the child. A reduction in the serum BUN and creatinine level is gradually appreciated.

Nutritional management for the child receiving hemofiltration is usually welcomed in the previously fluid-restricted child with large metabolic needs. Provision of optimal fluid volume and calories are best determined by the multidisciplinary team, which includes the critical care team, renal team, nutrition support services, and pharmacist. The replacement fluid, generally a modified solution of lactated Ringer's solution, can be a separate source of intake. In some systems, the volume varies to ensure that the desired volume of fluid removed matches the net volume of fluid removed. In other systems, the replacement fluid remains the same consistently, and net volume removed is based on other intake and output of the patient and desired net balance.

The critical process of addressing the high risk of infection associated with this therapy begins with strict adherence to aseptic technique. Surveillance cultures from the circuit are institution specific and may be done daily. Cannula care is the same as that given for any central line. Meticulous attention to preventing contamination is necessary, and any need to enter the circuit warrants careful consideration.

While receiving this therapy, the child's hematologic status may be compromised by anticoagulation. Frequent ACTs are necessary to evaluate the amount of heparin needed. After an appropriate rate for continuous infusion has been determined, the frequency of these tests may decrease, and a partial prothrombin time may be used for monitoring.[44] Assessment of the child's ability to establish and maintain hemostasis is ongoing. This assessment includes checking for guaiac-positive nasogastric drainage or stool, hematuria, oral/nasal or mucosal bleeding, petechiae, and oozing from wounds or venipuncture sites. Neurologic assessment is critical in the coagulation evaluation, especially in infants.

The impact of hemofiltration on the pharmacokinetics of all drugs the patient is receiving is evaluated. Clearance of nonprotein-bound drugs is enhanced with hemofiltration. Anticipating enhanced clearance is critically important, especially in the child who is vasopressor dependent. Enhanced clearance of insulin and some antibiotics, including the aminoglycosides and cefuroxime, also occurs. In general, because the extracorporeal circuit adds "body surface area" to the patient, the dosage of all nonprotein-bound drugs is increased (see Table 21-9). Both dosage and timing of medication administration are best determined by evaluation of peak and trough drug levels. Sieving coefficients, which describe the concentration gradient of a molecule in the UF as compared with that of plasma, can be used to calculate therapeutic dosages during hemofiltration (Table 21-13).

Hypothermia is another area of monitoring that is important to the child receiving CVVH therapy. Because no warming device is built into the commercially available systems, careful temperature monitoring is necessary.[45] This factor is especially important in the small infant who has yet to develop adequate thermoregulation.

The child's level of comfort is best evaluated with the patient and parents. Changes in the child's heart rate and blood pressure are integrated with assessments of behavior, facial expression, playfulness, and interaction with others. Hemofiltration should not cause pain. Use of analgesia is generally not indicated. Sedation, in an adjusted dose for renal failure, may be helpful in allowing the child to be less anxious, thereby maximizing rest and preventing accidental dislodgment of the cannula(s). Provision of some environmental control, the presence of parents, and a routine of day-night activities may serve to minimize the child's fear and lessen discomfort from unfamiliar physical and emotional feelings.

Using a complex technology to provide ultrafiltration at the bedside has specific implications for the care of the child and parents. The appearance of the blood circulating outside the body can be frightening and worrisome to families. Continuous observation and hourly monitoring may minimize the parents' sense of control and may maximize their feelings of helplessness. Because of the presence of a large central cannula, the child's mobility is usually restricted. It is a nursing challenge to help the child find a comfortable position and to include parents in the care of their child. Addition of child life therapy to the healthcare team can be invaluable for the mobility-restricted child.

Parents can best identify how much information they would like to receive about the care required of their child supported on CVVH. Knowledge about the need for hourly collection of data and the frequency of blood draws from the line may be helpful for some parents. The security precautions inherent in the circuit and anticipatory information about the expected necessity for routine circuit changes are examples of other kinds of information that some parents may find helpful.

Complications. Ongoing monitoring of the circuit requires skill and experience in troubleshooting complications. Unintentional decreases in ultrafiltration may be the result of changes within the child or circuit. As circuit flow diminishes, UFR decreases, and hemofilter patency is at risk.

Inadequate blood flow through the circuit can also result from cannulas that are too small, vascular access thrombosis, kinks in the tubing, or clotting of the hemofilter or cannulas. Occlusion can occur anywhere in the circuit. Inspecting the entire circuit for kinks and clots is a first step. Prefilter hemodilution at 30 to 50 ml/kg/hr may be helpful in preventing clot formation. Prefilter volume is easily removed by the filter.

When the hemofilter begins to clot, dark red streaks appear. Another hint that the filter is clotting is an increasing

TABLE 21-13 Drug Sieving Coefficients During Hemofiltration

Sieving Coefficients	Observed	Expected*	Sieving Coefficients	Observed	Expected*
Antibiotics			**Miscellaneous**		
Amikacin	0.95	0.95	Amrinone	0.80	0.70
Amphotericin B	0.35	0.10	Bromide	1.00	1.00
Ampicillin	0.69	0.80	Chlordiazepoxide	0.05	0.05
Cefmenoxime	0.54	0.58	Cisplatin	0.10	0.10
Cefoperazone	0.27	0.10	Clofibrate	0.06	0.04
Cefotaxime	1.06	0.62	Cyclosporine	0.58	0.10
Cefotiam	0.95	0.60	Diathybarbital	1.00	0.90
Cefoxitin	0.83	0.59	Diazepam	0.02	0.02
Ceftazidime	0.90	0.83	Digoxin	0.70	0.80
Ceftriaxone	0.20	0.15	Digitoxin	0.15	0.05
Cephapirin	1.48	0.55	Famotidine	0.73	0.85
Cilastatin	0.75	0.56	Glyburide	0.60	0.01
Ciprofloxacin	0.58	0.60	Glutethimide	0.02	0.50
Clindamycin	0.49	0.40	Lidocaine	0.14	0.36
Doxycycline	0.40	0.20	Lithium	0.90	1.00
Erythromycin	0.37	0.30	Metamizole	0.40	0.40
Fluconazole	1.00	0.88	N-Acetyl procainamide	0.92	0.90
Flucytosine	0.80	0.90	Nizatidine	0.59	0.65
Gentamicin	0.81	0.95	Nitrazepam	0.08	0.10
Imipenem	0.90	0.80	Nomifensin	0.70	0.40
Metronidazole	0.84	0.80	Oxazepam	0.10	0.10
Mezlocillin	0.71	0.68	Phenobarbital	0.80	0.60
Nafcillin	0.55	0.20	Phenytoin	0.45	0.10
Netilmicin	0.93	0.95	Phosphomycin	0.24	0.90
Oxacillin	0.02	0.05	Procainamide	0.86	0.86
Perfloxacin	0.80	0.80	Ranitidine	0.78	0.85
Penicillin	0.68	0.50	Theophylline	0.80	0.47
Piperacillin	0.82	0.80			
Streptomycin	0.30	0.65			
Sulfamethoxazole	0.30	0.60			
Teicoplanin	0.05	0.10			
Tobramycin	0.90	0.95			
Vancomycin	0.80	0.90			

From Golper TA, Marx MA: Drug dosing adjustments during continuous renal replacement therapies, *Int Soc Nephrol* 66:S165-168, 1998.
*The expected coefficient assumes that protein binding is the *sole* determinant of drug sieving and that protein binding is in healthy subjects. Observed coefficients correlate with expected coefficients with $r = 0.74$ and $P < 0.001$.

need for heparin to maintain ACTs between 180 and 200 seconds. To assess hemofilter patency, a rapid prefilter flush of normal saline solution or heparinized normal saline (1 U/ml) through the hemofilter into the collection bag with both lines clamped is administered. If an organized clot is present within the hemofilter, the dark streaks will not disappear with flushing.

Clotting within the hemofilter decreases the UFR and necessitates hemofilter change. If the hemofilter is totally occluded, the circuit is replaced immediately to preserve patency of the cannula. Once the new circuit is in place, fluid and heparin management is reevaluated. With the new circuit, improved ultrafiltration and fluid loss can be anticipated. An increase in the heparin infusion rate may be warranted to decrease the incidence of future clotting. If a new circuit cannot be placed immediately, the circuit is

disconnected, and the cannula preserved by packing with heparin (5000 U/ml).

The potential for a lethal occurrence of cannula disconnection warrants the frequent inspection of the entire circuit for tightly secured connections. Two major concerns include exsanguination and air emboli. If disconnection occurs, aseptic reconnection needs to rapidly occur. Immediate and temporary clamping of the circuit may prevent air entry. If air is present in a CVVH circuit, it is removed by syringe from the postfilter venous port before reconnecting and reestablishing flow through the circuit.

Hemofiltration systems require a postfilter bubble detection system. If air is detected, the pump is automatically stopped to halt the forward flow of blood. Air is then manually removed. An additional problem related to the actual circuit is spontaneous hemofilter capillary rupture.

Rupture of hemofilter capillary fibers occurs if the transmembrane pressure exceeds the manufacturer's guidelines. This problem is evidenced as a change in the UF color from clear pale yellow to pink or red and requires immediate removal and replacement of the hemofilter.

Documentation. Accuracy in documentation during hemofiltration is critical to evaluate the effectiveness of the therapy. Depending on the specific features of the therapy used, equipment involved, and flexibility of the standard PICU flow sheet, the documentation of hemofiltration can take on many appearances.

Documentation of the intake and output vary, based on institution documentation standards. Generally, sources of intake are recorded as intravenous (IV) fluid, including replacement fluid, dialysate (if used), nutritional infusions, vasopressor infusions, heparin infusions, and sources of gastrointestinal (GI) intake. Output includes ultrafiltrate, urine, blood, and GI losses. Intake and output per hour are recorded, as well as the net UF volume per hour.

Depending on the institution's documentation guidelines, calculation of intake and output sections will vary. When using the PRISMA system, calculation of the net fluid removal rate (i.e., net negative 20 ml/hr body balance) will be done, as opposed to calculation of the replacement fluid (Fig. 21-12). In this calculation, the replacement fluids are not calculated because the PRISMA automatically removes the replacement fluids. The following equation is used:

Amount of hourly fluid intake – Amount of hourly output
[+ (Net negative hourly balance) *or* – (Net positive hourly balance)] = Patient fluid removal rate to be set for that hour

Example: Prescribed net hourly balance is –20 ml) (the patient is fluid overloaded)

Intake	Output
Hyperalimentation = 100 ml/hr	Urine = 7 ml
Vasopressors = 5 ml/hr	Gastric drainage = 13 ml
Enteral feeds = 5 ml/hr	Blood loss = 5 ml

110 (Intake) – 25 (Output) + 20 (Net negative balance) = 105

When the machine is set to remove 105 ml for that hour, the patient will be net negative 20 ml.

Example: Using the same intake and output but the prescribed net hourly balance is +20 (the patient is dehydrated)

110 (Intake) – 25 (Output) – 20 (Net positive balance) = 65

When the machine is set to remove 65 ml for that hour, the patient will be net positive 20 ml.

Using other systems, however, may require calculation and hourly programming of replacement fluids. To do this, the following equation is used:

Amount of replacement fluid to be given over upcoming hour =
Total UF volume in bag – Total amount dialysate
infused over previous hour – Total fluid intake
for previous hour (not including last hour's
replacement fluid) – Desired net UF volume per hour

Confirming the calculation to be used with the healthcare team is imperative. Using the incorrect calculation may cause severe fluid imbalance and resultant hemodynamic instability in the critically ill child.

Routine documentation also includes the child's ACT results, the blood pump speed, the appearance of the hemofilter, and the UF color. Observations of the system and arming of bubble detector alarms for safety maintenance may be recorded in the form of a checklist.

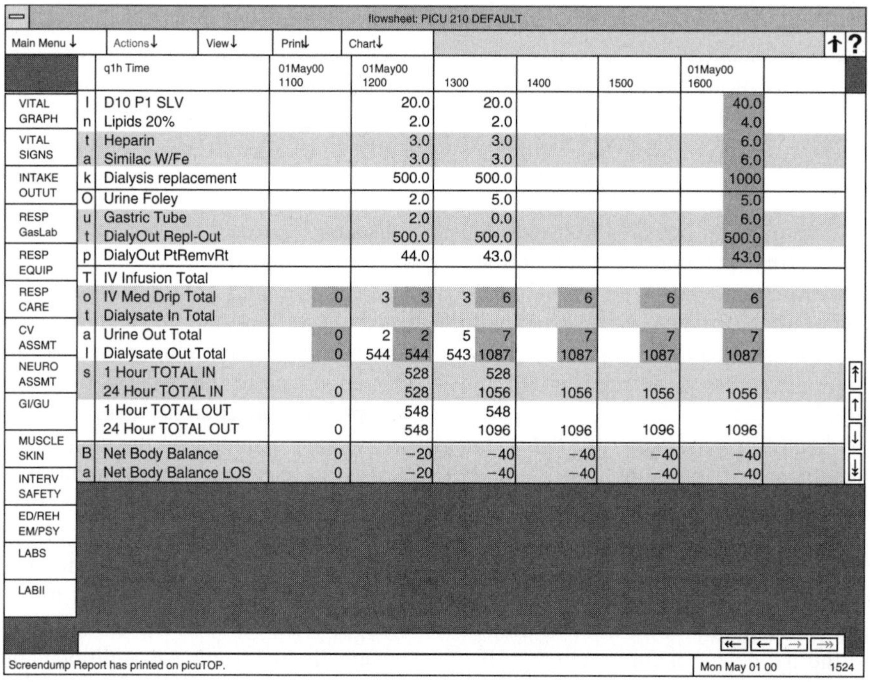

	q1h Time	01May00 1100	01May00 1200	1300	1400	1500	01May00 1600	
VITAL GRAPH	D10 P1 SLV		20.0	20.0			40.0	
	Lipids 20%		2.0	2.0			4.0	
VITAL SIGNS	Heparin		3.0	3.0			6.0	
	Similac W/Fe		3.0	3.0			6.0	
INTAKE OUTUT	Dialysis replacement		500.0	500.0			1000	
	Urine Foley		2.0	5.0			5.0	
RESP GasLab	Gastric Tube		2.0				6.0	
	DialyOut Repl-Out		500.0	500.0			500.0	
RESP EQUIP	DialyOut PtRemvRt		44.0	43.0			43.0	
	IV Infusion Total							
RESP CARE	IV Med Drip Total	0	3 / 3	3 / 6	6	6	6	
	Dialysate In Total							
CV ASSMT	Urine Out Total	0	2 / 2	5 / 7	7	7	7	
	Dialysate Out Total	0	544 / 544	543 / 1087	1087	1087	1087	
NEURO ASSMT	1 Hour TOTAL IN		528	528				
	24 Hour TOTAL IN	0	528	1056	1056	1056	1056	
GI/GU	1 Hour TOTAL OUT		548	548				
	24 Hour TOTAL OUT	0	548	1096	1096	1096	1096	
MUSCLE SKIN	Net Body Balance	0	–20	–40	–40	–40	–40	
INTERV SAFETY	Net Body Balance LOS	0	–20	–40	–40	–40	–40	

(flowsheet: PICU 210 DEFAULT — Main Menu, Actions, View, Print, Chart. Side menu: VITAL GRAPH, VITAL SIGNS, INTAKE OUTUT, RESP GasLab, RESP EQUIP, RESP CARE, CV ASSMT, NEURO ASSMT, GI/GU, MUSCLE SKIN, INTERV SAFETY, ED/REH EM/PSY, LABS, LABII. Vertical label "Intakes" and "Balance". Screendump Report has printed on picuTOP. Mon May 01 00 1524)

Fig. 21-12 CVVH flow sheet. (Courtesy The Children's Memorial Hospital, Chicago, Ill.)

Observations of the child's coagulation status, tolerance of the therapy, and the appearance of the catheter insertion sites are generally best documented in the nursing note. Education provided to the child and family and the identification of further learning needs are included in the record to ensure continuity of care for the child and family.

Modifications to Hemofiltration. Slow continuous ultrafiltration (SCUF) is one modification to hemofiltration. Ultrafiltration occurs according to the same principles described for CVVH but at a slower rate without replacement fluid. Thus solute clearance is both inefficient and ineffective. SCUF is used to prevent overhydration while maintaining intravenous fluids and nutritional balance. The desired hourly UFR is based on the patient's intake to maintain hemodynamic stability.

Another variation to therapy, continuous venovenous hemodiafiltration (CVVHD), differs from CVVH because it enhances solute clearance through diffusion. CVVHD is indicated for children with catabolic and uremic conditions complicating ARF. This system allows dialysate to flow over the outside surface of the filter countercurrent to blood flow on the inside surface of the filter. This provides optimal diffusion transport of solutes and urea from the patient's blood to the UF. CVVHD pulls larger molecules and proteins across the filter. Hourly measurements from the UF collection bag include the volumes of both dialysate infused and UF removed. Subtraction of the hourly dialysate volume infused from the volume collected in the UF collection bag results in the volume of actual UF removed.

The amount of UF produced can be altered through the interventions described under simple hemofiltration. Dialysate is usually prescribed by the nephrology team. High osmolar dialysate concentrations further increase UFR. Careful surveillance of the patient's hemodynamic status and routine monitoring of electrolyte levels are essential in evaluating the effectiveness of CVVHD for fluid and solute clearance.

CVVHDF is CVVHD with filtration. This technology uses both diffusion and convection to maintain fluid and electrolyte balance and control azotemia. It differs from CVVHD in that it uses a replacement fluid and CVVHD does not. The specific type of hemofiltration used depends on the clinical situation.

Hemodialysis

HD rapidly restores fluid, electrolyte, and acid-base balances and is more efficient in removing nitrogenous wastes than any other currently available form of therapy. More cumulative experience exists with HD than with any other therapeutic modality for management of acute renal failure. Newer single and dual-lumen vascular access permits HD in smaller infants and young children. HD monitoring equipment and blood lines with minimal extracorporeal blood volume make HD available for infants less than 5 kg.[34] HD may be the treatment of choice for several reasons. It is possible to calculate the amount of time necessary to remove a particular solute load for a given patient. This capability affords a sense of control and predictability in the management of life-threatening imbalances. In addition, depending on the availability of an HD team and appropriate system, HD can be rapidly initiated in the PICU. HD is also the only treatment available for certain toxic ingestions. The charcoal membrane used in HD removes some poisons, such as chloramphenicol and theophylline, that are not cleared by another type of membrane. Finally, HD may be the only available intervention when PD is contraindicated.

Principles of Therapy. PD and HD use the same principles that govern fluid and solute movement across a semipermeable membrane. Diffusion and osmosis occur relative to the concentrations and osmotic gradients present between the child's serum and the dialysate. Similar to PD, the goals of therapy determine which percentage of dialysate is used. Unlike PD, HD requires extracorporeal circulation. A dialyzer pumps blood and dialysate through the system in opposing directions. Countercurrent flow provides an efficient exchange of solutes. The rate of flow through the dialyzer and the length of each exchange can be controlled.

Urea, creatinine, and potassium are usually present in greater concentration in the patient's serum than in dialysate; therefore these solutes rapidly diffuse from the blood to the dialysate and are removed from the body. Diffusion is the predominant mechanism for effective clearance in hemodialysis. Bicarbonate, an alkalizing agent present in dialysate, moves from the dialysate to the blood and provides treatment for metabolic acidosis. Additional molecules can be removed through convective dialysis, where rapid fluid shifts from the blood to the dialysate tend to pull solutes along.

Procedure. Before HD, intravenous access is evaluated or obtained. Although in rare situations native arteriovenous (AV) fistulas are available, femoral vein or superior vena cava cannulation is common. Access usually requires a catheter with a larger bore and a shorter length than standard central venous catheters. The use of peripheral veins in the pediatric population necessitates the use of smaller catheters. Difficult volume and hemodynamic management may be the consequence. The smaller catheters result in increased resistance to flow from the dialyzer returning to the patient. This increased resistance results in an increase in hydrostatic pressure in the dialyzer, thereby increasing UF and fluid removal. Despite the associated risk of infection with the use of femoral vessels, this location may be the best choice. Venous cannulation of two separate locations or one with double-lumen capacity may be used.

Several dialyzers are commercially available. The choices for appropriate HD blood lines and dialyzer are dictated by the body surface area and intravascular blood volume of the child. When choosing a circuit, it is important to keep the extracorporeal volume (tubing plus dialyzer) less than 10% of the patient's total blood volume.[41] The smallest circuit volume currently available is 45 ml. This system, primed with whole blood, can be used in infants. In addition, there is a selection of membranes for desired effects. High-efficiency dialyzers employ membranes that have a larger surface area so that small solutes may diffuse more rapidly. High-flux dialyzers incorporate membranes that have larger pores and yield higher clearance of water and larger solutes.[36]

Maintenance. Determined by the goals of therapy, the HD team prescribes the length of exchange time. Amounts of glucose, acetate, sodium, calcium, and potassium are variably added to the dialyzing fluid, depending on the patient's situation. The length of one HD exchange usually extends over 2 to 6 hours. Some form of heparinization is required to prevent clot formation within the circuit, although 4-hour treatments may be undertaken heparin free with new biocompatible membranes.[46] If heparin is needed, baseline coagulation profiles are necessary before initiating HD. ACTs are monitored to ensure the maintenance of a therapeutic dose without toxic effects. ACTs between 150 and 200 seconds permit adequate anticoagulation with minimal bleeding risks.

Solute clearance depends on several factors, including the rates of blood and dialysate flow and the surface area and permeability of the membrane. The rate of urea and water removal can be calculated. Information about the patient's serum level of solute is an important component of this calculation. The actual serum value, the rate of urea production, the patient's metabolic rate, and the child's protein intake all play a part in determining the rate of urea clearance.

The acceptable rate of solute clearance is affected by how the child tolerates HD. Because solutes are rapidly removed from the serum but slowly removed from the brain, an osmolar gradient or disequilibrium between the intravascular and intracellular space may develop. This gradient results in fluid shifts and cerebral edema. The child with disequilibrium syndrome may exhibit confusion, irritability, headache, nausea, vomiting, and seizure activity. This syndrome seems to occur more when the BUN falls more than 35% with therapy. Consequently, initial treatments may be shortened to avoid this syndrome. Some centers use intravenous mannitol (0.5 g/kg) during the initial exchange to minimize disequilibrium effects.

Bedside HD of critically ill pediatric patients requires the collaborative expertise of both PICU and HD nurses. Before beginning HD, the expectations of each nurse are clarified. Usually the PICU nurse continues to manage ongoing care, the HD nurse manages the therapy, and together they collaboratively manipulate vasopressors, volume, and fluid and solute removal within established guidelines to manage the patient through the procedure. Communication between nurses is key because both will be continuously assessing the patient.

Monitoring. Assessment of the patient's intravascular volume status is an ongoing responsibility. When HD is initiated, a relative hypovolemia may develop owing to the external circulation of the child's blood in the amount of the circuit volume. Progressive hypovolemia and hypotension are possible as therapy progresses. It is not uncommon to initiate or increase the dose of vasopressors during HD. The treatment objective is usually to establish and maintain intravascular normovolemia, but expedient and/or large volume removal challenges this objective. Furthermore, the

flow rates may need to be decreased to maintain hemodynamic stability.

At the beginning of a HD session, hypoxemia may be seen with a decrease in the arterial Po_2 by as much as 20 mmHg. A potential cause for this phenomenon is activation of the complement system, which occurs when a cellulose membrane is used. Another potential cause for this phenomenon is hypoventilation, which may occur with either an acetate or bicarbonate bath. The effect usually peaks at 2 hours and usually recovers 1 to 2 hours after the dialysis session.[36] Patients already receiving oxygen therapy may require a higher percentage during this period. The use of acetate as a buffer in dialysate may contribute to the development of relative hypovolemia because acetate decreases systemic vascular resistance. Switching to a bicarbonate-based bath improves cardiovascular stability.

Hypervolemia may occur if too much fluid is returned to the patient. A common time for this imbalance is at the end of an exchange when the child may be receiving additional blood products. Additional HD time for fluid removal may be required.

Dysrhythmias may occur from electrolyte or acid-base imbalance. Hypotension, which decreases coronary perfusion pressure, and hypokalemia are two of the most common causes of dysrhythmias during HD.

Part of the routine surveillance of the patient's coagulation status includes following trends in the platelet count and monitoring ACTs. A relative thrombocytopenia may develop as platelets adhere to the dialyzer membrane over time.

Frequent monitoring of the dialysate and the child's temperature are important for several reasons. As for any patient with central vascular access, the risk of infection is increased. Daily surveillance cultures from dialysis tubing and dialysate are generally a part of institutional policy. Any elevation in temperature raises suspicion of infection, and a septic workup results. Urea may function as an antipyretic, and thus as the patient's serum urea begins to drop, an occult fever may appear, warranting further investigation. Hypothermia may also be identified, which can be improved by increasing the temperature of the dialysate bath. The standard dialysate bath is warmed to 37° C but may range between 35° C and 40° C depending on the clinical circumstance.[41]

Continuous monitoring of the child during HD includes observation of the blood in the circuit for color and clots and inspection of the circuit for leaks, loose connections, and the characteristics of flow. Nurses must assess the child's catheter insertion site or sites at each shift for skin integrity, bleeding, and signs of infection. The HD circuit uses pumps, thereby increasing the risk of air embolism. An air bubble detector alarm system is critical to safe care of the patient.

Documentation. Documentation during HD is a shared responsibility between the HD and PICU nurse. The HD nurse usually documents procedural information, for example, fluid intake, laboratory results, medication administration, and the amount of UF output. The PICU nurse usually documents the child's tolerance of the procedure and observations and assessments of the family, as well as identified needs and teaching. Documentation of information that is jointly monitored is institution specific. Optimal use of the record by the entire healthcare team essential.

Complications.   Although HD is the more familiar form of treatment for ARF, several potential complications can result. Complications may be exacerbated in a patient with small initial circulating volumes or hemodynamically instability. Common complications of HD include hemodynamic instability resulting from UF and osmolar losses, temperature irregularity, and complement activation.[41] The most common complication is hypotension, which may be corrected by UFR reduction. Other complications include dialysis disequilibrium syndrome and hypokalemia. The use of heparin leads to the possibility of bleeding. Circuit disconnection, infection, and transfusion reactions are other possible complications. Close monitoring is the cardinal rule. Communication between the bedside and the dialysis nurse is essential.

SUMMARY

Various therapies are now available to support the patient in ARF. Research in the identification of risk factors associated with ARF may allow earlier intervention, which may minimize the occurrence of ARF or limit mortality. Pediatric nursing research is needed to help guide practice related to the care of patients requiring renal replacement therapy.

Survival of the child with ARF who undergoes renal replacement therapy depends on the age of the child and the cause of the ARF. Children who are young or small have poorer survival rates than their older and larger counterparts.[46] The presence of such conditions as MODS makes the therapies available difficult to use because of the baseline hemodynamic instability of the child. Care of the patient in ARF is complex, requiring the combined expertise of an extensive multidisciplinary team. Collaboration within the team provides the best plan of care for each patient. The challenge for nursing is to help facilitate team communication and advocate for care that is in the best interest of the patient and family.

REFERENCES

1. Mendley SR, Langman CB: Acute renal failure in the pediatric patient, *Adv Ren Replace Ther* 4:93-101, 1997.
2. Robillard JE, Porter CC, Jose PA: Structure and function of the developing kidney. In Holliday MA, Barratt TM, Avner ED, eds: *Pediatric nephrology,* ed 3, Baltimore, 1994, Williams & Wilkins.
3. Carlson BM: *Human embryology and developmental biology,* St Louis, 1994, Mosby.
4. Moore KL: *Before we are born: basic embryology and birth defects,* ed 2, Philadelphia, 1983, WB Saunders.
5. Andrews M, Mooney K: Alteration of renal and urinary tract function in children. In McCance K, Heuther S, eds: *Pathophysiology: the biologic basis for disease in adults and children,* St Louis, 1990, Mosby.
6. Jose PA, Fildes RD, Gomez RA et al: Neonatal renal function and physiology, *Curr Opin Pediatr* 6:172-177, 1994.
7. Yao LP, Jose PA: Developmental renal hemodynamics, *Pediatr Nephrol* 9:632-637, 1995.
8. Seikaly MG, Arant BS: Development of renal hemodynamics: glomerular filtration and renal blood flow, *Clin Perinatol* 19:1-13, 1992.
9. Spitzer A, Berstein J, Boichis H et al: Kidney and urinary tract. In Fanaroff AA, Martin RJ, eds: *Neonatal-perinatal medicine: diseases of the fetus and infant,* ed 5, vol 2, St Louis, 1992, Mosby.
10. Gomez RA: The kidney in infants and children. In Greenberg A, Cheung AK, Falk RJ et al, eds: *Primer on kidney diseases,* ed 2, San Diego, 1998, Academic Press.
11. Briggs JP, Kriz W, Schnermann JB: Overview of renal function and structure. In Greenberg A, Cheung AK, Falk RJ et al, eds: *Primer on kidney diseases,* ed 2, San Diego, 1998, Academic Press.
12. Yarid A, Ichikawa I: Renal blood flow and glomerular filtration rate. In Holliday MA,

Barratt TM, Avner ED, eds: *Pediatric nephrology,* ed 3, Baltimore, 1994, Williams & Wilkins.
13. Sehic A, Chesney RW: Acute renal failure: diagnosis, *Pediatr Rev* 16:101-106, 1995.
14. Siegel NJ, Van Why SK, Boydsun II et al: Acute renal failure. In Holliday MA, Barratt TM, Avner ED, eds: *Pediatric nephrology,* ed 3, Baltimore, 1994, Williams & Wilkins.
15. Nissenson AR: Acute renal failure: definition and pathogenesis, *Kidney Int* 53:S7-S10, 1998.
16. Cole BR, Salinas-Madrigal L: Acute proliferative glomerulonephritis. In Holliday MA, Barratt TM, Avner ED, eds: *Pediatric nephrology,* ed 3, Baltimore, 1994, Williams & Wilkins.
17. Cadnapaphornchai P, Alvapati RK, McDonald FD: Differential diagnosis of acute renal failure. In Jacobson HR, Striker GE, Klahr S, eds: *The principles and practice of nephrology,* ed 2, St Louis, 1995, Mosby.
18. Andreucci VE, Fuiano G, Stanziale P et al: Role of renal biopsy in the diagnosis and prognosis of acute renal failure, *Kidney Int* 53(suppl 66):S91-S95, 1998.
19. Mindell JA, Chertow GM: A practical approach to acute renal failure, *Med Clin North Am* 81:731-748, 1997.
20. Koff SA: Obstructive uropathy: clinical aspects. In Holliday MA, Barratt TM, Avner ED, eds: *Pediatric nephrology,* ed 3, Baltimore, 1994, Williams & Wilkins.
21. O'Meara YM, Bernard DB: Clinical presentation, complications, and prognosis of acute renal failure. In Jacobson HR, Striker GE, Klahr S, eds: *The principles and practice of nephrology,* ed 2, St Louis, 1995, Mosby.
22. Safirstein R: Pathophysiology of acute renal failure. In Greenburg A, ed: *Primer on kidney diseases,* ed 2, San Diego, 1998, Academic Press.

23. Mucelli RP, Bertolotto M: Imaging studies in acute renal failure, *Kidney Int* 53:S102-S105, 1998.
24. Green T: Renal pharmacology. In Fuhrman B, Zimmerman J, eds: *Pediatric critical care,* ed 2, St Louis, 1998, Mosby.
25. St. Peter M, Halstenson C: Pharmacologic approach in patients with renal failure. In Chernow B, ed: *The pharmacologic approach to the critically ill patient,* Baltimore, 1994, Williams & Wilkins.
26. Johnson C, Simmons W: Dialysis of drugs, *Pharmacy Practice News* 26:17-22, Dec 1999.
27. Stewart C, Barnett R: Acute renal failure in infants, children, and adults, *Crit Care Clin* 13:575-590, 1997.
28. Chasse R: Diuretics, erythropoietin, and other medications used in renal failure. In Chernow B, ed: *The pharmacologic approach to the critically ill patient,* ed 3, Baltimore, 1994, Williams & Wilkins.
29. Gibson R: Management of the critically ill pediatric patient with acute renal failure, *Crit Care Nurs Q* 20:22-35, 1997
30. Eades SK, Christensen ML: The clinical pharmacology of loop diuretics in the pediatric patient, *Pediatr Nephrol* 12:603-616, 1998.
31. Luciani G, Nichani S, Chang A et al: Continuous versus intermittent furosemide infusion in critically ill infants after open heart operations, *Ann Thorac Surg* 64:1133-1139, 1997.
32. Carcoana O, Hines R: Is renal dose dopamine protective or therapeutic? *Crit Care Clin* 12:677-686, 1996.
33. Bergstein J: In Behrman R, Kliegman R, Jenson H, eds: *Nelson textbook of pediatrics,* ed 16, Philadelphia, 2000, WB Saunders.
34. Mentser M, Bunchman T: Nephrology in the pediatric intensive care unit, *Semin Nephrol* 18:330-340, 1998.

35. Mahnesmith R: Acute and chronic renal failure. In Bone R, ed: *Pulmonary and critical care medicine,* St Louis, 1998, Mosby.

36. Hebbar S, Muther R: Renal replacement therapies. In Civetta J, Taylor R, Kirby R, eds: *Critical care,* ed 3, Philadelphia, 1997, Lippincott-Raven.

37. Sorof J, Stromberg D, Brewer E et al: Early initiation of peritoneal dialysis after surgical repair of congenital heart disease, *Pediatr Nephrol* 13:641-645, 1999.

38. Vande Walle J, Raes A, Castillo D et al: New perspectives for PD in acute renal failure related to new catheter techniques and introduction of APD, *Adv Perit Dial* 13:190-194, 1997.

39. Flynn J: Causes, management approaches, and outcome of acute renal failure in children, *Curr Opin Pediatr* 10:184-189, 1998.

40. Hand MM, McManus ML, Harmon WE: Renal disorders in pediatric intensive care. In Rogers M, ed: *Textbook of pediatric intensive care,* Baltimore, 1996, Williams & Wilkins.

41. Smoyer W, Maxvold N, Remenapp R et al: Pediatric renal replacement therapy. In Fuhrman B, Zimmerman J, eds: *Pediatric critical care,* ed 2, St Louis, 1998, Mosby.

42. Reid M, Sawyer D: The human factors implications of peritoneal dialysis: cycler overfill incident reports, *Int J Trauma Nurs* 5:68-71, 1999.

43. Headrick CL: Adult/pediatric CVVH: the pump, the patient, the circuit, *Crit Care Nurs Clin North Am* 10:197-207, 1998.

44. Craig M: Continuous venous to venous hemofiltration, *Crit Care Nurs Clin North Am* 10:219-233, 1998.

45. McAlpine L: CAVH: principles and practical applications, *Crit Care Nurs Clin North Am* 10:179-189, 1998.

46. Maxvold N, Smoyer W, Gardner J et al: Management of acute renal failure in the pediatric patient: hemofiltration versus hemodialysis, *Am J Kidney Dis* 30:S84-S88, 1997.

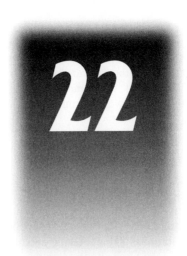

22 Gastrointestinal Critical Care Problems

Shari Simone

A wide variety of gastrointestinal (GI) problems occur in infants and children that may require intensive nursing care. Problems of the GI tract range from intussusception, treated by simple reduction with barium enema (BE), to fulminant liver disease with GI bleeding. GI disorders rarely occur in isolation but are often associated with other congenital defects or with multisystem dysfunction, placing infants and children with these disorders at high risk for morbidity and mortality.

GI problems result in the final common pathways of obstruction, GI and peritoneal inflammation, GI bleeding, and hepatic failure. The existence of one of these final common pathways often predisposes the child to the development of another. For example, the infant with an intestinal obstruction is at increased risk for developing perforation and/or necrosis of the bowel with peritoneal inflammation without prompt treatment. Critical care nurses play a vital role in the recognition and prevention of the progression of these final common pathways.

EMBRYOLOGY

The digestive tract and biliary passages develop from the primitive gut.[1] As early as the third week of gestation the primitive gut can be differentiated into the foregut, the midgut, and the hindgut. The pharynx, esophagus, stomach, duodenum (proximal to the opening of the bile duct), liver, pancreas, and bile duct system develop from the foregut.

The duodenum distal to the opening of the bile duct, jejunum, ileum, cecum, appendix, ascending colon, and proximal part of the transverse colon are derived from the midgut. Other parts of colon including the left one third to one half of the transverse colon, the rectum, and the superior part of the anal canal originate from the hindgut.

The esophagus and trachea are one tube until the fourth week of gestation, when the tracheoesophageal septum forms to separate the laryngotracheal tube and the esophagus. The esophagus is almost occluded by the proliferating epithelium during the fifth to sixth week of gestation. At about 7 weeks, the esophagus elongates and reaches its final length. By the end of the embryonic period, the esophagus hollows (recanalizes).

The stomach is first distinguished as a dilation of the gut during the fourth to fifth week of embryonic development. The stomach rotates clockwise longitudinally and moves from the neck region into the abdomen. The growth rate of the stomach wall varies, forming lesser and greater curvatures and giving the stomach its asymmetric appearance.

The liver, gallbladder, and biliary duct apparatus begin development during the fourth to fifth week of gestation from the hepatic diverticulum. The liver grows rapidly and soon fills most of the abdominal cavity. In the sixth week of gestation, hemopoiesis begins, giving the liver a bright red appearance. By the end of gestation, hemopoietic activity subsides, liver growth slows, and its size relative to body weight is reduced. The biliary apparatus is functional by the thirteenth to sixteenth week.

Bile formation by the hepatic cells begins during the twelfth week. Bilirubin (bile pigments) begins to form and enter the duodenum during the thirteenth to sixteenth week of development. Bilirubin gives duodenal contents a dark green or meconium color. The biliary apparatus is functional at the thirteenth to sixteenth week of gestation.

The pancreas is created from ventral and dorsal buds and fuse in its final form during the seventh week of gestation. Somatostatin-, glucagon-, insulin-, and pancreatic polypeptide-containing cells appear at or before the tenth week of gestation. Insulin secretion begins at about the twentieth week.

The duodenum begins to develop early in the fourth week of gestation, originating from the foregut and midgut. The duodenum rotates with the stomach. During the fifth and sixth weeks, the lumen of the duodenum narrows and may be occluded by epithelial cells. By approximately the sixth week, the gut lengthens rapidly and causes a U-shaped region of the future jejunum and the entire transverse colon to transiently herniate into the umbilical cord. The intestines continue to develop within the umbilical cord. At the tenth to twelfth week of gestation, while the intestines rotate counterclockwise 270 degrees, reentry of the intestines occurs. By the end of the embryonic period, the lumen hollows. Further positioning of the small intestine, appendix, and transverse and sigmoid colon continues until the GI tract assumes its final anatomic position at the twentieth week of gestation and becomes fixed to the posterior abdominal wall.

The colon is formed at the sixth week of gestation by division of the rectum and upper anal canal from the urogenital sinus. The rectum and the superior part of the anal canal are also separated from the exterior by the cloacal (anal) membrane. This anal membrane normally breaks down by the seventh to eighth week, forming the anal canal.

ESSENTIAL ANATOMY AND PHYSIOLOGY

Growth and maintenance of the human body is dependent on the digestion and absorption of nutrients and water. This process begins in the oral cavity and ends at the anal sphincter. The GI tract is supported by a rich blood supply, the lymphatic system, and intrinsic and autonomic nervous innervation, which allows for food to be moved through the body, where it is exposed to and absorbed by a large surface area. A review of the developmental physiology of the digestive tract is presented in Fig. 22-1.

The oral cavity includes the lips, tongue, cheeks, teeth, taste buds, and salivary glands. These structures decrease the size of food, stimulate saliva secretion, and move food into position for swallowing.

The pharynx provides for the movement of food into the esophagus. Food passes through the pharynx to the esophagus in approximately 1 second.

The esophagus is a channel for the passage of food from the pharynx to the stomach. Along the length of the esophagus are glands that secrete mucus to provide lubrication for the passage of food. The lower gastroesophageal sphincter is located at the distal 2 to 5 cm of the esophagus. This sphincter surrounds the opening of the stomach with increased amounts of muscle and remains narrowed until a wave of peristalsis moves through it.

The stomach is a pear-shaped organ with the esophagus at the top end and the duodenum at the lower end. The stomach is the most dilated part of the GI tract and is an easily distensible reservoir for food. In infancy, the stomach usually is transverse. By approximately age 7 years, it is the shape and position of the adult stomach. At birth, the stomach has the capacity to hold approximately 10 to 20 ml. By 3 months, the stomach's capacity is 150 to 200 ml, and by age 10 years it is about 750 to 900 ml. Stomach capacity is important to consider when providing enteral feedings for the critically ill infant. The lining of the stomach is made up of mucosal folds called rugae. Within these folds are chief, parietal, and mucous neck cells that secrete various elements of digestive juice. The newborn stomach mucosal wall is thinner than that of an adult.

The liver and pancreas empty into the small intestine. The pancreas lies parallel to and beneath the stomach and has the internal structure identical to that of the salivary gland. The major function of the pancreas is digestion and utilization of dietary nutrients. The liver assists with digestion by synthesizing bile acid.

The small intestine consists of the duodenum, jejunum, and ileum and extends from the pyloric sphincter at the bottom of the stomach to the ileocecal valve. The lining of the small intestine consists of folds called villi that project

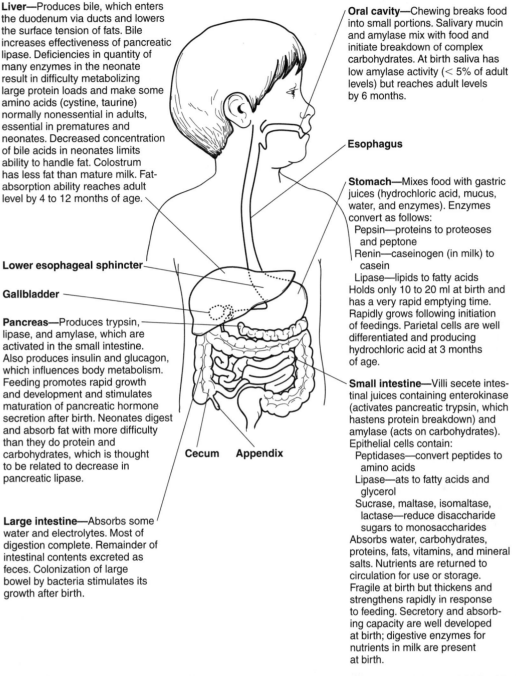

Liver—Produces bile, which enters the duodenum via ducts and lowers the surface tension of fats. Bile increases effectiveness of pancreatic lipase. Deficiencies in quantity of many enzymes in the neonate result in difficulty metabolizing large protein loads and make some amino acids (cystine, taurine) normally nonessential in adults, essential in prematures and neonates. Decreased concentration of bile acids in neonates limits ability to handle fat. Colostrum has less fat than mature milk. Fat-absorption ability reaches adult level by 4 to 12 months of age.

Lower esophageal sphincter

Gallbladder

Pancreas—Produces trypsin, lipase, and amylase, which are activated in the small intestine. Also produces insulin and glucagon, which influences body metabolism. Feeding promotes rapid growth and development and stimulates maturation of pancreatic hormone secretion after birth. Neonates digest and absorb fat with more difficulty than they do protein and carbohydrates, which is thought to be related to decrease in pancreatic lipase.

Large intestine—Absorbs some water and electrolytes. Most of digestion complete. Remainder of intestinal contents excreted as feces. Colonization of large bowel by bacteria stimulates its growth after birth.

Oral cavity—Chewing breaks food into small portions. Salivary mucin and amylase mix with food and initiate breakdown of complex carbohydrates. At birth saliva has low amylase activity ($< 5\%$ of adult levels) but reaches adult levels by 6 months.

Esophagus

Stomach—Mixes food with gastric juices (hydrochloric acid, mucus, water, and enzymes). Enzymes convert as follows:
  Pepsin—proteins to proteoses and peptone
  Renin—caseinogen (in milk) to casein
  Lipase—lipids to fatty acids
Holds only 10 to 20 ml at birth and has a very rapid emptying time. Rapidly grows following initiation of feedings. Parietal cells are well differentiated and producing hydrochloric acid at 3 months of age.

Cecum   Appendix

Small intestine—Villi secete intestinal juices containing enterokinase (activates pancreatic trypsin, which hastens protein breakdown) and amylase (acts on carbohydrates). Epithelial cells contain:
  Peptidases—convert peptides to amino acids
  Lipase—ats to fatty acids and glycerol
  Sucrase, maltase, isomaltase, lactase—reduce disaccharide sugars to monosaccharides
Absorbs water, carbohydrates, proteins, fats, vitamins, and mineral salts. Nutrients are returned to circulation for use or storage. Fragile at birth but thickens and strengthens rapidly in response to feeding. Secretory and absorbing capacity are well developed at birth; digestive enzymes for nutrients in milk are present at birth.

Fig. 22-1   Developmental physiology of the digestive tract. (From James SR, Mott SR: *Child health nursing: essential care of children and families,* Reading, Pa, 1988, Addison-Wesley.)

into the intestinal lumen. Microvilli cover the membranes of mature epithelial cells that make up the villus tip and form the brush border region. The brush border contains digestive enzymes and contributes to the transfer of nutrients and electrolytes. This area is highly specialized for absorption. Pitlike structures exist between villi called the crypts of Lieberkühn and are composed of absorptive cells and goblet cells that produce mucus. Three sets of lymph nodes also exist along the bowel.

The large intestine begins with the ileocecal valve at the cecum. It includes the appendix and extends through the ascending, transverse, and descending colon and ends at the rectum and anal canal. The internal and external sphincters are made up of the anorectal ring. In the large intestine, there is an increase in the number of goblet cells.

An infant's intestinal length is proportionately larger than that of an adult. This proportional increase allows for larger amounts of fluid to be lost by the infant.

The physiologic and biochemical functions of the GI tract are dependent on motility, secretion, digestion, and absorption. At birth, most of these functions are present, although some developmental differences in absorption, membrane permeability, and types of gastric secretions do exist (Box 22-1).

Motility

Movement within the GI tract is initiated by muscle contraction and is influenced by the nervous system, blood flow, temperature, and hormones.[2,3] The intestinal tract is stimulated by distension, most often from the presence of food. Peristalsis, the basic propulsive movement, is initiated and moves the digested material through the alimentary tract. Peristaltic movement occurs because a group of muscles encircle the lumen of the gut and contract around the digested material creating a pocket. As the muscles below the pocket relax, the longitudinal layers of the gut constrict and propel the contents forward.

During swallowing, food is transported from the posterior part of the mouth to the stomach. The process of swallowing is initiated by the central nervous system. Stimulation of receptors around the opening of the pharynx elicits the swallowing reflex and protects the trachea. The act of swallowing is primarily an automatic reflex for the first 3 months of life. Swallowing starts to become voluntary beginning at 6 weeks, and by 6 months it is fully voluntary. The primary peristaltic wave spreads into the stomach in 8 to 10 seconds. If this primary peristaltic wave does not move all the food to the stomach, secondary waves are initiated. During peristaltic contractions, the stomach and duodenum become relaxed and fill.

When the stomach is distended, peristaltic waves act to mix the food. During this time, the pylorus remains almost closed, allowing only water and other fluid to empty. Periodically, the waves of peristalsis become markedly stronger. The stronger pressure gradient results in the semiliquid food called "chyme" to move into the duodenum. The rate of gastric emptying is influenced by the osmolarity and volume of the food. Hypertonic feeds and high fat content delay emptying. Once peristalsis has developed in the newborn, the stomach empties in approximately 2 hours. The rapid transit time and small stomach capacity contribute to the frequency and amount of feeding and stools in infants. Human milk moves through the stomach faster than cow's milk.[4] In older infants and children, gastric emptying occurs in 3 to 6 hours.

As chyme enters the small intestine, contractions similar to those in the stomach occur. These peristaltic waves are weak and function to move some of the chyme toward the colon, spreading it along the intestine. Most of the chyme will stay in the duodenum until additional food is eaten and a new gastroenteric reflex intensifies peristalsis.

When chyme reaches the colon, contractions are poorly coordinated. These sluggish but persistent movements may occur several times each day. The result is a delay of 8 to 15 hours to move chyme from the ileocecal valve to the transverse colon.

Defecation is stimulated when feces enter the rectum. Peristaltic waves in the descending colon, sigmoid, and rectum are initiated. Relaxation of the internal sphincter results in contraction of the external sphincter. Voluntary control of the external sphincter allows a person to inhibit sphincter contraction, permitting defecation. Voluntary control of the external sphincter also allows for keeping the sphincter contracted.

Secretion

Throughout the GI tract, glands secrete enzymes and hormones used in digestion (Table 22-1). Mucus is also secreted to lubricate and protect the alimentary tract. The presence of food usually stimulates the glands in the region of the food and the surrounding areas to secrete digestive juices. The secretion of saliva by the parotid, submandibular, and sublingual glands begins the process of digestion and absorption. Gastric secretion is regulated by the parasympathetic fibers of the nervous system and by hormonal mechanisms. In the stomach, gastric pepsin initiates protein digestion. Gastric lipase affects fat hydrolysis.

Pancreatic juice is released into the duodenum mainly in response to the presence of chyme. The composition of the pancreatic juice varies depending on the food substances ingested. Large volumes of bicarbonate ions neutralize the acid from the stomach. Also contained in pancreatic juice are various enzymes that act on proteins, carbohydrates, and fat. Pancreatic secretion, like gastric secretion, is regulated by neural and hormonal mechanisms. Bile and bile salts (end product of cholesterol metabolism and the largest component of bile) are also released into the duodenum by way of the bile duct apparatus. Bile is produced and secreted by the liver and is essential for the absorption of fats and fat-soluble vitamins from the gut. Intestinal glands are stimulated by tactile stimulation, chemical irritation, distension, or motility within the gut.

Brunner glands and other cells of the intestinal mucosa secrete mucus. The crypts of Lieberkühn secrete pure extracellular fluid, supplying a vehicle for absorption of substances from chyme. The large intestine is lined with mucous cells that secrete only mucus.

Digestion and Absorption

Digestion and absorption by the GI tract provide the organic molecules of fat, carbohydrates, and protein to provide energy for the body to function. The gut prepares food by

TABLE 22-1 Selected Gastrointestinal Enzymes and Hormones

Organ	Enzyme	Action
Salivary glands	Ptyalin (salivary amylase)	Starch to smaller carbohydrates
Stomach	Pepsin (chief cells) intrinsic factor	Protein to polypeptides
	Gastric lipase	Triglycerides to glycerides and fatty acids
	Gastrin	Stimulates gastric acid secretion in the presence of stomach distension
	Somatostatin*	Inhibits various hormones, secretions, and motor effects
Pancreas	Elastase	Protein to amino acid
	Trypsin	Protein and polypeptides to amino acids
	Chymotrypsin	
	Nuclease	
	Carboxypeptidase A and B	
	Pancreatic lipase	Nucleic acids to nucleotides
	Pancreatic amylase	
	Cholesterol esterase	Polypeptides to smaller polypeptides
	Phospholipase A$_1$	Lipids to glycerol, glycerides, free fatty acids
		Starch to two disaccharide units (maltose)
		Hydrolysis of ester bonds in cholesterol and vitamins A, D, and E
		Phospholipid digestion
Intestines	Enteroglucagon	Inhibits gastric function
	Brush border enzymes:	
	Aminopolypeptidase	Polypeptides to smaller peptides
	Dipeptidase	Dipeptides to amino acids
	Maltase	Maltose to glucose
	Lactase	Lactose to glucose
	Sucrase	Sucrose, glucose, fructose
	Intestinal lipase	Fats to glycerides, glycerol, fatty acids
	Gastrone	Inhibits gastric secretion in presence of fats, sugars, and acids
	Secretin	Stimulates hepatic bile and pancreatic electrolyte and fluid secretion in the presence of polypeptides and acids
	Cholecystokinin-pancreozymin (CCK-PZ)	Stimulates pancreatic enzyme secretion and gallbladder contraction to release bile in the presence of fats

*Also found in the pancreas and small and large intestine.

chemical and mechanical means so it can be absorbed through the mucosal lining into the blood and lymph.

All major nutrients are absorbed in the small intestine. Bile salts and vitamin B$_{12}$ are absorbed only in the terminal ileum. The large intestine is primarily concerned with the absorption of water and electrolytes and functions in the synthesis of vitamin K and some B complex vitamins. The resultant feces usually consist of three-fourths water. The remaining one fourth is solid material, of which approximately 30% is dead bacteria. The brown color is the result of breakdown products of bilirubin called stercobilinogen. Table 22-2 lists the nutrients obtained through food and their site of absorption.

Carbohydrate digestion begins in the mouth where food mixes with ptyalin (also known as amylase), an enzyme contained in saliva. Ptyalin hydrolyzes starch into maltose and other small glucose polymers. Pancreatic amylase and

 TABLE 22-2 Nutrient Site of Absorption

Nutrient	Primary Sites of Absorption
Glucose	Duodenum, upper jejunum
Sucrose	Jejunum, ileum
Lactose	Jejunum, upper ileum
Amino acids	Duodenum, jejunum
Fats	Duodenum, upper jejunum
Sodium	Jejunum, ileum
Potassium	Jejunum, ileum
Calcium	Duodenum
Magnesium	Duodenum
Iron	Duodenum
Vitamin D	Jejunum, ileum
Vitamin B$_{12}$	Terminal ileum
Water	Stomach, small and large intestine

various other enzymes from the brush border of the intestinal epithelium are responsible for further digestion of carbohydrates in the small intestine. Carbohydrates are absorbed mostly in the form of a monosaccharide, such as glucose, galactose, and fructose. Glucose transport is related to the sodium-coupled glucose transport system. The glucose and galactose transport rate in infants is low compared with that in adults and apparently increases during the first year of life. The digested products are absorbed into the portal blood. Most of the carbohydrates are used for energy, although some excess glucose is stored as glycogen in the liver. Additional carbohydrates are changed into fat and stored as triglyceride.

The digestion of protein begins in the stomach with gastric acid secretion. These acids denature complex proteins, making them more conducive to the actions of proteolytic enzymes. Pepsin begins the digestion of protein in the stomach, providing approximately 10% to 30% of total protein digestion. Protein digestion continues in the small intestine under the influence of the pancreatic enzymes and mucosal enzymes. Protein absorption occurs mostly in the duodenum and jejunum in the form of amino acids. As with glucose transport, the sodium transport mechanism probably provides for amino acid transport. Amino acids are used in production of enzymes, in synthesis of plasma proteins, as components in liver structural proteins, in the gut, and in other organs and muscles. In certain conditions, amino acids are used in glyconeogenesis to make glucose when glycogen stores cannot meet the body's caloric needs. Valine, leucine, isoleucine, lysine, threonine, tryptophan, phenylalanine, and methionine are essential amino acids. Tyrosine and cysteine are semiessential because they can be synthesized only from essential precursors.

Newborn proteolytic activity and absorptive function is not fully developed. Intestinal permeability to whole proteins is increased in infants.[5] The increased permeability allows for cow's milk proteins and other allergens to traverse the intestinal wall. This may increase the infant's susceptibility to GI allergies.

Appropriate fat digestion and absorption depends on the proper functioning of the pancreas hepatobiliary system and the absorptive sites within the jejunum, ileum, and lymph nodes. Dietary fat is ingested primarily in the form of long-chain triglycerides. Other dietary lipids that are used by the body include small quantities of phospholipids, cholesterol, and cholesterol esters. Most digestion and absorption of fat occur in the small intestine, with the majority of fat absorbed by the middle one third of the jejunum. Lipolysis is dependent on the presence of bile acid, phospholipase A$_2$, and pancreatic lipases. Triglycerides are broken down to fatty acids and glycerol. Phospholipid envelops the triglyceride. Bile salts and fatty acids form micelles and attach themselves to the surface of epithelial cells. Fatty acids then diffuse into the cell and re-form to triglyceride molecules, which are released into the lymphatics and then to the systemic circulation. Medium-chain triglycerides are digested and transported through the intestinal lumen faster than long-chain triglycerides.

Medium-chain triglycerides do not require bile salts and pancreatic lipase for digestion.

In infants younger than 1 year of age, only 80% to 95% of triglycerides are absorbed.[6] A smaller pool of bile acid results in the inefficient absorption of fat. To minimize fat malabsorption, infants use alternative mechanisms to facilitate fat digestion.

Water absorption is dependent on movement of electrolytes. By diffusion water follows electrolytes across the intestinal membrane by passing through membrane pores. When chyme is dilute, water is absorbed through the intestinal mucosa into the blood. The greatest proportion of water absorption is in the jejunum and proximal part of the large intestine.

The information available regarding mineral, vitamin, and trace element absorption is limited. Electrolytes, like water, are absorbed through membrane pores or by transport into the blood. Greater absorption occurs in the proximal rather than the distal portion of the small intestine. Electrolytes are also absorbed in the large intestine. Sodium, chloride, potassium, and bicarbonate are more easily absorbed because they are monovalent, whereas polyvalent electrolytes, such as calcium and magnesium, are more difficult to absorb. Absorption of calcium occurs by active transport primarily in the duodenum, whereas phosphorus absorption takes place mostly in the jejunum. Calcium and phosphorus intake greatly affects phosphorus absorption. The absorption of trace elements is dependent on the milk source. Breast-fed infants are more efficient in absorbing trace elements than infants who are fed cow's milk–based formulas.[4]

GASTROINTESTINAL ASSESSMENT

Abdominal Examination

Nursing assessment of the GI system is fundamental to the care of infants and children who are critically ill, particularly when GI dysfunction is suspected or confirmed. Assessment is initiated with serial abdominal examinations, employing the basic techniques of inspection, auscultation, percussion, and palpation. Unlike other system assessments, auscultation is performed before percussion and palpation to prevent changes in bowel sounds. The examination is also performed with the patient in a completely supine position. The abdomen is inspected for the presence of bruises, wounds, scars, erythema, or discolorations; peristaltic waves and/or pulsations; visible asymmetry, masses, bowel loops, or protuberances; a flat, full, or scaphoid contour; distension; and umbilical and muscular abnormalities. Significant abdominal distension is a classic sign of intestinal obstruction.

Serial auscultation of the abdomen is performed in all four abdominal quadrants, noting the presence, or absence, and character of bowel sounds with particular attention to changes in sounds over time. Intestinal obstruction produces high-pitched, tinkling sounds; nasogastric (NG) intubation causes decreased or absent sounds. A quiet abdomen is present during paralytic ileus, and an ominously silent abdomen may indicate perforation with peritonitis. Other sounds, such as bruits, hums, and rubs, may also be heard with auscultation. A friction rub may indicate peritoneal inflammation.

Percussion is used to obtain information regarding abdominal contents, including air and fluid, as well as the size of intraabdominal organs and masses. Shifting dullness is elicited in the presence of intraperitoneal fluid. The normal liver and spleen are dull to percussion. Absence of dullness over the liver may be found with pneumoperitoneum, or may be elicited when an air-filled loop of bowel is located over the liver. Percussion of the liver more than 2 cm below the right costal margin (RCM) indicates hepatomegaly. Percussion of the spleen below the left costal margin (LCM) indicates splenomegaly.

Palpation is used to obtain information regarding abdominal pain and tenderness and data regarding the size, shape, and location of organs and masses. Palpation also is used to detect free fluid. Superficial palpation is performed first, followed by deep palpation. The liver is normally palpable at the RCM or is nonpalpable. The spleen is not normally palpable. Pain is the most common symptom in a patient with an "acute abdomen" (abdominal condition requiring urgent surgical evaluation). Deep palpation may be deferred in these patients and on any patient with a known or suspected abdominal mass because of the risk of rupturing the encapsulated mass.

The presence of rebound tenderness indicates peritoneal inflammation. The technique to elicit rebound tenderness consists of the examiner exerting firm pressure in an area away from the pain and then quickly releasing the pressure. A positive response is an unequivocally painful reaction. This technique is not used routinely with pediatric patients because it is unnecessarily painful for the child and does not reveal any new findings. Most children wince in response only to the change in pressure exerted, and children who have significant disease exhibit a painful reaction simply with light palpation.

Measurement of abdominal girth provides objective data regarding the degree of distension and is included in the assessment of the abdomen. Serial measurements are important to identify subtle changes, particularly in nonverbal children.

Monitoring all GI outputs, including emesis, gastric devices, ostomies, and stool, is essential in determining excessive output and potential electrolyte imbalances. Excessive gastric drainage can cause a metabolic alkalosis resulting from hydrochloric acid losses. Excessive losses from a new ileostomy or diarrhea can cause metabolic acidosis due to sodium bicarbonate losses. The color, character, and consistency of all GI output should be noted; the amount is estimated or measured and included in output calculations. Gastric drainage is tested for pH and blood, and stool is tested for blood. The character and content of emesis and stool are helpful in understanding the underlying disorder. Bilious vomiting is a significant finding, indicative of a proximal mechanical obstruction. Hematemesis indicates an upper GI bleeding site; hematochezia (bright red blood from the rectum) indicates brisk mid-GI or lower GI

tract bleeding. Melena is blood that has been digested during passage through the GI tract. Melanotic stools indicate slow upper or mid-GI tract bleeding.[7] Occult bleeding (heme test positive without visible blood) is the result of chronic blood loss.

Laboratory and Radiologic Assessment

Serial laboratory and diagnostic studies are obtained on all patients with a GI disorder. Table 22-3 summarizes common laboratory tests indicating GI dysfunction. Assessment of liver function includes the measurement of hepatocellular enzymes. The enzymes commonly measured are aspartate aminotransferase (AST), alanine aminotransferase (ALT), and alkaline phosphatase (ALP). Other enzymes that are more specific to liver function but less frequently measured include γ-glutamyltransferase (GGT) and 5'-nucleotidase.

AST is an enzyme found also in the heart, kidney, skeletal muscle, and brain and therefore not specific to liver function. However, the ALT enzyme is found primarily in the liver and is therefore more specific for liver function. It is important to remember that elevations in AST and ALT are seen with hepatocyte dysfunction or failure. Clinical assessment is correlated with diagnostic data to differentiate hepatic from nonhepatic disease. ALP is an enzyme active in the bone, intestine, and liver. An elevation in this enzyme is an indication of decreased biliary functioning or obstruction. The enzyme GGT is found in the hepatic and biliary system and other tissues. It is often assessed with the measurement of ALP to evaluate for biliary tract disease. Like GGT, 5'-nucleotidase is a liver-related enzyme used to investigate the origin of increased serum ALP.

Diagnostic studies include plain abdominal films, nuclear medicine scans, computed tomography (CT), magnetic resonance imaging (MRI), ultrasound, and endoscopy. Indications for these studies are presented in Table 22-4. Plain abdominal films are done in two views to identify air-fluid levels and provide an alternate view in addition to a flat plate x-ray film. Small infants and older children who are critically ill cannot be put in the upright position for a second view and require either a cross-table lateral or left lateral decubitus film. Chest radiographs are also obtained to rule out abnormalities within the thorax, or concurrent disease processes such as right lower lobe pneumonia, or complications of severe GI dysfunction such as pleural effusion. Contrast studies help define GI anatomy, aid in diagnosis (e.g., of gastroesophageal reflux), or are treatment measures, such as in the reduction of an intussusception with a hydrostatic BE. Additional diagnostic studies are warranted for specific disorders and are discussed specifically in the following sections.

GENERAL PRINCIPLES OF MANAGEMENT

In addition to ongoing assessment and monitoring, gastric decompression, intravascular volume replacement and maintenance, and pharmacologic management are general interventions indicated in response to GI pathologic events.

TABLE 22-3 **Indicators of Gastrointestinal Dysfunction**

Test	Pediatric Normal Value	Interpretation
Alanine aminotransferase (ALT)	Infant <54 units/L Child 1-30 units/L	Increases with hepatocellular injury
Aspartate aminotransferase (AST)	Infant 20-65 units/L Child 0-35 units/L	Increases with hepatocellular injury
Alkaline phosphatase (ALP)	Infant 150-420 units/L 2-10 yr 100-320 units/L 11-18 yr 100-390 units/L	Increases with biliary obstruction and cholestatic hepatitis
Lactate dehydrogenase (LDH)	Infant 150-360 units/L Child 150-300 units/L	Increases with rise in alkaline phosphatase
Gamma Glutamyl transferase (GGT)	All ages <120 IU/L	Increases with biliary obstruction and moderately increases with hepatocellular injury
Bilirubin		
Indirect	All ages 0.1-0.3 mg/dl	Increases with hemolysis
Direct	All ages 0.1-1.3 mg/dl	Increases with hepatocellular injury
Total	Infant <2 mg/dl Child 0.2-1.3 mg/dl	Increases with biliary obstruction
Prothrombin (PT)	Infant 10-15.9 sec Child 10.8-13.9 sec	Increases with vitamin K deficiency or hepatocellular injury
Albumin	All ages 3.8-5.4 g/dl	Reduces with hepatocellular injury (also dependent on protein intake)
Ammonia	Infant 29-70 µg/dl Child 0-50 µg/dl	Increases with hepatocellular injury
5′-Nucleotidase	All ages 5-10 units/L	Increases with biliary obstruction or cholestatic hepatitis
Lipase	All ages <200 units/L	Increases with pancreatitis (more sensitive and specific than amylase)
Amylase	Newborns have little amylase activity Children <2 yr have little pancreatic isoamylase >2 yr of age 23-85 units/L	Increases with acute pancreatitis; however, level includes salivary and pancreatic isoenzyme; therefore increase may be due to salivary inflammatory lesion (i.e., mumps)

From Jacobs DS et al, eds: *Laboratory test handbook.* Cleveland, 1996, Lexi-Comp.

Gastric Decompression

Decompression of the GI tract is one of the primary interventions indicated in patients with a GI abnormality. The goal of gastric decompression is to actively remove air and secretions from an injured GI tract. In GI obstruction, which often precedes perforation, there is dilation of the proximal bowel as peristalsis continues against the distal obstruction. In addition, air and secretions collect in the bowel lumen proximal to the obstruction. Decompression is employed either continuously or intermittently to actively remove air and secretions from the upper GI tract.

The preferred position for intubation and gastric decompression in a child is semiupright. An NG or orogastric (OG) tube is inserted into the stomach via the esophagus. The oral route may be preferred for young infants who are obligate nose-breathers. For the purpose of decompression, the largest possible double-lumen vented tube is used, such as the Salem sump tube or a Replogle tube, for neonates. Such tubes have a primary lumen to remove air and secretions; the other lumen serves as an air vent to keep the primary lumen from adhering to the stomach wall when suction is applied. It is important to note that the air vent lumen is not clamped off, and clogging with secretions needs to be prevented. A slight hissing sound signals that the tube is functioning properly. Patency may be maintained by instilling 5 to 30 ml of air (depending on the size of the child) into the air vent. The primary lumen can also be irrigated with saline. The child maintains a nothing-by-mouth (NPO) status, and excessive swallowing of air is discouraged.

Repositioning the tube, as well as irrigating as described earlier, may be indicated if there is doubt about the adequacy of gastric decompression. If inadequate, abdominal distension and diaphragmatic elevation can develop, which then compromise both respiratory and GI function. In addition to decompressing the GI tract, NG and OG tubes are used for gastric lavage, the administration of various medications, including antacids to prevent stress ulcer syndrome, and collection and analysis of gastric aspirate.

TABLE 22-4 Diagnostic Studies for Gastrointestinal Disorders

Procedure	Purpose/Comments	Examples of Abnormalities
X-ray Examination		
Abdominal flat plate Abdominal cross table Decubitus	Evaluate organ size, position, gas patterns (intraluminal and extraluminal), air/fluid levels	Pneumatosis intestinalis (air in bowel wall), TEF, small bowel obstruction, perforation, ileus, ascites
Fluoroscopy		
Barium swallow	Examine the esophagus and mucosal integrity; diagnose structural abnormalities	Malrotation, esophageal or small bowel strictures
Upper GI series	Examine the esophagus, stomach, and duodenum, diagnose structural abnormalities, motor disorders, delayed gastric emptying	Gastroesophageal reflux (GER), malrotation, volvulus, ulcerative disease
Upper GI with small bowel follow-through	Same as upper GI with follow-up spot films of esophagus, stomach, duodenum, and small intestines; diagnose small bowel abnormalities	Inflammatory disease (Crohn's and ulcerative colitis)
Barium enema	Examine the large intestine and mucosal integrity; diagnose structural abnormalities	Intussusception, Hirschsprung's disease, meconium ileus
Endoscopy		
Flexible upper endoscopy (esophagoscopy, gastroscopy, duodenoscopy)	Directly visualize the upper GI mucosa, diagnose mucosal injury, lesions, structural abnormalities, or source of GI bleeding	Esophageal varices, severe gastritis
Endoscopic retrograde cholangiopancreatography (ERCP)	Directly visualize the biliary pancreatic ducts	Pseudocyst, chronic pancreatitis, stones
Flexible sigmoidoscopy or colonoscopy	Directly visualize mucosa of large intestine, diagnose mucosal injury or source of lower GI bleeding	
Biopsy		
Percutaneous liver biopsy	Obtain liver specimen without laparotomy	Biliary atresia, hepatitis (when etiology and/or outcome uncertain)
Nuclear Scans		
Gastroesophageal scintigraphy (gastric emptying study)	Determine delayed gastric emptying (defined as 50% of isotope meal retained in stomach after 90 min in absence of obstruction)	GER
Liver-spleen	Determine liver and spleen size or presence of mass, abscess, or other abnormality (does not evaluate liver function)	
Hepatobiliary excretion scan (HIDA)	Determine liver excretory function	Biliary atresia
Meckel scan	Evaluate location of bleeding (radioactive isotope is taken up by gastric mucosal parietal cells)	Meckel's diverticulum
Other Imaging		
Magnetic resonance imaging (MRI)	Definitively image abdominal organs (deferred in hemodynamically unstable child)	Hepatic hemangioma (i.e., Kasabach-Merritt syndrome), hepatic arteriovenous malformation
Abdominal ultrasound	Visualize organ structure, diagnose tissue abnormalities rapidly and without patient transport	Hepatocellular disease, acute pancreatitis, hepatic arteriovenous malformation
Abdominal computerized tomography (CT) scan with contrast	Evaluate for vascular problems, definitive imaging of solid organs, evaluate for infection/abscesses, trauma	Pancreatitis, pseudocyst, hepatocellular disease

Intravascular Volume Replacement and Maintenance

Fluid administration takes into account insensible losses (supplied by maintenance fluids), estimated third-space losses, and measured losses, which include NG and OG tube secretions, ongoing GI bleeding, ostomy and fistula drainage, diarrhea, or losses from other tubes or drains and wounds.[8] Measured losses are calculated and replaced at specified intervals. Table 22-5 outlines electrolyte content of GI secretions and comparable intravenous (IV) replacement fluids.

If hypovolemia is severe, fluid resuscitation may be required to correct hypovolemia and maintain a urine output of 1 to 2 ml/kg/hour. As fluid returns to the intravascular space, fluid retention or overload can occur and the administration of diuretics may be indicated to aid in the excretion of excess fluid. Meticulous monitoring of intake and output is mandatory for these patients, as is ongoing assessment for signs and symptoms of fluid volume deficit or excess.

Pharmacologic Management

In most cases of actual or potential GI dysfunction, a variety of pharmacologic agents are employed. These agents are used to treat infection, excessive gastric acid secretion, and GI bleeding. Pharmacologic agents include antimicrobials to treat intraabdominal infection; histamine-receptor (H_2) antagonists and antacids to decrease and neutralize gastric acid secretion; and vasoconstrictive and sclerosing agents to decrease bleeding. The use of these medications are described in the following sections conjunction with treatment for specific clinical conditions.

GASTROINTESTINAL OBSTRUCTION

True GI obstructions occur most commonly in the newborn. Obstructions may be present in any portion of the gut from the esophagus to the anus and are related to a variety of causes (Table 22-6). The initial presentation, clinical findings, and patient management vary, depending on the type and location of the obstruction. A maternal history of polyhydramnios may indicate a proximal obstruction (i.e., esophageal atresia) because the fetus is unable to properly digest amnionic fluid. Small bowel obstruction commonly presents with bilious emesis and abdominal distension. Failure to pass a meconium stool in the first 24 hours of life is suggestive of a distal obstruction (i.e., Hirschsprung's disease). The pathophysiology of obstruction is depicted in Fig. 22-2.

Esophageal Atresia

Esophageal atresia is a congenital anomaly in which the esophagus is segmented with a blind pouch separating the upper and lower portion. In most instances, there is also a fistula connecting the distal esophagus and trachea. However, the use of the term "tracheoesophageal fistula" (TEF) to describe all anomalies of the esophagus is incorrect. There are several described types of tracheoesophageal deformities. The three main types (Fig. 22-3) include esophageal atresia with distal TEF, isolated esophageal atresia, and TEF without esophageal atresia (H-type). The most common is esophageal atresia with distal TEF, occurring in 85% of all cases.[9]

Pathogenesis. The esophagus and trachea develop embryologically at the same time. These structures are first

TABLE 22-5 Solution for Replacing Losses of Gastric Secretions

	Gastric Secretion (mEq/L)	Replacement Fluid D5%, 0.45 NS + 30 mEq/KCl/L
Sodium	60-75	77
Chloride	105-130	107
Potassium	5-30	30
H^+	0-65	0

From Filston HC: Fluid and electrolyte management in the pediatric surgical patient, *Surg Clin North Am* 72:1189-1205, 1992.

TABLE 22-6 Causes of Intestinal Obstruction

Mechanical Obstruction		Paralytic Ileus	
Intraluminal	**Extrinsic**	**Abdominal Conditions**	**Systemic Conditions**
Atresia or stenosis	Malrotation	Hirschsprung's disease	Trauma
Pyloric stenosis	Volvulus	Intestinal pseudoobstruction	Shock
Foreign body	Hernia	Severe gastroenteritis	Sepsis
Meconium	Annular pancreas	Perforation of viscus	Hypokalemia
Medications	Duplication cysts	Peritonitis	Drugs
Cholestyramine	Adhesions/bands	Pancreatitis	Diabetic acidosis
Antacid	Tumor	Necrotizing enterocolitis	General anesthesia
Kaolin	Granulomatous process	Toxic megacolon	Intussusception
Parasitic infection			

From Quan R: Bowel failure. In Levin DL, Morriss FC, eds: *Essentials of pediatric intensive care,* St Louis, 1990, Quality Medical Publishing.

recognized as a ventral diverticulum of the foregut at 22 to 23 days after fertilization.[9] The development of the esophagus and trachea is believed to occur by the proliferation of endodermal cells on the lateral walls of the diverticulum. Rosenthal theorized that these cell masses become ridges of tissue that divide the foregut into two separate channels, forming the esophagus and trachea.[10] This process is completed by 36 days after fertilization. During the fourth week of fetal life, interruptions in development may result in abnormalities of the esophagus with and without fistula formation between the two structures.

Associated Anomalies.   Deformities of the esophagus and trachea occur early in intrauterine development along with generalized organ differentiation and division. Mesodermal maldevelopment caused by some unknown intrauterine event is believed to be the cause for multisystem problems seen in many of these newborns. The majority of these defects are grouped under the name VACTERL (*V*-vertebral, *A*-anal, *C*-cardiac, *TE*-tracheoesophageal, *R*-renal, *L*-limb). Most series report the incidence of associated anomalies with esophageal atresia–TEF deformities to be between 30% and 55%. Cardiovascular disease is the most common associated anomaly, followed by limb and genitourinary defects.[11,12]

Clinical Presentation.   As with other causes of proximal obstruction, a maternal history of polyhydramnios is common. The infant typically presents with bubbly oral secretions and regurgitation of saliva, which cannot be swallowed because of the blind proximal esophageal pouch. Most babies with isolated esophageal atresia or esophageal atresia with TEF present with this problem soon after delivery. The diagnosis is made by careful placement of an NG tube into the blind pouch. A simple chest radiograph subsequently reveals a curled tube in the proximal esophageal pouch. With esophageal atresia and distal TEF, an abdominal film typically reveals a distended stomach with gas patterns throughout the small bowel. However, in the infant with isolated esophageal atresia, the abdominal film shows a gasless bowel pattern.

An infant with an H-type TEF usually presents at 3 to 4 months of age with a history of respiratory distress, pneumonia, and some degree of cyanosis with feedings. Direct bronchoscopic visualization is the diagnostic study of choice. The tracheal end of the fistula can usually be visualized through the membranous portion of the trachea.[9] Occasionally, a barium or water-soluble esophogram may be used for diagnosis, but often this does not demonstrate the fistula, and aspiration of the contrast material is a concern.

Critical Care Management.   Once a diagnosis of esophageal atresia with or without TEF is made, preoperative stabilization of the newborn is essential. Decompression of the proximal pouch is of utmost importance in the

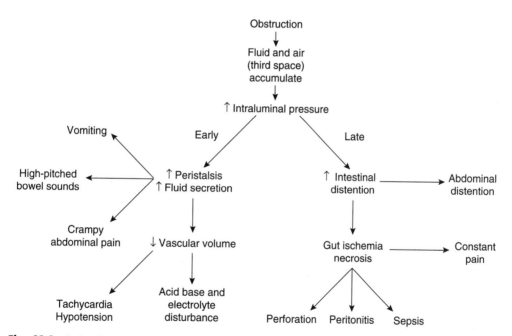

Fig. 22-2   Pathophysiology of intestinal obstruction. (From Quan R: Bowel failure. In DL Levin, FC Morris, eds: *Essentials of pediatric intensive care,* St Louis, 1990, Quality Medical Publishing.)

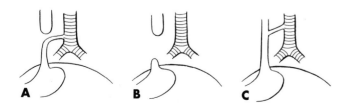

Fig. 22-3   Three forms of esophageal anomalies. **A** is the most common form of esophageal malformation; **B** is the next most common form; **C** is the classic "H" type fistula. (From Avery ME et al: *The lung and its disorders in the newborn infant,* ed 4, Philadelphia, 1981, WB Saunders.)

preoperative phase. This is accomplished using the general principles of gastric decompression described earlier, except that the Replogle tube is placed in the proximal esophageal pouch, thereby removing oral secretions and preventing pulmonary aspiration.

Operative Management for Esophageal Atresia With Distal TEF. Primary repair is the best surgical option and may be performed even in the small preterm infant.[13,14] The operative approach is through a right thoracotomy incision in which the fistula is first divided, and then the two segments of the esophagus are anastomosed.

Operative Management for Isolated Esophageal Atresia. In most cases of isolated esophageal atresia, there is a long gap between the proximal and distal segments of the esophagus, which precludes primary repair in the newborn period. For a full-term baby with no other abnormalities, usually only a feeding gastrostomy is placed. Over the next several months of life, it is believed that the esophageal segment will elongate spontaneously.[11] During this waiting period, the surgeon may choose to manually stretch the upper and lower segments of the esophagus.

The second stage of surgical intervention typically occurs when the chest x-ray film reveals overlapping of the esophageal segments (or less than a vertebral body apart). At this time, a primary end-to-end anastomosis of the esophagus is attempted. If for some reason the segments do not come together easily, a circular or spiral myotomy of the upper esophagus is performed. This procedure usually provides 1 to 2 mm of extra length by dividing the outer layer of the esophagus.

Conversely, for the sick preterm infant, this delayed type of primary closure may not be optimal. There also may be some infants in whom the gap between the esophageal segments is so wide that primary repair is impossible. In either of these cases, a cervical esophagostomy (exteriorizing the blind upper esophageal pouch in the neck region) and gastrostomy are performed in the newborn period. When the child reaches a weight of approximately 10 kg, an esophageal replacement procedure is performed using a piece of colon, small bowel, or stomach.

Operative Management of TEF. The operative approach to an isolated TEF is through a right thoracotomy or a right cervical incision. The fistula is divided primarily. Surgical complications are rare.

Postoperative Management. After esophageal atresia repair with or without TEF, the infant may require ventilatory support. The infant may require paralysis and prolonged mechanical ventilation if there is concern that the anastomosis is under tension. After extubation, if the child again requires assisted ventilation, the surgeon must be present to make sure the intubation does not interrupt the anastomosis. Oropharyngeal or nasopharyngeal suctioning is performed with a suction catheter that is measured and marked at the time of surgery to avoid the anastomosis site during the suctioning procedure.

An extrapleural chest tube and drain are placed at the time of surgery; an assessment of the color and consistency of the drainage is important. The presence of mucous in the collecting chamber may indicate a leak at the site of anastomosis.

Gastric decompression remains essential in the postoperative period. This can be accomplished with either an NG tube or a gastrostomy tube. If the surgeon has placed an NG tube, it is important to remember that it passes through the esophageal anastomosis. It is critical not to accidentally remove or replace the tube in the immediate postoperative period. Passage of saliva through the tube indicates that the infant is able to swallow and that the esophagus is patent.

Enteral alimentation may begin on the third to fourth postoperative day via the NG or gastrostomy tube. Care is taken not to overdistend the stomach or allow the feeding to back up into the esophagus. This may be accomplished by using a Y-connector attached to the NG or gastrostomy tube, allowing the stomach to be vented at the same time the feeding is delivered.

An esophagram is performed within 1 week postoperatively to evaluate the esophageal anastomosis. A leak is present in about 50% of cases; however, most are asymptomatic and seen only on the esophagram.[15] Infants with a significant anastomotic leak will have signs and symptoms of respiratory distress and may require intubation. If no leak is noted, the chest tube is removed and the baby may be allowed to attempt full nutrition by mouth. Successful transition to oral feedings usually takes several days to accomplish.

Stricture (narrowing at the anastomosis site) formation is common after repair of esophageal atresia with or without TEF.[16] Clinical symptoms include coughing, vomiting, and failure to gain weight. Diagnosis is confirmed with an esophagram. Infants commonly require several dilations to relieve the stricture.[16] Gastroesophageal reflux (GER) is a significant postoperative complication, with 20% of cases requiring antireflux surgery.[17] Tracheomalacia (collapsible trachea) is another common problem, which is thought to be due to an enlarged upper esophageal pouch or to inadequately formed or missing cartilage.[18] These infants may present to the pediatric intensive care unit (PICU) with a history of a chronic "barky" cough and respiratory distress, which has been exacerbated by a respiratory infection and potentially causing respiratory failure.

Duodenal Obstruction

Complete or partial duodenal obstruction may occur for a number of reasons. Atresia, stenosis, annular pancreas, and nonrotation or malrotation are the most common causes of duodenal obstruction. Each of these anomalies has unique characteristics that are important for optimal management.

Pathogenesis. During the fifth to sixth week of intrauterine development there is a rapid growth of the epithelial lining of the duodenum. However, the cross-section of the gut cannot accommodate this growth, which obliterates the duodenal lumen. By the eighth to tenth week of gestation, recanalization of the duodenal lumen occurs. The absence of this recanalization process causes duodenal atresia, stenosis, or intrinsic web formation.[19,20]

Atresia results in complete obstruction of the duodenal lumen by an intrinsic duodenal membrane made up of mucosa or submucosa. This maldevelopment may result in the formation of two blind ends of the duodenum connected by a short fibrous cord with an intact mesentery; or two blind ends with no fibrous cord and a V-shaped defect in the mesentery separating the two pieces of the duodenum (Fig. 22-4, *A*).

Duodenal stenosis is a partial obstruction of the lumen of the intestine. An intrinsic web or diaphragm can cause a partial obstruction. The child who has duodenal stenosis may not become symptomatic until well beyond the neonatal period.[21]

A congenital annular pancreas can create a situation of either atresia or stenosis, depending on the degree of pancreatic compression on the duodenum. The embryologic development of the pancreas occurs simultaneously with duodenal recanalization. The dorsal pancreas arises from the dorsal wall of the duodenum, and the ventral pancreas develops from the region between the duodenum and the hepatic diverticulum. As normal gut rotation occurs, the ventral pancreas grows around the right side of the duodenum until it meets with the dorsal pancreatic bud. An annular pancreas occurs when the tip of the ventral pancreas becomes fixed to the duodenal wall and during rotation

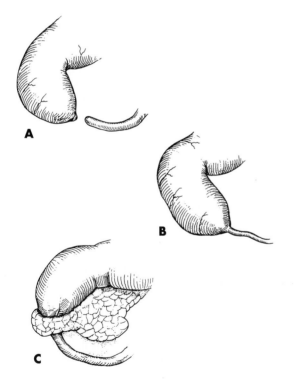

Fig. 22-4   Various types of duodenal atresia-stenosis. **A,** Complete duodenal atresia with discontinuity in the muscular wall of the bowel. **B,** Seromuscular layers may be in continuity with the atresia as represented by a complete membrane. **C,** An annular pancreas, which may create either atresia or stenosis depending on the degree of pancreatic compression on the duodenum. (From Ashcraft KW: *Atlas of pediatric surgery,* Philadelphia, 1994, WB Saunders.)

wraps around the right side of the duodenum to fuse with the dorsal pancreas.[22] The intestinal compression from the pancreatic wrap causes the obstruction, as small segments of pancreatic tissue partially or completely encircle the second portion of the duodenum (Fig. 22-4, *B*).

Another critical aspect of duodenal embryology is related to the positioning and fixation of the small bowel that may result in nonrotation or malrotation. Obstruction can occur when rotation and fixation do not occur correctly during fetal development. During the fourth week of gestation, the intestinal tract is elongating too rapidly for the abdominal cavity to accommodate its growth. The intestinal tract grows out of the abdomen into the umbilical cord. As the midgut begins to return to the abdomen at about 8 weeks' gestation, it rotates in a counterclockwise fashion around the superior mesentery artery. This rotation should be completed by the twelfth week. Fixation of the intestine inside the abdomen with the ligament of Treitz settling in the left upper quadrant and the cecum in the right lower quadrant should follow this rotation. When rotation and fixation do not occur or are incomplete, bowel obstruction as well as superior mesenteric artery (SMA) occlusion may ensue with resultant ischemia and volvulus (Fig. 22-5, *A, B, C*).

Associated Anomalies.   Diaphragmatic hernia and abdominal wall defects are associated anomalies thought to occur because development of the diaphragm and abdominal wall is related to the return of the small bowel into the abdominal cavity.[23] For example, if the pleuroperitoneal membranes have not closed completely before the gut reenters the abdominal cavity, the bowel is likely to pass through that opening and fill the space in the chest, resulting in a congenital diaphragmatic hernia. Omphalocele occurs when the bowel does not completely return to the abdominal cavity. Malrotation is always present with these defects.

Down's syndrome is found in 30% of infants born with duodenal obstruction.[19] The reason for this association is not known. Abnormalities of intestinal rotation are also associated with heterotaxia, an abnormal arrangement of body organs.[24] GI anomalies associated with heterotaxia include a midline liver, malpositioned stomach, and intestinal malrotation. In addition, major cardiac defects and asplenia or polysplenia are common.

Clinical Presentation.   A newborn with duodenal obstruction initially appears healthy, but quickly becomes symptomatic. An exception to this is the infant with an in-utero volvulus who presents with massive abdominal distension, respiratory distress, acidosis, and sepsis. A maternal history of polyhydramnios can alert the caregiver that an obstruction may be present. The infant with intestinal atresia or stenosis usually develops bilious vomiting within the first few days of life. Proximal small bowel obstructions result in earlier and more forceful vomiting, whereas abdominal distension is more pronounced with distal small bowel obstructions. Dehydration and signs of shock occur with delay in diagnosis. With pure duodenal atresia, the abdominal film usually reveals the classic "double-bubble" sign, in which the stomach and the first portion of the

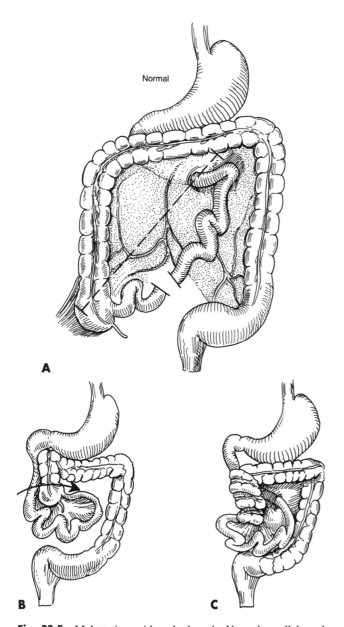

Fig. 22-5 Malrotation with volvulus. **A,** Normal small bowel mesenteric attachment (as demonstrated by line). This prevents twisting of the small bowel because of the broad fixation of the mesentery. **B,** Malrotation of the bowel with the cecum overlying the duodenum. **C,** Midgut volvulus around superior mesenteric artery caused by the narrow base of mesentery. (From Ross AJ III: Malrotation of the intestine. In PF Nora, ed: *Operative surgery,* ed 3, Philadelphia, 1990, WB Saunders.)

duodenum are dilated, and distal bowel gas is absent. This type of dilation can also be present with intestinal stenosis, but there is usually some air below the area of dilation. If air is seen below the double-bubble, a contrast upper GI is performed to rule out malrotation and volvulus.[18]

Critical Care Management. Surgical correction of most duodenal obstructions is accomplished by a duodeno-duodenostomy. Duodenoduodenostomy consists of excision of the atretic portion of the bowel and connection of duodenum to duodenum. In rare situations, to avoid atretic

bowel, duodenojejunostomy is performed, connecting duodenum to jejunum, leaving a portion of the duodenum connected to the pancreas with the ability to drain bile. An intrinsic duodenal web is repaired with duodenoplasty, excision of the web, and closure of the lumen of the bowel. Stabilization of infants with malrotation and volvulus by gastric decompression, airway stabilization, and fluid resuscitation must occur quickly with subsequent transport to the operating room. The twisting of the intestinal contents results in partial or complete occlusion of the superior mesenteric artery (SMA) and can rapidly cause ischemia if untreated. The Ladd's procedure, as described by Ladd and Gross, is required for correction of malrotation and volvulus.[25] The intestines are untwisted, assessed for viability, and resected in areas of necrosis or perforation. Occasionally the entire small bowel is necrotic, making chances of the infant's survival grim. Once a full assessment of the bowel is made, the Ladd's peritoneal bands are divided and the duodenum is mobilized and placed along the right side of the abdomen. An appendectomy is performed and the cecum and colon are placed on the left side. The appendix is removed to avoid a later misdiagnosis because the appendix is now located on the left rather than the right side. This type of abdominal placement allows for a broad base of mesentery, which prevents further volvulus.

Adequate decompression of the GI tract is the first goal of postoperative management. Placement of a gastrostomy tube for long-term decompression until bowel patency is demonstrated is somewhat controversial. Some surgeons believe this type of tube is essential, particularly in the preterm infant, whereas others favor decompression with an NG tube.[26] Decompression is required until the upper GI tract drainage decreases, the drainage changes in color from green to clear, and the baby begins to produce stool.

Adequate nutritional support can be provided with operative placement of a transanastomotic feeding tube for early enteral feedings with an elemental infant formula. Peripheral or central total parenteral nutrition (TPN) is a temporary alternative to enteral nutrition with the initiation of feedings as soon as is possible.

Jejunoileal Obstruction

Atresia of the jejunum or ileum is a complete congenital obstruction of the intestinal lumen at either location. Stenosis of the jejunum or ileum is very rare and will not be discussed.

Meconium ileus is one of the most common causes of obstruction in the small bowel and in the newborn is the earliest manifestation of cystic fibrosis.[27] Meconium ileus occurs when inspissated meconium becomes lodged in the small bowel, usually in the ileum, and complete obstruction occurs because of the tenacity of the meconium. The viscous nature of the meconium is usually caused by abnormal intestinal secretions and by pancreatic insufficiency related to cystic fibrosis.[27] There are two types of meconium ileus. Simple ileus exists when there is an obstruction in the ileum with dilated proximal bowel and microcolon below the obstruction. Complicated ileus results in the same obstruction and intestinal findings, plus volvulus, necrosis, and perforation.

Pathogenesis. Defects in the arteriomesenteric structure are thought to be primarily responsible for jejunoileal atresias. Atresia formation usually occurs early in gestation when a cordlike band separates the two ends of the bowel or when there is a total separation of the bowel resulting from a V-shaped deformity in the mesentery. This type of mesenteric vascular catastrophe, causing disruption of the bowel, can occur late in intrauterine life.[19]

Associated Anomalies. The relationship between meconium ileus and cystic fibrosis has been well established. There are no other consistent abnormalities seen in infants with jejunoileal atresia.[28] Rare reports of trisomy 21 have been associated with these atresias.

Clinical Presentation. An infant with jejunoileal atresia usually presents with bilious vomiting and abdominal distension within the first few days of life. A maternal history of polyhydramnios or amniotic bile staining may be present. Passage of meconium may or may not occur, depending on the level and extent of the obstruction.[20]

The clinical presentation of meconium ileus is similar to that of ileal atresia. An abdominal radiograph will reveal distended loops of bowel, and the mixture of abnormal meconium and air bubbles gives the intestines a ground-glass appearance.[27] A water-soluble contrast enema is the best diagnostic study and may be therapeutic in relieving the obstruction.

Critical Care Management. Infants with meconium ileus not complicated by peritonitis, bowel perforation, pseudocyst, or atresia may be treated nonoperatively with the use of a high hyperosmolar enema. Therefore it is essential that complications of meconium ileus be ruled out before performing the procedure. Bowel ischemia or peritonitis should be suspected in infants presenting with tenderness, rigidity, edema, or erythema of the abdominal wall. Fluid resuscitation must be initiated and hemodynamic stability achieved before transport to the operating room.

In simple meconium ileus, the hyperosmolar enema used for treatment usually employs gastrografin, a water-soluble contrast solution. The infant must receive intravenous fluids at twice maintenance to compensate for fluid drawn into the bowel lumen as a result of the hyperosmolar solution. The enema is administered with fluoroscopic guidance to prevent complications, especially perforation. With successful treatment, the infant passes a large amount of semisolid meconium for the next 24 to 48 hours. Failure to pass this meconium or progressive distension is an indication for operation.[27]

Surgical Management. Jejunal and ileal atresias are usually managed with end-to-end bowel anastomosis. The difficulty of the operative procedure is the result of the disparity in the size of the proximal dilated bowel and the small distal segment. The massively dilated segment is usually resected and the anastomosis is done in an oblique fashion to provide a wider opening.

Surgical repair of meconium ileus involves an enterostomy in the dilated segment of the ileum. The meconium is carefully expressed out of the proximal and distal segments,

using saline or *N*-acetylcysteine (Mucomyst) as irrigants to help liquefy the meconium. In rare cases, when complete removal of the meconium plug is possible, primary anastomosis is performed with a bowel that appears healthy. Residual thick meconium usually remains, requiring an ileostomy to vent the bowel. The technique of ileostomy formation with meconium ileus is a Bishop-Koop anastomosis, in which the end of the proximal bowel is anastomosed to the side of the distal segment, leaving the end of the distal area as a stoma. This vents the bowel but also allows for installation of *N*-acetylcysteine or other irrigants to flush out additional meconium or stool if needed. Because the normal fecal stream can continue with this operation, it is the procedure of choice for most surgeons.[29]

Postoperative Management. The postoperative infant requires an NG tube for proximal decompression, respiratory support as needed, fluid and electrolyte replacement, and antibiotics. Close monitoring of temperature, other vital signs, and urine output is essential. Abdominal distension, vomiting, evidence of peritonitis, and a pneumoperitoneum present for more than 24 hours after surgery suggests an anastomotic lead and requires immediate reexploration. The infant remains NPO and should receive parenteral nutrition until normal GI function returns; however, the more proximal the obstruction, the longer the period of postoperative intestinal dysfunction. Enteral alimentation usually begins with a predigested formula. The patient is observed closely for signs of malabsorption, such as increased gastric residuals, diarrhea, bloody stools, and presence of fecal-reducing substances.

If an ileostomy is present, *N*-acetylcysteine may be instilled into the stoma to evacuate fecal contents from the distal bowel. Initially, most of the stool is expelled through the ileostomy, but with time, the infant will have more output through the rectum. Once the meconium is cleared, an elemental enteral diet is started. Pancreatic enzymes are added when full-strength formula is begun, even if a firm diagnosis of cystic fibrosis has not yet been established. A complete cystic fibrosis workup is part of the postoperative management of any child with meconium ileus.

Intussusception

Intussusception is the telescoping or invagination of proximal bowel into distal bowel. It can be classified as idiopathic, associated with a specific lead point, postoperative, or chronic. The majority of cases are idiopathic, wherein the intussusception occurs at or near the ileocecal valve. Only approximately 5% of the cases have a specific lead point.[23] The most common lead point is a Meckel's diverticulum, followed by polyps, duplications, tumors, hemangiomas, and sutures lines or an appendiceal stump. Postoperative intussusception occurs within 2 weeks of a surgical procedure. It occurs most often in cases of intraabdominal or retroperitoneal procedures, although it has also been reported after thoracic and other procedures.[30] Intussusception is described as chronic when symptoms occur for 14 or more days and are less severe. This usually occurs in older children.[31] Patients with cystic fibrosis are prone to intussusception, and repeated reductions may be required.

The exact etiology of idiopathic intussusception is unknown. Possible causes include hypertrophied Peyer's patch (lymphoid tissue in the distal ileum), a localized area of hyperperistalsis, or viral gastroenteritis, with rotavirus and adenovirus being cited.[32-34] Older children with intussusception are usually found to have an anatomic abnormality, which is the associated lead point. Other types of lead points include the thick, inspissated fecal material seen in children with cystic fibrosis, or submucosal hemorrhage, exhibited in children with hemophilia and Henoch-Schönlein purpura.[35]

Pathogenesis.   When proximal bowel telescopes into distal bowel, it pulls the mesentery along with it (Fig. 22-6). The neck of the intussuscepted segment compresses the entrapped bowel. This compression, plus the traction on the mesentery, causes lymphatic and mesenteric venous obstruction, which eventually results in necrosis and gangrene of the entrapped bowel and subsequent perforation if treatment is delayed. Bowel dilation occurs proximal to the intussusception.

Clinical Presentation.   Typical presentation of intussusception is in an infant between 4 and 10 months of age, with a history of vomiting and acute, intermittent crampy abdominal pain. The child may stiffen and pull the legs up to the chest during the attacks. Initially, the child may appear normal between the episodes but becomes increasingly lethargic. Late in the course, the stools become blood tinged and progress to dark red mucoid clots or "currant jelly" stools. In some children, altered level of consciousness is the initial symptom, before GI signs or symptoms. In such cases, the differential diagnosis includes a postictal state and meningitis.[36] Occasionally, a sausage-shaped mass will be felt in the mid or upper abdomen. If symptoms persist longer than 6 to 12 hours, plain abdominal films will reveal an obstruction, which includes distended bowel loops and air-fluid levels. Abdominal ultrasound may be helpful in the workup of intussusception before BE. A positive or equivocal ultrasound identifies patients who should undergo BE for definitive treatment.[37]

In cases of postoperative intussusception, the presentation is not as straightforward. The child may appear to be doing well in the first few days postoperatively, then develops vomiting or increased NG aspirate, which may be attributed to a paralytic ileus. Plain abdominal films, however, reveal an obstruction, with dilated loops of bowel and air-fluid levels.

Critical Care Management.   Initial management includes NG decompression, intravenous fluid resuscitation, and intravenous antibiotics if symptoms have been present longer than 24 hours or there is evidence of fever and leukocytosis. The child is then adequately sedated before the BE is performed, which serves as a diagnostic as well as treatment measure. The air enema is gaining popularity because it has been shown to be as effective as barium in reducing the intussusception and is safer in the event of perforation during the procedure.[38] One to three attempts at hydrostatic reduction of the intussusception by controlled BE are made, with the operating room team on standby for surgical reduction if necessary. In idiopathic intussusception, BE reduction is successful in 65% to 75% of patients.[35] In cases in which there is a specific lead point, BE is less successful and surgical reduction is necessary. In children 6 years of age or older, where tumors (chiefly lymphosarcoma) and other abnormalities serve as a lead point, a BE may not be performed.

In patients who have had prolonged symptoms, bloody stools, severe distension and tenderness, and signs of shock, surgical intervention is warranted, after fluid resuscitation, gastric decompression, and antibiotic therapy. BE is not indicated in patients with postoperative intussusception because the site is high in the ileum or the jejunum. Most cases undergo successful manual reduction in the operating room.

Surgical reduction includes making a transverse right upper quadrant (RUQ) incision and then the surgeon "milks" the intussusception with his or her fingers, without applying traction on the bowel. The bowel is then examined for areas of necrosis or gangrene, perforations, and any abnormalities that could have served as a lead point. Resection is indicated if the intussusception is not reducible, if there is nonviable bowel, if there are any perforations, or if there is a specific lead point. An end-to-end anastomosis is performed in most cases. An appendectomy may be done.

Postoperative complications are rare and are related to the underlying pathology. The incidence of recurrence after surgical reduction is 0% to 3%.[38] Recurrent intussusception requires surgical reduction.

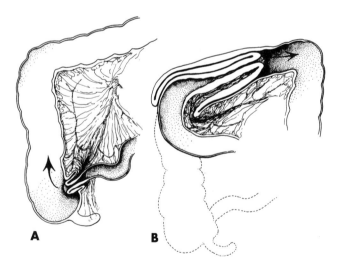

Fig. 22-6   Ileocolic intussusception. **A,** Beginning of an intussusception in which terminal ileum prolapses through the ileocecal valve. **B,** Ileocolic intussusception continuing through colon. This can be palpated as a mass in the right upper quadrant. (From Schnauffer LS, Marboubi S: Abdominal emergencies. In GR Fleischer, S Ludwig, eds: *Pediatric emergency medicine*, Baltimore, 1988, Williams & Wilkins.)

Toxic Megacolon

Pathogenesis.   Toxic megacolon is severe dilation of the colon. It is the most serious complication of ulcerative colitis, occurring in up to 5% of all patients with ulcerative colitis.[39] It is relatively rare in the pediatric population, however, it represents a medical and potentially surgical emergency.

Clinical Presentation. The clinical presentation of toxic megacolon consists of abdominal distension, abdominal tenderness, fever, signs of dehydration (secondary to third spacing), and electrolyte disturbances. High-dose steroid therapy, associated with treatment of ulcerative colitis, may mask some of the signs of toxic megacolon, specifically fever and abdominal tenderness. The child with toxic megacolon is at risk for colonic perforation, gram-negative sepsis, and massive hemorrhage. Diagnosis is made by clinical examination and confirming abdominal radiographs. Improper diagnosis or delays in treatment can lead to rapid clinical deterioration.[39]

Critical Care Management. Once the diagnosis of toxic megacolon is made, careful monitoring with serial radiographs of the abdomen and physical examinations are important. Gastric decompression is accomplished via an NG tube or, if necessary, a small bowel tube. The patient is NPO and parenteral nutrition is initiated. If aggressive medical management fails and the toxic megacolon persists longer than 48 hours, or if perforation and hemorrhage develop, surgical intervention and colectomy are necessary.[40]

GASTROINTESTINAL INFLAMMATION

Inflammation can occur anywhere along the GI tract or on the surface of the peritoneum and occurs with varying levels of severity. For example, a child may exhibit mild esophagitis as a result of GER or present with septic shock resulting from an intestinal perforation and resultant peritonitis. GI inflammation, seen in critically ill infants and children, results from GER, inflammatory bowel disease (ulcerative colitis or Crohn's disease), peritonitis, necrotizing enterocolitis (NEC), and pancreatitis.

Gastroesophageal Reflux

Pathogenesis. GER is the return of stomach contents into the esophagus as a result of incompetence of the lower esophageal sphincter (LES). It has been estimated that GER occurs in 1 in 500 live births and is one of the most common symptomatic clinical disorders affecting the GI tract in children.[41]

Clinical Presentation. The major features of the syndrome are effortless vomiting, failure to gain weight, and aspiration pneumonia. GER may exist without obvious vomiting, and may produce such complications as protein-losing enteropathy, neuropsychiatric syndromes, and apnea.

Half of all infants vomit or spit up at some time during the first 2 years of life, with only 5% having a significant underlying cause.[41] Most children with GER present by 6 weeks of age with symptoms of vomiting or failure to thrive, and outgrow the syndrome by approximately 18 months of age. The greatest improvement occurs at about 8 to 10 months of age when the child sits upright. Fifty percent of children with GER require medical evaluation and therapy

of some degree.[42] Symptoms that lead to a differential diagnosis of GER are presented in Box 22-2.

Critical Care Management. In a child with uncomplicated GER, the self-limiting factor of the disease may preclude the need for medical therapy. Traditional noninvasive therapy consists of three elements: upright positioning, thickened feedings, and frequent feeding. Positioning at a 45 to 60 degree angle in an infant seat or car seat has been standard procedure for many years, but poor truncal tone makes the seated, upright position detrimental because of increased abdominal pressure. Placing a child prone with the head of the crib elevated has been recommended. However, a large controlled study failed to show a significant benefit of head elevation when compared with prone flat positioning.[43] In addition to decreasing reflux, prone positioning improves gastric emptying, decreases aspiration, and decreases energy expenditure.[44] The right-side-down lateral position, although theoretically advantageous, has not been definitively compared with prone positioning. The American Academy of Pediatrics recommends that normal infants be placed supine or side-lying for sleep to minimize the risk of sudden infant death syndrome (SIDS), but specifically exempts infants with GER.[45]

Thickened feedings may be of benefit when significant emesis and poor weight gain are associated with GER. This

Box 22-2
Differential Diagnosis of Reflux Symptoms

Regurgitation, Vomiting
Pain, Esophagitis Symptoms

Cardiac pain
Pulmonary or mediastinal pain; chest wall pain (e.g., costrochondritis)
Nonesophagitis upper gastrointestinal inflammation (e.g., peptic ulcer disease)
Nonesophagitis dysphagia
Many possible causes of nonspecific irritability in infants
Functional; malingering

Respiratory Symptoms (Wheeze, Stridor, Cough, etc.)

Extrinsic compression (e.g., vascular ring)
Intrinsic obstruction (e.g., malformation, foreign body, cyst, tumor)
Airways reactive to other stimuli (e.g., allergens, infection)
Infection, inflammation, cystic fibrosis, pertussis, asthma, other
"Central" events (e.g., central apnea; "cough tic")

Neurobehavioral Symptoms (Sandifer's Syndrome, Seizurelike Spells)

Seizures
Dystonic reaction to drugs
Vestibular disorders
Early pertussis

Adapted from Orenstein SR: Gastroesophageal reflux. In Stockman JA, Winter RJ, eds: *Current problems in pediatrics*, Chicago, YearBook Medical Publishers, 21:223, 1991. Reprinted from Wyllie R, Hyams JS, eds: *Pediatric gastrointestinal disease: pathophysiology, diagnosis, management*, Philadelphia, 1993, WB Saunders.

measure does not reduce the incidence of reflux but may reduce the amount of emesis. Small, frequent feedings allow for adequate gastric emptying and may decrease the incidence of vomiting caused by gastric distension.

Diagnostic studies in addition to clinical examination are necessary to rule out causes of pathologic reflux. A barium study of the esophagus, stomach, and duodenum (upper GI series) is performed to rule out anatomical abnormalities such as malrotation. Esophageal pH monitoring is used to diagnosis and evaluate severity of reflux and is performed in patients who have experienced an apparent life-threatening event, reactive airway disease or recurrent pneumonias, intractable crying, unresponsiveness to medical measures, and GER symptoms after a fundoplication procedure.[46] A pH probe is inserted down a naris and positioned at the middle and lower thirds of the esophagus. The pH is continuously measured and recorded by a computer pH recorder for a 24-hour period. A pH of 4.0 denotes reflux of gastric contents. The frequency and duration are recorded including the number of episodes longer than 5 minutes, the longest episode, and the percentage of time the pH is less than 4.0. The nurse is instrumental in determining the relationship of reflux to various activities such as sleep, eating, position, and symptoms. These activities and symptoms are recorded on a bedside monitoring form.

Medications are added to the treatment regimen with evidence of pathologic reflux. Prophylactic pharmacotherapy may be indicated during exacerbations of severe respiratory disease, mechanical ventilation, or aggressive nutritional rehabilitation with gastric feedings.[47] Prokinetic agents, such as bethanechol and metoclopramide, are used to raise LES pressure and promote gastric emptying. Bethanechol is a cholinergic drug, and its potential for exacerbating bronchospasm limits its use in children with respiratory symptoms. Metoclopramide is a dopamine antagonist and has a narrow therapeutic range before central nervous system side effects such as dystonic reactions may be seen.[48] Cisapride, a prokinetic agent, which has been shown to be effective in treating children with GER, is no longer available because of reports of serious arrhythmias during concurrent use of some antibiotics.[49,50] H_2 antagonists are used successfully in children to prevent hydrochloric acid secretion in the stomach.[51] Cimetidine, ranitidine, and famotidine are the agents most commonly used. Omeprazole is an agent that blocks the parietal cell proton pump and effectively reduces acid secretion more completely than H_2 blockers. However, esophagitis relapse occurs with discontinuation and concerns about safety limit the use in children.[52,53] Antacids are best used as a supplemental therapy to H_2 blockade to neutralize gastric acid. Sucralfate is also beneficial as a mucosal barrier protectant.[54]

Overnight continuous NG feedings are used to treat GER in certain infants. This has proved effective in infants with poor weight gain and delayed gastric emptying. It provides for optimal caloric intake, and has a soothing effect on an irritated esophagus.

Failure to respond to medical therapy or failure to promptly diagnose GER may require surgical intervention. Antireflux procedures are typically performed for

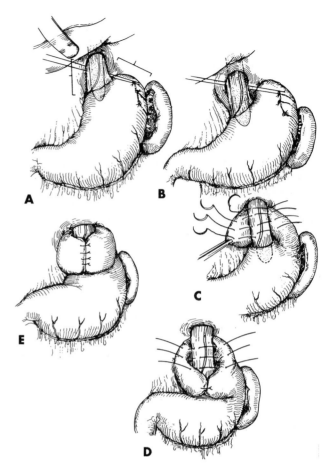

Fig. 22-7 **A,** A sizable bougie is placed in the patient's esophagus for the procedure to ensure that the wrap is not so tight that food passage is obstructed. **B,** The fundus is then drawn around behind the esophagus and **C,** interrupted sutures are used to construct the 360-degree wrap. **D,** When these sutures are tied, a cuff is formed around the lower esophagus. **E,** Distension of the stomach creates a valve that acts as a blood pressure cuff and can completely compress the lower esophagus. (From Ashcraft KW: *Atlas of pediatric surgery,* Philadelphia, 1994, WB Saunders.)

children who have not responded to medical management and who continue to be unable to gain weight appropriately. The Nissen fundoplication is the most commonly performed antireflux procedure in children, followed by the Thal fundoplication and the uncut Collis-Nissen fundoplication. Most pediatric studies report the reduction or elimination of reflux in more than 90% of patients after surgical fundoplication.[55,56]

The Nissen fundoplication involves a 360-degree wrap of the stomach around the distal esophagus, producing a tighter gastroesophageal junction, thereby decreasing the reflux of fluid back into the esophagus (Fig. 22-7). The Thal or "loose" fundoplication provides only a 180-degree wrap of the stomach, which is thought to provide adequate pressure, producing antireflux.[57,58] The uncut Collis-Nissen uses a neoesophagus that is created out of stomach, around which the fundus is wrapped.[59]

GI decompression using the gastrostomy tube that is typically placed during the operative procedure or an NG tube is of utmost importance. In some instances a transpyloric feeding tube is placed through the gastrostomy stoma to allow early introduction of enteral alimentation into the small bowel. Pain management and respiratory support are important aspects of postoperative care.

Peritoneal Inflammation

Peritoneal inflammation, or peritonitis, is associated with high morbidity and mortality. Peritoneal inflammation may occur with a rapid, abrupt onset or it may be the final outcome in a progression that begins with acute obstruction followed by necrosis and subsequent perforation. Peritonitis can be classified as either primary or secondary. Primary peritonitis is a condition wherein there is no obvious cause of contamination, but infection is indirectly introduced into the peritoneal cavity through the bloodstream or lymphatics. Common organisms include both gram-positive (*Streptococcus pneumoniae,* enterococcus) and gram-negative (*Escherichia coli, Klebsiella pneumoniae*) bacteria. If more than one organism is found, perforation must be suspected.[60]

Secondary peritonitis, also known as perforative peritonitis, occurs as a result of direct GI tract injury or contamination.[61] This can develop after an injury to a main intraabdominal blood vessel or solid organ, or after perforation of a hollow viscus. Secondary infection is relatively common and may include generalized peritonitis or localized abscess formation.

Pathogenesis. Peritoneal inflammation occurs as a result of either direct or indirect injury or contamination. Contaminants include chemicals, blood, meconium, bacteria, or foreign bodies. A localized area of inflammation usually occurs first. This local inflammatory process causes exudation of fluid into the peritoneal cavity. The exudate, rich in antibodies, complement, neutrophils, and macrophages, plays an important role in the body's defense mechanism. The release of exudate into the peritoneal cavity can successfully resolve the inflammatory process. Otherwise, contamination of the peritoneum extends with subsequent abscess formation or generalized peritonitis. In the state of generalized peritonitis, bacteria and toxins are absorbed by the peritoneal surface into the bloodstream, causing bacteremia and endotoxemia. Hypovolemia occurs as fluid shifts into the peritoneal cavity. Concurrent sepsis from bacteremia can lead to the catastrophic result of septic shock and death.

Clinical Presentation. The clinical presentation of primary peritonitis is not usually consist with typical signs of peritonitis but rather consists of more nonspecific signs including poor feeding, lethargy, abdominal distension, vomiting, and mild to moderate abdominal discomfort. Immunocompromised patients and those with indwelling catheters, such as a peritoneal dialysis catheter or ventriculoperitoneal shunt, are more susceptible.

Secondary peritonitis is associated with acute symptomatology. Abdominal pain is present and increases with movement and with breathing, often leading to shallow, rapid respirations. Abdominal wall spasm is exhibited, and it progresses from voluntary guarding in the early stages to involuntary spasm as the inflammation worsens. Very young infants do not exhibit abdominal wall spasm, but rather abdominal wall erythema, discoloration, or cellulitis. Abdominal distension and rigidity are also manifested, and the child is febrile and tachycardic. The complete blood count reveals leukocytosis with a left shift (increased immature neutrophils). Shifting dullness can be elicited on percussion because of the large amounts of free fluids in the peritoneal cavity. Anorexia, nausea, and vomiting are also exhibited, and bowel sounds may be decreased or absent. Occasionally diarrhea is present. As the inflammatory process progresses, signs of hypovolemia and sepsis become more apparent.

Abdominal CT is the gold standard in evaluating patients suspected of having an intraabdominal infection.[60] A diagnostic paracentesis may be performed if a chronic condition exists such as cirrhosis, nephrosis, and systemic lupus erythematosus or in a patient with a ventriculoperitoneal shunt. Fluid obtained with paracentesis is analyzed for cell count, protein concentration, pH, gram stain, and culture. Values consistent with intraabdominal infection include leukocytosis ($>300/mm^3$), low protein (<3.5 g/L because of hypoalbuminemia), and acidic fluid pH (<7.35). A positive gram stain of the peritoneal fluid is diagnostic but is more commonly negative. Frequently, the same organisms isolated from the peritoneal fluid are recovered in the blood.[62]

Critical Care Management. In addition to frequent physical examinations, serial abdominal girth measurements, laboratory monitoring and chest and abdominal radiologic studies are necessary. Supportive care includes ventilatory management, fluid resuscitation and inotropic support if hemodynamically unstable, gastric decompression, broad-spectrum antibiotic coverage, and early initiation of parenteral nutrition. Antibiotics must cover the most common organisms usually encountered with intraabdominal infection. These pathogens are those isolated in the lower GI tract, typically aerobic microorganisms such as *E. coli* (most common), *Klebsiella,* and occasionally, *Enterococcus.* Anaerobic microorganisms include *Bacteroides,* most often *B. fragilis.* Other anaerobes occasionally recovered include *Fusobacterium* and *Clostridium.* Infrequently, organisms such as *P. aeruginosa, S. aureus,* and *Candida* may be isolated and are more common in immunocompromised patients or patients receiving peritoneal dialysis. Antimicrobial agents must be started perioperatively and continued postoperatively to reduce the high frequency of wound infection that follows with peritonitis. Table 22-7 lists antibiotics frequently used for intraabdominal infection. Because of increased resistance of anaerobic organisms to clindamycin, metronidazole is recommended for anaerobic coverage. However, metronidazole is active against only anaerobes, and therefore coverage of the aerobic gram-negative organisms is also initiated. Antibiotic regimens may include (1) ampicillin, gentamicin and metronidazole; (2) ticarcillin-clavulanic acid and an aminoglycoside; or (3) imipenem and an aminoglycoside.[60]

If signs of perforation occur or if the child's clinical status deteriorates, surgery is warranted. Goals of surgery

TABLE 22-7 Antimicrobial Agents Frequently Used for Treatment of Intraabdominal Sepsis

Drug	Dosage (mg/kg)	Comments
Clindamycin	30 mg/kg divided q8h	Resistant *Bacteroides* species in some areas of country
Metronidazole	30 mg/kg divided q6h	Excellent activity against anaerobes; inactive against aerobes
Third-Generation Cephalosporins		
Cefotaxime	150 mg/kg divided q8h	Variable activity against anaerobes; inactive against *Pseudomonas* species
Ceftazidime	150 mg/kg divided q8h	Variable activity against anaerobes; very active against aerobic gram-negative rods
Ceftriaxone	50-75 mg/kg divided q12h	Variable activity against anaerobes; inactive against *Pseudomonas* species
Penicillins		
Ampicillin	100 mg/kg divided q6h	Active against *Enterococcus*
Piperacillin sodium and tazobactam (Zosyn)	240-400 mg/kg of piperacillin component divided q6-8h	Active against β-lactamase producing strains of *S. aureus, H. influenzae, B. fragilis, Klebsiella, E. coli,* and *Acinetobacter*
Ampicillin and sulbactam (Unasyn)	100-200 mg/kg of ampicillin q6h	Same as ampicillin and organisms producing β-lactamases such as *S. aureus, H. influenzae, E. coli, Klebsiella, Acinetobacter, Enterobacter,* and anaerobes
Vancomycin	40 mg/kg divided q6h	Active against all gram-positive cocci and bacilli, including *Staphylococcus aureus* and *Staphylococcus epidermidis* resistant to penicillins and cephalosporins, and activity against enterococci
Aminoglycosides		
Gentamicin	5-7.5 mg/kg divided q8h	Reduced activity at acid pH and in anaerobic environment of abscesses and deep tissue infections
Tobramycin	2.5 mg/kg divided q8h	Treatment of documented or suspected gram-negative bacilli including *Pseudomonas aeruginosa*
Amikacin	15-22.5 mg/kg divided q8h	Treatment of documented gram-negative enteric infection resistant to gentamicin
Imipenem	40-60 mg/kg divided q6h	Treatment of documented multidrug-resistant gram-negative infection
Aztreonam	90-120 mg/kg divided q6-8h	Treatment of documented multidrug-resistant aerobic gram-negative infection

From Takemoto CK, Hodding JH, Kraus DM: *Pediatric dosage handbook,* ed 6, Cleveland, 1999-2000, Lexi-Comp.

include closure of perforations, removal of necrotic tissue, drainage of abscesses, establishment of intestinal continuity, and preservation of intestinal length.

Necrotizing Enterocolitis

NEC is a condition of patchy or diffuse necrosis of the intestinal mucosa thought to result from a combination of decreased blood flow, hypoxia, and bacterial invasion.[63] The exact etiology of NEC remains unclear. It occurs most often in premature infants, but it has been reported in full-term babies and in infants and children whose preceding risk factors have included polycythemia, cyanotic heart disease, chronic diarrhea, or a prior anatomic GI obstruction.[64-66]

Pathogenesis. The pathogenesis of NEC is most likely related to several factors. Early theories proposed a relationship between enteral feeding, intestinal ischemia, and infection.[67] More recent studies advocate the role of these factors plus an immature GI function and immature immune mechanisms as inciting factors for neonatal intestinal mucosal injury.[68,69] Other predisposing factors include respiratory distress, hypothermia with associated stress response, patent ductus arteriosus, umbilical artery catheters, and exchange transfusions.[66]

In instances of hypoxic-ischemic injury, blood is shunted to the brain and heart and away from less vital organs such as the bowel. Vasoconstriction of the intestinal vasculature occurs, followed by bowel ischemia and mucosal damage.

Box 22-3
Staging Criteria for NEC

Stage 1 (Suspect)

History of perinatal stress

Systemic manifestations: temperature instability, lethargy, apnea, bradycardia

GI tract manifestations: poor feeding, increased gastric residuals, emesis (may be bilious or have positive results for occult blood), mild abdominal distension, occult blood in stool

Stage 2 (Definite)

Above history and signs and symptoms plus persistent occult or gross GI tract bleeding

Marked abdominal distension

Abdominal radiographs show significant intestinal distension with ileus, small bowel separation, pneumatosis intestinalis

Stage 3 (Advanced)

Same signs and symptoms as in stage 2 plus deterioration in vital signs

Evidence of septic shock or marked GI tract hemorrhage

Abdominal radiographs show pneumoperitoneum

Modified from Bell MJ, Ternberg JL, Reign RD et al: Neonatal necrotizing enterocolitis: therapeutic decisions based upon clinical staging, *Ann Surg* 1:187, 1978.

Bowel wall injury allows bacterial colonization and can lead to extensive tissue damage, including necrosis. Enteral feeding has been proposed as a contributing factor in NEC because more than 95% of infants with NEC have been fed enterally before its onset.[70] The volume of milk fed to infants may also be a contributing factor. The rate of feeding may exceed the infant's intestinal absorptive capability, resulting in malabsorption. Malabsorbed carbohydrates produce increased intestinal bacterial gas leading to abdominal distension. Abdominal distension may cause increased intraluminal pressure and result in reduced mucosal blood flow and ultimately intestinal ischemia. The bacterial gas penetrates the perforated intestinal wall, resulting in the diagnosis of free air on abdominal x-ray films. The entry of bacterial gas into the submucosal tissue (intraluminal wall) is called pneumatosis intestinalis.

Clinical Presentation. Any preterm infant should be considered at risk for developing NEC. A high level of suspicion is maintained even with subtle clinical changes, such as an increased feeding residual, increased abdominal distension, temperature instability, lethargy, and apnea. Later indications of NEC include Hemoccult-positive stools, discoloration of the abdominal wall, and visibly dilated bowel loops. On physical examination, the infant with NEC has abdominal tenderness, erythema, distension, and irritability along with respiratory compromise.

Staging criteria for NEC is outlined in Box 22-3. Stage I represents subclinical NEC in which clinical symptomatology is present but there are no radiographic findings. Stages II and III have radiographic findings consistent with disease.

Radiographic findings include pneumatosis, dilated loops of bowel, or pneumoperitoneum. Progression from one stage to another usually occurs within 24 to 48 hours after symptoms arise. Once the infant is stabilized, disease progression rarely occurs. Most episodes of perforation occur on presentation.[66,71]

Critical Care Management. The management of NEC is largely supportive. Certain measures are taken when the diagnosis is suspected. The patient is made NPO with NG decompression. Parenteral nutrition is provided while the patient is NPO. Duration of NPO status is dictated by the continued clinical and radiographic findings consistent with NEC. Abdominal radiographs (flat plate and cross-table lateral) are obtained when NEC is suspected and repeated every 6 hours during the acute phase to monitor for progression of disease. Laboratory studies include a complete blood count and differential to monitor for signs of sepsis and GI bleeding associated with the disease. Serial electrolyte and arterial blood gases (ABGs) are also obtained to monitor for metabolic acidosis and electrolyte disturbances associated with poor perfusion and advanced disease. Inflammation and edema of the intestine results in third spacing of fluid; which can cause significant fluid and electrolyte derangements if adequate replacement is not maintained. Infants generally require one and one half to two times maintenance levels of fluids to maintain adequate intravascular volume. Mechanical ventilation and inotropic support are often required to stabilize the critically ill infant in septic shock. Broad-spectrum antibiotic coverage is initiated immediately including anaerobic coverage (i.e., metronidazole) if perforation is observed on radiographic studies.

Indications for surgery include radiographic evidence of intestinal perforation or clinical deterioration despite aggressive medical management. Preparation for the operation includes stabilization with GI decompression, respiratory and cardiovascular support, thermoregulation, fluid resuscitation, and prevention of sepsis. The timing of surgical intervention for a child with NEC is critical but is a difficult management decision. Ideally the operation should take place when the bowel is truly necrotic but perforation has not occurred. If the operation occurs early, there may be a large gray, thin, edematous area of bowel that has no distinct boundaries, making surgical resection more difficult. On the other hand, if operation occurs too late the small bowel may be completely nonviable. Fig. 22-8 provides an algorithm for treatment of the neonate with NEC.

Infants with fulminant NEC experience all the clinical signs and symptoms previously described within hours and exhibit rapid deterioration and multisystem failure. Immediate surgical intervention is required.

Postoperatively, fluid loss through the ileostomy is closely monitored, noting the presence of blood. Fluid management can be difficult in these patients because of the increased fluid output coupled with third spacing of fluids. Parenteral nutritional support and broad-spectrum antibiotic coverage are continued. The reinstitution of enteral feeding following adequate bowel rest and stable radiographic

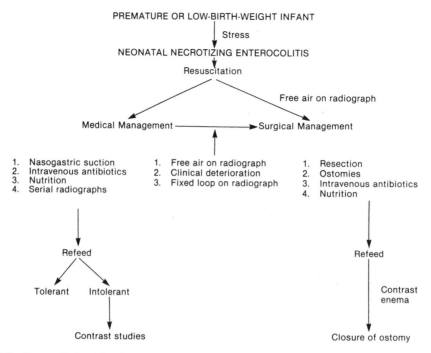

Fig. 22-8   Proposed algorithm for treatment of neonatal necrotizing enterocolitis. (From Ghoury MJ, Sheldon CA: Newborn surgical emergencies of the gastrointestinal tract, *Surg Clin North Am* 65:1083-1098, 1985.)

studies is performed slowly while monitoring for clinical symptoms of NEC.

Long-term prognosis for infants with NEC is good if they survive the initial critical period.[72] Stomal closure can occur between 6 weeks and 3 to 4 months of age, depending on the child's enteral feeding tolerance. In some children, the increased water loss from the ileostomy can force earlier closure of the stoma. Before stomal closure, all children undergo a BE to assess the distal segment of bowel for stricture formation, a complication occurring after some episodes of NEC. Stricture formation and acquired short bowel syndrome (SBS) are the two major complications that result from NEC.[73]

Short Bowel Syndrome

SBS is defined as the absence of more than 50% of the small bowel, which results in malabsorption of nutrients.[74,77] Wilmore reviewed cases of 50 infants younger than 2 months of age and defined SBS as residual jejunoileal length of less than 75 cm.[75] Thirty years ago children with this entity succumbed to the disease. Since that time, major advances in venous access, parenteral-enteral nutrition, understanding of bowel adaptation, and success with small bowel transplantation have greatly improved the patients' quality of life and chances for survival.[76]

Massive bowel loss can occur as a result of prenatal or postnatal causes. Before an infant is born, embryologic maldevelopment or vascular accidents necessitate emergent lifesaving surgery shortly after birth to correct the defect, but in many situations surgery leaves the child with a foreshortened small bowel. During infancy or childhood, disease processes, vascular thrombosis, or trauma can result in the same outcome. Volvulus and NEC are the two leading causes of SBS.[75,78-80]

Pathogenesis.   After major small bowel resection, there is a loss of intestinal mucosal absorptive surface area, along with rapid transit time of intestinal contents, resulting in inadequate ability of the gut to digest and absorb nutrients.[77,81] Depending on the severity of the symptoms, the child's nutritional rehabilitation course can be short and uncomplicated, or prolonged with multiple and severe complications, which ultimately lead to death.

With significant loss of small intestine, the bowel undergoes numerous changes. In many patients, there is excessive secretion of gastric acid, which can lead to diarrhea, decreased function of pancreatic enzymes, bacteria overgrowth, ulceration, hemorrhage, and denuded perianal skin.[82,83] Jejunal resection results in a loss of brush border enzymes, which impairs carbohydrate absorption. Stasis of carbohydrate substrate in the bowel further leads to bacterial overgrowth. Protein metabolism is hindered owing to malabsorption of peptides and amino acids. Loss of water-soluble vitamins including B_{12} is associated with a large jejunal resection. Ileal resection causes malabsorption of bile salts, which leads to excessive fatty stools and malabsorption of fat-soluble vitamins (A, D, E, and K).[77,83]

Because of the ileum's potential for adaptation and ability to transport bile acids and vitamin B_{12}, the ileum, rather than the jejunum, is the most critical area to leave intact.[20,83] The presence of the ileocecal valve aids in both slowing small intestinal transit time, thus improving absorption of nutrients, and decreasing the risk of colonization by colonic bacteria.[81,83] But in many cases, especially in patients with NEC, preservation of the valve is impossible. Studies have shown that long-term survival is possible with an 11- to 15-cm jejunoileum and an intact ileocecal valve or with 25- to 40-cm small bowel without an ileocecal valve.[75,84]

The exact length of the small bowel is difficult to ascertain but is thought to be approximately three times a person's linear length. The full-term neonate is estimated to have between 200 and 300 cm of small intestine.[85] Intestinal length increases to 600 to 800 cm by adulthood. For preterm infants, it is important to note that the small bowel doubles in length from the nineteenth to the thirty-fifth week of gestation. Thus resection of the small bowel in a preterm infant may have more severe consequences than for a full-term infant.[28]

Intestinal "adaptation" is the normal physiologic response of the small intestine after major resection. During this process, there is a gradual increase in surface area because of mucosal hyperplasia, villous lengthening, and increased depth of the intestinal crypts. Three mechanisms are involved in gut adaptation: luminal, hormonal, and cellular factors.[86]

Clinical Presentation.   Children with SBS regardless of cause will present with some degree of diarrhea and nutritional malabsorption. Significant diarrhea can result in dehydration and electrolyte disturbances. Other clinical findings may include vomiting, abdominal pain, and failure to thrive. In addition, signs and symptoms of protein-losing enteropathy such as edema (commonly periorbital, facial, abdominal, leg and ankle) and hypoalbuminemia may be evident. Protein-losing enteropathy is a pathophysiologic process in which there is excessive GI protein loss due to disruption of the intestinal lumen. Intestinal disruption allows serum proteins to be spilled into the lumen as a result of (1) mucosal erosion or ulceration, and (2) obstruction of the thoracic duct with transmission back to the small lymphatics in the small intestine.[87]

Critical Care Management.   After extensive bowel resection, nutrition is provided with TPN to ensure that nutrients, electrolytes, minerals, vitamins, and trace elements necessary for healing and growth are met. It is important to remember that the central line is the "lifeline" for a child with SBS. It is critical that the integrity and sterility of the catheter be maintained to prevent iatrogenic catheter loss.

Cholestatic liver disease is a common complication of long-term TPN, especially in the preterm infant. The cause for this is unknown but most likely is multifactorial. The responsible factors include toxicity of amino acids, bile acids, amino acid competition for transport across the canalicular membrane, toxins in the TPN solution, and lack of stimulation of biliary flow by the gut.[74,81] To reduce the risk of TPN-induced jaundice, early enteral alimentation is provided and the concentration of amino acids in the TPN is limited to 2.5 g/kg/day.

Surgical intervention may increase the small bowel absorptive surface. A bowel-lengthening procedure, which involves longitudinal division of a dilated segment of the bowel, tubularization of the two segments and end-to-end anastomosis, has been successful. This procedure, in theory, doubles the segmental length of bowel.[88] Other procedures include reversed small bowel segments, prejejunal isoperistaltic colonic interposition, and replacement of ileocecal value with a nipple valve intussusception.[89,90] Unfortunately, the success rate of these procedures has not been substantial. Small bowel transplantation is the procedure of choice to eliminate the problems associated with SBS.

Long-term survival of a child with SBS is dependent on transition from parenteral to enteral nutrition. Enteral nutrition is essential to stimulate small bowel adaptation and to prevent TPN-associated cholestasis.[91] The optimal nutrient composition of enteral feedings in short bowel patients is controversial. However, the initiation of enteral feeding should begin with an elemental formula (i.e., Pregestimil in children <1 year, Peptamen Junior >1 year) administered continuously and at a slow rate of infusion. Stool volume, pH, reducing substances, and daily weight measurements are closely monitored for feeding intolerance. As tolerance is observed, the child can be advanced to small bolus feeds during the day with resumption of continual NG or gastrostomy feeding at night. TPN is tapered with increasing enteral feeding volume while ensuring optimal caloric intake. However, the transition from parenteral to enteral nutrition is gradual and may take months or even years.

Byrne and colleagues described an approach to "rehabilitating" residual bowel with the administration of specialized nutrients (i.e., glutamine and long-chain triglycerides), growth factors (i.e., growth hormone, insulin-like growth factor-1), and a high-fiber diet.[92] The researchers reported improved caloric intestinal absorption and decreased stool output after a 3-week course of this therapy. A similar study performed by Scolapio and colleagues failed to demonstrate the same improvements. Experience in children is lacking. Further research in children and adults is needed to confirm these preliminary findings.[93]

The goals of drug therapy in patients with SBS are to reduce diarrhea, replace electrolytes, and treat complications. The most effective antidiarrheal agent for children with SBS is loperamide. It is used to reduce GI motility, thereby increasing nutrient contact time with the mucosa. However, this delay in intestinal transit time may also increase the child's risk for bacterial overgrowth. Bacterial overgrowth is a difficult problem to treat in SBS patients. The choice of antimicrobial therapy is largely empiric (i.e., metronidazole). Another agent used to treat high-volume secretory diarrhea is octreotide.[94] Octreotide is a somatostatin analogue that inhibits exocrine secretions from the stomach, pancreas, and small intestine; reduces splanchnic blood flow; and slows GI motility. Currently there are varying reports of its effectiveness in treating diarrhea.[81,83,86]

Other more long-term problems include the reduction in bile salt reabsorption, and malabsorption of fat-soluble vitamins, calcium, magnesium, and zinc. Cholestyramine is an ion-exchange resin that binds intraluminal bile acids and is often used to reduce the effects of malabsorbed bile salts on the colon. Supplementation of fat-soluble vitamins, calcium, and magnesium are imperative to prevent complications, such as rickets or tetany. Vitamin B_{12} supplementation is necessary in patients with a resected ileocecal valve. Folic acid, electrolytes, and trace elements are also essential if the levels are below normal.

The prognosis of children with SBS has dramatically improved since the introduction of parenteral nutrition. In addition, the success of small bowel transplantation may improve the outcome of patients with minimal residual bowel.

Pancreatitis

Pancreatitis is an acute inflammatory condition that results from an autodigestive process within the pancreas. It is relatively uncommon in children; however, it is being increasingly recognized in patients with multisystem disease.[95,96] Pancreatitis can present at any age and ranges in severity from a mild to fulminant inflammatory process.

The most frequent cause of childhood pancreatitis is blunt abdominal trauma, with child abuse identified in as many as one third of these cases.[22] In addition to traumatic pancreatitis, other common causes include viral infection, drugs, multisystem disease, and congenital anomalies.[96]

Pathogenesis. The exact mechanisms that initiate the sequence of enzymatic reactions resulting in acute pancreatitis are unclear. It is proposed that the autodigestive process results from premature activation of proteolytic enzymes within the pancreas, or from the reflux of activated enzymes into the pancreas from a distal obstruction.[22,96] Both processes cause a localized inflammatory response. If autodigestion is severe and extensive, vascular damage may occur, causing hemorrhagic pancreatitis. In addition, release of lipase into surrounding tissues can cause fat necrosis and breakdown of calcium. Local inflammation in and around the pancreas causes third spacing into the peritoneum and, if uncorrected, can lead to hypovolemia and cardiovascular collapse.

Clinical Presentation. Abdominal pain is the most common symptom observed in acute pancreatitis. It is described as sudden, constant, dull, epigastric, or periumbilical pain and may radiate to the back or is referred to the left shoulder. Diffuse peritoneal signs such as guarding, decreased or absent bowel sounds, and distension may also be present. However, unlike in adults, symptoms in children may be subtle with minimal abdominal pain or nonepigastric in origin.[95] In cases of hemorrhagic pancreatitis, a bluish discoloration may be seen in the flank area (Grey Turner's sign), indicating retroperitoneal bleeding. Periumbilical discoloration (Cullen's sign), indicating intraabdominal bleeding, may also be seen in cases of hemorrhagic pancreatitis. Patients are febrile and exhibit nausea and vomiting. In patients with fulminant pancreatitis, signs of shock may be exhibited.

Initial laboratory analysis reveals markedly elevated serum amylase and lipase, elevated transaminases (AST, ALT), leukocytosis, elevated hematocrit (as a result of hemoconcentration caused by intravascular fluid loss), and

hypocalcemia. Serum amylase level is typically elevated within hours and remains elevated for 4 to 5 days. It is important to remember that the serum amylase level reflects salivary and pancreatic components. Fractionation of the serum amylase can be readily performed in most clinical laboratories; however, it is not commonly ordered because of the specificity of the serum lipase level. Specificity is increased when the serum amylase and lipase levels increase at least threefold. Hypocalcemia is seen most often during the first few days of illness but rarely is associated with symptoms.

The plain abdominal radiograph may reveal a "sentinel loop" (dilated loop of bowel located near the pancreas), ileus, or a mass effect if a pseudocyst has developed. A pseudocyst is a cyst-like mass filled with pancreatic fluids extending out of the pancreas. Although a pseudocyst may develop from any of the causes of pancreatitis, it is most often a complication of traumatic pancreatitis. An abdominal ultrasound is useful in identifying both the presence and extent of pancreatic damage and complications resulting from acute pancreatitis. In addition to pseudocyst formation, other complications include abscess formation, splenic vein thrombosis, diabetes (usually temporary), and pancreatic enzyme insufficiency (in cases of chronic, recurrent pancreatitis). Endoscopic retrograde cannulation of the pancreatic ducts (ERCP) is helpful in defining abnormalities of the pancreatic and biliary ducts that result in structural/obstructive pancreatitis. Abdominal CT is usually reserved for more difficult patients or when the ultrasound results are unclear. Approximately 20% of patients with acute pancreatitis have a normal abdominal CT examination.[97]

Critical Care Management. Management of the patient with acute pancreatitis is multisystemic in approach, with the primary goal of suppressing or halting the autodigestive process. Strategies employed are aimed at decreasing the activity of the pancreas and include NPO, maintaining gastric decompression, and administering antacids and H_2 blockers that act to decrease gastric acid secretion.

Other goals of management include prevention of hypovolemia and shock with adequate fluid resuscitation, provision of respiratory and nutritional support, and restoration of normal pancreatic functions. Patients presenting with or progressing to a fulminant form of acute pancreatitis require comprehensive hemodynamic monitoring.

Frequent serial abdominal examinations, including abdominal girth measurement, and treating abdominal pain with analgesics are an integral part of care. Broad-spectrum antibiotics are also administered. While the patient is NPO, nutrition is provided with TPN.

Laboratory studies to be monitored include amylase and lipase, transaminases, electrolytes, albumin, complete blood count with differential, ABGs, and serum calcium levels. Hypocalcemia is a common metabolic complication of pancreatitis and assessing for signs and symptoms including irritability, muscle twitching, tetany, seizures, and the electrocardiogram for lengthening of the QT interval is imperative. Fever, tachycardia, and leukocytosis may occur in the patient with acute pancreatitis in the absence of infection. However, infection should be suspected with high fevers (greater than 39° C), significant leukocytosis (over 20,000/μL), or signs of clinical deterioration.[22] Abdominal CT with contrast is performed to identify pancreatic necrosis, pancreatic fluid collections, or pseudocyst. In addition, regular chest radiographs are obtained because patients are at risk for developing pleural effusions and acute respiratory distress syndrome (ARDS).

Efforts are made to treat acute pancreatitis medically and to avoid surgery. Surgical treatment is usually reserved for traumatic pancreatitis with ductal rupture, debriding necrotic and infected tissue, and draining of a pancreatic abscess when percutaneous drainage has failed.[98]

GASTROINTESTINAL BLEEDING

GI bleeding can vary in clinical presentation from acute life-threatening shock to asymptomatic bleeding with stools positive for occult blood. Bleeding can originate throughout the GI tract. Causes of upper and lower GI bleeding are listed in Tables 22-8 and 22-9.

Acute Gastritis

A common cause of upper GI bleeding, regardless of age, is acute gastritis. Acute gastritis, also referred to as erosive or

stress gastritis, is most commonly associated with severe stress in the critically ill patient. Patients may develop isolated gastroduodenal erosions or mucosal ulcerations in multiple sites within the stomach and duodenum. Acute gastritis occurs in critically ill children suffering from burns, severe head trauma, major surgical procedures, sepsis, multiple trauma, and respiratory failure. Critical care nurses play a key role not only in the early detection (by evaluating gastric aspirates) and treatment of upper GI bleeding but also in the prevention of upper GI bleeding by identifying children at risk and administering prophylactic medications (i.e., H_2 blocker) as ordered.

The etiology of acute gastritis secondary to stress is unknown but is, most likely, multifactorial. Potential causes include impaired blood flow, increased secretion of acid and pepsin, decreased production of mucus, decreased gastric somatostatin level, alterations in levels of adrenal steroids

TABLE 22-8   Upper Gastrointestinal Bleeding

Age Group	Common	Less Common
Neonates (0-30 days)	Swallowed maternal blood Gastritis Duodenitis	Coagulopathy Vascular malformations Gastric/esophageal duplication Leiomyoma
Infants (30 days-1 year)	Gastritis and gastric ulcer Esophagitis Duodenitis	Esophageal varices Foreign body Aortoesophageal fistula
Children (1-12 years)	Esophagitis Esophageal varices Gastritis and gastric ulcer Duodenal ulcer Mallory-Weiss tear Nasopharyngeal bleeding	Leiomyoma Salicylates Vascular malformation Hematobilia
Adolescents (12 years-adult)	Duodenal ulcer Esophagitis Esophageal varices Gastritis Mallory-Weiss tear	Thrombocytopenia Dieulafoy's ulcer Hematobilia

From Olson AD, Hillemeier AC: Gastrointestinal hemorrhage. In Wyllie R, Hyams JS, eds: *Pediatric gastrointestinal disease: pathophysiology, diagnosis, management,* Philadelphia, 1993, WB Saunders.

TABLE 22-9   Lower Gastrointestinal Bleeding

Age Group	Common	Less Common
Neonates (0-30 days)	Anorectal lesions Swallowed maternal blood Milk allergy Necrotizing enterocolitis Midgut volvulus	Vascular malformations Hirschsprung's enterocolitis Intestinal duplication Coagulopathy
Infants (30 days-1 year)	Anorectal lesions Midgut volvulus Intussusception (<3 yr) Meckel's diverticulum Infectious diarrhea Milk allergy (<4 yr)	Vascular malformations Intestinal duplication Acquired thrombocytopenia
Children (1-12 years)	Juvenile polyps Meckel's diverticulum Intussusception (<3 yr) Infectious diarrhea Anal fissure Nodular lymphoid hyperplasia	Henoch-Schönlein purpura Hemolytic-uremic syndrome Vasculitis (SLE) Inflammatory bowel disease
Adolescents (12 years-adult)	Inflammatory bowel disease Polyps Hemorrhoids Anal fissure Infectious diarrhea	Arteriovascular malformation Adenocarcinomas Henoch-Schönlein purpura Pseudomembranous colitis

From Olson AD, Hillemeier AC: Gastrointestinal hemorrhage. In Wyllie R, Hyams JS, eds: *Pediatric gastrointestinal disease: pathophysiology, diagnosis, management,* Philadelphia, 1993, WB Saunders.

and catecholamines, and impairment in the local production of prostaglandins.

Corticosteroid therapy has been implicated in causing acute gastritis; however, there is no evidence-based research to substantiate this claim. A large prospective descriptive study in pediatric patients revealed that 10.2% of 1006 admissions developed clinical signs of GI bleeding, only 1.6% were considered clinically significant.[99] Other reports demonstrate that patients with multitrauma, coagulopathy, respiratory failure, or pediatric risk of mortality score (PRISM) greater than 10 should receive prophylaxis to prevent upper GI bleeding.[100-102] Nonsteroidal antiinflammatory drugs (NSAIDs) are known to cause both gastritis and mucosal ulceration.[103]

Gastric acidity has also been associated with an increased risk of gastritis. Valentine and colleagues reported that patients with a gastric pH greater than 3.5 had only a 4% incidence of GI bleeding, and patients with a gastric pH greater than 5 had no overt GI bleeding.[104] However, increased gastric pH may increase the risk of nosocomial pneumonia by enhancing colonization of gram-negative bacteria. Therefore the current recommendation is to administer prophylaxis only to high-risk patients, which include those with respiratory failure requiring mechanical ventilation for more than 48 hours and/or in those with coagulopathy.[105]

The best gut protection is enteral feeding administered by the NG route. If this is not possible or if the patient is receiving transpyloric enteral feeding (and is identified as a high-risk patient), stress ulcer prophylaxis is indicated. Prophylaxis often will include an H_2 blocker (i.e., ranitidine, cimetidine) titrated to maintain gastric pH greater than 4. Patients receiving an H_2 blocker should be monitored for thrombocytopenia. Sucralfate may also be considered as adjunct therapy, which acts as a protective "barrier" by coating the gastric mucosa. This agent may be more convenient than an H_2 blocker because it does not affect the gastric pH and therefore does not require pH monitoring. Omeprazole is an agent that blocks the parietal cell proton pump and effectively reduces acid secretion more completely than H_2 blockers and has a longer duration of action (12 to 24 hours). The disadvantage of this drug is the method of administration. Omeprazole is supplied as capsules containing enteric-coated granules. The administration of the drug requires opening the capsule and dispersing the granules in a solution to prevent clogging of the feeding tube. However, obstruction of the feeding tube continues to be a commonly reported problem. The use of antacids is currently not supported secondary to the need for frequent administration to effectively maintain an increase in pH, leading to increased risk of reflux and microaspiration.[106]

Lower Gastrointestinal Bleeding

Lower GI hemorrhage is rare in the pediatric population. Individuals at risk are those with known coagulopathies, such as hemophilia A or B, chronic liver disease, and portal hypertension. Mucosal lesions, ulcers, polyps, arteriovenous malformations, and inflammatory bowel disease are also sources of lower GI tract bleeding.

TABLE 22-10   Signs and Symptoms in Gastrointestinal Hemorrhage

Sign	Indication	Site of Bleeding
Splenomegaly Jaundice	Portal hypertension	Esophageal varices Portal gastropathy
Hemangioma Telangiectasia	Multiple hemangioma syndrome	Vascular malformation of GI tract
Hematemesis	Bleeding from above the ligament of Treitz	Upper GI tract
Melena	Bleeding from above the ileocecal valve	Upper GI tract or small intestine
Hematochezia	Colonic bleeding, massive upper GI bleeding	GI tract
Nasogastric aspirate: gross blood	Bleeding from above the ligament of Treitz	Upper GI tract
Palpable purpura	Henoch-Schönlein purpura	GI tract

Modified from Olson AD, Hillemeier AC: Gastrointestinal hemorrhage. In Wyllie R, Hyams JS, eds: *Pediatric gastrointestinal disease: pathophysiology, diagnosis, management,* Philadelphia, 1993, WB Saunders.

Clinical Presentation.   GI hemorrhage can present in several distinct ways (Table 22-10). Hematemesis describes bright red vomiting or coffee ground-like emesis. This suggests a bleeding source above the ligament of Treitz (at the duodenojejunal junction in left upper abdominal quadrant). Hematochezia is the passage of bright red blood or maroon-colored stool from the rectum. It is most commonly associated with a colonic source of bleeding. Melena is the passing of dark, black, tarry stools, which occurs in patients bleeding from a site located above the ileocecal valve. The black color is the result of the action of the bacteria on the hemoglobin that has been converted to hematin. Borborygmi are deep rumbling abdominal sounds caused by the rapid transit of blood through the GI tract.

Critical Care Management.   Acute GI bleeding can result in massive exsanguination and shock. An NG tube is inserted in the case of upper GI bleeding to prevent aspiration of blood. Hemodynamic assessment guides administration of fluid, red blood cells (RBCs), and other blood products until the patient can be transported to the operating room for primary surgical intervention.

Radiographic studies play a limited role in the initial investigation of GI bleeding.

Esophageal Varices

Esophageal varices are the result of portal hypertension, which can occur at any stage of liver disease. In hepatic disease, portal hypertension is caused by cirrhotic changes (intrahepatic scarring) that collapse and distort the hepatic vasculature.

Pathogenesis. When blood flow through the liver is obstructed, portal venous pressure increases. The development of collateral circulation redirects the portal venous blood flow through vessels of lower resistance and avoids the obstruction. Collateral vessels develop in the abdominal wall, rectum, lower esophagus, and stomach. These low-pressure veins eventually become distended with blood, causing the veins to enlarge, developing into varices. The development of collateral portal circulation may reduce the portal pressure toward normal.

Clinical Presentation. The diagnosis of portal hypertension is based on clinical presentation, along with information obtained from a variety of studies. Splenomegaly is generally the first sign of portal hypertension in children. Hematemesis, melena, nosebleeds, or an unexplained decrease in hemoglobin level may also indicate portal hypertension, although massive hematemesis is often the first clinical sign in children. Barium studies can detect relatively large varices but are unable to provide additional clinically important information that can be obtained by an ultrasound or endoscopy. An abdominal ultrasound is useful in determining the presence and size of the portal vein and, with Doppler, can determine the direction of the blood flow through the portal system. An upper endoscopy is currently the best modality to determine the location and size of the varices.

Critical Care Management. Hemorrhaging esophageal varices are a true medical emergency and require prompt action. The cause of a bleeding episode is usually unknown, but factors suggesting rupture include a sudden increase in abdominal venous pressure as a result of physical exertion, coughing, sneezing, vomiting, or stool straining. The first priorities are stabilization of airway, breathing, and circulation. The child is turned on his or her side in a semi-Fowler position with suction at the bedside to protect the airway against possible aspiration or occlusion. In addition to suction, accessibility of supplemental oxygen and equipment for intubation and vascular access is ensured.

Close monitoring of vital signs and determination of blood loss indicate the amount of fluid replacement necessary. During the resuscitation phase, it is vital that the blood pressure be maintained. Isotonic crystalloid is administered in boluses of 20 ml/kg until systemic perfusion is restored or whole blood is available. As the child's condition stabilizes, the need for other blood products is determined by the complete blood count and coagulation indices. In general, fresh frozen plasma is administered to correct coagulation abnormalities or with every two to three units of packed RBCs (unless whole blood is used) to account for ongoing loss of coagulation factors. Platelet transfusions are reserved for patients whose platelet counts are less than 50,000 per cubic millimeter.

Simultaneous with fluid resuscitation, an NG tube is inserted to determine the volume of bleeding. Suspicion of esophageal varices is not a contraindication for the insertion of an NG tube. A large-diameter tube (10-16 French) is passed to provide access for gastric lavage with room-temperature normal saline. Room-temperature solutions prevent hypothermia and its associated side effects and are better tolerated by the patient.

Vasopressin is an antidiuretic hormone (ADH) that is naturally excreted by the posterior pituitary. Administration of this hormone produces a pharmacologic effect that reduces bleeding in 35% to 50% of cases.[7,107] Vasopressin acts directly on GI smooth muscle and induces systemic vasoconstriction. It also lowers portal venous pressure by reducing splanchnic arterial blood flow.

Vasopressin is given through a central venous line at a continuous infusion rate of 0.002 to 0.008 units/kg/minute or 0.2 to 0.4 units/minute. Vasopressin infusion is continued for as long as 24 to 36 hours and is slowly weaned if no evidence of rebleeding exists.

Because vasopressin vasoconstricts the coronary and renal arteries, it is important to closely monitor for arrhythmias and hypertension. If bleeding does not cease or if it reoccurs, further elevation of the vasopressin infusion creates increased intravascular pressure because of excessive vasoconstriction. The increased pressure on the portal system can precipitate greater blood loss.

Renal complications that accompany the use of vasopressin include fluid retention. Fluid intake should be limited to two-thirds maintenance requirements. Strict intake and output measurements are essential. Urine output of less than 0.5 ml/kg/hour in a child may be the result of fluid retention from the use of vasopressin requiring titration of the infusion.

Serum and urine laboratory values are obtained every 6 hours. Electrolyte and osmolality levels change significantly with fluid retention. Signs of fluid retention include decreased serum sodium and osmolality levels, whereas urine sodium and osmolality levels are increased. Liver dysfunction complicates the etiology of electrolyte disturbances. Low serum sodium may indicate hyponatremia resulting from vasopressin-induced free water retention. However, the total body sodium may actually be increased because of hepatorenal disease. The interpretation of serum sodium and the administration of replacement sodium require extreme caution.

Ascites and edema resulting from liver dysfunction may worsen as a result of vasopressin-induced water retention. Albumin may be administered in an effort to draw fluid from the extracellular space into the vasculature. A preparation of 25% albumin is used to decrease the total fluid volume administered. After the infusion of albumin, a dose of furosemide (1 mg/kg) is administered to facilitate diuresis. It may be necessary to repeat this procedure until the serum albumin and total protein levels normalize and fluid retention resolves.

Octreotide has largely replaced vasopressin in many pediatric centers because of its more favorable profile.[107-109] Octreotide is a synthetic analogue of somatostatin that has been proven in adults to be as effective as injection sclerotherapy in controlling acute bleeding.[108] Somatostatin reduces gastric blood flow and inhibits gastric acid and gastrin production. Like vasopressin, it reduces portal venous pressure by decreasing splanchnic blood flow; however, it does not produce major systemic side effects. Suggested dosing includes administering a 1 to 2 μg/kg intravenous bolus followed by a continuous infusion of 1 to 2 μg/kg/hour.[108] Currently there are no controlled studies on the use of somatostatin in children. Subsequent modes of therapy such as balloon tamponade and sclerotherapy are considered when medical therapy fails.

Balloon tamponade is performed with a Sengstaken-Blakemore tube (SBT). The availability of sclerotherapy has significantly reduced its use. The SBT is available in two sizes, pediatric and adult. The pediatric tube consists of three lumens: one for gastric aspiration, one for inflating the esophageal balloon, and one for inflating the gastric balloon. The adult SBT has the addition of a fourth lumen for aspiration of esophageal secretions. The SBT provides a tamponade effect to the bleeding varices. Inflation of the gastric balloon applies pressure to the vessels feeding the varices and thus decreases the blood flow. Inflation of the esophageal balloon allows pressure to be placed directly on the varices. In children, the gastric balloon is inflated first and if the bleeding continues, inflation of the esophageal balloon is considered.

Once balloon tamponading is initiated, it is necessary to keep children immobile. Activity can increase abdominal and intravascular pressures, causing increased bleeding activity. Therefore neuromuscular blockade may be necessary. Ventilatory support is necessary for as long as the SBT is in place.

Bleeding is monitored by the amount of blood aspirated with intermittent suction. The blood pressure and central venous pressure are continuously monitored and near-normal parameters are maintained by volume replacement. It is important that hypertension be avoided. Complete blood count levels are monitored every 4 hours until the hematocrit is stable. A hematocrit of 30 to 36 is adequate for these patients because hematocrits higher than 36 have been shown to stimulate rebleeding as a result of the increased intravascular pressure placing stress on the varices.[107] Packed RBCs are administered to raise the hematocrit. Coagulation indices and platelet counts are monitored and blood products, such as platelets and fresh frozen plasma, are given as described above. Vitamin K may also be administered to replace factors II, VII, IX, and X.

Complications commonly seen with the SBT are atelectasis and aspiration pneumonia. Atelectasis is the result of increased intrathoracic pressure from the balloon, whereas aspiration pneumonia occurs because of aspiration of esophageal secretions. To prevent respiratory complications, good pulmonary toilet is maintained. Balloon migration into the esophagus or airway can result in possible asphyxia and death. Esophageal perforation is a rare complication in children and is considered a surgical emergency.

Sclerotherapy is the current primary treatment of acute variceal bleeding in children.[109] The procedure is performed under general anesthesia through a flexible fiberoptic endoscope. A fine needle attached to a catheter is passed through the biopsy channel of the endoscope. After identifying the varices, the endoscopist injects the sclerosing agent into the varix or the surrounding tissue. The sclerosing agent rapidly induces thrombosis and sclerosis of the vein, and does minimal damage to the esophageal mucosa and muscle.

A complication of sclerotherapy is hemorrhage. The bleeding is often self-limiting, but it may be as severe as the original episode. Some oozing is to be expected after the procedure. Fever is a common complication, and alone is rarely considered serious. A persistent fever may indicate a bacteremia that is potentially lethal in the debilitated patient. Intense pain may indicate an erosion or perforation of the esophagus but, fortunately, is rarely seen.

The use of sucralfate after sclerotherapy for gastric cytoprotection has become common practice. Sucralfate has been demonstrated to be effective in the treatment of esophagitis with minimal side effects, by acting locally to form a protective barrier and increasing cytoprotection by

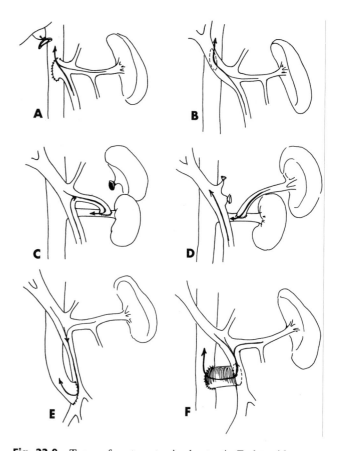

Fig. 22-9 Types of portosystemic shunts. **A,** End-to-side portocaval (all portal flow is diverted to systemic circulation). **B,** Side-to-side portocaval (the major direction of portal flow is to the systemic circulation, but the capacity for hepatic portal perfusion is retained, depending on the resistance within the liver. **C,** Proximal splenorenal (the principal direction of portal flow is to the systemic circulation; placing the shunt centrally minimizes the angulation of the splenic vein). **D,** Distal splenorenal (major direction of portal flow is to systemic circulation). **E,** Mesocaval (vena cava is transected and proximal cava is anastomosed to side of superior mesenteric vein. Major direction of visceral flow is toward vena cava). **F,** Interposition mesocaval (hemodynamically similar to mesocaval shunt. Autogenous vein graft is preferred for creation of this shunt in infants and children. (From Karrer F, Lilly JR, Hall RJ: Biliary tract disorders and portal hypertension. In KW Ashcraft, TM Holder, eds: *Pediatric surgery,* ed 2, Philadelphia, 1993, WB Saunders.)

stimulating prostaglandins and inactivating pepsin.[54,110] In addition, an H_2 blocker, such as ranitidine, is administered to decrease gastric acid secretion.

Surgical options are considered if medical therapy is ineffective. Shunting procedures divert the blood flow from the liver and allow for decompression of the portal system. Portacaval and splenorenal shunts are effective and control hemorrhage from esophageal varices (Fig. 22-9). In children, mesocaval and central splenorenal shunts have been successful even in very small infants. It was previously believed that the vessels needed for successful anastomosis and patent shunt were too small until a child was at least 7 years of age. It now seems that neither age nor size is a limitation to a successful shunt.[111]

Liver transplantation is a consideration for children with portal hypertension resulting from liver diseases known to progress to liver failure and death. Liver transplantation is discussed in Chapter 26.

ABDOMINAL WALL DEFECTS

Omphalocele and Gastroschisis

Omphalocele is a midline, umbilical defect of the ventral abdominal wall in which the intestines herniate into a sac consisting of peritoneum and amnion. Omphaloceles vary in size and can be extremely large, containing the entire midgut (distal duodenum, jejunum, ileum, ascending colon, and first portion of the transverse colon), liver, and spleen. The abdomen is, in this situation, small and scaphoid. If the sac remains intact, the appearance of the bowel may be fairly normal. Unfortunately in some cases the sac ruptures, leaving the organs exposed to the amniotic fluid or to the environment after birth.

Gastroschisis is an abdominal wall defect that usually occurs to the right of a normal umbilical cord. There is no sac covering the defect and the bowel usually appears thick, foreshortened, hemorrhagic, and matted. The defect is usually small and contains only the bowel. The clinical differences between gastroschisis and omphalocele are shown in Table 22-11.

Pathogenesis. The abdominal wall begins to develop by the fourth week of intrauterine life and is formed from cephalic, caudal, and lateral folds. Each of these folds is composed of somatic and splanchnic layers. It is theorized that if there is a failure of the normal embryonic folding and fusing of the somatic layers of the lateral folds, the anterior abdominal wall will not close completely.[112]

Omphalocele is thought to occur when the abdominal wall does not form completely as the midgut elongates out through the yolk sac, resulting in failure of the intestines to return to the abdominal cavity. There are many theories about the embryologic events resulting in gastroschisis, the most plausible explanation is that of Shaw.[113] The developing embryo initially has both a left and right umbilical vein as well as two arteries. By the eleventh week of gestation the right umbilical vein has been obliterated, leaving a weakness at this site in the abdominal wall. It is theorized that this weakness of the abdominal wall allows a rupture of the

lateral umbilical ring with bowel protruding through the defect, thus resulting in a gastroschisis.

Associated Abnormalities. Associated defects are more common with omphalocele than with gastroschisis. These can be divided into midline defects related to the failure of closure of the embryologic folds, chromosomal abnormalities, and other isolated abnormalities. Pentalogy of Cantrell occurs with the defective cephalic fold. This collection of defects includes intracardiac anomalies, ectopia cordis, sternal cleft, midline diaphragmatic hernia, and upper abdominal omphalocele. Lower midline abnormalities are related to defects in the caudal embryonic fold. These may include one or more of the following: cloacal exstrophy (severe abdominal wall defect also exposing the bladder), imperforate anus, colonic atresia, sacral vertebral abnormalities, and meningomyelocele. Omphalocele has been identified as a component of the Bechwith-Wiedemann syndrome. Chromosomal abnormalities, including trisomy 13 through 15, 16 through 18, and 21, many of which are incompatible with life, appear in approximately one third of patients with omphalocele, and cardiac malformations are present in up to 50%.[114] The most common cardiac defect is tetralogy of Fallot.

Clinical Presentation. Antenatal diagnosis of abdominal wall defects can usually be determined by ultrasound at approximately the fifteenth week of gestation. This

TABLE 22-11   Clinical Differential Diagnosis

Factor	Gastroschisis	Omphalocele
Location	Lateral to cord	Umbilical ring
Size of defect	Less than 4 cm	2-10 cm
Umbilical cord	Normal insertion	Inserts in sac
Sac	None	Present
Contents	Bowel, stomach	Bowel, liver, spleen, bladder, uterus, ovaries
Bowel appearance	Matted, fore-shortened	Normal
Malrotation	Present	Present
Small abdominal cavity	Present	Present
Associated anomalies	Unusual (15% atresia of the gut)	Common (37%-67%) GI, genito-urinary, CNS, cardiovascular, musculoskeletal
Coexisting syndromes	Not observed	Beckwith syndrome, cloaca, trisomy 13-15, trisomy 16-18, exstrophy of the bladder, pentalogy of Cantrell

Modified from Grosfeld JL, Weber TR: Congenital abdominal wall defects: gastroschisis and omphalocele, *Curr Probl Surg* 19:165, 1982.

prenatal determination assists the obstetrician to make a decision regarding transfer of the mother to a tertiary care setting. A cesarean section is usually indicated to prevent rupture of the sac or damage to the exposed viscera. If the defect has not been recognized before delivery, it is easily seen at birth, and thus treatment begins quickly.

Critical Care Management. If a sac is present, care is taken to prevent rupture. The defect is usually covered with sterile gauze and wrapped in a figure-of-eight bandage to prevent pressure on the exposed viscera. There are two options for managing the exposed viscera. A saline-soaked gauze pad covered with occlusive plastic dressing or a bowel bag that covers the child's legs and abdomen, or dry gauze soaked with saline before removal may be used. These options prevent radiant heat loss that can occur with saline-soaked gauze alone.

Respiratory assessment and stabilization are critical, especially in the preterm infant in whom assisted ventilation may be necessary. This is accomplished with endotracheal intubation. Any mask or blow-by ventilation allows excess air to enter the GI tract and should be avoided.

Gastric decompression is essential to empty the stomach and prevent GI distension. Active decompression is accomplished with intermittent or continual suctioning, using a large-bore NG or OG tube. Comfortable positioning also calms the infant and prevents excessive crying and air swallowing. The head of the crib is elevated when possible to facilitate drainage.

Fluids are administered at twice maintenance requirement because of the fluid loss from the exposed bowel. Antibiotics are administered and the child is prepared for the operating room. As part of the preoperative workup, assessment of associated anomalies is completed. Part of this workup may be delayed until after surgery, but the cardiac examination is completed before surgery, as well as evaluation of any anomalies that may require emergency surgical care.

Operative Management. Omphalocele and gastroschisis are repaired using one of two surgical approaches: a primary closure or a staged repair. The primary closure involves removing the sac from an intact omphalocele, and opening the defect circumferentially. The bowel is examined for areas of atresia or perforation. The abdominal wall is stretched, and the viscera are carefully placed into the abdominal cavity. Attempts to correct the malrotation are not performed. The primary closure is successful if the defect is small and the infant does not have other major problems. With the primary closure, care is taken to avoid compromise of respiratory status resulting from marked elevation of the diaphragm, compression of the vena cava resulting in impaired venous return, and impaired intestinal blood supply. During the surgical procedure, when a primary closure is being attempted, careful communication with the anesthesiologist is essential to evaluate difficulty with ventilation or perfusion. If either is significant, the primary closure is aborted and a staged repair is done.

A staged repair is the procedure of choice for a large defect, especially one in which the liver is involved. With this technique, a single layer of Silastic material is sutured to the abdominal wall around the defect and the viscera that

remains herniated. Over the next 7 to 10 days, the defect is slowly reduced, usually on a daily basis by squeezing down on the top of the Silastic silo, which pushes a small portion of the contents of the defect into the abdominal cavity.[115,116] During this process, the infant is maintained on intravenous antibiotics and the silo is bathed in an antibiotic solution. When the defect is almost completely reduced, the infant returns to the operating room for final closure. This process of slowly reducing the defect needs to be completed within 1 to 2 weeks or there is significant risk of wound infection. Regardless of surgical technique, the length of hospitalization, parenteral nutrition requirements, and rate of complications are similar.[116]

Postoperative Management. The goal of postoperative management includes maintaining a normothermic environment; restoration of fluid and electrolyte balance; provision of nutrition; and prevention of respiratory, circulatory, GI, and infectious complications. On return from the operating room, the infant is placed in an isolette or warmer bed to maintain normal temperature. Mechanical ventilation may be necessary regardless of whether a primary or staged repair is done. With primary closure, respiratory insufficiency is due to the significant pressure on the diaphragm from the expanded abdominal cavity. Between staged surgeries, the infant may have little need for ventilatory support but may require mechanical ventilation immediately after the reduction. Therefore the patient is often maintained on low ventilatory settings until the defect is completely closed.

The possibility of vascular compromise requires that the lower extremities be assessed for color and capillary refill. Pedal pulses are checked frequently. Elevating the infant's legs may facilitate venous return. The infant will have third space fluid loss, requiring twice-maintenance fluids and the administration of albumin to prevent intravascular hypovolemia.

Nutritional support is initially provided with TPN, but within 4 to 6 weeks, even those infants with a staged repair can begin elemental enteral feedings. The infant is observed for signs of feeding intolerance, including increased gastric residuals, abdominal girth, vomiting, and stool volume, and presence of reducing substances in stool sample.

Survival of those with omphalocele is largely related to the coexisting congenital anomalies, often necessitating other surgeries. Infants with gastroschisis, however, have increased incidence of residual bowel disease requiring reoperation in 25% of cases.[116] In addition, an increased incidence of GER has been observed in both gastroschisis and omphalocele patients on follow-up.[117]

HEPATIC FAILURE

Hepatic failure is the consequence of severe hepatocyte injury or dysfunction resulting in multisystem complications, which include encephalopathy, cerebral edema, coagulopathy, renal failure, and hemodynamic instability. The injury to the liver may be acute, resulting in fulminant injury to the hepatocytes and rapid development of the clinical signs of hepatic failure, without preexisting evidence of liver disease. Fulminant hepatic failure (FHF) results in rapid clinical deterioration. In other instances, hepatic failure is the result of chronic injury that has accumulated to cause serious compromise of hepatic function and results in end-stage disease. Regardless of the cause, the consequences and therapeutic modalities are the same. It is important that the clinical course of hepatic failure and the prognostic indicators be identified early to determine if spontaneous hepatic regeneration and recovery are likely with supportive therapies. Supportive therapies have been shown to be unsuccessful in those patients with clinical parameters suggesting progressive disease. Liver transplantation is the treatment of choice in these patients.[118,119]

Etiology

Hepatic failure is rare in childhood. The causes of hepatic dysfunction and failure in infants and children are divided into two categories: fulminant failure and failure from chronic liver disease. The incidence of any one etiology of liver failure is difficult to assess. One pediatric center reported 81 children dying of hepatic failure between 1976 and 1983.[120] Biliary atresia accounted for 20 cases, metabolic disorders (tyrosinemia, cystic fibrosis, α_1-antitrypsin deficiency, Wilson's disease, Zellweger syndrome) accounted for 22, and infectious causes were responsible for 15 cases. Cholestatic liver disease (Alagille's syndrome, TPN-associated disease) accounted for 12. Miscellaneous causes were cited for the remaining 5 cases.

The pediatric causes of liver disease are dependent on the age of the child.[121,122] In the neonate, biliary atresia and idiopathic hepatitis are the most common causes. In infants, metabolic causes (galactosemia, glycogen storage disease, tyrosinemia), except for Wilson's disease, occur more often. In older children, especially adolescents, chemical or acetaminophen intoxication, viral hepatitis, and Wilson's disease are more typical.

Biliary Atresia. Biliary atresia is the result of a progressive, idiopathic inflammatory process affecting the intrahepatic and extrahepatic bile ducts. This inflammatory process results in complete obliteration of the biliary tract. Obstruction to bile flow causes cholestasis and progressive fibrosis with eventual end-stage cirrhosis. Biliary atresia occurs in approximately 1 in 15,000 live births.[123] It can result in the development of end-stage liver disease within the first year of life and remains the leading indication for liver transplantation in children.[124] There are two forms of biliary atresia. The fetal type occurs in 10% to 35% of patients and is associated with congenital malformations and anomalies.[123] In this type of biliary atresia, there is no jaundice-free interval between the end of physiologic jaundice of the newborn and the onset of cholestasis.

The more common type of biliary atresia presents at 4 to 8 weeks of life with persistent cholestasis and jaundice and occurs in 65% to 90% of all cases.[123] These infants usually have a normal birth history, passed normal meconium stools, and had a jaundice-free interval.

Many etiologic agents have been explored. Biliary atresia is not thought to be an inherited disorder, although there are case reports of reoccurrences in families.[125,126] The role of viral infections as an etiologic mechanism has

been postulated. Preliminary studies have shown an association of biliary atresia and rotavirus but require further investigation.[127]

Infants with biliary atresia are generally full-term and appear healthy despite being jaundiced. The gestational history is unremarkable. Appetite and weight gain are initially normal, but stools progressively become pale and acholic (white, lacking bile pigment) during the first weeks of life. The infant initially may have physiologic unconjugated jaundice progressing to a conjugated hyperbilirubinemia. This is generally recognized between 4 and 8 weeks of age when the urine becomes dark and the stools acholic. The total serum bilirubin is between 6 and 12 mg/dl, with approximately 50% being conjugated.[128] Serum aminotransferases are mildly elevated, whereas ALP and GGT are markedly elevated. Physical examination may reveal hepatomegaly and, infrequently, splenomegaly.

No single test confirms the diagnosis of biliary atresia. An abdominal ultrasound is performed to exclude other causes of obstructive jaundice such as choledochal cyst. The patency of the extrahepatic biliary system is demonstrated by a nuclear scintiscan (HIDA scan). Evidence of radioactivity in the duodenum confirms a patent biliary system, thus eliminating the possibility of biliary atresia. When there is no evidence of excretion with the HIDA scan, further diagnostic evaluation is necessary in the form of a percutaneous liver biopsy. The histologic finding of intrahepatic bile duct proliferation suggests a mechanical obstruction, indicating the need for laparotomy and operative cholangiogram. If the extrahepatic system cannot be demonstrated by cholangiogram, surgical intervention is necessary.

The most common surgical procedure performed to establish bile flow is the Kasai hepatoportoenterostomy (Fig. 22-10). The residual biliary system is removed. The surface of the liver is dissected and an area through which bile can drain is exposed. A limb of jejunum is made into

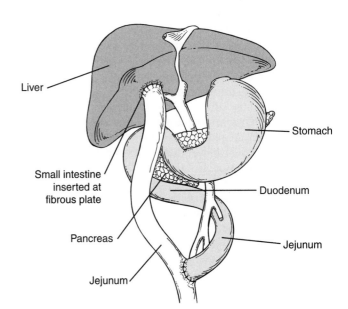

Fig. 22-10 Schematic representation of a hepatic portoenterostomy (Kasai procedure) providing bile drainage in a case of extrahepatic biliary atresia.

a Roux-en-Y intestinal conduit to maintain the patency of the intestine. Success of the procedure varies, depending on the age of the infant at the time of surgery and the center performing the surgery, with one fourth to one half of patients having inadequate drainage despite the surgical intervention. Improved outcomes have been shown when surgical intervention is performed before 2 months of age.[129]

The two postoperative problems of consequence are failure to establish bile flow and ascending cholangitis. Ascending cholangitis is a frequent and severe complication of a successful operation, occurring in 50% to 100% of patients with established bile flow after a Kasai procedure.[129] Surgical and medical approaches have been attempted to decrease the incidence of ascending cholangitis. Surgical modifications of the Kasai procedure have not had great success. Medical approaches include choleretic agents to improve bile flow, postoperative antibiotics, and long-term prophylactic oral antibiotics, all with limited success.

Long-term prognosis is guarded in infants with biliary atresia. Establishment of bile flow and resolution of the jaundice appears to be correlated with the best outcome. Patients who remain jaundiced experience hepatic failure between the ages of 2 and 10 years of age and require a liver transplant. Those with established bile flow and resolution of jaundice have a 90% chance of surviving past age 10 years. Survival to the third decade with a high quality of life has been reported.[130,131]

Arteriohepatic Dysplasia. Arteriohepatic dysplasia (Alagille's syndrome or syndromatic bile duct paucity) is characterized by a marked reduction of intrahepatic bile ducts and chronic cholestasis. It occurs in association with cardiac, vertebral, ocular, facial (frontal bossing, deep-set eyes, beaked nose, and pointed chin are typical facies), renal, and neurodevelopmental abnormalities. It is the most common form of familial intrahepatic cholestasis, with a wide variation in clinical symptoms in affected individuals.[132] The estimated incidence of Alagille's syndrome is 1 in 40,000 births.[129] It is a genetic disorder inherited as an autosomal-dominant trait, with the defective gene appearing to be on chromosome 20.[133] However, the majority of patients have no family history.

The number of interlobular bile ducts is often not decreased on initial liver biopsy in infants with Alagille's syndrome.[128] Over a variable period of months to years, the intrahepatic ducts are lost and the condition becomes more definable. Progressive liver disease develops in 10% to 20% of patients with Alagille's disease.[129] There is no way of predicting the progression of significant pathology. The cause of the bile duct paucity is unknown.[129] It has been suggested that an inability to secrete bile is related to the bile duct loss in Alagille's disease. The relationship of the liver disease to other systemic manifestations is unknown. Structural lesions involving the heart, eyes, kidneys, skeletal system, and genitalia are well described.

Alagille's syndrome generally presents in the first 3 months of life in the symptomatic patient. It is among the more common causes for cholestasis and jaundice in the newborn period and must be distinguished from biliary atresia and choledochal cyst. Nonsymptomatic adults are commonly undiagnosed until a related child with symptoms is identified. Biochemically, infants with Alagille's syndrome have moderately to markedly elevated bilirubin, ALP, GGT, and 5'-nucleotidase. There may also be mild to moderate elevations in serum transaminases. These elevations may persist through childhood. Serum triglyceride and cholesterol levels may be extremely elevated. Hepatomegaly is present in nearly all patients, whereas splenomegaly is rare initially.

Jaundice is present in the majority of patients with symptomatic disease. Pruritus is severe but rarely present before 3 to 5 months of age. Xanthomas resulting from cholestasis appear on the extensor surfaces of the fingers, palmar creases, nape of the neck, buttocks, and inguinal area. The formation of xanthomas is related to the severity of the cholestasis and correlates with elevated serum cholesterol levels. Diminished bile salt excretion results in fat malabsorption and deficiency of fat-soluble vitamins, which has profound systemic effects. Growth failure is common with delayed pubertal development. Progression of the disease to cirrhosis and hepatic failure was initially believed to be an uncommon event that is now being recognized more often.

Treatment goals include optimizing nutrition, preventing or correcting of fat-soluble vitamin deficiencies, and relieving pruritus and xanthomas. Infants may require specialized formulas with medium-chain triglycerides as the major fat component for improved absorption. Some infants may require continuous feeding to optimize caloric needs. Vitamins A, D, E, and K supplementation is often required secondary to fat-soluble vitamin malabsorption. Cholestyramine, a bile salt-binding resin, may be helpful in relieving associated pruritus. Surgical intervention is not effective. A small number of children progress to end-stage liver disease and benefit from liver transplantation.[131]

α_1-Antitrypsin Deficiency. α_1-Antitrypsin deficiency is the most common metabolic disease in children requiring liver transplantation. It is an autosomal-recessive disorder, specifically the mutant α_1-antitrypsin Z molecule. This molecule is synthesized normally but is retained within the endoplasmic reticulum of the hepatocyte. Although the pathogenesis still remains unclear, it is theorized that the accumulation of α_1-antitrypsin in the endoplasmic reticulum is directly related to the liver cell injury.[134] The consequences include premature pulmonary emphysema and chronic liver disease in infants and children. In the United States, the prevalence has been described as 1 in 2000 individuals. It is more common among Caucasians of Northern European ancestry.[135]

Infants with α_1-antitrypsin deficiency generally present in the first 2 months of life with persistent jaundice. The serum transaminases are slightly elevated and the liver may be enlarged. The liver disease may also be discovered later in childhood or adolescence with hepatosplenomegaly, ascites, or hemorrhage from esophageal varices. Many of these children experience progressive liver dysfunction requiring transplantation. The diagnosis is confirmed with a low (<70 mg/dl) serum α_1 concentration level and the

◆ **TABLE 22-12** **Clinical Profile of Viral Hepatitis**

Virus	Transmission	Active Immunization	Passive Immunization	Chronicity	Incubation Period
HAV	Fecal-oral, parenteral rare	Yes	Yes	No	15-49 days
HBV	Perinatal, sexual, parenteral	Yes	Yes	Common	60-180 days
HCV	Parenteral, perinatal rare, sexual infrequent	No	No	Common	14-160 days
HDV	Parenteral, sexual, perinatal rare	Indirect, against HBV	Indirect, against HBV	Common	21-42 days
HEV	Fecal-oral	No	No	No	21-63 days

From Fishman LN, Jonas MM, Lavine JE: Update on viral hepatitis in children, *Pediatr Clin North Am* 43:58, 1996.

determination of the α_1-antitrypsin phenotype (PiZZ).[136] α_1-Antitrypsin is an acute phase protein synthesized in the liver and will rise with tissue injury, inflammation, or infection. Therefore children with α_1-antitrypsin deficiency who suffer from pneumonia (for example) may have falsely normal levels during the acute illness.

There is no specific therapy for liver disease associated with α_1-antitrypsin deficiency. Children with progressive liver failure have been treated with liver transplantation.[137]

Wilson's Disease. Wilson's disease is an autosomal-recessive disorder of copper metabolism in which biliary excretion of copper is inadequate and the excess accumulates in the liver, brain, kidneys, cornea, and skeletal system. The disease has been recognized for approximately 60 years; however, the biochemical defect has yet to be identified. Hepatic disease occurs when the copper overload leads to the destruction of liver tissue. It occurs in 1 in 30,000 individuals.[136]

The clinical symptoms of Wilson's disease rarely present before the age of 6 years, more often in the second decade. Hepatic dysfunction is the most common presentation in children; however, the diagnosis is considered in older children and adolescents with a neurologic abnormality. Symptoms may be subtle initially and include malaise, anorexia, and lethargy. Signs of progressive liver disease such as jaundice, petechiae, hematemesis, and ascites may also be present at diagnosis. Presentation with fulminant hepatitis with progression to liver failure requiring transplantation does occur. Neurologic symptoms include gradual onset of clumsiness, dysarthria, drooling, tremors, loss of fine motor skills, and psychologic disturbances. Kayser-Fleischer rings, a greenish pigment encircling the cornea, (the result of copper deposits) is considered diagnostic of Wilson's disease. Its absence, however, does not rule it out.

The diagnosis of Wilson's disease may be difficult. The majority of children with Wilson's disease have a low serum level of the copper-binding protein ceruloplasmin, implying a homozygosity (disease state) or heterozygosity (carrier state). Urinary copper excretion is usually elevated. An ophthalmologic examination for Kayser-Fleischer rings is necessary. A liver biopsy may be necessary to determine the amount of copper in the liver. Asymptomatic siblings should also be screened for Wilson's disease. Treatment of Wilson's disease is aimed at improving the excretion of copper

through chelation with penicillamine and decreasing dietary intake of copper-containing foods.

Infection. Fulminant hepatic failure (FHF) is the syndrome of acute liver failure complicated by the development of hepatic encephalopathy within 8 weeks of the initial symptoms of liver disease without a history of previous or underlying liver dysfunction.[118,138] Early recognition is essential because a delay in diagnosis and treatment can often lead to a grave prognosis.

Viral hepatitis is the most common infectious cause of FHF.[138,139] Each of the five primary hepatotropic (affecting the liver) viruses (A through E) has been implicated in acute liver failure. Other agents (F, G), not yet identified, can also be responsible for clinically evident hepatitis.[140] Table 22-12 highlights the clinical profile of the viral hepatitis agents.

Hepatitis A virus (HAV) is a self-limited enteric infection and rarely leads to hepatic failure in children.[118,138] However, there are reports of HAV causing fulminant disease in intravenous drug users and the elderly.[118] HAV infection is diagnosed by the presence of anti-HAV IgM antibodies in the serum. The presence of anti-HAV IgG antibodies in the serum without anti-HAV IgM reflects immunity or past resolved infection.

Hepatitis B virus (HBV) is the most common form of hepatitis causing FHF worldwide.[139] HBV has been reported to cause FHF in infants vertically infected from their mothers and in older children from blood transfusions.[141] Fortunately, the number of reported cases is decreasing in the United States, which is most likely the result of a heightened awareness of associated risk factors and vaccination of high-risk groups.[138,142] The diagnosis of HBV infection is made by the presence of hepatitis B surface antigen (HBsAg) and hepatitis B core antibody IgM (anti-HBc IgM) in the serum. IgM antibody to hepatitis B core antigen must be present to differentiate between acute and chronic infection.

Hepatitis C virus (HCV), also known as non-A non-B hepatitis, has recently been implicated as a causative agent in FHF, although this presentation is rare.[143] The diagnosis is made by the presence of antibody to multiple HCV antigens (anti-HCV) in the serum.

Hepatitis D virus (HDV), or delta agent, requires the presence of coexisting HBV infection for its replication. Superinfection with HDV can lead to FHF.[139] The diagnosis of HDV infection is made by the presence of antibody to HDV (anti-HDV) in the serum.

Hepatitis E virus (HEV) is a self-limited enterically transmitted infection that rarely causes FHF.[139] The diagnosis is made by the presence of antibody to HEV (anti-HEV) in the serum.

Other viral agents that may cause FHF include Herpes simplex virus (HSV), Epstein-Barr virus (EBV), and Cytomegalovirus (CMV) but are more frequently seen in neonates or immunocompromised patients. HSV infection may be acquired at any one of three times: in utero, intrapartum, or postnatally. Neonates commonly exhibit disseminated disease in the first week of life with signs of multiple organ involvement. Clinical findings include irritability, seizures, respiratory distress, jaundice, coagulopathy, and shock. Viral recovery in the blood, cerebrospinal fluid, and bodily secretions may be difficult. Antiviral treatment is often administered based on clinical presentation, EEG, and MRI findings.

EBV is the principal cause of infectious mononucleosis but is also responsible for significant disease in immunocompromised children.[144] Clinical findings typically include exudative pharyngitis, lymphadenopathy, hepatosplenomegaly, atypical lymphocytosis on complete blood count, and elevated serum transaminases. The diagnosis is confirmed by the detection of EBV-specific antibodies in the serum.

CMV infections occur primarily in newborns and immunocompromised patients. The newborn presents with hepatosplenomegaly, jaundice, and less frequently purpura. The immunocompromised child typically contacts the virus after an organ transplant. The source of infection may be from the grafted organ, transfused blood products, or reactivation of a latent infection. Diagnosis is made with the CMV antigenemia serum test.

Less frequent viral agents that may cause FHF include adenovirus, enterovirus, parvovirus, and varicella-zoster virus. Immune deficiency is suspected when these viruses cause severe hepatic failure. Diagnoses are made by specific serologic or histologic analysis or by culture of blood, urine, stool, or liver tissue.

Drug-Induced Hepatic Failure. In children, drug-induced liver injury represents 15% to 20% of cases of FHF.[145] Drugs most commonly linked with hepatic failure are acetaminophen, anticonvulsants (phenytoin, valproate), halothane anesthesia, and isoniazid (INH).[146] Hepatitis may be caused by a direct injury or idiosyncratic process. Acetaminophen ingestion is an example of an agent that causes direct injury and can occur when taken in large single doses (exceeding 140 mg/kg). Agents that cause an idiosyncratic reaction (i.e., phenytoin, valproic acid, halothane) are thought to be the result of an immune-mediated hypersensitivity response and/or a reaction to the metabolites of the ingested agent.[146]

Consequences of Hepatic Failure

In children with hepatic disease, ongoing damage results in decreased function, which includes the metabolic and detoxification processes of the liver. The Kupffer cells' phagocytic process is significantly diminished with hepatic failure, resulting in decreased filtration of blood and placing the child at increased risk for infections. Decreased bile salt synthesis results in fat malabsorption. In children, fat accounts for a large percentage of calories consumed. Malnutrition and malabsorption of fat-soluble vitamins A, D, E, and K result. Vitamin A stores are long lasting, approximately to 2 years; thus a deficiency must be long-standing before ill effects are noted. Failure to absorb vitamin D results in demineralization of the bone leading to osteomalacia, rickets, and pathologic fractures. Vitamin E malabsorption has neurologic consequences, such as peripheral neuropathies and diminished deep tendon reflexes. Vitamin K deficiencies result in coagulopathies, which are discussed later in this section. Excessive accumulation of bile salts resulting from decreased extraction through the liver results in their deposition in the skin, causing intractable pruritus. Cholestasis (biliary obstruction) causes direct hyperbilirubinemia and jaundice.

The liver is crucial in the process of carbohydrate metabolism. Initially, serum glucose levels are elevated, but glycogen stores are decreased. If the liver is unable to store glycogen or generate new glucose, the kidneys assume the process of gluconeogenesis. As the hepatic failure progresses, hypoglycemia becomes a problem.

Protein metabolism is altered in hepatic failure. Altered albumin synthesis results in low serum albumin levels. Without adequate levels, the body is unable to maintain oncotic pressure. Consequently, fluid leaks from the blood vessels into the abdominal cavity and tissues, resulting in ascites and edema.

The liver's ability to manufacture clotting factors is impaired. Vitamin K absorption is influenced by the decreased synthesis of bile salts resulting in a decreased production of vitamin K-dependent clotting factors II, VII, IX, and X. Alterations in hemostasis are evidenced by prolonged prothrombin time, easy bruising, and bleeding.

A failing liver is also unable to remove activated clotting factors from the circulating serum. Hepatic necrosis causes an inflammatory response, thus activating clotting factors. Once activated, clotting factors circulate in the plasma, form microthrombi, and consume platelets and fibrinogen. Disseminated intravascular coagulation (DIC) results when fibrinolysis occurs and the liver is unable to synthesize clotting factors.

The liver's inability to detoxify hormones, drugs, and other harmful compounds results in a variety of clinical manifestations. Continued circulation of aldosterone and ADH contributes to the development of ascites and hepatorenal syndrome. Hepatorenal syndrome is a progressive renal failure directly related to liver disease. The mechanism causing the renal failure is unknown. The use of medications metabolized by the liver is avoided. In addition, with evidence of renal dysfunction, medications excreted by the kidneys are adjusted based on calculated creatinine clearance.

Complications of Hepatic Failure

Hepatic Encephalopathy. Hepatic encephalopathy is the change in mental status that accompanies hepatic failure. The encephalopathic agent responsible for these changes has not yet been identified. Generally it is assumed to be due to hyperammonemia; however, some patients with obvious hepatic encephalopathy have normal serum ammonia levels. The appearance of hepatic encephalopathy is variable. It depends on the extent of the liver damage, speed of injury, degree of portal-systemic shunting, and contributing factors. The child with FHF may progress to coma and unresponsiveness very rapidly, over several days, whereas the child with chronic liver disease may have intermittent alterations in mental status becoming more severe over time. Some children with chronic liver disease do well until a major insult occurs, such as a variceal hemorrhage, or until an infection precipitates the onset of encephalopathic changes.

Hepatic encephalopathy is traditionally divided into five stages, which are outlined in Table 22-13. Passage through the stages may be rapid. It is important to monitor the progression so that therapeutic support can be escalated. In cases of chronic liver dysfunction, the deterioration may be subtle. Changes in behavior, school performance, and handwriting are the most commonly noticed symptoms.

Four hypotheses postulate the pathophysiology of hepatic encephalopathy. No single hypothesis completely explains the process.[122] The *ammonia* hypothesis suggests that ammonia accumulation in the brain results in encephalopathic changes. The *synergistic neurotoxins* hypothesis suggests that encephalopathy and coma are a result of accumulating toxins with synergistic effects augmented by other metabolic abnormalities. An excessive production of the brain inhibitory neurotransmitter, serotonin, and the false neurotransmitter, octopamine, accompanied by a deficient synthesis of excitatory neurotransmitters, norepinephrine and dopamine, result in encephalopathy and coma and are the basis of the *false neurotransmitter* hypothesis. The final hypothesis is the activation of the gamma-aminobutyric acid *(GABA)–benzodiazepine inhibitory neurotransmitter.* GABA, the principal inhibitory neurotransmitter of the brain, is normally degraded in the liver;

◆ TABLE 22-13   Clinical Staging of Hepatic Encephalopathy

Category of Physical Signs	Stage I	Stage II	Stage III	Stage IV	Stage V
Mental status	Alert, oriented, slow mentation	Lethargic, confused, agitated	Stupor, arousal to voice	Unarousable	Unarousable
Behavior	Restless, irritable, short attention span, disordered sleep	Combative, sullen, euphoric	Sleeps most of time, marked confusion	None	None
Spontaneous motor activity	Incoordination, tremor, poor handwriting	Yawning, sucking, grimacing, intention tremor present, blinking	Decreased, marked intention tremor	Absent	None
Asterixis	Absent	Present	Present (if cooperates)	Absent	Absent
Muscle tone	Normal	Increased	Increased	Increased	Flaccid
Reflexes	Normal	Hyper-reflexic	Hyper-reflexic extensor plantars	Hyper-reflexic extensor plantars	Absent
Respirations	Regular or hyperventilation	Hyperventilation	Hyperventilation	Irregular	Apnea
Verbal response	Normal	Confused, dysarthric	Incoherent	None	None
Motor response	Obeys commands	Purposeful movements, may not respond to commands	Localized appropriately to pain	Abnormal flexor, abnormal extensor posturing	None
Pupils	Brisk	Brisk	Brisk	Sluggish	Fixed
Eye opening	Spontaneous	Verbal stimuli	Verbal stimuli	Noxious stimuli	None
Oculocephalic	Normal	Normal	Normal	Partial dysconjugate	Absent
Oculovestibular	Normal	Normal	Normal	Partial dysconjugate	Absent

From Treem WR: Hepatic failure. In Walker WA et al, eds: *Pediatric gastrointestinal diseases: pathophysiology, diagnosis, management,* Toronto, 1991, B.C. Decker. Reprinted by permission of Mosby.

however, during liver failure this process fails to occur, resulting in increased circulation of receptors.

Hepatic encephalopathy occurs as liver destruction progresses. The blood flow from the intestine is shunted around the liver completely, bypassing viable hepatocytes. Consequently, the filtration process of the liver does not occur. It is also believed that alterations in the function of the blood-brain barrier contribute to the development of hepatic encephalopathy. The blood-brain barrier is essential in preventing toxic substances in the systemic circulation from entering the brain.

Cerebral Edema. Cerebral edema is the major cause of mortality in patients with FHF, unlike chronic liver disease. The rapid increase in the water content of the brain in acute liver failure occurs from an alteration in the blood-brain permeability. Cerebral edema raises intracranial pressure (ICP) and can result in cerebral ischemia if not recognized and treated promptly. Therefore ICP monitoring is performed in some PICUs when patients reach stage III encephalopathy.

Impaired Coagulation. The liver is the site of synthesis for most of the coagulation factors (II, V, VII, IX, X), fibrinolytic agents, and inhibitors of coagulation. With the onset of hepatic failure, there are significant alterations in the coagulation process. Prothrombin time is often prolonged and is unresponsive to vitamin K. Coagulation factors are reduced; however, factor V, which is vitamin K *independent,* may be the most sensitive single indicator of outcome of FHF.[147] Factor V has a half-life of 12 to 24 hours; therefore a rapid decrease in this level reflects impaired synthesis resulting from rapidly developing hepatocellular injury. Fibrinogen levels are also reduced because of decreased synthesis and increased consumption. Thrombocytopenia is present, commonly less than 100,000 per cubic millimeter. Thrombocytopenia may be the result of platelet sequestration as a consequence of hypersplenism, or platelet-associated antibodies as seen in chronic active hepatitis, or DIC. With these coagulation abnormalities, patients with hepatic failure are at an increased risk for major hemorrhage, most commonly originating in the GI tract or the brain, potentially resulting in death.

Hepatorenal Syndrome. Oliguria is common in both acute and chronic liver failure. Hepatorenal syndrome is defined as unexplained progressive renal dysfunction without obvious histologic lesions. It is characterized by significant sodium retention without urinary sodium. Urinary sediment is present but without protein, cells, or casts, and the oliguria is unresponsive to intravascular volume expansion. Hepatorenal syndrome accounts for the majority of renal impairment in FHF and is often associated with a fatal outcome.[148]

Critical Care Management

The management of FHF is largely supportive therapy that requires a multisystem approach. Therapeutic measures are used to treat the complications of hepatic failure, including those outlined above plus metabolic derangements, hemodynamic instability, and respiratory dysfunction.

The laboratory evaluation of FHF is extremely broad and includes diagnostic tests to determine cause, assess liver function, and to assess function of other organs. The nurse plays a vital role in monitoring these laboratory values and performing serial assessments. Neurologic assessment is extremely vital for the detection of worsening encephalopathy and increased ICP and is initially performed every hour. The patient will also require emergent invasive hemodynamic monitoring and therapeutic measures. Frequently, these patients require intubation and mechanical ventilation to protect their airway. Routine care includes placement of a Foley catheter, strict intake and output, and appropriate isolation techniques if infectious etiology is suspected.

The patient is made NPO, and an NG tube is placed with evidence of GI bleeding or in the patient with stage III or IV encephalopathy. An H_2 blocker, such as ranitidine, is administered to prevent stress ulcers. The dose is adjusted based on evidence of renal dysfunction. An antacid is also administered with pH lower than 4.0. TPN is initiated when the patient is hemodynamically stable. However, the solution should contain a low amino acid concentration and trace minerals must be held because of the accumulation of copper and manganese in liver failure.

Deficits in intravascular volume are corrected and then total fluids are restricted. Overhydration is avoided because it may precipitate cerebral edema, ascites, and pulmonary edema. However, intravascular dehydration may cause hepatorenal syndrome, worsening encephalopathy, and hypotension. Therefore fluid management is best guided with central venous pressure trends. Dialysis or hemofiltration is indicated with severe renal insufficiency as evidenced by oliguria, elevated creatinine level, severe metabolic acidosis, hyperkalemia, hyperphosphatemia, and volume overload.

Respiratory distress and/or failure are associated with encephalopathy, and hepatorenal syndrome as evidenced by hypoxemia and respiratory acidosis. The child requires intubation for airway protection when stage III encephalopathy is reached. Hypoxemia may be exacerbated by the development of pulmonary edema and treatment includes increased positive end expiratory pressure.

Thrombocytopenia is treated when the platelet count drops to less than 50,000 per cubic millimeter with 1 unit/10 kg. Fresh frozen plasma transfusion is given for evidence of active bleeding. The hematocrit is maintained at 30% or greater with 15 ml/kg packed RBC transfusions. Cryoprecipitate infusion is given for fibrinogen levels less than 100 mg/dl. Vitamin K (up to 10 mg intravenously) is administered for 3 days to correct a prolonged prothrombin time (PT).

Hypoglycemia is common and may cause an altered level of consciousness. Hypoglycemia in the failing liver is the result of defective gluconeogenesis and increased peripheral insulin levels. Blood glucose is monitored closely and replaced with intravenous dextrose when levels are less than 60 mg/dl.

ICP monitoring may be warranted for patients with evidence of cerebral edema and increased ICP. However, emergent treatment includes intubation and hyperventilation (if not already performed) and mannitol to induce an osmotic diuresis. Hypotension is aggressively treated in order to ensure adequate cerebral perfusion pressure. Treatment of encephalopathy also includes the administration of Lactulose. Lactulose is used to reduce ammonia levels and is administered by an NG tube at a dose of 0.5 ml/kg/dose up to 30 ml/dose every 6 hours. The dose is adjusted to produce two to four loose stools per day. Strict intake and output are required to avoid dehydration.

Benzodiazepines and opiates are used judiciously because of the concern of the role of GABA-benzodiazepine receptor association with hepatic encephalopathy and the potential for drug accumulation secondary to decreased drug metabolism. The patient who requires sedation or analgesia is given small doses, which are titrated to effect. Continuous infusions are contraindicated.

Patients with acute liver failure are at increased risk for bacterial and fungal infections. Meticulous care of all indwelling catheters and assessing frequently for signs and symptoms of infection are crucial. Surveillance cultures and aggressive treatment of presumed infection are essential.

Various liver-assist therapies have been introduced as an alternative to the shortage of available donors for transplantation. Such therapies include plasmapheresis, hemodilu-tion, extracorporeal liver perfusion, and bioartificial liver. These assist devices have been used to provide a bridge to transplantation in case of irreversible damage or to gain time for regeneration of the hepatocytes. Temporary clinical improvement has been seen; however, further research is needed to achieve successful long-term outcomes.[149,150]

The appropriateness of orthotopic liver transplantation (OLT) is an important aspect of care for the patient with FHF. Survival rates for OLT approach 60% to 70% with transplantation. However, 25% of patients listed die before an organ becomes available.[150] This supports the urgency to list patients while in stage II or III encephalopathy. Outcome is dependent on prompt aggressive treatment of complications and early assessment for potential transplantation.

SUMMARY

GI problems in infants and children are extremely varied and can be complicated and severe. Although the pathology varies greatly, the nursing care and assessment follow common pathways. GI nursing assessment, gastric decompression, intravascular volume replacement and maintenance, and pharmacologic management are of critical importance to the survival of these infants and children.

FREFERENCES

1. Moore KL, Persaud TVN: *The developing human: clinically oriented embryology,* ed 6, Philadelphia, 1998, WB Saunders.
2. Bullock B, Rosendahl P: *Pathophysiologic adaptations and alterations in function,* ed 3, Philadelphia, 1992, JB Lippincott.
3. Hyman P, DiLorenzo C: Gastrointestinal motility. In Wyllie R, Hyams JS, eds: *Pediatric gastrointestinal disease: pathophysiology, diagnosis, management,* Philadelphia, 1993, WB Saunders.
4. Motil K: Development of the gastrointestinal tract. In Wyllie R, Hyams JS, eds: *Pediatric gastrointestinal disease,* Philadelphia, 1993, WB Saunders.
5. Urdall J, Walker W: The physiologic and pathologic basis for the transport of macromolecules across the intestinal tract, *J Pediatr Gastroenterol Nutr* 1:295-301, 1982.
6. Heubi J, Balistreri W, Suchy F: Bile salt metabolism in the first year of life, *J Lab Clin Med* 100:127-136, 1982.
7. McKenna CJ: Gastrointestinal bleeding in children: implications for nursing, *Nurs Clin North Am* 29:599-613, 1994.
8. Filston HC: Fluid and electrolyte management in the pediatric surgical patient, *Surg Clin North Am* 72:1189-1205, 1992.
9. Filston HC, Shorter NA: Esophageal atresia and tracheoesophageal malformations. In Ashcraft KW et al, eds: *Pediatric surgery,* Philadelphia, 2000, WB Saunders.
10. Rosenthal AA: Congenital atresia of the esophagus with tracheoesophageal fistula, *Arch Pathol* 12:756, 1931.
11. Ein SH, Shandling B, Wesson D et al: Esophageal atresia with distal tracheoesophageal fistula: associated anomalies and prog-nosis in the 1980's, *J Pediatr Surg* 24:1055-1059, 1989.
12. Mee RBB, Beasley SW, Auldist AW et al: Influence of congenital heart disease on management of osephageal atresia, *Pediatric Surgery International* 2:90-93, 1992.
13. Polson EC, Schaller RT, Tapper D: Improved survival with primary anastomosis in the low birth weight neonate with esophageal atresia and tracheoesophageal fistula, *J Pediatr Surg* 23:418-421, 1988.
14. Spitz L: Esophageal atresia: past, present, and future, *J Pediatr Surg* 31:19-25, 1996.
15. Ein SH: Congenital malformations of the esophagus. In Wyllie R, Hyams JS, eds: *Pediatric gastrointestinal disease: pathophysiology, diagnosis, management,* Philadelphia, 1999, WB Saunders.
16. Chittmittrapap S, Spitz L, Kiely EM et al: Anastomotic stricture following repair of esophageal atresia, *J Pediatr Surg* 25:508-511, 1990.
17. Ein SH, Shandling B, Heiss K: Pure esophageal atresia: outlook on the 1990's, *J Pediatr Surg* 28:1147-1150, 1993.
18. Jona JZ: Advances in neonatal surgery, *Pediatr Clin North Am* 45:605-617, 1989.
19. Gosche JR, Touloukian RJ: Congenital anomalies of the midgut. In Wyllie R, Hyams JS, eds: *Pediatric gastrointestinal disease: pathophysiology, diagnosis, management,* Philadelphia, 1999, WB Saunders.
20. Millar AJW, Rode H, Cywes S: Intestinal atresia and stenosis. In Ashcraft KW et al, eds: *Pediatric surgery,* ed 3, Philadelphia, 2000, WB Saunders.
21. Brown RA, Millar AJW, Linegar A et al: Fenestrated duodenal membranes: an analy-sis of symptoms, signs, diagnosis, and treatment, *J Pediatr Surg* 29:429, 1994.
22. Lerner A, Branski D, Lebenthal E: Pancreatic diseases in children, *Pediatr Clin North Am* 43:125-156, 1996.
23. Mason JD: The evaluation of acute abdominal pain in children, *Emerg Med Clin North Am* 14:629-643, 1996.
24. Chang J, Brueckner M, Touloukian RJ: Intestinal rotation and fixation abnormalities in heterotaxia: early detection and management, *J Pediatr Surg* 28:1281-1289, 1993.
25. Ladd WE, Gross RE: *Abdominal surgery of infancy and childhood,* Philadelphia, 1941, WB Saunders.
26. Clark LA, Oldham KT: Malrotation. In Ashcraft KW et al, eds: *Pediatric surgery,* ed 3, Philadelphia, 2000, WB Saunders.
27. Groff DB: Meconium disease. In Ashcraft KW et al, eds: *Pediatric surgery,* ed 3, Philadelphia, 2000, WB Saunders.
28. Touloukian RJ, Walker-Smith GJ: Normal intestinal length in preterm infants, *J Pediatr Surg* 18:720-723, 1983.
29. Lloyd DA: Meconium ileus. In Welch KJ, Randolph JG, Ravitch MM et al, eds: *Pediatric surgery,* ed 4, St Louis, 1986, Mosby.
30. Kiesling VJ Jr, Tank ES: Postoperative intussusception in children, *Urology* 33:387-389, 1989.
31. Reijan JA, Festen C, Joosten HJ: Chronic intussusception in children, *BrJ Surg* 76:815-816, 1989.
32. Ravitch MM: Intussusception. In Welch KJ et al, eds: *Pediatric surgery,* ed 4, St Louis, 1986, Mosby.

33. Raffensperger JG, ed: *Swenson's pediatric surgery,* ed 5, Norwalk, Conn, 1989, Appleton & Lange.

34. Montgomery EA, Pokek EJ: Intussusception, adenovirus, and children: a brief reaffirmation, *Hum Pathol* 25:169-174, 1994.

35. West KW, Stephens B, Vane DW et al: Intussusception: current management in infants and children, *J Pediatr Surg* 102:781-787, 1987.

36. Hickey RW, Sodhi SK, Johnson WR: Two children with lethargy and intussusception, *Ann Emerg Med* 19:390-392, 1990.

37. Verschelden P, Filiatrault D, Garel L et al: Intussusception in children: reliability of ultrasound in diagnosis a prospective study, *Radiology* 184:741-744, 1992.

38. West KW, Grosfeld JL: Intussusception in infants and children. In Wyllie R, Hyams JS, eds: *Pediatric gastrointestinal disease: pathophysiology, diagnosis, management,* Philadelphia, 1999, WB Saunders.

39. Markowitz JF: Ulcerative colitis. In Wyllie R, Hyams JS, eds: *Pediatric gastrointestinal disease: pathophysiology, diagnosis, management,* Philadelphia, 1999, WB Saunders.

40. Jackson WD, Grand RJ: Ulcerative colitis. In Walker WA, Durie PR, Hamilton JR et al, eds: *Pediatric gastrointestinal diseases: pathophysiology, diagnosis, management,* Toronto, 1991, BC Decker.

41. Fonkalsrud EW, Ament ME: Gastroesophageal reflux in childhood, *Curr Probl Surg* 23:10-70, 1996.

42. Glassman M, George D, Grill B: Gastroesophageal reflux in children, *Gastroenterol Clin North Am* 24:71-98, 1995.

43. Orenstein SR: Prone positioning in infant gastroesophageal reflux: is elevation of the head worth the trouble? *J Pediatr* 117:184-187, 1990.

44. Kawahara H, Den, J, Davidson G: Mechanisms responsible for gastroesophageal reflux in children, *Gastroenterology* 113:399-408, 1997.

45. Orenstein SR, Mitchell AA, Davidson Ward S: Concerning the American Academy of Pediatrics recommendation on sleep position for infants, *Pediatrics* 91:497-499.

46. Colletti RB, Christine DL, Orenstein SR: Indications for pediatric esophageal pH monitoring, *J Pediatr Gastroenterol Nutr* 21:253-262, 1995.

47. Orenstein SR: Gastroesophageal reflux. In Wyllie R, Hyams JS, eds: *Pediatric gastrointestinal disease: pathophysiology, diagnosis, management,* Philadelphia, 1999, WB Saunders.

48. Putman PE, Orenstein SR, Wessel HB et al: Tardive dyskinesia associated with metoclopramide use in a child, *Pediatrics* 121:983-985, 1992.

49. Lewin M, Bryant R, Fenrich A et al: Cisapride-induced long QT interval, *Pediatrics* 128:279-281, 1996.

50. Federal Drug Administration: Withdrawal of troglitazone and cisapride, *JAMA* 282:2228, 2000.

51. Kelly D: Do H_2 receptor antagonists have a therapeutic role in childhood? *J Pediatr Gastroenterol* 19:270-276, 1994.

52. Maton P: Omeprazole, *N Engl J Med* 324:965-975, 1991.

53. Gunasekaran T, Hassall E: Efficacy and safety of omeprazole for severe gastroesophageal reflux in children, *J Pediatr* 123:148-154, 1993.

54. McCarthy D: Sucralfate, *N Engl J Med* 325:1017-1025, 1991.

55. Johansson J, Johansson R, Joelsson B: Outcome 5 years after 360° fundoplication for gastro-oesophageal reflux disease, *Br J Surg* 80:46-49, 1993.

56. Kazerooni N, VanCamp J, Hirsch LR et al: Fundoplication in 160 children under 2 years of age, *J Pediatr Surg* 29:677-681, 1994.

57. Ashcraft KW, Goodwin CG, Amoury RW: Thal fundoplication: a simple and safe operative treatment for gastroesophageal reflux, *J Pediatr Surg* 13:643-647, 1978.

58. Boix-Ochoa J, Marhuenda C: Gastroesophageal reflux. In Ashcraft KW et al, eds: *Pediatric surgery,* ed 3, Philadelphia, 2000, WB Saunders.

59. Hoffman MA, Stylianos S, Jacir NN: Technique of the transabdominal uncut Collis-Nissen fundoplication, *Pediatric Surgery International* 5:471-472, 1990.

60. Johnson CC, Baldessarre J, Levison ME: Peritonitis: update on pathophysiology, clinical manifestations, and management, *Clin Infect Dis* 24:1035-1047, 1997.

61. Ohmann C, Hau T: Prognostic indices in peritonitis, *Hepatogastroenterology* 44:937-946, 1997.

62. Baetz-Greenwalt B, Goske M: Intraabdominal infection. In Wyllie R, Hyams JS, eds: *Pediatric gastrointestinal disease: pathophysiology, diagnosis, management,* Philadelphia, 1993, WB Saunders.

63. Albanese CT, Rowe MI: Necrotizing enterocolitis, *Semin Pediatr Surg* 4:200-206, 1995.

64. Polin RA, Pollack PF, Barlow B et al: Neonatal necrotizing enterocolitis in term infants, *J Pediatr* 89:460-462, 1975.

65. West KW, Rescorla FJ, Grosfeld JL et al: Pneumatosis intestinalis in children beyond the neonatal period, *J Pediatr Surg* 24:818-822, 1989.

66. Kliegman RM: Neonatal necrotizing enterocolitis. *Pediatric gastrointestinal disease: pathophysiology, diagnosis, management,* Philadelphia, 1999, WB Saunders.

67. Kliegman RM, Fanaroff AA: Necrotizing enterocolitis, *N Engl J Med* 310:1093-1103, 1984.

68. Kliegman RM, Walsh MC: Neonatal necrotizing enterocolitis: pathogenesis, classification, and spectrum of disease, *Curr Probl Pediatr* 17:213-288, 1987.

69. Kosloske AM: A unifying hypothesis for pathogenesis and prevention of necrotizing enterocolitis, *J Pediatr* 117:S68-S74, 1990.

70. Anderson DM, Kliegman RM: The relationship of neonatal alimentation practices to the occurrence of endemic necrotizing enterocolitis, *Am J Perinatol* 8:62-67, 1991.

71. Israel EJ: NEC. In Walker WA, Durie PR, Hamiltion JR, Walker-Smith JA et al, eds: *Pediatric gastrointestinal diseases: pathophysiology, diagnosis, management,* Philadelphia, 1991, BC Decker.

72. Ahmed T, Moore A: Early laparotomy improves survival in necrotizing enterocolitis (NEC), *Pediatr Res* 41:135A, 1997.

73. Horwitz JR, Lally KP, Cheu HW et al: Complications after surgical intervention for necrotizing enterocolitis: a multicenter review, *J Pediatr Surg* 30:994-999, 1995.

74. Vanderhoff JA, Langnas AN, Pinch LW et al: Short bowel syndrome, *J Pediatr Gastroenterol Nutr* 14:359-370, 1992.

75. Wilmore DW: Factors correlating with a successful outcome following extensive intestinal resection in newborn infants, *J Pediatr* 80:88-95, 1972.

76. Schroeder P, Goulet O, Lear PA: Small bowel transplantation: European experience, *Lancet* 336:110-111, 1990.

77. Ziegler MM: Short bowel syndrome in infancy: etiology and management, *Clin Perinatol* 13:163-173, 1986.

78. Cooper H, Floyd TS, Ross AJ et al: Morbidity and mortality of short bowel syndrome acquired in infancy: an update, *J Pediatr Surg* 19:711-718, 1984.

79. Grosfeld JR, Rescorla FJ, West KW: Gastrointestinal injuries in children: analysis of 53 patients, *J Pediatr Surg* 24:580-583, 1989.

80. Goulet OJ, Revillon Y, Jan D et al: Which patient needs a small bowel transplantation for neonatal short bowel syndrome, *Transplant Proc* 24:1058-1059, 1991.

81. Treem WR: Short bowel syndrome. In Wyllie R, Hyams JS, eds: *Pediatric gastrointestinal disease: pathophysiology, diagnosis, management,* Philadelphia, 1999, WB Saunders.

82. Hennessey K: Nutritional support and gastrointestinal disease, *Nurs Clin North Am* 24:373-384, 1989.

83. Wilmore DW, Byrne TA, Persinger RL: Short bowel syndrome: new therapeutic approaches, *Curr Probl Surg* 34:393-444, 1997.

84. Dorney SFA, Ament ME, Berquist WE et al: Improved survival in very short small bowel of infancy with use of long-term parenteral nutrition, *J Pediatr* 107:521, 1985.

85. Seibert JR: Small intestine length in infants and children, *Am J Dis Child* 134:593-595, 1980.

86. Webster TR, Tracy T Jr, Connors RH: Short-bowel syndrome in children, *Arch Surg* 126:841-846, 1991.

87. Gleason WA Jr: Protein-losing enteropathy. In Wyllie R, Hyams JS, eds: *Pediatric gastrointestinal disease: pathophysiology, diagnosis, management,* Philadelphia, 1999, WB Saunders.

88. Bianchi A: Intestinal loop lengthening: a technique for increasing small bowel length, *J Pediatr Surg* 15:145-151, 1980.

89. Garcia VG, Templeton JM, Eichelberger MR et al: Colon interposition for the short bowel syndrome, *J Pediatr Surg* 16:994-995, 1981.

90. Careskey J, Webster TR, Grosfeld JL: Ileocecal valve replacement, *Arch Surg* 116:618-622, 1981.

91. Mainous MR, Block EF, Dietch EA: Nutritional support of the gut: how and why, *New Horiz* 2:193-201, 1994.

92. Byrne TA, Morrissey TB, Nattakom TV et al: Growth hormone, glutamine, and a modified diet enhance nutrient absorption in patients with severe short bowel syndrome, *J Parenter Enteral Nutr* 19:296-302, 1995.

93. Scolapio JS, Camilleri M, Fleming CR et al: Effect of growth hormone, glutamine, and diet on adaptation in short-bowel syndrome: a randomized, controlled study, *Gastroenterology* 113:1074-1081, 1997.

94. Jaros W, Biller J, Green S et al: Successful treatment of idiopathic secretory diarrhea of infancy with the somatostatin analogue SMS, *Gastroenterology* 94:189-193, 1988.

95. Mader TJ, McHugh TP: Acute pancreatitis in children, *Pediatr Emerg Care* 8:157-161, 1992.

96. Werlin SL: Pancreatitis. In Wyllie R, Hyams JS, eds: *Pediatric gastrointestinal disease: pathophysiology, diagnosis, management,* Philadelphia, 1999, WB Saunders.

97. Balthazar EJ: CT diagnosis and staging of acute pancreatitis, *Radiol Clin North Am* 27:19-37, 1989.

98. Haddock G, Coupar G, Youngson GG et al: Acute pancreatitis in children: a 15-year review, *J Pediatr Surg* 29:719-722, 1994.

99. Chaibou M, Tucci M, Dugas MA et al: Clinically significant upper gastrointestinal bleeding acquired in a pediatric intensive care unit: a prospective study, *Pediatrics* 102:933-938, 1998.

100. Cochran EB, Phelps SJ, Tolley EA et al: Prevalence of, and risk factors for, upper gastrointestinal tract bleeding in critically ill pediatric patients, *Crit Care Med* 20:1519-1523, 1992.

101. Lacroix J, Nadeau D, Laberge S et al: Frequency of upper gastrointestinal bleeding in a pediatric intensive care unit, *Crit Care Med* 20:35-42, 1992.

102. Cook DJ, Fuller HD, Guyatt GH et al: Risk factors for gastrointestinal bleeding in critically ill patients, *N Engl J Med* 330:377-381, 1994.

103. Pearson SP, Kelberman I: Gastrointestinal effects of NSAIDs: difficulties in management and detection, *Postgrad Med* 100:131-143, 1996.

104. Valentine J, Turner WW, Borman KR et al: Does nasoenteral feeding afford adequate gastroduodenal stress prophylaxis? *Crit Care Med* 14:599-601, 1986.

105. Wilcox CM, Spenney JG: Stress ulcer prophylaxis in medical patients: who, what, and how much? *Am J Gastroenterol* 83:1199-1210, 1988.

106. Schepp W: Stress ulcer prophylaxis: still a valid option in the 1990s? *Digestion* 54:189-199, 1993.

107. Squires RH: Gastrointestinal bleeding, *Pediatr Rev* 20:1-14, 1999.

108. Alonso EM, Hackworth C, Whitington PF: Portal hypertension, *Clin Liver Dis* 1:1-18, 1997.

109. Fox VL: Gastrointestinal bleeding in infancy and childhood, *Gastroenterol Clin North Am* 29:37-65, 2000.

110. Chiang BL, Chiang MH, Lin MI et al: Chronic duodenal ulcer in children: clinical observation and response to treatment, *J Pediatr Gastroenterol Nutr* 8:161-165, 1989.

111. Evans S, Strovroff M, Heiss K et al: Selective distal splenorenal shunts for intractable variceal bleeding in pediatric portal hypertension, *J Pediatr Surg* 30:1115-1118, 1995.

112. Schuster SR: Omphalocele and gastroschesis. In Welch KJ, Randolph JC, Ravitch MM et al, eds: *Pediatric surgery,* ed 4, Chicago, 1986, YearBook Medical Publishers.

113. Shaw A: The myth of gastroschesis, *J Pediatr Surg* 10:973, 1975.

114. Tunell WP: Anterior abdominal wall defects. In. Wyllie R, Hyams JS, eds: *Pediatric gastrointestinal disease: pathophysiology, diagnosis, management,* Philadelphia, 1999, WB Saunders.

115. Nakayama DK, Harrison MR, Gross BH et al: Management of the fetus with an abdominal wall defect, *J Pediatr Surg* 19:408-413, 1984.

116. Tunell WP, Puffinbarger NK, Tuggle DW et al: Abdominal wall defects in infants: survival and implications for adult life, *Ann Surg* 221:525-528, 1995.

117. Fasching G, Huber A, Uray E: Late follow-up in patients with gastroschisis: gastroesophageal reflux is common, *Pediatric Surgery International* 11:103-106, 1996.

118. Lee WM: Acute liver failure, *N Engl J Med* 329:273-275, 1993.

119. Goss JA, Shackleton CR, Maggard M et al: Liver transplantation for fulminant hepatic failure in the pediatric patient, *Arch Surg* 133:839-846, 1998.

120. Lloyd-Still JD: Mortality from liver disease in children: implications for hepatic transplantation programs, *Am J Dis Child* 139:381-384, 1985.

121. D'Agata ID, Balistreri WF: Evaluation of liver disease in the pediatric patient, *Pediatr Rev* 20:376-395, 1999.

122. Kay MH, McDiarmid SV: Liver failure and transplantation. In Wyllie R, Hyams JS, eds: *Pediatric gastrointestinal disease: pathophysiology, diagnosis, management,* Philadelphia, 1999, WB Saunders.

123. Balistreri WF, Grand R, Hoofnagle JH et al: Biliary atresia: current concepts and research directions, *Hepatology* 23:1682-1692, 1996.

124. Busuttil RW, Seu P, Millis JM et al: Liver transplantation in children, *Ann Surg* 213:48-57, 1991.

125. Moore TC, Hyman PE: Extrahepatic biliary atresia in one human leukocyte antigen identical twin, *Pediatrics* 76:604-605, 1985.

126. Smith BM, Laberge JM, Schrebier R et al: Familial biliary atresia in three siblings including twins, *J Pediatr Surg* 26:1331-1333, 1991.

127. Riepenhoff-Talty M, Gouvea V, Evans MJ et al: Detection of group C rotavirus in infants with extrahepatic biliary atresia, *J Infect Dis* 174:8-15, 1996.

128. McEvoy CF, Suchy FJ: Biliary tract disease in children, *Pediatr Clin North Am* 43:75-98, 1996.

129. Whitington PF: Chronic cholestasis of infancy, *Pediatr Clin North Am* 43:1-26, 1996.

130. Laurent J, Gauthier F, Bernard O et al: Long-term outcome after surgery for biliary atresia: study of 40 patients surviving for more than 10 years, *Gastroenterology* 99:1793-1797, 1990.

131. Rosenthal P, Podesta L, Sher L et al: Liver transplantation in children, *Am J Gastroenterol* 89:480-492, 1994.

132. Alagille D, Estrada A, Hadchouel M et al: Syndromic paucity of interlobular bile ducts (Alagille syndrome or arteriohepatic dysplagia): review of 80 cases, *J Pediatr* 110:195-200, 1987.

133. Anad F, Burn J, Matthews D et al: Alagille syndrome and deletion of 20p, *J Med Genet* 27:729-737, 1990.

134. Schwarzenberg SJ, Sharp HL: Update on metabolic liver disease, *Pediatr Clin North Am* 43:27-56, 1996.

135. Perlmutter DH: Alpha 1–antitrypsin deficiency. In Walker WA et al, eds: *Pediatric gastrointestinal disease,* Toronto, 1991, B.C. Decker.

136. Teckman JH, Perlmutter DH: Metabolic disorders of the liver. In R Wyllie, JS Hyams, eds: *Pediatric gastrointestinal disease: pathophysiology, diagnosis, management,* Philadelphia, 1999, WB Saunders.

137. Casavilla FA, Reye J, Tzakis A et al: Liver transplantation for neonatal hepatitis as compared to the other two leading indications for liver transplantation in children, *Hepatology* 21:1035-1039, 1994.

138. Bernstein D, Tripodi J: Fulminant hepatic failure, *Critical Care Clinics* 14:181-197, 1998.

139. Pappas SC: Fulminant viral hepatitis, *Gastroenterol Clin North Am* 24:161-173, 1995.

140. Miyakawa Y, Mayumi M: Hepatitis G virus: a true hepatitis or an accidental tourist? *N Engl J Med* 336:795-796, 1997.

141. Fishman LN, Jonas MM, Lavine JE: Update on viral hepatitis in children, *Pediatr Clin North Am* 43:57-74, 1996.

142. Detre K, Belle S, Beringer K et al: Liver transplantation for fulminant hepatic failure in the United States: October 1987 through December 1991, *Clinical Transplant* 8:274-280, 1994.

143. Farci P, Alter HJ, Shimoda A et al: Hepatitis C virus-associated fulminant hepatic failure, *N Engl J Med* 335:631-634, 1996.

144. Evans JS: Acute and chronic hepatitis. In R Wyllie, JS Hyams, eds: *Pediatric gastrointestinal disease: pathophysiology, diagnosis, management,* Philadelphia, 1999, WB Saunders.

145. Devictor D, Tahiri C, Rousset A et al: Management of fulminant hepatic failure in children-an analysis of 56 cases, *Crit Care Med* 21:S348-349, 1993.

146. Lee WM: Drug-induced hepatotoxicity, *N Engl J Med* 333:1118-1127, 1995.

147. Pereira LM, Langley PG, Hayllar KM et al: Coagulation factor V and VII/V ratio as predictors of outcome in paracetamol induced fulminant hepatic failure: relation to other prognostic indicators, *Gut* 33:98-102, 1992.

148. Papper S: Renal failure in cirrhosis (the hepatorenal syndrome). In Epstein M, ed: *The kidney in liver disease,* ed 2, New York, 1983, Elsevier Science.

149. Stockmann H, Hiemstra CA, Marquet RL et al: Extracorporeal perfusion for the treatment of acute liver failure, *Ann Surg* 231:460-470, 2000.

150. Sundback CA, Vacanti JP: Alternatives to liver transplantation: from hepatocyte transplantation to tissue-engineered organs, *Gastroenterology* 118:438-447, 2000.

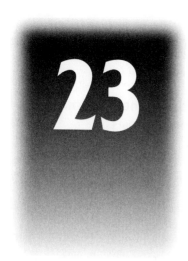

23 Endocrine Critical Care Problems

Tara Trimarchi

The endocrine system is a complex physiologic network that regulates growth, development, metabolism, and sexual differentiation. This integrated system of feedback loops depends on the stimulation or inhibition of glands that secrete hormones into the bloodstream.

Frequently encountered endocrine emergencies in children can be grouped into the final common pathways of alterations in fluid and electrolyte balance, circulatory failure, and alterations in glucose homeostasis. This chapter reviews the basic pathophysiology, diagnosis, and treatment of selected endocrine problems. Recommendations for the nursing management of the infant or child with a serious endocrine disturbance is discussed within the context of fluid deficit or excess with electrolyte imbalance, circulatory failure, and hypoglycemia or hyperglycemia.

MATURATIONAL ANATOMY AND PHYSIOLOGY

Endocrine Regulation of Water and Electrolyte Balance and Hemodynamic Stability

Water is distributed in the human body as intracellular fluid (70% of total body water) and extracellular fluid, which includes plasma and interstitial fluids (30% of total body water). Osmolality is an important factor regulating fluid balance between the intracellular fluid (ICF) and the extracellular fluid (ECF) compartments. Normal plasma osmolality ranges between 270 and 285 mOsm/L. Sodium is the major cation of the ECF and usually accounts for 90% of the plasma osmolality. Hormones, such as antidiuretic hormone, aldosterone, and atrial natriuretic hormone, act on the kidneys to influence the reabsorption and excretion of sodium and water, thereby regulating the concentration, composition, and volume of body fluids and maintaining osmolality within the normal range.

Antidiuretic Hormone (Vasopressin). Antidiuretic hormone (ADH) is formed in the supraoptic and paraventricular nuclei of the hypothalamus and is stored in the posterior pituitary. ADH increases the reabsorption of water in the collecting ducts of the kidneys. Through the action of ADH, water is returned to the vascular space, resulting in increased blood volume and decreased water loss in the urine. ADH secretion is regulated by plasma osmolality receptors located in the brain and by stretch receptors located in the ascending aorta and left atrium of the heart. When the plasma osmolality is higher than 285 mOsm/L, the osmoreceptors in the hypothalamus of the brain are stimulated, resulting in a sensation of thirst and ADH secretion. Through the ingestion of fluids and water reabsorption by the kidney, this response restores intravascular volume and maintains serum osmolality within the very narrow range of 282 to 295 mmol/kg.[1] Decreased blood pressure caused by hypovolemia or vasodilation stimulates stretch receptors located in the ascending aorta and left atrium and is also a stimulus for ADH secretion.

Mineralocorticoids (Aldosterone). Aldosterone is secreted by the adrenal cortex. Aldosterone acts on the renal tubules, resulting in the conservation of sodium and water and the excretion of potassium in the urine. Under the influence of aldosterone, sodium and water are returned to the vascular space and urine production is decreased. Aldosterone secretion is, in part, controlled by the renin-angiotensin system.

The renin-angiotensin system is stimulated by decreased renal perfusion, resulting from diminished blood volume and reduced arterial blood pressure. When the juxtaglomerular apparatus of the kidneys senses a state of low perfusion, the kidneys release renin. Renin stimulates the conversion of angiotensin I (a protein produced by the liver) to angiotensin II. Angiotensin II is a potent vasoconstrictor and stimulates aldosterone release. In addition to aldosterone release, some ADH is also released in response to angiotensin II. Vasoconstriction, in addition to the sodium and water retention induced by aldosterone and ADH, serves to restore blood pressure and volume.

Atrial Natriuretic Hormone (Atrial Natriuretic Peptide). Atrial natriuretic hormone (ANH), or atrial natriuretic peptide, is produced by the cells of the atria of the heart. ANH has vasoactive effects on blood vessels, including the glomerulus of the kidney, and acts to increase glomerular filtration rate. Increased glomerular filtration rate promotes increased urine production with an accompanying increase in salt excretion into the urine. ANH may also inhibit angiotensin II–mediated aldosterone and antidiuretic hormone release. The stimulus for the production of ANH and the role of ANH in sodium homeostasis are not completely understood. However, brain injury appears to be directly related to production of ANH. High atrial pressure resulting in stretching of atrial cells is also implicated as a stimulus for ANH production.[2]

Adrenal Hormones: Glucocorticoids and Catecholamines. Glucocorticoids (primarily cortisol) are produced and secreted by the adrenal cortex. Glucocorticoid production is regulated by the anterior pituitary. As circulating cortisol levels decrease, adrenocorticotropic hormone (ACTH) is secreted by the anterior pituitary gland. ACTH signals the adrenals to secrete cortisol. Glucocorticoids have the weak mineralocorticoid effect of enhancing water and sodium reabsorption in the kidney, resulting in the return of water to the vascular space.

In response to neuronal input, the adrenal medulla produces the catecholamines epinephrine and norepinephrine. Catecholamines maintain blood pressure by increasing vascular tone, heart rate, and myocardial contractility. Catecholamine production is also dependent on the presence of local cortisol in the adrenal cortex. During illness, surgery, and trauma, increased production of glucocorticoid hormones and catecholamines is essential for the mainte-

nance of the body's stress response. Inadequate cortisol and catecholamine production may result in profound hypotension because of volume loss, electrolyte imbalance, myocardial depression, and poor arterial tone.[3]

Endocrine Regulation of Energy Production by Cells: Glucose Homeostasis

Glucose is the main energy source for all body cells. Protein and fat are additional sources of energy. The endocrine system regulates the use of energy sources and the production of energy by cells. The hormones responsible for regulating energy production include insulin, glucagon, epinephrine, cortisol, and growth hormone.

Insulin is a hormone produced by the beta cells of the pancreas. Insulin regulates glucose, protein, and fat metabolism. Insulin also enhances glucose uptake by cells. This mechanism ensures that glucose is available for use as an energy-generating substrate. In addition, insulin stimulates protein synthesis and inhibits the breakdown of fat stores, or lipolysis.

Insulin is released in the postprandial state. As nutrients are absorbed by the gut, blood glucose rises. The release of insulin is stimulated by the rise in blood glucose. Insulin places the body in an anabolic state. Glucose, in excess of the needs of cells for energy production, is taken up and stored in the liver and skeletal muscles as glycogen. In addition, insulin stimulates the building of proteins from amino acids and the storage of fatty acids as adipose tissue.

Glucagon is produced by the alpha cells of the pancreas. Glucagon counterregulates insulin secretion and the anabolic effects of insulin. Glucagon raises blood glucose by stimulating the synthesis of glucose from glycogen stores in the liver. Glucagon also facilitates the breakdown of proteins, making amino acids available for gluconeogenesis, and stimulates lipolysis. Glucagon release is stimulated by hypoglycemia and neural impulses associated with the stress response.

Epinephrine is produced in the adrenal medulla and is released in response to sympathetic nervous system stimulation during stress. Epinephrine raises blood glucose by causing the breakdown of glycogen stores in the liver and skeletal muscle and by promoting gluconeogenesis, the synthesis of glucose from noncarbohydrate substrates, such as proteins and lipids. Epinephrine also induces lipolysis to make fat available as a substrate for energy production by cells.

Although relatively minor in importance, growth hormone and glucocorticoids (primarily cortisol) also regulate cellular energy production. *Cortisol* is produced by the adrenal cortex. Cortisol release is under the control of ACTH and is, in part, stimulated by a stress response. Glucocorticoids increase blood glucose and stimulate lipolysis.

Growth hormone, produced by the anterior lobe of the pituitary, stimulates protein synthesis, gluconeogenesis, and lipolysis. As with cortisol and epinephrine, growth hormone production increases during times of stress.

Glucose Stores in the Body. Hepatic glycogen stores are the initial glucose source in the fasting state. Healthy children typically possess glycogen stores sufficient for up to 8 hours of fasting. Infants' stores, however, are limited and may be sufficient to maintain blood glucose for approximately 4 to 6 hours of fasting. Following the depletion of glycogen stores, gluconeogenesis accounts for the primary glucose source. Well-nourished children can also maintain blood glucose in the normal range for approximately another 12 to 18 hours by converting to the oxidation of fatty acids as a primary energy source. During the process of oxidizing fatty acids, ketone bodies are produced (β-hydroxybutyrate and acetoacetate), which can be used as an energy source by muscle and brain cells.

DISTURBANCES OF WATER BALANCE: FLUID VOLUME DEFICIT

ADH Deficit (Diabetes Insipidus)

Neurogenic or central diabetes insipidus (DI) is a condition in which a deficit of ADH results in decreased reabsorption of water by the distal tubules of the kidneys and loss of free water in the urine. DI is typically associated with central nervous system disorders that damage or create pressure in the area of the hypothalamus, pituitary stalk, or posterior pituitary gland. Common causes of central DI in children include central nervous system lesions such as craniopharyngiomas, pituitary gland or suprasellar tumors, or the surgical resection of these tumors. Olson and colleagues[4] reported a 20% incidence of DI after transphenoidal pituitary surgeries, with the onset of the disorder occurring as late as 2 weeks after the procedure. Traumatic brain injury is also a common cause of DI. Finfer and co-workers[5] studied a series of 77 children with traumatic head injury that progressed to brain death. Seventy-eight percent of the children studied developed DI. Hypoxic-ischemic encephalopathy may result in DI as well.[6] In addition, Charmandari and Brook[7] reviewed a series of 120 children with DI who did not have brain tumors or known brain injury, and they reported that DI is associated with a small, but otherwise structurally normal pituitary gland and other hormone deficiencies, such growth hormone and ACTH deficiency. There are also familial degenerative disorders of the neurons that secrete ADH.[1]

DI may also be the result of a primary renal defect. Primary renal DI occurs when otherwise normal kidneys fail to respond to ADH. Secondary renal DI is loss of ADH sensitivity as a result of a known underlying renal disease or other factors that interfere with the kidney's ability to concentrate water, such as a protein deficiency, limited sodium intake, hypokalemia, hypercalcemia, and certain drugs (lithium, demeclocycline).

The signs and symptoms of central DI and underlying causes are outlined in Table 23-1. Urine output of approximately 40 ml/kg/day is typically encountered in cases of DI; however, up to 400 ml/kg/day of urine output related to DI has been reported.[1] Urinary water losses result in an ECF deficit that may be significant enough to precipitate hypo-

TABLE 23-1 Antidiuretic Hormone (ADH) Deficiency: Diabetes Insipidus

Signs and Symptoms	Underlying Mechanisms
Polyuria Urine hypoosmolar (clear in color)	ADH deficit with resulting diuresis
Hypernatremia Plasma hyperosmolarity	ECF volume depletion
Thirst, polydipsia	Dehydration
Dehydration or shock state	Hypovolemia secondary to ECF volume depletion
Irritability or change in mental status	Cerebral hypoperfusion caused by dehydration; changes in cerebral cellular function resulting from electrolyte abnormality

ECF, Extracellular fluid.

volemic shock. Serum sodium may be extremely high because of the ECF volume depletion. The child with an intact thirst mechanism who is allowed to drink may be able to orally replace urinary fluid losses and thereby maintain a normal serum sodium and serum osmolality. However, interference with drinking because of debilitating disease may rapidly precipitate volume depletion.

Diagnostic Presentation. Diagnostic findings in DI are outlined in Table 23-2. Low urinary osmolality (generally <100-200 mOsm/L) in conjunction with elevated serum osmolality (>285 mOsm/L) and elevated serum sodium (>145 mEq/L) is diagnostic of DI. These values reflect that water has been inappropriately lost in the urine with a resulting dehydration and plasma hyperosmolality. Stimulation tests such as the water deprivation test and vasopressin test may be used to confirm the diagnosis. The water deprivation test involves the restriction of all fluids until 3% to 5% of body weight has been lost. Because of the risk of hypovolemic shock, vital signs are monitored closely, along with hourly serum sodium, serum osmolality, urine osmolality, and body weight. At the completion of the test, vasopressin is administered subcutaneously or intranasally. A rise in urinary concentration and decreased urine output following the administration of vasopressin support the diagnosis of central DI. In cases of nephrogenic DI, no detectable improvement in the ability of the kidneys to concentrate urine is encountered after the administration of vasopressin.

Critical Care Management. Care of the child with central DI is outlined in Table 23-2. Interventions are directed at the prevention of complications associated with circulatory failure and hyperosmolar encephalopathy. Urinary losses in children with DI may be significant, and failure to replace losses may result in hypovolemic shock. High urine output may necessitate replacement on a half-hourly or hourly basis. Careful monitoring of the child's neurologic status is essential to detect early signs of

TABLE 23-2 Managing ADH Deficiency: Diabetes Insipidus (DI)

1. Participate in diagnostic workup	
History	Polyuria, enuresis, thirst, weight loss, fatigue, anorexia
Risk factors	Recent CNS trauma, infection or surgery, known midline cerebral defects, kidney disease (nephrogenic DI)
Physical examination	Dehydration: lethargy, increased skin turgor, lack of tears with crying, sunken fontanelle
	Hypovolemia/circulatory failure: tachycardia; weak, thready pulse; skin cold, clammy; delayed capillary refill; hypotension; depressed level of consciousness
	Irritability or altered mental status caused by hypernatremia
Laboratory tests	Serum osmolality increased (>290 mOsm/L)
	Serum sodium increased (>145 mEq/L)
	Urine osmolality decreased (<100-200 mOsm/L)
	Hypernatremia (<125 mEq/L)
	Urine specific gravity decreased (<1.010)
Stimulation tests	Water deprivation test
	Vasopressin test
2. Prevent complications associated with hypernatremia, hypovolemia, dehydration, and shock	Evaluate fluid balance:
	Compare urine output to fluid intake
	Measure urine specific gravity
	Monitor weight trends every 8 hr
	Assess orthostatic blood pressure, frequent vital sign assessments, neurologic checks, and physical examinations
Replace volume deficit and ongoing losses	Bolus with 10-20 ml/kg of normal saline if hypotensive
	Then 0.9% to 0.45% normal saline solution maintenance plus calculated replacement over 24-48 hours (rate of replacement and concentration of IV fluids dependent on serum sodium level)
	Replace urine losses
	Continue fluid replacement until vasopressin takes effect (urine specific gravity >1.010, and urine output decreased)
Replace ADH	Administer vasopressin
	Administer continuous infusion of vasopressin analog, such as aqueous arginine vasopressin, titrated repeatedly for maximum therapeutic effect. Typically, vasopressin doses of approximately 1.5 mU/kg/hr are required; however, doses may range from 0.5 to 10 mU/kg/hr
	Desired effect: urine volume decreased to <2 ml/kg/hr
	Urine specific gravity increased to >1.010
	Urine osmolality increased
	Normalization of serum sodium/osmolality
Observe for signs of water intoxication secondary to overtreatment (correction of hypernatremia should be no greater than a decrease of 2 mEq/L/hr)	Mental status changes, headache
	Nausea, vomiting
	Lethargy, weakness
	Seizures, coma

ADH, Antidiuretic hormone; *CNS*, central nervous system; *IV*, intravenous.

encephalopathy (headache, mental status changes) and potential seizures caused by altered serum sodium levels. In addition, encephalopathy is occasionally associated with overly rapid correction of hypernatremia. The child who presents with significant hypernatremia (>155 mEq/L) is at highest risk for hyperosmolar encephalopathy. Children with severe hypernatremia, particularly hypernatremic dehydration that develops rapidly, require slow correction, usually over a 36- to 48-hour period, to prevent hyperosmolar encephalopathy.

Vasopressin administration is also used to the treat central DI. The intravenous, subcutaneous, or intranasal routes are all viable options for vasopressin replacement. Desmopressin acetate (DDAVP), given intranasally, is a commonly used intermediate-acting preparation for home management. However, because of variability in absorption, it is not the preparation of choice in the critically ill patient. Children with DI who are receiving ADH replacement are at risk for both dehydration (because of inadequate replacement of both ADH and fluids) and water intoxication (because of overreplacement of water or overdoses of vasopressin). Critically ill children and children who cannot communicate are at increased risk for and often less able to tolerate sustained fluxes in intravascular fluid volume.

Therefore shorter-acting preparations such as vasopressin (Pitressin or aqueous arginine vasopressin) or lypressin (Diapid) are used to treat DI in the critically ill population. Continuous infusion of vasopressin analogs such as aqueous arginine vasopressin are most often used and are titrated repeatedly for maximum therapeutic effect.[8] Typically, a vasopressin dose of approximately 1.5 mU/kg/hr is required; however, doses may range from 0.5 to 10 mU/hr.[9,10]

A rise in urine specific gravity and decrease in urine output within 1 hour after the administration of a vasopressin analog indicate a therapeutic effect. Intravenous fluid rates are readjusted once antidiuresis has been achieved to prevent volume overload and water intoxication. Serum sodium and osmolality are useful indices of water balance and are usually obtained every 1 to 2 hours until an appropriate vasopressin dose and rate of intravenous fluid administration have been determined. Hourly monitoring of urine volume and specific gravity are also necessary for the determination of an appropriate vasopressin dose. Therapeutic goals that have been correlated with positive outcomes in the treatment of DI include a urine output of 2 to 3 ml/kg/hr, urine specific gravity of 1.010 to 1.020, and serum sodium of 140 to 145 mEq/L.[11] According to Lugo and colleagues,[11] urine specific gravity is the most sensitive marker of vasopressin responsivity and appropriateness of vasopressin dose, and urine output is the second most useful marker of therapeutic response. In addition, Lugo and co-workers[11] report a lag in serum sodium and osmolality normalization in relation to vasopressin administration.

Caution is exercised when administering vasopressin. Vasopressin causes local and systemic vasoconstriction. Children receiving vasopressin infusions must be monitored closely for signs of diffuse tissue ischemia, such as lactic acidosis, and local ischemia at the infusion site.[10]

Increased Atrial Natriuretic Peptide Production and Cerebral Salt Wasting Syndrome

Increased ANH production results in diuresis with loss of sodium in the urine. Central nervous system injury appears to be directly related to production of ANH and is the most common feature of children with salt wasting syndromes. Cerebral salt wasting syndrome typically occurs within the first week after brain injury. Evidence shows that hypovolemic states induced by DI and diabetic ketoacidosis; conditions that affect the myocardium, such as hypertension, congestive heart failure, and congenital heart defects; and chronic lung disease, such as bronchopulmonary dysplasia, may induce ANH production and a salt wasting syndrome. Furthermore, cases have been reported of elevated ANH levels in children with other endocrine disorders, such as Cushing's syndrome and hyperaldosteronism.[2]

Diagnostic Presentation. Cerebral salt wasting syndrome is defined by hyponatremia (serum sodium <130 mEq/L), in conjunction with normal or increased urine output and normal or slightly elevated urine specific gravity. In addition, increased sodium content (>80 mEq/L) is found in the urine of children with salt wasting syndromes.

Although not routinely monitored, serum ANH levels are high in children experiencing sodium loss from this cause.[2]

Because treatments for hyponatremia differ depending on the underlying cause, it is important to distinguish cerebral salt wasting syndrome from the syndrome of inappropriate antidiuretic hormone (SIADH) secretion in children who have a decreased serum sodium level. SIADH is the more common cause of hyponatremia, particularly in children with head injury. In contrast to cerebral salt wasting syndrome, SIADH results in a markedly decreased urine output and highly concentrated urine, along with fluid retention. In SIADH, the dilutional effect of fluid retention contributes to hyponatremia; thus fluid restriction, rather than sodium replacement, becomes the mainstay of therapy.[2]

Critical Care Management. Little research has demonstrated the best practices for treating cerebral salt wasting syndrome. Treatment usually includes replacement of any volume loss with an isotonic saline solution and sodium supplementation in the form of enteral sodium chloride administration, or intravenous infusion of a 3% sodium chloride solution.[2]

The use of 3% saline solution (a solution containing 0.513 mEq of sodium per milliliter of solution) for the treatment of hyponatremia warrants very careful calculation of the dose of sodium chloride required and close monitoring of the child during administration. Typically, the use of 3% saline solution is restricted to cases of symptomatic hyponatremia with serum sodium levels less than 125 mEq/L. The dose of 3% saline to be administered is based on the amount of sodium necessary to correct hyponatremia to a serum level of 125 mEq/L. The following calculation is often used to determine this dose:

Sodium deficit (amount to be administered) =
0.6 × (Body weight in kg) × (125 − Measured serum sodium level)

The total dose is administered slowly (often over 24 hours or more) to avoid causing encephalopathy associated with rapid correction of hyponatremia. Rises in serum sodium level that exceed 0.6 to 1 mEq/ hr are considered dangerous and contribute to the development of encephalopathy. Frequent monitoring of serum sodium levels to follow the rate of correction is necessary. Furthermore, because 3% saline is hyperosmolar, the site of intravenous administration is monitored closely for signs of phlebitis and subcutaneous tissue irritation indicative of extravasation.[10]

DISTURBANCES OF WATER BALANCE: FLUID VOLUME EXCESS

ADH Excess (SIADH Secretion)

SIADH secretion is a condition in which ADH is secreted despite serum hypo-osmolality, hyponatremia, and euvolemia. Inappropriate ADH secretion results in increased permeability of the renal distal tubules and collecting ducts, with a resulting increase in water reabsorption and intravascular fluid volume, and a decrease in urine production.

As with DI, SIADH may be due to traumatic or hypoxic ischemic brain injury or discrete diseases of the hypothala-

TABLE 23-3   ADH Excess (SIADH)

Signs and Symptoms	Underlying Mechanisms
Serum hypo-osmolality Serum hyponatremia	Dilutional hypervolemia from decreased urine production or increased fluid retention
Concentrated urine High urine sodium (>10-20 mEq/L) High fractional excretion of sodium	ADH concentrates urine by increasing permeability of renal collection tubule Decreased renin-angioten- sin II and aldosterone result in sodium excretion
Nausea, vomiting, weakness	Hyponatremia
Mental status changes Lethargy, irritability, headache (early) Pupillary changes, seizures, coma, death (late)	Cerebral edema resulting from fluid shift

ADH, Antidiuretic hormone; *SIADH,* syndrome of inappropriate ADH.

mus, pituitary stalk, or posterior pituitary. In cases of traumatic brain injury, the onset of SIADH may be delayed.[4,12] SIADH is also encountered in patients who have meningitis[13] and patients who have undergone spinal manipulation, such as spinal fusion for scoliosis.[14] In addition, nonneurologic disorders, such as hepatic disease, pulmonary diseases, high-dose chemotherapy, and bone marrow or peripheral stem cell transplants, are also associated with the development of SIADH.[15] The classic signs and symptoms of SIADH and the underlying mechanisms are outlined in Table 23-3. Hyponatremia (serum sodium <125 mEq/L) and hypo-osmolality (serum osmolality <260 mOsm/L) both result from the dilutional effect of the increased intravascular volume expansion. Worsening of the hypo-osmolar state may precipitate a shift of free water from the ECF to the ICF, which can result in cerebral edema.

Diagnostic Presentation.   Diagnostic findings are outlined in Table 23-4. The diagnosis of SIADH is made when urinary osmolality is high, with low serum osmolality and hyponatremia, in the face of a previously euvolemic state. Damaraju and colleagues[16] report that monitoring central venous pressure for the identification of increasing intravascular volume is helpful in the detection and management of SIADH.

TABLE 23-4   Managing ADH Excess (SIADH)

1. Participate in diagnostic workup	
History	Nausea, vomiting, headache, weakness
Risk factors	CNS infection, trauma, surgery
	Respiratory illness, positive pressure ventilation
Physical examination	Nausea, vomiting, weakness
	Urine output decreased
	Mental status changes (lethargy, irritability, headache, seizures, coma, pupillary changes)
	Hypertension (late)
Laboratory tests	Hyponatremia (<125 mEq/L)
	Serum osmolality decreased in the face of a high urine osmolality (<260 mOsm/L)
	BUN normal or decreased
	Increased fractional excretion of urine sodium
	Urine sodium increased
	Urine osmolality increased
2. Prevent complications associated with water intoxication or hyponatremia	
Evaluate fluid balance	Compare urine output to fluid intake
	Measure urine specific gravity
	Monitor weight trends every 8 hr
Evaluate for signs of water intoxication	Headache, nausea, vomiting
	Lethargy, weakness, irritability
	Mental status changes, pupillary changes, seizures, coma
Restrict fluids	Usually equal to the amount of insensible losses *or* one-half to three-fourths maintenance
Treat acute hyponatremia	Loop diuretic (furosemide) 0.5-1 mg/kg/dose
	Infusion of 3% NaCl solution: the dose of 3% saline to be administered is based on the amount of sodium needed to correct hyponatremia to a serum level of 125 mEq/L The following calculation is often used to determine this dose: Sodium deficit (amount to be administered) = 0.6 × (Body weight in kg) × (125 − Measured serum sodium level)
	The total dose is administered slowly (often over 24 hr or more) to avoid causing the encephalopathy associated with rapid correction of hyponatremia

ADH, Antidiuretic hormone; *SIADH,* syndrome of inappropriate ADH; *BUN,* blood urea nitrogen.

Critical Care Management. Treatment of the child with SIADH is outlined in Table 23-4. Interventions are focused on the prevention of complications associated with water intoxication and hyponatremia. Meticulous attention to fluid balance is essential. According to a study of spinal fusion patients by Brazel and McPhee,[14] administration of isotonic saline solutions, rather than half or quarter normal saline solutions, may help to prevent the development of hyponatremia associated with SIADH in at-risk populations. Once SIADH has developed, fluid restriction is the mainstay of treatment. Early detection of neurologic changes associated with water intoxication is critical. Children with SIADH are at risk for cerebral edema because the hyponatremic state allows free water to move from the ECF space to the ICF space (including brain cells), which may result in cerebral edema. Emergency treatment of hyponatremia may be necessary if it is accompanied by neurologic symptoms, such as depressed level of consciousness or seizure activity. The standard approach to treating SIADH is fluid restriction and, occasionally, the administration of a loop diuretic, such as furosemide (Lasix) 0.5 to 1 mg/kg/dose, and infusion of a 3% sodium chloride solution to correct the hyponatremia.[16]

ADRENOCORTICAL HYPOFUNCTION: FLUID VOLUME DEFICIT AND CIRCULATORY FAILURE

Adrenal Insufficiency/Adrenal Crisis

Adrenal insufficiency is associated with a variety of conditions in which there is a deficiency of glucocorticoids (primarily cortisol) and mineralocorticoids (aldosterone) and may also result in decreased catecholamine synthesis and release. The adrenal glands also produce androgens. Androgens, however, have a less important effect on fluid balance and hemodynamic stability.

Aldosterone deficiency causes decreased sodium and water reabsorption and increased potassium reabsorption in the renal distal tubules. Glucocorticoid deficits result in intravascular volume loss, electrolyte imbalance, and decreased responsiveness to and synthesis of catecholamines, which results in myocardial depression, poor arterial tone, and hypotension. Together, aldosterone and glucocorticoid deficiencies can cause profound hypotension. However, an isolated glucocorticoid deficit in the face of a significant stressor is sufficient to produce vasodilation and shock. Hypoglycemia may also ensue during states of adrenal insufficiency.

Primary adrenocortical deficiency (Addison's disease) is associated with conditions that impair the ability of the adrenals to produce cortisol or aldosterone. Diseases such as congenital adrenal hypoplasia, tuberculous adrenalitis, autoimmune adrenalitis, adrenoleukodystrophy, and adrenal hemorrhage cause primary adrenocortical dysfunction. Primary adrenal insufficiency, often caused by adrenal hemorrhage, is a known sequela of shock, particularly septic shock.[17] Adrenal hemorrhage precipitated by coagulopathy resulting from sepsis or a systemic inflammatory response is referred to as the Waterhouse-Friderichsen syndrome. Riorden and colleagues[18] studied 126 cases of meningococcemia in children and reported low cortisol levels and high ACTH levels, consistent with primary adrenal insufficiency, in patients who died of meningococcal disease. In addition, Briegel and associates[19] reported decreased requirement for vasopressors and earlier resolution of multiple organ dysfunction syndrome in adults with septic shock treated with stress dose hydrocortisone. Similarly, Hatherill and co-workers[20] reported a 52% incidence of adrenal insufficiency in children with septic shock on laboratory examination, but they did not find that the children with adrenal insufficiency experienced more organ system failure or higher morbidity. However, despite such studies, there is a risk of inducing immunosuppression with the use of corticosteroids, and not enough additional evidence supports the routine replacement of cortisol in patients with septic shock at the present time. In fact, earlier, large adult trials have not shown a clear benefit to the use of corticosteroids in patients with septic shock.[20-23] Shock states may also be confounded by decreased production of catecholamine resulting from damaged adrenal glands or by a phenomenon of diminished peripheral and myocardial catecholamine receptor responsivity.[19,24-26]

Secondary adrenocortical disease is due to intrinsic hypothalamic or anterior pituitary dysfunction in which there is low production or excretion of ACTH. Secondary diseases include hypothalamic or pituitary tumors or central nervous system trauma. Although adrenal function is intact, cortisol is not produced because the adrenal glands do not receive an ACTH signal from the pituitary gland to generate cortisol. In addition, as in primary adrenal insufficiency, shock states and sepsis, perhaps resulting from systemic inflammation, may induce secondary adrenal insufficiency.[27,28]

Adrenal crisis may be precipitated in the child with known adrenal insufficiency who is not given higher than maintenance doses of steroids during times of illness, surgery, or other significant stress. Adrenocortical insufficiency may also be iatrogenic, as seen with the administration of high-dose steroids over an extended period, resulting in the suppression of the hypothalamic-pituitary-adrenal axis. A fixed dose of exogenous cortisol (typically, cortisone acetate or hydrocortisone 7 mg/m^2/day or 0.5 to 0.75 mg/kg/day) is normally sufficient to meet normal physiologic requirements.[9] However, if exogenous steroids are abruptly withdrawn or if additional coverage is not provided during stress or illness, the adrenals are unable to respond to the demands for increased cortisol production because the hypothalamic-pituitary axis has been suppressed. Regardless of the underlying dysfunction (whether primary, secondary, or iatrogenic), adrenal crisis may be precipitated when the body is unable to respond to the demand for increased glucocorticoid production. Signs and symptoms of adrenocortical insufficiency and the underlying mechanisms are outlined in Table 23-5.[3,10]

Diagnostic Presentation. Diagnostic findings of adrenocortical dysfunction are outlined in Table 23-6. In general, presentation is often that of profound circulatory failure with components of hypovolemic, distributive, and cardiogenic shock. In fact, the recommendation is that

TABLE 23-5 Adrenal Insufficiency

Signs and Symptoms	Underlying Mechanisms
Serum hyponatremia	Mineralocorticoid effect (decreased sodium and increased potassium reabsorption in distal tubule)
Serum hyperkalemia	
	Glucocorticoid effect (decreased free water clearance)
Shock	Volume depletion
Tachycardia, hypotension, weak rapid pulse, cold clammy skin, decreased perfusion, fever	Vasodilation, myocardial depression, poor arterial tone, decreased responsiveness and synthesis of catecholamines
Nausea, vomiting, diarrhea, poor feeding, weakness, fatigue	Electrolyte imbalance
Mental status changes, irritability	Central nervous system changes resulting from fluid deficit, hypoglycemia, or electrolyte imbalance
Hypoglycemia	Decreased gluconeogenesis

 TABLE 23-6 Diagnosis and Treatment of Adrenocortical Dysfunction

1. Participate in diagnostic workup

History	Nausea, vomiting, diarrhea, fatigue, weakness, headache
Risk factors	Hypopituitarism, congenital adrenal hyperplasia, abrupt discontinuation of high-dose steroids, known adrenally insufficient child who was ill and failed to receive stress coverage, CNS lesions (trauma, tumor, hemorrhage, seizures, hydrocephalus), shock, sepsis or systemic inflammatory response syndrome
Physical examination	Dehydration, fever
	Mental status changes, headache, irritability
	Shock (tachycardia, weak thready pulse, cold clammy skin, decreased perfusion, hypotension)
Laboratory tests	Hyperkalemia
	Hyponatremia
	Hypoglycemia
	Serum cortisol level decreased
Stimulation tests	Cortrosyn (adrenal function)
	Metyrapone (pituitary function)

2. Prevent complications related to hypovolemic shock, hyperkalemia, hypoglycemia

Evaluate fluid balance	Compare urine output and fluid intake
	Monitor weight trends
	Measure urine specific gravity
	Assess orthostatic blood pressure
Monitor electrocardiogram for changes related to serum potassium level	
Treat acute hypovolemia, hyponatremia, or hypoglycemia	Normal saline bolus then 5% glucose in normal saline
	Vasopressors
	Plasma expanders
Treat acute hyperkalemia	Calcium gluconate 10 mg/ml IV (administered over 5 min)
	Sodium bicarbonate 1-2 mEq/kg IV
	Glucose and insulin: administer 1-2 g/kg of glucose, simultaneous with the administration of 0.3 U/kg of regular insulin, both given over 1 to 2 hr
	Sodium polystyrene sulfonate (Kayexalate) 1 g/kg PR (in a 30% sorbitol solution) or PO (in a 70% sorbitol solution)
	Severe cases may necessitate dialysis
Replace mineralocorticoids	Fludrocortisone (Florinef) 0.05-0.2 mg PO daily
Replace glucocorticoids	Emergency management and "stress dosing": cortisol replacement in the form of hydrocortisone at doses of 25-55 mg/m^2 or 2 to 4 times the normal physiologic replacement dose is given by continuous infusion or IV bolus every 4 to 6 hr
	Maintenance dosing: cortisone acetate or hydrocortisone 7 mg/m^2/day or 0.5-0.75 mg/kg/day
Observe for undertreatment	Dehydration, shock

CNS, Central nervous system; *IV,* intravenous; *PO,* by mouth; *PR,* per rectum.

adrenal insufficiency be considered in all patients with shock refractory to the administration of catecholamines.[3] In primary adrenal insufficiency, the skin and mucous membranes may appear darkened or "tanned" as a result of high levels of pituitary ACTH precursors that are also pigments. Pallor, however, may be seen in cases of secondary insufficiency. In addition, patients may experience gastrointestinal upset and generalized weakness and malaise. Associated electrolyte imbalances include hyponatremia and hyperkalemia. Hypoglycemia may also ensue. Interestingly, plasma cortisol levels may be within normal range in critically ill patients with adrenal insufficiency, making diagnosis on the basis of cortical level alone unreliable.[29]

Critical Care Management.   The treatment of the child with adrenal insufficiency is outlined in Table 23-6. Interventions are focused on the prevention of complications associated with shock and the correction of electrolyte imbalances. Emergency resuscitation usually includes the use of a solution of normal saline to expand the vascular volume. Vasoactive and positive inotropic agents, such as dopamine and epinephrine, may be used to increase peripheral vascular resistance, heart rate, and myocardial contractility. If the serum potassium exceeds 5.5 mEq/L, strategies outlined in Table 23-6 may be used to manage acute hyperkalemia.

Emergency replacement of glucocorticoids is achieved intravenously using a soluble cortisol preparation such as hydrocortisone, hemisuccinate, or 21-phosphate. Most often, cortisol replacement in the form of hydrocortisone at doses of 25 to 55 mg/m^2, or 2 to 4 times the normal physiologic replacement dose, is given by continuous infusion or intravenous bolus every 4 to 6 hours. When the child with primary disease can take medications orally, mineralocorticoid replacement is added by giving fludrocortisone acetate (Florinef) 0.05 to 0.2 mg daily. As with other endocrine disorders, meticulous attention to fluid and electrolyte balance is an important aspect of the nursing care of the child with acute adrenal insufficiency.[9]

DISTURBANCES OF GLUCOSE HOMEOSTASIS

Hypoglycemia

Hypoglycemia is defined as a blood glucose level less than 60 mg/dl in an infant or child. Premature infants often have blood glucose levels between 20 and 60 mg/dl. However, despite the fact that glucose levels are naturally lower in premature neonates, it is unclear if serum glucose levels in the 20 to 60 mg/dl range adequately meet the metabolic needs of their cells. Therefore in light of the profound effects of hypoglycemia on the developing brain, a blood glucose level less than 60 mg/dl should be considered hypoglycemic, even in the neonate. Hypoglycemia is induced by inadequate adaptation to fasting, as well as by disorders resulting in insulin excess or decreased production of hormones that counterregulate insulin. Typically, efforts are aimed at maintaining a child's blood glucose level above 65 mg/dl.

Inadequate glycogen storage resulting in decreased tolerance of fasting is a normal condition of infancy. It is particularly problematic in premature infants and infants who are small for gestational age, are septic, or have congenital heart disease. In addition, diseases that impair glycogen storage, glycogen use, or gluconeogenesis, such as hepatic failure, or inborn errors of metabolism, such as glycogen storage disease type I or fructose 1,6-diphosphatase deficiency, result in hypoglycemia during fasting states. Disorders of fatty acid metabolism, such as medium-chain acyl-dehydrogenase deficiency and carnitine deficiency, or disorders of protein metabolism may also precipitate hypoglycemia. Drugs that contribute to a reduction in glucose stores or the body's ability to use glucose stores include alcohol, sulfonamides, β-adrenergic antagonists, and salicylates.[30]

Hypoglycemia caused by hyperinsulinism or the overproduction of insulin is encountered in disorders such as beta cell hyperplasia (nesidioblastosis) and beta cell adenomas. Children with hyperinsulinism are also vulnerable to hypoglycemia because chronically high insulin levels inhibit counterregulatory responses and the use of the backup energy sources of glycogenolysis, gluconeogenesis, and fatty acid oxidation. In addition, increased insulin production is induced whenever a high concentration of glucose is administered to the body. Transient hypoglycemia may be encountered in any child when an infusion of high glucose concentration is abruptly discontinued because hyperinsulin production may persist after the sudden decrease in glucose supply. Newborns of diabetic mothers often manifest transient hypoglycemia because of hyperinsulin production extending beyond the in utero period of exposure to high glucose load.[31] Furthermore, any deficit of counterregulatory hormone production may induce a hypoglycemic state. Hypopituitarism and adrenal insufficiency are associated with deficiencies of cortisol, growth hormone, and epinephrine and also result in hypoglycemia.[32]

Diagnostic Presentation.   Because the brain has a very high obligatory glucose requirement, nervous system dysfunction is precipitated by hypoglycemia. A sensation of hunger quickly occurs during states of glucose deficit, and the stimulation of the adrenergic and cholinergic receptors of the nervous system results in weakness, tachycardia, tremor, and diaphoresis. Central nervous system abnormalities resulting from glucose deficit, such as headache, depressed level of consciousness, and seizure activity, ensue when hypoglycemia is persistent.

Accurate documentation of a blood glucose value less than 60 mg/dl may be all that is needed to diagnose transient hypoglycemia in the infant with a history of prenatal stress, sepsis, maternal diabetes, prematurity, or congenital heart disease or in the infant or child who becomes hypoglycemic after rapid discontinuation of high-concentration glucose infusions. Persistent hypoglycemia suspected to be associated with inborn errors of metabolism, hyperinsulinism, and adrenocortical hypofunction (hypopituitarism, or primary adrenal insufficiency) often requires confirmation by controlled fasting studies. A controlled fasting study can assist in determining the child's ability to use alternative cellular energy pathways and to diagnose the underlying problem of hyperinsulin production or counterregulatory hormone deficiency.

Critical Care Management.   The care of the child with hypoglycemia is outlined in Table 23-7. The primary goal in managing hypoglycemia is to prevent deleterious central nervous system manifestations, such as seizures. If the child is able to take fluids orally, treatment may simply involve the provision of carbohydrate-containing fluids such as glucose water, infant formula, or juice. Simple carbohydrates are most quickly absorbed and are therefore more desirable than more complex sugars, such those in processed foods or candy. If the child is unconscious or unable to take fluids orally, glucose is administered intravenously. Glucose 0.5 to 2 g/kg, given as a 10% to 25% dextrose solution, can be administered via continuous infusion or by bolus administration. Blood glucose is measured immediately after administering glucose to determine the effectiveness of treatment. Levels are repeatedly assessed until the blood glucose reaches the 80 to 120 mg/dl range.[30] Guidelines for the frequency of measuring blood glucose for the child at risk for hypoglycemia are outlined in Table 23-7.

Long-term treatment of the child with persistent hypoglycemia is determined by the underlying cause. Mild hyperinsulinism may be managed initially with oral diazoxide (Proglycem) 3 to 15 mg/kg/day and frequent feedings. If this regimen fails, a trial of a somatostatin analog octreotide (Sandostatin) 1 to 10 µg/kg/day given subcutaneously may be initiated. Children who do not improve on either of these regimens usually require a subtotal pancreatectomy. Children with inborn errors of metabolism are generally treated by limiting fasting periods and by providing small, frequent feedings or continuous nasogastric feedings of specialized formulas. Hypoglycemia related to

 TABLE 23-7   Managing Hypoglycemia

1. Participate in diagnostic workup

History	Child's age, length of fast
Risk factors	Infants: large or small for gestational age; history of maternal diabetes; preterm; hypoxic, stressed, septic, congenital heart disease
	Rapid discontinuation of high-concentration dextrose infusion
	Adrenocortical hypofunction (primary, secondary, iatrogenic)
Physical examination	Adrenergic response
	Signs of neuroglycopenia
Laboratory tests	Glucose (decreased)
Fasting study laboratory tests	Insulin, growth hormone, cortisol
	Serum ketones
	Lactates
	Free fatty acids
	Carnitine
	Urine ketones, organic acids

2. Prevent central nervous system complications associated with hypoglycemia

Measure blood glucose	Immediately if symptomatic (pallor, irritability, difficult to arouse, diaphoretic)
	q15min if blood glucose <50 mg/Dl
	q30min-q1h: until blood glucose is consistently in 80-120 mg/dl range *or* if making changes in glucose infusion rate/concentration
	q2-4h if blood glucose is consistently in 80-120 mg/dl range and child is receiving glucose infusion
	Before meals or feedings if blood glucose in 80-120 mg/dl range and child is no longer receiving glucose infusion doses
Manage acute hypoglycemia (blood glucose <60 mg/dl)	If no IV access and able to take PO/NG, give 4-6 oz formula, glucose water, juice
	If IV access, increase IV glucose rate/concentration (5-20 ml/kg 10% dextrose solution IV or 2 ml/kg 25% dextrose solution)
	If no IV access, symptomatic, and unable to take PO, give 1 mg glucagon intramuscularly, subcutaneously (Will not work with glycogen storage disease and children who are glycogen depleted)
Limit fasting demands	High-risk infant: provide glucose supplements orally or via IV infusion to maintain glucose levels
	Glycogen storage disease: Limit fasting to 3-4 hours (type 1) or 6-8 hours (type 3)
	Overnight nasogastric feedings
	Fatty acid oxygenation defects: limit fasting to 10-12 hours
Treat underlying problem	Hyperinsulinism: diazoxide, somatostatin, subtotal pancreatectomy
	Hypopituitarism: cortisol, growth hormone replacement

IV, Intravenous; *PO,* by mouth; *NG,* nasogastric.

cortisol or growth hormone deficiency is treated by replacing the deficient hormones.[9,31]

Hyperglycemia

Hyperglycemia is defined as a serum glucose level higher than 120 mg/dl. Blood glucose values that exceed the renal threshold (approximately 180 mg/dl) result in movement of glucose into the urine and glucosuria. The excretion of glucose in the urine may cause osmotic diuresis, leading to dehydration and cardiovascular collapse. Passive loss of sodium and potassium in the urine accompanies the osmotic diuresis, and hyponatremia and hypokalemia may ensue. However, in the case of osmotic diuresis, serum sodium levels may be normal or elevated as a result of hemoconcentration. Serum may become hyperosmolar because of the combined high solute loads from the hyperglycemia and hypernatremia.

Hyperglycemia Caused by Excess of Counterregulatory Hormones.
Adrenocortical hyperfunction (Cushing's syndrome) causes the overproduction of glucocorticoids and induces hyperglycemia. The underlying problem may be due to an abnormality of the pituitary gland, which results in an overproduction of ACTH, an abnormality of the adrenal glands, or severe stress response resulting in the overproduction of cortisol, or it may be iatrogenically triggered by the administration of exogenous corticosteroids. High levels of circulating catecholamines, which are also produced by the adrenal gland, may also cause hyperglycemia. Stimulation of the sympathetic nervous system during the stress response, adrenal overproduction, or ectopic production by a pheochromocytoma or neuroblastoma may increase circulating catecholamine levels. Furthermore, catecholamines administered exogenously may also induce hyperglycemia.

Diabetes: Syndromes of Insulin Deficit or Resistance.
Lack of insulin production is associated with beta cell injury. Autoimmune beta cell destruction is the pathophysiologic mechanism underlying most cases of type I diabetes mellitus. Acute pancreatitis may result in interference with beta cell function and temporarily decrease insulin production. In addition, sclerotic changes in the pancreas caused by cystic fibrosis may result in permanent type I diabetes. Type II diabetes mellitus, on the other hand, is a state of decreased cellular insulin receptor sensitivity. Type II diabetes is less common in children.

In cases of both underproduction and decreased sensitivity to insulin, glucose cannot enter cells. Decreased glucose uptake by cells results in increased blood glucose levels, the use of alternative metabolic pathways for energy production, such as fatty acid oxidation, and a generalized state of cellular energy deficit. Ketones, the byproducts of fatty acid oxidation, may accumulate and result in an acidemia known as diabetic ketoacidosis (DKA). DKA usually occurs in cases of type I diabetes. In addition to the risk of developing DKA, patients with diabetes also experience multiple system organ damage as a result of persistently high glucose load in the blood and chronic cellular energy deficit. Patients with diabetes may also become prone to infection. Children with type I diabetes almost always require regular injections of insulin to prevent hyperglycemia; however, type II diabetes may be managed with specialized diets or oral hypoglycemia agents.[33-35]

Severe Glucose Deficit: Diabetic Ketoacidosis.
Fig. 23-1 outlines the progression of DKA. Children with type I diabetes who are noncompliant with insulin administration and who are experiencing illness or severe stress are at risk for developing DKA. DKA evolves as insulin deficiency results in hyperglycemia and mobilization of fatty acids and when the relative excess of counterregulatory hormones stimulates gluconeogenesis. When gluconeogenesis occurs, body proteins and lipids are broken down, making amino acid and fatty acid substrates available for cellular energy production. In addition, relative lack of insulin in relation to epinephrine, growth hormone, and, to a lesser extent, cortisol further stimulates the mobilization of fatty acids, the production of ketone bodies, and resultant ketoacidosis.[33-35]

Significant hyperglycemia also results in a profound osmotic diuresis and urinary electrolyte loss. Acidosis may further compound electrolyte abnormalities, and dehydration may be severe enough to precipitate cardiovascular collapse. As perfusion status worsens, lactic acidosis contributes to the falling pH.[33-35]

DKA is accompanied by total body sodium and potassium deficits resulting from osmotic diuresis. However, fluid shifts between the ICF and ECF and significant hemoconcentration result in variable measured serum electrolyte values. Serum potassium and sodium levels may be high, normal, or low depending on the degree of intravascular fluid volume depletion and metabolic acidosis. Acidosis complicates the interpretation of the electrolyte values because it induces temporary shifts of potassium from the ICF to the ECF. Potassium may then move back out of the ECF and into ICF during correction of acidosis. Serum phosphorous levels follow a pattern similar to potassium in response to acidosis.[33,35]

Cerebral edema is a complication of the treatment of DKA. The precise cause of cerebral edema in children with DKA is unknown. It may occur at any time during the 24-hour period following the initiation of therapy. Risk factors believed to be associated with cerebral edema include a pH less than 7.0, glucose level higher than 800 mg/dl, hyperosmolality and hypernatremia, use of bicarbonate to correct acidosis, too rapid correction of blood glucose, and very young age.[33-35] Interestingly, in addition to cerebral edema, anasarca and pulmonary edema have been reported in patients receiving treatment for DKA.[33,36]

Diagnostic Presentation. Diagnostic findings in hyperglycemia and DKA can be found in Box 23-1 and Table 23-8. Urinary glucose measurements provide a useful initial screening device for identifying the patient at risk. When the urine test result is positive for glucose, a blood sample is obtained to estimate the blood glucose. Bedside estimates should be confirmed by a simultaneous laboratory measure. A history of polyuria, polydipsia, and weight loss with documented hyperglycemia assists in the diagnosis of diabetes mellitus, particularly when accompanied by a

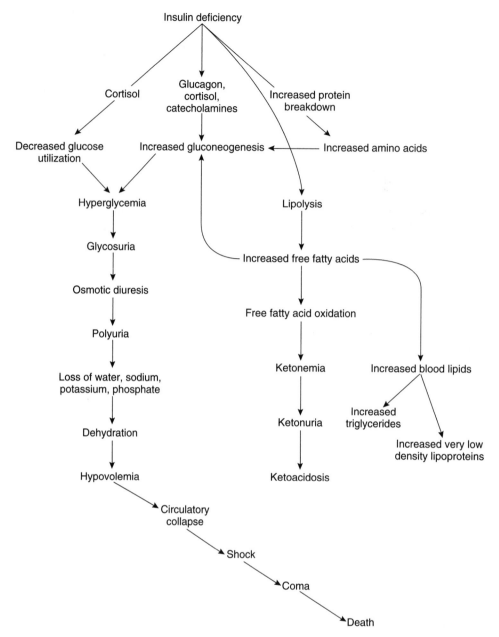

Fig. 23-1   Diabetic ketoacidosis. (Modified from Thompson JM: *Mosby's manual of clinical nursing,* ed 2, St Louis, 1989, Mosby, p 931.)

metabolic acidosis. Blood urea nitrogen (BUN) and creatinine levels provide an index of the degree of dehydration. Arterial pH, serum bicarbonate levels, and degree of base deficit reflect the degree of acidosis in the child with DKA. Urine ketones are also routinely measured in the child at risk for or experiencing DKA.

Critical Care Management

Hyperglycemia Without DKA.   Care of the child with hyperglycemia is outlined in Box 23-1. Definitive therapy involves the identification and treatment of the underlying cause of hyperglycemia. Nursing care is directed at the prevention of complications associated with acidosis and dehydration. A systematic process for screening patients at risk for hyperglycemia is also outlined in Box 23-1.

Mild dehydration (<5%) may be managed with oral fluid replacement of calorie-free liquids. More severe dehydration (>5%), or if the child who is unconscious or refusing to drink, requires intravenous fluid replacement.

Dietary management may be all that is required in some cases of transient and mild hyperglycemia. Feeding the child a low-concentrated carbohydrate diet may be sufficient to correct hyperglycemia. Otherwise, insulin may be given as four short-acting doses (before each meal and again at the time of a bedtime snack). A second option is a split-mixed dose of short- and long-acting insulin before breakfast and again before dinner. Frequent monitoring of blood glucose and monitoring for signs of hypoglycemia are essential with insulin administration and help to determine the most

Box 23-1
Diagnosing and Treating Hyperglycemia

1. Participate in diagnostic workup

   History: Polyuria, polydipsia, weight loss, fatigue

   Risk factors: Diabetes, significant stress, exogenous epinephrine, steroid or L-asparaginase administration, Cushing's syndrome, pheochromocytoma, glucagonoma

   Physical examination: Dehydration, mental status changes

   Laboratory tests: Hyperglycemia, hypernatremia, cortisol increased, glucagon increased, glucosuria

2. Detect hyperglycemia in patients at risk

   Measure urine for glucose q12h

   If urine test result is positive for glucose, measure blood glucose

   If blood glucose is >180 mg/dl, measure blood glucose qid until blood glucose consistently <180 mg/dl

   When blood glucose is consistently <180 mg/dl, resume measuring urine for glucose q12h

   If subcutaneous insulin being given, measure blood glucose 5 times per day (before breakfast, before lunch, before dinner, before bedtime snack, and at 2 AM)

   Additional measurements should be obtained as needed when clinical symptoms of hypoglycemia or hyperglycemia are detected

3. Prevent complications of hyperglycemia (dehydration, cerebral edema, weight loss)

   Correct fluid or electrolyte imbalance:

       Replace fluids lost as a result of osmotic diuresis orally or intravenously

       Low concentrated carbohydrate diet

       Administer insulin subcutaneously as ordered

   Evaluate fluid balance:

       Compare urine output to fluid intake

       Assess for orthostatic blood pressure

       Weigh daily while spilling glucose in urine

   Correct underlying cause:

       Surgery: Pheochromocytoma, glucagonoma

TABLE 23-8 Diabetic Ketoacidosis

Signs and Symptoms	Underlying Mechanisms
Hyperglycemia, dehydration, cardiovascular collapse	Osmotic diuresis secondary to hyperglycemia
Acidosis	Buildup of ketoacids and lactic acid in serum from lipolysis resulting in increased H^+ ion concentration in serum
Electrolyte imbalance	
Sodium	Total body hyponatremia because of passive loss of electrolytes as a result of osmotic diuresis; however, serum sodium may be high as a result of hemoconcentration
Potassium	In acidosis, potassium shifts from ICF to ECF; therefore initially serum potassium may increase, then decrease as a result of osmotic diuresis
Cardiac arrhythmia	Hypokalemia
	Hyperkalemia
Ketonuria	Serum ketone levels rise above the renal threshold and are spilled in the urine
Hyperpnea	Compensatory mechanism; effort to blow off excess CO_2 and thereby correct the degree of acidosis
Mental status changes/cerebral edema	Possibly related to rate of correction, level of acidosis, fluid shifts

ICF, Intracellular fluid; *ECF,* extracellular fluid; H^+, hydrogen.

---

appropriate insulin doses. Children receiving most or all of their calories intravenously are most easily managed using an intravenous insulin infusion titrated to maintain blood glucose values between 100 and 200 mg/dl.

Hyperglycemia With DKA. The prevention of complications related to dehydration, cardiovascular collapse, acidosis, electrolyte imbalance, and cerebral edema is the primary goal of the treatment of the child in DKA (Box 23-2). The first priority of care is to manage the dehydration. An initial fluid bolus (5 to 20 ml/kg of normal saline) is given over a 1- to 2-hour period. If the child continues to experience circulatory failure after the initial bolus, a second fluid bolus may be necessary. Remaining fluid deficits are usually replaced over a 24- to 48-hour period, often as 0.45% normal saline containing potassium supplements. (Potassium supplements are only added for children who are hypokalemic and have evidence of adequate renal function.)

However, some practitioners administer isotonic saline for extended periods to maintain an osmotic gradient that will prevent intracellular fluid shifts and cerebral edema. Ongoing urine losses caused by osmotic diuresis, in excess of 2 to 3 ml/kg/hr, may also be replaced with intravenous fluid.[33,35,37,38]

The second priority of care is to correct the acidosis and to prevent further lipolysis. Insulin has an inhibitory effect on ketone production; therefore the administration of insulin is the key to correcting metabolic acidosis. An intravenous infusion of regular insulin is the preferred method of administering insulin in children with DKA. Initial insulin doses are low; however, they are often be titrated to exceed normal physiologic requirements to decrease serum blood glucose levels and to inhibit further lipolysis and fatty acid oxidation. Infusions of 0.05 to 0.1 U/kg/hr of regular insulin are commonly administered. Hyperglycemia is always

---

Box 23-2
Treating Diabetic Ketoacidosis

1. Participate in diagnostic workup

   History: Polyuria, polydipsia, weight loss, fatigue, nausea, vomiting

   Physical examination: Dehydration, Kussmaul's respirations, facial flushing, abdominal tenderness, mental status changes

   Laboratory tests: Blood glucose, blood gas, electrolytes, BUN, creatinine, urine ketones and glucose

2. Prevent complications related to dehydration or cardiovascular collapse, acidosis, hypokalemia, hyperkalemia, cerebral edema

   Replace fluid or electrolytes lost as a result of osmotic diuresis:

   Resuscitate with 20 ml/kg of normal saline over a 1-hr period

   Repeat bolus if heart rate elevated or hypotensive after first bolus

   Replace remaining deficit over the next 24 to 48 hr with 0.9% or 0.45% normal saline

   While providing insulin infusion: Infusions of 0.05-0.1 U/kg/hr of regular insulin, titrated to effect

   Add 5% glucose to infusion when blood glucose reaches 300 mg/dl to prevent hypoglycemia

   Add 10% glucose to infusion when blood glucose reaches 200 mg/dl (and patient is receiving 5% dextrose) to prevent hypoglycemia

   Replace potassium losses in IV fluids

   Monitor ECG for signs of hyperkalemia and hypokalemia

   Correct acidosis: Insulin infusion

   Consider sodium bicarbonate for severe acidosis (pH <7.0) (controversial)

   Measure blood glucose:

   Every hour until insulin infusion is discontinued

   Every 2 hr until taking fluids orally and IV fluids are discontinued

   Five times per day after discontinuing IV fluids (before breakfast, before lunch, before dinner, before bedtime snack, and at 2 AM)

   Additional measurements should be obtained as needed when clinical symptoms of hypoglycemia are detected

   Monitor response to therapy: Vital signs (pulse, respirations, blood pressure)

   q30-60min while on insulin infusion

   q shift until ketones cleared

   Weigh daily

   Compare fluid intake to output

   Measure urine ketones/glucose whenever blood glucose >240 mg/dl

   Detect and treat cerebral edema in a timely fashion:

   Neurosigns hourly for 24 hr (mental status changes, pupillary response)

   Treat signs of cerebral edema immediately

BUN, Blood urea nitrogen; *IV*, intravenous; *ECG*, electrocardiogram.

---

corrected slowly (no more than a 10% decrease in serum glucose level every hour). Rapid correction of hyperglycemia is associated with the development of cerebral edema.[33,39] A 5% solution of glucose is added to the intravenous fluid as the blood glucose decreases to approximately 200 to 300 mg/dl. When the child's blood glucose decreases to approximately 200 mg/dl, the concentration of glucose is increased to 10%. Blood glucose is measured at least hourly while insulin is infused and should be measured within 30 minutes after a change in either the dose of insulin or concentration of glucose. The rate of the insulin infusion is usually held constant at a dose that achieves a normal serum glucose level and inhibition of further lipolysis, fatty acid oxidation, and ketone production. Monitoring of urine samples for ketones is used to identify the point at which fatty acid oxidation has ceased.

Infusion of sodium bicarbonate is occasionally used to correct severe acidosis (pH is less than 7.0) in children with DKA. Severe acidosis may cause myocardial depression and decrease the insulin sensitivity of cells.[40] However, the use of sodium bicarbonate in the treatment of DKA is controversial because bicarbonate administration may cause intracellular acidosis and worsens cerebral edema.[40] Research investigating the outcomes of adults with DKA who received bicarbonate therapy has demonstrated conflicting results. Recently Green and colleagues[40] retrospectively studied the use of bicarbonate for correction of acidosis associated with DKA in children. Green and co-workers[40] reported that administration of bicarbonate was unrelated to final outcome and that children with pH as low as 6.73 recovered without administration of bicarbonate. However, the study also did not find a correlation between adverse events, such as cerebral edema, and bicarbonate therapy. Sodium bicarbonate is administered intravenously in doses of 0.5 to 1 mEq/kg, or when the base deficit is known, according to the following formula:

$$mEq \text{ of bicarbonate} = 0.3 \times (\text{Body weight in kg}) \times (\text{Base deficit})[41]$$

Monitoring for life-threatening cardiac dysrhythmias precipitated by either hypokalemia or hyperkalemia is initiated for children undergoing treatment for DKA. Ventricular ectopic beats often are due to hypokalemia, and peaked T waves are indicative of hyperkalemia.

Monitoring for signs and symptoms of cerebral edema is indicated for children undergoing treatment for DKA. Indicators of cerebral edema and elevated intracranial pressure include mental status changes, decreased pupil reactivity, bradycardia, hypertension, and abnormal respiratory patterns. Cerebral edema in children with DKA may require acute intervention such as supported respiration and circulation, hyperosmolar therapy, moderate hypothermia, pharmacologically mediated reduction in cerebral metabolic rate, and appropriate positioning (such as head elevation).

SUMMARY

The endocrine system stimulates and inhibits the secretion of hormones into the bloodstream. Hormones regulate many metabolic processes of the body, including fluid and electrolyte balance and glucose homeostasis. Disorders of fluid and electrolyte balance and glucose homeostasis can cause hemodynamic instability and may progress to circulatory failure and shock. Care of the child with endocrine problems includes vigilant monitoring for the signs of frank hemodynamic instability and for the specific signs and symptoms of altered electrolyte levels, changes in fluid volume status, and states of abnormal glucose metabolism. Management of endocrine problems includes replacement or restriction of electrolytes and fluid, the replacement of hormones when appropriate, and support of circulation.

REFERENCES

1. Baylis PH, Cheetham T: Diabetes insipidus, *Arch Dis Child* 79:84-89, 1998.
2. Kappy MS, Ganong CA: Cerebral salt wasting in children: the role of atrial natriuretic hormone, *Adv Pediatr* 43:271-308, 1996.
3. Oekers, W: Current concepts: adrenal insufficiency, *N Engl J Med* 335:1206-1212, 1996.
4. Olson BR, Gumowski J, Rubino D et al: Pathophysiology of hyponatremia after transphenoidal pituitary surgery, *J Neurosurg* 87:499-507, 1997.
5. Finfer S, Bohn D, Colpitts D et al: Intensive care management of pediatric organ donors and its effect on post-transplant organ function, *Intensive Care Med* 22:1424-1432, 1996.
6. Lee YJ, Huang FY, Shen EY et al: Neurogenic diabetes insipidus in children with hypoxic encephalopathy: six new cases and a review of the literature, *Eur J Pediatr* 155:245-248, 1996.
7. Charmandari E, Brook CGD: 20 years of experience with idiopathic central diabetes insipidus, *Lancet* 353:2212-2213, 1999.
8. Lee YJ, Shen EY, Huang FY et al: Continuous infusion of vasopressin in comatose children with neurogenic diabetes insipidus, *J Pediatr Endocrinol Metab* 8:257-262, 1995.
9. Barone MA: *The Harriet Lane handbook,* ed 14, St Louis, 1996, Mosby.
10. Kohane DS, Tobin JR, Kohane IS: Endocrine, mineral and metabolic diseases. In Rogers MC, Helfaer MA, eds: *Handbook of pediatric critical care,* ed 3, Philadelphia, 1999, Williams & Wilkins.
11. Lugo N, Silver P, Nimkoff L et al: Diagnosis and management algorithm of acute onset central diabetes insipidus in critically ill children, *J Pediatr Endocrinol Metab* 10:633-639, 1997.
12. Taylor SL, Tyrrell JB, Wilson CB: Delayed onset of hyponatremia after transphenoidal surgery for pituitary adenomas, *Neurosurgery* 37:653-654, 1995.
13. Patwari AK, Singh BS, Manorama DE: Inappropriate secretion of antidiuretic hormone in acute bacterial meningitis, *Ann Trop Paediatr* 15:179-183, 1995.
14. Brazel PW, McPhee IB: Inappropriate secretion of antidiuretic hormone in post-operative scoliosis patients: the role of fluid management, *Spine* 21:724-727, 1996.
15. Abe T, Takaue Y, Okamoto Y et al: Syndrome of inappropriate antidiuretic hormone secretion (SIADH) in children undergoing high dose chemotherapy and autologous peripheral blood stem cell transplantation, *Pediatr Hematol Oncol* 12:363-369, 1995.
16. Damaraju SC, Rajshekhar V, Chandy MJ: Validation study of central venous pressure based protocol for the management of neurosurgical patients with hyponatremia and natriuresis, *Neurosurgery* 40:316-317, 1997.
17. Rao RH: Bilateral massive adrenal hemorrhage, *Med Clin North Am* 79:107-129, 1995.
18. Riordan FA, Thompson APJ, Ratcliff JM et al: Admission cortisol and adrenocorticotropic hormone levels in children with meningococcal disease: evidence of adrenal insufficiency? *Crit Care Med* 27:2257-2261, 1999.
19. Briegel J, Forst H, Haller M et al: Stress doses of hydrocortisone reverse hyperdynamic septic shock: a prospective, randomized, double-blind, single-center study, *Crit Care Med* 27:723-732, 1999.
20. Hatherill M, Tibby S, Hilliard T et al: Adrenal insufficiency in septic shock, *Arch Dis Child* 80:51-55, 1999.
21. Bollaert PE, Charpentier C, Levy B et al: Reversal of late septic shock with supraphysiologic doses of hydrocortisone, *Crit Care Med* 26:645-650, 1998.
22. Bone RC, Fisher CJ, Clemmer TP: A controlled trial of high-dose methylprednisolone in the treatment of severe sepsis and septic shock, *N Engl J Med* 317:653-658, 1987.
23. Veterans Administration Systemic Sepsis Cooperative Study Group: Effect of high dose glucocorticoid therapy on mortality in patients with clinical signs of systemic sepsis, *N Engl J Med* 317:659-665, 1987.
24. Bernard C, Tedgui A: Cytokine network and vessel wall: insights into septic shock pathogeneses, *Eur Cytokine Netw* 3:19-33, 1992.
25. Saito T, Takanashi M, Gallagher E et al: Corticosteroid effect on early beta-adrenergic down-regulation during circulatory shock: hemodynamic study and beta-adrenergic assay, *Intensive Care Med* 21:204-210, 1995.
26. Suba EA, McKenna TM, Williams TJ: In vivo and in vitro effects of endotoxin on vascular responsiveness to norepinephrine and signal transduction in the rat, *Circ Shock* 36:127-133, 1992.
27. Briegel J, Schelling G, Haller M et al: A comparison of adrenocortical response during septic shock and after complete recovery, *Intensive Care Med* 22:894-899, 1996.
28. Soni A, Pepper GM, Wyrwinski PM: Adrenal insufficiency occurring during septic shock: incidence, outcome and relationship to peripheral cytokine levels, *Am J Med* 98:266-271, 1995.
29. Vermes I, Beishuizen A, Hampsink RM et al: Dissociation of plasma adrenocorticotropin and cortisol levels in critically ill patients: possible role of endothelin and atrial natriuretic hormone, *J Clin Endocrinol Metab* 80:1238-1242, 1995.
30. Service FJ: Hypoglycemia, *Med Clin North Am* 79:1-7, 1995.
31. Schwitzgebel VM, Gitelman SE: Neonatal hyperinsulinism, *Clin Perinatol* 25:1015-1038, 1998.
32. Stanley CA: Hyperinsulinism in infants and children, *Pediatr Clin North Am* 44:363-374, 1997.
33. Brink SJ: Diabetic ketoacidosis, *Acta Paediatr* 427(suppl):14-24, 1999.
34. Klekamp J, Churchwell KB: Diabetic ketoacidosis in children: Initial clinical assessment and treatment, *Pediatr Ann* 25:387-393, 1996.
35. Salink M: Practical management of diabetic ketoacidosis in childhood and adolescence, *Acta Pediatr* suppl 425:63-66, 1998.
36. Martin YC: Simultaneous acute cerebral edema and pulmonary edema complicating diabetic ketoacidosis, *Diabetes Care* 18:1288-1290, 1995.
37. Fineberg L: Why do patients with diabetic ketoacidosis have cerebral swelling and why does treatment sometimes make it worse? *Arch Pediatr Adolesc Med* 150:785-786, 1996.
38. Harris GD, Fiordalisi I, Yu C: Maintaining normal intracranial pressure in a rabbit model during treatment of severe diabetic ketoacidemia, *Life Sci* 59:1695-16702, 1996.
39. Wagner A, Risse A, Brill HL et al: Therapy of severe diabetic ketoacidosis: zero mortality under very low dose insulin application, *Diabetes Care* 22:674-677, 1999.
40. Green SM, Rothrock SG, Ho JD et al: Failure of adjunctive bicarbonate to improve outcome in severe pediatric diabetic ketoacidosis, *Ann Emerg Med* 31:41-48, 1998.
41. Scheleien CL, Kuluz JW, Shaffner DH et al: Cardiopulmonary resuscitation. In Rogers MC, Helfaer MA, eds: *Handbook of pediatric critical care,* ed 3, Philadelphia, 1999, Williams & Wilkins.

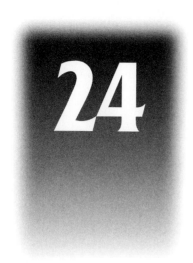

24 Hematologic Critical Care Problems

Debbie Brinker
Patricia A. Moloney-Harmon

Children in the pediatric intensive care unit (PICU) experience a variety of hematologic problems that vary in severity. This is partially because of the complex structure and function of blood and its components, which affect every cell and organ system in the body. In addition, organs of the hematopoietic system, such as bone marrow, are prone to the adverse effects of sepsis, trauma, shock, and drugs used for critical illnesses. The majority of hematologic problems seen in critically ill children are acquired and often present as an acute episode.[1] The more common problems include disseminated intravascular coagulation (DIC), vascular access thrombi, anemias, hemolytic uremic syndrome (HUS), and blood dyscrasias.

This chapter focuses on assessment of hematologic function, supportive and therapeutic interventions (i.e., blood product administration and apheresis), and alterations in hematologic function, including disorders of coagulation and oxygen-carrying capacity. Disorders will be discussed as final common pathways of altered hematologic function with emphasis on pathophysiology and nursing care of the patient with DIC, sickle cell anemia (SCA), and HUS.

ESSENTIAL EMBRYOLOGY

During embryologic development, blood formation can be recognized as early as 3 weeks after conception. By the sixth week of gestation, hematopoiesis (the production of red cells, white cells, and platelets) moves from the yolk sac to the liver, which is the main site of blood formation during the middle portion of fetal life. Following the twentieth week of gestation, hematopoiesis then moves to the bone marrow; and following birth, it takes place almost entirely in the bone marrow.

ESSENTIAL ANATOMY AND PHYSIOLOGY

Hematopoietic Organs

Bone marrow is the chief site for hematopoiesis. There are two types of bone marrow: yellow marrow, which contains a large percentage of fat cells; and red marrow, which contains mostly blood cells. The infant and young child have a larger proportion of red marrow because of the high

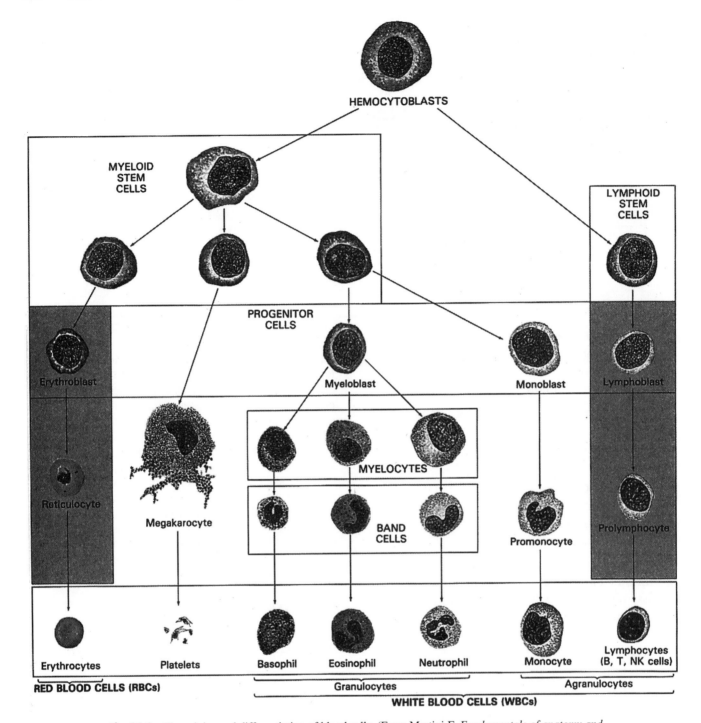

Fig. 24-1   The origins and differentiation of blood cells. (From Martini F, *Fundamentals of anatomy and physiology,* ed 3, Upper Saddle River, NJ, 1995, Prentice-Hall. Adapted by permission of Prentice-Hall, Upper Saddle River, NJ.)

requirements for red cell production. Early in life the red marrow is contained in the medullary cavities of the long bones. These cavities gradually fill with fat as the demands for red cell production decrease until the adult distribution of hematopoiesis (sternum, pelvis, vertebrae, cranium, ribs, and epiphyses of long bones) are reached at puberty. In disease states associated with anemias, hematopoiesis can return to its former sites, including the long bones, skull, liver, spleen, and lymph nodes. It may also take place in the adrenal glands, cartilage, adipose tissues, and kidneys. Fig. 24-1 illustrates the formation and maturation of blood cells.

Blood Stem Cell

Human bone marrow contains a pluripotent hematopoietic stem cell precursor that is capable of differentiating into erythroid, granulocytic, monocytic, megakaryocytic, and certain lymphoid cell lines. This cell gives rise to the marrow stem cell, which produces the precursor for erythrocytes, granulocytes, monocytes, and platelets. Stem cells are present in small numbers in blood and bone marrow. Their turnover depends on the needs of the body. It has been suggested that the structure of the stem cell is similar to that of the lymphocyte.

Composition of Blood

Blood is composed of plasma in which are suspended certain proteins (such as albumin, globulin), clotting factors, and the blood cells. These include leukocytes (white blood cells [WBCs]), erythrocytes (red blood cells [RBCs]), and thrombocytes (platelets).

Leukocytes. The main function of the leukocytes are to fight infection; defend the body against foreign organisms through phagocytosis; and produce, transport, and distribute antibodies in the immune system. Leukocytes are discussed in detail in Chapter 15.

Erythrocytes. Erythrocytes (RBCs) are the most abundant component in the blood. They have biconcave discs without nuclei and are extremely flexible. This allows them to travel extremely fast and bend and twist as they pass through tiny capillaries. Their elongated shape in the capillaries allows for more surface area for the exchange of oxygen and carbon dioxide.

After birth, the rate of hemoglobin (Hgb) synthesis and production of RBCs decreases dramatically during the first few days of life. Over the next few weeks, as the conversion occurs from fetal to adult Hgb, and the threshold of decreased venous oxygen saturation is reached, a physiologic nadir is created at about 7 to 10 weeks. A signal in the form of increased erythropoietin production is sent to the marrow, and erythropoiesis is stimulated, eventually leading to an increase in Hgb, at about 3 to 4 months of age. Premature infants reach their nadir earlier than term infants and require a longer period of time to recover.[2]

The main function of erythrocytes is the transport of oxygen and carbon dioxide, which is accomplished through Hgb, the major component of RBCs. Oxygen binds with Hgb and then is released at tissue sites where gas exchange takes place.

Fetal hemoglobin (Hb F) is present at birth and allows for more efficient binding of oxygen at lower surface tensions. Hb F constitutes 70% of the total Hgb at birth but declines rapidly. By 6 to 12 months of age, Hb F has been mostly replaced by adult Hgb, although levels of 1% to 2% of Hb F remain throughout life. Hb F shifts the oxyhemoglobin dissociation curve to the left so that oxygen bound to Hgb is not readily released to the tissues. This may compromise tissue oxygenation in newborns with diminished cardiovascular reserves.

RBCs are formed in the red bone marrow and progress through the stages of development outlined in Box 24-1.

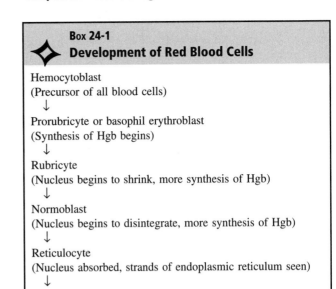

Box 24-1
Development of Red Blood Cells

Hemocytoblast
(Precursor of all blood cells)
↓
Prorubricyte or basophil erythroblast
(Synthesis of Hgb begins)
↓
Rubricyte
(Nucleus begins to shrink, more synthesis of Hgb)
↓
Normoblast
(Nucleus begins to disintegrate, more synthesis of Hgb)
↓
Reticulocyte
(Nucleus absorbed, strands of endoplasmic reticulum seen)
↓
Erythrocyte
(Mature RBC without nucleus or reticulum)

The mature erythrocyte is released into the circulation where the average lifespan is about 120 days. This time span represents the interval between the cell's release into the circulation from the bone marrow and its destruction. When the RBC ages, it is removed from the circulation by the spleen, liver, and red bone marrow. When the hematopoietic system is faced with a heavy demand for the production of RBCs, such as with hemorrhage, immature RBCs are released into the circulation. The number of immature cells and their degree of immaturity reflect the severity of stress placed on this body system. When the demand is great, the number of reticulocytes may increase by 30% to 50%. With an increased demand, the number of normoblasts may appear in large numbers. In severe anemias, the percentage of normoblasts may be as high as 5% to 20% of the circulating RBCs. Prorubricytes may also appear at this time. This information is also important in differentiating various types of anemias.

RBC production is also stimulated by decreased tissue oxygenation because RBC production depends not only on the actual number present in the circulation but also on their ability to carry oxygen and carbon dioxide. When tissue oxygenation is decreased, erythropoietin stimulates the stem cells in the bone marrow to produce mature RBCs. Erythropoietin is produced in the kidney and is released in response to hypoxia and anemia. Table 24-1 lists the normal RBC values at various ages.

Thrombocytes (Platelets). Platelet development takes place primarily in the bone marrow. Platelets are the smallest of the blood cell components. They are fragments of megakaryocytes. Megakaryocytes mature in the bone marrow and fragment, where each one releases approximately 5000 platelets into the blood. The lifespan of platelets is approximately 7 to 14 days. Approximately 10% to 15% of the circulating platelets are consumed in the daily repair of small vascular injuries.

TABLE 24-1	Red Blood Cell Studies		
Test	**Normal Values**	**Purpose**	**Clinical Significance**
Red blood count (RBC)	Millions of cells/mm^3	Measures total number of circulating RBCs	Increased in polycythemia, severe diarrhea, dehydration, acute poisoning, during and immediately following hemorrhage
	1 wk 3.9-6.3		Decreased in anemia, diseases of bone marrow function, hemolytic and pernicious anemia, subacute endocarditis
	2 wk 3.6-6.2		
	1 mo 3.0-5.4		
	2 mo 2.7-4.9		
	3-6 mo 3.1-4.5		
	0.5-2 yr 3.7-5.3		
	2-6 yr 3.9-5.3		
	6-12 yr 4.0-5.2		
	12-18 yr		
	M 4.5-5.3		
	F 4.1-5.1		
Hematocrit (Hct)	% of packed cells	Measures percentage of RBCs in a volume of blood	Increased in erythrocytosis, polycythemia, severe dehydration, shock—when hemoconcentration rises considerably
	3 days 44-72		Decreased in anemia, leukemia, acute massive blood loss, hemolytic reactions
	2 mo 28-42		Unreliable immediately after transfusions, hemorrhage
	6-12 yr 35-45		
	12-18 yr		
	M 37-49		
	F 36-46		
Hemoglobin (Hgb)	g/dl	Measures oxygen-carrying capacity of the blood	Increased in hemoconcentration of the blood, CHF
	1-3 days 14.5-22.5		Decreased in anemia; severe hemorrhage, hemolytic reactions
	2 mo 9.0-14.0		Unreliable immediately after transfusions, hemorrhage
	6-12 yr 11.5-15.5		
	12-18 yr		
	M 13.0-16.0		
	F 12.0-16.0		
Erythrocyte sedimentation rate (ESR)	0-10 mm/hr	Measures the rate at which RBCs settle out of unclotted blood in 1 hr	Increased values found in infections, inflammatory diseases, carcinomas, cell or tissue destruction, toxemia, nephritis, pneumonia, severe anemia
		Based on the fact that inflammatory and necrotic processes result in aggregation of RBCs, which makes them heavier and more likely to settle	Decreased values found in polycythemia vera, sickle cell anemia, CHF

Test	Subgroup	Value	Description	Interpretation
Reticulocyte count	Infants	2%-5% of total RBCs	Measures the number of immature RBCs (reticulocytes) compared with total RBCs. Indicates an increase in RBC production and/or a decrease in RBC destruction	Increased in hemolytic anemia, sickle cell disease, leukemia, 3-4 days following hemorrhage, after splenectomy, following treatment of anemia. Decreased levels indicate that the bone marrow is not producing enough erythrocytes and is seen in iron-deficiency anemia, aplastic anemia, chronic infection, radiation therapy
	Children	0.5-4.0% of total RBCs		
Mean corpuscular volume (MCV)		μm^3	Measures the volume occupied by a single RBC and indicates size of the cell: Normocytic—of normal size; Microcytic—smaller than normal; Macrocytic—larger than normal	Decreased in anemia, thalassemia. Increased in liver diseases, deficiency of folate or vitamin B_{12}
	1-3 days	95-121		
	0.5-2 yr	70-86		
	6-12 yr	77-95		
	12-18 yr M	78-98		
	F	78-102		
Mean corpuscular hemoglobin concentration (MCHC)		% Hgb/cell or g Hgb/dl RBC	Measure of the concentration of hemoglobin in an average cell	Most valuable in evaluating therapy for anemia because the two most accurate hematologic determinations (Hgb and Hct) are used in this test. Increased MCHC usually indicates spherocytosis. Decreased MCHC indicates that a unit volume of packed RBCs contains less hemoglobin than normal. May be seen in iron-deficiency anemia, thalassemia
	1-3 days	30-36		
	1-2 wk	29-37		
	1-2 mo	29-37		
	3 mo-2 yr	30-36		
	2-18 yr	31-37		
Mean corpuscular hemoglobin (MCH)		%/cell	Measure of the average weight of hemoglobin in the RBC. Less accurate than MCHC because uses RBC count in the calculation and that count may be inaccurate	Increased MCH associated with macrocytic anemia. Decreased value associated with iron-deficiency anemia
	1-3 days	31-37		
	1 wk-1 mo	28-40		
	2 mo	26-34		
	3-6 mo	25-35		
	0.5-2 yr	23-31		
	2-6 yr	24-30		
	6-12 yr	25-33		
	12-18 yr	25-35		

From Fischbach F: *A manual of laboratory diagnostic tests*, Philadelphia, 1980, JB Lippincott; Foster RL, Hunsberger MM, Anderson JJ: *Family-centered nursing care of children*, Philadelphia, 1989, WB Saunders.

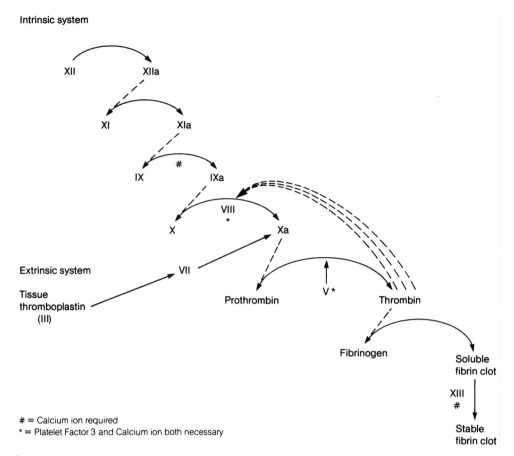

Intrinsic system

XII   XIIa

XI   XIa

IX   #   IXa

VIII
*

X   Xa

Extrinsic system   VII

Tissue
thromboplastin
(III)

Prothrombin   V *   Thrombin

Fibrinogen   Soluble
fibrin clot

XIII
#

Stable
fibrin clot

\# = Calcium ion required
* = Platelet Factor 3 and Calcium ion both necessary

Fig. 24-2   The coagulation sequence. (From Hudak C, Gallo B, Lohr T, eds: *Critical care nursing,*
Philadelphia, 1973, JB Lippincott.)

The rate of platelet production and the level of circulating platelets are thought to be controlled by thrombopoietin or thrombopoiesis-stimulating factor. The level of circulating catecholamines also has an effect on platelet levels. The administration of epinephrine can immediately produce a 20% to 50% increase in the platelet count. This response is likely to be the result of mobilization from the splenic pool. Hypoxia also increases the number of circulating platelets.

Platelets play a primary role in the process of hemostasis. Hemostasis is achieved by vascular spasm, formation of a platelet plug, formation of a blood clot, and formation of connective tissue, which permanently repairs the damaged vessel. Vascular spasm reduces blood flow through a damaged blood vessel to prevent further blood loss. When platelets come in contact with the damaged blood vessel, they adhere to the walls of the vessel at the site of damage. Other platelets in the area are activated, and aggregation occurs when these cells adhere to the first. Thus platelets group together to repair the damaged vessel.

Coagulation is a complex process involving an intricate series of reactions that include a number of different factors present in the blood or the tissues. These substances influence the mechanisms of clotting by promoting clotting with procoagulants (clotting factors) or inhibiting clotting with anticoagulants. Some are also involved in the removal of a clot once it is formed. Each clotting factor acts as an

enzyme, which, when activated, proceeds in a stepwise fashion to the next reaction. This is referred to as the *clotting cascade,* or more appropriately as a *clotting continuum,* because feedback is involved to activate and/or inhibit the coagulation process (Fig. 24-2).

The first step of coagulation is the formation of pro-thrombin activator. This step is the most complex because it involves a group of clotting factors involved in the extrinsic and intrinsic pathways. The extrinsic pathway is activated by trauma to the vascular walls and surrounding tissues. Factor III must be released from the endothelial cells and other tissues before activation can begin. When chemicals released into the tissues at time of injury (tissue factor) contact factor VII, sequential activation of factors X, V, II, and I take place. These factors then convert factor X to activated factor X.

When factor XII and platelets come in contact with collagen in the damaged wall of a vessel, the intrinsic pathway is activated. Factors XI, IX, VIII, X, II, and I are then activated, followed by the activation of factor X.

With the help of factor V, activated factor X forms prothrombin activator. Once this is formed, with the assistance of calcium ions, prothrombin is activated. Prothrombin is converted to thrombin with assistance of factor V. In the presence of thrombin and calcium ions, fibrinogen is converted into fibrin. The fibrin threads form a

◆ TABLE 24-2 Clotting Factors

Factor	Synonym
I	Fibrinogen
II	Prothrombin
III	Tissue thromboplastin
IV	Calcium
V	Proaccelerin
VII	Proconvertin
VIII	Antihemophilic factor A
IX	Christmas factor
X	Stuart-Prower factor
XI	Plasma thromboplastin antecedent
XII	Hageman factor
XIII	Fibrin stabilizing factor

From Eskenazi AE, Gordon JB, Bernstein ML: Hematologic disorders in the pediatric intensive care unit. In Rogers MC, ed: *Textbook of pediatric intensive care,* ed 3, Baltimore, 1996, Williams & Wilkins.

network over the damaged area of the vessel, which traps blood cells, platelets, and plasma. A blood clot is formed and prevents further leakage through the damaged vessel. Within minutes of formation, clot retraction pulls together the sides of the damaged vessel.

Once formed, the clot may be the basis for new connective tissue or it undergoes the processes of lysis and dissolution. After a few hours, fibroblasts invade the clot, and within 7 to 10 days, fibrous connective tissue is formed. Plasminogen and plasminogen activator, which are trapped within the clot with platelets and RBCs, ultimately produce plasmin, which lyses the clot.

The extrinsic pathway is activated when factor III gains access to the bloodstream; the intrinsic pathway is activated when blood comes in contact with an abnormal surface. Regardless of the initiating mechanism, the end is the same. Large amounts of thrombin are produced, which is then followed by the transformation of fibrinogen to fibrin. Table 24-2 lists the factors involved in the clotting mechanism.

ASSESSMENT AND DIAGNOSIS OF HEMATOLOGIC DISORDERS

On admission, infants and children may present with primary diagnoses of bleeding and/or coagulation disorders, or have coincidental findings discovered per history, physical examination, or laboratory results.

Clinical History

An admitting history includes questions regarding bleeding disorders (e.g., patient or family history of hemophilia or von Willebrand's disease), and whether a child bleeds or bruises easily. It is important for a parent/historian to distinguish "normal childhood bruising" over extremity bones and bony prominences versus soft-tissue bruising with no apparent cause.

Other important issues include symptoms from decreased or dysfunctional RBCs or WBCs. A history for anemia (decreased RBCs) includes fatigue, listlessness, decrease in activity or energy level, syncope, and pallor. An infectious history (e.g., frequent sinus infections, joint infections, and lacerations that do not heal) may be indicative of decreased (or dysfunctional) WBCs. Immunosuppressive conditions or therapies such as chemotherapy or antirejection drugs posttransplant are important to evaluate in terms of WBC and infection risk.

Assessment and Physical Examination

Physical examination of the child with a hematologic disorder begins with observation of the child's general appearance. The child may appear pale because of anemia. Jaundice may be present if the child has a potential clotting problem from hepatic dysfunction. Signs of clotting include petechiae, purpura (small, red/purple areas that may be flat in abnormal bleeding states such as DIC, or raised [palpable] areas in cutaneous vasculitis disorders such as Henoch-Schönlein purpura [HSP]), and ecchymosis.

Cardiovascular symptoms may manifest as massive bleeding secondary to trauma with hemodynamic instability and prolonged bleeding. Oozing from venipuncture, intravenous, or arterial puncture sites may also be present.

Pulmonary symptoms may include frank bleeding from endotracheal tube or prolonged nose bleeds. Signs of respiratory distress such as tachypnea and dyspnea (especially on exertion) correlated with a decreased Hgb value may also be present. Neurologic symptoms of hematologic dysfunction include signs of cerebral vascular accident (CVA) or a central nervous system (CNS) hemorrhage as evidenced by a change in the level of consciousness. The child may demonstrate unilateral changes in reflexes (including pupils), circulation, sensation, or movement (CSM).

The major gastrointestinal (GI) manifestation of hematologic dysfunction is frank or occult bleeding in GI contents. The presence of blood in the urine also may signal a bleeding disorder.

Monitoring Hematologic Function

Multiple laboratory tests are used to monitor hematologic function. The most common tests include the complete blood count (CBC) and coagulation studies. It is important to interpret the CBC based on age comparison normals because growth and developmental changes occur in the hematologic system. A summary of RBC studies is reviewed in Table 24-1 and coagulation studies are described in Table 24-3.

Bone marrow aspiration is a common procedure performed to assess hematologic status. The bone marrow is typically obtained from the posterior iliac crest. This diagnostic procedure allows for assessment of marrow cellularity, quantitative and qualitative changes in hematologic precursors (i.e., cytopenias), and evaluation for disorders such as acute leukemia (discussed in Chapter 25), and aplastic anemia.

TABLE 24-3 **Coagulation Studies**

Test	Normal Values*	Purpose	Clinical Significance
Platelet count	150,000-400,000/mm³	Measures total number of circulating platelets	Abnormally decreased in ITP; pernicious, aplastic, and hemolytic anemia; drugs, especially chemotherapeutic agents; bone marrow malignancies Abnormally increased after splenectomy and in certain cancers; may predispose to thrombotic episodes
Prothrombin time (PT) or INR (international normalized ratio)	11-15 sec <1.2	Indirectly measures the ability of the blood to clot and directly measures a defect in phase II clotting mechanisms (prothrombin, fibrinogen, factors V, VII, X)	Prolonged in prothrombin deficiency; vitamin K deficiency; deficiencies of fibrinogen; factors V, VII, X; anticoagulant therapy; severe liver disease; DIC
Activated partial thromboplastin time (APTT)	20-35 sec	Same as for PTT but more sensitive and faster to perform	Same as PTT
Fibrinogen D-Dimer	>150 mg/dl <0.5 μg/ml	Measures fibrinogen level Measure of degradation of cross-linked fibrin	Decreased in liver disease, DIC Increased in DIC
Thrombin time (TT); thrombin clotting time	9-13 sec	Measures fibrinogen to fibrin formation; detects stage III of fibrinogen abnormalities	Prolonged with low fibrinogen levels; anticoagulant therapy; liver disease; DIC

From Fischbach F: *A manual of laboratory diagnostic tests,* Philadelphia, 1980, J.B. Lippincott; Foster RL, Hunsberger MM, Anderson JJ: *Family-centered nursing care of children,* Philadelphia, 1989, W.B. Saunders; Jackson BS, Jones MB: Hematologic anatomy and physiology. In Kinney MR, Packa DR, Dunbar SB, eds: *AACN's clinical reference for critical-care nursing,* ed 2, New York, 1988, McGraw-Hill.
*Normal laboratory values vary by laboratory and are age dependent.

SUPPORT OF HEMATOLOGIC FUNCTION

There are a variety of interventions that are used to treat hematologic dysfunction. These include blood product transfusion therapy, pharmacologic interventions (i.e., anticoagulants and immune globulins), and mechanical interventions (i.e., apheresis).

Blood Product Transfusions

Critically ill pediatric patients may require blood product administration for a variety of reasons. Knowledge of special donor designation, modifications of the blood products including special processing procedures, and the potential risks of transfusions is essential for the provision of care. Table 24-4 presents blood products commonly used in the PICU, indications for these blood products, dosage, and nursing implications.

Special Donor Designation. Blood administration requires an understanding regarding donor-directed (designated) blood and human leukocyte antigen (HLA)-matched blood products. With the concern regarding safety of blood, most blood centers offer the ability for family and friends to donate blood for a specific patient. Although this is not possible for the emergent needs of a critically ill patient, parents may request information from the blood blank regarding donor-direction for postadmission transfusion needs. Directed donations, however, have not offered a

safety advantage over ordinary banked blood derived from anonymous volunteer donors.[3] There is a concern regarding the potential for increased clerical errors resulting from the additional steps in the donation process, as well as inaccurate history disclosure. Directed donation from parents to neonates is not recommended because of maternal alloantibodies and maternal antibodies in the infant's circulation.[3]

Another special donor situation occurs when HLA-matched platelets are required. Patients, especially after multiple platelet transfusions, may develop antibodies to antigens on platelets, and require HLA cross-matching to minimize chance of reaction to the donor platelets in order to receive an adequate rise in platelet count.

Patients who require ongoing (lifelong) transfusions (e.g., sickle cell disease [SCD]) may develop multiple alloantibodies to donor blood antigens, which make cross-matching difficult. This may cause a delay in availability of blood products for these individual patients.

Knowledge regarding special donor requirements for individual patients is important. It is vital to document the number of products available for immediate transfusion and to send patient blood samples when required for cross-matching to prevent a delay in product availability.

Modifications of Blood Products. Various methods are available to modify blood products before administration to minimize the risks of transfusions for patients with

TABLE 24-4   Blood Products Commonly Used in the PICU

Blood Product	Indication	Dosage	Must be ABO Compatible	Requires Compatibility Testing	Rate of Administration	Available Modifications	Special Considerations
Whole Blood	Symptomatic deficit of oxygen-carrying capacity plus hypovolemic shock; Massive blood loss; Exchange transfusions	20 ml/kg initially, followed by volume necessary to stabilize child's condition	Yes (must be ABO identical, Rh+ may receive Rh−)	Yes	As fast as tolerated	Warmed; Irradiated; Leukocyte-depleted; CMV neg, frozen, deglycerolyzed	Rarely used, usually for massive acute blood loss; Platelets, WBCs, and clotting factors within stored whole blood are not functional
Packed Red Blood Cells (PRBC)	Anemia/symptomatic deficit of oxygen-carrying capacity ± hypovolemia	10-20 ml/kg	Yes	Yes	2-4 hr (not greater than 6 hr)	Washed; Warmed; Irradiated; Leukocyte-depleted; CMV neg, frozen; Deglycerolyzed	Multiple transfusions may result in dilution of coagulation factors; Wait 4-6 hr after transfusion to check hematocrit
Platelets	Thrombocytopenia (usually platelet count <20,000 or <50,000 with active bleeding); Abnormal platelet function	1-2 units/10 kg	Yes (preferred)	No	As fast as tolerated, but usually not faster than 1 ml/kg/min	Irradiated; Leukocyte-depleted; CMV neg; Volume-reduced; Single donor; HLA matched	Do not use microaggregate filters; High risk of alloimmunization with repeated transfusions; Transfusion not indicated in platelet-destruction conditions, except with hemorrhage
Fresh Frozen Plasma	Deficit of plasma coagulation factors (prolonged PT, PTT)	Clotting deficiency: 10-15 ml/kg; Acute hemorrhage: 15-30 ml/kg	Yes	No	Depends on patient tolerance. Not faster than 1 ml/kg/min, not slower than 4 hr	Irradiated	Should not be used for hypovolemia/hypoproteinemia unless coagulation values are prolonged; Must be used within 6 hr of thawing
Cryoprecipitate	Hemophilia A; Hypofibrinogenemia; Factor XIII deficiency; Von Willebrand disease	1 unit/5 kg	Yes	No	As fast as tolerated, usually not faster than 1 ml/kg/min	Irradiated	Must be used within 6 hr of thawing
Albumin	Hypovolemia	5%: 10-20 ml/kg; 25%: 2-4 ml/kg	No	No	5%: As fast as tolerated; 25%: 20-60 min	NA	No infectious risk; Risk of circulatory overload secondary to increased osmotic pressure, especially with 25% albumin; Use within 6 hr of entering container

special needs. Modifications include leukodepletion and irradiation of blood products.

To reduce the risk of nonhemolytic febrile reactions, leukocyte-depleted blood products may be transfused, especially to patients receiving frequent transfusions. Leukocyte-depleted blood products are ordered primarily when it has been demonstrated or suspected that the patient has previously experienced a febrile transfusion reaction. Other indications for leukocyte-depleted blood products are to prevent alloimmunization in recipients of frequent platelet transfusions, to prevent cytomegalovirus (CMV) infection when CMV-negative blood products are not available, and in prospective renal allograft recipients. Leukocyte depletion is usually achieved by prestorage or bedside filtration—a process that removes 70% to 99% of WBCs. Leukocytes can also be removed by washing RBCs or by freezing and deglycerolyzing RBCs.[3-5]

Leukocytes present in the transfused blood component can react against an immunosuppressed patient, causing transfusion-associated graft-versus-host disease (TA-GVHD). Irradiation destroys the leukocytes' ability to engraft in the patient. Patients susceptible to TA-GVHD include transplant recipients, severely immunocompromised patients, and those with lymphoma or acute leukemia. The incidence of TA-GVHD is not known, but many oncology units and some neonatal centers routinely use irradiated blood.[6] It is generally recommended that patients at risk for TA-GVHD in the PICU receive irradiated blood products. Irradiated blood products pose no danger to healthcare personnel.[7] Filtration of blood products at the bedside includes use of a 170- to 260-micron filter, which is standard in blood administration and platelet recipient sets. These filtered tubing sets should hang no longer than 4 hours. Each set can be used for up to four units if total time is less than 4 hours. WBC filters (Pall filters) may also be used if leukofiltration is indicated and has not been accomplished prestorage at the blood bank.

Most transfusions can be administered without the use of a blood warmer. However, transfusions of more than one unit of blood every 10 minutes, and exchange transfusions in neonates, mandate the use of a blood warmer to prevent severe hypothermia, dysrhythmias, and cardiac arrest. Patients who are hypothermic before the transfusion, and those who have cold agglutinin disease, also require warmed blood products. When blood must be warmed, it is heated via an inline system. Because RBCs heated above 37° C. may hemolyze, only temperature-controlled devices designed specifically to warm blood should be used.[7]

Potential Complications.   The most important potential complication associated with blood product administration is transfusion reaction. Transfusion reactions are generally classified as hemolytic or nonhemolytic reactions. Each reaction has some characteristic signs and symptoms, but the type of reaction may be difficult to ascertain initially. Table 24-5 summarizes reactions, signs and symptoms, and treatments.

Acute Hemolytic Reactions.   Acute hemolytic reactions are potentially the most serious of transfusion reac-

tions. A hemolytic reaction occurs when the blood product recipient has antibodies to some antigen on the transfused RBCs. The most common etiology of this antibody-antigen reaction is ABO incompatibility. The most frequent source of hemolytic reactions is mismatched blood, usually as a result of clerical error.[4,5] Hemolytic reactions may be either immediate (fever, hematuria, etc.) or delayed. Delayed reactions may occur 3 to 5 days after the transfusion, with development of anemia and hematuria. Delayed reactions from low antigen titers undetected during cross-matching cause a slow build-up of antibody response; thus the delayed symptoms occur.

Nonhemolytic Reactions.   Nonhemolytic reactions are generally classified into febrile and allergic reactions. Febrile reactions, which are characterized by fever and possibly shaking chills, are the result of an immune response to infused WBCs or plasma proteins. Febrile reactions usually occur in frequently transfused patients and are rarely serious. However, because fever can be the initial manifestation of a life-threatening hemolytic reaction, the transfusion should be discontinued if the patient's temperature rises 1° C or more above baseline. Antipyretics may be administered to control the fever. Providing frequently transfused patients with leukocyte-depleted blood products can prevent febrile reactions.[3]

The other common type of nonhemolytic reaction is an allergic reaction. Most allergic reactions are mild, characterized by local erythema, pruritus, and urticaria. The transfusion is stopped temporarily, and an antihistamine preparation is administered. If the symptoms are mild and resolving, the transfusion may be restarted slowly. Patients who have had an allergic reaction to a transfusion may be pretreated with an antihistamine drug before subsequent transfusions.

Rarely, an anaphylactic reaction occurs. Features that distinguish an anaphylactic reaction are bronchospasm, hypotension, and absence of fever. These reactions, which are typically apparent after administration of only a few milliliters of the transfused blood product, occur almost exclusively in IgA-deficient recipients. Collaborative interventions include the administration of epinephrine, fluids, and corticosteroids.[3]

Alloimmunization.   Alloimmunization is another potential complication of receiving blood products, especially in patients who receive multiple transfusions. Such patients develop antibodies against antigens that they intrinsically lack, but that are present on the surface of the cells that have been transfused. Subsequent transfusions are affected; these newly formed antibodies may destroy future transfused cells that possess the targeted antigens. When platelets are transfused to a patient alloimmunized against platelets, there is no therapeutic effect; the patient is considered refractory to platelet therapy. Single-donor or HLA-matched platelets may offset the effects of alloimmunization. When RBCs are transfused to a patient alloimmunized against red cell antigens, hemolysis of the donor's cells may result. Appropriate cross-matching should prevent a serious hemolytic reaction. Using leukocyte-depleted blood components reduces the risk of alloimmunization.[3,5]

TABLE 24-5   Transfusion Reactions to Blood or Blood Products

Reaction	Cause	Signs and Symptoms	Treatment
Anaphylaxis (occurs with infusion of only a few ml of product)	Most often caused by antigen-antibody complexes involving antibodies to IgA	Bronchospasm Cough Respiratory distress Hypotension*	Discontinue transfusion Keep vein open with NS (completely new tubing set) Notify physician Administer epinephrine, steroids Provide respiratory support Use deglycerolized (washed) red cells in future transfusions
Acute hemolytic transfusion reaction	Transfusion of ABO-incompatible blood resulting in hemolysis of red cells	Fever, chills* Hypotension* Hemoglobinemia Hemoglobinuria Lumbar pain (classic sign) Shock Dyspnea Diaphoresis Anxiety (sense of impending doom) Chest pain Restlessness DIC	Stop transfusion Keep vein open with NS (completely new tubing set) Notify physician Treat shock and/or respiratory distress Produce osmotic diuresis to prevent acute tubular necrosis Treat DIC
Nonhemolytic	Recipients reacting to poorly defined transfused antigens or recipients' antibodies reacting to transfused leukocytes and/or plasma proteins	Fever (mild to severe)* Chills Headaches Palpitations Hives Local erythema Itching	Stop transfusion Keep vein open with NS (completely new tubing set) Notify physician Relieve symptoms (antipyretics, antihistamines) If reaction mild such as urticaria and/or slight fever and chills, may consider continuing transfusion after antihistamine. May also consider premedication and/or leukocyte-poor products for future transfusions.

*Consider bacterial contamination of product.

Circulatory Overload.   Circulatory overload is a potential complication of blood product administration, which occurs when the transfusion volume exceeds circulatory system capacity. Critically ill pediatric patients are at increased risk of circulatory overload because of their relatively small baseline blood volume and potentially compromised cardiovascular, pulmonary, and renal systems. This complication can usually be prevented by adjusting the transfusion volume and flow rate based on the patient's size and clinical status. The blood bank can divide packed cells into smaller aliquots and can provide "volume-reduced" platelets to fluid-sensitive patients. Increased respiratory support and diuretics may be necessary to treat circulatory overload.

Citrate Toxicity.   Citrate is a substance that is present in the anticoagulant preservative solution added to most blood products. In the body, citrate binds with serum calcium, potentially causing hypocalcemia. The patients most at risk for symptomatic citrate toxicity are those who receive very rapid transfusions, those who receive multiple transfusions over a relatively short period of time, and patients with existing hepatic or renal dysfunction because citrate is metabolized in the liver and excreted by the kidneys.[8]

The serum calcium level of patients at risk for citrate toxicity is checked before and during transfusions. When toxicity in the presence of hypocalcemia is anticipated, intravenous calcium chloride or calcium gluconate may be administered prophylactically.

Transmission of Infectious Diseases.   Transmission of infectious diseases is a potential complication of blood product administration. Although fear of acquiring HIV, which causes AIDS, is generally the dominant concern of transfusion recipients and their families, the chances of contracting other infectious diseases, such as hepatitis or CMV poses a more significant health risk.

Approximately 2.5% of adult AIDS cases reported to the Centers for Disease Control and Prevention (CDC) have been related to transfusions. However, pediatric AIDS cases have a much higher proportion of posttransfusion etiology. The vast majority of patients with transfusion-acquired AIDS were infected before 1985. Since 1985, all blood-collecting facilities have used the HIV antibody test to screen donated blood, which has significantly decreased the risk of HIV transmission. The current risk of acquiring HIV from a blood transfusion is unknown, but it is estimated to be 1 in 420,000. There is evidence that the risk is declining by 30% per year.[3]

The exact incidence of posttransfusion hepatitis is unknown. Hepatitis A virus (HAV) is usually transmitted by the fecal-oral route. At one time, it was believed that posttransfusion HAV infection was virtually nonexistent. More recently, there have been reports in the literature that document HAV transmission by transfusion. For example, several nursery-wide outbreaks of posttransfusion HAV infection among newborns have been reported. Fortunately, none of these studies has demonstrated significant morbidity from HAV.[9]

In contrast, hepatitis B virus (HBV) has long been known to produce posttransfusion infection, which can cause significant morbidity and mortality. Despite the fact that all blood is screened for hepatitis B surface antigen (HBsAg), several prospective studies have documented that up to 1.7% of transfusion recipients develop HBV infection. Possible explanations for this phenomenon include the presence of infectious donors who are in the incubation phase, before HBsAg testing would be positive, and infectious donors with a serum level below the limits of detectability with current assays.[9]

Non-A non-B hepatitis (NANBH) is the most common posttransfusion hepatitis, accounting for about 60% of all cases. Hepatitis C virus (HCV) has been confirmed to be the cause of most, if not all, cases of NANBH. In adults, the sequelae of NANBH are chronic active hepatitis in 40% to 50% of cases, and cirrhosis in 20%. Children who acquire HBV or HCV during infancy usually have a persistent viremia and chronic, mild liver disease, although cases of childhood cirrhosis and hepatocellular carcinoma have been reported. Adolescents may have a sustained neuroinflammatory activity that progresses into a more severe liver disease.[10]

Since May 1990, all units of blood and blood products have been tested for HCV antibody. Before routine testing, the risk of transfusion-associated HCV infection was estimated to be as high as 1 in 100. The estimate for transmitting HCV is 1 in 80,000.[11]

CMV transmission is another potential infectious risk of blood transfusions. Approximately 50% of the population are potential transmitters of CMV. Fortunately, in the majority of patients, CMV infection does not cause a clinical illness.

However, two populations at risk for serious complications from CMV infection are neonates and immunocompromised patients. In infants born to mothers without detectable CMV antibodies, acquired CMV infections can lead to atypical lymphocytosis, hepatosplenomegaly, pneumonia, or death. In immunosuppressed children, such as patients with oncologic disease and transplant recipients, CMV infection can cause life-threatening pneumonitis or hepatitis. Patients at risk for clinical CMV disease should receive blood that has been screened for antibodies to CMV.[8]

Coagulopathy. Coagulopathy can occur during massive transfusion, which is defined as the replacement of more than one blood volume.[12] During a rapid blood loss, the body cannot replace more than a small fraction of coagulation factors and platelets. Stored blood has also lost platelets and coagulation factors, such as factor VIII, which have become less active. When multiple transfusions are given over a short period of time, it is generally recommended that for every three units of packed RBCs administered, the child also receive one unit of fresh frozen plasma (FFP) and one unit of platelets.[13] Coagulation studies may be done to determine specific component replacement.

Pharmacologic Therapy

Growth Factors. The development and usage of engineered growth factors has dramatically changed the support provided for RBC, WBC, and platelet stimulation. Erythropoietin is a natural hormone produced by the kidneys to stimulate RBC production. The genetically engineered product (i.e., Procrit or Epo) is used for anemia secondary to chronic renal failure, chemotherapy-induced anemia, and for anemic Jehovah's Witness patients who will not accept blood product transfusions. The product is administered intravenously or subcutaneously.

WBC stimulation is promoted with granulocyte colony stimulating factor (G-CSF, i.e., Neupogen) or granulocyte macrocyte–colony stimulating factor (GM-CSF, i.e., Leukine). Its primary indication is prevention of chemotherapy-induced neutropenia. It also is administered for other causes of neutropenia, such as drug-induced neutropenia or sepsis. It may be administered intravenously or subcutaneously.

Other stimulating factors include platelet-stimulating factor (e.g, Neumega), which may be administered for postchemotherapy thrombocytopenia.

Immune Globulin Therapy. Indications for intravenous immune globulin (IVIg) administration in PICU patients include primary and secondary immunodeficiency states, immune thrombocytopenic purpura (ITP), and Kawasaki disease. Dosage and rate of administration of IVIg depends on the product used. Current standard dosage for ITP is 1 g/kg/day until therapeutic effect is noted (daily infusion, up to 5 days). Research regarding giving lower doses (e.g., 400 mg/kg/day) has proved efficacious for patients with ITP.[14]

Administration of IVIg requires an understanding of the starting rate of each product and recommended titration of the infusion rate to decrease the possibility of a severe allergic reaction. Patients are assessed and monitored closely for the spectrum of allergic reactions—mild to anaphylaxis. Many reactions are rate dependent and subside if the rate is slowed. If a patient has demonstrated a reaction, but has a continued need for IVIG therapy, premedication with diphenhydramine (Benadryl) and acetaminophen (Tylenol) may prevent an allergic response.

Anticoagulants. Anticoagulants administered in the PICU include heparin, low-molecular weight heparin (LMWH) (e.g., Enoxaprin), warfarin (e.g., Coumadin), tissue plasminogen activator (t-PA), or streptokinase (SK). Table 24-6 summarizes these medications, including indications, dosages, laboratory tests, and implications for nursing care. Specific information regarding heparin-induced thrombocytopenia (HIT) and care of patients with vascular access thrombi is discussed later in this chapter.

General nursing care for patients on anticoagulants includes careful monitoring of platelet count and coagulation studies, avoiding intramuscular injections and platelet-interfering drugs (i.e., ASA and NSAIDs), observation for frank and occult bleeding, and applying pressure (extended time) for all venipunctures and line insertion sites.

Mechanical Intervention

Apheresis. The term *apheresis* is derived from the Greek word for *removal.* Apheresis is a therapeutic process used to selectively extract abnormal blood components from the circulation. It is also used to harvest peripheral blood stem cells for storage and future transplantation, and for single-donor platelet concentrate collection.

All apheresis procedures have certain basic principles in common. Blood is withdrawn from the patient, pumped through a cell separator that removes the desired component by centrifugal force, and then returned to the patient. Each procedure is labeled according to the major component removed. Thus removal of leukocytes is termed *leukapheresis,* red cell removal is *erythropheresis,* and so forth. *Plasmapheresis,* which is also called *intensive plasma exchange,* refers to the removal of plasma.[15]

As with many advanced technologies, apheresis has been used more extensively in adults than in children. However,

---

◆ TABLE 24-6 Anticoagulants

Medication	Indication	Dosage	Laboratory Testing	Nursing Implications
Heparin	Prevention and/or treatment of DVT, pulmonary embolus, and venous or arterial thrombi	IV 0.75 mg/kg loading dose IV over 10 min. Initial maintenance dose <1 yr of age: 28 u/kg/hr >1 yr of age: 20 u/kg/hr Adjust heparin to maintain APTT at 60-85 sec	APTT 4 hr after loading dose; every 4 hr until therapeutic level then qid CBC, platelet count, and PT qd	If platelet count <150,000 or bleeding occurs, contact physician; may be secondary to HIT
Low Molecular Weight Heparin (LMWH)	Same as for heparin Patients in whom venous access for administration and monitoring for standard heparin is difficult	Treatment dose for enoxaparin (Lovenox) <2 mo: 1.5 mg/kg/dose q12h 2 mo: 1.0 mg/kg/dose q12h (Usual maximum dose is 2 mg/kg q12h)	CBC, PT, APTT at baseline Platelet count Anti-factor levels should be drawn 4-6 hr after SC dose qd × 2 days Weekly if therapeutic level is reached	For platelet count <150,000 or bleeding occurs contact physician
Warfarin (Coumadin)	Same as for heparin When patient has stable APTT and can be changed to oral dosing Patient who has mechanical valves	Oral Day 1: Loading dose 0.2 mg/kg (0.1 mg/kg following Fontan or liver dysfunction) Day 2-4 loading doses based on INR response (Dosage is age dependent and is adjusted based on INR [usual dose is 2.0-3.0 mg])	Protime/INR Measure daily for first 2-3 days, then weekly after therapeutic level reached. Consider monthly checks if patient is stable and on long-term therapy	Patient remains on heparin with warfarin until INR is stable Patients may require dosage adjustments because of dietary or drug interactions with warfarin

APTT, Activated partial thromboplastin time; *CBC,* complete blood count; *DVT,* deep vein thrombosis; *INR,* international normalized ratio; *IV,* intravenous; *PT,* prothrombin time; *SC,* subcutaneous.

pediatric apheresis use has increased substantially since the early 1980s, with documented safety and efficacy for a variety of conditions. Apheresis has been successfully performed on very young and critically ill patients, but the smaller and sicker the patient, the greater the risks involved.[15-18]

Indications. The indications for apheresis in the PICU patient are specific to the type of procedure. Plasmapheresis is indicated for the following conditions.

1. *HUS or thrombotic thrombocytopenic purpura (TTP).* Removal of circulating endotoxin and/or replacement of normal platelet aggregating factors. Outcome has variable success rate in HUS but has documented efficacy in TTP.[19,20]
2. *End-stage liver disease (immediately before transplant).* Removal of coagulant-poor plasma and replacement with coagulant-rich plasma and cryoprecipitate, keeping the patient euvolemic.
3. *Autoimmune (including hemolytic disorders), hyperacute GVHD posttransplant, Guillain-Barré syndrome,* and *acute hemolytic transfusion reaction.* Removal of deleterious antibodies and immune complexes.

Erythropheresis is utilized for SCD patients in acute crisis (especially acute chest syndrome) to remove sickled RBCs and replace with normal RBCs. Leukopheresis is primarily used for patients admitted with leukemia, with WBCs fewer than $150,000/mm^3$, at high risk for acute tumor lysis syndrome, before administration of chemotherapy. The procedure removes excessive leukocytes while leaving RBCs and plasma.

Procedure. The preparation and implementation of the apheresis procedure is typically the responsibility of the apheresis team (usually a hematologist and a specially trained apheresis nurse).

Vascular Access. The first, and often the most challenging, technical aspect to be considered in pediatric apheresis is the establishment of vascular access. A double-lumen catheter is necessary to simultaneously remove and return blood to prevent hypovolemia. Another line should be available for maintenance fluid and medication administration.

Priming and Anticoagulation. Priming of the apheresis tubing for pediatric patients is usually accomplished with albumin or packed RBCs (PRBCs) because the amount of extracorporeal blood necessary to fill the apheresis equipment may represent a significant proportion of the patient's blood volume (i.e., greater than 10%) and priming with saline would dilute the patient's hematocrit (Hct). Pediatric patients can become hypovolemic if the tubing is not primed with a solution to replace the blood being drawn off at the onset of the procedure.[15-17]

Anticoagulation with heparin and acid-citrate dextrose (ACD) is required to prevent thrombus formation in the tubing. It is crucial for nurses to monitor for side effects (i.e., bleeding from heparin [decreased perfusion; hypotension]) and hypocalcemia from ACD/citrate toxicity.

Complications. There are a number of potential complications associated with apheresis procedures in the PICU, including hypovolemia, circulatory overload, hypocalcemia,

hypothermia, and bleeding. Patients are monitored carefully for changes in condition to permit timely and appropriate intervention. The apheresis team is responsible to manage the apheresis procedure itself, whereas the critical care team is responsible for patient assessment and monitoring.

Hypovolemia can occur if an excessive amount of the child's blood is in the extracorporeal circuit, or from depletion of albumin, causing a shift of fluid out of the intravascular space. It is standard to have less than 15% of the child's circulating blood volume in the circuit at any given time.[21] The PICU nurse carefully monitors vital signs and assesses perfusion for signs of shock. The rate of blood removed may be slowed, albumin administered, and/or fluids infused to correct hypovolemia.

The child who receives a large volume of albumin or fluids in excess of amount infused may be at risk for circulatory overload. Assessment for signs of fluid excess includes increased central venous pressure (CVP), gallop rhythm, crackles from pulmonary edema, and/or increased postpheresis weight. The net fluid balance is calculated postpheresis. Fluids during the procedure may be adjusted or diuretics may be administered for symptomatic fluid overload.

Children are at risk for hypocalcemia resulting from loss of calcium in phered plasma and from citrate in the anticoagulant, which inactivates calcium. Ionized calcium is monitored during the procedure. Total calcium is inaccurate because of fluctuating albumin. Calcium gluconate or chloride is administered for clinical and/or laboratory signs of hypocalcemia.

Hypothermia may result from the blood being circulated in the extracorporeal circuit outside the body, exposed to room temperature. This may exacerbate the temperature instability of the critically ill child, especially those with sepsis or neurologic compromise. Temperature is monitored every 15 to 30 minutes and patients are assessed for other signs of hypothermia such as bradycardia and shivering. Caution is necessary when "cold" blood from the circuit is infused into a right atrial line, which can cause severe ventricular arrhythmias. Treatment includes increasing the ambient room temperature, applying warmed blankets, and potentially warming the circuit blood before returning it to the patient.

A number of factors put the pediatric apheresis patient at risk for bleeding complications, including preexisting coagulopathy, systemic anticoagulation, depletion of fibrinogen and platelets owing to the apheresis process, and the presence of a large intravascular line.

Prothrombin time (PT), partial thromboplastin time (PTT), fibrinogen level, platelet count, Hct, and activated clotting time (ACT) are measured before and after apheresis. These values help to determine the type and amount of anticoagulant used during the procedure. The apheresis nurse generally measures the ACT at the bedside at regular intervals, and the citrate and/or heparin doses are titrated accordingly. Normal ACT is 90 seconds; the desired ACT during apheresis is usually 150 to 180 seconds.[15-17]

The child is monitored for clinical signs of bleeding during and after the procedure. Platelets or other clotting factor transfusions may be necessary to replace those depleted during apheresis. In rare instances, protamine sulfate may be administered to reverse the anticoagulant effects of heparin. All hematologic values are rechecked 24 hours after the apheresis procedure.

DISORDERS OF COAGULATION

Immune Thrombocytopenic Purpura

Etiology/Incidence.   ITP is characterized by destruction of antibody-sensitized platelets by the reticuloendothelial system (RES), particularly the spleen. The child has normal laboratory results, except for moderate to severe thrombocytopenia (<50,000/µl).

ITP is acute in 80% of all pediatric cases, usually following a viral illness. About 60% of children recover within 4 to 6 weeks, and more than 90% recover within 3 to 6 months.[14] The true incidence is unknown, mostly because the disease is transient. Children in the PICU may present with primary ITP or secondary ITP from diseases such as systemic lupus erythematousus (SLE) or HIV.

Pathogenesis.   In most cases, ITP is mediated by antiplatelet antibodies, resulting in an increased rate of platelet destruction. The antibodies are also formed against donor platelets. The spleen plays a major role in platelet destruction; however, splenectomy is reserved for emergency treatment (e.g., uncontrollable hemorrhage in the PICU patient).

Although serious bleeding is rare despite severe thrombocytopenia (<30,000/µl), critically ill infants and children typically present with hemorrhagic symptoms, purpura, and signs of platelet bleeding (i.e., petechiae). Hemorrhagic blisters may be seen on the mucous membranes and lips. Epistaxis is common. Infrequently, patients will have GI or genitourinary (GU) bleeding. Intracranial hemorrhage is the most feared complication, which occurs in 0.5% to 1.0% of children, often at diagnosis.[22] Most children will have a normal bleeding time and minimal symptomatology from ITP alone when their platelet counts are greater than 30,000/µl.

The natural history of ITP is more benign in children than in adults. Treatment centers around conservative management until the condition improves sufficiently on its own. Treatment for symptomatic patients (and those with platelet counts less than 30,000/µl) consists of steroids and immunoglobulins to suppress the immune response and prevent platelet destruction. Splenectomy, although usually definitive therapy for ITP, is avoided because more cases of death from postsplenectomy sepsis have been reported than from hemorrhage in children with chronic disease.[22]

Hypervigilance is required in the assessment of children with ITP, especially those with platelet counts lower than 30,000/µl. Assessment includes observing for signs of oozing and hemorrhage, as well as occult bleeding. Neurologic status, including level of consciousness and changes in motor, sensation, and pupillary checks is monitored for signs of intracranial hemorrhage. Pulmonary secretions, GI content, and urine are observed and/or tested for occult or frank blood. If the patient has a distended abdomen, girth measurements may be trended, and the patient evaluated for GI bleeding. The skin and mucous membranes are assessed frequently for signs of new bleeding. Invasive line and venipuncture sites are observed for oozing and hemorrhage. Bleeding is controlled, with additional pressure and dressings provided for external bleeding sites. Epistaxis control measures are at the bedside. Protocols are institution specific, but may include Neo-synephrine nose drops and nasal packing material. In addition, ongoing monitoring is required for the patient's coagulation and CBC results, type and screen/cross-matching status, and availability of blood products for the patient who has an emergent need.

Critical Care Management.   ITP treatment includes administration of steroids, IVIg or IV anti-D (i.e., Rhogam, for Rh+ patients, or Winrho) to suppress the antibody response to platelets. Emergent treatment for hemorrhage includes transfusion of platelets because the patient may receive a transient rise before antibody destruction of the donor platelets. Transfusion of platelets is followed by steroid and immunoglobulin administration to enhance the platelet effect. Splenectomy is reserved for the emergently bleeding patient or the patient who is at high risk for bleeding and who is refractory after 24 to 48 hours of supportive management (steroids and immunoglobulins).[22]

High-dose steroid administration, (methylprednisolone 30 mg/kg/day, or Prednisone 1 to 2 g/kg/day), in divided doses and IVIg 1 g/kg/day are standard therapy for patients who are at high risk for bleeding. For patients who are Rh positive, intravenous Anti-D (Winrho), may be administered at an initial infusion dose of 25 to 50 µg/kg. Infusions of immunoglobulins may be repeated on subsequent days, following platelet counts closely. IV Anti-D has demonstrated a 48- to 72-hour delay before the platelet count increases, but has also demonstrated fewer reactions than IVIg.[23]

Patients are observed closely for signs of potential infection because the patient will be immunosuppressed on steroid therapy. Guidelines for the administration of IVIg are followed with close monitoring for the occurrence of allergic reactions.

Plasmapheresis may be considered in addition to steroid and immunoglobulin therapy to provide an acute effect. Plasmapheresis alone would be insufficient because the time required to have an effect on the platelet count rise would take about 2 to 5 days.[22]

Androgen therapy (i.e., danazol) and monoclonal antibodies have been used to decrease platelet antibody production. Currently, these agents are not standard therapy for the critically ill child with ITP.[22,23]

Disseminated Intravascular Coagulation

Etiology/Incidence.   DIC is not a distinct disease, but rather an abnormal coagulation syndrome which occurs secondary to another disease process.[19,24] It is characterized by excessive use of coagulation factors that exceeds the ability to replenish these factors and results in the rapid production of thrombin and activated factor X or excessive bleeding as a result of failure of clot formation. The onset of DIC is usually preceded by massive activation of the hemostatic processes. The leading cause is infection. Many bacterial processes invoke activating factors that initiate the intrinsic coagulation system. Endothelial and tissue damage also enhance intrinsic stimulation as well as activate the extrinsic coagulation pathway.

DIC may also occur secondary to shock, burns, malignancies, fat emboli, hemolytic transfusion reactions, or immune disease. Other precipitating factors are hypoxia, acidosis, and hypotension. DIC has actually been reported to complicate more than 100 clinical disorders.[25]

Pathogenesis. In DIC, there is acceleration of normal coagulation, but the end result is bleeding. Excessive production of thrombin and plasmin degrades fibrinogen to fibrin, leading to further activation of the coagulation system, deposition of fibrin in the microvasculature, activation of the fibrinolytic system, and platelet activation. Consumption of clotting factors and platelets occurs and, as the process continues, fibrin split products (FSPs) are produced. If FSPs are not cleared from the circulation by the RES, anticoagulation will be enhanced. Normally the RES removes fibrin, activated clotting factors, endotoxins, and FSPs from the circulation. Dysfunction of the RES owing to shock or liver disease impairs removal of these substances, leading to hypercoagulability and DIC. With an increase in circulating FSPs, there is decreased platelet function and adherence, inhibition of thrombin, activation of complement, and further endothelial damage. The development of microvascular thrombi and bleeding leads to cellular ischemia (Fig. 24-3).

The clinical presentation of DIC varies dramatically from one patient to another. Onset may be sudden or gradual. It may be difficult to differentiate clinical signs from those of the underlying disease state. DIC may be suspected only because of its known association with certain pathologic states. Bleeding is the most obvious clinical sign of DIC. In children, abnormal bleeding is often identified from ecchymoses or petechiae or in oozing from intravenous and venipuncture sites.[19]

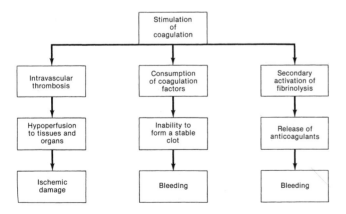

Fig. 24-3 The pathophysiology of DIC. (From Dressler DK: Patients with coagulopathies. In Clochesy JM et al, eds: *Critical care nursing,* Philadelphia, 1992, WB Saunders.)

In its most extreme case, the child with DIC shows pallor and circulatory failure, which is manifested by tachycardia and hypotension. Purpura and overt bleeding that may involve the pulmonary, cerebral, and intraventricular systems may be seen. In addition, thrombosis of the central and peripheral veins may lead to gangrene and tissue necrosis.

Abnormal serum coagulation values are an early indication of DIC. Typical findings include anemia with RBC fragmentation, thrombocytopenia, and prolonged PT, PTT, and thrombin time. An increase in FSPs is the cardinal sign of DIC. The greatest degree of diagnostic specificity is the measurement of the D-dimer FSP fragment, which is a breakdown product of cross-linked fibrin in either plasma or serum.[26,27] Fibrinogen levels are usually decreased but may be normal in some cases. Factors V and VIII are normal or may be extremely elevated. The presence of fragmented blood cells or schistocytes may be seen and indicates fibrin deposition in small vessels and a thrombolytic occurrence.

Many patients in the PICU are at risk to develop DIC. Thorough nursing assessment is essential in the prompt recognition and subsequent management of patients with DIC. The skin, mucous membranes, and all drainage or secretions are observed for obvious or occult bleeding.

Vital sign changes that may be indicative of bleeding and hypovolemia are tachycardia, tachypnea, and hypotension. It is important to remember that hypotension is a late sign in the child. Changes in mental status, such as irritability, restlessness, and lethargy, are signs of decreased cerebral perfusion related to hypovolemia and may present in the child with bleeding related to DIC.

Critical Care Management. Critical care management of patients with DIC is supportive, aimed at stabilization of cardiac status and restoration of fluid and electrolyte balance. Specific treatment of the underlying disorder includes correction of shock, acidosis, and electrolyte imbalance, and antibiotic therapy for bacterial infections. Replacement of coagulation factors is often necessary. PRBCs may be administered for active bleeding. In addition, if the child is actively bleeding and has a low platelet count (<20,000/μl), platelets are administered to increase the platelet count to 60,000/μl. If the platelet count is higher than 50,000/μl and the child is still bleeding, FFP 10 to 15 ml/kg body weight is administered to replace consumed clotting components. Cryoprecipitate is administered for fibrinogen levels below 75 g/dl to elevate fibrinogen levels. Table 24-4 presents specific implications associated with the use of these blood products.

Nursing care for the child receiving these blood products consists of monitoring for reactions to blood products, signs of fluid imbalance, and vital signs, including central venous pressure. Intake and output volumes are also strictly measured.

Controlling and preventing further bleeding is of paramount importance in caring for the critically ill child with DIC. Vital signs and laboratory studies are monitored frequently for changes that indicate bleeding. All output, including urine, stool, and nasogastric drainage, is tested for the presence of blood. All invasive sites are closely observed for oozing or active bleeding. Intramuscular injections and rectal procedures are avoided because of the increased risk for bleeding.

Heparin therapy for DIC is controversial because its efficacy has not been proven.[28] The rationale for administering heparin is the enhancement of antithrombin (AT) III activity, a major inhibitor of thrombin. With thrombin activity inhibited, degradation of fibrinogen to fibrin is impeded and further development of microvascular thrombi is slowed or halted. The concern about heparin therapy is the potential risk of further bleeding. When heparin is administered, the child receives an initial intravenous loading dose of 25 to 50 units/kg, followed by a continuous intravenous infusion of 5 to 10 units/kg/hour. Supportive therapy with platelet, FFP, and cryoprecipitate transfusions is continued.

The most valuable test for evaluating the effectiveness of heparin is the fibrinogen level. Even with a severe decrease in fibrinogen, the level should rise to a normal or near-normal level within 24 to 48 hours of effective heparin therapy.[19,29]

Assessing the child closely for the exacerbation of bleeding related to heparin is critical because this is the indication for discontinuation of heparin therapy. The child is also reevaluated regarding the need for further replacement of platelets and coagulation factors. Protamine sulfate may be administered to counteract the effects of heparin (1 mg for every 100 units of heparin). However, this is only rarely necessary owing to the short half-life of heparin.

The duration of heparin therapy for DIC may vary from 12 to 24 hours in conditions when the underlying disease may be treated effectively. Other conditions, such as leukemia, may require therapy for as long as 2 to 3 weeks.

Partial exchange transfusions with heparinized fresh blood or reconstituted FFP and PRBCs may be necessary if fluid overload becomes a persistent problem and the child continues to require large volumes of blood or clotting factors. Removal of selected mediators also may break the vicious, self-perpetuating cycle of DIC. Nursing responsibilities related to apheresis have been discussed previously.

Heparin-Induced Thrombocytopenia

Etiology/Incidence. HIT is typically characterized by a 50% or greater decrease in platelet count after 5 or more days of unfractionated (standard) heparin therapy. If a patient has been exposed to heparin in the recent past (less than 100 days), the presentation is often rapid, within the first 24 hours of reexposure. The platelet count nadir is usually around 50,000 µl; however, in some postoperative patients, mean platelet counts may remain above 300,000 µl.[30] The platelet nadir is not related to the risk of thromboemboli.

HIT is an uncommon complication of heparin therapy that can cause significant morbidity and mortality in the PICU patient. The incidence of HIT is about 5% in adult patients receiving unfractionated heparin, and unknown in pediatric patients. Twenty percent of patients with HIT can have paradoxically thrombotic complications, which can be devastating, including loss of limb or death.

HIT usually occurs in patients 5 to 15 days after beginning heparin therapy, but can occur earlier in patients with prior exposure to heparin. An unexplained drop in platelet count in a patient receiving heparin should raise the suspicion of HIT.

Pathogenesis. HIT is caused by an antibody-antigen reaction on the surface of platelets with unfractionated heparin. The mechanism by which HIT predisposes to thromboemboli is by the production of platelet-derived microparticles that are released in the circulation and activate the coagulation system. HIT is an intensely prothrombotic condition.

The pediatric patient suspected of having HIT needs to be assessed closely for signs of clotting (increased bruising, thrombus formation), or bleeding if the platelet count is extremely low. Blood samples from patients are tested for induction of platelet aggregation by heparin or serum evaluation for specific antibodies.

Critical Care Management. Any source of heparin, including LMWH (though it rarely causes HIT), is discontinued. This includes arterial and central line flush solutions. If there is no evidence of thrombosis and no indication for continuation of anticoagulants, discontinuation of heparin will result in the platelet count returning to normal.

If a thrombus is present and a need for continuation of anticoagulant therapy exists, medications such as danaparoid (Orgaran) and Ancrod may be administered because they have minimal cross-reactivity with heparin-induced antibody. Minimal data regarding drug selection exists for the pediatric population.

Vascular Access Thrombi

Etiology/Incidence. The small size of a central venous catheter lumen predisposes the infant and small child to the development of thrombi that can occlude the catheter. Central line occlusion can be caused by chemical-related thrombi, which develop from precipitates formed when incompatible solutions mix, and blood-related thrombi, which are caused by inadequate flow rate or flushing of the lumen, with subsequent platelet aggregation and thrombus formation.

Pathogenesis. Central venous catheters are thrombogenic because they are foreign to the body, they damage vessel walls and disrupt blood flow, and some infusions injure the vessels. Central venous catheter thrombotic complications include clots at the tips that impair infusion or withdrawal of blood, fibrin sleeves that are not adherent to vessel walls but may occlude lines, and deep venous thrombi that adhere to vessel walls with partial or complete obstruction.[30]

The most common presentation is the child with a central catheter from which blood cannot be withdrawn or into which fluids cannot be infused. The obstruction may be present in one or all lumens. Diagnostic work-up after failure to obtain line patency with antithrombotic instillation should include a venogram or Doppler ultrasound.

Emergent signs of superior vena cava syndrome may also be present if a large vessel thrombus occludes venous

TABLE 24-7 **Vascular Access Occlusion Therapy**

Drug	Local Instillation Amount	Guidelines
Alteplase (rTPA) (2 mg/ml)	2 ml to each lumen (or volume required to fill lumen)	Dwell × 1 hr Aspirate and flush with NS Repeat × 1 if needed
Streptokinase (3000 IU/ml)	3000 IU/ml to fill lumen (1.8-2.5 ml per each lumen)	Dwell × 1 hr Aspirate and flush with NS and attempt to aspirate blood Consider administering antihistamine and acetaminophen to decrease potential for allergic reaction

drainage from the upper body. Immediate diagnostic tests include a venogram, and possibly a V̇/Q̇ scan.

Critical Care Management. Prevention of central venous catheter occlusion requires adequate flushing, especially between incompatible medications, and adequate infusion rates to keep lumens patent. Early detection of line problems, including slow blood return, mandates an increase in flushing frequency for heparin-locked ports, or early instillation of an antithrombolytic agent.

Despite all efforts to maintain catheter patency, thrombi may develop. If the line is blocked without evidence of clinical compromise, an attempt is made to "dissolve" the clot, using SK, which has a high allergic reaction potential, or t-PA. Table 24-7 provides instillation guidelines for these agents. Small local occlusive thrombus (<1 cm) are treated with local low-dose thrombolytic infusion therapy for 24 to 72 hours, or more rapidly if immediate central line patency is required.

If the catheter is still not patent after local instillation, or if it has occluded a second time, further work-up is indicated. If a large vessel thrombus is suspected, a venogram or Doppler ultrasound evaluation is performed.[31]

Close monitoring of coagulation studies (PT, APTT, and fibrinogen) every 8 hours is performed after initiation of therapy. Assessment for signs of bleeding (frank and occult) and signs of movement of the thrombus (increased respiratory distress, or ECG changes secondary to pulmonary embolus) is essential.

If pulmonary embolus is suspected (or documented by V̇/Q̇ scan), the central line is either left in place or removed, depending on patient status, and heparin therapy (followed by 3 months of Coumadin), or LMWH is indicated.[33]

ANEMIAS

Anemia is defined as a deficiency in RBCs, Hgb, total volume, or any combination of the three, with the primary problem of insufficient oxygen transported on Hgb to meet cellular demand.[1,32] Patients with anemia may present to the PICU as an emergency or with an acute exacerbation of a chronic anemia. Overall, the main problems seen in children with anemia of any etiology are ineffective gas exchange, altered tissue perfusion, and altered fluid volume. Nursing care is directed toward assessment and management of these problems.

Anemia results from an excessive loss or destruction of blood, an inadequate production of Hgb and RBCs resulting from bone marrow failure or a deficiency state, or a combination of both.[34] The pathophysiologic process producing signs and symptoms of anemia primarily relates to the decreased oxygen-carrying capacity of the RBCs, resulting in inadequate oxygen to meet tissue demands. When a patient has excessive blood loss, pathophysiologic changes occur due to hypovolemia, with inadequate cardiac output for tissue perfusion.

The anemias seen in children are reviewed in Box 24-2 and discussed briefly in this section. SCA is discussed in more detail because children with this disease present to the PICU more frequently than do children with other types of chronic anemia.

Anemia Related to Blood Loss

Etiology/Incidence. Acute or chronic blood loss may produce anemia. With acute blood loss, the anemia is present after the loss of blood volume is replaced with extracellular fluid (ECF). Chronic blood loss produces anemia when the body has expended its iron reserve.

Pathogenesis. The clinical presentation of a child with anemia related to blood loss varies greatly. Those with chronic anemia often adapt to a low Hct and Hgb without compromise. On the other hand, a previously healthy child who has a sudden and dramatic reduction in Hct and Hgb may present as an acutely ill child in respiratory distress/failure and shock and require aggressive intervention. Clinical manifestations of acute hemorrhage include signs of shock (i.e., decreased level of consciousness, pallor, cool extremities, poor peripheral pulses, prolonged capillary refill, with a normal or low blood pressure, and possibly respiratory distress symptoms resulting from inadequate oxygenation). Bleeding may be obvious, with external hemorrhage, or hidden with internal bleeding until perfusion and oxygenation are severely compromised.

Laboratory tests to evaluate this type of anemia include a CBC with RBC indices, platelet count, PT, PTT, serum fibrinogen level, and FSP. During and shortly after an episode of bleeding, the platelet count and serum fibrinogen level may transiently decrease. The Hct and Hgb remain relatively stable in the acutely bleeding child because 24 to 72 hours are necessary for the Hct and Hgb levels to equilibrate and accurately reflect the total amount of blood loss.

Box 24-2

◆ **Classification of Anemias of Childhood**

A. Abnormal RBC production
   1. Disorder of proliferation/differentiation
      a. Aplastic anemia
      b. Pure red cell aplasia
      c. Erythropoietin deficiency
   2. Disorder of DNA synthesis
      a. Vitamin B_{12} deficiency
      b. Folate deficiency
   3. Disorder of Hgb synthesis
      a. Iron deficiency
      b. Thalassemia
B. Increased RBC destruction
   1. Intrinsic RBC abnormalities
      a. Membrane defects
         Hereditary spherocytosis
         Liver disease
      b. Abnormal red cell metabolism
         Glucose-6 phosphate dehydrogenase deficiency
         Pyruvate kinase deficiency
   2. Extrinsic abnormalties
      a. Mechanical destruction
         Microangiopathic hemolytic anemia
         Traumatic hemolysis (cardiac valve prosthesis)
      b. Infection
         Bacterial
         Viral
         Parasitic
      c. Antibody-mediated
         Alloimmune hemolytic disease of the newborn
         Drug reaction
         Autoantibody-mediated destruction of erythrocytes
      d. Hypersplenism
C. Blood loss
   1. Traumatic or gastrointestinal hemorrhage
   2. Surgical

From Nugent DJ, Tarantino MD: Hematology-oncology problems in the intensive care unit. In Fuhrman BP, Zimmerman JJ, eds: *Pediatric critical care,* St Louis, 1992, Mosby.

Critical Care Management.   Treatment for acute blood loss is aimed at restoring intravascular volume, initially with crystalloid solutions, followed by blood. The indication for RBC transfusion in the hemorrhaging patient is impaired oxygen delivery to end organs.[1] Patients primarily receive PRBCs as the component of choice. These may be given concurrently with FFP if plasma coagulation factors are also needed.

Chronic anemia is generally well tolerated, and transfusion is not usually necessary unless the Hgb falls below 6 to 7 g/dl. Because extracellular volume (ECV) is increased in the child with chronic anemia, caution is taken if the patient is transfused because volume overload is a potential risk. The child is assessed carefully for congestive heart failure and pulmonary edema during transfusion therapy.

Hemolytic Anemia

Etiology/Incidence.   The average lifespan of a RBC is 100 to 120 days. About 1% of RBCs are removed from the circulation each day and the same percentage is replaced by new red cells (reticulocytes) released from the bone marrow. Hemolytic anemia results when RBC destruction is abnormally high and the bone marrow compensatory mechanism cannot keep pace with the loss of RBCs. Hemolysis of RBCs may be caused by a variety of etiologies, as described in Box 24-2. Causes of hemolysis can be attributed to factors extrinsic to RBCs, such as in microangiopathic hemolytic anemias (e.g., HUS and TTP), infections, and autoantibodies (e.g., SLE). Intrinsic RBC defects may also cause hemolysis, including hemoglobinopathies such as glucose-6 phosphate dehydrogenase (G6PD), thalassemia, and spherocytosis.

Pathogenesis.   The child may have presenting symptoms, which vary from typical symptoms of mild anemia to life-threatening complications from acute loss of oxygen-carrying capacity and compromised tissue perfusion as previously discussed.

Because hemolysis of RBCs is the cause of this anemia, diagnosis is based on the fact that RBCs are undergoing premature disruption. A decreased (or often unmeasurable) haptoglobin, elevated lactate dehydrogenase (LDH), an elevated reticulocyte count, and elevated serum levels of unconjugated bilirubin are seen. Erythroid hyperplasia and a decrease in the granulocyte to erythrocyte level are revealed in examination of the bone marrow.

Critical Care Management.   If the child is experiencing critical signs of diminished oxygenation and/or tissue perfusion, PRBCs are administered. Blood products are not ordered based on a specific number, but based on clinical need for the patient with critical organ perfusion problems. If the child is experiencing an autoimmune hemolytic reaction owing to an underlying disorder such as lupus or lymphoma, a cross-match may be unreliable. There is an increased risk of severe transfusion reaction secondary to underlying alloantibodies that are not able to be detected. When required, transfusions should be given cautiously because the transfused RBCs are also subject to destruction. However, if the anemia is causing hemodynamic instability, the child is transfused with type-specific blood in a sufficient amount to stabilize the cardiovascular system, in spite of incompatibility. Close assessment for fluid overload is required because the child's ECF volume may be expanded as a result of compensatory mechanisms to meet oxygen and perfusion demands.

Aplastic Anemia

Etiology/Incidence.   Aplastic anemia refers to a pronounced reduction in the number of RBCs, WBCs, and platelets resulting from hypoplasia or aplasia of the bone marrow in the absence of malignant disease. This type of anemia may be congenital or acquired, resulting from medications, infections, chemical exposure, or radiation.

There are many specific etiologies for aplastic anemia, which include infections (e.g., Epstein-Barr virus and hepatitis), drugs (e.g., chloramphenicol), and idiopathic causes. The majority of cases are idiopathic.[1]

Pathogenesis.   Children show the classic signs of a low blood count. Anemia, pallor, and fatigue may be present because of a decreased RBC count; increased susceptibility to infections from a low WBC count; and ecchymosis, petechiae, and epistaxis resulting from a low platelet count. Bone marrow biopsy reveals a marked reduction in all cells. Children with severe aplastic anemia may present to the PICU with signs of decreased oxygenation resulting from a reduction in the oxygen-carrying capacity of the blood, cardiac failure, overwhelming infection, or massive bleeding.

Critical Care Management.   The treatment priority for the child with life-threatening complications of aplastic anemia is cardiopulmonary stabilization. RBC transfusions are administered and platelet transfusions are indicated for the child with signs of severe bleeding (e.g., GI bleeding). All blood products are irradiated and filtered before transfusion because of the risk of posttransfusion GVHD related to sensitization of the recipient to HLA antigens in the donated blood. Infections are treated with broad-spectrum antibiotics or antifungal agents, if a fungal infection is present.

Treatment specific to aplastic anemia includes androgen therapy, immunosuppressive therapy, and bone marrow transplantation. Bone marrow transplantation is the treatment of choice if a compatible donor is available. Chapter 25 provides information on the care of the child receiving a bone marrow transplant.

Sickle Cell Disease

Etiology/Incidence.   SCD refers to a group of hemoglobinopathies distinguished by the development of sickled cells in response to deoxygenation. SCA is the most common cause of SCD. SCA is an autosomal recessive disorder in which the child produces sickle hemoglobin (Hb S) rather than Hb A. The child with sickle cell trait has inherited a sickle gene (Hb S) from one parent and a normal hemoglobin gene (Hb A) from the other parent. This child is always a carrier of SCA, although the trait does not progress to anemia.

When the child inherits two Hb S genes, SCA results. The red cells of SCA contain up to 80% to 100% of Hb S. This is a potentially fatal disease that occurs predominantly in the black race.

Pathogenesis.   Sickling of the RBC describes the change of a normal round RBC to a sickle-shaped one. The sickling process begins with the substitution of valine for glutamic acid on the beta chain of the hemoglobin molecule. This process produces Hb S, which is less soluble than the normal cell when deoxygenated. The decreased solubility causes Hb S to become more viscous and change to the sickle shape.

Once RBCs sickle, they are more fragile and easily destroyed. They cannot flow easily through the capillary beds and tend to become clumped, causing obstruction and impediment to blood flow. Tissue hypoxia develops, which promotes further sickling. As the hypoxia worsens, infarctions and necrosis can develop (Fig. 24-4).

There are several factors that cause Hb S to sickle (Box 24-3). Hypoxia is a major determinant. Characteristics of blood flow can also increase the tendency toward sickling. Under normal circumstances, the cardiac output of the child with SCD is elevated. This compensatory mechanism ensures that the transit time of blood between the capillary and the lung is rapid so that sickling cannot occur. However, any pathophysiologic process that affects pressure (such as hypotension or pulmonary hypertension) or increases resistance (such as vasoconstriction or increased Hct) promotes sickling.

The clinical presentation of children with SCD varies greatly. The symptoms seen are usually the result of (1) hemolysis of the cells and the compensatory mechanisms invoked by the subsequent anemia, and (2) thrombi in the small vessels of various organs resulting from the sickling. General symptoms seen in the child with SCD include weakness, pallor, fatigue, tissue hypoxia, and jaundice, as the result of RBC hemolysis. The heart may become enlarged because of the higher cardiac output demanded by the chronic anemia. Thrombi from the sickled cells may cause progressive damage to multiple organs, including the eyes, liver, and lungs.

Box 24-3
Factors That May Promote Sickling

1. Pressure-related
   a. Hypotension
   b. Pulmonary hypertension
2. Resistance-related
   a. Vasoconstriction
   b. Increased Hct (>35%)
3. Desaturation-related
   a. Hypoxemia
   b. Acidosis

From Eskenazi AE, Gordon JB, Bernstein ML: Hematologic disorders in the pediatric intensive care unit. In Rogers MC, ed: *Textbook of pediatric intensive care,* ed 3, Baltimore, 1996, Williams & Wilkins.

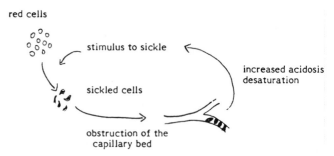

Fig. 24-4   The "vicious cycle" of progressive sickling causing intravascular occlusion. (From Eskenazi AE, Gordon JB, Bernstein ML: Hematologic disorders in the pediatric intensive care unit. In Rogers MC, ed: *Textbook of pediatric intensive care,* ed 3, Baltimore, 1996, Williams & Wilkins.)

Diagnosis of SCD and sickle cell trait are made through a variety of tests. The most commonly used is a hemoglobin electrophoresis. This assay separates the various types of hemoglobin and quantifies the percentages of various hemoglobins present. There are less sensitive tests that determine the presence or absence of Hb S; however, positive results require further screening with hemoglobin electrophoresis. Diagnosis may be made prenatally by using fetal blood obtained in placental aspiration or photoscope.

Critical Care Management. A PICU admission often signals a life-threatening episode with a high risk of morbidity and mortality for children with SCD. Outcome is often dependent on which organs are affected, the type of virus and/or bacteria causing the infection, if one is present, and the degree of progressive damage that has already occurred because of the disease. Nursing care is critical in managing the effects of the SCD crises.

The child with SCD may have signs of respiratory distress for a number of reasons. Pneumonia and pulmonary infarctions occur more often in this patient population. Splenic sequestration may also cause respiratory distress because the engorged spleen pushes up on the diaphragm. Hypoxemia causes increased sickling and, in turn, causes a vicious cycle of deoxygenation related to anemia and vaso-occlusive crisis.[35]

Assessment of breath sounds on a regular basis is imperative. The patient is observed for signs of respiratory distress, and the lungs are auscultated to detect decreased breath sounds along with abnormal sounds. Monitoring arterial blood gases on a regular schedule and continuous monitoring of oxygen saturation is essential. Oxygen by face mask or nasal cannula may be the only respiratory support that is needed. However, if the blood gases do not demonstrate improved oxygenation and the child's respiratory status continues to deteriorate, intubation and ventilatory support are necessary. Daily chest films are routinely performed to monitor progression or resolution of pulmonary complications.

Vaso-occlusive crises can vary in location, duration, and intensity. During a sickling event, vaso-occlusion prevents oxygen and nutrients from reaching the tissues. Pain is often the cardinal sign of a vaso-occlusive event. The pain has been described as being tremendously variable and unpredictable in onset, location, character, intensity, and duration.[36] Pain is the most common reason for emergency department visits and hospital admissions.[37] On admission to the PICU, the child's pain and level of analgesia is assessed. Pain assessment requires that the health care team, including the patient and family, be able to quickly differentiate between pain from vaso-occlusive crisis and pain from other complications of SCD.[36] Pain intensity is quantified by a chosen pain scale and documented on a flowsheet to monitor progression of the pain over time.

Drug therapy is the treatment of choice for pain associated with SCD. Ibuprofen or acetaminophen is used to initially manage mild to moderate pain. Codeine may be added if these are not effective. Severe pain may be treated with immediate-release or sustained-release morphine, oxycodone, hydromorphone, or methadone, given either orally or intravenously around the clock.[35] Another recommended regimen for pain management is intravenous morphine sulfate given every 1 to 2 hours around the clock.[38] A continuous narcotic infusion may be considered because bolus injections may not provide satisfactory analgesia because of the short plasma half-life of the narcotic. Patient-controlled analgesia (PCA) is an accepted method of pain management for children who are able to and want to manage their own pain relief. Two methods of PCA were compared in children with SCD. Children who received high-dose PCA with a low basal infusion required less morphine, had shorter lengths of stay, and had lower pain scores on day 2 of hospitalization when compared with children who received low-dose PCA with high basal infusions.[38]

Additional medications have been used to treat pain associated with a vaso-occlusive crisis. Intravenous methylprednisolone given in high doses has been shown to decrease the duration of severe pain.[39,40] A parenteral antiinflammatory drug (ketorolac) has been used for crisis pain and has the advantage of avoiding the risks associated with narcotics. However, one study did not demonstrate a synergistic analgesic effect for ketorolac; a lower morphine dose was not able to be used.[41] A case report presented the development of ketorolac-induced irreversible renal failure.[42] Further study is needed to evaluate the effectiveness of additional medications.

Hypovolemia is often seen in children with SCD in the PICU. Fluid replacement depends on the clinical condition and the results of the serum electrolytes, Hct, and coagulation studies. Children with splenic sequestration require crystalloid and RBCs immediately to restore circulating blood volume. Children in aplastic crisis require PRBCs because of their decreased Hct level. Crystalloids may be the only fluid replacement in vaso-occlusive crisis, depending on the degree of sickling and whether or not there is ischemia or infarction of the affected organ.

Patients with SCD tolerate a low Hct level extremely well, and transfusions should be initiated only when absolutely necessary. The Red Blood Cell Administration Practice Guideline Development Task Force of the College of American Pathologists recommends that RBC transfusions are indicated only to prevent recurrent refractory vaso-occlusive complications, stroke, or during certain illnesses (Box 24-4).[43] The potential for significant complications related to multiple transfusions include infection, iron overload, and alloimmunization. Iron overload results from the addition of 200 to 250 mg of iron added to the body's iron stores with each transfusion. This results in increased serum ferritin levels. If serum ferritin levels are greater than 2500 to 3500 mg/ml and the child still requires transfusions, chelation therapy is given.[44] Chelation therapy removes iron from body tissue and allows it to be excreted from the body. Deferoxamine is administered as a continuous subcutaneous infusion over 5 to 6 hours several times per week.[35]

Hydroxyurea has been used as an alternative to blood transfusions as a means to prevent recurrent stroke. Hydroxyurea reduces the frequency of vaso-occlusive crisis,

---

Box 24-4
Partial Exchange Transfusion in the PICU

1. Preparation
   a. Decision to transfuse
   b. Insertion of venous and arterial catheters (or two large-bore venous catheters, if possible)
   c. Blood sent to laboratory for:
      i. Complete blood count
      ii. Quantitative sickle cell preparation (this appears to correlate well with the quantity of Hb S noted at electrophoresis)
      iii. Electrolytes and calcium determination
      iv. Cross-match with PRBCs (sickle negative)
2. Procedure
   a. Volume of packed cells ($2 \times Hct \times 0.7 \times wt$ [kg])
   b. Rate
      i. Adjust intravenous line so transfusion occurs over 4 to 6 hr (more difficult if over 1000 ml are to be exchanged)
      ii. Withdraw blood at 10- to 15-min intervals from arterial line or large-bore venous catheter
      iii. Balance maintained within 5% of blood volume (blood volume, 80 ml/kg)
   c. Monitoring
      i. Heart rate and blood pressure (continuously)
      ii. Hematocrit (every 2 hr, and at last hour)
      iii. Electrolytes, calcium (at last hour)
   d. Endpoint
      i. Hematocrit 33% to 37% (add FFP to remainder of PRBCs if Hct is >35%)
      ii. % Hb S is <40% (initial screening by quantitative sickle cell preparation, followed by chromatography or electrophoresis)

From Eskenazi AE, Gordon JB, Bernstein ML: Hematologic disorders in the pediatric intensive care unit. In Rogers MC, ed: *Textbook of pediatric intensive care,* ed 3, Baltimore, 1996, Williams & Wilkins.

---

though the mechanism is unclear. It has been shown that there is an increase in the proportion of fetal Hgb cells within 8 to 12 weeks of beginning treatment.[45,46]

The nurse monitors for reactions to blood products and for signs of fluid imbalance. Children with SCD may require frequent transfusions during an acute episode, which increases the risk of volume overload. It is critical to closely monitor the patient for signs of fluid overload. The use of short-acting diuretics before or after the transfusion may help to prevent this complication. Other nursing responsibilities include monitoring vital signs and laboratory values and maintaining an accurate record of intake and output.

Exchange or partial exchange transfusions are often used for acute complications of SCA. The advantage of an exchange or partial exchange transfusion over a simple transfusion is that there is less risk for volume overload and a more rapid reduction in the percentage of cells containing Hb S. Preoperative exchange transfusions may be performed for children with SCD requiring surgery to reduce the risk of postoperative vaso-occlusive complications. Apheresis may also be used in the treatment of acute complications of SCD.

Prophylactic transfusions, done on a regular basis (every 3 to 6 weeks), are showing signs of promise in reducing complications associated with SCD.[47] Nursing responsibilities related to these procedures have been discussed in the previous section.

SCD is considered a multiorgan disease because of the risk of ischemia or infarction of many organs caused by sickling of RBCs and vaso-occlusion. The organs most commonly affected are the spleen, kidneys, and bone marrow; however, involvement of the lungs and the brain can also occur. Children with frequent episodes of intravascular sickling are at risk for progressive organ dysfunction because of decreased tissue perfusion, ischemia, and necrosis. All organs can be affected during an acute episode, as well as chronically. A complete and ongoing assessment of all organ systems during an intensive care admission is imperative.

A newer method of treating SCD is bone marrow transplantation. Transplantation changes the electropheresis pattern in the child's Hgb toward the donor's pattern.[35] It is considered a curative therapy. Patients can experience GVHD and some have died from this complication.

Complications of Sickle Cell Disease.   The most common clinical manifestations of SCD are vaso-occlusive crises, sequestration crises, and aplastic crises. These may lead to life-threatening complications such as acute chest syndrome, stroke, acute anemia, and sepsis, which require admission to the PICU.

Vaso-occlusive Crises.   The most common reason for admission to the PICU is vaso-occlusive crisis with ischemia or infarction of the occluded organ. Vaso-occlusive crisis is an acute, painful episode that is the result of intravascular sickling, occlusion of small vessels, and tissue ischemia and infarction. The onset is acute and may be precipitated by infection, hypoxia, fever, acidosis, dehydration, change in climate, and psychologic factors. However, a predetermining factor is often not identified. The joints and the extremities are most often affected.

Therapy for the child with vaso-occlusive crisis is aimed at removing the precipitating cause, treating complications, and preventing further crises. Treatment is supportive and includes hydration, antibiotics, and pain management, as discussed above. Oxygen is provided if the child is hypoxemic in order to prevent further sickling and possibly promote conversion of sickled RBCs to normal shape.

Acute Chest Syndrome.   Acute chest syndrome is the development of a new pulmonary infiltrate in combination with fever or respiratory symptoms in a patient with SCD.[48] It is the result of sickling of RBCs in the pulmonary vasculature, which may cause intrapulmonary shunting and abnormalities in gas exchange. These patients are also at high risk for pulmonary infarctions from recurrent sickling and pneumonia.

Signs and symptoms include pleuritic chest pain, hypoxia, tachypnea, retractions, and nasal flaring. The radiographic picture is consistent with pulmonary infiltrates. This may progress to a complete "whiteout" of lung fields and respiratory failure. Fever and an increased WBC count may be seen with both infection and infarction.

Box 24-5
Indications for Red Blood Cell Transfusion in Sickle Cell Disease

Acute Simple Transfusion

Symptomatic Anemias Resulting From Blood Loss

Complicated pain crisis not relieved by other medical therapy

Aplastic crisis

Splenic sequestration

Accelerated hemolysis (such as caused by delayed hemolytic transfusion reaction, warm autoimmune hemolytic anemia, or sickle crisis)

Preoperative preparation for most surgeries

Chronic Simple Transfusion

Prevention of recurrent occlusive stroke (<30% Hb S)

Selected sickle cell disease pregnancies (such as recurrent fetal loss, multiple gestations)

Possible role in recurrent chest syndrome and skin ulcers

Partial RBC Exchange Transfusions

Acute or impending stroke, including transient ischemic attack

Fat embolism syndrome

Unresponsive acute priapism

Acute, rapidly progressive chest syndromes

Preoperative preparation for some major surgeries and eye surgery

Simon TL, AuBuchon J, Cooper ES et al: Practice parameters for the use of red blood cell transfusions, *Arch Pathol Lab Med* 122:130-138, 1999.

Therapy for acute chest syndrome follows the general principles of therapy for vaso-occlusive crises. Pain relief is critical to allow effective pulmonary toilet and coughing. Antibiotics are recommended in any febrile child with acute chest syndrome because untreated bacterial infections can be devastating for children with SCD. Oxygen is necessary for the hypoxemic child to promote normal oxygenation and prevent further sickling. Partial exchange transfusion may be necessary even in the child with mild symptoms to halt progression of the disorder (Box 24-5). Recurrent acute chest syndrome is a criteria for bone marrow transplantation.[48]

Cerebrovascular Accident.   CVA is most often the result of thrombosis in the major cerebral arteries in younger children and hemorrhage in older children. CVA affects about 5% of children with SCD.[49]

The diagnosis of CVA is made on the basis of clinical signs. Unfortunately, warning signs of an impending CVA are rare. Some children may complain of headache or dizziness, but often the first signs are apparent only with the CVA itself. These signs may be hemiplegia, aphasia, speech difficulties, visual disturbances, seizures, or coma.

Upon admission of a child with neurologic signs suggesting CVA, assessment includes a history and a detailed neurologic examination. A CT or MRI is done to rule out a lesion such as subdural hematoma if the history (such as recent head trauma) suggests this. The CT is done without contrast materials because they may precipitate sickling by drying out the RBCs. If there are no signs of increased intracranial pressure, a lumbar puncture may be done to rule out an infectious process. Angiography is postponed until the child's condition is stable and the Hb S has been decreased to below 10% by exchange transfusion.

The most critical intervention for the child presenting with a CVA is a partial exchange transfusion to prevent progression of the CVA. Other therapy is supportive. If the child has experienced a large infarction, close monitoring for intracranial hypertension is necessary. Anticoagulant therapy is contraindicated. Bone marrow transplantation may benefit the child who experiences recurrent strokes.[50]

Splenic Sequestration.   Splenic sequestration is a life-threatening complication of SCD and one of the leading causes of death in children with this disease. There is massive engorgement of the splenic sinuses with blood and a significant amount of the RBC mass becomes trapped in the spleen. The result is an abrupt fall in hemoglobin levels, which may result in death from circulatory failure. The etiology of this complication is unknown and the severity of the crisis ranges from mild splenic enlargement with minimal decrease in hemoglobin level to substantial splenomegaly, life-threatening anemia, and shock.

Splenic sequestration is normally seen in infants and children younger than 6 years of age because these children have not yet undergone autosplenectomy. Autosplenectomy is a process by which repeated episodes of infarction reduce the spleen to fibrotic tissue with deposits of iron. By age 5 years, most patients with SCA have become permanently asplenic because of this process.[51]

Children with splenic sequestration have acute, severe left upper quadrant pain, vomiting, acute onset of anemia, a rapidly distending abdomen, and signs of hypovolemia. On physical examination, there is severe hypotension, cardiac enlargement, and splenomegaly. The Hct is often half the patient's normal value, and there is usually a rapid reticulocytosis with increased immature RBCs and moderate to severe thrombocytopenia.

Therapy for this crisis is the immediate transfusion of PRBCs to restore intravascular volume and oxygen-carrying capacity. Once the cardiovascular status stabilizes, the child usually improves rapidly. The spleen shrinks within a few days, and the thrombocytopenia resolves. Splenic sequestration may recur, usually within 4 months of the initial episode. Emergency splenectomy for an acute crises is not indicated so long as prompt attention to crisis is provided.

Aplastic Crisis.   Aplastic crisis is a condition that results from a primary erythropoietic failure often associated with a parvovirus infection. The cessation of bone marrow function causes the Hct to decrease dramatically. If the anemia is severe and the child is symptomatic or if general condition is compromised, an intensive care admission may be necessary.

The child with aplastic crisis usually appears listless and pale. Hemoglobin values are decreased and the reticulocyte count is less than 1%.

Most aplastic episodes are mild and require no treatment. Recovery is usually spontaneous with an elevated nucleated

RBC count, followed by reticulocytosis in 1 or 2 days. PRBCs may be administered to maintain a hemoglobin of 8 g/dl or more if the anemia is severe.

Sepsis.   Infection is the most common cause of death in children with SCD. These children are immunocompromised because of decreased splenic function with the loss of its filtering capabilities and diminished antibody function. Infections in children with altered splenic function are usually caused by organisms such as *Streptococcus pneumoniae, Haemophilus influenzae,* and *Neisseria meningitidis.*[52] Children with SCD seem to be at particular risk for septic shock caused by *S. pneumoniae.*

In children with SCD, a temperature higher than 38.5° C, band count greater than 1000/mm^3, or a high erythrocyte sedimentation rate (ESR) are treated with antibiotic therapy regardless of whether they appear septic. Children who appear septic are treated with antibiotics regardless of their temperature.

Other Crises.   The child admitted to the PICU with SCD may experience a variety of other crises. As with acute chest syndrome and CVA, any crisis may be precipitated by infection, dehydration, fatigue, and hypoxia.

Bony crises may involve the marrow or the cortex of the bone itself. The small bones of the hands and feet are commonly affected in infants and toddlers, giving rise to dactylitis or hand-foot syndrome. In all bony crises, pain, fever, and leukocytosis are present. With bone cortex involvement, pain, redness, and swelling over the affected area are seen.

Abdominal crises are often the result of occlusion of the mesenteric vessels or vessels of some of the viscera, such as the spleen or the kidney. These crises are characterized by acute abdominal pain, fever, malaise, anorexia, nausea, and an increased WBC count. These symptoms are often indistinguishable from an acute "surgical abdomen," and a thorough history and surgical evaluation are required. Patients with "crisis pain" usually remain in stable condition or improve slightly with supportive measures such as hydration and analgesics. Patients with an acute surgical abdomen do not improve with these measures, and instead become more acutely ill.

Therapy for other crises is supportive. Adequate hydration must be maintained. Antibiotic therapy is indicated if there is redness and swelling over a bone. Pain management is crucial with all crises. For the child with an abdominal crisis, pain management prevents atelectasis that occurs because of splinting of the abdomen.

MIXED DISORDERS

Hemolytic Uremic Syndrome

Etiology.   HUS is a clinical syndrome characterized by the triad of microangiopathic hemolytic anemia, thrombocytopenia, and acute renal failure. HUS is the most common cause of acquired renal failure in children. Although the primary systemic effects are hematologic and renal, there is potential for multisystem involvement, primarily of the GI and neurologic systems.

HUS does not appear to have a single etiology but is a syndrome of diverse causes. Numerous agents and predisposing factors have been associated with HUS, including infectious organisms, medications, and hereditary traits, but causality has not been definitively established.

Etiologic investigations of HUS have focused on infectious agents, specifically verotoxin-producing organisms such as *Escherichia coli.* One particular strain of *E. coli* (*E. coli* 0157:H7) has been identified as the most common pathogen associated with HUS; 80% to 90% of stools cultured from children with HUS are positive for *E. coli* 0157:H7. The most common source of contamination has been undercooked beef, although enterohemorrhagic strains of *E. coli* have also been found in unpasteurized juices and dairy products.[53-55]

Other infectious organisms that have been less commonly associated with HUS are *Shigella dysenteriae, Salmonella typhi, Camphylobacter jejuni, S. pneumoniae, Yersinia pseudotuberculosis,* and *coxsackie virus.*[53,55] HUS patients who have positive cultures for one of these enteropathogens (including *E. coli*) at the onset of their illness are "typical" HUS patients.

"Atypical" HUS etiologies may also include a familial form of HUS caused by a genetic deficiency of prostacyclin-stimulating hormone. Other potential precipitating factors include medications (e.g., cyclosporin A, mitomycin, chemotherapeutic agents, oral contraceptives), and conditions such as pregnancy, malignancy, lupus erythematosus, and malignant hypertension.[53,55] It is unclear which of these may cause HUS, which are chance simultaneous occurrences, or which are related to some third unidentified causal factor.

Incidence.   HUS most commonly affects children between the ages of 6 months and 4 years. Approximately 80% of the cases of HUS occur in children under the age of 5 years.[56,57] The majority of reported cases of HUS (75% to 80%) occur between the months of April and September.[56,57] No explanation for the age distribution or seasonal variation of HUS has been established.

The incidence of HUS in North America has been reported as two to four cases per 100,000 children younger than the age of 5 years.[57] Some studies have documented an increasing incidence of HUS since the early 1980s. The increased occurrence of HUS has coincided with an increased appearance of verotoxin-producing strains of *E. coli* as pathogens in humans.

Pathogenesis.   The major underlying mechanism of injury in HUS is vascular endothelial damage. In the postenteropathic (typical) form of HUS, the verotoxin, or shiga-like toxin (SLT) released by *E. coli* or other organisms initiates the endothelial damage.[53] The kidneys are the primary site of endothelial disruption, but thrombotic microangiopathy may be found in all organs.

Typically, damaged endothelial cells within the vasculature of the renal glomerulus swell and become separated from the basement membrane, creating a widened subendothelial space. Fibrin, platelets, and lipids are deposited in the subendothelial space, which when combined with the swollen endothelial cells, produce thickened glomerular capillary walls and thus reduced capillary lumen size. Small arterioles become thrombosed as a result of local intravascular coagulation activation. Thus the renal vasculature becomes obstructed by endothelial swelling and/or thrombi, resulting in a reduced filtering surface and renal ischemia. Consequently, the glomerular filtration rate is significantly diminished, and acute renal failure develops.[58] Histopathologic studies of renal tissue in children with HUS have demonstrated glomerular thrombotic microangiopathy and cortical necrosis.[58]

Thrombocytopenia in HUS is the result of both aggregation and destruction of platelets within the damaged microvasculature. Normally, an anticlumping substance released from the endothelium (prostacyclin) keeps platelet aggregation in check. However, there is evidence that in HUS, inappropriate platelet aggregation is facilitated by diminished prostacyclin activity. "Familial" HUS may be seen in patients who have a hereditary prostacyclin deficiency. The mechanism of prostacyclin inhibition in other forms of HUS is unknown. More recently, studies have demonstrated an increase in large von Willebrand factor multimers in the HUS patient, which may be responsible for systemic platelet aggregation and adherence. The result is that significant numbers of platelets are "trapped" in multiple microvascular thrombi or are injured and removed from the circulation by the spleen.[59] The pathogenesis of the hemolytic anemia of HUS is also related to renal endothelial disruption. Erythrocytes are mechanically damaged as they pass through the swollen and occluded arterioles. The spleen and liver remove these fragmented RBCs from the circulation, causing a progressive and severe anemia. An increase in von Willebrand factor multimers have also been implicated in causing hemolysis because they promote adhesion of young erythrocytes to endothelial cells.[59,60] The body attempts to compensate by accelerating RBC production, as evidenced by reticulocyte counts, which are often increased 2% to 20%.[53]

Although the kidneys are the primary location of pathologic changes in HUS, extrarenal involvement occurs in a significant proportion of patients. The GI system is actually the first site of physiologic derangement in most cases of "typical" HUS. Hemorrhagic colitis, frequently caused by *E. coli,* precedes the onset of HUS in up to 90% of patients. The mechanism of bowel injury is similar to the renal pathophysiologic process: endothelial disruption and thrombosis of the microvasculature, leading to ischemic/necrotic tissue damage. GI complications of HUS include perforation, obstruction, stricture, or intussusception of the bowel.[53] It has recently been recognized that in up to 20% of HUS patients, the pancreas suffers comparable hemorrhagic and necrotic damage. These microangiopathic changes are hypothesized to be endotoxin mediated. Similar hemorrhagic, thrombotic, and necrotic lesions have been documented in the CNS, lungs, adrenal glands, and hearts of some patients with HUS.[53,58]

HUS is not limited to renal, hematologic, and GI involvement. Approximately 30% of patients with HUS experience neurologic dysfunction because of involvement of the microvasculature of the brain and the direct neuro-logic effects of the toxins, similar to TTP, where the brain is the primary affected organ. Neurologic sequelae may include hemiparesis, cortical blindness, and a persistent state of altered consciousness.[53]

In the majority of HUS patients, the syndrome is preceded by a prodromal illness. Approximately 90% of children diagnosed with HUS have experienced gastroenteritis with some combination of diarrhea (usually bloody), vomiting, and/or abdominal pain at the onset of their illness. Less commonly, the diagnosis of HUS may be preceded by an upper respiratory infection or by no specific signs of illness at all. The average interval between onset of diarrhea and diagnosis of HUS is 1 week. Patients with nondiarrheal, "atypical" HUS are less likely to present with a prodromal illness condition and commonly have a more aggressive course.[53] Approximately one third of HUS patients are febrile in the prodromal period.[61]

Initial physical assessment of the child with HUS generally reveals a pale, lethargic, and/or irritable child, with evidence of abdominal pain or tenderness. Inspection of the skin may reveal hemorrhagic manifestations, such as bruising, petechiae, or purpura. Admission vital signs are usually within normal limits for age, although some children may have tachycardia and/or tachypnea if anemia is severe at presentation. Tachypnea may also reflect an attempt to compensate for metabolic acidosis resulting from renal failure. Hypertension may be present, but usually it develops later in the course of the disease.

Up to 10% of children with HUS present with seizure activity. The etiology of seizures at presentation is usually hyponatremia, but seizures may be the result of early CNS microangiopathy.[57]

Oliguria or anuria is present in more than 60% of children who develop HUS.[56] Urine is usually grossly hematuric. Laboratory analysis confirms acute renal failure, with rapidly increasing blood urea nitrogen (BUN) and creatinine levels. It is not unusual for a child with HUS to have a BUN level higher than 100 mg/dl and a creatinine level higher than 4 mg/dl within the first 2 days of diagnosis. Urinalysis reveals proteinuria and the presence of urinary casts. Serum electrolyte values may be initially normal, or consistent with acute renal failure (decreased sodium and calcium, increased potassium and phosphorus).[53]

Hematologic analysis helps to confirm the diagnosis of HUS. Microangiopathic hemolytic anemia is present, with a Hct typically less than 25%. Microscopic examination of the peripheral blood film reveals typical schistocytes (fragmented red cells). Thrombocytopenia (platelet count less than 100,000/μl) is present, but other coagulation values (PT, PTT) are typically within normal limits, differentiating this disorder from DIC. Commonly, the CBC also reveals leukocytosis upon presentation.[53]

If stool cultures are sent, the most common organism identified is *E. coli* 0157:H7. Other potential enteropathogens are listed within the discussion of HUS etiologies. Cultures from other sites are generally negative at presentation.

Diagnostic work-up of the patient with HUS is generally limited to laboratory analysis. Occasionally, abdominal pain and colitis lead to an exploratory laparotomy before the diagnosis of HUS is made, especially if the rest of the clinical picture is not consistent with "typical" HUS.[53]

Critical Care Management. Management of the child with HUS is primarily focused on rapid recognition, supportive care, and treatment of complications, which include acute renal failure, anemia, CNS dysfunction, and GI symptoms. Goals of management focus on restoration and maintenance of: (1) fluid and electrolyte balance, (2) renal function, (3) optimal cardiovascular function and blood pressure, (4) adequate RBC volume and functional platelets, (5) neurologic function, and (6) GI function and nutritional support.

Initially, the child with HUS may present with dehydration resulting from GI losses (diarrhea, vomiting) and decreased oral intake. As the disease progresses, GI losses generally diminish, and the child is at risk for fluid overload from acute renal failure. Treatment consists of strict intake and output with intravenous fluid adjustment, renal replacement therapy, and management of hypertension.

Initial fluid replacement with intravenous solutions is administered cautiously, with careful monitoring of serum electrolytes and an ongoing assessment for fluid overload. Subsequently, the patient with HUS is monitored closely for signs of hypervolemia, including peripheral edema, tachycardia, hypertension, pulmonary edema, and increased weight. In the oliguric or anuric patient, fluid intake is restricted to insensible losses (approximately 30% maintenance) plus urine output replacement.

Nursing responsibilities include assessing for signs of pulmonary edema, such as rales, hypoxemia, frothy sputum, tachypnea, and increased heart size and infiltrates, which are seen on chest radiographs. Serum electrolyte values are monitored closely (every 6 to 8 hours), along with assessment for complications of electrolyte imbalances (e.g., hyperkalemia, hyponatremia). Careful monitoring and treatment of hyponatremia with fluid restriction and dialysis are critical to electrolyte balance.

The majority of critically ill patients with HUS require dialysis during the acute phase of their illness. The decision to dialyze a patient is not based on absolute criteria, but on an overall assessment of the individual patient's status. Indications for dialysis include one or more of the following: anuria for longer than 24 hours, hypertension, pulmonary edema, hyperkalemia, and severe azotemia. Some clinicians initiate dialysis prophylactically for BUN concentrations greater than 100 to 150 mg/dl.[56]

Patients with HUS may receive peritoneal dialysis (PD) or hemodialysis (HD), or continuous veno-venous hemofiltration with dialysis (CVVHD). The advantages of PD are that fluid is removed gradually, so that hemodynamic stability is ensured, and that PD does not require vascular access. However, there are a number of disadvantages to PD as compared with HD or CVVHD for the HUS patient. The high glucose solutions used in PD may cause hyperglycemia, especially if the patient has pancreatic insufficiency caused by HUS. Probably the biggest disadvantage to PD in this population is the risk of precipitating or exacerbating the abdominal complications associated with HUS.

The main advantage of HD, aside from avoiding involvement of the GI tract, is that it provides more precise correction of fluid imbalance, electrolyte values, and acidosis. One disadvantage is that patients who are hemodialyzed must be systemically heparinized for each procedure, which may transiently increase their risk of bleeding.

CVVHD has been used with good results as a primary renal replacement therapy for HUS patients with severe GI inflammation and bleeding.[62] Primary advantages are that the GI tract is avoided, CVVHD can be accomplished in younger patients because of small filter sizes, and hemodynamic stability can be optimally maintained in comparison to HD.

Optimization of cardiovascular function may include antihypertensive medications, vasoactive therapy with inotropes and vasodilators, as well as treatment of severe anemia, bleeding, and fluid overload as previously discussed. Management of hypertension in the patient with HUS is a collaborative responsibility. In addition to fluid overload, hypertension is exacerbated by excessive renin release by the kidneys caused by decreased renal perfusion. Antihypertensives are required to control blood pressure in up to 40% of critically ill patients with HUS.[53]

The primary risk factor for bleeding in patients with HUS is thrombocytopenia. However, in addition to a decrease in the absolute number of platelets, there is evidence that the HUS patient's circulating platelets are hyporesponsive to aggregating agents, implying an additional platelet function abnormality.[59] It has been established that the platelets of uremic patients in general do not function properly; however, it is unclear whether there is an additional mechanism compounding this "malfunctioning" in HUS patients.

The child with HUS requires close monitoring for signs of bleeding, such as bruising, petechiae, oozing from invasive line sites, epistaxis, or upper and/or lower GI bleeding. Procedures that may promote bleeding, such as intramuscular injections and rectal instrumentation, are avoided. In addition, the child is assessed for signs of occult bleeding, such as increased abdominal girth, increased pulse and respiratory rate, diminished peripheral perfusion, a change in neurologic status, or hypotension (a late sign of hypovolemia).[53]

Blood component replacement is generally not aggressive in patients with HUS because there is evidence that transfused platelets and RBCs suffer the same damage in the microvasculature as the child's intrinsic blood components and may exacerbate the risk of thrombus formation. Consequently, RBCs are generally transfused only when the Hct falls below 15% to 20%, or sooner if the Hct is falling rapidly or if the patient is symptomatically anemic.[56] Most HUS patients receive at least one blood transfusion during the acute phase of their illness. Platelets are usually not administered until the platelet count is below 10,000 to 20,000/μl, or if there is active bleeding.

All blood products are administered slowly and timed to coincide with dialysis when possible, to minimize the risks of circulatory overload. All patients are monitored for signs of a transfusion reaction

There are a number of potential risk factors for neurologic dysfunction in the HUS patient. There is evidence that the microangiopathic process that obstructs perfusion in the renal vasculature can develop in the cerebral vasculature. Thus there is a risk of microthrombi or even large thrombus formation in the cerebral arterioles, potentially leading to infarction. In addition, thrombocytopenia coupled with hypertension puts the patient with HUS at significant risk for an intracranial hemorrhage.

Seizures, affecting about 10% of children with HUS, are treated with short-acting anticonvulsants, (i.e., benzodiazepines), followed by fosphenytoin or phenobarbital for sustained seizure control.[56]

Vigilance by the nurse is required to monitor for changes that may indicate neurologic damage. This can be challenging because patients are typically lethargic and/or irritable upon admission because of uremia, anemia, and/or a postictal state. Signs of focal infarction or hemorrhage include hemiparesis, seizures, change in motor strength, cranial nerve deficits, and a change in level of consciousness. Signs of increased intracranial pressure include decreased responsiveness to stimuli, pupillary changes, change in respiratory pattern, (late) decreased pulse, and increased blood pressure with widened pulse pressure. A brain CT or MRI may be required to identify infarctions, edema, or hemorrhage so that neurologic recovery can be optimized.

If there is clinical or radiologic evidence of neurologic deterioration, therapeutic modalities aimed at the removal of circulating endotoxin and the normalization of platelet-aggregating factors may be instituted. Fresh plasma infusion and plasmapheresis are the two most commonly employed therapies. Because plasmapheresis is so successful in treating TTP, which has similar pathophysiology to HUS, it may improve neurologic outcome. Case reports have shown efficacy, but studies have not demonstrated clinical significance in outcome.[59,60]

Collaborative interventions to optimize neurologic functioning include control of seizures with anticonvulsants and electrolyte balance. Standard interventions to reduce or prevent rises in intracranial pressure are instituted if the patient with HUS demonstrates cerebral edema on CT or MRI. The only modification for the anuric patient is that osmotic diuretics are not used because they draw fluid into the intravascular space, which can not be excreted, thereby exacerbating hypervolemia.

The patient with HUS is at risk for GI complications resulting from vascular endothelial damage, thrombi, and necrosis of bowel tissue. Careful monitoring of the patient is the cornerstone of managing GI complications. The child is assessed for abdominal tenderness, cramping, and distension, especially as compared with baseline status upon admission. Abdominal girth is measured and recorded each shift, and all gastric output is tested for the presence of blood. Ranitidine is administered to prevent gastric ulceration.

If a paralytic ileus or an acute abdominal process develops, the patient with HUS is kept on a nothing-by-mouth (NPO) status and a nasogastric tube is inserted to decompress the stomach. Approximately half the children with HUS require parenteral nutrition during the acute phase of their illness. The GI tract may require serial evaluation with kidney, ureter, and bladder (KUB) x-ray and/or abdominal ultrasound examination. Signs of an acute bowel infarction, perforation, obstruction, or necrosis include tachycardia, hypotension, acidosis, vomiting, and abdominal distension. Surgical intervention may be necessary.[56]

Nutritional support with total parenteral nutrition (TPN) is instituted early to stop catabolism present on admission, especially with the patient with diarrhea and vomiting. Once diarrhea and GI inflammation has resolved, enteral nutrition (nasoduodenal or jejunal) is instituted with formula requirements calculated in light of renal compromise.[53,56]

Pancreatitis, with both endocrine and exocrine involvement, has been recognized as a potential complication of HUS, presumably resulting from the same mechanisms that injure renal, GI, and cerebral tissue.[56] It may be difficult to evaluate the patient with HUS for pancreatitis because the clinical signs, abdominal pain and vomiting, may be present because of another etiology. Patients with these signs are made NPO regardless of whether a definitive diagnosis is made. Serum amylase and lipase levels are followed, but because these enzymes are partially excreted by the renal route, levels greater than four times normal are necessary to diagnose pancreatitis in patients with renal failure.[56] Abdominal ultrasound examinations may be performed; enlargement and sonolucence of the pancreas is consistent with pancreatitis.

The nurse assesses the patient with HUS for hyperglycemia resulting from pancreatic insufficiency, which may necessitate exogenous insulin administration. The anuric patient cannot be monitored for glycosuria; therefore serum glucose is measured every 4 to 8 hours. Serum glucose is maintained at 100 to 200 mg/dl with insulin administration carefully titrated by the nurse.

Antibiotic therapy for HUS and hemorrhagic colitis caused by *E. coli* 0157:H7 is controversial, with conflicting study results as to benefit, or even showing adverse effects.[56,58] Other therapies studied at various times include heparin, thrombolytic agents, prostacyclin infusion, gamma globulin, and vitamin E. None of these therapies has consistently proved effective for HUS, but some are still used in cases of severe disease, especially with cerebrovascular involvement.

The mortality rate from HUS is approximately 5%.[57,63] Of children with a one-time occurrence of HUS, 60% to 80% recover completely. Another 10% to 30% are left with long-term sequelae, which include hypertension, chronic renal failure, and neurologic complications such as hemiparesis, seizures, blindness, and cognitive deficits. Currently, less than 5% of all patients studied progressed to end-stage renal disease and renal transplantation, but recent long-term studies show evidence that in some post-HUS patients, renal function declines after apparent recovery.[53,57]

Extensive analysis has been done to identify patients at high risk for a poor outcome from HUS. Poor outcome is generally defined as chronic renal failure, neurologic sequelae, or death. Some investigators differentiate between typical (or classic) and atypical HUS when discussing prognosis. The typical form, which has a better prognosis, affects young children (usually younger than 3 years old), has a prodrome of bloody diarrhea, occurs during the summer, and is nonrecurrent. Hereditary and other atypical forms of HUS have a poorer prognosis in terms of morbidity and mortality.[56]

Other factors that have been statistically correlated with a poor outcome are high neutrophil count upon admission (which may reflect the degree of endotoxin exposure), short diarrhea prodrome before admission (which may reflect a higher infectious dose of circulating toxin), higher Hgb count upon admission (more invasive disease may prompt admission before hemolysis has occurred), seizures upon admission, bowel necrosis during the acute phase, and longer duration of anuria during the acute phase.[57] Although it is still difficult to predict the long-term outcome for an individual patient, even limited prognostic information may be useful in guiding therapies and in counseling parents of patients with HUS in the intensive care unit.

Thrombotic Thrombocytopenic Purpura

Etiology/Incidence. TTP has traditionally been considered an "adult" counterpart to HUS, very similar in pathophysiology, but with the CNS being the primary affected organ in TTP.

TTP has been reported rarely in children, with 16 case reports in a 1998 MEDLINE search.[64] The disorder can present in infancy or childhood, and relapses can occur at varying intervals. Etiology is similar to HUS, with a viral prodrome before presenting symptoms. Case reports of TTP secondary to HIV infection have been reported.[65]

Pathogenesis. The basic process in both HUS and TTP is the deposition of fibrin in the microcirculation with subsequent microangiopathic hemolysis and thrombocytopenia. The pathophysiology is unclear; however, the most consistent hematologic feature is platelet aggregation with the presence of unusually large von Willebrand factor multimers.[59,65]

Thrombocytopenia is the major complication in TTP, followed by hemolysis. Pathophysiologic changes in the brain and microvasculature of other organs cause the presenting signs and symptoms.

Children most commonly (about 50%) present with neurologic symptoms, ranging from dizziness, weakness, lethargy to obtundation, and hemiparesis.[65] Other symptoms

include fever and bleeding (epistaxis and/or bruising). Hematuria, oliguria (or anuria), and bloody diarrhea are seen less often. Laboratory values are similar to HUS, with a low Hct and low platelet count.

Despite excellent assessment and critical care management, the outcome for TTP in children is discouraging, with 38% mortality in the 16 reported cases. Microthrombi were demonstrable in all major organs at autopsy. No pretreatment characteristics were identified as prognostic indicators of relapse.[65]

The critically ill child usually presents with profound neurologic impairment, along with hemorrhage and, often, renal impairment. Assessment and nursing care include neurologic system observation for changes in level of consciousness and/or signs of hemorrhage, respiratory assessment for adequate oxygenation and ventilation, close observation for signs of renal failure with strict intake and output and urine testing, and hypervigilant assessment for signs of frank and occult bleeding. CBC and coagulation studies are monitored frequently and interpreted with the clinical assessment to determine the need for blood product administration.

Critical Care Management. The mainstay of treatment for TTP is plasmapheresis and excellent supportive care. Plasmapheresis has been shown to be much more beneficial in treating patients with TTP, as opposed to treating HUS.[19] Treatment with blood products, including PRBCs, platelets, and fresh frozen plasma are the mainstay of supportive therapy.[61,65] Recognizing the consumptive nature of the pathophysiology of TTP, in the presence of active hemolysis, transfused RBCs are hemolyzed in the same manner as native RBCs. Transfused platelets may also be destroyed and cause more microthrombi. Other therapies that have been used with varying success include corticosteroids, high-dose IVIg, vincristine, antiplatelet agents, and splenectomy.[19]

IVIg and antiplatelet agents and steroids are also administered with the goal of halting the peripheral platelet aggregation. Remission has been demonstrated with the prophylactic use of FFP without plasmapheresis.[65] Children with renal impairment who need dialysis are treated in the same manner as those with HUS—with peritoneal dialysis, HD, or CVVHD being the therapeutic modalities.

Care of the TTP patient requires the same level of nursing expertise that is required for any child with multisystem failure. The child with TTP is usually very critical, with profound neurologic, renal, and other system dysfunction or failure. Nurses require skills in caring for the patient undergoing pheresis and/or dialysis therapies as discussed in previous sections. Line placement for dialysis/pheresis is difficult in terms of access and bleeding status of the patient. Hemodynamic monitoring of the patient with impaired cardiovascular function may be required, especially for the unstable child during dialysis/pheresis procedures. Cardiovascular support with titration of vasoactive infusions to optimize cardiac output may be needed. Intubation and mechanical ventilation is often required for airway protection and to provide optimal oxygenation and ventilation in the neurologically impaired child.

SUMMARY

Critically ill children may experience a wide range of hematologic problems related to a variety of causes. Anemia and thrombocytopenia also may be part of the pathologic process that brings children to the PICU. Children's response to medical and nursing interventions depends on their preexisting state, the severity of their illness, and length of time before treatment is initiated.

Caring for these children requires a collaborative approach. It is imperative that the nurse caring for these children be vigilant for subtle but significant signs that occur because of the complexity of the patient's needs and the potential for rapid changes in the patient's condition. Expert nursing management is essential to maximize the potential for a positive outcome.

REFERENCES

1. Nugent D, Tarantino MD: Hematology-oncology problems in the intensive care unit. In Fuhrman BP, Zimmerman JJ, eds: *Pediatric critical care,* St Louis, 1998, Mosby.
2. Walters MC, Abelson HT: Interpretation of the complete blood count, *Pediatr Clin North Am* 43:599-622, 1996.
3. Manno CS: What's new in transfusion medicine? *Pediatr Clin North Am* 43:793-808, 1996.
4. Folkes ME: Transfusion therapy in critical care nursing, *Crit Care Nurs Q* 13:15-28, 1990.
5. National Blood Resource Education Program's Nursing Education Working Group Choosing blood components and equipment, *Am J Nurs* 91:42-50, 1991.
6. Luban NLC, DePalma L: Transfusion therapy in the pediatric intensive care unit. In Holbrook PR, ed: *Textbook of pediatric intensive care,* Philadelphia, 1993, WB Saunders.
7. American Association of Blood Banks: *Technical manual,* Bethesda, Md, 1997, The Association.
8. Bonato J: Blood transfusions: are they safe? *Crit Care Nurse* 9:40-44, 1989.
9. DePalma L, Luban NLC: Transfusion-transmitted diseases: AIDS and hepatitis, *Contemp Pediatr* 8:22-39, 1991.
10. Utili R, Zampino R, Bellopede P et al: Dual or single hepatitis B and C virus infections in childhood cancer survivors: long-term follow-up and effect of interferon treatment, *Blood* 94:4046-4052, 1999.
11. Dodd R: The risk of transfusion-transmitted infection, *N Engl J Med* 327:419, 1992.
12. Fosburg M, Kevy SV: Red cell transfusion. In Nathan DG, Oski FA, eds: *Hematology of infancy and childhood* (Vol. 2), Philadelphia, 1987, WB Saunders.
13. Mehta P, Gross S, Kao K: Transfusion with packed red blood cells. In Blumer JL, ed: *A practical guide to pediatric intensive care,* St Louis, 1990, Mosby.
14. Warrier I, Bussel JB, Valdez L et al: Safety and efficacy of low-dose intravenous immune globulin (IVIG) treatment for infants and children with immune thrombocytopenic purpura. Low-dose IVIG study group, *J Pediatr Hematol Oncol* 19:197-201, 1997.
15. Kevy S, Fosburg M: Therapeutic apheresis in childhood, *J Clin Apheresis* 5:87-90, 1990.

16. Kasprisin D: Clinical considerations in pediatric apheresis, *Plasma Therapy Transfusion Technology* 5:207-212, 1984.
17. Kasprisin D: Guidelines for performing therapeutic apheresis in children, *Plasma Ther Transfusion Technology* 5:213-218, 1984.
18. Kasprisin D: Techniques, indications, and toxicity of therapeutic hemapheresis in children, *J Ther Apheresis* 5:21-24, 1989.
19. Parker RJ: Etiology and treatment of acquired coagulopathies in the critically ill adult and child, *Crit Care Clin* 13:591-609, 1997.
20. Bell W: Thrombotic thrombocytopenic purpura, *JAMA* 265:91-93, 1991.
21. Headrick CL: Adult/pediatric CVVH: the pump, the patient, the circuit, *Crit Care Nurs Clin North Am* 10:197-207, 1998.
22. Bussel JB: Autoimmune thrombocytopenic purpura, *Hematol Oncol Clin North Am* 4:179-191, 1990.
23. Vesely S, Buchanan GR, Cohen A et al: Self-reported diagnostic and management strategies in childhood idiopathic thrombocytopenic purpura: results of a survey of practicing pediatric hematology/oncology specialists, *J Pediatr Hematol Oncol* 22:55-61, 2000.
24. Young L: DIC: the insidious killer, *Crit Care Nurse* 10:26-33, 1990.
25. Esparaz B, Green D: Disseminated intravascular coagulation, *Crit Care Nurse Q* 13:7-13, 1990.
26. Kruskal JB, Commerford PJ, Franks JJ et al: Fibrin and fibrinogen-related antigens in patients with stable and unstable coronary artery disease, *N Engl J Med* 317:1361-1365, 1987.
27. Wada HL, Wakita Y, Nakase T et al: Increased plasma-soluble fibrin monomer levels in patients with disseminated intravascular coagulation, *Am J Hematol* 51:255-260, 1996.
28. Bray GL: Inherited and acquired disorders of homeostasis. In Holbrook PR, ed: *Textbook of pediatric intensive care,* Philadelphia, 1993, WB Saunders.
29. Lusher JM: Diseases of coagulation: the fluid phase. In Nathan DG, Oski FA, eds: *Hematology of infancy and childhood,* ed 3, Philadelphia, 1987, WB Saunders.
30. Andrew M, Monagle P, Brooker L, eds: *Thromboembolic complications during infancy and childhood,* Hamilton, Ontario, 2000, BC Decker.

31. Michelson AD, Bovill E, Monagle P, Andrew M: Antithrombotic therapy in children, *Chest* 114(suppl 5):7485-7695, 1998.
32. Pascucci RC: Pediatric intensive care. In Gregory G, ed: *Pediatric anesthesia,* Vol 2, New York, 1989, Churchill Livingstone.
33. Andrew M, deVeber G: *Pediatric thromboembolism and stroke protocols,* Hamilton, Ontario, 1997, BC Decker.
34. Platt OS, Nathan DG: Hematology. In Avery ME, First L, eds: *Pediatric medicine,* Baltimore, 1989, Williams & Wilkins.
35. Simon K, Lobo, ML, Jackson S: Current knowledge in the management of children and adolescents with sickle cell disease. Part I, Physiological issues, *J Pediatr Nurs* 14:281-295, 1999.
36. Beyer JE, Platt AF, Kinney TT et al: Practice guidelines for the assessment of children with sickle cell pain, *JSPN* 4:61-73, 1999.
37. Shapiro BS, Cohen DE, Howe CJ: Patient-controlled analgesia for sickle-cell-related pain, *J Pain Symptom Manage* 8:22-28, 1993.
38. Trentadue NO, Kachoyeanos MK, Lea G: A comparison of two regimens of patient-controlled analgesia for children with sickle cell disease, *J Pediatr Nurs Care: Nurs Care Child Fam* 13:15-19, 1998.
39. Benini JC, Rogers ZR, Sandler ES et al: Beneficial effect of intravenous dexamethasone in children with mild to moderately severe acute chest syndrome complicating sickle cell disease, *Blood* 92:3082-3089, 1998.
40. Griffin TC, McIntire D, Buchanan GR: High-dose intravenous methylprednisolone therapy for pain in children and adolescents with sickle cell disease, *N Engl J Med* 330:733-737, 1994.
41. Hardwick WE, Givens TG, Monroe KW et al: Effect of ketorolac in pediatric sickle cell vaso-occlusive pain crisis, *Pediatr Emerg Care* 15:179-182, 1999.
42. Simckes AM, Chen SS, Osorio AV et al: Ketroloac-induced irreversible renal failure in sickle cell disease: a case report, *Pediat Nephrol* 13:63-67, 1999.
43. Simon TL, AuBuchon J, Cooper ES et al: Practice parameters for the use of red blood cell transfusions, *Arch Pathol Lab Med* 122:130-138, 1999.

44. Charache S, Lubin B, Reid CD: *Management and therapy of sickle cell disease.* Washington, DC, 1992, U.S. Department of Health and Human Services, Public Health Service, National Institutes of Health.

45. Charache S: Experimental therapy of sickle cell disease: use of hydroxyurea, *Am J Pediatr Hematol Oncol* 16:62-66, 1994.

46. Ware RE, Zimmerman SA, Schultz WH: Hydroxyurea as an alternative to blood transfusions for the prevention of recurrent stroke in children with sickle cell disease, *Blood* 94:3022-3026, 1999.

47. Reed WF, Vichinsky EP: Transfusion practice for patients with sickle cell disease, *Curr Opin Hematol* 6:432-438, 1999.

48. Golden C, Styles L, Vichinsky E: Acute chest syndrome and sickle cell disease, *Curr Opin Hematol* 5:89-92, 1998.

49. Ohene-Frempong K, Weiner SJ, Sleeper LA et al: Cerebrovascular accidents in sickle cell disease: rates and risk factors, *Blood* 1:288-294, 1998.

50. Kinney TR, Sleeper LA, Wang WC et al: Silent cerebral infarcts in sickle cell anemia: a risk factor analysis, *Pediatrics* 103:640-645, 1999.

51. Eskenazi AE, Gordon JB, Bernstein JL: Hematologic disorders in the pediatric intensive care unit. In Rogers MC, ed: *Textbook of pediatric intensive care,* ed 3, Baltimore, 1996, Williams & Wilkins.

52. Hoppe C, Styles L, Vichinsky E: The natural history of sickle cell disease, *Curr Opin Pediatr* 10:49-52, 1998.

53. Haws RM, Baum M: Hemolytic-uremic syndrome. In Levin DL, Morriss FC, eds: *Essentials of pediatric intensive care,* ed 2, New York, 1997, Churchill Livingstone.

54. Hilborn ED, Mshar PA, Fiorentino TR et al: An outbreak of *Escherichia coli* 0157:H7 infections and haemolytic uraemic syndrome associated with consumption of unpasteurized apple cider, *Epidemiol Infect* 124:31-36, 2000.

55. Siegler RL, Griffin PM, Barrett TJ et al: Recurrent hemolytic uremic syndrome secondary to *Escherichia coli* 0157:H7 infection, *Pediatrics* 91:666-668, 1993.

56. Siegler RL: The hemolytic uremic syndrome, *Pediatr Clin North Am* 42:1505-1529, 1995.

57. Siegler RL, Pavia AT, Christofferson RD et al: A 20 year population-based study of postdiarrheal hemolytic uremic syndrome in Utah, *Pediatrics* 94:35-40, 1994.

58. Foerster J: Red cell fragmentation syndromes. In Lee GR, Foerster J, Lukens J et al, eds: *Wintrobe's clinical hematology,* Vol. 1, Baltimore, 1999, Williams & Wilkins.

59. Baker KR, Moake JL: Thrombotic thrombocytopenic purpura and the hemolytic-uremic syndrome, *Curr Opin Pediatr* 12:23-28, 2000.

60. Wick TM, Moake JL, Udden MM et al: Unusually large von Willebrand factor multimers preferentially promote young sickle and nonsickle erythrocyte adhesion to endothelial cells, *Am J Hematol* 42:284-292, 1993.

61. Dervenoulas J, Tsirigotis P, Bollas G et al: Thrombotic thrombocytopenic purpura/hemolytic uremic syndrome (TTP/HUS): treatment outcome, relapses, prognostic factors: a single-center experience of 48 cases, *Ann Hematol* 79:66-72, 2000.

62. Cavagnaro F, Ronco R, Verdaguer M et al: Continuous hemofiltration in children with abdominal complications of hemolytic-uremic syndrome in a renal allograft recipient, *Nephron* 74:238, 1996.

63. Hand MM, McManus ML, Harmon WE: Renal disorders in pediatric intensive care. In Rogers MC, Nichols DG, eds: *Textbook of pediatric intensive care,* ed 3, Baltimore, 1996, Williams & Wilkins.

64. Andrew M, Montgomery RR: Acquired disorders of hemostasis. In Nathan DG, Orkin SH, eds: *Nathan and Oski's hematology of infancy and childhood,* ed 5, Philadelphia, 1998, WB Saunders.

65. Andrew M, Michelson AD, Bovill E et al: Guidelines for antithrombotic therapy in pediatric patients, *J Pediatr* 132:575-588, 1998.

Multisystem Problems

This section addresses the needs of patients experiencing multiple system dysfunction and their complicated demands and unique needs. Because these patients' illnesses involve more than a single body system, they present a distinctive challenge to the care team.

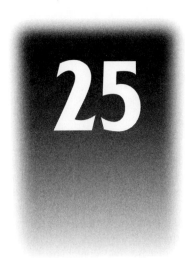

25 Oncologic Critical Care Problems

Tammara L. Jenkins

Cancer has been perceived by many people, health professionals included, as a "terrible, hopeless disease that leads to certain death."[1] But today a degree of optimism prevails. The treatment of childhood cancers has made tremendous strides in recent years, with 65% of children with cancer now surviving more than 5 years after diagnosis.[2] Many childhood malignancies that were once universally fatal are now potentially curable, such as acute lymphoblastic leukemia (ALL).

In the past, few children with malignancy were admitted to critical care units because there seemed to be little benefit to providing aggressive care. However, with the remarkable advances made in pediatric oncology, critical care technologies, immunology, and the treatment of infectious diseases, more children are recovering from cancer and complications related to malignancies and aggressive treatment modalities.[3]

Children with oncologic or hematologic disease are typically admitted to the pediatric intensive care unit (PICU) for complications resulting from either local or systemic manifestations of malignant tumor or disease, or effects of antineoplastic therapy.[3,4] To fully appreciate the unique care needs of a child with malignancy, critical care nurses require an understanding of the child's underlying malignancy, as well as the likely causes of life-threatening complications.

Children with malignancy may present to the PICU with dysfunction of one or several organ systems. This chapter provides an overview of general complications associated with malignancies and their treatment, as well as complications specifically related to solid tumors, leukemias, and bone marrow transplantation (BMT). Because many of these complications may have other etiologies not related to cancer, this chapter focuses on how complications may manifest and be treated differently in children with oncologic disease.

CARE OF THE NEUTROPENIC PATIENT

The neutropenic child presents a unique challenge to the intensive care unit (ICU) team. Children who receive chemotherapeutic agents or radiation therapy or who undergo BMT typically become both neutropenic and thrombocytopenic at some point during the course of their disease or treatment regimen. The risk of infection has been shown to increase when the number of circulating neutrophils is less than 1000/mm^3, with the risk of infection being directly related to the extent and duration of the neutropenic state.[5] Severe neutropenia, defined as an absolute neutrophil count (ANC) of 500/mm³ or less, is the single most important risk factor predisposing them to infection.[6]

The decreased number of neutrophils that occurs in children with malignancy may be the result of the production of inadequate neutrophils by the bone marrow, as seen in acute leukemias, or the production of abnormal granulocytes that are incapable of participating in phagocytosis. Antineoplastic chemotherapy, radiation therapy, and other pharmacologic interventions used in the treatment of malignancies, such as steroid administration, may contribute to immunosuppression and neutropenia.[6] In addition, the myelosuppression that causes neutropenia typically causes concurrent thrombocytopenia, placing the patient at additional risk for hemorrhage and coagulopathies. Children with neutropenia and thrombocytopenia are at high risk for serious and life-threatening complications. Box 25-1 out-

lines assessment parameters and care considerations for the child in the ICU with neutropenia and thrombocytopenia.

GENERAL COMPLICATIONS OF MALIGNANCY

Infection and Sepsis

Despite progress made in the treatment of children with cancer, complications related to infection remain a leading cause of morbidity and mortality.[6] As more aggressive treatments are used in the treatment of childhood cancer, more children become immunocompromised for a longer period of time and subsequently become more susceptible to infection. In addition to treatment intensity, the type of tumor and the state of the disease also contribute to the

---

Box 25-1
Assessment Parameters and Care Considerations for the Child With Neutropenia and Thrombocytopenia

Assessment Parameters

Vital Signs

- Temperature at least q2h; in febrile patients increase to q1h

Skin

- Assess for breakdown, lesions, pain, and rashes, especially in less visible areas (e.g., skin folds of buttocks, axilla, perineum, perianal area, breasts, and scrotum)
- Assess any incision, wounds, or biopsy sites for drainage, odor, erythema, inflammation, and pain

Neurologic

- Assess for complaints of headache, neck stiffness, orthostatic dizziness, changes in LOC, visual disturbances
- Assess for complaints of sinus pressure, pain, congestion, or drainage

Pulmonary

- Assess respirations and breath sounds for presence, absence, or change in pattern, effort, or rate
- Assess for changes in amount and color of sputum

Genitourinary

- Assess for changes in genitourinary function, e.g., frequency, color, and appearance of urine; dysuria

Gastrointestinal

- Assess bowel function, e.g., consistency, pain, frequency, color, amount
- Assess mouth and throat for presence of stomatitis, ulcers, white patches, dryness, erythema, and dental problems
- Assess mouth and throat for complaints of pain and dysphagia

Vascular Access Devices

- Assess catheter exit, entrance, suture, and tunnel sites for signs of infection (e.g., skin breakdown, erythema, pain, tenderness, discharge, swelling, or warmth)

- Assess for presence of fever (*Reminder:* the clinical signs and symptoms of a normal immune response may be suppressed in severely neutropenic patients or patients receiving steroid therapy; fever may be the only presenting sign of a VAD infection)

Special Care Considerations

- STRICT HANDWASHING
- Monitor CBCs with differential count every day and calculate ANC
- Limit contact with individuals with signs and symptoms of a suspected transmissible illness or disease
- Avoid contact with persons recently immunized with live vaccinations
- Maintain skin integrity and excellent hygiene
- Use lotion to prevent dry, cracking skin, and bathe with only mild, nondrying soap
- Prevent rectal trauma by avoiding rectal temperatures, enemas, suppositories, or digital examinations
- Administer stool softeners as necessary to prevent straining during bowel movements
- Avoid injections whenever possible, because of the risk of abscess formation in the skin
- Avoid use of tampons in adolescent females
- Evaluate potential for CNS infection
- Perform meticulous mouth and skin care using only soft sponge toothbrushes in conjunction with frequent oral rinses, even in the critically ill and intubated child
- Maintain use of strict aseptic technique when performing all invasive procedures or manipulating invasive tubes or catheters
- Avoid patient contact with fresh flowers, soil, potted plants, or contact with stagnant water
- Avoid contact with foods that may introduce pathogens into the GI tract (e.g., raw or undercooked meats, unwashed raw fruits or vegetables, tap or unfiltered water)

frequency and types of infection that occur.[6] The immuno-compromised child presenting to the ICU with infection typically demonstrates clinical manifestations of sepsis or septic shock. Prompt recognition of signs of infection and sepsis, and timely interventions, may significantly decrease the risk of mortality associated with septic shock.

Pathogenesis.   The development of infection in children with cancer may be related to compromise in a variety of host defenses. The nature of the disease and the myelosuppressive action of chemotherapy and radiation therapy result in immune alterations that compromise a child's ability to combat infection. Tumors themselves may predispose children to infection. Primary or metastatic tumors may cause obstruction that promotes infection by the colonizing of organisms at the site of the obstruction. For example, a child with Wilms' tumor may experience an increased incidence of urinary tract infections as a result of urinary obstruction caused by the tumor.[6] The tumor may erode through the body's protective barriers, such as the skin and mucosal surfaces, and permit the entrance of pathogens into the bloodstream. These protective barriers may also be broken by the numerous invasive diagnostic and therapeutic procedures performed on critically ill children with cancer. Venous access devices, biopsies, pressure monitoring devices, respiratory care equipment, and indwelling catheters all provide direct access to the bloodstream for a variety of pathogens.

Defects in cellular or humoral immunity further increase the susceptibility to infection in children with certain malignancies. Children with Hodgkin's disease and non-Hodgkin's lymphoma are known to have impaired T-cell and monocyte function as well as diminished B-cell function. Patients with leukemia may have defective cell-mediated immunity. Children who have undergone splenectomies are found to experience diminished antibody responses, the loss of specific phagocytosis factors, and loss of the spleen's filtering functions. These factors increase the susceptibility to infection with encapsulated organisms. Corticosteroids can alter leukocyte mobilization, diminish cell-mediated immunity, and impair phagocytosis.[6] Chemotherapy and radiation therapy regimens before BMT contribute to impairment of cellular and humoral immunity. The special aspects of infection in the pediatric BMT patient are discussed in the Complications of Bone Marrow Transplantation section of this chapter.

Cancer treatment may contribute to new sources of infection. Stomatitis is a common side effect of certain chemotherapeutic agents, such as methotrexate (MTX), actinomycin-D, adriamycin, and transplant chemotherapy. Under certain conditions, septicemia can develop from stomatitis. Damage that occurs to the gastrointestinal (GI) mucosa from antineoplastic therapy may be the reason that enteric organisms are often isolated in the cancer patient with infection. Rectal fissures may occur and can be a source of fulminant infection, usually by gram-negative bacteria.[3,7,8]

Malnutrition that often occurs in children with malignancies can increase susceptibility to infection by causing impaired phagocytosis, decreased macrophage mobilization,

and depressed lymphocyte function. Broad-spectrum antibiotic therapy, which is often used, can lead to alterations in microbial colonization and overgrowth of resistant organisms present in the critical care environment.[6] In addition, any critically ill child will be at an increased risk for infection from the mere fact of being in a debilitated state and in a critical care environment.[8]

All of these factors put children with cancer at a significant risk for bacterial, fungal, viral, and parasitic infections. Box 25-2 identifies the most common pathogens known to cause infection in neutropenic pediatric patients. Bacterial infections, particularly caused by gram-negative enteric bacilli, are often the most serious acute infections occurring in children with cancer. Gram-positive organisms isolated in serious infections are most likely associated with venous access devices.[6]

Fungal infections are particularly troublesome in children with cancer. The most commonly encountered fungal infections in affected children include those from *Candida* and *Aspergillus* species.[9] *Candida* infections may range from local infections, such as thrush, to widespread dissemination. Mucosal lesions, which often occur as a result of cancer therapy, may provide a portal for *Candida* septicemia. *Aspergillus* is a ubiquitous fungus that aggressively invades the sinuses, lungs, and brain and is extremely

---

Box 25-2
Potential Causative Organisms in the Septic Child With Malignancy

Bacterial Infections

Any gram-negative or gram-positive organism, including:
Escherichia coli
Klebsiella pneumoniae
Pseudomonas aeruginosa
Bacteroides fragilis
Clostridium difficile
Mycobacterium spp.
Nocardia spp.

Viral Infections

Cytomegalovirus
Respiratory syncytial virus
Adenovirus
Herpes simplex virus
Varicella zoster virus

Parasitic Infections

Pneumocystis carinii
Strongyloides stercoralis

Fungal Infections

Candida spp.
Aspergillus spp.

Adapted from Freifeld AG, Walsh TJ, Pizzo PA: Infectious complications in the pediatric cancer patient. In Pizzo PA, Poplack DG, eds: *Principles and practice of pediatric oncology,* ed 3, Philadelphia, 1997, Lippincott-Raven Publishers, pp. 1069-1114.

difficult to eradicate from the body.[9-11] It is often fatal in severely immunocompromised children, such as those who have undergone BMT or those who are severely neutropenic following high-dose chemotherapy. Diagnosis of *Aspergillus* infection is often problematic because of difficulties in culturing the organism.[8]

Viral infections may cause significant morbidity and mortality in children with cancer because they have the potential for rapid dissemination in immunocompromised hosts. In addition, exposure to seasonal viruses, such as respiratory syncytial virus (RSV) and adenovirus, may cause severe upper and lower respiratory tract disease in the immunocompromised patient.[12] The herpes virus group can be responsible for a variety of infections. Herpes simplex infections are usually more severe and prolonged in children with malignancies. Dissemination can occur with mucosal lesions, cellulitis, or pneumonia. Abnormalities in T-cell function and diminished cell-mediated response to varicella zoster can cause fulminant varicella, which may disseminate to the liver, lung, and central nervous system (CNS). In children who have had varicella zoster infection, herpes zoster infection (shingles) can occur as a reactivation of this virus. Children with lymphomas appear to have the greatest risk for development of herpes zoster infection.[6]

The most common cause of viral pneumonia in the immunocompromised host is cytomegalovirus (CMV), especially in those who have undergone BMT. Pneumonitis is the most common clinical consequence of CMV infection in these children. The parainfluenza virus may also cause significant respiratory failure.[6,7] Parasitic infections in children with cancer are most commonly attributed to *Pneumocystis carinii*. This organism is responsible for serious pneumonitis in this population, and if left untreated is usually fatal.[3,6]

Although the pathogenesis of infection and sepsis may be different in the pediatric patient with malignancy, the clinical progression and final common pathway of septic shock is the same for any pediatric patient; hemodynamic instability, circulatory collapse, and intractable lactic acidosis. Chapter 27 provides a detailed account of the pathogenesis, clinical presentation, and clinical management of septic shock.

Clinical Presentation. Because shock may rapidly ensue in these children, and host responses may be subtle, early recognition and prompt treatment of infections are imperative.[6] If infection is undetected and left untreated in a patient with malignancy, especially one who is neutropenic, it may prove to be fatal in a very short course. Detection of infection requires strong clinical judgment and a careful search for signs and symptoms, which are often covert.[8] Fever is the single most consistent indicator of infection, in the neutropenic patient because the lack of an inflammatory response prevents many of the classic signs and symptoms of infection from appearing. In fact, fever may be the only sign of an active infection in the severely neutropenic patient, and may be crucial to diagnosis.[13]

Diagnosis requires thorough physical examination, radiologic and laboratory evaluation (blood counts, electrolyte levels, and coagulation studies), and cultures of any potential source of infection. Surveillance bacterial and fungal culture results of throat, urine, stool, and blood are often routinely monitored twice weekly to allow for early detection of infection. In addition, these same cultures are typically obtained at a maximum of once per day if the child develops a fever. If invasive lines are in place when the child becomes febrile, they are considered potential sources of infection.[6] Routine viral screenings during RSV season are also recommended.

Critical Care Management. The only true treatment for infection, sepsis, and septic shock is the administration of antiinfectious agents, specific to the causative pathogen. However, the inability to obtain blood cultures should never preclude the timely administration of antiinfectious agents. Broad-spectrum coverage begins immediately as soon as sepsis is suspected. Empiric antibacterial therapy, generally using a cephalosporin, aminoglycoside, and extended-spectrum penicillin, is initiated until culture and sensitivity reports are available. When the child has a venous access device, coverage for gram-positive organisms, such as vancomycin, is usually added.[4] Typically, gram-positive coverage will be initiated until culture reports are obtained. Once blood cultures rule out the existence of a gram-positive organism, coverage for such organisms is discontinued because of the increasing development of resistant organisms. There are a variety of antimicrobial agents available for use, and numerous complex antimicrobial regimens have been developed by various institutions for treatment of fever in the neutropenic child. Ultimately, the choice of agents and regimens should be dependent on predominant organisms, sensitivity patterns, and experience of the ordering practitioner.[6]

In children with persistent fever and neutropenia, antifungal treatment should be added. Amphotericin B has typically been the treatment of choice for fungal infections.[9,10] Unfortunately, amphotericin B is associated with serious complications, most notably anaphylaxis and nephrotoxicity.[9] If renal function is impaired, it may be necessary to lower the dose of amphotericin B or administer the drug on alternate days.[9] Fever, chills, and rigors that commonly accompany amphotericin B administration may be minimized by the administration of intravenous diphenhydramine, meperidine, and oral acetaminophen, as needed. When side effects are severe, hydrocortisone may be added to the infusion. The use of new antifungal agents, such as appropriately engineered lipid formulations of amphotericin B, may preserve the antifungal efficacy with fewer adverse effects. One such agent is amphotericin B lipid complex (ABLC). ABLC, while not uniformly efficacious for all fungal infections, has shown great promise in clinical trials and is indicated for use in the treatment of invasive fungal infections in patients who are refractory to or intolerant of traditional amphotericin B therapy.[9]

Viral and parasitic organisms are also suspected, especially in the event of pulmonary infection. For suspected viral infections, ganciclovir in combination with intravenous immunoglobulin (IVIg) or acyclovir may be administered.[6] Acyclovir is often used for the treatment of varicella zoster, herpes simplex, and herpes zoster infections. It is also administered prophylactically to prevent stomatitis in BMT patients who are seropositive for herpes simplex.

Although the use of aerosolized ribavirin has fallen out of favor for the treatment of RSV infection in the general pediatric population, it has been used with some success in several studies of immunocompromised patients presenting with RSV infection.[12,14-17] Proponents of this therapy in the immunocompromised patient advocate early use of ribavirin to prevent the progression of RSV infection to the lower respiratory tract. In addition, the increasing use of RSV-immunoglobulin (RSVIg), both prophylactically in the at-risk patient and in combination with aerosolized ribavirin for infected patients, holds promise in decreasing mortality related to RSV infection.[17] However, despite these encouraging reports, further studies are necessary to determine effective therapy for RSV infection in the BMT patient.

Prophylactic therapy against respiratory viruses, using either respiratory syncytial virus immune globulin intravenous (RSV-IGIV) or palivizumab (an intramuscular monoclonal antibody), has recently been advocated for severely neutropenic patients, such as BMT patients. Although neither medication has been evaluated in randomized trials in immunocompromised children, children with severe immunodeficiencies may benefit from this prophylaxis. The American Academy of Pediatrics recommends that if severely immunocompromised children are receiving standard immune globulin intravenous (IGIV) monthly, physicians may consider substituting RSV-IGIV during the RSV season.[18] RSV-IGIV may also provide prophylaxis against other non-RSV respiratory infections that palivizumab does not.

Parasitic infections are routinely treated with trimethoprim-sulfamethoxazole (TMP-SMX). TMP-SMX may also be given prophylactically in neutropenic patients to prevent the onset of *Pneumocystis carinii* pneumonia (PCP). Pentamidine isethionate is commonly administered prophylactically to prevent PCP in immunodeficient (particularly HIV positive) and immunosuppressed patients.[4,6]

The use of granulocytes in the management of sepsis, although still controversial, is used for the neutropenic child whose white blood cells (WBCs) have been suppressed. Proponents of granulocyte transfusions believe that because the child lacks intrinsic neutrophils to combat infection, administration of granulocytes may provide an extrinsic bridge of WBCs available to fight infection until the patient's own WBCs return. Saarinen and colleagues administered granulocyte transfusions to 10 children suffering from documented life-threatening infections during profound, prolonged neutropenia.[19] They reported prompt and vigorous bone marrow myeloid recovery immediately after granulocyte transfusion in all 10 patients. However promising this mode of therapy may be, further studies are warranted before granulocyte transfusions become part of standard therapy. There are significant complications that have been associated with granulocyte transfusions, namely fever and chills, pulmonary complications such as pneumonitis with the potential for respiratory failure, transmission of blood-borne infections such as CMV, and the induction of alloimmunization, which may jeopar-

dize all future platelet transfusions.[19] In addition, there are case reports of respiratory failure when granulocytes were administered in close proximity to amphotericin B administration. Because there have been no large generalizable clinical studies demonstrating improved outcomes resulting from granulocyte transfusions, and given the risk of respiratory failure, many practitioners continue to avoid granulocyte transfusions. Instead, granulocyte-macrophage colony-stimulating factor (GM-CSF) and granulocyte colony-stimulating factor (G-CSF) have been used as an alternative therapy to accelerate granulocyte recovery. These cytokines, which accelerate hematopoiesis when given following chemotherapy-induced neutropenia, have been shown to reduce the severity and duration of neutropenia for some children.[19]

Should sepsis progress to septic shock, the shock state is managed as for any other patient presenting with sepsis or septic shock. The only caveat to management of the pediatric oncology patient with septic shock is that repeated administration of chemotherapeutic agents, or administration of certain cardiotoxic chemotherapeutic agents, may cause myocardial dysfunction, which in conjunction with sepsis, may decrease the child's tolerance for fluid loading and fluid resuscitation. Fluid management and inotropic support in such cases may need to be augmented and guided via hemodynamic monitoring, including pulmonary artery pressure monitoring.

Pericardial Tamponade

The etiology of pericardial tamponade in children with cancer may be much different than that in other children who present to the ICU with this clinical syndrome. Pericardial tamponade may occur as a direct result of a primary tumor invasion into the pericardium, metastatic invasion (such as with Hodgkin's disease or ALL), infection or severe inflammation, or as a sequelae to radiation therapy, manifesting as either pericardial effusions or constrictive fibrosis. Pericardial effusions may also be seen in children with Wilms' tumor in whom a thrombus may extend into the heart.[3,4]

Pathogenesis. Acute pericardial tamponade is a rare presentation for children with malignancies. More often, chronic accumulation of fluid permits the pericardium to stretch gradually over time and allows it to accommodate large fluid volumes before cardiac tamponade occurs.[3,4]

Clinical Presentation. The classic signs and symptoms of acute pericardial tamponade do not differ from other patient populations presenting with this clinical picture. For a complete discussion of these classic signs and symptoms, as well as pathogenesis and diagnostic techniques, please refer to Chapter 18 (Cardiovascular Critical Care Problems). Clinical presentation in the pediatric oncology patient may be rapid, but more commonly is insidious in onset. Chronic accumulation of fluid may present with more subtle signs and symptoms, such as fatigue, dyspnea, cough, chest pain, abdominal distention, and signs and symptoms of right-sided congestive heart failure. Early recognition of impending tamponade and intervention is important.

Critical Care Management. The management of pericardial tamponade is dictated by the degree of existing circulatory compromise. Emergent care consists of pericardiocentesis, preferably performed via echocardiographic guidance. For those children who are thrombocytopenic or have evidence of other coagulopathies, platelets and fresh frozen plasma may be needed before pericardiocentesis. Pericardiocentesis in children with cancer is not only therapeutic but also allows collection of a specimen for malignancy diagnosis. Depending on the cause of the pericardial tamponade, a "pig-tailed" catheter may be placed after pericardiocentesis to allow for drainage of any reaccumulated pericardial fluid.[4,20] Obviously, placement of such a catheter places the child at great risk for infection and resultant myocarditis. Meticulous care, including use of strict aseptic or sterile technique, for both the catheter and catheter site is provided.

Supportive care includes hydration, oxygen, and positioning to achieve maximum patient comfort. Definitive therapy is directed toward treating the underlying cause. Hematologic malignancies are treated with chemotherapy. Solid tumors are removed or may be diminished by local radiation or sclerosing therapy. In situations in which prolonged palliation is warranted, a pericardial window may be placed. A pericardiectomy may be considered if the above treatments fail, if there is an associated constrictive pericardial disease, or if a pericardial window is not technically feasible.[4]

Acute Respiratory Failure

The development of acute respiratory failure in the child with an oncologic disease commonly requires critical care resources. The inability to ventilate and adequately oxygenate may occur from a variety of infectious and noninfectious insults, including pulmonary opportunistic infections and chemotherapy or radiation therapy-induced pulmonary disorders. Primary pulmonary malignancies are rare in children and do not account for many ICU admissions, with the exception of tracheal compression from a mediastinal mass.[3,6] Pleural effusions and pulmonary infiltrates are two of the more common causes of acute respiratory failure and the need for mechanical ventilation in children with malignancy.

Pleural Effusions. Pleural effusions in the child with cancer may occur for a variety of reasons, including irritation of the pleural membrane by cancer cells, infection, an extension of the tumor itself, or lymphatic or venous obstruction of the pleura by a mediastinal mass. In addition, chylous effusions may occur from obstruction of the lymphatics.[3] Children at risk for pleural effusions include those with leukemia, Hodgkin's disease and non-Hodgkin's lymphoma, sarcomas, neuroblastoma, and Wilms' tumor.[3,6]

Signs and symptoms of a pleural effusion include dyspnea, cough, pleuritic chest pain, tachypnea, and tachycardia. Physical examination may reveal dullness on percussion over the infected area. Diagnosis of a pleural effusion involves techniques similar to those used for pleural effusions from other disease processes. Chest radiographs help confirm the presence of fluid in the pleural space. Pleural fluid can also be examined for the presence of malignant cells or to rule out infection.[6]

Thoracentesis and possibly chest tube placement are indicated to drain the fluid when it is causing respiratory distress, or to make a diagnosis. In addition, sclerotherapy may be necessary to prevent or delay formation of a new effusion.[3] Sclerotherapy employs agents such as tetracycline, talc, or bleomycin to cause adhesions and irritation in the pleural or pericardial spaces. The procedure consists of injecting these agents into the respective spaces, and may be repeated for several days as needed. Ultrasound examination may be helpful to guide the physician to the effusion area, especially when the effusion is loculated. Therapy specific to the disease process should be instituted.

Careful respiratory assessment and monitoring are necessary for the child with a pleural effusion. In addition, the nurse needs to be aware of the procedure and possible side effects of various sclerotherapy techniques. These side effects are dependent on agents used but can include pain, nausea and vomiting, infection, inflammation, hypoxia, pneumothorax, and hemothorax.

Pulmonary Infiltrates. In a nonneutropenic host, respiratory infections may be attributed to the usual causes of community-acquired pneumonia. However, in the child with malignancy who is neutropenic, bacterial pneumonias may be one of the most common causes of pulmonary infiltrates and can cause significant mortality. Gram-negative organisms are the most likely etiologic pathogens; however, viral, fungal, or parasitic organisms should also be considered because they are a common cause of infectious pneumonitis in patients with prolonged neutropenia.[3]

The incidence of protozoal PCP, which was once quite common, has decreased greatly because of the use of prophylactic TMP-SMX, although it still does occur in immunocompromised hosts.[6] Fungal pneumonitis is most commonly diagnosed in a neutropenic host who has received prolonged antibacterial agents without evidence of clinical improvement. *Aspergillus* and *Candida* are the most common causative organisms.[6]

As previously mentioned, pulmonary injury can be attributed to a variety of chemotherapeutic agents (Box 25-3) and radiation therapy. Lung damage from chemotherapeutic agents is often difficult to detect because such damage is usually insidious in onset and is caused by the presence of other sources of pulmonary injury such as infection,

Box 25-3
Chemotherapeutic Agents Associated With Pulmonary Injury

Adriamycin
Bleomycin
Busulfan
Cyclophosphamide
Cytosine arabinoside
Methotrexate

radiation, or metastatic lung disease, which can complicate diagnosis. Some chemotherapy agents may cause dose-dependent pulmonary changes, whereas others, such as MTX, may actually cause an inflammatory-type hypersensitivity reaction. Drug-associated lung injury appears histologically as diffuse alveolar damage.[21] Radiation to the lung fields can cause an acute inflammatory response of the lung tissue (Fig. 25-1). Radiation damage to the lungs is related to the total dose received, the dose rate, and the volume of lung tissue irradiated. The more radiation that is administered to the lung fields, the greater the damage.[21]

Clinical manifestations of acute respiratory failure resulting from pulmonary infiltrates include fever, cough (usually dry and hacking), rales, dyspnea, hypoxia, cyanosis, and tachypnea. The chest radiograph typically demonstrates a diffuse infiltrative pattern[3,4,8] (Fig. 25-2).

Differential diagnosis of respiratory dysfunction in the child with cancer can be difficult and often requires invasive techniques. Diagnostic testing includes cultures, serology, radiologic studies including x-ray and chest computerized tomography (CT) scans, arterial blood gas analysis, and ventilatory function tests. Bronchoalveolar lavage (BAL) may be used to obtain samples for testing and isolate the causative organism. If this is unsuccessful, an open lung biopsy may be necessary to differentiate infectious and noninfectious causes.[6]

Management of the child with cancer in acute respiratory failure focuses on the support of respiratory and circulatory function, minimizing the risk of pulmonary edema, and aggressively identifying and treating infectious processes. Broad-spectrum antibiotics are started immediately in the child who develops fever and pulmonary symptoms. These are instituted even before receiving results of diagnostic testing because rapid progression to an overwhelming pneumonia and sepsis can occur.[6]

Supplemental oxygen is an essential aspect of therapy. The amount of oxygen that is required can be determined by usual methods of arterial blood gas monitoring and pulse oximetry. The child with cancer has the potential for enhanced oxygen toxicity as a consequence of previous chemotherapy or radiation therapy, and thus is maintained on the lowest amount of oxygen that results in sufficient oxygenation.[7,8]

Most children with malignancy have limited energy reserves resulting from disease progression, malnutrition, and the toxic effects of chemotherapy and radiation therapy. Any stress to the body places them at risk for sudden deterioration in pulmonary function and respiratory failure, necessitating the use of mechanical ventilation. The indications for mechanical ventilation in the child with malignancy are similar to those for any child suffering from respiratory failure (see Chapter 19 for a complete discussion of respiratory failure). There are, however, some unique problems to consider in the population with cancer if intubation is required.

The trauma of intubation may cause upper airway bleeding in the child with malignancy because of thrombocytopenia, coagulation abnormalities, or mucositis that already exists. Platelets, fresh frozen plasma, or vitamin K may be necessary before intubation to minimize the risk of bleeding.[8] If intubation needs to be performed as an emergency, the oral route is preferred to the nasal route to diminish the risk of serious bleeding. Intubation can also increase the risk of infection in the immunosuppressed patient population.[3] An increased awareness of the need for strict aseptic technique when performing an invasive procedure, such as suctioning, is necessary for the immunocompromised child. Tracheal aspirate cultures are obtained at least twice weekly, and as needed if any changes in the color, odor, or amount of secretions are detected.

Once the child has an artificial airway in place, positive end-expiratory pressure (PEEP) is used at a level high enough to maintain the oxygen concentration at 40% to 50% or less to minimize the risk of toxicity.[7,8] High airway

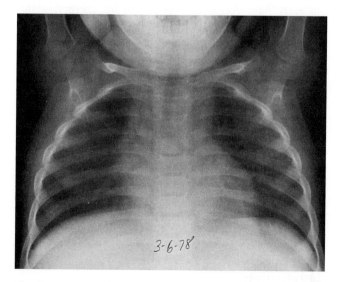

Fig. 25-1 Bilateral peritracheal and parahilar infiltrates resulting from radiation pneumonitis.

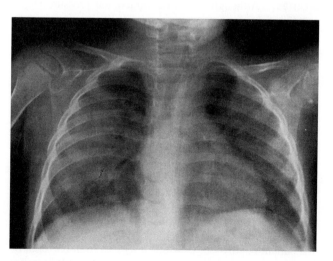

Fig. 25-2 Bilateral diffuse peripheral infiltrates in a 2-year-old boy with lymphoma proven to be PCP, which is sparing the central portions of the lung that are involved with radiation fibrosis.

pressures and rapid ventilatory rates, although not preferred, may be necessary to maintain adequate gas exchange. In such cases, it is imperative that the child be adequately sedated in order to optimize oxygenation and ventilation.[8] If the child with acute respiratory failure is still receiving potentially toxic chemotherapy or radiation therapy, these treatments may need to be discontinued or modified to prevent further lung damage.[21] High-dose corticosteroids may also be added to the treatment regimen to decrease lung inflammation.

Neurologic Complications

Seizures.   As with many oncologic emergencies, seizures may occur in the child with malignant disease for a variety of reasons, including tumor involvement, metastatic disease, or as sequelae of either drug therapy or disease progression. Astrocytomas, ependymomas, and malignant gliomas may occur in the central hemisphere and create seizures.[4] Lymphomas, retinoblastomas, and rhabdomyosarcomas may metastasize and lead to seizures.[4,7,8] Chemotherapeutic agents, such as intrathecal MTX, L-asparaginase, and vincristine, may actually induce seizure activity. Metabolic abnormalities associated with organ dysfunction, such as hypocalcemia, hypoglycemia, hyponatremia, and uremia, may also cause seizures.[3] And finally, neutropenia and thrombocytopenia may place the child at risk for CNS infections, such as meningitis or brain abscesses, or intracerebral hemorrhage.

Regardless of the cause, seizures in the child with malignant disease should be treated the same as seizures in any other child. Maintenance of airway patency and adequate ventilation should be the priority because most seizures are self-limiting. However, progression to status epilepticus warrants emergent intervention and management in the critical care environment. See Chapter 20 for management of seizures and status epilepticus in the pediatric patient.

Increased Intracranial Pressure/Herniation Syndromes.   Although increased intracranial pressure (ICP) and the risk of cerebral herniation is concerning in any pediatric patient, it is of particular concern in the patient with malignancy. The reader is referred to Chapters 10 and 20 for detailed discussion of the pathophysiology, clinical manifestations and current management of increased ICP and herniation syndromes in children. However, it is important to note that the causes of increased ICP may be different in the pediatric oncology patient, and the onset may be either rapid or insidious.

Obviously, the child with a space-occupying lesion in the brain is at risk for developing increased ICP. However, children with any malignancy are at risk for increased ICP because of the effects of either acquired or induced neutropenia and/or thrombocytopenia.[3,4] CNS infections, with resultant cerebral edema, may lead to increased ICP in this patient population. Cerebral abscesses from bacterial or fungal sources are common causes of increased ICP in the neutropenic patient. However, perhaps the most devastating cause of increased ICP is intracerebral hemorrhage caused by thrombocytopenia (Fig. 25-3). Massive bleeding into the

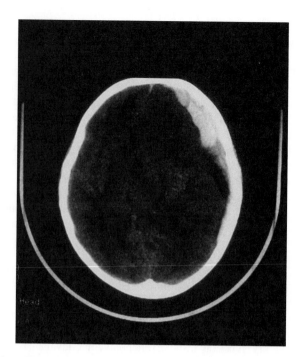

Fig. 25-3 Intracerebral hemorrhage in a 12-year-old female, approximately 100 days after BMT for CML.

cranial vault may lead to rapid onset of intracerebral herniation and brain death.

Symptoms of increased ICP and herniation syndrome are no different in the pediatric oncology population than in the general PICU population. However, there are subtle changes in clinical presentation in the neutropenic and thrombocytopenic patient. Any subtle changes in level of consciousness or complaints of headache, nausea, or vomiting are thoroughly investigated to rule out intracranial pathology.[22] This is particularly challenging in the patient with malignancy because many therapies for malignancy routinely cause sedation, nausea, and vomiting. Astute recognition and early intervention are paramount for preventing the catastrophic sequelae of increased ICP in these patients.

Definitive treatment is aimed at treating the underlying cause of the increased ICP. Emergent surgical intervention to debulk or remove space-occupying lesions or evacuate intracerebral bleeds may be necessary, although these patients are high surgical risks and there is a significantly increased morbidity and mortality associated with surgical intervention.[4,22] CNS infections are treated with anti-infection therapy, and at times, emergent whole brain irradiation may be necessary to reduce a rapidly growing intracranial tumor. If bleeding is suspected, platelet or fresh frozen plasma administration may be warranted. The use of ICP monitoring devices is very controversial because of the increased risk of bleeding and infection in neutropenic and thrombocytopenic patients.

Hemorrhage

Hemorrhage in the pediatric patient with malignancy is most often the result of thrombocytopenia, coagulopathies, or a combination of both. Although the precipitating factors for

TABLE 25-1   Indications for Platelet Transfusion Support in Children with Cancer

In the Presence of Significant Hemorrhage*	In the Absence of Significant Hemorrhage
Thrombocytopenia of any severity (usually significant hemorrhage does not occur if the platelet count is >20,000/mm³ unless other factors are present, i.e., infection, local anatomic lesion)	Before major surgical procedure if platelet count is <50,000/mm³
Suspected platelet count dysfunction (e.g., aspirin) irrespective of platelet count (a rare occurrence in today's practice)	Before lumbar puncture or minor surgical procedure if platelet count is <20,000/mm³ In febrile patient with platelet count <20,000/mm³, especially in a child with ANLL or who is extremely ill Platelet count <5,000/mm³ with little likelihood of imminent (1-2 days) rise

From Buchanan GR: Hematologic supportive care of the pediatric cancer patient. In Pizzo PA, Poplack DG, eds: *Principles and practice of pediatric oncology,* ed 3, Philadelphia, 1997, Lippincott-Raven.
*Significant hemorrhage is defined as recurrent or severe epistaxis, gingival bleeding, extensive buccal blood blisters, gross GI hemorrhage (not just occult blood in stool), retinal bleeding, extensive new cutaneous bleeding, suspected or proven internal hemorrhage. Bruises and scattered petechiae are *not* considered clinically significant hemorrhage.

hemorrhage in this patient population may be somewhat unique to the patient with malignancy, the final common pathway is similar to any pediatric patient with disruption of normal hematopoiesis and hemostasis. Thrombocytopenia is one of the most common bleeding problems for patients with malignancies. Bleeding may be easily managed or may constitute a life-threatening emergency with catastrophic insults to organ systems and the potential for circulatory collapse.

Pathogenesis.   Thrombocytopenia, defined as a platelet count less than 175,000/mm³, occurs as a result of tumor involvement of the bone marrow, myelosuppression from chemotherapy or radiation therapy, increased platelet destruction, or hypersplenism.[23] Coagulopathies, such as disseminated intravascular coagulation, may occur as a result of chemotherapy, vitamin K-dependent factor deficiency, liver insult or failure, or a variety of other causes. See Chapter 24 for a complete discussion of both normal and abnormal hematopoiesis and hemostasis.

Clinical Presentation.   The clinical presentation of hemorrhage in the pediatric patient with malignancy is essentially no different than in any other child with acute bleeding and/or coagulopathies. Signs may be overt, such as severe epistaxis or frank blood from a nasogastric tube, or may be subtler, such as an increasing abdominal girth or changes in level of consciousness. The critical care nurse identifies patients at risk through close monitoring of laboratory data and is alert to any changes in clinical presentation that may signify bleeding to prevent loss of circulating blood volume that would predispose the child to circulatory collapse.

Critical Care Management.   Care of the thrombocytopenic patient is augmented to prevent breaks in skin integrity or increased risk of spontaneous bleeding. Administering platelet transfusions to maintain a platelet count above 20,000/mm³ seems to be an accepted practice for pediatric patients. Table 25-1 provides guidelines for platelet transfusion in the pediatric oncology patient. However, despite these guidelines, indications for platelet transfusions remain a subject of great debate in the pediatric

literature. Because most instances of intracranial hemorrhage seem to occur with platelet counts lower than 5000/mm³, proponents of prophylactic platelet transfusions believe that maintaining a platelet count of greater than 20,000/mm³ provides a degree of protection against catastrophic events.[23] Opponents, on the other hand, advocate that transfusions are reserved for children with platelet counts either below 5000/mm³ or between 5000 and 20,000/mm³ who present with warning signs, such as sudden increases in cutaneous bleeding, oral blood blisters, or retinal hemorrhage.[23]

Typhlitis

Children with malignancy may develop an acute abdomen for much the same reasons as children without malignancy. However, in the majority of cases, acute abdomen in these children is directly related to the underlying malignant disease. Immunodeficient states put these children at the unique risk of developing esophagitis, gastric hemorrhage, perirectal abscess, hemorrhagic pancreatitis, or acute hepatic enlargement from tumor.[3,8] Other causes of GI complications include complications of therapy, such as chemotherapy-induced ileus, and direct or indirect effects of tumor mass, such as obstruction by a tumor or metastatic involvement of the GI tract. One of the most worrisome abdominal processes unique to the immunodeficient host is typhlitis.

Pathogenesis.   Typhlitis is a necrotizing colitis in the cecum that typically occurs after administration of chemotherapeutic agents or disease-induced neutropenia. Although it is most often associated with treatment for leukemias, typhlitis may occur in any neutropenic patient. The pathophysiology appears to be multifactorial, involving loss of bowel wall integrity, invasion of the cecal mucosa by bacteria (most commonly *Clostridium septicum* or gram-negative bacteria such as *Pseudomonas aeruginosa*), and decreased host immune defenses. This sequence of events leads to bacteremia, and bowel wall inflammation, progressing to necrosis, full-thickness infarction, hemorrhage, and potential perforation.[3,24,25]

TABLE 25-2   Causes of Acute Renal Impairment in the Child With Malignancies

Primary Causes	Secondary Causes
1. Renal tumor	1. Chemotherapeutic/supportive agents
2. Malignant infiltration	Cyclosporine A
3. Postrenal obstruction	Cisplatin
4. Renal vessel obstruction	Methotrexate
5. Tumor Lysis Syndrome	Amphotericin B
6. Paraneoplastic syndrome	Ifosfamide
7. Hypertension	2. Radiation therapy

From Rossi R, Kleta R, Ehrich JHH: Renal involvement in children with malignancies, *Pediatr Nephrol* 13:153, 1999.

Clinical Presentation. Right lower quadrant pain is typically the first presenting symptom of typhlitis. For this reason, typhlitis is suspected in all children with malignancy who present with such pain. Fever may or may not be present. Other signs and symptoms include nausea, vomiting, or watery or bloody diarrhea. Blood cultures may be helpful in identifying causative organisms and directing therapy. However, diagnosis is typically based on physical examination and imaging studies, with computed tomography and ultrasonography providing the most sensitive identification of typhlitis.[25,26]

Critical Care Management. Treatment of typhlitis is centered around medical management with the administration of broad-spectrum antiinfective agents.[24,26] Surgical intervention is controversial, with mortality rates ranging from 20% to 100%.[3] Because of the potential increase in mortality, specific criteria for surgical intervention have been recommended (Box 25-4). If left untreated, typhlitis will progress to overwhelming sepsis and death.

COMPLICATIONS OF SOLID TUMORS

Acute Tumor Lysis Syndrome

Although renal failure in the child with malignant disease may result from a variety of primary and secondary causes (Table 25-2), one of the most dramatic causes of renal failure is acute tumor lysis syndrome (ATLS). ATLS results directly from malignant cell degradation and the inadequate ability of the kidneys to excrete the large quantities of uric acid, phosphorus, and potassium released during cell lysis. The syndrome, consisting of a metabolic triad of hyperuricemia, hyperkalemia, and hyperphosphatemia, is most commonly associated with the presence of rapidly proliferating tumors, such as Burkitt's lymphoma and T-cell leukemia/lymphoma.[27,28] Patients most at risk for developing ATLS are those who present with bulky abdominal tumors (such as with Burkitt's lymphoma), elevated serum uric acid and lactic dehydrogenase levels before treatment, and oliguria.

Serum uric acid levels may be elevated because of obstructive uropathy, whereas lactic dehydrogenase levels may be elevated because of decreased venous return resulting from compression by the tumor mass.[22,29] Oliguria before treatment is most often caused by tumor obstruction.

Pathogenesis. ATLS may occur either before therapy, as a result of spontaneous cell lysis, or it may occur 1 to 5 days after initiation of specific cytotoxic chemotherapy.[8,27] Chemotherapy administration causes a profound lysis of malignant cells in tumors with high growth fractions, such as Burkitt's lymphoma, which has a doubling time of anywhere from 38 to 116 hours.[3] Cell lysis causes a rapid release of the intracellular components uric acid, phosphorus, and potassium, all of which are normally excreted by the kidney. Elevated uric acid, or hyperuricemia, results from the breakdown of nucleic acids from the cells and the resultant release of purines. Uric acid, which may also be promoted by lactic acidosis secondary to poor tissue oxygenation in patients with high leukocyte counts, precipitates in the collecting ducts and renal tubules, leading to decreased renal clearance.[3,7]

Hyperphosphatemia occurs as a result of the release of phosphates during tumor cells lysis. Lymphoblasts have up to four times the phosphate content of normal lymphocytes.[3,22] Hyperphosphatemia causes both precipitation of calcium phosphate salts (which precipitate in the renal tubules), and a resultant hypocalcemia. These huge quantities of intracellular metabolites released during cell lysis, in addition to the precipitation of both uric acid and calcium-phosphate salts in the renal system, overwhelm the ability of the kidneys to clear them, leading to acute renal failure.[4,7]

The third part of the metabolic triad, hyperkalemia, occurs because of the release of potassium from the cells during tumor lysis and is accentuated by the onset of renal failure and the presence of acidosis.[22] Hyperkalemia is an ominous sign, placing the child at risk for life-threatening ventricular dysrhythmias and possibly cardiac arrest.

Clinical Presentation. Early recognition of the metabolic abnormalities and renal failure associated with ATLS

TABLE 25-3   Clinical Manifestations of Acute Tumor Lysis Syndrome

Hyperuricemia	Hyperphosphatemia	Hypocalcemia (resultant)	Hyperkalemia
Lethargy	Pruritic tissue changes	Anorexia	Muscles weakness
Nausea	Inflammation of the eyes and joints	Vomiting	Paresthesia
Vomiting		Cramps	Nausea
Renal colic		Tetany	Diarrhea
Flank pain		Altered level of consciousness	Abdominal cramps
Hematuria		Neuromuscular irritability	Acidosis
Oliguria		Seizures	Asystole
Azotemia		Lethargy	Elevated T waves
		Numbness	Prolonged PR intervals
		Tingling of the extremities	Depressed ST segments
		Prolonged QT intervals	Widened QRS

---

is crucial to preventing possible life-threatening complications. Clinical manifestations reflect these metabolic abnormalities and are outlined in Table 25-3.

Diagnostic evaluation begins with laboratory analysis, including a CBC with differential to monitor the leukocyte count, serum chemistries (including sodium, potassium, chloride, bicarbonate, calcium, phosphorus, uric acid, blood urea nitrogen, and creatinine), and urinalysis. An ultrasound of the abdomen and retroperitoneum is performed immediately if abdominal mass lesions or renal failure are present.[3,4] Continuous ECG monitoring of children with ATLS will signal widened QRS complexes or peaked T waves characteristic of hyperkalemia. However, in the presence of high leukocyte counts, serum potassium levels may be falsely elevated because of spontaneous lysis of leukocytes, platelets, and erythrocytes. This pseudohyperkalemia differs from true hyperkalemia in that there are no ECG changes, and actual potassium concentrations may be determined from plasma analysis rather than serum.[3]

Critical Care Management. The key to management of patients at risk for ATLS is prevention and early identification of those who are most at risk for its development. Children with identified risk factors for renal failure resulting from ATLS may be admitted to the ICU for early intervention, either before or after initiation of chemotherapy.

Prevention of renal failure in children with normal urine output, regardless of serum uric acid levels, involves hydration, alkalinization, and allopurinol administration.[3,27] Hydration is achieved with the administration of crystalloids (normal saline or D5W.45NS) at two to four times that of maintenance fluid, roughly 3000 ml/m²/day. Such aggressive fluid replacement serves to maintain hydration as well as enhance renal excretion of uric acid and phosphates.

Sodium bicarbonate is added to maintenance fluids to increase urine pH and limit or prevent the formation of uric acid crystals in the collecting ducts that normally would occur in an acidic environment. Alkalinization is adequately achieved when urine pH is between 7.0 and 7.5, and is discontinued when uric acid levels are normalized, usually within 24 hours of starting therapy.[3,27] If levels have not normalized within this timeframe, bicarbonate administra-

tion may continue, but only until chemotherapy is started to prevent the phosphates released during tumor lysis from precipitating as calcium phosphate salts in the kidneys.[4,7] Over-alkalinization to a urine pH greater than 7.5 may aggravate symptoms of hypercalcemia by shifting ionized calcium to its non-ionized form.[22] Because of the increased risk of hyperkalemia, potassium is not added to the hydration fluid. Diuretics may be administered to maintain a urine output of at least 1 ml/kg/hour.

Allopurinol is administered to decrease uric acid production. It accomplishes this by inhibiting the enzyme xanthine oxidase, which is responsible for the formation of uric acid from the purine breakdown products hypoxanthine and xanthine.[3,30] However, because allopurinol is excreted solely by the kidneys, doses are decreased if renal failure develops. Hyperphosphatemia may be prevented by the oral administration of binding resins such as aluminum hydroxide, which enhances phosphate excretion in the stool. Calcium supplements are used with caution because an increase in serum calcium while the patient is hyperphosphatemic may accelerate calcium-phosphorus precipitation.[3,22]

For children presenting with oliguric renal failure and increased serum uric acid levels, management is centered on treatment of acute renal failure. Renal obstruction is ruled out before initiating therapy. Once obstruction is ruled out, and the child's volume status is determined, definitive treatment may begin with the initiation of renal replacement therapy (RRT). Choice of RRT will be dependent on the child's hemodynamic stability and the severity of metabolic abnormalities.[4,8,27]

Immediate intervention for hyperkalemia is necessary if serum potassium levels are greater than 6.5 mEq/L or characteristic ECG changes occur. Chapter 11 outlines the appropriate management of hyperkalemia. Emergent dialysis may be necessary in situations in which hyperkalemia and renal failure cannot be managed with the measures described. It may also be used in cases when neurologic symptoms develop.[3,4,7] Regardless of the presence of renal failure, certain interventions are important for the management of any child with ATLS. Hemodynamic monitoring, including arterial and central venous pressure monitoring is necessary to guide and monitor fluid therapy. In the presence of renal failure and/or cardiopulmonary dysfunction, placement of a pulmonary artery catheter may be useful in monitoring fluid balance for complications of aggressive hydration, such as congestive heart failure or pulmonary edema.[4] Additional nursing interventions are similar to those for critically ill children who are experiencing acute renal failure from any cause. Attentive monitoring includes hourly urine outputs, urine pH and urine specific gravity with each void, and frequent electrolyte levels (at least every 4 hours for the first 24 hours, and then every 6 to 8 hours). Because ATLS often occurs in the presence of a high leukocyte count, some practitioners have advocated the use of leukopheresis, exchange transfusions, or low-dose steroids as treatment modalities to reduce the consequences of massive tumor lysis. However, these modalities have not been subject to any controlled analysis and are therefore not recommended as standard therapy.[3]

Superior Vena Cava Syndrome/Superior Mediastinal Syndrome

The presence of thoracic tumors may pose a variety of severe complications in the child with malignancy. Most commonly, these complications are related to the presence of anterior mediastinal masses. Anterior mediastinal masses occur most commonly in children with metastatic diseases, such as Hodgkin's disease and non-Hodgkin's lymphomas.[22] Other related malignancies include acute T-cell lymphoblastic leukemia, mediastinal granulomas, neuroblastoma, rhabdomyosarcoma, and Ewing's sarcoma.[3,7]

Pathogenesis.   Two distinct clinical syndromes have been associated with the presence of anterior mediastinal masses: superior vena cava syndrome (SVCS) and superior mediastinal syndrome (SMS). SVCS develops because of either extrinsic compression of the superior vena cava (SVC) by tumor invasion into surrounding anatomic structures, or by intrinsic obstruction of the SVC from tumor or thrombotic complications of venous access devices.[4,22] True SVCS without tracheal compression is a relatively rare condition in children, occurring in approximately 12% of children with malignant anterior mediastinal tumors at presentation[3] (Fig. 25-4). More often, anterior mediastinal tumor masses cause not only compression of the SVC, but concomitant compression of the trachea or mainstem bronchus and life-threatening airway obstruction. This combination of SVCS and airway obstruction is termed *superior mediastinal syndrome.*[3]

Both the SVC and pediatric airway are very susceptible to obstruction and do not resist extrinsic mechanical compression. The SVC is a thin-walled, potentially collapsible vessel with a relatively low intraluminal pressure that is located within a tight compartment formed by the mediastinum and sternum. The location of the lymph nodes, which surround the SVC, and the thymus may also cause compression of the vena cava when involved with tumor or infection.[3,4,22] Similarly, the pediatric airway is small and compliant, making it highly vulnerable to collapse if compressed by a mediastinal mass. In addition, certain nonneoplastic states, such as infection or bleeding into the retropharyngeal space, may lead to tracheal compression or obstruction.[3,8]

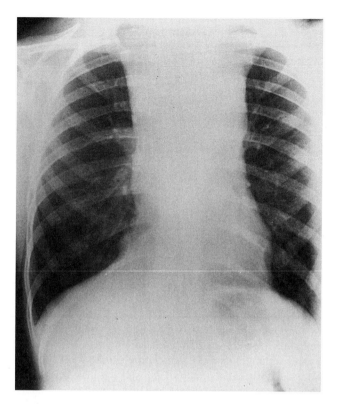

Fig. 25-4   Superior mediastinal mass with SVCS in a child with lymphosarcoma.

Because of the close proximity of the SVC to the trachea and other airway structures, the potential for SVCS or SMS should be considered in all children presenting with anterior mediastinal masses until proven otherwise. In SVCS, both compression and obstruction of the SVC decrease venous return from the head, neck, and upper thorax. The decrease in venous return leads to a decrease in ventricular volume and filling pressures, which in turn leads to a decrease in ventricular output, creating a cycle of cardiac compromise and shock.[4,7] However, the onset of pronounced cardiac compromise and shock may be varied in the pediatric oncology patient. Similarly, compression of the pediatric airway leads to inadequate oxygenation and ventilation, progressing from respiratory distress to complete respiratory failure.

SVCS or SMS resulting from rapidly growing tumors may demonstrate a rapid onset of signs and symptoms. Yet, if the obstruction has occurred over time, such as with a slow accumulation of blood around the SVC or compression or invasion by a slow-growing tumor, collateral blood flow may have developed to allow for some degree of venous return. The child may be able to compensate for some time with collateral blood flow, yet eventually this flow will prove ineffective and the child will exhibit more pronounced symptoms of SVCS.[3] Inadequate venous drainage from the head and the development of cerebral edema may cause seizures and increased ICP.[3,4,7]

Clinical Presentation.   Clinical manifestations of SVCS and SMS are dependent on both the degree and duration of obstruction. If the compression has increased slowly over time, signs and symptoms of these syndromes may be more subtle and difficult to attribute to an exact cause. Presenting signs and symptoms may be tachypnea, wheezing, cough, and stridor. Acutely, a child may present with fever, cough, and mild shortness of breath, progressing to signs and symptoms of respiratory distress. Additional clinical manifestations for both rapid or insidious onset include hoarseness, dyspnea, chest pain, diaphoresis, jugular venous distension, upper extremity edema, conjunctival edema, and plethora and cyanosis of the face, neck, and upper extremities.[3,7,22] Fullness may be noted in the brachial veins if the right arm is raised above the chest and evidence of collateral venous circulation on the chest and abdomen may also be present when SVCS develops over time.

Critical Care Management. SVCS and SMS are potentially life-threatening emergencies that require prompt diagnosis and recognition of signs and symptoms. In emergent cases, diagnosis of SVCS or SMS is possible through the history and physical examination, with confirmation via chest radiograph. If time allows, a CT scan or magnetic resonance imaging (MRI) scan of the chest and/or echocardiographic imaging assists in determining both the location and extent of the tumor, as well as the degree of obstruction. In addition, venograms may be useful if SVCS is thought to be caused by a suspected thrombus within a central catheter.[3,4,22]

A CBC yields helpful information and is the least invasive means of determining whether or not a leukemia-lymphoma syndrome exists. Diagnosis is attempted by the least invasive means possible. A histopathologic diagnosis via bone marrow biopsy or tumor biopsy is obtained as soon as possible to initiate definitive treatment. However, in an emergent situation in which airway compromise or cardiovascular instability may be present or impending, the risk-versus-benefit ratio is assessed before performing such procedures.

Initial management is centered on maintaining airway patency and cardiovascular stability. The aggressiveness of initial management is dependent on the child's presenting clinical condition. The child is positioned in a semi-Fowler position to improve gas exchange with supplemental oxygen administered as needed.[7] However, intubation and mechanical ventilation may be required to protect the airway against potential or actual obstruction until the tumor bulk decreases. Children with SVCS or SMS are at a much higher risk for complications, including death, during intubation. They may suffer respiratory and/or cardiac arrest when placed in a supine position for sedation and/or anesthesia caused by further impedance of venous return and airflow.[3,7,22]

Neuromuscular blockade agents are avoided during intubation of the child with actual or potential airway obstruction, because the child will be unable to breathe spontaneously should the practitioner not be able to pass the endotracheal tube past the level of obstruction. In addition, general anesthesia causes an increase in abdominal muscle tone, a decrease in respiratory muscle tone, diminished lung volumes and bronchial smooth muscle relaxation, and absent caudal movement of the diaphragm. These changes may exacerbate the effects of extrinsic compression of the vena cava and airway.[3] General anesthesia is avoided

whenever possible, and reserved for use with difficult intubations.[3,8] Halothane is the preferred inhalational anesthetic agent for intubation of a child with a mediastinal mass and severe airway obstruction.[8] Furthermore, in cases of critical airway obstruction, elective or emergent intubation is best achieved via fiberoptic bronchoscopy because the bronchoscope may more easily be guided past the level of obstruction, with the endotracheal or nasotracheal tube being inserted over the bronchoscope.

Radiation therapy and chemotherapy tailored to the histopathologic reports are the primary and preferred modes of treatment. However, in emergent situations involving airway compromise, empiric radiation therapy and/or chemotherapy may be instituted.[3,22] In addition, surgical removal or debulking of the tumor mass may be warranted. Steroids may be given for cytoreduction of the tumor and to reduce inflammation caused by tumor invasion or compression, providing symptomatic relief.[7,22] Thrombolytic therapy is instituted in those situations when SVCS is associated with intracaval thrombosis. Lange and colleagues describe success with infusion of urokinase at 200 mg/kg/hour.[3]

Frequent and careful assessment of cardiopulmonary function is key to the management of the child with SVCS or SMS. In addition, because of the risk of cerebral edema and neurologic compromise, frequent neurologic assessment, including pupil size and reactivity, and level of consciousness are performed. If swelling of the upper extremities exists, the upper extremities are elevated to promote venous return and the lower extremities are used for venous access and blood pressure measurements. Diuretics, if ordered to reduce edema, are administered with caution to prevent dehydration and further decrease in blood flow and cardiac output.

Spinal Cord Compression

Spinal cord compression (SCC), while typically not life-threatening to most patients, causes severe neurologic morbidity. Prolonged cord compression may cause irreversible paralysis, sensory loss, and sphincter incompetence.[22] Primary spinal cord tumors are rare in children. More often, SCC is due to extrinsic tumor or metastatic tumor involvement that erodes the spinal column. Occasionally, the development of a spinal dural bleed related to lumbar puncture in a thrombocytopenic patient may cause signs of compression.[3,8] Lange and associates report that 4% of children with cancer develop spinal cord dysfunction, usually related to tumor compression.[3]

Pathogenesis. Most SCC in children with cancer is due to epidural compression from extension of paravertebral tumor through the intervertebral foramina[22] (Fig. 25-5). Metastatic spread to the cord parenchyma, as well as secondary edema and ischemia, may also injure the spinal cord. Metastatic spinal cord disease in children is most commonly associated with sarcomas; however, neuroblastomas, lymphomas, leukemias, Wilms' tumor, or primary tumors of the CNS have also been implicated.[3,4,8] Although most SCC occurs during the terminal metastatic phase of disease, it may be a presenting symptom in neuroblastomas or lymphomas.

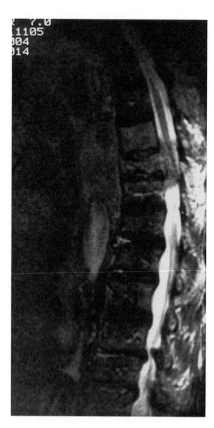

Fig. 25-5   Metastatic tumor at T9 with epidural disease and SCC.

Clinical Presentation.   Signs and symptoms of SCC are dependent on tumor location and the age of the child. Back pain, both localized and radicular in nature, is seen in up to 80% of children with SCC and may be exaggerated by activities such as coughing and sneezing, straining, flexion of the back, and leg raising.[4,22] Motor weakness is common, yet rarely a presenting symptom. Sensory deficits are seen less often, or when present are difficult to document, especially in young children.[22] When present, sensory losses typically manifest as numbness, tingling, and loss of sensation. Identification of the level of sensory loss may help determine the extent of spinal cord involvement. Changes in bowel or bladder habits may also indicate spinal cord involvement, typically below the level of the second lumbar vertebrae.[4]

Critical Care Management.   Any child with neoplastic disease and complaints of back pain is presumed to have SCC until proven otherwise. Diagnostic evaluation includes obtaining spine radiographs, although fewer than half of children with SCC present with abnormal films. Although lumbar myelography was the most useful diagnostic tool for SCC, MRI is now the diagnostic study of choice for determining tumor location and the degree of cord block.[22]

Children presenting with back pain and neurologic deficits or a history of progressive spinal cord dysfunction receive an immediate intravenous bolus of dexamethasone at a dose of 1 to 2 mg/kg, followed by emergent MRI study. If there are no signs of neurologic deficit, nor signs of progression of mild deficits, a lower dose of corticosteroids is administered, followed by MRI study within 24 hours.[3,4,22] If the SCC is thought to be epidural in origin, the spinal cord is decompressed immediately. Decompression may be achieved via administration of high-dose dexamethasone, followed by emergent radiation therapy or surgical decompression. Although there are no studies to support one therapy over the other, both radiation therapy and surgical intervention have unique benefits. Some tumors, such as lymphomas and neuroblastomas, are particularly radioresponsive, providing a less invasive mode of treatment. On the other hand, surgical decompression may be useful in identification of tumor histology.[3,4] Once tumor histology is identified, the administration of tumor-specific chemotherapy may be of benefit.

Initial care of the child with SCC is centered on relief of the compression by the methods discussed above. In addition, adequate pain assessment and management is necessary because SCC may be very painful. Once spinal cord decompression is achieved, patient management is similar to the care of any child with spinal cord injury. Chapter 28 provides complete information on the unique care needs of the child with spinal cord injury. The prognosis for children with SCC typically reflects the level of involvement at the time treatment is initiated. Patients who are ambulatory upon presentation usually remain ambulatory. However, although most adults who present nonambulatory rarely regain function, more than half of children presenting nonambulatory regain the ability to walk after emergent intervention.[3,22]

COMPLICATIONS OF LEUKEMIC DISEASE

Childhood leukemias may be classified as either acute or chronic malignancies, and are thought to be due to the malignant transformation of a single abnormal progenitor cell with the ability to expand by indefinite self-renewal.[31] The causes of this transformation are highly complex, multifactorial, and are not yet fully understood. There are both different types and subtypes of acute and chronic leukemias, which are thought to occur as the malignant transformation occurs at various points along the myeloid or lymphoid stem cell lineages.

Hyperleukocytosis

Hyperleukocytosis is defined as a peripheral WBC count exceeding 100,000/mm^3.[3] The high numbers of circulating blasts cause capillary obstruction, microinfarction, and organ dysfunction. Leukocyte counts greater than 300,000/mm^3 are associated with a high risk of morbidity and mortality. Hyperleukocytosis is most often associated with the myeloid leukemias, as compared with the lymphoid leukemias. Lange and colleagues describe hyperleukocytosis as occurring in 9% to 13% of children with ALL, in 5% to 22% of children with acute nonlymphoblastic leukemia (ANLL), and in most children with chronic myelogenous leukemia (CML) in chronic phase.[3]

Pathogenesis. The complications of hyperleukocytosis occur as sequelae of leukostasis, which causes increased blood viscosity and impaired blood flow to many organ systems. The aggregation of blast cells causes sludging in the vascular system. Thrombus formation occurs as a result of plasma being trapped between large blast cells. Although this disruption to blood flow may occur in any organ system, the small vessels of the lung and brain are most at risk for devastating effects of hyperleukocystosis.[3,7,22]

Leukostasis in the capillary beds of the brain or lung can cause life-threatening complications. In the cerebral vasculature, local cell proliferation damages cerebral vessels, leading to intracerebral hemorrhage and thrombus formation. In the lungs, alveolar damage occurs as blast cells degenerate in the pulmonary vessels and interstitium, releasing their intracellular contents. Respiratory failure may ensue because of decreased numbers of functional alveoli. Lactic acidosis may occur because of the poor perfusion at the microcirculatory level, with resultant anaerobic metabolism of the blast cells. And finally, impairment of renal blood flow may lead to the same metabolic consequences as previously discussed for ATLS, namely hyperuricemia, hyperphosphatemia, hyperkalemia, and potential renal failure.[3,22]

Clinical Presentation. The clinical presentation is most often manifested in the pulmonary system and CNS, although presenting symptoms may be subtle or indistinguishable from other clinical states. Signs and symptoms are generally dependent on the area of microcirculatory involvement. Pulmonary leukostasis can lead to a variety of clinical manifestations, from dyspnea to cyanosis and hypoxia requiring intubation. Both hypoxemia and lactic acidosis may be present and identified via laboratory analysis. CNS involvement may be observable by mental status changes progressing from agitation and confusion to delirium or stupor. Signs of increased ICP, such as blurred vision, ataxia, retinal distention, or papilledema, may also be present.[3]

Diagnostic evaluation for children with suspected hyperleukocytosis includes a CBC with clotting times, arterial blood gas analysis, chest radiograph, and CT scan. In addition, a venogram or arteriogram may be performed if vessel thrombosis is suspected.

Critical Care Management. Because of the potential for devastating CNS or pulmonary injury, establishment and maintenance of effective oxygenation, ventilation, and perfusion should immediately occur, especially in children with WBC counts of greater than 300,000/mm^3. Treatment for hyperleukocytosis is aimed at rapidly reducing the number of circulating leukocytes. Management includes the immediate institution of hydration, alkalinization, and allopurinol administration, as discussed in ATLS management, as well as the prompt initiation of specific cytoreductive therapy.[3,7,22] Cytoreductive therapy is discussed at the end of this section.

As with any child with an oncologic disorder, these children may require platelet and red blood cell (RBC) transfusions. Platelet transfusions are administered when the platelet count falls below 20,000/mm^3 to minimize the risk

of cerebral hemorrhage. Platelets are not known to significantly increase blood viscosity. However, RBC transfusions are used cautiously because this therapy may cause a further increase in blood viscosity, precipitate leukostasis, and lead to further organ dysfunction. It is often recommended that RBC transfusions be given only for hemoglobin levels less than 7 to 8 g/dl. Hemoglobin levels should not be raised to greater than 10 g/dl.[3,22]

The approach to treating the child with a potentially fatal WBC count remains controversial. Leukopheresis is one treatment modality that is thought to be beneficial in reducing a large tumor cell burden and decreasing the metabolic load on the kidneys. Advocates of this form of therapy believe it may reduce the WBC count by 20% to 60% while waiting for the effects of cytoreductive therapy to occur.[7,22] The disadvantages of leukopheresis include the need for anticoagulation therapy to perform the procedure and risk of bleeding, as well as difficulty obtaining vascular access in small children, and the limited availability and expertise for this intervention in many institutions. In small children, exchange transfusion is often less difficult than leukopheresis and may be performed instead. However, as with leukopheresis, there are no studies to support the effectiveness of either of these therapeutic modalities.[22] Some centers also recommend the use of emergent cranial irradiation to prevent intracranial hemorrhage.

Children with leukostasis require careful pulmonary and neurologic assessment for the development of complications such as respiratory failure and cerebrovascular accident. In addition, hematologic laboratory data is monitored frequently. Ventilatory management may be needed in situations of severe neurologic or respiratory deterioration.

There are various types of childhood leukemias and current therapies for each malignancy. Numerous treatment protocols exist for childhood leukemias. Both single and a variety of multiple drug regimens have been developed to treat childhood leukemias, with the choices of drugs being highly dependent on the type of leukemia being treated. However, despite the wide variety of chemotherapeutic drug regimens available, the common goal in the treatment of childhood leukemias (particularly those presenting with hyperleukocytosis) is to induce and maintain remission, or lack of evidence of disease. The ability to achieve complete remission quickly and to maintain remission is directly correlated to overall prognosis and degree of long-term survivability.[31] Because of the desire to quickly induce remission, a child presenting with hyperleukocytosis may require the administration of chemotherapeutic agents while in the PICU. Because the administration of chemotherapeutic agents requires specialized training, the critical care nurse collaborates with pediatric oncology specialists and is aware of institutional regulations regarding the administration of cytotoxic agents.

An example of cytoreductive therapy during the induction phase of treatment of ALL is the administration of vincristine and prednisone. This combination induces remission in approximately 85% of children with ALL. However, the addition of L-asparaginase, an anthracycline (such as daunorubicin), or both has been shown to improve the rate of remission from induction therapy to 95%.[31]

Although certain side effects, or toxicities, are inherent to particular chemotherapeutic agents, there are several common toxicities that may manifest after the administration of all chemotherapeutic agents. Even though chemotherapeutic agents are meant to target malignant cells, they most often cannot differentiate normal host tissue cells from malignant cells. Certain normal host tissue cells, such as bone marrow and mucosal epithelial cells, are particularly sensitive to the cytotoxic effects of chemotherapeutic drugs, even when these drugs are given in therapeutic doses. Common toxic effects, because of this increased tissue sensitivity, include myelosuppression (with resultant pancytopenia), nausea and vomiting, alopecia, both oral and intestinal mucositis, and liver dysfunction.[32] Ongoing research is focused on minimizing toxic effects of chemotherapeutic agents through the development of new chemotherapy drugs and newer therapeutic means for blunting these toxic responses.

COMPLICATIONS OF BONE MARROW TRANSPLANTATION

Special Considerations in the Bone Marrow Transplant Patient

BMT is a burgeoning therapy that is no longer reserved for the treatment of hematologic and oncologic malignancies. Clinical trials have either been conducted, or are in progress, to study the efficacy of BMT for a wide variety of nonneoplastic diseases, such as severe aplastic anemia, chronic granulomatous disease, severe combined immunodeficiency, and autoimmune diseases, such as multiple sclerosis, systemic lupus erythematosus, and juvenile rheumatoid arthritis.[33-35] In addition, although the term "BMT" is still used as a general term to describe the collection of hematopoietic precursor cells from bone marrow, these cells may also be obtained from peripheral blood stem cells (PBSC) or umbilical cord blood (UCB). These newer methods of transplantation are used in the hopes of preventing some of the complications of traditional BMT. Discussion of the differences between these newer methods is beyond the scope of this chapter. Recognizing the vast complexity of state-of-the-art transplantation, this section will review fundamental principles of BMT and common complications associated with BMT.

There are two primary forms of BMT: allogeneic and autologous. A third form of transplant is a syngeneic transplant from an identical twin. Allogeneic transplantation occurs when a designated donor contributes healthy bone marrow, PBSCs or UCB to a patient with malignancy. The preferred donor is a human leukocyte antigen (HLA)-matched sibling, although unrelated HLA-matched donors matched through an international registry or unmatched related donors may be used. In order to accept the donor marrow or cells, a sufficient degree of immunosuppression must be provided to prevent acute rejection of the cells and allow a "graft" to occur. This immunosuppression occurs via a "conditioning" or "preparative" regimen in which the patient's own marrow is either partially or fully ablated using high-dose chemotherapy, with or without total body irradiation (TBI).[8,36] Once the patient's marrow is ablated, the donor's marrow is intravenously administered to the recipient with the hope that the donor's cells will engraft and eventually become the patient's new marrow. Simply stated, engraftment refers to the point at which the donor cells have sufficiently established themselves as the patient's new hematopoietic system. The point of engraftment is determined by laboratory analysis of the recipient's marrow, with the exact number of cells required for engraftment dependent on the underlying disease and type of transplantation performed. After transplantation, the recipient's hematopoietic system may be completely from the donor (known as donor chimerism), completely from the recipient (known as graft rejection with autologous recovery), or a mixture of donor and recipient cells (referred to as mixed chimerism). The most favorable outcomes occur with donor chimerism; however, some degree of mixed chimerism may be present with a clinical remission of disease.[37]

Autologous BMT refers to the process in which patients donate their own bone marrow or PBSCs for use later in their treatment. This form of BMT is typically used for patients with lymphomas or solid tumors.[8,36,38] Preferably, the marrow is collected when the patient is in complete remission. Once collected, the marrow may be treated in the laboratory with specific antitumor monoclonal antibodies or selected chemotherapeutic agents, and then is cryopreserved. After receiving the conditioning regimen, the patients' marrow is thawed and intravenously administered back to the patient.[8,36]

Complications of allogeneic BMT include infections, respiratory failure resulting from infectious or noninfectious pneumonitis, acute and chronic graft-versus-host diseases (GVHDs), and veno-occlusive disease (VOD).[8,36] Although autologous BMT does not have the same complications associated with allogeneic BMT, it is associated with a higher rate of recurrent disease.

Infection

Infection is the leading cause of morbidity and mortality in patients who have undergone a BMT. The risk of life-threatening infections is most worrisome during the first 3 months after transplantation, with the greatest risk occurring during the first month. As the transplanted marrow engrafts, the immune system recovers. Mature blood cells are usually produced within 3 to 4 weeks. The initial month of severe neutropenia is typically characterized by bacterial and candidal infections.[36] Vigilant attention to both the prevention and prompt recognition of infections is crucial during this time of pancytopenia and increased susceptibility (see Box 25-1 for a review of assessment parameters and care considerations for the child with neutropenia and thrombocytopenia). Although the use of full-protective isolation for allogeneic transplant patients has fallen out of favor, many facilities require the use of hepafilter rooms for fully ablated BMT patients during the first month posttransplant.

In the 1- to 3-month period after transplantation, infections from viruses, fungi, and protozoans develop, especially in patients with GVHD. Serious viral infections, particularly as a result of CMV or reactivated herpes simplex virus, are a major concern. The risk of infection progressively declines 3 months after transplantation. Autologous BMT patients and allogeneic BMT patients without chronic GVHD are at a lower risk of infection. However, allogeneic BMT patients who have developed chronic GVHD are at great risk for recurrent bacterial infections.[36] Prophylactic antiinfection medications are typically administered to transplant patients as discussed earlier in this chapter.

Pulmonary Complications

Pulmonary complications occur in approximately 10% to 15% of pediatric BMT patients.[39] These complications are often described according to the time that they occur in the transplant process. Initially, lung damage may occur as a sequelae of the conditioning regimen, most commonly as a result of the irradiation. The lungs, more specifically the interstitium, are particularly sensitive to the cytotoxic medications and irradiation used during conditioning.[39] Scar tissue may form in the interstitial space during the healing process, interfering with gas exchange and respiratory mechanics.

As with other infections, the most common pulmonary infections during the first month posttransplantation manifest as gram-negative bacterial or fungal pneumonias. Pulmonary edema, associated with pulmonary endothelial cell damage caused by chemotherapy and radiation, is another respiratory complication that can occur in the second and third week after BMT. During the 1- to 6-month posttransplant period, interstitial pneumonias are common. Causative organisms during this time include CMV as well as idiopathic lung problems. After 6 months, pulmonary dysfunction can be related to chronic GVHD or continued immunologic deficiencies. Bacterial pneumonias continue to occur during this time.

The most common form of interstitial pneumonitis (IP) used to be CMV infection. However, with the routine administration of prophylactic ganciclovir, this incidence is decreasing. Instead, the most current form of IP is now idiopathic IP in which no causative organism can be identified. This increase in idiopathic disease may represent unrecognized infections or the toxic effects of chemotherapy or radiation therapy that has been administered as part of the conditioning regimen.[37]

RSV infection is of particular concern in the pediatric BMT patient. A major factor for morbidity and mortality seems to be whether the RSV infection has progressed to the lower respiratory tract or remains in the upper respiratory tract. Mortality rates for BMT patients with lower respiratory tract RSV infection, progressing to respiratory failure, ranges between 31% and 100%. Mortality depends on factors such as the choice of treatment used, when the treatment was initiated, and whether or not the patient was engrafted at the onset of infection and disease.[14,17]

Regardless of the cause of respiratory dysfunction and/or failure, once mechanical ventilation is required, the risk of morbidity and mortality significantly increases. Primary pulmonary parenchymal disease, in the setting of multisystem organ failure and/or hemodynamic compromise, has been associated with very high mortality rates in both adults and children.[40,41] Price and colleagues report an 18.8% survival rate for intubated BMT patients, compared with a 65.7% survival rate in nonintubated BMT patients.[42] Likewise, Huaringa and associates report an 18% survival rate in adult BMT patients who developed pulmonary complications and required mechanical ventilation.[43] Nichols and colleagues reported a 9% survival rate for pediatric BMT patients with respiratory failure.[44] Most recently, Keenan and colleagues reported a 16% survival rate for intubated pediatric BMT patients who survived for 30 days postextubation.[45] In addition, this study identified major risk factors for death for pediatric patients undergoing mechanical ventilatory support. The risk factors included respiratory failure as the reason for intubation, the presence of pulmonary infection, and impairment of more than one organ system, and were associated with survival rates of 4%, 6%, and 2%, respectively. The authors further reported that the 2% survival rate applied if more than one organ system was dysfunctional 7 days after intubation, and that no children in their study survived if the combination of acute respiratory distress syndrome, hepatic failure, and renal failure were present.[45]

Acute Graft-Versus-Host Disease

Acute GVHD remains a significant cause of morbidity and mortality after BMT.[46] This form of acute rejection occurs in up to 80% of patients after allogeneic BMT.[8,47]

Pathogenesis. Although acute GVHD is defined as occurring within the first 100 days of transplantation, it typically manifests within the first 2 to 5 weeks after transplantation.[47] This disorder, which primarily affects the immune system, skin, liver, and GI tract, results from allogeneic donor cytotoxic T lymphocytes recognizing the immunocompromised recipient, or host, as foreign and attempting to reject the host.[8,36,46] The severity of GVHD seems to be directly related to the number of T cells transferred during transplantation, to the degree of HLA differences between donor and recipient, and to the degree of immunocompromise in the recipient.[47]

Clinical Manifestations. Manifestations of acute GVHD may occur as early as 1 to 3 weeks after transplantation. Skin manifestations usually begin with a maculopapular rash involving the palms and soles, which is often intensely pruritic. This rash may resolve spontaneously or, in the most severe forms, progress to bullae formation, and severe sloughing and desquamation of the skin.[36,46]

Liver involvement may range from minimal jaundice and mild elevations in liver function test values to complete liver dysfunction; however, hepatic failure with encephalopathy resulting from GVHD is rare.[36] Intestinal manifestations include severe diarrhea, nausea, vomiting and crampy abdominal pain. The diarrhea is commonly green, watery, mucoid stool mixed with fecal casts formed

TABLE 25-4 **Criteria for Severity Index for Acute Graft-versus-Host Disease**

| Index* | Skin Involvement | | | Liver Involvement | | | Gastrointestinal Involvement | |
	Stage (Max.)	Extent of Rash		Stage (Max.)	Total Bilirubin (mg/l00 ml)		Stage (Max.)	Volume of Diarrhea (ml/Day)
A	1	<25%		0	<2.0		0	<500
B	2	25%-50%	Or	1-2	2.0-6.0	Or	1-2	500-1500
C	3	>50%	Or	3	6.1-15.0	Or	3	>1500
D	4	Bullae	Or	4	>15.0	Or	4	Severe pain and ileus

From Rowlings PA, Przepiorka D, Klein JT et al: IBMTR Severity Index for grading acute graft-versus-host disease: retrospective comparison with Glucksberg grade, *Br J Haematol* 97:855-864, 1997.
*Assign Index based on maximum involvement in an individual organ system.

by the mix of stool and sloughed intestinal cells. In 13% of patients, the diarrhea may be accompanied by anorexia and dyspepsia.[36,47]

A histologic diagnosis is usually necessary to rule out other causative factors for the clinical signs and symptoms, including chemotherapy, radiation, or infection. Diagnosis is accomplished by biopsy of the involved organ, although liver biopsies are often not possible in the immediate period following BMT because of severe thrombocytopenia. The severity of GVHD is graded on a scale of I to IV based on the extent of damage to the organ (Table 25-4). The original grading system, based on criteria developed in 1975, was a subject of debate in the transplant community because of considerable interobserver variation. In 1997 the International Bone Marrow Transplantation Registry (IBMTR) proposed revised guidelines for grading of GVHD, and validated the guidelines through retrospective analysis, although no analysis has been performed in the pediatric patient.[48] For example, the volume of diarrhea must be adjusted by body surface area. Nonetheless, these guidelines are used for determining treatment and predicting outcomes. Children presenting with grade II GVHD or above are at a higher risk of developing life-threatening infections and complications.[36,46]

Critical Care Management. The preferred treatment for GVHD is prevention. Matching the donor and recipient at the major histocompatability complex significantly reduces the incidence of acute GVHD. However, even when a sibling donor and recipient have fully matched HLA typing, moderate to severe GVHD may still occur because of the presence of minor transplantation antigens not detectable by current typing technology.[36,46] In addition, patients needing BMT may not have a matched sibling donor. The use of matched or mismatched unrelated donors is increasing in frequency, although such transplants remain controversial. Newer BMT protocols are attempting to use T-depleted marrow, in which T-cells are removed from the marrow before transplantation in an effort to reduce the immunologic response in the recipient.[36,49,50] The T cells may then be reinfused at a later time, especially if needed to fight infection. However, the use of T-replete marrow has been associated with a higher incidence of acute GVHD, and the combination of T-depleted and T-replete marrow has

an increase in graft failure compared with BMT from a matched sibling donor.[50] This increased risk of graft failure and relapse may be due to the immune-mediated antileukemic effect of GVHD.[51]

The use of medications to suppress, remove, or inactivate T lymphocytes is also important in prevention. Immunosuppressive agents may include MTX, cyclosporine (CSP), antithymocyte globulin (ATG), and prednisone.[8,36] The use of two agents, typically MTX and CSP, may result in significantly less acute GVHD and are generally administered for at least several months posttransplantation.[8,36] Prevention of GVHD also includes the irradiation of all blood products administered to transplant patients to prevent the transfusion of active T lymphocytes from product donors.

Should GVHD develop despite prophylaxis, immunosuppression may need to be intensified. Mild (grade I) cases may not always require intervention, but more extensive disease typically involves both increasing the dose of cyclosporine and the addition of methylprednisolone to the MTX and CSP prophylactic regimen. In severe cases, medications such as ATG or thalidomide may need to be added, although studies have not yet proven their efficacy in children with acute GVHD.[8,52] Mehta and colleagues report efficacy of thalidomide in at least 50% of children with chronic GVHD, but little or no efficacy in children with exclusively acute GVHD.[52]

The skin is assessed at least every 8 hours. In cases of grade I and II GVHD of the skin, minor maculopapular rashes, dry skin, and itching can be treated with meticulous skin care and lubrication with lotions and creams. In addition, mild nonirritating soaps are used. Antihistamines may be administered for pruritus. More severe cases of GVHD are rare, but total body sloughing may occur and is treated similarly to thermal injuries or diseases such as Stevens-Johnson syndrome or toxic epidermal necrolysis. As such, these cases may require skin debridement. Awareness of high infection risk to these children because of the loss of skin integrity is critical. The skin is kept clean and dry, and adhesive tape is avoided. Skin lesions are cultured as indicated. In addition, the presence of severe GVHD skin involvement will require vigilant pain assessment and management, typically using continuous narcotic infusions. See Chapter 29 for discussion of the special care needs of children with severe loss of skin integrity.

GVHD of the GI tract requires strict intake and output records, frequent (usually twice daily) weights, monitoring of electrolytes because stool output may be excessive, control of nausea and vomiting with antiemetics, meticulous rectal care after each stool, and nutritional support with hyperalimentation to allow for bowel rest. The perianal area is assessed at least every 8 hours for redness, fissures, or signs of abscess formation. The stool is assessed for amount, color, and consistency. Because of the potential blood loss through the GI tract, all stool is tested for blood and frequent monitoring of hematocrit and platelet values may be necessary. These children are also at an increased risk for infection because of GI mucosal breakdown.

Severe oropharyngeal mucositis may be present with acute GVHD, although it may also occur as a result of chemotherapy administration, radiation therapy, and infection. The degree of mucosal damage may range from mild inflammation to severe ulceration, bleeding, and potential airway obstruction.[53] Regardless of the degree of mucosal damage, pain and dryness are typically present, causing a significant impact on quality of life. Because there are no effective primary treatments for severe oropharyngeal mucositis, management is focused on relief of symptoms. Although there are differing opinions across institutions on the specific management of mucositis, current general management principles include pretransplant dental consultation (to eliminate dental problems that may exacerbate mucositis) and basic routine oral care. In addition, the use of topical anesthetic agents (such as lidocaine), mucosal coating agents (such as antacid solutions or hydroxypropyl cellulose), antiinflammatory agents (such as topical benzydamine), and saliva replacement agents may provide relief of pain and dryness. Prevention of secondary infection is crucial and may include the administration of topical antibacterial and antifungal agents or systemic prophylactic antiviral agents.[53]

Veno-occlusive Disease

In the early days of BMT, veno-occlusive disease (VOD) went essentially unrecognized as a separate disease process because liver problems were common in the posttransplant period. Patients often suffered from viral hepatitis, bacterial and fungal infections, GVHD, and liver complications from hyperalimentation. This is no longer the case, and VOD is now recognized as a major complication of BMT, accompanied by significant morbidity and mortality.[8,54]

Important risk factors for the development of VOD include preexisting liver disease or dysfunction, and the use of busulfan (BU) as part of the conditioning regimen. In 1996, Rozman and colleagues, on behalf of the IBMTR, examined risk factors for hepatic VOD in 1717 recipients of HLA-identical sibling transplants.[55] The authors reported that the relative risk of developing VOD after the use of BU for conditioning was 2.8 compared with the

use of TBI. In a subsequent study, the IBMTR reported that deaths from VOD were more frequent in patients receiving BU/CSP versus CSP/TBI for the conditioning regimen.[56]

Pathogenesis. VOD is characterized by deposits of fibrous materials that block small venules of the liver, causing an obstruction to blood flow from the liver.[8] Sinusoidal outflow obstruction causes the fluid content of the blood to be drained through the lymphatic system and into the peritoneal cavity, leading to ascites.

Clinical Manifestations. Symptoms typically develop 1 to 3 weeks after BMT and are initially the result of intrahepatic portal hypertension. Not all symptoms may occur in all children. Clinical characteristics depend on the degree of obstruction of hepatic blood flow. They include sudden weight gain, right upper quadrant pain, hepatomegaly, ascites, jaundice, encephalopathy, increased total bilirubin with normal or mildly elevated liver function tests, and coagulopathy. Some cases of VOD are self-limited with spontaneous resolution, whereas others are progressive and lethal.[54] Other liver diseases that may have more specific treatments, such as hepatitis or GVHD, must be ruled out. Typically, jaundice appears later in GVHD, and ascites is not common in liver dysfunction caused by GVHD, hepatitis, and viral or fungal infections.[54]

Critical Care Management. Diagnostic testing includes ultrasound and CT scanning, which may reveal a congested liver, ascites, or an enlarged portal vein. Doppler detection of reduced portal vein blood flow in VOD has also been described.[57] Liver biopsies may be performed, although they may be associated with a significant risk in the oncology population because of thrombocytopenia.[54]

Management of VOD is primarily supportive to provide time for the liver to heal. This is achieved by treating the side effects of liver failure, including fluid overload, third spacing, electrolyte imbalances, and coagulation abnormalities. The administrations of anticoagulants and thrombolytic agents have been only marginally successful when used to prevent and/or treat VOD.[8] Orthotopic liver transplantation and thrombolytic therapy with agents such as tissue plasminogen activator have been suggested as treatment options.[54,58] Prophylactic use of prostaglandin E_1 has also been described.[59] The prognosis of VOD is variable, with most patients with mild to moderate VOD (maximum serum bilirubin <10 mg/dl) recovering from disease. However, 95% of patients with severe VOD die as a result of multisystem organ failure.[8]

SUMMARY

New cancer treatment modalities are increasingly complex and aggressive. With refinement of these treatment regimens, the use of high-dose intensive chemotherapy and BMT will find broader application in cancer patients and patients with impaired host defenses or immunodeficiencies. Children receiving these regimens will more likely need, and benefit from, critical care resources at various points during their illness and treatment regimen. Only by careful observation and frequent clinical updates will the care of these patients be managed successfully.

The transition to the critical care unit can often be a difficult one. Most children have been hospitalized often. Families are familiar with the oncology unit staff and routines. This transition can be facilitated by the primary nurse who can disseminate information regarding the child's previous history and response to procedures to the entire critical care team before the child's arrival, when time allows. Parents should be empowered to remain involved in their child's care to the fullest extent possible, especially given the chronic nature of malignant disease. Multidisciplinary patient care conferences can be useful to discuss treatment plans and allow expression of concerns regarding therapy.

Ethical concerns, such as aggressiveness of therapy in a "terminal" patient, end-of-life decisions, and even allocation of resources, may arise among the members of the multidisciplinary team. Critical care nurses play a key role in facilitating discussion regarding such concerns and seeking appropriate consultation from experts, such as ethicists. The abundance of biomedical research on the treatment of pediatric malignancies demonstrates the hope that such patients will no longer be labeled as having a "terminal" disease. It is essential that critical care nurses strive to incorporate knowledge of the complexities of care of the child with malignancy into their practice. The nursing contribution to the team approach is a central one that will lead to improvement in outcomes for these children.

REFERENCES

1. Fanslow J: Attitudes of nurses toward cancer and cancer therapies, *Oncol Nurs Forum* 12:43-47, 1985.
2. Robison LL: General principles of the epidemiology of childhood cancer. In Pizzo PA, Poplack DG, eds: *Principles and practice of pediatric oncology,* ed 3, Philadelphia, 1997, Lippincott-Raven Publishers.
3. Lange B, O'Neill JA Jr, Goldwein JW et al: Oncologic emergencies. In Pizzo PA, Poplack DG, eds: *Principles and practice of pediatric oncology,* ed 3, Philadelphia, 1997, Lippincott-Raven Publishers.
4. Ognibene FP, Pizzo PA: Oncologic issues. In Holbrook PR, ed: *Textbook of pediatric critical care,* Philadelphia, 1993, W.B. Saunders.
5. Albano EA, Pizzo PA: Infectious complications in childhood acute leukemias, *Pediatr Clin North Am* 35:873-901, 1988.
6. Freifeld AG, Walsh TJ, Pizzo PA: Infectious complications in the pediatric cancer patient. In Pizzo PA, Poplack DG, eds: *Principles and practice of pediatric oncology,* ed 3, Philadelphia, 1997, Lippincott-Raven Publishers.
7. Derengowski S, O'Brien E: Critical care of the pediatric oncology patient, *AACN Clinical Issues* 7:109-119, 1996.
8. Eskenazi AE, Mogul MJ, Yeager AM et al: Management of the child with malignant disease in the pediatric intensive care unit. In Rogers MC, ed: *Textbook of pediatric intensive care,* ed 3, Baltimore, 1996, Williams & Wilkins.
9. Walsh TJ, Seibel NL, Arndt C et al: Amphotericin B lipid complex in pediatric patients with invasive fungal infections, *Pediatr Infect Dis J* 18:702-708, 1999.
10. Denning DW: Invasive aspergillosis, *Clin Infect Dis* 26:781-805, 1998.
11. Trigg ME, Morgan D, Burns TL et al: Successful program to prevent aspergillus infections in children undergoing marrow transplantation: use of nasal amphotericin, *Bone Marrow Transplant* 19:43-47, 1997.
12. Adams RH, Christenson JC, Petersen FB et al: Pre-emptive use of aerosolized ribavirin in the treatment of asymptomatic pediatric marrow transplant patients testing positive for RSV, *Bone Marrow Transplant* 24:661-664, 1999.
13. Pizzo PA, Robichaud KJ, Wesley R et al: Fever in the pediatric and young adult patient with cancer: a prospective study of 1001 episodes, *Medicine* 61:153-165, 1982.
14. Bowden RA: Respiratory virus infections after marrow transplant: the Fred Hutchinson Cancer Research Center experience, *Am J Med* 102:27-30, 1997.
15. Ljungman P: Respiratory virus infections in bone marrow transplant recipients: the European perspective, *Am J Med* 102:44-47, 1997.
16. McColl MD, Corser RB, Bremner J et al: Respiratory syncytial virus infection in adult BMT recipients: effective therapy with short duration nebulized ribavirin, *Bone Marrow Transplant* 21:423-425, 1998.
17. Whimbey E, Englund JA, Couch RB: Community respiratory virus infections in immunocompromised patients with cancer, *Am J Med* 102:10-18, 1997.
18. American Academy of Pediatrics, Committee on Infectious Diseases and Committee on Fetus and Newborn: Prevention of respiratory syncytial virus infections: indications for the use of palivizumab and update on the use of RSV-IGIV, *Pediatrics* 102:1211-1216, 1998.
19. Saarinen UM, Hovi L, Vilinikka L et al: Reemphasis on leukocyte transfusions: induction of myeloid marrow recovery in critically ill neutropenic children with cancer, *Vox Sanguinis* 68:90-99, 1995.
20. Medary I, Steinherz LJ, Aronson DC et al: Cardiac tamponade in the pediatric oncology population: treatment by percutaneous catheter drainage, *J Pediatr Surg* 31:197-199, 1996.
21. Alberts WM: Pulmonary complications of cancer treatment, *Cur Opin Oncol* 9:161-169, 1997.
22. Kelly KM, Lange B: Oncologic emergencies, *Pediatr Clin North Am* 44:809-830, 1997.
23. Buchanan GR: Hematologic supportive care of the pediatric cancer patient. In Pizzo PA, Poplack DG, eds: *Principles and practice of pediatric oncology,* ed 3, Philadelphia, 1997, Lippincott-Raven Publishers.
24. Kaste SC, Flynn PM, Furman WL: Acute lymphoblastic leukemia presenting with typhlitis, *Med Pediatr Oncol* 28:209-212, 1997.
25. Sloas MM, Flynn PM, Kaste SC et al: Typhlitis in children with cancer: a 30-year experience, *Clin Infect Dis* 17:484-490, 1993.
26. Wu SF, Peng CT, Tsai FJ et al: Typhlitis in acute childhood leukemia, *Acta Paed Sin* 37:208-210, 1996.
27. Rossi R, Kleta R, Ehrich JHH: Renal involvement in children with malignancies, *Pediatr Nephrol* 13:153-162, 1999.
28. Stapleton FB, Strother DR, Roy S et al: Acute renal failure at onset of therapy for advanced stage Burkitt lymphoma and B cell acute lymphoblastic lymphoma, *Pediatrics* 82:863-869, 1988.
29. Larsen G, Loghman-Adham M: Acute renal failure with hyperuricemia as initial presentation of leukemia in children, *J Pediatr Hematol Oncol* 18:191-194, 1996.
30. Smalley RV, Guaspari A, Haase-Statz S et al: Allopurinol: intravenous use for prevention and treatment of hyperuricemia, *J Clin Oncol* 18:1758-1763, 2000.
31. Margolin JF, Poplack DG: Acute lymphoblastic leukemia. In Pizzo PA, Poplack DG, eds: *Principles and practice of pediatric oncology,* ed 3, Philadelphia, 1997, Lippincott-Raven Publishers.
32. Balis FM, Holcenberg JS, Poplack DG: General principles of chemotherapy. In Pizzo PA, Poplack DG, eds: *Principles and practice of pediatric oncology,* ed 3, Philadelphia, 1997, Lippincott-Raven Publishers.
33. Burt RK, Traynor AE: Hematopoietic stem cell transplantation: a new therapy for autoimmune disease, *Stem Cells* 17:366-372, 1999.
34. Horn B, Viele M, Mentzer W et al: Autoimmune hemolytic anemia in patients with SCID after T cell-depleted BM and PBSC transplantation, *Bone Marrow Transplant* 24:1009-1013, 1999.
35. Leung TF, Chik KW, Li CK et al: Bone marrow transplantation for chronic granulomatous disease: long-term follow-up and review of literature, *Bone Marrow Transplant* 24:567-570, 1999.

36. Sanders JE: Bone marrow transplantation in pediatric oncology. In Pizzo PA, Poplack DG, eds: *Principles and practice of pediatric oncology,* ed 3, Philadelphia, 1997, Lippincott-Raven Publishers.

37. Atkinson K: Interstitial pneumonitis. In Atkinson K, ed: *Clinical bone marrow and blood stem cell transplantation,* ed 2, Cambridge, Mass, 2000, Cambridge University Press.

38. Rauck AM, Grovas AC: Bone marrow transplantation in adolescents, *Adoles Med* 10:445-449, 1999.

39. Fisher VL: Long-term follow-up in hematopoietic stem-cell transplant patients, *Pediatric Transplant* 3:122-129, 1999.

40. Jackson SR, Tweeddale MG, Barnett MJ et al: Admission of bone marrow transplant recipients to the intensive care unit: outcome, survival and prognostic factors, *Bone Marrow Transplant* 21:697-704, 1998.

41. Todd K, Wiley F, Landaw E et al: Survival outcome among 54 intubated pediatric bone marrow transplant patients, *Crit Care Med* 22:171-176, 1994.

42. Price KJ, Thall PF, Kish SK et al: Prognostic indicators for blood and marrow transplant patients admitted to an intensive care unit, *Am J Respir Crit Care* 158:876-884, 1998.

43. Huaringa AJ, Leyva FJ, Giralt SA et al: Outcome of bone marrow transplantation patients requiring mechanical ventilation, *Crit Care Med* 28:1014-1017, 2000.

44. Nichols DG, Walker LK, Wingard JR et al: Predictors of acute respiratory failure after bone marrow transplantation in children, *Crit Care Med* 22:1485-1491, 1994.

45. Keenan HT, Bratton SL, Martin LD et al: Outcome of children who require mechanical ventilatory support after bone marrow transplantation, *Crit Care Med* 28:830-835, 2000.

46. Dickinson AM, Hromadnikova I, Sviland L et al: Use of a skin explant model for predicting GVHD in HLA-matched bone marrow transplants—effect of GVHD prophylaxis, *Bone Marrow Transplant* 24:857-863, 1999.

47. Deeg HJ, Yamaguchi M: Acute graft-versus-host disease. In Atkinson K, ed: *Clinical bone marrow and blood stem cell transplantation* ed 2, Cambridge, Mass, 2000, Cambridge University Press.

48. Rowlings PA, Przepiorka D, Klein JT et al: IBMTR Severity Index for grading acute graft-versus-host disease: retrospective comparison with Glucksberg grade, *Br J Haematol* 97:855-864, 1997.

49. Aversa F, Terenzi A, Carotti A et al: Improved outcome with T-cell-depleted bone marrow transplantation for acute leukemia, *J Clin Oncol* 17:1545-1550, 1999.

50. Green A, Clarke E, Hunt L et al: Children with acute lymphoblastic leukemia who receive T-cell–depleted HLA mismatched marrow allografts from unrelated donors have an increased incidence of primary graft failure but a similar overall transplant outcome, *Blood* 94:2236-2246, 1999.

51. Nimer SD, Giorgi J, Gajewski JL et al: Selective depletion of CD8+ cells for prevention of graft-versus-host disease after bone marrow transplantation, *Transplantation* 57:82-87, 1994.

52. Mehta P, Kedar A, Graham-Pole J et al: Thalidomide in children undergoing bone marrow transplantation: series at a single institution and review of the literature, *Pediatrics* 103:44, 1999.

53. Schubert MM: Oro-pharyngeal mucositis. In Atkinson K, ed: *Clinical bone marrow and blood stem cell transplantation,* ed 2, Cambridge, Mass, 2000, Cambridge University Press.

54. Baglin TP: Veno-occlusive disease of the liver complicating bone marrow transplantation, *Bone Marrow Transplant* 13:1-4, 1994.

55. Rozman C, Carreras E, Qian C et al: Risk factors for hepatic veno-occlusive disease following HLA-identical sibling bone marrow transplantation for leukemia, *Bone Marrow Transplant* 17:75-80, 1996.

56. Davies SM, Ramsay NKC, Klein JP et al: Comparison of preparative regimens in transplants for children with acute lymphoblastic leukemia, *J Clin Oncol* 18:340-347, 2000.

57. Zieger MH, Koscielniak E: Diagnosis and follow-up of veno-occlusive disease of the liver by use of Doppler ultrasound, *Pediatr Radiol* 23:137-139, 1993.

58. Nimer SD, Milewicz AL, Champlin RE et al: Successful treatment of hepatic venoocclusive disease in a bone marrow transplant patient with orthotopic liver transplantation, *Transplantation* 49:819-821, 1990.

59. Gluckman E, Jolivet I, Scrobohaci ML et al: Use of prostaglandin E1 for prevention of liver veno-occlusive disease in leukaemic patients treated by allogeneic bone marrow transplantation, *Br J Haematol* 74:277-281, 1990.

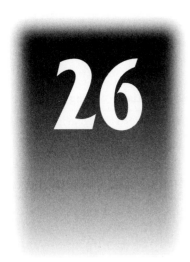

26

Organ Transplantation

Peggy Slota
Lynn Seward
Patricia O'Brien
Christine Angeletti

Solid organ transplantation has become accepted therapy for end-stage failure of the heart, liver, kidney, lung, and intestine. Generally, successful transplantation in adult patients preceded widespread application of these procedures in the pediatric population. Transplantation has been performed in newborns, infants, and children and appears to parallel the successful outcomes reported in adults (Table 26-1). However, many concerns of nurses caring for infants and children are of little consequence in adult programs. These include differences in technical detail related to the small size of children; availability of appropriate-sized organs; the urgency of transplantation to maximize neurologic, psychologic, and physical growth; and awareness of the psychologic changes patients undergo when making developmental transitions from infancy through adolescence.

This chapter discusses heart, lung, liver, intestine, renal, and multivisceral transplantation in the pediatric population, with a brief discussion of pancreas transplantation and the future of islet cell transplantation research. The surgical procedures for transplantation of different organs are described, as well as the critical care nursing of the patient in the immediate postoperative period. The quality of life and long-term outcomes in pediatric solid organ transplantation are discussed, including growth and development,

TABLE 26-1   Transplants by Solid Organ and Age Group*

Age Group	Kidney Cadaveric	Kidney Living Related	Liver Cadaveric	Liver Living Related	Pancreas	Kidney-Pancreas	Intestine†	Heart	Heart-Lung	Lung	Totals
<1 yr	15	52	1,301	191	8	3	29	953	9	39	2,600
1-5 yr	551	770	2,019	146	14	3	91	556	35	49	4,234
6-10 yr	786	769	796	31	7	1	27	329	17	68	2,831
18-34 yr	18,614	10,993	3,515	10	450	2,704	42	2,007	232	1,065	39,632
35-49 yr	31,052	10,358	12,802	6	742	3,835	26	5,734	238	1,772	66,565
50-64 yr	24,153	5,747	12,480	11	74	363	8	12,231	60	2,742	57,869
≥65 yr	4,553	782	1,936	3	2	1	0	1,195	0	163	8,635
Unknown ages	15	4	11	0	0	6	0	3	0	2	41
GRAND TOTAL	81,959	31,539	35,951	409	1,309	6,921	249	23,767	639	6,132	188,875

*Data from United Network of Organ Sharing (UNOS) 1999 Annual Report; reporting from 1988 through 1998.
†Intestine data began being reported as of April 19, 1994.

psychosocial adjustment, and physiologic concerns of chronic rejection, immunosuppression, infections, and other postoperative complications.

HISTORY

The history of solid organ transplantation spans only about 50 years. The first successful solid organ transplant performed in humans was a kidney transplant between twin brothers in 1954 by Merrill and Murray in Boston. In 1963, the first patient to undergo liver transplantation was a 3-year-old with extrahepatic biliary atresia who died of hemorrhage on the day of transplantation. Subsequent attempts in Denver, Boston, and Paris were unsuccessful until 1967, when Starzl achieved the first human liver transplant with extended survival. This 18-month-old child with hepatocellular carcinoma survived for 13 months before dying of metastatic disease despite good graft function.[1] After extensive experimental work by Shumway and Lower at Stanford University, Barnard in South Africa performed the first successful cardiac transplant in 1967. Demekov performed the first recorded orthotopic experimental pulmonary transplant in 1947 without immunosuppression. However, the longest survival period achieved was 10 days. Generally, experience with single lung transplants was unsuccessful before the introduction of cyclosporine. As early as 1959, Lillehei of Minnesota developed the surgical techniques for small bowel transplantation. Intestinal allografts were found not only to be subject to rejection but also to be able to mount a graft-versus-host (GVH) reaction. The first pancreas transplant in a human was performed in 1966; however, relatively few have been performed in children.

In the early 1960s, several events occurred that changed the course of human clinical transplantation. First, the development of tissue typing established methods to enhance histocompatibility. Second, methods for regular dialysis treatment were developed that could be integrated with transplantation. Third, methods for organ preservation and cooling were developed. Finally, new, potent immunosuppressant drugs were developed.

Pioneering work during this time vastly increased knowledge of the immune system. From a greater understanding of the immune system came a description of the process of rejection and then attempts to alter the immune response to promote tolerance and prevent rejection. Hitchings and Elion of the Burroughs Wellcome Research Laboratories, working to synthesize purine and pyrimidine derivatives to act as antimetabolites, developed azathioprine (Imuran), which quickly replaced 6-mercaptopurine and continues in clinical use today.[2] The combination of steroids with azathioprine treatment was reported by Starzl[1] to have a synergistic immunosuppressive effect.

Over the years, other immunosuppressive treatments were introduced. In the mid-1970s, Jean Borel discovered the fungal peptide cyclosporin A, which is a powerful immunosuppressant that has been found to be particularly effective when combined with azathioprine and steroids. Following the availability of cyclosporine in the early 1980s, improved survival led to a rapid increase in the number of transplants. The use of this drug ushered in the present era of transplantation.

The monoclonal antibody OKT3 was introduced to treat rejection episodes in 1983. The potent immunosuppressive agent, tacrolimus (Prograf; formerly FK506), was approved by the Food and Drug Administration in April 1994, after a clinical trial at the University of Pittsburgh.[3] The ability to wean and withdraw steroids in pediatric patients is a significant benefit of tacrolimus therapy. Many other pharmaceuticals, such as sirolimus, rituximab, mycophenolate mofetil, and daclizumab are currently being explored for their efficacy in immune suppression.

CURRENT CHALLENGES

Although organ transplantation has been lifesaving for many children, it has also raised many questions and concerns. The shortage of donor organs is the primary limiting factor in treating patients who could benefit from the procedure. The imbalance between donor supply and patient demand necessitates a procedure for selecting patients for transplantation considered most likely to benefit from the operation. Selection criteria vary between organs and between transplant programs and include both medical and psychosocial considerations.

Currently, approximately 2100 children, ranging from newborns to 18 years of age, are awaiting organ transplants.[4] Over the past 10 years, the percentage of cadaveric pediatric donors has decreased from 26% to 19%.[4] Many of these children will die because of the shortage of organs; thus other solutions have been proposed. Living related donor transplantation is becoming a successful option for transplantation of kidneys, liver segments, and lung lobes. Segmental organ-sharing between recipients has also been explored with some success.[5] Xenograft transplantation, however, has historically been unsuccessful, raising ethical and infectious disease concerns and provoking protests from the public and animal rights groups.[6] Anencephalic infants have been proposed as potential organ donors for infants, and this possibility has raised many ethical questions. The balance of risks and benefits for donors and recipients, ability to obtain informed consent for these innovative procedures, consideration of human and animal rights, and equitable access and distribution of needed organs are challenging issues.

Transplantation is the embodiment of high technology and therefore high-cost medical care. The average hospital charge for solid organ transplants runs well into the hundreds of thousands of dollars. The financial requirements for transplantation can be prohibitive if adequate funding or insurance coverage is not available. Each candidate must meet the financial requirements to maintain financial stability of the institution's transplant program. Currently, private health insurance, the Federal Government's medical program, and combined Federal/State Medicaid programs cover the cost of most transplants.[4]

EVALUATION PROCESS

A multidisciplinary approach is used in evaluating infants and children for transplantation. The evaluation process has several goals: (1) to determine that transplantation is the only treatment option; that is, other conventional therapies and treatment options are not likely to be successful; (2) to rule out major systemic diseases or permanent damage in other organ systems that would increase risk or preclude transplantation; (3) to assess the ability of the child and family to cope with the stresses of transplantation and comply with the complex medical regimen; (4) to educate the child and family to enable an informed decision concerning transplantation; and (5) to establish rapport between the child and family and the transplant team. Developing a trusting relationship between the transplant team and family, educating the family and child (at the appropriate developmental level) to enable an informed choice, and incorporating the family as members of the child's caregiving and decision-making team are important nursing goals that are initiated during the evaluation period.

A thorough evaluation of the clinical status of the patient and of the failing organ is undertaken to establish severity of disease and prognosis. The principal indications for organ transplantation in children are discussed in the introduction to each organ section. Generally, contraindications to organ transplantation include active infection; malignancy; active substance abuse; and severe, permanent damage in another major organ system that would result in the patient's demise or poor quality of life.

An adequate social support system is crucial in considering transplantation in children because they are dependent on others to provide care and nurturing. A dedicated caregiver who will take responsibility for the child's care after the transplant must be identified; ideally, two or more caregivers share responsibility. Generally, every effort is made to support the family in coping with the stress of transplantation and providing adequate care for the child. Psychosocial assessment and ongoing support and intervention by social services and child psychiatry services are important.

Maintaining an optimal level of physical and emotional wellness in the transplant candidate facilitates the necessary strength to tolerate the evaluation and waiting phase of transplantation and contributes to a successful outcome. Ongoing physical assessment, educating the patient and family about signs and symptoms of illness or progressive failure, and promotion of health-related activities are nursing interventions.

An important part of a transplant evaluation, particularly in renal transplantation, involves tissue typing in an attempt to match a recipient with the most compatible donor. The body identifies the transplanted organ as foreign and initiates a number of physiologic mechanisms to destroy the new organ. Histocompatibility testing is performed to match donor and recipient as closely as possible to reduce the immune system response to foreign antigens and reduce the incidence of rejection.

Histocompatibility testing varies with each organ. Organs vary in their immunogenicity (likelihood of inducing rejection). The lungs and bowel are most immunogenic, but the heart is most likely to develop acute rejection. Some organs, like the heart, exist singly, and the entire organ must be used, so donations must come from cadaveric donors. The kidney and segments of the liver and lungs may be removed from living related donors, so tissue typing can be more exact. Most organs can now be preserved for many hours outside of the body, which allows tissue typing to be performed. Other organs, the heart and lung in particular, have shorter preservation times, which precludes routine tissue typing.

The less antigenic the graft, the less the host will react against it. In human transplantation when the donor and recipient are identical twins and there is no antigenic difference, the tissue is accepted without immunosuppressive agents. When the donor and recipient are siblings or when a parent donor is used for an offspring, there is greater statistical likelihood for antigen sharing between the donor and the recipient than when a cadaveric or unrelated donor is used. Patient outcomes are better when either a sibling graft or a parent-child graft is used as compared with a cadaveric transplant. The improved outcome may also be related to the shorter ischemic times when a living-related donor graft is used.

The ABO and human lymphocyte antigen (HLA) systems are the main antigen systems in the body. Both tissue typing and tissue matching procedures may be performed before transplantation. The *ABO system* identifies the presence or absence of antibodies on most body tissues and on red blood cells. The major blood groups are O (universal donor), A, B, and AB (universal recipient). Transplants are performed within blood groups but may be done with donors from a compatible blood group; for example, B recipient receives an O heart. Because O-type organs can be used by any blood type and type O patients can only receive O organs, public policy dictates that O-type organs be used in O patients first. Some evidence shows that liver transplants may cross ABO-compatible groups.[7] *RHO antigens,* positive or negative, appear to have no role in graft rejection. Therefore an O-recipient may receive an O+ donor organ.

The *HLA* molecules are present on most cells and allow the body to distinguish self from nonself (foreign antibodies). The presence of these antigens plays an important role in graft rejection. The major histocompatibility complex is the HLA genetic complex for each individual. HLA molecules are divided into class I antigens (HLA, A, B, and C antigens) and class II antigens (HLA-DR, DQ, and DP antigens).

Matching procedures are performed to identify the recipient's preformed circulating antibodies to donor antigens. Cross-matching can be done between a specific donor and recipient before transplant to identify compatibility. Cross-matching is also performed between a recipient and a randomly selected panel of donor lymphocytes to measure recipient level of antibody reactivity. This is known as a percentage panel reactive antibody (PRA) and is established as part of the evaluation process. A positive cross-match denotes the presence of antibodies in the recipient serum against donor lymphocytes and is a predictor of hyperacute rejection. A high PRA means the recipient has been sensitized to one or more foreign HLAs and makes finding a suitable donor much more difficult. Serums from recipients with preformed antibodies indicated by a high PRA are cross-matched against donor lymphocytes before transplant. The transplant can occur if the cross-match is negative.

The *United Network for Organ Sharing (UNOS)* is a nonprofit organization under contract with the U.S. Department of Health and Human Services to operate the Organ Procurement and Transplantation Network (OPTN). In accordance with government guidelines administered by the Health Care Finance Administration (HCFA) in 1988, regional organ procurement organizations (OPOs) were designated to coordinate identification of potential donors and organ recovery with transplant centers and participate in public and professional educational activities to increase organ donation. OPOs are involved in the procurement of all solid organs in the United States. All organ transplant candidates are listed in the UNOS computer. In collaboration with UNOS, each solid organ group has agreed on a national organ distribution scheme to match organs with recipients based on criteria such as ABO compatibility, patient weight, recipient medical status, HLA compatibility, presensitization, waiting time, and distance between donor and recipient. There are specific criteria for each organ to ensure equitable allocation of cadaveric organs among qualified potential organ recipients.[4]

The major factor that limits organ transplantation for all that could benefit is the lack of donors. The percentage of pediatric donors has decreased over time, although the percentage of pediatric thoracic recipients has increased.[4] The shortage of donor organs has prompted some innovative changes in practice in recent years. The age and weight range for pediatric transplants has been broadened. Improvements in organ preservation have increased the length of time that the organ remains viable outside the body and therefore allows organs to be transported greater distances. A preservation solution containing hydroxyethyl starch was developed at the University of Wisconsin and has lengthened kidney and liver preservation times. Cardiac assist devices are used at some centers to provide a bridge to pediatric heart transplantation. Segmental liver transplants increase the donor pool for young infants. Patients with end-stage renal disease can be managed with dialysis until a donor becomes available, but patients needing a heart or liver often have little time to wait and may die before a donor organ is found.

All pediatric cadaveric organ donors are declared dead before removal of any vascular organ. Most states have enacted brain death legislation in accordance with the Uniform Determination of Death Act (see Chapter 20 for brain death criteria).[8] Federal Required Request legislation requires that all family members be given the option to donate or refuse to donate the organs of their loved one. In addition, the OPO in the region must be notified by every hospital of every death. Critical care nurses play a vital role in identifying and caring for potential donors, participating with the healthcare team and OPO in approaching family members about organ donation, and in supporting the family's ultimate decision.

The period spent waiting for an appropriate donor and for the transplant to occur is one of great stress and anxiety for patients and their families. Children normally regress in the face of serious illness and return to their previous developmental level following recovery. Older children and adolescents may grieve the loss of their good health and former lifestyle, especially if their illness has had a sudden onset. The forced dependence and lack of control are very difficult during the waiting period. All feel a sense of being interminably "on hold," unable to make future plans. Although many organ transplant candidates are stable and can wait at home, some are critically ill and require hospitalization. The fear that an organ will not be found in time is heightened for these patients and families. The need for invasive procedures, intravascular lines, ventilators, and other mechanical support increases the risk of infection. Serious infection may temporarily place a patient's candidacy on hold until the infection is treated. Critically ill patients may develop multisystem organ failure that would preclude organ transplantation.

Children and families need emotional support and reassurance during the waiting period. Critically ill children waiting for organ transplantation require constant monitoring and frequent adjustment of treatment to maintain their tenuous hold on life, as well as meticulous care to prevent complications. The critical care team's efforts are temporizing, at best, because the therapeutic answer to the patient's problem is organ transplantation.

PROMOTION OF GRAFT TOLERANCE

The clinical evolution of transplantation of foreign tissue or organs has been successful because of development of surgical technique, preservation technology, evaluation of histocompatibility, immunosuppression, and induction of donor-specific nonreactivity (tolerance).[9] Investigation of tolerance has been a key, multidecade research initiative. As recognized early on in research related to bone marrow transplantation, an immunologically active graft could turn around and reject the new host, provoking graft-versus-host disease (GVHD). For the defenseless recipient, the risk of the disease was found to be proportional to the extent of histocompatibility variance between the graft and recipient. Investigation continued with all avenues of research, including HLA matching, preconditioning in the form of total body irradiation or myelotoxic drugs, cell-mediated immunity, experimentation with chemical suppression, and the eventual adaptation of double- or triple-drug immunosuppression.[9]

Examination of long-term survivors in 1992 demonstrated that allograft acceptance may have been facilitated by the presence of a small fragment of extramedullary donor marrow, including stem cells, which had been assimilated into the larger immunologic network of the recipient. Movement was in both directions, so residual leukocytes (chimeric leukocytes) were in both the donor graft and the host.[9] Because of the observation, the interaction was seen as bidirectional and mutually canceling (graft versus host and host versus graft); perhaps explaining why all patients do not develop GVHD after immunologically active organ transplantation or why HLA matching is sometimes so poorly predictive of outcome. Cell survival, then, depends on immunosuppression that protects both cell populations equally. The discovery of this "spontaneous leukocyte chimerism" led researchers to believe that it occurred naturally after whole organ transplantation. Chimerism is not synonymous with tolerance, but it is a requirement for acceptance of the graft and a requirement for eventual tolerance. In fact, the long-term survival of a graft indicates that donor leukocyte chimerism has occurred and explains why immunosuppressant drugs can be eventually and permanently stopped in some cases.[9]

Although, historically, occasional attempts had been made to improve graft outcome by infusing donor bone marrow, the belief was that the donor cells would be destroyed without preconditioning with radiation or myelotoxic drugs. The discovery in 1992 recognized a window of opportunity in which donor bone marrow could be safely infused into the recipient, without preconditioning or deviation from normal immunosuppression practices. Recently this approach was used in a number of kidney, heart, liver, and lung recipients who were given donor bone marrow cells during organ transplantation after revascularization occurred. Chimerism was produced, which was estimated as 1000 times greater than that naturally occurring in whole organ transplants. Data indicated persistent chimerism, a trend toward donor-specific nonreactivity, and improved patient and graft survival.[9] Weaning from long-term immunosuppressive therapy would be of obvious benefit to organ recipients. Although an immunosuppressant drug-free state may never be obtained, the goal is to move in that direction in inducing tolerance.

Pharmacologic Immunosuppressant Therapy

Pharmacologic immunosuppressive therapy is initiated during the transplant procedure and maintained thereafter to suppress the natural immune response of the host and prevent or limit rejection of the transplanted organ. Although the rationale for immunosuppressive therapy has remained the same through the years, the immunosuppressive protocols continue to vary according to the transplanted organ, the transplant center, and the continuous research and introduction of new improved agents. Maintenance immunosuppression refers to the medications that are used on a long-term basis to prevent rejection. Other medications are used on a short-term basis to treat acute rejection episodes.

Immunosuppressant regimens continue to vary between transplant institutions, but combination therapy using double- or triple-drug protocols remains the practice of choice. Combination therapy provides enhanced immunosuppression, as well as reduced drug toxicity because of the lower dosages of each specific drug. As Fig. 26-1 depicts, the immunosuppressive drugs act on different sites in the immune system, therefore having varying effects on the process of rejection and the extent of systemic side effects experienced by the patient.

Ongoing research is exploring new approaches to standard immunosuppressive protocols that result in optimum graft function by inhibiting the immune system and decreasing the incidence of rejection, subsequently increasing the long-term quality of life for the child with a transplanted organ. The most common immunosuppressive agents used alone or in combination protocols to prevent rejection and optimize graft function are cyclosporine, tacrolimus, azathioprine, mycophenolate mofetil, and corticosteroids. Many complications are associated with immunosuppression, including hypertension, renal insufficiency, posttransplant lymphoproliferative disorders, viral or opportunistic infections, drug toxicity, steroid-related complications (obesity, growth failure, bone disease), nephritis, and cervical lymphadenopathy.

As with any pharmacologic therapy, knowledge is required about the immunosuppressant medications and other pharmacologic agents used to combat the adverse

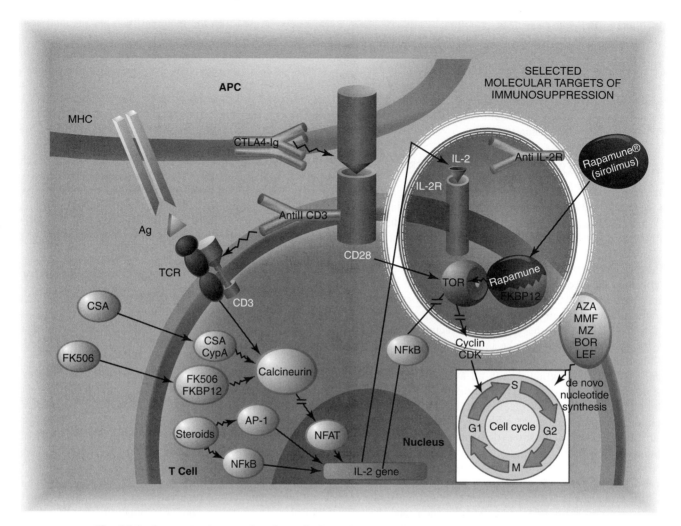

Fig. 26-1 Immunosuppressant functions. Cyclosporine and tacrolimus function as calcineurin inhibitors. Sirolimus inhibits target of rapamycin *(TOR)*, which is a regulatory enzyme critical to immune function and is the first agent in this distinct class of immunosuppressants. TOR inhibitors alter T cell proliferation largely through their inhibition of responsiveness to proliferative cytokines such as interleukin-2. *Ag,* Antigen; *APC,* antigen-presenting cell; *AZA,* azathioprine; *BQR,* brequinar sodium; *CDK,* cyclin-dependent kinase; *CSA,* cyclosporine; *CTLA4-Ig,* cytotoxic T-lymphocyte antigen −4 immunoglobulin; *Cyp,* cyclophilin; *FK506,* tacrolimus; *FKBP12,* FK506 binding protein; *IL-2,* interleukin-2; *IL-2R,* interleukin-2 receptor; *MHC,* major histocompatibility complex; *LEF,* leflunomide; *MMF,* mycophenolate mofetil; *MZ,* mizoribine; *NFAT,* nuclear factor of activated T cells; *NFkB,* nuclear factor Kb; *TCR,* T cell receptor; *TOR,* target of rapamycin. (Courtesy Wyeth-Ayerst Laboratories. From Sehgal SN: Rapamune (RAPA, rapamycin, sirolimus): mechanism of action immunosuppressive effect results from blockade of signal transduction and inhibition of cell cycle progression, *Clin Biochem* 31:335-340, 1998.)

effects of immunosuppression, including the action, dosage and administration, adverse effects, drug interactions, assessment parameters, and nursing implications. Because of the many medical problems of transplant patients, complex immunosuppressant protocols, and the large number of medications each patient receives, correctly administering medications and assessing patients for side effects become a challenging and vital responsibility for nurses and families. Pharmacologic agents used with transplant patients, including their indications, side effects, and nursing implications, are detailed in Table 26-2.

Cyclosporine Modified (Neoral) and Cyclosporine (Sandimmune). Cyclosporine is a potent immunosuppressive medication that is a metabolite of a soil fungus. Introduced in 1978, it revolutionized immunosuppression, substantially improving patient survival following transplantation. The drug's main mechanism of action is calcineurin inhibition, similar to tacrolimus. Cyclosporine does cause anemia but has minimal effect on neutrophil response; therefore some infection-fighting mechanisms remain intact. A correspondingly lower incidence of severe infections in cyclosporine-treated patients is found in some reports.

Text continued on p. 885

TABLE 26-2 Pharmacologic Agents Used in Solid Organ Transplant Recipients: Immunosuppressants and Antiviral Agents

Drug*	Side Effects	Nursing Implications

Immunosuppressants
Cyclosporine (Sandimmune)
Cyclosporine-modified (Neoral)
• Immunosuppressant
• Inhibits T cell proliferation
• Metabolized by liver
• Excreted through bile in feces
• Oral absorption is highly variable
Availability:
  Oral: Capsule, oral solution
  Injection
Dosage:
  Oral:
    Initial: 14-18 mg/kg/day
    Maintenance: 5-10 mg/kg/day
    Based on blood levels
  IV: 5-6 mg/kg/day continuous infusion or divided dose
Cyclosporine monoclonal TDX trough: 300-700 ng/ml
	• CNS toxicity: tremors, seizures, headaches, paresthesia, flushing, and confusion
	• Nephrotoxicity; ↑ BUN, ↑ serum creatinine; ↓ creatinine clearance, ↑ K, ↑ uric acid
	• Hypomagnesemia
	• Hypertension
	• Hepatotoxicity
	• Infection
	• GI: anorexia, nausea, vomiting, diarrhea
	• Dermatology: gum hyperplasia and hirsutism
	• Lymphoma
		1. Observe for CNS symptoms.
		2. Seizures managed with antiseizure medication and correction of other derangements.
		3. Tremors more pronounced at higher doses.
		4. Headache is treated as symptoms demand.
		5. Monitor renal function and intake and output closely.
		6. Monitor cyclosporine levels: Levels should be drawn at trough just before the next dose is given.
		7. Monitor blood pressure; patient may need antihypertensive medications.
		8. Monitor liver function tests (LFTs)
		9. Observe for signs and symptoms of infection.
		10. Treat for GI symptoms as needed; adjust dose if possible.
		11. Provide good oral hygiene along with routine dental care.
		12. May use depilatory cautiously to remove hair if desired for aesthetic reasons.
		13. Monitor chest x-ray film and do frequent physical examination.
		14. Cyclosporine level is increased by some calcium channel blockers, antifungal agents, corticosteroids, and various antibiotics (e.g., erythromycin, clarithromycin).
		15. Cyclosporine level is decreased by phenobarbital, phenytoin, rifampin, and carbamazepine.

Data from Armitage JM, Fricker FJ, del Nido P et al: A decade (1982-1992) of pediatric cardiac transplantation and the impact of FK506 immunosuppression, *J Thorac Cardiovasc Surg* 105:464-472, 1993; Asante-Korang A, Boyle GJ, Webber SA et al: Experience of FK506 immune suppression in pediatric heart transplantation: a study of long-term adverse effects, *J Heart Lung Transplant* 15:415-422, 1996; Green M, Michaels M, Webber S et al: The management of Epstein-Barr virus associated post-transplant lymphoproliferative disorders in pediatric solid-organ transplant recipients, *Pediatr Transplant* 3:271-281, 1999; Jain A, Mazariegos G, Kashyap R et al: Comparative long-term evaluation of tacrolimus and cyclosporine in pediatric liver transplantation, *Transplantation* 70:617-625, 2000; McAlister V, Gao Z, Peltekian K et al: Sirolimus-tacrolimus combination immunosuppression, *Res Let* 355:9201, 2000; McGhee B, Howrie D, Kraisinger M et al: *Pediatric drug therapy handbook & formulary,* Department of Pharmacy, Children's Hospital of Pittsburgh, 1997, Lexi-Comp; Robinson BV, Boyle GJ, Miller SA et al: Optimal dosing of intravenous tacrolimus following pediatric heart transplantation, *J Heart Lung Transplant* 18:786-791, 1999; Sehgal SN: Rapamune (RAPA, rapamycin, sirolimus): mechanism of action immunosuppressive effect results from blockade of signal transduction and inhibition of cell cycle progression, *Clin Biochem* 31:335-340, 1998; Webber SA, Green M: Post-transplantation lymphoproliferative disorders: advances in diagnosis, prevention, and management in children, *Prog Pediatr Cardiol* 00:1-13, 2000.

*Most dosages used for immunosuppressant and antiviral therapy are highly variable. Dosages depend on concurrent usage of other immunosuppressant agents or other pharmacologic therapies, risk or severity of rejection, risk of viral exposure, medication blood levels, responsiveness to therapy, and specific transplant center research protocols. Dosages given above are intended as reference points and are presented as either initial dosages or as ranges of dosages currently used. Therapeutic peak and trough levels are highly variable based on organ transplanted, time posttransplant, and rejection status.

BP, Blood pressure; *CNS,* central nervous system; *IV,* intravenous; *BUN,* blood urea nitrogen; *GI,* gastrointestinal; *CVM,* cytomegalovirus; *EBV,* Epstein-Barr virus; *ELISA,* enzyme-linked immunosorbent assay; *CBC,* complete blood count; *WBC,* white blood cell; *IM,* intramuscular; *SC,* subcutaneous.

Continued

TABLE 26-2 Pharmacologic Agents Used in Solid Organ Transplant Recipients: Immunosuppressants and Antiviral Agents—cont'd

Drug*	Side Effects	Nursing Implications

Tacrolimus (Prograf; formerly FK506)
• Potent immunosuppressant
• Inhibits T cell proliferation
• Inhibits interleukin-2 (IL-2) production
• Suppresses lymphokine production
• Metabolized and excreted in bile
• Oral absorption is highly variable
Availability:
  Oral: capsule
  Injection
Dosage:
  Oral: 0.2 mg/kg/day divided bid
  IV: 0.05 mg/kg/day as continuous
    infusion
Tacrolimus ELISA whole blood trough:
  5-20 ng/ml
	• Headaches
	• Irritability
	• Insomnia
	• Nausea, vomiting
	• Tremors
	• Hyperkalemia
	• Nephrotoxic effects
	• Hypomagnesemia
	• Seizures
	• Ileus
	Side effects increase with intravenous administration or high blood levels.
		1. Follow BUN and creatinine.
		2. Do not mix with $NaHCO_3$ in IV form.
		3. Administer as a constant infusion.
		4. Give 4 hours apart from alkalizing drugs (such as $NaHCO_3$) if given orally.
		5. Tacrolimus adheres to plastic surfaces; levels should be drawn from a site not used for administration.
		6. Tacrolimus should not be mixed or given with bicarbonate or Bicitra or Carafate.
		7. Tacrolimus levels are increased by erythromycin, antifungal agents, verapamil, cimetidine, diltiazem, and some antidepressants.
		8. Tacrolimus levels are decreased by carbamazepine, rifampin, phenobarbital, and phenytoin.
		9. Monitor tacrolimus trough levels.

Sirolimus (Rapamune)
• Newest of the immunosuppressive agents
• Indicated as primary immunosuppression with cyclosporine or for tacrolimus rescue in liver, small bowel, and heart recipients showing signs of neurotoxicity, nephrotoxicity, or other complications
• Structurally similar to tacrolimus
• Macrolide antibiotic that inhibits T and B cell activity
• Synergistic effects with cyclosporine and tacrolimus
Availability: oral administration only; liquid, premeasured foil pouch, pill form available soon
Dosage: variable
  1-10 mg/day; dosage calculated
    based on other immunosuppressants
    in use
	• Anemia
	• Thrombocytopenia
	• Diarrhea
	• Hypercholesterolemia and hypertriglyceridemia (responds to existing cholesterol-lowering agents)
	• Rash
	• Acne
	• Hypokalemia
	• Joint pain
		1. Mix with 2 oz of water or orange juice only. Do not administer the drug without dilution.
		2. After administering the medication, rinse the container with at least 2 more oz and administer to patient to be sure entire dose was taken.
		3. Sirolimus should be kept refrigerated, not frozen.
		4. Dose should be consistently taken with or without food.
		5. Dosage is administered once daily. Dose should be given 4 hr after cyclosporine or tacrolimus.
		6. Prolonged half-life; therapeutic levels are reached in 7-10 days. Blood levels are not used clinically at the present time.

Data from Armitage JM, Fricker FJ, del Nido P et al: A decade (1982-1992) of pediatric cardiac transplantation and the impact of FK506 immunosuppression, *J Thorac Cardiovasc Surg* 105:464-472, 1993; Asante-Korang A, Boyle GJ, Webber SA et al: Experience of FK506 Immune suppression in pediatric heart transplantation: a study of long-term adverse effects, *J Heart Lung Transplant* 15:415-422, 1996; Green M, Michaels M, Webber S et al: The management of Epstein-Barr virus associated post-transplant lymphoproliferative disorders in pediatric solid-organ transplant recipients, *Pediatr Transplant* 3:271-281, 1999; Jain A, Mazariegos G, Kashyap R et al: Comparative long-term evaluation of tacrolimus and cyclosporine in pediatric liver transplantation, *Transplantation* 70:617-625, 2000; McAlister V, Gao Z, Peltekian K et al: Sirolimus-tacrolimus combination immunosuppression, *Res Let* 355:9201, 2000; McGhee B, Howrie D, Kraisinger M et al: *Pediatric drug therapy handbook & formulary*, Department of Pharmacy, Children's Hospital of Pittsburgh, 1997, Lexi-Comp; Robinson BV, Boyle GJ, Miller SA et al: Optimal dosing of intravenous tacrolimus following pediatric heart transplantation, *J Heart Lung Transplant* 18:786-791, 1999; Sehgal SN: Rapamune (RAPA, rapamycin, sirolimus): mechanism of action immunosuppressive effect results from blockade of signal transduction and inhibition of cell cycle progression, *Clin Biochem* 31:335-340, 1998; Webber SA, Green M: Post-transplantation lymphoproliferative disorders: advances in diagnosis, prevention, and management in children, *Prog Pediatr Cardiol* 00:1-13, 2000.

TABLE 26-2 Pharmacologic Agents Used in Solid Organ Transplant Recipients: Immunosuppressants and Antiviral Agents—cont'd

Drug*	Side Effects	Nursing Implications

Azathioprine (Imuran)
• Immunosuppressant
• Antimetabolite depresses antibody production
• Metabolized by the liver to the active drug (6-mercaptopurine)
• Excreted in the urine
Availability:
  Oral: tablet
  Injection
Dosage: oral, IV
  Initial: 3-5 mg/kg/day
  Maintenance: 1-3 mg/kg/day
	• Bone marrow suppression
	  Leukopenia
	  Thrombocytopenia
	  Anemia
	• Hepatotoxicity
	• Infection
	• GI: nausea, vomiting, diarrhea, mouth ulcers
	• Pancreatitis
	• Muscle wasting
		1. Monitor CBC and platelet counts.
		2. May hold dose if WBC count <3000.
		3. Monitor for signs of bleeding.
		4. Monitor for signs of infection.
		5. Administer blood products as directed.
		6. Monitor LFTs.
		7. Observe for signs of liver dysfunction.
		8. Administer with food.
		9. Provide good oral hygiene.
		10. Monitor serum amylase and lipase levels.

Mycophenolate mofetil (CellCept) • Immunosuppressant • Used in conjunction with other immunosuppressant agents for the prophylaxis and treatment of organ rejection in patients receiving allogeneic heart, liver, renal, and small bowel grafts, in management of graft-versus-host disease in bone marrow transplant patients, and as an add-on agent in place of azathioprine. Availability: capsules Dosage: 1200 mg/m^2/day divided q8-12h *or* 30-45 mg/kg/day divided q8-12h Mycophenolate mofetil trough: ≥1.0 µg/ml mycophenolic acid (MPA)	• Increased susceptibility to infections and malignancies, especially cutaneous • Fever • Headache • Hypercholesteremia • Diarrhea • Nausea • Vomiting • Dyspepsia • Leukopenia • Neutropenia • Anemia • Thrombocytopenia • Myalgia • Hematuria • Cough	1. Antacids decrease mycophenolate absorption. 2. Acyclovir and ganciclovir compete with mycophenolate for renal tubular secretion resulting in increased concentrations of both drugs. 3. Some children may require every-8-hr dosing to achieve adequate trough levels of >1.0 µg/ml. 4. Capsules should not be opened or crushed. 5. Inhalation of the drug or direct contact of the drug with the skin or mucous membranes should be avoided. 6. Dose adjustments are not necessary in patients with renal dysfunction.

Corticosteroids
Prednisone, methylprednisolone
• Immunosuppressants
• Antiinflammatory
• Suppress T and B lymphocytes
• Metabolized by liver
• Excreted in the urine
Availability:
  Oral: tablet
  Injection
Dosage:
  Prednisone: 0.05-2 mg/kg/day
  Methylprednisolone: 0.5-10 mg/kg/day
  (highly variable)
	• Infection
	• Fluid retention: ↑ weight, ↑ Na reabsorption, ↑ BP, ↑ uric acid, edema, moon facies, cushingoid appearance
	• Osteoporosis: ↓ calcium absorption; leaches calcium from bone
	• Increased appetite
	• Mood swings, depression, irritability
	• Psychosis
	• Fragile, sun-sensitive skin
	• Slow wound healing
	• Stomatitis
	• Acne and hirsutism
	• Muscle weakness—proximal more pronounced
	• Nausea, vomiting, peptic ulcer
		1. Steroids may increase glucose levels in the blood and urine, requiring insulin or oral hypoglycemics.
		2. Cataracts or glaucoma may occur with long-term treatment; provide ophthalmic examinations.
		3. Monitor serum electrolytes, glucose, and blood pressure.
		4. Doses should not be discontinued or decreased abruptly without physician's supervision.
		5. High-dose steroids given IV push over fewer than 10 min has resulted in sudden death.

Continued

TABLE 26-2   Pharmacologic Agents Used in Solid Organ Transplant Recipients: Immunosuppressants and Antiviral Agents—cont'd

Drug*	Side Effects	Nursing Implications

Polyclonal Antilymphocyte Antibodies
Antithymocyte globulin-equine (Atgam)
Antithymocyte globulin-rabbit (Thymoglobulin)
• Immunosuppressants
• Cytotoxic antibody directed against antigens expressed on human T lymphocytes
• Indicated for allograft rejection in kidney, liver, small bowel, and heart transplant recipients
Availability: injection
Dosage:
  Atgam: 15 mg/kg/day
  Thymoglobulin: 1.5 mg/kg/day
	• Fever, chills
	• Leukopenia, thrombocytopenia
	• Rash, pruritus, urticaria
	• Arthralgia, chest or back pain
	• Diarrhea, nausea, vomiting
	• Dyspnea
	• Headache
	• Hypotension
	• Night sweats
	• Pain at infusion site, thrombophlebitis
	• Anaphylaxis
	• Dizziness, weakness, faintness
	• Edema
	• Seizures
	• Tachycardia, pulmonary edema, laryngospasm
	• Systemic infection
		1. Monitor vital signs frequently during infusion and every 4 hr after medication.
		2. Premedicate with acetaminophen and diphenhydramine; also may give hydrocortisone.
		3. Patient should remain on a monitor.
		4. Administer via central or large-bore peripheral line; use of high-flow line will minimize the occurrence of phlebitis or thrombosis. Observe site frequently.
		5. Record weight on chart.
		6. Monitor baseline CBC, differential, and platelets.
		7. Infuse slowly over 2-6 hr; concentration should not exceed 1 mg/ml.
		8. Filter infusion with 0.2-5 micron filter.
		9. Do not keep in diluted form more than 12 hr.
		10. Do not infuse simultaneously with blood products or other medications.
		11. Have emergency crash cart and drugs available.

Monoclonal Antibody **Muromonab-CD3 (Orthoclone OKT3)** • Potent immunosuppressant • Treatment of acute allograft rejection • Effective in reversing acute hepatic and cardiac rejection episodes Availability: injection Dosage: <30 kg: 2.5 mg/day >30 kg: 5 mg/day Alternative dosing: 0.1 mg/kg/day up to 5 mg	• Cytokine release syndrome • Headache • Tachycardia • Hypertension • Hypotension • Tremor • Aseptic meningitis • Seizures • Pruritus • Rash • Diarrhea, nausea, vomiting • Increased BUN, creatinine • Joint pain • Photophobia • Pulmonary edema • Fever	1. Severe pulmonary edema has occurred in patients with fluid overload. 2. Drug is contraindicated in patients with known hypersensitivity, those in fluid overload, or patients with >3% weight gain within prior week and high fever. 3. Store in refrigerator; do not freeze. Drug should not be used if left out of the refrigerator for more than 4 hr. 4. Dosage of concomitant immunosuppressants may need to be reduced. 5. First dose effect (flulike symptoms, anaphylactic-type reaction) may occur within 30 min to 6 hours, up to 24 hr after the first dose. Cardiopulmonary resuscitation may be needed. 6. Corticosteroid administration is required before infusion to decrease incidence of reactions. Use for 3-5 days. 7. Patient temperature should not exceed 37.8° C at time of administration.

Data from Armitage JM, Fricker FJ, del Nido P et al: A decade (1982-1992) of pediatric cardiac transplantation and the impact of FK506 immunosuppression, *J Thorac Cardiovasc Surg* 105:464-472, 1993; Asante-Korang A, Boyle GJ, Webber SA et al: Experience of FK506 Immune suppression in pediatric heart transplantation: a study of long-term adverse effects, *J Heart Lung Transplant* 15:415-422, 1996; Green M, Michaels M, Webber S et al: The management of Epstein-Barr virus associated post-transplant lymphoproliferative disorders in pediatric solid-organ transplant recipients, *Pediatr Transplant* 3:271-281, 1999; Jain A, Mazariegos G, Kashyap R et al: Comparative long-term evaluation of tacrolimus and cyclosporine in pediatric liver transplantation, *Transplantation* 70:617-625, 2000; McAlister V, Gao Z, Peltekian K et al: Sirolimus-tacrolimus combination immunosuppression, *Res Let* 355:9201, 2000; McGhee B, Howrie D, Kraisinger M et al: *Pediatric drug therapy handbook & formulary,* Department of Pharmacy, Children's Hospital of Pittsburgh, 1997, Lexi-Comp; Robinson BV, Boyle GJ, Miller SA et al: Optimal dosing of intravenous tacrolimus following pediatric heart transplantation, *J Heart Lung Transplant* 18:786-791, 1999; Sehgal SN: Rapamune (RAPA, rapamycin, sirolimus): mechanism of action immunosuppressive effect results from blockade of signal transduction and inhibition of cell cycle progression, *Clin Biochem* 31:335-340, 1998; Webber SA, Green M: Post-transplantation lymphoproliferative disorders: advances in diagnosis, prevention, and management in children, *Prog Pediatr Cardiol* 00:1-13, 2000.

TABLE 26-2   Pharmacologic Agents Used in Solid Organ Transplant Recipients: Immunosuppressants and Antiviral Agents—cont'd

Drug*	Side Effects	Nursing Implications

Monoclonal Antibody
Daclizumab (Zenapax)
Basiliximab (Simulect)
• Induction immunosuppressant
• Monoclonal antibody that prevents IL-2 from binding to the IL-2 receptor and inhibits the proliferation of activated T cells
• Indicated in the prophylaxis of acute rejection in transplant recipients
Availability: injection
Dosage:
  Daclizumab: 1 mg/kg × 5 doses 2 weeks apart each
  Basiliximab: 12 mg/m² administered on day 0 and day 4 following transplant
	Uncommon adverse reactions:
	• GI: constipation, nausea, diarrhea, vomiting, abdominal pain
	• Edema
	• Headache
	Very rare adverse reactions:
	• Chest or back pain
	• Fever
	• Fatigue
	• Hypotension
	• Dyspnea
	• Insomnia
	• Tachycardia
	• Bleeding
		1. Daclizumab and basiliximab do not cause the cytokine release syndrome characteristic of OKT3 or antilymphocyte globulin use.
		2. Filtering is not necessary.
		3. No premedications are necessary.

Immune Globulin
Cytomegalovirus immune globulin intravenous, human (CMV-IGIV; Cytogam)
• Attenuation of CMV or EBV disease associated with solid organ transplant
Availability: injection
Dosage:
  Prophylaxis: 150 mg/kg every 2 weeks × 8 weeks (4 doses), 100 mg/kg at weeks 12 and 16 (2 additional doses)
  Treatment: 100 mg/kg every other day × 3 doses then 100 mg/kg weekly; reevaluate; repeat
	• Flushing of the face
	• Diaphoresis
	• Muscle cramps
	• Back pain
	• Nausea and vomiting
	• Wheezing
	• Dizziness
	• Fever
	• Headache
	• Tightness in the chest
	• Hypersensitivity reactions
	• Chills
	• Hypotension
	• Arthralgia
		1. Administer IV only.
		2. Administer as separate infusion.
		3. Filters are not necessary.
		4. If minor side effects occur, slow rate or temporarily stop the infusion.
		5. If anaphylaxis or hypotension occur, discontinue infusion and use a pharmacologic agent such as diphenhydramine.

Intravenous immune globulin (IVIG) • Used in conjunction with appropriate antiinfective therapy to prevent or modify acute bacterial or viral infections in patients with immunodepression • Immunodeficiency syndrome Availability: injection Dosage: highly variable 500 mg/kg/dose every other day × 7 days	• Flushing of the face • Hypotension • Dizziness • Fever • Headache • Nausea and vomiting • Hypersensitivity reactions • Chills • Diaphoresis • Tightness in the chest	1. Do not administer IM or SC. 2. Follow package insert for rate of administration. 3. Monitor platelet count. 4. Monitor vital signs closely. 5. Have epinephrine available. 6. Slowing or stopping the infusion often allows minor symptoms to disappear. 7. Uncommonly used in solid organ transplant patients.

Continued

Cyclosporine is metabolized by the liver and excreted via bile into the feces.

Cyclosporine is available in an oral form (a liquid in an olive oil base and capsules) and in an intravenous solution. Absorption of the drug after oral administration varies widely, and it is usually given on an empty stomach to reduce the interference of food with absorption. Cyclosporine is fat soluble, so its bioavailability in patients with severe liver dysfunction is reduced. Children metabolize cyclosporine more rapidly than adults and thus require higher doses per kilogram of body weight and occasionally a more frequent dosing schedule to maintain adequate levels of immunosuppression. Many medications interfere with cyclosporine metabolism (see Table 26-2).

TABLE 26-2 Pharmacologic Agents Used in Solid Organ Transplant Recipients: Immunosuppressants and Antiviral Agents—cont'd

Drug*	Side Effects	Nursing Implications
Antiviral Agents		
Ganciclovir (DHPG, Cytovene)		

• Antiviral agent
• Treatment of CMV, EBV infection
• Prophylaxis of CMV, EBV infection
Availability:
  Oral: capsule
  Injection
Dosage:
  Initial: 10 mg/kg/day IV divided bid
  Maintenance: 5 mg/kg/day
  Oral: 700 mg/m^2 q8h
	• Confusion, seizure, coma
	• Rash
	• Reversible neutropenia and thrombocytopenia
	• Myelosuppression
	• Azoospermia
	• Nausea and vomiting
	• Pancreatitis
	• Phlebitis
	• Potential long-term carcinogenic effect
	• Peripheral extremity pain
		1. Monitor CBC, differential, platelets, and serum creatinine.
		2. Handle and dispose of according to guidelines issued for cytotoxic drugs.
		3. Administer by slow IV infusion over at least 1 hr.
		4. Infuse through large vein to minimize risk of phlebitis.
		5. Maintain patient's hydration status.
		6. Use 0.22- or 5-micron filter.
		7. Patient should have regular ophthalmologic examinations for worsening CMV disease.
		8. Dosage adjustment may be necessary in patients with neutropenia, thrombocytopenia, or impaired renal function

Acyclovir (Zovirax)		

• Antiviral agent
• Used in the treatment of herpes simplex and herpes zoster, varicella zoster, and EBV infections
Availability:
  Oral: capsule, suspension
  Injection
Dosage: variable
  IV: 750-1500 mg/m^2/day
  Oral: 20 mg/kg qid
	• Abnormal renal function
	• Lethargy
	• Tremor
	• Seizure
	• Confusion, hallucinations, delirium
	• Agitation, insomnia, dizziness
	• Coma
	• Skin rash, diaphoresis
	• LFTs
	• Nausea, vomiting
	• Phlebitis at injection site
	• Nephrotoxicity
	• Pain, sore throat
		1. Administer over 1 hour intravenously, not to exceed a final concentration of 7 mg/ml.
		2. Use with caution in those with renal disease or receiving other nephrotoxic drugs concurrently. Maintain adequate urine output during first 2 hr after IV infusion.
		3. Use with caution in children with underlying neurologic abnormalities.
		4. Monitor urinalysis, BUN, serum creatinine, liver enzymes, and CBC.
		5. Drug is incompatible with blood products and protein-containing solutions.

Cyclosporine is often administered intravenously in the immediate posttransplant period. It is given as an infusion over 2 to 6 hours or as a continuous infusion (preferred.) Whole blood assays for cyclosporine may be falsely elevated if blood samples are drawn through the same line through which the drug is infused; therefore intravenous (IV) lines used for administration of the drug should not be used to draw samples for drug levels. IV cyclosporine may be given until adequate levels of the drug are reached with the oral preparation. Cyclosporine dosages are adjusted based on trough levels, evidence of nephrotoxicity or other major side effects, and during rejection. Generally, trough levels are maintained at a higher level in the early posttransplant period, and then doses are gradually tapered to a lower long-term maintenance level.

Cyclosporine (and tacrolimus) administration, especially at high blood levels, may also predispose patients to seizures. Seizures associated with cyclosporine administration are more prevalent in children than in adults following transplantation. Posttransplant patients are at risk for seizures as a result of infection, metabolic derangements (e.g., hypomagnesemia), fluid overload, use of steroids, or hypertension. A decrease in cyclosporine dose or temporary discontinuation of the drug may stop seizure activity. Seizure activity should still be treated with antiseizure medications and correction of electrolyte imbalances or other treatable derangements. Long-term morbidity from cyclosporine-related seizures is unusual.

Other adverse effects from cyclosporine administration include other symptoms of central nervous system (CNS) toxicity, such as headache, paresthesia, flushing, and confusion; nephrotoxicity; hypomagnesemia; hypertension; hepatotoxicity; infection; gastrointestinal (GI) symptoms, such as anorexia, nausea, vomiting, and diarrheas; gum hyperplasia; hirsutism; and lymphoma.

Tacrolimus (Prograf). Tacrolimus is a potent, selective anti–T cell immunosuppressant drug, whose mode of action is similar to that of cyclosporine.[10] Tacrolimus is a novel macrolide antibiotic derived from the soil fungus *Streptomyces tsukubaensis,* found in the Tsukuba region of northern Japan. Tacrolimus, cyclosporine, and sirolimus belong to a class of compounds whose cellular activity depends on binding to specific cytosolic binding proteins, called immunophilins. Tacrolimus and cyclosporine inhibit calcineurin, a phosphatase required for early T cell activation.[11]

Tacrolimus holds promise for transplant recipients because of associated potency and action. The first human trials of tacrolimus were conducted as rescue therapy for liver graft rejection unresponsive to conventional immunosuppressive therapy.[12] The efficacy of tacrolimus has been demonstrated with pediatric cardiac, liver, intestinal, and renal transplant recipients. Results of long-term study have indicated that tacrolimus-based immunosuppression provides significant long-term benefits, including improved graft and patient survival, reduced rate of rejection, less hypertension, and lower steroid dosage requirements.[13]

Clinical studies indicate that tacrolimus has very similar side effects to cyclosporine. Hypertension may still occur but to a lesser extent than with cyclosporine; hirsutism and gingival hyperplasia are not seen with tacrolimus use.[14] In a study of 49 pediatric heart transplant recipients who received tacrolimus as the primary immunosuppressant, the common cyclosporine side effects of hypertension, gingival hyperplasia, coarsening of facial features, and hirsutism were not seen.[14] Results of another study in pediatric liver transplant recipients suggested that tacrolimus-based therapy may prove to have long-term benefits related to improved patient and graft survival, reduced rates of rejection, less hypertension, and the decreased requirement for steroids. Reported toxicities in children are dose related and include impaired renal function, headaches, nausea, vomiting, paresthesias, and insomnia.

Absorption of tacrolimus appears to occur more rapidly than cyclosporine, with peak plasma concentrations of tacrolimus achieved in 0.5 to 4 hours. Tacrolimus is metabolized and excreted in the bile with an associated half-life of 4 to 14 hours.[15] Current tacrolimus pediatric IV dosing is 0.02 to 0.05 mg/kg/day via a 24-hour continuous infusion. The drug is administered through central or peripheral IV access. Because tacrolimus adheres to plastic surfaces, IV lines used for administration of the drug should not be used to draw the drug level. Also, administration sets should not contain polyvinyl chloride. Once whole blood levels of approximately 10 to 20 ng/ml are achieved with the child tolerating oral intake, oral doses are prescribed. As increased side effects of tacrolimus have been reported with intravenous use, the child is switched to oral dosing as soon as tolerated. The initial oral dose is 0.2 to 0.3 mg/kg/day in two divided doses. Monotherapy with tacrolimus has been achieved in 70% to 80% of patients by 1 year in one center.[16]

Sirolimus (Rapamune). Sirolimus, the newest of the immunosuppressive agents, is structurally similar to tacrolimus and has synergistic effects with both tacrolimus and cyclosporine. Unlike cyclosporine and tacrolimus, which are calcineurin inhibitors, sirolimus inhibits the mammalian target of rapamycin (m-TOR), which is a regulatory enzyme critical to immune function within the cytotoxic T cell. Sirolimus is a macrolide antibiotic that inhibits T cell proliferation chiefly through the inhibition of responsiveness to proliferative cytokines such as interleukin-2. Sirolimus may cause significant bone marrow suppression, bone pain, and serum lipid elevations. It has been used as a rescue agent in liver, small bowel, or heart recipients experiencing neurotoxicity, nephrotoxicity, or persistent rejection with the use of other immunosuppressants. Dosage is based on the indication and the amount of other immunosuppressant agents in use and ranges from approximately 1 to 10 mg once daily. It is usually used in addition to cyclosporine or tacrolimus.

Sirolimus is available in a liquid form, with the capsule form soon to be available. It is mixed only with orange juice or water for administration and is kept refrigerated. Absorption is affected by food; therefore the drug should be consistently taken either with or without food 4 hours after the dose of cyclosporine or tacrolimus. Because of the prolonged half-life of sirolimus, therapeutic levels may not be achieved for 7 to 10 days after initiating the drug. Complete blood count (CBC), differential, platelets, liver function tests, and serum lipids should be monitored closely. Acetaminophen may be used in management of the associated bone pain. Elevated cholesterol or triglycerides can be managed by 3-hydroxy-3-methylglutaryl coenzyme A (HMG-COA) reductase inhibitors or fibric acid derivatives.

Azathioprine (Imuran). Azathioprine, an antimetabolite to DNA synthesis, is metabolized into 6-mercaptopurine (6-MP), the active form of the drug. It was first used as an immunosuppressant with renal transplant patients in 1963. The combination of corticosteroids and azathioprine was found to be more effective than either drug alone and became the basic therapy for patients receiving other grafts as well. Subsequently, many other drugs were added to this combination, but they generally failed to improve the therapeutic index until the development of cyclosporine. Azathioprine prevents the rapid cell division that occurs in the immune response, thus limiting the ability of the body to generate cytotoxic T cells. Azathioprine is toxic primarily to the bone marrow, and its use may cause leukopenia. This effect results in an increased risk of infection when azathioprine is used in higher doses.

Azathioprine is metabolized by the liver and excreted by the kidney. It is available in oral and intravenous forms. The oral form is readily absorbed from the GI tract.

Mycophenolate mofetil (CellCept). Mycophenolate mofetil is an immunosuppressant used in conjunction with other immunosuppressant agents for the prophylaxis and treatment of organ rejection in patients receiving allogeneic heart, liver, renal, and small bowel grafts; in management of GVHD in bone marrow transplant patients; and as an add-on agent in place of azathioprine. Mycophenolate mofetil is a prodrug metabolized into its active form mycophenolic acid by the liver.

Immunosuppression with mycophenolate may cause increased susceptibility to infections and malignancies, especially cutaneous. Side effects include hypertension, fever, headache, hypercholesteremia, diarrhea, nausea, vomiting, dyspepsia, leukopenia, neutropenia, anemia, thrombocytopenia, myalgia, hematuria, and cough. Antacids decrease mycophenolate absorption. Acyclovir and ganciclovir may compete with mycophenolate glucuronide for renal tubular secretion, resulting in increased concentrations of both drugs. Other drugs that inhibit renal tubular secretion may increase mycophenolic acid concentration.

Dosage for children is 1200 mg/m^2/day divided every 8 to 12 hours. Alternative dosing is 30 to 45 mg/kg/day divided every 8 to 12 hours. Trough levels should be 1 μg/ml. Children often require dosing every 8 hours to achieve therapeutic trough levels because of their rapid clearance of the drug. Capsules should not be opened or crushed. Inhalation of the drug or direct contact of the drug with skin or mucous membranes should be avoided because this agent may have teratogenic effects.[17]

Corticosteroids. Corticosteroids are potent antiinflammatory agents that exert widespread systemic pharmacologic effects. Included in this group of agents are the endogenous glucocorticoids, cortisol, and the exogenous agents prednisone and methylprednisolone (Solu-Medrol). Steroids have several immunosuppressive properties and are used both to prevent rejection and to treat acute rejection episodes. Steroids interfere with macrophage function, impairing antigen recognition. They inhibit both interleukin-1 (IL-1) and interleukin-2 (IL-2), causing a decrease in the production of cytotoxic T cells. At high doses (e.g., bolus doses of 500 to 1000 mg), corticosteroids have a profound negative effect on the function of lymphocytes. The ability to recognize their target antigens is impaired, and circulating lymphocytes are redistributed into lymphoid compartments, where they avoid contact with the transplanted organ.

Steroids are predominantly metabolized by the liver and excreted by the kidney. Steroids are commonly given intravenously at the time of surgery (as Solu-Medrol) and then orally (as prednisone) following transplantation. The oral preparation is usually well absorbed from the GI tract. High doses of corticosteroids are given immediately after the transplant to prevent rejection and then tapered to lower maintenance levels over several days or weeks. Eventually, attempts are made to wean the steroids altogether. Because of the many toxic side effects of steroids, especially their negative effect on linear growth in prepubertal children, low maintenance doses are advantageous. The goal is to reach a very low maintenance dose, or ideally, an every-other-day dose schedule to improve growth in prepubertally children and eventually wean steroids completely. Prednisone inhibits normal adrenocorticoid production of cortisol, so the drug dosage is tapered before discontinuation to avoid symptoms of adrenal corticoid insufficiency that occur if the drug is abruptly stopped.

High-dose steroid therapy is usually the initial treatment for rejection episodes. A 1- to 3-day "pulse" of high-dose methylprednisolone given intravenously followed by an oral prednisone taper to maintenance levels over 5 to 10 days is a common treatment option. Most rejection episodes are successfully treated with steroid treatment in addition to optimizing the use of cyclosporine or tacrolimus.

Polyclonal Antilymphocyte Antibodies: Antithymocyte Globulin-Equine (Atgam), Antithymocyte Globulin-Rabbit (Thymoglobulin). Immune globulin preparations are produced by injecting an animal with human thymocytes. The animal produces antibodies to the human thymocytes, which are then separated and purified into an immune globulin preparation. The antilymphocyte sera is then infused into the patient, and the immunosuppressive effect is achieved through antigen-antibody binding and the depletion of circulating lymphocytes.

This therapy has been used primarily to treat allograft rejection episodes that are resistant to corticosteroid treatment. In addition, it may be used as an induction therapy to delay cyclosporine or tacrolimus therapy for 2 to 4 weeks posttransplant, thus minimizing potential nephrotoxicity from calcineurin antagonism immediately after the operation. It is also used as an adjunct to other immunosuppressive therapy to delay the onset of the first rejection episode.

Before administration, prior sensitization to the heterologous globulin is assessed by giving a subcutaneous test dose diluted with normal saline (Atgam only.) During daily administration, premedication with an antihistamine and acetaminophen will decrease the incidence of toxic reactions such as flushing, chills, fever, occasional anaphylactic reactions, and serum sickness. Maintenance dose is regulated by monitoring T cell subsets.

Monoclonal Antibodies: Muromonab-CD3 (Orthoclone OKT3). Monoclonal antibodies are produced by a hybridization technique that joins sensitized B cell lymphocytes with murine myeloma cells and produces monoclonal antibodies. The antibodies are targeted to react with a specific subset of lymphocytes defined by surface cell antigens.[18] Monoclonal antibodies are derived from a single clone, so each molecule is an identical, highly specific antibody to a specific antigen. In the case of OKT3, the antigen is the CD3 cell surface receptor of the T lymphocytes.

OKT3 acts on the immune system causing an immediate decline in circulating T cells (as soon as 8 to 12 hours). This prevents the lymphocytes from reacting with foreign antigens from the transplanted organ and inhibiting T cell function. Because of its potency, OKT3 has different toxic effects than the other immunosuppressant antibodies. Experience in renal, liver, and cardiac transplantation has demonstrated its efficacy in treating rejection.

OKT3 has also been used prophylactically in the immediate transplant period by some heart and renal transplant programs.[19] The efficacy of prophylactic use of OKT3 in decreasing rejection has not been established. Some evidence now shows that prophylactic use of OKT3 may be associated with an increased risk of lymphoma following heart transplantation in adults.[20]

OKT3 comes as an IV preparation and is given once daily as an IV bolus infusion over 1 minute. Treatment for rejection is determined by biopsy results, but it is usually a 10- to 14-day course. Premedication, of acetaminophen, diphenhydramine, and corticosteroids, is given to decrease adverse reactions, especially common with the first dose. OKT3 administration has been associated with an increased incidence of cytomegalovirus (CMV) infection. Therefore many patients receive CMV prophylaxis concomitant with a course of OKT3. Because OKT3 is a murine-derived protein, patients may develop antibodies to the drug, which could limit the potency of the drug in the future treatment of the patient. The manufacturer (Ortho Pharmaceutical Co.) offers an immunoassay service to measure antibody titers to OKT3. OKT3 is contraindicated in patients with known hypersensitivity, those with fluid overload, or patients who have had a greater than 3% weight gain within the prior week. Serious side effects may occur, including pulmonary edema and cytokine release syndrome.

Daclizumab (Zenapax) and Basiliximab (Simulect). Daclizumab and basiliximab are immunosuppressive monoclonal antibody products produced by recombinant technology. They prevent IL-2 from binding to the IL-2 receptor and inhibit the proliferation of activated T cells. Daclizumab and basiliximab are used as induction therapy in the prophylaxis of acute rejection, as part of an immunosuppressive regimen that includes other immunosuppressant agents. Daclizumab is given at the time of surgery (usually 1 mg/kg) and every 2 weeks thereafter, for a total of 5 doses. Basiliximab is administered on the day of surgery (day 0) and on day 4.

Daclizumab and basiliximab do not cause the cytokine release syndrome characteristic of OKT3 or antilymphocyte globulin, which often leads to a combination of fever, respiratory difficulty, and hypotension. Adverse effects are uncommon, and when they occur, they are mild and include GI symptoms such as constipation, nausea, vomiting, diarrhea, and abdominal pain. Other adverse effects, such as edema, tremor, headache, oliguria, chest pain, fever, fatigue, hypotension, dyspnea, insomnia, back pain, tachycardia, and bleeding, are very rare. They do not appear to alter the pattern, frequency, or severity of adverse reaction or infectious complications associated with other immunosuppressants.

Immune Globulins. Immune globulins are sometimes used in conjunction with appropriate antiinfective or antiviral therapy to prevent bacterial or viral infections in patients with immunosuppression. For example, specific immune globulins, such as hyperimmune CMV immune globulin, may be used to attenuate CMV or Epstein-Barr virus (EBV) infections. Rituximab (Rituxan) is a genetically engineered human monoclonal antibody directed against the CD20 antigen found on the surface of normal and malignant B lymphocytes. Rituximab is indicated for the treatment of patients with relapsed or refractory, low-grade or follicular, CD20-positive, B cell non-Hodgkin's lymphoma. Preliminary case reports suggest rituximab may be beneficial in some patients with EBV-related posttransplantation lymphoproliferative disorder (PTLD), refractory to other treatment.[17]

Antiviral Agents. Antiviral agents, such as ganciclovir and acyclovir, are used as prophylaxis or treatment of specific viruses, including CMV, EBV, and herpes simplex and zoster, for immunosuppressed patients who are more susceptible to devastating viral infections in the postoperative period.

Other Agents. Several other treatments have been tried to prevent or treat rejection following transplantation. Some centers have used the anticancer agents cyclophosphamide (Cytoxan) and vincristine in patients with severe rejection. Total lymphoid irradiation (TLI) has been used in small groups of patients. With renal transplant patients, it was used before transplantation in an attempt to induce immune tolerance to the donor organ and decrease later rejection.[21] It has also been used after heart transplantation to treat intractable rejection.[22] New monoclonal antibodies are being sought. Ideally, scientists hope to find a method for inducing a state of true tolerance to the transplanted organ.

Long-Term Immunosuppression. Long-term immunosuppression can lead to other problems, most often hypertension, renal insufficiency, cutaneous malignancies, neurologic symptoms or findings, infections, and steroid-related complications such as obesity, growth failure, bone disease, and diabetes.

Rejection of the Organ Allograft

Because all the physiologic properties of the human immune system have not been fully explained, the phenomenon of rejection is not completely understood. Rejection is the result of a series of complex immunologic responses in which the recipient recognizes the donor organ as being different from itself. Foreign antigens on the donor organ are recognized by the host organism, and then through a number of pathways, destruction of the donor graft occurs. This process involves lymphocyte infiltration, cellular edema, eventual cellular necrosis leading to organ dysfunction, and later, if untreated, graft loss. A more complete discussion of the immune system is found in Chapter 15.

Hyperacute rejection is a humoral-mediated immune response, which occurs within minutes or hours of transplantation as the result of preformed circulating antibodies to the donor. The organ sustains intense endothelial damage with interstitial edema and clotting of the microvasculature. The kidney appears most prone to hyperacute rejection, whereas the liver and heart appear more tolerant of transplant antigen incompatibility.[7] Using ABO-compatible donors and avoiding implants in cross-match–positive recipients are standard practices to prevent hyperacute rejection in renal and cardiac transplantation.

Acute rejection is a T cell–mediated immune response, which may occur 1 to 2 weeks after transplantation and any time thereafter. The T lymphocytes of the recipient are activated by the surface antigens of the donor organ, causing cellular infiltration of the transplanted organ with resultant interstitial edema and cellular necrosis. Because of cellular damage, acute rejection may interfere with normal organ function. Immunosuppressive therapy after transplantation is designed to prevent and treat acute rejection episodes.

Chronic rejection is a combination of both humoral and cellular immune responses, which may occur 3 months after transplantation but is more common after the first year. It has an insidious onset, appears to be progressive, and results in vascular damage to the organ, eventually leading to organ failure. Retransplantation is the only known treatment.

The diagnosis of acute rejection is different for each solid organ transplant. In the following sections, the clinical signs of rejection and the use of specific procedures to diagnose rejection are described and discussed for each organ.

HEART, HEART-LUNG, AND LUNG TRANSPLANTATION

Heart Transplantation. The treatment of end-stage heart disease in infants and children with heart transplantation became available in the early 1980s following improved outcomes in adults and the introduction of cyclosporine. Heart transplantation is now a well-established therapy for infants and children with end-stage heart disease who have failed conventional medical and surgical therapies or for whom no other therapies are possible.

The International Society of Heart and Lung Transplantation (ISHLT) provides a wealth of information about cardiac transplantation in the annual report.[19,23] A rapid increase in the total number of pediatric heart transplants occurred in the 1980s, reaching 324 transplants in 1990. Since then, there has been a plateau in the total number of transplants and a recent decline in the yearly total. These data reflect a limit in available donor organs, yet the number of potential recipients continues to increase. Heart transplants in children 18 years of age and younger make up about 10% of the total number of heart transplants performed annually in the United States.

Infants make up about 25% of the pediatric heart transplant population, with patients of ages 1 to 10 years and those 11 to 18 years equally composing the rest of the group. The main indications for pediatric heart transplantation are congenital heart disease (75% of the infant group) and cardiomyopathy (65% of the 11- to 18-year-old group).

The pediatric registry contains data on more than 4000 heart transplants performed from 1983 to 1999.[19] The actuarial survival for this period was 78% at 1 year and 64% at 5 years. Recent data from 1995 to 1998 suggest improved early survival with a 1-year actuarial survival of 82%. In experienced centers, significantly better survival has been observed. In all eras, the greatest mortality is in the first few months after transplantation. Infant actuarial survival is lower than that of other age groups because of a higher incidence of early death. Primary graft failure is the most common cause of early death in the first month after the transplant. For those infants who survive the first year, late survival is similar to that of other age groups. Some data suggest that newborn recipients may have a long-term survival advantage.[24]

Acute rejection, followed by infection, is the leading cause of death 1 month to 1 year posttransplant in children, as in adults. After 3 years, chronic rejection/posttransplant coronary artery disease is the leading cause of late mortality in children. The conditional half-life (for patients surviving more than 1 year posttransplant) for all pediatric recipients is now estimated at 14.4 years, suggesting that many children will survive to reach adulthood after heart transplantation.[19]

Powerful arguments have been made on both sides of the "palliate or transplant" controversy for infants with hypoplastic left heart syndrome (HLHS). Those who argue in favor of palliation cite the relative scarcity of donors, the high incidence of early graft failure in this group of patients, and the long-term morbidity and mortality risks after transplantation. They propose that using pieces of an infant's own heart to fashion some form of circulation capable of sustaining life is preferable to using someone else's tissue (i.e., a transplanted organ), with its attendant need for immunosuppression. These patients would still be potential transplant candidates if the palliative repair failed. Many believe that the limited supply of donors should go to infants with no other treatment options. Proponents of transplantation believe it is a better alternative for infants with HLHS, which requires several high-risk palliative procedures without achieving normal cardiac structure or function. They argue that having a normal heart offsets the risks of chronic immunosuppression.

Several factors are considered in evaluating treatment strategies. Ninety percent of mortality in both groups occurred in the first year of life. The limited infant donor supply and resultant longer waiting times are likely to increase the number of infants who die while waiting for a transplant. This pretransplant mortality negatively impacts the outcome statistics for infants in the transplant option group. Even with that fact in mind, a study comparing outcomes at 1 year and 5 years for both treatment strategies on patients from 1989 to 1994 reported better outcomes with transplantation in both periods.[25] However, the true incidence of late transplant complications, such as PTLD and posttransplant coronary artery disease, will become more apparent as pediatric survivors live 10 or more years after transplant. With recent improvements in the surgical outcomes for stage I repairs in large referral centers, palliative repair may become a more attractive option, and there may be fewer infant transplants as a primary procedure for HLHS in the future. Heart transplantation for infants with no other treatment options will continue.

Heart-Lung and Lung Transplantation. Pediatric combined heart-lung and lung transplantation have been available since 1985, when the first successful pediatric heart-lung transplant was performed at the University of Pittsburgh.[10] The Registry of the International Society for Heart and Lung Transplantation has received data on more than 11,608 heart-lung and lung transplants *worldwide* (all age groups), including 2510 combined heart-lung procedures from 124 centers, 5347 single-lung procedures from 153 centers, and 3751 double-lung procedures from 140 centers.[26] Children have received heart-lung, double-lung, sequential bilateral single-lung, and single-lung transplants. The 1998 data reported 15 heart-lung transplants in children and 75 lung transplants in children.[26]

The number of heart-lung procedures has declined steadily over the past 6 years, primarily related to limitations in pediatric donor availability but also because of the expansion of single- and double-lung transplants and the strict, but necessary, criteria set for recipient eligibility.[4]

(For example, potential recipients with cystic fibrosis who have *Pseudomonas cepacia* in their airways or sinuses are no longer placed on waiting lists in many centers.[27]) Cardiac repair and simultaneous bilateral or single-lung transplantation have been performed in some centers, which allows a scarce donor heart to be used in a different recipient.[28] Single-lung transplantation offers a therapeutic option for patients with lung disease without infection and for selected patients with pulmonary hypertension and adequate cardiac reserve. In some cases, a double-lung transplant may be preferred over heart-lung transplant for children with adequate cardiac function and inadequate pulmonary function. In addition, procurement of a cadaveric lung allograft for a recipient requiring only a single or double lung provides the use of the heart for standard orthotopic heart transplantation in another recipient. Donors deemed unsuitable for heart-lung transplantation on the basis of a unilateral lung pathologic condition, including trauma, atelectasis, and even pneumonia, may be suitable for single-lung and orthotopic heart graft procurement. Furthermore, selected donors with excessive vasopressor requirements, cardiac contusions, or arrhythmias may be viewed as potential double-lung or single-lung donors. With the increased success of lung transplantation, the fact that only 1 in 20 donors has suitable lungs for transplantation has prompted some surgeons to consider living-related segmental lung donors.

Children who are candidates for lung transplantation have end-stage parenchymal or vascular lung disease causing a significant impact on their daily activities. The major indications for combined heart-lung procedures have been primary pulmonary hypertension; pulmonary vascular disease secondary to congenital heart disease, including Eisenmenger's syndrome; and cardiomyopathy with pulmonary vascular disease. The major indication (almost 50% of cases) for lung procedures has been cystic fibrosis. Congenital disease and primary pulmonary hypertension necessitate other lung procedures. Other indications include interstitial lung disease, arteriovenous malformations, GVHD, and rheumatoid lung.

The operative mortality (less than 30 days) associated with lung transplantation is approximately 18%. Early mortality in lung transplantation has not been higher in the pediatric age group, but fewer children under 2 years of age have had lung transplantation.

Causes of death in lung recipients are similar for all forms of lung transplantation. As in heart transplantation, intraoperative technical complications (including primary graft failure and hemorrhage) and cardiac complications account for about one third of all deaths. Infections have been reported in an additional one third of deaths, which is higher than heart recipient rates. Most infections causing mortality are related to viral and fungal infections. Antiviral prophylaxis is used for at least 4 weeks after transplantation. Cystic fibrosis patients are also at higher risk for severe bacterial infections. They are often colonized with resistant organisms. In addition, they may be malnourished, with chronic subacute infections, such as sinusitis. In general,

cystic fibrosis in children is challenging to manage. Triple drug immunosuppression is avoided in these patients, and aggressive, extended antimicrobial therapy is used. More thorough pulmonary toilet is required to prevent or treat pulmonary infections.

Rejection has not been as significant a cause of death as in previous years, primarily because of new and innovative immunosuppressive agents. However, most patients will suffer one or two episodes of acute rejection in the first 3 months posttransplant. The most significant long-term complication of lung transplantation is chronic rejection, characterized by obliterative bronchiolitis.

Posttransplantation lymphoproliferative disease is also a potential complication, particularly in children with no exposure to EBV and in children receiving lungs or intestines, which have a more significant quantity of donor-derived lymphatic tissue. Often, the infection occurs in the recipient's lung within the first year after transplantation.

Survival in lung recipients has been lower than that in heart recipients. Currently, little difference in survival rate is apparent between the specific types of lung transplant procedures. One-year survival is 66% for heart-lung, 68% for single lung, and 74% for double-lung transplantation. The 5-year survival rate for heart-lung transplantation has been 41%.[26]

Transplantation Procedures

Heart Transplantation Procedure. The operative technique for cardiac transplantation in infants and children is similar to that in adults except for modifications in those with congenital cardiac anomalies. The operation is performed through a median sternotomy using cardiopulmonary bypass. *Standard orthotopic* heart transplantation involves removing the recipient's diseased heart, retaining the great arteries and back wall of the atria, and performing biatrial anastomoses. The recipient's remaining atrial chambers may be large, and the donor and recipient atria may contract asynchronously.

Bicaval anastomoses are becoming more common, especially in recipients with congenital heart disease. *Total cardiac* transplantation leaves a small cuff of the recipient left atrial tissue (the area receiving the pulmonary veins) in place, but the right atrium is removed. The donor right atrium is left intact, and the donor superior and inferior vena cava are anastomosed to the recipient cava.[29] This technique requires less dissection if the recipient atria have been involved in previous operations and is less likely to damage the sinus node.

Heterotopic heart transplantation leaves the recipient's own heart in place and attaches the donor heart, via conduits to the great arteries as a "piggyback" heart. Rarely performed in children, heterotopic transplantation has a role in patients with increased pulmonary vascular resistance (PVR) as an alternative to heart-lung transplantation or when the donor organ is too small for the recipient, but transplantation is necessary because death is imminent.[29]

Donor selection and organ recovery require some adjustments for infants and younger children. Hearts can come from donors larger than the recipient, sometimes more than double the recipient's body weight. The recipient's failing heart is often markedly dilated, so the mediastinum can accommodate a larger heart. This may be especially advantageous if increased PVR is present. Surgeons usually remove extra donor aorta and pulmonary artery to use in reconstruction of these vessels in patients with congenital heart disease. Surgical techniques for cardiac transplantation in patients with many congenital cardiac anomalies have been described.[29,30]

Heart-Lung and Lung Transplantation Procedures. Transplant techniques have been refined over the past 20 years. In the past, bronchial anastomosis disruption was an early cause of death. Use of steroids sometimes impeded vascular supply to the transplanted donor bronchus, leading to bronchial air leaks, bleeding, stenosis, mucosal necrosis with aspiration pneumonia, and infection.[31] Consequently, steroid dosages have been greatly reduced, and triple-drug immunosuppression is used for most heart-lung and lung recipients.

Removal of the diseased heart and lung(s) without causing phrenic, recurrent laryngeal, or vagus nerve injury is technically challenging.[29] The trachea is divided immediately above the carina, or the division is made on the recipient's right and left mainstem bronchi as they emerge from the mediastinum.[32] The donor heart and lungs are prepared and removed en bloc after core cooling and administration of cardioplegia to the heart. Reimplantation of the heart-lung graft is accomplished by sequential tracheal, caval, and aortic anastomoses.

The single-lung transplant is performed through a thoracotomy. Choice of which lung to transplant is affected by previous surgery, such as lobectomy (the opposite lung is then chosen for transplant because no scar tissue is present), size of the donor (if a relatively large lung is to be transplanted, the left side is preferred because the left hemidiaphragm is easier to mobilize downward to accommodate the lung tissue; however, oversized grafts are avoided), and lung condition (the most diseased or damaged lung is replaced).

When a single lung is transplanted or sequential transplantation of bilateral lungs is performed, the recipient's pulmonary artery is clamped to determine if the patient can tolerate the implantation without the use of cardiopulmonary bypass. This avoids the potential issue of platelet destruction and other complications associated with bypass. Once oxygenation has been established, the diseased organ is removed with cauterization of bleeding and preservation of essential nerves. The donor organ is placed, and three major anastomoses are completed. First, the bronchial anastomosis is completed. Second, the two major pulmonary veins from the one lung of the donor are attached to the recipient's left atrium (larger children), or a section of the atrial wall with pulmonary vein insertion points is implanted. Last, the pulmonary artery is anastomosed. The recipient and donor pulmonary arteries are spread, and an anastomosis is performed with very small "bites" through all the layers of the vessel, using continuous sutures.[32]

In a bilateral lung transplant, a "clamshell incision" or a bilateral thoracosternotomy is used to provide full exposure of the operative field. Patients over 20 kg are intubated with a double-lumen endotracheal tube to allow selective, unilateral lung ventilation. A pulmonary artery (PA) catheter is placed to provide continuous assessment of PA pressures and cardiac output. After cannulation of the PA, right ventricular tolerance of both left and right PA clamping is assessed, as well as identification of the "best lung" by sequential ventilation and assessment of arterial blood gases. If there is any question of right ventricular dysfunction, cardiopulmonary bypass is used to support the patient through the transplant. If the patient is able to tolerate unilateral lung ventilation and pulmonary artery clamping, each lung is sequentially implanted.

Postoperative Care Following Heart and Heart-Lung Transplantation

Many aspects of postoperative nursing care following transplantation of thoracic organs are similar to the care of infants and children after cardiopulmonary surgery (see Chapter 18). Postoperative recipients require close monitoring and physical and hemodynamic assessment. A PA catheter is often used to monitor right ventricular performance and PA pressures, especially if preoperative high PVR is present. Cardiac output is assessed noninvasively by the quality of peripheral pulses, capillary refill, skin temperature and color, and urinary output. Serum electrolyte levels, arterial blood gases, and chest tube drainage are documented. Careful evaluation of heart and respiratory sounds is necessary. Maintaining hemodynamic stability is important while minimizing fluid overload and pulmonary edema. Strict monitoring of intake and output (often while maintaining a negative fluid balance) is required to avoid fluid overload or hypovolemia.

Of particular interest in the postoperative lung transplant patient is the reimplantation response. This is defined as the morphologic, radiologic, and functional changes that occur in a transplanted lung in the early postoperative period as the result of surgical trauma, ischemia, denervation, lymphatic interruption, and other injurious processes (exclusive of rejection) that are unavoidable aspects of the transplant operation. Functionally, the reimplantation response produces a temporary impairment of the ventilation/perfusion ratio in the transplanted lung. Some transient impairment of blood flow may also occur. The patient may present with symptoms of adult respiratory distress syndrome (ARDS), manifested as defects in pulmonary gas exchange, compliance, and vascular resistance, as well as an inability of the disrupted lymphatic system to clear interstitial fluid. Subjectively, the patient becomes very anxious and complains of shortness of breath. Examination of the patient reveals diffuse rales, and chest x-ray film demonstrates pulmonary edema. Treatment includes vigorous diuresis, chest physiotherapy, and reintubation if necessary. In addition to reimplantation response, differential diagnoses include rejection and infection. Distinguishing among these diagnoses, though often difficult, is essential to formulating a treatment and nursing care plan. The incidence and severity of the reimplantation response seem to be decreasing, possibly because of better preservation techniques.

Assessing for clinical signs of infection and rejection is a primary nursing function. A small increase in temperature can indicate infection. Fevers greater than 38° C require prompt and aggressive workup. Persistent or productive cough with or without fever or decrease in forced expiratory volume in 1 second (FEV_1) require further investigation by chest x-ray film and, frequently, bronchoscopy. (See also sections on infection and rejection.) CMV and *Pneumocystis carinii* are important opportunistic infections in heart-lung or lung transplant recipients. The risks of infection by any organism are directly related to potency and duration of immunosuppression, donor selection, operating room technique, and postoperative exposure to pathogens.

Significant Postoperative Issues and Complications

Organ-Specific Rejection

Organ-Specific Rejection: Heart. The principal mediators of cardiac allograft rejection are T lymphocytes.[29] Humoral mechanisms are thought to be less significant except in sensitized patients or perhaps in chronic rejection. Clinical signs of acute rejection of the heart in infants and children are often subtle and nonspecific and may be absent until rejection is severe. Signs and symptoms of rejection in infants include irritability, lethargy, poor feeding, tachypnea, and tachycardia. Children may demonstrate decreased exercise tolerance, marked fatigue, elevated temperature, and signs of congestive heart failure. On auscultation, a gallop or pericardial friction rub may be appreciated, and dysrhythmias may be detected. Rejection may impair contractility and result in low cardiac output.

Additional diagnostic tests for acute rejection may be helpful. Cardiomegaly may be seen on chest x-ray film. Electrocardiogram (ECG) may show atrial or ventricular dysrhythmias. Summation of ECG voltages may be decreased from the patient's baseline in severe rejection. Hemodynamic data obtained via intracardiac lines or during cardiac biopsy procedures may show increased filling pressures, decreased right atrial saturation, increased right ventricular end-diastolic pressure (RVEDP), and decreased cardiac output during rejection episodes.

Echocardiograms are a useful noninvasive test in monitoring for rejection. The presence of increased posterior wall thickness, decreased left ventricular volumes, decreased ventricular function, and pericardial effusion suggests rejection and warrants further investigation. Systolic dysfunction occurs late and usually indicates severe cellular rejection. Boucek and colleagues[33] described an increase in left ventricular mass and other parameters on the echocardiogram as reliable markers for rejection in infants. Another recent study by Santos-Ocampo and associates[34] found echocardiogram indices of rejection less reliable early after transplant when compared with biopsy results and significant variability in observations depending on the value measured. Echocardiogram detection of diastolic dysfunction may not be a reliable indicator of graft rejection.[29]

Despite a number of possible noninvasive parameters, right ventricular endomyocardial biopsy remains the "gold standard" in the diagnosis of cardiac rejection. Histologic grading for rejection is standardized based on criteria from the ISHLT.[29] Mild rejection is characterized by minor perivascular and interstitial infiltrates. Moderate rejection involves increased infiltrates and focal myocyte necrosis. Severe rejection is manifested by increased inflammatory infiltrates, multiple sites of myocyte necrosis, and interstitial edema with or without hemorrhage. Although endomyocardial biopsy is the most reliable method currently available to diagnose cardiac rejection, it is not infallible. There are many anecdotal reports of patients with clinical signs of severe rejection who had a negative cardiac biopsy result and, conversely, patients who appeared well but had a biopsy demonstrating rejection. The importance of experience and clinical judgment in weighing all available data to reach a diagnosis and prescribe appropriate treatment cannot be overemphasized in the field of transplantation, especially when dealing with infants and children.

Biopsies are performed most frequently in the first few months (as often as weekly in the first month) following transplantation because risk of rejection is highest. The length of time between biopsies is gradually increased over the first 2 years. Many programs perform a biopsy on patients once or twice a year for an indefinite period. After patients require treatment for rejection, follow-up biopsies are performed 1 to 2 weeks later to confirm resolution of rejection.[29]

The endomyocardial biopsy involves advancing a bioptome catheter into the right ventricle under fluoroscopy or echocardiographic guidance and obtaining four to five tissue samples for microscopic analysis. The procedure is usually performed on an outpatient basis and takes approximately one-half hour. In most centers, vascular access is through the right internal jugular in all ages. Femoral veins may be used in infants and young children. EMLA cream and local anesthetic are often used at the puncture site. Some older children may cooperate for the procedure without sedation, but most children need some form of procedural sedation. Uncooperative or highly anxious patients may require anesthesia. Pneumothorax and bleeding at the puncture site are possible complications. Damage to the tricuspid valve is possible after multiple biopsies, resulting in a flail tricuspid valve. Perforation of the heart muscle is rare. Overall, the procedure has low associated morbidity.[29]

The endomyocardial biopsy technique and the size of the bioptomes used have been modified so that endomyocardial biopsies can be performed in neonates, as well as in older children. However, endomyocardial biopsy has some disadvantages in children: (1) a sampling error is inherent in the technique; (2) it is an invasive technique, which is more difficult to repeat in young children; and (3) anesthesia is an added risk that is sometimes required. Researchers continue to seek a more reliable, noninvasive test to identify rejection.

Acute rejection, along with infection, remains the leading cause of death in the first year after cardiac transplantation.[19] Despite the initiation of triple-immunosuppression therapy, most patients will have at least one rejection episode, usually within the first 3 months after transplantation. Data from a prospective, multiinstitutional study conducted by the Pediatric Heart Transplant Study Group showed that the peak hazard for first rejection was at 2 months posttransplant, and the actuarial freedom from rejection was 61% at 1 month and 37% at 6 months. Furthermore, the same study showed that although infants younger than 6 months of age had similar rates of rejection compared with older children, the mortality caused by rejection was lower, suggesting that rejection may be a less aggressive process in infants.[35] The critical care nurse plays a vital role in monitoring infants and children for signs of rejection in the early postoperative period. Prompt recognition of rejection and the institution of immunosuppressive therapy increase the likelihood of successful treatment.

Treatment of episodes of rejection usually involves a 3-day pulse of methylprednisolone. If the rejection episode is associated with graft dysfunction or is resistant to steroid treatment, other agents, such as OKT3, are used. Therapy tends to be aggressive because persistent rejection increases the risk for chronic rejection.

Chronic rejection of the cardiac allograft is characterized by posttransplantation coronary artery disease, which represents a growing concern in the long-term survival of pediatric recipients. Pathologic findings in this condition are different from atherosclerotic coronary artery disease. This is a diffuse process of coronary artery luminal narrowing, believed to be immune mediated, resulting in ischemia and ventricular failure. The incidence of coronary artery disease in children is less than adults, but children need to live with the graft for a much longer period, and it may be that the onset of the coronary artery disease is simply delayed. Reviews have estimated the incidence of coronary artery disease in children who have survived 1 year posttransplant as 10% to 30%.[24,36,37] In a multicenter study including 815 patients, 58 had angiographic or autopsy evidence of coronary artery disease, and 49 patients died, including 5 of 10 who had undergone retransplantation.[38] Diagnosis can be difficult, and some patients who die suddenly were found to have coronary disease on autopsy. Coronary angiography is known to be insensitive in diagnosis. Currently, no effective medical therapies are known, and the only treatment is retransplantation.

Organ-Specific Rejection: Lung.   Rejection is common in the early weeks following transplantation. Lung allografts initiate much stronger immune responses than cardiac allografts alone. Rejection of the heart after heart-lung transplantation is unusual; the lung suffers most of the host immune response.[29] In the early period after transplantation, clinical manifestations of lung rejection may include fever, increased work of breathing, new pulmonary infiltrates, and hypoxemia. However, mild or even moderate rejection often is clinically silent or is characterized just by mild dyspnea. Results of plain chest x-ray film and ventilation scans may be completely normal, although in the later stages, some abnormalities caused by alveolar involvement may appear. Radiographically and functionally, alveolar rejection is associated with transplant opacification and decreased ventilation without a corresponding reduction in blood flow.

Bronchiolitis obliterans (obliterative bronchiolitis [OB]) represents chronic rejection of the lung allograft. It is often associated with a history of recurrent acute rejection episodes or sometimes with strong immunologic response to CMV. Onset is usually 6 months to 3 years after transplantation. It manifests as dyspnea with progressive small airway obstruction and decreased function, often refractory to augmented immunosuppression, which ultimately results in respiratory failure. Clinically, the FEV_1 may also decline rapidly and progressively. Secondary infection is common.[32] OB occurs in about 50% of lung transplant recipients by 4 years posttransplantation[28] and becomes the main cause of death after the first year posttransplantation.[29] Diagnosis is based on history, clinical presentation, chest radiographs, and pulmonary function testing.

Definitive diagnosis of lung rejection, essential in asymptomatic rejection, is accomplished by transbronchial biopsy (TBB.) Severity of acute cellular rejection is classified by the amount and distribution of lymphocytic infiltrates around the blood vessels and airways. Sensitivity of TBB in the diagnosis of OB is poor because OB is characterized by fibrous obliteration of small airways and TBB samples from small airways are usually not obtained.[29] Biopsies are performed for routine surveillance for asymptomatic acute rejection and when clinical manifestations of rejection are present. The initial routine biopsy is done before hospital discharge and then every 3 months for 2 years.[29] For long-term monitoring, patients can be provided with a handheld peak flowmeter, which measures peak expiratory flow (PEF). Decreased PEF may be an indicator of chronic rejection (OB). Exercise tolerance is monitored as well; earlier desaturations with exercise may occur with rejection.

Because of the increased incidence of rejection with lung transplantation, children require higher levels of immunosuppression initially, resulting in increased toxicity and other effects from the immunosuppressant drugs. Triple-drug immunosuppression is routinely used, yet early rejection still occurs often. Achieving monotherapy over time in heart transplant patients is more common than in patients who have received lungs.[29] Increased immunosuppression and use of other pharmacologic agents may be successful in treating acute cellular rejection. Augmented immunosuppression is often not effective in treating OB, but it may slow the decline of small airway function. Even though the heart is rarely involved in acute rejection in a heart-lung transplant, the diagnosis of OB presents increased risk for posttransplant coronary artery disease.

Infection.   Infections are one of the leading causes of morbidity and mortality in the immunocompromised child after organ transplantation. The risk of infection is highest in the first few months following transplantation, when immunosuppression is greatest. The incidence of infection has declined in the past decade as a result of the continuous development of new immunosuppressive agents. These agents are very specific in altering the immune response that causes rejection while sparing other immunologic functions that defend against infection. Using these new pharmaceuticals enables the steroid dose to be decreased, reducing the risk of infection. In addition, increased knowledge about posttransplant infections allows improved detection and treatment. Also, the development of more effective antiviral agents has aided in the prevention and treatment of viral infections.

Improvements in the diagnosis and management of rejection have decreased the time interval of intense immunosuppression, which was often associated with infections. It is recognized that the greater the amount and duration of immunosuppression, the greater the likelihood of infection. The following section reviews the risk factors for infection in the child after transplantation; describes the types of infections, their presentation and treatment; and outlines the vital role of the nurse in prevention and surveillance.

Risk factors for infection include the use of intense immunosuppression, host characteristics, and the pediatric intensive care unit (PICU) environment. Immunosuppression is at its highest level in the immediate posttransplant period because this is when the risk of acute rejection is highest. At the present time, all pharmacologic therapies disturb normal immune defenses to some extent; none are specific enough to block only the processes that cause rejection.

Many patients, before transplantation, are immunocompromised secondary to their debilitating chronic illness, poor nutrition, or end-stage organ failure. A weakened host then undergoes a major operation and requires complex postoperative care involving the use of invasive equipment and procedures that further compromise the body's defenses. The presence of an endotracheal tube, multiple invasive lines, catheters, and drainage tubes breach the normal external defense mechanism of the body and carry a risk of infection. The PICU environment also predisposes transplant patients to an infectious risk with exposure to multiple organisms common in the hospital environment and to numerous caregivers. Immunosuppression, a compromised host, and environmental concerns combine to make infection a significant risk for the child recovering from transplantation (see also Chapter 15).

Significant infections occur most often in the first 6 months following transplantation. Specific organisms are typically responsible for infections occurring immediately after transplantation, up to 6 months posttransplant, and after 6 months posttransplant (Table 26-3). Most infections in the first month are nosocomial infections, primarily involving bacteria, and occur as a result of multiple lines and invasive procedures or are related to preexisting disease conditions and surgical manipulation. From 1 month to 6 months, opportunistic infections are most common and may cause significant morbidity and mortality.

Opportunistic infections are caused by organisms common in the environment that rarely cause disease in an immunocompetent host. In the immunosuppressed patient, however, these organisms are capable of causing illness. Infection can also result from exposure to an exogenous source of a virulent pathogen, such as meningococcal

---

◆ TABLE 26-3   Infectious Complications Within the First 180 Days of Transplantation*

Early (0-1 Month)	Middle (0-6 Months)	Late (>6 Months)
Bacterial	**Viral**	**Viral**
Gram-negative enteric bacilli (small bowel, liver, neonatal hearts)	Cytomegalovirus (all transplant types and seronegative recipients of seropositive donors)	Epstein-Barr virus (all transplant types; less than middle period)
Pseudomonas/Burkholderia spp. (lung—cystic fibrosis)	Epstein-Barr virus (all transplant types and seronegative recipients; small bowel—highest risk)	Varicella-zoster virus (all transplant types)
Gram-positive organisms (all transplant types)	Varicella-zoster virus (all transplant types)	Community-acquired viruses (all transplant types)
Fungal	**Opportunistic Organisms**	**Bacterial**
All transplant types	*Pneumocystis carinii* (all transplant types)	*Pseudomonas/Burkholderia* spp. (lung—cystic fibrosis; lung recipients with chronic rejection)
Viral	*Toxoplasma gondii* (seronegative recipient of a seropositive donor heart)	Gram-negative bacillary bacteremia (small bowel)
Herpes simplex (all transplant types)	**Bacterial**	**Fungal**
Nosocomial respiratory (all transplant types)	*Pseudomonas/Burkholderia* spp. (lung—cystic fibrosis)	*Aspergillus* spp. (lung transplants with chronic rejection)
	Pneumonia—gram-negative organisms	

From Green M, Michaels M: Infections in solid organ transplant recipients. In Long SS, Pickery LK, Prober CG, eds: *Principles and practice of pediatric infectious diseases,* New York, 1997, Churchill Livingstone, pp 626-634.
*Infections are listed from most to least common for each time period.

meningitis; reactivation of an organism, such as herpes or CMV; or endogenous invasion of a normally present organism, such as overgrowth of GI flora. Sites of infection after transplant include the lungs, CNS, wounds, skin, mucous membranes, GI tract, and urinary tract.

Bacterial Infections. Bacterial infections are most common in the first month after transplantation and are similar to the organisms found in the postoperative surgical patient. Gram-negative bacilli including *Pseudomonas aeruginosa*, *Proteus* species, *Klebsiella* species, and *Escherichia coli* are common infecting organisms, and both *Staphylococcus epidermidis* and *S. aureus* are seen. Bacterial infections usually arise from organisms already colonizing the patient. Because of a disruption of anatomic and mechanical defense systems, such as the skin, mucous membranes, cilia, and mucosa of the GI tract, bacteria are able to enter the body and cause infection. Common types of bacterial infections are pneumonia, wound infections, line sepsis, and urinary tract infections.

Unusual bacterial infections include *Legionella*, an aquatic organism that causes pneumonia, and *Nocardia*, commonly present in soil and decaying matter that enters the body by inhalation and can cause pneumonia and infections of the CNS. Both are often associated with environmental hazards, such as construction or contamination in air filtration systems.

Most surgical patients receive prophylactic antibiotics at the time of surgery and for a short period after surgery to prevent bacterial infection. The antibiotic chosen is a broad-spectrum agent effective against the common organisms causing wound infections in a particular healthcare setting. Prolonged use of prophylactic antibiotics raises concerns about the growth of antibiotic-resistant bacteria and fungi. Equally important in the prevention of bacterial infections is removal of all invasive monitoring lines, tubes, and catheters as soon as possible.

Viral Infections. Viruses comprise an important group of infecting organisms after transplantation and include herpes simplex viruses, varicella-zoster, CMV, EBV, hepatitis virus, and the human immunodeficiency virus (HIV). Viral infections can be primary or secondary. Primary infections are caused the first time the individual is exposed to the organism, including those that can be transmitted from donor to recipient. A secondary infection is a reactivation of the virus. Infants and young children are more likely to have primary infections, whereas adolescents and adults are more likely to have been exposed to most common viruses and have a reactivation of a previous infection. Prospective recipients and donors are carefully screened for negative titers to the more common viral agents to assist with the prevention of infection.

Herpes simplex viruses are divided into two types: HSV-1 is responsible for most herpes infections above the waist, most commonly of the lips, face, and mouth; HSV-2 is responsible for herpes genitalia. HSV-1 infections are usually acquired during childhood and establish a permanent residence in most hosts. Herpes genitalia is acquired through sexual activity.

HSV-1 is usually a localized infection of recurrent vesicles and low ulcerations on the lips and oral mucosa. It can be diagnosed by its classic appearance, but viral cultures provide the definitive diagnosis. HSV-1 infection is common in the first month following transplantation. Treatment of both HSV-1 and HSV-2 infections is with acyclovir.

Varicella-zoster can be a dangerous infection for children recovering from transplantation. Immunization before transplantation may be helpful in prevention of active disease later. Outbreaks of chickenpox are common in childhood, and transplant patients may be exposed many times. The disease is likely to be more virulent in the immunocompromised host and can cause pneumonitis and significant respiratory compromise. Children may be given varicella immune globulin (VZIg) upon exposure to provide them with antibodies to fight the disease. Treatment of active infection is with IV acyclovir and reduction of immunosuppressant drug dosages in severe cases.

CMV is a significant viral infection that occurs after transplantation. Infection with CMV can be a primary infection in which a seronegative recipient receives a CMV-positive blood transfusion, a CMV-positive donor organ, or is exposed to infected individuals. Reactivated, or secondary, infection occurs when a seropositive patient then becomes immunosuppressed. Primary infections appear to be associated with more serious and symptomatic morbidity and may vary in intensity with the organ transplanted. CMV is associated with rejection or acute glomerular injury in renal transplants and with hepatitis and hepatic failure in liver transplant recipients.

CMV is also a significant pathogen following thoracic organ transplantation. There appears to be an association between CMV and accelerated development of arterial atherosclerosis in cardiac transplant recipients.[39] Generally, CMV infection is more of a problem in lung recipients than in heart recipients.[29]

The symptoms and severity of CMV infection are variable. Patients who are most susceptible are seronegative and receive a seropositive organ, have prolonged fever and hematologic abnormalities, or have intense immunosuppressive therapy. Infection usually occurs 1 to 3 months posttransplantation. Common clinical findings include prolonged (may be high-grade) fever and hematologic abnormalities, including leukopenia, thrombocytopenia, and atypical lymphocytosis. Some patients may present with malaise, anorexia, myalgias, and arthralgias. Disseminated disease can affect many organ systems, including the lung, liver, pancreas, kidneys, stomach, intestine, and brain, and is associated with significant mortality. CMV was traditionally regarded as the major infectious agent to complicate transplantation. However, the introduction and effectiveness of prophylactic use of ganciclovir (DHPG), a derivative of acyclovir, has resulted in a dramatic decrease in morbidity related to CMV.

Diagnosis is based on clinical presentation and confirmed through viral culture, serology, and histology.[40] CMV-pp65 is a rapid diagnostic method currently used that detects CMV-specific antigens in peripheral polymorphonuclear cells with a mixture of monoclonal antibodies.[41]

In addition to infection with CMV, transplant patients may develop superinfections, most often in the lung. CMV infection has been shown to suppress cell-mediated immunity, further impairing the body's ability to fight infection. Superinfections with opportunistic organisms such as *P. carinii* may occur simultaneously.

Ganciclovir has led to improved outcomes for CMV-infected patients, with a clinical response evident 5 to 7 days after initiation of therapy.[42] Because of the high morbidity and mortality associated with CMV infection following transplant and, until recently, a lack of treatment for the disease, there is much interest in preventing the infection. The use of acyclovir for CMV prophylaxis with high-dose oral therapy is supported in some protocols. The efficacy of prophylactic use of CMV immune globulin in patients who are seronegative and receive a seropositive organ has been demonstrated.

EBV presents as a continuum of illness, and benign symptoms may progress to more serious syndromes. EBV is known to cause mild infections similar to mononucleosis in patients following transplantation and more serious EBV-associated malignant lymphoma (Burkitt's lymphoma), but, most importantly, it is the major risk factor for the development of PTLD months to years after organ transplantation. PTLD represents a spectrum of diseases characterized by the EBV-driven B lymphocyte proliferation ranging from a mononucleosis-like illness to monoclonal B cell lymphoma.[43]

EBV disease is diagnosed in pediatric solid organ recipients via clinical history and physical examination findings in combination with laboratory confirmation.[44] Risk factors include young age, EBV seronegative status before transplantation of an organ from a seropositive donor, and multiple episodes of rejection requiring treatment. The child may have a history of lethargy or malaise usually associated with febrile periods and anemia. Diarrhea (which may be guaiac positive), protein-losing enteropathy, and weight loss may suggest GI involvement. Patients may be asymptomatic but more often present with findings of peripheral adenopathy, hepatosplenomegaly, or exudative tonsillitis. Less often, children present with neurologic symptoms indicating CNS involvement.[44]

Early diagnosis is vital for effective treatment. Diagnosis is based on clinical manifestations, histopathology, laboratory studies, and radiographic findings. Radiologic examinations (including computed tomography) of the chest and abdomen are performed to evaluate enlarged lymph nodes and to look for occult foci of the EBV disease. Pulmonary nodules are the most common macroscopic finding in heart and heart-lung recipients.[29] Biopsy is done if the lesion is safely accessible to provide information on histology. Laboratory data using the EBER-1 probe, which labels EBV-encoded RNA in infected cells, is the most reliable histologic stain for diagnosis of EBV infection. EBV titers are not specific for active EBV disease. Some children who were seronegative before transplant will have positive EBV titers related to passive immunization with blood products.

The EBV-PCR (polymerase chain reaction) is a blood test that identifies increased levels of circulating EBV-infected lymphocytes or EBV viral load. This test shows promise in predicting risk of EBV infection before clinical disease and in detecting disease in patients with symptomatic presentation. Elevated viral load in combination with typical EBV symptoms appears to be diagnostic of EBV disease and PTLD.[44] However, use of the EBV viral load is limited, in that the viral load may be comparable in children with EBV viral infections to those with EBV-PTLD and some children may have an elevated viral load without signs of active infection.[44]

Starzl was the first to suggest withdrawal or reduction in the patient's immunosuppression in the 1980s. Since that time, it has become standard in the treatment of patients with PTLD and is often effective. However, rebound rejection may then occur. Beyond the temporary discontinuation or drastic reduction of the immunosuppressive therapy, the optimal management of EBV disease and PTLD in the solid organ transplant remains controversial and varies among centers. Depending on the transplant center and individual strategies, other treatments include antiviral therapies (e.g., acyclovir or ganciclovir), antibody therapies (e.g., IVIg, CMV-IVIg [Cytogam]), interferon (may induce aggressive rejection), radiation, chemotherapy, and surgical resection of tumors in localized disease. Rituximab, a genetically engineered, anti-CD20 monoclonal antibody, is indicated for the treatment of certain CD-20 positive, B cell non-Hodgkin's lymphomas and may prove effective in treating CD20-positive, B cell PTLD.

Fungal Infections. The most common fungal infections following transplantation are those caused by the *Candida* species of organisms; these infections occur in the mouth, GI tract, and vagina. Oral candidiasis, known as thrush, is a common infection in infants and also prevalent in immunocompromised patients and those receiving broad-spectrum antibiotics. Thrush appears as wet, white lesions on the tongue and mucous membranes of the mouth, which are painful and can impair oral nutritional intake. The infection can spread through the GI tract, causing esophagitis, and can cause a *Candida* diaper rash. Transplant patients often receive the topical antifungal drug nystatin prophylactically to prevent *Candida* infections. Vaginal infections caused by *Candida* present symptoms of itching, irritation, and a malodorous white discharge. The offending organism must be identified through appropriate diagnostic tests because *Trichomonas* has a similar presentation. The treatment of choice is clotrimazole suppositories.

Candida can become disseminated throughout the body, usually through the GI mucosa, and cause serious infection. The diagnosis can be difficult, and signs and symptoms include a disseminated rash and swollen tender muscles, persistent fever, eye pain, and eventual signs of CNS disease. Treatment involves administration of IV antifungal agents.

Several unusual fungal infections can present later in the posttransplant period and are generally community acquired. All have an insidious onset and are difficult to diagnose. *Aspergillus* can cause pneumonia, pulmonary infarction, GI bleeding, and brain abscesses. *Cryptococcus* enters the body through the lungs and disseminates to the

CNS. Coccidioidomycosis disseminates to the lungs, CNS, joints, and liver. Histoplasmosis causes disease in lungs and CNS, liver, spleen, and lymph nodes. All these fungal infections are treated with systemic antifungal agents.

Parasitic Infections. The most common parasitic infections seen after transplantation are pneumonia caused by *Pneumocystis carinii* (PCP) and infections with toxoplasmosis. Symptoms of *Pneumocystis* include an abrupt onset of dyspnea, cough, hypoxemia, and fever. Bilateral alveolar infiltrates are seen on chest x-ray film, and definitive diagnosis is made with bronchoalveolar lavage or transbronchial biopsy. Treatment is with IV trimethoprim-sulfamethoxazole (Bactrim) or IV pentamidine. Prophylaxis is maintained as long as necessary. When immunosuppressive therapy is significantly decreased, prophylaxis may be decreased or eliminated. If patients are allergic to trimethoprim, they may be able to be desensitized or may receive pentamidine inhalation therapy once per month.

Management of Infections. The critical care nurse plays a vital role in the assessment of transplant patients for infection. All caregivers must have a very high index of suspicion for infection in this patient population. Signs of infection may be subtle; may be masked by the use of immunosuppressive agents, especially steroids; or may be confused with rejection or other problems. An aggressive approach to diagnosis is warranted because the consequences of untreated infection can be life threatening.

A complete head-to-toe physical assessment specifically focused on possible signs or symptoms of infection should be performed daily. All fevers should be taken seriously, although many serious infections may present with little or no fever. Complaints of headache, subtle mental status changes, and fever are important signs of potential CNS infection. Assessment of mental status, evidence of impairment of cranial nerves or sensory or motor function, and the presence of meningeal signs are all critical elements of a neurologic assessment. The mouth, tongue, and oral mucosa should be carefully examined for evidence of thrush or herpetic lesions. The lymph node chains of the head and neck should be examined for signs of infection and inflammation. Alterations in respiratory function can be key signs of an infectious process, especially because pneumonia is a common type of infection following transplantation. Tachypnea, dyspnea, cough, labored respirations, retractions, hypoxia, and rales and rhonchi on auscultation are all important observations. Tachycardia, pulsus paradoxus, a new murmur, and signs of pericardial effusion can sometimes be associated with an infectious process. Abdominal distension, cramping and pain, nausea, vomiting, diarrhea, and changes in the stool may be a result of infection. Cloudy urine, burning on urination, or a change in the frequency of urination may suggest a urinary tract infection. Pain or inflammation of the joints should be noted. All skin surfaces and mucous membranes should be examined closely for any signs of infection.

Preventing infection is a critical nursing responsibility. Isolation techniques after transplantation vary between institutions and organ types, but the mainstay of all prevention is good handwashing. A recent study comparing strict handwashing to gown and glove isolation techniques in children undergoing solid organ transplantation reported a significant decrease in nosocomial acquisition of infections in both the handwashing group and the gown and glove isolation group, despite an infection rate in the overall PICU population that was not significantly different from the year before the study throughout the year following the study.[45] These data indicate that some infections may be preventable in the solid organ transplantation population and that implementation of interventions that may prevent nosocomial acquisition of organisms is beneficial to patients. Surveillance of visitors and caregivers to prevent contact with anyone actively infected and to observe for breaks in handwashing technique is important. All invasive lines are cared for with aseptic technique and discontinued as soon as possible. Patients are extubated as early as possible, and aggressive pulmonary toilet is carried out. Early ambulation is an important goal. Meticulous skin and mouth care are crucial to prevent further breaks in the body's defensive barrier. The physical environment is kept clean. The importance of nutritional status in preventing and treating infection is recognized.

Decreased Cardiac Output Related to Ventricular Dysfunction. Ventricular dysfunction leading to low cardiac output after cardiac transplantation can be caused by several factors. An ischemic injury to the donor heart causing poor contractility can occur during retrieval, during the cold ischemic time while the heart is being transported, or during the implantation. Inadequate preservation and prolonged ischemia times (longer than 6 hours) can contribute to global ventricular dysfunction, although long ischemia times have not been correlated with increased early mortality.[46] Ventricular dysfunction can be acute and present in the operating room with poor cardiac effort, difficulty weaning from bypass, and increased filling pressures. More common is worsening ventricular function over 1 to 3 days postoperatively with low cardiac output, fluid overload, and ventricular dilation.

Treatment includes optimizing inotropic support, aggressive use of vasodilators, and measures to reduce PVR, including use of nitric oxide. Ultrafiltration or dialysis may be needed early after transplantation to manage fluid overload and acute renal dysfunction caused by low cardiac output and the nephrotoxic effects of cyclosporine or tacrolimus. Assist devices such as extracorporeal membrane oxygenation (ECMO) or left ventricular assist devices (LVADs) should be considered for acute ventricular dysfunction when elevated PVR and other organ dysfunction is thought to be reversible.

Decreased Cardiac Output Related to Increased Pulmonary Vascular Resistance. Increased PVR in the heart or heart-lung recipient resulting from long-standing congestive heart failure before transplantation can cause acute right ventricular failure in the immediate postoperative period. The donor heart, already stressed by a period of cold arrest and cardiopulmonary bypass, must attempt to pump against elevated PVR and may not be able to meet the challenge. Right ventricular dilation and signs of right-sided heart failure ensue with elevated right atrial pressures, tachycardia, dilated neck veins, hepatomegaly, pericardial and pleural effusions, a gallop rhythm or tricuspid regurgitation murmur, and marked right ventricular dysfunction on echocardiography.

Early and aggressive treatment to decrease PVR is critical after transplant to limit right ventricular distension and dysfunction. Patients who are known to have a high PVR before transplant have usually been tested in the catheterization laboratory for their response to drug therapy, oxygen, and nitric oxide. Therapy is begun in the operating room or early in the postoperative period to keep pulmonary pressures as low as possible. Afterload reducers, such as amrinone or milrinone, nitroprusside, and possibly prostaglandins, are used along with inotropic agents. Nitric oxide is increasingly used in this setting. Other measures to reduce PVR include sedation with or without chemical paralysis, careful suctioning, good pulmonary toilet to prevent atelectasis, and avoidance of acidosis and hyperventilation. Nursing interventions to decrease cardiac workload include maintaining normal temperature, ensuring adequate pain control, reducing environmental stressors, providing emotional support to decrease anxiety, providing proper nutrition, and ensuring adequate rest.

Decreased Cardiac Output Related to Bleeding, Hypovolemia, or Hypothermia.

Postoperative mediastinal bleeding and the risk of cardiac tamponade are of particular concern after heart or heart-lung transplantation. The native pericardium is often stretched by severe cardiac dilation. The donor heart may be smaller than the patient's native heart, resulting in a large potential space in the pericardial sac. Blood can easily accumulate and may contribute to hypovolemia, decreased cardiac output, and possible tamponade. Patients may also bleed in the absence of a stretched pericardium. Chest tube drainage is closely monitored, and measures to ensure adequate drainage of the mediastinum are followed. Coagulopathies are monitored and corrected. The patient is closely observed for signs of tamponade, and prompt treatment is instituted if tamponade is suspected. Reoperation for bleeding is sometimes necessary.

Hypovolemia and hypothermia are commonly seen following cardiopulmonary bypass and may contribute to decreased contractility in the newly transplanted heart. Careful assessment of fluid balance and temperature is followed by appropriate fluid replacement and rewarming.

Decreased Cardiac Output Related to Alterations in Heart Rate and/or Rhythm.

Change in heart rate because of denervation of the donor heart and rhythm disturbances may also lead to alterations in cardiac output after transplantation. Because nervous system connections to the heart are permanently severed during transplantation, there is no autonomic control of heart rate. In the absence of parasympathetic control, the resting heart rate is elevated. The Valsalva maneuver and carotid massage are no longer effective following transplantation. The sympathetic nervous system normally acts to increase heart rate. Loss of sympathetic control impairs the ability to respond quickly to the need for increased cardiac output. Slower mechanisms that increase cardiac output include the Starling response,

which increases stroke volume in response to increase in venous return and the release of endogenous catecholamines with both inotropic and chronotropic properties. Changes in heart rate in response to increased metabolic demands such as fever or exercise occur more slowly and depend on an appropriate circulating blood volume to provide adequate preload and normal contractility. The absence of a normal compensatory reflex tachycardia may cause orthostatic hypotension because of venous pooling. Vasodilation (especially resulting from vasodilating drugs or rewarming early postoperatively) may lead to hypotension and a rapid decrease in cardiac output because of reduced preload or decreased afterload.

Medications that act on the autonomic nervous system are ineffective. Digoxin loses much of its influence on heart rate and rhythm but may be a useful inotropic agent and may slow the sinus node. Atropine has no effect on heart rate in the transplanted heart. Adenosine may have a more profound effect, so a lower dose is used initially. Calcium channel blockers such as verapamil, which have negative inotropic effects, are used cautiously. Because β-blockers inhibit circulating catecholamines, which are important in increasing heart rate in the transplanted heart, they may blunt the heart rate response and are used with caution.

The ECG following cardiac transplantation will demonstrate two P waves representing both the donor sinoatrial (SA) node and the recipient SA node, if the recipient's wall of the right atrium containing the SA node remains in place (Fig. 26-2). (This will not occur if the recipient's right atrium is removed during transplantation.) Because the impulse from the recipient SA node cannot cross the suture line, there is no further stimulation of the conduction system or cardiac contraction. The donor SA node initiates the electrical stimulation through the conduction system, which results in contraction.

Dysrhythmias are often seen in the early postoperative period. After cardiac transplantation, children depend on an adequate heart rate to maintain cardiac output; therefore any dysrhythmia can have a negative consequence on cardiac output. Bradydysrhythmias may be due to SA node dysfunction related to surgical trauma or ischemic injury during preservation. These difficulties usually resolve with time. Use of a temporary external pacemaker or continuous intravenous isoproterenol will provide a faster heart rate and enhance cardiac output. Ventricular and supraventricular tachydysrhythmias may occasionally be seen and are more difficult to manage. Pharmacologic therapy is limited because the heart is denervated. Tachycardia limits the use of many inotropic agents, and the negative inotropic effects of most antidysrhythmics can have a deleterious effect on contractility in the early postoperative period. Drug therapy is used cautiously. Overdrive pacing or cardioversion may be used as alternatives. The development of arrhythmias after the first week posttransplant may be an early symptom of rejection.

Prevention of Ventilation/Perfusion Mismatch.

Pulmonary perfusion and ventilation are closely monitored in the postoperative period for patients who have received a heart-lung or single- or double-lung transplants. Pulmonary

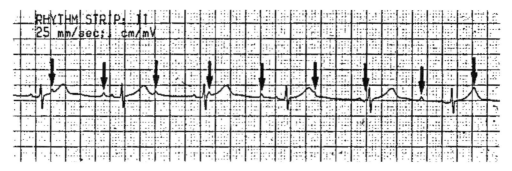

Fig. 26-2   Rhythm strip after cardiac transplant. Arrows indicate recipient's native (but unconducted) P waves.

perfusion can be assessed by monitoring end-tidal CO_2. Ventilation can be assessed through evaluation of breath sounds and arterial blood gases. To improve perfusion to the transplanted lung, patients may be positioned with the operative side down, as flow is related to gravity. Ventilation to transplanted lungs can be enhanced by positioning the isolated transplanted lung up. Variable positions may be effective in improving ventilation, as airflow is compliance dependent. If unilateral pulmonary edema is present, positioning the patient affected side down will help to optimize arterial blood gases. When gases have improved, repositioning frequently will help to maintain ventilation.

Frequent assessment of airway clearance and provision of thorough pulmonary toilet are essential. Suctioning is only done above the level of the anastomosis. The patient's ability to cough and clear the airway, chest x-ray film, breath sounds, and characteristics of the sputum are used to guide pulmonary care. Increased FIO_2 may be required to facilitate pulmonary care. Incentive spirometer or other aids may help in normalizing pulmonary function.

Alteration in Comfort.   Postoperative pain management is essential to allow the child to gradually assume independent airway control and ventilation. Pain medication and alternative therapies (e.g., epidural catheters) are provided in addition to supporting the parents' coping and their ability to comfort their child. Providing rest periods and a semblance of day-night cycling help to promote sleep. Although isolation rooms are not required, placement of the patient in a private room may be helpful both in the prevention of infection and in providing a quiet, more restful environment.

LIVER TRANSPLANTATION

Liver transplantation for children with end-stage liver disease is currently available in many centers worldwide. Approximately 400 children undergo liver transplantation each year. Since 1983, liver transplantation has been recognized as a nonexperimental treatment option for children with end-stage liver disease. In the precyclosporine era, 5-year survival statistics for children treated with azathioprine were a dismal 30%.[1] With advances in preservation methods, refined surgical techniques, and improved immunosuppression protocols, some centers are reporting better than 90% 1-year survival rates.

Indications for pediatric liver transplantation include biliary atresia, metabolic diseases (α_1-antitrypsin deficiency, tyrosinemia), familial cholestasis (Byler's disease, Indian childhood cirrhosis, Alagille's syndrome), fulminant hepatic failure, biliary hypoplasia, infectious hepatitis, idiopathic cirrhosis, neonatal hepatitis, sclerosing cholangitis, congenital hepatic fibrosis, and carcinomas such as hepatoma and hepatoblastoma. Biliary atresia is the most common indication for liver transplantation in the child (over 50% of the cases per center).

The UNOS system for classifying liver transplant candidates by status has three categories.[4] Patients may be assigned to status I (highest priority) when they are being cared for in the intensive care unit and have a life expectancy (without transplantation) of less than 7 days or are hospitalized with OTC deficiency or Crigler-Najjar disease type I. In addition, status I patients must have at least one of the following criteria: fulminant hepatic failure, mechanical ventilation, continuing or recurrent upper GI bleeding, stage III or IV encephalopathy, refractory ascites or hepatohydrothorax, biliary sepsis requiring vasopressor support, primary nonfunction or hepatic artery thrombosis of a graft, acute decompensated Wilson's disease, or hepatorenal syndrome. Status IIB patients must have documented, unresponsive GI bleeding, hepatorenal syndrome, bacterial peritonitis, refractory ascites or hepatohydrothorax, recurrent cholangitis, growth failure, ornithine transcarbamoylase (OTC) deficiency, or Crigler-Najjar disease type I. All other patients are listed as status III.

Although the number of livers available to be transplanted has remained about the same in recent years, the number of UNOS-listed patients continues to climb every year.[47] The shortage of pediatric-sized organs and concerns related to preventing unnecessary deaths has led researchers to explore methods for expanding the donor pool.[47] Deviations from the standard orthotopic liver transplantation procedure have been developed by producing volume-reduced grafts based on segmental anatomy. These modifications are referred to as technical-variant liver transplantation. Currently, four procedures are being practiced for liver grafts, including the standard orthotopic whole liver transplant, reduced-sized liver transplantation (RSLT), split-liver transplantation (SLT), and living-related transplantation (LRT). The use of University of Wisconsin (UW) solution has lengthened acceptable cold preservation time to 18 to 24 hours, providing recovering surgical teams additional time required to prepare recovered organs for RSLT and SLT procedures.[48] All of these procedures are orthotopic procedures, which means replacement of the native liver with the allograft. Back table preparation of the newly recovered liver includes identifying vessels, reducing graft size, and sending tissue for pathology examination of graft quality before the recipient operation.

Liver Transplantation Procedures

The *standard orthotopic liver transplant* procedure involves removal of the diseased organ and replacement with a donor organ in three stages: recipient hepatectomy phase, anhepatic phase (recipient liver is removed and graft is implanted), and reperfusion phase (achievement of hemostasis and reconstruction of the hepatic artery and biliary tract). After the child has been anesthetized and positioned, a bilateral subcostal incision with xiphoid extension and removal of the xiphoid process are performed. The suprahepatic inferior vena cava (IVC), the infrahepatic IVC, the portal vein, the hepatic artery, and, when present, the common bile duct are isolated and then clamped, after which the native liver is removed. This begins the anhepatic phase, which ends when the donor liver is reperfused. For children over 25 to 30 kg, venovenous bypass is sometimes used to provide more stability during the anhepatic phase.[48] As an alternative, vena cava flow can be preserved by ligating the hepatic veins individually and preserving the vena cava for segmental or "piggyback" implantation.[48]

During the hepatectomy and anhepatic phases of a standard transplant, four vascular anastomoses are completed: (1) suprahepatic IVC, (2) infrahepatic IVC, (3) portal vein, and (4) hepatic artery. After completion of the infrahepatic IVC anastomosis, the donor liver is flushed with cold lactated Ringer's solution to remove air and the preservation solution. The reperfusion phase occurs once the portal vein anastomosis is completed and portal venous blood flow is reestablished to the graft. A color change in the allograft can be observed. Patchy areas of poorly perfused parenchyma may persist until the hepatic artery anastomosis is completed. Hemostasis is achieved during this operative phase by suture ligation and cautery.[48]

Currently, transplantation of the liver in children is done most often using a procedure called the piggyback hepatectomy, whereby the recipient's IVC is preserved. The native liver is removed with preservation of the recipient IVC. The graft is connected to a confluence of recipient hepatic veins (end-to-side "piggyback" to the skeletonized recipient vena cava) and then to the arterio-aortic anastomosis.

After arterial reconstruction, biliary anastomosis is done. Biliary reconstruction in pediatric recipients is typically performed with a Roux-en-Y limb of intestine (choledocho-

jejunostomy), as the patient's native bile duct is usually absent or inadequate in most children undergoing transplant. In children with an adequate common bile duct, duct-to-duct anastomosis may occur using a T tube to stent the bile duct of the recipient. Vascular anomalies may require complex arterial reconstructions or interposition grafts to the aorta. Jackson-Pratt drains are placed under the diaphragm, and the incision is then closed.

RSLTs involve cutting a whole liver and using the left lobe for pediatric recipients. Although RSLT provides an appropriate-size graft for the pediatric population, it does not increase the number of recipients. Reducing the size simply transfers it from the adult recipient pool to the pediatric pool without increasing the overall supply of organs.

The first transplantation with a reduced-size donor organ liver graft was performed by Bismuth and Houssin in 1984.[49] The procedure requires two surgical teams: one to perform the graft reduction and one to perform the recipient hepatectomy. Preparation of the graft involves dissection of the bile duct system, followed by the hepatic artery, portal vein, and hepatic veins. The recipient procedure parallels standard orthotopic liver transplantation, except when there is significant disproportion in donor organ size, in which case the recipient IVC is preserved and the donor liver is placed in a "piggyback" position with only one caval anastomosis to the recipient hepatic veins.[48]

The *SLT* technique evolved from reduced-size liver transplants. The first SLTs occurred in 1988 simultaneously in the United States and Europe.[50] Initial results were discouraging, and the procedure was almost abandoned; however, the European clinicians continued to modify their techniques. The advances included improved microsurgical techniques using high magnification to repair blood vessels and radiologic assessment of the graft using dyes to facilitate the mapping of the vessels. Livers may be removed from the donor and split into the right and left lobes or split in situ in the donor. The right side of the liver is almost always large enough for an adult recipient, and the smaller left side is given to the pediatric recipient. The donor liver graft is prepared in the recipient operating room, where hepatic resection is performed through the principal fissure between the right and left lobes. The right lobe graft is identical to that prepared for a reduced-sized graft, retaining the portal vein and hepatic artery. The left lobe graft usually requires vascular interposition grafts.[50]

LRT has evolved from the SLT procedure. Using a living donor increases the donor pool of available organ segments and allows intense and thorough evaluation of the donor organ, thereby reducing the risk of graft nonfunction.[5] The donor (usually a parent) undergoes a left lateral segment hepatectomy, which is prepared as in SLT. Implantation of the graft is similar to the split-liver procedure (Fig. 26-3). The procedure usually requires venous grafts to bridge the gap between the donor and recipient hepatic arteries and portal veins.[48] The donor evaluation is usually conducted by a physician who is not a member of the transplantation team.

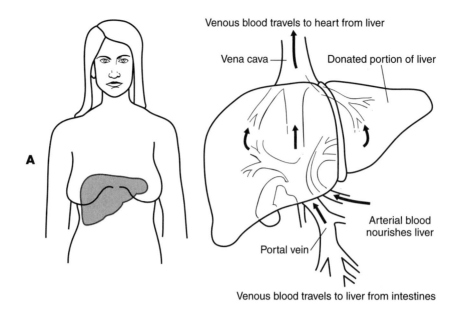

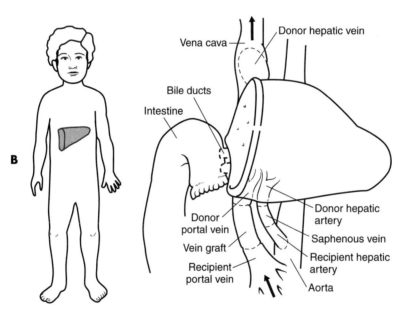

Fig. 26-3 Living donor liver transplant procedures. **A,** Left lateral segment of donor is divided at the falciform ligament. Left hepatic vein and short segments of left portal vein (or branch) and left hepatic artery (or branch) are transected. **B,** To provide tension-free vascular anastomoses, parenteral or cryopreserved donor veins are used as the portal vein and hepatic artery. Orientation of grafts with choledochojejunostomy on the right is similar to cadaveric segmental implants. (From Colombani P: Liver transplantation. In O'Neill JA, Rowe MI, Grosfeld JL et al, eds: *Pediatric surgery,* St Louis, 1998, Mosby, p 598.)

The initial screening includes a comprehensive assessment of the potential donor and morphologic assessment of the potential graft, including informed consent, medical and psychiatric examinations, computed tomography volumetrics, and arteriography.[48]

Living-related grafts have been used most often as primary grafts for stable (non-PICU patients) recipients under the age of 1 year. Segmental grafts have had outcomes comparable with size-matched whole pediatric liver grafts for survival rates.[51] In a consecutive series of 97 pediatric recipients, no differences were seen in patient and graft survival observed between patients who received a standard, full-size graft and those who received a technical-variant transplantation. However, those with technical-variant grafts experienced more biliary complications, increased sepsis, and higher postoperative intervention rates.[52] The regenerative capacity of the liver is such that the donor liver is restored to its ideal mass in about 6 weeks.[47] A significant consideration in the use of living-related grafts is the inherent risk of death for the donor. In many centers, the frequency of LRTs has decreased with the increase in success of SLTs.[50]

Postoperative Care Following Liver Transplantation

A preliminary nursing assessment is completed before admitting the patient to the PICU. This assessment includes an evaluation of preexisting disease factors and significant psychosocial information. At the time of transplant, the child may have numerous physical signs and symptoms, including bleeding, severe ascites, pruritus, hepatorenal syndrome, malnutrition, and hepatic encephalopathy. Knowledge of the child's developmental status and family dynamics at the time of transplant assist with meeting identified psychosocial needs.

The admission process for the postoperative liver transplant patient is similar to patients with any major abdominal surgical procedure. Isolation procedures are required only with those patients known to have preexisting, colonized, drug-resistant body flora (e.g., methicillin-resistant *S. aureus* [MRSA], vancomycin-resistant enterococcus [VRE]). Standard PICU monitoring is used. A central line is used to continuously monitor central venous pressure (CVP); PA catheters are infrequently inserted.

"Liver ABCs" are completed first. *A* is for aeration. As with any patient, airway management is the first priority. All patients will return to the PICU intubated and supported on a ventilator. *B* is for blood pressure. A cuff blood pressure check is a priority; hypertension or hypotension is a common postoperative assessment finding. *C* is for coagulopathies. All drains and incision sites are carefully assessed for bleeding. The patient's prothrombin time (PT), partial thromboplastin time (PTT), and platelet counts are assessed at admission.

Coagulopathies and technical aspects of liver transplantation can precipitate the need for massive intraoperative transfusions. The lengthy 4- to 18-hour operation, or the use of massive volume exchange, and prolonged bowel exposure can predispose the patient to hypothermia. Normothermia can be achieved with heating lamps or a warming blanket.

After the liver ABCs, a quick system check is performed. The incision and Jackson-Pratt drainage are assessed. The incision is often covered with an occlusive dressing. The dressing should be dry and intact. The patient returns from the operating room with Jackson-Pratt drains in place, strategically positioned to prevent or allow early recognition of complications. The lateral drain on the right side of the patient is placed posteriorly in the right subdiaphragmatic space. This drain allows the dome of the right lobe to seal against the diaphragm. The second drain on the right is placed under the right hepatic lobe, leading up to the area of the bile duct anastomoses. This drain allows the assessment of a bile leak. The third drain, on the patient's left side, is positioned in the posterior aspect of the left subdiaphragmatic space. Initially, drainage is bloody. Later, unusual bloody drainage could be observed in any of the Jackson-Pratt drains. Drains are emptied every 2 hours. The

hematocrit of the drain contents is checked if drainage is excessive.

Laboratory tests are drawn expediently. Routine laboratory tests include hematology studies, a coagulation profile, electrolytes, liver function tests, and an arterial blood gas. A chest radiograph is obtained as well.

The admitting nurse receives a complete report from anesthesia. The report includes organ ischemic time, the length of surgery, current laboratory values, and a summary of the operative course, including complications. The intraoperative use of venovenous bypass is included in the operative report. If a reduction hepatectomy was performed, assessment for signs of increased bleeding, biliary fistulas, and infection from the raw surface is appropriate because the incidence of these complications is greater with reduced-sized grafts.[52] If a LRT is performed, the nurse should receive information about the donor's condition.

The most significant and life-threatening immediate complication that can occur is primary nonfunction of the graft. Poor initial function may be associated with a phenomenon called primary graft dysfunction from ischemia-reperfusion injury in the donor organ during the preservation period. In some of these cases of primary graft failure, an urgent need arises for retransplantation.

Report on the visible condition of the liver is useful information. The allograft should change from a pale tan color to reddish-brown after anastomoses are complete. After the arterial grafts are anastomosed, bile production should occur. If hyperbilirubinemia exists preoperatively, the urine appears dark orange in the early postoperative period. The presence of these signs are excellent early prognostic indicators of graft function.

For the first 5 consecutive days after placement, graft function is assessed by ultrasound and liver biopsy (when necessary). The ultrasound is used to assess vessel patency and bile duct dilation. Concern is raised if the resistive index of the hepatic artery is estimated to be less than 0.5 on ultrasound. Other signs of poor graft function may include hypotension, hyperkalemia, hypoglycemia, coagulopathies, and decreased level of consciousness.

Liver function tests are helpful in assessing graft function as well (Table 26-4). Alanine aminotransferase (ALT), which is present in liver, kidney, heart, and skeletal tissue, should be less than 40 in children. Increased ALT may indicate acute hepatic rejection. Elevated aspartate aminotransferase (AST) (present in liver, heart, kidney, pancreas, and brain tissue) may indicate ischemic injury, such as that occurring with hepatic artery thrombosis. AST is the last enzyme level to return to normal following injury. γ-Glutamyl transpeptidase (GGTP), present in liver, kidney, prostrate, and spleen tissue, is normally less than 44 in children. Elevation of GGTP may indicate bile duct obstruction. Alkaline phosphatase (ALP) varies with age because of increases during periods of rapid growth but may also indicate hepatobiliary tract obstruction if elevated. Because bilirubin is metabolized in the liver, elevations of total bilirubin indicate liver disease or bile duct obstruction. (See further discussion of liver failure and liver function testing in Chapter 22.)

TABLE 26-4   Liver Function Tests

Biochemical Indices	Newborn/Infant Values	Child Values
Alanine amino-transferase (ALT)/(SGPT)	<50 IU/L	<40 IU/L
Aspartate amino-transferase (AST)/(SGOT)	<50 IU/L	<40 IU/L
Alkaline phospha-tase (ALP)	Newborn: <310 IU/L 1 mo-1yr: <360 IU/L	1-9 yr: <290 IU/L 10-14 yr: <400 IU/L >14 yr: <125 IU/L
γ-Glutamyl transpeptidase (GGTP)	<120 IU/L	<44 IU/L
Ammonia	42-51 μmol/L	9-38 μmol/L
Direct bilirubin	0.0-0.6 mg/dl	0.0-0.3 mg/dl
Total bilirubin	1-12 mg/dl	0.2-1.3 mg/dl
Prothrombin time (PT or protime)		10-12.8 seconds
Activated partial thromboplastin time (APTT or PTT)		24.4-33.2 seconds
Total protein	4.4-7.3 g/dl	6-8 g/dl
Albumin	2.9-5.5 g/dl	3.8-5.4 g/dl

From UPMC Health System, Department of Pathology: *Laboratory information manual,* Pittsburgh, 1998, Clinical Laboratories.
SGPT, Serum glutamic-pyruvic transaminase; *SGOT,* serum glutamic-oxaloacetic transaminase.

With a well-functioning graft, the patient may be normotensive or hypertensive. Laboratory values may reveal normoglycemia and resolving hypokalemia, hypocalcemia, and coagulopathies. The child should wake up 4 to 6 hours after admission to the PICU. Some patients who were encephalopathic before transplant require more intensive neurologic examinations. The patient's fluid status is reviewed. Because of third-space loss, the need for intraoperative fluid resuscitation is common. Several blood volume replacements may need to be administered. Within 48 hours after admission to the PICU, the patient should have diuresis.

Intraoperative medications are reviewed. The transplant operation is lengthy, and changes in anesthesia personnel often occur. During report, immunosuppressive medications and doses are double-checked by the nurse and operating room personnel. Pharmacologic therapy is extensive and includes immunosuppressive agents, PCP prophylaxis, antacids, antibiotic prophylaxis for several days, *Candida* prophylaxis, hepatic artery thrombosis (HAT) prophylaxis, and, possibly, selective decontamination of the digestive tract. (See promotion of graft tolerance and immunosuppression.)

Significant Postoperative Issues or Complications

Organ-Specific Rejection: Liver.   Acute and chronic rejection can occur after hepatic transplantation. Acute, or cellular, rejection is characterized by the invasion of mononuclear cells in the portal triads. (See discussion of promotion of graft tolerance and rejection also.)

Symptoms of rejection are variable and often vague. Symptoms commonly include fever, abdominal pain, and graft tenderness; flushed skin, tachypnea, distended abdomen, irritability, loss of appetite, diarrhea, myalgia, and septic appearance also occur. Subsequent swelling and edema of the graft with increased vascular resistance may lead to variceal bleeding or hepatic artery or portal vein thrombosis. Changes in liver function laboratory studies may provide the first indication that rejection is occurring (see Table 26-4). An early but nonspecific indicator of rejection may be a rapid increase in GGTP levels. A subsequent increase in serum bilirubin and ALP and variable changes with ALT and AST levels may be observed. A liver biopsy may be performed if rejection is suspected and the patient is unresponsive to medical therapy. With acute rejection, some degree of mononuclear cellular infiltrate in the portal tracts is found on biopsy.

With chronic rejection, there is disappearance of the intrahepatic bile ducts with varying degrees of bridging fibrosis. However, the liver has significant regenerative capacity and may recover function even after severe rejection. Therefore chronic rejection occurs less often in liver recipients (less than 10% of pediatric patients) than in heart, kidney, and lung recipients.[48]

Because acute rejection is usually cell mediated, episodes can be managed with increased immunosuppression. Some centers also use induction therapy, with monoclonal antibodies or polyclonal globulins, for treatment of rejection. Although acute rejection is common early in the posttransplantation period, triple-therapy immunosuppression has helped to reduce the number and severity of acute rejection episodes.

Infection.   Infectious complications continue to be a very significant cause of postoperative morbidity and mortality in pediatric liver recipients, with up to 50% of children affected.[48] Posttransplant infections are discussed in detail in the sections on heart-lung postoperative issues. In liver transplant patients, early infections are often bacterial and may originate in the abdomen related to local ischemia, the incision, associated bleeding, or bowel contamination or are from indwelling catheter infections, the lungs, or the urinary tract. Children with a failed Kasai procedure are prone to recurrent episodes of cholangitis.[42] As most children undergo Roux-en-Y choledochojejunostomy, intraoperative infectious complications include contamination of the bile ducts with yeast and bacteria.[42]

Infectious complications associated with HAT generally occur within the first 30 days after transplant.[42] HAT can precipitate areas of necrosed liver, abscesses, and bacteremia. Bile duct strictures with resultant cholangitis can occur following HAT. Technical difficulties may necessitate reexploration of the abdomen with associated increased incidence of fungal infection.

Viral, protozoal, and fungal infections, including CMV, EBV, and PTLD, are also common infectious agents in the liver transplant recipient. As a result of effective prophylaxis, PCP and CMV infections in transplant recipients has declined.[53] PTLD occurs in 5% to 20% of liver transplant recipients.[48] Incidence appears to relate to exposure history of the donor and recipient and the type and amount of immunosuppression. Mortality is high; patients are treated with significant reduction or withdrawal of immunosuppression and antiviral agents.

Most posttransplant infections can be treated. Antibiotic and antiviral prophylaxis and early recognition of symptoms of infection have contributed to a decrease in morbidity and mortality in transplant recipients in the last decade.[48]

Ineffective Airway Clearance and Breathing Patterns Resulting in Impaired Gas Exchange.

Pulmonary assessment includes frequent auscultation of breath sounds, interpretation of arterial blood gases, and monitoring of chest x-ray films. The child's coagulation status determines the appropriateness of chest physiotherapy. Gentle chest physiotherapy is performed if coagulopathies persist. Once hemostasis is achieved, aggressive chest physiotherapy is initiated.

Because of the liver-lung relationship, patients with fulminant and chronic hepatic failure may manifest pulmonary signs of the failing liver. The pulmonary effects of chronic liver disease are more prevalent in the adult population; however, such complications have been reported in children.[54] Pleural effusions and arteriovenous collateral vessels with ventilation/perfusion mismatch and resultant intrapulmonary shunting are reported complications.

Ineffective airway clearance is related to the long abdominal procedure, large transverse abdominal incision, and postoperative pain. Ineffective breathing patterns may be related to diaphragm paralysis and abdominal distension secondary to ascites, large donor liver, or bleeding. The goal is to wean ventilator support within the first postoperative day; at least 50% of the patients are extubated by the end of the second postoperative day. However, many of the children experience collapse of the right upper and right middle lobes of the lung. Phrenic nerve paresis caused by clamping of the upper vena cava and right mainstem bronchus intubation contribute to lobar collapse. Also, the potential for diaphragmatic paralysis exists if the right phrenic nerve is injured during surgery. An elevated diaphragm, seen on chest x-ray film, and decreased expansion of the right lower lobe with spontaneous respiration may indicate phrenic nerve damage. Generally, if the child is unable to tolerate extubation twice, an ultrasound examination is used to confirm the suspected diagnosis. In addition, poor nutritional status preoperatively may contribute to delayed weaning.

Persistent ascites may also limit tidal volume and impair ventilation. A large donor liver, as well, may reduce intrathoracic space and tidal volume. Emergent indications for liver transplantation may necessitate widening the candidate's weight range with an increased mismatch in donor to recipient size. Inability to close the abdominal incision may further impair the patient's respiratory effort because supportive musculature and associated resistance will not assist the patient's ventilatory efforts.

Impaired gas exchange may be related to right pleural effusion and intrapulmonary shunting. Preoperative ascites may promote rapid fluid accumulation postoperatively. The sympathetic response observed with acute rejection may increase ascites accumulation.[55] Treatment measures include the use of diuretics, albumin administration with diuretics, and drainage of the accumulated pleural fluid by thoracentesis or insertion of a pigtail catheter in the pleural space.

Pulmonary infection is common. Common viral organisms include CMV, respiratory syncytial virus, adenovirus, herpes simplex, and herpes zoster. Pulmonary *Aspergillus* and systemic candidiasis may contribute to pulmonary dysfunction.

Alterations in Tissue Perfusion.

Beyond evaluation of airway and ventilation, close monitoring of vital signs, hemodynamics, hemoglobin and hematocrit, intake and output, and peripheral perfusion (including postoperative evaluation of pretransplant encephalopathy) and careful observation for signs and symptoms of hemorrhage are vital.

Park and colleagues[56] described the hemodynamic profile of 73 children with chronic liver disease. Eighty-two percent of the children had high cardiac output with a cardiac index greater than 4 $L/min/M^2$. In four of the children, there was evidence of intrapulmonary and arteriovenous shunting. After transplant, cardiac index decreased by a mean of 35% ($P < .001$). The authors concluded that transplantation improved chronic hemodynamic abnormalities (hyperdynamic state) in children with chronic liver disease.

Greater than 70% of liver transplant recipients experience hypertension, with approximately 10% of these patients requiring long-term antihypertensive medications.[55] Mean arterial blood pressure in excess of 90 mmHg or systolic blood pressure greater than 140 mmHg requires treatment. Severe hypertension is most problematic within the first postoperative week.

Several hypotheses exist regarding the cause of hypertension in liver transplant patients. These include alterations in renin levels and immunosuppressant administration. Vigilant nursing assessment of blood pressure will ensure prompt treatment and minimize associated side effects, which include seizures, subarachnoid hemorrhage, intraparenchymal hemorrhage, and coma.

Pharmacologic treatment of hypertension is institution specific. Initially, the use of a nitroprusside infusion may be necessary. Intravenous and oral drug therapy may include use of renin-angiotensin inhibitors, peripheral vasodilators, β-blockers, and α-adrenergic blockers. Commonly used antihypertensives include nifedipine (Procardia), hydralazine (Apresoline), captopril (Capoten), and labetalol (Normodyne). Combination therapy is often prescribed. (See management of hypertension in Chapter 18.)

Hypotension is infrequently seen and is usually associated with complications, for example, hemorrhage, graft failure, or sepsis. Patients may bleed from anastomotic sites or the cut edges of segmental grafts. With graft dysfunction, coagulopathies will persist despite ongoing administration of fresh-frozen plasma, platelets, and crystalloids. Blood is drained from the abdomen using multiple drains while coagulopathies are corrected. Hypotension in the presence of primary graft dysfunction is associated with alterations in blood chemistry. Hypotension after the first 72 hours may be an indication of intraabdominal sepsis. Hematology laboratory tests, coagulation profile, and serum pH are monitored if hypotension exists.

Abdominal drainage and incisional oozing are carefully assessed. The abdominal girth is assessed as frequently as every hour. If drainage from the Jackson-Pratt is excessive, a hematocrit of the drainage is obtained. Drainage of greater than 80 ml/kg/hr and decreased hemoglobin and hematocrit values usually indicate surgical bleeding. Intraabdominal bleeding and increased abdominal girth impede venous return and may impair effective ventilation and oxygenation. If the patient was already extubated, mechanical ventilation may need to be reestablished. Blood and fluid replacement is ongoing. Often vasopressor therapy is prescribed to maintain an acceptable blood pressure. If surgical bleeding is suspected, the child returns to the operating room for an exploratory laparotomy. If findings suggest graft failure, the patient is relisted for a replacement graft. Fluid resuscitation may be ongoing until retransplantation occurs.

HAT occurs in 5% to 30% of pediatric patients and can lead to graft failure if adequate collateral circulation is not established. HAT is suspected if liver function studies do not begin to decrease within the first 48 hours after transplantation. HAT may cause biliary tract necrosis and secondary cholestasis, biliary stricture, and recurrent sepsis. In one third of the cases, the patient may be asymptomatic.[57] Symptoms occur in three forms: fulminant hepatic failure with liver gangrene, biliary complications such as a bile leak or biliary stricture, or chronic bacteremia with visible intrahepatic abscesses. Portal vein thrombosis may also occur.

Several causes of HAT are documented. Tzakis and Starzl[57] report that HAT is usually caused by technical problems, with contributing nontechnical factors. A lower incidence of HAT is associated with transplantation of liver fragments resulting from the larger size hepatic artery.

Treatment measures are initiated in the immediate postoperative period to prevent HAT. Within 12 hours after transplantation, daily ultrasound and Doppler examinations are initiated to evaluate vessel patency. Additional diagnostic studies such as angiogram and liver biopsy may be performed. Patients at risk because of technical difficulties or other factors are placed on a protocol to maintain and enhance blood flow through anastomoses. If a patient is believed to be at high risk for development of HAT, a heparin infusion may be initiated early in the postoperative period. Subclinical anticoagulation is achieved with intravenous dextran 40 (Gentran 40), subcutaneous low-dose heparin, oral aspirin, or dipyridamole (Persantine.) Dextran 40 draws water from the extravascular space, decreasing blood viscosity and platelet adhesiveness. Rapid corrections of coagulopathies are avoided. The patient's hematocrit is maintained at 30% to minimize the incidence of HAT.

In some centers, hyperbaric oxygen (HBO) therapy is used as an adjunct to anticoagulation. The hyperoxygenation associated with this therapy is thought to decrease ischemic-reperfusion injury or minimize the effects of any decreased blood flow to the liver. Patients with HAT in one study were treated within 24 hours of diagnosis with HBO therapy twice daily for 2 weeks or until symptoms resolved. Perhaps by aiding collateral development, HBO significantly delayed retransplantation but did not significantly affect survival or retransplantation rates.[58] If medical management is unsuccessful, HAT is treated in the operating room with reanastomosis or retransplantation in primary graft failure.

Altered Renal Function. Impairment in renal function is common postoperatively as a result of fluid shifts; persistent hypoproteinemia; diuretics; tense abdominal pressure affecting renal filtration pressure; and numerous nephrotoxic agents, such as immunosuppressants and antibiotics. Patients are at risk for intravascular volume depletion related to massive ascites or significant blood loss caused by abnormal coagulation. In the immediate postoperative period, fluids are restricted. Fluid balance and blood urea nitrogen (BUN)/creatinine ratio should be monitored closely.

Oliguria is reported in over 50% of liver transplant recipients on postoperative day 1 or 2.[55] Management of the patient includes fluid restriction, diuretics, and low-dose dopamine. Crystalloid replacement may be useful for ensuring adequate intravascular volume; however, rarely is urine output increased. Additional fluids are administered with caution because fluid overload may precipitate edema and ascites and worsen hypertension. Both cyclosporine and tacrolimus are known to have nephrotoxic effects, so careful monitoring of drug levels is important.

Polyuria rarely occurs but may be seen in patients recovering from hepatorenal failure or acute tubular necrosis. Hepatorenal syndrome is associated with liver failure and is usually irreversible.

Metabolic and Nutritional Deficits. Common electrolyte derangements seen after transplant include hypocalcemia, hypokalemia or hyperkalemia, hypoglycemia or hyperglycemia, and hypomagnesemia. Electrolyte, calcium, and serum glucose levels are obtained every 6 hours. Hourly glucometer readings are obtained until normoglycemia is achieved.

Hypokalemia occurs more often, but hyperkalemia may also be present after surgery. Potassium is usually not added to intravenous fluids because of the risks of renal failure and possible graft necrosis with a resultant increase in serum potassium.

Hypocalcemia occurs frequently in patients. Causes of hypocalcemia include citrate intoxification from the large quantities of blood products administered, hypoproteinemia, and liver membrane damage with subsequent shift of calcium from the extracellular to the intracellular space and decreased ionized calcium resulting from metabolic or respiratory alkalosis.

A "syndrome" of hypertension, metabolic alkalosis, hypernatremia, hypokalemia, and relative oliguria has been described.[59] Proposed causes include large citrate load, multiple doses of diuretics, and nasogastric suction. However, none of these adequately explains the "syndrome," because it is short lived. Preoperative respiratory alkalosis may be replaced by postoperative metabolic alkalosis as a result of the citrate load in the blood products, nasogastric drainage, fluid restriction, and diuretic therapy.

Hypomagnesemia is common with end-stage renal disease and can be exacerbated in the early postoperative period. Magnesium-containing antacids, oral magnesium gluconate, and intravenous magnesium sulfate may be prescribed. Effects of magnesium on blood pressure may be direct or through the influences on the internal balance of potassium, sodium, and calcium. Hypophosphatemia may be observed. Increased phosphate needs of the allograft for the repletion of adenosine triphosphate may be the contributing factor.

Total parenteral nutrition is usually initiated within 24 hours postoperatively. Feedings are initiated as soon as postoperative ileus resolves. Malabsorption and diarrhea are common problems experienced postoperatively. Causes of infectious diarrhea include CMV, *Clostridium difficile,* and other enteric organisms. The malabsorption syndrome may be transient, with an unclear etiology. Hypothesized causes include manipulation of the bowel during surgery and immunosuppressive drugs.

Biliary Tract Complications. Complications of biliary tract anastomosis occur in up to 20% of patients.[48] Strictures may occur, resulting in biliary obstruction. Hepatic abscesses can occur if biliary obstruction is not detected. Cholangitis and bile leaks also occur. Bile leakage results most often from the cut edges of segmental grafts or at the jejunal anastomosis. Symptoms of bile leakage include fever, bacteremia, alteration in liver function tests (LFTs), and evidence of fluid collection on ultrasound. Treatment involves reoperation to repair or revise the biliary tract anastomosis.

HAT should be suspected in patients with biliary complications because arterial blood is the principal blood supply to the bile duct graft. In the patient with a T tube, the nurse may observe biliary sludge in the drainage. Sludge is a chalklike substance composed of organic fibrous matrix from the sloughing of the bile duct lining. Cholangitis and biliary tract obstruction can occur with severe biliary sloughing.

Altered Skin Integrity-Skin and Wound Issues. The skin and visceral layers are generally closed. Normally, the abdominal dressing is removed after 24 hours ,and the incision is left open to air to promote healing. If donor liver size or bowel edema precludes surgical closure, complex wound care is required. An enterostomal therapy consult can assist the bedside nurse and surgeons in providing optimal wound care. Dressing changes over draining wounds are required frequently and are accomplished with the use of Montgomery straps to limit patient discomfort associated with tape removal (see Chapter 16).

For the majority of pediatric patients, a Roux-en-Y biliary reconstruction is indicated; therefore a T tube is not usually inserted. If present, T tube drainage is carefully assessed, with normal drainage appearing bilious. Absence of a color change in the drainage may indicate graft dysfunction.

Alterations in Comfort. After liver transplantation, the goal of pain management is to achieve a balance between comfort and ability to assess the patient's level of consciousness, as hepatic metabolism of pain medication may be impaired. The importance of evaluating mental status is crucial because graft function is imperative for metabolizing narcotics. Small IV narcotic doses are preferable to the use of benzodiazepines or phenothiazines because in an emergency, narcotic antagonists can be used to reverse the narcotics and permit evaluation of hepatic encephalopathy.

Variations in narcotic dosing for pain management are found among transplant centers. In some centers, the administration of narcotics is generally avoided, and when they are used, they are prescribed in reduced doses. Once the liver demonstrates adequate functioning, with the patient awake and complaining of pain, narcotics can be administered safely.

INTESTINAL AND MULTIVISCERAL TRANSPLANTATION

Intestinal failure is described as the inability to maintain nutritional intake and normal fluid and electrolyte balance without artificial means or total parenteral nutrition (TPN). Usually, failure occurs following significant loss of GI absorptive function (massive resection) or major functional abnormalities of the enterocytes, smooth muscle, or enteric nervous system.[60] The most common cause of intestinal failure in the pediatric population is short bowel syndrome resulting from surgical correction of congenital or acquired defects such as gastroschisis, midgut volvulus, intestinal atresia, or necrotizing enterocolitis. Functional causes for intestinal failure include disorders of motility such as chronic pseudoobstruction or Hirschsprung's disease resulting from disorders of smooth muscle, enteric nervous system, or total aganglionosis or disorders caused by abnormal enterocyte function, such as microvillus inclusion disease and radiation enteritis.

Although TPN has been a lifesaving therapy enabling children with intestinal failure to survive many more years, lifelong TPN may initiate a host of serious complications, including sepsis, TPN-induced hepatic dysfunction, metabolic disorders, loss of venous access, and pulmonary embolism. Thus far, the majority of candidates have required liver and small bowel transplants because of the resultant cholestasis from long-term hyperalimentation use.

Intestinal transplantation is viewed as a procedure that improves the quality of life, similar to kidney transplantation.[60] Intestinal transplantation, either alone or as a composite graft with other intraabdominal organs, is reserved for children with irreversible intestinal failure who develop life-threatening complications related to TPN or anatomic defects.[61]

Intestines may be transplanted as an isolated intestinal graft (intestinal failure alone), as a combined intestine and liver graft (intestinal failure with hepatic dysfunction), or as part of an abdominal multivisceral graft (extensive abnormalities of the GI tract and other organs). The status of the other abdominal organs determines which organs will need to be implanted in a multiorgan graft. Multivisceral transplants may include the stomach, liver, pancreas, spleen, duodenum, and small bowel. Segments of the large bowel may also be implanted but have been discontinued in at least one center because of colon-related complications, including severe graft rejection and increased incidence of infection[60] (Fig. 26-4). The combination of advanced surgical techniques and the introduction of the immunosuppressant tacrolimus (formerly FK506) into clinical use greatly increased survival rates for the liver and small bowel graft or isolated small bowel transplant recipients. Data concerning small bowel transplantation began to be reported to UNOS in 1994. From 1994 to 1998, 173 of 249 intestine

transplants were reported to have been performed in children ages 0 to 17 years.[4]

Each candidate is unique, and evaluation is tailored by the transplant team following confirmation of the diagnosis of intestinal failure. A thorough, multidisciplinary evaluation is done. Evaluation includes intestinal assessment (anatomy, upper and lower GI barium and motility studies, bowel histology), hepatic assessment (LFTs, albumin, alpha-fetoprotein, PT, PTT, ultrasound, histology), vascular access (Doppler ultrasound of central veins), nutritional evaluation, infection screening, and other studies (CBC, type and cross, BUN, creatinine, chest radiography, echocardiogram, ECG, ventilation/perfusion scan). Contraindications for small bowel transplantation include uncontrolled sepsis; malignancy elsewhere in the body; HIV infection; and severe cerebral, cardiac, or respiratory disease.

Many children who require a combined liver and small bowel transplant will die from liver failure while awaiting a donor because of the shortage of age- and size-matched donor organs.[61] These candidates are listed according to current UNOS intestine criteria. Status 1 patients have liver dysfunction and line access problems as evidenced by no

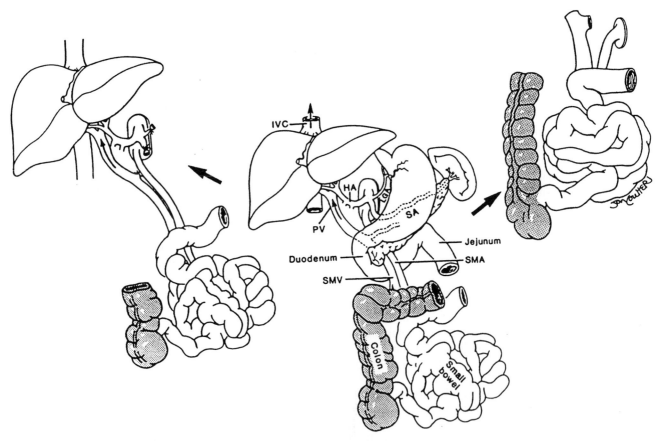

Fig. 26-4 Types of intestinal transplantation. Combined intestine and liver graft *(left);* abdominal multivisceral graft *(middle);* isolated intestinal graft *(right).* Large bowel *(shaded area)* could be included as a composite of intestinal graft, although rarely done because of colon-related complications leading to poor patient outcome. *IVC,* Inferior vena cava; *PV,* portal vein; *HA,* hepatic artery; *SA,* splenic artery; *SMA,* superior mesenteric artery; *SMV,* superior mesenteric vein. (From Todo S, Reyes J: Intestinal transplantation. In O'Neill JA, Rowe MI, Grosfeld JL et al, eds: *Pediatric surgery,* St Louis, 1998, Mosby, p 607.)

access through the subclavian, jugular, or femoral veins. Status 2 patients have no liver dysfunction and have line access available in standard sites. The candidate may be listed for an isolated intestinal graft, if cholestatic liver disease is not present. If the child needs a liver graft, the child is also listed with UNOS as a liver candidate. The ideal donor is of the same blood type and of the same size or up to 25% variance from the recipient. HLA matching is random and not considered in recipient selection. Transplantation of CMV-positive liver and small bowel into a CMV-negative recipient is not even considered unless the recipient is dying of liver failure.

Intestine and Multivisceral Transplantation Procedures

Grafts used in intestinal and multivisceral transplantation are cadaveric with the exception of rare living-related isolated intestinal transplantation.[60] Donor selection is similar to the criteria for other organs. Because intestinal mucosa is sensitive to ischemia, transplant surgeons are cautious in using donors with a history of prolonged hypotension or cardiac arrest. Donors receive gut decontamination through a nasogastric tube, as well as intravenous antibiotics. After graft retrieval, the lumen is irrigated again for decontamination if the colon is included in the graft.

Recipients require routine gut decontamination and antibiotic prophylaxis as well. In an isolated intestinal transplantation, the graft is revascularized by an anastomosis of the superior mesenteric artery of the graft to the infrarenal aorta. Donor vein grafts may be used for venous reconstruction. Each end of the graft is anastomosed to the recipient bowel. A jejunostomy tube is placed for venting and eventual initiation of enteral feeding. A terminal ileostomy is used to facilitate endoscopic examinations and biopsies.

Procurement of an abdominal multivisceral composite graft takes approximately 3 to 4 hours. The graft is separated as a back table procedure into separate intestinal, pancreas, and liver allografts, which are then preserved before reimplantation. Composite grafts are first connected to a common conduit of the recipient's hepatic veins and then are arterialized by anastomosis of the coeliac and superior mesenteric arteries to the infrarenal aorta using a conduit or homograft. Intestinal continuity requires an anastomosis with both the native proximal and distal gut. A "chimney allograft ileostomy" is accomplished to provide for surveillance of the intestinal allograft during the first few postoperative months. When stable immunosuppression has been accomplished, without rejection creating the need for frequent endoscopic examination, the ileostomy can be closed.[61] A jejunostomy feeding tube is placed at the time of the operation for venting and initiation of enteral feedings. The surgical procedure can be challenging when the child has had numerous previous surgical procedures, especially if adhesions and portal hypertension are present. In addition, when the child requires the implantation of multiple donor organs, the surgical procedure is quite lengthy and the

number of complications can increase. Surgical procedures vary depending on the organs transplanted and the condition of the donor organs.

Postoperative Care Following Intestinal and Multivisceral Transplantation

Care of children after intestine or multivisceral transplant is similar to the care required of a liver transplant patient. The main principles of the critical care management in the postoperative period are immunosuppression and prevention of rejection, prevention of infection, fluid balance, maintenance of nutritional status, assessment of graft function, and long-term rehabilitation.[61] Because the number and type of organs transplanted vary, assessment of each organ's function and engraftment are required. Additional concerns include care of the large abdominal incision and the ileostomy. Consultation with an enterostomal therapist in the immediate postoperative period is helpful in preventing impairment of skin integrity. Lengthy recovery periods are anticipated because time is needed for the intestine to become functional.

Significant Postoperative Issues or Complications

Immunosuppression.   The same protocols for postoperative immunosuppression are used in both isolated or composite intestinal allograft recipients. A combination protocol of tacrolimus and steroids is often used. Tacrolimus is often initiated in the operating room via continuous infusion, preferably peripherally. A trough level of 20 to 25 ng/ml is the initial goal, with reduction to 8 to 12 ng/ml after 6 to 12 months. Oral tacrolimus is started once GI motility is observed.

Initial dosing of methylprednisolone is tapered over the next 5 days to 1 mg/kg/day. Cyclophosphamide may be given for 4 weeks and then switched to mycophenolate mofetil or azathioprine. Prostaglandin is administered for the first 5 postoperative days because of its beneficial vasodilatory effects on renal and splanchnic vasculature that may prevent microvascular thrombosis.

Organ-Specific Rejection: Intestines.   Despite improved immunosuppression, rejection is still a major problem. (See also sections with discussion of promotion of graft tolerance and rejection.) Rejection of the transplanted intestine is assessed by clinical examination, endoscopic observation, radiologic examination, and histologic evaluation of mucosal biopsies.[60] There are no biochemical indices that reflect rejection of the intestinal allograft. Functional studies and serologic assays are not reliable indicators of rejection because graft dysfunction also occurs with preservation injury, hypoperfusion injury, and enteritis.[60] Clinical signs of acute rejection include fever, abdominal distension, abdominal pain, increased or decreased enteric output, and watery diarrhea. Dusky stomal mucosa, mucosal edema, and decreased peristalsis may be associated endoscopic findings. Severe, acute rejection is characterized by severe diarrhea, abdominal pain, abdominal distension, and metabolic acidosis. Endoscopic findings with severe acute rejection include ulceration, mucosal sloughing, bleeding, and loss of peristalsis. Chronic rejection is characterized by chronic diarrhea, malabsorption, and weight loss. Gastric emptying times may be evaluated radiologically, with prolonged emptying times indicating rejection.

Endoscopic examinations are performed on a periodic basis and if intestinal rejection is suspected from clinical observations. The endoscopic examination yields valuable information about the appearance of the graft's mucosa and intestinal motility.

Infection.   Infection is a common complication. (See section on posttransplant infection in heart-lung.) Translocation of bacteria from the intestine to the bloodstream can occur if bacteria seeps through damaged intestinal mucosa into the bloodstream. Causes of translocation include intestinal overgrowth, sloughing of the mucosa, rejection, and PTLD. Therefore broad-spectrum antibiotic prophylaxis is ordered for the first 7 days, and bowel decontamination is continued for the first 4 postoperative weeks to minimize translocation caused by overgrowth. Frequent blood and body fluid cultures are done, and surveillance stool cultures are performed weekly. Quantitative culture with colonies of greater than 10 organisms are considered significant only in the presence of systemic sepsis or ongoing acute cellular rejection of the intestinal allograft and are treated appropriately.[62]

CMV disease is also a risk, especially when a recipient with CMV-negative serologic status receives an organ from a CMV-positive donor. Prophylaxis for all patients is important in the prevention of active disease, with antiviral agents and CMV immunoglobulin (Ig) used for high-risk patients. Early identification of CMV disease can also facilitate more effective treatment. Routine ileoscopy, biopsies of both the small bowel and liver as needed, and routine serum antigen testing (PP65) are performed. Treatment consists of ganciclovir and CMV Ig as first-line agents and foscarnet and cidofovir as second-line agents, along with cautiously lowered immunosuppression. Treatment is continued until the patient is symptom free and the PP65 is normal. Monitoring should include BUN, creatinine clearance, urine output, urine proteins, CBC, differential, platelets, LFTs, electrolytes, and observation for allergic reactions.

Assessment of Graft Function.   Graft function and viability are assessed in the operating room immediately following graft reperfusion. Because the allograft may be of varying lengths of the GI tract and different anatomic structures or organs (may include stomach, small intestine, duodenum, colon, liver), the assessment must be thorough, aggressive, and multidisciplinary. There are not good biochemical markers to indicate function. (See other sections for assessment of graft function for other abdominal organs.)

Serum nutritional markers (transferrin, albumin, and retinoic acid) and the absorption studies (D-xylose testing and fecal fat content) are performed to evaluate intestinal absorption abilities, assessing carbohydrate absorption and fat metabolism. Motility is evaluated by barium GI series with determination of duration of gastric emptying and intestinal transit time. Most recipients experienced delayed gastric emptying during the early postoperative period with the initiation of oral feedings. This problem usually resolved in about 3 months, but gastrostomy is required to alleviate symptoms.[60]

All intestine recipients suffer high stomal output and diarrhea, sometimes requiring readmission for fluid and nutritional management. Pharmacologic measures, including the administration of antidiarrheal agents, are used to decrease GI motility, but high stomal output may continue for years in patients with rapid intestinal transit. Graft dysmotility may be related to graft denervation. Recently, enteric ganglia at the roots of the celiac and mesenteric arteries have been preserved in an attempt to slow intestinal transit. Evaluation of the outcomes of ganglia preservation requires additional follow-up.[60] Many children requiring intestinal transplant have never eaten before surgery, so during the postoperative period an occupational therapist or feeding specialist assists these children with mastery of this task.

Maintenance of Fluid and Electrolyte Balance. The fluid shifts between the graft, lungs, and peripheral tissues in the first 2 to 3 days can result in generalized fluid retention combined with intravascular volume depletion. Careful measurement of enteric output is essential, with early surgeon notification of extremes of output. Assessment of stomal output for volume, consistency, reducing substances, and bacterial overgrowth is performed. Excessive output may indicate rejection and reflects poor absorption. Enteral feedings are introduced to stimulate absorption as soon as tolerated in the postoperative period. Total caloric intake is maintained with parenteral nutrition, which is decreased once enteral feedings are tolerated. The goal is to achieve independence from TPN in all functioning grafts within 4 to 6 weeks. Initiation of enteral feedings through the jejunostomy tube is a gradual process, and the goal is to wean TPN and tube feedings to an exclusive oral diet. Enteral feeding is weaned by reducing daily duration of administration as oral intake improves.

Graft-Versus-Host Disease.   GVHD is another potential complication caused by the large quantities of lymphoid tissue present in the intestine. Recipients of a liver and intestine graft and isolated intestine transplants have been treated with increased immunosuppression for GVHD, which is diagnosed by the presence of a fine intermittent pink skin rash and histologic diagnoses per intestinal and skin biopsy. GVHD develops in about 10% of recipients, is usually nonlethal, and occurs most often after reduction or discontinuation of immunosuppression therapy.[60]

KIDNEY TRANSPLANTATION

Substantial experience has been gained in providing care and treatment to children with end-stage renal disease (ESRD). These developments have allowed this patient population the opportunity to live far longer than was previously expected. Experience has demonstrated that infants and very small children are not only acceptable candidates for treatment but are also favored candidates when outcome and quality of life are measured. During the last decade, patient and graft survival rates have improved significantly related to more effective immunosuppressive regimens, improved pretransplant dialysis, and current postoperative monitoring and care.[63]

In 1999, UNOS reported survival rates of cadaveric kidney transplants in 1- to 5-year-olds to be 97.4%, 90.2%, and 88.8% at 1, 3, and 5 years, respectively, with living related donation (LRD) transplant survival rates being slightly higher. Overall survival rates of all types of kidney transplant recipients steadily remain greater than 90% after 5 years in children of ages 1 to 18 years.[4]

About 900 children are diagnosed with ESRD each year.[63] The five most common diagnoses requiring transplantation were hypoplastic or dysplastic kidneys, obstructive uropathy, focal segmented glomerulosclerosis, reflux nephropathy, and systemic immunologic disease. The cause of ESRD in children also varies depending on age groups, according to data reported to the North American Pediatric Renal Transplant Cooperative Study (NAPRTCS).[64] In children younger than 5 years of age, congenital anomalies and congenital nephrotic syndrome are the most common causes. In adolescents, chronic glomerulonephritis is most common. On the average, there is an interval of about 4 to 5 years between the onset of glomerular disease and the onset of ESRD. The cause of each child's renal failure is important information for the healthcare team and the family. The identification of a hereditary renal disease has implications for family members who may wish to be considered as kidney donors. Because certain renal diseases tend to recur in the transplanted kidney, this information can influence the timing of the transplant, as well as the choice of LRD versus a cadaveric donor.

Timing of transplantation takes into account patient age, progressive growth failure and associated deterioration of CNS structure and function, and the cause of the ESRD. Historically, outcomes for small infants were not as successful as older children, but improvements in surgical technique and patient care now allow surgery in infants weighing at least 6 kg or older than 6 months of age.[65] One study in long-term mortality has shown no significant difference in the 5-year patient survival of those treated with hemodialysis (95%), LRD renal transplant (88%), and cadaveric renal transplant (85%).[66] This is important to consider in caring for the newborn or infant for whom increased linear growth is preferred before transplantation. However, almost all children with ESRD will not grow and develop along normal curves. Because muscle mass is normally more limited in children than adults, serum creatinine levels will not correlate as well with the degree of renal failure. Growth retardation may occur with serum creatinine levels of less than 3 mg/dl. Children with congenital nephrotic syndrome may suffer growth failure despite aggressive medical management with serum creatinine as low as 1 mg/dl. They may require nephrectomy 6 weeks before transplantation to correct nutritional and coagulation abnormalities. Children with oxalosis are often transplanted early (kidney graft or liver and kidney graft) to avoid prolonged renal insufficiency or dialysis that may cause extrarenal accumulation of oxalate.[63]

Preemptive transplantation (transplantation before the initiation of dialysis in the child with ESRD), although controversial, will maximize growth; minimize social, educational, and psychologic impacts of chronic illness; and decrease the complications of dialysis. LRD can facilitate optimal timing of preemptive transplantation. Better outcomes are possible for both the donor and recipient because surgery can occur when both are optimally healthy, kidney ischemic times are short, the allograft function is usually immediate, and immunosuppression may be initiated before the transplant.[63]

The principles of conservative medical management of ESRD in children are based on maintaining metabolic balance and growth and development by diet and drug therapy. When conservative management can no longer relieve the symptoms of uremia and permit the child to function in peer, school, or family life, an alternative form of treatment is necessary. With the availability of dialysis and transplantation, conservative treatment should exclude the need for drastic limitations on diet and activity.

Treatment options include chronic hemodialysis (usually using Brescia-Cimino arteriovenous fistula on the forearm or polytetrafluoroethylene graft if inadequate veins), chronic continuous ambulatory peritoneal dialysis (CAPD) or continuous cycling peritoneal dialysis (CCPD), and transplantation. Although many patients are brought to an optimal metabolic state with dialysis before transplantation, undergoing transplantation without dialysis is not unusual. Dialysis allows time for the child's medical, surgical, and urologic abnormalities, including metabolic derangements, bladder outlet obstruction, bone deformities, immunizations, and dental care, to be corrected. A voiding cystourethrogram is used to evaluate the bladder. Many children whose bladders were thought to be unusable may in fact be surgically augmented so that these children may void normally. Every effort is made to use the bladder; however, when it absolutely cannot be used, diversion to an ileal or colonic conduit may be performed. Central venous access is initiated at the time of nephrectomy, dialysis, or transplantation. Bilateral nephrectomy, before or at the time of transplant, is indicated in malignant hypertension that has failed to respond to maximal antihypertensive therapy and ultrafiltration by dialysis, for persistent infections, for structural upper tract uropathies, and in congenital nephrotic syndrome.

Pretransplantation evaluation is done by a multidisciplinary team. Standard evaluation includes the history and physical examination and laboratory tests including hematology, coagulation studies, chemistry, urine analysis, and blood bank screening. Blood bank screening includes ABO type, hepatitis profile, HIV screen, HLA type, and antileukocyte antibody screening. As a minimum, the donor and recipient should be ABO compatible and have a negative T cell cross-match. Ensuring that the recipient does not have preformed antibodies against antigens on the donor's T lymphocytes will prevent hyperacute rejection, which results in rapid, irreversible loss of graft function. Screening may be repeated monthly while patients are on the waiting list. Contraindications for transplantation include malignancy and active infection. Relative contraindications include major systemic disease and profound disability.

The decision to use a living-related or cadaver donor is dependent on the philosophy of the transplant center, as well as the availability of a living-related or living nonrelated donor (LNRD) and the family's wishes. LRD should be used when possible, considering the improved graft and patient survival rates. LRDs or LNRDs must be at least 18 years of age, have two healthy kidneys, be highly motivated, and meet the center's immunologic, medical, and psychosocial parameters. Donors must also have ABO compatibility, preferably share at least one haplotype for the serologically detectable antigens, and have a negative T cell cross-match. Medical evaluation confirms the health and renal function status of the donor and is usually performed by a physician other than the transplant surgeon.

When an LRD or LNRD cannot be identified, the child is placed on the waiting list for a cadaveric kidney. The waiting list has grown as the number of candidates has increased, related to the surgical techniques available currently for smaller infants. Patients in particular blood groups are assigned points based on the quality of the antigen match and the time of waiting. Extra points are assigned for recipients with a PRA greater than 80% (broader spectrum of anti-HLA antibodies), pediatric patients, previous donors who need a transplant, and medical urgency.[67] With all else being equal, patients with the longest waiting time on the list are given priority. Some patients are listed at more than one center, which increases their chances of receiving an organ sooner by 86%.[68] Allowing multiple listing may discriminate against patients with less resources for travel and medical care or patients in other geographic regions. In addition, follow-up care may be more difficult for out-of-state patients.

While on the waiting list, monthly determinations of sensitivity against a representative panel of lymphocytes are made. Donor organs that match a recipient in ABO compatibility and have an identical HLA match are offered nationally first, then locally. Generally, the donor kidney is selected on the basis of a negative cross-match between the recipient's serum and lymphocytes from the donor. Other criteria include current sensitization, length of time waiting, and recipient's age. The donor should be older than 6 and younger than 65 years old, normotensive, and otherwise healthy and free of transmissible disease. Donors have been declared brain dead and are maintained on life support systems until the kidneys can be recovered.

Kidney Transplantation Procedures

Once the selection has been determined, recipients undergo a final T cell cross-match and dialysis, if necessary. When required, preoperative transfusions are administered at the same time as dialysis to remove the potassium load from the banked blood. They also receive a thorough evaluation of current fluid and electrolyte status. Central venous access is established, if not already available. The bladder is filled with an antibiotic solution. Medications, including antibiotic prophylaxis, corticosteroids, and immunosuppression induc-

tion, are administered. Because the primary immunosuppressants, cyclosporine and tacrolimus, are potentially nephrotoxic, immunosuppression may be induced with monoclonal or polyclonal antibodies or other agents and administration of primary immunosuppressants delayed until function of the new organ is ensured.

Transplantation in the very small child poses different challenges because the donor kidney is usually relatively large. The abdomen must expand to accommodate a new, larger organ, which while consuming much of the infant's cardiac output, may impede venous return form the lower extremities and impede respiratory efforts. On release of the venous and arterial clamps following anastomoses of vessels, the lower extremities and donor organ are reperfused, which may result in hypovolemia and acidosis. The new organ may initially sequester blood and may produce urine close to the infant's blood volume on a hourly basis, resulting in hypotension.[63] It is essential that the CVP and blood pressure are adequate when the vascular clamps are removed. In addition, washout of the preservation solution from the large organ into the infant recipient may result in life-threatening hyperkalemia and hypothermia.[63] Therefore in infants and children receiving a large kidney, the CVP is increased to 15 to 20 mmHg with infusion of crystalloids, albumin, or packed red blood cells; sodium bicarbonate is administered to counteract acidosis; the kidney is warmed; urine output is replaced aggressively; and serum electrolytes are monitored closely.[63]

Arterial and venous anastomoses are completed in implantation of the donor organ; then the clamps are removed when CVP is adequate. Maintaining blood pressure and filling pressures during reperfusion is vital. Transfusions of blood and colloid may be necessary to provide a circulating blood volume that is adequate to perfuse the new kidney; ongoing, aggressive volume replacement may be required if the donor organ is large. The donor's ureter is anastomosed to the bladder mucosa of the recipient. A ureteral stent may be required in small bladders. The kidney and anastomoses are inspected and irrigated, and the abdomen is closed. If the donor organ is making urine at the end of the procedure, the peritoneal catheter (if in place preoperatively) may be removed.

The surgical placement of the transplanted kidney in the older child is generally similar to that in adults. Placement of the anastomoses depends on the size of the child and the size of the vessels.

Large adult kidneys that are transplanted into children will decrease in size with time but will function adequately. Conversely, cadaveric kidneys from small children that are transplanted into adolescents undergo hypertrophy and increase in function.

Postoperative Care Following Kidney Transplantation

The patient usually is transferred directly from the operating room to the PICU, where monitoring continues. A chest x-ray film confirms central line placement. A renal ultrasound is obtained to serve as a baseline for future comparison, as is a radionuclide scan, which confirms perfusion to the newly grafted kidney.

It is not unusual to keep small infants, who have received a large adult kidney placed intraperitoneally, intubated and supported on a ventilator for several days. A central line is usually inserted to monitor the effects of fluid loss on circulating blood volume and to determine replacement therapy. Fluid and electrolyte status is measured meticulously, and output is replaced milliliter per milliliter. The intravenous solution is adjusted frequently based on the serum and urine electrolytes. Calcium losses can cause problems. Immediate functioning of adult kidneys placed in infants will necessitate larger amounts of fluid replacement. Intraoperative bowel manipulation usually results in an ileus. The patient will require a nasogastric tube and parenteral nutrition until bowel function returns. A bladder catheter is placed for bladder decompression and urine output measurement.

Significant Postoperative Issues and Complications

Organ-Specific Rejection: Kidney. Hyperacute rejection is currently uncommon because of screening of blood type and antigens. When present, this rejection occurs immediately postoperatively. Accelerated rejection is also rare and is thought to be a secondary response resulting in antibody formation after contact with an antigen to which recipients were sensitized. This occurs 3 to 5 days after transplantation and presents as a severe, sudden graft dysfunction. (See also sections on promotion of graft tolerance and rejection.)

Acute rejection is the most common (40% of LRD recipients and 50% of cadaver recipients) and occurs most often during the first 6 months (especially with cadaver donors) but can occur at any time during the life of the graft.[63] It is usually reversible when identified and treated early. Clinical manifestations can be subtle. In the infant or small child who received a large kidney, early diagnosis of rejection may be difficult because of the abundance of renal parenchyma. By the time the BUN or creatinine level is elevated, rejection may be severe. In one study, hypertension and fever were significantly predominant in the rejection group; the creatinine level was elevated in only 45% of those with rejection.[69]

In addition to monitoring serial creatinine, ultrasound, radionuclide scans, and percutaneous renal biopsy are often necessary to confirm the diagnosis of rejection. Renal biopsy is important in the confirmation and management of acute rejection, as the histologic severity of rejection can be used to determine the optimal therapy for the patient. The parameters for diagnosing acute rejection in renal transplantation include fever, decreased urinary output, graft pain and tenderness, increased BUN and creatinine levels, malaise, weight gain, and hypertension. The use of cyclosporine and tacrolimus has made the diagnosis of acute rejection more difficult because of potential nephrotoxicity. A biopsy may be required to differentiate between immunosuppressant nephrotoxicity and early recurrence of the original disease.

Other differential diagnoses for symptoms of rejection, such as urinary obstruction, acute tubular necrosis (ATN), and urinary extravasation, can usually be ruled out by ultrasound and radionuclide scan.

Chronic rejection may occur after an episode of severe acute rejection as early as the first few weeks posttransplantation, but often, it is a disorder characterized by progressive ischemic loss of nephron mass secondary to vascular lesions. Chronic rejection is characterized by a gradual decline in glomerular filtration and an increase in permeability of the glomerulus to protein. The most common signs of chronic rejection are hypertension, proteinuria, edema, gradual rise in BUN and creatinine levels, and decreased creatinine clearance. Clinical manifestations of chronic rejection may not be evident until filtration rates are less than 25% of normal.

Treatment for rejection may include increasing the level of immunosuppression, adding adjunctive immunosuppressants or antibody therapy depending on the severity of rejection, and increasing the dose of corticosteroids or providing steroid boluses and recycling. Renal ultrasounds are used to monitor rejection, but percutaneous renal biopsy is the most reliable indicator of rejection. The rare patient who demonstrates rejection refractory to treatment may be treated with dialysis and antilymphocyte preparations.

Infection. Infection is a frequent cause of morbidity and mortality in the renal transplant recipient.[63] (See discussion of infection in heart-lung section for details regarding posttransplant infections.) Prominent among these infections are those with a large number of pathogens, mainly gram-negative bacteria (greater in younger patients and more prevalent in the first month) and opportunistic organisms such as PCP and CMV. The type of infection generally varies by the time after transplant and the recipient's age. Varicella-zoster, fungal infections, and protozoal infections may also occur. Trimethoprim prophylaxis is initiated early and is usually maintained as long as the immunosuppressants continue.

CMV disease is the major pathogen in the first 1 to 3 months posttransplant.[63] Ninety percent of the time, acquisition is by transplantation of a CMV-positive organ. Patients who are CMV seronegative and are the recipient of a kidney from a CMV-positive donor may be treated with prophylactic CMV-specific immunoglobulin. The first dose must be administered within 72 hours of the transplant, then subsequent doses are given up to 16 weeks after the transplant. Symptoms of CMV disease in these patients include prolonged episodes of fever, fatigue, cold or flulike symptoms, leukopenia, thrombocytopenia, abnormal LFTs, hepatomegaly or splenomegaly, decreased renal function, and elevated BUN or creatinine level.

EBV infection may also occur in renal recipients. The use of immunosuppressants to block interleukin-2 synthesis can decrease the number of virus-specific cytotoxic T cells, which then allows viral replication and proliferation of transformed B cells. Symptoms of tonsillitis, fever, hepatocellular dysfunction, focal brain or pulmonary disease, focal GI tumors with bleeding, or perforation or infiltration of the allograft may occur. Diagnosis is through EBV-PCR, titers, imaging, and renal biopsy. Treatment is with CMV-specific immunoglobulin and ganciclovir (DHPG), decrease or withdrawal of immunosuppressants, and chemotherapy, reserved for ganciclovir-resistant patients. Many tumors that occur in transplant recipients are lymphomas, specifically non-Hodgkin's, B cell origin with EBV implicated. Treatment may include decreased immunosuppression, local excision of masses, and chemotherapy. Cutaneous and other tumors also occur.

The patient who tolerates the graft poorly and requires large amounts of immunosuppressive drugs is the one most likely to develop serious infections. For this reason, vigorous immunosuppressive therapy is not pursued. Instead, rejection is allowed to proceed, and the kidney is then removed and later replaced with a second transplant.

Fluid and Electrolyte Imbalance. After surgery, the kidney may produce a massive diuresis, may remain totally anuric, or may produce urine volumes between these extremes. Serum and urine electrolytes are determined frequently (as often as every 6 hours for the first 2 days). IV fluids are administered based on the serum electrolyte levels and urine volumes. Inadequate fluid and electrolyte replacement may precipitate hyponatremia, hypokalemia, and hypotension. This response is especially important in the very small child, in whom fluid shifts occur very rapidly. Hypotension heralding hypovolemia must be prevented to maintain adequate perfusion to the new graft and prevent possible graft thrombosis.

Most patients with good allograft function will have normal BUN and serum creatinine levels by the third or fourth postoperative day. At this time, their management includes routine fluid volumes. Often these patients have been receiving hemodialysis before transplantation with concomitant fluid intake restriction. Hypocalcemia, except in the patient with severe hyperparathyroidism, usually ceases to be a problem in the presence of good renal function. Phosphorus regulation, however, may continue to be problematic for the patient, now in the form of hypophosphatemia. It is not unusual for the newly grafted kidney to develop a "phosphate leak," requiring oral phosphate supplementation for an indefinite period.

Decreased Urine Output. Graft function must be evaluated when decreased urine output occurs postoperatively. The differential diagnosis for decreased output is mechanical obstruction of the Foley catheter, hypovolemia, ATN, rejection, and technical events such as vascular or urologic complications. Posttransplant oliguria or anuria is commonly caused by ATN or rejection (discussed earlier.) If the transplanted kidney is experiencing ATN, it may produce diuresis for a day and then become anuric and may not secrete urine for days or weeks. This is more common as the result of prolonged ischemia during cadaveric organ retrieval. The reversibility of this ischemic disease is difficult to predict, and anuria may persist for several weeks before adequate renal function begins. The child is maintained on dialysis until the ATN has resolved. If hemodialysis is used, it is important not to aggressively ultrafiltrate because excessive fluid loss could result in thrombosis of the

allograft. Careful regulation of immunosuppressive agents and other drugs excreted by the kidney is especially important during this period.

Other causes for oliguria and anuria cannot be overlooked and are equally investigated. Diminished urinary flow may be caused by obstruction of the bladder catheter or stent by a simple kink or a clot. To rule out mechanical obstruction, very gentle irrigation may be necessary to ensure drainage.

Hypovolemia may be due to surgical blood loss or third spacing of fluids, and it is particularly common when patients previously had been receiving peritoneal dialysis. Fluid boluses may be required. Occasionally, a very small child returns from the operating room oliguric and in congestive heart failure after having received a substantial amount of fluids and colloids within a few hours. Careful fluid replacement, diuretics, or dialysis are necessary until the intravascular volume status has normalized. Ultrasound will rule out hemorrhage or graft compression.

An unusual and potentially preventable complication is graft thrombosis. Renal artery or vein stenosis or thrombosis may occur, as well as arteriovenous fistulas. Preliminary data suggest that graft thrombosis may be an increased risk for recipients younger than 6 years of age who have not had prior dialysis, as well as children who receive cadaveric grafts from young donors. Renal artery thrombosis is a devastating complication, which demonstrates sudden anuria. Diagnosis is made by ultrasound, renal scan, or exploratory surgery. Nephrectomy may be required. Venous occlusion is less common; graft swelling, tenderness, hematuria, and oliguria occur. Ultrasound will demonstrate no venous flow, obstructed arterial flow, and swelling. Venous thrombectomy may relieve the occlusion, but nephrectomy may be required.

Occasionally the distal ureter, which is minimally vascularized, becomes necrotic from ischemia, causing obstruction and subsequent extravasation of urine into the lower abdomen. Analysis of the leaking fluid may aid in diagnosis. A renal scan will confirm this diagnosis. If the leak is very small, a bladder catheter may be able to provide adequate drainage until the leak has healed. Placement of a nephrostomy tube or ureteral stent or reimplantation of the ureter may be necessary.

Although rare, obstruction of the ureter or ureteropelvic junction may also be caused by a clot, kidney stone, edema, or stenosis. Swelling of the graft, increased serum creatinine, pain, and drainage may occur. Edema may resolve spontaneously with resolution of the obstruction. Stenosis may be treated successfully with percutaneous transluminal dilation, a procedure with low morbidity and successful long-term effects. If not successful, surgery may be required.

Hypertension. Hypertension often occurs in children who have received a renal transplant. The multiple risk factors include acute or chronic rejection; side effects of corticosteroids and cyclosporine; recurrence of primary renal disease, arterial stenosis, and ischemia of native kidneys; volume loading and forced diuresis; and excessive sodium and fluid retention. Effective treatment for hypertension is essential because poor control can cause seizures and intracerebral bleeding, as well as accelerated deterioration of the graft. Hypertension may be severe and require nitroprusside infusion. (See discussion of hypertension management in Chapter 18.)

Posttransplant Erythrocytosis. Overproduction of erythropoietin by the allograft occurs for an unknown reason. Treatment is with angiotensin-converting enzyme (ACE) inhibitors such as enalapril (Vasotec) or captopril (Capoten.)

Gastrointestinal Complications. Prolonged ileus after an intraabdominal transplant is not uncommon. Nasogastric drainage is important, and oral feedings should be initiated as soon as bowel function is reestablished. If feeding is delayed beyond 5 days, TPN may be initiated.

Transplant recipients have an increased risk of peptic ulcer disease and hemorrhage with the administration of high doses of corticosteroids. Gut prophylaxis is continued until the corticosteroid doses are decreased.

Recurrence of Renal Disease. The recurrence of the primary renal disease in the allograft is of great concern in the pediatric recipient. Steroid-resistant nephrotic syndrome with focal segmental glomerulosclerosis, hemolytic-uremic syndrome (with diarrheal prodrome—low incidence of recurrence; without prodrome—more likely recurrence), oxalosis, and membranoproliferative glomerulonephritis have all been reported to recur. Rapid damage to grafts from oxalate deposition in oxalosis may occur, leading some to consider oxalosis as a contraindication to kidney transplant alone. In some cases, a liver and kidney graft is used during transplantation. The liver is not damaged by the primary disease, but implantation of a new liver cures the disease and prevents recurrence of the kidney damage. Cystinosis, another inherited metabolic disorder, results in the reappearance of cystine crystals in the allograft, but graft dysfunction, related to the recurrence of kidney disease resulting from cystinosis, does not occur. Unfortunately, the extrarenal manifestations of cystinosis, such as deposition of cystine crystals in other major organs, continue to persist after successful transplantation.

PANCREAS AND ISLET CELL TRANSPLANTATION

The number of pancreas transplantations performed for the treatment of diabetes mellitus, especially in adults, has increased dramatically in the last few years. More than one half of the transplants reported to the International Pancreas Transplant Registry have been performed since 1991.[4] In 1995 a total of 3900 pancreas transplants were performed. However, only 11 transplants were reported in the age group of 5 years and younger and 9 transplants in the age group of 6 to 18 years. Since 1995 the number of annual isolated pancreas transplants in all ages has more than tripled, increasing to 368 in 1999.[4] However, from 1994 to 1998, a total of only 40 pancreas transplants have been performed in children ranging from newborn to age 18 years.[4] The

survival data from October 1987 to December 1997 shows a 1-year graft survival rate of 76.6% and a 4-year survival rate of 63.9%.[4]

Diabetes is a chronic disease that affects more than 12 million Americans and is associated with permanent and irreversible functional and structural changes in body cells. The financial impact of this disease is staggering both to the patient and to society. The goals of pancreas transplantation are to improve the quality of life: to restore glucose control, permit independence from insulin, and halt the progression of complications. Pancreatic transplantation procedures are performed in rigorously selected diabetic patients at this time, very few of whom are children. Because generalized immunosuppression (with its inherent risk of toxicity, infections, and malignancy) is necessary to prevent rejection, pancreas transplantation has been limited to patients whose secondary complications of diabetes are, or predictably will be, more serious than the potential side effects of antirejection therapy. Patients who require or who have had a kidney transplant and who are obligated to immunosuppressive therapy meet this criterion. However, some nonuremic, non–kidney transplant patients are also in this category, such as those with preproliferative retinopathy who are at great risk for loss of vision or those with albuminuria who have early but progressive diabetic nephropathy. Currently, most pancreas transplants are performed in adult uremic patients either simultaneously with or 6 months to 1 year following renal transplantation. The rationale is that an endocrine-functioning pancreas may protect the renal graft and stabilize diabetic complications and may also assist in monitoring pancreatic rejection. Acute rejection is common. Renal biopsies can be performed to monitor rejection, but pancreatic biopsies are not indicated because the pancreas is highly vascular.

Because of the morbidity of the pancreas transplant procedure, the future for restored pancreatic function in children may rest with islet cell transplantation. This alternative to whole organ pancreaticoduodenal transplant is attractive because it is simpler and may facilitate immunoalteration pretransplant.[70] In addition, successful islet transplantation enables children with diabetes to avoid the chronic and sometimes devastating complications of lifelong diabetes. Though not yet successful in adults (only 20 of 140 documented cases of insulin independence have occurred), research is continuing.[70] Successful islet transplants require procurement of a sufficient number of islets from a single pancreas, improvement of islet preparation and preservation techniques, employment of techniques to alter graft immunogenicity without alloimmunity and long-term immunosuppression to enable engraftment into the recipient liver, and establishment of insulin independence after the transplant. In March of 2000, the Juvenile Diabetes Foundation awarded a 10 million dollar grant to explore the possibility of islet cell transplantation in conjunction with gene therapy to prevent rejection (Dr. Massimo Trucco of Children's Hospital of Pittsburgh) In addition, research will focus on the development of a vaccine to be used to prevent diabetes in genetically susceptible children.

QUALITY OF LIFE AND FOLLOW-UP CARE ISSUES

The commitment to transplant in children with end-stage organ failure can be one of the most challenging yet rewarding programs undertaken by a transplant center. It provides many avenues for highly skilled and sensitive nursing care. Solid organ transplantation is a viable therapeutic option for critically ill children who will be limited in either their lifestyle or their lifespan.

Children and families facing the process of transplantation deal with multiple issues. The developmental level of the child, the family dynamics, and the fact that many of the children are very young and have little or no participation in or control over their own care necessitate increased family and medical community commitment.

Children with organ failure are at risk of experiencing physical and emotional problems similar to those of children with other chronic or life-threatening illnesses. Although it presents new challenges and requirements for care, transplantation offers the chance of long-term survival and rehabilitation. Before transplantation, children often incur repeated hospitalizations, which may involve separation from family members, school, friends, and familiar environments. Throughout the process of transplantation, the child is influenced by previous experiences with hospitals and healthcare professionals and ongoing developmental changes.

Severe stress for patients, family, and staff occurs during the posttransplant period if rejection, infection, or other complications delay or interrupt the progress of recovery. Quality of life is affected by clinical problems such as chronic rejection and noncompliance. Certain special programs, such as weaning steroids, withdrawing immunosuppressant therapy, and switching from cyclosporine to tacrolimus in cases of severe hirsutism, have helped to address these issues. Constant efforts at reassurance, support, and promotion of normal life patterns for child and family must be provided. The PICU and acute care staff must be aware of the individual family's coping patterns, as well as their need to participate in the patient's care. When living related donation occurs, the donor who needs to mourn the loss of a body part can easily feel unappreciated and ignored while the recipient is the focus of care. When the donor is the child's parent, these are significant issues.

Other parenting issues are key in the immediate postoperative period. Weichler[71] reported an exploratory study determining information needs of mothers of liver transplant recipients. A 13-item, open-ended interview guide was completed by eight mothers. The most prominent maternal emotions were fear of the child's death and fear of organ rejection. In the PICU phase, mothers reported feelings of guilt over seeing their child with numerous invasive tubes in place. The mothers perceived that the most important way for parents to cope with these fears was to be as prepared as possible for the transplant process. In the PICU, mothers reported the following five consistent information needs: (1) the purpose of the tubes, (2) liver enzyme laboratory values, (3) child's blood pressure, (4) medications, and (5) child's overall well-being. Three of the eight mothers

reported that they were too stressed to seek information during the PICU phase.

Supervised viewing of the native organ with pathology personnel may provide support to the parents. Parents have reported that seeing their child's liver relieved the lingering question of the necessity of the transplant at the time. If the diagnosis or cause of liver failure (or other organ failure) is unknown, meeting with the pathologist allows parental questions to be asked, although they may go unanswered.

Returning the transplant patient to his or her home and community may prove to be very stressful. The very small child tends to be overactive for a few months until the excitement of being well becomes exhausting and normal childhood activity resumes. The adolescent, who is already in a period of structural ego alteration, may have conflicts about body image, identity, and dependency. A cushingoid appearance and struggles with weight gain may make returning to school difficult.

The family, having previously cared for the ill patient, may find it difficult to let go and permit independent activity. Previously submerged intrafamilial tensions may become overt with the stresses of chronic illness, and the family structure may disintegrate. Consideration must also be given to the financial stresses that burden families of transplant patients. With the exception of some specific federal legislation for renal transplantation, the costs of transplants must usually be covered by each individual family's resources or private insurance.

Discharge planning should be initiated early in the course of hospitalization. In addition to teaching the child and family about the medications and required procedures, discussion should be initiated around home issues such as attending school or day care, travel and vacations, camps, and pets.[72]

Families should be aware that transplant staff need to be notified when certain physical symptoms or changes occur. These include fever, diarrhea lasting longer than 24 hours (or 12 hours for intestine recipients), enlarged lymph nodes, seizures, tremors, abdominal pain, headache, irritability, disorientation, GI bleeding, fatigue or lethargy, abnormal laboratory results, or new medications prescribed by other healthcare providers. Patients and families should be taught when to call with information and when it is appropriate to take the child to the emergency department.

Routine immunization schedules are initiated 3 months after transplantation. Live, attenuated viral vaccines are usually not administered to immunosuppressed children, but well-child care may include inactivated vaccines as recommended by the transplant team. Influenza vaccine is given annually. When possible, hepatitis B immunizations should be administered before transplantation. Routine childhood illnesses may be serious in immunosuppressed transplant recipients. The transplant team must be made aware of exposures so that decisions for care, such as immunoglobulins, can be made when appropriate and in a timely fashion.

Survival and quality of life issues have been examined in several studies. Over the past 15 years, marked improvement has been seen in outcomes for pediatric heart, heart-lung, and lung recipients, although there is a lower rate of survival for heart-lung and lung recipients than cardiac recipients.[26] Most patients resume physical normal function, although peak exercise performance may be compromised.[29] Chronic rejection appears to be the principal factor that limits survival in both groups.

Uzark and colleagues[73] conducted a multicenter study involving 52 heart recipients, ages 8 to 16 years, who had survived more than 3 months posttransplant. Using several measures, they assessed family stress, resources, parental coping, and child adaptation. They found that patients experienced a dramatic improvement in functional status but may be at increased risk for problems in psychosocial adaptation. They noted an increase in behavior problems, which were highly correlated with family stress. DeMaso and colleagues[74] studied 23 patients of ages 3 to 20 years and assessed psychologic functioning using the Children's Global Assessment scale before transplant and at 1-year posttransplant. They also evaluated the impact of pretransplant psychologic function, family function, and posttransplant medical severity. Seventy-eight percent of patients had good psychologic function posttransplant. Pretransplant emotional status and family function correlated more with posttransplant psychologic function than medical severity. Two studies focusing on long-term outcomes in children following heart transplantation report that rehabilitation and quality of life have been good or excellent.[75,76] In general, quality of life for children after heart transplantation is improved compared to pretransplant status, and recipients cope well with the stressors of transplantation. One significant issue, particularly for adolescents, is noncompliance with immunosuppressive therapy, which may have dire consequences.

Quality of life issues in children following liver transplantation have also been reported.[77,78] Zitelli and associates[78] noted that objective lifestyle changes in 65 children had improved from their pretransplant status and that overall the children attended school, took fewer medications, and experienced fewer days of hospitalization. Zamberlan[77] interviewed 20 school-age children 3 to 6 years after liver transplantation who perceived their quality of life to be good; however, many negative feelings about physical appearance were expressed. The 20 children expressed feelings of insecurity and loneliness, had difficulties in peer relations, and had higher anxiety scale scores as compared with a normal group on the Piers-Harris Self-Concept Scale.

One of the key issues in quality of life for renal transplant recipients is growth and development. As mentioned previously, children with ESRD do not have normal growth and development before transplantation. After transplantation, some children have an accelerated period of growth (catch-up growth), others demonstrate some improvement in growth, and others continue to fall behind on growth charts. Data suggest that normal or accelerated growth after transplantation is more likely to occur in infants or young children, that growth may continue to be impaired if graft function is not normal, that growth improves with less steroid usage, and that other endocrine factors may affect growth patterns.[63] Follow-up of renal transplant recipients continues to focus on growth patterns. Manipulation of steroid administration, including alternate-day dosing and withdrawal of steroids, is continuing to be investigated. Some investigators have reported improved growth, especially in prepubertal children, with administration of recombinant growth hormone.[63]

Studies of long-term outcomes in renal recipients have been done, but outcomes would probably be better currently with the improvement in immunosuppression therapy.[63] Four studies of rehabilitation of pediatric renal recipients were reviewed, and the majority of patients were leading functional lives in terms of employment, family life, and education.[79] Children studied with greater than 10 years of allograft function demonstrated high achievement in education, participation in sports and other extracurricular activities, and employment and generally were satisfied with the quality of their lives. The major issue identified was dissatisfaction with their appearance, especially in terms of stature.[80] This is an issue that may begin to resolve with earlier transplantation (and less growth disruption) and decreased use of long-term steroids.

Further examination of the long-term effects on growth and development, school performance, and emotional status of children must occur now that there is a larger surviving population of pediatric transplant patients. Future patient issues of sexual maturation, fertility, and long-term drug effects during the first and second generations will become important. Creative approaches to facilitate treatment compliance must be developed and tested.

REFERENCES

1. Starzl TE, Esquivel C, Gordon R et al: Pediatric liver transplantation, *Transplant Proc* 19:3230-3235, 1987.
2. Hitchings GH, Elion GB: Chemical suppression of the immune response, *Pharmacol Rev* 15:365, 1963.
3. Armitage JM, Fricker FJ, Kurland G et al: Pediatric transplantation: the years 1985 to 1992 and the clinical trial of FK506, *J Thorac Cardiovasc Surg* 105:337, 1993
4. UNOS: 1999 Annual Report of the U.S. Scientific Registry of Transplant Recipients and the Organ Procurement and Transplantation Network: Transplant Data 1988-1998. Rockville, Md, and Richmond, Va, February 21, 2000.
5. Emond JC, Leib M: The living related liver transplant evaluation: linking risk factors and outcome, *Liver Transpl Surg* 2(suppl 1):57, 1996.
6. Caplan A: Must I be my brother's keeper? Ethical issues in the use of living-related donors as sources of liver and other solid organs, *Transplant Proc* 25:1997, 1993.
7. Gordon RD, Iwatsuki S, Esquivel CO et al: Liver transplantation across ABO groups, *Surgery* 100:342-348, 1986.
8. Uniform Determination of Death Act: President's Commission for the Study of Ethical Problems in Medicine and Biomedical and Behavioral Research: *Defining death: medical, legal and ethical issues in the determination of death,* Washington, DC, 1981, US Government Printing Office.
9. Reyes J, Starzl TE: Principles of transplantation. In O'Neill JA, Rowe MI, Grosfeld JL, eds: *Pediatric surgery,* ed 5, St Louis, 1998, Mosby.
10. Armitage JM, Fricker FJ, del Nido P et al: A decade (1982-1992) of pediatric cardiac transplantation and the impact of FK506

immunosuppression, *J Thorac Cardiovasc Surg* 105:464-472, 1993.

11. Sehgal SN: Rapamune (RAPA, rapamycin, sirolimus): mechanism of action immunosuppressive effect results from blockade of signal transduction and inhibition of cell cycle progression, *Clin Biochem* 31:335-340, 1998.

12. Starzl TE, Todo S, Fung J et al: FK-506 for liver, kidney, and pancreas transplantation, *Lancet* 2:1002-1004, 1989.

13. Jain A, Mazariegos G, Kashyap R et al: Comparative long-term evaluation of tacrolimus and cyclosporine in pediatric liver transplantation, *Transplantation* 70:617-625, 2000.

14. Asante-Korang A, Boyle GJ, Webber SA et al: Experience of FK506 immune suppression in pediatric heart transplantation: a study of long-term adverse effects, *J Heart Lung Transplant* 15:415-422, 1996.

15. Venkataramanan R, Jain A, Warty VW et al: Pharmacokinetics of FK-506 following oral administration: a comparison of FK-506 and cyclosporine, *Transplant Proc* 23:931-933, 1991.

16. Webber SA: 15 Years of pediatric heart transplantation at the University of Pittsburgh: lessons learned and future prospects, *Pediatr Transplant* 1:8-21, 1997.

17. McGhee B, Howrie D, Kraisinger M et al: *Pediatric drug therapy handbook & formulary,* Department of Pharmacy, Children's Hospital of Pittsburgh, 1997, Lexi-Comp.

18. Goldstein G: An overview of orthoclone OKT-3, *Transplant Proc* 18:927, 1986.

19. Boucek M, Faro A, Novick RJ et al: The Registry of the International Society for Heart and Lung Transplantation: Third Official Pediatric Report-1999, *J Heart Lung Transplant* 18:1151-1172, 1999.

20. Swinnen LJ, Costanzo-Norton M, Fisher SG et al: Increased incidence of lymphoproliferative disorder after immunosuppression with the monoclonal antibody OKT3 in cardiac transplant recipients, *N Engl J Med* 324:1437-1439, 1990.

21. Levin B, Hoppe RT, Collins G et al: Treatment of cadaveric renal transplantation recipients with total lymphoid irradiation, antithymocyte globulin, and low dose prednisone, *Lancet* 2:1321, 1998.

22. Hunt S, Strober S, Hoppe R et al: Use of total lymphoid irradiation for therapy of intractable cardiac allograft rejection, *J Heart Transplant* 8:104, 1989.

23. Hosenpud JD, Bennet L, Keck BM et al: The Registry of the International Society for Heart and Lung Transplantation: Sixteenth official Report-1999, *J Heart Lung Transplant* 18:611-640, 1999.

24. Chinnock RE: Pediatric Heart Transplantation at Loma Linda: 1985-1996; In Cecka M, Terasaki P, eds: *Clinical transplants 1996,* Los Angeles, Calif, 1996, UCLA Tissue Typing Laboratory.

25. Jenkins PC, Flanagan M, Jenkins K et al: Comparison of survival in transplantation and staged surgery for hypoplastic left heart syndrome. *Circulation* 100(suppl 1):I-672, 1999.

26. International Society for Heart and Lung Transplantation: Sixteenth Annual Data Report, April 1999.

27. Armitage JM, Kurland G, Michaels M et al: Critical issues in pediatric lung transplantation, *J Thorac Cardiovasc Surg* 109:60, 1995.

28. Spray TL, Mallory GB, Canter CB et al: Pediatric lung transplantation: indications, techniques, and early results, *J Thorac Cardiovasc Surg* 107:990, 1994.

29. Webber SA, Griffith BP: Heart and heart-lung transplantation. In O'Neill JA, Rowe MI, Grosfeld JL et al, eds: *Pediatric surgery,* ed 5, St Louis:, 1998, Mosby.

30. Franco KL, ed: *Pediatric cardiopulmonary transplantation,* Armonk, NY, 1997, Futura.

31. Veith F, Kamholz S, Mollenkopf F et al: Lung transplantation, *Transplantation* 35:271-278, 1983.

32. Griffith BP, Hardesty RL, Armitage JM et al: A decade of lung transplantation, *Ann Surg* 218:310-318, 1993.

33. Boucek M, Mathis C, Kanakriyeh M et al: Echocardiographic evaluation of cardiac graft rejection after infant heart transplantation, *J Heart Lung Transplant* 12:824-831, 1993.

34. Santos-Ocampo S, Sekarski T, Saffitz J et al: Echocardiographic characteristics of biopsy-proven cellular rejection in infant heart transplant recipients, *J Heart Lung Transplant* 15:25-34, 1996.

35. Rotondo K, Naftel D, Boucek R et al: Allograft rejection following cardiac transplantation in infants and children: a multiinstitutional study, *J Heart Lung Transplant* 15:S80, 1996.

36. Gajarski RJ, Smith EO, Denfield SW et al: Long-term results of triple drug based immunosuppression in nonneonatal pediatric heart transplant recipients, *Transplantation* 65:1470-1476, 1998.

37. Kanter K, Tam V, Vincent R et al: Current results with pediatric heart transplantation, *Ann Thorac Surg* 68:527-531, 1999.

38. Pahl E, Zales VR, Fricker FJ et al: Posttransplant coronary artery disease in children. a multicenter national survey. *Circulation* 90(suppl 2):56-60, 1994.

39. MacDonald K, Rector TS, Braulin EA et al: Association of coronary artery disease in cardiac transplant recipients with cytomegalovirus infections, *Am J Cardiol* 64:359, 1989.

40. Kosmach B, Webber SA, Reyes J: Care of the pediatric solid organ transplant recipient: the primary care perspective. *Pediatr Clin North Am* 45:1395-1418, 1998.

41. Halwachs G, Zach R, Pogglitsch H et al: A rapid immunocyto-chemical assay for CMV detection in peripheral blood of organ-transplant patients in clinical practice, *Transplant* 56:2, 1993

42. Green M, Michaels M: Infections in solid organ transplant recipients. In Long SS, Pickery LK, Prober CG, eds: *Principles and practice of pediatric infectious diseases,* New York, 1997, Churchill Livingstone.

43. Boyle GJ, Michaels MG, Webber SA et al: Posttransplantation lymphoproliferative disorders in pediatric thoracic organ recipients, *J Pediatr* 131:309-313, 1997.

44. Green M, Michaels M, Webber S et al: The management of Epstein-Barr virus associated post-transplant lymphoproliferative disorders in pediatric solid-organ transplant recipients, *Pediatr Transplant* 3:271-281, 1999.

45. Slota M, Green M, Farley A et al: The role of gown and glove isolation and strict hand-washing in the reduction of nosocomial infection in children with solid organ transplantation, *Crit Care Med* 29, 2001 (in press).

46. Shaddy RE, Naftel DC, Kirklin JK et al: Outcome of cardiac transplantation in children: survival in a contemporary multi-institutional experience, *Circulation* 94(pt 2):69-73, 1996.

47. Lucey MR: New trends in liver transplantation, American Association for the Study of Liver Diseases 50th Annual Meeting, Medscape, 1999.

48. Colombani P: Liver transplantation. In O'Neill JA, Rowe MI, Grosfeld JL et al, eds: *Pediatric surgery,* St Louis, 1998, Mosby.

49. Bismuth H, Houssin D. Reduced-size orthotopic liver transplantation in children, *Surgery* 95:127, 1995.

50. Reyes J, Gerber D, Mazariegos GV et al: Split-liver transplantation: a comparison of ex vivo and in situ techniques, *J Pediatr Surg* 35:283, 2000.

51. Sindhi R, Rosendale J, Mundy D et al: Impact of segmental grafts on pediatric liver transplantation: a review of the United Network for Organ Sharing registry data (1990-1996), *J Pediatr Surg* 34:107, 1999.

52. Sieders E, Peeters PM, TenVergert EM et al: Analysis of survival and morbidity after pediatric liver transplantation with full-size and technical-variant grafts. *Transplantation* 68:540-545, 1999.

53. Singh N: Infectious diseases in the liver transplant recipient, *Semin Gastrointest Dis* 9:136-146, 1998.

54. Mews CF, Dorney SF, Sheil AG et al: Failure of liver transplantation in Wilson's disease with pulmonary arteriovenous shunting, *J Pediatr Gastroenterol Nutr* 10:230-233, 1990.

55. Whitington P: Advances in pediatric liver transplantation. In Barnes LA, ed: *Advances in pediatrics,* St Louis, 1990, Mosby.

56. Park SC, Beerman LB, Gartner JC et al: Echocardiographic findings before and after liver transplantation, *Am J Cardiol* 55:1373-1378, 1985.

57. Tzakis A, Starzl TE: Pediatric liver transplantation. In Ashcraft KW, Holder TM, eds: *Pediatric surgery,* ed 2, Philadelphia, 1992, WB Saunders.

58. Mazariegos GV, O'Toole K, Mieles LA et al: Hyperbaric oxygen therapy for hepatic artery thrombosis after liver transplantation in children, *Liver Transplant Surg* 5:429-436, 1999.

59. Shaw BW, Stratta R, Donovan JP et al: Postoperative care after liver transplantation, *Semin Liver Dis* 9:202-230, 1989.

60. Todo A, Reyes J: Intestinal transplantation. In O'Neill JA, Rowe MI, Grosfeld JL et al, eds: *Pediatric surgery,* ed 5, St Louis, 1998, Mosby.

61. Reyes J, Bueno J, Kocoshis S et al: Current status of intestinal transplantation in children, *J Pediatr Surg* 33:243-254, 1998.

62. Reyes J, Fishbein T, Bueno J et al: Reduced-size orthotopic composite liver-intestinal allograft, *Transplantation* 66:489-492, 1998.
63. Matas AJ, Najarian JS: Kidney transplantation. In O'Neill JA, Rowe MI, Grosfeld JL et al, eds: *Pediatric surgery,* ed 5, St Louis, 1998, Mosby.
64. McEnery PT, Alexander SR, Sullivan K et al: Renal transplantation in children and adolescents: the 1992 annual report of the North American Pediatric Renal Transplant Cooperative Study, *Pediatr Nephrol* 7:711-720, 1993.
65. Najarian JS, Almond PS, Mauer M et al: Renal transplantation in the first year of life: the treatment of choice for infants with end-stage renal disease, *J Am Soc Nephrol* 2:S228-233, 1992.
66. Kim MS, Jabs K, Harmon WE: Long-term patient survival in a pediatric renal transplantation program, *Transplantation* 51:413-417, 1991.
67. Maxfield A: The workings of the transplant waiting list, *Nephrol News Issues* 13:28-30, 1999.

68. Bell J: Viewpoint: why multiple listing is wrong, *Nephrol News Issues* 13:28-30, 1994.
69. Bunchman TE, Fryd DS, Sibley RK et al: Manifestations of renal allograft rejection in small children receiving adult kidneys, *Pediatr Nephrol* 4:255-258, 1990.
70. Sutherland DER, Wahoff DC. Pancreatic Transplantation. In O'Neill JA, Rowe MI, Grosfeld JL et al, eds: *Pediatric surgery,* ed 5, St Louis, 1998, Mosby.
71. Weichler NK: Information needs of mothers of children who have had liver transplants, *J Pediatr Nurs* 6:88-96, 1990.
72. Kosmach B, Corbo-Richert B, Pike N: Organ transplantation. In Jackson PL, Vessey JA, eds: *Primary care of the child with a chronic condition,* ed 3, St Louis, 1999, Mosby.
73. Uzark K, Sauer S, Lawrence K et al: The psychosocial impact of pediatric heart transplantation, *J Heart Lung Transplant* 11:1160-1167, 1992.
74. DeMaso D, Twente A, Spratt E et al: Impact of medical severity and family functioning on adjustment following pediatric heart transplantation, *J Heart Lung Transplant* 14:1102-1108, 1995.

75. Baum D, Bernstein D, Starnes V et al: Pediatric heart transplantation at Stanford: results of a 15 year experience, *Pediatrics* 88:203-214, 1991.
76. Sigfusson G, Fricker FJ, Bernstein D et al: Long term survivors of pediatric heart transplantation: a multi-center report of sixty-eight children who have survived longer than five years, *J Pediatr* 130:862-871, 1997.
77. Zamberlan K: Quality of life in school-age children following liver transplantation, *Dissertation Abstracts International* SO:150-Osb, 1989.
78. Zitelli B, Miller J, Gartner J et al: Changes in lifestyle after liver transplantation, *Pediatrics* 82:173-180, 1988.
79. Potter DE: Long term results of renal transplantation in children, *Nephron* 63:373, 1993.
80. Morel P, Almond PS, Matas AJ et al: Long-term quality of life after kidney transplantation in childhood, *Transplantation* 52:47-53, 1991.

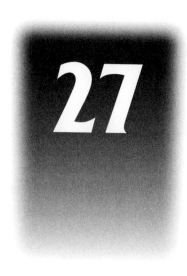

Shock

Cathy H. Dichter
Martha A.Q. Curley

Shock, along with its associated reduction in effective tissue perfusion, results from the loss of integrity of one or more of the four essential components of circulation: blood volume, cardiac pump, vascular tone, and cell function (Table 27-1). Regardless of the cause, the final common pathway of shock is cell destruction caused by either ineffective tissue delivery or impaired use of essential cellular substrates.

The extent to which shock contributes to morbidity and mortality among critically ill infants and children is directly related to the ability of caregivers to (1) rapidly recognize the cluster of symptoms characteristic of shock; (2) vigilantly attend to the administration and titration of collaborative management strategies intended to interrupt the numerous pathophysiologic cascades associated with shock; and (3) efficiently provide intensive nursing care.

CATEGORIES OF SHOCK

Although classified in a variety of ways, shock can be divided into two major categories. Based on characteristic blood flow, the categories are low-flow shock and maldistributive shock. Low-flow shock states are characterized by decreased cardiac output. The low-flow state may be due to hypovolemia, cardiac failure, or critical obstruction of blood flow from the heart. Maldistributive shock states are characterized by normal or increased cardiac output but an abnormal distribution of blood flow. This category of shock includes neurogenic shock, anaphylaxis, and, most commonly, septic shock. Clustering all shock states into these two hemodynamically based categories provides clinically relevant information. Not only do these two categories of shock present differently from one another, but also the primary interventions in each are different. However, it is crucial to note the mixed nature of most forms of clinical shock. For example, septic shock presents as maldistributive shock but may progress to low-flow shock secondary to myocardial depression.

One of the most challenging clinical problems in pediatric critical care is caring for the patient in shock. Shock is a "state in which profound and widespread reduction of effective tissue perfusion leads first to reversible, and then, if prolonged, to irreversible cellular injury."[1]

◆ TABLE 27-1   Shock States

Altered Component of Circulation	Shock
Blood volume: insufficient circulating blood volume in relation to vascular space	**Low-flow: hypovolemic**
Cardiac pump: insufficient cardiac output despite adequate ventricular preload	**Low-flow: cardiogenic**
Vascular tone: inappropriate systemic or pulmonary vascular tone	**Maldistributive: distributive**
Cellular function: ineffective tissue use of oxygen and nutrients	**Maldistributive: septic**

Box 27-1
◆ Causes of Shock

Low-Flow Shock (Hypovolemic)

Blood Loss

Trauma (e.g., splenic rupture)
Gastrointestinal bleeding
Inadequate replacement

Plasma Loss

Capillary leak syndrome
Hypoproteinemia
Nephrotic syndrome
Burns
Peritonitis
Bowel obstruction

Water Loss

Vomiting and diarrhea
Diabetes mellitus
Diabetes insipidus

Low-Flow Shock (Cardiogenic)

Metabolic

Hypoxemia, acidosis, hypoglycemia, severe electrolyte imbalance

Dysrhythmias

Drug toxicity

Cardiac Tamponade

Coexisting Disorders

Cardiac failure secondary to congenital or acquired heart disease

Maldistributive Shock

Neurogenic

Anesthesia, spinal cord injury

Anaphylactic

Immune or nonimmune induced

Septic Shock

Any infectious organism

Low-Flow Shock

The most common shock syndrome in infants and children is low-flow shock resulting from acute hypovolemia. Any illness or injury that results in an acute reduction in

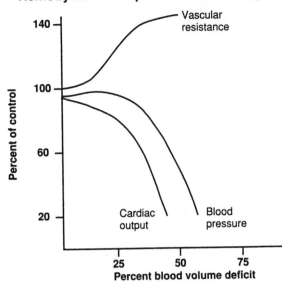

Hemodynamic Response to Hemorrhage

Fig. 27-1 Model for cardiovascular response to hypovolemia from hemorrhage. (Reproduced with permission from *Textbook of pediatric advanced life support,* 1990. Copyright by American Heart Association.)

circulating blood volume—that is, severe blood, plasma, or body fluid loss—can cause hypovolemia and shock. The decrease in intravascular volume can be absolute, as in hemorrhage after trauma, or relative, as in nephrotic syndrome when plasma moves out of the vascular space into the interstitial space. Other common causes of hypovolemic and low-flow shock in infants and children are listed in Box 27-1.

The progressive pathophysiologic effects of intravascular volume loss include decreased venous return, decreased ventricular filling, decreased stroke volume, decreased cardiac output, and then ineffective tissue perfusion. Following the loss of volume, a series of cardiac and peripheral hemostatic adjustments are stimulated in an attempt to support myocardial and cerebral perfusion pressures. In previously healthy hypovolemic patients, systolic and mean arterial blood pressures are often maintained until the blood volume deficit reaches 25% (Fig. 27-1). The degree to which compensatory mechanisms succeed in maintaining blood pressure is determined by the infant's or child's preexisting health status, particularly cardiac reserve, as well as the volume and rate of blood or fluid loss and resuscitation attempts.

Insufficient cardiac output despite adequate and at times increased ventricular preload is the second cause of low-flow shock. In addition to congenital or acquired heart disease, other important causes of cardiogenic low-flow shock in the pediatric population include hypoxemia, acidosis, posthypoxic-ischemic arrest, hypoglycemia, severe electrolyte imbalance, dysrhythmias, drug intoxication, chest trauma (myocardial contusion), and outflow obstructions. The term *obstructive shock* is sometimes used to describe the low-flow state that results from mechanical obstruction to ventricular outflow from either decreased diastolic filling (tension pneumothorax, tension pneumo-pericardium, pericardial effusion, cardiac tamponade) or increased ventricular afterload (massive pulmonary embolus). Compensatory mechanisms designed to support perfusion pressures often contribute to the progression of cardiogenic shock.

Maldistributive Shock

Maldistributive shock results from an abnormal distribution of blood volume. Hemodynamically, its defining feature is an overall decrease in systemic vascular resistance (SVR). Vasomotor paralysis, increased venous capacity, or abnormal shunting of blood past capillary beds results in the abnormal apportionment of circulating blood volume that is characteristic of maldistributive shock. In infants and children, maldistributive shock may be neurogenic, anaphylactic, and, most commonly, septic shock (see Box 27-1).

Neurogenic maldistributive shock is characterized by massive vasodilation from loss of sympathetic vasomotor tone. Alterations in the regulation of vasomotor tone may be due to either pharmacologic blockade (anesthetic agents, morphine, barbiturates, antihypertensives) or traumatic damage to the sympathetic nervous system (spinal cord transection above T1). The resulting vasodilation leads to increased vascular capacity in affected body parts, usually the extremities, depriving vital organs of oxygen and nutrients.

Anaphylactic maldistributive shock is caused by massive release of mediators from tissue mast cells and circulating basophils resulting from anaphylaxis or an anaphylactoid reaction. Anaphylaxis, an immediate hypersensitivity reaction, may occur after sensitized individuals are exposed to drugs, especially antibiotics, food, or insect venom. Mediated by the interaction of immunoglobulin E (IgE) antibodies (on the surface of mast cells and basophils) and the antigen, primary mediators of anaphylaxis are released, including histamine, serotonin, and others. Subsequently, secondary mediators, such as bradykinin and prostaglandins, are synthesized and released. Although clinically indistinguishable from anaphylaxis, an anaphylactoid reaction results from nonimmunologic release of mediators from mast cells and basophils. Anaphylactoid reactions may occur as a result of various medical agents, such as contrast dye, protamine, muscle relaxants, and anesthetics.[2] Anaphylactic shock is hemodynamically very similar to septic shock with profound vasodilation and capillary leak. In addition, patients often demonstrate urticarial rash, laryngeal edema, and severe bronchospasm. Unlike in the emergency department, anaphylactic shock is an uncommon phenomenon in the ICU.

The most common maldistributive shock in pediatrics is septic shock. Zimmerman and Dietrich[3] describe septic shock as a disease of intermediary metabolism induced by an infectious agent (microorganism), which results in physiologic and destructive host responses and corresponding fuel energy deficits. All organisms (gram-negative bacteria, gram-positive bacteria, viruses, fungi, rickettsiae, spirochetes, protozoa, and parasites) can initiate the multi-

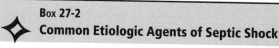

Box 27-2
Common Etiologic Agents of Septic Shock

Neonate
β-Hemolytic streptococci
Escherichia coli
Herpes simplex virus

Older Infant and Child
Haemophilus influenzae, type B*
Neisseria meningitidis
Streptococcus pneumoniae
β-Hemolytic streptococci

Nosocomial
Staphylococcus aureus
Staphylococcus epidermidis
Pseudomonas
Candida

*As a result of immunization with conjugated vaccines in the United States, microbial causes of sepsis in immunocompetent children are limited.

system, subcellular metabolic derangements associated with septic shock, but etiologic agents vary according to age and immunologic status of the patient and the place of microbial acquisition (community vs. hospital setting) (Box 27-2). In pediatrics, gram-negative and gram-positive nosocomial infections occur in almost equal proportions; the foci primarily include skin and lungs.[4] Endotoxin release from gram-negative bacteria (Fig. 27-2) or exotoxin release from gram-positive bacteria are two prominent exogenous mediators that serve as triggers to this complex process.[5]

The normal inflammatory immune response is triggered when the microorganism gains access to the body's internal environment. The inflammatory immune response is triggered in an effort to eliminate or neutralize the microorganism and its toxins, contain the microorganism invasion and prevent its systemic access (bloodstream), and promote rapid healing of involved tissues.[6] When the ability to serve these functions is overwhelmed, there is systemic release of the microorganism (and associated toxins) and subsequent activation and release of various endogenous mediators and cytokines, referred to as the systemic inflammatory response syndrome (SIRS).

The interrelationship among SIRS, sepsis, septic shock, and organ dysfunction was originally conceptualized by Bone[7] and later adopted by the American College of Chest Physicians and the Society of Critical Care Medicine[8] (Box 27-3). An important conceptual outcome of this work was that inflammation (with or without infection) was identified as a major pathogenic factor in the development of SIRS, sepsis, septic shock, and multiple organ dysfunction syndrome (MODS). In addition, establishing consensus on the use of terminology and diagnostic criteria facilitates clarity and consistency so that clinicians can compare the results of clinical research studies related to sepsis.

To determine the incidence of SIRS, sepsis, severe sepsis, septic shock, and MODS in critically ill children, Proulx and

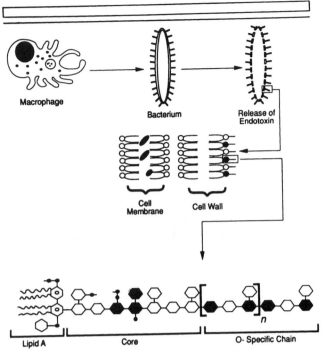

Fig. 27-2 Phagocytosis of gram-negative bacteria releases endotoxin, which is a component of the bacterial cell wall. Endotoxin is a lipopolysaccharide molecule with three components: lipid A, a polysaccharide core, and an O-specific chain. Lipid A contains most of the biologic effects of endotoxin, and O-specific chain is a major antigen recognized by the body. (From Klein DM, Witek-Janusek L: Advances in immunotherapy of sepsis, *Dimens Crit Care Nurs* 11:79, 1992. Copyright 1992 by Hall Johnson Communications. Reproduced with permission. For further use, contact the publisher at 9737 West Ohio Avenue, Lakewood CO 80226.)

colleagues[9] conducted a prospective cohort study involving 1058 consecutive pediatric intensive care unit (PICU) admissions. SIRS occurred in 82% of PICU admissions; 23% had sepsis, 4% had severe sepsis, 2% had septic shock; 16% had primary MODS, and 2% had secondary MODS. Compared with patients with primary MODS, secondary MODS was associated with a longer duration of organ dysfunction, longer length of stay after MODS diagnosis, and a higher risk of mortality.

The hallmarks of septic shock are a maldistribution of circulating blood flow, imbalance of oxygen supply and demand, alterations in metabolism, and cardiac dysfunction, resulting in a myriad of pathophysiologic events (Box 27-4).

Two specific causes of septic shock that require specific mention are meningococcemia and toxic shock syndrome. Meningococcemia, caused by the gram-negative diplococcus *Neisseria meningitidis,* is a particularly virulent infection in children. Clinical presentation is often dramatic, with death often ensuing in a matter of hours. Classic presentation includes purpura fulminans, initially described as petechiae coalescing to diffuse purpuric ecchymotic lesions (Fig. 27-3). Poor prognostic indicators include purpura fulminans along with hypothermia, seizures, or hypotension on presentation; white blood cell (WBC) count of less than

Box 27-3

Definitions of SIRS, Sepsis, Septic Shock, and Multiple Organ Dysfunction Syndrome

Infection

Microbial phenomenon characterized by an inflammatory response to the presence of microorganisms or the invasion of normally sterile host tissue by those organisms

Bacteremia

Presence of viable bacteria in the blood

Systemic Inflammatory Response Syndrome (SIRS)

Systemic inflammatory response to a variety of severe clinical insults. The response is manifested by two or more of the following conditions:
Temperature >38° C or <36° C
Tachycardia
Tachypnea
WBC >12,000 cells/mm^3, <4000 cells/mm^3, or >10% immature (band) forms

Sepsis

Presence of SIRS with infection. This systemic response is manifested by two or more of the following conditions *as a result of infection:*
Temperature >38° C or <36° C
Tachycardia
Tachypnea
WBC >12,000 cells/mm^3, <4,000 cells/mm^3, or >10% immature (band) forms

Severe Sepsis

Presence of sepsis associated with organ dysfunction, hypoperfusion, or hypotension (e.g., lactic acidosis, oliguria, an acute change in mental status)

Septic Shock

Presence of sepsis with hypotension, despite adequate fluid resuscitation, along with the presence of perfusion abnormalities that may include, but are not limited to, lactic acidosis, oliguria, or an acute alteration in mental status. Patients who are receiving inotropic or vasopressor agents may not be hypotensive at the time that perfusion abnormalities are measured.

Multiple Organ Dysfunction Syndrome (MODS)

Presence of altered organ function in an acutely ill patient such that homeostasis cannot be maintained without interventions

From the American College of Chest Physicians/Society of Critical Care Medicine Consensus Conference: Definitions for sepsis and organ failure and guidelines for the use of innovative therapies in sepsis, *Crit Care Med* 20:864-874, 1992.
WBC, White blood cell.

5000 mm^3; and platelet count of less than 100,000 mm^3.[10] Fulminant disease is often associated with bilateral adrenal hemorrhage referred to as Waterhouse-Friderichsen syndrome. The severe, rapidly progressive cardiovascular collapse associated with meningococcemia is thought to be a result of endotoxin-induced myocardial depression.

Box 27-4
Major Pathophysiologic Changes Associated With Septic Shock

Maldistribution of Circulating Blood Flow	Imbalance of Oxygen Supply and Demand	Alterations in Metabolism	Cardiac Dysfunction
Increased capillary permeability	$\dot{V}/\dot{Q}$ mismatching	Hypermetabolism	Decreased coronary artery blood flow
Vasodilation	Intrapulmonary shunting	Inadequate substrate metabolism	Myocardial depressant factor
Selective vasoconstriction	Maldistribution of blood volume	Protein catabolism	Decreased LV ejection fraction
Loss of autoregulation	Microcirculatory abnormalities	Liver dysfunction	LV dilation
Microvascular thrombi	Oxygen extraction defects	Resistance to exogenous medication administration	Abnormal ventricular compliance
Vascular obstruction	Increased demand	Peripheral cell dysfunction	
Tissue edema	Pain, fever		
Cellular aggregation	Tachycardia		
Microthrombi	Increased work of breathing		
Fluid imbalances	Restlessness or anxiety		

Modified from Secor VH: Primary events and mediator release. In Secor VH, ed: *Multiple organ dysfunction and failure,* ed 2, St Louis, 1996, Mosby, Table 1-2, p 12.
$\dot{V}/\dot{Q}$, Ventilation-perfusion ratio; *LV,* left ventricular.

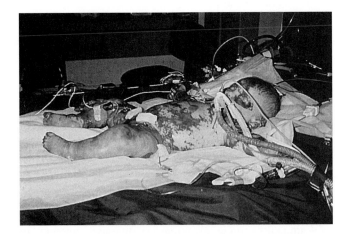

Fig. 27-3 Infant with purpura fulminans associated with meningococcemia.

Close contacts of all patients with invasive meningococcal disease are at risk and should receive prophylaxis within 24 hours of the diagnosis of the primary case. Close contacts include anyone who had contact with the patient's oral secretions during the 7 days before the onset of disease in the primary case. The chemoprophylactic drug of choice for pediatric contacts continues to be rifampin.[11] Ciprofloxacin, in a single oral dose, may be given to nonpregnant adults older than 18 years of age.

Toxic shock syndrome (TSS), septic shock resulting from toxin-producing strains of *Staphylococcus aureus,* can occur in nonmenstruating women and in males. Risk factors include surgical wound infections or focal (sinusitis, pneumonia, etc.) and systemic *S. aureus* infection. TSS is probable when at least four of the five major diagnostic criteria are fulfilled. Diagnostic criteria, defined by the Centers of Disease Control and Prevention, are included in Table 27-2. Individualized treatment includes antistaphylococcal antibiotics and control of the focus of infection.

TABLE 27-2   Diagnostic Criteria of Toxic Shock Syndrome

Fever	>38.9° C
Rash	Diffuse macular erythroderma
	Desquamation (palms and soles) 1-2 weeks after onset of illness
Hypotension	Systolic pressure less than the 5th percentile for children <16 yr

Three or More Organ System Involvement Is Required:

Gastrointestinal	Vomiting or diarrhea or both
Muscular	Severe muscle pain or creatine phosphokinase over twice upper normal
Mucous membrane	Hyperemia (conjunctival, oral, vaginal)
Renal	BUN over twice upper normal and increased WBC in urine (without UTI)
Hepatic	Total bilirubin, AST (SGOT), or ALT (SGPT) over twice upper normal
Hematologic	Platelets <100,000/mm³
Central nervous system	Change in consciousness when fever and hypotension absent
Laboratory results	Sterile blood, throat, CSF cultures (except for *Staphylococcus aureus*); serologic test for Rocky Mountain spotted fever, leptospirosis, or measles must be negative

From American Academy of Pediatrics: *1997 Red Book: Report of the Committee on Infectious Diseases,* ed 24, Elk Grove Village, Ill, 1997, American Academy of Pediatrics.
BUN, Blood urea nitrogen; *WBC,* white blood cell; *UTI,* urinary tract infection; *AST,* aspartate aminotransferase; *SGOT,* serum glutamic-oxaloacetic transaminase; *ALT,* alanine aminotransferase; *SGPT,* serum glutamic-pyruvic transaminase; *CSF,* cerebrospinal fluid.

TRAJECTORY OF ILLNESS

Shock is a syndrome that reflects the body's attempt to adapt to an insult and preserve vital organ function. The trajectory of adaptation in shock can be divided into three phases: a compensated stage during which blood pressure is maintained, although there is evidence of ineffective tissue perfusion; an uncompensated stage that reflects the inadequacy of compensatory mechanisms in the maintenance of blood pressure; and a refractory stage. Response to therapy varies during these stages.

In the *first phase,* the body's intrinsic supportive mechanisms can generally maintain normal vital organ function. Systemic blood flow is usually normal or increased. Hemodynamic values and vital signs may be normal or enhanced, reflecting the physiologic attempt to maintain vital organ perfusion. Although some parameters may appear enhanced, the body's total metabolic needs are not met, as evidenced by lactic acidosis and oliguria.[12] The success of the body's intrinsic supportive mechanisms is determined by the patient's preexisting state (e.g., volume status and myocardial function), illness, time elapsed, and treatment provided.

In the *second phase,* compensatory mechanisms are insufficient to maintain blood pressure and effective oxygen and nutrient delivery to the tissues. Delayed or inadequate maintenance of intravascular volume or other iatrogenic causes may play some role in the patient's deterioration. More often, though, the body simply lacks sufficient substrate for metabolic processes, or the cellular damage sustained is such that available substrate cannot be used. During this uncompensated period, clear evidence of poor perfusion is seen both in clinical parameters, such as skin, kidney, and brain, as well as in hemodynamic parameters, such as blood pressure, oxygen saturation, and filling pressures. Various tissues and organ systems experience insults, and multiple organ dysfunction, such as acute respiratory distress syndrome (ARDS) or disseminated intravascular coagulation (DIC), may develop and hasten the onset of the final stage and preclude recovery.

In the *third phase,* shock becomes irreversible. Damage to vital organs such as the heart and brain cannot be reversed with either time or therapeutic maneuvers.

Refractory or unresponsive septic shock has been described as progressing through three phases: a hyperdynamic-compensated phase, a hyperdynamic-uncompensated phase, and a hypodynamic or cardiogenic shock phase.[13] A previous assumption was that the hyperdynamic state ("warm shock") was consistently followed by the hypodynamic state ("cold shock"); however, research has shown two flaws with this assumption. First, with more generous use of hemodynamic monitoring and vigorous volume expanders, the incidence of hypodynamic septic shock is not as common. In fact, in adults with septic shock, approximately only 10% die of progressively deteriorating cardiac output (hypodynamic).[14] Second, the terms *warm* and *cold* shock did not always correlate accurately with true hemodynamic findings. Bone[7] therefore advises against using the terms *warm* and *cold* shock. Although fluid-resuscitated adults rarely display hypodynamic septic shock, hypodynamic septic shock (low cardiac output rather than low SVR) appears more common in fluid-resuscitated children.[15] In fact, low cardiac output, rather than low SVR, is associated with pediatric septic shock mortality.[16-18] In refractory septic shock, decreased SVR persists, but cardiac output falls because of unresponsive myocardial depression.

PHYSIOLOGIC RESPONSES TO SHOCK

Although physiologic responses to the different types of shock vary, patterns do exist within each category. The common physiologic characteristic of all early shock states is either reduced or ineffective oxygen supply relative to tissue demand. Physiologic mechanisms such as increased oxygen extraction in low-flow shock and increased cardiac output in maldistributive shock attempt to compensate for the uncoupling of oxygen supply and demand. Autoregulation maintains perfusion to the brain and heart by diverting blood flow from the nonessential areas of the skin, gut, and kidneys. With time, ongoing redistribution of blood flow can lead to progressive dysfunction, and, ultimately failure of major organ systems.

Neuroendocrine Activation

The neuroendocrine response, also known as the stress response, consists of sympathetic nervous system (SNS) and endocrine activation. The effects of SNS activation are diverse and serve one of two primary functions: maintenance of cardiovascular and respiratory function and energy and substrate mobilization.

Cardiac centers in the brainstem stimulate most of the sympathetic nerves at once, causing an increase in cardiac output, heart rate, and blood pressure. This stimulation results in a tenfold increase in norepinephrine, producing vasoconstriction in all vascular beds. With SNS stimulation, the adrenal medulla also releases massive amounts of catecholamines; epinephrine levels increase fiftyfold. Epinephrine increases both heart rate and myocardial contractility (unless limited by reduced or impaired myocardial function) and increases tissue perfusion pressure by direct vasoconstriction of all vascular beds except those in skeletal muscle and the liver.

A fall in mean arterial pressure or pulse pressure results in baroreceptor stimulation. Baroreceptor stimulation leads to diminished parasympathetic stimulation and enhanced sympathetic stimulation of the heart, producing positive cardiac inotropy and chronotropy and arterial and venous vasoconstriction. Low capillary hydrostatic pressure relative to plasma oncotic pressure shifts interstitial fluid into the intravascular compartment. The benefits of this "autotransfusion" are self-limiting because dilution of the hematocrit and plasma oncotic pressure eventually results. Because extracellular fluid volume is higher in children than in adults, this mechanism may play a greater role in pediatric shock than in adult shock.

When cerebral perfusion pressures reach very low levels (below cerebral autoregulation—about 40 mmHg in older children), a sympathetic surge produces massive vasoconstriction and a temporary arrest in the decline of blood pressure and cardiac output. The central nervous system (CNS) ischemic reflex maintains blood pressure by doubling SVR and producing a fivefold increase in pulmonary vascular resistance (PVR).

Metabolic alterations also result from neuroendocrine activation, initially aimed at meeting increased body demands. Metabolic alterations are characterized by hypermetabolism, hyperglycemia, and hypercatabolism.[19] Fig. 27-4 illustrates the myriad effects on metabolism. Importantly, hyperglycemia may be initially present because of epinephrine secretion. However, hypoglycemia develops, as hepatic glycogen stores are depleted (usually in less than 12 hours) and gluconeogenesis fails. Hypoglycemia should be care-

fully scrutinized as a sign of adrenal insufficiency. Adrenal insufficiency most commonly occurs in patients who have purpura fulminans or those with a history of chronic steroid use. In addition, any patient whose perfusion and blood pressure is unresponsive to vigorous volume resuscitation and vasoactive support should be evaluated for adrenal insufficiency.[20]

Anaerobic Metabolism

By definition, shock is congruent with hypoperfusion and tissue ischemia. This results in local tissue acidosis caused by decreased carbon dioxide clearance and anaerobic metabolism. At a time when oxygen demands are greatest

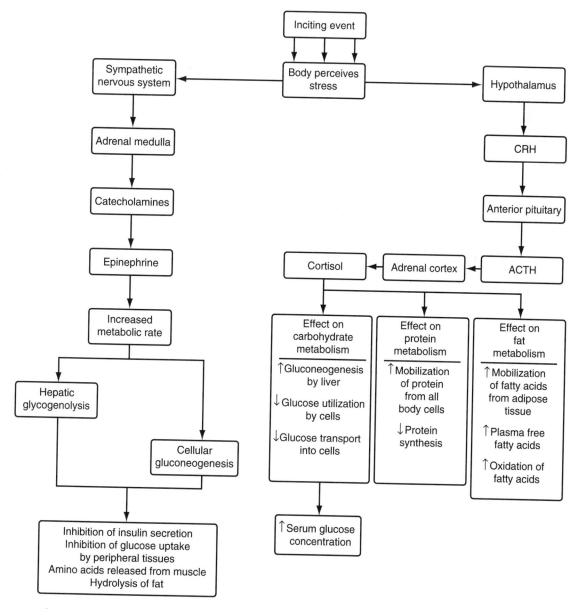

Fig. 27-4 Neuroendocrine effects on metabolism. As the body perceives stress or insult, neuroendocrine compensatory mechanisms are triggered to provide more energy to meet the body's needs. *ACTH,* Adrenocorticotropic hormone; *CRH,* corticotropin-releasing hormone. (From Kimbrell JD: Alterations in metabolism. In Secor VH, ed: *Multiple organ dysfunction and failure,* ed 2, St Louis, 1996, Mosby, p 149.)

for tissue repair, effective oxygen delivery is insufficient. Cellular processes therefore occur without oxygen (anaerobic metabolism), lactic acid accumulates, and metabolic acidosis develops. Decreased oxygen consumption ($\dot{V}O_2$) occurs secondary to reduced blood flow or maldistribution of flow. Arterial pH and base deficit determination serve as readily available markers of effective tissue perfusion and oxygenation.

Lactate levels may help to determine the degree of tissue perfusion. Lactate levels greater than 2 mmol/L are generally considered to be indicative of shock.[21] However, the use of lactate levels is limited by the fact that it is a late marker of tissue perfusion. Significant tissue ischemia is present by the time lactate is elevated.[2] In addition, because the liver clears lactate, liver hypoperfusion or dysfunction may markedly increase elevated lactate levels. Serial determinations of lactate have been used to assess the adequacy of resuscitation interventions in shock.

Gastric intramucosal pH monitoring may also provide a noninvasive method for the indirect measurement of tissue oxygenation.[22] Gastrointestinal tonometry uses a standard vented nasogastric tube combined with a silicone balloon system permeable to CO_2. When the saline-filled balloon is placed in close proximity to the gastric mucosa, CO_2 gas diffuses from the gastrointestinal mucosa into the balloon tonometer. The CO_2 measurement, used in conjunction with the arterial blood bicarbonate, serves as an indirect estimate of the intramucosal pH of the gut. Mucosal acidosis correlates well with the onset of anaerobic metabolism in response to sepsis or hypoxia.[23] Casado-Flores and colleagues[24] report that low gastric pH (<7.30) was associated with an increased risk of mortality in PICU patients; however, no relationship was found between gastric pH and the development of MODS.

Fluid Shifts

Some category-specific hemodynamic changes and responses to shock also occur. Hypovolemic shock is characterized by low circulating blood volume and decreased preload. Compensatory, generalized vasoconstriction takes place, decreasing venous capacity and translocating venous blood to the central circulation, thereby increasing preload. A rise in blood pressure and cardiac output may follow.

The renin-angiotensin-aldosterone system (RAAS) and antidiuretic hormone (ADH) also help restore intravascular volume within minutes after hemorrhage or trauma. Renal vasoconstriction and hypoperfusion activate the RAAS with increased production and secretion of renin. Increased plasma renin activity stimulates the release of angiotensin I. Angiotensin I is converted to angiotensin II by the angiotensin-converting enzyme (ACE) in the vascular epithelium of the lungs and in other tissues, including the heart, adrenals, kidneys, and brain. Angiotensin II is a potent vasoconstrictor that also stimulates the production of aldosterone by the adrenal gland, increasing sodium and water reabsorption in the renal tubules. Stimulated by an increase in serum osmolality, vasopressin (ADH) secretion from the posterior pituitary gland results in peripheral vasoconstriction and increased reabsorption of water from the renal tubules and collecting ducts. Stress precipitates the release of adrenocorticotropic hormone (ACTH) from the anterior pituitary, which then stimulates the adrenal glands to release cortisol. Cortisol sensitizes arteriolar smooth muscle to the effects of catecholamines.

In contrast to the low ventricular filling pressures seen in patients with hypovolemic shock, the ventricular filling pressures in those with cardiogenic shock are high. This is a consequence of both myocardial dysfunction and loss of ventricular diastolic compliance and the additional venous return brought about by the compensatory venous constriction.

Mediator Release

A myriad of mediators is triggered in all shock states and during their associated resuscitative interventions. The release of mediators comes from not only the body's normal protective host response but also endothelial damage and ischemia or reperfusion injury. The endothelium, an active metabolic organ, is subject to damage in shock, as well as by other factors such as mechanical disruption, hypoxemia, acidosis, and microorganisms.[25] When damaged, the endothelium is unable to perform its normal functions, that is, anticoagulation and vasoregulation. Normally integral to maintaining the fluidity of blood, damaged endothelium displays procoagulant activity leading to thrombin formation and fibrin deposition. Vasoregulatory properties of the endothelium, through nitric oxide production (among others), are also influenced. Damaged endothelium results in widespread capillary permeability and massive fluid loss to tissues and organs. The result of both endothelial malfunctions is further obstruction of blood flow and ischemia, especially in the microvasculature.

Arachidonic acid, a normal constituent of all cell membranes (except red blood cells), is released in a variety of circumstances. Cytokines, catecholamines, neuroendocrine responses, tissue injury, hypoxia, or endotoxin can liberate arachidonic acid from cell membranes.[26] Arachidonic acid is metabolized through two major pathways: the cyclooxygenase and lipoxygenase pathways. Metabolism of arachidonic acid through the cyclooxygenase pathway results in the formation of the cytokines thromboxane A_2, prostacyclin, and prostaglandins E_2 and D_2. Thromboxane produces pulmonary and systemic vasoconstriction and enhances platelet aggregation. Prostacyclin decreases SVR and PVR, increases vascular permeability, and inhibits platelet aggregation. Prostaglandins decrease SVR, inhibit platelet aggregation, increase vascular permeability, activate production of cyclic adenosine monophosphate (cAMP), and increase gastrointestinal smooth muscle contraction. The metabolism of arachidonic acid through the lipoxygenase pathway results in the formation of leukotrienes that stimulate neutrophil and eosinophil chemotaxis and lysosomal release. The leukotrienes also increase SVR, produce smooth muscle contraction, and increase vascular permeability. In total, arachidonic acid metabolism increases capillary permeability, platelet dysfunction, maldistribution

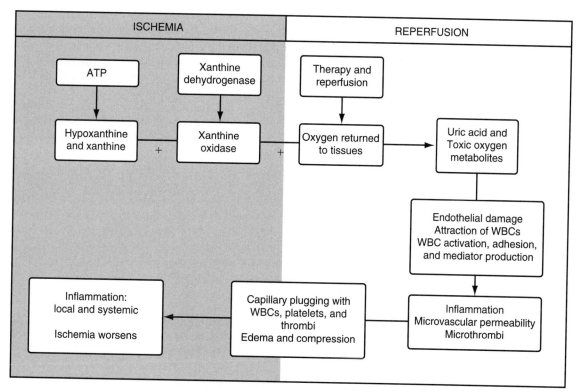

Fig. 27-5   Toxic oxygen metabolite (TOM) formation in ischemia and reperfusion injury. TOMs produced during reperfusion injury attract and activate white blood cells (WBCs), which can produce more TOMs and other inflammatory mediators such as proteases. (From Huddleston VB, ed: *Multiple organ failure: a pathophysiological approach,* Boston, 1991.)

of blood flow, and organ ischemia; causes pulmonary edema and intrapulmonary shunting; and thus contributes significantly to MODS associated with shock. The kidney, gastrointestinal tract, liver, lungs, and brain are at particular risk. Dysfunction of any of these organs may preclude successful treatment of shock.

Mediator release from ischemia or reperfusion injury represents a shift in the traditional view that the pathophysiologic state of shock is a result of ischemic cellular damage. New research reveals that tissue injury following shock is not solely due to hypoxia but due to reperfusion and subsequent inflammation.[27] Toxic oxygen metabolites and neutrophils primarily mediate ischemia or reperfusion injury. Tissue enzymes and substances undergo "transformations" during ischemia. When blood and oxygen in these tissues are restored, molecular oxygen (O_2) reacts with these "transformed" tissue enzymes and substances to produce superoxide radicals[25] (Fig. 27-5). Reperfused tissues release free radicals, lactic acid, potassium, and other substances that are toxic to endothelium and the tissues and potentiate the damage already experienced in the initial ischemic state.

Numerous mediators released are unique to septic shock. The influential mediators of gram-negative septic shock include endotoxin, tumor necrosis factor, and interleukin-1.[27] Endotoxin is one of the most powerful triggers of the inflammatory immune response. A component of the gram-negative bacteria cell wall, this lipopolysaccharide is shed when the bacteria multiplies or dies. Most prominent of

endotoxin's effects is the simultaneous stimulation of the complement and coagulation cascades. Unremitting activation of the complement cascade with associated histamine activation contributes to common clinical findings of septic shock. Continued activation of the complement cascade results in increased capillary permeability, vasodilation, and lysosome release. Histamine, derived from mast cells in damaged tissues and from basophils in the blood, decreases SVR, increases vascular permeability, and augments gastrointestinal motility.

Activation of the coagulation cascade occurs when both the complement system and the inflammatory immune response are triggered. The Hageman factor (factor XII) has a pivotal role in the interdependency between the coagulation cascade and the inflammatory immune response, as well as other plasma enzyme cascades, such as kallikrein and kinin. Activation of the coagulation and fibrinolytic systems contributes to the high incidence of clotting abnormalities and increases the incidence of vascular obstruction, tissue ischemia, and organ dysfunction. The Hageman factor also stimulates the production of bradykinin, a potent vasoactive peptide found in plasma or tissue fluid. Bradykinin causes venodilation, increased vascular permeability, bronchoconstriction, and constriction of gastrointestinal smooth muscle.

Tumor necrosis factor (TNF; cachectin), a cytokine released from macrophages, leukocytes, and other immune cells, is thought to be the major mediator of sepsis and MODS.[5,27] TNF enhances the inflammatory immune response, including fever, tachypnea, tachycardia, increased vascular permeability, metabolic acidosis, and altered blood distribution to organs, such as the gut and kidney.[28] TNF also stimulates the release of interleukin-1 (IL-1), arachidonic acid metabolism, and the production of platelet-activating factor (PAF). In the presence of TNF, complement and clotting cascades are activated.[29] The net result is sequestration of platelets, vasodilation, increased capillary permeability, and microvascular constriction.

IL-1 is a cytokine that is released by monocytes and macrophages and works synergistically with TNF to perpetuate the inflammatory immune response and to release PAF. The predominant effects of PAF produce vasodilation, activate platelet aggregation, and increase tissue permeability.

Patients in septic shock typically exhibit reduced left ventricular ejection fraction and left ventricular dilation.[30] In addition to adrenergic receptor dysfunction and impaired myocardial intracellular calcium flux, myocardial dysfunction occurs secondary to the negative inotropic effects of numerous chemical mediators, including myocardial depressant factors, endotoxin, TNF, complement products, and leukotrienes. Myocardial depressant factors are hemodynamic inhibitory peptides released secondary to ischemia to the splanchnic region. As in other organs, eventually myocardial perfusion and oxygen consumption are disrupted in septic shock.

CLINICAL ASSESSMENT: RED FLAGS OF CARDIOVASCULAR COLLAPSE

Shock is a dynamic process that requires vigilant assessment and continuous patient monitoring and reevaluation. Clinical or physical assessment findings reflect the consequences of ineffective tissue perfusion. Early recognition of patients both at risk and with the earliest indications of shock ensures the best outcomes.

Unexplained and persistent tachycardia, that is, tachycardia not related to fever, anemia, pain, or agitation, is a common but nonspecific finding in shock. Increased heart rate is an attempt to compensate for inadequate stroke volume. In addition, dysrhythmias, which impair cardiac function, are not uncommon in pediatric patients with electrolyte imbalance, metabolic acidosis, and hypoxemia. All of these symptoms can occur in all shock states.

Unexplained persistent tachypnea, that is, tachypnea not related to fever, anemia, pain, or agitation, is also a valuable and early sign of shock. The evolving metabolic acidosis associated with shock is compensated by an increase in alveolar ventilation. Decreased CNS pH is a potent stimulus to chemoreceptors located in the medulla to increase minute ventilation. The rise in minute ventilation, through an increase in respiratory rate, results in respiratory alkalosis in the early stages of shock. When respiratory alkalosis is present, the seriousness of a patient's condition may be underestimated.

Low-Flow Shock

The red flags of low-flow shock are the signs of increased SVR and decreased cardiac output. To maintain blood pressure in low-flow states, SVR increases, as blood pressure (BP) is the product of cardiac output (CO) and SVR (BP = CO × SVR). Because of a higher sympathetic tone and an ability to maintain vasoconstriction for a long time, children exhibit a remarkable ability to maintain blood pressure in low-flow shock states. Peripheral vasoconstriction and an increase in SVR is an attempt to compensate for the decrease in cardiac output.[31] Symptoms of increased SVR can be assessed in three major organ systems: the skin, kidneys, and brain.

Impairment of peripheral circulation is assessed by examination of capillary refill, skin color and temperature, and peripheral pulses. Normally, a child's extremities are warm and pink with brisk capillary refill (<2 seconds). The child in low-flow shock, however, has poor peripheral perfusion illustrated by the hallmark signs of low cardiac output—delayed capillary refill (>2 seconds), cool extremities, and diminished peripheral pulses.[32] To accurately assess capillary refill from the arterial side of the circulation, the extremity should be slightly elevated above heart level. Although capillary refill is widely used, recent studies[33,34] have questioned its value.

Skin color changes may progress from pink, to pale, to mottled, and then to a marbleized appearance. Pale skin may be noted when the hemoglobin and hematocrit levels are decreased. A core-to-skin temperature gradient greater than 2° C is considered significant. The temperature gradient widens with progressive decreases in peripheral perfusion.[35] Proximal-to-distal skin temperature gradients—that is, changes in the position of the demarcation line between warmth and coolness—can be trended as well.

In low-flow shock, peripheral pulses are difficult to palpate. Weak pulses result from the narrow pulse pressure characteristic of a diminished stroke volume and increased SVR. The narrow pulse pressure occurs before systolic pressures fall. Stroke volume and SVR determine systolic blood pressure, whereas SVR reflects diastolic blood pressure. When cardiac output falls, SVR increases to maintain the blood pressure. The increased SVR increases the diastolic component of the blood pressure and maintains the systolic component. Because pulse pressure is a sensitive indicator of stroke volume, it is an important parameter to monitor.

Urine output, a reflection of kidney perfusion, is an important assessment parameter in infants and children experiencing shock. Particularly in hypovolemic patients, urine output may decrease long before other signs of ineffective tissue perfusion are evident. Renal blood flow is dependent on cardiac output. Sudden decreases in renal blood flow or pressure decrease the glomerular filtration rate and result in decreased urine output and increased urine specific gravity. Low urine output is defined as less than 0.5 to 1 ml/kg/hr in infants and children and less than 1 to 2 ml/kg/hr in newborns.

Signs and symptoms of inadequate cerebral perfusion are often subtle in the early stages of shock. Level of consciousness is assessed developmentally. Infants frequently exhibit a weak cry or poor suck. Infants normally do not tolerate missed feedings or wet or soiled diapers, especially if they have a diaper rash. Toddlers normally do not tolerate their parents' absence in a foreign environment for any period. The child's sensorium may be clouded; response to stimuli may be limited; and anxious, irritable, or lethargic behavior may be present. As shock progresses, somnolence advances to obtundation and is an ominous sign.

Unique to hypovolemic shock, physical signs may vary between hypovolemic shock caused by dehydration, resulting in both intravascular and interstitial hypovolemia, and hypovolemic shock caused by hemorrhage, resulting in intravascular hypovolemia and interstitial euvolemia or even hypervolemia.[31] Children with dehydration display classic signs of interstitial hypovolemia. A sunken anterior fontanelle, sunken eyes, dry mucous membranes, poor skin turgor, decreased capillary refill, cool extremities, and mental status changes are exhibited. The degree to which these signs are evident depends on the degree of dehydration (see Table 11-8).

The condition of a patient in cardiogenic low-flow shock contrasts sharply to the patient with hypovolemic low-flow shock in that intravascular volume is adequate or even increased. In cardiogenic shock secondary to congestive heart failure, the patient often appears "wet" and may have a gallop rhythm. For example, diaphoresis, periorbital/sacral or dependent edema, hepatomegaly, jugular venous distension, and rales with increased work of breathing are present. In cardiogenic shock secondary to an outflow obstruction, the patient may exhibit a low-voltage electrocardiogram (ECG) and electromechanical dissociation (EMD). If cardiac tamponade is present, a significant pulsus paradoxus, greater than 10 mmHg, may be present.

Late signs and symptoms of low-flow shock include progressive neurologic deterioration, hypotension, and bradycardia. The presence of even mild hypotension denotes decompensated shock; therefore an observed fall of 10 mmHg in systolic blood pressure should prompt aggressive intervention.[12] The lower limit (5th percentile) of normal systolic blood pressure can be estimated with the following formula: 70 mmHg + (2 × age in years).[12]

Maldistributive Shock

The red flags of maldistributive shock are the signs of decreased SVR and increased cardiac output. To maintain blood pressure in low SVR states, cardiac output must increase. Cardiac output is unevenly distributed, with some tissues effectively and some tissues ineffectively perfused. Low SVR results in increased skin blood flow, resulting in septic shock patients having warm and dry skin. Patients experiencing septic shock often appear flushed and well perfused, with normal or brisk capillary refill despite the ominous nature of their illness. They are often febrile (>38° C) but may be hypothermic (<36° C). Because neutrophil activation produces many of the early signs of infection and the inflammatory response, septic patients who are neutropenic may not present symptoms in the typical fashion.

In patients with high cardiac output, pulses are easily palpated. Bounding pulses, a rare finding in a pediatric physical examination, reflect a widened pulse pressure occurring secondary to an increased stroke volume and decreased SVR. Urine output may initially be normal or increased, despite a relative hypovolemia. Subtle changes in mental status (e.g., confusion) may be present.

Late symptoms include those present in low-flow shock states, as well as evidence of MODS. The patient manifests signs and symptoms of low cardiac output. A narrowed pulse pressure is present and correlates with reduced stroke volume; progressive hypotension accompanies decreased cardiac output. Clot and interstitial edema obstruct blood flow through the periphery. Tissue acidosis causes arterioles to dilate and venules to constrict, causing further pooling and stasis of blood. Marked capillary leak and interstitial and pulmonary edema are present. See Table 27-3 for phases and clinical manifestations of septic shock.

Hemodynamic and Oxygenation Profiles

Table 27-4 provides a summary of the numerous hemodynamic and oxygenation profile changes associated with low-flow and maldistributive shock states. Currently, a lack of pediatric research is available to help guide collaborative practice. Normal values are not necessarily optimal values in shock.[17]

Heart rate increases in all shock states. Mean arterial pressure remains normal when compensatory mechanisms are effective but falls when compensatory mechanisms fail. Right atrial pressures (RAPs) and pulmonary artery wedge pressures (PAWP) reflect right and left ventricular preload, respectively. Both are decreased in hypovolemic shock, because circulating blood volume is inadequate. As ventricular function deteriorates in cardiogenic shock, RAP and PAWP increase. RAP and PAWP are initially decreased in early septic shock as vasodilation leads to venous pooling and decreased venous return. Both RAP and PAWP increase in late septic shock, reflecting myocardial failure.

Pulmonary vascular resistance index (PVRI), reflecting right ventricular afterload, is high in all shock states. In septic shock, many factors, including pulmonary vasoconstriction, microembolic occlusion, and lung injury, necessitate the use of high positive end-expiratory pressure (PEEP). All these factors increase PVRI and may contribute to right ventricular dysfunction, placing the requisite hyperdynamic state at risk. Systemic vascular resistance index (SVRI), reflecting left ventricular afterload, increases to maintain blood pressure in low-flow shock. SVRI remains low in septic shock.

The cardiac index (CI) is decreased in low-flow states, is high in early septic shock, but falls in late septic shock. Skin temperature is directly proportional to cardiac output and inversely proportional to SVRI. Even though cardiac output is increased in septic shock, the left ventricular ejection fraction (LVEF) is significantly decreased. The increased cardiac output in septic shock is secondary to an increase in heart rate and ventricular dilation, not an increase in contractility. Overall myocardial performance is often compromised by diffuse myocardial edema, circulating myocardial depressant factor from splenic hypoperfusion, adrenergic receptor dysfunction, and impaired sarcolemma calcium flux.[5]

TABLE 27-3 Phases and Clinical Manifestations of Septic Shock

Organ System	Sepsis	Hyperdynamic Septic Shock*	Hypodynamic Septic Shock†
Central nervous system	Change in activity Change in feeding Change in response	Clouded sensorium Irritability Disorientation Lethargy	Disorientation Lethargy Obtundation
Cardiovascular	Sinus tachycardia Bounding pulses	Sinus tachycardia Bounding pulses Warm, dry, flushed skin Widened pulse pressure ± Diminished perfusion ± Mottled extremities ↑↓ Capillary refill Generalized edema Relative hypovolemia Progressive hypotension	Sinus tachycardia Weak, thready pulse Dysrhythmias Narrowed pulse pressure Diminished perfusion Mottled extremities ↓ ↓ Capillary refill Generalized edema Hypotension
Pulmonary	Tachypnea	Tachypnea Progressive hypoxemia	Pulmonary edema
Metabolic	Fever or hypothermia Respiratory alkalosis	Fever or hypothermia Hyperglycemia or hypoglycemia Progressive metabolic acidosis	Fever or hypothermia Hyperglycemia or hypoglycemia Severe metabolic acidosis
Hematology/ immunology Renal	Leukocytosis/leukopenia ↑ Immature neutrophils (bands)	Leukocytosis/leukopenia ↑ Immature neutrophils (bands) ↓ Urine output	Leukocytosis/leukopenia ↓ Urine output

Data from Carcillo JA: Management of pediatric septic shock. In Holbrook PR, ed: *Textbook of pediatric critical care,* Philadelphia, 1993, WB Saunders, pp 114-142; Robbins EV: Maldistribution of circulating blood volume. In Huddleston VB, ed: *Multisystem organ failure: pathophysiology and clinical implications,* St Louis, 1992, Mosby, pp 85-108; Rosenthal-Dichter C: Septic shock. In Slota, MC, ed: Core *curriculum for pediatric critical care nursing,* Philadelphia, 1998, WB Saunders, p 638.

*Hyperdynamic septic shock is characterized by increased cardiovascular findings and seemingly 'good' perfusion, the body's demands are still not adequately met.

†Hypodynamic septic shock may be accompanied by signs and symptoms of deteriorating organ dysfunction(s).

TABLE 27-4 Hemodynamic and Oxygenation Profile Changes in Shock

Parameter	Norms	Hypovolemic	Cardiogenic	Septic Early	Septic Late
Heart rate (beats/min)	Newborn-3 mo: 85-205 3 mo-2 yr: 100-190 2-10 yr: 60-140 >10 yr: 60-100	Increased			
MAP	>60 mmHg	Normal$_{\text{Compensated}}$ then decreased$_{\text{Decompensated}}$			
CI	2.5-5.5 L/min/M^2	Decreased	Decreased	Increased then decreased	
RAP/PAWP	2-6 mmHg/6-12 mmHg		Increased	Decreased then increased	
PVRI	PVRI = Mean PA - PCWP/CI × 80 Norm: 80-240 dyne-sec/cm^5/M^2	Normal or increased			
SVRI	SVRI = MAP − RAP/CI × 80 Norm: 800-1600 dyne-sec/cm^5/M^2	Increased		Decreased then increased	
$\dot{D}o_2$	$\dot{D}o_2 = Cao_2 \times CI \times 10$ Norm: 620 ± 50 ml/min/M^2	Decreased		Increased then decreased	
$\dot{V}o_2$	$\dot{V}o_2$ = arterial $\dot{D}o_2$ − venous $\dot{D}o_2$ Norm: 120-200 ml/min/M^2	Increased then decreased			
OER	$Cao_2 − C\bar{v}o_2/Cao_2 \times 100$ Norm: 25 ± 2%	Increased then decreased		Normal/Increased then decreased	
Svo_2	Norm: 75% (60%-80%)	Decreased then increased		Normal/Decreased then increased	

MAP, Mean arterial blood pressure; *CI,* cardiac index; *RAP,* right atrial pressure; *PAWP,* pulmonary artery wedge pressure; *PVRI,* pulmonary vascular resistance index; *SVRI,* systemic vascular resistance index; $\dot{D}o_2$, oxygen delivery; $\dot{V}o_2$, oxygen consumption; *OER,* O$_2$ extraction ratio.

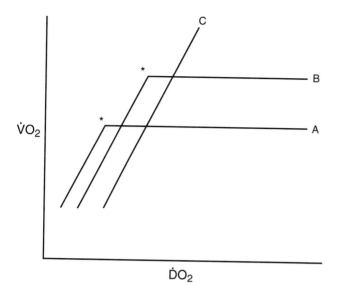

Fig. 27-6 Abnormal $\dot{V}O_2$ in sepsis. Sepsis may result in a hyper-utilization state *(B)* with increased $\dot{V}O_2$ and intact oxygen extraction ratio (OER) or in *(C)* a pathologic supply-dependence state in which OER is nonexistent. *Critical $\dot{D}O_2$ range; *A*, normal $\dot{V}O_2/\dot{D}O_2$ curve; *B*, elevated critical $\dot{D}O_2$ range; *C*, supply-dependent $\dot{V}O_2$. (Adapted from Carcillo JA: Management of pediatric septic shock. In Holbrook PR, ed: *Textbook of pediatric critical care*, Philadelphia, 1993, WB Saunders, p 130.)

Considering that shock represents an imbalance of oxygen supply and demand, oxygenation profile monitoring provides data necessary for informed individualized titration of therapy. Oxygen delivery ($\dot{D}O_2$) and oxygen extraction ratio (OER) balance to maintain tissue oxygen consumption ($\dot{V}O_2$) over a very wide range (Fig. 27-6). When $\dot{D}O_2$ decreases in low-flow states, OER increases to maintain $\dot{V}O_2$. This continues until a critical $\dot{D}O_2$ range is reached, after which $\dot{V}O_2$ depends on $\dot{D}O_2$. This is referred to as supply-dependent $\dot{V}O_2$. Patients in septic shock require higher $\dot{D}O_2$ to maintain adequate tissue perfusion and to avoid anaerobic metabolism.[21] Associated with poor outcome, a pathologic supply-dependent $\dot{V}O_2$ may exist in patients with septic shock. In this state, $\dot{V}O_2$ is abnormally supply dependent at normal or supernormal $\dot{D}O_2$ rates.[36] Late in septic shock, there may be an uncoupling of the $\dot{D}O_2$-$\dot{V}O_2$ relationship.

Supply-independent $\dot{V}O_2$ occurs secondary to an endotoxin-induced impairment of oxidative metabolism, a redistribution of blood flow away from the microcirculation, and a severe impairment of mitochondrial oxygen use. Although controversial, there may be no benefit to increasing $\dot{D}O_2$ beyond the point of $\dot{V}O_2$ plateau.[15]

Continuous mixed venous oxygen saturation monitoring ($S\bar{v}O_2$) provides valuable on-line information about tissue perfusion. In low-flow shock, the $S\bar{v}O_2$ is low, reflecting decreased cardiac output and an increased OER. In septic shock, the $S\bar{v}O_2$ reflects the adequacy of the cardiac output to maintain the hyperdynamic state and tissue extraction of oxygen.

Like $S\bar{v}O_2$, the arteriovenous difference in oxygen (a-$\bar{v}DO_2$) gradient is inversely related to cardiac output. The a-$\bar{v}DO_2$ gradient increases in low-flow states because tissues extract more oxygen. In late septic shock, decreased $\dot{D}O_2$ and a narrow a-$\bar{v}DO_2$ are ominous signs.

Pollack, Fields, and Ruttimann[16] identified several pediatric predictors of outcome from septic shock. Survivors of septic shock were able to maintain a normal or hyperdynamic state, that is, increased CI (3.3 to 6 L/min/M$_2$), higher $\dot{V}O_2$ (>200 ml/min/M^2), and higher OER (>28%), and did not experience significant pulmonary disease. On the other hand, nonsurvivors demonstrated low CI (<3.3 L/min/M^2) and low and poor O$_2$ use (<$\dot{V}O_2$, <a-$\bar{v}DO_2$, and lower OER), had lower temperatures (<37° C), and experienced pulmonary disease. In adult survivors of septic shock, the characteristic hyperdynamic state (increased heart rate and cardiac output with decreased SVR) begins to resolve within 24 hours. Nonsurvivors develop unresponsive hypotension and progressive MODS.[37] Pediatric patients who are fluid resuscitated, unlike their adult counterparts, more commonly experience low cardiac output (vs. low SVR).[16-18] In addition, oxygen delivery (vs. oxygen extraction) appears to be the major determinant of oxygen consumption.[38] Implications for management of septic shock include supporting factors associated with positive outcomes and eliminating factors associated with negative outcomes.

Interpreting and predicting hemodynamic and oxygenation profile changes in any shock state are done cautiously. Changes may be due to the disease process, interventional strategy (e.g., inadequate fluid resuscitation, catecholamine selection), or the impact of the two on system maturation. Patients may exhibit one hemodynamic picture and may progress to another. For instance, children with persistent shock often progress to worsening cardiac failure but may resolve their shock state, requiring an alteration in hemodynamic support.[15] More clinical research is definitely needed in this area.

COLLABORATIVE MANAGEMENT

Patient management requires an appreciation of the overall treatment perspective[38a,39]; that is, essential treatment includes both definitive treatment and supportive treatment. Definitive treatment is directed toward resolution of the primary problem, whereas supportive treatment is directed toward achieving an optimal physiologic, oxygenation, and hemodynamic state. Optimal states may not reflect "normal" values but values that meet the dynamic individual needs of the patient. The primary focus of therapy is on improving tissue perfusion and oxygenation. Objective criteria may include supporting supply-independent $\dot{V}O_2$ and a normal OER while preventing metabolic acidosis.

An integral component of the management of patients experiencing shock is monitoring. Continuous patient assessment and noninvasive and invasive monitoring are essential to adequately manage patients in shock. Changes in the patient's physiologic status occur rapidly, and mechanisms to quickly evaluate the effectiveness of therapy are invaluable. Vigilant and repeated assessments of the same clinical parameters facilitate trending and allow optimal titration of therapies. Titration of pharmacologic agents to collaboratively determined clinical and hemodynamic end points is necessary.

Alterations in tissue perfusion may affect the accuracy of several of the standard noninvasive monitoring modalities available in the PICU, that is, end-tidal CO_2 (ET_{CO_2}) and pulse oximetry monitors. For example, the ET_{CO_2} reading may not correlate with the Pa_{CO_2}; however, ET_{CO_2} reflects pulmonary capillary blood flow. Alterations in pulmonary perfusion associated with shock and the effectiveness of therapy can be evaluated by assessment and trending of the ET_{CO_2}-Pa_{CO_2} gradient. Pulse oximetry depends on a reliable pulse, which may not be present in low-flow shock states.

To provide and titrate optimal therapy in maldistributive shock states, hemodynamic and oxygenation variables require quantification. The RAP normally quantifies right ventricular preload, the equivalent of circulating blood volume. Because ventricular compliance affects atrial pressure, an abnormal relationship between ventricular preload and work is seen. Pulmonary artery (PA) catheters are necessary to evaluate left ventricular filling pressures and cardiac output and provide a route to obtain true mixed venous blood samples or provide continuous $S\bar{v}_{O_2}$ monitoring. Strategies to enhance successful PA catheter insertion during low cardiac output states include stiffening the 5 Fr PA catheter with iced saline through the PA port and planning PA catheter insertion after a fluid bolus.

Sequential echocardiograms are also helpful in monitoring cardiac function. Echocardiography quantifies ventricular ejection fraction (normal 65%), quantifies the disparity between right and left ventricular function, and determines whether pericardial effusions are present.

Supportive Treatment

When prioritizing the care of the critically ill patient in shock, the ABCs of resuscitation are the supportive component of essential treatment. Immediate therapy includes assessing for and establishing a patent airway, maintaining oxygenation and ventilation, and improving perfusion while the underlying cause of shock is determined. Although children usually have an adequate airway, as many as 80% of children with septic shock may eventually require mechanical ventilation.[40] Once elective endotracheal intubation and assisted ventilation are initiated, additional interventions can be directed at circulatory support.

Establishing and maintaining vascular access is a priority in treating shock. If venous access is not present, a protocol for the establishment of venous access is recommended.[12] The preferred location of vascular access is the largest vein that may be rapidly accessed without interrupting emergent management. Although multilumen central lines are preferred because they allow simultaneous monitoring of central venous pressure and a direct access to the central circulation while minimizing the risk of tissue extravasation with administration of vasoactive and caustic medications, peripheral access can be initially used if already in place. Previous adult and animal research has suggested a benefit of supradiaphragmatic access versus infradiaphragmatic access.[41] The limited research involving young animals has

not shown the preference for supradiaphragmatic locations. In fact, Gaddis and colleagues[42] report that a fluid bolus of at least 5 ml effectively increases the delivery of peripherally injected medications into the central circulation. Besides intravenous routes of drug administration, the intraosseous (IO) route is effective for rapid fluid and drug delivery and should be considered for children younger than 6 years of age.

Definitive Treatment

Identification and treatment of the patient's primary problem are of critical importance. These interventions constitute the definitive component of essential treatment. For example, controlling hemorrhage, cardioverting the tachydysrhythmia, or providing appropriate broad-spectrum antibiotic coverage as soon as possible if sepsis is suspected or documented is considered definitive treatment. Other definitive interventions in sepsis include locating, excising, draining, and removing the focus of the infection, that is, draining an abscess or replacing the central line.

Enhance Substrate Delivery

The therapeutic goal in any shock state is to enhance substrate delivery ($\dot{D}_{O_2}$) to the tissues. This is of heightened importance given that research shows that oxygen delivery, rather than oxygen extraction, is the major determinant of oxygen consumption is pediatric patients.[38] This goal is accomplished by maximizing cardiovascular performance and optimizing arterial oxygen content (Ca_{O_2}). The major emphasis is to improve tissue perfusion.

Maximize Cardiovascular Performance

Optimize Preload. Rapid intravascular volume expansion is guided by clinical parameters (noting end-organ perfusion, including urine output) and hemodynamic parameters (most prominently central venous pressure [CVP] monitoring). Early and aggressive correction of intravascular volume deficit is necessary to increase cardiac output and to reestablish microcirculatory flow. Maintenance of the hyperdynamic septic state and improvement of oxygen consumption are critically dependent on vigorous fluid administration.[40] Improvement in perfusion pressure and oxygen delivery and consumption indicates successful fluid resuscitation.

Fluid selection for optimizing preload is determined by the source of the fluid loss and the child's clinical condition. As a general rule, isotonic crystalloids or colloids are initially administered. Table 27-5 reviews the different recommendations for fluid selection based on the cause of the loss of fluid.

A long-standing controversy exists regarding the most suitable fluid for shock resuscitation—crystalloids versus colloids. Both have inherent advantages and disadvantages. Crystalloid solutions (0.9% sodium chloride or lactated Ringer's solution) are readily available and cost effective, but approximately only one fourth of the volume infused remains in the intravascular space. This necessitates the

TABLE 27-5   Recommended Therapies for Hypovolemic Shock by Etiology

Cause	Therapy
Dehydration*	20 ml/kg of 0.9% sodium chloride bolus.
	Reassess for continuing signs of end-organ hypoperfusion (increased heart rate, decreased capillary refill, depressed mental status, decreased urine output).
	Repeat 20 ml/kg boluses until signs of shock abate.
Diabetic ketoacidosis*	If signs of end-organ hypoperfusion: follow recommendations as for dehydration.
	If no signs of end-organ hypoperfusion: 20 ml/kg of 0.9% sodium chloride over 2 hours, followed by more specific electrolyte-containing fluid.
Thermal injuries†	If signs of end-organ hypoperfusion: follow recommendations as for dehydration.
	If no signs of end-organ hypoperfusion: Parkland formula (begin with D5LR): total fluids (first 24 hours) = maintenance + (4 ml/kg × %BSA burn) + other losses.
	Administer ½ of the fluids in the first 8 hours and the rest in the next 16 hours.
	Reassess every 6-8 hours.
Sepsis/Septic shock†‡	40-60 ml/kg of 0.9% sodium chloride bolus.
	Reassess for continuing signs of end-organ hypoperfusion (increased heart rate, decreased capillary refill, depressed mental status, decreased urine output).
	May require 80-100 ml/kg of fluid to stabilize.
Hemorrhage§	20 ml/kg of whole blood or components bolus.
	Reassess for signs of anemia or continued bleeding and monitor hematocrit.

From Thomas NJ, Carcillo JA: Hypovolemic shock in pediatric patients, *New Horiz* 6:126, 1998.
In cases of fluid-refractory shock:
*May have ongoing fluid losses (stool loss, urine output) greater than resuscitation fluids administered.
†May require addition of inotropic support.
‡May require exogenous steroid therapy if history of chronic steroid use or purpura fulminans.
§May have unrecognized ongoing blood loss.
BSA, Body surface area; *D5LR*, 5% dextrose lactated Ringer's solution.

administration of large quantities of crystalloid solution to restore intravascular volume (potentially 4 to 5 times the deficit). Note that the use of lactated solutions in patients with impaired liver function is not recommended because it increases blood lactate concentrations and renal loss of sodium and potassium.[13]

Colloids (albumin; synthetic plasma substitutes, such as hetastarch and dextran; whole blood; packed cells; and fresh frozen plasma [FFP]) contain relatively large molecules that are impermeable to capillary membranes and therefore are more likely to remain in the intravascular space. However, these solutions are more expensive and may cause sensitivity reactions. Colloids are important for maintaining plasma osmotic pressure and minimizing interstitial edema. In treating shock, the ideal solution would expand the intravascular space but limit interstitial accumulation. Prevention of interstitial pulmonary edema is critically important to prevent alterations in gas exchange.

With that being said, Schierhout and Roberts[43] recently conducted a meta-analysis of randomized clinical trials of volume replacement with colloids compared with crystalloids in critically ill adults. Twenty-six studies (1622 patients) were included. Resuscitation with colloid solutions was associated with a 4% increase in the absolute risk of mortality (4 extra deaths for every 100 patients resuscitated). Because colloids are considerable more expensive and are associated with a higher mortality in adults, their continued use for volume replacement is not supported.

Blood is administered as soon as possible to replace whole blood loss or to correct anemia. However, careful attention to large-volume and rapid administration of blood products is imperative because the patient is at risk for hypothermia and poor metabolism of citrate, potentially leading to ionized hypocalcemia. Both of these factors may result in significant myocardial dysfunction. Autotransfusion devices, for example, cell-saving devices, scavenge then return blood lost during spinal fusion and intrathoracic surgical cases (when no enteric contamination has occurred). Albumin is commonly used if the hematocrit is adequate. FFP and platelets are administered if clotting abnormalities or thrombocytopenia exists. Synthetic plasma substitutes (dextran and hetastarch) are relatively inexpensive but cause diminished platelet function.

Equally important as the type of fluid is the amount of fluid administered. The most common error made in fluid resuscitation is the inadequate or delayed volume administration.[31] The amount and rate of infusion depend on the child's condition; 20 ml/kg of an isotonic crystalloid infused over several minutes is a reasonable starting point. Repeated boluses of the same amount are infused if no improvement is seen in the child's clinical and hemodynamic parameters, for example, improved perfusion, increased urine output, decreased acidosis, and increased mean arterial pressure.

Fluids should be given with the goal of attaining normal perfusion and blood pressure, recognizing that the average fluid requirement in the first hour for septic shock patient is 60 ml/kg but may be as high as 200 ml/kg.[15] Carcillo, Davis, and Zaritsky[40] reported that aggressive fluid administration in excess of 40 ml/kg in the first hour after presentation to the emergency department is associated with improved survival, decreased occurrence of persistent hypovolemia, and no increase in the risk of cardiogenic pulmonary edema or ARDS in pediatric patients in septic shock. The researchers did not control for type of fluid used, crystalloids were used preferentially, and colloids were used if the blood pressure was unresponsive to crystalloids. Blood products were also used if coagulation was a problem.

If patients with nonhemorrhagic hypovolemic shock fail to respond to the initial 60 ml/kg of crystalloid fluid, they are said to have fluid refractory shock. This subset of patients may require a combination of large amounts of fluid resuscitation, as well as catecholamine support.[31] In addition, other possible complicating factors include pneumothorax, pericardial effusion, ongoing intraabdominal fluid loss (e.g., from volvulus, intussusception), gastrointestinal ischemia, brainstem dysfunction, adrenocortical insufficiency, and pulmonary hypertensive crisis.

When managing children with cardiogenic or septic shock, efforts to improve cardiac output and tissue perfusion by volume augmentation are carefully monitored. The volume of fluid that can be safely administered is contingent on ventricular compliance. Monitoring of ventricular enddiastolic pressure (i.e., CVP or PAWP) permits early detection of cardiac decompensation and provides an important guide for fluid replacement. The vascular congestion associated with cardiogenic shock may be improved by concurrent administration of albumin with diuretics (furosemide [Lasix]).

Perkin and Levin[43a] described a helpful method of evaluating the effectiveness of volume replacement. Fluid is administered until the patient's hemodynamic status is corrected or the CVP exceeds the preinfusion value by 2 mmHg or the PCWP within 3 mmHg. A CVP greater than 7 to 10 mmHg indicates myocardial dysfunction, excessive right ventricular afterload, or volume overload. The authors note that the absolute limitation to fluid administration is persistent increase in ventricular filling pressure without improvement in cardiac output.

Research indicates that outcome may be influenced when aggressive fluid resuscitation (60 ml/kg in the first hour) is coupled with goal-directed therapies. Ceneviva and colleagues[44] examined 50 children with fluid-refractory (60 ml/kg in the first hour) dopamine-resistant shock. After fluid resuscitation, inotropes, vasopressors, and vasodilators were administered to target and maintain normal CI and SVR. An 18% mortality was reported as compared with other studies with a reported 58% mortality that used goal-directed therapies without aggressive fluid resuscitation.[17]

Emergency autotransfusion to maintain an adequate perfusion pressure is enhanced by elevating the patient's limbs or by gentle compression on the liver. The Trendelenburg position is used cautiously, especially when cerebral perfusion pressures are questionable.

Optimize Contractility.   Before, or concurrent with, the administration of positive inotropic medications, negative inotropic states—for example, hypoxia, acidosis, hypoglycemia, hypokalemia, and hypocalcemia—must be rectified (Fig. 27-7). Acidosis depresses myocardial function and

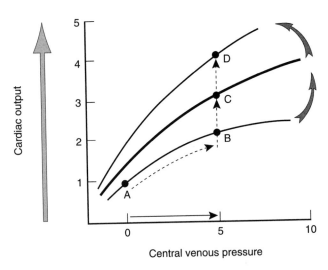

Fig. 27-7   Starling's law. Stroke volume and cardiac output are increased in the hypovolemic, acidotic child (point A) by increasing preload through volume infusion (point B), by restoring ventricular function curve to a more normal one (point C), and by correcting acidosis and metabolic abnormalities. Myocardial function curve (and cardiac output) can potentially be shifted to a supranormal value (point D) with infusion of a positive inotropic agent. (Modified from Crone RK: Acute circulatory failure in children, *Pediatr Clin North Am* 27:525-537, 1980.)

renders sympathomimetic drugs ineffective. Poor outcomes have been associated with a base deficit greater than 10 mEq/L in patients with cardiogenic or septic shock. Base deficits greater than a negative 6 require correction. The primary correction for metabolic acidosis secondary to cardiovascular collapse is restoration of tissue perfusion. With adequate tissue perfusion and oxygenation, metabolic acidosis will self-correct. When the arterial pH is less than 7.20 and adequate ventilation has been established (i.e., $Paco_2$ in the normal range for the patient), correction with $NaHCO_3$ is indicated. The dose is calculated from the base deficit (mEq $NaHCO_3$ = 0.3 [weight in kg] × base deficit). The calculated dose usually approximates 1 to 2 mEq/kg. If the serum sodium is greater than 150, tris-hydroxymethyl-amino-methane (THAM), a non-CO_2-generating buffer, can be used with cautious evaluation of hypoglycemia and hyperkalemia.

Electrolyte shifts will occur when correcting metabolic acidosis. As the pH increases, ionized calcium levels fall, and potassium shifts into the intracellular space, decreasing the serum potassium level. Calcium replacement may be necessary to correct hypocalcemia (ionized calcium level less than 1.3 mg/dl), occurring frequently in circulatory failure, especially after administration of large amounts of albumin, whole blood, or FFP.

After vigorous fluid resuscitation, pharmacologic therapy is then used to enhance cardiovascular performance (Table 27-6). Sympathomimetics stimulate α-, β-, and dopaminergic receptors throughout the body, causing a variety of effects. There is appreciable interpatient variability in dose and pharmacodynamic effect with most catecholamines. Also, stress may deplete endogenous catecholamine stores and down-regulate α-adrenergic receptor sites.[45] Individual

TABLE 27-6   Pharmacologic Therapy Used in Shock

Drug	Site of Action	Dose (μg/kg/min)	Primary Effect*	Secondary Effect
Dopamine	Dopaminergic	2-5	Increase renal perfusion	Dysrhythmias
	Dopaminergic and β_1	2-10	Inotropy	
			Chronotropy	
	α	10-20	Increase renal perfusion	
			Vasoconstriction	
Norepinephrine	$\alpha > \beta$	2-10	Vasoconstriction	>MVO$_2$
			Inotropy	Dysrhythmias
				<Renal BF
Epinephrine	α and β	0.05-1.5	Vasoconstriction	>MVO$_2$
			Inotropy	Dysrhythmias
			Chronotropy	<Renal BF
Dobutamine	β_1	5-20	Inotropy	Tachycardia
				Dysrhythmias
				Vasodilation
				Hypotension
Sodium nitroprusside	NA	0.5-10 (light-sensitive)	Vasodilation (balanced)	<PVR
				>V̇/Q̇ mismatch
				Cyanide toxicity
Nitroglycerin	NA	0.2-20	Vasodilation (venous)	<PVR
				>ICP
Amrinone	NA	5-10 μg/kg/min (load with up to 3 mg/kg over 20 min)	Inotropy Vasodilation	Dysrhythmias <PVR Thrombocytopenia
Milrinone	NA	0.75 to 1.0 μg/kg/min (load with 75 μg/kg over 20 min)	Inotropy Vasodilation Improves diastolic function	Dysrhythmias <PVR

*Difficult to predict the dose-response effect. Management requires individual titration at the bedside.
MVo$_2$, Myocardial oxygen consumption; *BF,* blood flow; *PVR,* pulmonary vascular resistance; V̇/Q̇, ventilation/perfusion; *ICP,* intracranial pressure.

dose and drug titration are performed at the bedside and based on both desired and observed clinical and hemodynamic outcomes. Frequently, more than one catecholamine is administered at a time; finding the best combination and dosage requires continuous assessment of clinical and invasive hemodynamic parameters.

The rapid onset, controllable dosage, and ultra-short half-life of catecholamines make them effective for treating shock, especially in patients thought to have a vascular component to hypotension. Dopamine, epinephrine, and norepinephrine are the most often used exogenous catecholamines or vasopressors. Alternatively, patients with myocardial depression in the face of hypotension may benefit from a β_1-inotrope, such as dobutamine. See Fig. 27-8 for an example of the medical management for hemodynamic support of the pediatric patient experiencing septic shock.[15]

Dopamine is an endogenous catecholamine whose effects depend on the patient's own endogenous catecholamine response (related to maturation) and releasable norepinephrine stores (related to stress levels). Dopamine activates the dopaminergic and adrenergic receptors in a dose-dependent manner. Dopamine's major advantage is that at low doses (1 to 5 μg/kg/min) it produces splanchnic and renal vasodilation and a decrease in SVR. The dopaminergic effect on

renal blood flow results in increased urine output. Dopamine stimulates β_1-adrenergic receptors at moderate doses (5 to 10 μg/kg/min), resulting in a moderate positive inotropic effect in patients with normal myocardial function. At high doses (>10 μg/kg/min), dopamine is primarily an α-adrenergic agonist that causes tachycardia, renal vasoconstriction, and increased SVR. The resulting increased afterload may decrease cardiac output. When dopamine infusions greater than 20 μg/kg/min are required to maintain blood pressure, an epinephrine drip is preferable.[12] Dopamine is often used either in patients requiring no greater than 10 μg/kg/min or at low doses for its selective effect on renal and splanchnic perfusion in patients who require other inotropes. Dopamine depresses prolactin and thyroid hormone release, although the effect on thyroid function over prolonged infusion of dopamine is uncertain. Importantly, differential diagnoses of sick euthyroid syndrome and dopamine-induced hypothyroidism should be considered in chronically critically ill children.[46,47]

Epinephrine, also an endogenous catecholamine, mimics SNS stimulation by providing a perfect balance of both α and β stimulation. Epinephrine increases myocardial and cerebral perfusion pressures. Its most pronounced action is on the β-receptors of the heart, vascular, and other smooth

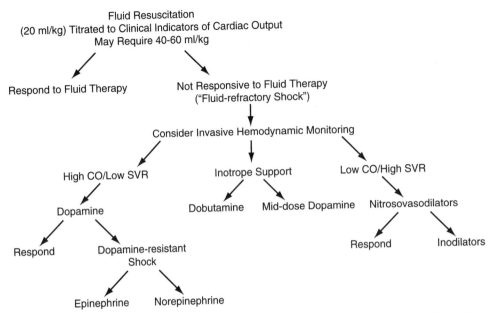

Fig. 27-8 Proposed management of septic shock (American College of Critical Care Medicine Clinical Practice Parameters). *CO*, Cardiac output; *SVR*, systemic vascular resistance.

muscle. Epinephrine may be particularly helpful in infants and children because of its direct action on adrenergic receptors rather than through a release of stored norepinephrine (depleted norepinephrine stores have been noted in the pediatric population). Epinephrine is effective in shock states in which SVR is significantly low (septic shock and anaphylaxis). Hypotensive septic patients may not respond to α agents in a normal manner, so higher doses (1 to 1.5 μg/kg/min) may be needed.[12] Renal blood flow will improve if perfusion pressure improves. Because catecholamines increase myocardial oxygen consumption, signs of myocardial hypoxia or ischemia, such as ST segment and T wave changes on the ECG, may occur during administration.

Norepinephrine (Levophed) has been repopularized, especially in the treatment of septic shock. Also an endogenous catecholamine, norepinephrine's potent vasoconstrictor effects overshadow its positive inotropic effects. Starting dosage is 0.05 to 0.1 μg/kg/min. β Effects predominate at the lower dosage, whereas α effects predominate at the higher dosage. Norepinephrine has been reported to reverse hypotension in patients with septic shock who have not responded to dopamine or combination dopamine-dobutamine. It is thought to be particularly helpful in patients with low SVR and high cardiac output shock states (hyperdynamic septic shock).[15]

Dobutamine, a synthetic catecholamine, is a β$_1$-stimulant that increases cardiac contractility but causes only a slight increase in heart rate. Because the α- and β$_2$-adrenergic receptors are not stimulated by dobutamine, SVR is usually decreased, and only minimal vasoconstriction is occasionally observed. Effects do not depend on releasable norepinephrine stores. Dobutamine is very effective as a selective inotropic agent in the normotensive patient with poor perfusion secondary to diminished cardiac performance.

The starting dose is 5 to 10 μg/kg/min; if greater than 20 μg/kg/min is required to maintain blood pressure, epinephrine should be considered. Dobutamine is not as effective as dopamine in infants younger than 1 year of age and in patients with septic shock.[12] In cardiogenic shock, dobutamine will increase cardiac output, while decreasing CVP, PAWP, PVR, and SVR.[46] In a volume-depleted or hypotensive patient, dobutamine may cause systemic and pulmonary vasodilation and increased right-to-left intrapulmonary shunting and thus decrease cardiac output and oxygen delivery despite improved contractility.[46]

Optimize Afterload. In low-flow states, blood pressure is usually supported by an increase in SVR. However, in cardiogenic low-flow shock, the increased SVR may further compromise myocardial function and further limit cardiac output (Fig. 27-9). When heart failure coexists with increased resistance to ventricular outflow (as evidenced by increased SVRI or PVRI), the use of vasodilators, often in combination with a positive inotropic agent, is indicated. Factors that increase afterload—for example, hypothermia, acidosis, hypoxia, pain, and anxiety—should be managed before considering vasodilator therapy. By reducing the resistance to left ventricular outflow, arterial vasodilators increase the cardiac ejection fraction and increase stroke volume. In contrast, venous vasodilators shift blood into the periphery and reduce right and left ventricular end-diastolic volume. Decreased end-diastolic volume reduces myocardial wall stress and improves myocardial perfusion. Most vasodilators are classified as "balanced" and exert both arterial and venous effects. Nitrosovasodilators (nitroprusside and nitroglycerine) are recommended as first-line vasodilators. Inovasodilators, those agents with both inotrope and vasoactive properties, such as amrinone and milrinone, are reserved for patients with vasodilator-

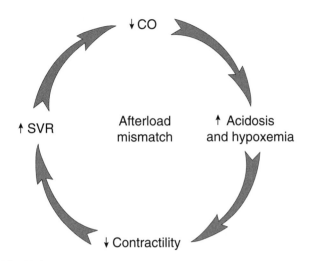

Fig. 27-9 "Afterload mismatch" present in low-flow cardiogenic shock. *CO,* Cardiac output; *SVR,* systemic vascular resistance.

resistant low cardiac output or with cyanide or methemoglobin toxicity.[15] Regardless of the vasodilator chosen, note that hypotension will result if administered to a hypovolemic patient. Fluids should be readily available at the bedside.

Sodium nitroprusside is a direct-acting vasodilator that relaxes both arteriolar and venous smooth muscle. The subsequent fall in afterload and preload improves cardiac output only when the reduction of outflow resistance predominates over the effects of the reduced venous return. The dose range for nitroprusside is 0.5 to 8 µg/kg/min. Manifestations of toxicity (headache, nausea, palpitations, hyperventilation, metabolic acidosis, and unexplained elevation of venous oxygen tension) have occurred at relatively low doses, leading some to suggest a maximum infusion rate of 4 to 8 µg/kg/min for adults and less for infants and young children. Some precautions are necessary when the drug is administered: monitor serum levels of thiocyanate and cyanide and the toxic metabolites of nitroprusside; protect the 5% dextrose infusion containing the drug from light.

Nitroglycerine also relaxes both arteriolar and venous smooth muscle and is helpful in cardiogenic shock by reducing left ventricular filling pressures and SVR. Compared with nitroprusside, nitroglycerine produces a smaller reduction in preload and afterload and a smaller increase in cardiac output. Intravenous administration is initiated at 0.1 µg/kg/min and gradually increased to achieve hemodynamic and clinical effect, usually up to 10 µg/kg/min. Nitroglycerine is administered in specialized tubing (polypropylene or polyethylene) as it is adsorbed in polyvinyl chloride tubing, especially in new tubing sets or at slow infusion rates.

The inodilators, amrinone and milrinone, are nonglycoside, nonadrenergic, phosphodiesterase inhibitors that produce positive inotropic and vasodilator effects. An initial bolus of amrinone 0.75 to 3 mg/kg is required, followed by a continuous infusion of 5 to 10 µg/kg/min. In this dose range, amrinone reduces afterload and preload by its direct effect on vascular smooth muscle. In children with de-

pressed myocardial function, amrinone produces a prompt increase in cardiac output. Because amrinone is a nonsympathomimetic inotropic agent, it may be of particular value in patients with clinical problems that down-regulate adrenergic receptor sites, such as septic shock. A close analog of amrinone, milrinone has a greater positive inotropic potency with the bone marrow suppressive effects of amrinone. Recommended initial loading dose is 75 µg/kg with initial infusion rates of 0.75 to 1 µg/kg/min. Lindsay and colleagues[48] recommend that for every increase of 0.25 µg/kg/min, a 25-µg/kg bolus be administered. Because the median half-life is 1.47 hours, immediate hemodynamic effects may not be seen unless appropriate loading doses and infusion adjustments are made. Both inodilators have long half-life elimination compared with nitrosovasodilators.

Optimize Heart Rate and Rhythm. Changes in heart rate directly affect cardiac output. However, increasing the heart rate to optimize cardiac output is usually not an option among pediatric patients. When tissue perfusion is inadequate, heart rate is usually at or near peak capacity. Excessively rapid heart rates associated with fever, volume depletion, and endogenous catecholamine release secondary to the stress response may limit ventricular diastolic filling and compromise stroke volume and cardiac output. Aggressive management of dysrhythmias that occur secondary to electrolyte imbalance and metabolic acidosis is warranted.

Maximize Substrate Transport

Arterial Oxygen Content. Although much clinical attention is appropriately focused on optimizing cardiovascular performance in patients with shock, an equal amount of attention must also be placed on the oxygen content of blood perfusing the cardiovascular bed. Oxygen content is optimized by maintaining adequate hemoglobin levels (National Institutes of Health [NIH] guidelines recommend greater than 10 g/dl), that is, a hematocrit that optimizes $\dot{D}o_2$. Blood administration is required to correct both whole blood loss and severe anemia.

Lucking and colleagues,[49] studying children in hyperdynamic septic shock after volume loading and pharmacologic support, found that despite an initial low OER, $\dot{V}o_2$ could be increased by augmenting $\dot{D}o_2$ through packed red blood cell (RBC) transfusion. The researchers noted that because $\dot{V}o_2$ correlates with survival, consideration should be given to enhancing $\dot{V}o_2$ despite an initial low OER and high $\dot{D}o_2$. Mink and Pollack[50] reported a similar study but found that although $\dot{D}o_2$ significantly increased after a similar RBC transfusion, $\dot{V}o_2$ did not change.

Not only are adequate levels of hemoglobin important, but also hemoglobin saturation with oxygen is ensured by providing adequate oxygenation and ventilation. Extreme shifts in the oxyhemoglobin dissociation curve are avoided by maintaining normal pH and body temperature.

Minimize Energy Expenditure

In addition to enhancing substrate delivery to the tissues, an adjunctive strategy is to limit the patient's metabolic demands. Early identification of clinical states that increase demand and initiation of interventions to decrease physiologic work benefit patients with little or no metabolic reserve. Interventions include providing adequate support of ventilation to decrease the work of breathing, early identification of both heat and cold stress (for each degree Celsius, the metabolic demands change 13%), prevention of shivering, and providing periods of rest and adequate sedation and analgesia. Nurses play an invaluable role in reducing the anxiety and fear that patients and families experience during critical illness and intensive care. The unfamiliar environment, painful procedures, and the potential for death that accompany advanced shock are issues that nurses are in a unique position to address.

Optimize Nutrition

Critically ill infants and children are at risk for malnutrition because their metabolic needs far exceed their nutritional stores and also because of the nature and duration of their illnesses. Previously well-nourished infants and children may develop nutritional deficiencies after 3 to 5 days of serious illness and intensive care; infants and children who have been hospitalized for some time before the development of shock may already be malnourished. Providing nutritional support demands the same priority as providing definitive treatment of shock.[51] In fact, Pollack, Ruttimann, and Wiley[52] have noted that critically ill children who receive better nutritional support display improvement in physiologic stability and outcome.

Data suggest that there are advantages to using enteral over parenteral nutrition to meet the nutritional requirements of the critically ill patient. Critical illness is associated with gut atrophy and increased mucosal permeability to bacteria and macromolecules such as endotoxin. The theory is that the translocation of these products, or at least the relative ischemia and subsequent reperfusion of the splanchnic organs, are somehow implicated in the development of single or multiple organ failure. Food in the lumen of the gut is cytoprotective.[53] Animal studies demonstrate that enteral nutrition maintains mucosal integrity and the immunologic function of the gastrointestinal tract, decreases bacterial translocation, blunts the systemic inflammatory response to a toxin load, and improves survival in experimental hemorrhage and peritonitis.[54]

Although little data is available to guide the nutritional support of pediatric critical care patients, Curley and Castillo[51] recommend the initiation of enteral nutrition as soon as possible. The transpyloric versus gastric route of feeding is preferred because critical illness impairs gastric emptying. The efficacy of enteral nutritional support in critically ill children has not been subjected to prospective randomized clinical trials. However, Chellis and colleagues[55] demonstrated that early transpyloric feedings were feasible and safe in the PICU, even with mechanically ventilated patients receiving vasoactive support. Patients achieved caloric goals within 48 hours after initiating enteral feedings, tolerated feedings, and demonstrated no complications such as aspiration or abdominal distension. In addition, enteral feedings proved to be cost effective in critically ill pediatric patients.

Parenteral feeding is reserved for the patient with a nonfunctional gastrointestinal tract. Renal replacement therapies, such as continuous venovenous hemofiltration (CVVH), can be used to facilitate caloric delivery in patients who are fluid restricted or in acute renal failure (see Chapter 21).

PROACTIVE CARE: VIGILANCE

Preventing or minimizing the often lethal complications of shock through anticipatory monitoring of evolving problems is an important nursing activity. All organ systems are at risk of hypoxia and acidosis, thus increasing the risk of organ dysfunction and the development of MODS.

Newborns

Shock in the newborn period presents additional challenges to the pediatric critical care nurse. Shock-induced acidosis and hypoxia can increase pulmonary artery pressures and precipitate right-to-left shunting through fetal channels (foramen ovale or ductus arteriosus), resulting in significant hypoxemia. The newborn in stress is often hypothermic because of immature thermoregulation and has low serum glucose and calcium levels as a result of limited intracellular stores. Because of their large surface area/volume ratio, infants lose heat rapidly to the environment. Alterations in carbohydrate metabolism occur secondary to endogenous epinephrine release. Epinephrine produces an initial increase in serum glucose levels that decreases rapidly with depletion of hepatic glycogen stores and failure of gluconeogenesis. Anaerobic glycolysis elevates blood lactate and pyruvate levels, contributing to acidosis. Stressed neonates are at high risk for apnea, necrotizing enterocolitis as blood is shunted away from the gut, and seizures caused by hypoglycemia and hypocalcemia.

Multiple Organ Dysfunction Syndrome

MODS causes 97% of the deaths that occur in the pediatric critical care unit.[56] The mortality associated with MODS is directly related to the number of organ systems involved in the dysfunction process. Failure of one system is associated with 1% mortality, whereas failure of two systems is associated with 11% to 26% mortality. Three- and four-system involvement is associated with 50% to 62% and 75% mortality, respectively.[56,57] The most common organ system involved in MODS is the respiratory system, followed by the cardiovascular and neurologic systems. Criteria for pediatric patients with MODS are detailed in Table 27-7.

Organ system dysfunction such as ARDS, DIC and purpura fulminans, acute tubular necrosis (ATN), gastrointestinal hemorrhage, and hepatic dysfunction is not uncommon in critically ill children with shock.

Ongoing assessment of pulmonary function is important so that early detection and management of respiratory

TABLE 27-7 Criteria for Pediatric Patients With MODS

Organ System	Criteria
Respiratory	RR >90/min (infants <12 months)
	RR >70/min (children ≥12 months)
	Pao_2 <40 mmHg (in absence of cyanotic heart disease)
	$Paco_2$ >65 mmHg
	Pao_2/Fio_2 <250 mmHg
	Mechanical ventilation (>24 hr if postoperative)
	Tracheal intubation for airway obstruction or acute respiratory failure
Cardiovascular	MAP <40 mmHg (infants <12 months)
	MAP <50 mmHg (children ≥12 months)
	HR <50 beats/min (infants <12 months)
	HR <40 beats/min (children ≥12 months)
	Cardiac arrest
	Continuous vasoactive drug infusion for hemodynamic support
Neurologic	Glasgow coma scale score <5
	Fixed, dilated pupils
	Persistent (>20 min) intracranial pressure (>20 mmHg or requiring therapeutic intervention)
Hematologic	Hemoglobin <5 g/dl
	WBC count <3000 cells/mm^3
	Platelets <20,000/mm^3
	Disseminated intravascular coagulation (PT >20 sec or aPTT >60 sec in presence of positive FSP assay)
Renal	BUN >100 mg/dl
	Serum creatinine >2 mg/dl
	Dialysis
Gastrointestinal	Blood transfusion >20 ml/kg in 24 hr because of gastrointestinal hemorrhage (endoscopic confirmation optional)
Hepatic	Total bilirubin >5 mg/dl and SGOT or LDH more than twice normal value (without evidence of hemolysis)
	Hepatic encephalopathy ≥grade II

From Wilkinson JD, Pollack MM, Glass NL et al: Mortality associated with multiple organ system failure and sepsis in pediatric intensive care, *J Pediatr* 111:324-328, 1987.
BUN, Blood urea nitrogen; *FSP,* fibrin split products; *HR,* heart rate; *LDH,* lactic dehydrogenase; *MAP,* mean arterial pressure; *MODS,* multiple organ dysfunction syndrome; *PT,* prothrombin time; *aPTT,* activated partial thromboplastin time; *RR,* respiratory rate; *SGOT,* serum glutamic-oxaloacetic transaminase; *WBC,* white blood cell.

failure can be ensured. Oxygen reserve is limited, and compensatory mechanisms are maximized in shock states, sharply decreasing the patient's tolerance of even brief periods of hypoxia and respiratory acidosis. In patients who develop ARDS, the mechanism of injury may involve activation of complement proteins that promote aggregation of granulocytes in the lung. Granulocytes release proteolytic enzymes and toxic oxygen radicals that cause direct lung injury. Decreased pulmonary compliance and altered ventilation/perfusion ($\dot{V}/\dot{Q}$) relationship result in increased intrapulmonary shunting and venous admixture. In cardiogenic shock, left ventricular end-diastolic pressure of approximately 20 to 25 mmHg directly results in the development of pulmonary edema. In septic shock, damage to the alveolar pulmonary capillary epithelium produces a protein fluid leak into the interstitium and alveoli. Early and appropriate intervention in either case includes oxygen administration and colloid-diuretic therapy. Endotracheal intubation, mechanical ventilation, and PEEP are used to support an adequate functional residual capacity and limit intrapulmonary shunting (see Chapter 8).

DIC and purpura fulminans are both states associated with systemic microvascular thrombosis. DIC results from an activation of the coagulation cascade with subsequent generation of thrombin. Because DIC often accompanies shock states, blood coagulation studies are assessed early in the patient's course. The primary strategy is to treat the underlying process causing DIC, but when DIC is rapidly progressing, the approach is to support the patient's hemostatic system with blood component therapy as indicated. The acceptable minimum platelet count may vary from one institution to another. FFP and cryoprecipitate are used to correct prolonged prothrombin time, activated partial thromboplastin time, and abnormal fibrinogen levels when necessary.

Purpura fulminans specifically describes the extensive, patchy, purpuric, and ischemic areas of the extremities and buttocks noted in patients with fever, septic shock, and DIC,[58] often associated with meningococcal or *Haemophilus influenzae* infection. The pathophysiology involves endotoxemia, vasculitis, DIC, and a low blood flow state, resulting in widespread thrombosis of the venules and capillaries, particularly of the superficial vascular plexus.[10] Numerous therapies intended to limit tissue loss and prevent gangrene are under investigation. Current therapies include heparinization,[59] plasmapheresis,[60,61] sympathetic blockade,[62] plasma protein concentrates such as antithrombin III (AT-III)[63] and activated protein C,[64] tissue plasminogen activator[65,66] and nitroglycerin. Irazuzta and McManus[58] reported an increase in skin perfusion with the use of topical nitropaste 2% (15 mg/2.5 cm; total 15 cm; every 6 hours).

Renal hypoperfusion reduces glomerular filtration and stimulates aldosterone and antidiuretic hormone secretion, which contribute to progressive azotemia with or without oliguria. In shock, acute renal failure occurs on a continuum from ATN to cortical necrosis. Albumin with diuretics and low-dose dopamine augment renal perfusion and urine output. Progressive hyperkalemia, refractory acidosis, and hypervolemia may require renal replacement therapy.

Gastrointestinal hypoperfusion can lead to ulceration of the stomach and intestines and increases the risk of bleeding. Stress ulcer prevention with histamine (H_2)–receptor antagonist administration may control gastric acidity and prevent gastric bleeding. In addition, gastrointestinal hypoperfusion disrupts the patient's gut barrier

Box 27-5

Unconventional Treatment for Systemic Inflammatory Response Syndrome and Shock

Anticytokine Therapy

Monoclonal antibodies
   Tumor necrosis factor
   Interleukin-1
   Complement fragment C5a
Receptor antagonists
   Tumor necrosis factor
   Interleukin-1
   Platelet-activating factor
   Thromboxane
   Bradykinin

Antiendotoxin Therapy

Endotoxin monoclonal antibodies
Lipid A derivatives
Peptides and lipoproteins that bind endotoxin

Antioxidant Therapy

Allopurinol
Mannitol
Catalase
Superoxide dismutase
Iron chelators

Miscellaneous Antiinflammatory Therapy

Complement inhibitors
   C1 inhibitor
Arachidonic acid inhibitors
   Ibuprofen (cyclooxygenase pathway)
   Imidazole (thromboxane pathway)
   Diethylcarbamazine (lipoxygenase pathway)
   Leukotriene inhibitor
Protease inhibitors

Modulators of Coagulation

Antithrombin III
Aprotinin
Protein C
Heparin
Plasminogen activators
Anticlotting factor monoclonal antibodies
Nitric oxide

Miscellaneous Therapies

Gut decontamination
Antihistamines
Naloxone
Calcium channel blockers

Adapted from Bone RC: A critical evaluation of new agents for the treatment of sepsis, *JAMA* 266:1686-1691, 1991. Copyright 1989 by American Medical Association; Secor VH: Multiple organ dysfunction syndrome: overview and conclusions. In Secor VH, ed: *Multiple organ dysfunction and failure,* ed 2, St Louis, 1996, Mosby, p 416.

function, leading to the translocation of bacteria and endotoxin to the systemic circulation. Given that no current therapies can increase mesenteric blood flow or prevent ischemia or reperfusion-mediated gut injury, the alternative is to provide at least tropic enteral feedings (full-strength formula at 0.5 ml/kg/hr) to limit bacterial overgrowth.[67]

The liver may also fail to perform many functions, for example, metabolism of drugs and hormones and conjugation of bilirubin. Medications, especially those metabolized by the liver, are dosed with careful attention to drug plasma levels and physiologic effect. Doughty and colleagues[68] noted that children with multiple organ dysfunction can have up to 90% reduction in their drug-metabolizing ability.

UNCONVENTIONAL THERAPIES

Numerous therapies related to the care and treatment of patients in shock are currently under investigation. Therapies range from tube feeding for decreasing the risk of translocation to innovative immunotherapy for minimizing the inflammatory immune response and decreasing mediator activity and damage. Given the conceptual shift recognizing the role in the inflammatory immune response in all shock states, therapies once thought only applicable to septic shock may have more of a role in other shock states because of their final common pathway—ineffective tissue perfusion and cellular ischemia and death.

Unconventional therapies can be organized into (1) anticytokine therapy (including monoclonal antibodies); (2) antiendotoxin therapy; (3) antioxidant therapy; (4) antiinflammatory therapy; (5) modulators of coagulation; and (6) miscellaneous therapy. Many of the mediator therapies focus on either neutralizing the mediator in the circulation or blocking the interaction between the mediator and its cell-surface receptors, thereby preventing the mediator from affecting its particular target[69] (Box 27-5).

Monoclonal antibodies (MoAbs) to a myriad of mediators, as well as to endotoxin, have been developed. Although two antiendotoxin antibodies (HA-1A and E5) showed initial promise,[70,71] results were suggestive rather than conclusive.[72] In addition, concerns were raised regarding the studies' methods and the efficacy and therapeutic potential of the MoAbs. Given that overwhelming inflammation without a septic source is common in shock states, other MoAbs, such as anti-TNF or anti-TNF–receptors, have been developed and are under investigation. A number of individual therapies used in combination will likely prove to be beneficial for patients in shock states, especially septic shock.[73]

Antioxidant therapies are pivotal in the research arena given the recent recognition that WBC activation and tissue and reperfusion injury are related to overwhelming inflammation.

Endogenous endorphins play an important role in modulating SNS responses in all types of shock. Peripheral endorphin effects may involve vascular and myocardial depression, calcium transport, and modulation of macrophage responses. The opioid antagonist naloxone has been found to rapidly reverse hypotension secondary to endotoxin and blood loss in animals. Naloxone has been used successfully in some children with septic shock who failed to respond to conventional therapy. The response to naloxone therapy has been inconsistent, and severe reactions may occur.

Similar variable results have been obtained with the use of corticosteroids in treating shock. Despite adverse effects (superinfection, electrolyte imbalance, hyperglycemia, and gastrointestinal bleeding),[74] corticosteroid administration may improve *short-term* survival and permit reversal of shock in certain subgroups of septic shock patients. The theory is that in septic shock, steroid administration before antibiotic administration may help attenuate the inflammatory response secondary to endotoxin release.[3] Bollaert and colleagues[75] examined the effect of steroid administration on the reversal of shock, hemodynamics, and survival in adult patients with late shock treated with catecholamines. In this prospective, randomized clinical trial, the administration of steroids for greater than 96 hours resulted in significant improvement in hemodynamics and survival. Compared with 21% of placebo-treated patients, 68% of steroid-treated patients achieved a 7-day reversal of shock. Long-term mortality (28 day) was also lower in the steroid-treated group (32% vs. 63%). Rates of complications between the two groups were not significantly different. Replication of this study is needed in the pediatric population.

Bactericidal/permeability-increasing protein (BPI) has shown promise in the treatment of severe meningococcal sepsis. BPI is proposed to kill meningococci and to bind and clear the bacterial endotoxin, thus minimizing the systemic inflammatory process.[76] Phase II and phase III clinical trials, including pediatric trials, are underway and suggest that BPI may have a therapeutic benefit in the treatment of life-threatening infections and conditions associated with bacteremia and endotoxemia.[77,78] Specifically, when administered early in the course of meningococcal sepsis, BPI may limit the severity of purpura fulminans and improve limb salvage.

With regard to nutrition, immunonutrition may be associated with a reduction of ICU morbidity. Atkinson and colleagues[79] examined the effects of enteral immunonutrition on hospital mortality and length of stay in critically ill adults ($N = 369$). In a prospective, randomized clinical trial, patients either received enteral feeds supplemented immune-enhancing ingredients (arginine, purine nucleotides, and ω-3 fatty acids) or a control enteral feed. Although no significant differences occurred in hospital mortality (even though the immunonutrition group was sicker), a significant reduction in the length of mechanical ventilation and length of hospital stay was noted in the immunonutrition group of patients. This study reflects the future trend in examining immune-enhancing nutrition that may be clinically significant in a patient's recovery from shock.

Plasmapheresis (removal of the child's blood, separation of the plasma and blood cells, and reinfusion of the packed cells in fresh plasma) and continuous renal replacement therapies (continuous arteriovenous/venovenous hemofiltration [CAVH/CVVH]) have also been used to remove septic shock mediators, endotoxin, or bacterial byproducts. McManus and Churchwell[80] identified coagulopathy (defined as PTT >50 seconds and fibrinogen <150 mg/dl) as a poor prognostic indicator in meningococcemia and purpura fulminans. The authors used plasmapheresis in severely coagulopathic patients as a means of restoring normal clotting factors without fluid overload. Although the sample size was small, plasmapheresis was found to be safe and effective in correcting coagulopathy and stabilizing hemodynamics. Also, evidence shows that plasma levels of some mediators are lowered with the use of continuous renal replacement therapies (CRRTs),[81] but the clinical significance remains uncertain.

In summary, clinical investigations are underway on numerous therapies. Inherent research challenges to these trials are coupled with the difficulty in sorting out the therapeutic benefit. Therapies may be deemed statistically and clinically insignificant merely because of the timing of administration. Secor[25] points out that timing may be as critical as the therapy itself. Second, it is very unlikely that a single therapy will "fix" or minimize the overwhelming inflammatory response, given its intricacy and complexity.

SUMMARY

In summary, care of the pediatric patient in shock requires multidisciplinary collaboration. Recognizing the child's condition early, diligently tending to the administration and evaluation of treatment, and preventing the onset of common complications compose a challenging nursing role.

REFERENCES

1. Kumar A, Parrillo JE: Shock: classification, pathophysiology, and approach to management. In Parrillo JE, Bone RC, eds: *Critical care medicine: principles of diagnosis and management,* St Louis, 1995, Mosby.
2. Bochner BS, Lichtenstein LM: Anaphylaxis, *N Engl J Med* 324:1785-1790, 1991.
3. Zimmerman JJ, Dietrich KA: Current perspectives on septic shock, *Pediatr Clin North Am* 34:131-163, 1987.
4. Jarvis WR: Epidemiology of nosocomial infections in pediatric patients, *J Pediatr Infect Dis* 6:344-351, 1987.
5. NIH Conference: Parrillo JE (Moderator): Septic shock in humans, advances in the understanding of pathogenesis, cardiovascular dysfunction, and therapy, *Ann Intern Med* 113:227-242, 1990.
6. Rosenthal-Dichter C: Septic shock. In Slota MC, ed: *Core curriculum for pediatric critical care nursing,* Philadelphia, 1998, WB Saunders.
7. Bone RC: Let's agree on terminology: definition of sepsis, *Crit Care Med* 19:973-976, 1991.
8. American College of Chest Physicians/Society of Critical Care Medicine Consensus Conference: Definitions for sepsis and organ failure and guidelines for the use of innovative therapies in sepsis, *Crit Care Med* 20:864-874, 1992.
9. Proulx R, Fayon M, Farrell CA et al: Epidemiology of sepsis and multiple organ dysfunction syndrome in children, *Chest* 109:1033-1037, 1996.
10. Wong VK, Hitchcock W, Mason W: Meningococcal infection in children: a review of 100 cases, *J Pediatr Infect Dis* 8:224-227, 1989.
11. Committee on Infectious Diseases: American Academy of Pediatrics: *1997 Red Book: Report of the Committee on Infectious Diseases,* ed 24, Elk Grove Village, Ill, 1997, The Academy.
12. Chameides L, Hazinski MF: *Pediatric advanced life support,* Dallas, 1997, American Heart Association.

13. Perkin RM, Levin DL: Shock in the pediatric patient. Part I. *J Pediatr* 101:163-169, 1982; Shock in the pediatric patient. Part II. Therapy, *J Pediatr* 101:319-332, 1982.

14. Ognibene FP, Parker MM, Natanson C et al: Depressed left ventricular performance: response to volume infusion in patients with sepsis and septic shock, *Chest* 93:903-910, 1988.

15. Task Force of the American College of Critical Care Medicine (ACCM): ACCM clinical practice parameters for hemodynamic support of pediatric septic shock (in press).

16. Pollack MM, Fields AI, Ruttimann UE: Sequential cardiopulmonary variables of infants and children in septic shock, *Crit Care Med* 12:554-559, 1984.

17. Pollack MM, Fields AI, Ruttimann UE: Distributions of cardiopulmonary variables in pediatric survivors and nonsurvivors of septic shock, *Crit Care Med* 13:454-459, 1985.

18. Ferdman B, Jureidini SB, Mink RB: Severe left ventricular dysfunction and arrhythmias as a complication of gram positive sepsis: rapid recovery in children, *Pediatr Cardiol* 19:482-486, 1998.

19. Kimbrell JD: Alterations in metabolism. In Secor VH, ed: *Multiple organ dysfunction and failure*, ed 2, St Louis, 1996, Mosby.

20. Carcillo JA, Cunnion RE: Septic shock, *Crit Care Clin* 13:553-574, 1997.

21. Tuchschmidt J, Oblitas D, Fried FC: Oxygen consumption in sepsis and septic shock, *Crit Care Med* 19:664-671, 1991.

22. Clark CH, Gutierrez G: Gastric intramucosal pH: a noninvasive method for the indirect measurement of tissue oxygenation, *Am J Crit Care* 1:53-60, 1992.

23. Gutierrez G, Palizas F, Doglio G et al: Gastric intramucosal pH as a therapeutic index of tissue oxygenation in critically ill patients, *Lancet* 339:195-199, 1992.

24. Casado-Flores J, Mora E, Perez-Corral F et al: Prognostic value of gastric intramucosal pH in critically ill children, *Crit Care Med* 26:1123-1127, 1998.

25. Secor VH: Multiple organ dysfunction syndrome: background, etiology, and sequence of events. In Secor VH, ed: *Multiple organ dysfunction and failure*, ed 2, St Louis, 1996, Mosby.

26. Secor VH: The systemic inflammatory response syndrome: role of inflammatory mediators in multiple organ dysfunction syndrome. In Secor VH, ed: *Multiple organ dysfunction and failure*, ed 2, St Louis, 1996, Mosby.

27. Waxman K: Shock: ischemia, reperfusion, and inflammation, *New Horiz* 4:153-160, 1996.

28. Secor VH: The inflammatory/immune response in critical illness: role of the systemic inflammatory response syndrome, *Crit Care Clin North Am* 6:251-264, 1994.

29. Hazinski MF, Iberti TJ, MacIntyre NR et al: Epidemiology, pathophysiology and clinical presentation of gram negative sepsis, *Am J Crit Care* 2:224-237, 1993.

30. Natanson C, Hoffman WD, Parrillo JE: Septic shock: the cardiovascular abnormality and therapy, *J Cardiothorac Anesth* 3:215-227, 1989.

31. Thomas NJ, Carcillo JA: Hypovolemic shock in pediatric patients, *New Horiz* 6:120-129, 1998.

32. Joly HR, Weil MH: Temperature of the great toe as an indication of the severity of shock, *Circulation* 39:131-138, 1969.

33. Baraff LJ: Capillary refill: is it a useful clinical sign? *Pediatrics* 92:723-724, 1993.

34. Gorelick MH, Shaw KN, Baker MD: Effect of ambient temperature on capillary refill in healthy children, *Pediatrics* 92:699-702, 1993.

35. Fagan MJ: Relationship between nurses' assessments of perfusion and toe temperature in pediatric patients with cardiovascular disease, *Heart Lung* 17:157-165, 1988.

36. Schumacker PT, Cain SM: The concept of a critical oxygen delivery, *Intensive Care Med* 13:223-229, 1987.

37. Parrillo JE: Septic shock in humans: advances in the understanding of pathogenesis, cardiovascular dysfunction, and therapy, *Ann Intern Med* 111:227-242, 1990.

38. Carcillo JA, Pollack MM, Ruttimann UE: Sequential physiologic interactions in cardiogenic and septic shock, *Crit Care Med* 17:12-16, 1989.

38a. Natanson C, Hofffman WD, Parrillo JE: Septic shock and multiple organ failure. In Parrillo JE, Bone RC, eds: *Critical care medicine: principles of diagnosis and management*, St Louis, 1995, Mosby

39. Bone RC: Sepsis, the systemic inflammatory response syndrome, and multiple organ dysfunction syndrome: recent advances. *Sepsis and septic shock: current issues and recent development* (abstract brochure), Anaheim, Calif, 1993, National Teaching Institute, AACN.

40. Carcillo JA, Davis AL, Zaritsky A: Role of early fluid resuscitation in pediatric septic shock, *JAMA* 266:1242-1245, 1991.

41. Dalsey W, Barsan W, Joyce S et al: Comparison of superior vena cava and inferior vena cava access using a radioisotope technique during normal perfusion and cardiopulmonary resuscitation, *Ann Emerg Med* 13:881-884, 1984.

42. Gaddis GM, Dolister M, Gaddis ML: Mock drug delivery to the proximal aorta during cardiopulmonary resuscitation: central vs peripheral intravenous infusion with varying flush volumes, *Acad Emerg Med* 2:1027-1033, 1995.

43. Schierhout G, Roberts I: Fluid resuscitation with colloid or crystalloid solutions in critically ill patients: a systematic review of randomised trials, *BMJ* 316:961-964, 1998.

43a. Perkin RM, Levin DL: Shock. In Levin DL, Morriss FC, eds: *Essentials of pediatric intensive care*, St Louis, 1990, Quality Medical Publishing.

44. Ceneviva G, Paschall JA, Maffei F et al: Hemodynamic support in fluid refractory pediatric septic shock, *Pediatrics* 102:e19, 1998

45. Zaritsky A, Chernow B: Use of catecholamines in pediatrics, *J Pediatr* 105:341-350, 1984.

46. Zaritsky AL: Recent advances in pediatric cardiopulmonary resuscitation and advanced life support, *New Horiz* 6:201-211, 1998.

47. Van den Berghe G, de Zegher F, Lauwers P: Dopamine suppresses pituitary function in infants and children, *Crit Care Med* 22:1747-1753, 1994.

48. Lindsay C, Barton P, Lawless S et al: Pharmacokinetics and pharmacodynamics of milrinone lactate in pediatric patients with septic shock, *J Pediatr* 132:329-334, 1998.

49. Lucking SE, Williams TM, Chaten FC et al: Dependence of oxygen consumption on oxygen delivery in children with hyperdynamic septic shock, *Crit Care Med* 18:1316-1319, 1990.

50. Mink RB, Pollack MM: Effect of blood transfusion on oxygen consumption in pediatric septic shock, *Crit Care Med* 18:1087-1091, 1990.

51. Curley MAQ, Castillo L: Nutrition and shock in pediatric patients, *New Horiz* 6:212-225, 1998.

52. Pollack M, Ruttimann U, Wiley J: Nutritional depletion in critically ill children: associations with physiological instability and increased quantity of care, *J Parenter Enteral Nutr* 9:309-313, 1985.

53. Frost P, Edwards N, Bihari D: Gastric emptying in the critically ill: the way forward, *Intensive Care Med* 23:243-245, 1997.

54. Heyland DK, Cook DJ, Guyatt GH: Enteral nutrition in the critically ill patient: a critical review of the evidence, *Intensive Care Med* 19:435-442, 1993.

55. Chellis MJ, Sanders SV, Webster HW et al: Early enteral feeding in the pediatric intensive care unit, *J Parenter Enteral Nutr* 20:71-73, 1996.

56. Wilkinson JD, Pollack MM, Glass NL et al: Mortality associated with multiple organ system failure and sepsis in pediatric intensive care, *J Pediatr* 111:324-328, 1987.

57. Wilkinson JD, Pollack MM, Ruttiman UE et al: Outcome of pediatric patients with multiple organ system failure, *Crit Care Med* 14:271-274, 1986.

58. Irazuzta J, McManus ML: Use of topically applied nitroglycerin in the treatment of purpura fulminans, *J Pediatr* 117:993-995, 1990.

59. Kupperman N, Inkelis SH, Saladino R: The role of heparin in the prevention of extremity and digit necrosis in meningococcal purpura fulminans, *Pediatr Infect Dis J* 13:867-873, 1994.

60. Churchwell KB, McManus ML, Kent P et al: Intensive blood and plasma exchange for treatment of coagulopathy in meningococcemia, *J Clin Apheresis* 10:171-177, 1995.

61. Van Deuren M, Santman FW, van Dalen R et al: Plasma and whole blood exchange in meningococcal sepsis, *Clin Infect Dis* 15:424-430, 1992.

62. Chiafery MC, Stephany RA, Holliday KJ: Epidural sympathetic blockade to relieve vascular insufficiency in an infant with purpura fulminans, *Crit Care Nurse* 13:71-76, 1993.

63. Cobcroft R, Henderson A, Solano C et al: Meningococcal purpura fulminans treated with antithrombin III concentrate: what is the optimal replacement therapy? *Aust N Z J Med* 24:575-576, 1994 (letter).

64. Rivard GE, David M, Farrell C et al: Treatment of purpura fulminans in meningococcemia with protein C concentrate, *J Pediatr* 126:646-652, 1995.

65. Aiuto L, Barone SR, Cohen PS et al: Recombinant tissue plasminogen activator restores perfusion in meningococcal purpura fulminans, *Crit Care Med* 25:1079-1082, 1997.

66. Zenz W, Muntean W, Gallisti S et al: Recombinant tissue plasminogen activator treatment in two infants with fulminant meningococcemia, *Pediatrics* 96:44-48, 1995.

67. Deitch EA, Rutan R, Waymack JP: Trauma, shock, and gut translocation, *New Horiz* 4:289-299, 1996.

68. Doughty LA, Carcillo JA, Frye R: *Decreased P450 metabolism in pediatric sepsis and multiple organ failure,* San Diego, Calif, 1997, Society of Critical Care Medicine Symposium.

69. Secor VH: Multiple organ dysfunction syndrome: overview and conclusions. In Secor VH, ed: *Multiple organ dysfunction and failure,* ed 2, St Louis, 1996, Mosby.

70. Greenberg RN, Wilson KM, Kunz AY et al: Observations using antiendotoxin antibody (E5) as adjuvant therapy in humans with suspected, serious gram negative sepsis. *Crit Care Med* 20:730-735, 1992.

71. Ziegler EJ, Fisher CJ, Sprung CL et al: Treatment of gram-negative bacteremia and septic shock with HA-1A human monoclonal antibody against endotoxin, *N Engl J Med* 324:429-436, 1991.

72. Warren HS, Danner RL, Munford RS: Sounding board: anti-endotoxin monoclonal antibodies, *N Engl J Med* 326:1153-1156, 1992.

73. Giroir BP: Mediators of septic shock: new approaches for interrupting the endogenous inflammatory cascade, *Crit Care Med* 21: 780-789, 1993.

74. Bone RC, Fisher CJ, Clemmer TP et al: A controlled clinical trial of high-dose methylprednisolone in the treatment of severe sepsis and septic shock, *N Engl J Med* 317:653-658, 1987.

75. Bollaert P, Charpentier C, Levy B et al: Reversal of late septic shock with supraphysiologic doses of hydrocortisone, *Crit Care Med* 26:645-650, 1998.

76. Giroir BP, Quint PA, Barton P et al: Preliminary evaluation of recombinant amino-terminal fragment of human bactericidal/permeability-increasing protein in children with sever meningococcal sepsis, *Lancet* 350:1439-1443, 1997.

77. Elsbach P: The bactericidal/permeability-increasing protein (BPI) in antibacterial host defense, *J Leukoc Biol* 64:14-18, 1998.

78. Elsbach P, Weiss J: Role of the bactericidal/permeability-increasing protein in host defense, *Curr Opin Immunol* 10:45-49, 1998.

79. Atkinson S, Siefert E, Bihari D: A prospective, randomized double blind controlled clinical trial of enteral immunonutrition in the critically ill, *Crit Care Med* 26:1143-1146, 1998.

80. McManus ML, Churchwell KB: Consumptive coagulopathy as predictor of outcome in purpura fulminans, *Anesthesiology* 75:A286, 1991.

81. Silvester W: Mediator removal with CRRT: complement and cytokines, *Am J Kidney Dis* 30:s38-s43, 1997.

28 Trauma

Patricia A. Moloney-Harmon
Patricia Adams

Trauma remains the leading cause of death in children. In children between the ages of 1 and 19 years, injuries cause more deaths than all diseases combined and are a leading cause of disability.[1] The single largest cause of trauma-related death is motor vehicle incidents. Approximately 24% of pediatric motor vehicle deaths involve alcohol. A recent study found that the majority of alcohol-related child passenger deaths involve a child riding unrestrained with a driver who has been drinking.[2] Nonintentional injury is not the leading cause of death in children under 1 year of age; however, a recent study demonstrated 32.1 injury deaths per 100,000 infant years.[3] Other causes of death include homicides, suicides, drownings, burns, and falls. In the United States, it is estimated that more than 30,000 children suffer permanent disabilities from injury every year.[1]

Blunt trauma accounts for 80% of all accidental injuries. Blunt injuries are associated with rapid deceleration, which occurs with motor vehicle incidents; or from direct blows, the result of contact sports or child abuse. Penetrating trauma accounts for the other 20% of injuries. Penetrating trauma is most commonly the result of firearms or stab weapons. If the late teenage years are included in the pediatric population, blunt and penetrating trauma are almost equal as the cause for injury.

Head injury is the most common injury seen in children and accounts for 80% of all pediatric trauma deaths, due to the larger proportion of body weight that the head of a child provides. Skeletal injuries usually involve the long bones, especially of the lower limbs. Other common injuries include abdominal and thoracic. The kidneys, spleen, and liver are not well protected in the child and thus are more susceptible to trauma.

Regardless of the type of injury, the final common pathways of trauma are tissue hypoxia secondary to inadequate oxygenation and ventilation, hypovolemia, and cerebral hypertension. The goal of pediatric trauma care is to stabilize the effects of traumatic injury before irreversible damage occurs. Often, children will survive the initial insult only to die later because of complications such as malignant intracranial hypertension, sepsis, respiratory failure, or multiple organ dysfunction syndrome (MODS). Vigilance by the nurse will help to prevent these complications.

INITIAL RESUSCITATION

Primary Survey

The initial resuscitation of the pediatric trauma victim is guided by the principles of the primary and secondary survey. The primary survey allows for the rapid identification of any life-threatening injuries and takes place when the child is initially evaluated. The primary survey focuses on the initial stabilization of the cardiopulmonary system, which is covered in Chapter 31.

However, there are some specific points for the pediatric trauma patient.

The child is assumed to have a cervical spine injury until proven otherwise, so that manual in-line immobilization is a critical aspect of airway management. An appropriately sized rigid cervical collar can be applied, but immobilization is maintained manually if a collar is not available. To determine the correct size, the collar is measured in width from the top of the shoulder to the chin with the head in neutral position. There are several collars available that take pediatric cervical spine anatomy into account (Fig. 28-1).

While in-line manual cervical immobilization is maintained, the airway is opened using the jaw-thrust method. The jaw-thrust maneuver alone may relieve airway obstruction. If the child does not respond, vomit, blood, or broken teeth may be obstructing the airway. Severe maxillofacial injuries or injuries to the larynx may also produce airway obstruction.

If the child does not respond to positioning and suctioning, artificial ventilation with 100% oxygen and intubation is indicated. A rapid-sequence intubation is appropriate for the child with a full stomach or in the child with the potential for increased intracranial pressure (ICP). All pediatric trauma victims are assumed to have a full stomach, and a rapid-sequence intubation will minimize the possibility of regurgitation (Fig. 28-2).[4]

The application of cricoid pressure (Sellick's maneuver) is performed during a rapid-sequence intubation to prevent passive regurgitation of stomach contents into the pharynx. In this technique, the upper esophagus is compressed against the cervical vertebral column by applying anteroposterior pressure on the cricoid cartilage (Fig. 28-2).[4] Cricoid pressure is maintained until correct placement of the endotracheal tube has been confirmed.

In some uncommon instances, the child will require a needle cricothyroidotomy. This technique is indicated in the child with an obstruction below the larynx or with a significant maxillofacial or airway injury. A 14- or 16-gauge needle is inserted through the cricothyroid membrane to establish the airway. If this is not possible, a surgical tracheostomy is performed.

Assessment of the child's breathing status includes observation for signs of respiratory distress, especially once the airway is established. Significant thoracic injury may be present even with minimal outward signs of trauma. If respiratory distress, unequal breath sounds, and unstable vital signs are present, a pneumothorax or hemothorax is suspected and warrants immediate intervention. For a pneumothorax, needle decompression of the chest is performed without waiting for confirmation of the diagnosis by chest roentgenogram. A 14- to 20-gauge needle is inserted into the fourth or fifth intercostal space at the midaxillary line. After the initial rush of air occurs, a chest tube is inserted into the same space.

If a hemothorax is suspected, a large-bore needle is inserted at the same site used for evacuation of a pneumothorax. Fluid resuscitation is started before evacuation of the hemothorax to prevent exsanguination. Excessive bleeding through the chest tube may require clamping of the tube to tamponade bleeding. If bleeding persists at a rate of equal to or greater than 2 ml/kg/hr, an emergency thoracotomy is indicated.[4] A small amount of blood loss can quickly produce hypovolemic shock in the child. Table 28-1 presents the four classes of hemorrhage, with clinical signs and initial treatment for each stage.

The most crucial aspect of treatment for the hypotensive pediatric trauma victim is restoration of the circulating blood volume. An intravenous line is inserted, although this may be difficult in the hypovolemic child. If venous access cannot be obtained quickly, intraosseous access may be attempted. If the response to an initial bolus of lactated Ringer's solution or normal saline at 20 ml/kg is inadequate, a second fluid bolus is given, also at 20 ml/kg. If shock still persists, packed red blood cells (PRBCs) are administered at 10 ml/kg. Fluids are warmed by a fluid warmer before administration to prevent hypothermia. Once shock has been controlled, fluids can be delivered at the maintenance rate.

If shock continues despite all interventions, other causes are considered. The child may have developed a tension pneumothorax, which requires immediate intervention. If muffled heart sounds and pulsus paradoxus are present, the child may have developed pericardial tamponade, which

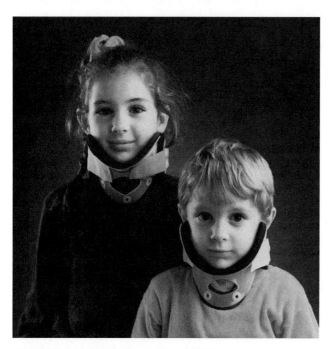

Fig. 28-1 Pediatric cervical spine immobilization collar. The NecLoc Extrication Collar, Jerome Medical, is designed for prehospital extrication and transport of children, taking into account cervical spine anatomy difference between children and adults.

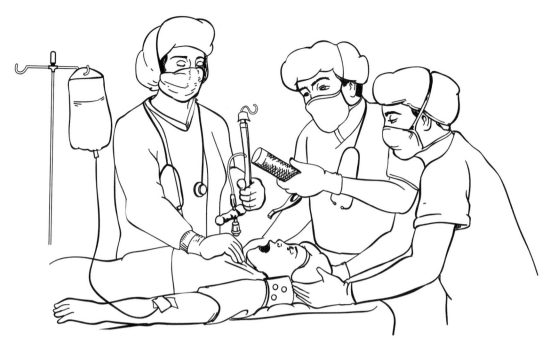

Fig. 28-2 Technique for oral endotracheal intubation in the pediatric trauma patient using cricoid pressure and "manual in-line axial traction." The technique generally requires three individuals. The individual on the left is applying cricoid pressure while the individual on the right holds the patient's head in a neutral position with two hands using manual in-line traction. Before intubation and after in-line traction is applied, the anterior portion of the cervical collar is removed. (From Tobias JD, Rasmussen GE, Yaster M: Multiple trauma in the pediatric patient. In Rogers MC, ed: *Textbook of pediatric intensive care,* ed 3, Baltimore, 1996, Williams & Wilkins.)

TABLE 28-1 Classes of Hemorrhage for Children

Class	Blood Loss	Signs	Treatment
Class I	15% or less 40-kg child = 500 ml blood	Pulse: slight increase BP: normal Respiration: normal Capillary refill: normal Tilt test:* normal	Crystalloids Rule 3:1 (3 ml of RL:1 ml blood loss), e.g., 500 mL blood loss = 1200-1500 ml RL
Class II	20%-30% 40-kg child = 800 ml blood	Tachycardia >150 BP: systolic decreased, decreased pulse pressure Tachypnea >35-40 Delayed capillary refill Positive tilt test Urine output normal (1 ml/kg/hr)	Crystalloids Rule 3:1 as above, e.g., 800 ml blood loss = 2100-2400 ml RL
Class III	30%-35% 40-kg child = 1200 ml blood	Blood pressure drop Narrow pulse pressure Urine output affected	Crystalloids 20 ml/kg Packed red cells 10 ml/kg
Class IV	40%-50% 40-kg child = 1600 ml blood	Nonpalpable blood pressure and pulse No response to verbal or painful stimuli	Crystalloids 20 ml/kg Packed red cells

From Widner-Kolberg MR, Moloney-Harmon PA: Pediatric trauma. In Cardona VD, Hurn PD, Mason PJB et al, eds: *Trauma nursing: from resuscitation through rehabilitation,* ed 2, Philadelphia, 1994, WB Saunders.
*A tilt test is performed by sitting the child upright. The test is normal if the child can stay up longer than 90 seconds and maintain blood pressure.
BP, Blood pressure; *RL,* Ringer's lactate.

requires an immediate pericardiocentesis. If these are not present and shock persists, immediate surgical intervention, such as an exploratory laparotomy, is warranted.

Once airway, breathing, and circulation have been stabilized, a rapid assessment for neurologic injury takes place. Head injuries are common in children, and carry a high incidence of mortality and morbidity.

Neurologic assessment during the primary survey consists of observation of the level of consciousness, pupil size and reaction, and motor response. The Glasgow Coma Scale (GCS) or the AVPU (alert, verbal, pain, unresponsive) scale can be used to determine initial level of consciousness. The AVPU scale is defined in Box 28-1.

Control of intracranial hypertension, maintenance of adequate cerebral perfusion and prevention of hypoxia are the goals of stabilization for the child with a neurologic injury. A secure airway is critical because hypoxia and hypercapnia must be avoided. If the child is hypotensive, fluids are given at the resuscitation dose, even if neurologic injury is present. However, an isolated head injury rarely causes shock. If shock is present, a high index of suspicion for another source of bleeding should exist.

Once the cervical spine has been cleared by roentgenography, the head of the bed may be elevated. This will help to decrease cerebral venous pressure and control intracranial hypertension.

Exposure is an important component of the primary survey. The child is completely exposed, to examine for life-threatening injuries. This does, however, place the child at risk for hypothermia. Hypothermia produces various physiologic consequences, such as metabolic acidosis and dysrhythmias, and can interfere with resuscitation efforts.

Radiant warmers and warmed intravenous fluids and blood are used with pediatric trauma patients during resuscitation. The child's core temperature is maintained between 36° C and 38° C. If the child is hypothermic on arrival to the unit, a warming blanket on the bed and warm, humidified oxygen are used. See Chapter 14 for more information on the management of hypothermia in the child.

Secondary Survey

The secondary survey follows the primary survey and the initial stabilization of the cardiorespiratory system. The secondary survey is the systematic evaluation of each body system for injury. The order of the examination may vary but normally proceeds in descending order of urgency.[4] The examination of the abdomen and perineum occurs last unless otherwise indicated because this assessment produces pain and the child's response may obscure other findings. As the secondary survey is initiated, it is important to remember that any child with one injury is assumed to have another until proven otherwise. The examination is as gentle as possible, and reassessment is continuous. In-depth assessment of each system is covered under system-specific injuries later in this chapter.

TRAUMA SCORES

Reliable means of measuring injury severity and resulting disability are necessary to scientifically assess care provided to injured children.[5] Numerous scoring systems that use measures of anatomic or physiologic derangements to quantify severity of injury have been developed. These scores include the GCS; Trauma Score (TS); Circulation, Respiration, Abdomen, Motor, Speech (CRAMS) Scale; Revised Trauma Score (RTS); Abbreviated Injury Scale (AIS); Pediatric Risk of Mortality (PRISM); and Injury Severity Score (ISS). These scores are used for field triage, quality assessment, scientific comparison of trauma patients, and epidemiologic research.[5]

A Pediatric Trauma Score (PTS) was developed in the 1980s because the existing scores did not take into account normal pediatric physiologic parameters. The PTS considers the unique anatomic and physiologic characteristics of the child and uses these measures to predict childhood injury severity.[6] Table 28-2 illustrates the PTS. A score of 8 or less

---

Box 28-1
AVPU Scale

A = Patient is alert
V = Patient responds to verbal commands
P = Patient responds to pain
U = Patient is unresponsive

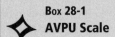 **TABLE 28-2   Pediatric Trauma Score**

| | Category | | |
Component	+2	+1	-1
Size	>20 kg	10-20 kg	<10 kg
Airway	Normal	Maintainable	Unmaintainable
Systolic BP	>90 mmHg	50-90 mmHg	<50 mmHg
CNS	Awake	Obtunded/LOC	Comatose
Skeletal	None	Closed fracture	Open/multiple fractures
Cutaneous	None	Minor	Major
		Sum _____	

From Tepas JJ, Ramenofsky ML, Mollitt DL et al: The pediatric trauma score as a predictor of injury severity: an objective assessment, *J Trauma* 28:427, 1988.
BP, Blood pressure; *CNS,* central nervous system; *LOC,* loss of consciousness.

warrants transport to a pediatric trauma center.[6] In addition to predicting severity of injury, the PTS identifies children who are at immediate risk of mortality. Tepas and colleagues found that a score of less than 6 predicted mortality.[6] Orliaquet and associates determined that a score of less than 4 was associated with immediate risk of mortality.[7]

Most trauma scoring systems are based on anatomic or physiologic dysfunction. The Trauma Injury Severity Score (TRISS) methodology combines anatomic injuries and physiologic dysfunction, using the RTS and ISS. The RTS identifies the degree of neurologic and cardiovascular dysfunction, and the ISS assesses multiple injuries. TRISS methodology calculates the probability of survival for an injured patient.[8] The most widely used method to assess mortality in critically ill children is the PRISM score. Both the ISS using TRISS methodology and the PRISM are useful in pediatric trauma. PRISM stratifies patients into low- and high-risk groups, which allows for accurate prediction of resource utilization. PRISM also predicts mortality risk in pediatric trauma, though not as accurately as the TRISS methodology.[9]

SYSTEM-SPECIFIC INJURIES

Head Injury

Etiology/Incidence.   Head injury is a common pediatric injury and the most common cause of traumatic death in children.[10] Each year, approximately 22,000 acute brain-injured children in the United States die, and another 29,000 are left with a permanent disability. Mortality in children with severe head injuries is 6% to 10%, as opposed to 30% to 50% in the adult with severe head injuries.[11]

Anatomic and physiologic differences in children make them more susceptible to head injury and its consequences. The cranial bones are thinner in children and offer less protection to the growing brain. In addition, the size of the infant head is large in proportion to body size. These anatomic considerations predispose children to head injury. Children's response to head injury differs in that they have a lower incidence of mass lesions but a higher one of intracranial hypertension.[11] Because children experience intracranial hypertension more frequently, they are more susceptible to a secondary head injury rather than a primary head injury.

Pathogenesis.   Traumatic brain injury (TBI) is characterized by primary and secondary injury. Primary injury is produced by the trauma itself. It occurs immediately following impact and may cause damage and/or death of the neuronal cells. Axonal injuries, laceration of brain tissue, contusions, skull fractures, and scalp injuries are examples of a primary head injury. Hypoxic injury may also cause a primary head injury if any of the neurons or astrocytes is injured by hypoxia or ischemia. Secondary injury is produced by the brain's response to trauma. It is a dynamic process that evolves over a period of hours to days and generally peaks 3 to 5 days after injury. Loss of cerebral autoregulation, development of extracellular and intracellular edema, and a breakdown of the blood-brain barrier are components of secondary injury, which is compounded by systemic hypertension and hypotension, hypoxia, and hypercapnia. Recent work has identified the mechanisms that produce the components of secondary injury after TBI. These include ischemia, excitotoxicity, energy failure and resultant cell death cascades, secondary cerebral swelling, axonal injury, and inflammation and regeneration (Fig. 28-3).[12]

Previous work identified cerebral hyperemia as an important factor in the development of intracranial hypertension in the head-injured child. However, Kochanak and colleagues focused on the development of early posttraumatic hypoperfusion.[12] Adelson and colleagues used stable xenon-computed tomographic (CT) method to assess cerebral blood flow in infants and children after severe TBI.[13] Patients were assessed early after injury, and posttraumatic hypoperfusion was common. In addition, ischemia, defined as global cerebral blood flow less than 20 ml/100 g/min, was associated with a poor outcome. Loss of vasodilators and amplification of vasoconstrictors may be mechanisms that produce early posttraumatic hypoperfusion (Fig. 28-4).[12]

Specific Head Injuries.   There are a number of specific head injuries that may be seen in children. Even though these are discussed separately, each one may be an element of a more serious brain injury.

Scalp lacerations are common in infants and young children and usually do not require a hospital stay for treatment. Because of the vascularity of the scalp, a large amount of bleeding may result from a laceration. Once underlying pathology has been ruled out, treatment is minimal and consists of stopping bleeding and inspecting, irrigating, and suturing the wound. Palpation and possibly a skull film may rule out an underlying skull fracture.

Many children with head trauma have a concomitant *skull fracture.* Most of these children have linear fractures. The majority of linear fractures are uncomplicated and heal spontaneously in 2 to 3 months. However, there are some linear fractures that are considered serious, based on their location. A fracture that crosses a major vascular structure, such as the middle meningeal artery or the dural venous sinus, has the potential of bleeding into the subdural or epidural space. A complication of a linear fracture seen in children is the growing fracture. With this complication, a portion of the arachnoid membrane becomes trapped between two edges of the fractured bone, producing a leptomeningeal cyst. The child may present with a soft and pulsating skull defect, seizures, and other neurologic defects.[14] This defect may resolve with age, or surgical intervention may be necessary.

A depressed skull fracture is a fracture in which the inner table of the skull is displaced by more than the thickness of the entire bone. This represents a more severe injury because a great deal of force is required to produce this situation. The treatment of a depressed skull fracture is debridement and elevation of the fragment within 4 hours.[15]

A basilar skull fracture is a common type of skull fracture in children and represents a significant blow to the head. A basilar skull fracture usually involves a break in the base of the frontal, ethmoid, sphenoid, temporal, or occipital bone. The diagnosis is generally made on clinical presentation.

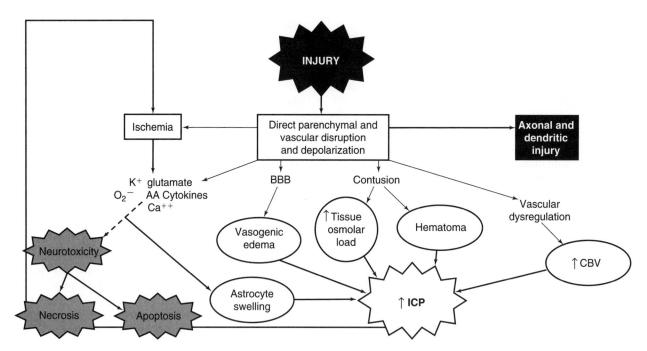

Fig. 28-3 Categories of mechanisms proposed to be involved in the evolution of secondary damage after severe traumatic brain injury (TBI) in infants and children. Three major categories for these secondary mechanisms include ischemia, excitotoxicity, energy failure, and cell death cascades; cerebral swelling; and axonal injury. A fourth category, inflammation and regeneration, contributes to each of these cascades. *AA,* Amino acids; *BBB,* blood-brain barrier; *CBV,* cerebral blood volume; *ICP,* intracranial pressure. (From Kochanek PM, Clark RSB, Ruppel RA et al: Biochemical, cellular, and molecular mechanisms in the evolution of secondary damage after severe traumatic brain injury in infants and children: lessons learned from the bedside, *Pediatr Crit Care Med* 1:4-19, 2000.)

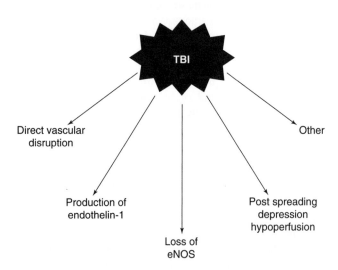

Fig. 28-4 Schematic outlining putative mediators involved in the production of early posttraumatic hypoperfusion and ischemia after severe traumatic brain injury (TBI). *eNOS,* Endothelial nitric oxide synthase. (From Kochanek PM, Clark RSB, Ruppel RA et al: Biochemical, cellular, and molecular mechanisms in the evolution of secondary damage after severe traumatic brain injury in infants and children: lessons learned from the bedside, *Pediatr Crit Care Med* 1:4-19, 2000.)

A history of impact at the back of the head raises the index of suspicion. There may also be a loss of consciousness, seizures, or other signs of neurologic deficit. On physical examination, the child may show certain findings that are indicative of a basilar skull fracture. Rhinorrhea, raccoon eyes (periorbital ecchymosis), anosmia, and ocular motor palsies may occur with anterior fossa fractures. Hematotympanum, otorrhea, vertigo, Battle's sign (mastoid ecchymosis), or unilateral hearing loss may occur with middle fossa fractures. Hypotension, tachycardia, and changes in the respiratory pattern may be indicative of brainstem compression that can occur with posterior fossa fractures.[14] Cerebrospinal fluid (CSF) leakage from the ear indicates disruption of the leptomeninges, and CSF leakage from the nose indicates leakage through the perinasal sinuses. Clear drainage from the ears or nose is tested for the presence of glucose because glucose is present in CSF. However, because CSF is often mixed with blood and blood contains glucose, the presence of glucose does not always confirm that the fluid is CSF. If CSF is mixed with blood, as the blood dries, an xanthochromic (yellow) halo will appear on a dressing. The presence of a halo confirms the presence of CSF. A serious potential complication of CSF leakage is the development of meningitis. This is unusual, however, and

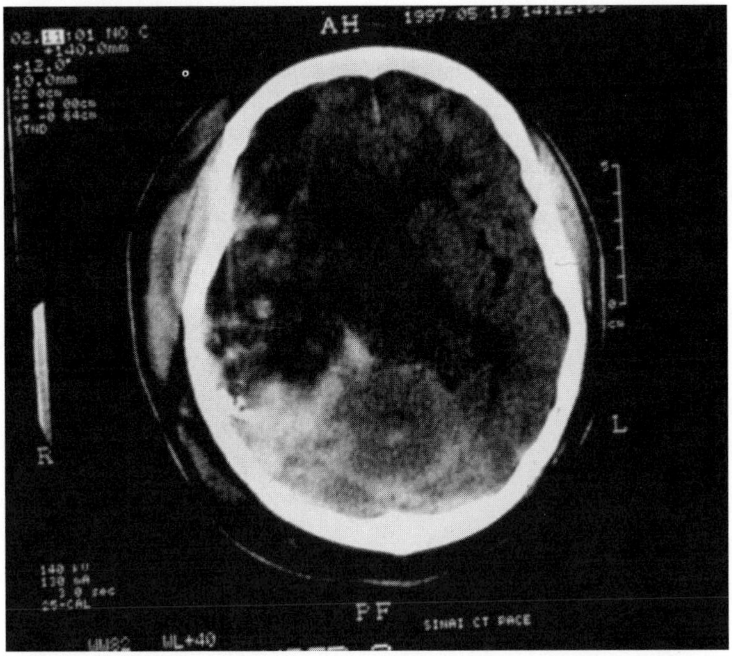

Fig. 28-5 Cerebral contusion with mass effect and midline shift.

the use of prophylactic antibiotics is controversial. The trend has been to treat only documented cases of meningitis.[15]

In general, most basilar skull fractures are uncomplicated. Skull films identify basilar skull fractures in only 10% of cases. CT scans are indicated to identify the area of the fracture and any underlying brain injury. Because the cribriform plate is disrupted, insertion of nasotracheal and nasogastric tubes is avoided. Most children with basilar skull fractures require only 24 to 48 hours of observation with frequent neurologic checks and can expect a full recovery.

Concussion is the mildest form of traumatic injury to the brain. With a concussion, the child momentarily loses consciousness at the time of injury. The loss of consciousness is the result of the stretching and shearing forces in the brainstem.[15] Diagnosis is usually made on a historical basis based on a temporary loss of consciousness.

The nature of concussion is varied based on the age group. Infants tend to have a less specific clinical presentation. They usually exhibit benign posttraumatic seizures, vomiting, diaphoresis, pallor, and lethargy and do not usually experience a loss of consciousness.[15] In the older child, posttraumatic amnesia becomes an important finding. The child may also complain of headaches, dizziness, and fatigue and may show some behavioral changes. The child's neurologic function usually normalizes in about 1 week, though some symptoms may persist for months or even to 1 year. This postconcussive syndrome is expected to resolve completely.

Cerebral contusion is defined as an actual bruising or microscopic bleeding of the brain, associated with temporary or permanent structural damage. A contusion is similar to a concussion in that a transient or actual loss of consciousness may occur; however, a contusion causes an actual disruption of cerebral tissue to varying degrees, often

accompanied by parenchymal hemorrhage and focal edema. The contusion may occur at the site of impact (coup injury) or at a site opposite the impact (contrecoup injury). The degree of injury is reflected by alterations in the child's mental status. In a mild contusion, the return of consciousness is not as rapid as with a concussion and there is retrograde amnesia. With mild retrograde amnesia, the memory loss is only that of exact details of events occurring immediately before impact. More severe amnesia manifests itself by the memory loss extending for a period of hours before the impact occurred. Children with more severe amnesia often have some disorientation, slowed reaction, headache, vomiting, and other mild neurologic abnormalities. Diagnosis of contusion is made based on focal neurologic signs and CT scan. The most common pattern seen on CT is that of multiple small hemorrhages surrounded by varying degrees of edema (Fig. 28-5).

Return to consciousness following rapid neurologic deterioration may be seen in children with a cerebral contusion. The cause in children is usually the result of diffuse generalized cerebral swelling. The most common CT scan finding among all children with an acceleration/deceleration injury is diffuse cerebral swelling.

The incidence of cerebral contusion in infants is rare compared with older children. This is attributed to several factors. The skull of the infant is more pliable, and there are less convolutional markers on the inner table. Because the surface between bone and brain tissue is smoother, there is less resistance to movement and surface injury is minimized. Also, the infant's brain is less myelinized; and demyelinized brain tissue has a softer consistency, which may reduce injury.[16]

Treatment of a cerebral contusion depends on the severity of the contusion. Treatment may be supportive medical therapy, involving treatment of increased ICP if it

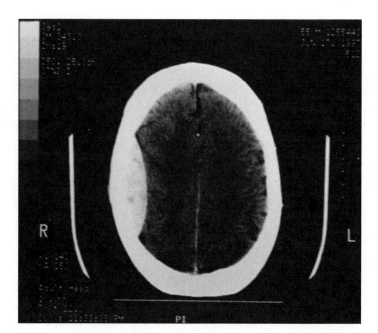

Fig. 28-6 Epidural hematoma with mass effect and small midline shift.

exists. Surgical treatment (removal of the contused tissue) may be necessary if medical management does not control increased ICP or if significant shifts are seen on CT scan.

An *epidural hematoma* refers to a collection of blood above the dura. Epidural hematomas are less common in children, especially infants, because of several reasons. The dura is tightly adherent to the inner table of the skull, especially at suture lines in infants and young children. Also, the fixation of the middle meningeal artery does not occur until approximately 2 years of age. Because the artery is not embedded into the temporal bone until fixation occurs, it can rotate and possibly avoid injury.

An epidural hematoma is a readily correctable lesion if identified and removed before secondary injury to the brainstem occurs. The classic lucid interval between the initial loss of consciousness and subsequent rapid neurologic deterioration is much less common in children.[15] More often, the symptoms tend to be vague depending on the age of the child and the location of the bleeding. Infants may experience bulging fontanelles, separation of the sutures, decreased hematocrit, and shock with significant bleeding. In older children, an enlarging hematoma may cause herniation into other areas of the brain, producing corresponding signs. The child may exhibit hemiparesis, hemiplegia, ipsilateral pupil dilation, posturing, or contralateral limb weakness. Symptoms may be delayed for hours or days if the source of bleeding is venous rather than arterial. If the hematoma continues to enlarge and the compensatory mechanisms of the brain become exhausted, temporal lobe herniation and brainstem compression occurs. A progressive decrease in the level of consciousness is the most significant diagnostic sign for all age groups. If time permits, a CT scan is performed, which will show a localized, high-density lesion with mass effect (Fig. 28-6). If the child demonstrates rapid clinical deterioration, immediate surgical intervention without the benefit of a CT scan is necessary.

Treatment of choice is surgical evacuation of the hematoma. This is performed as quickly as possible to avoid increasing morbidity or mortality. Evacuation of the hematoma is by craniotomy with removal of the clot and control of bleeding. Burr holes are technically difficult but may be useful as a diagnostic procedure in the absence of CT scan evaluation.[15] With prompt surgical intervention, the prognosis for the child with an epidural hematoma is good.

A *subdural hematoma* is a collection of blood in the subdural space, often with associated cortical damage from lacerated vessels or direct contusion. Acute subdural hematomas are almost always caused by a traumatic incident. They are usually associated with a high mortality and morbidity because of the fact that the lesion is often caused by disruption of a cortical artery or a large bridging vein. The impact required to produce this type of injury is significant and is associated with severe contusion of the underlying vein. Common causes of a subdural hematoma are high-speed motor vehicle accidents, falls, assaults, and violent shaking. One study demonstrated that subdural hematomas were more likely to occur with inflicted head injury rather than accidental injury.[17]

The clinical presentation of a child with a subdural hematoma is routinely that of a youngster who has sustained a major head injury. The lucid interval seen with epidural hematoma is not seen because the brain is so severely injured. The child presents with profound neurologic deterioration, and because of the force of impact, the mental status is almost always affected.

Confirmation of the diagnosis of subdural hematoma is made with CT scan (Fig. 28-7). The most effective treatment is evacuation of the clot with control of bleeding and possible resection of damaged brain tissue.[15] Even with aggressive treatment, the prognosis for the child with a subdural hematoma is less favorable than for the child with an epidural hematoma. This is because of the associated damage to the underlying brain tissue.

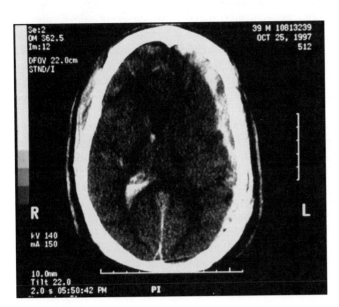

Fig. 28-7 Left subdural hematoma with mass effect, midline shift, and intraventricular hemorrhage.

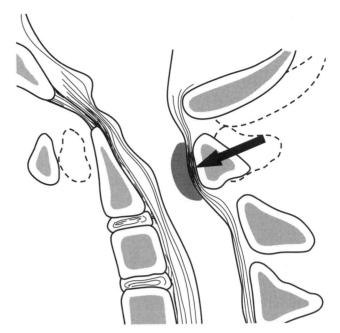

Fig. 28-8 A lateral view depicting compression from displaced bony elements causing spinal injury. This is a common mechanism of primary spinal cord injury in children because of their hypermobile vertebral column. (From Allen EM, Boyer R, Cheney WB et al: Head and spinal cord injury. In Rogers MC, ed: *Textbook of pediatric intensive care*, ed 3, Baltimore, 1996, Williams & Wilkins.)

Because a large number of children experience intracranial hypertension following severe TBI, collaborative management focuses on controlling increased ICP. Chapter 20 provides in-depth information regarding care of the child with a head injury.

Spinal Cord Injury

Etiology/Incidence. Spinal cord injury is relatively rare in children. Approximately 1100 children with spinal cord injury are reported annually.[18] Motor vehicle accidents are the leading cause of spinal cord injury in children. In addition to occupant motor vehicle accidents, pedestrian and bicycle motor vehicle accidents are common causes of spinal injury in children.[18] Sports-related and recreational injuries, child abuse, falls, and birth-related injuries also account for a large proportion of pediatric spinal cord injuries.[19]

The type and severity of injuries seen in children differ than from those seen in adults.[18] Children experience a higher incidence of cervical injuries and spinal cord injury without radiographic abnormality (SCIWORA). There are a number of factors related to this, but the most significant factor is the inherent differences between the pediatric and adult spine. The development of the pediatric spine is a continuous, dynamic process. Development is characterized by changes in the geometric configuration of the vertebrae; development of the ossification centers; closure of the epiphyseal plates; changes in the characteristics of the ligaments and soft tissues; and changes in osseous shape, size, strength, and integrity.[20] Even though the epiphyses fuse at different ages, most epiphyseal plates are fused by 8 years of age. Multiple ossification centers are present at

birth but continue to develop throughout childhood. The vertebral bodies are wedge-shaped, and the vertebrae are mostly cartilaginous. The vertebral facets tend to have a horizontal orientation, and they become more vertical and ossify between 7 and 10 years of age. Before this time, they provide minimum stability to the vertebral column. The head of the infant and young child is large in relation to the neck, and the paraspinous muscles are not well developed. The vertebral ligaments and soft tissue are more elastic than in adults. These features all contribute to creating hypermobility of the neck and a tendency toward SCIWORA, severe ligamentous injury, and upper cervical spine injuries (Fig. 28-8).[21]

These differences make the children susceptible to different patterns of injury compared with adults. The types of injuries change as the biomechanical and anatomic features of the spine become more adult-like; however, the adult spinal characteristics and patterns of injury are not fully seen until after the age of 15 years.[21]

Pathogenesis. Younger children between the ages of 0 and 8 years often sustain soft tissue injury without fractures. This is related to hypermobility and osseous immaturity. Manifestations of soft tissue injuries include SCIWORA, ligamentous dislocations, subluxation without fracture, growth plate injuries, and epiphyseal separations. In contrast, adolescents experience more "true" fractures than ligamentous or growth plate injuries.

Hypermobility of the child's spine is the most critical determinant of injury.[21] Hypermobility protects the spinal cord from injury because force is dispersed over multiple vertebral levels. Hypermobility also accounts for the low incidence of spinal injury in the child and the patterns of injury. When spinal injury does occur, it is usually severe and accounts more often for complete loss of function in the child than in any other age group.[21]

Sixty percent to eighty percent of vertebral injuries in the first 10 years of life involve the cervical region, especially the upper portion (occiput through C-3).[18] Significant ligamentous injuries have a propensity for the upper cervical spine. Atlanto-occipital dislocation (separation of the occipital condyles from the atlas) results in severe craniovertebral junction instability and can cause fatal neurologic injury. Immediate internal fixation is necessary to preserve neurologic function because halo immobilization may not maintain alignment and traction with tongs may cause distraction of the craniovertebral junction, even with a small amount of weight.

Atlantoaxial dislocations (subluxations) are usually not fatal. Subluxation at the C1-C2 level is better tolerated than subluxation at the lower levels because the spinal canal is larger at C-1. Rotatory subluxation occurs with injury to the capsular ligaments. Anterior subluxations often occur in conjunction with rupture of the transverse ligament of the atlas and with relaxation of other atlantoaxial ligaments. Posterior subluxations occur with injury to the dens.

Anterior or posterior instability is seen best on flexion and extension radiographs. Rotatory subluxations are apparent with a CT scan. Rotatory subluxations greater than 40 degrees cause facet interlock and require external reduction and internal fixation.[23]

Young children are susceptible to dislocations without fractures at all levels of the vertebrae, though this tends to occur mostly in the cervical region. Fracture characteristics change with vertebral maturation. Younger children tend to experience epiphyseal separations and growth plate fractures, whereas adolescents usually sustain more adult-like fracture patterns. Most cervical spine injuries in adolescents, like adults, occur at the C5-C6 level.

Occipital condyle fractures are extremely rare in children. These fractures are usually stable, though they can cause cranial nerve dysfunction. Fractures of the atlas or axis are also uncommon in young children; these fractures tend to occur more often in adolescence.

Fractures of the thoracic or lumbar spine in children often occur in the T11-L2 region where the rigid thoracic segments join the more mobile lumbar segments. Again, these injuries tend to involve the soft tissues and the ligaments, which result in cartilaginous or growth plate injuries. Children restrained by lap belts involved in motor vehicle accidents may sustain fractures in the midlumbar region.

As previously mentioned, a group of children experience SCIWORA. The hallmark of this entity is the presence of a spinal cord injury even though radiographic studies are normal. Flexion-extension views and CT scans are also normal. The injury occurs because of the immature pediatric spine where momentary intersegmental damage causes disruption of the cord without disrupting bones or ligaments.

Four mechanisms are proposed for SCIWORA. These include longitudinal distraction, hyperflexion, hyperextension, or ischemic spinal cord damage.[24] The inherent elasticity of the spinal column can cause the spinal cord to be susceptible to a longitudinal distraction mechanism. The horizontally oriented facet joints result in greater mobility but less stability. Forward movement of the upper cervical spine is facilitated, causing a flexion injury. Hyperextension of the cervical spine causes inward bulging of the ligamentum flavum and increased thickness in the spinal cord. This can reduce the diameter of the spinal canal by as much as 50% and allow for direct damage to the spinal cord. In addition, the anatomy and biomechanics of the occipitoatlantal junction cause the vertebral arteries to be susceptible to compression during hyperextension. This can result in temporary occlusion leading to ischemia and infarction.[25]

Injuries experienced by children with SCIWORA tend to be devastating. Children with SCIWORA often present with delayed onset of neurologic deficit, although the reasons for this are not known. The delayed onset follows what appears to be an insignificant injury but once onset ensues, it progresses rapidly to a severe, permanent neurologic deficit. This may occur several hours to days after injury; however, in retrospect, a history of subtle neurologic symptoms is often elicited.[24]

Critical Care Management. Any child who has experienced head or facial trauma or who complains of neck pain is suspected of having a spinal cord injury. Clearance of the cervical spine requires anteroposterior, lateral, and open-mouth views of the cervical spine.[18] It is critical that the cervical spine films include views of C7 and T1. These views are obtained by gently pulling the shoulders downward to visualize the seven cervical vertebrae.

Because of the possibility of SCIWORA, occult fractures and vertebral malalignment are ruled out by CT scan. In addition, children with head and neck injuries are questioned for the presence of transient neurologic symptoms that may indicate SCIWORA.

There are some considerations when evaluating cervical spine films in the child. The vertebral bodies of the child are less rectangular than those of the adult. These bodies have a biconcave appearance, which can give the impression of a compression fracture. This can be ruled out by comparing all the vertebral bodies, because the normal vertebral bodies will all appear the same. In addition, angulation in the infant spine is more extreme than in the adult. This is due to the fact that the infant spine is very cartilaginous and, especially at the C2-C3 level, vertebral offsets may appear. These may give the impression of subluxation.

Initial management of spinal cord injury begins with appropriate resuscitation and stabilization of the spine. Data indicate that a high proportion of children younger than 15 years of age with spinal cord injury die immediately or within the first hour after injury.[18] As many as 50% of children with spinal cord injuries may die in the field, and among the children who survive the initial injury, another 25% will die during the initial period of hospitalization.[26] Children who do survive the initial 3 months have a better chance of survival after 5 years compared with other age

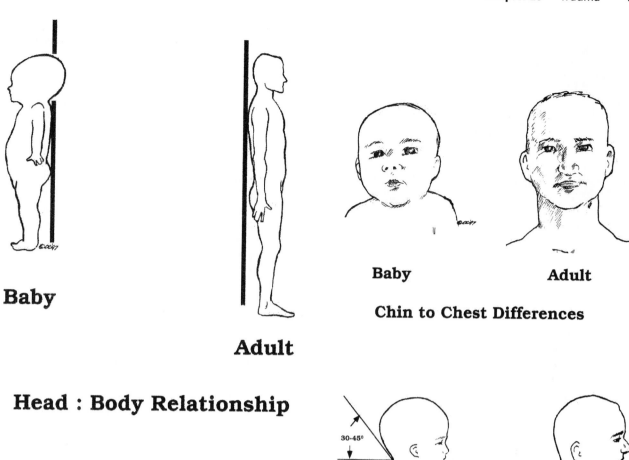

Baby

Adult

Head : Body Relationship

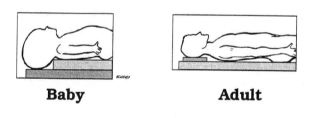

Baby   ## Adult

Spinal Alignment

Fig. 28-9 Children vs. adults: Differences in pediatric head-to-body relationship and spinal alignment. (Courtesy Jerome Medical.)

Baby   ## Adult

Chin to Chest Differences

30-45°

Baby   ## Adult

Differences in Head Shape and Location of Ear

Fig. 28-10 Children vs. adults: The anterior neck length, measured from chin to chest, is negative in infancy and peaks in preadolescence. The occipital angle (the angle between the occiput and the neck) is very steep in infancy compared with the adult. (Courtesy Jerome Medical.)

groups with spinal cord injury.[26] The high initial mortality suggests that critically injured children do not tolerate severe neurologic injury or multisystem trauma.

Initial immobilization of the child with suspected spinal cord trauma is standard. However, using a standard backboard to achieve immobilization may be problematic. Young children have a disproportionately large head (the head represents 25% of total body length in infancy and only 14% in adulthood), and when positioned on a flat surface, the head may be forced forward, causing it to flex. This difference is demonstrated in Fig. 28-9. Therefore when immobilizing the young child, the occiput is lower than the

body. In determining the correct size collar, it is also important to take into account chin to chest differences and differences in head shape and location of the ear (Fig. 28-10). New pediatric spinal immobilization devices that take these differences into account are made especially for children (Fig. 28-11).

Initial management includes attention to airway, breathing, and circulation. Hypotension is assumed to result from bleeding until proven otherwise. Spinal neurogenic shock, often resulting from complete upper spinal cord injury, may

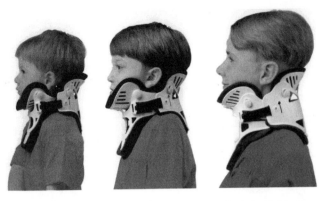

Fig. 28-11 The Miami Jr. collar, Jerome Medical, is designed to address the growth transition of the head, neck, and upper body from birth through preadolescence. The collar is available in three sizes specifically designed for children: P1 (ages 0 to 2), P2 (ages 2 to 6), and P3 (ages 6 to 12).

occur at the time of injury. The triad of symptoms are hypotension, bradycardia, and hypothermia. These symptoms result from the sudden loss of sympathetic outflow from the cervicothoracic region. The loss of vasomotor tone is treated with a low dose norepinephrine (Levophed) infusion at 0.1 to 1.0 µg/kg/min. Atropine, 0.01 to 0.02 mg/kg/dose, may be used to treat increased parasympathetic tone. Atropine may be repeated every 5 to 10 minutes as necessary, used alternatively or concurrently with norepinephrine.[27] Volume expansion is also appropriate. In addition, with spinal shock, there is a temporary but complete loss of segmental reflex activity.[22] These children have flaccid, areflexic limbs with no sensory or sphincter function. Priapism may also be present. Gradually, after 7 to 21 days, segmental reflex function returns and spasticity occurs.[22]

The administration of methylprednisolone may have significant benefit if administered within the first 8 hours after injury. An intravenous bolus of 30 mg/kg followed by a continuous infusion of 5.4 mg/kg/hr for 23 hours has been recommended.[15]

The use of external orthotic devices depends on the nature of the injury and the age of the child. A stiff molded collar may be useful to restrict cervical movement and is suitable for muscular injuries, atlantoaxial rotatory subluxation, and nondisplaced atlas fractures. However, these collars are not truly effective in immobilizing the cervical spine but serve more as a reminder not to move the neck.

Complete reduction and immobilization of the cervical spine may be accomplished by the use of traction. However, the halo jacket is considered the preferred immobilization device because it completely stabilizes the head, yet allows for patient mobility (Fig. 28-12). Care focuses on prevention of dislodgment, loosening, and pin protrusion, especially in young children. Other potential complications are decubitus ulcers, brain abscesses, and pin site infection.

Treatment of thoracic and lumbar spine injuries is based on the characteristic of the fracture and the presence of pain, spinal deformity, or neurologic deficits. Children with more than 50% compression of the height of the vertebral body,

spinal instability, kyphotic deformity, or severe intractable pain are treated with open reduction and internal fixation. Children with less than 50% compression are treated with surgical decompression of the spinal cord and/or nerve roots.[22]

Unstable fractures and dislocations, progressive neurologic deficits with an incomplete cord injury, or compound wounds are treated surgically. Persistent instability despite the use of external orthotic devices requires internal fixation.

Ongoing care of the child with a spinal cord injury revolves around supporting the child's physiologic and psychosocial needs. In addition to managing the initial resuscitation and care of the stabilization device, attention is focused on supporting the child's oxygenation and ventilation status, if necessary. The child with a spinal cord injury will suffer neuromuscular failure if the lesion is at C4 or above. Injuries above the T1 level result in paralysis of the intercostal muscles, and injuries above T10-T12 result in paralysis of the abdominal muscles. This may have implications for younger children who are abdominal breathers. Also, abdominal muscle involvement will limit effective coughing.

Assessment of ventilatory parameters is important, especially vital capacity. Once baseline vital capacity has been obtained, values are obtained at least every 4 hours. If vital capacity decreases over time, diaphragmatic failure is occurring and ventilatory support is necessary. Ventilatory support may be permanent or temporary, depending on the level of the injury. If the injury is at C3-C4 or above, lifelong ventilatory support will be necessary.

The psychosocial needs of the child with a spinal cord injury and the family of the child are tremendous. Especially with a high cord injury, the child no longer has control over the most basic bodily functions. For the adolescent, a time of developing complete independence has now become a time of complete dependence. Interventions revolve around sensitivity to the needs of children or adolescents as they experience changes in their ability to interact and be independent.

Family needs are also enormous as they face the prospects of a permanent change in their lives as well as the life of the child. The family is assisted with coping with the change and with regaining their preinjury level of functioning or attaining a higher level of functioning.

Early involvement in a rehabilitation program is critical. If the child is in a center that has a rehabilitation program, involvement may begin on the day of injury. Concentration on a bladder and bowel program, prevention of contractures and decubitus ulcers, and relief of spasticity are three major areas focused on by the rehabilitation program.

Thoracic Injury

Etiology/Incidence. Thoracic trauma accounts for one of the highest mortality rates in children, second only to head injury.[28] Morbidity associated with thoracic injury is also an issue. Peclet and colleagues found that children who suffered thoracic injury were more severely injured than those who did not.[29] Seventy percent of the children in this

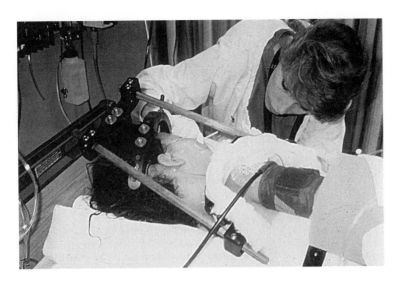

Fig. 28-12   Halo traction.

study required admission to the intensive care unit, and twenty percent required surgical intervention. Thoracic injury, when combined with injuries to other systems, increases the severity of injury and requires extensive resource use.

A unique feature of the child who has sustained thoracic trauma is the compliant thorax resulting from the flexibility of the bony and cartilaginous structures. It is not unusual, therefore, for the child to have major internal injury from compression of the chest without fracture of the bony thorax. A child's mediastinum is freely mobile and capable of wide anatomic shifts. This creates the potential for life-threatening situations such as dislocation of the heart, angulation of the great vessels, compression of the lung, and angulation of the trachea. Children with any type of traumatic injury experience aerophagia, which results in gastric dilation that limits diaphragmatic excursion and leads to reflex ileus. In a small child, this also can compromise ventilation and gas exchange.

Serious thoracic injury is most commonly the result of blunt trauma. Motor vehicle-related and bicycle-related injuries account for the majority of thoracic trauma.[18] Falls and child abuse are also common causes of thoracic injury in children. The presence of serious thoracic injury increases the potential for mortality by a factor of 10.

Pathogenesis.   The pathogenesis of thoracic injury is related to the specific injury. Regardless of the injury, the pathogenesis may include impaired oxygenation and ventilation, and/or decreased cardiac output.

Rib Fractures.   The incidence of rib fractures in children is less than in the adult. The decreased incidence can be attributed to the incomplete ossification of the pediatric skeleton, which results in more flexibility in the bones. The presence of rib fractures in a child suggests severe traumatic force. Fractures of multiple ribs have been directly correlated with an increase in mortality.[30]

Injuries associated with rib fractures vary according to the fracture site. The four upper ribs are protected by the shoulder girdle and are less likely to fracture. Fractures of ribs one through four suggests injury to the bronchial, tracheal, or great vessels.

The most commonly fractured ribs are the middle ones (four through nine). Often, these ribs penetrate lung tissue, causing serious damage. Pneumothorax and hemothorax often accompany middle rib fractures.

The lowest three ribs are not attached to the sternum and can withstand a great deal of force without breaking. Fractures of these free-floating ribs are often accompanied by liver, spleen, or kidney laceration.

Signs of rib fractures are localized pain on movement or deep breathing and crepitus on palpation. The child may breathe shallowly to decrease pain, leading to hypoventilation. Treatment of rib fractures is aimed at rest and pain relief.

Flail Chest.   Flail chest occurs when there are multiple fractures of the same rib, or when there are fractures of the rib and sternum. The configuration of the fractures results in a floating rib segment. The chest wall becomes unstable as the flail segment moves paradoxically to the rest of the chest wall (Fig. 28-13).

As the diaphragm descends with inspiration, subatmospheric pressure allows the flail segment to move inward toward the negative pressure. The flail segment moves outward as the diaphragm rises with expiration. The paradoxic movement causes a decrease in tidal volume by preventing the lung from fully expanding and causing atelectasis. Ventilation/perfusion mismatch results. Children with a flail chest often have an accompanying pulmonary contusion. Hypoventilation, combined with the contusion and shunting, accounts for the morbidity associated with a flail chest.

Treatment of an uncomplicated flail chest is similar to that of rib fractures. Rest, analgesia, and meticulous pulmonary toilet are the primary treatments. Children with significant impairment of gas exchange may require pneumatic stabilization, which consists of intubation and positive pressure ventilation. Judicious use of intravenous fluid and good pulmonary toilet are also recommended.

Traumatic Asphyxia.   Traumatic asphyxia occurs almost exclusively in children because of their compliant chest wall and absence of valves in the superior and inferior vena cava. Direct compression against a closed glottis

INJURY

ACTIVE BREATHING

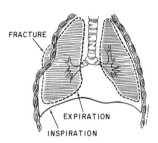

FRACTURE

EXPIRATION

INSPIRATION

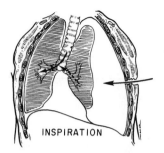
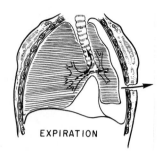

INSPIRATION   EXPIRATION

Fig. 28-13   Flail chest. There is a paradoxic segment of the chest wall and loss of the normal bellows mechanism. (From Jones KW: Thoracic trauma. In Mayer TA, ed: *Emergency management of pediatric trauma,* Philadelphia, 1985, WB Saunders.)

Fig. 28-14   Open pneumothorax results in ipsilateral lung collapse, mediastinal shift, and impaired ventilation of the opposite lung. (From Jones KW: Thoracic trauma. In Mayer TA, ed: *Emergency management of pediatric trauma,* Philadelphia, 1985, WB Saunders.)

causes an acute increase in intrathoracic pressure with accompanying obstruction of vena caval drainage. A marked increase in venous pressure occurs, causing extravasation from the capillary bed and hemorrhage from the brain and other organs. Traumatic asphyxia may occur as the result of automobile wheels passing over the chest of the child or when the child is trampled. Often the child is lying on soft ground, which allows for compression without sternal or rib fractures.

Signs and symptoms of traumatic asphyxia include cyanosis of the face and neck; petechiae of the head, neck, and chest; and retinal and subconjunctival hemorrhages. Signs of disorientation and respiratory distress may be present. Pulmonary contusion and pneumothorax often accompany traumatic asphyxia.

Treatment for traumatic asphyxia and associated injuries is symptomatic. Increased ICP may result from prolonged asphyxia and is treated accordingly.

Pneumothorax.   Pneumothorax is the most common manifestation of thoracic injury, caused by blunt or penetrating trauma. Pneumothorax can range from a small, single pneumothorax to a life-threatening tension pneumothorax or open pneumothorax.

Simple pneumothorax occurs when air enters the pleural space, secondary to tears in the tracheobronchial tree, the esophagus, or the chest wall itself. Because the thorax is flexible, a pneumothorax may be present without rib fractures. Symptoms of a pneumothorax range from none to severe respiratory distress. Physical examination may reveal decreased breath sounds and hyperresonance to percussion over the injured area. If the child is stable, a chest roentgenogram is obtained to confirm the diagnosis.

Treatment of a pneumothorax varies. The child in severe respiratory distress requires needle thoracostomy first, followed by tube thoracostomy. The child who is stable requires only a tube thoracostomy. A very small pneumothorax (<15%) in the asymptomatic child may require only observation.

Tension pneumothorax results when air enters the pleural space but is unable to exit. The trapped air accumulates,

increasing intrapleural pressure, which causes the affected lung to collapse. The air continues to accumulate, causing the mediastinum to shift and compress the contralateral lung. Excessive shift in the mediastinum results in vena cava compression, a decrease in venous return to the right side of the heart, and, ultimately, a decrease in cardiac output. If tension pneumothorax is not corrected immediately, cardiovascular collapse and death occurs.

Signs of tension pneumothorax include severe respiratory distress, absence of breath sounds and hyperresonance over the affected lung, cardiovascular instability, and tracheal shift to the unaffected side. A needle thoracentesis is the immediate treatment of choice. This relieves the tension, allowing the mediastinum to shift back. Once the air is evacuated, a chest tube insertion is performed.

The third type of pneumothorax is an open pneumothorax. An open pneumothorax occurs when there is an opening in the chest wall, usually resulting from penetrating trauma. The opening allows air to move freely in and out of the pleural space. With a large wound, the mediastinum moves to one side or the other, depending on the phase of respiration. During inspiration, air moves through the wound. The lung collapses, and the mediastinum moves toward the functioning lung. During expiration, air exits through the wound, the lung partially reexpands, and the mediastinum shifts back (Fig. 28-14).

The child with an open pneumothorax often shows signs of restlessness, cyanosis, subcutaneous emphysema, and mediastinal shift. In addition, a sucking sound may be heard as air moves through the open wound. The open wound is covered immediately with an airtight seal. Sterile towels or a gloved hand can be used until a dressing is applied. Once the patient has stabilized, a petroleum jelly gauze is applied.

Hemothorax.   Hemothorax occurs when blood accumulates in the pleural space, causing collapse of the affected lung. Hemothorax can occur secondary to blunt or penetrating injury. Blood collects in the pleural space, causing the affected lung to collapse. Injury to the heart, great vessels, or other thoracic structures may lead to the development of a hemothorax.

Signs and symptoms of hemothorax include respiratory distress, decreased or absent breath sounds, and dullness to percussion over the affected area. Shock may develop because children can lose up to 40% of their total blood volume into a hemothorax.[28]

Treatment of a hemothorax varies slightly from that of a pneumothorax. Blood is immediately evacuated from the pleural space with a chest tube; however, intravenous access is established before evacuation to allow for fluid resuscitation. The chest tube is placed in the seventh or eighth intercostal space, which drains the hemothorax, reexpands the lung, and allows for monitoring of ongoing bleeding. Blood volume is rapidly replaced. Any child who exhibits blood loss of more than 1 to 2 ml/kg/hr is prepared for a thoracotomy.

Pulmonary Contusion.   Pulmonary contusion is one of the most common thoracic injuries seen in the child and is the most common cause of potentially fatal chest injury. It is often seen in the absence of bony injury. Pulmonary contusion is suspected whenever the child has a thoracic injury, especially if there is bruising noted on the chest.

Pulmonary contusion occurs when the lung is traumatized, causing bleeding from the capillary endothelium. Resultant increased capillary permeability allows for the development of both alveolar and interstitial edema. Impaired gas exchange results, causing ventilation/perfusion mismatch and decreased compliance.

Signs and symptoms of pulmonary contusion may not initially be evident. Signs of respiratory distress may develop within several hours after injury and may include wheezing, hemoptysis, fever, rales, and signs of hypoxemia. Chest roentgenograms will demonstrate patchy densities, but this may not occur for 24 to 48 hours after the initial injury (Fig. 28-15). Tyburski and colleagues demonstrated that the severity of pulmonary contusion on x-ray films combined with Pao_2/Fio_2 ratio was valuable in determining the need for ventilatory assistance and predicting outcome.[31]

Treatment of pulmonary contusion is dependent on the severity. Mild contusions may be managed with oxygen, analgesia, pulmonary toilet, and judicious fluid management to prevent large increases in interstitial pulmonary edema. Severe pulmonary contusions, which significantly alter respiratory function, may require intubation and mechanical ventilation. A pulmonary artery catheter is often placed to monitor pulmonary capillary wedge pressure to closely monitor fluid status. Albumin may be used for osmotic purposes; serum osmolarity is maintained at 300 mOsm. Diuretics may also be used to decrease the amount of pulmonary interstitial fluid.

Ventilatory interventions include the use of high-flow oxygen and positive end-expiratory pressure (PEEP). The pulmonary status is continuously evaluated with serial monitoring of arterial blood gases and continuous monitoring of Spo_2 and end-tidal CO_2. Because the child may be on a high amount of PEEP, close monitoring for the development of airleak syndrome is critical.

Other interventions for the child with a pulmonary contusion include positioning, observation for signs of

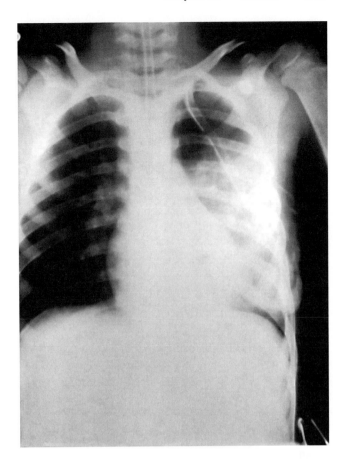

Fig. 28-15   Pulmonary contusion.

infection, and meticulous pulmonary toilet. Optimal position to enhance matching of ventilation to perfusion in patients with a pulmonary contusion is best determined at the bedside with the aid of Spo_2 monitoring.

The child with pulmonary contusion may be at risk for the development of acute respiratory distress syndrome (ARDS), although one study demonstrated a low incidence of ARDS following pulmonary contusion or multiple trauma.[32] A recent study demonstrated the effectiveness of pressure control inverse ratio ventilation (PCIRV) in patients who develop ARDS following blunt chest trauma.[33] PCIRV was shown to be an effective mode of ventilation in patients with ARDS following blunt chest trauma; however, there are complications, including auto-PEEP and decreased cardiac output.[33] Intermittent prone positioning has been shown to recruit collapsed lung tissue and improve gas exchange in trauma patients with blunt chest trauma and severe ARDS.[34]

Cardiac Tamponade.   Cardiac tamponade occurs when blood accumulates in the pericardial sac, increasing pericardial pressure. The increase in pressure alters the pumping mechanism of the heart, resulting in a decrease in cardiac output. Stab wounds are the most common cause of tamponade in the trauma patient. Firearms can also produce tamponade and cause sudden death. Blunt trauma rarely results in tamponade. Signs and symptoms of acute tamponade are the classic triad of jugular venous distension, hypotension, and muffled heart sounds, although these may be difficult to detect in the child. The short, fat neck of the child makes assessment of venous distension difficult. Also, the thin chest wall allows for increased transmission of sound. Another classic sign is the presence of a pulsus paradoxus of greater than 10 mmHg. Tamponade is suspected in children with persistent hypotension despite fluid resuscitation. In the absence of hypovolemia, an increased central venous pressure may be noted. Initial treatment of pericardial tamponade is pericardiocentesis. If pericardiocentesis is not successful, or if tamponade reoccurs, operative intervention is warranted.

Commodio Cordis. Commodio cordis occurs in children and is the result of the sudden impact to the precordium. It results in cessation of normal cardiac function. The child may experience a life-threatening dysrhythmia that is refractory to resuscitation.[35] Most children do recover; however, some patients require long-term antiarrhythmic drugs, pacemakers, inotropic drugs, or intraaortic balloon pumps. Significant mortality and morbidity are associated with this injury.[18]

Myocardial Contusion. Myocardial contusion occurs when traumatic forces cause local injury to the myocardium. Dysrhythmias may occur secondary to injury.[36] Children suffering from myocardial contusion are less likely than adults to have dysrhythmias or alterations in cardiac function.[37]

Signs of myocardial contusion are chest pain and alteration in cardiac function. Chest wall bruising and tenderness may not be present, making a high suspicion of injury an important diagnostic factor. A 12-lead echocardiogram is obtained on all patients with a suspected contusion. One third of children with nonpenetrating myocardial trauma will develop S-T segment and T-wave changes during the first 24 to 48 hours after injury like those seen with myocardial ischemia and infarction.[38]

Significant elevations in serum glutamic-oxaloacetic transaminase (SGOT) and lactate dehydrogenase (LDH) occur with hemorrhagic shock, so these alterations are not significant for myocardial contusion.[38] Two-dimensional echocardiography may be used to detect ventricular wall motion abnormalities and determine ventricular ejection fraction.

Using serial cardiac isozyme studies may be helpful in making the diagnosis of contusion, but there are questions about the value of enzyme use.[39] For example, the myocardial band of creatine kinase (CK-MB) may be elevated, but false-positive results are often seen in trauma patients.[40] Increases in serum levels of CK-MB also occur in patients with chronic renal failure or skeletal muscle damage.[41] Elevations in CK-MB have been shown to correlate poorly with the extent of myocardial injury. Serum levels of greater that 4% to 6% may be indicative of damage.[42]

Measurement of levels of cardiac troponin I (cTnI) may be more useful because levels correlate more closely with myocardial contusion than do CK-MB.[43] cTnI is a specific biochemical marker of myocardial injury. Measures of this marker may help to indicate myocardial contusion because serum levels are not increased in patients with severe acute or chronic skeletal muscle injury. The normal level for cTnI is 0.03-0.14 ng/ml; levels of greater than 0.15 ng/ml indicate cardiac injury.[42]

Treatment of myocardial contusion involves treatment of symptoms. Long-term sequelae of myocardial contusion in children are unknown. Aneurysm, myocardial rupture, and postcontusion pericarditis have been reported in adults.

Aortic Rupture. Aortic rupture, although rare in the pediatric population, can occur secondary to blunt trauma. Common sites of injury are the descending aorta distal to the level of the ligamentum arteriosum, which is associated with horizontal deceleration injuries; and disruption of the ascending aorta, secondary to vertical deceleration injuries.[44]

Injuries may vary from a small tear in the intimal lining to complete transection. Signs and symptoms of injury will range from no external sign of injury to cardiopulmonary arrest. Discrepancies between pulse in the upper and lower extremities and between blood pressure in the limbs are suggestive of aortic trauma.

Interventions for the patient with aortic injury include assisting with diagnostic procedures such as an aortogram. Fluid resuscitation is started immediately, and the patient is prepared for immediate thoracotomy.

Diaphragmatic Rupture. Rupture of the diaphragm occurs most commonly following blunt trauma in which there is a sudden increase in intraabdominal or intrathoracic pressure against a fixed diaphragm. The left hemidiaphragm is most commonly injured. The diagnosis is often missed when the child is asymptomatic.

The most common presenting symptoms are chest pain and shortness of breath. Unilateral diaphragm dysfunction accompanied by herniation of intraabdominal contents into the chest cavity causes these symptoms. Physical examination may reveal decreased breath sounds or auscultation of bowel sounds over the affected lung. The mediastinum may shift to the contralateral side and the abdomen will appear scaphoid in the infant and young child. Chest roentgenogram may reveal diaphragmatic displacement, loops of bowel in the thorax, or the presence of a nasogastric tube in the thoracic cavity (Fig. 28-16). Surgical repair of the diaphragmatic tear is required.

Tracheobronchial Injury. Tracheobronchial tree injury is rare in the child because of the elasticity of the thorax and the mobility of the mediastinum. Blunt tracheobronchial injury can result from a variety of forces, including shearing, compression, and vertical stretch. Injuries most commonly occur at the take-off point of a mainstem or upper lobe bronchus.

Signs of a tracheobronchial disruption include mediastinal or subcutaneous emphysema, hemoptysis, airway obstruction, pneumothorax with persistent airleak, and massive atelectasis refractory to treatment. Bronchoscopy is the most reliable means of diagnosing the site and extent of injury. Treatment is variable, depending on the thoracic injury, tolerance of the child, and associated lesions. Surgical repair of the lesion may be indicated; however,

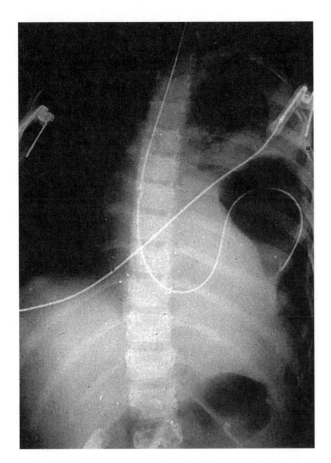

Fig. 28-16 X-ray film positive for diaphragmatic hernia.

conservative treatment by thoracic drainage or lesion intubation has been effective.[45]

Critical Care Management. Critical care management of the child with thoracic trauma is injury specific. Chapters 7, 8, 18, and 19 provide information about assessment and management of children who develop the final common pathways of respiratory failure and low cardiac output.

Abdominal Injury

Etiology/Incidence. Abdominal injuries in children are not common; however, the failure to promptly diagnose these injuries and successfully manage them accounts for increased mortality and morbidity. Usually, serious injury to the head or limbs is obvious, whereas serious abdominal injury tends to be subtle.

Features of a child's physical maturity may place the youngster at increased risk for injury. For a number of reasons, the abdomen of a child is at greater risk for injury than an adult's abdomen. The smaller size of the abdomen predisposes the child to multiple rather than single injuries because energy from the impacting force is dissipated. The large solid organs, which are most often injured, are covered with only a very flexible rib cage and a less developed abdominal musculature, which provide little protection.[46]

Abdominal trauma continues to be the leading cause of morbidity and mortality in children, with blunt trauma accounting for the majority of injuries. Examples of mechanisms that result in intraabdominal injury include falls, pedestrian accidents, bicycle accidents, and motor vehicle crashes.[47] The mechanism of injury is similar in these examples and results in blunt trauma, better defined as injury occurring when kinetic energy is transferred to the intraabdominal organs through the abdominal wall.

Penetrating injuries are often caused by gunshot, stabbings, or impalement on an object. These mechanisms may cause injury to any or all of the abdominal organs and vessels. Hollow viscus injuries are more common with penetrating trauma.[4]

Pathogenesis. The pathogenesis of abdominal trauma is related to the specific abdominal organ injured. The most frequent final common pathway is severe bleeding.

Spleen. The spleen is the most commonly injured abdominal organ in childhood. Splenic injury usually follows blunt trauma to the upper abdomen or lower thorax. Recent advances in understanding splenic function have revolutionized the treatment of splenic injuries; pediatric surgeons in particular have championed nonoperative management of this injury type.[48]

The spleen is located in the left hypochondrium, where in older children and adolescents, the lower rib cage covers the spleen entirely. In infants and small children, the rib cage does not extend down far enough and is also more pliable than the ossified adult rib cage. Therefore the pediatric spleen is not adequately protected by the rib cage.

The child with a splenic injury usually receives a blow to the left upper quadrant with or without an associated rib fracture. The child often experiences pain in the left shoulder, in the left upper quadrant, or in the left part of the chest with breathing. Bruising, abrasions, nausea, and vomiting may be present. Heart rate and blood pressure may be normal, or mild tachycardia and hypotension may occur. A mass may be palpable in the left upper quadrant. The child may have a positive Kehr sign (pain in the left shoulder), Turner sign (ecchymosis in the left flank), and/or Cullen sign (ecchymosis around the umbilicus). Ecchymosis in the left upper quadrant or left flank is a strong indication of injury.[48]

Laboratory analysis is often normal in a child with splenic injury, but if abnormalities are seen, they are usually a decreased hematocrit and leukocytosis in the 20,000 to 30,000 mm^3 range. Both chest and abdominal x-ray films may be suggestive of splenic trauma; Box 28-2 presents these findings. An abdominal x-ray film alone will not confirm the diagnosis of splenic trauma. It will, however, provide evidence to confirm the clinical findings. CT is used to evaluate splenic injuries. CT is also used to increase the use of nonoperative management of splenic injuries and splenic salvage.[49]

Treatment is aimed toward splenic preservation. The spleen has three main functions: clearance and phagocytosis of particulate matter from the blood, antibody formation, and hematopoiesis. It performs these functions through a

Box 28-2
X-ray Examination Findings Suggestive of Splenic Injury

Chest X-ray Findings

Lower left rib fractures
Elevation of the left hemidiaphragm
Pleural effusion

Abdominal X-Ray Findings

Raised left hemidiaphragm
Stomach dilation or medial displacement
Opacification of the left hypochondrium
Downward displacement of the transverse colon
Fluid between coils of intestines

From Scorpio RJ, Wesson DE: Splenic trauma. In Eichelberger MR, ed: *Pediatric trauma: prevention, acute care, rehabilitation,* St Louis, 1993, Mosby.

TABLE 28-3   Spleen Injury Scale

Grade	Injury Description
I	
Hematoma	Subcapsular, nonexpanding, <10% surface area
Laceration	Capsular tear, nonbleeding, <1 cm parenchymal tear
II	
Hematoma	Subcapsular, 10%-50% surface area, intraparenchymal, nonexpanding, <5 cm diameter
Laceration	Capsular tear, 1-3 cm parenchymal depth, does not involve a trabecular vessel
III	
Hematoma	Subcapsular, >50% surface area or expanding; ruptured subcapsular or parenchymal hematoma; intraparenchymal hematoma >5 cm or expanding
Laceration	>3 cm parenchymal depth or involving trabecular vessels
IV	
Hematoma	Ruptured intraparenchymal hematoma with active bleeding
Laceration	Laceration involving segmental or hilar vessels producing major devascularization (>25% of spleen)
V	
Laceration	Completely shattered spleen
Vascular	Hilar vascular injury that devascularizes spleen

From Lynch JM, Meza MP, Newman B et al: Computed tomography grade of splenic injury is predictive of the time required for radiographic healing, *J Pediatr Surg* 32:1093-1096.

combination of specific microanatomy and a high rate of blood flow. Originally thought to be expendable, it is now realized that the spleen plays a critical role in combating infection. Appreciation of the increased risk of overwhelming postsplenectomy sepsis in children has led to a heightened awareness of the importance of splenic preservation, especially in the pediatric age group. Currently, postsplenectomy sepsis is a well-recognized syndrome that can occur days to years following removal of the spleen.

More specifically, the spleen is recognized as a source of antibodies against *Haemophilus influenzae,* pneumococcus, and meningococcus. Preservation of even a portion of the spleen provides some protection against postsplenectomy infection. As a result, strategies for splenic conservation have been developed and splenorrhaphy, which refers to suturing of the spleen, is often performed when operative management is necessary.[48]

The spleen may be preserved by nonoperative means as well; in fact, most children with splenic trauma can be treated this way. Nonoperative management is recommended for the child who maintains stable vital signs, requires less than one-half blood volume replacement, and is free of other abdominal injuries that require surgery.[49] If the child is monitored nonoperatively, close monitoring in the intensive care unit is required for at least 24 hours. Vital signs are assessed frequently, and hematocrit and hemoglobin are measured at least daily. Strict bedrest is maintained until there have been no requirements for blood for 48 hours. At this point, ambulation can occur and the child can be discharged home. Discharge is determined by the severity of injury based on the splenic injury scale. Complications of nonoperative management are primarily associated with rebleeding. This complication is indicated by unstable vital signs, decreasing hematocrit and hemoglobin, and worsening findings on abdominal examination.

After discharge, the child may return to school but should refrain from vigorous activities for a period of time, depending on the severity of the splenic injury. A case report

recently described a boy who experienced splenic trauma, which was managed nonoperatively. Thirty-eight days postinjury, he experienced splenic rupture after low intensity swimming and one dive from the side of the pool.[50] Lynch and colleagues determined that the time to radiographic healing is directly proportional to the severity of splenic injury, based on the Spleen Injury Scale (Table 28-3).[51] Based on Lynch's work, the mean time to radiographic healing in Grade I, II, III, and IV injuries is 3.1, 8.2, 12.1, and 20.7 weeks, respectively.

If the child requires operative management and splenic preservation is not possible, a splenectomy is required. Standard principles of postoperative care will apply; however, because these children are at risk for overwhelming postsplenectomy infection (OPSI), protection from infection is critical. This is accomplished through vaccination and prophylactic antibiotics. Vaccines available are those against pneumococcus, *H. influenzae* type B (HIB), and *Neisseria meningitidis.* The use of the pneumococcal and HIB vaccines is strongly recommended. These vaccines are administered in the postoperative period.

Even with vaccines, antibiotic prophylaxis is suggested, especially in infants and young children. Penicillin prophylaxis is recommended to continue until adolescence. Amoxicillin is advocated by some instead of penicillin because it is effective against HIB. Erythromycin may be used as an alternative to penicillin for children with a penicillin allergy.[48]

Not surprisingly, patient compliance with antibiotic regimen prophylaxis is poor. In addition, infections can still occur. Therefore it is critical that parent teaching include recognition of signs of infection and prompt medical attention for initiation of antibiotics.

Liver.   Liver injuries are a major cause of death in children with blunt trauma. Severe liver injuries are associated with significant blood loss, and exsanguination is the most common cause of death. A shearing force results from sudden deceleration and consequently, the pattern of injury in the liver parenchyma can vary widely and be very diffuse. Right lobe injury is more prevalent than left; fortunately, the majority of right-sided injuries are superficial and simple. In contrast, left-sided injuries tend to be deeper and more complex.[52]

Children with liver injuries experience pain in the right upper shoulder or right upper quadrant tenderness. They may also have bruising, seatbelt markings, and abrasions. Hypotension may be present if major bleeding is occurring. Fractured ribs are a common concomitant finding.

Initial laboratory tests include a complete blood count (CBC), urinalysis, aspartate aminotransferase (AST), alanine aminotransferase (ALT), and amylase. Elevations in AST and ALT appear to correlate with hepatic injury.[52]

Management of children with hepatic injuries is similar to the treatment for splenic injuries. Nonoperative management for the hemodynamically stable child is the treatment of choice. Nonoperative management, however, mandates that the child be followed closely in the intensive care unit with frequent monitoring of blood work. Hematocrit levels are assessed every 4 hours or more often, if indicated by clinical condition. Once the liver transaminase normalizes, the child can ambulate; however, activity is restricted until complete healing has occurred. Delayed bleeding has been reported to occur as late as 1 month after injury.[52]

Operative management is indicated if the child exhibits hemodynamic instability, transfusion requirements of greater than 33% to 50% of the circulating blood volume in 24 hours, signs of peritoneal irritation, or a pneumoperitoneum or other abdominal injuries that require surgical repair.[52,53] In the case of a severely injured liver, such as a lobar fracture, the initial management is to control the massive bleeding. Hemodynamic instability, defined by the need for a blood transfusion in excess of 25 ml/kg within the first 2 hours, is a strong indicator of major hepatic vascular injury which is associated with a high mortality rate.[53] If liver resection is required, it also carries a high mortality rate.[52]

Pancreas.   Pancreatic injury is relatively uncommon in children. Because of its relative protection in the retroperitoneum, occurrence of injury is documented in only 3% to

---

Box 28-3	
Classification of Pancreatic Injury	
Class I	Contusion or laceration without duct injury
Class II	Ductal transection or parenchymal injury with probable duct injury
Class III	Proximal transection or parenchymal injury with probable duct injury
Class IV	Combined pancreatic and duodenal injury

From Jobst MA, Canty TG, Lynch FP: Management of pancreatic injury in pediatric blunt abdominal trauma, *J Pediatr Surg* 34:818-823, 1999.

12% of all cases of severe abdominal trauma. The diagnosis of pancreatic injury, short of intraoperative inspection, is often difficult and given the current preference of nonoperative management of most pediatric abdominal injuries, delays are common.[54] Traumatic pancreatitis commonly results from blunt trauma compressing the pancreas over the body of the vertebral column, causing contusion and/or parenchymal disruption with or without ductal disruption (Box 28-3). Because of the retroperitoneal location of the pancreas, associated injuries involving the duodenum, stomach, extrahepatic biliary system, and the spleen are common. Injury resulting from pancreatic trauma is usually devastating because of extensive bleeding and tissue damage from pancreatic and biliary secretions.

Children who have experienced pancreatic trauma usually have diffuse abdominal tenderness, abdominal pain, vomiting, and findings of associated injuries. Hemodynamic instability may be present, resulting from massive retroperitoneal bleeding or massive sequestration of third space fluid losses.

Although serum amylase level remains one of the most useful indicators in detecting pancreatic injury, elevated levels also occur with other diagnoses or injuries such as appendicitis, bowel perforation, mesenteric thrombosis, and salivary gland trauma. In addition, initial serum amylase levels do not correlate with the severity of pancreatic injury.[55] An important consideration is the trend of amylase elevations. Although a single elevated level may not be indicative of pancreatic injury, a trend of increasing levels may be. Also, a high level followed by decreasing levels may indicate pancreatic contusion without ductal injury.[56] Other diagnostic methods, including serum lipase levels, CT scan, and ultrasound, are limited by low sensitivity and specificity for acute injury when performed as part of the initial evaluation.[54]

The preferred treatment of traumatic pancreatitis is nonoperative, if there is no evidence of ductal disruption. The use of nasogastric suction to rest the gastrointestinal (GI) system is a major treatment modality. Also, total parenteral nutrition is important and is continued for at least 3 weeks to allow for bowel rest. In addition, serial physical examinations are important and the child is monitored for signs of infection. Complications include the development of pancreatic fistulas and pseudocyst formation.

Operative management is indicated for patients who have pain, fever, ileus, or elevated serum amylase levels that persist or develop. Also, external drainage or partial or total pancreatectomy may be performed for children who have findings of traumatic pancreatitis at the time of operative exploration for other intraabdominal injuries.

Gastric and Intestinal Injury. Hollow visceral injury is uncommon and occurs in less than 2% of the children evaluated for blunt abdominal trauma.[57] In recent years, however, the incidence is increasing as a result of improved recognition and societal influences such as urban violence and child abuse. Also, the widespread availability of guns has led to an increase in penetrating injury, which most commonly affects the hollow visceral organs.[58]

Hollow viscus injuries are difficult to diagnose. The only early sign of this type of injury may be a subtle degree of abdominal tenderness. Specific solid-organ injuries are useful indicators for hollow viscus injuries. Injury to the pancreas is associated with hollow viscus injury because the C-loop of the duodenum encircles the head of the pancreas and is at high risk when the pancreas is injured.[59]

Abrasions or contusions in the upper abdomen should raise the index of suspicion for stomach injury. Bloody gastric drainage, tympanic sounds when percussion is performed over the liver, detection of free air, and a nasogastric tube in abnormal position on an x-ray film are all indicative of stomach injury. If the stomach perforates, the child develops a board-like abdomen with intense pain. Peritonitis develops within hours, and surgery is always required.

The small intestine can be ruptured by even mild abdominal trauma. Perforation of the small intestine may result from compression, such as that which occurs with lap belts. The child with ruptured intestines may have minimal symptoms, yet frank peritonitis is inevitable. Surgical repair is always required. Perforation of the small bowel has low mortality and complication rates if surgery takes place within 24 hours of injury.[60]

The colon and rectum are rarely injured, and when they are, injury is usually due to penetrating trauma.[61] The child presents with signs of free air or peritonitis on x-ray films. Surgical repair is necessary.

Critical Care Management. Assessment of the child with a suspected intraabdominal injury includes a careful history of the incident including mechanism of injury, consideration of the child's subjective complaints, and meticulous physical examination. In addition, appropriate and accurate diagnostic evaluations are essential. Caring for a child with an intraabdominal injury necessitates a multidisciplinary approach. Essential team members include, but are not limited to, surgeons, intensivists, pediatric nurses, and radiographic specialists.[62]

Evaluation of children with blunt abdominal trauma continues to present a significant challenge. Physical examination alone does not allow for enough sensitivity for accurate diagnosis; thus clinicians need to rely on more objective diagnostic methods for a more thorough assessment. With respect to penetrating trauma, however, this is rarely an issue because exploratory laparotomy is indicated in nearly all cases.[63]

TABLE 28-4 Peritoneal Lavage Results

	Result	Indication
Aspirate	Gross blood >20 ml	Positive
	Pink fluid	Intermediate*
	Clean	Negative
Lavage fluid	Bloody	Positive
	Clear	Negative
RBC	>100,000 cells/mm^3	Positive
	50,000-100,000 cells/mm^3	Intermediate*
WBC	>500 cells/mm^3	Positive
	100-500 cells/mm^3	Intermediate*
Amylase	>175 U/dl	Positive
	75-175 U/dl	Intermediate*
	<75 U/dl	Negative
Bacteria	Present	Positive
Fecal material	Present	Positive
Bile	Present	Positive
Food particles	Present	Positive

From Mason PJB: Abdominal injuries. In Cardona VD, Hurn PD, Mason PJB et al, eds: *Trauma nursing: from resuscitation through rehabilitation,* ed 2, Philadelphia, 1994, WB Saunders.
*Intermediate lavage results require further observation of the patient, possible repeat lavage, and interventions based on clinical presentation.

Historically, diagnostic peritoneal lavage (DPL) and CT have been considered the standard methods for evaluating blunt abdominal trauma. DPL is helpful for deciding if laparotomy is indicated in hemodynamically unstable patients (Table 28-4). CT provides more precise information about the severity of injuries if the patient can tolerate the scanning procedure. More recently another diagnostic tool, ultrasonography (US), has been used for evaluating blunt abdominal trauma. US has been used in Europe and Japan since the 1980s, and its usefulness has recently been acknowledged in the United States.[64] The decision as to which diagnostic method to apply, however, is often controversial.

Advocates of US propose that it is a quick and efficient method for evaluating patients who have sustained blunt abdominal trauma. US can be performed simultaneously with ongoing resuscitation measures in the emergency department, thus eliminating the need to transport the child to radiology. It is also safe, inexpensive, and noninvasive and can easily be repeated. US involves no radiation or contrast use and causes minimal discomfort. It is also the method of choice for patients with clotting disorders or adolescents who may be pregnant. Ultrasound waves are transmitted well in abdominal organs, soft tissue, and fluids, such as urine, bile, blood ascites, and pleural fluid; they are not transmitted in air-containing organs such as the lungs and the GI tract. Direct localization and grading of the organ injury by US is not possible in most cases and time should not be spent attempting to quantify the severity of the lesion. The goal is to demonstrate the presence of a significant hemoperitoneum in an unstable patient, which establishes the need for immediate laparotomy.[63]

Despite enthusiastic support for US as a diagnostic tool for evaluating blunt abdominal trauma, many clinicians recommend a cautious approach when considering its use. Although abdominal US can be a very powerful tool to rapidly triage a sick and unstable child in the emergency department, it can also have a high false-negative rate; thus many clinicians strongly advise against relying solely on abdominal US for definitive management.[65] US is a valuable screening method to determine the need for further diagnostic testing; however, it is often believed that it should not replace DPL or CT in the evaluation of intraabdominal injury.

The management of blunt abdominal trauma in children has changed significantly in the past decade as a result of advances in diagnostic imaging and an improved understanding of the healing processes in the spleen and liver. In the past, mandatory laparotomy was the accepted mode of treatment for proven or suspected hemoperitoneum. Such treatment modalities have been replaced with intensive observation of patients able to be stabilized with supportive therapy. Numerous pediatric centers throughout the country have experienced very high success rates with nonoperative management of blunt abdominal trauma. As a result, a concomitant reduction in morbidity and mortality has occurred.[66] In addition, nonoperative management has been shown to decrease risks associated with blood transfusions and the length of hospital stay.[67]

Although nonoperative management of abdominal injuries is the most frequent and preferred treatment of choice, it is essential to clarify that "nonoperative" is not synonymous with "nonsurgical." Expert surgical consultation is required in all but the most trivial of abdominal injuries. If nonoperative management is to be successful, meticulous observation in an intensive care setting is essential.

Immediate treatment focuses on cardiopulmonary stabilization, if appropriate. If the child is hemodynamically unstable, an intravenous line is placed, ideally above the diaphragm in case of rupture of the hepatic vein and the inferior vena cava. Resuscitation fluids are administered. If the child is managed nonoperatively, close monitoring of vital signs (especially trends) and appropriate serum levels is mandatory. Indications for laparotomy include massive bleeding, unstable vital signs in spite of aggressive fluid resuscitation, requirements for more than one half of the child's circulating blood volume for replacement, severe abdominal distension associated with hypotension, penetrating injuries, and some blunt injuries.

Penetrating wounds of the abdomen require surgical intervention. Penetrating injuries often result in bleeding or perforation of the hollow viscera; therefore peritoneal irritation or hemorrhagic shock appears early. If signs are not evident, significant injury may still exist and surgical exploration is still indicated. Penetrating wounds may result in evisceration of the abdominal contents. The organs are not replaced into the abdomen and are not allowed to kink or twist. The abdominal organs are covered with moist, sterile dressings until surgical repair can take place.[4]

Genitourinary Injuries

Etiology/Incidence. Genitourinary injuries occur often in children, with 90% the result of blunt abdominal trauma. Trauma to the genitourinary tract is strongly suspected in the patient with multiple injuries, because symptoms may be obscured by concomitant injuries.

Unique anatomic features of the child's genitourinary system allow for an increased risk of renal and bladder injury. A child's bladder lies higher in the abdomen, as compared with an adult's bladder that rests in the pelvic region; weaker abdominal muscles in the child are thus less protective of the bladder. In addition, underdeveloped abdominal musculature along with decreased perirenal fat offers less protection to the kidney. The kidney is proportionately larger in relation to the rest of the body. Also, the kidney may retain fetal lobulations, which allows for easier parenchymal disruption because these lobulations are less resistant to blunt forces.[68]

Children with congenital renal abnormality are more vulnerable to injury from blunt trauma than other children. The hydronephrotic, ectopic, or diseased kidney is prone to injury from even minor trauma. The incidence of renal injury in children who have a preexisting anomaly or disease is between 5% and 21%.[69]

Pathogenesis. Approximately 80% of genitourinary injuries result from blunt trauma and the remaining 20% from penetrating trauma. The mechanism of renal injury as a result of blunt abdominal trauma may be direct or indirect. With a direct injury, the kidney is crushed against adjacent viscera, ribs, spinal column, or abdominal wall. An indirect injury, or decelerating injury, primarily causes contusion or laceration. Renal injuries as a result of indirect mechanisms are difficult to detect, and only an accurate description of the injury will lead to the correct diagnosis.

A variety of classifications of renal injuries are described in the literature—some in terms of minor and major; others in terms of degree of contusions, lacerations, and tears. A classification of renal injuries is presented in Fig. 28-17.

A child who has sustained blunt trauma may be asymptomatic or complain of abdominal or flank pain. Hematuria, which is the hallmark sign of renal injury, may occur in 90% of cases, yet there is no correlation between the magnitude of injury and the degree of hematuria. Also, the absence of hematuria does not exclude the possibility of renal injury if there are other findings that strongly suggest it. Plain abdominal x-ray films are rarely helpful; up to 85% are normal in spite of proven kidney injury. Instead, the excretory urogram (IVP) is the standard for diagnosis of renal injury. However, hypotension with low perfusion can cause poor upper urinary tract visualization and may make the IVP a limited imaging technique.

US provides anatomic, not functional, information. Ease of use because of its portability and absence of radiation make it a helpful tool with respect to locating a kidney if it is not visualized with IVP. Doppler-enhanced US may provide information on renal perfusion and verify the integrity of the vascular pedicle of the kidney. CT continues to be the standard imaging study for acute renal trauma in children, primarily because there is more accurate display of

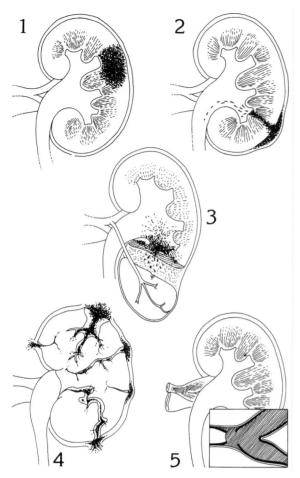

Fig. 28-17 Composite of the five classes of blunt renal injury: *1,* contusion; *2,* laceration; *3,* transection; *4,* fragmentation; *5,* pedicle injury. (From Hensle TW, Dillon P: Renal injuries. In Touloukian RJ, ed: *Pediatric trauma,* ed 2, St Louis, 1990, Mosby.)

renal injury and better visualization of nonvascularized areas of renal tissue.[69]

Although significant controversy exists with regard to the management of renal trauma, the ultimate goals are to prevent mortality, reduce immediate and long-term morbidity, and preserve as much functioning renal parenchyma as possible.[70] Considering that patients with renal trauma often have associated injuries, the immediate management of the patient is determined more by the patient's general clinical state than by the renal injuries. Renal injuries, in and of themselves, are rarely life threatening; hypovolemic shock in patients with renal injury is nearly always due to associated trauma.

The management of blunt kidney injury in children is dependent on the stability of the child and the extent of the injury. Approximately 85% to 95% of renal injuries are best managed nonoperatively.[71] Injuries in this category include contusions and simple lacerations. Successful results can be anticipated with nonoperative management if the child is maintained on bed rest with monitoring of laboratory studies, vital signs, and urinary status. The remaining 5% to

15% of clinically stable patients with major renal trauma elicit controversial opinions with regard to operative versus nonoperative treatment. Some centers advocate routine exploration and repair of such injuries, whereas others advocate conservative management. There is less controversy concerning management of penetrating trauma than there is about management of blunt renal trauma. Most penetrating renal injuries require surgical exploration during laparotomy for associated intraabdominal injury. A minor renal stab wound without associated intraabdominal injury may be observed in a child with stable vital signs and with radiographic evidence of parenchymal function. In contrast, gunshot wounds almost always require surgical exploration.[69]

The incidence of ureteral trauma in children is low but is suspected after severe blunt trauma or penetrating injury to the abdomen. When ureteral injury does occur, the most common is the separation of the ureter at its junction with the renal pelvis. This may occur as a result of a sudden extreme flexion of the trunk that stretches the ureter. This injury is more likely in children because of their hyperextensible and hypermobile spine.[72]

Attention to the description of injury is essential for a correct diagnosis. IVP is the best screening test for ureteral injury; it will be manifested as urinary extravasation or a decrease in collecting system visualization or both. Operative repair is required for such injuries, and recovery is usually without sequelae if the injury is recognized early and treated appropriately.[72]

In the child, the bladder is considered an abdominal organ and therefore vulnerable to external trauma. As the bony pelvis grows, the bladder eventually becomes a pelvic organ and more protected from injury. Although penetrating trauma to the bladder, such as from a gunshot or stab wound, can occur, blunt trauma to the abdomen is the more common cause of injury. Blunt injury most commonly results from motor vehicle accidents, falls, crushing injuries, or blows to the abdomen.[72] Bladder rupture is most often defined as extraperitoneal or intraperitoneal. Intraperitoneal rupture of the bladder occurs following a sudden rise in the intravesical pressure resulting from a blow to the pelvis or lower abdomen (seat belt injury). The increased pressure ruptures the dome of the bladder, which is the weakest and most mobile part of the organ. Treatment of intraperitoneal rupture requires surgical intervention because continued intraperitoneal spillage of urine leads to metabolic derangements, such azotemia and acid-base disorders, which potentially lead to death of the child.[72]

Extraperitoneal bladder ruptures are seen almost exclusively in association with pelvic fractures. The bladder is usually sheared on its anterior lateral wall, near the bladder base. Treatment of extraperitoneal bladder rupture is best accomplished through a selective approach. The extent of the injury and the sex of the child are important considerations when formulating a treatment plan. With the exception of large or complicated extraperitoneal rupture, bladder catheter drainage permits complete healing in most cases. This approach is advantageous because it does not convert a closed pelvic fracture to an open one. If the suspected injury is due to penetrating bone fragments, surgical exploration to remove or reduce the bone fragments is preferable in order to prevent persistent leakage and sepsis.[69]

Urethral injuries in the female are rare because of a short urethra. Urethral injuries are seen most often in males because the male's urethra is longer and less well protected. In males, urethral injuries are generally divided into two types: posterior and anterior. Posterior injuries include those of the prostatic and membranous urethra, above and including the urogenital diaphragm; anterior injuries include those of the bulbous and penile, or pendulous, urethra below the urogenital diaphragm. Almost all injuries of the posterior urethra in males occur in conjunction with fracture of the bony pelvis. Most of these injuries are due to motor vehicle accidents involving automobiles, motorcycles, or pedestrians. Shearing forces of the bony disruption cause urethral injury. Most injuries of the anterior urethra are due to blunt trauma to the perineum. The bulbous urethra is crushed against the pelvic arch as the patient falls astride an object. Common mechanisms of injury include straddling a fence, having a foot slip from the rung of a ladder, or hitting a bump in the road while riding a bicycle and coming down hard on the seat or the crossbar.[72]

Management of urethral injuries is individualized depending on the severity and extent of injury. Minor and incomplete anterior injuries may be able to be managed with temporary suprapubic diversion; more severe anterior injury may require diversion and staged urethroplasty. A common complication of this type of injury is stricture formation. Posterior injury, usually caused by pelvic fracture, is more difficult to manage. Most clinicians agree that posterior urethral tears require suprapubic diversion and delay of treatment of any resultant stricture. Although some clinicians favor early operative intervention, many advocate treatment delay because complications such as stricture, incontinence, and impotence are infrequent.[69]

Injuries to the male genitalia may be the result of blunt trauma or penetrating injury. Examples of blunt trauma include falls or kicks, whereas penetrating injuries may be due to falls onto sharp objects such as glass, fences, sticks, and so on. Injury to the penis may be caused by a falling toilet seat in a child being toilet trained; zipper injuries are also common, particularly in uncircumcised males who catch the redundant foreskin in the zipper of their pants. Testicular trauma in males can also occur during sporting events if the child is hit or kicked in the scrotum. Management of such injuries depends on the type and severity of the injury.

Perineal injuries of young females may occur as a result of falls on sharp or blunt objects or straddle injuries. It is important to pay careful attention to the history; if it is not consistent with the type and degree of injury, sexual abuse is suspected. In any injury to the female vulva or vagina, urethral or rectal injuries are also considered. Management of the injury will depend on the extent and severity of the injury.

Critical Care Management. The abdomen and flank are examined carefully to detect the presence of pain,

masses, abrasions, contusions, or flank ecchymosis (Grey Turner's sign), all of which may suggest retroperitoneal bleeding. Considering that genitourinary injuries are rarely life threatening, knowledge about the location, type, and extent of injury is necessary as a guide to determine appropriate treatment. A detailed history and physical examination are critical. Details of the method of injury are elicited from the patient, family, or others who may have been present. Signs and symptoms of genitourinary trauma will vary depending on severity, location, presence of associated injuries, and the child's general condition. Urinalysis is performed early in the evaluation of every child who suffers significant trauma.

Some form of radiographic investigation is necessary to exclude injury to the urinary tract if a child presents with hematuria, a history of a deceleration injury, or abdominal trauma. The specific imaging method may vary depending on the clinical status of the patient, the capability of the institution, and practitioner preference. Radiographic imaging may include IVP, renal scan, cystogram, US, CT scan, and renal angiography. The type and role of radiographic evaluation is a controversial subject. In the past, IVP was recommended for all patients with hematuria; currently, many practitioners are reluctant to expose all children to a potentially serious reaction to contrast medium, and unnecessary radiation and expense. Instead, they recommend that IVP be used in children with physical findings of renal injury, evidence of significant blood loss or hematuria, or when renal artery injury is suspected. CT scans have become more widely used and are often the procedure of choice for many practitioners. The major benefit of CT scan is that all organs in the upper abdominal and retroperitoneal areas can be simultaneously evaluated.[72]

The management of genitourinary injury is primarily nonoperative and is aimed at prevention of complications and maintenance of function.[69] Management involves close monitoring for signs of complications and progress of healing.

Orthopedic Injury

Etiology/Incidence. Musculoskeletal trauma is common in children; it occurs in approximately 20% of all trauma sustained by children.[73] Skull and clavicle fractures are most common at birth; however, during the first year of life, fractures are rare. Fractures that occur during the first 2 years of life may be an indication of skeletal problems, bone disease, or child abuse. In children 2 years of age through adolescence, fractures of the upper extremity occur more often than fractures of the lower extremity.[73] Fractures of the femoral shaft peak during toddler and adolescent years with the primary mechanisms also being age dependent. Falls are the primary mechanism of injury for children younger than 6 years of age, motor vehicle-pedestrian incidents for children 6 to 9 years old, and motor vehicle incidents for adolescents.[74]

Motor vehicle incidents are a common cause of fractures and are associated with the more serious injuries. For example, the unrestrained child in a car can be tossed around the inside in a crash and actually ricochet off the interior structures multiple times. A child pedestrian can be thrown a long way with significant force upon impact.

Falls are another common cause of fractures. Children may fall from great heights, resulting in numerous fractures along with other injuries. Additional causes of fractures include sports-related trauma, penetrating injuries, and child abuse. With child abuse, fractures are a common manifestation, second only to skin injuries.

Children are susceptible to fractures because of the types of activities they engage in and because of their immature skeleton. Many fractures, such as hairline or greenstick fractures, are not serious, but intraarticular or epiphyseal plate fractures have serious potential for growth plate disruption.

Children have different complications from fractures than adults. Growth disturbances will follow epiphyseal plate fractures. Osteomyelitis resulting from an open fracture or an open reduction from a closed fracture tends to be more extensive in a child. This infection has the potential to damage the epiphyseal plate, resulting in growth disturbance. Volkman ischemia (resulting from vascular compromise) of the nerves and muscles, posttraumatic myositis ossificans, and refracture are more common in children.[75]

Torn ligaments and dislocation are less common in children. The ligaments are strong and resilient; in fact, the ligaments are stronger than the associated epiphyseal plates. A sudden extension on a ligament at the time of injury results in the separation of the epiphyseal plate rather than a torn ligament.

This is also true of the fibrous joint capsule. The type of injury that would produce a traumatic dislocation of the shoulder in an adult will produce a separation fracture of the proximal humeral epiphysis in a child.

Children's fractures heal more rapidly because of the osteogenic activity of the periosteum and endosteum. The osteogenic activity is very active at birth, decreases progressively throughout childhood, and remains constant from adulthood to old age.

Pathogenesis. The mechanism of bone injury involves external forces acting on the body and the bony structures (direct impact) or internal forces caused by muscle contraction or ligament stress (bending force). Bone breakage is produced by loading forces where the ability of the bone to store and dissipate energy by temporary deformation has been exceeded. Loading forces include bending, tension, compression, torsion, and combined loading. These forces can be applied along the bone's long axis or along the traverse axis. The magnitude and rate of loading will determine the extent of bone deformation.

Epiphyseal fractures are of particular concern in children. As mentioned earlier, these injuries have the potential to produce growth disturbances in children by causing progressive angular deformity and limb length discrepancies.[76] Epiphyseal fractures have been classified according to the Salter-Harris classification (Table 28-5).

Type	Description	Management	Prognosis
I	Complete epiphyseal separation without fracture; most common in younger children with thick epiphyseal plates	Closed reduction and cast immobilization	Excellent unless the blood supply to the epiphysis is compromised
II	Most common epiphyseal fracture; separation of epiphyseal plate with a fracture through the metaphysis, producing a triangular fragment	Closed reduction and cast immobilization	Excellent unless the blood supply to the epiphysis is compromised
III	Fracture through part of the epiphyseal plate and extending into the joint	Open reduction and internal fixation usually required	Good, with restoration of normal joint surface and vascularity
IV	Fracture completely through the epiphyseal plate and extending through a portion of the metaphysis	Open reduction and internal fixation	At risk for interrupted longitudinal growth unless there is perfect anatomic alignment, which must be maintained until complete healing
V	Crush injury to an area of the epiphyseal plate that is nondisplaced with no fracture line visible on roentgenography	Immobilization and non–weight bearing for a minimum of 3 weeks to prevent further compression	Poor. Injury is frequently identified only in retrospect after growth disturbance has occurred

TABLE 28-5 Salter and Harris Classification of Epiphyseal Plate Fractures

Joy C: Musculoskeletal trauma. In Joy C, ed: *Pediatric trauma nursing.* Rockville, Md, 1989, Aspen Publishers.

Types of fractures seen in children are presented in Fig. 28-18. Greenstick fractures are common in small children and are characterized by an incomplete fracture of the bone with a portion of the cortex and periosteum still intact. Transverse fractures are seen in infants and small children with the fracture line across the bone at a right angle to the longitudinal axis of the bone. Spiral fractures are caused by torsional forces, such as when the extremity rotates while the body remains in a fixed position. This injury is commonly associated with child abuse. Comminuted fractures are seen more often in older children and adolescents and are the result of a high-impact force such as a fall from a high height or a high-speed motor vehicle accident.

Pelvic fractures may occur as the result of a severe injury, such as that associated with a motor vehicle accident. The most important aspect of the fracture is not the fracture itself but associated complications such as internal bleeding from torn vessels and extravasation of urine from bladder rupture or urethral injury. Pelvic fractures are classified as stable or unstable, depending on whether the fracture interferes with the stability and integrity of the pelvic ring. Stable fractures do not transgress the pelvic ring, therefore they do not interfere with the stability of the pelvis in relation to weight bearing and do not require reduction. Unstable fractures include separation of the symphysis pubis, an opening in the pelvic ring, movement of one half of the pelvis, or a bucket handle fracture, in which the fractured half of the pelvis rolls forward and inward.[75] Usually these fractures result from a crush injury that occurs when the child is run over by a vehicle.

Transverse – Results from angulation force or direct trauma.
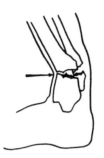

Oblique – Results from twisting force.
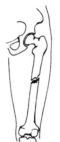

Spiral – Results from twisting force with firmly planted foot.
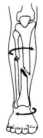

Comminuted – Results from severe direct trauma; has more than two fragments.
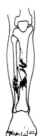

Impacted – Results from severe trauma causing fracture ends to jam together.
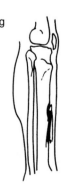

Compressed – Results from severe force to top of head or os calcis or acceleration/deceleration injury.
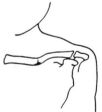

Greenstick – Results from compression force; usually occurs in children under 10 years of age.
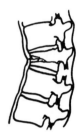

Avulsion – Results from muscle mass contracting forcefully, causing bone fragment to tear off at insertion.
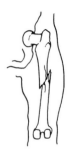

Fig. 28-18 Types of fractures. (From Budassi-Sheehy S, ed: *Manual of emergency care,* St Louis, 1990, Mosby.)

Box 28-4
**Abnormalities Associated
With Musculoskeletal Trauma**

Blood loss associated with a specific injury
Neurologic or vascular deficit distal to the injury
Visible deformity, shortening, or angulation of a limb
Partial or complete loss of a digit or limb
Increase in limb circumference that worsens
Manifestations of pelvic fracture
Crush injury
Any injury suspected of resulting in compartment syndrome
Abnormal muscle or tendon function
Point tenderness or muscle spasms
Bruising
Swelling
Crepitus
Abnormal movement between joints or a joint

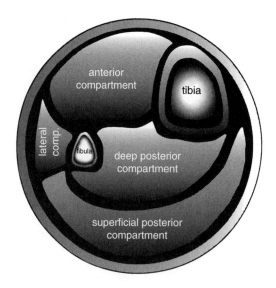

Fig. 28-19 The four compartments of the lower leg. (From Robertson WW: Crush injury and compartment syndrome. In Eichelberger MR, ed: *Pediatric trauma: prevention, acute care, rehabilitation,* St Louis, 1993, Mosby.)

Box 28-5
Components of a Neurovascular Assessment

Circulation

Color
Temperature
Capillary refill
Edema
Pulses above and below the injury

Sensation

Numbness
Tingling
Level of pain

Motion of Extremities

Coordinated
Symmetric
Strength

A serious musculoskeletal injury that may be seen is an amputation. Amputations may occur as the result of power tools, farm machinery, railroad accidents, or sharp objects. Amputations are classified as partial or complete with varying degrees of tissue and bone injury. A guillotine type of amputation involves a wound that has clean, well-defined edges, and has the best prognosis for reimplantation. A crush amputation is the separation of the body part with extensive damage to the soft tissue, bone, nerve, and blood vessels. This wound has a poor prognosis for limb salvage.

Patient Management. As with any trauma patient, the first focus is on the ABCs (airway, breathing, and circulation). A detailed musculoskeletal assessment takes place during the secondary survey. Observation along with palpation of each bone and joint will help to identify abnormalities. These abnormalities are listed in Box 28-4 and are documented once identified. Observation for spontaneous movement always takes place before manipulation of the extremity. Manipulation of the injured extremity may inflict pain and interfere with further examination.

Once the injuries are recognized, the first priority is to estimate blood loss and then follow with a neurovascular assessment. Components of the neurovascular assessment are included in Box 28-5. Extremities are compared bilaterally. Neurovascular status is monitored frequently for the first 24 hours after injury, after application of a cast or traction, after surgery, and after any treatment, including temporary splinting.

Assessment after an amputation injury also first focuses on the ABCs. Blood loss is estimated, but with a complete amputation, the severed blood vessels retract and clamp down, resulting in effective clotting and minimal bleeding.

The child with an orthopedic injury requires monitoring for the development of compartment syndrome. Compartment syndrome is progressive vascular compromise caused by an increase in pressure within an anatomic space that causes circulatory impairment and compromised tissue function within that space. Direct bleeding and inflammation may cause increased pressure within a compartment. In

addition, a decrease in the size of the compartment caused by the constriction of a splint or cast may produce compartment syndrome. This syndrome can occur anywhere in which fascia binds muscle groups however, it tends to occur most often in the four components of the lower leg (Fig. 28-19).

The manifestations of compartment syndrome are seen with the "five P's":

1. Pain, which is described as extreme, occurs out of proportion to the apparent injury. Pain may also occur with passive movement of the affected extremity.
2. Paresthesia, specifically numbness or tingling, may occur. The child may also exhibit a decreased ability

to discriminate between two points on the affected extremity.

3. Pallor is a late sign, and delayed capillary refill may be present.
4. Paralysis or a progressively weakening muscle is another late sign.
5. Pulselessness occurs only after compartment pressures are extremely high because the larger arteries remain open until then. Therefore an injured extremity with a strong pulse does not rule out compartment syndrome.

Diagnosis of compartment syndrome is based on the presence of these symptoms and on increased interstitial pressure. This pressure can be directly measured using a variety of systems that use a needle or a catheter connected to a pressure transducer and monitor. Interstitial pressures exceeding 30 to 35 mmHg are indicative of compartment syndrome.

The initial treatment of fractures involves controlling bleeding, assessing neurovascular status, and then applying splints or traction. A closed fracture will require anatomic alignment and splinting. An open fracture requires wound irrigation, debridement, fracture alignment, and stabilization in the operating room. Continuous monitoring for signs of complications, such as infection or compartment syndrome, is critical.

Amputations require special attention. Initially, if severe bleeding is occurring, direct pressure with a soft dressing is applied and the extremity is elevated. If there is minimal bleeding, a sterile dressing is applied to the stump, which is then splinted and elevated. Tourniquets and clamps are contraindicated because they may cause tissue ischemia and vessel damage. Intravenous access is obtained for fluid resuscitation and antibiotics.

The goal of care for the amputated body part is to reduce ischemia time. The body part is gently rinsed with normal saline to remove visible dirt. It is then wrapped in moist, sterile gauze, placed in a sealable plastic bag, and then put on ice for transport to the operating room or to another center. The body part is never placed directly in saline or ice because moisture absorbed by the tissue will result in swelling and necrosis.

Postoperatively, the child's neurovascular status is frequently assessed. Leech therapy alleviates venous engorgement that may compromise the graft (Chapter 16 provides information on leech therapy). Spo$_2$ monitoring of the reimplanted body part provides early information about the development of arterial compromise. Anticoagulants may be given to prevent hemostasis in the reimplanted vessels, so measures to prevent bleeding are initiated. Antibiotics are administered to prevent or treat infection. Psychosocial support is crucial, especially if the child loses the body part, to help the child and family cope with a changed body image.

Compartment syndrome requires immediate treatment if pressures exceed normal limits. The limb is placed in a neutral position because elevation results in further compromise of arterial flow. Cast or constricting bandages are opened and removed. If the symptoms and excessive pressures continue, a fasciotomy may be performed to release pressure and maintain extremity circulation. The incision will be left open for a period of time with the limb splinted in a functional position. A dressing is applied to the open wound, and, if after 24 hours the muscle is considered viable, saline dressings are applied and changed daily until the wound is closed.[77]

Pain management is an important issue for those caring for children with musculoskeletal injuries. Results of a study examining pain in children suggest that children hospitalized with orthopedic conditions experience a higher number of painful occurrences and symptoms than children hospitalized with other conditions.[78] Occurrences such as postoperative pain, pain with moving, and pain associated with traction and pins were rated as causing more pain than injections, venipuncture, and intravenous insertion. Recommended methods for pain control include oral or intravenous medication, patient-controlled analgesia, and nonpharmacologic methods.[79] Chapter 17 provides in-depth information regarding pain management.

PRIORITIES FOR MULTIPLE TRAUMA

Airway management and maintenance of adequate oxygenation is of critical importance in the child with multiple injuries. Many children with multiple trauma have an unmaintainable airway or inadequate respiratory effort. Also, shock and the child's physiologic response to trauma leads to an oxygen debt. Definitive airway control is obtained through intubation while maintaining cervical spine immobilization. Children with evidence of tension pneumothoraces or hemothoraces require emergent decompression before, or with, intubation.

Priorities in addressing circulation include controlling bleeding and stabilizing hemodynamic status. Aggressive fluid resuscitation is necessary for the hypotensive child, even in light of a potential head injury. Maintaining cerebral blood flow and oxygen delivery adequately minimizes neurologic injury. Hypotension and decreased cerebral oxygen delivery have been shown to potentiate secondary injury and worsen outcomes in head injury.[80] Fluids have been shown to reduce mortality and improve neurologic outcomes.[81]

Patients with severe thoracoabdominal injuries and concomitant head trauma provide a challenge to prioritization. Patients with severe bleeding who are unresponsive to fluid and blood administration require emergent surgical intervention. Assessment and management of chest and abdominal injuries is generally prioritized based on the assumption that correction of hemorrhagic shock is the optimal treatment for head trauma.[82]

Orthopedic injuries are of secondary importance in the resuscitation of the child with multiple injuries. However, appropriate treatment is necessary to prevent long-term disability and may be life saving. Fractures require splinting with emergent reduction if there is evidence of neurovascular compromise. Open fractures require surgical intervention, but treatment does not defer resuscitation of more serious injuries. Potentially life-threatening fractures that require urgent treatment are femur and pelvic fractures.

Delayed treatment of these injuries has been associated with poor outcomes.[83]

CHILD MALTREATMENT

History

Varying forms of child abuse have been accepted by society for many centuries. In earlier times, children who were considered undesirable for religious or economic reasons or because they were defective or female were often destroyed; such actions were culturally sanctioned. During the fourteenth century, unwanted children were thrown into the Thames; during the Industrial Revolution, young children were forced to work long hours in hazardous settings with unhealthy conditions.

The first legal intervention on behalf of a child occurred in 1874 in the United States. Ironically, the case was brought to court by the American Society for the Prevention of Cruelty to Animals (SPCA). The SPCA was able to demand legal protection for a child who was regularly beaten by her adoptive parents on the basis that she belonged to the Animal Kingdom. Most states did not adopt laws requiring reporting of abuse until the 1960s and 1970s. Today, all 50 states have laws requiring the reporting of child abuse. The public became more acutely aware of this concern when Dr. Henry Kempe coined the phrase "battered-child syndrome" in 1962. Despite the progress that has been made in this area, child maltreatment continues to be a serious social problem.

The Spectrum of Child Abuse

Children of any race, age, religion, sex, and socioeconomic group can be victims of child maltreatment. Compared with other medical conditions during childhood, the data indicate that more children are affected by maltreatment than all other serious illnesses combined. There are also many cases of abused and neglected children that do not come to the attention of social service agencies.[84] Over the years, the issue of child maltreatment has evolved such that it is now a multidisciplinary problem requiring contributions and interventions from medicine, nursing, public health, sociology, psychology, law, and social work. Although it is generally beneficial to have a variety of disciplines involved, this can also be a cause for concern. Efforts in problem solving may be uncoordinated, and fields that may have historically been at odds with one another need to cooperate with the common goal of preventing and eliminating child abuse.[84]

Incidence of Abuse

Almost four decades have passed since Kempe and colleagues published their landmark description of the battered child. Since that time there continue to be many challenges, including gaining an understanding of the problem and striving to develop better systems for improved reporting and more effective intervention. Despite the fact that all 50 states have laws that require the reporting of abuse, under-recognition continues to be a problem.[85] Although the true incidence of child abuse is unknown, the data indicate that the numbers have increased significantly in the last 15 years. This increase, however, is controversial as to whether the numbers represent increasing societal recognition of the problem or real changes in the rates of maltreatment.[84] Flaws in the existing data collection systems exist because every state uses its own definitions of abuse and neglect and applies its own standards of proof when substantiating whether maltreatment occurred.

A recent study examined children who were victims of abuse over a 10-year period. Children injured by child abuse compared with nonintentional injury were more likely to be younger and to have a preinjury medical history. They were more likely to be injured by battering and shaking and to sustain intracranial injury. They also were more likely to be admitted to intensive care and have a longer length of stay.[86]

Defining Child Maltreatment

Child abuse can take on many forms and is difficult to define and standardize. Physical abuse is a form that is often easy to identify and recognize; other forms such as emotional and psychologic abuse are just beginning to be acknowledged. Still other forms of abuse such as child pornography and prostitution remain difficult to identify and manage.

Unfortunately, the term *child maltreatment* is subject to a variety of interpretations and definitions. In addition to a lack of clear definitions, inadequate professional experience, and lack of training and motivation to report, disagreement exists about how responsible parents should be for the safety of their children. A general definition of child maltreatment may be described as an act that endangers a child such that substantial risk to his or her health, safety, development, or mental well-being is created. Various forms of child maltreatment exist, including physical abuse and neglect, sexual abuse, and emotional abuse and neglect.

Physical Abuse. The physical abuse of children is a concept that remains difficult to define. Although the definition depends largely on the mores and values of the times, most health care workers agree that physical abuse involves the nonaccidental injury of the child at the hands of the caregiver.[87] When making an assessment of physical injury, two elements are essential to consider. First is whether the explanation given is plausible as a means of causing the injury, and second is whether the developmental level of the child is consistent with the history.[84] Physical injuries labeled by the parents as self-inflicted accidents require certain motor skills on the part of the child; thus knowledge of child development is essential.

Physical Neglect. Identifying the scope of the problem of neglect is nearly impossible because of the inability to give clear and consistent answers to the question of what constitutes neglect of a child. Typically defined as an act of omission rather than commission, neglect may or may not be intentional. It is sometimes obvious and other times nearly invisible.[88] Although neglect can result in obvious physical signs such as malnutrition, other forms, such as

Box 28-6
Examples of Neglect

Delaying or failing to provide physical or mental health care
Inadequate supervision
Lack of protection from household/environmental hazards
Poor personal hygiene
Poor nutrition
Inappropriate substitute child care

emotional neglect, can have a destructive impact on a child's future development. Neglect may also be fatal as a result of inadequate physical protection, failure to provide the essential necessities of life, and inadequate health care (Box 28-6). A note of caution, however, is not to define as willful neglect a case in which an impoverished or uneducated family is providing, in truth, the best care possible within their means.

Sexual Abuse. Sexual abuse refers to contacts or interactions between a child and an adult when the child is being used for sexual stimulation of the perpetrator or another person. Sexual abuse may also be committed by a person under the age of 18 if that person is significantly older than the victim or when the perpetrator is in a position of power or control over the victim. Subsequent sexual activity is defined as abusive because the child does not have the cognitive ability to understand the deviance of the act nor of age to give consent. Most sexual abuse is neither disclosed immediately nor reported to authorities subsequent to disclosure. Many times victimization comes to light because of an unintentional report from the child victim, such as confiding in a friend.[89]

Sexual abuse can be assaultive or nonassaultive. Assaultive abuse produces physical injury and, often, severe emotional trauma. Nonassaultive abuse often results in little or no physical injury, yet the child who is chronically sexually misused often suffers a severe disruption in the development of his or her own sexuality. Sexual abuse is the least reported form of child abuse, particularly nonassaultive, chronic abuse.

Munchausen Syndrome by Proxy. Munchausen syndrome by proxy (MSBP) is a form of child abuse that has been recognized for approximately 20 years. The syndrome occurs when a child's parent or guardian falsifies a medical history or actually causes an illness or injury to the child in order to gain attention from hospital medical staff. The child's mother usually manifests the induction or fabrication of illness; however, fathers or other guardians may also demonstrate the behavior. Additional elements of MSBP include denial of responsibility for illness and resolution of symptoms when the child is separated from the perpetrator. Generally, clinicians regard MSBP as different from other forms of child abuse for three reasons: (1) it seems that MSBP may be symptomatic of a psychiatric disturbance in the perpetrator, (2) mortality and morbidity rates are higher, and (3) MSBP seems to be premeditated rather than motivated by acute frustration and impulsive behavior.[90] Although difficult to differentiate who has the condition,

parent or child, MSBP is a complex interaction between parent, child, and the medical establishment. The priority is to ensure the child's safety and to prevent further harm.

Histories Suggestive of Child Maltreatment

Obtaining an accurate history in cases of pediatric injury is usually challenging but even more so in the case of suspected child maltreatment. To make the correct diagnosis, nurses, physicians, and other members of the team need to be suspicious for its possible occurrence. When a clinician is concerned about the mechanism of injury, the extent of the injury, or the timing, child abuse is considered.[85] Physicians and nurses are often dependent on family members for an explanation of an injured child's condition because many children may be too frightened, too young, or too ill to give an explanation. Even when they are able to do so, many children are unwilling to accuse the adult who cares for them of abuse. Also, it is rare for an adult to spontaneously admit to inflicting injuries.

Other clues or presentations suggestive of child abuse include denial of the existence of injuries or how they occurred, an explanation inconsistent with the physical findings, and a marked delay in seeking medical attention. A history of prior trauma is important to note, and review of the medical record may reveal a pattern indicative of prior abuse. All details of the elected history are carefully evaluated in the context of their consistency or discrepancy with the physical findings.

Physical Examination

The physical examination of the battered, sexually abused, or neglected child is critical. Sometimes, physical injuries not revealed in the history may be discovered. The absence of external injury, however, does not rule out abuse. Children with significant head or abdominal trauma may not have any outward visible signs of trauma. Documentation of physical findings is an important component of the examination. Physical signs of possible abuse are listed in Box 28-7.

Radiographic Examination

Radiographic studies are invaluable in the diagnosis of intentional injuries. Skeletal surveys, CT scans, bone scans, and magnetic resonance imaging (MRI) scans are all useful. Radiographic evidence of intentional injuries is presented in Box 28-8.

Psychosocial Interventions

Maltreatment of children is a family problem. The effects reach much further than the abused child and his or her perpetrator. Issues revolve around partners or spouses who allow the abuse to occur, and many times the partners abuse one another as well. Siblings of abused children may also be abused or be witnesses to the maltreatment. Many parents were maltreated in their own childhood. Because it is a

---

Box 28-7

Physical Signs of Possible Abuse in the Child

Skin and Subcutaneous Tissue

Cradle cap, diaper rash, uncleanliness, and other evidence of unconcern or unawareness of infant needs

Cigarette burns, bite marks (human, insect, etc.; infected or not), grab marks, belt lashes (also the characteristic loop lamp cord welts)

Ecchymosis, hematomas, abrasions, and lacerations unusual for the child's developmental age

Injury to the external genitalia, anus, and rectum

Marks on the neck from strangling by hand or rope

External ears traumatized by pinching, twisting, or pulling

Unusual skin rashes that defy dermatologic diagnosis

Burns, particularly of the soles of the feet, hands, or buttocks

Skeletal System

Tenderness, swelling, and limitation of motion of an extremity

Periosteal swelling

Deformities of the long bones

Head

Cephalhematomas

Irregularities of contour resulting from skull fractures

Signs of intracranial trauma

Eyes

Subconjunctival hemorrhages

Traumatic cataracts

Retinal hemorrhages

Papilledema

Ears

Ruptured eardrums from blows to the head

Face

Periorbital ecchymosis

Displaced nasal cartilages

Bleeding from the nasal septum

Fracture of the mandible

Mouth

Lacerated frenulum of the upper lip

Loosened or missing teeth

Burns of the lips or tongues

Chest

Deformity of the chest and limitation of motion due to fracture of the ribs

Subcutaneous edema

Hemothorax

Abdomen

Signs of peritoneal irritation from ruptured organs

Abdominal masses from hematomas

Central Nervous System

Lower motor neuron paralysis from spinal cord injury

Upper motor neuron paralysis from intracranial injury

Neurologic signs varying with location and extent of the injury

From Widner-Kolberg MR: Recognizing child abuse and neglect and what to do about it. Presented at Pediatric Issues in Multisystem Trauma Conference, Walnut Creek, CA, 1991, Symposia Medicus.

Box 28-8
Radiographic Evidence of Intentional Injuries

Multiple Fractures

In different stages of healing, including:

Single blow fractures in infant

Epiphyseal separation

Spiral fracture in the young

Fractured ribs

Fractured spine*

Cortical Metaphyseal Fragmentation

"Chip" fractures or "corner spurs" partially separated from the metaphysis

Traumatic Involucrum†

Exuberant calcifying new bone formation secondary to subperiosteal forces and hematoma (grasping, shaking, and torsion forces); may produce "bucket-handle" images (extension of hematoma beyond the end of the shaft)

Skull Fracture‡

With† or without subdural hematoma

Suture Separation†

Hemorrhage* without fracture

Increasing head circumference in infant—whiplash forces from shaking alone can cause

From Widner-Kolberg MR: Recognizing child abuse and what to do about it. Presented at Pediatric Issues in Multisystem Trauma Conference, Walnut Creek, CA, 1991, Symposia Medicus.

*Cerebrospinal injury, subdural, intraventricular, and/or intracerebral hemorrhage are most serious complications and principle causes of death and permanent crippling.

†Not visible radiographically until 7 to 18 days after trauma.

‡Evident immediately after trauma.

family problem, the issue is understood, treated, and prevented in the context of families.[91]

The child victim of abuse and the family need comprehensive psychosocial intervention. This intervention is best provided by a trained mental health professional, such as a clinical nurse specialist, social worker, or psychologist who specializes in the care of child maltreatment victims. The status of the child and the parent-child relationship are assessed and treatment is based on that assessment. The approach is one of nonjudgmental support and probing for relevant information. Even though the nurse caring for the child will probably not do the in-depth psychosocial intervention, it is still essential that the parent or caretaker be treated in a nonjudgmental manner. Although difficult, partnership with the parent (should he or she be the perpetrator) is still possible so long as it is made explicit that the focus of all work is the child's welfare. Professional style is mutually respectful and as inclusive of parents as possible while still maintaining the child's safety.[92]

Considerations for the Practitioner in Suspected Child Maltreatment Cases

Reporting Child Maltreatment.   All 50 states have enacted laws requiring practitioners and other persons to report child maltreatment. Some states are more specific than others as to those who are mandated to report, but states that list these professionals usually include physicians, nurses, other medical professionals, counselors, social workers, and school personnel.[87] These laws also have a number of provisions designed to remove legal impediments to reporting. These provisions include immunity from civil and criminal liability for reporting, abolition of doctor-patient privilege in situations of suspected maltreatment, and penalties varying from nominal fines to imprisonment for failure to report.[93]

Protection for the Child.   Abused and neglected children are often too young and too frightened to seek help themselves. Because of their physical and psychologic immaturity, they are helpless against the cruelty of their caregivers. In the instance of suspected abuse, a decision is made whether it is safe to return the child to his or her home. If hospitalization is required due to a medical condition, the matter is temporarily solved. If hospitalization is not medically warranted, the practitioner, in concert with a social worker or protective services worker, makes the decision. The custody and possible placement of children during the investigative process is often controversial and

therefore entails careful scrutiny of a number of factors such as age of the child, nature of the injury, past treatment of injuries, and family characteristics. Such a decision is not made lightly because it could result in additional harm to the child, even a potentially fatal injury. Severity of abuse is not always the contributing factor to removal, instead, perceived future risk is of greater significance.[87]

Documentation.   Inadequate documentation of pediatric injuries often makes the diagnosis of child abuse difficult. Thorough, well-documented histories and complete physical examinations are essential, as well as information about the presence of witnesses to the injury. Even minor injuries require thorough evaluation and history because bruises are a common occurrence in children who have been maltreated. The inadequacy of documentation points to the need for concrete tools to improve documentation and continued education about the signs of child abuse. The abused child's hospital record is part of the substantive evidence that is used in court; thus detailed descriptions are critical. Failure to recognize and document, in accurate detail, the presence of injuries and the pattern of illnesses that are possibly related to child abuse may lead to recurrent trauma or death.[94]

SUMMARY

Pediatric trauma is a national epidemic. It is the leading killer of children between the ages of 1 and 14 years and is a major cause of disabling injuries. This is a major concern to society when one considers the tragedy to the family, in addition to the implications of the loss of work potential, the length and cost of rehabilitation, and the effects on growth and development.

Children have been shown to have a better potential for recovery than adults from traumatic injury.[7,95] Expert care can maximize this potential. Expert care includes precise assessment, formulation of diagnoses based on assessment, and collaborative interventions guided by appropriate diagnoses. Research has demonstrated the positive impact nursing care has on the trauma patient; however, more study is needed, especially in the pediatric population. Research priorities for trauma nursing have been identified.[96]

Nurses are in a key position to provide leadership in the area of pediatric injury prevention. They can educate legislators and the public about how to manage this public health epidemic. Children can be protected by further research in all areas of pediatric trauma, including trauma prevention, resuscitation, and nursing interventions to further maximize outcome.

REFERENCES

1. National Center for Health Statistic: *Healthy people 2000–review 1997.* Hyattsville, 1999, Department of Health and Human Services.
2. Quinlan KP, Brewer RD, Sleet DA et al: Characteristics of child passenger deaths and injuries involving drinking drivers, *JAMA* 283:2249-2252, 2000.
3. Scholer SJ, Hickson GB, Ray WA: Sociodemographic factors identify US infants at high risk of injury mortality, *Pediatrics* 103:1183-1188, 1999.
4. Tobias JD, Rasmussen GE, Yaster M: Multiple trauma in the pediatric patient. In Rogers MC, ed: *Textbook of pediatric intensive care,* ed 3, Baltimore, 1996, Williams & Wilkins.
5. Furnival RA, Schunk JE: ABCs of scoring systems for pediatric trauma, *Pediatr Emerg Med* 15:215-223, 1999.
6. Tepas JJ, Ramenofsky ML, Mollitt DL et al: The pediatric trauma score as a predictor of injury severity: an objective assessment, *J Trauma* 28:425-429, 1988.

7. Orliaquet GA, Meyer P, Blanot S et al: Predictive factors of outcome in severely injured children, *Anesth Analg* 87:537-542, 1998.

8. Boyd CR, Tolson MA, Copes WS: Evaluating trauma care: the TRISS method, *J Trauma* 27:370-378, 1987.

9. Castello MV, Cassano A, Gregory P et al: The pediatric risk of mortality (PRISM) score and injury severity score (ISS) for predicting resource utilization and outcome of intensive care in pediatric trauma, *Critical Care Medicine* 27:985-988, 1999.

10. Ghajar J, Hariri RJ: Management of pediatric head injury, *Pediatr Clin North Am* 39:1093-1125, 1992.

11. Mansfield RT: Head injuries in children and adults, *Critical Care Clinics* 13:611-627, 1997.

12. Kochanek PM, Clark RSB, Ruppel RA et al: Biochemical, cellular, and molecular mechanisms in the evolution of secondary damage after severe traumatic brain injury in infants and children: Lessons learned from the bedside, *Pediatr Crit Care Med* 1:4-19, 2000.

13. Adelson PD, Clyde B, Kochanek PM et al: Cerebrovascular response in infants and young children following severe traumatic brain injury: a preliminary report, *Pediatr Neurosurg* 26:200-207, 1997.

14. Vernon-Levett P: Head injuries in children, *Crit Care Nurs Clin North Am* 3:411-421, 1991.

15. Allen EM, Boyer R, Cheney WB et al: Head and spinal cord injury. In Rogers MC, ed: *Textbook of pediatric intensive care,* ed 3, Baltimore, 1996, Williams & Wilkins.

16. Walker ML, Storrs BB, Mayer TA: Head injuries. In Mayer TA, ed: *Emergency management of pediatric trauma,* Philadelphia, 1985, WB Saunders.

17. Reece RM, Sege R: Childhood head injuries: Accidental or inflicted? *Arch Pediatr Adolesc Med* 154:11-15, 2000.

18. Cantor RM, Leaming JM: Evaluation and management of pediatric major trauma, *Emerg Med Clin North Am* 16:229-256, 1998.

19. Apple DF, Anson CA, Hunter JD et al: Spinal cord injury in youth, *Clin Pediatr* 34:90-95, 1995.

20. Jarosz DA: Pediatric spinal cord injuries: a case presentation, *Crit Care Nurs Q* 22:8-13, 1999.

21. Dickman CA, Rekate HL, Sonntag VKH et al: Pediatric spinal trauma: vertebral column and spinal cord injuries in children, *Pediatr Neurosci* 15:237-256, 1989.

22. Dickman CA, Rekate HL: Spinal trauma. In Eichelberger ME, ed: *Pediatric trauma: prevention, acute care, rehabilitation,* St Louis, 1993, Mosby.

23. Godersky JC, Menezes AH: Optimal management for children with spinal cord injury, *Contemp Neurosurg* 11:1-6, 1989.

24. Pang D, Pollack IF: Spinal cord injury without radiographic abnormality in children—the SCIWORA syndrome, *J Trauma* 29:654-664, 1989.

25. Kriss VM, Kriss TC: SCIWORA (spinal cord injury without radiographic abnormality) in infants and children, *Clin Pediatr* 35:119-124, 1996.

26. Kewalramani LS, Kraus JF, Sterling HM: Acute spinal cord lesions in a pediatric population: epidemiological and clinical features, *Paraplegia* 18:206-219, 1980.

27. Lindzon RD: Spine and spinal cord trauma. In Barkin RM, Rosen P, eds: *Emergency pediatrics: a guide to ambulatory care,* ed 5, St Louis, 1999, Mosby.

28. Eichelberger MR: Trauma of the airway and thorax, *Pediatric Annals* 16:307-316, 1987.

29. Peclet M, Newman K, Eichelberger M et al: Patterns of injury in children, *J Pediatr Surg* 25:85-91, 1990.

30. Garcia VF, Gotschall CS, Eichelberger MR: Rib fractures in trauma: a marker of severe trauma, *J Trauma* 30:697-698, 1990.

31. Tyburski JG, Collinge JD, Wilson RF et al: Pulmonary contusions: quantifying lesions on chest x-ray films and factors affecting prognosis, *J Trauma* 46:833-838, 1999

32. Davis SL, Furman DF, Costarino AT: Adult respiratory distress syndrome in children: associated disease, clinical course, and predictors of death, *J Pediatr* 123:35-45, 1993.

33. McCarthy MC, Cline AL, Lemmon GW et al: Pressure control inverse ration ventilation in the treatment of adult respiratory distress syndrome in patients with blunt chest trauma, *Am Surg* 65:1027-1030, 1999.

34. Voggenreiter G, Neudeck F, Aufmkolk M et al: Intermittent prone positioning in the treatment of severe and moderate posttraumatic lung injury, *Crit Care Med* 27:2375-2382, 1999.

35. Futterman LG, Lemberg L: Commodio cortis: sudden cardiac death in athletes, *Am J Crit Care* 8:270-272, 1999.

36. Lofland GK: Thoracic trauma in children. In Ashcraft KW, ed: *Pediatric surgery,* ed 3, Philadelphia, 2000, WB Saunders.

37. Mueller-Dickinson C: Thoracic trauma in children, *Crit Care Nurs Clin North Am* 3:423, 1991.

38. Othersen HB: Cardiothoracic injuries. In Touloukian RJ, ed: *Pediatric trauma,* ed 2, St Louis, 1990, Mosby.

39. Manolis AS, Vassilikos V, Mauonis T et al: Detection of myocardial injury during radiofrequency catheter ablation by measuring serum cardiac troponin I levels: procedural correlates, *J Am Coll Cardiol* 34:1099-1105, 1999.

40. Tellelz DW, Harden WD, Takehaski M et al: Blunt cardiac injury in children, *J Pediatr Surg* 22:1123-1128, 1987.

41. Adams JE, Bodor GS, Davila-Roman VG et al: Cardiac troponin I: a marker with high specificity for cardiac injury, *Circulation* 88:101-106, 1997.

42. Nicholson JF, Pesce MA: Reference ranges for laboratory tests and procedures. In Behrman RE, Kliegman RM, Jensen HB, eds: *Nelson's textbook of pediatrics,* ed 16, Philadelphia, 2000, WB Saunders.

43. Flynn MB, Bonini S: Blunt chest trauma, *Crit Care Nurse* 19:68-77, 1997.

44. Stiles QR, Cohlemia GS, Smith JH: Management of injuries to the thoracic and abdominal aorta, *Am J Surg* 150:133, 1985.

45. Slimane MA, Becmeur F, Aubert D et al: Tracheobronchial ruptures from blunt thoracic trauma in children, *J Pediatr Surg* 34:1847-1850, 1999.

46. Horwitz JR, Andrassy RJ: Considerations unique to children. In Ford EG, Andrassy RJ, eds: *Pediatric trauma: initial assessment and management,* Philadelphia, 1994, WB Saunders.

47. Patrick DA, Bensard DD, Moore EE et al: Ultrasound is an effective triage tool to evaluate blunt abdominal trauma in the pediatric population, *J Trauma* 45:57-63, 1998.

48. Scorpio RJ, Wesson DE: Splenic trauma. In Eichelberger MR, ed: *Pediatric trauma: prevention, acute care, rehabilitation,* St Louis, 1993, Mosby.

49. Brasel KJ, DeLisle CM, Olson CJ et al: Splenic injury: trends in evaluation and management, *The Journal of Trauma: Injury, Infection, and Critical Care* 44:283-286, 1998.

50. Brown RL, Irish MS, McCabe AJ et al: Observation of splenic trauma: when is a little too much? *J Pediatr Surg* 34:1124-1126, 1999.

51. Lynch JM, Meza MP, Newman B et al: Computed tomography grade of splenic injury is predictive of the time required for radiographic healing, *J Pediatr Surg* 32:1093-1096, 1997.

52. Torres AM, Garcia VF: Hepatobiliary trauma. In MR Eichelberger, ed: *Pediatric trauma: prevention, acute care, rehabilitation,* St Louis, 1993, Mosby.

53. Gross M, Lynch F, Canty T et al: Management of pediatric liver injuries: 13-year experience at a pediatric trauma center, *J Pediatr Surg* 34:811-817, 1999.

54. Keller MS, Stafford PW Vane DW: Conservative management of pancreatic trauma in children, *J Trauma* 42:1097-1100, 1997.

55. Jobst MA, Canty TG, Lynch FP: Management of pancreatic injury in pediatric blunt abdominal trauma, *J Pediatr Surg* 34:818-823, 1999.

56. Rescorla FJ, Grosfeld JL: Pancreatic injury. In Eichelberger MR, ed: *Pediatric trauma: prevention, acute care, rehabilitation,* St Louis, 1993, Mosby.

57. Canty Sr. TG, Canty Jr. TG, Brown C: (1999), Injuries of the gastrointestinal tract from blunt trauma in children: a 12-year experience at a designated pediatric trauma center, *J Trauma* 46:234-240, 1999.

58. Newman KD: Gastric and intestinal injury. In Eichelberger MR, ed: *Pediatric trauma: prevention, acute care, rehabilitation,* St Louis, 1993, Mosby.

59. Allen GS, Moore FA, Cox CS et al: Hollow visceral injury and blunt trauma, *The Journal of Trauma: Injury, Infection, and Critical Care* 45:69-75, 1998.

60. Fang JF, Chen RJ, Lin BC: Small bowel perforation: is urgent surgery necessary? *The Journal of Trauma: Injury, Infection, and Critical Care* 47:515-520, 1999.

61. Rouse TM: Colonic, rectal, and perineal injury. In Eichelberger MR, ed: *Pediatric trauma: prevention, acute care, rehabilitation,* St Louis, 1993, Mosby.

62. Halow KD, Ford EG: Abdominal injury. In Ford EG, Andrassy RJ, eds: *Pediatric trauma: initial assessment and management,* Philadelphia, 1994, WB Saunders.
63. Fernandez L McKenney MG, McKenney KL et al: Ultrasound in blunt abdominal trauma, *J Trauma* 45:841-848, 1998.
64. Yoshii H, Sato M, Yamamoto et al: Usefulness and limitations of ultrasonography in the initial evaluation of blunt abdominal trauma, *J Trauma* 45:45-51, 1998.
65. Teitelbaum DH: Letters to the editor, *J Trauma* 46:357-358, 1999.
66. Fallat ME, Casale AJ: Practice patterns of pediatric surgeons caring for stable patients with traumatic solid organ injury, *J Trauma* 43:820-824, 1997.
67. Patrick DA, Bensard DD, Moore EE et al: Nonoperative management of solid organ injuries in children results in decreased blood utilization, *J Pediatr Surg* 34:1695-1699, 1999.
68. Brown SL, Elder JS, Spirnak JP: Are pediatric patients more susceptible to major renal injury from blunt trauma? A comparative study, *J Urol* 160:138-140, 1998.
69. Allshouse MJ, Betts JM: Genitourinary injury. In Eichelberger MR, ed: *Pediatric trauma: prevention, acute care, rehabilitation,* St Louis, 1993, Mosby.
70. Quinlan DM, Gearhart JP: Blunt renal trauma in childhood: features indicating severe injury, *Br J Urol* 66:526-531, 1990
71. Lebet RM: Abdominal and genitourinary trauma in children, *Crit Care Nurs Clin North Am* 3:433-444, 1991.
72. Corriere JN Jr: In Ford GE, Andrassy RJ, eds: *Pediatric trauma: initial assessment and management,* Philadelphia, 1994, WB Saunders.
73. Thomas MD: Musculoskeletal injury. In Eichelberger MR, ed: *Pediatric trauma: prevention, acute care, rehabilitation,* St Louis, 1991, Mosby.
74. Hinton RY, Lincoln A, Crockett MM et al: Fractures of the femoral shaft in children: incidence, mechanisms, and socioeconomic risk factors, *J Bone Joint Surg* 81-A:500-509, 1999.
75. Salter RB: Musculoskeletal injuries. In Mayer TA, ed: *Emergency management of pediatric trauma,* Philadelphia, 1985, WB Saunders.
76. Campbell LS, Campbell JD: Musculoskeletal trauma in children, *Crit Care Nurs Clin North Am* 3:445-456, 1991.
77. Willis RB, Rorabeck C: Treatment of compartment syndrome in children, *Orthop Clin North Am* 21:401-412, 1990.
78. Wong D, Baker C: Pain in children: comparison of assessment scales, *Pediatric Nursing* 14:9-17, 1988.
79. McCarty EC, Mencio GA, Green NE: Anesthesia and analgesia for the ambulatory management of fractures in children, *J Am Acad Orthop Surg* 7:81-91, 1999.
80. Chestnut RM, Marshall LF, Klauber MR: The role of secondary brain injury in determining outcome from severe head injury, *J Trauma* 34:216, 1993.
81. Shapira Y, Artru A, Qassam N et al: Brain edema and neurological status with rapid infusion of 0.9% saline or 5% dextrose after head trauma, *J Neurosurg Anesth* 7:17, 1995.
82. Wright MM: Resuscitation of the multitrauma patient with head injury, *AACN Clinical Issues* 10:32-45, 1999.
83. Melio FR: Priorities in the multiple trauma patient, *Emerg Med Clin North Am* 16:29-43, 1998.
84. Theodore AD, Runyan DK: A medical research agenda for child maltreatment: negotiating the next steps, *Pediatrics* 104:168-177, 1999.
85. Leventhal JM: The challenges of recognizing child abuse: seeing is believing, *JAMA* 281:657-659, 1999.
86. DiScala C, Sege R, Li G et al: Child abuse and unintentional injuries: a 10-year retrospective, *Arch Pediatr Adolesc Med* 154:16-22, 2000.
87. Crosson-Tower C: *Understanding child abuse and neglect,* ed 4, Boston, 1999, Allyn and Bacon.
88. Erickson MF Egeland B: Child neglect. In Briere J, Berliner L, Bulkley JA et al, eds: *APSAC handbook on child maltreatment,* London, 1996, Sage Publications.
89. Berliner L, Elliott DM: Sexual abuse in children. In Briere J, Berliner L, Bulkley JA et al, eds: *ASPAC handbook on child maltreatment,* London, 1996, Sage Publications.
90. Donald T, Jureidine J: Munchausen syndrome by proxy: child abuse in the medical system, *Arch Pediatr Adolesc Med* 159:753-758, 1996.
91. Crittendon PM: Research on maltreating families: implications for interventions. In Briere J, Berliner L, Bulkley JA et al, eds: *ASPAC handbook on child maltreatment,* London, 1996, Sage Publications.
92. Jones DPH, Lynch MA: Diagnosing and responding to serious child abuse: confronting deceit and denial is vital if children are to be protected, *Br Med J* 317:484-484, 1998.
93. Zellman GL, Faller KC: Reporting of child maltreatment. In Briere J, Berliner L, Bulkley JA et al, eds: *APSAC handbook on child maltreatment,* London, 1996, Sage Publications.
94. Boyce MC, Melhorn KJ, Vargo G: Pediatric trauma documentation: adequacy for assessment of child abuse, *Arch Pediatr Adolesc Med* 150:730-732, 1996.
95. Li G, Tang N, DiScala C et al: Cardiopulmonary resuscitation in pediatric trauma patients: survival and functional outcome, *J Trauma* 47:1-7, 1999.
96. Bayley EW, Richmond T, Noroian EL et al: A Delphi study on research priorities for trauma nursing, *Am J Crit Care* 3:208-216, 1994.

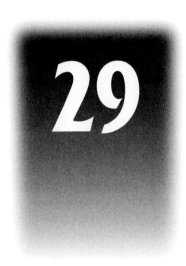

Thermal Injury

Patricia M. Lybarger
Patrick Kadilak

Fire and burn injuries are second only to motor vehicle accidents as the leading cause of death in children of ages 1 to 4 years in the United States. They are among the leading causes of injury and death in children of ages 1 to 19 years. Severe burns are considered the most catastrophic injury a person can survive, resulting in disfigurement, pain, emotional distress, and tremendous economic costs.[1]

Burn care has progressed dramatically in the last 20 years, in large part as the result of the establishment of specialized burn centers. Advances in fluid and electrolyte resuscitation, early excision and wound closure,[2,3] and nursing care in this area have increased the probability of surviving massive burns.

Burn injury is divided into three phases. The emergent or shock phase begins at the time of injury and extends until fluid resuscitation is complete. The acute phase lasts until wound closure is achieved. The rehabilitative and reconstructive phase can continue for the rest of the individual's life. Every organ system is affected by an injury to the skin that involves 25% total body surface area (TBSA) or more. Burns affecting more than 50% TBSA have a prolonged critical care phase that may last weeks or months.

ETIOLOGY OF PEDIATRIC BURN INJURIES

Most childhood burn deaths occur as a result of house fires, in which children are unable to escape the heat and smoke. Many causes, including careless handling of smoking materials, unsafe cooking and heating practices, faulty wiring, use of candles, and match play have been associated with these fatal fires. The causes of injury are varied, and most are unintentional injuries. However, the possibility of intentional injury is a major concern because it has been reported that between 8% and 24% of admissions to burn units are related to child abuse by burning.[4,5]

Children at greatest risk are those who cannot protect themselves. An infant relies totally on others for protection, whereas a preschooler can be taught to tell an adult when matches or lighters are found and to "stop, drop, and roll." Children with neurologic disorders, disabilities, and developmental delays also present a higher risk from inability to protect themselves and have a higher incidence of preventable injuries, have extended hospitalizations, and bear significantly higher mortality risks.[6]

Overall, burn injuries in children tend to follow patterns related to both developmental level and the socioeconomic environment of the child. Scalds are the leading cause of burn injury for young children and account for 58% to 67% of all burn injuries.[7,8] Most scald injuries are related to the handling and consumption of hot food and liquids. Food prepared in microwave ovens, as well as hot coffee and soup, are often involved. The pattern of splash and dripping is a common finding across the upper body and lap. These wounds are painful and may be very deep, depending on the nature of the scalding liquid and the time that the skin was exposed to it. Grease scalds from kitchen fryers can produce

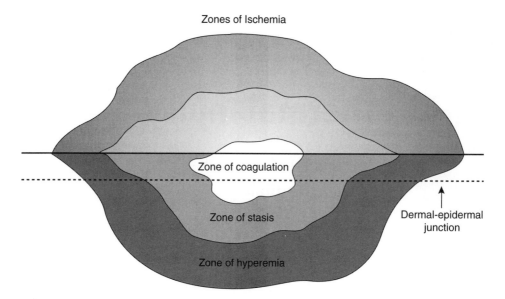

Fig. 29-1 Zones of ischemia.

serious injury because the hot grease cools slowly and is difficult to remove.

Hot household tap water is an important cause of lower body scald injuries, especially in the bath. Because children's skin is thinner than that of a young adult, even short exposure to water at 140° F, a common setting for home water heaters, can cause tissue destruction in fewer than 5 seconds in children and in less time in small infants.[9] Children may unintentionally turn on the hot water faucet when left unattended in the bathtub and be unable to get away from it. Adult supervision, setting water heaters between 120° and 130° F, and checking bath water temperature before placing a child in the tub are key to preventing these injuries.

As children become more mobile and curious, their exposure to household burn hazards expands. Electrical burns to the oral cavity are seen in infants and toddlers after chewing on the connection between appliances and extension cords. Contact burns from hot irons, ovens, wood stoves, and radiators occur in all ages. Ingestion of household chemicals can lead to devastating gastrointestinal damage, and even when diluted, cutaneous contact with these chemicals can cause full-thickness burns.

Match and fire play are a problem for the school-age population but have been recognized in children as young as 2 years of age. Flame burns associated with clothing ignition can cause serious injury from both heat and melting fabrics. Ignition of flammable liquids is seen in children old enough to work on their bikes or mow the lawn. Flash burns involving flammable liquids and explosives add a chemical component to the burn. Cigarette smoking and other risk-taking behaviors contribute to the burn problem for adolescents. With the increasing availability of the Internet, adolescents have found recipes for a variety of explosive and flammable mixtures.

There are seasonal and regional differences that affect the pattern of burn injury. Summer brings fireworks, barbecues, and sunburn. Winter brings alternative heating sources, such as electric space heaters, kerosene heaters and wood stoves. Traditional birthday celebrations may involve lighted candles. Cultural and socioeconomic factors, such as housing, heating, and cooking traditions, may also influence the risk and patterns of burn injury in any community.

Most people who die in house fires are overcome by the smoke and are unable to escape. Those that survive are at high risk for an inhalation injury as are those who are burned in an enclosed space or have burned facial areas. Inhalation injury continues to be the number-one cause of death in thermally injured patients and can occur with or without associated burns.[10] Inhalation injury may not always be evident initially, but carbon monoxide poisoning, thermal damage, and inhaled toxic chemical damage all affect survival.

PATHOPHYSIOLOGY

Burn severity depends both on the intensity of the heat and the duration of its contact with the skin. The magnitude of the physiologic response depends on the type, size, location, and depth of the burn. All body systems are potentially affected as the body adapts to compensate for the alterations in normal function.

Zones of Injury

Thermal damage to tissue is described in three zones (Fig. 29-1). The area of superficial damage is the *zone of hyperemia,* appearing warm and red. The middle area of damage is the *zone of stasis,* where the microcirculation is damaged and changes in capillary permeability allow fluids to leak from the vascular system into the interstitial space. This leads to local edema and shock when extensive wounds are present. The deepest area is the *zone of coagulation,* wherein heat-damaged cells occlude blood vessels. The

◆ TABLE 29-1   Burn Depth Categories

	Superficial Partial Thickness (First Degree)	Partial Thickness (Second Degree)	Full Thickness (Third Degree)
Cause	Scald, flash, flame, contact, chemical, ultraviolet light	Scald, flash, flame, contact, chemical, ultraviolet light	Scald, flash, flame, contact, chemical, electrical
Surface appearance	Dry, no blisters Minimal or no edema Erythematous	Moist blebs, blisters Underlying tissue mottled pink and white Good capillary refill	Dry, leathery eschar Mixed white, waxy, pearly Khaki, mahogany, soot-stained
Pain and temperature	Very painful Rapid heat loss	Very painful	Rapid heat loss Insensate Less rapid heat loss
Histologic depth	Epidermal layers only	Epidermis, papillary and reticular layers of dermis May include fat domes of subcutaneous layer	Down to and may include subcutaneous tissue May include fascia, muscle, and bone
Healing time	2 to 5 days with no scarring May have some discoloration	Superficial, 5-21 days with no grafting Deep partial, 21-35 days with no infection If infected, converts to full thickness	Small areas may heal from the edges after weeks Large areas require grafting

obstructed microcirculation prevents the humoral components of the immune response from reaching the burned tissue.

Classification of Burn Wounds

Classification of burn depth requires skilled clinical judgment. Surface appearance provides only a clue to the actual tissue damage below. Burns are rarely of uniform depth throughout. Appearance, pain, and tissue pliability are all used to assess wound depth. The type of burning agent and the extent of skin exposure combine to form challenging clinical presentations.

Burn depth is classified as partial thickness or full thickness (Table 29-1). Superficial partial-thickness burns involve only the epidermis. Deep partial-thickness burns involve the epidermis and the dermis but spare epidermal appendages necessary for epidermal regeneration. Full-thickness burns involve the epidermis, dermis, epidermal appendages, and sometimes subcutaneous tissues, such as fat, muscle, and bone. Any burn wound can be converted to a deeper thickness if infection, hypoxia, desiccation, or further mechanical tissue damage develops.

Burns are also described by measuring the size of the TBSA burned. For children, this size is determined using a Lund and Browder or Berkow chart, which takes into account the proportional body changes that occur during growth (Fig. 29-2). Deep partial- and full-thickness burns on body parts are charted as a percent of the whole. Superficial partial-thickness injuries are not part of the calculation because the integrity of the skin is not broken.

Affected areas are measured and combined to determine TBSA burned. This percent TBSA becomes important in calculating fluid resuscitation and nutritional needs after burns.

A number of other methods are used for determining TBSA burned in children. The palmar method may be used in smaller or more scattered burns. This method equates the palm of the child's hand with 1% of the body surface area. Another method is the baby rule of nines (Fig. 29-3). This method is used primarily in children younger than 3 years of age and allows for the relative difference in head size and lower extremity size in children compared with adults. Of all the methods, the Lund and Browder chart is preferred for children because it takes into account the variation in distribution of body surface area in children of different ages.[11]

INJURY TYPES

Thermal Injuries

Thermal injuries include three subclassifications: scald injuries, contact injuries, and flame injuries. All three types are governed by the principles of thermodynamics; thus the depth and severity of injury are dependent on the duration of contact and properties of heat or cold transference of the injury source. This becomes particularly relevant when examining a scald injury because the transference of heat by a liquid results in a greater zone of stasis. This zone will evolve over the first 72 hours, resulting in a more significant injury than on first assessment.

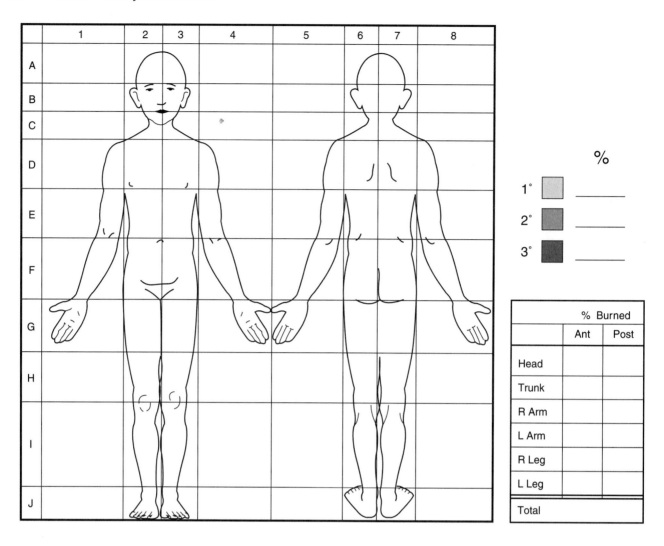

| | | 1 | 2 | 3 | 4 | 5 | 6 | 7 | 8 |

%
1° _____
2° _____
3° _____

	% Burned	
	Ant	Post
Head		
Trunk		
R Arm		
L Arm		
R Leg		
L Leg		
Total		

	Newborn	3 Years	6 Years	12+ Years
Head	18%	15%	12%	6%
Trunk	40%	40%	40%	38%
Arms	16%	16%	16%	18%
Legs	26%	29%	32%	38%

Fig. 29-2   Lund and Browder chart.

Electrical Injuries

Electrical injuries are caused by the conversion of electrical energy into heat energy, which coagulates body tissues. Electrical injuries can be divided into two categories based on the voltage to which the tissue was exposed. Low-voltage injuries are those sustained with contact with less than 1000 volts, including house current (115 to 220 volts). High-voltage injuries are those with contact with greater than 1000 voltage lines and include high-tension wires (up to 250,000 volts).

Electrical injuries in children occur most often in the infant and toddler and adolescent age groups. Infants and toddlers, while exploring their environment, often put everything they find into their mouth. Saliva, which serves as an excellent conductor, creates a current pathway from the electrical source and through the child's tissues. Thus the majority of these injuries are low-voltage injuries from plugs or cords and result in oral commissure burns.[12] The structure of extension cords, including holiday light sets, is a neglected area in legislation and federal standards for injury prevention. Voluntary standards are maintained by most manufacturers via independent laboratory approval and have contributed to some solutions, such as extension cords being manufactured with safety caps for unused plugs. However, this precaution is not universal and does not address cord-biting or cord-sucking injuries.[13]

The adolescent usually comes in contact with electricity as an unintentional sequela of risk-taking behavior such as climbing power poles or trees, as a result of tangled kites in high-tension wires, from lightening strikes, from contact

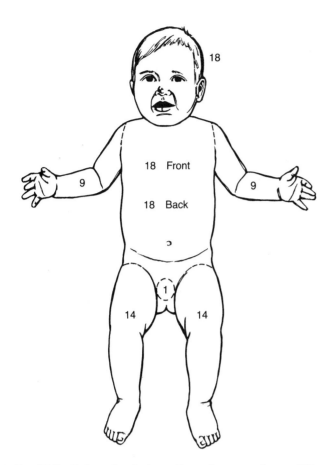

Fig. 29-3 Baby rule of nines allows for proportionate difference in head size related to lower extremity size in children younger than 3 years of age compared with adults. Note that head is 18% of the total body surface area (TBSA) in children versus 9% TBSA in adults. Lower extremity is then 14%, rather than 18% in adults. (From Kravitz M: Thermal injuries. In Cardona V et al, eds: *Trauma nursing: resuscitation through rehabilitation,* Philadelphia, 1994, WB Saunders, p 710.)

with transformers, or from household electrical appliances. Of the injuries seen in the adolescent group (11 to 18 years of age), 76% to 90% are high-voltage injuries, resulting in amputation, deep muscle involvement, fasciotomy, and significant morbidity. In addition, 60% to 90% of the adolescents sustaining high-voltage injuries are male.[12,13] Prevention of high-voltage injuries as a result of adolescent risk-taking behavior remains an ongoing challenge to prevention educators.

Although most injuries occur because of direct physical contact with an electrical source, the child may not have to actually touch the current source to sustain injury. Electrical current has been known to jump or "arc" from the source to electrically conductive substances in its search for a path in which to "ground." This holds true for current flowing through the body, because it may arc from one area of the body to another (e.g., across flexed joints). Additional injury can occur by electrical contact with clothing causing ignition, resulting in surface burns from burning fabrics and inhalation injury from the smoke and toxic chemicals produced by the burning clothing.

The physiologic impact of an electrical injury on the body is very unpredictable, causing damage by three mechanisms: (1) direct injury caused by the effect of the electricity on the body, (2) thermal damage as electricity is converted into heat, and (3) trauma resulting from a fall or severe muscle contraction following the electrical injury.[12,14] Direct injury caused by electrical contact includes vascular aneurysms and destruction of muscle and red blood cells, resulting in myoglobinuria and hemoglobinuria. In addition, vascular thrombosis formation; cardiac arrhythmias; myocardial damage; neurologic impairment; ophthalmologic injuries; rupture of the tympanic membrane; and, with forceful tetanic contractions, fractures and tendon rupture are other sequelae of direct injury by electrical contact. Extensive cellular destruction can also result in massive infusion of intracellular potassium into the circulation. The resulting hyperkalemia can rapidly reach toxic levels or produce lethal dysrhythmias.

Thermal damage caused by the electrical injuries is often difficult to assess. Where the current enters the body, there may be only a small entrance wound. The current then follows a path of least resistance and explodes out of the body where the body is in contact with a grounding source, resulting in one or more exit wounds. Massive tissue edema can result in compartment syndrome with further tissue destruction. Because the extent of tissue destruction is often hidden under normal-appearing skin, fluid loss into the interstitial spaces may go undetected. This can lead to inadequate restoration of the circulating blood volume during fluid resuscitation. The sum of these effects may result in local tissue destruction and intravascular coagulation so severe that amputation of the necrotic tissue becomes essential.

Management of pediatric electrical injuries begins with a detailed understanding the history of the injury, including type and strength of voltage, duration of contact, presence or absence of water, and associated trauma workup for suspected fall or injury. Blood chemistry abnormalities are monitored, including serum electrolytes, as well as skeletal and cardiac enzymes indicative of skeletal or cardiac muscle destruction. Cardiac rhythm, regardless of voltage level, is monitored for dysrhythmias. Assessment for myoglobinuria and compartment syndrome, including circulation sensation and movement distal to the injury, is essential.

Chemical Injuries

Chemical injury results from the thermal energy produced when strong acids or alkalis come in contact with body tissue. Strong acids and alkalis are the most common causes of chemical burns in children. In infants, injury is common from household cleaning chemicals, such as lye, ammonia, sulfuric acid, and laundry detergents. Older children are injured in school laboratory accidents or when "experimenting" at home. In addition, older children may be injured by gasoline-soaked clothing or by exposures related to their first jobs or home activities.

Chemicals destroy skin by coagulation necrosis, which may progress over time. The severity of the injury is dependent on the chemical properties, the concentration of the chemical, and the duration of contact with skin or mucous membranes. Care for children with chemical injuries includes obtaining a thorough history of the accident with the type and duration of contact and rinsing the affected area with copious amounts of water until a burn center consult can be obtained, as well as frequent assessment of the affected area.

Inhalation Injury

Inhalation injury, often called smoke inhalation, is a condition associated with exposure to the heat and toxic fumes produced by fire conditions in a closed space. Complete and incomplete combustion of materials commonly found in the everyday environment produces extreme heat, toxic fumes, and a reduction in the environmental oxygen concentration, often reducing it to 16% or less.

The identification of a person who has sustained an inhalation injury is often difficult. Clinically, a person who is at risk has the following characteristics:

- Burned in a closed space or standing upright as their clothing burned
- Burns of the face or neck
- Singed eyebrows, nasal hairs, and hairline or facial hair
- Carbon particles in the mouth or nose or carbonaceous sputum
- Brassy cough, hoarseness, or stridor
- Significant serum carboxyhemoglobin level (greater than 15%)[9]

These children warrant close observation and immediate intervention if respiratory distress develops. Early or prophylactic intervention, particularly in young children, is essential for survival.

The inhalation injury produced by fire conditions has four components. First, thermal injury occurs in the upper airways because of exposure to high environmental temperatures and superheated gases. Direct heat damage is usually limited to the upper airway because the moist mucous membranes act as a heat exchanger, lowering the temperature of the inhaled gases before they cross the vocal cords. In fire conditions, the upper airway extracts excess heat from inhaled gases. This protects the lower airway (below the vocal cords) from thermal damage. The sole exception to this is the inhalation of steam. Steam has a heat-carrying capacity that is approximately 400 times the capacity of ambient air. This allows the steam to pass through the vocal cords with little heat loss in the upper airway, thus creating thermal burns below the vocal cords. The exposure to hot gases produces diffuse edema throughout the upper airway, resulting in airway obstruction. The edema rapidly advances and peaks at about 6 to 12 hours after injury.

Extensive burns of the head and neck or hot liquid aspiration can produce such massive edema in local tissues that the airway is compromised. Although not a true inhalation injury, these injuries may present with similar clinical signs and symptoms. Suspicion of aspiration or

extensive head or neck burns is treated by protecting the airway with an endotracheal tube (ETT) until the edema resolves. Because of the small comparative size of children's airways, intervention in the form of endotracheal intubation is often required.[15]

Another aspect of inhalation injury occurs when carbon monoxide (CO) combines with the hemoglobin molecule to reduce the oxygen-carrying capacity of red blood cells. CO is a clear, colorless, odorless gas produced by the incomplete combustion of organic materials, such as wood, paper, cotton, gasoline, and others. Incomplete combustion occurs because insufficient oxygen is available in fire conditions. Depending on the carboxyhemoglobin levels, the child may experience symptoms ranging from mild intellectual dysfunction to apnea and cardiac arrest (Table 29-2). The binding of CO to hemoglobin can be reversed by the administration of 100% oxygen. Experiments attempting to quantify the elimination half-life of CO by nonrebreathing face mask or by ETT intubation demonstrate a range of 26 to 146 minutes.[16]

Hyperbaric oxygen (HBO) therapy may also be indicated for the child with CO poisoning, although its use remains controversial. A child undergoing HBO treatment is put into a hyperbaric chamber and is exposed to 100% oxygen at a pressure higher than atmospheric pressure. This method has shown to aid in displacing CO from the hemoglobin molecule, thus providing increased amounts of available oxygen and reversing the toxic effects of CO.[17]

Another sequela of inhalation injury is hypoxia caused by exposure to fire conditions wherein environmental oxygen is rapidly consumed by combustion. This results in environmental oxygen concentrations that reduce the FIO_2, so PaO_2 levels of 50 to 60 mmHg are commonplace. Combined with CO exposure, the reduced FIO_2 worsens the tissue hypoxia and its consequences.

The inhalation of toxic gases from the fire may produce a chemical pneumonitis. The combustion of commonly found materials liberates toxic gases, which can include

TABLE 29-2 Physiologic Effects of Carbon Monoxide Exposure

Carboxyhemoglobin Level (%)	Physiologic Effects
<20	Headache, dyspnea, confusion, lapse of attention, loss of peripheral vision
20-40	Irritability, faulty judgment, dim vision, nausea, vomiting, easily fatigued
40-60	Tachycardia, tachypnea, confusion, hallucinations, ataxia, syncope, convulsions, coma
>60	Often fatal

Adapted from Cohen MA, Guzzardi W: Inhalation of products of combustion, *Ann Emerg Med* 12:628-632, 1983.

hydrogen sulfide, hydrogen cyanide, hydrogen chloride, acrolein, mustard gas, nerve gas, and many others. When these gases come in contact with the epithelium lining the tracheobronchial tree, they form corrosive acids that destroy the cilia and underlying tissue. Toxic materials also adhere to soot particles that are inhaled, providing an additional source of toxic exposure and debris that must be cleared. Toxins are absorbed into the general circulation, where they can have systemic effects (e.g., production of hydrogen cyanide, which causes immediate respiratory dysfunction). The initial response of the lung is bronchorrhea followed by a sloughing of necrotic tissues. The increased debris formation plus the loss of the cilia results in atelectasis. The clinical symptoms may present hours to 7 days later.

There are three time periods following injury when the damage caused by these toxic agents occur. Immediately after the exposure to fire conditions, hypoxia associated with decreased environmental oxygen concentrations, CO poisoning, and airway edema from exposure to hot gases develops. During the 24 to 48 hours following injury, pulmonary edema is associated with the toxicity of inhaled gases and fluid resuscitation. After 48 hours, the effects of atelectasis and pneumonia become evident as a clinical picture similar to acute respiratory distress syndrome (ARDS) develops.

The presence of skin involvement further complicates the management of inhalation injury. Skin damage that involves more than 25% TBSA results in diffuse capillary leak throughout the body, including the lung. The increase in interstitial water surrounding the alveoli reduces effective gas exchange and increases the patient's volume requirements. Inhalation injury can increase the body's fluid requirement up to 37% over calculated fluid resuscitation needs. The assessment of fluid balance becomes increasingly complicated, and pulmonary edema is a common complication. The treatment of pulmonary edema is usually reduction of the infused fluid volume in increments until symptoms disappear.[18]

Full-thickness, circumferential surface burns of the neck and chest wall can compromise pulmonary function even further. When inelastic eschar surrounds the chest, a corsetlike effect is created. Edema continues to occur in the burn wound, compressing the tissues of the chest wall inward and compromising the vital capacity. Relief is provided by escharotomies (incisions through the eschar) that allow the chest wall to expand. Escharotomies to relieve chest compression are usually performed within the first 24 hours after injury, but extensions of the escharotomies may need to be done as the edema continues through the emergent phase.

Surviving the initial inhalation injury is not the end of the child's pulmonary problems. The child may develop ARDS following hypoxic or hypovolemic insult or as a component of septic shock associated with bacteremia from wound debridement, intravascular lines, urinary tract infections, or pneumonia.

The long-term sequelae of inhalation injury include bronchiolitis obliterans, cylindrical bronchiectasia, and tracheal stenosis associated with prolonged intubation or tracheostomy. Children whose respiratory units are destroyed at a young age have a better prognosis for long-term respiratory function than do school-age children or adolescents. As the young child grows after the injury, the remaining respiratory units can increase in surface area more than would normally be expected to compensate for the units that were destroyed.

Circumferential Burns

Full-thickness circumferential burns of the torso or extremity present a special problem for the child. As mentioned earlier, circumferential burns to the torso may impede a child's ability to ventilate. Similarly, circumferential areas of full-thickness burns to extremities are nonelastic and produce a tourniquet effect that diminishes blood flow to the affected area. As edema occurs in the affected area and the tissue cannot stretch, the child experiences numbness and tingling distal to the injured area, loss of motor function and sensation, and severe pain. Release of pressure must occur and requires surgical intervention by escharotomy or fasciotomy (Fig. 29-4). An escharotomy involves an incision through the burned tissue down to the subcutaneous fat layers to restore blood supply. A fasciotomy is necessary when the escharotomy has not restored adequate perfusion and the injury has extended into the muscle. This procedure involves a deeper incision through the fascia covering the muscle compartments and allows the expansion of compressed or edematous areas of muscle.

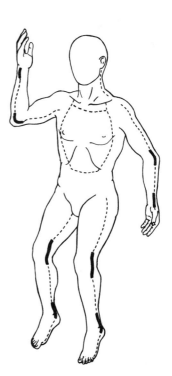

Fig. 29-4 Diagram shows preferred site of escharotomy incisions. (From Finkelstein JL, Schwartz SB, Madden MR et al: Pediatric burns: an overview, *Pediatr Clin North Am* 39:1145-1163, 1992.)

The best time to perform an escharotomy varies and is based on frequent assessment of the affected area, distal circulation, sensory motor function, and pulses, as well as respiratory effort and peak inspiratory pressures with torso burns. If an escharotomy is performed, blood loss may be a problem as circulation is restored and is monitored. If the escharotomy is performed too late, necrosis of the entire extremity distal to the injury site, compartment syndrome, and gangrene can develop.

Exfoliative Disorders

Although not considered thermal injuries, several diseases including toxic epidermal necrolysis (TEN), epidermolysis bullosa, and purpura fulminans are increasingly being treated in burn units. Burn units have been demonstrated to coordinate resources to manage these large complex wounds and reduce mortality.[19-21]

TEN is a rare, severe form of epidermal sloughing occurring most often as a result of a severe drug-induced reaction. In addition to epidermal sloughing, the epithelial linings of the gastrointestinal tract and respiratory tract and the mucous membranes of the eye and oropharynx may also slough. TEN is manifested by fever (all cases), conjunctivitis (32% of cases), sore throat (25% of cases), pruritus (28% of cases), malaise, and a rash with a positive Nikolsky's sign (a sloughing of sheets of epidermis in response to light touch).[22] Drugs that often trigger TEN include sulfonamides, nonsteroidal antiinflammatory drugs, anticonvulsants, penicillins, and allopurinol. Milder forms of the same disease process include erythema multiforme and an intermediate form known as Stevens-Johnson syndrome.

Staphylococcal scalded skin syndrome (SSSS), a syndrome clinically similar to TEN, is caused by a staphylococcal skin infection usually occurring in children younger than 5 years of age. Some strains of staphylococci produce an epidermolytic toxin that causes the epidermis to cleave at the upper malpighian and granular layers. The presentation of SSSS is very similar to TEN, also presenting with a positive Nikolsky's sign. Differentiation between these two diseases is generally done by histologic examination of a skin biopsy or sample.

CRITICAL CARE MANAGEMENT

Emergent (Shock) Phase

As with any other trauma, initial management priorities focus on support of airway, breathing, and circulation (ABCs). For the burned patient, the first priority is to stop the burning process, then proceed with the ABCs.

Thorough and ongoing assessment of the airway is key in the initial nursing care. Immediate intubation is considered if a facial burn, upper airway edema, or an inhalation injury is present. Ensuring an adequate airway is crucial because delay may make intubation difficult or impossible as a result of massive swelling.

Maintenance of a stable airway may require creativity, including the use of tracheal ties or other nonadhesive

stabilization techniques because traditional adhesives do not stick to slippery, wet, edematous skin. With oral intubation, care is taken to protect the commissures of the mouth from erosion by the ties used to hold the ETT in place. Creativity and nursing vigilance to ensure the protection of these areas can significantly reduce the need for difficult oral or lip reconstruction. This may include the use of elastomer oral commissure pads; the use of double tracheostomy ties to secure the tube; or additional padding with dressings or 4 × 4's under the ties, above the ears, or at the back of the head (Fig. 29-5).

Ventilatory support is provided as needed. Oxygen at 100% is continued for any child with CO poisoning until carboxyhemoglobin levels are below 15%. In cases of inhalation injury, conventional mechanical ventilation modes may not provide sufficient ventilatory support and necessitate the use alternative ventilatory therapies.[23-25]

Maintenance of fluid balance is an important component of the emergent phase. Establishment of intravenous access with a large-caliber catheter is essential because fluid resuscitation is vital to the initial management

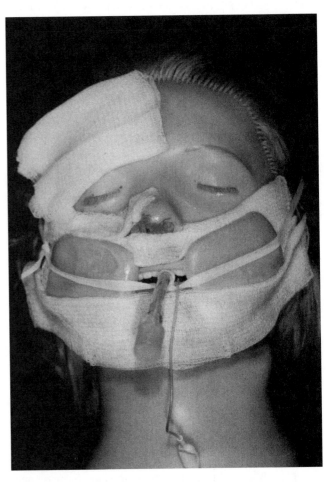

Fig. 29-5 Securing oral endotracheal tubes requires creativity and attention to prevent oral commissure erosion, as well as possible accidental extubation. Pictured here, elastomer oral commissure pads are used to prevent injury, with two tracheostomy cotton twill ties providing stability and ensuring tube security. (Photo courtesy Topliffe L and Lopez A, 1999.)

of a major burn. A urinary catheter is inserted to evaluate the patient's response to the burn and fluid resuscitation efforts.

A nasogastric tube is placed for gastric decompression and monitoring in patients with major injuries. Children with major burns are at risk for postinjury paralytic ileus. Thus the nasogastric tube is critical to prevent vomiting and aspiration.[9] Enteral feeding should begin as soon as possible after the injury to promote normal function of the gut and to decrease potential for bacterial translocation across the gastric mucosa.

Pertinent information about the circumstances of the injury is obtained, and a secondary survey for other injuries is performed. Other important data include weight; known allergies; medical history; chronic medication, drug, or alcohol use; and tetanus prophylaxis within the past 5 years.[9]

Cardiovascular Response. In large body surface area (BSA) burns, profound vascular changes lead to fluid shifts in burned and unburned tissue. There is a loss of intravascular volume into the interstitium. Local increases in vascular permeability are the result of direct heat damage that causes large fluid and protein losses through the wound itself. Mediator-induced cell damage appears to contribute to changes in cellular function in nonburned tissue, contributing to the overall edema that occurs after a large burn injury. The fluid and protein shifts are most pronounced in the first several hours because of the combined effect of increased permeability and an imbalance in osmotic pressures. If not treated, these changes lead to burn shock, characterized by hypovolemia, hypoproteinemia, decreased oxygen tension, and increased tissue pressure.

Cardiac compromise is a factor in burn injury, although compared with the adult population, the issue is minimized by the child's ability to compensate with an increased heart rate. Initially, cardiac output falls abruptly but returns to 30% of the preburn level within 30 minutes of injury. If resuscitation is adequate, cardiac output returns to preburn levels within 36 hours.[26] Thereafter cardiac output increases to supernormal levels and may remain elevated for some time, which is typical of the hypermetabolic response to thermal injury. Both metabolic and immune factors play a role in myocardial dysfunction following burn injury, but the exact mechanism has not been identified.[11]

Metabolic Response. Immediately following thermal injury, the emergent (shock) phase ensues. This phase, lasting for 24 to 48 hours, is characterized by decreases in cardiac output, oxygen consumption, and body temperature. After the emergent phase is the acute phase, during which the metabolic rate increases and persistent tachycardia, tachypnea, hyperpyrexia, and body wasting are seen.[1] The metabolic rate increases in proportion to burn size in a linear relationship up to 1.55 times basal levels.[1,27] Maximal levels are attained between the fifth and twelfth postburn day; however, increased metabolic output remains until wound closure occurs.[11] It is unclear whether the metabolic rate returns to baseline even at complete wound closure or how protracted the elevated levels remain in terms of weeks, months, or years.

Hypermetabolism mandates increased cardiac output and oxygen use, which produces an increase in blood flow to the visceral organs and burn wound. The visceral organs do not increase oxygen consumption; however, the burn wound requires increased blood flow to provide nutrients for wound healing to occur.

Immune Response. Infection is the leading cause of morbidity for burn patients. Persistently open wounds, increased metabolic needs, decreased nutritional intake, loss of plasma protein, and suppression of the host defense mechanism all contribute to the burned patient's susceptibility to infection. An altered immune response follows thermal injury, with defects related to both the altered host environment and the injury-triggered host deficiency state. The skin barrier is lost, providing an open portal of entry for microorganisms. Neutrophil function is diminished, and opsonization is decreased, leaving the child increasingly susceptible to local and systemic infections. Thus in the critical care management of a burned patient, emphasis is placed at maintaining as aseptic an environment as is feasible.

Fluid Resuscitation. Fluid requirements for the first 24 hours vary between 2 and 4 ml/kg of body weight multiplied by the percent TBSA burn. Various formulas are used for determining the volume of fluid resuscitation (Table 29-3). These calculations are only guidelines; rate increases or decreases in fluid resuscitation are based entirely on the individual patient's response (urinary output, hemodynamics, and ventilatory status). Rate and fluid choices vary depending on the type of fluid used, patient age, size of burn, and the presence of associated injury. The rate of infusion is systematically decreased over the first 24 to 48 hours to adjust for expected fluid shifts to the intravascular space. Insensible losses and maintenance needs are added above the rates established by these formulas to accurately meet patient requirements.

Fluid overload has serious consequences for children, resulting in pulmonary, cerebral, and local tissue edema. Tissue oxygenation is compromised because of extracellular edema, particularly in burned tissue. Individual patient response is monitored closely, and fluid replacement is optimized. Cardiac filling pressures and cardiac index can be used to titrate vasopressors during the resuscitative phase. Fluid replacement and circulatory support are planned to adjust for anticipated fluid shifts. Changes in electrolyte balance, hematocrit level, or osmolality are treated in the context of known burn pathophysiology. Colloid solutions may be included in the resuscitation therapy, generally after the first 24 hours, in an attempt to maintain fluids in the intravascular space or provide necessary plasma elements.

Evaluation of Fluid Resuscitation. The adequacy of fluid resuscitation for the burned child can be monitored by assessment of urine output, cardiovascular status, acid-base changes, mental status, and body temperature. Hourly urine output is a critical criterion for the evaluation of fluid resuscitation. A gauge for the resolution of burn shock is the point at which the child is able to maintain adequate urine output for 2 hours while receiving fluids at the calculated maintenance rate.[28] The goal for urine output is 1 to 2

TABLE 29-3 Fluid Resuscitation Formulas

Formula	Type and Volume of Fluid	
	First 24 Hours	**Second 24 Hours**
Brooke	Colloid: 0.5 ml/kg/% burn	0.25 ml/kg/%
	Crystalloid: Lactated Ringer's	Lactated Ringer's 0.75 ml/kg/% burn
	1.5 ml/kg/% burn	1500-2000 ml
	D5W: 2000 ml/m²	Same
	Urine: 30-50 ml/hr (adult); 1-2 ml/kg/hr (child)	½ of first 24 hour's colloids
	Rate: ½ in first 8 hr	+ crystalloids
	¼ in next 8 hr	
	¼ in last 8 hr	
	Calculation of volume: use burn area up to 50% TBSA,	
	>50% TBSA calculate at 50% TBSA	
Parkland	Colloid: none	700-2000 ml (adult) as needed to
	Crystalloid: lactated Ringer's	maintain urine output
	4 ml/kg/% burn	None
	D5W: none	Sufficient to maintain urine output
	Urine: 50-70 ml/hr (adult); 1-2 ml/kg/hr (child)	Same
	Rate: ½ in first 8 hr	½ of first day's lactated Ringer's
	¼ in next 8 hr	
	¼ in last 8 hr	
	Calculation of volume: use total burn area for *all* size burns	
Hypertonic saline	Colloid: none	None
	Crystalloid: Na⁺ 250 mEq/L	D5W
	Cl⁻ 150 mEq/L	
	lactate 100 mEq/L	
	D5W: "liberal" free water by mouth	
	Urine: 30-40 ml/hr (adult); 1-2 ml/kg/hr (child)	
	Rate: average 30 ml/hr	
	Calculation of volume: titrate to urine output not burn size	

D5W, 5% dextrose in water; *TBSA,* total body surface area.

ml/kg/hr in the child and 30 to 50 ml/kg/hr in patients greater than 50 kg.

A mild metabolic acidosis occurs with burn shock but usually resolves within 18 to 24 hours of injury. Children younger than 2 years of age, because of their inadequately developed buffer system, are especially prone to the development of metabolic acidosis.[29] Serum pH is monitored closely, and bicarbonate is given if the acidosis becomes severe or if circulating blood volume is restored without resolution of acidosis.

Mental status is a critical guide to evaluate the adequacy of fluid resuscitation. A child in an obtunded state requires a thorough assessment because the burn injury itself does not directly affect mental status. If obtunded because of shock, fluid resuscitation should restore the child's normal sensorium. If this is not the case, other causes of altered level of consciousness are considered, including concurrent trauma issues that might have occurred during the accident, as well as hypoglycemia.

Pediatric burn patients are particularly affected by alteration in temperature because of their greater BSA. In addition, they are less able to shiver because of relatively small muscle mass, which limits their ability to generate heat.[9] Patients with large burns are at risk for hypothermia

until skin coverage is achieved. Exposure during procedures and dressing changes may produce rapid hypothermia. Efforts by patients to maintain temperature increase oxygen consumption and energy expenditure and add to the stress of the burn injury.

The environment is kept free of drafts and warmer than normal to allow a normal temperature (37° to 37.5° C) to be maintained. Use of warm blankets, head covering, reflective blankets, and warming shields are nursing measures that effectively raise the body temperature. Increasing environmental humidity can decrease evaporative losses from wet dressings and exposed body surfaces. Continuous monitoring with a rectal probe may be appropriate initially. Warmed intravenous and irrigation solutions and a warming blanket may be considered if profound hypothermia develops.

Wound Care. As the child's respiratory and cardiovascular status is stabilized, attention can be directed toward the management of the burn wounds. Immediately following injury, clothing is removed, and a total survey of the body is performed in a clean, warm environment. In children with large burns, assessing only a portion of the body at a time may be necessary to maintain the child's temperature. This approach becomes increasingly important in the infant and young child because heat loss is rapid and physiologic consequences are significant. Classification of depth and determination of TBSA involvement are verified. Less obvious areas of injury, such as the scalp and oropharynx, are examined for evidence of thermal injury. Regular assessment of peripheral pulses is performed on involved extremities.

Surgical escharotomies may be required during the resuscitation phase to restore effective circulation to extremities and digits. After the escharotomy has been performed, the neurologic status of the affected limb is assessed frequently because peak edema formation does not occur until 24 hours after the burn.[28]

Wounds are cleansed with antibacterial soap and sterile water or normal saline. Loose tissue is mechanically debrided, and the prescribed topical agent is applied. Topical agents are not applied if the child is to be transferred to a burn center; instead the wounds are wrapped in clean dry dressings. The initial dressings are wrapped loosely, particularly in the hands and feet, to allow anticipated swelling. The head and extremities are elevated for comfort and to minimize fluid accumulation. Access to peripheral pulses is anticipated, so dressings are wrapped to allow periodic assessment of circulation. Wound management varies with physician preference, but current therapy generally involves total removal of all devitalized tissue as soon as feasible.

Comfort Management. Most extensive burn injuries have components of superficial and partial- and full-thickness injuries. Superficial and partial-thickness injuries are very painful. Full-thickness injuries initially are anesthetic, but as the wounds are debrided, the nerve endings in the deeper layers of tissue become exposed, resulting in very painful lesions. In addition, wound contraction inhibits joint mobility, so range-of-motion exercises, activities of daily living, and dressing changes are painful and anxiety producing. Intravenous narcotics are indicated for the pain associated with burns. The medications of choice are morphine sulfate and fentanyl. Anxiolytic medications such as midazolam or lorazepam are especially important for comfort management and when providing ventilatory support. Medications are given in small doses and titrated to relieve distress without complicating ventilation. The recommended approach is that all medications be given intravenously during the emergent phase because of unreliable uptake from edematous tissues when given subcutaneously or intramuscularly.

In addition to pharmacologic management of pain, interventions such as relaxation techniques and distraction may be appropriate. These approaches also provide a means for family members to be involved in the care of the child. Every effort is made to meet the patient's need for comfort and psychologic support. Consideration is given to associated injuries, past medical history, and the developmental needs of the child.

Psychologic Support. During the resuscitative phase of care, patients may be awake and alert. Survival, loss of control, and adaptation to an unfamiliar environment are the focus of psychosocial support systems. The ability to communicate needs is impaired as a result of the treatment of pain, anxiety, and respiratory function.

> **Box 29-1**
> **American Burn Association Criteria for Patient Transfer to a Burn Center**
>
> 1. Partial-thickness burns greater than 10% total body surface area (TBSA)
> 2. Burns that involve face, hands, feet, genitalia, perineum, and major joints
> 3. Full-thickness burns in any age group
> 4. Electrical burns, including lightning injury
> 5. Chemical burns
> 6. Inhalation injury
> 7. Burn injury in patients with preexisting medical disorders that could complicate management
> 8. Burn patients with concomitant trauma in which the burn injury poses the greatest risk of morbidity or mortality
> 9. Burned children in hospitals without qualified personnel or equipment for the care of children
> 10. Burn injury in patients who will require special social, emotional, or long-term rehabilitative intervention

The child and family should be informed of the procedures taking place and included in the overall plan of care. Efforts to reassure and calm the family are important components. Social services, psychiatry, chaplaincy, and other hospital resources can be involved as needed.

Transfer and Referral Priorities

The American Burn Association has identified the type of injuries that require referral to a specialized burn center (Box 29-1). The patient with electric, chemical, or thermal injury requires immediate assessment and stabilization at the closest appropriate hospital. There, hospital personnel complete a primary and secondary assessment and evaluate the patient for potential transfer. Clear documentation of procedures and care provided accompany the patient to the receiving hospital. The use of transfer agreements between regionalized burn centers and outlying community hospitals are considered to facilitate orderly transfers and to meet continuing education needs.[9] Some suggest that the early transfer of the child with acute burns may shorten the length of hospitalization and reduce complications.[30]

Acute Phase

Wound Care and Coverage. After stabilization has been achieved in the emergent phase, attention is directed toward closing the burn wound. The first step in this process is the assessment of wound depth and the surface area involved. The depth and extent are variable, depending on the intensity of the source and the duration of contact with the source of injury. Over the first 48 to 72 hours after injury, the wounds continue to evolve. The ultimate depth of the injury, especially in scald and chemical injuries, may not be evident until this evolution is complete.

The goals of wound care become the preservation of as much viable tissue as possible, removal of all necrotic tissue, control of the growth of microorganisms on the wound, and creation of an environment that is conducive to wound healing. Where extensive full-thickness skin loss occurs, the deficit must be replaced by some form of autograft or permanent skin substitute. These goals are achieved in a myriad of ways, but the ultimate outcome is the same—wound closure with intact, durable skin.

The first step in the preservation of viable tissue is the recognition of that which is viable. Viable tissue is pink, moist, warm, and sensate (depending on the depth of the wound). Viability is a reflection of the degree of perfusion of the tissue, the availability of adequate substrates for tissue repair, and the degree of exposure to such noxious agents as bacteria and fungus, some topical agents, and cleansing solutions. Debriding dressings, mechanical trauma, shearing forces caused by movement, and desiccation (drying) of the wound bed contribute to loss of viable tissue. Episodes of hypotension, hypoxia, and poor perfusion of the wound bed can also reduce tissue viability.

The activities of the burn care team are directed toward the preservation of viable tissue. Specifically, the focus of care is to maintain adequate tissue perfusion, provide adequate nutritional resources, prevent desiccation, reduce shear and mechanical trauma, and critically evaluate dressing materials that are being used on a particular wound. In addition, keeping the wound free of debris and necrotic tissue, reducing the exposure of the wound to toxic topical agents and cleansing solutions, and providing permanent wound closure by early excision of eschar and grafting as soon as possible are the tenets of the burn care team.

Controlling all of the variables that influence tissue viability is not possible, but care should be taken to reduce known risks to tissue survival while considering the requirements of the whole child. When the viability of a specific tissue is uncertain, it is often best to allow the body to demarcate the line between viable and nonviable. This dilemma often occurs when the viability of fingers or toes is in question.

Debridement of necrotic tissue is the second component in wound care. It can be achieved in a number of ways, including dressings, blunt and sharp debridement with hydrotherapy or showers, and primary excision under anesthesia. Regardless of the methods selected by the burn team for the individual patient, providing adequate pain and anxiety relief is essential. Intravenous or oral narcotics and anxiolytic agents must be given in adequate doses during these procedures. Assessment of the child's pain and anxiety is performed throughout the procedure, and additional medication is administered, as needed.[30a]

Many dressing materials are on the market, with new ones being introduced often. The specific properties and recommended uses for a product must be understood by caregivers. Inappropriate use of a product can actually be detrimental to the wound. The choice of material is generally directed by the goal of the therapy. If debridement of the wound is the goal, one of the least expensive and most commonly available materials is wide mesh gauze (WMG). WMG is laid in a single layer over the wound. It may be impregnated with a cream topical agent before application

or soaked with a liquid topical agent after a bulky outer dressing has been applied.

Many biologic dressings are available. These materials include human cadaver allografts, porcine xenografts, and several biosynthetic materials (manufactured materials impregnated with collagen). The biologic dressings must be applied to clean wound beds because they decrease evaporative water loss from the wound and create a warm moist environment. Biologic dressings placed over contaminated wounds facilitate the growth of microorganisms and result in deepening of the wound. At the first sign of purulent drainage, increasing local inflammation, or systemic signs of sepsis, the biologic dressing that is not adherent to the wound bed is removed, and the wound is inspected and cultured.

The ideal coverage of the debrided full-thickness burn wound is skin grafts from the child's own body. Autologous skin grafts, the patient's own skin, remains the only permanent, durable closure for the burn wound. Autografts may be harvested from unburned areas of the body. Split-thickness autografts include both epidermal and dermal elements and vary in thickness from 0.015 to 0.04 cm. Epidermal appendages are spared so that the donor site will heal in 10 to 14 days. The donor site is then available for reharvesting.

Full-thickness grafts include epidermis, dermis, and sometimes fat and muscle tissue. Because no epidermal appendages remain, the donor site must be either primarily closed or grafted with a split-thickness skin graft. Full-thickness grafts in large surface area burns are a very limited resource. They are therefore reserved for hand and facial reconstruction and for coverage of open joints.

Several artificial skin replacement products are in the research and development phases or newly available on the market. These products, in whole or part, remain integrated with the patient's body or are gradually replaced by the body's own tissue.[31] One such artificial skin, Integra, developed by Burke and Yannis, provides a dermal template with a temporary "epidermal" membrane. The artificial skin consists of a collagen mat with a Silastic membrane (temporary epidermis) on one side. The full-thickness burn wound is excised and Integra is sutured in place with the collagen side down. Over about 4 weeks the collagen mat is replaced by the body's own collagen. The Silastic membrane, which until this time has reduced evaporative water losses from the wound, is removed at 3 weeks. A very thin split-thickness skin graft or epithelial cell cultures are then applied to the neodermis. The neodermis and split-thickness graft form a durable skin replacement with a cosmetically acceptable appearance.

Epithelial cell cultures (e.g., Genzyme) are additional commercially available products that can be used as part of the coverage plan for the extensively burned child. A postage stamp–sized skin biopsy of normal skin is obtained and sent to specific tissue culture laboratories. In the laboratory, the epidermis is mechanically separated from the dermis. Enzymes are then added to the epidermal tissue to produce a single-cell suspension. The single-cell suspension is then inoculated into special tissue culture media. In about

10 days, the epidermal cells have grown into confluent sheets. These sheets are treated with an enzyme, Dispase, to release them from their attachments to the plastic flasks. At this time they can be transferred to the patient's tissue; however, in most instances, the surface that they would cover would be insufficient to meet the patient's needs. These primary cultures are then treated with enzymes to produce a single-cell suspension that is again inoculated into tissue culture media and incubated for another 10 days. The cultured epithelial sheets are then Dispase-released from the flasks, clipped to Vaseline gauze carriers with surgical clips, and transported to the operating room for application to the patient.

This process requires approximately 21 days. At this time, the equivalent of 2 m^2 of epithelial cell cultures become available to the patient. During this waiting period, the wounds are excised and covered with some form of biologic or temporary dressing.

The epithelial cell cultures are applied to the excised wound beds and are secured in place with either sutures or surgical staples. Care is taken to handle the cultures as little as possible because even minor mechanical trauma results in the death of the epithelial cells involved. Postoperatively, the wounds are dressed with dry dressings, and the areas are immobilized. In approximately 7 days, the Vaseline gauze backings are gently removed. Thin glistening sheets of epithelial cells can be seen as the backings are very gently removed from the tissue. The coverage remains very fragile for several weeks, requiring nonadherent dressings and great care in handling.

The durability of epithelial cell cultures is never the same as normal skin but rather is like that of thin split-thickness grafts. They can, however, provide lifesaving coverage for the child with extensive full-thickness burns. With any method of wound coverage selected by the burn team, coverage must be pursued aggressively if the child is to survive and avoid systemic sepsis and shock.

Regardless of the type of wound covering, it is critical that the child's wound be assessed at least daily for signs of deterioration. Signs of wound infection must be identified early before systemic infection develops. Clinical manifestations include discoloration of eschar (dark red, brown, or black), conversion of a split-thickness injury to a full-thickness one, rapid acceleration of the eschar, reddened necrotic lesions in unburned skin, discoloration of unburned skin at the wound edge, and accelerated circular subcutaneous edema with central necrosis.

Infection Control.   The goals for the burned child related to infection control include the following:

- Prevent the transmission of microorganisms from the child to the environment and other patients.
- Prevent the transmission of microorganisms from the environment and other patients to the child.
- Control or eradicate microorganisms that are not part of the child's normal flora.

Creating physical barriers between the burned child and the environment helps to prevent the transmission of microorganisms from the child to the environment and other patients

and from the environment and other patients to the child. These barriers can be created in a number of ways, depending on the architecture and resources of the individual unit. The child can be cared for in a single room or in a laminar flow unit on an open ward. Barriers can include plastic aprons, gauntlets, gloves, hats, and masks or isolation gowns, gloves, hats and masks. Standard precautions require the addition of goggles or face shields if a reasonable risk exists for splash and splatter of body fluids or tissues.

An environment that is conducive to wound healing is warm and moist and has sufficient substrates for cell maturation and division.[32] Unfortunately, this environment is also conducive to the growth of microorganisms. These organisms compete with the body's cells for available substrate and produce toxins that inhibit the repair of the damaged tissue. The wound, therefore, is kept warm, moist, and as clean as possible, if wound healing is to be facilitated.[32] Topical agents are applied to the wounds to control the growth of microorganisms on the wound until permanent coverage is achieved. The appropriateness of a specific agent for a specific wound depends on the characteristics of the topical agent, the wound, and the clinical experience or preference of the burn team. Table 29-4 lists the properties of the various agents and their limitations.

Nutritional Management.   The burned child has increased nutritional requirements related to the hypermetabolic state and the energy needed to heal wounds. Calculated nutritional needs are based on basal metabolic rate, physical activity, and stress-induced energy needs (Table 29-5). Caloric requirements are estimated based on the BSA involved in a burn injury, as well as the child's daily requirements based on growth needs, and may range from 1.2 to 1.5 times their basal metabolic rate.[33,34] A nutritional consult is planned on admission to determine caloric, carbohydrate, and protein goals with a systematic plan to meet these goals. Formulas vary for determining the exact nutritional needs, and some may calculate as much as twice the normal caloric and protein requirements. Adequacy of nutritional support can be evaluated from calorie counts; laboratory values, including prealbumin and albumin levels; metabolic cart measurements; biweekly weights; and the status of wound healing.

Oral nutrition is the preferred method of feeding; however, oral intake is often insufficient because of anorexia, intubation, and an inability to voluntarily take in all the calories required. Providing supplemental enteral feedings via flexible feeding tubes is often indicated in these situations to achieving calorie and protein goals. Feeding tubes can be placed into the small bowel via the gastric pylorus to minimize issues with decreased gastric motility or high gastric residuals. Some burn centers continue enteral postpyloric feedings during surgical procedures to make it possible to achieve nutritional goals.[34] Other centers successfully use a program of intragastric feedings, sometimes combined with a limited intravenous hyperalimentation program.[2,35]

The use of a limited intravenous hyperalimentation program may be required in patients with prolonged

TABLE 29-4   Topical Agents

Topical Agent	Effectiveness	Side Effects	Ease of Use	Pain	Cost
Silver sulfadiazine (Silvadene, Flamazine) 1% in water-miscible cream base	Broad-spectrum Minimal eschar penetration	Dose-related neutropenia Sulfa allergies *Do not use* in patients with toxic epidermal necrolysis Development of pseudoeschar	Semiclosed dressings Changed bid-qid Residue *must* be washed off with each dressing change	Cooling; least painful	$34.35 (400 g)
Silver nitrate solution 0.5% in water	Broad-spectrum Only penetrates 2-4 mm into burn wound	Hypoallergenic Leaches electrolytes from wound, especially sodium and potassium Methemoglobinemia Environmental staining	Bulky (½-inch thick), wet dressings Changed bid-qid Must be soaked q2h to maintain wetness Stains skin and environment black Surrounding normal skin must be protected from staining with petrolatum-based gauze	Stings briefly on application or soaking	$ 9.75 (liter)
Mafenide acetate (Sulfamylon) 10% in water-miscible cream base	Broad-spectrum including *Pseudomonas* Rapid and deep wound penetration	Inhibits spontaneous epithelial regeneration Carbonic anhydrase inhibitor causing metabolic acidosis as a result of HCO_3 wasting Sensitivity rash	Semiclosed dressings Changed bid-qid Residue *must* be washed off with each dressing change	Burning feeling for 15-20 min	$126.00 (453 g)
Povidone iodine (Betadine) 1%	Broad-spectrum, including fungi	Iodine absorption through wound increasing serum iodine levels Iodine allergies Environmental staining	Semiclosed or wet dressings Changed bid-qid	Stinging pain	$3.86 (480 ml)
Hypochlorite Dakin's Eusol	Broad-spectrum in concentrations of 0.025%-0.125% Safe for use as a wet dressing over tendons and open joints (used rarely in United States)	Can macerate normal tissue Unstable, use fresh Keep in a dark place Drying to tissue	Wet-wet dressings Wet-dry dressings (debriding) Changed bid-qid Soak q2h	Stings	<$1.00 (gal)
Collagenase (Santyl) and polysporin powder	Broad-spectrum but no fungi coverage	Sensitivity rash to sulfa drugs	Dressing can be removed moist or dry Changed qd	None	Collagenase: $29.95 (15 g) Polysporin: $10.00 (10 g)
Normal saline 0.45% or 0.9%	No antimicrobial properties Keeps wound moist	Can macerate tissue	Wet-wet dressings Wet-dry dressings (debriding) Changed bid-qid Soak q2h	Stings	A few cents

Data from Medical Economics Company: *The red book,* Montvale, NJ, 1999, Medical Economics.

TABLE 29-5   Nutritional Support for Pediatric Burns*

Basal Metabolic Rates: Infants and Children							
Age 1 wk to 10 mo		**Age 11 to 36 mo**			**Age 3 to 16 yr**		
	Metabolic Rate (kcal/hr)		**Metabolic Rate (kcal/hr)**			**Metabolic Rate (kcal/hr)**	
Weight (kg)	**Male or Female**	**Weight (kg)**	**Male**	**Female**	**Weight (kg)**	**Male**	**Female**
3.5	8.4	9.0	22.0	21.2	15	35.8	33.3
4.0	9.5	9.5	22.8	22.0	20	39.7	37.4
4.5	10.5	10.0	23.6	22.8	25	43.6	41.5
5.0	11.6	10.5	24.4	23.6	30	47.5	45.5
5.5	12.7	11.0	25.2	24.4	35	51.3	49.6
6.0	13.8	11.5	26.0	25.2	40	55.2	53.7
6.5	14.9	12.0	26.8	26.0	45	59.1	57.8
7.0	16.0	12.5	27.6	26.9	50	63.0	61.9
7.5	17.1	13.0	28.4	27.7	55	66.9	66.0
8.0	18.2	13.5	29.2	28.5	60	70.8	70.0
8.5	19.3	14.0	30.0	29.3	65	74.7	74.0
9.0	20.4	14.5	30.8	30.1	70	78.6	78.1
9.5	21.4	15.0	31.6	30.9	75	82.5	82.2
10.0	22.5	15.5	32.4	31.7			
10.5	23.6	16.0	33.2	32.6			
11.0	24.7	16.5	34.0	33.4			

From Altman PL, Dittner DS, eds: *Metabolism,* Bethesda, Md, 1968, Federation of American Societies for Experimental Biology.
*To calculate basal metabolic rate (BMR), determine the age and weight of the patient, read across to appropriate sex, identify metabolic rate (kcal/hr), and multiply metabolic rate by 24 hours. For burn patients, multiply BMR by 1.2 to 1.5 to account for hypermetabolic state of burn injury.

paralytic ileus, an inability to meet caloric needs by other routes, or other gastrointestinal abnormalities making the enteral route impractical. Consideration is given to providing necessary proteins, vitamins, trace elements, and lipids necessary for wound healing and growth.[1]

Comfort Management.   Comfort management is an essential issue in the acute phase, as it was in the emergent phase. Comfort management for the acutely ill child with a large surface area burn is complicated by many factors. The hypermetabolic state of the patient accelerates use of narcotic and anxiolytic medications.[36] Assessing the severity of the child's pain and fear is often difficult because of the child's growth and developmental level, level of consciousness, and ability to communicate. All of these factors influence the nurse's ability to assess the level of discomfort and the child's responses to interventions. Pain assessment tools are useful in helping the alert child to express pain.

Often the child is too ill to express discomfort, and the nurse can only rely on physiologic parameters. This is particularly true if the child has been chemically paralyzed to facilitate mechanical ventilation. Liberal amounts of analgesics and anxiolytic medications are provided. A child with planned interventions including dressing changes, positioning, physical therapy, and chest physiotherapy receives appropriate premedication based on the response to previous interventions.

Intravenous narcotics, particularly morphine sulfate and fentanyl, have become the standard for pain management.

Severe pain requires continuous infusions of intravenous narcotics. For very painful procedures, such as dressing changes, when premedication may not provide adequate comfort or analgesia, bolus doses of narcotics and anxiolytic drugs are used. For the alert school-age child and adolescent, patient-controlled analgesia is effective. Nonpharmacologic pain management strategies, such as distraction, guided imagery, hypnosis, music, and providing the child with opportunities to exercise control, can be effective in the acute phase, as well as in the resuscitative phase. These have been found to be successful adjuncts to the traditional pharmacologic management of pain and anxiety.[36] Their application for a specific child should address the child's growth and developmental level, level of consciousness, and willingness to participate in these strategies, as well as the skill of the nurse or caregiver.

Mobility.   Patients with burns are often immobilized for periods of time, placing them at risk for associated complications. Movement is restricted initially by pain, bulky dressings, and splints. Bed rest and sedation also place the burned child at risk for the hazards of immobility. Later, scar contractures, discomfort of healed wounds, muscle wasting from disuse, and loss of stamina affect the ability to move about comfortably. To maintain optimal physical functioning, the patient's mobility is considered from admission. Active and passive range-of-motion (ROM) exercises are done with every dressing change and throughout rehabilitation and recreational therapy activities. Nursing care involves routine position changes for the patient on bed rest, comfort and protection from nerve damage, and maintenance of joints in extended functional positions.

Physical and occupational therapy consultation and participation in their own daily care can maximize burned children's functioning through the hospital stay and beyond. Involvement in exercise and self-care activities has important short- and long-term benefits for the child. Patients benefit from being out of bed as soon as feasible. Pressure wraps or garments must be applied to grafted legs to help compensate for vascular instability in the newly grafted skin when the child is out of bed or ambulating. Many problems of wound contracture, hypertrophic scarring, and impaired mobility can be limited when these issues are addressed early.

Psychosocial Issues.   Emotional support for the family and patient is critical throughout this prolonged critical illness. Nurses are instrumental in providing this support and in coordinating support from others. The early involvement of social service and mental health professionals is essential in supporting the child and family. Maintaining contact with the child's peers, school teachers, and other members of the community ultimately eases the child's return to a normal life.[2]

As the child begins to recover and passes through critical illness toward rehabilitation, the concerns of the child and family shift toward the child's ability to physically function and the child's ultimate appearance. Children with facial and hand scars have the most difficult time dealing with their changed appearance. The child's body image changes with growth and development, producing new challenges to coping through the different developmental stages. Parents and siblings share these struggles.

For the child who is unable to survive the injury, support for the family becomes the focus of resources. The team's goals are to help them grieve for their lost child and begin to rebuild their lives as they heal their own emotional scars.[37]

Nursing staff and other caregivers need to support themselves and each other through this emotionally draining experience. Establishment of clear boundaries and involvement with patients and families may aid to prevent vicarious trauma and maintain objectivity. Support groups, workshops, and individual discussions help professionals to support the family and care for themselves. Open discussions surrounding the ethical issues that often surround the care of these children are an invaluable resource to the staff who participate.

BURN OUTCOMES

Successive improvements in burn care, technology, regionalization of burn centers, and improved fluid and electrolyte resuscitation have substantially increased survivability of major burn injuries, especially in children. The costs of this improved treatment, in terms of allocation of scarce resources, economic, as well as ethical, have called into question the wisdom of providing maximum care instead of comfort care in patients with massive burn injuries.

Outcomes research, a strategy to provide benchmarks to compare future results with care provided, has recently begun to examine this question. Physical appearance and functional outcomes examined in patients with greater than 80% TBSA burns found that over 80% were independent in basic activities of daily living, indicating that most pediatric burn survivors satisfactorily adapt to their functional limitations even after severe injuries.[38] In addition, the massively burned patients have a quality of life comparable with the age-matched population. This finding also suggests that although the cosmetic and functional impairments may be irreparable and life-lasting, high-quality acute care, skillful multidisciplinary aftercare, and family support can yield positive long-term outcomes for these children.[39]

SUMMARY

The child who sustains a major burn injury faces and overcomes multisystem assault with the help of an interdisciplinary team. A vast array of professionals participates in the effort to restore the child's physiologic and emotional integrity. An essential part of this team is the child's parents, who must help the child with integration into the community and development into a productive member of society. Today, physical survival from devastating burn injury can almost be ensured. The challenge for professionals in the future is to ensure that survival is meaningful for the child, family, and the community.

REFERENCES

1. Herndon DN: *Total burn care,* London, 1996, WB Saunders.
2. Sheridan R, Prelack K, Kadilak P et al: Supplemental parenteral nutrition does not increase mortality in children, *J Burn Care Rehabil* 21:S234, 2000.
3. Tompkins RG, Remensnyder JP, Burke JF et al: Significant reductions in mortality for children with burn injuries through the use of prompt eschar excision, *Ann Surg* 208:577-585, 1988.
4. Bennett B, Gamelli R: Profile of an abused burned child, *J Burn Care Rehabil* 19:88-94, 1998.
5. Hultman CS, Priolo D, Cairns BA et al: Return to jeopardy: the fate of pediatric burn patients who are victims of abuse and neglect, *J Burn Care Rehabil* 19:367-376, 1988.
6. Ramirez RJ, Behrends LG, Blakeney P et al: Children with sensorimotor deficits: a special risk group, *J Burn Care Rehabil* 19:124-127, 1998.
7. Forjuoh SN: The mechanisms, intensity of treatment, and outcomes of hospitalized burns: issues for prevention, *J Burn Care Rehabil* 19:456-460, 1998.
8. Sheridan RL, Ryan CM, Petras L et al: Burns in children younger than two years of age: an experience with 200 consecutive admissions, *Pediatrics* 100:721-723, 1997.
9. American Burn Association: *The advanced burn life support course,* Chicago, 2000, The Association.
10. Nguyen TT, Gilpin DA, Meyer NA et al: Current treatment of severely burned patients, *Ann Surg* 223:14-25, 1996.
11. Rieg LS, Jenkins M: Burn injuries in children, *Crit Care Nurs Clin North Am* 3:457-470, 1991.
12. Rai J, Jeschke M, Barrow RE et al: Electrical injuries: a 30 year review, *J Trauma* 46:933-936, 1999.

13. Rabban JT, Blair J, Rosen CL: Mechanisms of pediatric electrical injury: new implications for product safety and injury prevention, *Arch Pediatr Adolesc Med* 151:696-700, 1997.

14. Zubair M, Besner GE: Pediatric electrical burns: management strategies, *Burns* 23:413-420, 1997.

15. Sheridan RL: Recognition and management of hot liquid aspiration in children, *Ann Emerg Med* 27:89-91, 1996.

16. Weaver LK: Carbon monoxide poisoning, *Crit Care Clin* 15:297-317, 1999.

17. Thorp JW: Hyperbaric oxygen therapy. In Holbrook PR, ed: *Textbook of pediatric critical care,* Philadelphia, 1993, WB Saunders.

18. Demling RH, LaLonde C: *Burn trauma,* New York, 1989, Thieme Medical Publishers.

19. McGee T, Munster A: Toxic epidermal necrolysis syndrome: mortality rate reduced with early referral to regional burn center, *Plastic Reconstr Surg* 102:1018-1022, 1998.

20. Brown DL, Greenhalgh DG, Warden GD: Purpura fulminans: a disease best managed in a burn center, *J Burn Care Rehabil* 19:119-123, 1998.

21. Sheridan RL, Briggs SE, Remensnyder JP et al: The burn unit as a resource for the management of acute nonburn conditions in children, *J Burn Care Rehabil* 16:62-64, 1995.

22. Becker DS: Toxic epidermal necrolysis, *Lancet* 351:1417-1420, 1998.

23. O'Toole G, Peek W, Jaffe D et al: Extracorporeal membrane oxygenation in the treatment of inhalation injuries, *Burns* 24:562-565, 1998.

24. Reper P, Dankaert R, van Hille P et al: The usefulness of combined high-frequency percussive ventilation during acute respiratory failure after smoke inhalation, *Burns* 24:34-38, 1997.

25. Sheridan RL, Huford WE, Kacmarek R et al: Inhaled nitric oxide in burn patients with respiratory failure, *J Trauma* 42:629-634, 1997.

26. Aikawa N, Martyn JAJ, Burke JF: Pulmonary artery catheterization and thermodilution cardiac output determination in the management of critically burned patients, *Am J Surg* 135:811-817, 1978.

27. Goran MI, Broemeling L, Herndon DN et al: Estimating energy requirements in burned children: a new approach derived from measurements of resting energy expenditure, *Am J Clin Nutr* 54:35-40, 1991.

28. Kravitz M: Thermal injuries. In Cardona V, Hurn P, Bastnagel-Mason P et al, eds: *Trauma nursing: from resuscitation through rehabilitation,* ed 2, Philadelphia, 1994, WB Saunders.

29. Helvig E: Pediatric burn injuries, *AACN Clin Issues Crit Care Nurs* 4:433-442, 1993.

30. Sheridan R, Weber J, Prelack K et al: Early burn center transfer shortens the length of hospitalization and reduces complications in children with serious burn injuries, *J Burn Care Rehabil* 20:347-350, 1999.

30a. Sheridan RL, Hinson M, Nackel A et al: Development of a pediatric burn pain and anxiety management program, *J Burn Care Rehabil* 18:455-459, 1997.

31. Monafo WW: Current concepts: initial management of burns, *N Engl J Med* 335:1581-1586, 1996.

32. David JA: *Wound management: a comprehensive guide to dressing and healing,* Springhouse, Pa, 1986, Springhouse Corporation.

33. Prelack K, Cunningham JJ, Sheridan RL et al: Energy and protein provisions for thermally injured children revisited: an outcome-based approach for determining requirements, *J Burn Care Rehabil* 18:177-181, 1997.

34. Rodriguez D: Nutrition in patients with severe burns: state of the art, *J Burn Care Rehabil* 17:62-70, 1996.

35. Hansbrough WB, Hansbrough JF: Success of immediate intragastric feeding of patients with burns, *J Burn Care Rehabil* 14:512-515, 1995.

36. Osgood PF, Szyfelbein SK: Management of burn pain in children, *Pediatr Clin North Am* 36:1001-1013, 1989.

37. Arnold JH, Gemma PB: *A child dies: a portrait of family grief,* Rockville, Md, 1983, Aspen Publications.

38. Meyers-Paal R, Blakeney P, Robert R et al: Physical and psychologic rehabilitation outcomes for pediatric patients who suffer 80% or more TBSA, 70% or more third degree burns, *J Burn Care Rehabil* 21:43-9, 2000.

39. Sheridan RL, Hinson MI, Liang MH et al: Long-term outcomes of children surviving massive burns, *JAMA* 283:69-73, 2000.

30

Toxic Ingestions

Maureen A. Madden

Poisoning continues to be a significant cause of pediatric injury. Five percent of all accidental childhood deaths are related to poisoning. Methods of exposure to toxic agents vary, with ingestions accounting for the majority of exposures.[1] The 1998 Annual Report of the American Association of Poison Control Centers Toxic Exposure Surveillance System reported more than 2 million human exposures to toxins that year. Fifty-three percent of the cases involved children younger than 6 years of age. Males predominated in the ingestions under age 13, whereas teenage cases involved more females.[1] The majority of the 755 fatalities were associated with ingestion and inhalation exposures. Children younger than 6 years accounted for 2.1% of the fatalities, whereas adolescents accounted for 5.9%.

The substances involved most often in human exposure are not the most toxic but the most readily accessible. Some of the more common agents involved in pediatric exposures are cosmetics, cleaning fluids, analgesics, plants, and cough and cold preparations. Toxic effects do not often occur with these substances because children usually do not ingest amounts sufficient to produce toxicity.

Other agents ingested less often but that do not require large exposures to produce toxic effects are barbiturates, clonidine, iron, theophylline, antidepressants, alcohols, cocaine, and caustics. The ingestion of these substances causes the greatest percentage of hospitalizations, intensive care unit (ICU) admissions, and fatalities in pediatric poisonings. Table 30-1 compares the most common with the most toxic substances ingested.

Characteristics that place children at risk of ingestions differ for various age groups. Toddlers are newly mobile, curious, and anxious to explore their environment through reaching, climbing, and tasting. They are without suicidal intent. Usually only one substance is

TABLE 30-1 Most Common Versus Most Toxic Agents Ingested

Most Common*	Most Toxic†
Cosmetics	Analgesics
Cleaning substances	Antidepressants
Analgesics	Stimulants/street drugs
Plants	Cardiovascular drugs
Foreign bodies	Sedatives/Hypnotics
Cough/cold preparations	Alcohols
Topicals	Chemicals
Pesticides/Insecticides	Gases and fumes
Vitamins	Cleaning substances
Antimicrobials	Anticonvulsants
GI preparations	Asthma therapies
Arts/Crafts/Office supplies	Antihistamines
Hydrocarbons	Hydrocarbons
Antihistamines	Automotive products
Hormones and hormone antagonists	Hormones/Hormone antagonists
	Insecticides/Pesticides

From Litovitz TL, Klein-Schwartz W, Caravati EM et al: 1998 Annual Report of the American Association of Poison Control Centers Toxic Exposure Surveillance System, *Am J Emerg Med* 17:435-487, 1999.
*Most common in pediatric exposures for younger than 6 years of age.
†Listed in order of frequency in human exposures.

involved, and the amount ingested tends to be small and nontoxic. Toddlers often present for evaluation soon after ingestion.

An increasing number of significant pediatric exposures in children younger than 6 years of age involve ingestion of a grandparent's or other elderly caretaker's medicine. These agents, often in sustained-release dosage forms, tend to be more toxic to children.

Most adolescent ingestions occur in the home and are intentional rather than accidental. They are associated with academic difficulties, social adjustment problems, failed romances, family issues, or the death of a loved one. Adolescent ingestions commonly involve multiple substances, they are a result of either suicide attempts or substance abuse, and commonly a delay occurs between ingestion and when medical attention is sought.

At present, 65 poison control centers serve 257.5 million of the estimated 270.3 million people living in the United States.[1] Poison control centers have streamlined the most efficient methods of diagnosing and treating poisonings. Other significant contributions made by the centers include education, prevention, research, and legislation. For example, the development of child-resistant containers (resulting from the Poison Prevention Act of 1970) is credited with significant reduction in morbidity and mortality from accidental ingestions, particularly aspirin products.[2]

COMMON PRINCIPLES OF EMERGENCY AND CRITICAL CARE MANAGEMENT

Initial evaluation of the patient in whom a toxic ingestion is known or suspected includes establishing a patent airway, effective ventilatory pattern, and adequate perfusion. Primary measures to stabilize the patient's condition are based on the priorities of resuscitation. In the secondary phase of evaluation, clinical signs that identify the toxin are observed, and appropriate treatment is initiated. Fig. 30-1 provides an algorithm for management of the patient with a known or suspected toxic ingestion.

Toxidromes

After initial evaluation and stabilization, the examination focuses on the assessment of the central and autonomic nervous system; eye findings; changes in skin, oral, and gastrointestinal (GI) mucosa; and odors. These areas represent the ones most likely affected in toxic syndromes. The clinical syndromes, called toxidromes, comprise a constellation of signs and symptoms that suggest a specific class of poisoning. Toxidromes help identify the toxin so that appropriate treatment can be initiated in a timely manner. The most common toxidromes are sympathomimetic, theophylline, sedative/hypnotic, opiate, anticholinergic, and cholinergic.[3-4] Table 30-2 presents the toxidromes with associated symptoms and causative agents.

Identification of Toxin

The goal of identification is to determine which patients are at risk for toxic effects. An additional goal is to minimize intervention for children not at risk for toxic effects because the majority of pediatric ingestions result in no harm to the child.[5] For the vast majority of patients, the clinical condition rather than the specific ingredients of the ingestion directs the management. This approach does not preclude treating specific toxins or toxidromes, but rather enforces the concept of basic clinical management and resuscitation techniques.[6]

A thorough history is obtained, including type and amount of ingestion if known; the possibility of multiple agents; time of ingestion; time of presentation; any history of vomiting, choking, coughing, or alteration in mental status; and any interventions performed before presentation at the medical facility. Regardless of the history of the substance ingested by a child or adolescent, serum and urine toxicology screens may be necessary to rule out the possibility of unknown ingestants. Appropriate laboratory studies include basic serum chemistry studies in symptomatic patients, confirmation of suspected toxins, and the determination for the need of specific antidotal therapy. Toxicologic analysis in children is most valuable to identify serum drug levels, but unexpected findings rarely lead to changes in management.[7,8] Suicide attempts include evaluation for unreported agents, including salicylates and acetaminophen, because most adolescents with suicidal intent are unreliable when reporting ingested

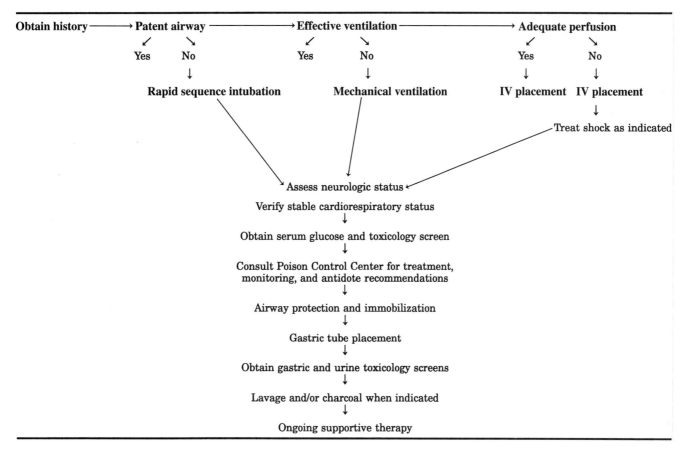

Fig. 30-1   Management of the patient with a suspected toxic ingestion.

TABLE 30-2 Toxidromes		
Toxidrome	**Symptoms**	**Causative Agent**
Sympathomimetic (stimulant)	Restlessness, excessive speech and motor activity, tremor, insomnia, tachycardia, hyperthermia, mydriasis, hallucinations	Amphetamines Phencyclidine (PCP) Cocaine Other stimulants
Theophylline (specific sympathomimetic)	Tachycardia, hypotension, cardiac dysrhythmias, tachypnea, agitation, seizures, vomiting with epigastric pain	
Sedative/Hypnotic	Sedation, confusion, delirium, hallucinations, coma, paresthesia, diplopia, blurred vision, slurred speech, ataxia, nystagmus	Barbiturates Benzodiazepines
Opiate	Altered mental status, miosis, unresponsiveness, shallow respiration, bradypnea, bradycardia, hypotension, decreased bowel sounds, hypothermia	All narcotic agents Heroin Clonidine
Anticholinergic	Fever, flushing, tachycardia, urinary retention, dry skin, blurred vision, mydriasis, decreased bowel sounds, ileus, myoclonus, psychosis, hallucinations, seizures, coma	Some mushrooms Cyclic antidepressants Antihistamines Atropinics Over-the-counter sleep preparations
Cholinergic	Salivation, lacrimation, urination, defecation, emesis, diarrhea, bradycardia	Organophosphates Insecticides Some mushrooms Severe black widow spider bites

agents. There is limited data and information to distinguish lethal concentrations of certain drugs and toxic substances in children.[5,9,10]

The Unknown Toxin

When the name or the amount of a poison ingested is unknown, the incident is unwitnessed, or the history is vague, the child is treated as though a harmful substance was consumed. If elements of the history provided are contradictory or questionable, it is especially important to rule out the possibility of trauma as a cause of the patient's physical injuries. Physical assessment focuses on the potential for unreported traumatic injuries, as well as significant details related to the ingestion, and a clinical presentation that suggests a toxidrome. The availability of antidotes such as naloxone (Narcan), glucose, oxygen, diphenhydramine (Benadryl), physostigmine, digoxin immune Fab (Digibind), methylene blue, deferoxamine, N-acetylcysteine (NAC) (Mucomyst), calcium gluconate, and glucagon is necessary when the ingestion of a toxic substance is suspected.[10,11] The local poison control center can provide details regarding the indications and guidelines for use of these antidotes. Further emergency and critical care management is guided by the principle of simultaneous stabilization, diagnosis, and treatment.

Further management focuses on GI decontamination. Once the ingestant is correctly identified, the management can focus specifically on principles related to that toxin.

Gastrointestinal Decontamination

Reducing the life-threatening potential of an ingested substance is an early treatment goal and depends on the effectiveness of several different treatment modalities. These modalities may include decreasing absorption of the toxin, altering metabolism, increasing elimination of the ingested substance, or administering a specific antidote or other suitable therapy.[12]

Decreasing Absorption

Gastric Emptying. The best gastric emptying technique to employ depends on clinical status. An individualized approach based on the timing of ingestion, type of substance, and amount of the ingested substance in conjunction with the clinical status will dictate treatment decisions.

Gastric emptying is performed when a benefit is anticipated and one of the following conditions exist: the substance does not bind to activated charcoal, it is difficult to remove by gastric lavage (e.g., large pills), the opportunity to use activated charcoal is significantly delayed, or the child presents within 1 hour of ingestion with significant central nervous system (CNS) symptoms. Gastric emptying has limited benefit if attempted more than 1 hour after ingestion because most toxins have already been absorbed or passed through the pylorus. Ipecac-induced emesis and gastric lavage are two techniques used for gastric emptying.

Ipecac, when recommended, is the agent of choice for forced emesis. Ipecac is very useful in the home for immediate treatment of accidental ingestions. However, it is no longer favored in the clinical setting because it causes significant delay in the administration of activated charcoal because of prolonged vomiting. Ipecac acts as both a local gastric irritant and a central stimulant, triggering the vomiting center in the reticular formation. The result is coordinated muscular activity of the stomach and small intestine, producing emesis. Dosages of 10 ml for infants older than 6 months, 15 ml for children 1 to 12 years, and 30 ml for children older than 12 years usually produce emesis in 20 minutes.[13]

Ipecac is contraindicated in infants younger than 6 months of age, with the ingestion of strong caustics (acids or alkalis) or hydrocarbons, and in the presence of neurologic impairment. Other contraindications are loss of the gag reflex and ingestion of agents likely to cause rapid onset of CNS depression or seizures (e.g., clonidine, cyclic antidepressants, lindane, cocaine, and isoniazid).

Gastric lavage evacuates the stomach and augments decontamination in the presence of residual toxins. The substance is flushed through a large-bore nasogastric or orogastric tube (28 to 38 Fr) with room temperature fluids until the yield is clear. The tube size required for effective lavage may be too large for pediatric patients; the largest bore tube, known as an Ewald tube, can be placed only in adolescents. Tracheal intubation precedes lavage for patients in whom the gag reflex is diminished and ability to protect the airway is compromised to avoid the hazards of vomiting and subsequent aspiration.

Gastric lavage is no longer considered the standard of care in pediatric patients. There is a lack of strong clinical evidence supporting the efficacy of lavage in improving outcomes of poisoned patients. But gastric lavage is still recommended if the amount ingested is very large, if presentation takes place within 1 to 2 hours of ingesting agents that delay gastric emptying (e.g., barbiturates, anticholinergic drugs), if sustained-release and insoluble compounds have been ingested, or if the agent is particularly toxic.[2,13,14] Because activated charcoal is very effective, it is given at the initiation of the lavage procedure and possibly repeated at its conclusion. Gastric lavage is contraindicated with caustic and hydrocarbon ingestions.

Activated Charcoal. Activated charcoal reduces absorption of a toxin by binding with it in the GI tract. It is best administered by nasogastric or orogastric tube to small children who may refuse to drink it because of its poor palatability and gritty texture. The commonly recommended dose of 1 g/kg may result in undertreatment with pediatric ingestions, but alternative recommendations depend on knowledge of the amount ingested. If the amount ingested is known, a total charcoal dose is administered, determined by a charcoal to ingestant ratio of 10 g:1 g. The total volume of fluid required to achieve this dose may require division into smaller aliquots (15 to 25 g) given every 1 to 2 hours. The extended dosing regimen may provide for increased efficacy in preventing absorption of sustained-release agents. When the amount of the ingestant is unknown, then a dose of 1 g/kg is recommended. Preparations of 15 g, 25 g, or 50 g of activated charcoal are commercially available. Administration of the entire premixed preparation that most closely approximates the child's weight is reasonable and often meets or exceeds the recommended 1 g/kg dose.

Activated charcoal binds all organic substances but is not effective with alcohols and glycols, hydrocarbons, caustics, heavy metals such as lead, mercury, lithium, and arsenic, or agents with rapid onset.[15] Ideally, charcoal is administered within 2 hours of the ingestion. The first dose of activated charcoal is most effective in children when combined with a properly dosed cathartic such as sorbitol. Once bound to the charcoal, sorbitol propels the toxin rapidly through the intestinal tract, decreasing intestinal transit time. Subsequent doses of activated charcoal are administered without cathartics to avoid severe diarrhea, fluid shifts, and electrolyte abnormalities, resulting in complications such as hypernatremia and seizures.

The patient's ability to tolerate charcoal varies. Charcoal administration is usually followed by periods of vomiting, especially when it has been preceded by ipecac or when given with sorbitol. It is difficult to determine whether nausea has subsided in young children who are unable to completely describe physical symptoms. The potential hazards of vomiting and aspiration are significant for patients with diminished ability to protect the airway, and intubation is indicated before administration of charcoal.

Priorities for patients who receive charcoal include positioning in left lateral decubitus with the head of the bed elevated, ensuring that suction is readily available to protect the airway if vomiting occurs, and immobilizing the child to maintain intravenous patency and the position of the gastric tube. The presence of bowel sounds is assessed before administering charcoal because absent bowel sounds may indicate development of an ileus or obstruction. Charcoal is contraindicated in these situations.

Enhancing Elimination. Multiple-dose activated charcoal has been shown to enhance elimination of certain agents. This is a separate role for activated charcoal in addition to preventing absorption. Repeated dosing has been shown to enhance elimination of toxins by interrupting hepatic recirculation of the ingested drug or its metabolites, adsorbing after initial absorption, or adsorbing toxins secreted across the gastric membrane into the bowel lumen by a GI dialysis effect. This role is well described for several drugs, such as theophylline, phenobarbital, salicylates, carbamazepine, and phenytoin. Drugs in a bound state adsorbed to activated charcoal are nontoxic.[15]

Whole Bowel Irrigation. Whole bowel irrigation has emerged as a new modality to augment gastric decontamination, particularly for sustained-release or enteric-coated preparations, drug-filled packets, and ingestions not adsorbed to activated charcoal (i.e., heavy metals). A polyethylene glycol-balanced electrolyte solution (Golytely or Colyte) hastens the evacuation of substances from the GI tract without creating fluid and electrolyte shifts. The irrigating solution is infused via a nasogastric tube at a rate of 15 to 40 ml/kg/hr and continued until the rectal effluent is clear or until radiopaque toxins disappear or pass into

the cecum on a kidney-ureter-bladder film. Whole bowel irrigation is contraindicated with bowel obstruction, perforation, or ileus.[5]

Alkaline Diuresis. Forced diuresis with alkalinization of urine pH may enhance the removal of toxins that are weak acids via ion trapping. Alkalinization of urine will shift the acid-base equilibrium of weak acids from the uncharged state to ions that do not readily cross cell membranes. This causes the ions to be trapped in the renal tubular lumen, reducing reabsorption and enhancing excretion. Urinary alkalinization is accomplished by administering intravenous sodium bicarbonate until the urine pH approaches 7.5. The intravenous solution is infused at a rate of 1.5 to 2 times maintenance volume for the patient to maintain urine output at a minimum of 2 ml/kg/hr. Alkaline diuresis has been predominately used to enhance elimination of salicylates and phenobarbital.[5,12] This technique is limited by the risk of intravascular volume depletion and potential for excessive alkalinization.

Extracorporeal Methods. Extracorporeal methods of drug removal are useful in certain life-threatening ingestions when substantial absorption of the toxin has already occurred. Methods of extracorporeal drug removal include peritoneal dialysis, hemodialysis, hemoperfusion, and plasmapheresis. The decision to use extracorporeal removal techniques is based on the clinical features of the poisoning. Dialysis or hemoperfusion is considered when the child's condition progressively deteriorates despite intensive supportive therapy. These techniques are highly invasive and have proven to be beneficial with a limited number of toxins.

Dialysis eliminates toxic substances by movement of solutes across a semipermeable membrane as a result of a concentration gradient. The effectiveness of peritoneal dialysis and hemodialysis depends on the molecular weight, lipid-water solubility, protein-binding properties, time of ingestion, and plasma concentration of the toxin. Peritoneal dialysis is far less effective than hemodialysis and is used only occasionally in acute ingestions. Hemodialysis has proven to be effective in enhancing elimination of salicylates, ethylene glycol, methanol, lithium, and isopropanol.[13]

Hemoperfusion involves the passage of blood over an adsorbent matrix material of charcoal or resin. Although hemoperfusion is preferred over hemodialysis for several toxins, hemodialysis is more readily initiated and is often used instead. Hypotension and thrombocytopenia are potential complications of hemoperfusion. Plasmapheresis separates harmful substances from the plasma by continuous centrifugation. Substances that are eliminated best by this method have small volumes of distribution and tight plasma protein-binding properties.

The sections that follow detail the care of children who have ingested potentially harmful toxic substances. Pharmaceutical agents include acetaminophen, barbiturates, carbamazepine, clonidine, iron, theophylline, and cyclic antidepressants. Nonpharmaceutical agents discussed are the alcohols (methanol, ethylene glycol, isopropanol, and ethanol), drugs of abuse (cocaine, heroin, methadone, and phencyclidine [PCP]), and household toxins (caustics and

TABLE 30-3 Systems Most Commonly Affected by Pharmaceutical Toxins

Agent	Systems Involved
Acetaminophen	Hepatic
Barbiturates	Neurologic
	Cardiovascular
	Renal
Carbamazepine	Neurologic
	Cardiovascular
	Hepatic
	Renal
Clonidine	Neurologic
	Cardiovascular
Iron	Cardiovascular
	Neurologic
	Metabolic
	Hepatic
	Renal
	Gastrointestinal
Theophylline	Cardiovascular
	Neurologic
	Gastrointestinal
	Metabolic
Cyclic antidepressants	Neurologic
	Cardiovascular

TABLE 30-4 Systems Most Commonly Affected by Nonpharmaceutical Toxins

Agent	Systems Involved
Alcohols	
Methanol	Neurologic
Ethanol	Neurologic
Isopropyl alcohol	Neurologic
	Cardiovascular
	Gastrointestinal
	Renal
Ethylene glycol	Neurologic
	Cardiovascular
	Respiratory
	Renal
Caustics	Gastrointestinal
Hydrocarbons	Respiratory
	Neurologic
	Cardiovascular
	Hepatic
	Renal

hydrocarbons). Tables 30-3 and 30-4 list these substances and also indicate the body system(s) most often affected.

PHARMACEUTICAL TOXINS

Acetaminophen

Etiology/Incidence. Acetaminophen is used commonly as an antipyretic and analgesic in the pediatric population and is contained in more than 100 products. Its availability in the home makes it more accessible to children than other household products. It is one of the most common drugs associated with intentional and accidental overdoses. Acetaminophen ingestions are potentially more harmful in adolescents than in young children because the quantity consumed is usually greater. Therefore adolescents are two times more likely to manifest toxic blood levels and six more times more likely to develop hepatotoxicity than are young children.[16]

Pathogenesis. Acetaminophen reaches peak serum levels 30 minutes to 4 hours after administration.[17] However, peak plasma levels may not occur with an overdose until 4 or more hours after ingestion, especially with extended release or combination products that include agents that slow gastric motility.

The toxic dose of acetaminophen after a single acute ingestion is 150 mg/kg for children and approximately 7 g for adults. Acetaminophen is rapidly absorbed from the stomach and small intestine and is normally metabolized by

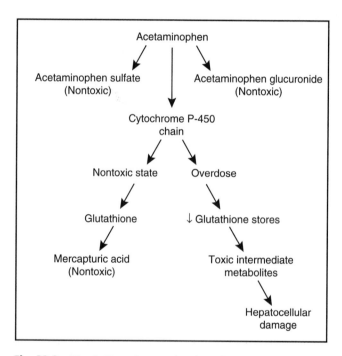

Fig. 30-2 Metabolism of acetaminophen. (From Agran PF, Zenk KE, Romansky SG: Acute liver failure and encephalopathy in a 15 month old infant, *Am J Dis Child* 137:1107-1114, 1983. © American Medical Association.)

conjugation in the liver to nontoxic agents, via sulfate and glucuronide conjugates, which are then eliminated in the urine (Fig. 30-2). Toxic amounts overwhelm the normal pathway of metabolism, resulting in metabolism in the liver through the mixed function oxidase cytochrome P-450 system to a toxic metabolite, *N*-acetyl-p-benzoquinone-imine (NAPQI). Normally, NAPQI, a free radical, is detoxified by conjugation with glutathione to form the nontoxic and renally eliminated mercapturic acid. In overdose, the sulfation increases ultimately causing depletion of glutathione stores. The depletion of glutathione inhibits normal formation of the nontoxic mercapturic acid; the toxic NAPQI accumulates and binds to vital proteins and the lipid bilayer of hepatocytes. This results in hepatocellular death and subsequent centrilobular liver necrosis.[18] Hepatotoxicity becomes evident when aspartate transaminase (AST), alanine aminotransferase (ALT), bilirubin, and prothrombin time (PT) are elevated. There is a delayed toxicity associated with acetaminophen and the elevation in liver function studies is usually not evident until 24 to 72 hours after ingestion.

The course of acetaminophen toxicity is generally divided into four phases. Phase 1 occurs up to the first 24 hours following ingestion. The patient is usually asymptomatic during this phase. The physical assessment of the patient may reveal symptoms including anorexia, nausea, vomiting, malaise, and diaphoresis. Young children often vomit earlier than older children and rarely exhibit diaphoresis. Abnormalities in AST, ALT, bilirubin, PT, or international normalized ratio (INR) are not seen. The risk of toxicity can be determined by plotting a 4-hour-after-ingestion acetaminophen level on the Rumack-Matthew nomogram (Fig. 30-3). This nomogram should not be relied on to accurately assess the risk of toxicity following multiple acetaminophen ingestions, extended-release formulations, chronic ingestions, or coingestion of multiple agents.

Phase 2 occurs 24 to 72 hours after ingestion. The patient may appear to feel better and exhibit decreasing symptoms of phase 1. However, AST, bilirubin, and PT/INR begin to increase and right upper quadrant abdominal pain may occur if antidotal treatment has been delayed or not initiated.

Phase 3 begins 72 to 96 hours after ingestion. Jaundice, coagulopathy, hepatic encephalopathy, recurrence of nausea and vomiting occur with a tender hepatic edge present. Hepatotoxicity is indicated by significantly elevated AST (>1000 IU/L), ALT, bilirubin, PT, and INR. Peak elevation of AST occurs during this phase.

Phase 4 has complete resolution of symptoms or complete resolution of organ failure, occurring typically 7 days to 3 weeks after ingestion. The majority of patients with acetaminophen overdose survive with supportive care in conjunction with antidotal therapy. However, approximately 4% of patients who develop severe hepatotoxicity go on to develop hepatic failure, with less than half resulting in death or transplantation.[18]

Critical Care Management. A reliable history is obtained to determine the time of the poisoning and to rule out the possibility of coingestants. Activated charcoal with sorbitol is recommended to prevent development of a toxic serum level. A serum acetaminophen level is drawn 4 hours after ingestion. If the time of ingestion is unknown or exceeds 8 hours, a level is drawn and empiric antidotal therapy with NAC is initiated.

If the serum level of acetaminophen exceeds 150 mg/L at 4 hours after ingestion (possible hepatic toxicity on the nomogram), NAC (Mucomyst) is administered. NAC acts

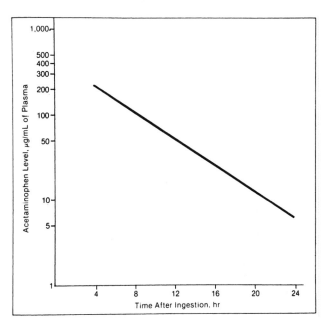

Fig. 30-3 Acetaminophen toxicity nomogram. Area above line indicates probable hepatotoxic reaction. Area below line indicates no hepatotoxic reaction. (From Rumack BH, Peterson RC, Koch CG et al: Acetaminophen overdose, *Arch Intern Med* 141:380, 1981. ©1981, American Medical Association.)

as a chemical substitute for glutathione by providing sulfhydryl groups to detoxify NAPQI so it does not bind to hepatic macromolecules. NAC is diluted to a 5% concentration before administration. It can be mixed with a citrus or carbonated beverage to decrease its pungent smell and is administered orally or by lavage tube. Small children may be at risk of fluid overload or hyponatremia with the 5% dilution. If vomiting occurs within 1 hour after administration, the dose is repeated.

NAC is very effective when administered within 24 hours of toxic acetaminophen ingestion, with optimal benefits seen when administered within 8 hours of ingestion. The initial enteral dose of NAC is 140 mg/kg, followed by 70 mg/kg every 4 hours for a total of 17 doses.[19] It has recently been shown to reduce morbidity and mortality, even if presenting greater than 24 hours postingestion with evidence of hepatotoxicity. The optimal dose or dosing frequency in this situation is unknown, so the conventional dosing guidelines are used. The endpoint of maintenance (70 mg/kg every 4 hours) dosing is resolution of laboratory abnormalities or death. For extended-release acetaminophen, levels are obtained at 4 and 8 hours after ingestion. NAC is initiated if either level is above the lower line on the nomogram. An intravenous form is available in Canada and Europe but is available only as an investigational drug in the United States. Intravenous administration may be indicated if persistent vomiting exists. The 20% NAC enteral preparation may be diluted to a 3% solution with D5W and administered intravenously by filtration through a 0.22-micron filter.[18]

Liver function studies and neurologic status are monitored to assess for signs of hepatic encephalopathy. Altered mental status in the presence of elevated liver enzymes can progress to hepatic coma and death in severe acetaminophen ingestions.

Barbiturates

Etiology/Incidence. Barbiturates are a class of sedative-hypnotic agents and include phenobarbital and pentobarbital. Indications for prescribed use include induction of sleep, sedation, and inhibition of epileptiform activity. Barbiturates are classified according to their duration of action: ultrashort, short, intermediate, or long acting (Table 30-5). In this drug class, barbiturates that are highly lipid soluble have a more rapid onset and a shorter duration of action, as well as a greater degree of hypnotic activity compared with those that are less lipophilic. Duration of action, however, does not correlate with the serum half-life of these medications.[20]

CNS effects are related to the brain tissue concentration of barbiturate. The effect of barbiturates is primarily on the CNS through inhibition of neurotransmission across neuronal and neuroeffector junctions. Therapeutic doses of barbiturates do not produce toxic effects unless used in combination with other medications or alcohol. Approximately three times the therapeutic dose of a barbiturate is necessary to produce the side effects of overdose.

Pathogenesis. Barbiturates have a very narrow therapeutic index (i.e., the difference between an effective dose and a lethal dose is small). Barbiturates are usually taken orally. When taken with liquids, absorption is hastened; when taken with food, absorption is slowed. Serum levels are only somewhat indicative of toxicity because of the discrepancy between plasma and brain tissue concentration. Patients most at risk for death are those who are not treated despite elevated serum levels: greater than or equal to 3 mg/dl for short-acting barbiturates, greater than or equal to 7 mg/dl for intermediate-acting barbiturates, and greater than or equal to 10 mg/dl for long-acting barbiturates.[21] Short-acting barbiturates, particularly those with high lipid solubility, are considered more toxic than the longer-acting forms.[20] Short-acting agents are absorbed in the small intestine and transformed in the liver to inactive metabolites, which are excreted predominantly in urine. Phenobarbital, a long-acting agent, is only partly metabolized in the liver.

TABLE 30-5 Classification of Barbiturates by Duration of Action

Long Acting	Short to Intermediate	Ultrashort
Phenobarbital	Amobarbital	Hexobarbital
Mephobarbital	Butabarbital sodium	Methohexital sodium
Metharbital	Pentobarbital sodium Secobarbital	Thiopental sodium

From Bertino JS, Reed MD: Barbiturate and nonbarbiturate sedative hypnotic intoxication in children, *Pediatr Clin North Am* 33:705, 1986.

At toxic levels, barbiturates primarily act as depressants of the CNS and cardiovascular system. The medication, dose, and route of ingestion influence the effect of the overdose on the child. In addition, children metabolize barbiturates faster than adults. The initial signs and symptoms of toxicity are slurred speech, ataxia, lethargy, nystagmus, headache, and confusion or coma. As toxicity becomes more severe, deep tendon and brain stem reflexes may be depressed, but this usually occurs well after respiratory depression occurs. Shock may occur secondary to medullary depression, peripheral vasodilatation, or diminished myocardial contractility. Other findings may include hypoglycemia, hypothermia, and bullous skin lesions.[20] The child may demonstrate miosis early, with a common late presentation of dilated pupils unresponsive to light. Early deaths occur as a result of respiratory arrest, cardiovascular dysrhythmias, and circulatory collapse, whereas delayed deaths are due to acute renal failure, aspiration pneumonitis, pulmonary edema, and cerebral edema.

Respiratory dysfunction results from depression of the respiratory control centers in the brainstem. The neurogenic drive to breathe may be obliterated and the mechanisms that affect respiratory rhythm may be altered. As respiratory depression continues, hypoxemia and hypercarbia develop. The cough reflex may be suppressed, and the child may experience laryngospasm resulting from inhibition of smooth muscle activity.

Critical Care Management. Management of a patient with a suspected barbiturate overdose, as with any CNS depressant, begins with an assessment and stabilization of the airway. Once the airway is protected, whether with intubation or an active gag reflex, gastric emptying by lavage can be attempted, followed by administration of activated charcoal and a cathartic. If phenobarbital is identified as the toxic agent, multiple doses of activated charcoal may be administered.

If warranted by inadequate gas exchange, the unconscious patient is placed on mechanical ventilation. For the patient who presents in shock, aggressive intravascular volume replacement is begun with crystalloid fluid (20 ml/kg). Assessment for adequate renal function is essential.

Cardiovascular and nervous system dysfunction is treated primarily with supportive care. Temperature is assessed regularly to prevent hypothermia-induced ventricular fibrillation. If the child is hypothermic, the first line of treatment is to prevent further heat loss.

Respiratory dysfunction is managed by ensuring a patent airway and adequate gas exchange. Assessment of arterial blood gases and serum pH guides intervention. The presence of aspiration pneumonitis requires treatment with antibiotic therapy.

Cardiovascular dysfunction treatment includes volume replacement as needed. If volume replacement does not resolve hypotension, continuous infusion of dopamine (1 to 20 μg/kg/min) or dobutamine (2 to 12 μg/kg/min) may be required.

With phenobarbital, alkalinization of the urine (maintaining urine pH >7.5) with sodium bicarbonate is helpful with excretion. This is best accomplished by intravenous administration of 1 to 2 mEq/kg of sodium bicarbonate followed by 2 to 4 mEq/kg over the next 6 to 12 hours. Although, alkalinization without forced diuresis remains common, recent studies comparing multiple-dose activated charcoal to alkalinization have shown that multiple-dose activated charcoal is far more effective in shortening the elimination half-life.[20] It is important to maintain urine output at greater than 1 ml/kg/hr; therefore forced diuresis may be necessary in renal dysfunction. Forced diuresis is accomplished by administration of one or more fluid challenges followed by intravenous furosemide (1 to 2 mg/kg). Overdose of long-acting barbiturates (phenobarbital) may respond well to hemodialysis or hemoperfusion because the lower protein-binding capability allows them to be removed via these techniques. Extracorporeal elimination is considered only for patients whose clinical condition is deteriorating despite aggressive therapy.[22]

Carbamazepine

Etiology/Incidence. Carbamazepine (Tegretol) is used for treatment of partial complex and tonic-clonic seizures, trigeminal neuralgia, and bipolar affective disorder. Carbamazepine inhibits sodium channels by reducing their ability to recover from inactivation, preventing another action potential, thereby raising the seizure threshold. It is structurally related to cyclic antidepressants, exhibiting similar clinical symptoms including CNS and respiratory depression, anticholinergic symptoms, and cardiac conduction abnormalities. Carbamazepine is available for oral administration in tablets, caplets, extended-release, and suspension formulations.

Pathogenesis. A normal therapeutic loading dose of carbamazepine is 5 to 10 mg/kg. Any ingestion above this range is considered toxic. Carbamazepine is lipophilic with an erratic absorption. There is no simple correlation between drug dose and plasma concentration. Peak levels usually do not occur for 3 to 8 hours after ingestion and may occur as long as 24 hours after ingestion with a large overdose. The length of therapy (single dose versus long-term therapy), the patient's age, and interactions with other medications influence plasma drug concentration. Also, children metabolize carbamazepine more rapidly than adults. Carbamazepine metabolism is increased when administered with phenobarbital and phenytoin and decreased with erythromycin. Therapeutic serum concentrations differ, depending on whether carbamazepine is used alone or in conjunction with other medications. For single-drug therapy, a therapeutic level of carbamazepine is 4 to 12 µg/ml. When used with other antiepileptic medications, a serum concentration of 4 to 8 µg/ml is the therapeutic range.[23] Serum levels poorly correlate with toxicity. Treatment of overdose is based on the patient's clinical condition rather than the serum level. Table 30-6 correlates the stages of intoxication with serum levels and signs and symptoms.

Carbamazepine is metabolized by the liver via oxidation and conjugation, into a pharmacologically active metabolite with some inactive products, and excreted in the urine. Carbamazepine exerts some anticholinergic effects, delay-

ing gastric emptying time. Following acute ingestion, the CNS and cardiovascular systems are the most affected, with some hepatic and renal system involvement.

Carbamazepine toxicity produces prominent neurologic signs and symptoms. In mild to moderate toxicity, nystagmus, drowsiness, and ataxia are common.[24] At higher serum concentrations, symptoms in children include dystonia, choreoathetosis, seizures, and stupor. Other clinical symptoms of toxicity include nausea, vomiting, respiratory depression, hypothermia, and coma. The patient's neurologic status may wax and wane following carbamazepine overdose, with increased absorption in stage 4, when normal peristalsis resumes.

Cardiac conduction delays, dysrhythmias, and hypotension indicate cardiovascular system dysfunction. These effects are the result of the fact that carbamazepine chemical structure is similar to that of cyclic antidepressants.

Acute hepatic dysfunction occasionally occurs following carbamazepine overdose. Alteration in renal function may include hyponatremia and syndrome of inappropriate antidiuretic hormone (SIADH). These side effects can be present with long-term administration of carbamazepine and aggravated by overdose.

Critical Care Management. Upon presentation, assessment of the airway is made and stabilization with intubation is performed, especially if CNS depression is present. Emesis is not used with carbamazepine, but gastric lavage may be performed once a secure airway is present and if the child presents within 1 hour of ingestion. Multiple-dose activated charcoal is the therapy of choice in carbamazepine overdose. Repeated doses are recommended because the serum half-life of carbamazepine may be reduced by as much as 50% with this therapy, which decreases enterohepatic recirculation and increases elimination.[25] Catharsis is not recommended because of the potential for increased systemic absorption as a result of increased drug distribution throughout the GI tract.[26]

 TABLE 30-6 Stages of Carbamazepine Overdose With Serum Level and Clinical Signs

Stage	Serum Level	Clinical Signs
I	>25 µg/ml	Stupor or coma, abnormal pupillary reaction to light, respiratory depression
II	15-25 µg/ml	Irritability, combativeness, choreiform movements, hallucinations
III	11-15 µg/ml	Nystagmus, drowsiness, ataxia
IV	<11 µg/ml	Normal mental examination, mild ataxia, may relapse to earlier stages

From Weaver DF, Camfield P, Fraser A: Massive carbamazepine overdose: clinical and pharmacologic observations in five episodes, *Neurology* 38:756-757, 1988.

The need for intensive monitoring is anticipated following significant ingestions of carbamazepine. Children are monitored in the ICU until their condition has remained stable for 24 hours because of the risk of relapse during stage 4 with increased reabsorption. Concretions of carbamazepine are suspected when plasma levels rise or the manifestation of symptoms is delayed.[23] An abdominal radiograph is performed to confirm this diagnosis, and surgical intervention with gastrotomy may be necessary.

Neurologic dysfunction with respiratory depression may require tracheal intubation and mechanical ventilation. The combative patient is protected from injury. Paradoxic seizures may occur with toxic carbamazepine levels and are treated with benzodiazepines or phenobarbital.[27]

Cardiovascular dysfunction is assessed by ECG monitoring for conduction delays and dysrhythmias and hemodynamic monitoring for hypotension. Hypotension is treated with fluid boluses, and if unresponsive to fluid, vasopressors are initiated.

Alteration in hepatic function is assessed by liver function studies. Conventional therapy, including monitoring serum glucose levels and administration of clotting factors for prolonged clotting time, is recommended for hepatic dysfunction. Carbamazepine can be removed by charcoal hemoperfusion, but this therapy is reserved for patients who are not responding to multiple doses of activated charcoal or who are clinically worsening even with aggressive management.[4]

At high carbamazepine levels, vasopressin secretion can be stimulated, leading to fluid retention, SIADH, and hyponatremia. Monitoring of serum electrolytes, particularly sodium and for adequate urinary output, is necessary to identify SIADH. Treatment with water restriction and sodium supplementation is initiated promptly.

Clonidine

Etiology/Incidence. Clonidine is the most commonly used centrally acting antihypertensive and is now indicated for migraine headache prophylaxis; attention deficit/hyperactivity disorder; Tourette's syndrome; and management of opioid, ethanol, and nicotine withdrawal. Clonidine can cause significant toxicity in children. Clonidine centrally stimulates postsynaptic α-adrenergic receptors, which inhibits sympathetic discharge and produces decreased peripheral vascular tone, heart rate, stroke volume, and cardiac output.[28] Clonidine also inhibits uptake of norepinephrine by neuronal tissues, producing CNS depression. Clonidine is available in 0.1-, 0.2-, and 0.3-mg tablets and transdermal patches. The transdermal patches contain 2.5, 5.0, or 7.5 mg of clonidine and are designed to release 0.1, 0.2, or 0.3 mg of clonidine per day over a period of 1 week.[29]

Pathogenesis. Clonidine is well absorbed from the GI tract, metabolized by the liver, and excreted unchanged primarily in urine. Its effects are evident 30 to 60 minutes after ingestion and peak approximately 2 to 3 hours following oral administration, with effects up to 8 hours. Antihypertensive effects are present for as long as 24 hours

following an oral dose. Overdose in children has been documented with as little as a 0.1-mg dose or by dermal exposure, mouthing, or ingestion of a transdermal patch. A discarded transdermal patch contains enough clonidine to produce overdose symptoms in a child.

Clonidine overdose involves an exaggeration of the clonidine pharmacologic properties primarily affecting the CNS and the cardiovascular systems. The majority of children develop symptoms within 1 hour of a clonidine overdose. There is no progression or development of symptoms or toxic effects more than 4 hours after presentation to the hospital.[30]

CNS dysfunction mimics narcotic overdose, where miosis, coma, and respiratory depression are the hallmarks. Symptoms vary from lethargy, somnolence, stupor, or coma, and are postulated to be from inhibition of the uptake of norepinephrine by the neurons, which then blocks noradrenergic activity.[31] Patients who are severely obtunded may have decreased ventilatory effort and hypoxia and may require intubation and mechanical ventilation to maintain adequate respiratory effort. Other CNS symptoms include hypothermia, which is attributed to α-adrenergic receptor stimulation of the serotonin-acetylcholine pathways, causing decreased metabolic heat production and increased heat loss.[29] Cool, pale skin is presumed to be the result of vasoconstriction. Hypotonia, hyporeflexia, and irritability may also be seen.

Cardiovascular system dysfunction depends on the plasma level of clonidine. Serum levels of higher than 10 to 15 mg/ml stimulate the release of norepinephrine, which causes the peripheral α-receptors to vasoconstrict, resulting in transient hypertension. The hypertensive phase is short-lived because clonidine overdose triggers a centrally mediated sympathetic inhibition causing hypotension. Patients with a serum level lower than 10 mg/ml present with normotension or hypotension. Sinus bradycardia, a known side effect, is commonly noted in children with clonidine overdose.[30] Conduction abnormalities including first-degree heart block and second-degree atrioventricular block are seen in both overdose and therapeutic dosing. Patients with underlying conduction dysfunction and the very young are most at risk for sinus bradycardia and conduction delays.[28]

Critical Care Management. If clonidine ingestion is suspected, emesis is contraindicated because of the risk of rapid CNS and respiratory depression. Activated charcoal administration with or without prior gastric lavage can be considered if instituted early. Gastric lavage has limited utility because clonidine is rapidly absorbed and patients typically present following the onset of symptoms.

Appropriate therapy focuses on respiratory and hemodynamic status. Most clonidine overdoses respond well to supportive measures. If hypotension and shock are present, the child is treated with infusion of 20 ml/kg of intravenous fluid and placed in the Trendelenburg position. If signs of shock do not resolve with those measures, an infusion of dopamine (5 to 10 µg/kg/min) is begun.

Patients usually require supportive and symptomatic treatment in the critical care setting for less than 24 hours following clonidine overdose. Careful monitoring of vital signs, including temperature, is necessary. Hypothermia is treated with passive rewarming to maintain a normal body temperature. Tracheal intubation and mechanical ventilation are instituted if respiratory effort is absent or inadequate to maintain normal serum oxygen and carbon dioxide levels. Control of the airway protects the child from aspiration and subsequent respiratory compromise.

Cardiovascular dysfunction treatment is based on the child's symptoms. Bradycardia associated with cardiovascular compromise is responsive to intravenous atropine (0.10 mg/kg); although repeated doses may be necessary because of the long half-life of clonidine.[28,30] Hypotension is treated first with volume infusion, and then with dopamine infusion, as described in the initial management section. Treatment with a nitroprusside infusion (0.5 to 0.8 µg/kg/minute) is instituted for a hypertensive phase only if end-organ compromise is noted. Dysrhythmias resolve with decreasing serum clonidine levels and usually do not require treatment.

Naloxone (Narcan) is recommended for treatment of all patients with clonidine overdoses in which CNS, cardiovascular, or respiratory depression is present.[32] Naloxone was first used because of the similarity in clonidine overdose symptoms to opioid toxicity. The interaction between clonidine and opioid receptors is poorly understood, but several patients experiencing clonidine overdose have responded well to naloxone. The initial naloxone dose is 0.01 mg/kg, and if no response is noted, a repeat dose of 0.1 mg/kg is administered. A continuous infusion of naloxone may be necessary secondary to its short half-life.

Iron

Etiology/Incidence. Iron ingestion is one of the more common childhood ingestions because of the availability of iron and iron-containing compounds in the household. The similarity of colors, shapes, and flavorings between multivitamins and other iron-containing products and candy makes them especially enticing to children. Iron supplementation is prescribed for pregnant women, and iron is a common component in both pediatric and adult multivitamins. Elemental iron is available in combination with gluconate, sulfate, or fumarate salts; each preparation has varying amounts of elemental iron. Cases of iron ingestion rarely require intensive care management if toxicity is recognized and treated promptly. Iron supplements used to be the leading cause of fatal ingestions in children, but the incidence is now declining. The Food and Drug Administration (FDA) mandates that all iron-containing preparations display a warning label to inform of potential toxicity for children with accidental overdose.

After ingestion in normal doses, 10 to 15 mg of iron is absorbed daily through the GI tract.[33] Ferrous iron is absorbed into the mucosal cells of the duodenum and jejunum and is oxidized to ferric iron, where it is bound to ferritin, an iron storage protein. It is then released into the plasma, where it is bound to transferrin, an iron-specific binding globulin. Iron bound to transferrin is nontoxic.

With acute iron overdose, the total serum concentration of iron exceeds the total iron-binding capacity. Excess free iron is directly toxic to the vasculature and leads to the release of vasoactive substances including serotonin and histamine. Excess quantities of ferritin lead to vasodilation resulting in increased vascular permeability and fluid loss, with subsequent hypotension and metabolic acidosis.[34] The free iron is deposited in the liver, spleen, and kidneys. These iron deposits cause pathophysiologic changes in the mitochondria, result in free radical formation and lipid peroxidation that contribute to necrosis, cell death, and tissue injury.[4] Metabolic acidosis develops as a result of poisoning of the mitochondria, compromising cellular respiration and producing lactic acidosis. Serum iron levels peak 2 to 4 hours following ingestion, and begin to fall 6 hours after ingestion. Table 30-7 shows the correlation between serum iron levels and toxicity. An iron concentration higher than 350 µg/dl is indicative of moderate to severe toxicity.[35]

Pathogenesis. The pathophysiology of iron toxicity is related to the development of metabolic acidosis. Iron toxicity is mediated through both local and systemic effects. Acute iron poisoning in children follows the classic five clinical stages of iron toxicity. The initial stage begins from 30 minutes after ingestion to no later than 6 hours and is the result of the corrosive effects of iron on the GI mucosa. The child complains of nausea and moderate to severe abdominal pain and presents with vomiting, diarrhea, or GI hemorrhage. Vomitus and stools may be dark gray or black because of the presence of iron. In severe poisoning, the child may present with hypotension, shock, and coma. If a child presents in coma shortly following an iron ingestion, the prognosis for neurologic recovery is poor.[36]

The second phase of iron toxicity is described as the latent stage. The child is asymptomatic, with mild lethargy present. It is a deceptive period that occurs 6 to 24 hours postingestion, but this phase may be absent in children with severe poisoning.

Profound toxicity is evident with patients who progress to the third phase, 12 to 48 hours after ingestion. Shock results from the free iron, causing venous pooling, which creates relative hypovolemia, vasodilatation, and poor

Table 30-7 Serum Iron Level and Potential Severity of Intoxication

Serum Iron Level	Potential Toxicity
<100	None
100-350	Minimal toxicity
350-500	Moderate toxicity; chelation usually not necessary
500-1000	Severe toxicity; start chelation immediately
>1000	Potentially lethal; start maximum chelation immediately

From Henretig FM, Temple AR: Acute iron poisoning in children. *Clin Lab Med* 4:579, 1984.

cardiac output. Subsequent poor perfusion and ischemia results in a worsening metabolic acidosis. An iron-induced coagulopathy may cause increased bleeding and exacerbate hypovolemia. Systemic signs of toxicity include lethargy, hyperventilation, hypoglycemia, seizures, and coma.

The fourth stage of iron toxicity consists of hepatic injury or failure. This may occur 2 to 3 days after severe iron ingestion. It is thought to be a direct result of uptake of iron by the liver's reticuloendothelial system. Alterations in glucose metabolism, coagulopathies, and hepatic encephalopathy accompany hepatic failure.

The final stage occurs days to weeks after the iron overdose and only rarely occurs. The initial gastric insult can progress to gastric outlet obstruction secondary to development of strictures, stenosis, or scarring.[34]

Critical Care Management. Toxicity is dependent on the amount of elemental iron ingested. Ingestion of more than 20 mg/kg of elemental iron produces GI effects; ingestion of more than 60 mg/kg causes systemic toxic effects; and ingestion more than 250 mg/kg is potentially lethal. Iron levels may not correlate with amount ingested and clinical symptoms. Children who ingest greater than 20 mg/kg or who are symptomatic, regardless of serum level, need to be treated. Following stabilization of the airway, breathing, and circulation, GI decontamination procedures are considered. Activated charcoal does not bind to iron and therefore is not utilized. Gastric emesis may have limited benefit in a child who has already vomited several times and may obscure the severity of toxicity based on GI symptoms. Gastric lavage to remove pills and fragments may be ineffective if the tablets are large or several hours have elapsed since ingestion. If lavage is used, only normal saline or tap water is used. Other compositions, including sodium bicarbonate, have been studied as lavage solutions. They have not shown any greater benefit, and potential risks with electrolyte imbalances have limited their utility.[34]

Whole bowel irrigation has become the standard of care for severely poisoned patients with large GI burdens of iron. After lavage, an abdominal radiograph is obtained to document the presence of retained iron tablets in the stomach and pylorus. If present, irrigation with polyethylene glycol electrolyte lavage solution (Golytely) enhances stooling while quickly emptying iron from the GI tract.[37] This solution is instilled at room temperature into the stomach via nasogastric tube at 250 to 500 ml/hour for children younger than 5 years and up to 2 L/hour for adolescents. Whole bowel irrigation continues until diarrhea is produced and the effluent resembles the infusate. If lavage and whole bowel irrigation are unsuccessful in removing intact iron tablets, emergency gastrotomy may be considered.[35]

Chelation therapy, which binds iron into a soluble complex, is initiated in the emergency department after a baseline urine sample is obtained, with intravenous deferoxamine at a maximum dose of 15 mg/kg/hour for children in whom severe intoxication is suspected. The daily maximum recommended dose is 360 mg/kg/day, with a limit of 6 g. Hypotension may occur with the infusion of deferoxamine and may limit the rate of infusion. Deferoxamine combines with iron to form ferrioxamine, which is excreted by the renal system; it appears that deferoxamine cannot remove iron once bound to transferrin but can chelate free iron and iron being transported between transferrin and ferritin.[33,34] The urine changes to "vin rose," a pink color, shortly after chelation begins. Serum iron levels are followed during chelation therapy. Chelation is discontinued when the serum iron level falls below 100 µg/dl, the child appears clinically well, the anion-gap acidosis has resolved, and there is no further urine color change.[36]

Initial laboratory studies include complete blood count (CBC); serum electrolytes including glucose, renal, and hepatic function; blood type and cross-match; total iron-binding time; a serum iron level 2 to 6 hours after ingestion; and coagulation studies. These values help to guide management, especially for the child who is asymptomatic at presentation. Initial management also includes close monitoring for the known side effects of iron toxicity. Intravenous access is obtained in any child with suspected moderate to severe toxicity so that hypotension, metabolic acidosis, hypoglycemia, and blood dyscrasias can be treated promptly. Continuous monitoring of the adequacy of the child's airway, breathing, and circulation, particularly blood pressure, is necessary.

Patients who manifest clinical signs and symptoms of toxicity, such as metabolic acidosis, hemodynamic instability, and lethargy, are managed in an ICU and are discharged only after 24 hours of clinical stability following therapy. Cardiovascular assessment includes central venous pressure monitoring to provide a guide to the patient's volume status and fluid management. Periodic assessment of serum hemoglobin and hematocrit levels is necessary to track blood loss via the GI tract. All stools and emesis are tested for presence of blood. Blood loss via stools or emesis is replaced. Volume replacement with blood components or other fluids is initiated early in the treatment of hypotension. Intravenous infusion of catecholamines, such as epinephrine (0.2 to 2.0 µg/kg/min) or dopamine (1 to 20 µg/kg/min), may be required to treat hypotension that is refractory to volume replacement.

Neurologic dysfunction management is primarily supportive. If the child has inadequate cough or gag reflexes, tracheal intubation is performed and mechanical ventilation instituted. Acid-base balance is assessed by serial measurement of serum pH and bicarbonate ions. Intravenous sodium bicarbonate is administered as necessary to treat metabolic acidosis.

Hepatic failure requires assessment and treatment of hypoglycemia and coagulopathy. Hypoglycemia is treated with intravenous infusion of dextrose-containing solutions, the concentrations of which are titrated to maintain the serum glucose level above 80 to 100 mg/dl. Increased PT, partial thromboplastin time (PTT), or clinical signs of bleeding are treated with infusion of the appropriate clotting factors.

Renal function is assessed by hourly measurement of urine output and periodic monitoring of specific gravity, blood urea nitrogen (BUN), and serum creatinine. If acute renal failure occurs, continuous hemofiltration or hemodialysis can be used to remove ferrioxamine, as well as other metabolic end products.[34] Renal transplantation may be necessary if the renal system does not recover following iron toxicity.

GI dysfunction is monitored by serial assessment of abdominal girth and tenseness and for the presence of blood in gastric contents and stool. H_2 blockers may be administered to protect the upper GI tract. If GI perforation is suspected, the child requires an exploratory laparotomy to identify and manage areas of necrosis. Peritonitis is treated with appropriate antibiotic therapy. All severe iron overdoses require follow-up several weeks after ingestion to evaluate for GI complications, such as strictures and stenosis, which may require surgical intervention.

Theophylline

Etiology/Incidence. Theophylline is most commonly used in children as a bronchodilator to relieve bronchospasm associated with asthma. The therapeutic serum level ranges from 10 to 20 mg/L. Each 1 mg/kg of theophylline raises the serum level by 2 mg/L. Theophylline is available in liquid, capsule, tablet, and suspended-release preparations. Maintenance dosages vary with each child based on weight, concentration of the preparation, and extent of illness. Theophylline toxicity is characterized by serum levels higher than 20 mg/L. Acute toxicity is affected by the type of preparation ingested, route of exposure, age-related clearance rate, and drug and nondrug interactions. The toxic effects following chronic overdose do not correlate with serum drug levels. Precipitating factors associated with theophylline overdoses include dosage errors, accidental ingestions, suicide attempts, respiratory tract infections, or erythromycin administration.[38]

Pathogenesis. Pharmacologic properties of theophylline include CNS stimulation, positive chronotropic and inotropic effects, antagonizing adenosine activity, reduction of peripheral arteriolar resistance, relaxation of bronchial smooth muscle, inhibition of mast cell degranulation, increase in renal blood flow and glomerular filtration rate, and increases in gastric acid and pepsin secretion. These processes are accelerated in situations when theophylline toxicity occurs. Theophylline toxicity primarily affects the GI tract, CNS, and cardiovascular system.[4] The most common symptoms of theophylline toxicity include nausea and vomiting, tachydysrhythmias, seizures, hypotension, metabolic acidosis, and hypokalemia. Severe toxicity will also produce hematemesis and bloody diarrhea.

Patients are at risk from the cardiac effects with severe overdoses secondary to excessive catecholamine stimulation of the myocardium exacerbated by hypokalemia, hypocalcemia, hypophosphatemia, metabolic acidosis, and an increased myocardial oxygen demand. Altered cardiac output results from supraventricular dysrhythmias such as sinus tachycardia, atrial tachycardia, atrial flutter, and atrial fibrillation. Ventricular dysrhythmias may develop, but sustained dysrhythmias that require prolonged therapy are rare. Serious dysrhythmias occur most often in young patients with acute theophylline overdoses when serum levels exceed 50 µg/ml.[39] Theophylline's β_2 effects, which

reduce peripheral vascular resistance, are responsible for severe hypotension and reduced myocardial perfusion associated with toxicity.

CNS disturbances include agitation, headache, confusion, tremulousness, hyperreflexia from cerebral excitation, and seizures. In acute intoxication, seizures are infrequent and are usually focal and brief. Theophylline causes an increase of cyclic adenosine monophosphate (cAMP) by inhibiting the activity of phosphodiesterase, the enzyme responsible for metabolizing cAMP. This results in smooth muscle relaxation, peripheral vasodilation, myocardial stimulation, and CNS excitation.

Other metabolic disorders that may result from theophylline overdose are hyperglycemia from increased gluconeogenesis, and glycogenolysis caused by catecholamine release. Hypokalemia occurs early and is the result of potassium moving into the cells secondary to hyperglycemia, loss of potassium through vomiting, and the diuretic action of theophylline. All of these may contribute to the cardiac dysrhythmias.[38]

Critical Care Management. In severe overdose, gastric lavage and activated charcoal with a cathartic may both be used, up to 4 hours after ingestion with regular preparations and up to 8 to 12 hours after ingestion of sustained-release preparations. Emesis is not typically employed because of rapid onset of seizures and protracted vomiting caused by toxicity. If vomiting inhibits the instillation of activated charcoal, an antiemetic may be administered because activated charcoal is very effective in reducing serum theophylline levels. For severe intoxication, multiple-dose charcoal has been indicated. Initial laboratory studies necessary are theophylline level at presentation, followed by repeat levels in 2 to 4 hours, serum electrolytes, glucose, calcium, and baseline coagulation studies. Seizures are treated with a benzodiazepine followed by phenobarbital if the seizure does not resolve. It may be necessary to intubate the child and to provide ventilatory support and neuromuscular blockade to help control the seizure activity.[38]

Priorities include monitoring for cardiac dysrhythmias. The patient's electrolytes are carefully evaluated over time and rapidly corrected if a dysrhythmia develops. These dysrhythmias usually resolve spontaneously as the theophylline level returns to the therapeutic range. If the patient is unstable or not tolerating the dysrhythmia, treatment with low doses of propranolol (0.02 mg/kg IV) repeated every 5 to 10 minutes (with a maximum of 0.1 mg/kg IV) is recommended.[40] The desired response to propranolol when treating hypotension, sinus tachycardia, atrial fibrillation, and rapid ventricular rates is a return to the patient's baseline parameters for blood pressure and cardiac rhythm. Esmolol is another effective agent currently under investigation for use with theophylline toxicity.[38] One case study reports effective treatment of tachycardia and hypotension with administration of intravenous esmolol, an ultra–short-acting β-blocker, in a 500-µg/kg bolus over 1 minute, followed by a 50-µg/kg/min continuous infusion.[41] Propranolol and other nonselective β-blockers are used cautiously in asthmatic patients because they may cause bronchospasm.

Maintaining seizure precautions and ongoing assessment of level of consciousness is necessary to limit the degree of cerebral anoxia caused by seizure activity. Because a correlation exists between the length of seizure activity and morbidity and mortality, seizures are controlled as soon as possible. Lorazepam (0.05 mg/kg IV) is indicated for immediate cessation of seizure activity and is administered with phenobarbital (10 mg/kg) for continued seizure control.

The effectiveness of antiemetics in theophylline toxicity is variable. Recommendations include the use of metoclopramide (2 mg/kg IV) or ranitidine (1 to 2 mg/kg/day IV) to control vomiting and increase the tolerance of charcoal. Metoclopramide and ondansetron may be more beneficial because they promote gastric motility and do not lower the seizure threshold. Multidose activated charcoal is typically used rather than whole bowel irrigation because of the risk of irrigation decreasing the effectiveness of the charcoal. However, whole bowel irrigation is beneficial with ingestion of sustained-release preparations.

Hemoperfusion is effective at enhancing the elimination of theophylline and is instituted early in treatment, when patients with protracted vomiting do not allow the instillation of charcoal. Indications for hemoperfusion include unstable hemodynamics, uncontrolled seizures, inability to give charcoal despite antiemetic therapy with persistent elevation in theophylline levels after 6 to 8 hours, extensive hematemesis, serum theophylline levels between 40 and 60 µg/ml in chronic overdoses or 90 and 100 µg/ml in acute overdoses.[4] In some circumstances, it may be beneficial to perform whole bowel irrigation and charcoal hemoperfusion simultaneously. The patient is assessed for signs of thrombocytopenia, hypocalcemia, and infection at the catheter insertion site when hemoperfusion is in progress.

Other interventions include administration of potassium, phosphate, and sodium bicarbonate with subsequent monitoring of laboratory values to evaluate the resolution of toxic effects.

Cyclic (Tricyclic) Antidepressants

Etiology/Incidence. The cyclic antidepressants are the most widely prescribed pharmacologic treatment for depression in adults and children. Tricyclic antidepressants are one type of this class of drugs. The cyclic antidepressants can be divided into the first-generation and second-generation antidepressants. The first-generation, or tricyclic, antidepressants were developed in the 1960s. The second-generation cyclic antidepressants were released during the 1980s and 1990s to improve the therapeutic index, decrease side effects and adverse reactions, and reduce the incidence of serious toxicity. As the mechanisms of action have become more selective, the incidence of cardiac and neurologic toxicity has decreased. In addition to depression, children also are prescribed cyclic antidepressants for treatment of hyperkinesis, sleep disorders, school phobias, and enuresis. Adults are prescribed cyclic antidepressants for depression, chronic pain, and sleep disorders. The more com-

mon tricyclics include amitriptyline (Elavil), desipramine (Norpramin), imipramine (Tofranil), whereas the second-generation antidepressants include amoxapine (Asendin), fluoxetine (Prozac), sertraline (Zoloft), paroxetine (Paxil), and bupropion (Wellbutrin).

Pathogenesis. When ingested, cyclic antidepressants are initially rapidly absorbed from the GI tract, unless anticholinergic effects decrease the rate of absorption by slowing GI motility. The drugs have large volumes of distribution and are largely protein bound. The drugs bind to proteins at a certain pH, typically a more alkaline pH; therefore acidemia may increase the amount of unbound or free drug in the plasma. Serum levels are of little use in overdose because of the extent of protein binding and volume of distribution. These drugs are highly lipid soluble, sparingly water soluble and extensively metabolized on the first pass through the liver.[42] Cyclic antidepressant toxicity primarily affects the central nervous and cardiovascular systems accompanied by anticholinergic crisis. Toxicity is mediated by anticholinergic effects, quinidine-like effects on cardiac function, direct α-receptor blockade, and inhibition of catecholamine reuptake in the CNS and peripheral nervous system. A quinidine-like effect is the membrane depressant effect on the myocardium through inhibition of sodium channels. Symptoms of toxicity develop within 4 to 6 hours but may be delayed for up to 24 hours.[43]

Cyclic antidepressant toxicity may progress rapidly, initially presenting with anticholinergic signs and progressing to lethal dysrhythmias and hypotension. Anticholinergic effects on the CNS include respiratory depression, agitation, lethargy, hallucinations, hyperthermia, ataxia, choreoathetoid movements, seizures, and coma. Peripheral anticholinergic effects include hypotension, decreased GI motility, dry and flushed skin, urinary retention, sinus tachycardia, mydriasis, and hyperreflexia.[42,44,45] Seizures occur in 10% to 20% of patients with tricyclic antidepressant overdose and are most likely to occur in comatose patients.[46]

Cardiovascular dysfunction often accompanies cyclic antidepressant overdose because of the increase in the polarization period. Decreased cardiac output may occur as a result of myocardial depression or dysrhythmias. Cyclic antidepressant's quinidine-like effects slow cardiac conduction and causes myocardial depression, prolonging the PR and QRS interval. These measurements should use the standard lead for pediatric QRS measurement, the precordial lead V_5. The widened QRS interval provides the best measurement of tricyclic antidepressants, with an interval of more than 100 milliseconds seen as evidence of serious overdose (Fig. 30-4). Increased repolarization time facilitates ventricular tachycardia, ventricular fibrillation, or asystole.[44] Decreased inotropy is evidenced with general signs of decreased cardiac output and hypotension.

Seizures and coma with severe overdose dominate neurologic dysfunction. Respiratory failure can occur from CNS depression, seizure-related apnea, upper airway obstruction, or pulmonary edema. Because acidosis increases the amount of free drug in the serum, even mild hypoventilation may potentiate dysrhythmias and aggravate the poor inotropic performance of the myocardium.

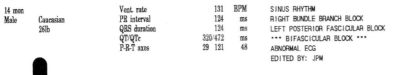

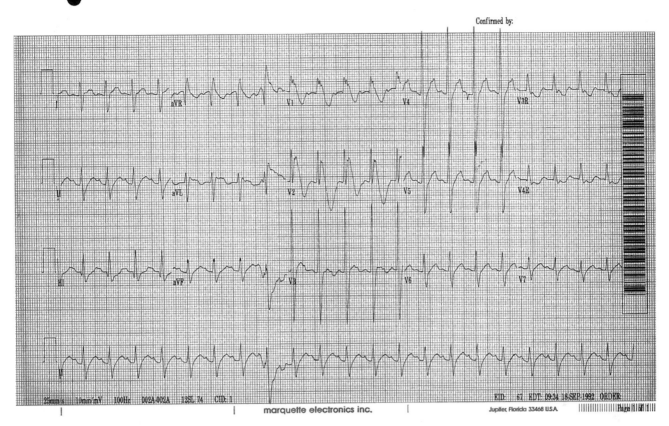

Fig. 30-4 Electrocardiogram in a patient with a prolonged QT interval following tricyclic antidepressant overdose.

Critical Care Management. Cyclic antidepressant overdose is suspected if a child presents in coma or with symptoms compatible with anticholinergic crisis. Initial interventions are to secure an airway and stabilize vital signs. Symptoms of toxicity develop rapidly after ingestion with deterioration in clinical status occurring within 1 hour after ingestion and life-threatening events most often occurring within 2 hours.[42] Emesis is contraindicated because of the rapid onset of CNS depression or seizures. Lavage is indicated for patients with altered level of consciousness. Following lavage, activated charcoal and a cathartic are recommended. Intubation is recommended before gastric decontamination to minimize the risk of aspiration. Because of the tight protein binding, hemoperfusion, hemodialysis, and forced diuresis have no role in the management. Alkalinization of the serum is the preferred method for reducing acute cardiovascular side effects. A sodium bicarbonate infusion alters the pH, increasing protein binding of the drug and reducing the amount of free drug available, resulting in decreased toxicity.

Primary treatment of respiratory dysfunction is directed toward achieving and maintaining the patency of the airway. Intubation and mechanical ventilation are initiated promptly for patients in whom oxygenation and ventilation are at risk. Arterial blood gases are assessed for both hypoxia and acidosis because these problems are known to increase the frequency and recurrence of dysrhythmias.

Cardiovascular dysfunction may result in hypotension. Treatment begins with a 20 ml/kg fluid bolus of normal saline or lactated Ringer's solution. If these measures are ineffective in returning the blood pressure to normal range, a continuous infusion of phenylephrine (0.1 to 0.5 µg/kg/min), norepinephrine (0.05 to 1.0 µg/kg/min), or dopamine (5 to 30 µg/kg/min) may be required.[42,44] These medications exert predominantly direct α-agonistic effects and counteract the α-adrenergic blockade of the cyclic antidepressants.

Treatment of dysrhythmias begins with ensuring adequate ventilation, followed by sodium bicarbonate infusion. Mild metabolic alkalosis (pH >7.45 to 7.55) has proven to be effective in narrowing widened QRS complexes, correcting hypotension, and in decreasing the incidence of dysrhythmias in cyclic antidepressant overdoses.[4,33] Hyperventilation to induce respiratory alkalosis is thought to be less effective for controlling dysrhythmias. Serum sodium levels are monitored during and following administration of sodium bicarbonate. If sodium bicarbonate therapy is ineffective for controlling dysrhythmias, lidocaine (1 mg/kg IV) is given as a bolus and followed with a continuous infusion (10 to 50 μg/kg/minute).

Seizures or coma can manifest neurologic dysfunction. Diazepam (100 to 250 μg/kg IV over 3 minutes) is the drug of choice for immediate use in cyclic-related seizures. Seizures are usually brief and respond to benzodiazepines. If the patient fails to respond to benzodiazepines, barbiturates or propofol may be used. Phenytoin is not recommended because of its limited efficacy and data suggesting prodysrhythmic effects. Coma usually resolves within 24 hours of ingestion.

Parasympathetic nervous system dysfunction requires intervention as necessary. Urinary retention, evidenced by bladder distension, may require placement of an indwelling catheter. Constipation may result from slowed peristalsis, although the use of activated charcoal and cathartics may promote elimination and relieve this symptom. It is important to assess the patient for the presence of active bowel sounds before the administration of charcoal because paralytic ileus is common and is a contraindication to its use. Patients are monitored in an intensive care setting on a cardiac monitor until symptom free for 24 hours.

NONPHARMACEUTICAL TOXINS—THE ALCOHOLS AND DRUGS OF ABUSE

Methanol

Etiology/Incidence.   Methanol, also known as wood alcohol, is a colorless, flammable liquid with a distinctive, somewhat pleasing odor. It is a common component of household substances such as windshield washer fluid, antifreeze, carburetor fluid, Sterno fuel, varnishes, solvents, gasohol, moonshine, duplicating fluids, and paint stripper or remover. Methanol itself is not toxic but its metabolites are; therefore early recognition of toxicity is imperative. Methanol is potentially toxic with ingestion of only a single mouthful.

Pathogenesis.   Methanol is completely absorbed by the GI tract with peak levels 30 to 90 minutes after ingestion. Once absorbed, approximately 85% to 90% of methanol is metabolized in the liver and the remainder is excreted unchanged through the lungs and kidneys. Methanol is metabolized by the hepatic alcohol dehydrogenase pathway and creates the toxic metabolites, formaldehyde, and formic acid. Formic acid, the principal metabolite, inhibits mitochondrial respiration, which results in tissue hypoxia and lactic acidosis. The toxic formic acid accounts for the majority of the anion gap, metabolic acidosis, and ocular toxicity. Formaldehyde has a short half-life, lasting only minutes. Formic acid is much more slowly metabolized and degradation is folate dependent, so it bioaccumulates and is responsible for the toxic effects seen.[17,47,48] Methanol

toxicity produces a triad of symptoms affecting the GI, CNS, and ocular systems.

There is an asymptomatic latent period of 24 to 72 hours after methanol ingestion, which is shortened when large amounts are ingested. The latent period occurs while the toxic metabolites accumulate and it may be prolonged with coingestion of ethanol. The initial symptoms include headache, lethargy, dizziness, nausea, vomiting, and abdominal pain. Visual disturbances and severe acidosis develop after these initial symptoms. The visual complaints include decreased visual acuity, hazy vision, photophobia, and snowstorm-like "snowflakes" in the visual field.

Initially, there is little CNS depression and the child may appear anxious with dyspnea or Kussmaul's breathing. If untreated, the metabolites increase, causing severe metabolic acidosis and the patient's level of consciousness deteriorates from lethargy progressing to coma.

The vision dims with advanced optic nerve toxicity, and hyperemia of the optic disks, retinal edema, and fixed dilated pupils may be present. The accumulation of formic acid causes optic papillitis, retinal disease, and optic atrophy, all of which can result in permanent blindness.[27]

Patients who develop coma, convulsions, and apnea have a poor prognosis. Death usually results from circulatory collapse or respiratory arrest.

Critical Care Management.   Methanol ingestion results in an elevation in the osmolal gap because it alters the volume of water in serum accompanied by an increased serum anion gap and hypoglycemia.[47] Osmolal gap is defined as the difference between measured and calculated osmolality. Early in a patient's clinical course (under 12 to 24 hours), before methanol has been completely metabolized, rapid diagnosis of methanol toxicity can be made on the basis of the presence of an osmolal gap (Box 30-1). Calculated osmolality is subtracted from measured osmo-

---

Box 30-1
Calculation of Anion and Osmolal Gaps

Anion gap = (Na + K) − (Cl + HCO$_3$)
   (Normal anion gap = 12-16 mmol/L)
Example: (135 + 4) − (102 + 22)
   = 139−124
   = 15
Elevated anion gap: (148 + 4) − (100 + 18)
   = 152−118
   = 34
Osmolal gap = Measured osmolality − Calculated osmolality
   (Normal osmolal gap ≤10 mOsm/kg)
   Normal measured osmolality = 285-290 mOsm/kg
   Calculated osmolality = (2Na) + (glu/18) + (BUN/2.8)
Example: (2 × 138) + (108/18) + (14/2.8)
   = 276 + 6 + 5
   = 287
Elevated osmolal gap: >10 mOsm/kg
   = measured − calculated osm
   = 299 − 287
   = 12

lality and normally does not exceed 10 mOsm/kg. The elevated osmolal gap gradually resolves as methanol is metabolized, toxic metabolites form, and an anion gap metabolic acidosis develops.[48]

Under normal circumstances, the anion gap is 12 to 16 mmol/L. An elevated anion gap occurs later in the clinical course of patients with methanol ingestion because of retention of nonvolatile organic acids. Calculation of the osmolal and anion gap is useful for the initial management of patients in whom methanol ingestion is suspected because it identifies the presence of harmful substances, therefore eliminating delay in treatment while specific laboratory levels are awaited. For a patient who is symptomatic, is acidotic, or has a peak level of 20 mg/dl of methanol, treatment is initiated with an ethanol infusion.

Patients who appear neurologically impaired are intubated to ensure an adequate airway and effective ventilation. Although the benefits of charcoal administration are unknown in methanol ingestions, charcoal is usually recommended, especially if ingestion of multiple substances is suspected.

Treatment of metabolic acidosis includes correction of pH and base deficit by administration of sodium bicarbonate. Although acidosis may be reversed, ocular damage associated with the toxic effects of methanol metabolism often persists.

Alcohol dehydrogenase has a greater affinity for ethanol than methanol, therefore ethanol infusions are used to inhibit methanol metabolism to toxic metabolites of formaldehyde and formic acid, which promotes its excretion unchanged by the lungs and kidneys. Ethanol is administered in a 5% to 10% solution intravenously or orally in a 20% to 30% solution. A loading dose (7.6 to 10 ml/kg) is administered intravenously in 10% dextrose solution over 30 minutes. Maintenance dosage is 0.15 ml/kg/hr orally of 95% ETOH solution or 1.4 ml/kg/hr intravenously of a 10% ethanol solution, until a serum level of 100 mg/dl is achieved.

Alcohol dehydrogenase inhibitors (ADHs) are generally maintained until methanol levels are less than 20 mg/dl. The FDA recently approved fomepizole (4-MP, Antizol) for ethylene glycol poisoning, and it is being researched for its utility with methanol toxicity. Fomepizole has a greater affinity for alcohol dehydrogenase versus ethanol or methanol and has a better safety profile than ethanol.[47] In addition, folic acid is being recommended to enhance the folate-dependent metabolism of formic acid. The pediatric dose of sodium folate is 1 mg/kg every 4 to 6 hours.

Hemodialysis enhances the elimination of methanol and its toxic byproducts and is indicated in patients with a serum level of 50 mg/dl, severe metabolic acidosis, ingestion of more than 40 ml or in the presence of neurologic or visual disturbances.[33,48] Higher doses of ethanol are required during hemodialysis because ethanol is easily dialyzed.[49] Maintenance doses of 250 to 350 mg/kg/hour are required to achieve and maintain the necessary serum level.

Patient monitoring includes evaluating arterial blood gases, blood alcohol level, and serum glucose level to assess the effectiveness of ethanol administration. Glucose is

monitored closely because glycogen stores are depleted rapidly after methanol ingestion. Complications of dialysis, such as infection and hypoglycemia, are recognized and treated early.

Ethylene Glycol

Etiology/Incidence. Ethylene glycol is a colorless, sweet-tasting liquid with a faint odor found in permanent types of antifreezes and coolants. It is also contained in latex paint, glass cleaners, stains, dyes, waxes, inks, and a variety of household cleaners, including floor waxes and polishes, shoe polishes, and surface cleaning solutions. Ethylene glycol ingestions have been attributed to its bittersweet taste. Ethylene glycol poisonings usually occur as isolated instances with children. In adolescents and adults, toxicity commonly occurs when ethylene glycol is ingested as an ethanol substitute.

Pathogenesis. Ethylene glycol is rapidly absorbed, peaking in the bloodstream within 1 to 4 hours of ingestion. Once absorbed, a significant amount is eliminated by the kidneys; however, renal toxicity is acute and progressive. Once renal compromise is present, almost all of the ethylene glycol is then metabolized in the liver by alcohol dehydrogenase to glycolaldehyde, glyoxylic acid, oxalic acid, and formic acid. As with methanol, the toxicity of ethylene glycol results from its metabolites. Ethylene glycol produces CNS depression, and its metabolites cause metabolic anion gap acidosis, hypocalcemia, further CNS depression, and tissue damage.[48] After a delay of 12 to 24 hours, oxalate crystals may appear in the urine (when oxalic acid chelates serum calcium) and is deposited in the tissues, causing acute renal failure, metabolic acidosis, and cardiac and CNS toxicity. Ingestion of an amount as small as 1.4 to 1.6 ml/kg can be lethal.

Three clinical stages of poisoning have been described. Progression and severity of signs in these stages depend on the ingested dose. Stage 1 occurs from 1 to 12 hours after ingestion and is characterized by nausea, vomiting, metabolic acidosis, oxalate crystalluria, and progressive central nervous signs including elation, slurred speech, confusion, nystagmus, depressed deep tendon reflexes, myoclonic jerks, and seizures without the characteristic ethanol odor on the breath. Hyperemia of the CNS produces symptoms of inebriation, such as ataxia, stupor, and coma. A result of calcium oxalate crystal deposition in the leptomeninges, vessel walls, and perivascular spaces is meningoencephalitis.

After the first 12 to 18 hours, tachycardia, tachypnea, mild hypertension, congestive heart failure, cyanosis, and pulmonary edema leading to cardiorespiratory failure characterize the second stage. Myocardial and pulmonary dysfunction occur as a result of accumulation of the toxic intermediate and deposition of calcium oxalate crystals in the heart and lungs.

The third stage occurs 1 to 3 days after ingestion and is marked by flank pain, hematuria, proteinuria, oliguria, acute tubular necrosis, and renal failure. Damage to the renal tubules is thought to be caused by the byproducts glycolaldehyde, glycolic, and glyoxylic acid, during ethylene glycol metabolism.[33]

Critical Care Management. Ventilatory support, if needed, is initiated immediately. Emesis is contraindicated because of the risk for CNS depression. Gastric lavage is indicated for patients presenting within several hours after ingestion of massive amounts or if gastric motility is slowed by another ingestant or coma. Activated charcoal does not bind to ethylene glycol and is not used.

Ethanol administration blocks ethylene glycol metabolism and development of toxic metabolites through alcohol dehydrogenase binding. A loading dose of ethanol is given when there are clinical signs and a history of ethylene glycol ingestion, severe or persistent metabolic acidosis, or a blood ethylene glycol level of 25 mg/dl or higher. Ethanol loading is also recommended for patients who are awaiting ethylene glycol serum determinations or hemodialysis. The antidote, fomepizole, is a potent inhibitor of ADH and was approved by the FDA for the treatment of ethylene glycol poisoning. Reports indicate that the intravenous administration of fomepizole every 12 hours prevents renal damage and metabolic abnormalities associated with the metabolism of ethylene glycol to its toxic metabolites.[50]

In cases when ethylene glycol concentration is higher than 50 mg/dl or renal failure exists, hemodialysis is recommended. Thiamine (0.25 to 0.5 mg/kg) and pyridoxine (1 to 2 mg/kg) administration are thought to decrease oxalate production. The prevention of oxalate crystal formation and subsequent deposition in the kidney are benefits of forced diuresis in the treatment of ethylene glycol intoxication.

Priorities for critical care management include meticulous assessment of intake and output to ensure adequate hydration despite forced diuresis. Care is aimed toward enhancing clearance of ethylene glycol and its metabolites. If hemodialysis is required, care is focused on the maintenance of normal hemodynamics and fluid and electrolyte balance during therapy. Ethanol administration is continued until the ethylene glycol level reaches zero.

Close monitoring of blood gas and calcium determinations are necessary for early detection and treatment of metabolic acidosis and hypocalcemia. Intravenous sodium bicarbonate (1 to 2 mEq/kg) is indicated because ethylene glycol is metabolized faster than methanol, resulting in a more profound metabolic acidosis. Calcium chloride (10 to 20 mg/kg/dose) is required to reverse the hypocalcemia effects of calcium oxalate precipitation in the serum.

Isopropanol

Etiology/Incidence. Isopropyl alcohol is a clear, colorless solution, found in rubbing alcohol, antifreeze, skin lotions, and glass cleaners. Parents may use isopropanol for sponging a child to reduce fever with isolated cases resulting in stupor or coma. Consequently, this practice is strongly discouraged.

Pathogenesis. The peak absorption of isopropanol occurs in about 30 minutes because of rapid GI absorption with complete absorption in 2 hours. Isopropanol is a CNS and cardiac depressant. Approximately 20% to 50% of

isopropanol is excreted unchanged by the kidneys. The liver is responsible for about 50% to 80% of isopropanol metabolism converting it to acetone. The kidneys primarily excrete acetone with some excretion through the lungs. The half-life of isopropanol is 4 to 6 hours and that of acetone is 16 to 20 hours. Acetone acts as a CNS depressant and the prolonged CNS depression seen with isopropanol ingestion is related in part to the acetone's effect.

Isopropanol toxicity produces CNS effects including depression, ataxia, confusion, stupor, and coma. The depression has been described to be 2 to 3 times more profound than ethanol ingestions.[47] Patients may appear intoxicated but do not smell like alcohol; rather they have the fruity odor of acetone. Hyperglycemia, inconsistent pupil size, miosis, and depressed or absent deep tendon reflexes are other CNS manifestations characteristic of isopropanol toxicity.

As a myocardial depressant, acetone causes altered cardiac function with profound hypotension and has been noted to be a poor prognostic sign. Patients may have sinus tachycardia but usually no other cardiac dysrhythmias. Impaired GI system function results from the effects of isopropanol as a local irritant. GI symptoms such as gastritis, abdominal pain, vomiting, and hematemesis usually occur as a result of isopropanol ingestion. Renal tubular necrosis, myopathy, and hemolytic anemia have also developed after ingestion of isopropanol.

Critical Care Management. Supportive care is the primary treatment. Airway protection is crucial to prevent aspiration should vomiting occur. Emesis is not recommended because of the rapid CNS depression associated with isopropanol. Gastric lavage is recommended because it may limit absorption and helps to decrease the local irritation in the lining of the stomach. Serum isopropyl alcohol level confirms and quantitates alcohol level, but the clinical presentation is a better indicator of prognosis.

Therapy for isopropanol ingestion is fairly nonspecific, focusing mostly on general supportive care. Maintaining adequate ventilation and normotension is the primary goal. Care of children with isopropanol toxicity necessitates close monitoring for and correction of fluid and electrolyte imbalances. If hypoglycemia develops, the patient will require adjustment of intravenous glucose infusions to maintain serum glucose in the normal range of 80 to 120 mg/dl.

Hypotension is treated with fluid boluses (20 ml/kg IV) and vasopressor support if needed. Hemodialysis is used when serum isopropyl alcohol levels are greater than 400 mg/dl or hypotension is refractory to treatment.

Ethanol

Etiology/Incidence. Ethanol is found in alcoholic beverages, perfumes, cologne, cold preparations, aftershave, mouthwash, and antiseptics. Blood ethanol levels less than 50 mg/dl can produce mild intoxication in children; however, a lethal dose has been estimated at 3 mg/kg equivalent (e.g., 5 to 10 ounces of mouthwash or 1 to 2 ounces of cologne).[4] Ethanol is more likely to be ingested than some other substances because these products are used daily and are usually within reach of young children.

Pathogenesis. Ethanol is rapidly absorbed from the gastric tract, peaking in the serum 30 to 60 minutes after ingestion when the stomach is empty. Absorption is delayed when food is present in the stomach and total absorption may take up to 6 hours. A total of 90% is metabolized in the liver by alcohol and aldehyde dehydrogenases with some oxidation. The kidney excretes the remainder. Ethanol affects the reticular activating system, causing direct CNS depression, decreased motor function, and decreased level of consciousness. At high concentrations, ethanol is an anesthetic and can cause autonomic dysfunction, hypothermia, and hypotension with subsequent coma and death from respiratory depression and cardiovascular collapse.

Ethanol ingestion may be manifested clinically by flushed face, diaphoresis, agitation, or ebullient and loquacious speech resulting from early disinhibition. This may progress to ataxia, slurred speech, blurred or double vision, drowsiness, stupor, depression, or coma. Significant intoxication is characterized by the presence of an osmolal gap (see Box 30-1). Ethanol metabolism causes impaired gluconeogenesis during the Krebs cycle. Profound hypoglycemia can ultimately lead to convulsions and coma in the pediatric patient, but the prognosis for children who ingest ethanol is generally good.

Critical Care Management. The initial treatment for ethanol intoxication involves providing supportive measures such as airway protection, oxygen, and monitoring fluids. Emesis is contraindicated because of rapid CNS depression. Gastric lavage may be recommended when the child is seen within 30 to 60 minutes after ingestion and CNS depression is present. Charcoal and forced diuresis are ineffective because the liver is the primary metabolic pathway. Cardiac and respiratory support is necessary in addition to the initiation of an intravenous infusion of 10% dextrose if hypoglycemia exists.

Supportive therapy with ongoing monitoring of vital functions until toxic effects subside is the primary focus of intensive care. Children who ingest ethanol require frequent serum glucose and ethanol determination and assessment for changes in mental status. Reassuring parents by noting signs of improvement in clinical status is helpful as the child progresses through the recovery period. The patient needs to be protected against aspiration. If hypoxia develops, the patient may require intubation and mechanical ventilation. Intravenous fluids are administered to replace urinary losses and correct electrolyte imbalance, acidemia, and hypotension. If hypotension is refractory, vasopressors may be necessary. Hypothermia is treated with passive rewarming; and normothermia is the goal. Maintaining seizure precautions is necessary until symptoms of neurologic toxicity abate. If the blood ethanol level is greater than 300 to 350 mg/dl and clinical deterioration progresses despite supportive care, hemodialysis is used.[4]

Cocaine

Etiology/Incidence. Grown in Peru and Bolivia, cocaine is an alkaloid that is extracted from the leaves of the *Erythroxylum* coca plant. It is crystallized as hydrochloride salt, prescribed as a local anesthetic and mucous membrane

vasoconstrictor, and used illicitly as a CNS stimulant. The adulterants with which cocaine is diluted for illicit use include local anesthetics, sugars, stimulants, toxins, and inert compounds and may also exert toxic effects.[51]

Cocaine may be injected intravenously, sniffed intranasally, ingested, or applied to the mucous membranes. Cocaine can also be smoked in its free-base form known as "crack." Children may be exposed to cocaine by passive transmission via the placenta in utero, or in breast milk, or by inhalation of crack vapors.[52] Cocaine is well absorbed by all mucous membranes, metabolized by liver esterases and plasma cholinesterase, degraded nonenzymatically, and excreted in the urine as its primary metabolite, benzoylecgonine.[53] Cocaine levels in blood may be detected within several minutes of ingestion. They peak in 15 to 30 minutes and persist for up to 8 hours.[54] Cocaine may be detected in urine within 1 hour of ingestion or administration and persists for up to 3 days in children and 5 days in neonates following exposure.

Pathogenesis. Three systems primarily affected by cocaine's toxic effects are the neurologic system, the cardiovascular system, and the respiratory system. Cocaine stimulates the sympathetic nervous system, and an overdose is especially toxic to the brain and heart. Cocaine stimulates the presynaptic release of dopamine, norepinephrine, serotonin, and acetylcholine in the CNS. It alters normal intraneural communication by augmenting the effects of the catecholamines, norepinephrine, and dopamine. Cocaine stimulates the "fight or flight" mechanism, evidenced by clinical signs of stimulation of norepinephrine secretion. Signs and symptoms are dose related, with low doses producing euphoria and CNS stimulation and high doses producing anxiety, agitation, paranoid delusions, mydriasis, hypertension, hyperthermia, tachycardia, and cardiac dysrhythmias.[4] As cocaine continues to stimulate norepinephrine and dopamine release, the cardiovascular and neurologic systems demonstrate progressive stimulation that may progress to exhaustion, producing coma and cardiopulmonary arrest.

Cardiovascular dysfunction is first manifested by sinus tachycardia or supraventricular dysrhythmias followed by hypertension, peripheral vasoconstriction, ventricular ectopy, and occasionally, ventricular fibrillation or asystole. These signs may occur as a result of the toxic action cocaine exerts on the tissues of the myocardium directly, or because of its effect of sensitizing the heart to the actions of norepinephrine and dopamine.[44] Evidence of a toxic dose is seen when heart rate and blood pressure peak and begin to fall, ventricular dysrhythmias become more frequent, and the patient begins to show signs of shock with decreased peripheral perfusion and cyanosis. Progression of signs includes ventricular fibrillation, circulatory collapse, and an ashen appearance before cardiac arrest. Cocaine-induced coronary artery vasoconstriction may also cause myocardial ischemia or infarction related to increased myocardial oxygen demand and cocaine's thrombogenic potential.[53]

Neurologic dysfunction begins as the cerebral cortex is stimulated. Dysfunction is further evident with talkativeness, hyperalertness, mydriasis, and nausea and/or vomiting occurring. As stimulation continues and cocaine affects the functions of the medulla, the child becomes hyperthermic, develops hyperreflexia, and may have seizures. As the CNS becomes exhausted, the child becomes comatose with flaccid paralysis.

Tachypnea and increased depth of respiration evidence the early stimulation phase of the CNS. Later, depression of the medullary respiratory center occurs, the child becomes more dyspneic and may progress to cyanosis and respiratory failure. Seizures, or respiratory depression secondary to antiepileptic medications, may also contribute to respiratory failure in cocaine toxicity. Cerebral vascular accidents, including subarachnoid hemorrhage, cerebral infarction, transient ischemic attacks, and seizures have been reported with cocaine toxicity. Seizures may develop secondary to infarction or hemorrhage, and the majority are single, generalized, and not associated with any lasting neurologic deficits.[53]

Critical Care Management. Because cocaine is absorbed quickly with smoking, snorting, or injection, no treatment can decrease its absorption or enhance its excretion. If cocaine is ingested, GI decontamination may be considered after initial stabilization of airway, breathing, and circulation. Initial management of cocaine exposure depends on the phase at which the patient presents for care. Adequate cardiovascular and respiratory function is ensured. Assessment of cardiovascular function includes heart rate and rhythm, blood pressure, and peripheral perfusion. Respiratory evaluation includes assessment of both respiratory rate and depth, with pulse oximetry or arterial blood gas analysis as needed. Intravenous access is obtained promptly and vital signs are monitored frequently. Continuous core temperature monitoring is initiated to assess for hyperthermia. Emesis is not used, but activated charcoal and a cathartic may be given for oral ingestions. Whole bowel irrigation has been used safely to remove packets and crack vials in drug smugglers.

Cardiovascular dysfunction is initially treated with fluid resuscitation. There is significant controversy regarding the use of antidysrhythmics with cocaine ingestion. The majority of antidysrhythmic agents are contraindicated because they exacerbate the problems of coronary artery spasm, ischemia, infarction, and ventricular arrhythmias. A lidocaine bolus (1 mg/kg) and continuous infusion (10 to 50 µg/kg/min) may be required to suppress ventricular arrhythmias if no other alternatives are present. Benzodiazepines slow the heart rate, may have an additive antiarrhythmic effect, and are added, if not already used, only to offer protection against the combined proconvulsant effect of lidocaine and cocaine. If unable to determine whether the dysrhythmia is from ischemia or sodium channel blockade with QRS widening, sodium bicarbonate and benzodiazepines are given first, followed by lidocaine if dysrhythmias persist.[53] Nitroglycerin may be used to relieve chest pain and angina. Severe hypertension resulting from vasoconstriction is best treated with sedatives such as diazepam (40 to 200 µg/kg IV) or lorazepam (30 µg/kg/day in three or four doses intravenously) in an effort to control hypertension, calm the patient, prevent seizures, and decrease hypertonicity. If these measures fail to control hypertension,

a continuous infusion of nitroprusside (0.2 to 10 µg/kg/min) may be necessary. Pulmonary artery pressure monitoring may be indicated to estimate the left heart filling pressures and to guide management.

Use of a tool such as the Glasgow coma scale or the Pediatric Coma Scale guides neurologic assessment. Seizures may be treated with diazepam (100 to 250 µg/kg) or lorazepam (50 µg/kg) given intravenously over 3 minutes. Hyperpyrexia is aggressively treated with cooling blankets or tepid baths, avoiding shivering, which increases body temperature. Respiratory dysfunction management includes maintenance of a patent airway as the first priority. Oxygen may be administered to prevent complications of hypoxemia. Intubation is considered if the child is unable to maintain a patent airway, adequate cough, or gag reflexes; if seizures compromise respiratory function; or if arterial blood gas analysis demonstrates hypercarbia. Mechanical ventilation may be required to treat respiratory insufficiency or respiratory failure.

Heroin

Etiology/Incidence. Heroin is an illicit semisynthetic narcotic agent initially developed as a less-addicting morphine substitute. It originally gained popularity in the 1970s, but now a resurgence of heroin use and abuse has occurred in the 1990s. Heroin has become cheaper and more readily available in the past few years, and a new generation of young heroin users has developed novel patterns of abuse.

Heroin acts as a pro-drug that allows for rapid CNS absorption, providing euphoric and toxic effects. All routes of administration rapidly absorb heroin with intravenous heroin at serum peak levels within 1 minute. Intranasal and intramuscular heroin reach peak levels in 3 to 5 minutes, and subcutaneous heroin reaches peak levels within 5 to 10 minutes. Heroin is seven times more toxic than intravenous morphine and the route of administration strongly affects the drug's potential for overdose or death. The majority of nonfatal and fatal heroin overdoses occur when injected intravenously.

Pathogenesis. Heroin is highly lipid soluble with rapid and complete uptake into the CNS that produces a feeling of intoxication. Heroin produces opiate intoxication syndrome consisting of altered mental status, miosis, and respiratory depression. It reacts with three types of receptors, mu, kappa, and delta, to produce a wide range of changes in the CNS. Initial effects include euphoria, sedation, impaired thinking, miosis, and mild decrease in blood pressure and urinary retention. Toxic ingestions produce hypotension, bradycardia, depressed respiration, agitation, uncontrolled muscle movements, hallucinations, headache, nausea and vomiting, stupor, coma, seizures, or death.[54]

The mu receptors are responsible for most of the analgesic effects, respiratory depression, delayed GI motility, miosis, and euphoria, whereas kappa agonists, independent of the mu receptors, produce analgesia, respiratory depression, and dysphoria. Delta receptors work to mediate spinal analgesia. Centrally mediated respiratory depression is caused by a direct effect on the brainstem, reducing responsiveness to carbon dioxide. Respiratory depression is the dominant symptom and the most common cause of death in heroin overdose. Heroin crosses the blood-brain barrier within 15 to 20 seconds and achieves a high brain level of both heroin and its metabolites. In the CNS, heroin is quickly hydrolyzed to a substrate that is metabolized over 20 to 30 minutes to morphine. Heroin and its metabolites both have significant agonist and analgesic effects on the CNS. Any circulating heroin can be hydrolyzed in the peripheral tissues of the kidneys and liver to morphine. The by-products of morphine are water soluble and readily excreted in urine and bile.[55]

Critical Care Management. Heroin intoxication is usually witnessed, and identification of the toxin is known. Initial management includes assessment of adequacy of ventilation and airway stability. The majority of patients will present with inadequate respiratory effort and require assistance with bag-valve-mask breathing and oxygen delivery. If ingestion of heroin is confirmed, parenteral naloxone therapy is initiated. If the patient does not respond to naloxone within 10 minutes, or the airway is unstable, then intubation is performed. If the patient is breathing well without support, naloxone is not administered, and the patient is observed. Emesis is contraindicated because of rapid absorption of heroin and CNS depression.

Gastric decontamination with whole bowel irrigation and activated charcoal is used in cases of body packers or "mules" who attempt to smuggle large numbers of concentrated drug packets by ingesting them. These individuals are typically asymptomatic but are at risk for delayed and prolonged toxicity from packet rupture. If symptomatic, a continuous infusion of naloxone can be administered in conjunction with gastric decontamination.

Ongoing management typically consists of supportive care, primarily of the respiratory system with assisted ventilation, until the CNS depressive effects are no longer present. In the hypoventilating patient suspected of heroin overdose, an initial dose of naloxone (0.1 mg/kg) may be given, followed by a higher dose (maximum 2 mg) if no response is seen in 3 to 5 minutes. The short duration of action of naloxone may require multiple doses until respiratory compromise is no longer present. A chest radiograph is obtained for patients who clinically present with a significant cough or poor oxygenation.

Naloxone treatment of heroin overdose is associated with complications, including seizures, tachycardia, severe agitation, nausea and vomiting, diaphoresis, and hypertension. Heroin has a 1% to 3% associated risk of inducing noncardiogenic pulmonary edema, whereas naloxone is associated with a 1.6% rate of complications, including seizures and arrhythmias.[55] Patients with heroin overdose and respiratory compromise require observation and cardiorespiratory monitoring until cessation of clinical symptoms. Patients are carefully evaluated to rule out coingestion, especially benzodiazepines, which contribute to a much higher complication rate.

Methadone

Etiology/Incidence. Methadone is a synthetic narcotic that is used in the treatment of heroin addiction and withdrawal. Methadone is unrelated to morphine but is similar in mu effect. It replaces the illicit substance with a legal, oral, and long-acting agent, but excessive dosing may cause toxicity. Methadone will produce symptoms similar to heroin intoxication and overdose. Children are particularly susceptible to the effects of methadone overdose, with respiratory depression and death potentially occurring with a 10-mg dose.

Pathogenesis. Methadone is very lipid soluble and well absorbed from the GI tract into the blood stream with a long elimination half-life of 15 to 20 hours in children. Methadone is 70% to 90% bound to albumin and plasma proteins. The oral duration of action is 6 to 8 hours initially and 22 to 48 hours after repeated doses. It is hydrolyzed with a fairly extensive metabolism on first pass through the liver. Methadone is excreted in sweat and saliva, and 10% is excreted unchanged along with metabolites in urine and stool.[54]

Methadone can produce mild side effects such as drowsiness, lightheadedness, weakness, euphoria, dry mouth, and urinary retention with proper dosing. Symptoms of methadone overdose include marked drowsiness, confusion, tremors, nausea and vomiting, cold and clammy skin, hypotension, hypothermia, bradycardia, miosis, seizures, stupor leading to coma, and severe respiratory depression.[56]

Critical Care Management. Methadone has a slow onset of action and a very long duration of effect. All patients who present with methadone toxicity require hospitalization and monitoring. Initial management consists of assessment and stabilization of respiratory effort. Intubation is performed for all patients with significant respiratory depression. If respiratory depression is not immediately addressed, cyanosis, hypoxia, and apnea may develop. The major cause of death in methadone toxicity is respiratory arrest.

Emesis is contraindicated. Activated charcoal may be worthwhile because gastric motility is slowed by methadone.

The majority of critical care management is supportive in nature. The child may require intubation and mechanical ventilation support until respiratory depression subsides. The patient is initially NPO, and intravenous fluid is given for hydration. Naloxone is given intravenously as a continuous infusion, starting with a loading dose (0.005 mg/kg) followed by an infusion of 0.0025 mg/kg/hr, tapering gradually as symptoms resolve to avoid relapse. Hypotension is treated with fluid boluses (20 ml/kg) and if refractory may require inotropic support.

Phencyclidine

Etiology/Incidence. Phencyclidine (PCP) was developed in the 1950s as a dissociative anesthetic-analgesic. It was the prototype of a drug combining analgesic and anesthetic actions without respiratory or cardiovascular depression. PCP produced dysphoric effects and was rapidly adapted as a street drug after being removed from the pharmaceutical market. PCP is easily and cheaply synthesized from readily obtainable ingredients. It typically used by polydrug abusers.[57]

PCP can be smoked, snorted, or ingested. It has a rapid onset of action and may elicit drug-induced psychosis with flashbacks lasting for weeks.

Pathogenesis. PCP is a highly lipid-soluble drug, which is also soluble in water and alcohol. It is metabolized by the liver to hydroxyl and glucuronide and then excreted in the urine as an inactive complex within 12 hours of ingestion. PCP is thought to block the calcium channel influx, which results from glutamate binding.

PCP primarily affects the CNS, stimulating α-adrenergic receptors and potentiating catecholamines. The major effects are psychologic, sympathomimetic, cholinergic, and cerebellar. People may have sharply contrasting responses to PCP. It has profound effects on thinking, alters time perception and sense of reality, affects mood, and may create a dreamlike, euphoric, or depressed state. Intoxication with PCP may produce negative effects including disorientation, confusion, anxiety, irritability, paranoid states, hostility, or belligerence. Dangerously violent behavior may develop.[58] At high doses, PCP abuse may produce nystagmus, hypertension, tachycardia, salivation, flushing, sweating, dizziness, blurred vision, ataxia, and CNS stimulation or depression. The symptoms are quite variable, and children present with miosis, choreoathetosis, and seizures more often than adults.[57] The presence of hypertension, abnormal behavior, and miosis in children strongly suggest PCP poisoning. Most fatalities associated with PCP poisoning are related to violent actions rather than the toxicity of the dose.[19]

Critical Care Management. Initial management consists of assessing and maintaining adequate respiration, circulation, and thermoregulation. To prevent self-injury, the patient is safely restrained, using physical and chemical methods as necessary. If the patient has a history of recent ingestion of PCP, GI decontamination is initiated. Gastric lavage may be performed once the patient's anxiety or agitation is well controlled. Activated charcoal effectively absorbs PCP and increases its nonrenal clearance. Unless there are specific contraindications, sorbitol is administered with the activated charcoal. Alkaline diuresis, hemoperfusion, and hemodialysis are not beneficial because of the substantial protein binding, high lipid solubility, and limited renal excretion of PCP.

The continuation of supportive treatment until resolution of symptoms is the primary treatment. If seizures occur, benzodiazepines can be used in addition to treating agitation. Hyperthermia is treated with passive cooling techniques. The patient is kept well hydrated to lessen the effects of rhabdomyolysis and prevent deposition of pigment in the kidneys, which could lead to renal failure.

The majority of patients rapidly regain normal CNS function within several hours of using PCP. However, some patients may remain comatose or exhibit bizarre behavior for days or even weeks after ingesting high doses. Patients who may have an underlying psychiatric disorder may also have symptoms for an extended period.

The major complication of PCP is from injuries related to behavior, including self-inflicted injuries, injuries from exceptional physical exertion, or injuries from resisting physical restraints. Patients who have ingested PCP appear to be unaware of their surroundings and pain because of PCP's dissociative anesthetic effects.

HOUSEHOLD TOXINS

Caustics

Etiology/Incidence. A caustic is a substance that causes functional and cellular damage on contact with body surfaces. The injury results as neutralization of the substance takes place at the expense of the tissues, releasing thermal energy and causing burns. Caustics are classified as strong acids or alkalis and can be found in most homes. The incidence of caustic injuries to the esophagus has increased significantly since the use of concentrated liquid alkaline cleansers became popular. In addition, many accidental childhood ingestions occur as a result of the substances being placed or stored in easily accessible and familiar containers such as milk cartons and soda cans. Common sources of acid exposure include toilet bowel cleaner, swimming pool products, and battery fluid. Household sources of alkali agents include drain openers, lye, hair permanent products, and oven cleaners. The skin, eyes, respiratory tract, and GI tract are all systems affected by caustic injury. Ingestion of caustics causes the most life-threatening and long-term morbidity.[59]

The majority of caustic burns to the esophagus are a result of sodium hydroxide or lye ingestions and most often occur in children younger than 5 years of age.[60] Commercial ammonia is an alkali that causes ulcers or full-thickness burns to the esophagus after ingestion and irritation to the lungs or pulmonary edema after inhalation. Toilet bowl cleaners that contain sulfuric, hydrochloric, or phosphoric acid burn the oropharyngeal mucosa and are usually spit out on contact. Detergents and bleach are commonly ingested by children and produce local irritation without causing necrosis.

Pathogenesis. Esophageal burns produced by the ingestion of caustic agents are classified as first-degree burns, which produce hyperemia and superficial desquamation; second-degree burns, which result in blisters and shallow mucosal ulcers; and third-degree burns, which produce deeper ulceration into the esophageal muscle. Caustics can affect a variety of regions along the GI tract in addition to the esophagus because of the agents' low surface tension and ability to spread to a large surface area.

The location of the injury varies but can involve the cricopharyngeal area, impression of the aortic arch and left bronchus, lower esophageal sphincter, and stomach. Greater damage occurs in these locations because the ingested agent may become stagnant. Granular agents may imbed in the tissues of the oropharynx or proximal esophagus, whereas liquid agents produce damage along the entire esophagus to the stomach lining. When the lower esophageal sphincter is involved, the resting pressure decreases, causing reflux of the agent back and forth between the esophagus and stomach. This is usually followed by violent regurgitation.

Acids produce a coagulating necrosis in the stomach and esophagus, resulting in eschar formation. This limits deep penetration into the tissue, but leads to metabolic acidosis and pooling of acids in the stomach.

Alkaline agents usually affect the mouth, esophagus, and stomach. However, it is possible to have esophageal burns without oral involvement if the agent is swallowed rapidly. The alkali acts as a solvent on the lipoprotein lining, causing a liquefaction necrosis with inflammation and deep penetration into the mucosal, submucosal, and muscular layers of the esophagus and stomach. This is followed several days later by saponification of mucosal fats and proteins, thrombosis of adjacent blood vessels, cell necrosis, and tissue degeneration. Sloughing develops 4 to 7 days after ingestion when bacteria invade the injured areas. The development of strictures can occur anytime between 21 and 42 days after exposure.[61]

Critical Care Management. The identity, concentration, pH, and amount of substance ingested are important to ascertain. Depending on the severity of injury, the patient may present with physical findings of impending airway obstruction. If possible, gentle or fiber-optic intubation is preferred over blind nasotracheal because of the increased risk of soft-tissue perforation. Emesis is contraindicated because of the reexposure to the caustic agent. Gastric lavage is also contraindicated for both acid and alkali ingestions. Large liquid acid ingestions may benefit from nasogastric suction because pyloric sphincter spasm may prolong the contact time with the gastric mucosa. Activated charcoal is relatively contraindicated because of poor adsorption and endoscopic interference. If the gag reflex is intact, dilution may be beneficial in the ingestion of solid or granular alkaline material if performed within 30 minutes of ingestion. The child can be given a small amount of tap water (5 ml/kg) to dilute the substance, but the risk of inducing emesis is weighed against the benefit of dilution. Acids are not diluted with water because of excessive heat production. All small children, symptomatic patients, and those with altered mental status are admitted for observation and subsequent endoscopy to evaluate the extent of injury.

Hydration accompanied by NPO for 12 to 24 hours until the extent of the injuries has been determined is initiated. The child requires close observation for drooling or the presence of lesions in the oral mucosa, stridor, hoarseness, subcutaneous air, respiratory distress, acute peritonitis, and hematemesis in the early stages of hospitalization. Airway edema or obstruction may occur up to 48 hours after an alkaline exposure, and delayed perforation may occur up to 4 days after an acid exposure.

The child who has sustained first-degree burns is assessed for the ability to tolerate liquids and slowly advanced to a regular diet. For children with second-degree and third-degree burns or evidence of perforation, the administration of antibiotics and antacids may be indicated. These children may also need parenteral nutrition and an endoscopy 2 to 3 weeks after the ingestion to evaluate the extent of esophageal dysmotility or stricture formation. Repeated esophageal dilations may be required if strictures develop.[59,61] Long-term sequelae may require surgical intervention to repair the severely damaged esophagus.

Hydrocarbons

Etiology/Incidence. Fully 60% of all hydrocarbon exposures involve children and 90% of hydrocarbon-related deaths involved children, younger than 5 years of age. Hydrocarbons are defined as all-organic compounds made of predominately carbon and hydrogen molecules, including those derived from petroleum distillation. Hydrocarbons are classified into four different categories: aliphatics (paraffins), aromatics, alicyclics or cycloparaffins, and halogenated products. Aliphatic hydrocarbons are found in the form of petroleum distillates such as furniture polish, lamp oil, lighter fluid, propane, and isobutane. Aromatic hydrocarbons, such as benzene, toluene, and xylene, are found in glues, nail polish, paints, and paint removers. Alicyclic hydrocarbons are otherwise known as turpentine, cyclopropane, and cyclohexane. Halogenated hydrocarbons, such as carbon tetrachloride, chloroform, methylene chloride, Freon, and trichloromethane, are particularly harmful because they produce various forms of systemic toxicity.

Pathogenesis. The pulmonary system is predominately affected by hydrocarbon ingestion. The CNS, GI, cardiac, and dermatologic systems are also commonly affected with rare hematologic, hepatic, and renal effects. Aliphatic hydrocarbons produce minimal systemic toxicity but may cause pulmonary injury, depending on their viscosity and ease of aspiration. Alicyclics can produce pulmonary aspiration and direct CNS depression. Aromatic and halogenated hydrocarbons can cause cardiac arrhythmias in addition to aspiration and CNS depression (Box 30-2).

The risk of aspiration depends on the viscosity, surface tension, and volatility of the substance. The lower the viscosity and surface tension and the higher the volatility, the greater the risk of aspiration.[62] Products with low viscosity pose a high aspiration hazard because of the tendency to spread over a large surface area. Chemical pneumonitis may develop from as little as a few milliliters of a hydrocarbon. Aspiration usually occurs at the time of ingestion or upon emesis. Large amounts of most alicyclic and aromatic hydrocarbons can be tolerated by ingestion if not aspirated. Agents that are not aspirated easily but that cause systemic toxicity (i.e., the halogenated hydrocarbons) induce neurotoxicity. Benzene, in addition, is associated with aplastic and acute myeloblastic anemia because of its ability to injure bone marrow.

The ingestion of a hydrocarbon causes irritation of the mouth, pharynx, and gastric mucosa and is usually followed by vomiting. Aspiration of these substances, which are lipid solvents, leads to hydrocarbon pneumonitis within 12 to 24 hours after exposure and is typically accompanied by rapid development of low-grade fever.[62]

Hydrocarbons disrupt surfactant, cause direct injury to the epithelium and pulmonary capillaries and create bronchospasm, alveolar instability, and collapse resulting in atelectasis and pulmonary edema. Symptoms exhibited include coughing, retractions, grunting, tachypnea, dyspnea, cyanosis, and severe hypoxia. Physical examination is characterized by rales on auscultation, rhonchi, wheezing, or decreased breath sounds. Positive radiographic findings, such as perihilar densities, basilar pneumonitis, atelectasis, and consolidation, have been noted as early as 2 hours after ingestion.[63] Other pulmonary complications include pneumatoceles, emphysema, pleural effusion, pneumothorax, pneumomediastinum, and pneumopericardium.

Halogenated and aromatic hydrocarbons are well absorbed by the GI tract and pulmonary system. This enables them to cause direct CNS depression resulting in headache, dizziness, ataxia, lethargy, changes in mental status, and seizures. Patients can also exhibit signs of narcosis, inebriation, or coma.[4]

Inhalation of halogenated hydrocarbons has been known to cause fatal ventricular dysrhythmias resulting from myocardial sensitization to catecholamines. The pathophysiologic effect of inhalation of these substances causes increased ventricular irritability, predisposing the heart to ventricular fibrillation.

All hydrocarbons produce symptoms of GI distress including nausea, vomiting, hematemesis, and diarrhea. Absorption varies, depending on the type of hydrocarbon. Aliphatic hydrocarbons have minimal absorption, whereas alicyclic, aromatic, and halogenated hydrocarbons can have significant GI absorption.

Halogenated hydrocarbons have been known to produce centrilobular necrosis. Specific types include carbon tetra-chloride and chloroform, which induce fatty degeneration of the liver, resulting in necrosis.[64]

Many halogenated hydrocarbons that produce hepatic dysfunction also cause renal tubular acidosis. Damage occurs directly to the proximal tubule and the loop of Henle from carbon tetrachloride. This leads to acute renal failure between 1 and 7 days after exposure.[64]

Critical Care Management. Ingestion of hydrocarbons commonly leads to gagging with pulmonary aspiration. Aspiration may lead to the rapid development of chemical pneumonitis and intubation, and mechanical ventilation is initiated quickly, preferably using a cuffed endotracheal tube. Once initial stabilization is achieved, consideration of gastric decontamination is considered. Gastric emptying remains a controversial recommendation. Because the majority of hydrocarbons do not cause systemic toxicity but have significant risk for causing pulmonary injury, emesis and gastric lavage are not recommended. When there are no contraindications, gastric emptying may be helpful for hydrocarbons that have inherent toxicity, have been ingested with a toxin, or have been used to stabilize a toxin or when a large volume of hydrocarbon is ingested. Hydrocarbons that have inherent toxicity include CHAMP: C—camphor, H—halogenated hydrocarbons, A—aromatic hydrocarbons, M—hydrocarbons associated with metals, and P—hydrocarbons associated with pesticides.[65]

Children with a history of hydrocarbon ingestion are monitored for signs of pulmonary aspiration, including coughing, choking, or gagging and oxygen desaturation on pulse oximetry. If these signs are present, a chest radiograph is necessary to evaluate potential parenchymal injury. Clothes are removed, copious bathing is done, and eye irrigation performed if necessary to reduce absorption by other routes.

Admission to the ICU is warranted in children with severe parenchymal injury and pneumonia. Care of these patients includes mechanical ventilation and close attention to maintenance of a patent airway, effective pulmonary toilet, and routine monitoring of arterial blood gases until symptoms of respiratory compromise subside. Pulmonary dysfunction and radiographic changes determine the degree of mechanical support required in the acute phase of parenchymal injury. Severe injuries may require the use of extracorporeal membrane oxygenation.

SUMMARY

Children who have ingested pharmaceutical or nonpharmaceutical toxins are a critical care nursing challenge in the emergency department and the ICU. The effects of a toxic ingestion may be systemic, involving many organ systems. Finely tuned collaboration between nurses, physicians, and poison experts is necessary for a positive outcome for these patients. Intentional ingestions necessitate the involvement of psychiatry. Accidental ingestions require education and reinforcement by the health care team for caregivers and children to decrease the probability of a reoccurrence.

REFERENCES

1. Litovitz TL, Klein-Schwartz W, Caravati EM et al: 1998 Annual Report of the American Association of Poison Control Centers Toxic Exposure Surveillance System, *Am J Emerg Med* 17:435-487, 1999.
2. Liebelt EL, DeAngelis CD: Evolving trends and treatment advances in pediatric poisonings, *JAMA* 282:1113-1115, 1999.
3. Aks SE: Toxidromes. In Toxicon, 2000, at http://toxicon.er.uic.edu/toxidro.htm.
4. Rodgers GC, Matayunas NJ: *Handbook of common poisonings of children,* ed 3, Elk Grove, Ill, 1994, American Academy of Pediatrics.
5. Bond GR: The poisoned child: evolving concepts in care, *Emerg Med Clin North Am* 13:343-355, 1995.
6. Goldfrank LR, Flomenbaum NE, Lewin NA et al: Principles of managing the poisoned patient or overdosed patient: an overview. In Goldfrank LR, Flomenbaum NE, Lewis NA et al, eds: *Goldfrank's toxicologic emergencies,* ed 6, Stamford, Conn, 1998, Appleton & Lange.
7. Belson MG, Simon HK, Sullivan K et al: The utility of toxicologic analysis in children with suspected ingestions, *Pediatr Emerg Care* 15:383-387, 1999.
8. Sugarman JM, Rodgers GC, Paul RI: Utility of toxicology screening in a pediatric emergency department, *Pediatr Emerg Care* 13:194-197, 1997.
9. Hanzlick R: National Association of Medical Examiners Pediatric Toxicology (Pedtox) Registry Report 3. Case submission summary and data for acetaminophen, benzene, carboxyhemoglobin, dextromethorphan, ethanol, phenobarbital, and pseudoephedrine, *Am J Forensic Med Pathol* 16:270-277, 1995.
10. Woolf AD, Chrisanthus K: On-site availability of selected antidotes: results of a survey of Massachusetts hospitals, *Am J Emerg Med* 15:62-66, 1997.
11. Gill F: Pediatric poisonings. In Joy C, ed: *Pediatric trauma nursing,* Rockville, Md, 1989, Aspen Publishers.
12. Prybys KM, Tomassoni AJ: Principles of pediatric toxicology, *Top Emerg Med* 18:56-72, 1996.
13. Gorelick M: Gastric emptying. In Dieckman R, Fiser D, Selbst S, eds: *Pediatric emergency and critical care procedures,* St Louis, 1997, Mosby.
14. Olson KR, Roth B: Update on the management of the patient with overdose, the PedsCCM-Teaching Files, 1997, at http://www.chestnet.org/pccu/lesson9-12.html.
15. Lovejoy FH: Childhood poisonings: what role for ipecac and charcoal? *Contemp Pediatr* 12:99-108, 1992.
16. Rumack BH: Acetaminophen overdose in children and adolescents, *Pediatr Clin North Am* 33:691-701, 1986.
17. 1. Madsen M: Poisonings, ingestions and overdoses, the PedsCCM-Teaching Files, 1996, at http://www.peds.umn.edu/divisions/pccm/acp/poison.html.
18. Farrell SE: Toxicity, acetaminophen. In MC Fernandez, JT VanDeVoort, MJ Burns et al, ed: *Emedicine online medical reference textbooks,* 2000, at http://www.emedicine.com/emerg/topic819.htm.
19. Madsen M: Specific toxins. In the PedsCCM-Teaching Files, 1996, at http://www.ped.umn.edu/divisions/pccm/teaching/acp/toxin.html.
20. Osborn HH: Barbiturates and other sedative-hypnotics. In Goldfrank LR et al, ed: *Goldfrank's toxicologic emergencies,* ed 6, Stamford, Conn, 1998, Appleton & Lange.
21. Bertino JS, Reed MD: Barbiturate and non-barbiturate sedative intoxication in children, *Pediatr Clin North Am* 33:703-722, 1986.
22. Hofert SM: Poisonings. In Siberry GK, Iannone R, eds: *The Harriet Lane handbook,* ed 15, St Louis, 2000, Mosby.
23. Doyen S: Carbamazepine. In Goldfrank LR, Flomenbaum NE, Lewin NA, eds: *Goldfrank's toxicologic emergencies,* ed 6, Stamford, Conn, 1998, Appleton & Lange.
24. Lifshitz M, Gavilov V, Sofer S: Signs and symptoms of carbamazepine overdose in young children, *Pediatr Emerg Care* 16:26-27, 2000.
25. Wason S, Baker RC, Carolan P et al: Carbamazepine overdose—the effects of multiple dose activated charcoal, *Clin Toxicol* 30:39-48, 1992.
26. Weaver DF, Camfield P, Fraser A: Massive carbamazepine overdose: clinical and pharmacologic observations in five episodes, *Neurology* 38:755-759, 1988.
27. Goldfrank LR, Flomenbaum NE: Toxic alcohols. In Goldfrank LR, Flomenbaum NE, Lewin NA et al, eds: *Goldfrank's toxicologic emergencies,* ed 6, Stamford, Conn, 1998, Appleton & Lange.
28. DeRoos F: Clonidine. In Goldfrank LR, Flomenbaum NE, Lewin NA et al, eds: *Goldfrank's toxicologic emergencies,* ed 6, Stamford, Conn, 1998, Appleton & Lange.
29. Roberts JR, Zink BJ: Clonidine. In Haddad LM, Winchester JF, eds: *Clinical management of poisoning and drug overdose,* ed 2, Philadelphia, 1990, WB Saunders.
30. Wiley JF II, Wiley CC, Torrey SB et al: Clonidine poisoning in young children, *J Pediatr* 116:654-658, 1990.
31. Mack RB: Clonidine overdose—kingdom of the temporarily infirm, *Contemp Pediatrics* 5:149-154, 1988.
32. Lewin NA, Howland MA: Antihypertensive agents: including beta blockers and calcium channel blockers. In Goldfrank LR, Flomenbaum NE, Lewin NA et al, eds: *Goldfrank's toxicologic emergencies,* ed 4, Norwalk, Conn, 1990, Appleton & Lange.
33. Woolf AD, Berkowitz ID, Liebelt E et al: Poisoning and the critically ill child. In Rogers MC, ed: *Textbook of pediatric intensive care,* Baltimore, 1996, Williams & Wilkins.
34. Perrone J: Iron. In Goldfrank LR, Flomenbaum NE, Lewin NA et al, eds: *Goldfrank's toxicologic emergencies,* ed 6, Stamford, Conn, 1998, Appleton & Lange.
35. Mann KV, Picciotti MA, Spevack TA et al: Management of acute iron overdose, *Clinical Pharmacy* 8:428-440, 1989.
36. Henretig FM, Temple AR: Acute iron poisoning in children, *Clin Lab Med* 4:575-586, 1984.
37. Everson GW, Bertoccini EJ, O'Leary J: Use of whole bowel irrigation in an infant following iron overdose, *Am J Emerg Med* 9:366-369, 1991.
38. Weisman RS: Theophylline. In Goldfrank LR, Flomenbaum NE, Lewin NA et al, eds: *Goldfrank's toxicologic emergencies,* ed 6, Stamford, Conn, 1998, Appleton & Lange.
39. Gaudreault P, Wason S, Lovejoy Jr. FH: Acute pediatric theophylline overdose: a summary of 28 cases, *J Pediatr* 102:474-476, 1983.
40. Gaudreault P, Guay J: Theophylline poisoning: pharmacologic considerations and clinical management, *Medical Toxicology and Adverse Drug Exposures* 1:169-191, 1986.
41. Seneff M et al: Acute theophylline toxicity and the use of esmolol to reverse cardiovascular instability, *Ann Emerg Med* 19:671-673, 1990.
42. Weisman RS: Cyclic antidepressants. In Goldfrank LR, Flomenbaum NE, Lewin NA et al, eds: *Goldfrank's toxicologic emergencies,* ed 6, Stamford, Conn, 1998, Appleton & Lange.
43. McFee RB, Mofenson HC, Caraccio TR: A nationwide survey of the management of unintentional low dose tricyclic antidepressant ingestions involving asymptomatic children: implications for the development of an evidenced-based clinical guideline, *J Toxicol Clin Toxicol* 38:15-19, 2000.
44. Bauman LA: Poisoning in the traumatized pediatric patient, *Int Anesthesiol Clini* 32:103-121, 1994.
45. Bosse GM, Matyunos NJ: Delayed toxidromes, *J Emerg Med* 17:679-690, 1999.
46. Braden NJ, Jackson JE, Walson PD: Tricyclic antidepressant overdose, *Pediatr Clin North Am* 33:287-297, 1986.
47. Egland AG, Landry DR: Alcohols. In Bowman JG et al, ed: *Emedicine online medical reference textbooks,* 2000, at http://www.emedicine.com/emerg/topic19.htm.
48. Dies DF, Guidry SA, McMartin KE et al: Methanol & ethylene glycol intoxication: diagnosis and management, *Resident and Staff Physician* 43:12-21, 1997.
49. Jacobsen D, McMartin KE: Methanol and ethylene glycol poisonings: mechanism of toxicity, clinical course, diagnosis and treatment, *Med Toxicol* 1:309-334, 1986.
50. Barceloux DG, Krenzelok EP, Olson K et al: American academy of clinical toxicology practice guidelines on the treatment of ethylene glycol poisoning, *J Toxicol Clin Toxicol* 37:537-560, 1999.
51. Hollander JE, Hoffman RS: Cocaine. In Goldfrank LR, Flomenbaum NE, Lewin NA et al, eds: *Goldfrank's toxicologic emergencies,* ed 6, Stamford, Conn, 1998, Appleton & Lange.
52. Bateman DA, Heagerty MC: Passive freebase cocaine ("crack") inhalation by infants and toddlers, *Am J Dis Child* 143:25-27, 1989.
53. Hoffman RS, Hollander JE: Evaluation of patients with chest pain after cocaine use, *Critical Care Clinics* 13:809-828, 1997.

54. Nelson LS: Opioids. In Goldfrank LR, Flomenbaum NE, Lewin NA et al, eds: *Goldfrank's toxicologic emergencies,* ed 6, Stamford, Conn, 1998, Appleton & Lange.

55. Sporer KA: Acute heroin overdose, *Ann Intern Med* 130:584-590, 1999.

56. Preston A: Extract from the methadone briefing, ISDD, London, 1996, at http://www.drugtext.com.

57. Goldfrank LR, Lewin NA: Phencyclidine. In Goldfrank LR, Flomenbaum NE, Lewin NA et al, eds: *Goldfrank's toxicologic emergencies,* ed 6, Stamford, Conn, 1998, Appleton & Lange.

58. Berger P: Phencyclidine, Encarta online Encyclopedia, 2000, at http://www.ncbi.nln.nih.gov.encarta.

59. Rao RB, Hoffman RS: Acetaminophen toxicity in an urban county hospital, *N Engl J Med* 338:544-545, 1998.

60. Rothstein FC: Caustic injuries to the esophagus in children, *Pediatr Clin North Am* 33:665-689, 1986.

61. Kardon E: Caustic ingestions. In Kreplick L, VanDeVoot JT, Burns MJ et al, eds: *Emedicine online medical reference textbooks,* 2000, at http://www.emedicine.com/emerg/topic86.htm.

62. Henretig FM, Shannon M: Toxicologic emergencies. In Fleisher G, Ludwig S, eds: *Textbook of emergency medicine,* ed 3, Baltimore, 1993, Williams & Wilkins.

63. Litovitz TL: The alcohols: ethanol, methanol, isopropanol, ethylene glycol, *Pediatr Clin North Am* 33:311-323, 1986.

64. Keaton BF: Chlorinated hydrocarbons. In Haddad LM, Winchester JF, eds: *Clinical management of poisoning and drug overdose,* ed 2, Philadelphia, 1990, WB Saunders.

65. Shih RD: Hydrocarbons. In Goldfrank LR, Flomenbaum NE, Lewin NA et al, eds: *Goldfrank's toxicologic emergencies,* ed 6, Stamford, Conn, 1998, Appleton & Lange.

31

Resuscitation and Transport of Infants and Children

Mary Fallon Smith
Aimee Lyons

Pediatric resuscitation offers a challenge to the pediatric critical care nurse. Participating in resuscitation attempts requires specialized knowledge and skills. Consideration of the potential impact of the child's developmental maturity integrated with nursing's humanistic approach to supporting families in crises is a vital aspect of care.

Educational programs in advanced pediatric life support are now widely available, including the Emergency Nursing Pediatric Course (ENPC) and Trauma Nursing Core Course (TNCC) from the Emergency Nurses Association and Pediatric Advanced Life Support (PALS) provider course from the American Heart Association. These courses provide an excellent means of preparing nurses to manage emergent situations when caring for children. Consistent use of the techniques taught in these courses can greatly improve the success rate of pediatric resuscitation efforts.

This chapter begins with a discussion of the epidemiology of cardiopulmonary arrest in infants and children. Research that influenced standards of pediatric resuscitation are discussed. The standards for pediatric advanced life support are reviewed, emphasizing nursing care issues. Management and coordination of the transport of critically ill children are then outlined.

EPIDEMIOLOGY OF CARDIOPULMONARY ARREST IN CHILDREN

Intentional and nonintentional injuries remain the most common cause of death in children over 1 year of age, followed by cancer and congenital anomalies.[1] Half of all infant deaths are caused by one of four diagnoses: congenital anomalies, prematurity or low birth weight, sudden infant death syndrome (SIDS), and respiratory distress syndrome.[2] The data show a much higher incidence of deaths in the infant population (711 per 100,000) than in all other pediatric ages combined (38 per 100,000).

The average age of children requiring cardiopulmonary resuscitation (CPR) reported from a large urban pediatric center was 1.98 years of age with a median age of 5 months.[3] Children under the age of 1 year accounted for roughly half of all cases reported in a review by Young and Seidel.[4] The incidence of adolescent CPR was shown to be intermediate between that of children and adults. These statistics are helpful in identifying age groups at higher risk for cardiopulmonary arrest.

ETIOLOGY OF CARDIOPULMONARY ARREST

Cardiac arrest resulting from primary cardiac dysfunction is a rare occurrence in the pediatric population.[5] Pediatric cardiac arrests occur after a prolonged disruption in homeostasis produced by the final common pathways of *respiratory failure* or *cardiovascular collapse*.

TABLE 31-1 Survival Rates in Pediatric CPR

Patient Characteristic	Survival Rate (%)
Prehospital	8.4
Inpatient	24
Intensive care unit	20
Drowning	26
Asystole	5
VT/VF	30
Age <1 year	6

Adapted from Young KD, Seidel JS: Pediatric cardiopulmonary resuscitation: a collective review, *Ann Emerg Med* 33:195-204, 1999. *CPR,* Cardiopulmonary resuscitation; *VF,* ventricular fibrillation; *VT,* ventricular tachycardia.

In a secondary cardiac arrest, widespread organ dysfunction occurs not only during the arrest but also during the period preceding the arrest. Pediatric resuscitation attempts are often very difficult and prolonged because the precipitating events, such as a prolonged period of hypoxemia, acidosis, and organ hypoperfusion, must be corrected, and ongoing secondary organ dysfunction must be reversed. Secondary cardiac arrest also predisposes patients to severe or irreversible organ damage, for example, poor neurologic outcome or multiorgan dysfunction syndrome (MODS).

Respiratory failure is imminent when the respiratory system is unable to fulfill its role in gas exchange. The causes of respiratory failure are varied and result from both intrinsic and extrinsic factors. Any shock state can contribute to insufficient tissue perfusion and cardiovascular collapse. In contrast, a small segment of the pediatric population suffers from significant cardiac disease such as complex congenital heart disease (CHD), post–cardiac surgery myocardial/conduction system dysfunction, myocarditis, and cardiomyopathy.

One of the major features that distinguishes pediatric patients suffering cardiac arrest from adults is that the causes in children are diverse. Young and Seidel[4] conducted a collective review of the current body of knowledge regarding survival rates and outcomes in pediatric CPR. The review encompassed data from 44 studies over 27 years for a total of 3094 patients. A summary of their findings, outlined in Table 31-1, reflects the diverse characteristics regarding pediatric cardiopulmonary arrest. A noteworthy finding was that patients in respiratory arrest who did not deteriorate into cardiac arrest had a 75% hospital discharge rate.

In a series of pediatric CPR cases occurring in the hospital, Ludwig[3] found that the most common diagnoses of hospitalized patients requiring resuscitation involved the respiratory system. Cardiac and central nervous system abnormalities occurred at relatively the same rates but half as often as respiratory disorders. Other causes included gastrointestinal and multisystem disorders. In their experience, 80% of children who arrested followed the pathway of respiratory distress, respiratory failure, and then cardiac arrest.

Regardless of the setting, one dramatic finding in pediatric resuscitation research is that the type of arrest significantly influences outcome. Although the causes of pediatric cardiac arrest vary across settings, the outcomes are equally dismal. The survival rate and long-term neurologic outcome for children who suffer pure respiratory arrest with timely intervention are dramatically better than those of secondary cardiac arrest, even when intervention is rapidly initiated. There was a 25% mortality rate for children who experienced a respiratory arrest and an 87% mortality rate when cardiac arrest occurred.[4] An exception to this is the near-drowning patient. Children who receive rapid early advanced life support have a survival rate closer to 35%.[6]

RED FLAGS OF IMPENDING CARDIOPULMONARY ARREST

Nurses, by early recognition of the prearrest state, can significantly affect patient outcome. This intervention requires expertise in recognizing the *red flags* of impending cardiopulmonary arrest. These include clinical signs of compensation for respiratory distress and cardiovascular collapse that are present in the clinically unstable pediatric patient. Many believe that "children deteriorate rapidly," but in reality, they are exquisitely capable of compensating until they can no longer support vital organ function. The clinical manifestations of compensation are related to failure of oxygen delivery to end organs, such as the skin, brain, kidney, and cardiovascular system.

Even if vital signs are within the normal range for the patient's age, if they are incongruent with the child's clinical need, they are considered red flags. Faster heart rates can be expected when, for example, the patient is active, anxious, anemic, dehydrated, febrile, or in pain. Faster respiratory rates can be expected, for example, in the active, febrile child or when there is significant past medical history of chronic pulmonary disease. Faster heart and respiratory rates indicate a need for increased cardiac output or minute ventilation. Rates incongruent with need are considered red flags.

Manifestations of oxygen deprivation to the skin include circumoral pallor, mottling, grayish color, cyanosis, diaphoresis, and decreased capillary refill time. Pallor and mottling are earlier indicators of decreased oxygenation and deteriorate to cyanosis once compensatory reserves are depleted.

Red flags of respiratory distress are listed in Box 31-1. Tachypnea, a salient symptom, occurs as the patient attempts to maintain minute ventilation when tidal volume is compromised. Retractions become more pronounced when lung compliance continues to decrease within the highly compliant chest wall of the pediatric patient.

Airway problems often precipitate pediatric arrests because pathologic processes that cause airway narrowing exponentially compromise gas flow within the airway. Patients position themselves to maximize their airway; they

Box 31-1
Respiratory Distress: Red Flags

Early Signs

Tachypnea
Mechanics of breathing
  Retractions
  Nasal flaring
  Head bobbing
  Grunting on exhalation
  Air entry: stridor or wheezing
Change in breath sounds
  Prolonged inspiratory time—stridor
  Prolonged expiratory time—wheezing

Late Signs

Skin color changes—dusky or cyanotic
Apnea or irregular respirations
Change in level of consciousness or activity
Bradycardia

Box 31-2
Cardiovascular Collapse: Red Flags

Early Signs

Tachycardia
Altered perfusion
  Skin
    Prolonged capillary refill
    Increased core-to-skin temperature gradient
  Brain
    Altered level of consciousness or activity
    Decreased response to parents
    "Worried" appearance
  Kidneys
    Decreased urine output
Decrease in pulse quality

Late Signs

Decreased response to pain
Flaccid tone
Hypotension
Bradycardia

sit up, lean forward, and extend their neck. Inspiratory stridor is present with upper airway disease, whereas wheezing may be heard on auscultation in lower airway disease. Inspiratory times are prolonged in upper airway disease; the opposite is true in lower airway disease. Grunting on expiration occurs as an infant attempts to maintain functional residual capacity (FRC).

Changes in the patient's level of consciousness or activity depend on the patient's primary alteration in gas exchange. With hypoxia the patient usually becomes restless, agitated, and irritable. Hypercapnia usually produces opposite symptoms; the patient usually becomes somnolent and lethargic, has decreased muscle tone, loses interest in the environment, or, even more ominous in a toddler, is less reactive to a parent's departure.

Late signs of respiratory distress often include apnea and decreasing level of consciousness or activity, followed by bradycardia. Much energy is expended trying to maintain oxygenation and ventilation. Infants, especially, tire and exhibit periods of apnea.

Arterial blood gases (ABGs) that are incongruent with the patient's clinical presentation serve to quantify the patient's ominous status. When a patient begins to tire, $Paco_2$ levels climb despite tachypnea, and Pao_2 falls despite increasing Fio_2. Pulse oximeters have facilitated rapid detection and intervention during transient periods of arterial desaturation. The end-tidal CO_2 ($ETco_2$) increases with the $Paco_2$, then precipitously falls as pulmonary perfusion becomes compromised.[7]

Red flags of cardiovascular compromise include tachycardia and alterations in perfusion to the skin, brain, and kidneys (Box 31-2). Tachycardia, the first sign of a stressed cardiac state, serves to maintain cardiac output when stroke volume is compromised by inadequate preload, increased afterload, or myocardial dysfunction. The smaller the child, the more reliant on heart rate to maintain cardiac output. Blood pressure is usually not helpful as an early sign of

deterioration because increased systemic vascular resistance (SVR) maintains blood pressure when the cardiac output is decreased.

Hypotension is not evident until approximately 25% of the intravascular volume is lost. The estimated circulating blood volume in children represents approximately 8% of the body weight or 80 ml/kg. For example, a 5-kg infant may be expected to have a circulating blood volume of 400 ml; 8% of 5 kg is equal to 400 g or ml (1 g = 1 ml). A 25% blood loss in a 5-kg infant is 100 ml.

Early symptoms of low cardiac output are the signs of increased SVR and are best assessed in end-organ perfusion of the skin, brain, and kidney. Signs include capillary refill longer than 2 seconds, a mottled or marbleized skin appearance, an increased core-to-skin temperature gradient, an altered level of consciousness, a worried appearance, and decreased urine output (less than 1 ml/kg in an infant or 0.5 ml/kg in a child older than 2 years).

Infants' temperatures drop, and serum glucose and calcium levels fall when infants are stressed. Late symptoms of cardiovascular collapse include decreased response to pain, flaccid muscle tone, hypotension, and bradycardia. These symptoms are directly related to progressive intracellular acidosis and hypoxia.

Severe hypoglycemia may also lead to cardiac compromise. The clinical manifestations are similar to cerebral hypoxia. Hypoglycemia may also lead to secondary failure of oxygen delivery as a result of hypoperfusion.

STRATEGIES FOR PREVENTION OF CARDIOPULMONARY ARREST

Although the outcome for pediatric patients who suffer cardiac arrest is grim, existing research has identified a number of factors that may improve outcome. These factors include prevention, early recognition, and monitoring of children in distress.[8]

Prevention of a pulseless state is critical. Early application of both basic and advanced life support to prevent a pulseless state has been related to improved outcome.[3,4] This intervention is especially critical in the prehospital phase of care. Pediatric patients are often brought to the emergency department with minimal treatment in the field.[9] Many emergency medical service (EMS) systems train and equip their emergency medical technicians (EMTs) primarily to provide adult life support. This leads to prolonged periods of hypoxia and hypoperfusion in children who are critically ill during transport. This issue is being addressed through emergency medical services for children (EMS-C) programs across the country.[10] Advanced training in prehospital critical care should lead to the prevention of a significant number of cardiopulmonary arrests in children.

Prevention strategies also apply to the emergency department setting. Pediatric resuscitation is challenging for emergency department staff because of the diverse range in the age and size of the children who come to the hospital with impending cardiopulmonary arrest. Lanoix and Golden[11] recommend enhancing pediatric resuscitation rooms in emergency departments by color coding all equipment, displaying a simplified wall chart of pediatric parameters, and suspending monitoring equipment from the ceiling. A weight-based quick reference for pediatric emergency medications and infusion drip rates can be used to expedite drug administration. A sample is shown in Fig. 31-1. Implementing any of these recommendations will save time and anxiety during resuscitation efforts.

The emergency team can also take steps to improve outcomes of patients who come to the hospital with multiple trauma. Data have shown that delays in the provision of definitive care for children who have been critically injured increase mortality and morbidity rates.[12] Implementation of a formal pediatric trauma team that can be rapidly mobilized expedites treatment and facilitates early involvement of the necessary specialists.

In all settings, the key factor in preventing the deterioration of respiratory failure or shock to cardiopulmonary arrest is in being prepared. Nurses play a crucial role in this area. Nurses ensure that the emergency equipment of the correct size is available and operating, in case it is needed. This equipment includes a resuscitation bag and mask, suction set up with both tonsil tip and endotracheal suction catheters, laryngoscope handle and blade, a stylet and an endotracheal tube (ETT) (including one size above and below). Resuscitation and intubation drugs can also be prepared in case they are needed.

One major factor influencing outcome in the pediatric population that has probably received the least amount of empiric review is the role nurses play in the recognition of the prearrest state. Nurses play a critical role by recognizing the *red flags* of respiratory distress and cardiovascular compromise that are present in the clinically unstable pediatric patient. The mark of a true nursing expert is skill in assessing these red flags, anticipating deterioration in

patient status, and advocating for changes in collaborative management when early signs of distress are evident.

COLLABORATIVE MANAGEMENT

The alphabetical approach to resuscitation is the same for all age groups, but pediatric resuscitation requires an emphasis on support of ventilation, as well as an awareness of the influence of maturation on respiratory and cardiovascular system performance. The goal is to restore stability as soon as possible by reestablishing vital organ perfusion and oxygenation, especially to the brain. Neurologic outcome appears to be directly related to the child's response to initial resuscitation efforts rather than postresuscitation interventions.

Very little clinical research on resuscitation of pediatric patients exists, largely because the overall incidence of cardiopulmonary arrest in infants and children is low. Much of the data that guide pediatric practice are derived from animal models with ventricular fibrillation (VF) that are not reflective of causes most commonly seen in pediatric arrests.[13] As new research becomes available, revisions to the existing standards can be anticipated.

Airway Management and Breathing

Positioning is the first step in airway management. Infants should be placed in the "sniffing position" by a head tilt–chin lift or jaw-thrust maneuver that brings the angle of the chin up 90 degrees from the bed (Figs. 31-2 and 31-3). This maneuver prevents hyperextension of the airway and allows maximal ventilation. In contrast to the neutral head position in the infant, a child's head is positioned slightly farther back. Roth and colleagues[14] found the jaw-thrust maneuver to be more effective than the head tilt–chin lift maneuver in maintaining an open airway in unconscious children. If any secretions, blood, or vomitus are noted in the posterior pharynx when the airway is positioned, they should be immediately suctioned with a rigid tonsil-tip suction device to clear the child's airway.

Airway adjuncts may be required to maintain a patent airway in children who are spontaneously breathing. An oropharyngeal airway is indicated for unconscious patients to relieve obstruction from the tongue. It is sized by placing it next to the patient's face with the flange at the corner of the mouth and the tip at the angle of the jaw.[15] The airway is placed by using a tongue depressor to displace the tongue downward. It is then inserted into the mouth following the natural contour of the tongue.

A nasopharyngeal airway is indicated for conscious patients with intact gag reflexes. It is also useful in children with nasopharyngeal edema. The length should approximate the distance between the nares and the tragus of the ear. Its diameter should be slightly smaller than that of the nares. It is inserted by lubricating and gently passing it along the floor of the nostril into the nasopharynx.

Once a patent airway is established, the spontaneously breathing patient with compromised ventilation or perfusion

Weight = 19 Kilograms			
Resuscitation	Standard Dose /kg	Dose mg	Dose cc's
Atropine (0.4 mg/cc)	0.02 mg/kg	0.38 mg	0.95 cc's
Bicarbonate (1 mEq/cc)	1 mEq/kg	19 mEq	19 cc's
Calcium Chloride	0.1 cc/kg	190 mg	1.9 cc's
Calcium Gluconate	0.5 cc/kg	950 mg	9.5 cc's
Dextrose 25% (0.25 gm/cc)	0.25-1 gm/kg	4.75-19 gm	19-76 cc's
Dextrose 50% (0.5 gm/cc)	0.25-1 gm/kg	4.75-19 gm	9.5-38 cc's
Epinephrine (1:10,000)	0.1 cc/kg	190 mcg	1.9 cc's
* High Dose (1:1,000)	0.1 cc/kg	1900 mcg	1.9 cc's
Lidocaine (20 mg/cc)	1 mg/kg	19 mg	0.95 cc's
Naloxone (Narcan) (0.4 mg/cc)	0.1 mg/kg	1.9 mg	4.8 cc's
Bretylium (50 mg/cc)	5 mg/kg	95 mg	1.9 cc's
Adenosine (3 mg/cc)	0.1 mg/kg	1.9 mg	0.63 cc's
Sedative/Anticonvulsive			
Lorazepam (Ativan) (2 mg/cc)	0.1 mg/kg	1.9 mg	0.95 cc's
Diazepam (Valium) (5 mg/cc)	0.1-0.3 mg/kg	1.9-5.7 mg	0.38-1.1 cc's
Midazolam (Versed) (1 mg/cc)	0.1 mg/kg	1.9 mg	1.9 cc's
Midazolam (Versed) (5 mg/cc)	0.1 mg/kg	1.9 mg	0.38 cc's
Phenytoin (Dilantin) (50 mg/cc)	10 mg/kg	190 mg	3.8 cc's
Fentanyl (50 mcg/cc)	2 mcg/kg	38 mg	0.76 cc's
Phenobarb (65 mg/cc)	10 mg/kg	190 mg	2.9 cc's
Muscle Relaxants			
Succinylcholine (Quelicin) (20 mg/cc)	1.5 mg/kg	28.5 mg	1.4 cc's
Pancuronium (Pavulon) (1 mg/cc)	0.1 mg/kg	1.9 mg	1.9 cc's
Atracurium (Tracrium) (10 mg/cc)	0.5 mg/kg	9.5 mg	0.95 cc's
Vecuronium (Norcuron) (1 mg/cc)	0.1 mg/kg	1.9 mg	1.9 cc's
ANESTHETICS			
Methohexital (Brevital) (10 mg/cc)	1-2 mg/kg	19-38 mg	1.9-3.8 cc's
**Thiopental (Pentothal) (25 mg/cc)	4 mg/kg	76 mg	3 cc's
Ketamine (Ketalar) (10 mg/cc)	1-2 mg/kg	19-38 mg	1.9-3.8 cc's

* High dose epinephrine (1:1,000), to be used for ETT route and as a second dose I.V. (First ETT dose in newborns should be a standard dose)
**Per anesthesia request a full 10 cc syringe of the above thiopental dilution shall be drawn up during an elective intubation.

Medication	How to Mix Infusion	Rate		
*DOPAMINE	Mix 60 mgs. (1.5 cc's)	FACTOR = .95		
40 mgs/cc	Dopamine with 48.5 cc's	4.8 ccs/hr =	5	mcg/kg/min
	D5W	9.5 ccs/hr =	10	mcg/kg/min
		11.9 ccs/hr =	12.5	mcg/kg/min
		14.3 ccs/hr =	15	mcg/kg/min
		16.6 ccs/hr =	17.5	mcg/kg/min
		19 ccs/hr =	20	mcg/kg/min
*EPINEPHRINE	Mix 3 mgs. (3 cc's)	FACTOR = 19		
1 mg/ml	Epi. with 47 cc's	1.9 ccs/hr =	0.1	mcg/kg/min
(1:1000)	D5W	3.8 ccs/hr =	0.2	mcg/kg/min
		5.7 ccs/hr =	0.3	mcg/kg/min
		7.6 ccs/hr =	0.4	mcg/kg/min
		9.5 ccs/hr =	0.5	mcg/kg/min
*LIDOCAINE	Mix 200 mgs. (5 cc's)	FACTOR = .285		
40 mg/cc	Lidocaine with 45 cc's	5.7 ccs/hr =	20	mcg/kg/min
	D5W	7.1 ccs/hr =	25	mcg/kg/min
		8.6 ccs/hr =	30	mcg/kg/min
		10 ccs/hr =	35	mcg/kg/min
		11.4 ccs/hr =	40	mcg/kg/min
*DOBUTAMINE	Mix 60 mgs. (4.8 cc's)	FACTOR = .95		
250 mg/20 cc	Dobutamine with 45.2 cc	4.8 ccs/hr =	5	mcg/kg/min
	D5W	9.5 ccs/hr =	10	mcg/kg/min
		11.9 ccs/hr =	12.5	mcg/kg/min
		14.3 ccs/hr =	15	mcg/kg/min
		16.6 ccs/hr =	17.5	mcg/kg/min
		19 ccs/hr =	20	mcg/kg/min

Fig. 31-1 Pediatric emergency medications reference guide sample: 19 kilograms. (Courtesy Children's Hospital, CPR Committee, 1999.)

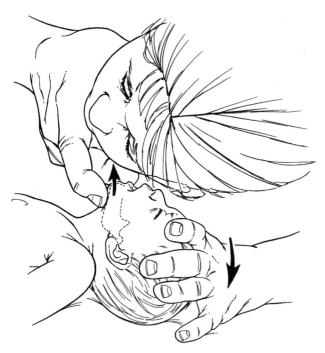

Fig. 31-2 Opening airway with head tilt–chin lift maneuver. One hand is used to tilt the head, extending the neck. Index finger of rescuer's other hand lifts the mandible outward by lifting on the chin. Note that the angle of the chin is 90 degrees from the bed. Head tilt should not be performed if cervical spine injury is suspected. (From *Textbook of pediatric advanced life support*, Dallas, 1994, American Heart Association.)

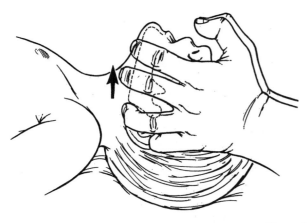

Fig. 31-3 Opening airway with jaw-thrust maneuver. Airway is opened by lifting the angle of the mandible. Rescuer uses two or three fingers of each hand to lift the jaw while other fingers guide the jaw upward and outward. (From *Textbook of pediatric advanced life support*, Dallas, 1994, American Heart Association.)

requires oxygen to be delivered at the highest possible concentration. A nonrebreather mask is the preferred method unless the patient requires assisted ventilation.[16]

Patients who are not breathing spontaneously require manual ventilation with a bag-valve-mask and 100% oxygen. The mask should be fitted as close as possible to the size of the child's face. A properly fitted mask provides an airtight seal and minimizes rebreathing. Effective ventila-

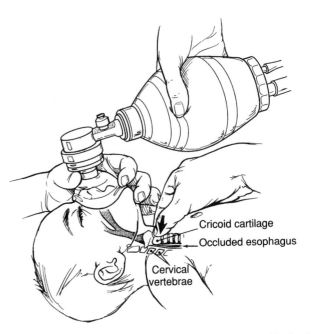

Fig. 31-4 Cricoid pressure (Sellick maneuver). (From *Textbook of pediatric advanced life support*, Dallas, 1994, American Heart Association.)

tion with 100% oxygen should be consistently maintained because children do not tolerate even short periods of hypoxia. When pressures greater than 15 cm H_2O are necessary to adequately ventilate the patient, the Sellick maneuver (pressure over the larynx on the anterolateral surface of the cricoid cartilage) can be used to collapse the esophagus against the cervical vertebrae (Fig. 31-4). This maneuver may prevent aspiration in the unintubated patient.

Healthy lungs of infants and children are normally very compliant and accept large tidal volumes (V_T) at low pressures. The delivered V_T is the amount needed to provide normal chest excursion, usually 7 to 10 ml/kg. Care is taken because most pediatric resuscitation bags are capable of delivering volumes in excess of the individual needs of the patient. Self-inflating bags deliver volume until the pressure exceeds that of the pop-off valve, which is usually 30 to 35 cm H_2O. Self-inflating bags only deliver an FIO_2 of 0.5 to 0.6 unless a gas reservoir is present. In contrast, anesthesia bags refill with fresh gas, thus delivering an FIO_2 of 1.0. Anesthesia bags are also capable of a wider range of peak inspiratory pressures (PIPs) and positive end-expiratory pressure (PEEP) and thus are useful in patients with poor lung compliance. Use of excessive pressures places the patient at risk for barotrauma; therefore anesthesia bags should be operated by experienced personnel, with pressures monitored and controlled using an attached pressure gauge and gas escape valve.

Children have a greater propensity for air swallowing when distressed. This, along with increased tracheal-esophageal proximity, places the child at risk for gastric distension during positive pressure bag-valve-mask ventilation. In addition to the risk of pulmonary aspiration, gastric

Box 31-3
Steps in Rapid-Sequence Induction Process

1. Organize equipment and personnel
2. Administer 100% oxygen
3. Administer premedications
4. Administer sedatives and paralytics
5. Intubate
6. Confirm endotracheal tube placement

TABLE 31-2 Guidelines for Rapid-Sequence Intubation (RSI) Medications

Patient Condition	RSI Medication
Nonhead trauma	A. Pentothal
	B. Succinylcholine
	C. Atropine (under age 7)
Head trauma	A. Lidocaine
	B. Pentothal
	C. Pancuronium 0.01 mg/kg (defasciculating dose) followed by succinylcholine OR: Rocuronium 1.2 mg/kg
	D. Atropine
Asthma	A. Ketamine
	B. Succinylcholine
	C. Atropine
Hypotension	A. Midazolam
Contraindications to succinylcholine (hyperkalemia, renal disease, muscular disease, burns)	A. Pentothal
	B. Rocuronium
	C. Atropine
Postintubation	A. Pancuronium
	B. Lorazepam
Pain control	A. Fentanyl

Courtesy Collaborative Practice Group, Emergency Department, Children's Hospital, Boston.

distension elevates the diaphragm, compromising lung expansion and tidal volume. Gastric decompression, using the largest nasogastric tube that the nares can accommodate comfortably, should be accomplished early in the resuscitation effort.

Patients requiring assisted ventilation need to be intubated as soon as possible by a provider who is skilled in pediatric intubation. Early endotracheal intubation is recommended because it secures the airway, facilitates the use of PEEP, and provides a route for the administration of select resuscitation drugs when venous access is delayed. However, for children who require intubation in out-of-hospital settings, effective bag-valve-mask ventilation may be preferable. Gaushe and colleagues[17] found that scene time was prolonged and fatal complications more likely when children were intubated in this setting. They recommended that emergency medical systems should focus training on providing effective bag-valve-mask ventilation, along with prompt transport, and defer endotracheal intubation until the patient arrives in the emergency department.

The safest method for intubating when there is risk of aspiration of gastric contents is by rapid-sequence induction (RSI). This method is performed following a sequence of steps involving preparation, preoxygenation, premedication, sedation, and paralysis. Box 31-3 outlines the steps in the procedure. Indications for RSI are respiratory arrest, need for airway control, Glasgow coma scale score of less than 8, shock, and respiratory failure. The RSI medications are selected based on the child's hemodynamic status, preexisting conditions, and institution-specific policies. Guidelines for medication selection in RSI are outlined in Table 31-2. Once RSI is accomplished, the patient is intubated.

Various methods for determining correct ETT size have been proposed. Appropriate ETT size often approximates the diameter of the patient's little, or fifth, finger, but this method is somewhat inaccurate and does not offer an opportunity to anticipate equipment needs before a patient's arrival in the emergency department or critical care unit. The following formula also accurately predicts correct ETT size: (Age in years + 16) ÷ 4.

Clearly, the ETT size chosen should be the largest that adequately ventilates the lungs while fitting comfortably through the glottis and the cricoid cartilage. Smaller sizes increase airway resistance, result in excessive air leaks, plug easily with secretions, and by themselves may ultimately cause respiratory failure. The nurse may anticipate anatomic variation by choosing three ETT sizes (one larger and one smaller than the calculated size).

Stylets are used to provide rigidity and direct the tip of the ETT up through the glottic opening. To avoid airway trauma, caution is taken to ensure that the stylet does not extend beyond the Murphy's eye or the tip of the ETT during intubation.

Confirmation of ETT placement is achieved most accurately by exhaled CO_2 detection (Fig. 31-5). Auscultating breath sounds high along the midaxillary line, the axillas, and the stomach further confirms ETT placement. Because of the thin chest wall and subsequent prevalence of referred breath sounds, slight change in the pitch of the patient's breath sounds may indicate right mainstem intubation in infants and children. Right mainstem intubation is a common problem in the pediatric population because of the standard length of ETTs and the variation in sizes of children. Additional clinical indicators of correct ETT placement include the presence of condensation in the ETT on expiration and symmetric chest excursion with manual ventilation. On chest radiographs, the ETT should be 1 to 2 cm above the carina or halfway between the carina and clavicles. The carina approximates the level of the fourth rib; therefore the tube should approximate the level of the third.

In rare instances, alternative methods to establish an airway may be necessary. Laryngeal mask airways may be

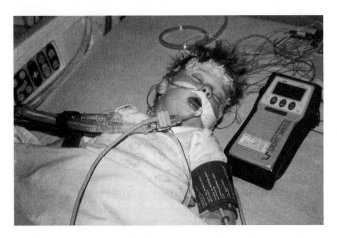

Fig. 31-5 End-tidal CO_2 monitor and endotracheal tube taping technique.

inserted as an alternative to a tracheal tube. They are available in sizes to accommodate infants and children. Surgical airways include cricothyrotomy and tracheostomy. Because of the close proximity of the cricoid cartilage to the vocal cords, a cricothyrotomy is always considered as a last resort, especially in children younger than age 12. Emergency tracheostomy is rarely performed.

Once intubated, the ETT is held firmly in place, and markings on the ETT in relation to the nares or lip line are noted while the tube is taped in place. The most common method of securing the ETT involves cutting two pieces of 1-inch tape that are torn in half and spiraling one half of each piece up the ETT. The other half of each piece is secured to the upper lip (see Fig. 31-5). The head is positioned at midline or maintained in a neutral position, particularly during radiographic determination of placement. Excessive flexion of the patient's neck may force an uncuffed ETT down onto the carina, and extension of the neck or rotation of the head may dislodge the ETT completely.

Continuous assessment of the adequacy of ventilation is always a priority. The magnitude and duration of hypoxia sustained during a period of respiratory distress or arrest adversely affect the myocardium, ultimately influencing myocardial response to resuscitation if cardiac arrest develops. Spontaneous breaths are supported with humidified oxygen at an FIO_2 of 1.0.

Short-term hyperventilation may be advantageous in the initial management of hypercapnia, and it provides a compensatory alkalosis in the patient with metabolic acidosis. However, sustained hyperventilation should be avoided because it may compromise cerebral blood flow and promote cerebral anoxia.

Circulation

In case of cardiac arrest, the primary goal in resuscitation is restoration of hemodynamic stability. After stabilization of the airway and establishment of adequate ventilation, pulses are immediately assessed to determine the need for cardiac compressions. This section expands on the traditional concept of circulation to include measures focused to improve tissue perfusion: vascular access and the administration of intravenous fluids, followed by resuscitation medications.

Cardiac Compressions. Cardiac compressions are indicated if pulses are absent or the pulse rate is less than 60/min with inadequate perfusion. Compression rates are recommended based on studies that have demonstrated a relationship between the faster rates and higher mean arterial pressures, cardiac index, and cerebral blood flow.[18]

Many studies are investigating the mechanism of blood flow and techniques to improve blood flow during CPR. However, controversy continues regarding the precise mechanism of blood flow during closed chest cardiac compression. Recent studies suggest that open cardiac compression produces better coronary and cerebral perfusion pressures.[19] This technique is most commonly reserved for resuscitation of trauma patients. Interposed abdominal compression and active compression-decompression CPR techniques are currently being evaluated in children.[20]

Establishing Vascular Access. Establishing vascular access to administer fluids and drugs is a priority once adequate oxygenation, ventilation, and compressions have been addressed. Obtaining venous access can be difficult and frustrating in the hemodynamically stable pediatric patient and worse in a patient in an arrest situation. During an arrest, the largest and most accessible vein that does not interrupt resuscitation is the preferred site for vascular access.

Establishment of percutaneous peripheral access is limited to three attempts or 90 seconds, whichever occurs first. The team then needs to consider other techniques and routes of administration. Several methods of venous access are commonly used in children. The steel needle (butterfly) is adequate for infants whose condition is stable but is not recommended during resuscitation because of the risk of infiltration, especially when administering caustic medications and fluids at high rates. Over-the-needle catheters are preferred because they can be inserted deep into the vein, thereby decreasing the risk of infiltration. Larger sizes that facilitate more rapid infusion rates are recommended.

Central lines provide access for volume replacement, rapid medication administration close to effector sites, and central venous pressure (CVP) measurement. Complications associated with this access option are reported more often in the pediatric age group. Therefore this procedure should be delegated to the more experienced provider to limit the iatrogenic complications of hemorrhage, pneumothorax, hemothorax, embolism, cardiac injury, or infection.[18]

Supradiaphragmatic central lines, the jugular and subclavian veins, are preferred, based on the theory that higher and more rapid peak serum drug concentrations are produced when medications are administered via this route than via more peripheral sites. However, neckline placement often interferes with the resuscitation attempt, and data are insufficient to support improved outcomes. Current recommendations still consider long catheters placed above the diaphragm from the femoral vein to be adequate.[18]

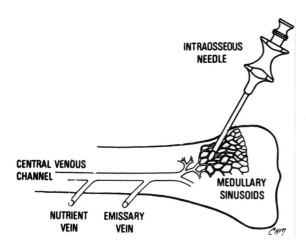

Fig. 31-6   Intramedullary venous system demonstrates position of intraosseous needle in medullary sinusoids. Blood may be aspirated from sinusoids to confirm position of needle. (From Spivey WH: Intraosseous infusions, *J Pediatr* 111:639-643, 1987.)

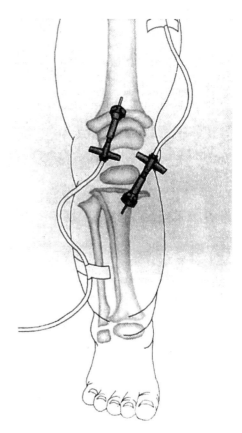

Fig. 31-7   Recommended sites for intraosseous infusion. (From Manley L, Haley K, Dick M: Intraosseous infusion: rapid vascular access for critically ill or injured infants and children, *J Emerg Nurs* 14:63-68, 1988.)

The intraosseous route for fluid and drug administration has regained popularity. An intraosseous infusion is recommended as an alternative means to deliver intravenous fluids and medications in children when vascular access is inadequate or unavailable within three attempts or 90 seconds, whichever comes first.[18] The success rate for this method in older children is lower; however, it is a reasonable alternative.[20a] Intraosseous infusion is accomplished by insertion of a bone marrow needle with stylet into the medullary cavity in a direction away from the epiphyseal plate (Fig. 31-6). The preferred site is the broad flat portion of the anteromedial surface of the tibia approximately 1 to 2 cm below the tibial tuberosity or above the femur's external condyles (Fig. 31-7). Successful insertion is demonstrated by (1) loss of resistance from the bony cortex, (2) aspiration of bone marrow, and (3) free flow of fluid without extravasation. The intraosseous route is acceptable for volume expansion with blood, plasma, colloids, or crystalloid. Average gravity flow rates of 100 ml/hr can be accomplished in the infant, whereas much higher flow rates have been reported when a pressure infuser is used. Drug levels achieved via the intraosseous route are similar to the peripheral venous route.

Complications associated with intraosseous infusion are rare. These complications may be prevented by limiting the amount of time they are in place and by avoiding the use of hypertonic solutions. The only absolute contraindication for the use of intraosseous access is placement within a recently fractured bone.

Fluid Resuscitation.   Most children suffering cardiopulmonary arrest require volume restoration or expansion because of excessive losses, venous pooling, vasodilation, and capillary leaking. Often, because of hesitancy in administering large volumes of fluid rapidly to small children, too little fluid is administered too late.

Volume restoration precedes the use of vasoactive drugs in resuscitation. The amount of volume administered depends on the extent of fluid deficit based on an estimate of

volume lost and presence of ongoing losses. It is not uncommon for children to require large amounts of fluid for resuscitation.[21] Several 20 ml/kg fluid boluses are required before any improvement in the patient's clinical response is appreciated. Controversy surrounds the type of fluid that should be administered during a resuscitation attempt. Colloids and synthetic colloids, such as 5% albumin and hetastarch, are true volume expanders and generally remain within an intact vascular space after administration. Colloids are not used in patients with capillary leak syndrome (e.g., those patients with trauma, sepsis, or burns) because of the high associated risk of respiratory distress syndrome. Approximately 20% to 25% of isotonic crystalloids, such as normal saline and Ringer's lactate, leak from the intravascular space shortly after administration; therefore volume replacement with crystalloid may require 20% to 25% more than the estimated loss. The advantage of using crystalloids is that they are relatively inexpensive and readily available.

The routine use of large volumes of high dextrose–containing fluids during fluid resuscitation for hypovolemic shock is avoided. This may result in significant hyperglycemia with resultant osmotic diuresis.

When hemorrhage occurs, the volume of red blood cell administration can be approximated by multiplying 4 ml/kg by the difference, in grams, between actual and desired hemoglobin. In cases in which the hemoglobin is unknown,

TABLE 31-3 Physiologic Approach to Resuscitation

A: Airway
B: Breathing (oxygenation + ventilation)
C: Circulation (perfusion)

Heart rate and rhythm	Asystole	Oxygen
	Bradycardia	Epinephrine (bolus and infusion)
		Atropine
	AV block	Oxygen
		Atropine or isoproterenol
		Epinephrine infusion
		Pacemaker
	PVCs	Oxygen
		Lidocaine
		Procainamide
	Ventricular tachycardia	Oxygen
		Cardioversion at 0.5-1 J/kg
		Amiodarone
		Lidocaine
		Magnesium
	Ventricular fibrillation	Oxygen
		Shocks at 2 J/kg
		May repeat doubling joules
		Consider: epinephrine
		Amiodarone
		Lidocaine
		Magnesium
Preload		Volume restoration
		Decrease excessive intrathoracic pressure
		Relieve cardiac tamponade
		Correct asynchronous cardiac rhythms
Afterload		Correct hypoxemia, acidosis, hypothermia
		Question congenital outflow obstruction
		Treat sepsis, drug overdose, anaphylaxis
		Consider vasodilators if CHF is present
Contractility		Correct hypoxemia, hypoglycemia, K^+ and Ca^+
		Correct acidosis: ventilation ($NaHCO_3$)
		Positive inotropic agents: epinephrine, dobutamine, dopamine, amrinone
		Primary management includes correction of hypoxemia, acidosis, hypoglycemia, potassium and calcium imbalance, hypothermia, vagal stimulation, and drug toxicity

AV, Atrioventricular; *CHF,* congestive heart failure; *PVCs,* premature ventricular contractions.

10 ml/kg of packed red blood cells or 20 ml/kg of whole blood is administered to restore blood volume.

Resuscitation Medications. Patients with persistent hypotension and poor perfusion following aggressive fluid resuscitation may require catecholamine support to restore effective cardiac output. Table 31-3 outlines a physiologic approach to resuscitation that helps to organize intervention priorities. Drugs, compared with airway and breathing, are often less essential in resuscitation of infants and children. Correction of hypoxemia and acidosis and the restoration of tissue perfusion are primary goals. However, the child's response to resuscitation efforts is poor in the face of uncorrected imbalances, such as pH, glucose, potassium, and calcium. Hypothermia further contributes to metabolic acidosis, which renders the myocardium refractory to electrical and pharmacologic intervention. Vagal stimulation may result in refractory bradydysrhythmias. In addition, toxic ingestions may compromise respiratory and cardiac function, requiring immediate intervention. Successful resuscitation depends on correction of such factors, with interventions beyond restoring adequate ventilation.

A great deal of individual physiologic variation, depending on system maturity, is present in the pediatric population. Children and adolescents are able to maintain cardiac output when heart rate decreases by increasing stroke volume. However, sick infants have relatively fixed stroke volumes, so cardiac output depends primarily on heart rate and rhythm. A relatively fixed stroke volume, characteristic of the infant for the first 6 to 12 months of life, is the result of limited ventricular compliance and contractility. Both are less than in the mature heart because of the greater proportion of noncontractile myocardial tissue relative to contractile myocardial mass.[22] In addition, increased interventricular interaction is especially evident in the small infant; that is, the degree of filling of one chamber affects the degree of filling of another.[22] Therefore if a large volume of fluid loads the right ventricle or if pulmonary hypertension is present, the interventricular septum will bulge toward the left and compromise left ventricular filling. Knowledge that infants lack myocardial function sufficient to respond to volume loading or overcome excessive afterload is important.

Sympathetic nervous system immaturity is another factor that requires consideration in seriously ill infants. Sympathetic innervation of the myocardium is incomplete at birth; therefore infants are less responsive to endogenous and exogenous stimulation of the sympathetic nervous system.[23] As a result, the use of catecholamines in infant resuscitation does not reliably produce the same effect as in the older child. Moreover, predicting the cardiovascular effect of any dose of any agent is difficult. Infants may require higher doses per kilogram of infused catecholamines, but their use requires continuous monitoring and titration of individual hemodynamic affects. Because of sympathetic immaturity, infants are more sensitive to parasympathetic stimulation and experience more vagal-induced bradydysrhythmias than older children.

In summary, determination of how best to individualize the use of catecholamines to improve cardiac output is based on the maturity of the patient. Receptor density and responsiveness, ventricular compliance, and stroke volume all improve with age.

The primary resuscitation drugs used in pediatric advanced life support are outlined in Table 31-4. All dosages are based on kilograms of body weight. It is important to closely estimate body weight using a reference chart or a

TABLE 31-4   Primary Pediatric Resuscitation Drugs

Drug	Dose	Nursing Implications
Epinephrine	IV/IO: 0.01mg/kg (1:10,000) ET: 0.1 mg/kg (1:1,000) Repeat doses: 0.1 mg/kg (1:1000)	Instill 2-3 ml normal saline following ET administration
Atropine	0.02 mg/kg (min 0.1 mg)	Masks hypoxia induced brady-cardia: monitor O_2 saturation Causes pupillary dilation
Sodium bicar-bonate	1 mEq/kg	Flush with normal saline before and after admin-istration
Calcium chloride	20 mg/kg	Administer slowly
Naloxone	<20 kg: 0.1 mg/kg >20 kg: 2 mg	Short duration may result in return of symptoms
Adenosine	0.1-0.2 mg/kg (max 12 mg)	Give rapid IV push Follow with imme-diate normal saline flush May cause tran-sient bradycardia
Amiodarone	5 mg/kg Repeat dose: 5 mg/kg Max: 15 mg/kg/day	Monitor for hypo-tension
Lidocaine	1 mg/kg	Give rapid bolus
Magnesium	25-50 mg/kg Max: 2 g	Use for presence of torsades de pointes

IV, Intravenous; *IO,* intraosseous; *ET,* endotracheal.

Broselow tape. The Broselow method bases dosages on patients' length. The tape is placed along the patient's side, and the appropriate drug dosages for the patient are preprinted on it. Suggested emergency cart medications are found in Appendix IV.

Epinephrine. During an asystolic arrest, the *initial* beneficial effect of any catecholamine is mediated through its alpha effect.[18] Epinephrine is the catecholamine of choice during resuscitation because it is direct acting and provides a perfect balance of alpha and beta stimulation. Alpha stimulation causes peripheral vasoconstriction that improves myocardial perfusion pressure generated during closed chest compressions, thus enhancing oxygen delivery to the heart. Epinephrine dramatically increases myocardial blood flow, cerebral blood flow, and subsequent cerebral oxygen uptake. Its effect redistributes carotid blood flow to the cerebral circulation and coronary blood flow to the myocardium, which then stimulates spontaneous cardiac contractions. Restoration of coronary artery perfusion pressures is essential for the return of spontaneous circulation. This effect is critical in infants and children because most arrest rhythms are unstable slow rhythms not related to heart block.

Guidelines for administering an epinephrine infusion are outlined in Chapter 27. Side effects of a peripheral epinephrine infusion include compromised skin and extremity blood flow.

Atropine. Atropine, a parasympathetic nervous system blocker, produces both positive chronotropic and dromotropic effects. It is indicated for slow arrest-related rhythms, that is, bradycardia and atrioventricular blocks resulting from structural heart disease.[18]

Slow rhythms during resuscitation most often occur as a result of hypoxemia. As a consequence, atropine is unlikely to be efficacious in this situation. Atropine also blocks hypoxemia-induced bradycardia. Therefore careful monitoring of oxygen saturation through pulse oximetry is indicated, and prolonged attempts at intubation are avoided.

Inadequate atropine doses stimulate vagal nuclei and produce paradoxical bradycardia. This affect is avoided by using the full vagolytic dose.

Sodium Bicarbonate. During an arrest, poor ventilation and low-flow states produce mixed respiratory and metabolic acidosis. Inadequate tissue perfusion results in anaerobic metabolism and subsequent lactic acid production. In addition, the circulation of poorly oxygenated blood further contributes to tissue hypoxia and subsequent ischemia. The priority in managing acidosis is restoration of ventilation and tissue perfusion. An in-depth discussion of acid-base imbalance is included in Chapter 9.

Sodium bicarbonate ($NaHCO_3$) serves as a buffer by combining with the hydrogen ion (H^+) to form carbonic acid (H_2CO_3), then CO_2 and H_2O. It is not a first-line drug in resuscitation. It is indicated when severe acidosis is documented related to prolonged cardiopulmonary arrest. It is also indicated for treatment of hyperkalemia and tricyclic antidepressant overdose.

Because CO_2 crosses the blood-brain barrier and cell membranes more rapidly than HCO_3, transient increases in CO_2 produced by $NaHCO_3$ administration can paradoxically worsen cerebrospinal fluid and intracellular acidosis. In hypoxic states, $NaHCO_3$ administration decreases myocardial contractility, cardiac index, and blood pressure and may worsen electromechanical dissociation. Because respiratory failure is often the precipitating event in cardiopulmonary arrest among infants and children, this population is at greater risk of severe intracellular acidosis because of impaired CO_2 elimination.

Many other physiologic disturbances occur with excessive $NaHCO_3$ administration. Potassium shifts into the intracellular space; a 0.1 rise in pH typically results in a 0.5 mEq/L decrease in serum potassium. Hypernatremia and hypocalcemia result. Hyperosmolar states may also result from increased serum sodium produced by $NaHCO_3$ administration. The intravascular shift of free water that results from hyperosmolarity may be lethal because it has been implicated in intracranial hemorrhage in infants. To prevent this, $NaHCO_3$ is diluted 1:1 with sterile water in infants younger than 3 months unless 4.2% infant $NaHCO_3$ is available (0.5 mEq/ml). $NaHCO_3$ *is not recommended* until the patient has been adequately oxygenated and ventilated, CPR has been initiated, epinephrine has been administered without success, and a venous pH of 7.0 or less or an arterial pH of 7.2 or less has been documented.[18]

Calcium. Calcium increases myocardial contractility, increases ventricular excitability, and increases conduction velocity through the ventricles. It is indicated in the management of documented total or ionized hypocalcemia (commonly seen in stressed infants) and in the management of the adverse cardiac effects associated with hyperkalemia, hypermagnesemia, and calcium channel blocker overdose. It may also be indicated for children who have received blood with citrate-phosphate-dextran used as a preservative.

Glucose. Glucose is indicated to treat documented hypoglycemia. Infants have limited glycogen reserves and when stressed, particularly in the presence of sepsis, experience acute marked hypoglycemia. Hypoglycemia depresses cardiac contractility and may precipitate seizure activity. Symptoms of hypoglycemia, which include decreased perfusion, diaphoresis, tachycardia, and hypotension, mimic those of hypoxemia.

Conversely, some evidence shows that hyperglycemia worsens neurologic outcome.[24] Rapid-response blood glucose screening methods should be used to guide administration of glucose.

Naloxone. Naloxone is an opiate antagonist that reverses the effects of narcotics, such as respiratory depression and hypoperfusion. It is indicated when narcotic overdose is suspected to be the cause of cardiopulmonary arrest. It is rapid acting and has a short half-life. For cases in which complete reversal is not desired, such as with patients on morphine drips, naloxone may be titrated to the desired effect.

Adenosine. Adenosine is an endogenous purine nucleoside. It exerts a strong depressant effect on the sinus and atrioventricular (AV) nodes. It slows conduction through the AV node and causes interruption of the reentry pathway. It is indicated for the treatment of supraventricular tachycardia (SVT). If the cause of the tachyarrhythmia is not a reentry mechanism, adenosine will not terminate it but may assist with identifying the underlying rhythm by producing a transient AV blockade. The half-life of adenosine is less than 10 seconds with duration of less than 2 minutes.

Amiodarone. Amiodarone is a lipid-soluble antiarrhythmic that may be used for atrial and ventricular arrhythmias. It produces vasodilatation and AV nodal suppression. It also inhibits the outward potassium current, which prolongs the QT interval. Amiodarone also inhibits sodium channels, which slows ventricular conduction. Its most acute side effect is hypotension. It is a highly complex pharmacologic agent with potential for long-term complications. Its long-term use should be directed by an expert such as a pediatric cardiologist.

Lidocaine. Lidocaine increases the fibrillation threshold by reducing the automaticity of ventricular pacemakers. It is indicated for ventricular fibrillation and ventricular tachycardia, which are rare events in children. Once the bolus doses of lidocaine have been effective, a lidocaine infusion is initiated. Guidelines for administration of a lidocaine drip are outlined in Chapter 27.

Lidocaine is metabolized by the liver. Therefore its dose is modified for children with inadequate liver function or decreased perfusion to the liver. Symptoms of lidocaine toxicity that initially appear are alterations in the central nervous system such as nausea, decreased mental status, and seizures. Depression of cardiac function may occur later as a result of toxicity.

Magnesium. Magnesium is a major intracellular cation. It inhibits calcium channels and causes smooth muscle relaxation. It is used in the treatment of torsades de pointes or documented hypomagnesemia.

Routes of Drug Administration. Routes of drug administration for resuscitation include central venous, endotracheal, intraosseous, and intracardiac. Ideally, resuscitation drugs are administered close to adrenergic receptor sites located on the arterial side of the circulation. To ensure that a bolus medication is delivered into the central circulation rapidly, each medication is followed with a rapid 2- to 5-ml normal saline flush. Continuous infusions of vasoactive medications can be initiated at 5 to 10 times the usual rate while heart rate and blood pressure are continuously monitored. When the desired effect is evident, the infusion rate is decreased. Another option is to administer the continuous infusion through a Y connector with a faster running intravenous line. Care is taken when titrating either line.

The intraosseous route is acceptable when venous access is delayed. The intraosseous route, considered similar to a peripheral venous route, is acceptable for all resuscitation drugs.

Although data in humans are limited, several resuscitation drugs defined by the acronym *LEAN* (lidocaine, epinephrine, atropine, and naloxone) may be administered by the tracheal route if intravenous access is unavailable. These drugs are rapidly absorbed when given by the tracheal route, having a direct cardiac effect. Ten times the standard intravenous dose is recommended via the tracheal route (i.e., 0.1 mg/kg of the 1:1000 solution).[18] Both epinephrine and atropine have a prolonged effect after tracheal administration; thus less frequent administration may be required.

All tracheal drugs should be diluted with 2 to 3 ml of normal saline and injected deeply into the tracheobronchial tree using a needleless syringe and attached suction catheter or feeding tube. Injection is accomplished after passive exhalation, and a resuscitation bag is used to distribute the drug throughout the lung periphery. Sterile normal saline is the only diluent recommended for this procedure, in volumes not to exceed 5 ml in infants or 10 ml in adolescents.

The intracardiac route for drug administration is a last resort, primarily because the procedure interrupts cardiopulmonary resuscitation. Other iatrogenic complications include cardiac tamponade, pneumothorax, and coronary artery laceration. If a drug is inadvertently injected into the myocardium, it may cause intractable VF.

Cardiac Dysrhythmia Management. During cardiopulmonary arrest in infants and children, hypoxic and acidotic blood circulates through normal coronary arteries under extremely low perfusion pressure. As a consequence, the majority of pediatric cardiopulmonary arrest-related dysrhythmias occur as a result of metabolic dysfunction and not from coronary artery disease. Therefore the emphasis in pediatric resuscitation is on reestablishing adequate oxygenation, ventilation, and tissue perfusion, *not* on complex rhythm analysis and its drug management.

Unstable rhythms that require treatment are those that compromise cardiac output and those that have the potential to deteriorate into a lethal rhythm. Extremes in heart rate are of no concern unless the effective cardiac output does not match the patient's clinical need. The clinical assessment parameters of blood pressure, heart rate, and end-organ perfusion (specifically to the brain, skin, and kidneys) provide rapid measures of the adequacy of cardiac output and effectiveness of intervention strategies.

Slow Rhythms. Slow rhythms are the most common arrest-related rhythm disturbance in infants and children. Because of heart rate dependency, the hemodynamic effect of bradydysrhythmias may be significant in an infant or child. Slow arrest-related dysrhythmias are related to either hypoxic-ischemic insults or structural heart disease.[18] Occasionally, primary bradycardic arrests occur in children with congenital complete heart block or in an infant during procedures that cause vagal stimulation (e.g., oral-pharyngeal stimulation or a Valsalva maneuver related to painful procedures).

Slow rhythms associated with hypoxic-ischemic insults are often wide QRS complex without P waves. Slow rhythms associated with structural heart disease are often related to heart block or sinus node dysfunction. Priorities for managing bradydysrhythmias start with the resuscitation ABCs (airway, breathing, and circulation) and then progress if severe cardiopulmonary compromise is present (Fig. 31-8).

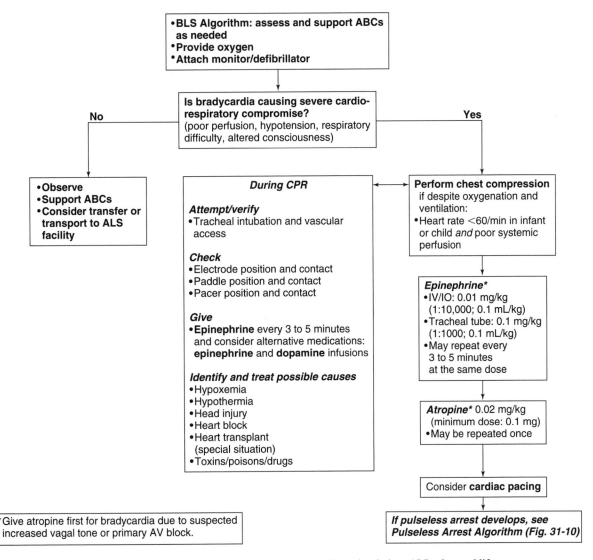

Fig. 31-8 PALS bradycardia algorithm. *ABCs,* airway, breathing, circulation; *ALS,* advanced life support; *IV,* intravenous. (From American Heart Association: Guidelines 2000 for cardiovascular care, *Circulation 2000,* 102(suppl):I291-I342, 2000.)

In an arrest, cardiac pacing may be helpful in managing patients with slow rhythms resulting from structural heart disease. Pacing can be accomplished by external (transcutaneous), transvenous, or epicardial electrodes. Pacing in the hypoxic-ischemic cardiac arrest patient is rarely successful. Even if ventricular capture is accomplished, pacing does not improve myocardial contractility and tissue perfusion.

Fast Rhythms. Fast rhythms are expected in critically ill pediatric patients. Unstable fast rhythms fall into two main categories: those with narrow QRS complexes and those with wide QRS complexes. The differential for narrow fast rhythms include sinus tachycardia (ST), supraventricular tachycardia (SVT), atrial flutter (AF), or atrial fibrillation (Af). One can easily mistake a rapid ST for SVT. Key diagnostic features of ST include rhythm variability and a heart rate that is congruent with the patient's need for increased cardiac output. Key diagnostic features of SVT include a monotonous rhythm and a heart rate in excess of the patient's clinical need. ST is a symptom reflecting the patient's need for increased cardiac output, whereas unstable SVT is a primary cardiac rhythm disturbance requiring primary intervention. AF and Af are rare cardiac rhythms in groups other than pediatric patients with complex CHD.

The differential for wide-complex fast rhythms is aberrantly conducted SVT or VT. Distinguishing between the two may be impossible in a patient whose condition is unstable. Because wide-complex SVT is extremely rare in the pediatric age group, *all wide-complex fast rhythms are considered to be VT until proven otherwise.*

Pediatric groups at risk for ventricular tachydysrhythmia as a terminal rhythm include children requiring prolonged resuscitation, infants beyond the neonatal period, older children, and children with CHD. A critical cardiac mass along with sympathetic maturity characteristic of infants beyond 6 to 12 months of age is thought to be necessary for ventricular tachydysrhythmias to occur. During prolonged resuscitation attempts, many doses of catecholamines, which stimulate the sympathetic nervous system, are often administered. Children with CHD who have arrests more often exhibit bradycardia but are 3 times more likely than those without CHD to exhibit ventricular tachydysrhythmias. Supporting the critical mass theory, many children with CHD usually have cardiac enlargement. Metabolic causes of ventricular dysrhythmias include hyperkalemia, hypoglycemia, hypothermia, and tricyclic antidepressant overdose.

Treatment of all unstable fast rhythms includes synchronized cardioversion at 0.5 J/kg (Fig. 31-9). If unsuccessful, the joules are doubled, and cardioversion is repeated.

In VT, lidocaine administration before cardioversion may result in a higher conversion rate. Lidocaine is administered in a dose of 1 mg/kg every 10 to 15 minutes. A continuous lidocaine infusion of 20 to 50 µg/kg/min is useful after conversion to normal sinus rhythm (NSR) if the patient has structural heart disease, has multiple premature ventricular contractions (PVC), or recurrent VT or VF.

Absent (Collapse) Rhythms. Absent (collapse) rhythms include asystole, VF, and pulseless electrical activity (PEA). These rhythms are considered hemodynamically significant because all three fail to produce cardiac output.

Asystole, like bradycardia, is a common pediatric arrest rhythm. The management goal is to improve oxygenation and perfusion (Fig. 31-10).

VF and pulseless VT, which are managed in a similar manner, are uncommon pediatric rhythms. The overall frequency of VF and VT is 10%.[4] *Immediate* shocks at 2 J/kg is the *most important* determinant of successful conversion to NSR. The pulse and cardiac rhythm are reevaluated after each shock attempt. If unsuccessful, the joules are doubled, and the patient is defibrillated twice in rapid succession. With the advent of automated external defibrillators (AED), shocks in the field are more readily available. AEDs are recommended for use in children older than 8 years old. Their use in the field has shown to be as effective for children as for adults.[25]

Epinephrine may improve coronary artery perfusion pressure, increasing the effectiveness of shocks. The epinephrine dose is increased after the first dose as for asystole and repeated every 3 to 5 minutes. Lidocaine may be used to increase the fibrillation threshold but should not delay defibrillation. Metabolic problems, such as calcium, potassium, magnesium, or glucose imbalance, and hypothermia or drug intoxication (e.g., with digitalis or tricyclic antidepressants), are continually reassessed and corrected. If VF reoccurs, the previous successful energy level for shocks are used.

Amiodarone is the next medication of choice for treating VF. Lidocaine may be used as an alternative. Magnesium is indicated for VF with a torsades de pointes pattern.

PEA is characteristic of organized cardiac electrical activity without effective cardiac output. PEA is usually a slow wide-complex rhythm, for example, junctional or idioventricular rhythm. When PEA is caused by hypovolemia, tension pneumothorax, or pericardial tamponade, a narrow-complex, rapid heart rate may be seen. Causes also include hypoxia and acidosis.

Evaluation of Interventions

Patients require thorough and frequent reassessment of their airway, breathing, and circulation throughout the resuscitation process. Initial improvement in a patient's condition may not be sustained because of underlying causes. The child's response to the interventions must be closely monitored. Reestablishment of end-organ perfusion is a positive indicator of successful patient outcome.

If the patient does not respond despite aggressive efforts to resuscitate, a decision to terminate the resuscitation must be made. This is a very difficult decision and is most often made collaboratively by the resuscitation team. Several laboratory and clinical findings influence the decision to terminate resuscitation efforts. These include

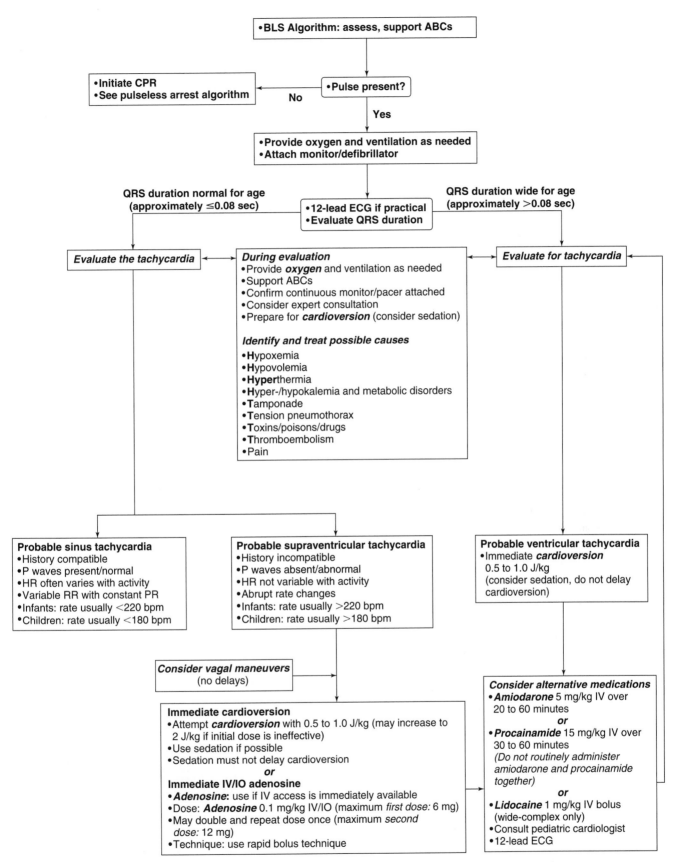

Fig. 31-9 Algorithm for pediatric tachycardia with poor perfusion. *CPR,* Cardiopulmonary resuscitation; *NS,* normal saline; *ECG,* electrocardiogram; *IV,* intravenous. (From American Heart Association: Guidelines 2000 for cardiovascular care, *Circulation 2000,* 102(suppl):I291-I342, 2000.)

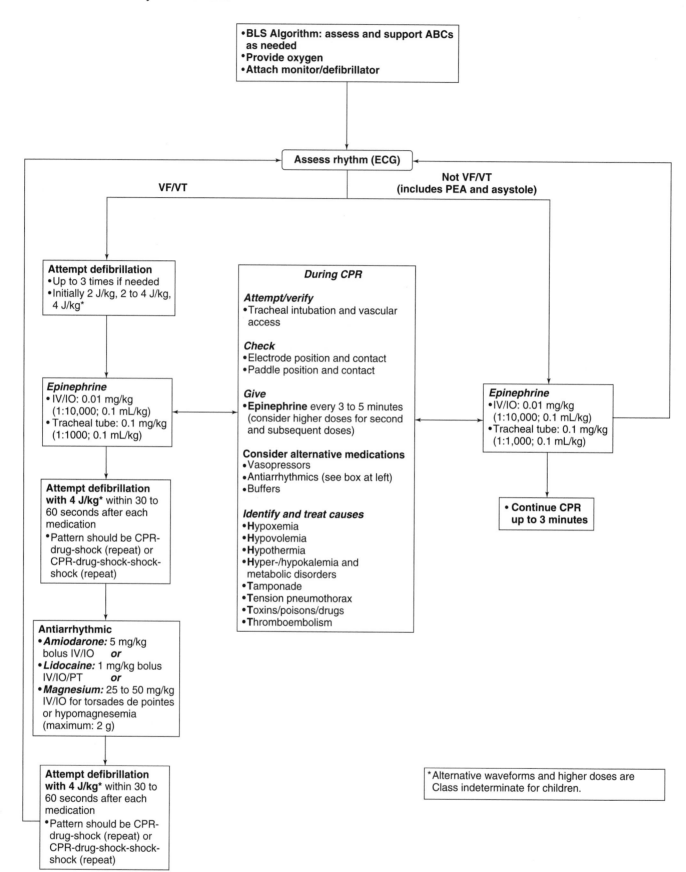

Fig. 31-10 Algorithm for asystole and pulseless arrest. *CPR,* Cardiopulmonary resuscitation; *IV,* intravenous; *IO,* intraosseous. (From American Heart Association: *1999 Handbook of emergency cardiovascular care for healthcare providers,* Dallas, 1999, AHA.)

prolonged acidosis, iatrogenic causes of arrest, and the absence of spontaneous circulation after 30 minutes of resuscitation.[26]

Diagnostic Studies

For patients who are responsive to resuscitation interventions, a variety of laboratory and radiologic studies are indicated during and following successful resuscitation depending on the child's underlying diagnosis. Laboratory studies may include a complete blood count, serum glucose, electrolytes, blood culture, blood typing, and arterial or venous blood gases. Other laboratory studies commonly completed are urinalysis, urine culture, and cerebrospinal fluid analysis.

The most common radiographic study indicated is a chest radiograph to identify any cardiac or pulmonary problems, as well as to identify ETT placement. Other radiographs, computed tomography (CT), and magnetic resonance imaging (MRI) may be indicated to identify any other injuries or pathologic processes that may be suspected.

Family Care

Throughout the crisis of resuscitation, parents require information and support. Information is best provided according to the individual needs of the parents. For example, some parents may want updates every 5 minutes, whereas others may want to know only the outcome when resuscitation attempts are over. A critical nursing intervention is to keep families accurately informed and assured that everything possible is being done to assist their child.

Providing parents with a private place is essential, both for them and for parents of other critically ill children. A member of the team who has an established relationship with the parents, such as the nurse, member of the clergy, or social worker, ideally stays with the parents, especially if they are alone.

Whether stabilization occurs or attempts to resuscitate are unsuccessful, parents should be given options to see, touch, or hold their child as soon as possible. Some parents may wish to remain at their child's bedside during the resuscitation attempt. Although this may seem difficult for caregivers, each family is assessed individually. Elements of protocols for parental presence may include educating staff in resuscitation methods *and* in providing options for parents, especially parents of children whose conditions have been deteriorating over time and in whom CPR can be expected. When death is imminent, the child is allowed to die in the presence or in the arms of parents.

A movement is underway fostering parental presence during resuscitation because of nursing's moral imperative to preserve the wholeness, integrity, and dignity of the family unit.[27] The Emergency Nurses Association position statement supports this philosophy.[28] It seems reasonable to initiate flexible programs to facilitate parental presence during pediatric CPR, especially with parents of chronically critically ill patients.

Documentation

Ongoing documentation of resuscitation events is crucial. Accuracy is enhanced if the person responsible for documentation has no other role in the resuscitation attempt and is positioned in close proximity to the code leader and patient. Fig. 31-11 illustrates an example of a resuscitation flow sheet that facilitates documentation. Effective resuscitation flow records provide precise information about code events, include the patient's response to therapy, and minimize the time required for documentation during and after the code.

Postresuscitation documentation has a summary statement that includes the time and duration of the arrest, ETT size and markings compared with the lip or nares line, catheter sizes and length of insertion, all intravenous fluid administered, blood work and blood loss, drugs and dosages administered, and the patient's and family's response to therapy.

POSTRESUSCITATION MANAGEMENT

Patient care goals after cardiopulmonary resuscitation include further stabilization of oxygenation, ventilation, cardiac output, and tissue perfusion. These goals are vital for neurologic preservation. Two major concerns include the potential of iatrogenic trauma from the resuscitation attempt and multisystem dysfunction resulting from organ hypoperfusion with hypoxic and acidotic blood.

The ABCs are also useful in organizing postarrest stabilization measures. Assessment starts with an evaluation of the adequacy of the airway. Assessment parameters include the airway size, presence of an ETT leak, and the security of the ETT. If a cuffed ETT is placed, cuff volume and pressures are checked. This is important in pediatrics because cuffed ETTs are infrequently used and can potentially cause a significant amount of airway damage in a short period. The placement and patency of the nasogastric tube (NGT) is also assessed. After decompressing the stomach with a large-volume syringe, the NGT is connected to intermittent suction. A chest radiograph is usually indicated to evaluate pulmonary disease, assess for iatrogenic injury, and check tube placement, that is, ETT, central lines, or chest tube positioning.

Serial ABGs are assessed throughout the resuscitation attempt. Exhaled CO_2 detection is continuously monitored as well. Saturation monitoring resumes when the patient's pulse pressure is adequate. Once the airway is stable, optimal ventilator parameters are identified. Airway pressures sufficient to provide adequate chest excursion and at least 95% saturation are noted during hand ventilation. Keeping the patient's F_{IO_2} at 1.0, airway pressures are matched with the ventilator. Once the patient is supported on the ventilator, the patient's ABGs are reanalyzed in 20 minutes, and further adjustments in PIPs and PEEPs, tidal volume, and F_{IO_2} are made.

Vascular access is reassessed for adequacy, patency, and security. Additional vascular access may be indicated and, after fluid resuscitation, can be accomplished in a controlled manner. Intraosseous lines are discontinued as

USE PLATE OR PRINT

PT. NAME _____
LAST   FIRST

DATE _____ DIV. _____

MEDICAL REC. NO. _____

Children's Hospital
CODE BLUE RECORD

Page _____ of _____

Date _____ Weight _____ Location _____

Admission Diagnosis _____ DNR / Advance Directive ☐ Yes ☐ No

TIME (make entries at least every 5 minutes)	VITAL SIGNS						CARDIAC RHYTHM	ASSESSMENT / INTERVENTIONS (NOTE BY WHOM) LAB RESULTS / X—RAYS	MEDICATIONS
	HR	RR	BP	SpO$_2$	T	EtCO$_2$			

Resuscitation Team:

RN _____
RN _____
MD _____   RN _____   Anesthesia _____
MD _____   RN _____   COPP _____
MD _____   Security _____
RT _____

Time of Arrest / Emergency _____
Time Code Team Called _____
Time Code Team Arrived _____

CPR initiated at _____ by _____
ET intubation at _____ by _____
Vascular access at _____ by _____
First defibrillation at _____ by _____

Disposition: ☐ Survived
                ☐ Expired

Transfer Location:
☐ OR   ☐ Floor
☐ ICU   ☐ ED
☐ Other _____

Code Leader's Name _____ MD
Code Leader's Signature _____ MD

Recorder's Name _____ RN
Recorder's Signature _____ RN

1st COPY – Patient Record   2nd COPY – Nurse Manager   3rd COPY – CPR Committee (MICU Office, Farley 517)

03031 25/PKG 3/99

Fig. 31-11   Code blue record. (Courtesy Children's Hospital, CPR Committee, Boston, 1999.)

soon as possible after adequate direct vascular access has been obtained. The skin surrounding peripheral intravenous sites requires particular attention. The potential for iatrogenic injury from intravenous infiltration is high. Immediate consultation to plastic surgery may be indicated.

The initial set of vital signs includes temperature assessment. Patient exposure and administration of large quantities of unwarmed intravenous solutions during the arrest place the patient at risk for postarrest hypothermia. The hypothermic patient benefits from rewarming measures, for example, warm blankets and overhead radiant warmers or lights.

As soon as possible after resuscitation, a baseline neurologic examination is performed and documented. The neurologic examination is placed in context of the prearrest neurologic status and drugs used during or immediately after resuscitation (e.g., atropine, dopamine, and chemical paralyzing agents). Atropine and dopamine act synergistically to cause pupillary dilation, the duration of which cannot be accurately determined because routine half-life calculations are probably invalid following resuscitation.

In addition to ABGs, initial postresuscitation blood work includes studies to evaluate oxygen-carrying capacity, fluid balance, system function (especially renal and liver function), and coagulation profiles. Urine output is evaluated, and if not already present, a Foley catheter is placed.

Patients are usually poorly perfused, acidotic, and hypotensive after a cardiac arrest. The most common reason for poor perfusion in this case is cardiogenic shock, the result of arrest-related myocardial ischemia. Patients may benefit from a 10- to 20-ml/kg fluid bolus administered over several minutes. If ventricular or pulmonary compliance is poor, a fluid bolus is administered with caution. Continuous infusions of inotropic agents (e.g., epinephrine, dopamine, and dobutamine) can be used to augment contractility and enhance tissue perfusion. Drug therapy is based on clinical presentation. Management of shock is discussed in depth in Chapter 27.

INTERFACILITY TRANSPORT

Following resuscitation, some patients may require transport to a pediatric facility that can best meet their evolving needs. Interfacility transport offers a system to ensure that all patients receive an appropriate level of care. According to the American Academy of Pediatrics (AAP),[29] the goal of pediatric interfacility transport is to improve outcomes in critically ill or injured neonates, infants, and children who are not in proximity to a hospital that provides the required level of care.

History

With the development of critical transport services throughout the country, the AAP developed guidelines for air and ground transportation of pediatric patients. These guide-lines provide a framework for minimum goals for pediatric and neonatal critical care transport programs. Federal guidelines also govern interfacility transports. The Consolidated Omnibus Reconciliation Act of 1985 (COBRA)[30] and the Emergency Medical Treatment and Active Labor Act (EMTALA)[31] regulations state that interfacility transport cannot be used as a method to avoid initial assessment, stabilization, or intervention, especially with regard to a patient's ability to pay. All necessary means to stabilize the patient are attempted before transport. Regionally, hospitals should have written interfacility transfer agreements outlining the level of responsibility of both receiving and referring facilities throughout the transport process. Thus when a transport occurs, preset agreements are already in place, and compliance with federal guidelines is ensured.

Transport Process

Once the healthcare team at the referring institution recognizes the need for specialty services, a decision to transport to a tertiary facility is made. Once an interfacility transport team is activated, the patient is prepared.

The goal is optimal stabilization of the patient. The patient's condition and the trajectory of the disease process are considered. The ABCs of stabilization help to ensure that the patient is physically prepared for transport. Airway patency is checked. If any question remains concerning the ability of the patient to maintain a patent airway, a transport team will intubate the patient. Once the airway is stabilized, adequate ventilation and oxygenation are ensured. Circulation is then assessed and stabilized. Obtaining intravenous access is critical. In most instances, at least two patent intravenous lines are preferred during transport. Necessary measures are taken to prevent thermal instability. While patient stabilization is underway, the patient's medical record, laboratory reports, radiographs, and CT scans are copied. Fig. 31-12 provides the standard approach for each patient requiring transport.

Team Composition. Transport programs have various team compositions, which include physicians, nurses, respiratory therapists, paramedics, and EMTs. All pediatric teams have members who are experts in the management of critically ill infants and children. A wide variety of team compositions exist, and to date, no single composition is preferred over the other.

Patient safety and available medical care during transport are factors to consider in composing the team for a particular transport. There are multiple team compositions to choose from, depending on a hospital's location to the tertiary center. Local basic life support (BLS) and advanced life support (ALS) systems offer rapid response times, but they are adult oriented and have a limited ability for advanced pediatric resuscitation techniques. Adult-based critical care transport services offer both flight and ground resources but often have limited expertise in the care of the neonatal and pediatric patient. Specialized pediatric and neonatal transport systems offer experienced nurses, respiratory therapists, physicians, and emergency medical

---

Children's Hospital Transport Program Patient Care Protocols
Standard Approach to the Patient

1. Follow universal precautions. If a contagious disease is suspected or there is potential for exposure to blood or body fluids, take appropriate measures to protect the transport team members and the patient.
2. Perform a primary survey to identify, and initiate treatment for, life-threatening problems with airway, breathing and circulation.
3. Obtain additional history from health care providers, the patient, and the family.
4. Perform a physical assessment, including vital signs.
5. Initiate patient monitoring, to include:
   a. ECG and respiratory rate
   b. Pulse oximetry (SpO_2)
   c. Non-invasive blood pressure (NIBP)
   d. Additional monitoring as indicated based on the patient's condition
6. Monitor and maintain the patient's body temperature.
7. Perform appropriate diagnostic tests.
8. Provide treatment to stabilize prior to transport based on the applicable Children's Hospital Transport Program Patient Care Protocol(s) and/or orders from the medical control physician.
   a. Unless otherwise specified, follow the Children's Hospital Intensive Care Unit Nursing Policies and Procedures for nursing care and medication administration
9. Obtain informed consent from parent(s) or guardian(s) for treatment and transport. If no parent or guardian is available, refer to the administrative policy.
10. Obtain copies of the medical records and x-rays. For neonatal patients, also obtain copies of the mother's records.
11. Provide psychosocial support for the patient and the family.
12. Contact the medical control physician to discuss patient management and/or disposition.
13. Contact the receiving nursing unit and provide a focused report on the patient's condition.
14. Initiate transport as soon as the patient's condition permits.
15. Apply passenger safety restraints to the patient to the extent that the patient's condition permits.
16. Continuously monitor the patient's condition and provide appropriate treatment during transport. Notify the medical control physician of any significant changes in the patient's condition.
17. Document pertinent data and events using the transport flow sheet; document adverse events on a Children's Hospital incident report.

Fig. 31-12 Sample patient care protocol. (Courtesy Children's Hospital Transport Program, Boston, 1999.)

---

personnel skilled in the care of critically ill infants and children.

The patient's severity of illness and the risk for deterioration determine the team composition and their level of expertise. A child who is currently stable but has a potential to deteriorate during the transport necessitates a team that is not only capable of caring for this child in a mobile environment but has the expertise necessary to restabilize the patient.

Regardless of the composition, the transport nurse is often considered the team leader. The transport nurse's role is to coordinate the stabilization of the child before transport, provide continuous evaluation and monitoring of the patient's physiologic status, and provide patient management under guidelines throughout the transport. The nurse is responsible for patient and team safety at all times. The transport nurse maintains awareness of the potential risks involved and is able to react accordingly in a mobile environment. Pediatric or neonatal transport nurses maintain certifications in pediatric advanced life support (PALS), Neonatal Resuscitative Program (NRP), critical care certification (CCRN), BLS, and the trauma nurse certification course (TNCC) or advanced trauma life support (ATLS).

Education of Team Members. Education and training for transport team members are intense. Didactic and interactive skill sessions are part of many training programs. Not only are team members expected to manage multiple medical and surgical emergencies, but they are also trained to perform advanced technical procedures. Didactic sessions build on the clinician's knowledge base and introduce

specific aspects of transport management, such as air flight physiology, interpreting radiographs, and providing care in a mobile environment. Procedure skill stations for the development of advanced skills such as bag-mask ventilation; tracheal intubation; intravenous, intraosseous, and central venous line placement; shocks; cardioversion; and arterial puncture are implemented in many programs. Simulated cases consisting of computer-controlled mannequins that imitate crisis situations are often part of the education process. Team building and communication skills are also important components of the education program.

Didactic sessions, simulation, and procedure skill stations introduce team members to transport protocols. Protocols provide the standard of care for the transport team when working outside of the hospital setting. An example of a protocol for management of respiratory distress and failure can be found in Fig. 31-13. If team members need to deviate from the established protocols the medical control physician (MCP) is called for advice.

Team Safety. A major consideration for a transport team is the safety of the team members and patient. Team orientation to ground and air safety, protective clothing, physical fitness, emergency planning, wilderness survival, stress management, and debriefing sessions are aspects that are imperative to safe team performance.[29] Without safety training, the team can be unaware and unprepared for the potential risks that can occur during transport. For example, team members must know how to use the emergency exits in the planes and rotor-wing aircraft, avoid

Children's Hospital Transport Program
Patient Care Protocols
Pediatric Respiratory
Distress and Failure

Definition: Respiratory distress describes a patient's efforts to increase minute ventilation in order to compensate for impaired gas exchange secondary to pulmonary or other systemic disease. Respiratory failure occurs when compensatory mechanisms fail, and oxygenation and ventilation become inadequate. Respiratory failure may occur without the presence of respiratory distress.

Clinical presentation:
1. History: Dyspnea, rapid and/or labored breathing, difficulty speaking or swallowing, diaphoresis, fever, cough, drooling.
2. Physical exam: Tachypnea, grunting, nasal flaring, retractions, tachycardia, anxiety, pallor (respiratory distress); head bobbing, paradoxical movement of the abdomen and chest, decreased responsiveness, decreased respiratory effort and rate, gasping respirations, cyanosis (respiratory failure). The exam should include assessment for stridor, wheezing, asymmetry of breath sounds, rales, and rhonchi.
3. Laboratory data: Arterial blood gas, chest x-ray films, plus lateral and anteroposterior neck films.

Differential diagnosis:
1. Upper airway obstruction: croup, epiglottitis, foreign body obstruction, bacterial tracheitis, smoke inhalation
2. Lower airway obstruction: status asthmaticus, foreign body aspiration, bronchiolitis, bronchiectasis
3. Parenchymal or interstitial lung disease: pneumonia, pulmonary edema, pulmonary hemorrhage, pulmonary contusion

Evaluation and Treatment:
1. Assess the airway, and provide management as indicated according to the Airway Management protocol.
2. Assess breathing, including respiratory rate, effort, air entry, and breath sounds. Provide intervention as follows:
   a. Provide supplemental oxygen to any patient with respiratory distress, according to the Oxygen Therapy protocol.
   b. Assist ventilations using a bag and mask with $FiO_2 = 1.0$ for patients with respiratory failure or impending respiratory failure as evidenced by decreasing level of consciousness, decreasing respiratory rate and/or effort, head bobbing, paradoxical abdominal movement, deep retractions, and/or cyanosis.
   c. Utilize a pressure manometer when delivering positive-pressure ventilations unless using a device with a pop-off valve.
   d. Perform endotracheal intubation when indicated according to the *Airway Management* protocol.
   e. Perform cricothyrotomy when indicated according to the *Cricothyrotomy* protocol.
3. For patients with signs of upper airway obstruction and suspected airway edema:
   a. Administer **racemic epinephrine** 2.25% solution 0.5 ml in 3 ml 0.9% NaCl by nebulizer.
   b. If croup is suspected, administer **dexamethasone** (Decadron) 0.5 mg/kg IV. Dexamethasone may be administered IM if vascular access is not available.
   c. If epiglottitis is suspected, contact the medical control physician.
4. If anaphylaxis is suspected, administer:
   a. **Epinephrine** 0.01 mg/kg (0.01 ml/kg) of 1:1,000 solution SC (maximum dose 0.3 mg [0.3 ml])
   b. **Diphenhydramine** (Benadryl) 1 mg/kg IV
   c. **Methylprednisolone** (Solumedrol) 2 mg/kg IV
5. For patients with signs of bronchospasm, administer bronchodilator therapy as follows:
   a. For acute, severe distress, administer **epinephrine** 0.01 mg/kg (0.01 ml/kg) of 1:1,000 solution SC (maximum dose 0.3 mg [0.3 ml]).
   b. Administer **albuterol** 2.5-5 mg in 3 ml 0.9% NaCl by nebulizer or two to four "puffs" by MDI, and repeat as needed.
   c. Administer **ipratroprium bromide** (Atrovent) by nebulizer or MDI, up to three doses.
   d. If reactive airway disease is suspected, administer **methylprednisolone** (Solumedrol) 2 mg/kg IV. Do not administer if the patient has already received steroids at the referring hospital within the past 6 hours, unless a lower dose was administered or the patient experienced vomiting after administration of oral prednisone.
   e. If the patient remains significantly bronchospastic, consult with the medical control physician regarding administration of continuous **albuterol** by nebulizer or **terbutaline** by continuous intravenous infusion.
6. For patients who have chronic respiratory insufficiency and are maintained on noninvasive ventilation, continue CPAP or BiPAP as per the patient's usual settings, and consult with the medical control physician regarding adjustment of ventilatory support for transport.
7. For patients who are chronically dependent on mechanical ventilation:
   a. Consult with the medical control physician regarding use of the patient's portable ventilator for transport and adjustment of settings.
   b. If the patient deteriorates, remove the patient from mechanical ventilation and provide manual ventilations using a resuscitation bag.
   c. Consider obtaining a blood gas (venous or arterial) prior to transport, if clinical assessment of oxygenation and/or ventilation cannot be reliably performed.
   d. Monitor the patient with continuous pulse oximetry and capnography during transport.
8. For patients who require initiation of ventilatory support via endotracheal tube or tracheostomy on transport:
   a. Provide ventilatory support using FiO_2 of 1.0 except as outlined in the Oxygen Therapy protocol, using the following:
      1. A resuscitation bag using an inflating pressure to produce adequate chest rise, a PEEP of 3 to 5 cm H_2O, and a rate that provides adequate ventilation; OR
      2. A transport ventilator using an inflating pressure to produce adequate chest rise, a PEEP of 3 to 5 cm H_2O, and a rate that provides adequate ventilation.
      3. Consult with the medical control physician if higher levels of PEEP are required.
   b. If the patient deteriorates, remove the patient from mechanical ventilation and provide manual ventilations using a resuscitation bag.
   c. Consider obtaining a blood gas (venous or arterial) prior to transport, if clinical assessment of oxygenation and/or ventilation cannot be reliably performed.
   d. Monitor the patient with continuous pulse oximetry and capnography during transport.

Fig. 31-13 Respiratory distress and failure protocol. (Courtesy Children's Hospital Transport Program, Boston, 1999.)

a spinning tail rotor, and troubleshoot equipment failures in any mode of transport. Many teams do not share patient information with the pilots until acceptance or denial of the transport has been determined. Pilots do not need patient status information to cloud judgment when making decisions about the ability to fly safely based on weather conditions.

Mode of Transport. Response time, weather, and team capabilities are factors that are carefully considered when choosing the mode of transport. Modes available for transport include ground ambulances, rotor-wing aircraft (helicopters), and fixed-wing aircraft (propeller planes and jets). In some cases, weather may necessitate that a ground ambulance be used even if the distance is significant. Time of day and traffic conditions may necessitate a rotor-wing transport to save time because of traffic delays on the ground.

Time is another factor that influences the mode of transport chosen for a particular patient. A 2-hour ground transport of a child who is thought to have a rapidly expanding intracranial bleed is not appropriate, and the referring hospital team chooses the most rapid means of transporting the child safely to the tertiary facility. Another factor to keep in mind is the number of transfers required if the patient is air transported. The more often a patient is transferred to and from different vehicles (i.e., emergency department to ambulance, ambulance to helicopter, helicopter to ambulance, ambulance to receiving unit), the higher the likelihood of adverse effects, accidental extubation, and displacement of intravenous lines. Altitude may also increase the risk of adverse affects. However, the time that is saved by flying may compensate for the potential risks.

Equipment. Each transport program requires specialized equipment to safely transport the pediatric or neonatal patient. Essential for every team is pediatric-sized airway and intravascular access supplies (Fig. 31-14). Monitoring equipment requires pediatric or neonatal modes. Pediatric- or neonatal-size ECG leads, oxygen saturation probes, and immobilization equipment such as c-spine collars and back boards are essential for safe and efficient patient transport. Pocket-sized pediatric or neonatal drug cards are helpful for quick reference. Transport equipment also includes specialized comfort measures for this unique population, including pacifiers, stuffed animals, and security objects. Many pediatric or neonatal transport teams have configured ambulances to include TVs and VCRs and CD players to create a relaxing and nontraumatic transport environment for the child.

Communication. Team communication begins with the call from the referring hospital, clinic, doctor's office, or local 911 emergency system. Any referring physician should have rapid and direct access to a transport team. For many programs, this point of contact is usually accomplished by a toll-free number, which is answered in the transport program's dispatch center. Initial information, such as patient name, age, weight, referring physician, referring facility, phone number, and diagnosis, is gathered by the dispatcher or communication specialist who then transfers the call to the MCP (Fig. 31-15).

At the same time the transport team is notified, mobilization begins. Once the MCP has discussed the patient's current condition with the referring institution and given any medical advice necessary for stabilization, the MCP then contacts the transport team to update them on the child's status.

Cell phones and long-range alpha pagers are used to maintain communication between the transport team and the MCP when out in the field. Dispatchers can also link the team to the MCP by land radio access. The communication method must be continuous and reliable. A backup communication system should be available in case the primary system malfunctions. Continuous verbal contact between the transport team and MCP is essential in case medical direction is necessary when the team is out on a transport.

Communication between the team and referring institution is also essential. Many transport teams contact the referring institution en route to obtain reports from the nurses or physicians who are caring for the child, which accomplishes two goals. First, the team has an up to-date picture of the patient so that they can adequately prepare the equipment and medication needed en-route, and, second, critical scene time is decreased when the report has been given before arrival. When the team arrives, only a brief update is necessary, and patient care can begin immediately.

The transport team is also responsible for communicating patient status and estimated time of arrival to the unit at the accepting facility. This can be done through the dispatcher or other communication system. Before leaving the referring institution, the team communicates with the MCP about patient status and the plan for transport.

On arrival to the accepting unit, the team is responsible for ensuring that the accepting physicians and nurses receive a comprehensive report on the child's condition and care to date. Once the patient's care has been transferred to the accepting medical team, a follow-up call is made to the referring physician stating the patient's condition on arrival. This is the final piece of communication from the team to the referring institution.

Communication between the transport team and the patient's family is extremely important. The team must fully inform the parent or guardian about the risks and benefits of transporting their child, the differential diagnosis, and what is to be expected from the transport team. The parent or legal guardian must sign or verbally give consent for medical treatment and transport. Transport of a child is traumatic to many parents, and open communication from the team can help parents deal with the process.

The decision to have a parent ride with the team to the receiving facility is governed by state laws and team policies. If the parent rides with the team, two goals can be accomplished. The child may be less anxious with the parent in the ambulance, and the parent's anxiety level may be decreased. The parent will also be available immediately at

---

**BLACK SUPPLEMENTAL PACK—CHILDREN'S HOSPITAL
TRANSPORT TEAM**

VENOUS ACCESS:
1 5.5F Arrow CVL kit
1 guide wire
2 intraosseous needles
2 each 3.5, 5.0 umbilical catheters
1 each 3.5, 5.0 dbl lumen umbilical catheters
1 transport instruments tray
2 3.0 silk sutures
2 #11 blades

**THORACOTOMY/
THORACENTESIS:**
2 each 10F, 12F chest tubes
1 sterile Kelly clamp
2 thoracentesis kits:
  23G butterfly
  19G butterfly
  3-way stopcock
  60cc syringe
Xeroform gauze
1 Y-connector
2 5-in-1 connectors
2 Hemlich values
1 roll 3" foam tape

RESPIRATORY:
1 self inflating resuscitation bag with PEEP valve
1 each neonatal, pediatric ventilator circuit
1 meconium aspirator
1 "premie" kit
1 Survanta kit

**IV
SUPPLIES:**
1 each:
500cc NS
500cc D5¼
500cc D10W
250cc 5% albumin

blood tubing
pressure bag

**RED MEDICATION PACK—CHILDREN'S HOSPITAL
TRANSPORT TEAM**

| 1 pediatric emergency medication reference guide | 1 calculator |

2 methylprednisolone 62.5 mg/ml—2 ml	2 ampicillin 1 gm/vial	2 gentamicin 40 mg/ml—2 ml	1 clindamycin 150 mg/ml—6 ml	2 vancomycin 500 mg/vial	1 cefotaxime 1 gm/vial	1 NaCHO₃ 1 meq/ml—50 ml
1 dexamethasone 10 mg/ml—10 ml						
1 phytonadione 2 mg/ml—1 ml / 1 erythromycin opthalmic 3.5 gm						
1 ondansetron 2 mg/ml—2 ml / 2 xylocaine 2%—2 ml amps	1 D25W 250 mg/ml—10 ml	1 D50W 500 mg/ml—50 ml	1 mannitol 250 mg/ml—50 ml	2 NS 10 ml vials	4 NaHCO₃ 0.5 meq/ml—5 ml	
1 heparin 1000 µ/ml—10 ml						
1 naloxone 1 mg/ml—2 ml / 2 phenytoin 50 mg/ml—5 ml						

2 dobutamine 12.5 mg/ml—20 ml	2 dopamine 40 mg/ml—5 ml	3 nifedipine UDL brand 10 mg/0.38 ml	1 hydralazine 20 mg/ml—1 ml	1 nitroprusside 25 mg/ml 2 ml **with** 10 ml sterile H₂O for dilution	6 digoxin 100 mcg/ml—1 ml	4 atropine 0.4 mg/ml—1 ml	2 adenosine 3 mg/ml—2 ml	2 epinephrine 1:1000—1 ml

8 phenobarbitol 130 mg/ml	**1** diphenhydramine 50 mg/ml—1 ml	**2** lidocaine 20 mg/ml—5 ml
		1 epinephrine 1:1000—30 ml

2 mag SO₄ 500 mg/ml —2 ml	1 CaCL 100 mg/ml —10 ml	2 CaGluc 100 mg/ml —10 ml	1 NaCl 14.6%— 20 ml	1 K⁺ acetate 2 meq/ml— 20 ml	1 K⁺ phosphate 4.4 meq/ml —15 ml	1 KCL 2 meq/ml— 5 ml	1 furosemide 10 mg/ml— 10 ml

12 1cc syringes	**4** 30cc syringes	**12** 18G needles	IV drip labels
12 3cc syringes	**4** 60cc syringes	**4** 25G needles	**1** glucagon kit
12 10cc syringes		**4** 27G needles	
		12 interlink needles	

Fig. 31-14 Transport equipment pack list. (Courtesy Children's Hospital Transport Program, Boston, 1999.) *Continued*

**ORANGE TRANSPORT PACK—CHILDREN'S HOSPITAL
TRANSPORT TEAM**

rubber bands, tourniquet
black pen
oral airways (1 each): 5, 6, 7, 8, 9
nasal trumpets (1 each): 14, 16, 18, 20, 22, 24, 26

1 neonatal nasal cannula
1 pediatric nasal cannula
1 pediatric NRB mask
1 adult nasal cannula
1 adult NRB mask

1 500cc anesthesia bag
1 1L anesthesia bag
2 O₂ supply tubings
1 manometer with tubing and adaptor

Anesthesia face masks
(1 each):
neonate
infant
toddler
pediatric
small adult
large adult

Nebulizer Kit:
1 20cc btl ventolin 5 mg/cc
1 15cc btl racemic epinephrine
3 single dose Atrovent 0.5 mg/2.5cc
5 amps terbutaline 1 mg/cc
4 saline "bullets"
1 neb setup with mask and ett adaptor

Syringes (5 each):
1cc
3cc
10cc

2 armboards
6 18G needles
6 interlink needles

IV Catheters
(4 each):
14G
16G
18G
20G
22G
24G

Interlink:
5 hep lock caps
5 blue connectors
3 slip-adaptor T-connectors

Butterflies:
(2 each):
19G
21G
23G
24G

Thermometer

Tegaderm
4×4 gauze
alcohol pads
betadine pads

(6 each)

(5) 10cc vials
NS

1 roll each:
1" adhesive tape
1" silk tape
Co-flex

Blood culture bottle
(5) lancets
1 each:
large red, green, blue, purple lab tubes, green/purple microtainers

2 3-way stopcocks

1 set ECG leads
1 each neo, pedi, adult sat probe
1 each Critikon BP cuffs: #1, #2, #3, #4, #5
1 each HP BP cuffs:#1, #2, #3

1 each pedi, adult Easy cap
EtCO₂ supplies (**1** each):
ett adapter, supply tubing, pedi, adult cannulas

CPAP prongs (**1** each):
small
medium
large

Suction catheters (**2** each): 6, 8, 10, 12
1 tonsil tip suction
1 each 5, 8 feeding tubes
1 each 6, 8 Vigon sumps
1 10F Replogyle
1 each 8, 10, 12, 14 Salem sumps
1 each: anti-reflux valve, Lubifax, specimen trap, catheter tip syringe

Intubation roll:

1 roll 1" adhesive tape
2 bezoin applicators
1 10cc syringe
1 each neo, pedi McGill forceps
2 laryngoscope handles
laryngoscope blades (1 each):
　　Miller 0, 1, 2, 3
　　W-H 1.5
　　MacIntosh 1, 2, 3, 4
1 each pedi, adult stylets
extra laryngoscope bulbs (small and large)
2 AA batteries
2 C batteries
swivel adapter

Endotracheal tubes (uncuffed up to size 5, cuffed ≥5.5):

2 each: 2.0, 2.5, 3.0, 3.5, 4.0, 4.5, 5.0, 5.5, 6.0, 6.5
1 each: 7.0, 7.5, 8.0

4 microbore tubing sets
2 large bore tubing sets
1 Ivion pump set
1 arterial line set
2 trifuse adaptors
1 luer lock T-connector
2 60cc syringes

Fig. 31-14, cont'd For legend see p. 1047.

CHILDREN'S HOSPITAL PEDIATRIC/NEONATAL TELEPHONE CONSULTATION/TRANSFER RECORD

DATE: ___/___/___ TIME(MILITARY): _____
PERSON PROCESSING CALL: _____

PT NAME:_____
SEX: ☐ ♂ ☐ ♀   DOB: ___/___/___
AGE:_____ IF NEONATE, GEST. AGE:_____
PRELIM DIAGNOSIS:_____
_____
REFERRING MD:_____
REFERRING HOSPITAL:_____
☐ED ☐PEDS ☐DR ☐SCN ☐OTHER_____
CITY, STATE:_____
CALL BACK #:_____
PCP:_____ PHONE:_____
ALLERGIES:_____
EXPOSURES: _____

HISTORY/COURSE/INTERVENTIONS:

WGT:____kg T____ HR____ RR____ BP____
O2 DELIVERY:_____ O2 SAT:_____
☐ETT/TRACH SIZE:_____ CUFFED YES/NO
ACCESS:☐PIV X___ SIZE:___ ☐IO ☐UAC
☐UVC 1 2 LUMEN ☐CVL 1 2 3 LUMEN☐ALINE
IVF: TYPE:_____ RATE:_____
        TYPE:_____ RATE:_____
        TYPE:_____ RATE:_____

NEURO STATUS:_____

USE PLATE OR PRINT
PT NAME: _____
MR #:_____

LABS: Diff %:
                                             P___ B___
                                             L___ M___

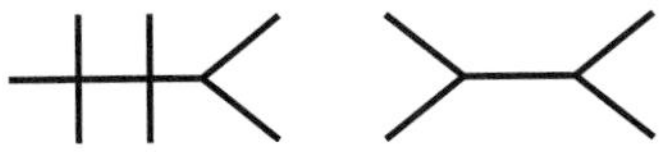

OTHER:_____
BLOOD GAS #1:_____ A☐ V☐ C☐

BLOOD GAS #2:_____ A☐ V☐ C☐

XRAY RESULTS:_____
_____

RECOMMENDATIONS:

SIGNATURE:_____

☐ CONSULT, REFERRED TO:_____
NOTIFIED: ☐TEAM ☐AMBULANCE ☐COPP
☐ ATTENDING ☐RECEIVING CHARGE RN/MD

TEAM COMPOSITION: ☐RN/RN ☐RN/RN/HO ☐
RN/RN/BACK-UP MD ☐BMF ☐CH RN/BMF
☐REF HOSP TEAM ☐OTHER _____

ACCEPTING SERVICE/FIRM: _____

ATTENDING: _____
UNIT: ☐7N ☐P5 ☐P6 ☐ED ☐OTHER:_____

IF NO TRANSPORT, REASON: _____

IF NO CH BED, ALTERNATIVE ARRANGEMENT:
_____

Fig. 31-15 Transport intake form. (Courtesy Children's Hospital Transport Program, Boston, 1999.)

the receiving hospital to give the child's medical history and to sign any consents for treatment. If the parent or parents are driving to the receiving facility, the team should supply directions to the facility and advise them not to follow the ambulance.

According to the Joint Commission on Accreditation of Healthcare Organizations (JCAHO).[33] The transport medical record serves as a basis for evaluating the patient's condition and treatment. The transport medical record should contain the patient's medical evaluation at the referring facility, during transport, and on arrival at the receiving facility. Treatment efforts and the patient's ongoing clinical status are documented throughout the entire transport process, beginning at the referral facility and continuing to the accepting facility.

The line of responsibility to the patient is blurred when a transport team is called.[34] There is no clear point in the transport process that separates the responsibilities of care among the referring facility, the transport team, and the

Children's Hospital Transport Team In Patient Tracking Form

For QUALITY ASSURANCE

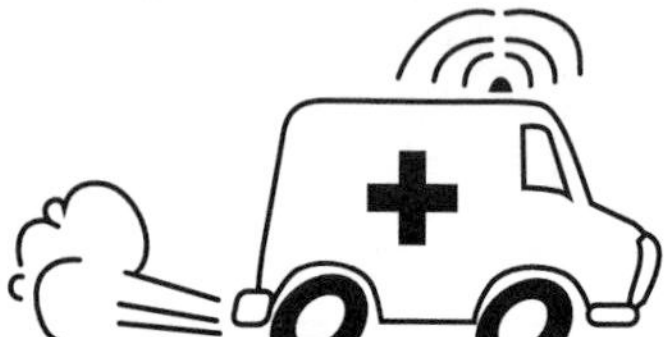

Call: _____
DCH: _____
ARH: _____
DRH: _____
ACH: _____

Database: ☐

Charges: ☐

Date of Transport: _____

Time of Transport: _____

Referring Physician: _____

Nurse: _____

Referral Center: _____

Address: _____

Phone Number: _____

Preliminary Diagnosis: _____

Age/Gestational Age: _____

Brief History: _____
_____
_____
_____

Significant Events/Procedure done on transport *(by whom/# of attempts)*: _____
_____
_____

Transport Team Members:
RN/RN: _____
Resident: _____
MD to "make" team: _____
Ref Hosp. Req. MD: _____
MD per Medical Control: _____

In-Patient Unit admitted to: _____
Transferred to: _____
Date of Transfer: _____

APGARS: ___1___   ___3___   ___5___

ETT Placement by CXR: _____ Taped at: _____ CXR on arrival: _____
Transport Opportunities for Improvement   Follow-up _____
_____
Initial ABG on Admission to CH   _____
Final Diagnoses and Disposition   _____

Quality Assurance Surveillance Indicators
☐ Hyperventilation—$PaCO_2$ <30
☐ Initial ABG hypoventilation pH <7.25
☐ Accidental extubation en-route
☐ Loss of IV access
☐ Hypothermia/rectal temp <35.5°C
☐ Departure from receiving hospital >1 hour

☐ Failure to bring equipment
☐ Ran out of O_2 or Air
☐ Right main intub. on arrival CXR
☐ Broken equipment _____
☐ Departure from CH >30 minutes
☐ Transfer to ICU within 24 hours

Fig. 31-16   Transport team quality assurance form. (Courtesy Children's Hospital Transport Program, Boston, 1999.)

accepting facility. The amount of responsibility tends to gradually shift throughout the transport process. The accepting facility begins to take some responsibility when they agree to accept the child and give treatment recommendations. The transport team and receiving facility become more responsible as the team becomes more involved in the patient care. Once the patient arrives at the receiving facility, the responsibility of the referring facility continues to diminish. Transport agreements between referring facilities and transport teams can help clarify some of the haziness of liability. All recommendations, arrangements, and interventions are documented in the medical record throughout the transport process.

Evaluation. A continuous performance improvement (PI) program is an important component of any transport program. A PI program ensures delivery of quality patient care and safe team performance. The PI process can identify potential system problems, resolve identified problems related to patient care and program operations, and provide ongoing evaluation of strategies implemented to resolve the problem (Fig. 31-16).

Keys to a successful transport, regardless of mode or team composition, include careful and continuous monitoring of patient status. ETTs are well secured before transport to decrease the risk of accidental extubation. Continuous $ETco_2$ measurements during transport provide ongoing information about the child's airway status. Intravenous lines require protection so that turbulence, rough driving conditions, or patient transfers do not cause inadvertent displacement. In addition to being secured, intravenous sites are visible and easily accessible during transport to monitor for infiltration and to access quickly in emergency situations. Keys to remember in emergency situations (arrest, extubation) are to have emergency equipment easily accessible. Having at least one round of code medications in an easily accessible place like a chest or arm uniform pocket will enhance immediate administration if the child requires pharmacologic intervention. Protocols and reference materials must be easily accessible during transport. In addition, all transport equipment must have a 4-hour battery life in case of power failure.

RESUSCITATION PERFORMANCE IMPROVEMENT

Nurses with specialty education in pediatric emergency and critical care are a valuable asset to pediatric resuscitation teams. Their positive impact can be further enhanced through coordinated training programs within institutions that focus on the code team approach to pediatric resuscitation. Monthly interdisciplinary mock codes in which objective criteria are used to evaluate knowledge acquisition and skill performance are excellent ways to assess the program. As part of a system-wide quality improvement plan, pediatric mock codes help to perfect skills while also helping to consolidate individual and team roles. In addition, system deficiencies, such as availability of personnel, paging difficulties, impossible

---

QA/QI VARIABLES:

Level of response requested

☐ Code Blue
☐ "STAT" (Specify:_____)

Were there issues with:

☐ **Locating the site of the emergency**
Describe:_____

☐ **Identifying medical leadership**
Comments:_____

☐ **Obtaining emergency equipment**
Comments:_____

☐ **Equipment function**
Comments:_____

☐ **Transfer of patient after resuscitation**
Comments:_____

☐ **Family members**
Comments:_____

Comments on any factors which could be improved:

EVENT VARIABLES:

Witnessed

☐ Yes
☐ No

Types of monitoring at time of event

☐ ECG
☐ SpO2
☐ Arterial Pressure
☐ CVP

Immediate Cause

☐ Dysrhythmia
☐ Shock/hypotension
☐ Respiratory failure/arrest
☐ Neurologic event
☐ Other

Initial Condition

Conscious?	☐ Yes	☐ No
Breathing?	☐ Yes	☐ No
Pulse?	☐ Yes	☐ No

Initial Rhythm

☐ VF
☐ VT
☐ PEA
☐ Bradycardia
☐ SVT
☐ Asystole
☐ NSR
☐ ST
☐ Other _____

_____
_____
_____
_____
_____
_____

To be completed by nurse recorder
For QI Purposes only - not to be placed in the medical record

Fig. 31-17 Code blue quality improvement tool. (Courtesy Children's Hospital, CPR Committee, Boston, 1999.)

drug dilutions, and malfunctioning equipment, can be identified in a benign setting. Mock codes also ensure that resuscitation team members are familiar with crash cart contents. Appendix IV (Emergency Cart Contents) contains a list of PICU crash cart contents. It is important that crash cart contents reflect the patient population of the unit because items that may be appropriate for a pediatric cardiovascular surgical unit may be inappropriate for a multidisciplinary PICU. However, standardizing in-patient pediatric unit crash carts is essential so that code team members can work rapidly from any crash cart in any location. Specialty items, such as cast cutters on an orthopedic unit, can be accommodated in boxes attached to the generic crash cart.

Every resuscitation attempt requires evaluation as a potential opportunity for system-wide improvement. Survival rates and patient outcomes should be an integral part of the resuscitation team's PI program. Strategies that proved successful can be highlighted through retrospective review. Fig. 31-17 illustrates an example of a performance improvement assessment tool used by a CPR committee to evaluate resuscitation events. A child's potential death represents one of the most stressful experiences any staff member can encounter. Team conferences after successful *and* unsuccessful resuscitation attempts provide the entire healthcare team with an opportunity for mutual support.

SUMMARY

Three major characteristics distinguish cardiopulmonary arrest in infants and children. These are the diverse causes of the arrest, the fact that most cardiopulmonary arrests can be prevented in infants and children, and certainty that primary cardiac arrest is unusual. Research demonstrates significant differences in overall survival and neurologic outcome in children depending on the type of arrest; survival is better in those who experience only respiratory arrest. Therefore early recognition and intervention to prevent a pulseless state are critical. Survival rates have been shown to be higher when the interval between cardiac arrest and intervention is shorter. Despite these factors, which would provide the infant and child an apparent advantage, survival among pediatric patients experiencing cardiopulmonary arrest is poor.

Critical care nurses, working collaboratively with other healthcare professionals, are in a unique position to appreciate the anatomic, physiologic, and maturational factors that affect the pediatric patient's response to resuscitation efforts. The essence of caring for the critically ill pediatric patient includes the ability to rapidly identify signs of compensation, intervene, and prevent cardiopulmonary arrest. Nurses are in a key position to make a critical difference in improving the currently dismal pediatric outcomes.

REFERENCES

1. Guyer B, MacDorman MF, Martin JA: Annual summary of vital statistics-1997, *Pediatrics* 102:1333-1348, 1998.
2. MacDorman MF, Atkinson JO: Infant mortality statistics from the 1996 period linked birth/infant death data set, *Mon Vital Stat Rep* 46(suppl 2):1-22, 1998.
3. Ludwig S: Resuscitation-pediatric basic and advanced life support. In Fleisher GR, Ludwig S, eds: *Textbook of pediatric emergency medicine,* ed 4, Philadelphia, 2000, Lippincott-Williams & Wilkins.
4. Young KD, Seidel JS: Pediatric cardiopulmonary resuscitation: a collective review, *Ann Emerg Med* 33:195-204, 1999.
5. Mott S: Cardiac emergencies. In Kelley S, ed: *Pediatric emergency nursing,* ed 2, Norwalk, Conn, 1994, Appleton & Lange.
6. Sachdeva RC: Near drowning, *Crit Care Clin* 15:281-296, 1999.
7. Curley MAQ, Thompson JE: End-tidal CO_2 monitoring in critically-ill infants and children, *Pediatr Nurs* 16:397-403, 1990.
8. Nadkarni V, Hazinski MF, Zideman D et al: Pediatric resuscitation, *Circulation* 8:2185-2195, 1997.
9. Reisdorff EJ, Howell KA, Saul J et al: Prehospital interventions in children, *Prehosp Emerg Care* 2:180-183, 1998.
10. Weintraub B: Emergency medical services for children, *J Emerg Nurs* 23:274-275, 1997.
11. Lanoix R, Golden J: The facilitated pediatric resuscitation room *J Emerg Med* 17:363-366, 1999.

12. Vernon DD, Furnival RA, Hansen KW et al: Effect of a pediatric trauma response team on emergency department treatment time and mortality of pediatric trauma victims, *Pediatrics* 103:20-24, 1999.
13. Ushay HM, Notterman DA: Pharmacology of pediatric resuscitation, *Pediatr Clin North Am* 44:207-233, 1997.
14. Roth B, Magnusson J, Johansson I et al: Jaw lift: a simple and effective method to open the airway in children, *Resuscitation* 39:171-174, 1998.
15. Manley LK: Procedures involving the respiratory system. In Berdardo LM, Bove MA, eds: *Pediatric emergency nursing procedures,* Boston, 1994, Jones & Bartlett, pp 63-81.
16. Yaster M, Maxwell LG: Airway management. In Nicholas DG, Yaster M, Lappe DG et al, eds: *Golden hour: the handbook of advanced pediatric life support,* ed. 2, St Louis, 1996, Mosby.
17. Gaushe M, Lewis RJ, Stratton SJ et al: Effect of out-of-hospital pediatric endotracheal intubation on survival and neurological outcome, *JAMA* 283:783-790, 2000.
18. Chameides L, Hazinski MF, eds: *Pediatric advanced life support,* Dallas, 1997, American Heart Association.
19. Torres A, Pickert CB: Long-term functional outcome of inpatient pediatric cardiopulmonary resuscitation, *Pediatr Emerg Care* 13:369-373, 1997.
20. Zaritsky AL: Recent advances in pediatric cardiopulmonary resuscitation and advanced life support, *New Horiz* 6:201-211, 1998.

20a. American Heart Association: Guidelines 2000 for cardiopulmonary resuscitation and emergency cardiovascular care, *Circulation 2000,* 102(suppl):I291-I342.
21. Thomas NJ, Carcillo JA: Hypovolemic shock in pediatric patients, *New Horiz* 6:120-129, 1998.
22. Friedman WF: The intrinsic physiologic properties of the developing heart, *Prog Cardiovasc Dis* 15:87-111, 1972.
23. Burke SS: Neonatal topics. In Soud TE, Rogers, JS, eds: *Manual of pediatric emergency nursing,* St Louis, 1998, Mosby.
24. Hazinski MF, Mahmoudi S: Pediatric and neonatal resuscitation. In Soud TE, Rogers JS, eds: *Manual of pediatric emergency nursing,* St Louis, 1998, Mosby.
25. Atkins DL, Hartley LL, York DK: Accurate recognition and effective treatment of ventricular fibrillation by automated external defibrillators in adolescents, *Pediatrics* 101: 393-397, 1998.
26. Scribano PV, Baker MD, Ludwig S: Factors influencing termination of resuscitative efforts in children: a comparison of pediatric emergency medicine and adult emergency medicine physicians, *Pediatr Emerg Care* 13:320-324, 1997.
27. Eichhorn DJ, Meyers TA, Mitchell TG et al: Opening the doors: family presence during resuscitation, *J Cardiovasc Nurs* 10:59-70, 1996.
28. Emergency Nurses Association: ENA Position Statement: Family presence at the bedside during invasive procedures and/or resuscitation, Des Plaines, Ill, 1998.

29. MacDonald M, Ginzburg H, eds: *American Academy of Pediatrics Task Force on Interhospital Transport: guidelines for air and ground transport of neonatal and pediatric patients,* Elk Grove Village, Ill, 1999, American Academy of Pediatrics.

30. Consolidation Omnibus Budget Reconciliation Act (COBRA) of 1985, (42 USC 1395cc), as amended by the Omnibus Budget Reconciliation Acts (OBRA) of 1987, 1989 and 1999.

31. Emergency Medical Treatment and Active Labor ACT 1395dd, 42USC, 1994.

32. Meyer-Pahoulis E, Williams SL, Davidson SI et al: The pediatric patient in the postanesthesia care unit, *Nurs Clin North Am* 28:519-530, 1993.

33. Joint Commission on Accreditation of Healthcare Organizations: *Accreditation manual for hospitals,* Oakbrook Terrace, Ill, 1991, JCAHO.

34. Youngberg BJ: Legal issues related to transport. In McCloskey K, Orr R, eds: *Pediatric transport medicine,* St Louis, 1995, Mosby.

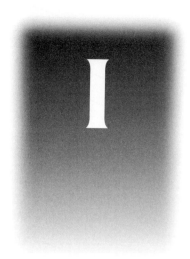

Normal Blood Pressure

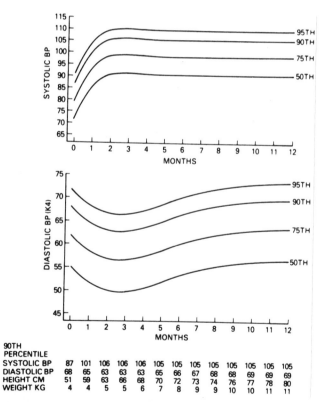

90TH PERCENTILE												
SYSTOLIC BP	87	101	106	106	106	105	105	105	105	105	105	105	105
DIASTOLIC BP	68	65	63	63	63	65	66	67	68	68	69	69	69
HEIGHT CM	51	59	63	66	68	70	72	73	74	76	77	78	80
WEIGHT KG	4	4	5	5	6	7	8	9	9	10	10	11	11

Fig. A1-1 Age-specific percentiles of blood pressure (BP) measurements in boys—birth to 12 months of age; Korotkoff phase IV (K4) used for diastolic BP. (From National Heart, Lung, and Blood Institute, Bethesda, MD: Report of the second task force on blood pressure control in children—1987. Reproduced with permission of *Pediatrics,* vol. 79, p. 1. Copyright © 1987.)

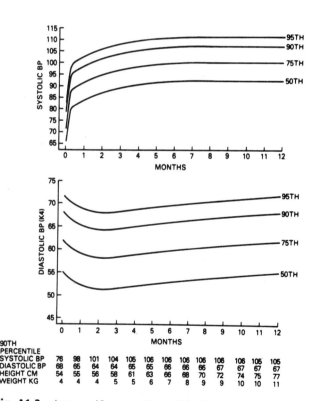

90TH PERCENTILE												
SYSTOLIC BP	76	98	101	104	105	106	106	106	106	106	106	105	105
DIASTOLIC BP	68	65	64	64	65	65	66	66	66	67	67	67	67
HEIGHT CM	54	55	56	58	61	63	66	68	70	72	74	75	77
WEIGHT KG	4	4	4	5	5	6	7	8	9	9	10	10	11

Fig. A1-2 Age-specific percentiles of blood pressure (BP) measurements in girls—birth to 12 months of age; Korotkoff phase IV (K4) used for diastolic BP. (From National Heart, Lung, and Blood Institute, Bethesda, MD: Report of the second task force on blood pressure control in children—1987. Reproduced with permission of *Pediatrics,* vol. 79, p. 1. Copyright © 1987.)

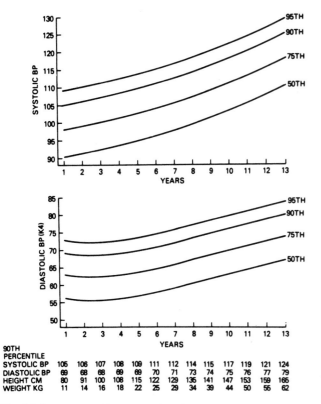

90TH PERCENTILE													
SYSTOLIC BP	105	106	107	108	109	111	112	114	115	117	119	121	124
DIASTOLIC BP	69	68	68	69	69	70	71	73	74	75	76	77	79
HEIGHT CM	80	91	100	108	115	122	129	135	141	147	153	159	165
WEIGHT KG	11	14	16	18	22	25	29	34	39	44	50	55	62

Fig. A1-3 Age-specific percentiles of blood pressure (BP) measurements in boys—birth to 1 to 13 years of age; Korotkoff phase IV (K4) used for diastolic BP. (From National Heart, Lung, and Blood Institute, Bethesda, MD: Report of the second task force on blood pressure control in children—1987. Reproduced with permission of *Pediatrics,* vol. 79, p. 1. Copyright © 1987.)

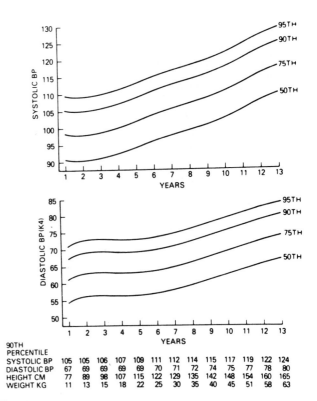

90TH PERCENTILE													
SYSTOLIC BP	105	105	106	107	109	111	112	114	115	117	119	122	124
DIASTOLIC BP	67	69	69	69	69	70	71	72	74	75	77	78	80
HEIGHT CM	77	89	98	107	115	122	129	135	142	148	154	160	165
WEIGHT KG	11	13	15	18	22	25	30	35	40	45	51	58	63

Fig. A1-4 Age-specific percentiles of blood pressure (BP) measurements in girls—birth to 1 to 13 years of age; Korotkoff phase IV (K4) used for diastolic BP. (From National Heart, Lung, and Blood Institute, Bethesda, MD: Report of the second task force on blood pressure control in children—1987. Reproduced with permission of *Pediatrics,* vol. 79, p. 1. Copyright © 1987.)

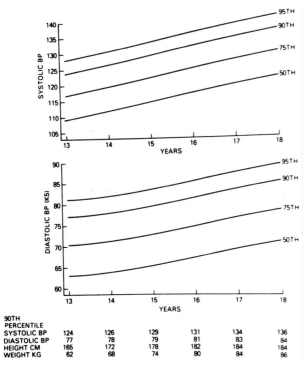

90TH PERCENTILE						
SYSTOLIC BP	124	126	129	131	134	136
DIASTOLIC BP	77	78	79	81	83	84
HEIGHT CM	165	172	178	182	184	184
WEIGHT KG	62	68	74	80	84	86

Fig. A1-5 Age-specific percentiles of blood pressure (BP) measurements in boys—birth to 13 to 18 years of age; Korotkoff phase IV (K4) used for diastolic BP. (From National Heart, Lung, and Blood Institute, Bethesda, MD: Report of the second task force on blood pressure control in children—1987. Reproduced with permission of *Pediatrics,* vol. 79, p. 1. Copyright © 1987.)

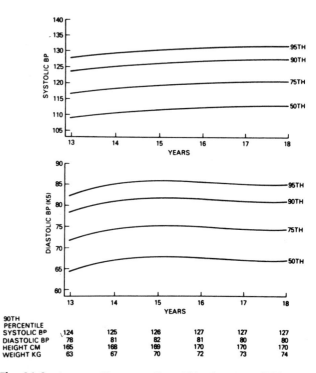

90TH PERCENTILE						
SYSTOLIC BP	124	125	126	127	127	127
DIASTOLIC BP	78	81	82	81	80	80
HEIGHT CM	165	168	169	170	170	170
WEIGHT KG	63	67	70	72	73	74

Fig. A1-6 Age-specific percentiles of blood pressure (BP) measurements in girls—birth to 13 to 18 years of age; Korotkoff phase IV (K4) used for diastolic BP. (From National Heart, Lung, and Blood Institute, Bethesda, MD: Report of the second task force on blood pressure control in children—1987. Reproduced with permission of *Pediatrics,* vol. 79, p. 1. Copyright © 1987.)

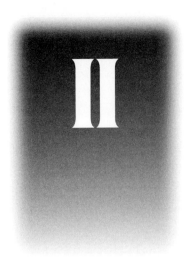

Growth Charts

GIRLS: BIRTH TO 36 MONTHS
PHYSICAL GROWTH
NCHS PERCENTILES*

NAME _____ RECORD # _____

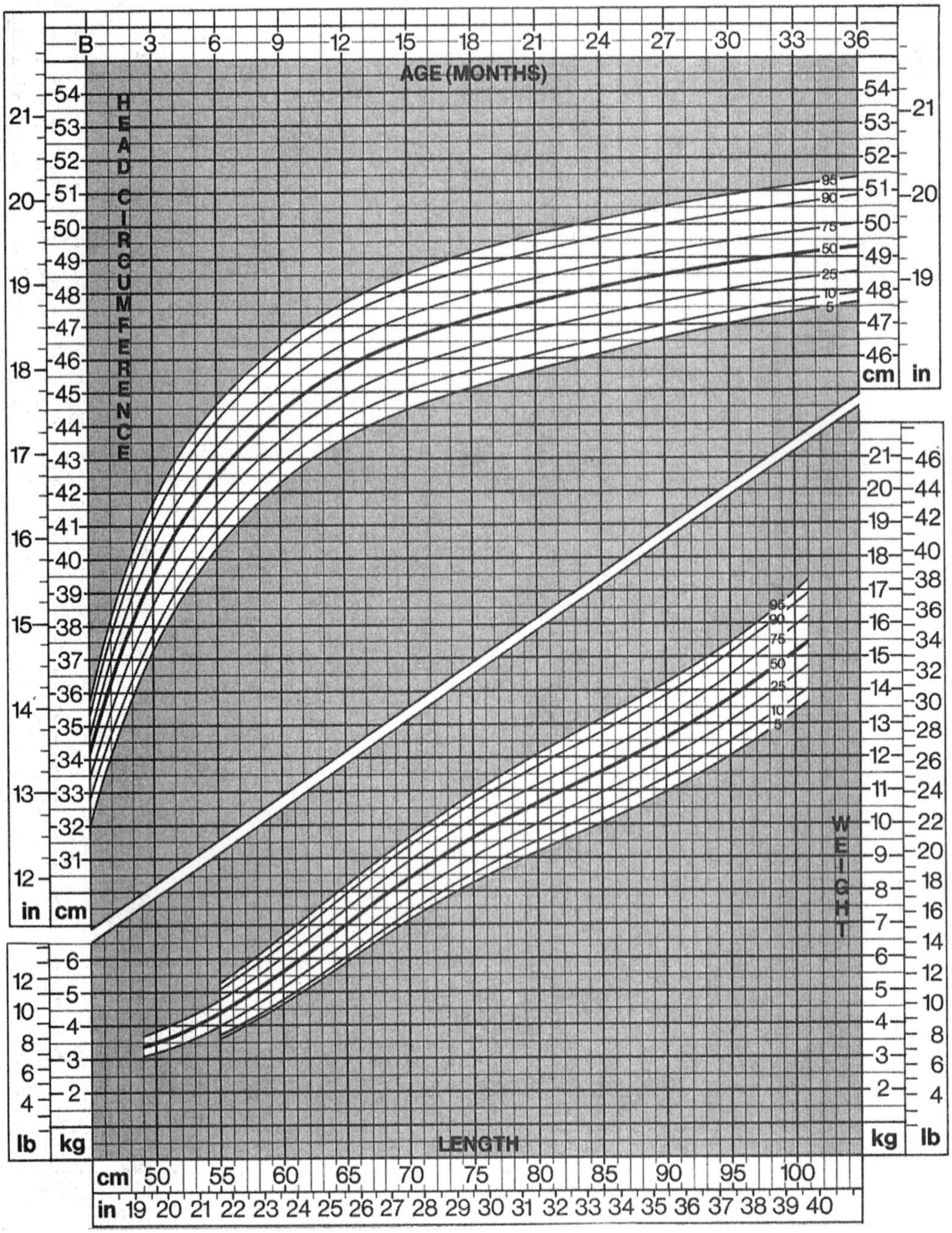

HEAD CIRCUMFERENCE

AGE (MONTHS)

B 3 6 9 12 15 18 21 24 27 30 33 36

WEIGHT

LENGTH

cm 50 55 60 65 70 75 80 85 90 95 100
in 19 20 21 22 23 24 25 26 27 28 29 30 31 32 33 34 35 36 37 38 39 40

*Adapted from: Hamill PVV, Drizd TA, Johnson CL, Reed RB, Roche AF, Moore WM: Physical growth: National Center for Health Statistics percentiles. AM J CLIN NUTR 32:607-629, 1979. Data from the Fels Longitudinal Study, Wright State University School of Medicine, Yellow Springs, Ohio.

© 1982 Ross Laboratories

DATE	AGE	LENGTH	WEIGHT	HEAD CIRC.	COMMENT

ROSS ROSS PRODUCTS DIVISION
ABBOTT LABORATORIES
COLUMBUS, OHIO 43215-1724

51208 09890WB
(0.05)/SEPTEMBER 1993   LITHO IN USA

GIRLS: BIRTH TO 36 MONTHS
PHYSICAL GROWTH
NCHS PERCENTILES*

NAME _____

RECORD # _____

Ross
Growth &
Development
Program

AGE (MONTHS)

LENGTH

WEIGHT

AGE (MONTHS)

MOTHER'S STATURE _____

FATHER'S STATURE _____

GESTATIONAL

AGE _____ WEEKS

DATE	AGE	LENGTH	WEIGHT	HEAD CIRC.	COMMENT
	BIRTH				

* Adapted from: Hamill PVV, Drizd TA, Johnson CL, Reed RB, Roche AF, Moore WM: Physical growth: National Center for Health Statistics percentiles. AM J CLIN NUTR 32:607–629, 1979. Data from the Fels Longitudinal Study, Wright State University School of Medicine, Yellow Springs, Ohio.

© 1982 Ross Laboratories

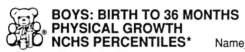

BOYS: BIRTH TO 36 MONTHS PHYSICAL GROWTH NCHS PERCENTILES*

Name_____ Record #_____

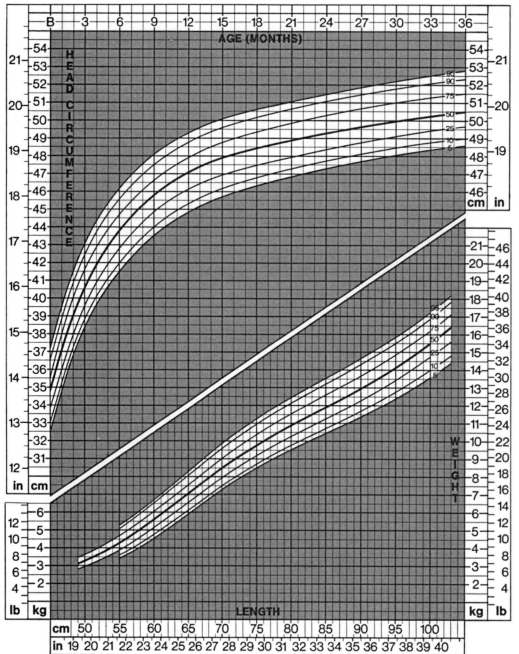

DATE	AGE	LENGTH	WEIGHT	HEAD CIRC.	COMMENT

ROSS ROSS PRODUCTS DIVISION
ABBOTT LABORATORIES
COLUMBUS, OHIO 43215-1724

51208 09890WB
(0.05)/SEPTEMBER 1993   LITHO IN USA

BOYS: BIRTH TO 36 MONTHS
PHYSICAL GROWTH
NCHS PERCENTILES*

Name_____ Record #_____

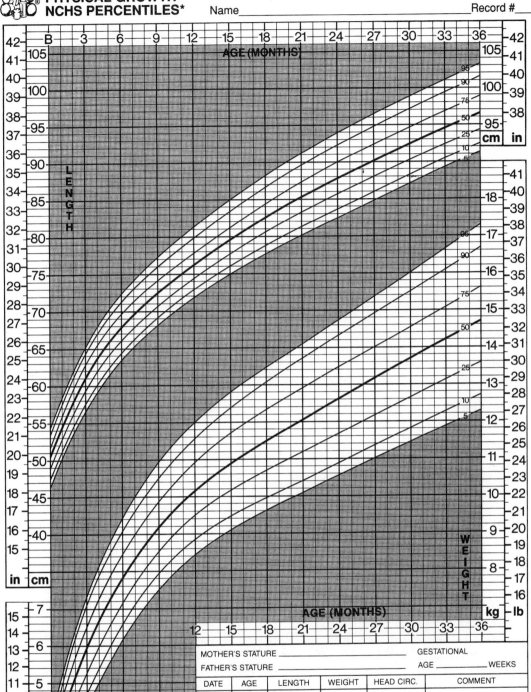

ROSS
PEDIATRICS

MOTHER'S STATURE _____ GESTATIONAL
FATHER'S STATURE _____ AGE _____ WEEKS

DATE	AGE	LENGTH	WEIGHT	HEAD CIRC.	COMMENT
	BIRTH				

*Adapted from: Hamill PVV, Drizd TA, Johnson CL, Reed RB, Roche AF, Moore WM: Physical growth: National Center for Health Statistics percentiles. AM J CLIN NUTR 32:607-629, 1979, Data from the Fels Longitudinal Study, Wright State University School of Medicine, Yellow Springs, Ohio.

© 1982 Ross Products Division, Abbott Laboratories

GIRLS: 2 TO 18 YEARS
PHYSICAL GROWTH
NCHS PERCENTILES*

Name_____   Record #_____

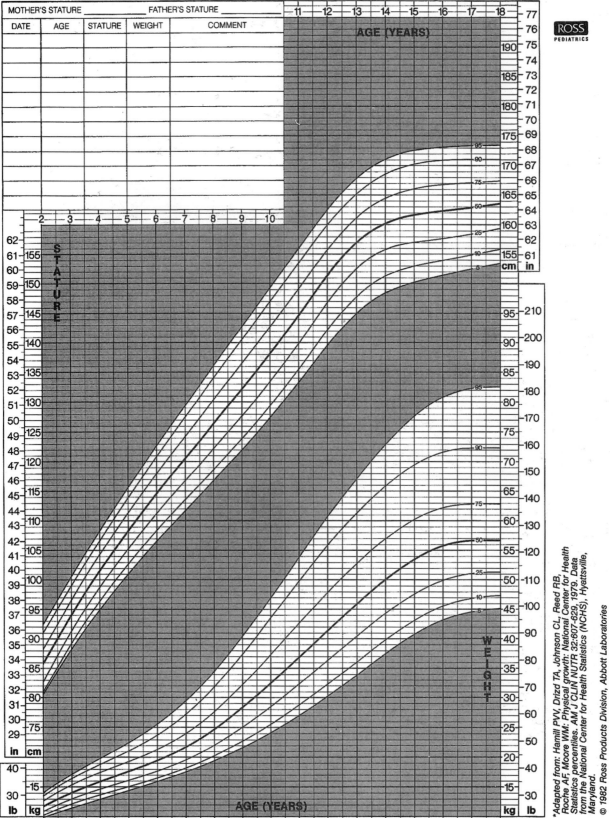

*Adapted from: Hamill PVV, Drizd TA, Johnson CL, Reed RB, Roche AF, Moore WM.: Physical growth: National Center for Health Statistics percentiles. AM J CLIN NUTR 32:607-629, 1979. Data from the National Center for Health Statistics (NCHS), Hyattsville, Maryland.

© 1982 Ross Products Division, Abbott Laboratories

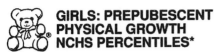

GIRLS: PREPUBESCENT PHYSICAL GROWTH NCHS PERCENTILES*

Name_____ Record #_____

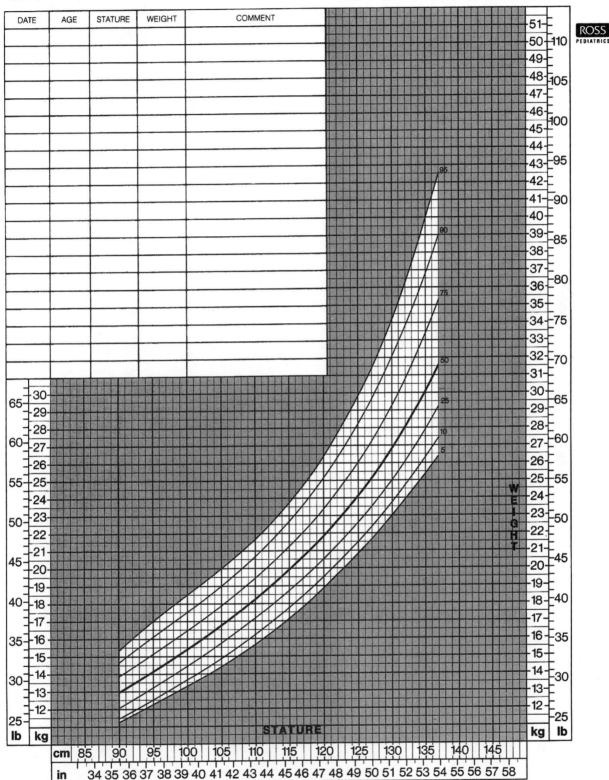

51214 09893WB
(0.05)/SEPTEMBER 1993

ROSS PRODUCTS DIVISION
ABBOTT LABORATORIES
COLUMBUS, OHIO 43215-1724

LITHO IN USA

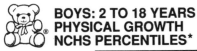

BOYS: 2 TO 18 YEARS
PHYSICAL GROWTH
NCHS PERCENTILES*

Name_____   Record #_____

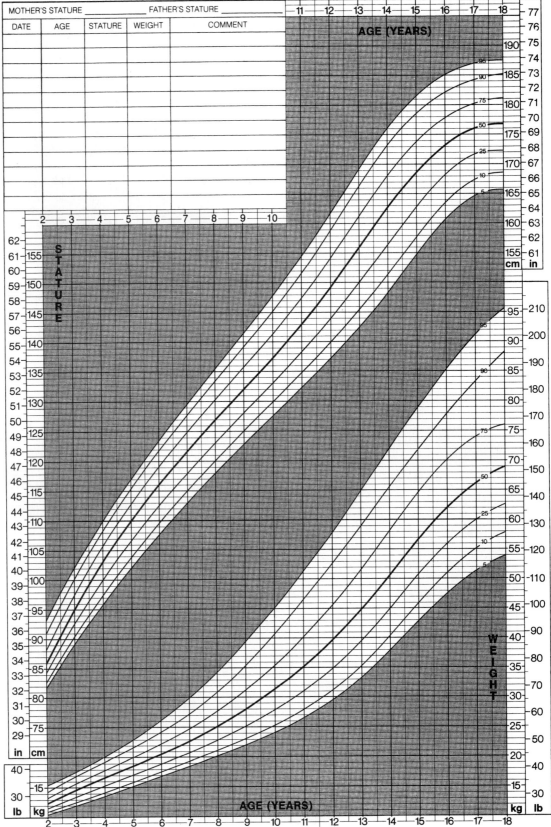

*Adapted from: Hamill PVV, Drizd TA, Johnson CL, Reed RB, Roche AF, Moore WM: Physical growth: National Center for Health Statistics percentiles. AM J CLIN NUTR 32:607-629, 1979. Data from the National Center for Health Statistics (NCHS), Hyattsville, Maryland.

© 1982 Ross Products Division, Abbott Laboratories

BOYS: PREPUBESCENT
PHYSICAL GROWTH
NCHS PERCENTILES*

Name_____ Record #_____

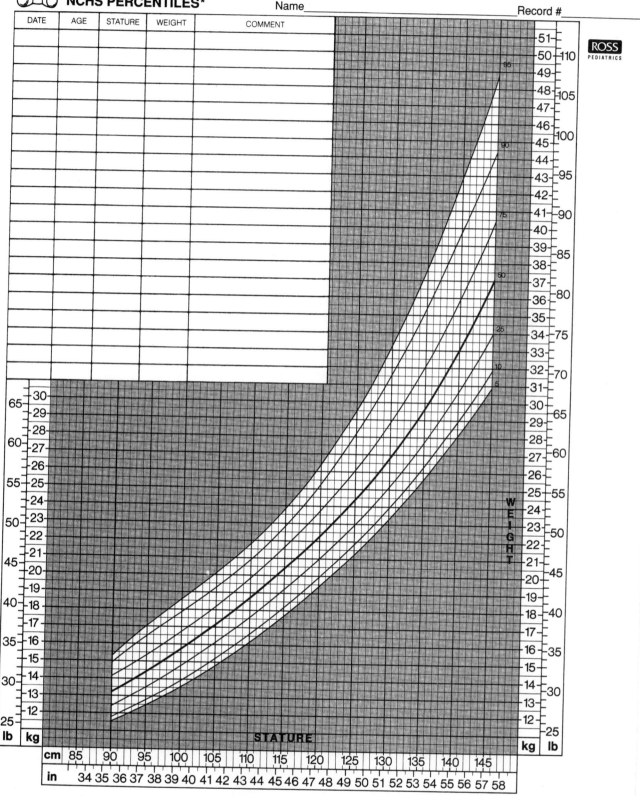

DATE	AGE	STATURE	WEIGHT	COMMENT

ROSS
PEDIATRICS

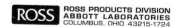

WEIGHT

STATURE

51212 09892WB
(0.05)/JUNE 1994

ROSS PRODUCTS DIVISION
ABBOTT LABORATORIES
COLUMBUS, OHIO 43215-1724

LITHO IN USA

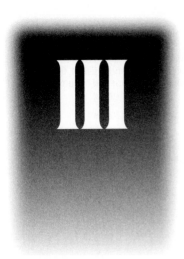

III Normal Immunization Schedule

Fig. A3-1 Recommended Childhood Immunization Schedule. (Approved by the Advisory Committee on Immunization Practices [ACIP], the American Academy of Pediatrics [AAP], and the American Academy of Family Physicians [AAFP].)

Recommended Childhood Immunization Schedule
United States, January-December 2001

Vaccines[1] are listed under routinely recommended ages. [Bars] indicate range of recommended ages for immunization. Any dose not given at the recommended age should be given as a "catch-up" immunization at any subsequent visit when indicated and feasible. (Ovals) indicate vaccines to be given if previously recommended doses were missed or given earlier than the recommended minimum age.

Information in bold has been added by the American Academy of Family Physicians (AAFP).

Age ▶ / Vaccines ▼	Birth	1 mo	2 mos	4 mos	6 mos	12 mos	15 mos	18 mos	24 mos	4-6 yrs	11-12 yrs	14-16 yrs
Hepatitis B[2]	Hep B #1	Hep B #1	Hep B #2		Hep B #3						(Hep B)	
Diphtheria, Tetanus, Pertussis[3]			DTaP	DTaP	DTaP		DTaP[3]			DTaP	Td	
H. influenzae type b[4]			Hib	Hib	Hib	Hib						
Inactivated Polio[5]			IPV	IPV	IPV[5]					IPV[5]		
Pneumococcal Conjugate[6]			PCV	PCV	PCV	PCV						
Measles, Mumps, Rubella[7]						MMR				MMR[7]	(MMR[7])	
Varicella[8]						Var					(Var[8])	
Hepatitis A[9]									Hep A—in selected areas[9]			

Approved by the Advisory Committee on Immunization Practices (ACIP), the American Academy of Pediatrics (AAP), and the American Academy of Family Physicians (AAFP).

[1]This schedule indicates the recommended ages for routine administration of currently licensed childhood vaccines as of November 1, 2000, for children through 18 years of age. Additional vaccines may be licensed and recommended during the year. Licensed combination vaccines may be used whenever any components of the combination are indicated and its other components are not contraindicated. Providers should consult the manufacturers' package inserts for detailed recommendations.

[2]Infants born to mothers who are negative for hepatitis B antigen (HB-Ag) should receive the first dose of hepatitis B (Hep B) vaccine by age 2 months. The second dose should be at least 1 month after the first dose. The third dose should be administered at least 4 months after the first dose and at least 2 months after the second dose, but not before 6 months of age for infants.

Infants born to HB-Ag–positive mothers should receive hepatitis B vaccine and 0.5 ml hepatitis B immune globulin (HBIG) within 12 hours of birth at separate sites. The second dose is recommended at 1 to 2 months of age and the third dose at 6 months of age.

Infants born to mothers whose HB-Ag status is unknown should receive hepatitis B vaccine within 12 hours of birth. Maternal blood should be drawn at the time of delivery to determine the mother's HB-Ag status; if the HB-Ag test is positive, the infant should receive HBIG as soon as possible (no later than 1 week of age).

All children and adolescents who have not been immunized against hepatitis B should begin the series during any visit. Special efforts should be made to immunize children who were born in or whose parents were born in areas of the world with moderate or high endemicity of hepatitis B virus infection.

[3]The fourth dose of DTaP (diphtheria and tetanus toxoids and acellular pertussis vaccine) may be administered as early as 12 months of age, provided 6 months have elapsed since the third dose and the child is unlikely to return at age 15 to 18 months. Td (tetanus and diphtheria toxoids) is recommended at 11 to 12 years of age if at least 5 years have elapsed since the last dose of DTP (diphtheria, tetanus, and pertussis), DTaP, or DT. Subsequent routine Td boosters are recommended every 10 years.

[4]Three Haemophilus influenzae type B (HIB) conjugate vaccines are licensed for infant use. If PRP-OMP (Pedvax-HIB or ComVax [Merck]) is administered at 2 and 4 months of age, a dose at 6 months is not required. Because clinical studies in infants have demonstrated that using some combination products may induce a lower immune response to the HIB vaccine component, DTaP/HIB combination products should not be used for primary immunization in infants at 2, 4, or 6 months of age unless approved by the Food and Drug Administration for these ages.

[5]An all-IPV (poliovirus vaccine inactivated) schedule is now recommended for routine childhood polio vaccination in the United States. All children should receive four doses of IPV at 2 months, 4 months, 6 to 18 months, and 4 to 6 years of age. Oral polio vaccine (OPV) should be used only in selected circumstances. (See *MMWR*, May 19, 2000/49 (RR-5); 1-22.)

[6]The heptavalent conjugate pneumococcal vaccine (PCV) is recommended for all children 2 to 23 months of age. It is also recommended for certain children 24 to 59 months of age. (See *MMWR*, Oct. 6, 2000/49 (RR-9); 1-35.) **The full AAFP Clinical Policy on Pneumococcal Conjugate Vaccine is available at www.aafp.org/policy/camp/24.html.**

[7]The second dose of measles, mumps, and rubella (MMR) vaccine is recommended routinely at 4 to 6 years of age, but may be administered during any visit provided at least 4 weeks have elapsed since receipt of the first dose and that both doses are administered on or after the first birthday. Those who have not previously received the second dose should complete the schedule by the 11- to 12-year-old visit.

[8]Varicella (Var) vaccine is recommended at any visit on or after the first birthday for susceptible children; that is, those who lack a reliable history of chickenpox (as judged by a health care provider) and who have not been immunized. Susceptible persons 13 years of age or older should receive 2 doses, given at least 4 weeks apart.

[9]Hepatitis A (Hep A) is shaded to indicate its recommended use in selected states or regions, and for certain high-risk groups; consult your local public health authority. (See *MMWR*, 48(RR-12); 1-37, Oct 01, 1999.)

For additional information about the vaccines listed above, please visit the National Immunization Program Home Page at http://www.cdc.gov/nip/ or call the National Immunization Hotline at 800-232-2522 (English) or 800-232-0233 (Spanish).

Full AAFP immunization policies can be found at the AAFP website, www.aafp.org/clinical.

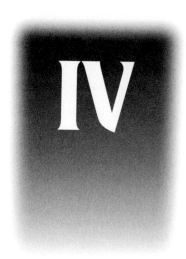

Emergency Cart Contents

TABLE A4-1   Standard Code Cart Supplies

Cart Exterior

Medication labels
Extension cord
Gloves, nonsterile
Backboard
Equipment checklists
Code-Blue forms
Sharps container
Oxygen tank with regulator
Self-inflating resuscitation bag with masks (adult, child, infant)

Drawer #1: MEDICATIONS

Small medication tray (see attached contents list)
Large medication tray (see attached contents list)
Reference book
Calculator

		Number
Drawer #2: NEEDLES/SYRINGES		
Syringes	TB 3 ml (3 cc), 10 ml (10 cc)	10 each
	Heparinized	4
Needles	18, 22, 25 gauge	4 each
Microtainers		4
Alcohol wipes		1 box
Gauze, 2 × 2 in		1 box
Sterile 0.9% NaCl	10 ml	10
InterLink cannula		4
IV catheters	24-14 gauge	4 each
Butterfly needles	21, 23, 25 gauge	4 each
T-connectors		4
Super STAT forms		4

		Number
Drawer #3: AIRWAY		
Intubation Tray		
Benzoin		4
Cloth tape, 1 in, latex-free		1 roll
Stylettes	Pedi, adult	1 each
Lidocaine jelly		1 tube
Lubafax jelly		1 packet
Afrin spray		1
Magill forceps	Infant, adult	1 each
Yankauer suction		2
Laryngoscope handle		2
Laryngoscope blades	Miller 0, 1, 2, 3	1 each
	Macintosh 2, 3	1 each
	WisHipple 1.5	1
Endotracheal tubes	2.5-5.5 uncuffed 5.0–8.0 cuffed	2 each
Batteries	C, D, AA	2 each
Laryngoscope bulbs	Small, large	2 each
Ambu masks	Neonate, infant, toddler, child, small adult, adult	1 each
Oral airways	Size 5-9	1 each
Nasal airways	Assorted sizes	
Tongue depressors		2
Mapleson F resuscitation bag with oxygen tubing	500, 1000 cc	1 each
Oxygen flowmeter with nipple adapter		1

Continued

TABLE A4-1 **Standard Code Cart Supplies—cont'd**

		Number
Drawer #4: IV THERAPY		
Syringes	30 ml (30 cc), 60 ml (60 cc)	4 each
Blood collection tubes	Red, purple, blue, green, large red	2 each
Intraosseous needles	15 g, 18 g	2 each
Medfusion tubing		4
Extension tubing		4
Stopcocks, 3-way		4
Solusets	Mini, macrodrip	1 each
Gauze sponges, 2 × 2 in		1 box
Silk tape	½ in, 1 in, 2 in	1 roll each
Tourniquets, latex-free		1 roll
Armboards	Small, med, large	1 each
IV spike		4
Suture on curved needle	3-0 silk	4
Kelly clamp		2
Bandaids, assorted		1 each
Betadine wipes		1 box
Biooclusive dressing		4
InterLink T-connector		4
IV solutions	LR, NS, D5W, D51/2NS, 500 ml	1 each
Albumin	250 ml	1

		Number
Drawer #5: MISCELLANEOUS		
Suction Supplies		
Suction canister with tubing		1
Suction catheters	6, 8, 10, 12, 14 Fr	1 each
0.9% NaCl for instillation	3-ml ampules	4
Gastric drainage		
Feeding tubes	5, 8 Fr	1 each
Salem Sump tubes	10, 14, 18 Fr	1 each
Catheter tip syringe	60 ml	2
Catheters		
Central venous, Arrow	4 Fr, 8 cm double lumen	1
	7 Fr, 12 cm triple lumen	1
Pressure, Cook	3.0 Fr single lumen	1
	5.0 Fr single lumen	1
Oxygen/Nebulizer Therapy		
Nonrebreather oxygen mask	Adult, pediatric	1 each
Hand-held nebulizer with ETT adapter		1
MDI chamber for ETT		1
Oxygen tank key		1
Other		
Betadine		1 bottle
Blood pressure cuffs	Infant, child, adult	1 each
Face shields		4
Flashlight		1

STANDARD CODE MEDICATIONS

◆ Table A4-2   Small Code Cart Tray

Generic Name	Brand Name	Strength/Concentration	Volume	Number	Comments
Atropine sulfate		0.4 mg/ml	1 ml	5	
Calcium Chloride		10% (100 mg/ml)	10 ml	3	
Dextrose		25% (250 mg/ml)	10 ml	2	
Dextrose		50% (500 mg/ml)	50 ml	2	
Epinephrine		1:1000 (1 mg/ml)	30 ml	1	
Epinephrine		1:10,000 (0.1 mg/ml)	10 ml	4	Prefilled syringe
Lidocaine	Xylocaine	2% (20 mg/ml)	5 ml	2	Prefilled syringe
Sodium bicarbonate	Neut	4.2% (0.5 mEq/ml)	5 ml	4	
Sodium bicarbonate		8.4% (1 mEq/ml)	50 ml	2	

◆ Table A4-3   Large Code Cart Tray

Generic Name	Brand Name	Strength/concentration	Volume	Number	Comments
Adenosine	Adenocard	3 mg/ml	3 ml	2	
Albuterol MDI	Ventolin	90 µg/puff		1	For inhalation only
Albuterol	Ventolin	0.5% (5 mg/ml)	20 ml	1	For inhalation only
Amiodarone	Cordarone	50 mg/ml	3 ml	6	
Bretylium	Bretylol	50 mg/ml	10 ml	1	
Dexamethasone	Decadron	5 mg/ml	5 ml	2	
Diphenhydramine	Benadryl	50 mg/ml	1 ml	2	
Dobutamine	Dobutrex	12.5 mg/ml	20 ml	2	
Dopamine	Inotropin	40 mg/ml	5 ml	3	
Epinephrine, racemic	Vaponefrin	2.25%	20 ml	1	For inhalation only
Furosemide	Lasix	10 mg/ml	2 ml	4	
Hydralazine	Apresoline	20 mg/ml	1 ml	2	
Insulin, regular	Humulin	100 u/ml	10 ml	1	
Mannitol	Osmitrol	20% (20 g/100 ml)	500 ml	1	
Naloxone	Narcan	0.4 mg/ml	1 ml	5	
Nitroprusside	Nipride	25 mg/ml	2 ml	1	
Pancuronium	Pavulon	1 mg/ml	10 ml	1	
Phenylephrine	Neo-Synephrine	10 mg/ml	2 ml	3	
Phenytoin	Dilantin	50 mg/ml	2 ml	5	
Succinylcholine	Anectine	20 mg/ml	10 ml	1	

Revised 8/15/00.

TABLE A4-4   PICU Code Cart Medication Drawer Layout

CODE CART MEDICATION DRAWER LAYOUT

ANTIBIOTICS	STEROIDS	INDUCTION AGENTS	MISCELLANEOUS	INOTROPES/PRESSORS

ANTIBIOTICS
- Ampicillin 1 g × 3
- Cefotaxime 1 g × 3
- Gentamicin 10 mg/ml, 2 ml × 4

STEROIDS
- Dexamethasone 4 mg/ml, 1 ml × 3
- Hydrocortisone 100 mg × 1
- Methylprednisolone 40 mg × 3

INDUCTION AGENTS
- Etomidate 2 mg/ml, 10 ml × 2
- Propofol 10 mg/ml, 20 ml × 1
- Rocuronium 10 mg/ml, 5 ml × 1 (exp 2 mos)
- Succinylcholine 20 mg/ml, 10 ml × 1 (exp 6 mos)
- Glycopyrrolate 0.2 mg/ml, 1 ml × 5
- Neostigmine 5 mg/ml, 2 ml × 1

MISCELLANEOUS
- Dantrolene 20 mg × 1
- Diphenhydramine 50 mg/ml, 1 ml × 2
- Fosphenytoin 50 mg PE/ml, 2 ml × 10 (exp 2 mo)
- Furosemide 10 mg/ml, 10 ml × 1
- Heparin 1000 units/ml, 10 ml × 2

INOTROPES/PRESSORS
- Dobutamine 12.5 mg/ml, 20 ml × 3
- Milrinone 1 mg/ml, 10 ml × 2
- Dopamine 40 mg/ml, 5 ml × 2
- Ephedrine 50 mg/ml, 1 ml × 2
- Norepinephrine 1 mg/ml, 4 ml × 2
- Phenylephrine 10 mg/ml, 1 ml × 1

ANTIHYPERTENSIVES
- Esmolol 100 mg/ml, 10 ml × 1
- Hydralazine 20 mg/ml, 1 ml × 2
- Labetolol 5 mg/ml, 20 ml × 2
- Nitroglycerin 5 mg/ml, 10 ml × 2
- Nitroprusside 25 mg/ml, 2 ml × 2

RESUSCITATION MEDS
- Epinephrine 1:10,000 Bristojet (0.1 mg/ml), 10 ml × 3
- Epinephrine 1:1000 (1 mg/ml), 30 ml × 2
- Epinephrine 1:1000 (1 mg/ml), 1 ml × 5
- Atropine 0.4 mg/ml, 1 ml × 5
- Sodium bicarbonate Neut 4.2% (0.5 mEq/ml), 5 ml × 4
- Sodium bicarbonate 8.4% (1 mEq/ml), 50 ml × 4
- Sodium bicarbonate 8.4% Bristojet (1 mEq/ml), 50 ml × 1

- Naloxone 0.4 mg/ml, 1 ml × 5
- Normal saline 10 ml × 10
- Sterile water for injection 10 ml × 10

- Calcium chloride 100 mg/ml, 10 ml × 4
- Calcium gluconate 100 mg/ml, 10 ml × 4
- Magnesium sulfate 500 mg/ml, 2 ml × 4

ANTIARRYTHMICS
- Adenosine 3 mg/ml, 2 ml × 2
- Amiodarone 50 mg/ml, 3 ml × 6
- Lidocaine 1% (10 mg/ml), 2 ml × 5
- Lidocaine 2% (20 mg/ml), 2 ml × 5
- Lidocaine 4% (40 mg/ml), 50 ml × 1
- Procainamide 100 mg/ml, 10 ml × 2
- Verapamil 2.5 mg/ml, 2 ml × 2

MANNITOL
- Mannitol 25% (0.25 g/ml), 50 ml × 2

DEXTROSE
- Dextrose 25% bristojet (0.25 g/ml), 10 ml × 2
- Dextrose 50% (0.5 g/ml), 50 ml × 2

SECOND DRAWER

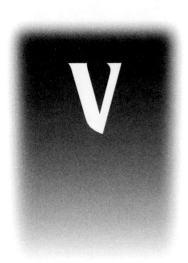

Drug Compatibility Chart

A GUIDE TO DRUG COMPATIBILITY

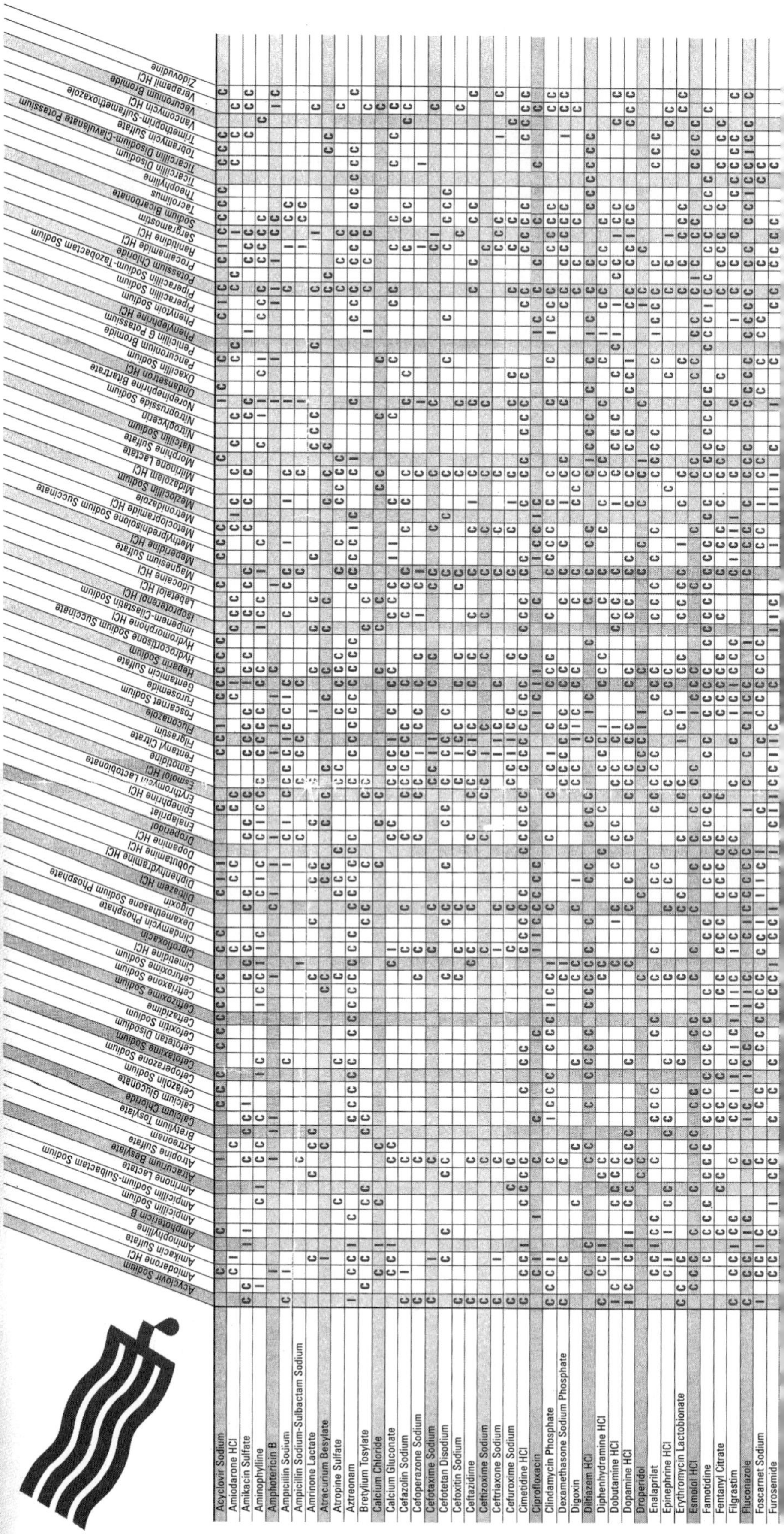

Row headings (left axis, top to bottom):

- Acyclovir Sodium
- Amiodarone HCl
- Amikacin Sulfate
- Aminophylline
- Amphotericin B
- Ampicillin Sodium
- Ampicillin Sodium–Sulbactam Sodium
- Amrinone Lactate
- Atracurium Besylate
- Atropine Sulfate
- Aztreonam
- Bretylium Tosylate
- Calcium Chloride
- Calcium Gluconate
- Cefazolin Sodium
- Cefoperazone Sodium
- Cefotaxime Sodium
- Cefotetan Disodium
- Cefoxitin Sodium
- Ceftazidime
- Ceftizoxime Sodium
- Ceftriaxone Sodium
- Cefuroxime Sodium
- Cimetidine HCl
- Ciprofloxacin
- Clindamycin Phosphate
- Dexamethasone Sodium Phosphate
- Digoxin
- Diltiazem HCl
- Diphenhydramine HCl
- Dobutamine HCl
- Dopamine HCl
- Droperidol
- Enalaprilat
- Epinephrine HCl
- Erythromycin Lactobionate
- Famotidine
- Fentanyl Citrate
- Filgrastim
- Fluconazole
- Foscarnet Sodium
- Furosemide

Column headings (top axis):

- Amikacin Sulfate
- Aminophylline
- Amphotericin B
- Ampicillin Sodium
- Ampicillin Sodium–Sulbactam Sodium
- Atracurium Besylate
- Atropine Sulfate
- Aztreonam
- Bretylium Tosylate
- Calcium Chloride
- Calcium Gluconate
- Cefazolin Sodium
- Cefoperazone Sodium
- Cefotaxime Sodium
- Cefotetan Disodium
- Cefoxitin Sodium
- Ceftazidime
- Ceftizoxime Sodium
- Ceftriaxone Sodium
- Cefuroxime Sodium
- Cimetidine HCl
- Ciprofloxacin
- Clindamycin Phosphate
- Dexamethasone Sodium Phosphate
- Digoxin
- Diltiazem HCl
- Diphenhydramine HCl
- Dobutamine HCl
- Dopamine HCl
- Droperidol
- Enalaprilat
- Epinephrine HCl
- Erythromycin Lactobionate
- Famotidine
- Fentanyl Citrate
- Filgrastim
- Fluconazole
- Foscarnet Lactobionate
- Furosemide
- Gentamicin Sulfate
- Heparin Sodium
- Hydrocortisone Sodium Succinate
- Hydromorphone HCl
- Imipenem–Cilastatin Sodium
- Isoproterenol HCl
- Labetalol HCl
- Lidocaine HCl
- Magnesium Sulfate
- Meperidine HCl
- Methylprednisolone Sodium Succinate
- Metoclopramide HCl
- Metronidazole
- Midazolam HCl
- Milrinone
- Morphine Sulfate
- Nafcillin Sodium
- Nitroglycerin
- Nitroprusside
- Norepinephrine Sodium
- Ondansetron HCl
- Oxacillin Sodium
- Pancuronium Bromide
- Penicillin G Potassium
- Phenylephrine HCl
- Phenytoin Sodium
- Piperacillin Sodium
- Piperacillin Sodium–Tazobactam Sodium
- Potassium Chloride
- Procainamide HCl
- Ranitidine HCl
- Sargramostim
- Sodium Bicarbonate
- Tacrolimus
- Theophylline
- Ticarcillin Disodium
- Ticarcillin Disodium–Clavulanate Potassium
- Tobramycin Sulfate
- Trimethoprim–Sulfamethoxazole
- Vancomycin HCl
- Vecuronium Bromide
- Verapamil HCl
- Zidovudine

- Heparin Sodium
- Hydrocortisone Sodium Succinate
- Hydromorphone HCl
- Imipenem-Cilastatin Sodium
- Isoproterenol HCl
- Labetalol HCl
- Lidocaine HCl
- Magnesium Sulfate
- Meperidine HCl
- Methylprednisolone Sodium Succinate
- Metoclopramide HCl
- Metronidazole
- Mezlocillin Sodium
- Midazolam HCl
- Milrinone Lactate
- Morphine Sulfate
- Nafcillin Sodium
- Nitroglycerin
- Nitroprusside Sodium
- Norepinephrine Bitartrate
- Ondansetron HCl
- Oxacillin Sodium
- Pancuronium Bromide
- Penicillin G Potassium
- Phenylephrine HCl
- Phenytoin Sodium
- Piperacillin Sodium
- Piperacillin Sodium-Tazobactam Sodium
- Potassium Chloride
- Procainamide HCl
- Ranitidine HCl
- Sargramostim
- Sodium Bicarbonate
- Tacrolimus
- Theophylline
- Ticarcillin Disodium
- Ticarcillin Disodium-Clavulanate Potassium
- Tobramycin Sulfate
- Trimethoprim-Sulfamethoxazole
- Vancomycin HCl
- Vecuronium Bromide
- Verapamil HCl
- Zidovudine

The matrix cells contain the values **C** (Compatible), **I** (Incompatible), and blank (No information available or conflicting information).

LEGEND

I **Incompatible**

C **Compatible**

blank **No information available or conflicting information. The primary literature should be consulted.**

Compatibility should not be assumed.

Abbott Laboratories
Hospital Products Division
Abbott Park, IL 60064

REFERENCES

1. Trissel, LA: Handbook on Injectable Drugs, ninth edition, American Society of Health-System Pharmacists, Bethesda, MD, 1996.
2. King, JC: Guide to Parenteral Admixtures, Pacemarq, Inc., St. Louis, 1996.

REVIEWERS

1. David DiPersio, Pharm D., Critical Care Pharmacist, Vanderbilt University Medical Center, Nashville, TN.
2. Jim Pierce, Pharm D., Clinical Specialist, Trauma Critical Care, University of Tennessee, Knoxville, TN.

Compatibility may be affected by numerous factors including temperature, drug concentration, other medications present, diluent and contact time.
This chart is not intended to be an exhaustive review. The clinician is encouraged to compare conditions in their institutions with conditions tested in the literature. All clinicians involved in the prescribing, compounding and administration of medications have the responsibility of ensuring that medications delivered are compatible. Abbott Laboratories cannot be responsible for events arising from use of this chart.

96-4457/R2-10-Jun, 98

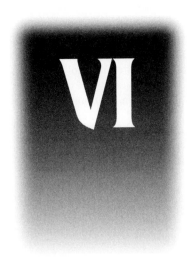

VI Critical Care Registered Nurse (CCRN) Certification Examination Blueprint— Pediatric Program

I. CLINICAL JUDGMENT (80%)

Assess, plan, intervene/implement, and evaluate a plan of care for a patient with each of the following conditions:

A. Cardiovascular (19%)
1. Myocardial conduction system defects (e.g., congenital heart block, Wolff-Parkinson-White syndrome, prolonged QT interval)
2. Acute congestive heart failure/pulmonary edema
3. Hypertensive crisis
4. Cardiogenic shock
5. Congenital heart defect/disease
6. Hypovolemic shock
7. Acute inflammatory disease (e.g., myocarditis, endocarditis, pericarditis)
8. Arrhythmias (e.g., supraventricular tachycardia, Vtach, Vfib, atrial fib, atrial flutter, acquired heart blocks, junctional rhythms, 2nd- and 3rd-degree block)
9. Cardiomyopathies (e.g., hypertrophic, dilated, restrictive)
10. Cardiac trauma

B. Pulmonary (24%)
1. Acute respiratory failure
2. Respiratory distress syndrome (e.g., acute respiratory distress syndrome)
3. Acute respiratory infections (e.g., acute pneumonia, croup, strep pneumonia, epiglottitis, respiratory syncytial virus, cystic fibrosis)
4. Status asthmaticus
5. Pulmonary hypertension
6. Thoracic trauma (e.g., lung contusions, fractured ribs, hemothorax, pulmonary hemorrhage)
7. Pulmonary aspirations (e.g., aspiration pneumonia, foreign-body aspiration)
8. Air-leak syndromes (e.g., pneumothorax)
9. Bronchopulmonary dysplasia
10. Apnea of prematurity (e.g., infant apnea, reflux apnea)
11. Congenital anomalies (e.g., sequelae of diaphragmatic hernia, diagnosis and management of tracheoesophageal fistula, tracheal malacia, tracheal stenosis)

C. Endocrine (4%)
1. Diabetes insipidus
2. Syndrome of inappropriate secretion of antidiuretic hormone
3. Diabetic ketoacidosis
4. Acute hypoglycemia
5. Adrenal disorders (e.g., adrenal insufficiency, inborn errors of metabolism, hyperthyroidism, hypothyroidism)

D. Hematology/Immunology (4%)
1. Organ transplantation (e.g., liver, bone marrow, kidney, heart, pancreas)
2. Life-threatening coagulopathies (e.g., disseminated intravascular coagulation, idiopathic thrombocytopenia purpura, hemophilia)
3. Immunosuppression (e.g., congenital [severe combined immunodeficiency syndrome], acquired [human immunodeficiency virus, acquired immunodeficiency syndrome, neoplasms])

E. Neurology (10%)
1. Encephalopathy (e.g., hypoxic-ischemic, metabolic, infectious, edema)
2. Head trauma (including shaken baby)
3. Spinal fusion
4. Acute spinal cord injury
5. Space-occupying lesions (e.g., brain tumors)
6. Hydrocephalus
7. Intracranial hemorrhage/intraventricular hemorrhage (including stroke)
8. Neurologic infectious diseases (e.g., meningitis)
9. Seizure disorders
10. Congenital neurological abnormalities (e.g., spina bifida, myelomeningocele, arteriovenous malformation)
11. Neuromuscular disorders (e.g., muscular dystrophy, Werdnig-Hoffman)

F. Gastrointestinal (5%)
   1. Acute gastrointestinal (GI) hemorrhage
   2. Hepatic failure/coma (e.g., portal hypertension, fulminant hepatitis, biliary atresia, hyperbilirubinemia)
   3. GI abnormalities (e.g., volvulus, malrotation, intussusception, short bowel syndrome, Hirschsprung's disease)
   4. Bowel infarction/obstruction/perforation (e.g., necrotizing enterocolitis)
   5. Acute abdominal trauma
G. Renal (3%)
   1. Acute and chronic renal failure (e.g., acute tubular necrosis)
   2. Life-threatening electrolyte imbalances (e.g., potassium, sodium, phosphorus, magnesium, calcium)
   3. Renal trauma

H. Multisystem (11%)
   1. Septic shock/systemic immune response syndrome (e.g., meningococcemia)
   2. Toxic ingestions (e.g, drug/alcohol overdose, poisoning)
   3. Asphyxia (e.g., near drowning, traumatic)
   4. Burns
   5. Hemolytic uremic syndrome
   6. Multisystem trauma (e.g., child abuse)
II. PROFESSIONAL CARING AND ETHICAL PRACTICE (20%)
   A. Advocacy/Moral Agency (4%)
   B. Caring Practices (4%)
   C. Collaboration (4%)
   D. Systems Thinking (2%)
   E. Response to Diversity (2%)
   F. Clinical Inquiry (2%)
   G. Facilitator of Learning (2%)

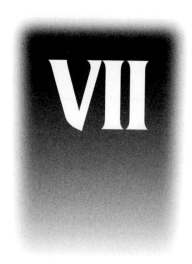

Multidisciplinary ICU, Children's Hospital, Boston, Clinical Practice Guideline

Enteral Nutrition Support

Advances in enteral feeding techniques, venous access, and enteral and parenteral nutrition have made it possible to provide nutritional support to almost all critically ill pediatric patients. Despite the abundant literature and widespread use of nutritional therapy, areas of nutritional support remain controversial and wide variations in practice exist. Therefore a multidisciplinary task force was convened to critically appraise the literature and make recommendations on enteral nutrition and gut protection practices to the Multidisciplinary Intensive Care Unit (MICU) Committee.

Whenever possible, prospective randomized clinical trials (PRCTs) were evaluated. Published reports were also reviewed when PRCTs were unavailable. Each conclusion is graded on the strength of evidence:

A: Supported by PRCT or metaanalysis of PRCT
B: Supported by well-designed, nonrandomized, prospective, retrospective, or case cohort-controlled studies
C: Supported by uncontrolled published experiences, case reports, or expert opinion

The following three topical areas of enteral nutritional support were addressed:

I. When and where should enteral feedings be started in the various patient populations cared for in the MICU?
II. Which enteral feeding tubes should we be using in the MICU? What is "best practice" in maintaining these enteral feeding tubes in the MICU?
III. What enteral feedings should be administered and how should they be started and advanced? How is enteral feeding tolerance best assessed?

I. When and where should enteral feedings be started in the various patient populations cared for in the MICU?

A. Critically ill patients are often hypermetabolic early in their illness, especially when it is complicated by sepsis. The hypothesis that nutritional support is clinically beneficial has not been supported by well-designed clinical trials.[1]
B. The rationale for nutritional support is based on clinical judgment. Nutritional support is often considered in patients who are unlikely to consume adequate nutrients for a prolonged period. In adults, the data suggest that critical depletion of lean tissue occurs after 14 days of starvation.[1]
C. Pediatric patients, because of higher metabolic rates and energy needs for growth, are more susceptible to under-nutrition than adults. The younger the patient, the more rapid and severe the clinical consequences of under-nutrition and starvation. The current standard of care is to initiate nutritional support in adults who will or have had 7 days of inadequate energy intake. Studies of pediatric body composition and energy reserves suggest a 5-day cutoff for well-nourished children, and 3 days for malnourished children and premature infants.[1,2]
D. Data suggest that there are advantages to using enteral over parenteral nutrition to meet the nutritional requirements of the critically ill patient. Critical illness is associated with gut atrophy and increased mucosal permeability to bacteria and macromolecules such as endotoxin. It has been postulated that the translocation of these products,

or at least the relative ischemia and subsequent reperfusion of the splanchnic organs, are somehow implicated in the development of single- or multiple-organ failure. Food in the lumen of the gut is cytoprotective.[3] Animal studies demonstrate that enteral nutrition maintains mucosal integrity and the immunologic function of the gastrointestinal tract, decreases bacterial translocation, blunts the systemic inflammatory response to a toxin load, and improves survival in experimental hemorrhage and peritonitis.[4]

E. Trauma patients fed by enteral nutrition have fewer complications than patients given parenteral nutrition (B). However, it is not clear whether enteral nutrition support provides a specific benefit or whether total parenteral nutrition (TPN) itself or overfeeding with TPN is associated with increased infections.[1]

F. The efficacy of enteral nutritional support in critically ill children has not been subjected to PRCTs. Chellis and colleagues demonstrated that early transpyloric feedings were feasible, well-tolerated without complication of aspiration or abdominal distension, and cost effective in critically ill pediatric patients (B).[5] All patients were mechanically ventilated; 76% were on one or more vasoactive agents.

Recommendations

Unless contraindicated, all MICU patients should receive enteral nutritional support as soon as possible after admission.

Enteral feedings are contraindicated in the following patients:

- Patients who may require endotracheal intubation or extubation within 4 hours.
- Hemodynamically unstable patients requiring escalation of therapy.
- Patients with a postoperative ileus.
- Patients with active upper gastrointestinal bleeding.
- Patients at risk for necrotizing enterocolitis or other causes of intestinal ischemia (as suspected on abdominal film or in patients post–major anoxic injury with renal and liver dysfunction).
- Patients with intestinal obstruction.
- Patients post–allogenic BMT (bone marrow transplantation) who have graft-versus-host disease or post-BMT patients before gut recontamination.
- Patients whose care is being redirected.

When enteral feedings are indicated, patients should be fed by the following routes:

- **Oral route,** if the patient is alert, unintubated, with a strong cough and gag reflex
- **Nasogastric route,** if the oral route is inaccessible and the patient has a strong cough and gag reflex
- **Nasojejunal route,** if the patient is at *high* risk for aspiration, such as those with a depressed gag reflex, delayed gastric emptying, and gastroesophageal reflux

The risk of aspiration determines whether feedings are placed in the stomach or jejunum. Gastric feeding is preferable (even in the intubated patient) because it allows the normal digestive process and hormonal responses to continue. Gastric acid secretion may be important for bactericidal effect. When compared with jejunal feeding, gastric feeding allows tolerance to large osmotic loads with less frequent cramping, distension, diarrhea, and a lower likelihood of dumping syndrome.

Transpyloric feeding is indicated in patients at *high* risk for aspiration, such as those with a depressed gag reflex, delayed gastric emptying, and gastroesophageal reflux.[6] Small-bowel feedings can usually be performed even in the presence of gastric atony and colonic ileus. Concomitant gastric decompression may be required.[7] If jejunal feedings are selected, patients at risk for gastric ulceration should also receive gut protection.

Of note, Montecalvo and others reported that adult patients fed by nasojejunal tubes (NJTs) received a significantly higher proportion of their daily caloric goal, had a significantly greater increase in serum prealbumin concentrations, and had a lower rate of pneumonia than in similar patients fed by continuous nasogastric tubes (NGTs).[8] Ibanez and others also reported a high incidence of gastroesophageal reflux (GER) in adult patients with orotracheal intubation and NGTs.[9] The presence of a 7F NGT was a risk factor for GER. Semirecumbency did not prevent GER, but the incidence rate was lower than in the supine position.

If enteral feedings are contraindicated, parenteral nutrition should be initiated.

IIa. Which enteral feeding tubes should we be using in the MICU?

Name	Size	Stylet	Weighted	Cost/ea
Corpak	6 Fr (22 in)	Yes	No	$9.19
	8 Fr (36 in)	Yes	No	$11.07
Kangaroo	6 Fr (20 in)	No	No	$7.32
	8 Fr (36 in)	Yes	Yes	$8.36
Accusite pH	6 Fr (30 in)	Yes	No	$45.00
Zinetics	8-10 Fr (48 in)			

Krafte-Jacobs and others compared transpyloric feeding tube placement using a pH-assisted placement versus standard placement in critically ill children.[10] Results indicated that 97% of patients in the pH-assisted group had successful placement after the first attempt, compared with 53% in the standard group. The average time for successful placement was 6 minutes. If placement was not successful, a second placement attempt was made after metoclopramide (Reglan) administration. All patients in the pH-assisted group had successful placement after the second attempt, compared with 78% of patients in the standard group. The pH-assisted method was associated with decreased radiation exposure and cost savings when compared with a standard placement technique (A).

Weighted enteral tubes are used by the GI service in patients with a history of vomiting.

Recommendations

Use nonweighted enteral feeding tubes (EFTs) for gastric placement and pH-guided EFTs for jejunal placement. Although the pH-guided NJT is more expensive, it may reduce hospital and patient costs by eliminating the use of fluoroscopy.

Metoclopramide (Reglan) may be used to facilitate transpyloric intubation. Metoclopramide accelerates gastric emptying and intestinal transit from the duodenum to the ileocecal valve by increasing the amplitude and duration of esophageal contractions, the resting tone of the lower esophageal sphincter, and the amplitude and tone of the gastric (antral) contractions, and by relaxing the pyloric sphincter and duodenal bulb, while increasing the peristalsis of the duodenum and jejunum. These effects help coordinate gastric, pyloric, and duodenal motor activity. Following IV administration, the onset of action on the gastrointestinal tract is 1 to 3 minutes; effects persist for 1 to 2 hours. A single IV dose is 0.1 to 0.2 mg/kg in patients under 6 years; 2.5 to 5.0 mg in patients 6 to 14 years; and 10 mg in patients 14 years and older.

When pH-guided EFT are used the pH should only be rechecked if there is potential dislodgment. All EFTs should be replaced on a monthly basis.

IIb. What is "best practice" in maintaining these enteral feedings tubes in the MICU?

Recommendations

A systemwide policy and procedure should be developed to address the following issues[11]:

A. Flush EFT before and after medication administration
   1. Rationale
      a. Evaluate the patency of the tube
      b. Clear formula residue or inadequately crushed medications
      c. Prevent physical and pharmacokinetic incompatibilities
   2. Flush solution: water or normal saline (to avoid dilutional hyponatremia)
   3. Flush volume
      a. 3 ml minimum plus 1 ml per year of age up to 10 years
      b. 10 to 30 ml after age 10 years (more fluid can be used if desired)
B. Dilute liquid medications before administration (A)
   1. Rationale
      a. Prevent obstruction by viscous solutions
      b. Prevent physiologic consequences of undiluted medications
         1) Irritation to the gastric mucosa
         2) Gastric distension and diarrhea resulting from hyperosmolar drugs
   2. Diluent solution: water or normal saline
   3. Diluent volume
      a. Dependent on medication volume (e.g., 2 to 3 times medication volume)
      b. 10 to 30 ml after age 10 years (more fluid can be used if desired)

C. Crush and dissolve tablets thoroughly before administration (C)
   1. Rationale: Prevent tube obstruction
   2. Methods: Crush tablet to a fine powder within unit-dose packet using mortar and pestle or Kelly clamps, or crush between two medication cups
   3. Diluent solution: warm water
   4. Diluent volume
      a. 1 ml/yr of age to 10 years
      b. 10 to 30 ml after age 10 years (more fluid can be used if desired)
   5. Do not crush enteric-coated, sustained-release, chewable, sublingual, or buccal formulations (C)
      a. Rationale
         1) Prevent tube occlusion from incompletely dissolved medications
         2) Prevent altered drug efficacy
            a) Sustained-release: avoid potential adverse effects associated with higher than expected peak concentration followed by subtherapeutic levels
            b) Enteric-coated: avoid stomach irritation or destruction of drug by gastric acids
            c) Chewable tablets: difficult to crush and uneven particles can block feeding tubes
            d) Sublingual and buccal drugs: lose effectiveness when delivered by an unintended route
      b. Use alternative drug formulation or therapeutically similar drug
         1) In some instances, the injectable form of the medication may be given orally. Factors impacting this decision include:
            a) Type of salt
            b) Drug stability in the gastric pH
            c) First past metabolism (enteral dose may require a large volume of parenteral medication for equivalent effect)
            d) Oral form may require a prodrug to ensure bioavailability
D. Administer each medication separately, flushing with water between medications (C)
   1. Rationale
      a. Prevent pharmacokinetic incompatibilities
      b. Prevent tube occlusion
   2. Flush solution: warm water or normal saline
   3. Flush volume
      a. 3 ml minimum then 1 ml/yr of age to 10 years
      b. 10 to 30 ml after age 10 years (more fluid can be used if desired)
E. Avoid adding medications to enteral feeding formula
   1. Rationale: prevent physical and pharmacokinetic incompatibilities
      a. Changes in drug potency and bioavailability
      b. Viscosity, consistency, and particle size
      c. Avoid formula contamination
F. If medications are best absorbed on an empty stomach and patients are receiving continuous feedings, hold

feedings for a time before and after medication administration
1. Rationale: to optimize drug absorption
2. Time interval
   a. 15 minutes (C)
   b. some drugs, such as phenytoin, may require 1 to 2 hour formula-free intervals before and after administration
G. Consult pharmacy about medication administration via EFTs (C)
1. Rationale
   a. Prevent tube obstructions (C)
   b. Optimize medication efficacy
2. Availability of liquid dosage form
   a. Use liquid dosage form when available (C)
   b. Not all liquid medications are suitable for EFT delivery
      1) Acidic liquid medications (e.g., elixirs) tend to clump in enteral formula
      2) Liquid medications with sweeteners often contain sorbital, which is also a cathartic
      3) Concentrated liquid medications tend to be thick and need to be diluted with water, especially in NJ tube fed patients
3. Optimal routes: NGT, NJT
4. Drug-formula compatibilities: Unlike IV-TPN drug coadministration guidelines, the effects of mixing drugs and enteral formulas have not been well defined. The routine mixing of medications in enteral feeding formulations should be discouraged.
5. Alternative therapeutic equivalents

Guidelines for Maintaining EFTs

1. Flush EFTs before and after checking for residual gastric contents (C)
   a. Rationale: Aspiration of gastric contents causes coagulation (especially with low pH of gastric fluid and with caseinate-based formulas)
   b. Flush solution: water or normal saline
   c. Flush volume
      1) 3 ml minimum plus 1 ml/yr of age to 10 years
      2) 10 to 30 ml after age 10 years (more fluid can be used if desired)
2. Flush all EFTs routinely (C)
   a. Rationale: Retrograde migration of gastric juices can occur (low pH causes increased obstruction)
   b. Frequency options
      1) Every 4 to 6 hours regardless of continuous feeding
      2) Every 4 to 6 hours if NOT on continuous feeding
      3) Whenever feedings are interrupted or feeding rates are decreased
   c. Flush solution: water or normal saline
   d. Flush volume
      1) 3 ml minimum then 1 ml/yr of age to 10 years
      2) 10 to 30 ml after age 10 years (more fluid can be used if desired)

3. Guidelines for managing obstruction of EFTs
   a. Irrigation solution
      1) Room-temperature or warm water is the preferred agent (A)
      2) Coca-Cola (or other carbonated beverage) or cranberry juice is seldom effective and should not be used
      3) If water fails to clear the EFT, use the following enzyme solution:
         a) In a medication cup, prepare a slurry consisting of the contents of 1 viokase capsule, 1 sodium bicarbonate tablet, and approximately 10 to 30 ml of warm water (viokase, a pancreatic enzyme, needs a basic environment to be active)
         b) Instill the slurry into the EFT; wait about 1 hour to ensure that the enzyme solution has maximal contact with the obstruction
         c) Withdraw the contents from the EFT (slurry and obstruction), avoiding excess force to prevent catheter damage
         d) Irrigate the EFT with warm water before resuming use

IIIa. What enteral feedings should be administered and how should they be started and advanced?

The following recommendations are considered "best practice" and are supported by uncontrolled published experiences, case reports, or expert opinion.

A. What to feed (specific formulas are examples)
   1. Resume previously established schedule or follow the recommendations in the following table:

	Premature (<2 kg)	<1yr	1 to 10 yr	>10 yr
Normal intact gut	Breast milk, Enfamil Premature	Breast milk, Enfamil with Iron	Pediasure, Nutren Jr	Isocal, Ensure
Lactose intolerant		Lacto-free, Prosobee	Pediasure, Nutren Jr	Isocal, Ensure
History of constipation or diarrhea, neuromuscular disease, or immobility			Pediasure with Fiber	Ensure with Fiber, Jevity
Fluid restricted		Kcal dense	KCal dense	Ensure Plus, Nutren 1.5 or 2.0
Renal disease		PM 60/40	Osmolite	
Impaired gut perfusion	Semi-elemental	Pregestimil, Alimentum	Pepta-men Jr	Peptamen, Vital HN
	Elemental	Neocate	Neocate +1, Pediatric Vivonex	Vivonex

B. How to Feed: Bolus versus Continuous
   1. If possible, resume previously established feeding method and schedule

2. Gastric route
   a. Use bolus feedings (more "physiologic")
      1) <6 months: every 3 hours
      2) >6 months: every 4 hours
   b. Use continuous gastric-tube feedings if an intermittent bolus poses a significant risk of respiratory distress, reflux, and aspiration[12]
3. Transpyloric route: use continuous feedings
C. How to initiate feedings
   1. Establish the goal of therapy
      a. Enteral nutrition: calculate full caloric requirements and advancement plan
      b. Trophic feeding: stimulate gut mucosal integrity and function, begin feeding within 24 hours of admission at low rates[4]
   2. For nutrition
      a. Strength
         1) If the patient's ability to protect airway is questionable begin with clear liquids
         2) Start with full strength feeding UNLESS the patient:
            a) Is receiving a hypertonic feeding (>600 mOsm)
            b) Has been NPO (nothing by mouth) for more than 2 weeks
            c) Was malnourished before admission
            d) Is at risk for gut ischemia
         3) If starting with ½ strength, increase to full strength after 24 hours
      b. Starting volume
         1) Bolus: calculate half the volume of full-strength formula needed to meet maintenance caloric requirements, then divide by the number of feedings per day (C)[6]
         2) Continuous 5 to 20 ml/kg/day; start low in patients at risk for gut ischemia
      c. How to advance
         1) Bolus: increase by 25% each feeding as tolerated
         2) Continuous: <1 yr: 1 to 5 ml per hour every 3 to 4 hours; >1 yr: 5 to 20 ml per hour every 4 hours
      d. Consider the use of free H_2O
         1) As per routine before admission
         2) If constipation an issue
         3) If the patient is receiving calorically dense feedings
         4) To meet total fluid requirements
         5) Volume, if intake is not a concern: 30 to 50 ml bolus
            a) After tube medications OR
            b) After bolus feedings OR
            c) Every 4 hours
   3. Tropic feedings
      a. Use full-strength formula as above
      b. 1 to 2 ml/hr
      c. Route: NGT or NJT

IIIb. How is enteral feeding tolerance best assessed?

Although the process is poorly understood, critical illness can seriously impair gastric emptying. Despite the presence of a functioning, intact small bowel, gastroparesis and duodenogastric reflux can lead to feeding intolerance. In addition, gastroparesis and gastroesophageal reflux can lead to nosocomial pneumonia. Separately, opiate administration also contributes to altered intestinal motility.

Erythromycin is a well-known prokinetic, but concerns regarding the use of an antibiotic in another role, with the risks of generating bacterial resistance, make it an unpopular choice.[3]

Only one PRCT was relevant to pediatric feeding intolerance.[13] Only two issues—diarrhea and residuals—were addressed.

A. What to assess
   1. Bolus gastric feedings: check and refeed residual before each feeding while advancing
      a. If more than half the previous bolus feeding or twice the hourly rate
      b. If transitioning to jejunal feedings
   2. Jejunal feedings: check abdominal girth every 12 hours while advancing; increasing abdominal distension may indicate feeding intolerance
   3. Eliminate the practice of routine checking of gastric residuals; the practice is not research-based and precipitates feeding tube obstruction and the unnecessary cessation of feedings. Do check residuals if abdominal distension or retching occurs[14,15]
B. Expect loose stools (<15 to 20 ml/kg/day)
   1. If diarrhea is present, check other etiologies before stopping feedings (e.g., H_2 antagonist, antacids—especially magnesium-containing, antibiotics, serum albumin level, *Clostridium difficile*, sorbital content of current medications). Before stopping feedings, send stool for reducing sugars and fat.
   2. Consider the use of antidiarrheal agents (for nonseptic patients)

REFERENCES

1. Klein S, Kinney J, Jeejeebhoy K et al: Nutritional support in clinical practice: review of published data and recommendations for future research directions, *Am J Clin Nutr* 66:683-706, 1997.
2. American Society for Parenteral and Enteral Nutrition (ASPEN): Standards for nutritional support—hospitalized pediatric patients, *Nutr Clin Pract* 4:33-37, 1989.
3. Frost P, Edwards N, Bihari D: Gastric emptying in the critically ill: the way forward, *Intensive Care Med* 23:243-245, 1997.
4. Heyland DK, Cook DJ, Guyatt GH: Enteral nutrition in the critically ill patient: a critical review of the evidence, *Intensive Care Med* 19:435-442, 1993.
5. Chellis MJ, Sanders SV, Webster HW et al: Early enteral feeding in the pediatric intensive care unit, *JPEN J Parenter Enteral Nutr* 20:71-73, 1996.
6. Wilson SE, Dietz WH, Grand RJ: An algo-

rithm for pediatric enteral alimentation, *Pediatr Ann* 16:233-240, 1987.

7. Cerra FB, Blackburn GL, Jeejeebhoy K et al: Applied nutrition in ICU patients: a consensus statement of the American College of Chest Physicians, *Chest* 111:769-778, 1997.

8. Montecalvo MA, Steger KA, Farbar HW et al: Nutritional outcome and pneumonia in critical care patients randomized to gastric versus jejunal tube feedings, *Crit Care Med* 20:1377-1387, 1992.

9. Ibanez J, Penafiel A, Raurich JM et al: Gastrointestinal reflux in intubated patients receiving enteral nutrition: effect of supine and semirecumbent positions, *JPEN J Parenter Enteral Nutr* 16:419-422, 1992.

10. Krafte-Jacobs B, Persinger M, Carver J et al: Rapid placement of transpyloric feeding tubes: a comparison of pH-assisted and standard insertion techniques in children, *Pediatrics* 98:242-248, 1997.

11. Belknap DC, Seifert CF, Petermann M: Administration of medications through enteral feeding catheters, *Am J Crit Care* 6:382-391, 1997.

12. ASPEN: Pediatric guidelines: critical care pediatric, *JPEN J Parenter Enteral Nutr* 17:48-49SA, 1995.

13. Gottschlich MM, Jenkins M, Warden GD et al: Differential effects of three enteral dietary regimens on selected outcome variables in burn patients, *JPEN J Parenter Enteral Nutr* 14:225-236, 1990.

14. Fuchs GJ: Enteral support of the hospitalized child. In Suskind RM, Lewinter-Suskind L, editors: *Textbook of pediatric nutrition*, ed 2, New York, 1993, Raven Press.

15. Lin HC, Van Citters GW: Stopping enteral feeding for arbitrary gastric residual volume may not be physiologically sound: results of a computer simulation model, *JPEN J Parenter Enteral Nutr* 21:286-289, 1997.

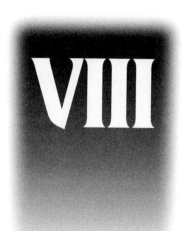

VIII Children's Hospital Neonatal/Pediatric Transport Data Base

CHILDREN'S HOSPITAL NEONATAL / PEDIATRIC TRANSPORT DATA BASE

(PRINT / SIGN / INITIAL BELOW)   ***INITIAL EACH SECTION OF DB AS COMPLETED

NAME: _____

DATE: ____/____/____

AGE: _____ DOB: ____/____/____ WGT: _____ KG

REF. HOSP./UNIT: _____

REPORT RECEIVED FROM: _____

TIME CALL RECEIVED: _____ TEAM MOBILIZED: _____

ARRIVE RH: _____ DEPART RH: _____ ARRIVE CH: _____

TEAM MEMBERS

RN: _____

RN: _____

MD: _____

EMT: _____

EMT: _____

MCP: _____

VITAL SIGNS								NEURO		MEDICATIONS	CONTINUOUS INFUSIONS			
TIME	ISOL. TEMP	PT TEMP.	HR	RESP	NIBP	ABP	MAP	PUPILS L / R	GCS		A	B	C	D

REFERENCE TABLES

Age Based Estimates for Vital Signs and Weight

AGE	Weight (kg)	Heart Rate	Resp. Rate	Systolic BP*	Diastolic BP*
premature	1	145/min	- 40	42 ± 10	21 ± 8
premature	1 - 2	135	- 40	50 ± 10	28 ± 8
newborn	2 - 3	125	- 40	60 ± 10	37 ± 8
1 month	4	120	24 - 35	80 ± 16	46 ± 16
6 month	7	130	24 - 35	89 ± 29	60 ± 10
1 year	10	120	20 - 30	96 ± 30	66 ± 25
2-3 years	12 - 14	115	20 - 30	99 ± 25	64 ± 25
4-5 years	16 - 18	100	20 -30	99 ± 20	65 ± 20
6-8 years	20 - 26	100	12 - 25	100 ± 15	60 ± 10
10-12 yr	32 - 42	75	12 - 25	110 ± 17	60 ± 10
> 14 yr	>50	70	12 - 18	118 ± 20	60 ± 10

*mean ± 2 standard deviations

Resuscitation Equipment / Drugs Based on Length, Weight, or Age

Length (cm)	58-70	70-85	85-95	95-107	107-124	124-138	138-156
Weight (kg)	5-7	8-11	12-14	15-17	18-24	25-32	33-40
Age (years)	0.5	1	2	3	5	8-10	>12
Bag mask	infant	child	child	child	child	child/adult	adult
Oral airway	infant	small child	child	child	child	small adult	adult
Oxygen mask	newborn	peds	peds	peds	adult	adult	adult
ET Tube	3.0/3.5	3.5/4.0	4.0/4.5	4-5	5.0	5.5	6.0
Laryngoscope	1 Miller	1 Miller	2 Miller	2*	2*	2-3*	3*
Suction catheter	8F	8-10F	10F	10F	10F	10F	12F
Stylet	6F	6F	6F	6F	14F	14F	14F
Nasogastric tube	5-8F	8-10F	10F	10-12F	12-14F	14-18F	18F
Urine Catheter	5-8F	8-10F	10F	10-12F	10-12F	12F	12F
Chest Tube	10-12F	16-20F	20-24F	20-24F	24-32F	28-32F	32-40F

03703 100/PKG. 6/99

ET tube size estimate (mm) = [16 + age in years] / 4
1. Use uncuffed ET tube under age 8. If cuffed subtract 0.5 size
2. ET tube depth of placement estimation
 1. Distance in cm from trachea to incisors/gum line = 3 x (ET tube size)
 2. Distance in cm from midtrachea to incisors/gum line = 12 + (age in years) / 2

Pediatric Glasgow Coma Scale*

Eye Opening	Best Motor	Best Verbal
0-1 years	0-1 year	0-2 years
4. spontaneous	6. —	5. normal cry, smile, coo
3. to shout	5. localizes pain	4. cries
2. to pain	4. flexion withdrawal	3. inappropriate cry, scream
1. no responce	3. flexion/decorticate	2. grunts
	2. extension/decerebrate	1. no response
	1. no response	
0-1 years	>1 year	2-5 years
4. spontaneous	6. obeys	5. appropriate words
3. to shout	5. localizes pain	4. inappropriate words
2. to pain	4. flexion withdrawal	3. cries or screams
1. no responce	3. flexion/decorticate	2. grunts
	2. extension/decerebrate	1. no response
	1. no response	> 5 years
		5. oriented
		4. disoriented but converses
		3. inappropriate worda
		2. incomprehensible
		1. no response

Total score indicates that injury is mild (13-15), moderate (9-12), or severe (≤8).

Pediatric Trauma Score*

Patient Features	Score +2	Score +1	Score -1
Size (kg)	>20	10 - 20	< 10
Airway	normal	maintainable	Non-maintainable
Systolic BP (mmHg)	>90	50-90	<50
Mental status	awake	oblunded	comatose
Open wound	none	minor	major
Extremity fractures	none	closed	open or multiple

*A total score of ≤8 suggests the need for a specialized trauma center. A score of < 1 predicts a mortality rate of > 98%, a acorn of 4 predicts – 50% mortality, and a score of > 8 predicts < 1% mortality.   *Ramnofsky: J Trauma 1988; 28:1038*

8 mm
7 mm
6 mm
5 mm
4 mm
3 mm
2 mm

LINES	SITE	SOLUTION	UAC TAPED @ _____	UVC TAPED @ _____
A	/			
B	/			
C	/			
D	/			

	REF. HOSPITAL	TRANSPORT	TOTAL
INTAKE			
OUTPUT			

SAFETY CHECK:

RESPONSE PRIORITY 1 / 2 / 3   RETURN PRIORITY 1 / 2 / 3

PATIENT SAFETY RESTRAINTS ☐   INFANT SEAT ☐

MONITOR ALARMS: CARDIAC ____/____ ; O2 SAT ____/____

VENTILATOR ALARMS ☐

GROUND PROVIDER _____ VECH. # _____

AIR PROVIDER _____ FIXED WING ☐ HELICOPTER ☐

VENTILATION						BLOOD GASSES			NOTES / TRANSPORT EVENTS
O2 PRE/POST	ETCO2	FiO2 MODE	PIP PEEP	iT PAW	Vt RATE	SITE pH	PCO2 TCO2	PO2 02SAT	

1. Procedure _____   Indication _____

Analgesia / Sedation _____

_____

_____

1. Procedure _____   Indication _____

Analgesia / Sedation _____

_____

_____

1. Procedure _____   Indication _____

Analgesia / Sedation _____

_____

_____

PATIENT

STAMP

CHIEF COMPLAINT: _____

HPI: _____
_____
_____
_____

REF. HOSP. MEDS & TIMES: _____

REF. HOSP. PROCEDURES: _____

PERINATAL: MAT. AGE___ G__ P___ SAB___ TAB__ BLOOD TYPE__ AB__ GBS__ HEP__ HIV__ CHLY__ GC__ RUBELLA__

SEROLOGY__ PRENATAL STEROIDS Y / N

SIG. MAT. PMHx: _____

LABOR	**PERINATAL COMPLICATIONS**	**ROUTE OF DELIVERY**	**ANESTHESIA**
☐ NO	☐ MAT FEVER	☐ VAGINAL ☐ VBAC	☐ GENERAL
☐ YES	☐ MAT HTN	☐ SPONTANEOUS	☐ SPINAL / EPIDURAL
☐ SPONTANEOUS	☐ FETAL DISTRESS	☐ FORCEPS/VACUUM	☐ LOCAL
☐ SPONT / AUGMENTED	☐ ABRUPTION / PREVIA	☐ CESAREAN SECTION	☐ NONE
☐ INDUCED	☐ PRECIPITOUS DELIVERY	☐ PRIMARY	
RUPTURE OF MEMBRANES	☐ OTHER_____	☐ REPEAT	**PRESENTATION**
☐ AROM ___ HRS / DAYS PTD	**AMNIOTIC FLUID**	☐ EMERGENCY	☐ VERTEX
☐ SROM ___ HRS / DAYS PTD	☐ CLEAR ☐ MECONIUM ☐ BLOODY		☐ BREECH
			☐ TRANSVERSE

NEONATAL: GEST. AGE._____ wks (dates ☐ u/s ☐ exam ☐) VITAMIN K ☐ HEP B VAC ☐ EYE CARE ☐ STATE SCREEN ☐

DATE OF DELIVERY _____/_____/_____ TIME OF DELIVERY_____ APGARS: ___ 1 ___ 3 ___ 5 ___ 10

DR RESUSCITATION: ☐ NONE ☐ BLOWBY 02 ☐ SUCTION BELOW CORDS ☐ BAG/MASK ☐ BAG/ETT ☐ CPR ☐ MEDS

PMH: _____
_____

CURRRENT PT. MEDS: _____

ALLERGIES: _____ **IMMUNIZATIONS:** UTD N / Y _____ **EXPOSURES:** N / Y _____

SIGNIFICANT FAMILY HISTORY: _____

SPIRITUAL / SOCIAL/CULTURAL: _____

IMPRESSION: _____

PRIMARY CARE PROVIDER: _____ PHONE (____) _____ - _____

PARENT / GUARDIAN(S): _____ PHONE (____) _____ - _____

_____ PHONE (____) _____ - _____

CHECKLIST:
☐ CHART COPY (IES)
☐ XRAY COPIES
☐ LABWORK

☐ PARENTAL CONSENT(S)
☐ INFO SHEET TO PARENT (S)
☐ CALLBACK TO MCP
☐ COPP NOTIFIED

RECEIVING HOSPITAL: ☐ CHILDRENS ☐ OTHER_____
RECEIVING FIRM _____ UNIT _____ NOTIFIED ☐
RECEIVING SERVICE _____ NOTIFIED ☐
REPORT GIVEN TO _____

CONTROLLED SUBSTANCES:	AMOUNT TAKEN	AMOUNT USED	AMOUNT WASTED	AMOUNT RETURNED	INITIALS
MSO4					
FENTANYL					
MIDAZOLAM					
LORAZEPAM					
PENTOTHAL					
OTHER					

NEUROLOGICAL / MUSCULOSKELETAL

FONTANEL
- ☐ FLAT
- ☐ FULL/SOFT
- ☐ DEPRESSED
- ☐ BULGING

HEAD CIRC.
_____ CM

TONE
- ☐ JITTERY / SPASTIC
- ☐ HYPERTONIC
- ☐ NORMAL
- ☐ HYPOTONIC
- ☐ FLOPPY

LOC
- ☐ ALERT/ ORIENTED
- ☐ ALERT/ DISORIENTED
- ☐ LETHARGIC
- ☐ OBTUNDED
- ☐ STUPOROUS
- ☐ COMATOSE
- ☐ PHARMACOLOGICAL
    SEDATION/PARALYSIS

MOTOR STRENGTH
- ☐ RESISTS FORCE R/ L
- ☐ MIN. RESISTANCE R/ L
- ☐ RESISTS GRAVITY R/L
- ☐ NO RESISTANCE R / L

RANGE OF MOTION
- ☐ NORMAL
- ☐ CONTRACTURES:
  _____

REFLEXES
- ☐ COUGH
- ☐ GAG
- ☐ SUCK
- ☐ MORO

OTHER
- ☐ NUCHAL RIGIDITY
- ☐ CSF RHINORRHEA
- ☐ CSF OTORRHEA
- ☐ CAPUT
- ☐ CEPHALOHEMATOMA
- ☐ VP SHUNT
- ☐ HIP CLUNKS L / R

COMMENTS: _____

RESPIRATORY

AIRWAY
- ☐ ORAL   ☐ NASAL
- ☐ CPAP: PRONGS / NPT
- ☐ ETT: SIZE ___ CUFF Y/N
    TAPED AT ___ CM ☐ SECURE

TRACH: SIZE ____ TYPE _____

CHEST TUBES
- ☐ LEFT: SIZE _____ ☐ SX ☐ HV
- ☐ RIGHT: SIZE _____ ☐ SX ☐ HV

PATTERN
- ☐ REGULAR
- ☐ IRREGULAR
- ☐ APNEA
- ☐ KUSSMAUL
- ☐ CH-STOKES

EFFORT
RETRACTIONS:
- ☐ NONE
- ☐ MILD
- ☐ MOD
- ☐ SEVERE

- ☐ SUBSTERNAL
- ☐ SUPRASTERNAL
- ☐ SUBCOSTAL
- ☐ INTERCOSTAL

- ☐ GRUNTING
- ☐ FLARING

CXR REPORT: _____
_____

BREATH SOUNDS
- ☐ STRIDOR
- ☐ WHEEZES INSP / EXP

LEFT	*RIGHT*
☐ CLEAR	☐ CLEAR
☐ RALES	☐ RALES
☐ RHONCHI	☐ RHONCHI
☐ DIMINISH.	☐ DIMINISH.
☐ ABSENT	☐ ABSENT

COMMENTS: _____

CARDIOVASCULAR

SKIN COLOR
- ☐ PLETHORIC
- ☐ PINK
- ☐ PALE
- ☐ ASHEN
- ☐ MOTTLED
- ☐ JAUNDICED
- ☐ CYANOTIC

PERFUSION / SKIN
CAP REFILL___ SEC
- ☐ EDEMA 1+ 2+ 3+
  - ☐ DEPENDENT
  - ☐ GENERAL
- ☐ DRY
- ☐ MOIST
- ☐ DIAPHORETIC
- ☐ WARM
- ☐ COOL

PULSES

	LFT	RGT
RADIAL		
FEMORAL		
PEDAL		

FOUR EXTREMITY BPS

RA	LA
RL	LL

MURMUR
- ☐ NO
- ☐ YES

DESCRIBE:
_____
_____

- ☐ GALLOP
  S3 S4

OTHER
- ☐ JVD   LIVER ____CM BELOW RCM
- SPLEEN TIP PALPABLE   ☐ NO ☐ YES ____CM

EKG
- ☐ REGULAR   ☐ IRREGULAR   ☐ SINUS   ☐ PACED

OTHER: _____
_____
_____

COMMENTS: _____

GASTROINTESTINAL

ABDOMEN
- ☐ SOFT   ☐ NONTENDER
- ☐ FLAT   ☐ TENDER AT _____
- ☐ ROUND   ☐ VISIBLE LOOPS
- ☐ DISTENDED ☐ ERYTHEMA
- ☐ FIRM

GIRTH _____ CM

BOWEL SOUNDS
- ☐ ABSENT
- ☐ HYPOACTIVE
- ☐ ACTIVE
- ☐ HYPERACTIVE

STOOL: HEM +/-

- ☐ EMESIS: HEM +/-
- ☐ BILIOUS
- ☐ PROJECTILE

NUTRITION
- ☐ NPO SINCE
  _____ HR

DIET: _____
  _____
  _____

BREAST ☐
BOTTLE ☐

GASTRIC TUBES
- ☐ NGT: SIZE ___ TYPE ____
- ☐ NJT: SIZE ___ TYPE ____
- ☐ OGT: SIZE ___ TYPE ____
- ☐ GT: SIZE ___ TYPE ____
- ☐ PATENT
- ☐ PLACEMENT CONFIRMED
- ☐ DRAINAGE _____

GENITOURINARY

- ☐ AMBIGUOUS
- ☐ NORMAL MALE
- ☐ NORMAL FEMALE
- ☐ FOLEY: SIZE _____

URINE:
- ☐ CLEAR
- ☐ SEDIMENT
- ☐ AMBER
- ☐ YELLOW
- ☐ HEMATURIA

COMMENTS: _____

LABORATORY RESULTS

CULTURES:
- ☐ BLOOD
- ☐ CSF   ☐ URINE
- ☐ TRACH ASP
- CX @ RH/CH

☐ CSF:
  GLUCOSE_____
  PROTEIN _____
  RBC _____
  WBC _____
  P___ L___ M___

BLOOD TYPE:
_____

COOMBS:
_____

CHEMISTRIES:

CBC:

DIFF %:
P ___   B ___
L ___   M ___

CA: _____ PT: _____ PTT: _____
BILI: _____ AMYL: _____ LIPASE: _____

OTHER LABS: _____
_____

RADIOLOGY: _____
_____
_____

INTEGUMENT

KEY:
AB – ABRASION
L – LACERATION
C – CONTUSION
I – INCISION
FX – FRACTURE
B – BURN
R – RASH
D – DRESSING
T – TENDERNESS

COMMENTS: _____

INDEX

A

A-delta fibers, 550
A waves, 355
AACN, 6, 7
AACN Certification Corporation, 7, 8
ABCX model of crisis, 50
Abdominal injury, 963-967
Abdominal palpation, 153
Abdominal response, 345
Abdominal wall defects, 793, 794
Abducens nerve, *327, 333*, 335t
ABG analysis, 262
Abnormal autonomic responses, 585
Abnormalities of body temperature regulation
  drug fever, 452
  hyperthermia, 450-452
  hypothermia, 454-455
  malignant hypothermia, 452-453
Abnormal respiratory patterns, 252t
ABO system, 878
Absent (collapse) rhythms, 1038
Absolute neutrophil count (ANC), 480, 481t
Absorption, 770
Accentuated heart sounds, 154
Accessory nerve, *327, 333*, 337t
Accommodation, 20, 73
Accountability, 82
ACE inhibitors (ACEIs), 199, 200
Acetaminophen
  fever treatment, in, 451, 452
  nonopioid, as, 567
  overdose, 1004-1006
  pain management, 565t, 567-568
Acetazolamide, 586t, 713
Acetylcholine, 142
Acetylcysteine, 282t
Acid-base balance, 309-321
  analyzing, 314
  base excess/deficit, 314
  buffer system, 310, 311
  electrolytes, 312-314
  metabolic acidosis, 317t, 318, 319
  metabolic alkalosis, 317t, 319, 320
  mixed disturbances, 320, 321
  renal system, 312
  respiratory acidosis, 314-317
  respiratory alkalosis, 317, 318
  respiratory system, 311, 312
  triple acid-base disorders, 321
Acid-base disturbances, 314-320
Acoustic nerve, *327, 333*, 336t
Acquired immune response (specific immunity), 473-480
Acrania, 325t

Page references in *italics* denote figures; page references
followed by "t" denote tables.

ACTH, 806
Actinomycin D, 533t
Activated charcoal, 1002, 1003
Activated partial thromboplastin time (APTT), 828t
Active immunity, 474t
Active transport, 373
Acute chest syndrome, 842, 843
Acute gastritis, 789, 790
Acute GVHD, 869-871
Acute hemolytic transfusion reaction, 831t
Acute hypoxia, 588
Acute inflammatory demyelinating polyneuropathy
  (AIDP), 684
Acute interstitial nephritis (AIN), 740
Acute lung injury (ALI), 672-681
Acute lymphoblastic leukemia (ALL), 866, 867
Acute motor axonal neuropathy (AMAN), 684
Acute myocarditis, 629-631
Acute poststreptococcal glomerulonephritis (APSGN), 739
Acute renal failure (ARF), 735, *736*; *see also*
  Renal critical care problems
Acute respiratory distress syndrome (ARDS), 672-681
Acute respiratory failure (ARF), 498, 858-860
Acute tubular necrosis (ATN), 580, 737, 740
Acute tumor lysis syndrome (ATLS), 862-864
Acyclovir
  antiinfective agent, as, 856-857
  antidote, as, 533t
  antiviral agent, as, 886t
  renal failure, 747t
Adaptation, 20
ADCC, 479
Addison's disease, 811
Adenosine
  cardiac arrest, 205
  dosage/administration, 205
  resuscitation drug, as, 1035t, 1036
  side effects, 205
ADH, 374, 805
ADH deficiency, 807-809
ADH excess, 809-811
Admission criteria, 656
Adolescents
  developmental care, 41
  developmental characteristics, 37-40
  hospitalization, and, 40, 41
Adrenal insufficiency/adrenal crisis, 811-813
β-Adrenergic blocking agents, 200, 203
Adrenergic receptors, 192, 193t
Adrenocorticotropic hormone (ACTH), 806
Adriamycin, 534t, 858
Adult CCRN examination, 7
Adult learning theory, 96, 99
Advanced life support; *see* Resuscitation efforts
Advocacy, 119
Advocacy/moral agency, 9, 10
Aerosol therapy, 281, 282, 282t

PALS Medications for Cardiac Arrest and Symptomatic Arrhythmias

Drug	Dosage (Pediatric)	Remarks
Adenosine	0.1 mg/kg Repeat dose: 0.2 mg/kg Maximum single dose: 12 mg	Rapid IV/IO bolus Rapid flush to central circulation Monitor ECG during dose
Amiodarone for pulseless VF/VT	5 mg/kg IV/IO	Rapid IV bolus
Amiodarone for perfusing tachycardias	Loading dose: 5 mg/kg IV/IO Maximum dose: 15 mg/kg per day	IV over 20 to 60 minutes Routine use in combination with drugs prolonging QT interval is *not* recommended; hypotension is most frequent side effect
Atropine sulfate*	0.02 mg/kg Minimum dose: 0.1 mg Maximum single dose: 0.5 mg in child, 1.0 mg in adolescents; may repeat once	May give IV, IO, or ET Tachycardia and pupil dilation may occur but *not* fixed dilated pupils
Calcium chloride 10% = 100 mg/ml (=27.2 mg/ml elemental Ca)	20 mg/kg (0.2 ml/kg) IV/IO	Give slow IV push for hypocalcemia, hypermagnesemia, calcium channel blocker toxicity, preferably via central vein. Monitor heart rate; bradycardia may occur
Calcium gluconate 10% = 100 mg/ml (=9 mg/ml elemental Ca)	60-100 mg/kg (0.6-1.0 ml/kg) IV/IO	Give slow IV push for hypocalcemia, hypermagnesemia, calcium channel blocker toxicity, preferably via central vein
Epinephrine for symptomatic bradycardia*	IV/IO: 0.01 mg/kg (1:10,000, 0.1 ml/kg) ET: 0.1 mg/kg (1:1000, 0.1 ml/kg)	Tachyarrhythmias, hypertension may occur
Epinephrine for pulseless arrest*	First dose: IV/IO: 0.01 mg/kg (1:10,000 0.1 ml/kg) ET: 0.1 mg/kg (1:1000, 0.1 ml/kg) Subsequent doses: Repeat initial dose or may increase up to 10 times (0.1 mg/kg, 1:1000, 0.1 ml/kg) Administer epinephrine every 3 to 5 min IV/IO/ET doses as high as 0.2 mg/kg of 1:1000 may be effective	
Glucose (10% or 25% or 50%)	IV/IO: 0.5-1.0 g/kg • 1-2 ml/kg 50% • 2-4 ml/kg 25% • 5-10 ml/kg 10%	For suspected hypoglycemia; avoid hyperglycemia
Lidocaine*	IV/IO/ET: 1 mg/kg IV/IO: 20-50 µg/kg per minute	Rapid bolus 1 to 25 ml/kg per hour of 120 mg/100 ml solution or use "Rule of 6" (see back cover)
Lidocaine infusion (start after a bolus)		
Magnesium sulfate (500 mg/ml)	IV/IO: 25-50 mg/kg; maximum dose: 2 g per dose	Rapid IV infusion for torsades or suspected hypomagnesemia; 10- to 20-min infusion for asthma that responds poorly to α-adrenergic agonists
Naloxone*	≤5 years or ≤20 kg: 0.1 mg/kg >5 years or >20 kg: 2.0 mg	For total reversal of narcotic effect. Use small repeated doses (0.01 to 0.03 mg/kg) titrated to desired effect
Procainamide for perfusing tachycardias (100 mg/ml and 500 mg/ml)	Loading dose: 15 mg/kg IV/IO	Infusion over 30 to 60 min; routine use in combination with drugs prolonging QT interval is *not* recommended
Sodium bicarbonate (1 mEq/ml and 0.5 mEq/ml)	IV/IO: 1 mEq/kg per dose	Infuse slowly and only if ventilation is adequate

From The American Heart Association in Collaboration with the International Liaison Committee on Resuscitation (ILCOR): Guidelines 2000 for Cardiopulmonary Resuscitation and Emergency Cardiovascular Care: An International Consensus on Science, *Circulation* 102(Suppl I):I-308, 2000.
ET, Endotracheal; *IO,* intraosseous; *IV,* intravenous.

*For endotracheal administration, use higher doses (2 to 10 times the IV dose); dilute medication with normal saline to a volume of 3 to 5 ml and follow with several positive-pressure ventilations.